CW01572897

# Drug Information Handbook *for* Physician Assistants

## 1999-2000

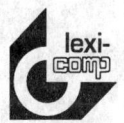

lexi-comp

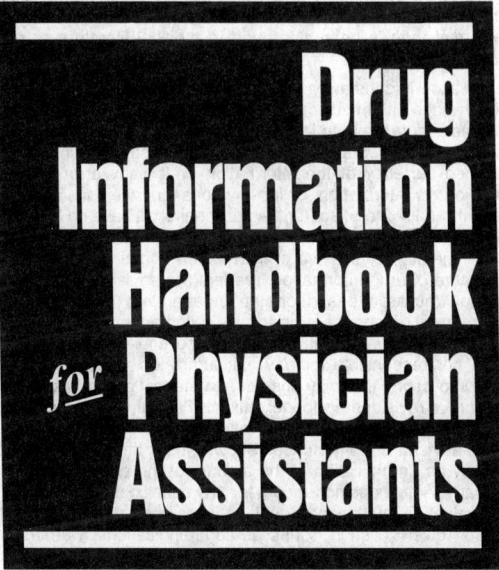

# Drug Information Handbook for Physician Assistants

*1999-2000*

Edited by:

**Michael J. Rudzinski, RPA-C, RPh**
*Physician Assistant*
Promedicus Health Group
Buffalo, New York

**J. Fred Bennes, RPA, RPh**
*Clinical Professor of Pharmacy*
University of Buffalo School of Pharmacy
*Director of Quality and Resource Management*
Promedicus Health Group
Buffalo, New York

**LEXI-COMP, INC**
Hudson (Cleveland)

## NOTICE

This handbook is intended to serve the user as a handy quick reference and not as a complete drug information resource. It does not include information on every therapeutic agent available. The publication covers commonly used drugs and is specifically designed to present certain important aspects of drug data in a more concise format than is generally found in medical literature or product material supplied by manufacturers.

Drug information is constantly evolving because of ongoing research and clinical experience and is often subject to interpretation. While great care has been taken to ensure the accuracy of the information presented, the reader is advised that the authors, editors, reviewers, contributors, and publishers cannot be responsible for the continued currency of the information or for any errors, omissions, or the application of this information, or for any consequences arising therefrom. Therefore, the author(s), editors, and/or the publisher shall have no liability to any person or entity with regard to claims, loss, or damage caused, or alleged to be caused, directly or indirectly, by the use of information contained herein. Because of the dynamic nature of drug information, readers are advised that decisions regarding drug therapy must be based on the independent judgment of the clinician, changing information about a drug (eg, as reflected in the literature and manufacturer's most current product information), and changing medical practices. The editors are not responsible for any inaccuracy of quotation or for any false or misleading implication that may arise due to the text or formulas as used or due to the quotation of revisions no longer official. Further, the *Drug Information Handbook for Physician Assistants* is not offered as a guide to dosing. The reader, herewith, is advised that information shown under the heading **Usual Dosage** is provided only as an indication of the amount of the drug typically given or taken during therapy. Actual dosing amount for any specific drug should be based on an in-depth evaluation of the individual patient's therapy requirement and strong consideration given to such issues as contraindications, warnings, precautions, adverse reactions, along with the interaction of other drugs. The manufacturers most current product information or other standard recognized references should always be consulted for such detailed information prior to drug use.

The editors and contributors have written this book in their private capacities. No official support or endorsement by any federal agency or pharmaceutical company is intended or inferred.

If you have any suggestions or questions regarding any information presented in this handbook, please contact our drug information pharmacist at

## 1-800-837-LEXI (5394)

This manual was produced using the FormuLex™ Program – a complete publishing service of Lexi-Comp Inc.

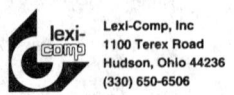

**Lexi-Comp, Inc**
1100 Terex Road
Hudson, Ohio 44236
(330) 650-6506

ISBN 0-916589-83-8

# TABLE OF CONTENTS

# TABLE OF CONTENTS *(Continued)*

# ABOUT THE EDITORS

### Michael J. Rudzinski, RPA-C, RPh

Michael (Mike) Rudzinski received his Bachelor's of Science degree in Pharmacy from the State University of New York at Buffalo in 1975 and his Bachelor's of Science degree as a Physician Assistant from the University of Oklahoma in 1979.

Mike started working in his local neighborhood pharmacy in 1967, and has been active in pharmacy ever since. He has practiced as a clinical pharmacist in hospital and retail settings for 24 years, and is currently practicing in a community pharmacy. In addition to his pharmacy work, Mike has been practicing as a physician assistant in a staff model HMO for 19 years, in primary care, and orthopedic medicine. He is currently employed with Promedicus Health Group.

Mike gives presentations yearly at the national American Academy of Physician Assistants Annual PA Conference and serves on the editorial board for the *Clinician Reviews Journal*. He is a clinical preceptor for D'Youville College's physician assistant program, Daemen College's physician assistant program, and the State University of New York at Buffalo Schools of Pharmacy, Nurse Practitioners, and Medicine. He also serves as adjunct faculty for the D'Youville College PA program. He is a member of the American Academy of Physician Assistant (AAPA), the New York State Society of Physician Assistants (NYSSPA), and the Pharmacist Society of the State of New York (PSSNY). Mike would also like to acknowledge all the help and guidance he has received throughout his career from family, friends, and colleagues.

### J. Fred Bennes, RPA, RPh

Fred Bennes received a Bachelor of Science in Pharmacy (1973) from the University of North Carolina, Chapel Hill and a Physician Associate Certificate (1974) from Duke University. Since then he has practiced as a primary care physician assistant in rural, inner city, and suburban settings both in North Carolina and New York. Additionally, Fred has been on the faculty of the State University of New York at Buffalo for the Schools of Pharmacy, Graduate Nursing, and Medicine. Besides clinical practice and didactic teaching, he has developed and directed a seven pharmacy practice at a staff model HMO and served as the Practice Administrator for an 85-physician medical group.

Currently, Fred is Clinical Professor of Pharmacy at the University of Buffalo School and Pharmacy and the Director of Quality and Resource Management at Promedicus Health Group, a large multispecialty group practice with designs on the innovative practice of healthcare. Fred was an early supporter of certification for Physician Assistants, being so certified from 1976-1998 when he retired from active practice to pursue teaching and administrative challenges.

# ABOUT THE AUTHORS

## Charles F. Lacy, RPh, PharmD

Dr Lacy received his doctorate from the University of Southern California School of Pharmacy. With over 17 years of clinical experience at one of the nation's largest teaching hospitals, he has developed a reputation as an acknowledged expert in drug information and critical care drug therapy.

In his current capacity as Coordinator of Drug Information Services at Cedar-Sinai Health System in Los Angeles, Dr Lacy plays an active role in the education and training of the medical, pharmacy, and nursing staff. He coordinates the Drug Information Center, the Medical Center's Intern Pharmacist Clinical Training Program, the Department's Continuing Education Program for Pharmacists; maintains the Medical Center Formulary Program; and is editor of the Medical Center's *Drug Formulary Handbook* and the drug information newsletter *Prescription*.

Presently, Dr Lacy holds teaching affiliations with the University of Southern California School of Pharmacy, the University of California at San Francisco School of Pharmacy, the University of the Pacific School of Pharmacy, and the University of Alberta at Edmonton, School of Pharmacy and Health Sciences. Additionally, Dr Lacy is the current Director of the Center for International Health Care Practitioners at Western University of Health Sciences, where he plays a leading role in the advanced training of postgraduate pharmacists from areas throughout the Pacific rim, including Japan, Hong Kong, New Zealand, and Korea.

Dr Lacy is an active member of numerous professional associations including the American Society of Health-System Pharmacists (ASHP), the California Society of Hospital Pharmacists (CSHP), the American Society of Consultant Pharmacists (ASCP), and the American College of Clinical Pharmacy (ACCP).

## Lora L. Armstrong, RPh, BSPharm, BCPS

Lora L. Armstrong received her bachelor's degree in pharmacy from Ferris State University. With over 17 years of clinical experience at one of the nation's most prominent teaching institutions, she has developed a reputation as an acknowledged expert in drug information. Her interests involve the areas of critical care, hematology, oncology, infectious disease, and pharmacokinetics. Ms. Armstrong is a Board Certified Pharmacotherapy Specialist (BCPS).

In her current capacity as Director of Drug Information at the University of Chicago Hospitals (UCH), Ms Armstrong plays an active role in the education and training of the medical, pharmacy, and nursing staff. She coordinates the Drug Information Center, the medical center's Adverse Drug Reaction Monitoring Program, and the department's Continuing Education Program for Pharmacists. She also maintains the hospital's strict formulary program and is editor of the *UCH Formulary of Accepted Drugs* and the drug information newsletter "Topics in Drug Therapy." Ms. Armstrong also serves on the Editorial Advisory Board of the *Journal of the American Pharmaceutical Association*.

Ms Armstrong is an active member of the American Society of Health-System Pharmacists (ASHP), the American Pharmaceutical Association (APhA), the American College of Clinical Pharmacy (ACCP), and the Society of Critical Care Medicine (SCCM). She is the APhA designated author for this handbook.

## Morton P. Goldman, PharmD, BCPS

Dr Goldman received his bachelor's degree in pharmacy from the University of Pittsburgh, College of Pharmacy and his Doctor of Pharmacy degree from the University of Cincinnati, Division of Graduate Studies and Research. He completed his concurrent 2-year hospital pharmacy residency at the VA Medical

Center in Cincinnati. Dr Goldman is presently the Assistant Director of Pharmacotherapy Services for the Department of Pharmacy at the Cleveland Clinic Foundation (CCF) after having spent over 3 years at CCF as an Infectious Disease pharmacist and 4 years as Clinical Manager. He holds faculty appointments from Case Western Reserve University, College of Medicine; The University of Toledo, College of Pharmacy; and The University of Cincinnati, College of Pharmacy. Dr Goldman is a board-certified Pharmacotherapy Specialist.

In his capacity as Assistant Director of Pharmacotherapy Services at CCF, Dr Goldman remains actively involved in patient care and clinical research with the Department of Infectious Disease, as well as the continuing education of the medical and pharmacy staff. He is an editor of CCF's *Guidelines for Antibiotic Use* and coordinates their annual Antimicrobial Review retreat. He is a member of the Pharmacy and Therapeutics Committee and many of its subcommittees. Dr Goldman has authored numerous journal articles and lectures locally and nationally on infectious diseases topics and current drug therapies. He is currently a reviewer for the *Annals of Pharmacotherapy* and the *Journal of the American Medical Association*, an editorial board member of the *Journal of Infectious Disease Pharmacotherapy*, and coauthor of the *Drug Information Handbook* and the *Drug Information Handbook for the Allied Health Professional* produced by Lexi-Comp, Inc. He also provides technical support to Lexi-Comp's Clinical Reference Library™ publications.

Dr Goldman is an active member of Cleveland's local clinical pharmacy society, the Ohio College of Clinical Pharmacy, the Society of Infectious Disease Pharmacists, the American College of Clinical Pharmacy, and the American Society of Health-Systems Pharmacy.

## Leonard L. Lance, RPh, BSPharm

Leonard L. (Bud) Lance has been directly involved in the pharmaceutical industry since receiving his bachelor's degree in pharmacy from Ohio Northern University in 1970. Upon graduation from ONU, Mr Lance spent four years as a navy pharmacist in various military assignments and was instrumental in the development and operation of the first whole hospital I.V. admixture program in a military (Portsmouth Naval Hospital) facility.

After completing his military service, he entered the retail pharmacy field and has managed both an independent and a home I.V. franchise pharmacy operation. Since the late 1970s Mr Lance has focused much of his interest on using computers to improve pharmacy service and to advance the dissemination of drug information to practitioners and other health care professionals.

As a result of his strong publishing interest, he serves in the capacity of pharmacy editor and technical advisor as well as pharmacy (information) database coordinator for Lexi-Comp. Along with the *Drug Information Handbook for the Allied Health Professional* edition, he provides technical support to Lexi-Comp's *Pediatric Dosage Handbook*, *Laboratory Test Handbook*, *Diagnostic Procedure Handbook*, *Infectious Diseases Handbook*, *Poisoning & Toxicology Handbook*, and *Geriatric Dosage Handbook* publications. Mr Lance has also assisted approximately 120 major hospitals in producing their own formulary (pharmacy) publications through Lexi-Comp's custom publishing service.

Mr Lance is a member and past president (1984) of the Summit Pharmaceutical Association (SPA). He is also a member of the Ohio Pharmacists Association (OPA), the American Pharmaceutical Association (APhA), and the American Society of Health-System Pharmacists (ASHP).

# EDITORIAL ADVISORY PANEL

**Matthew A. Fuller, PharmD, MBA**
*Clinical Pharmacy Specialist*
Psychiatry
*Cleveland Department of Veterans Affairs Medical Center*
Brecksville, Ohio

**Mark Geraci, PharmD**
*Department of Pharmacy Practice*
University of Illinois
Chicago, Illinois

**Harold J. Grady, PhD**
*Director of Clinical Chemistry*
Truman Medical Center
Kansas City, Missouri

**Larry D. Gray, PhD**
*TriHealth Clinical Microbiology Laboratory*
Bethesda Oak Hospital
Cincinnati, Ohio

**Martin D. Higbee, PharmD**
*Associate Professor*
Department of Pharmacy Practice
The University of Arizona
Tucson, Arizona

**Jane Hurlburt Hodding, PharmD**
*Supervisor, Children's Pharmacy*
Miller Children's Hospital at Long Beach Memorial
Long Beach, California

**Rebecca T. Horvat, PhD**
*Assistant Professor of Pathology and Laboratory Medicine*
University of Kansas Medical Center
Kansas City, Kansas

**Carlos M. Isada, MD**
Department of Infectious Disease
Cleveland Clinic Foundation
Cleveland, Ohio

**David S. Jacobs, MD**
*President, Pathologists Chartered*
Overland Park, Kansas

**Bernard L. Kasten, Jr, MD**
*Vice-President/Medical Director*
Corning Clinical Laboratories
Teteroboro, New Jersey

**Polly E. Kintzel, PharmD**
*Clinical Pharmacy Specialist*
Bone Marrow Transplantation, Detroit Medical Center
Harper Hospital
Detroit, Michigan

**Donna M. Kraus, PharmD**
*Assistant Professor of Pharmacy Practice*
Departments of Pharmacy Practice and Pediatrics
*Clinical Pharmacist*
Pediatric Intensive Care Unit
University of Illinois at Chicago
Chicago, Illinois

## EDITORIAL ADVISORY PANEL *(Continued)*

**Lowell L. Tilzer MD**
*Associate Medical Director*
Community Blood Center of Greater Kansas City
Kansas City, Missouri

**Beatrice B. Turkoski, RN, PhD**
*Professor, Advanced Pharmacology and Applied Therapeutics*
Kent State University School of Nursing
Kent, Ohio

**Richard L. Wynn, PhD**
*Professor and Chairman of Pharmacology*
Baltimore College of Dental Surgery
Dental School
University of Maryland at Baltimore
Baltimore, Maryland

# PREFACE

Physician assistants, other nonphysician primary care providers, pharmacists, and physicians are increasingly confronted with information that is becoming more intense. The need to access basic drug information in an efficient manner that is relevant to your practice is a challenge that is equally as intense.

This book was created for working healthcare practitioners who need clinically applicable information in a practical format. It is focused on the primary care environment where the majority of patient activity occurs. Our goal was to produce a comprehensive and concise presentation that still remained portable.

In surveying the needs of practitioners, we realized there was a need for a reference that could be used at the point of the patient encounter. Thus, there is a new annotated organization to the material that is pertinent and logical. Some of the additional features include herbal drug monographs, dosing information for adults/pediatrics/geriatrics for each monograph, and appendices with updated guidelines, unique categorical listings, and clinical calculation tools.

A portable text cannot allow for information on every therapeutic agent available. We believe, though, that you will find the consistent and comprehensive format to be useful in your therapeutic decision making. We would welcome any comments to improve future editions.

# ACKNOWLEDGMENTS

The *Drug Information Handbook for Physician Assistants* has been extracted from the *Drug Information Handbook*, 7th ed, by Lacy, Armstrong, Goldman, and Lance (also published by Lexi-Comp, Inc) and adapted to the specific information needs of physician assistants. Special acknowledgment is also extended to the *Drug Information Handbook for Nursing,* Turkoski B and Lance B (Lexi-Comp, Inc), for information related to Patient Education.

The *Drug Information Handbook for Physician Assistants* exists in its present form as the result of the concerted efforts of the following individuals: Robert D. Kerscher, publisher and president of Lexi-Comp Inc; Lynn D. Coppinger, managing editor; Barbara F. Kerscher, production manager; David C. Marcus, director of information systems.

Other members of the Lexi-Comp staff whose contributions deserve special mention include Diane M. Harbart, MT (ASCP), medical editor; Jeanne E. Wilson, production/systems liaison; Leslie J. Ruggles, Julie A. Katzen, Jennifer L. Rocky, Stacey L. Hurd, Kathleen E. Schleicher, and Linda L. Taylor, project managers; Alexandra J. Hart, composition specialist; Jackie L. Mizer, Ginger S. Conner, and Kathy Smith, production assistants; Tracey J. Reinecke, graphic designer; Cynthia A. Bell, CPhT; Edmund A. Harbart, vice-president, custom publishing division; Jack L. Stones, vice-president, reference publishing division; Jay L. Katzen, director of marketing and business development; Jerry M. Reeves, Marc L. Long, and Patrick T. Grubb, regional sales managers; Brad F. Bolinski, Kristin M. Thompson, Matthew C. Kerscher, Tina L. Collins, Kelene A. Murphy, and Leslie G. Rodia, sales and marketing representatives; Paul A. Rhine and Jason M. Buchwald, academic account managers; Kenneth J. Hughes, manager of authoring systems; Sean M. Conrad and James M. Stacey, system analysts; Thury L. O'Connor, vice-president of technology; David J. Wasserbauer, vice-president, finance and administration; Elizabeth M. Conlon and Rebecca A. Dryhurst, accounting; and Frederick C. Kerscher, fulfillment manager.

Much of the material contained in this book was a result of pharmacy contributors throughout the United States and Canada. Lexi-Comp has assisted many medical institutions to develop hospital-specific formulary manuals that contain clinical drug information as well as dosing. Working with clinical pharmacists, hospital pharmacy and therapeutics committees, and hospital drug information centers, Lexi-Comp has developed an evolutionary drug database that reflects the practice of pharmacy in these major institutions.

In addition, the authors wish to thank their families, friends, and colleagues who supported them in their efforts to complete this handbook.

# DESCRIPTION OF SECTIONS AND FIELDS USED IN THIS HANDBOOK

The *Drug Information Handbook for Physician Assistants* is divided into four sections.

The first section is a compilation of introductory text pertinent to the use of this book.

The drug information section of the handbook, in which all drugs are listed alphabetically, details information pertinent to each drug. Extensive cross-referencing is provided by U.S. brand names, Canadian brand names, and synonyms. Commonly-used natural products have also been included. The fields of information in each monograph have been carefully chosen by the editors to reflect the professional responsibilities and decisions of physician assistants. Many combination-product monographs have been condensed with only brand names and forms available; for more information, see the individual components.

The third section is an invaluable appendix which offers a compilation of tables, guidelines, nomograms, algorithms, and conversion information which can be helpful when considering patient care.

The last section of this handbook contains two indices, a Pharmacologic Index and an Alphabetical Index which includes U.S. and Canadian brand names, synonyms, and major topics in the appendix.

The **Alphabetical Listing of Drugs** is presented in a consistent format and provides the following fields of information:

| | |
|---|---|
| Generic Name | U.S. adopted name |
| Pronunciation | Phonetic pronunciation guide |
| Pharmacologic Class | Unique systematic classification of medications |
| U.S. Brand Names | U.S. trade names (manufacturer-specific) |
| Mechanism of Action | How the drug works in the body to elicit a response |
| Use | Information pertaining to appropriate indications of the drug. Includes both FDA approved and non-FDA approved indications. |
| Usual Dosage | The amount of the drug to be typically given or taken during therapy for children and adults; also includes any dosing adjustment/comments for renal impairment or hepatic impairment and other suggested dosing adjustments (eg, hematological toxicity) |
| Dosage Forms | Information with regard to form, strength, and availability of the drug. The field is strung with the forms bolded and uses the following abbreviations: Aero = aerosol; Cap = capsule; Crm = cream; Inf = infusion; Inh = inhalation; Inj = inject; Liq = liquid; Oint = ointment, Soln = solution; Supp = suppository; Susp = suspension; Syr = syrup; Tab = tablet; Top = topical. |
| Contraindications | Information pertaining to inappropriate use of the drug |
| Warnings/ Precautions | Precautionary considerations, hazardous conditions related to use of the drug, and disease states or patient populations in which the drug should be cautiously used |
| Pregnancy Risk Factor | Five categories established by the FDA to indicate the potential of a systemically absorbed drug for causing birth defects |

| | |
|---|---|
| Pregnancy Implications | Information pertinent to or associated with the use of the drug as it relates to clinical effects on the fetus, breast-feeding/lactation, and clinical effects on the infant |
| Adverse Reactions | Side effects are grouped by percentage of incidence (if known) and/or body system; in the interest of saving space, <1% effects are grouped only by percentage |
| Drug Interactions | If a drug has demonstrated involvement with cytochrome P-450 enzymes, the initial line of this field will identify the drug as an inhibitor, inducer, or substrate of specific isoenzymes (ie, CYP1A2). A summary of this information can also be found in a tabular format within the appendix section of this handbook. The remainder of the field presents a description of the interaction between the drug listed in the monograph and other drugs or drug classes. May include possible mechanisms and effect of combined therapy. May also include a strategy to manage the patient on combined therapy (ie, quinidine). |
| Onset | The time after drug administration when therapeutic effect is observed. May also include time for peak therapeutic effect. |
| Duration | Length of therapeutic effect |
| Half-life | The reported half-life of elimination for the parent of metabolites of the drug. |

**Special PA Issues**

| | |
|---|---|
| Patient Education | Specific information pertinent for the patient |
| Dietary Considerations | Information is offered, when appropriate, regarding food, nutrition, and/or alcohol |
| Monitoring Parameters | Laboratory tests and patient physical parameters that should be monitored for safety and efficacy of drug therapy |
| Reference Range | Therapeutic and toxic serum concentrations listed including peak and trough levels |
| Related Information | Cross-reference to other pertinent drug information found elsewhere in this handbook |

# FDA PREGNANCY CATEGORIES

Throughout this book there is a field labeled Pregnancy Risk Factor (PRF) and the letter A, B, C, D or X immediately following which signifies a category. The FDA has established these five categories to indicate the potential of a systemically absorbed drug for causing birth defects. The key differentiation among the categories rests upon the reliability of documentation and the risk:benefit ratio. Pregnancy Category X is particularly notable in that if any data exists that may implicate a drug as a teratogen and the risk:benefit ratio is clearly negative, the drug is contraindicated during pregnancy.

These categories are summarized as follows:

A      Controlled studies in pregnant women fail to demonstrate a risk to the fetus in the first trimester with no evidence of risk in later trimesters. The possibility of fetal harm appears remote.

B      Either animal-reproduction studies have not demonstrated a fetal risk but there are no controlled studies in pregnant women, or animal-reproduction studies have shown an adverse effect (other than a decrease in fertility) that was not confirmed in controlled studies in women in the first trimester and there is no evidence of a risk in later trimesters.

C      Either studies in animals have revealed adverse effects on the fetus (teratogenic or embryocidal effects or other) and there are no controlled studies in women, or studies in women and animals are not available. Drugs should be given only if the potential benefits justify the potential risk to the fetus.

D      There is positive evidence of human fetal risk, but the benefits from use in pregnant women may be acceptable despite the risk (eg, if the drug is needed in a life-threatening situation or for a serious disease for which safer drugs cannot be used or are ineffective).

X      Studies in animals or human beings have demonstrated fetal abnormalities or there is evidence of fetal risk based on human experience, or both, and the risk of the use of the drug in pregnant women clearly outweighs any possible benefit. The drug is contraindicated in women who are or may become pregnant.

# SAFE WRITING PRACTICES

Health professionals and their support personnel frequently produce handwritten copies of information they see in print; therefore, such information is subjected to even greater possibilities for error or misinterpretation on the part of others. Thus, particular care must be given to how drug names and strengths are expressed when creating written healthcare documents.

The following are a few examples of safe writing rules suggested by the Institute for Safe Medication Practices, Inc.*

1. There should be a space between a number and its units as it is easier to read. There should be no periods after the abbreviations mg or mL.

| Correct | Incorrect |
|---------|-----------|
| 10 mg | 10mg |
| 100 mg | 100mg |

2. Never place a decimal and a zero after a whole number (2 mg is correct and 2.0 mg is **incorrect**). If the decimal point is not seen because it falls on a line or because individuals are working from copies where the decimal point is not seen, this causes a tenfold overdose.

3. Just the opposite is true for numbers less than one. Always place a zero before a naked decimal (0.5 mL is correct, .5 mL is **incorrect**).

4. Never abbreviate the word unit. The handwritten U or u, looks like a 0 (zero), and may cause a tenfold overdose error to be made.

5. IU is not a safe abbreviation for international units. The handwritten IU looks like IV. Write out international units or use int. units.

6. Q.D. is not a safe abbreviation for once daily, as when the Q is followed by a sloppy dot, it looks like QID which means four times daily.

7. O.D. is not a safe abbreviation for once daily, as it is properly interpreted as meaning "right eye" and has caused liquid medications such as saturated solution of potassium iodide and Lugol's solution to be administered incorrectly. There is no safe abbreviation for once daily. It must be written out in full.

8. Do not use chemical names such as 6-mercaptopurine or 6-thioguanine, as sixfold overdoses have been given when these were not recognized as chemical names. The proper names of these drugs are mercaptopurine or thioguanine.

9. Do not abbreviate drug names (5FC, 6MP, 5-ASA, MTX, HCTZ, CPZ, PBZ, etc) as they are misinterpreted and cause error.

10. Do not use the apothecary system or symbols.

11. Do not abbreviate microgram as µg; instead use mcg as there is less likelihood of misinterpretation.

## SAFE WRITING PRACTICES *(Continued)*

12. When writing an outpatient prescription, write a complete prescription. A complete prescription can prevent the prescriber, the pharmacist, and/or the patient from making a mistake and can eliminate the need for further clarification. The legible prescriptions should contain:

    a. patient's full name

    b. for pediatric or geriatric patients: their age (or weight where applicable)

    c. drug name, dosage form and strength; if a drug is new or rarely prescribed, print this information

    d. number or amount to be dispensed

    e. complete instructions for the patient, including the purpose of the medication

    f. when there are recognized contraindications for a prescribed drug, indicate to the pharmacist that you are aware of this fact (ie, when prescribing a potassium salt for a patient receiving an ACE inhibitor, write "K serum leveling being monitored")

*From "Safe Writing" by Davis NM, PharmD and Cohen MR, MS, Lecturers and Consultants for Safe Medication Practices, 1143 Wright Drive, Huntington Valley, PA 19006. Phone: (215) 947-7566.

# ALPHABETICAL LISTING OF DRUGS

♦ **A-200™ Shampoo [OTC]** *see* Pyrethrins *on page 783*

# Abacavir (a BAK a veer)

**Pharmacologic Class** Antiretroviral Agent, Reverse Transcriptase Inhibitor (Nucleoside)

**U.S. Brand Names** Ziagen®

**Mechanism of Action** Nucleoside reverse transcriptase inhibitor. Abacavir is a guanosine analogue which is phosphorylated to carbovir triphosphate which interferes with HIV viral RNA dependent DNA polymerase resulting in inhibition of viral replication.

**Use** Treatment of HIV infections in combination with other antiretroviral agents

**USUAL DOSAGE** Oral:

Children: 3 months to 16 years: 8 mg/kg body weight twice daily (maximum 300 mg twice daily) in combination with other antiretroviral agents

Adults: 300 mg twice daily in combination with other antiretroviral agents

**Dosage Forms Soln, oral (strawberry-banana flavored):** 20 mg/mL (240 mL); **Tab:** 300 mg

**Contraindications** Prior hypersensitivity to abacavir (or carbovir) or any component of the formulation; do not rechallenge patients who have experienced hypersensitivity to abacavir

**Warnings/Precautions** Should always be used as a component of a multidrug regimen. Fatal hypersensitivity reactions have occurred. **Patients exhibiting symptoms of fever, skin rash, fatigue, and GI symptoms (eg, abdominal pain, nausea, vomiting) should discontinue therapy immediately and call for medical attention. Ziagen® SHOULD NOT be restarted because more severe symptoms may occur within hours, including LIFE-THREATENING HYPOTENSION AND DEATH. To report these events on abacavir hypersensitivity, a registry has been established (1-800-270-0425).** Use with caution in patients with hepatic dysfunction; prior liver disease, prolonged use, and obesity may be risk factors for development of lactic acidosis and severe hepatomegaly with steatosis.

**Pregnancy Risk Factor** C

**Pregnancy Implications** Health professional are encouraged to contact the antiretroviral pregnancy registry to monitor outcomes of pregnant women exposed to abacavir (1-800-258-4263)

Clinical effects on the fetus: Administer during pregnancy only if benefits to mother outweigh risks to the fetus

Breast-feeding/lactation: HIV-infected mothers are discouraged from breast-feeding to decrease potential transmission of HIV

**Adverse Reactions Note:** Hypersensitivity reactions, which may be fatal, occur in ~5% of patients (see Warnings). Symptoms may include anaphylaxis, fever, rash, fatigue, diarrhea, abdominal pain, nausea and vomiting. Less common symptoms may include edema, lethargy, malaise, myalgia, shortness of breath, mouth ulcerations, conjunctivitis, lymphadenopathy, hepatic failure and renal failure.

Rates of adverse reactions were defined during combination therapy with lamivudine. Adverse reaction rates attributable to abacavir alone are not available.

Adults:

Central nervous system: Insomnia (7%)

Gastrointestinal: Nausea (47%), vomiting (16%), diarrhea (12%), anorexia (11%), pancreatitis

Neuromuscular & skeletal: Weakness

Endocrine & metabolic: Hyperglycemia, hypertriglyceridemia (25%)

Miscellaneous: Elevated transaminases

Children:

Central nervous system: Fever (19%), headache (16%)

Dermatologic: Rash (11%)

Gastrointestinal: Nausea (38%), vomiting (38%), diarrhea (16%), anorexia (9%)

**Half-Life** 0.8-1.5 hours

**Special PA Issues**

**Patient Education:** This is not a cure for AIDS or AIDS complex, nor will it reduce the risk of transmission to others. Long-term effects are not known. You will need frequent blood tests to adjust dosage for maximum therapeutic effect. Take as directed, for full course of therapy; do not discontinue (even if feeling better). You may experience headache or muscle pain or weakness. Report skin rash, acute headache, severe nausea or vomiting, or difficulty breathing.

♦ **Abbokinase® Injection** *see* Urokinase *on page 948*

♦ **Abenol®** *see* Acetaminophen *on page 21*

♦ **Abitrate®** *see* Clofibrate *on page 221*

♦ **Absorbine® Antifungal [OTC]** *see* Tolnaftate *on page 915*

♦ **Absorbine® Antifungal Foot Powder [OTC]** *see* Miconazole *on page 604*

♦ **Absorbine® Jock Itch [OTC]** *see* Tolnaftate *on page 915*

♦ **Absorbine Jr.® Antifungal [OTC]** *see* Tolnaftate *on page 915*

## Acarbose (AY car bose)
**Pharmacologic Class** Antidiabetic Agent (Miscellaneous)
**U.S. Brand Names** Precose®
**Mechanism of Action** Competitive inhibitor of pancreatic α-amylase and intestinal brush border α-glucosidases, resulting in delayed hydrolysis of ingested complex carbohydrates and disaccharides and absorption of glucose; dose-dependent reduction in postprandial serum insulin and glucose peaks; inhibits the metabolism of sucrose to glucose and fructose

**Use**
Monotherapy, as indicated as an adjunct to diet to lower blood glucose in patients with noninsulin-dependent diabetes mellitus (NIDDM) whose hyperglycemia cannot be managed on diet alone
Combination with a sulfonylurea, metformin, or insulin in patients with NIDDM when diet plus acarbose do not result in adequate glycemic control

**USUAL DOSAGE** Oral:
Adults: Dosage must be individualized on the basis of effectiveness and tolerance while not exceeding the maximum recommended dose
**Initial dose:** 25 mg 3 times/day with the first bite of each main meal
**Maintenance dose:** Should be adjusted at 4- to 8-week intervals based on 1-hour postprandial glucose levels and tolerance. Dosage may be increased from 25 mg 3 times/day to 50 mg 3 times/day. Some patients may benefit from increasing the dose to 100 mg 3 times/day.
Maintenance dose ranges: 50-100 mg 3 times/day.
**Maximum dose:**
≤60 kg: 50 mg 3 times/day
>60 kg: 100 mg 3 times/day
**Patients receiving sulfonylureas:** Acarbose given in combination with a sulfonylurea will cause a further lowering of blood glucose and may increase the hypoglycemic potential of the sulfonylurea. If hypoglycemia occurs, appropriate adjustments in the dosage of these agents should be made.
**Dosing adjustment in renal impairment:** $Cl_{cr}$ <25 mL/minute: Peak plasma concentrations were 5 times higher and AUCs were 6 times larger than in volunteers with normal renal function; however, long term clinical trials in diabetic patients with significant renal dysfunction have not been conducted and treatment of these patients with acarbose is not recommended

**Dosage Forms Tab:** 50 mg, 100 mg

**Contraindications** Known hypersensitivity to the drug and in patients with diabetic ketoacidosis or cirrhosis; patients with inflammatory bowel disease, colonic ulceration, partial intestinal obstruction or in patients predisposed to intestinal obstruction; patients who have chronic intestinal diseases associated with marked disorders of digestion or absorption and in patients who have conditions that may deteriorate as a result of increased gas formation in the intestine

**Warnings/Precautions** Hypoglycemia: Acarbose may increase the hypoglycemic potential of sulfonylureas. Oral glucose (dextrose) should be used in the treatment of mild to moderate hypoglycemia. Severe hypoglycemia may require the use of either intravenous glucose infusion or glucagon injection.

Elevated serum transaminase levels: Treatment-emergent elevations of serum transaminases (AST and/or ALT) occurred in 15% of acarbose-treated patients in long-term studies. These serum transaminase elevations appear to be dose related. At doses >100 mg 3 times/day, the incidence of serum transaminase elevations greater than 3 times the upper limit of normal was 2-3 times higher in the acarbose group than in the placebo group. These elevations were asymptomatic, reversible, more common in females, and, in general, were not associated with other evidence of liver dysfunction.

When diabetic patients are exposed to stress such as fever, trauma, infection, or surgery, a temporary loss of control of blood glucose may occur. At such times, temporary insulin therapy may be necessary.

**Pregnancy Risk Factor** B
**Pregnancy Implications** Breast-feeding/lactation: It is not known whether acarbose is excreted in human milk
**Adverse Reactions**
>10%:
Gastrointestinal: Abdominal pain (21%) and diarrhea (33%) tend to return to pretreatment levels over time, and the frequency and intensity of flatulence (77%) tend to abate with time
Hepatic: Elevated liver transaminases
<1%: Sleepiness, headache, vertigo, erythema, urticaria, severe gastrointestinal distress, weakness
**Drug Interactions** Decreased effect: Thiazides and other diuretics, corticosteroids, phenothiazines, thyroid products, estrogens, oral contraceptives, phenytoin, nicotinic acid, sympathomimetics, calcium channel-blocking drugs, isoniazid, intestinal adsorbents (eg, charcoal), digestive enzyme preparations (eg, amylase, pancreatin)
(Continued)

## Acarbose *(Continued)*

### Special PA Issues

**Patient Education:** Take this medication exactly as directed, with the first bite of each main meal. Do not change dosage or discontinue without first consulting prescriber. Do not take other medications with or within 2 hours of this medication unless so advised by prescriber. It is important to follow dietary and lifestyle recommendations of prescriber. You will be instructed in signs of hypo-/hyperglycemia by prescriber or diabetic educator. If combining acarbose with other diabetic medication (eg, sulfonylureas, insulin), keep source of glucose (sugar) on hand in case hypoglycemia occurs. You may experience mild side effects during first weeks of acarbose therapy (eg, bloating, flatulence, diarrhea, abdominal discomfort); these should diminish over time. Report severe or persistent side effects, fever, extended vomiting or flu, or change in color of urine or stool.

**Monitoring Parameters:** Postprandial glucose, glycosylated hemoglobin levels, serum transaminase levels should be checked every 3 months during the first year of treatment and periodically thereafter

### Related Information

Hypoglycemic Drugs *on page 1020*

♦ **Accolate®** *see* Zafirlukast *on page 969*

♦ **Accupril®** *see* Quinapril *on page 788*

♦ **Accutane®** *see* Isotretinoin *on page 499*

♦ **ACE** *see* Captopril *on page 146*

## Acebutolol *(a se BYOO toe lole)*

**Pharmacologic Class** Antiarrhythmic Agent, Class II; Beta Blocker (with Intrinsic Sympathomimetic Activity)

**U.S. Brand Names** Sectral®

**Mechanism of Action** Competitively blocks beta$_1$-adrenergic receptors with little or no effect on beta$_2$-receptors except at high doses; exhibits membrane stabilizing and intrinsic sympathomimetic activity

**Use** Treatment of hypertension, ventricular arrhythmias, angina

**USUAL DOSAGE** Oral:

Adults:

Hypertension: 400-800 mg/day (larger doses may be divided); maximum: 1200 mg/day
Ventricular arrhythmias: Initial: 400 mg/day; maintenance: 600-1200 mg/day in divided doses
Elderly: Initial: 200-400 mg/day; dose reduction due to age related decrease in Cl$_{cr}$ will be necessary; do not exceed 800 mg/day

**Dosing adjustment in renal impairment:**
Cl$_{cr}$ 25-49 mL/minute/1.73 m$^2$: Reduce dose by 50%
Cl$_{cr}$ <25 mL/minute/1.73 m$^2$: Reduce dose by 75%

**Dosing adjustment in hepatic impairment:** Use with caution

**Dosage Forms** Cap: 200 mg, 400 mg

**Contraindications** Hypersensitivity to beta-blocking agents, avoid use in uncompensated congestive heart failure; cardiogenic shock; bradycardia or heart block; sinus node dysfunction; A-V conduction abnormalities. Although acebutolol primarily blocks beta$_1$-receptors, high doses can result in beta$_2$-receptor blockage. Use with caution in bronchospastic lung disease and renal dysfunction (especially the elderly).

**Warnings/Precautions** Abrupt withdrawal of beta-blockers may result in an exaggerated cardiac beta-adrenergic responsiveness. Symptomatology has included reports of tachycardia, hypertension, ischemia, angina, myocardial infarction, and sudden death. It is recommended that patients be tapered gradually off of beta-blockers over a 2-week period rather than via abrupt discontinuation.

**Pregnancy Risk Factor** B

**Pregnancy Implications** Enters breast milk/use caution

**Adverse Reactions**

>10%: Central nervous system: Fatigue
1% to 10%:
Cardiovascular: Chest pain, edema, bradycardia, hypotension
Central nervous system: Headache, dizziness, insomnia, depression, abnormal dreams
Dermatologic: Rash
Gastrointestinal: Constipation, diarrhea, dyspepsia, nausea, flatulence
Genitourinary: Polyuria
Neuromuscular & skeletal: Arthralgia, myalgia
Ocular: Abnormal vision
Respiratory: Dyspnea, rhinitis, cough
<1%: Ventricular arrhythmias, heart block, heart failure, facial edema, Xerostomia, anorexia, impotence, urinary retention, cold extremities

**Drug Interactions**

Decreased effect of beta-blockers with aluminum salts, barbiturates, calcium salts, cholestyramine, colestipol, NSAIDs, penicillins (ampicillin), rifampin, salicylates, and sulfinpyrazone due to decreased bioavailability and plasma levels; decreased effect of sulfonylureas with beta-blockers

Increased effect/toxicity of beta-blockers with calcium blockers (diltiazem, felodipine, nicardipine), oral contraceptives, flecainide, haloperidol (propranolol, hypotensive effects), H$_2$-antagonists (metoprolol, propranolol only by cimetidine, possibly ranitidine), hydralazine (metoprolol, propranolol), loop diuretics (propranolol, not atenolol), MAO inhibitors (metoprolol, nadolol, bradycardia), phenothiazines (propranolol), propafenone (metoprolol, propranolol), quinidine (in extensive metabolizers), ciprofloxacin, thyroid hormones (metoprolol, propranolol, when hypothyroid patient is converted to euthyroid state)

Beta-blockers may increase the effect/toxicity of flecainide, haloperidol (hypotensive effects), hydralazine, phenothiazines, acetaminophen, anticoagulants (propranolol, warfarin), benzodiazepines (not atenolol), clonidine (hypertensive crisis after or during withdrawal of either agent), epinephrine (initial hypertensive episode followed by bradycardia), nifedipine and verapamil lidocaine, ergots (peripheral ischemia), prazosin (postural hypotension)

Beta-blockers may affect the action or levels of ethanol, disopyramide, nondepolarizing muscle relaxants and theophylline although the effects are difficult to predict

**Onset** 1-2 hours

**Duration** 12-24 hours

**Half-Life** 6-7 hours average

**Special PA Issues**

Patient Education: Take exactly as directed. Do not increase, decrease, or adjust dosage without consulting prescriber. Take pulse daily, prior to medication and follow prescriber's instruction about holding medication. Do not take with antacids. Do not use alcohol or OTC medications (eg, cold remedies) without consulting prescriber. If diabetic, monitor serum sugars closely (may alter glucose tolerance or mask signs of hypoglycemia). May cause fatigue, dizziness, or postural hypotension; use caution when changing position from lying or sitting to standing, when driving, or when climbing stairs until response to medication is known. May cause alteration in sexual performance (reversible). Report unresolved swelling of extremities, difficulty breathing or new cough, unresolved fatigue, unusual weight gain, unresolved constipation, or unusual muscle weakness.

Monitoring Parameters: Blood pressure, orthostatic hypotension, heart rate, CNS effects, EKG

**Related Information**

Beta-Blockers *on page 1002*

- ♦ **Acebutolol Hydrochloride** *see Acebutolol on previous page*
- ♦ **ACE Inhibitors** *see Chart on page 995*
- ♦ **Aceon®** *see Perindopril Erbumine on page 711*
- ♦ **Acephen® [OTC]** *see Acetaminophen on this page*
- ♦ **Aceta® [OTC]** *see Acetaminophen on this page*

# Acetaminophen (a seet a MIN oh fen)

**Pharmacologic Class** Analgesic, Miscellaneous

**U.S. Brand Names** Acephen® [OTC]; Aceta® [OTC]; Apacet® [OTC]; Arthritis Foundation® Pain Reliever, Aspirin Free [OTC]; Aspirin Free Anacin® Maximum Strength [OTC]; Children's Silapap® [OTC]; Feverall™ [OTC]; Feverall™ Sprinkle Caps [OTC]; Genapap® [OTC]; Halenol® Childrens [OTC]; Infants Feverall™ [OTC]; Infants' Silapap® [OTC]; Junior Strength Panadol® [OTC]; Liquiprin® [OTC]; Mapap® [OTC]; Maranox® [OTC]; Neopap® [OTC]; Panadol® [OTC]; Redutemp® [OTC]; Ridenol® [OTC]; Tempra® [OTC]; Tylenol® [OTC]; Tylenol® Extended Relief [OTC]; Uni-Ace® [OTC]

**Mechanism of Action** Inhibits the synthesis of prostaglandins in the central nervous system and peripherally blocks pain impulse generation; produces antipyresis from inhibition of hypothalamic heat-regulating center

**Use** Treatment of mild to moderate pain and fever; does not have antirheumatic effects (analgesic)

### Acetaminophen Dosing

| Age | Dosage (mg) | Age | Dosage (mg) |
|---|---|---|---|
| 0-3 mo | 40 | 4-5 y | 240 |
| 4-11 mo | 80 | 6-8 y | 320 |
| 1-2 y | 120 | 9-10 y | 400 |
| 2-3 y | 160 | 11 y | 480 |

(Continued)

## Acetaminophen *(Continued)*

**USUAL DOSAGE** Oral, rectal (if fever not controlled with acetaminophen alone, administer with full doses of aspirin on an every 4- to 6-hour schedule, if aspirin is not otherwise contraindicated):

Children <12 years: 10-15 mg/kg/dose every 4-6 hours as needed; do **not** exceed 5 doses (2.6 g) in 24 hours; alternatively, the following doses may be used. See table.

Adults: 325-650 mg every 4-6 hours or 1000 mg 3-4 times/day; do **not** exceed 4 g/day

**Dosing interval in renal impairment:**

$Cl_{cr}$ 10-50 mL/minute: Administer every 6 hours

$Cl_{cr}$ <10 mL/minute: Administer every 8 hours (metabolites accumulate)

Hemodialysis: Moderately dialyzable (20% to 50%)

**Dosing adjustment/comments in hepatic impairment:** Appears to be well tolerated in cirrhosis; serum levels may need monitoring with long-term use

**Dosage Forms Caplet:** 160 mg, 325 mg, 500 mg; Extended: 650 mg; **Cap:** 80 mg; **Drops:** 48 mg/mL (15 mL); 60 mg/0.6 mL (15 mL); 80 mg/0.8 mL (15 mL); 100 mg/mL (15 mL, 30 mL); **Elix:** 80 mg/5 mL, 120 mg/5 mL, 160 mg/5 mL, 167 mg/5 mL, 325 mg/5 mL; **Liq, oral:** 160 mg/5 mL, 500 mg/15 mL; **Soln:** 100 mg/mL (15 mL); 120 mg/2.5 mL; **Supp, rectal:** 80 mg, 120 mg, 125 mg, 300 mg, 325 mg, 650 mg; **Susp, oral:** 160 mg/5 mL, **Oral drops:** 80 mg/0.8 mL; **Tab:** 325 mg, 500 mg, 650 mg; Chewable: 80 mg, 160 mg

**Contraindications** Patients with known G-6-PD deficiency; hypersensitivity to acetaminophen

**Warnings/Precautions** May cause severe hepatic toxicity on overdose; use with caution in patients with alcoholic liver disease; chronic daily dosing in adults of 5-8 g of acetaminophen over several weeks or 3-4 g/day of acetaminophen for 1 year have resulted in liver damage

**Pregnancy Risk Factor** B

**Adverse Reactions** Percentage unknown: May increase chloride, bilirubin, uric acid, glucose, ammonia, alkaline phosphatase; may decrease sodium, bicarbonate, calcium <1%: Rash, nausea, vomiting, blood dyscrasias (neutropenia, pancytopenia, leukopenia), anemia, analgesic nephropathy, nephrotoxicity with chronic overdose, hypersensitivity reactions (rare)

**Drug Interactions** CYP1A2 enzyme substrate (minor), CYP2E1 and 3A3/4 enzyme substrate

Decreased effect: Rifampin can interact to reduce the analgesic effectiveness of acetaminophen

Increased toxicity: Barbiturates, carbamazepine, hydantoins, sulfinpyrazone can increase the hepatotoxic potential of acetaminophen; chronic ethanol abuse increases risk for acetaminophen toxicity; effect of warfarin may be enhanced

**Onset** <1 hour

**Duration** 4-6 hours

**Half-Life** Adults: Normal renal function: 1-3 hours; End-stage renal disease: 1-3 hours

**Special PA Issues**

**Patient Education:** Take exactly as directed (do not increase dose or frequency); most adverse effects are related to excessive use. Take with food or milk. While using this medication, avoid alcohol and other prescription or OTC medications that contain acetaminophen. Maintain adequate hydration (2-3 L/day of fluids unless instructed to restrict fluid intake). This medication will not reduce inflammation; consult prescriber for anti-inflammatory, if needed. Report unusual bleeding (stool, mouth, urine) or bruising; unusual fatigue and weakness; change in elimination patterns; or change in color of urine or stool.

**Dietary Considerations:**

Food: May slightly delay absorption of extended-release preparations; rate of absorption may be decreased when given with food high in carbohydrates

Alcohol: Excessive intake of alcohol may increase the risk of acetaminophen-induced hepatotoxicity; avoid or limit alcohol intake

**Monitoring Parameters:** Relief of pain or fever

**Reference Range:**

Therapeutic concentration: 10-30 µg/mL

Toxic concentration: >200 µg/mL

Toxic concentration with probable hepatotoxicity: >200 µg/mL at 4 hours or 50 µg/mL at 12 hours

## Acetaminophen and Codeine *(a seet a MIN oh fen & KOE deen)*

**Pharmacologic Class** Analgesic, Narcotic

**U.S. Brand Names** Capital® and Codeine; Phenaphen® With Codeine; Tylenol® With Codeine

**Mechanism of Action** Inhibits the synthesis of prostaglandins in the central nervous system and peripherally blocks pain impulse generation; produces antipyresis from inhibition of hypothalamic heat-regulating center; binds to opiate receptors in the CNS, causing inhibition of ascending pain pathways, altering the perception of and response to pain; causes cough supression by direct central action in the medulla; produces generalized CNS depression

**Use** Relief of mild to moderate pain

**USUAL DOSAGE** Doses should be adjusted according to severity of pain and response of the patient. Adult doses ≥60 mg codeine fail to give commensurate relief of pain but merely prolong analgesia and are associated with an appreciably increased incidence of side effects. Oral:

Children: Analgesic:
    Codeine: 0.5-1 mg codeine/kg/dose every 4-6 hours
    Acetaminophen: 10-15 mg/kg/dose every 4 hours up to a maximum of 2.6 g/24 hours for children <12 years
        3-6 years: 5 mL 3-4 times/day as needed of elixir
        7-12 years: 10 mL 3-4 times/day as needed of elixir
        >12 years: 15 mL every 4 hours as needed of elixir
Adults:
    Antitussive: Based on codeine (15-30 mg/dose) every 4-6 hours
    Analgesic: Based on codeine (30-60 mg/dose) every 4-6 hours
        1-2 tablets every 4 hours to a maximum of 12 tablets/24 hours

**Dosing adjustment in renal impairment:** Refer to individual monographs for Acetaminophen and Codeine

**Dosage Forms Cap:** #2: Acetaminophen 325 mg and codeine phosphate 15 mg (C-III); #3: Acetaminophen 325 mg and codeine phosphate 30 mg (C-III); #4: Acetaminophen 325 mg and codeine phosphate 60 mg (C-III); **Elix:** Acetaminophen 120 mg and codeine phosphate 12 mg per 5 mL with alcohol 7% (C-V); **Susp, oral, alcohol free:** Acetaminophen 120 mg and codeine phosphate 12 mg per 5 mL (C-V); **Tab:** Acetaminophen 500 mg and codeine phosphate 30 mg (C-III); acetaminophen 650 mg and codeine phosphate 30 mg (C-III); **Tab:** #1: Acetaminophen 300 mg and codeine phosphate 7.5 mg (C-III); #2: Acetaminophen 300 mg and codeine phosphate 15 mg (C-III); #3: Acetaminophen 300 mg and codeine phosphate 30 mg (C-III); #4: Acetaminophen 300 mg and codeine phosphate 60 mg (C-III)

**Contraindications** Hypersensitivity to acetaminophen, codeine phosphate, or similar compounds

**Warnings/Precautions** Use with caution in patients with hypersensitivity reactions to other phenanthrene derivative opioid agonists (morphine, hydrocodone, hydromorphone, levorphanol, oxycodone, oxymorphone); tablets contain metabisulfite which may cause allergic reactions

**Pregnancy Risk Factor** C

**Adverse Reactions**
>10%:
    Central nervous system: Lightheadedness, dizziness, sedation
    Gastrointestinal: Nausea, vomiting
    Respiratory: Shortness of breath
1% to 10%:
    Central nervous system: Euphoria, dysphoria
    Dermatologic: Pruritus
    Gastrointestinal: Constipation, abdominal pain
    Miscellaneous: Histamine release
<1%: Palpitations, hypotension, bradycardia, peripheral vasodilation, increased intracranial pressure, antidiuretic hormone release, biliary tract spasm, urinary retention, miosis, respiratory depression, physical and psychological dependence

**Drug Interactions** Increased toxicity: CNS depressants, phenothiazines, tricyclic antidepressants, guanabenz, MAO inhibitors (may also decrease blood pressure); effect of warfarin may be enhanced

**Special PA Issues**
    **Monitoring Parameters:** Relief of pain, respiratory and mental status, blood pressure, bowel function

♦ **Acetaminophen and Hydrocodone** *see* Hydrocodone and Acetaminophen *on page 449*
♦ **Acetaminophen and Oxycodone** *see* Oxycodone and Acetaminophen *on page 688*

# Acetaminophen, Isometheptene, and Dichloralphenazone
    (a seet a MIN oh fen, eye soe me THEP teen, & dye KLOR al FEN a zone)
**Pharmacologic Class** Analgesic, Miscellaneous
**U.S. Brand Names** Isocom®; Isopap®; Midchlor®; Midrin®; Migratine®
**Dosage Forms Cap:** Acetaminophen 326 mg, isometheptene mucate 65 mg, dichloralphenazone 100 mg

♦ **Acetasol® HC Otic** *see* Acetic Acid, Propylene Glycol Diacetate, and Hydrocortisone *on page 25*
♦ **Acetazolam®** *see* Acetazolamide *on this page*

# Acetazolamide (a set a ZOLE a mide)
**Pharmacologic Class** Anticonvulsant, Miscellaneous; Carbonic Anhydrase Inhibitor; Diuretic, Carbonic Anhydrase Inhibitor; Ophthalmic Agent, Antiglaucoma
*(Continued)*

## Acetazolamide *(Continued)*

**U.S. Brand Names** Diamox®; Diamox Sequels®

**Mechanism of Action** Reversible inhibition of the enzyme carbonic anhydrase resulting in reduction of hydrogen ion secretion at renal tubule and an increased renal excretion of sodium, potassium, bicarbonate, and water to decrease production of aqueous humor; also inhibits carbonic anhydrase in central nervous system to retard abnormal and excessive discharge from CNS neurons

**Use** Lowers intraocular pressure to treat glaucoma, also as a diuretic, adjunct treatment of refractory seizures and acute altitude sickness; centrencephalic epilepsies (sustained release not recommended for anticonvulsant)

**USUAL DOSAGE Note:** I.M. administration is not recommended because of pain secondary to the alkaline pH

Neonates and Infants: Hydrocephalus: To slow the progression of hydrocephalus in neonates and infants who may not be good candidates for surgery, acetazolamide I.V. or oral doses of 5 mg/kg/dose every 6 hours increased by 25 mg/kg/day to a maximum of 100 mg/kg/day, if tolerated, have been used. Furosemide was used in combination with acetazolamide.

Children:
Glaucoma:
Oral: 8-30 mg/kg/day or 300-900 mg/m$^2$/day divided every 8 hours
I.M., I.V.: 20-40 mg/kg/24 hours divided every 6 hours, not to exceed 1 g/day
Edema: Oral, I.M., I.V.: 5 mg/kg or 150 mg/m$^2$ once every day
Epilepsy: Oral: 8-30 mg/kg/day in 1-4 divided doses, not to exceed 1 g/day; sustained release capsule is not recommended for treatment of epilepsy
Adults:
Glaucoma:
Chronic simple (open-angle): Oral: 250 mg 1-4 times/day or 500 mg sustained release capsule twice daily
Secondary, acute (closed-angle): I.M., I.V.: 250-500 mg, may repeat in 2-4 hours to a maximum of 1 g/day
Edema: Oral, I.M., I.V.: 250-375 mg once daily
Epilepsy: Oral: 8-30 mg/kg/day in 1-4 divided doses; **sustained release capsule is not recommended for treatment of epilepsy**
Altitude sickness: Oral: 250 mg every 8-12 hours (or 500 mg extended release capsules every 12-24 hours)
Therapy should begin 24-48 hours before and continue during ascent and for at least 48 hours after arrival at the high altitude
Urine alkalinization: Oral: 5 mg/kg/dose repeated 2-3 times over 24 hours
Elderly: Oral: Initial: 250 mg twice daily; use lowest effective dose
**Dosing adjustment in renal impairment:**
Cl$_{cr}$ 10-50 mL/minute: Administer every 12 hours
Cl$_{cr}$ <10 mL/minute: Avoid use → ineffective
Hemodialysis: Moderately dialyzable (20% to 50%)
Peritoneal dialysis: Supplemental dose is not necessary

**Dosage Forms Cap, sustained release:** 500 mg; **Inj:** 500 mg; **Tab:** 125 mg, 250 mg

**Contraindications** Hypersensitivity to sulfonamides or acetazolamide, patients with hepatic disease or insufficiency; patients with decreased sodium and/or potassium levels; patients with adrenocortical insufficiency, hyperchloremic acidosis, severe renal disease or dysfunction, or severe pulmonary obstruction; long-term use in noncongestive angle-closure glaucoma

**Warnings/Precautions** Use in impaired hepatic function may result in coma; use with caution in patients with respiratory acidosis and diabetes mellitus; impairment of mental alertness and/or physical coordination may occur
I.M. administration is painful because of the alkaline pH of the drug
Drug may cause substantial increase in blood glucose in some diabetic patients; malaise and complaints of tiredness and myalgia are signs of excessive dosing and acidosis in the elderly

**Pregnancy Risk Factor** C

**Pregnancy Implications**
Clinical effects on the fetus: Despite widespread usage, no reports linking the use of acetazolamide with congenital defects have been located
Breast-feeding/lactation: The American Academy of Pediatrics considers acetazolamide to be **compatible** with breast-feeding

**Adverse Reactions**
>10%:
Central nervous system: Malaise
Gastrointestinal: Anorexia, diarrhea, metallic taste
Genitourinary: Polyuria
Neuromuscular & skeletal: Muscular weakness
1% to 10%: Central nervous system: Mental depression, drowsiness

<1%: Fever, fatigue, rash, hyperchloremic metabolic acidosis, hypokalemia, hyperglycemia, black stools, GI irritation, dryness of the mouth, dysuria, bone marrow suppression, blood dyscrasias, paresthesia, myopia, renal calculi

**Drug Interactions**
Decreased effect: Increased lithium excretion and altered excretion of other drugs by alkalinization of urine (such as amphetamines, quinidine, procainamide, methenamine, phenobarbital, salicylates); primidone serum concentrations may be decreased
Increased toxicity: Cyclosporine trough concentrations may be increased resulting in possible nephrotoxicity and neurotoxicity; salicylate use may result in carbonic anhydrase inhibitor accumulation and toxicity including CNS depression and metabolic acidosis; digitalis toxicity may occur if hypokalemia is untreated

**Onset** Extended release capsule: 2 hours; peak effect: 3-6 hours; I.V.: 2 minutes; peak effect: 15 minutes; Tablet, peak effect: 1-4 hours

**Duration** Extended release capsule: 18-24 hours; Tablet: 8-12 hours; I.V.: 4-5 hours

**Half-Life** 2.4-5.8 hours

**Special PA Issues**
**Patient Education:** Take as directed; may be taken with food to reduce GI upset. Do not chew or crush long-acting capsule (contents may be sprinkled on soft food). Arrange for periodic ocular examinations while taking this medication (may affect intraocular pressure). You may experience drowsiness, dizziness, or weakness; use caution when driving or engaging in hazardous tasks until response to medication is known. If you experience nausea, loss of appetite, or altered taste, small frequent meals, frequent mouth care, or sucking on lozenges may help. Monitor serum glucose closely (may cause substantial increase in blood glucose in some diabetic patients). You may experience increased sensitivity to sunlight; use sunblock, wear protective clothing, and avoid exposure to direct sunlight. Report unusual and persistent tiredness; numbness, burning, or tingling of extremities or around mouth lips or anus; muscle weakness; or excessive depression.

**Monitoring Parameters:** Intraocular pressure, potassium, serum bicarbonate; serum electrolytes, periodic CBC with differential

## Acetic Acid (a SEE tik AS id)
**Pharmacologic Class** Antibacterial, Otic; Antibacterial, Topical
**U.S. Brand Names** VōSol®
**Use** Irrigation of the bladder; treatment of superficial bacterial infections of the external auditory canal and vagina
**USUAL DOSAGE**
Irrigation (note dosage of an irrigating solution depends on the capacity or surface area of the structure being irrigated):
For continuous irrigation of the urinary bladder with 0.25% acetic acid irrigation, the rate of administration will approximate the rate of urine flow; usually 500-1500 mL/24 hours
For periodic irrigation of an indwelling urinary catheter to maintain patency, about 50 mL of 0.25% acetic acid irrigation is required
Otic: Insert saturated wick; keep moist 24 hours; remove wick and instill 5 drops 3-4 times/ day
Vaginal: One applicatorful every morning and evening
**Dosage Forms Jelly, vaginal (Aci-jel®):** 0.921% with oxyquinolone sulfate 0.025%, ricinoleic acid 0.7%, and glycerin 5% (85 g); **Soln:** Irrigation: 0.25% (1000 mL); Otic (VōSol®): Acetic acid 2% in propylene glycol (15 mL, 30 mL, 60 mL)
**Contraindications** During transurethral procedures; hypersensitivity to drug or components
**Warnings/Precautions** Not for internal intake or I.V. infusion; topical or irrigation use only; use of irrigation in patients with mucosal lesions of urinary bladder may cause irritation; systemic acidosis may result from absorption
**Pregnancy Risk Factor** C
**Adverse Reactions** <1%: Systemic acidosis, urologic pain, hematuria

## Acetic Acid, Propylene Glycol Diacetate, and Hydrocortisone
(a SEE tik AS id, PRO pa leen GLY kole dye AS e tate, & hye droe KOR ti sone)
**Pharmacologic Class** Antibiotic/Corticosteroid, Otic
**U.S. Brand Names** Acetasol® HC Otic; VōSol® HC Otic
**Dosage Forms Soln, otic:** Acetic acid 2%, propylene glycol diacetate 3%, and hydrocortisone 1% (10 mL)

## Acetophenazine (a set oh FEN a zeen)
**Pharmacologic Class** Antipsychotic Agent, Phenothiazine, Piperazine
**U.S. Brand Names** Tindal®
**Use** Management of manifestations of psychotic disorders
**USUAL DOSAGE** Adults: Oral: 20 mg 3 times/day up to 60-120 mg/day
Hospitalized schizophrenic patients may require doses as high as 400-600 mg/day
Hemodialysis: Not dialyzable (0% to 5%)
(Continued)

## Acetophenazine *(Continued)*

**Dosage Forms** Tab, as maleate: 20 mg

**Contraindications** Blood dyscrasias and bone marrow suppression, patients in coma or brain damage, known hypersensitivity to acetophenazine

**Pregnancy Risk Factor** C

**Onset** 2-4 hours

**Duration** ~24 hours

**Half-Life** 20-40 hours

**Related Information**
Antipsychotic Agents *on page 1001*

♦ **Acetophenazine Maleate** *see* Acetophenazine *on previous page*

♦ **Acetoxymethylprogesterone** *see* Medroxyprogesterone Acetate *on page 561*

## Acetylcholine *(a se teel KOE leen)*

**Pharmacologic Class** Cholinergic Agonist; Ophthalmic Agent, Miotic

**U.S. Brand Names** Miochol-E®

**Mechanism of Action** Causes contraction of the sphincter muscles of the iris, resulting in miosis and contraction of the ciliary muscle, leading to accommodation spasm

**Use** Produces complete miosis in cataract surgery, keratoplasty, iridectomy and other anterior segment surgery where rapid miosis is required

**USUAL DOSAGE** Adults: Intraocular: 0.5-2 mL of 1% injection (5-20 mg) instilled into anterior chamber before or after securing one or more sutures

**Dosage Forms** Powder, intraocular, as chloride: 1:100 [10 mg/mL] (2 mL, 15 mL)

**Contraindications** Hypersensitivity to acetylcholine chloride and any components; acute iritis and acute inflammatory disease of the anterior chamber

**Warnings/Precautions** Systemic effects rarely occur but can cause problems for patients with acute cardiac failure, bronchial asthma, peptic ulcer, hyperthyroidism, GI spasm, urinary tract obstruction, and Parkinson's disease; open under aseptic conditions only

**Pregnancy Risk Factor** C

**Pregnancy Implications** Acetylcholine is used primarily in the eye and there are no reports of its use in pregnancy; because it is ionized at physiologic pH, transplacental passage would not be expected

**Adverse Reactions** <1%: Bradycardia, hypotension, flushing, headache, altered distance vision, decreased night vision, transient lenticular opacities, dyspnea, diaphoresis

**Drug Interactions**
Decreased effect possible with flurbiprofen and suprofen, ophthalmic
Increased effect may be prolonged or enhanced in patients receiving tacrine

**Special PA Issues**
**Patient Education:** May sting on instillation; use caution while driving at night or performing hazardous tasks, do not touch dropper to eye

♦ **Acetylcholine Chloride** *see* Acetylcholine *on this page*

## Acetylcysteine *(a se teel SIS teen)*

**Pharmacologic Class** Antidote; Mucolytic Agent

**U.S. Brand Names** Mucomyst®; Mucosil™

**Mechanism of Action** Exerts mucolytic action through its free sulfhydryl group which opens up the disulfide bonds in the mucoproteins thus lowering mucous viscosity. The exact mechanism of action in acetaminophen toxicity is unknown; thought to act by providing substrate for conjugation with the toxic metabolite.

**Use** Adjunctive mucolytic therapy in patients with abnormal or viscid mucous secretions in acute and chronic bronchopulmonary diseases; pulmonary complications of surgery and cystic fibrosis; diagnostic bronchial studies; antidote for acute acetaminophen toxicity

**USUAL DOSAGE**

Acetaminophen poisoning: Children and Adults: Oral: 140 mg/kg; followed by 17 doses of 70 mg/kg every 4 hours; repeat dose if emesis occurs within 1 hour of administration; therapy should continue until all doses are administered even though the acetaminophen plasma level has dropped below the toxic range

Inhalation: Acetylcysteine 10% and 20% solution (Mucomyst®) (dilute 20% solution with sodium chloride or sterile water for inhalation); 10% solution may be used undiluted

Infants: 1-2 mL of 20% solution or 2-4 mL 10% solution until nebulized given 3-4 times/day

Children: 3-5 mL of 20% solution or 6-10 mL of 10% solution until nebulized given 3-4 times/day

Adolescents: 5-10 mL of 10% to 20% solution until nebulized given 3-4 times/day

**Note:** Patients should receive an aerosolized bronchodilator 10-15 minutes prior to acetylcysteine

Meconium ileus equivalent: Children and Adults: 100-300 mL of 4% to 10% solution by irrigation or orally

**Dosage Forms Soln, as sodium:** 10% [100 mg/mL] (4 mL, 10 mL, 30 mL); 20% [200 mg/mL] (4 mL, 10 mL, 30 mL, 100 mL)

**Contraindications** Known hypersensitivity to acetylcysteine

**Warnings/Precautions** Since increased bronchial secretions may develop after inhalation, percussion, postural drainage and suctioning should follow; if bronchospasm occurs, administer a bronchodilator; discontinue acetylcysteine if bronchospasm progresses

**Pregnancy Risk Factor** B

**Pregnancy Implications** Clinical effects on the fetus: There are no adequate and well controlled studies in pregnant women; use if only clearly needed

**Adverse Reactions**
>10%:
  Gastrointestinal: Vomiting
  Miscellaneous: Unpleasant odor during administration
1% to 10%:
  Central nervous system: Drowsiness, chills
  Gastrointestinal: Stomatitis, nausea
  Local: Irritation
  Respiratory: Bronchospasm, rhinorrhea, hemoptysis
  Miscellaneous: Clamminess
<1%: Skin rash

**Onset** Oral: Peak plasma levels 1-2 hours; Inhalation: Mucus liquefaction occurs maximally within 5-10 minutes

**Duration** Oral: Can persist for >1 hour

**Half-Life** Oral: Reduced acetylcysteine: 2 hours; Total acetylcysteine: 5.5 hours

**Special PA Issues**
  **Patient Education:** Pulmonary treatment: Prepare solution (may dilute with sterile water to reduce concentrate from impeding nebulizer) and use as directed. Clear airway by coughing deeply before using aerosol. Wash face and face-mask after treatment to remove any residual. You may experience drowsiness (use caution when driving) or nausea or vomiting (small frequent meals may help). Report persistent chills or fever, adverse change in respiratory status, palpitations, or extreme anxiety or nervousness.

  **Reference Range:** Determine acetaminophen level as soon as possible, but no sooner than 4 hours after ingestion (to ensure peak levels have been obtained); administer for acetaminophen level >150 µg/mL; toxic concentration with probable hepatotoxicity: >200 µg/mL at 4 hours or 50 µg at 12 hours

♦ **Acetylcysteine Sodium** see Acetylcysteine *on previous page*
♦ **Acetylsalicylic Acid** see Aspirin *on page 80*
♦ **Aches-N-Pain® [OTC]** see Ibuprofen *on page 466*
♦ **Achromycin® Ophthalmic** see Tetracycline *on page 885*
♦ **Achromycin® Topical** see Tetracycline *on page 885*
♦ **Aciclovir** see Acyclovir *on next page*
♦ **Acidulated Phosphate Fluoride** see Fluoride *on page 383*
♦ **Aclovate® Topical** see Alclometasone *on page 36*

# Acrivastine and Pseudoephedrine (AK ri vas teen & soo doe e FED rin)

**Pharmacologic Class** Antihistamine

**U.S. Brand Names** Semprex®-D

**Mechanism of Action** Refer to Pseudoephedrine monograph; acrivastine is an analogue of triprolidine and it is considered to be relatively less sedating than traditional antihistamines; believed to involve competitive blockade of $H_1$-receptor sites resulting in the inability of histamine to combine with its receptor sites and exert its usual effects on target cells

**Use** Temporary relief of nasal congestion, decongest sinus openings, running nose, itching of nose or throat, and itchy, watery eyes due to hay fever or other upper respiratory allergies

**USUAL DOSAGE** Adults: 1 capsule 3-4 times/day
  **Dosing comments in renal impairment:** Do not use

**Dosage Forms Cap:** Acrivastine 8 mg and pseudoephedrine hydrochloride 60 mg

**Contraindications** MAO inhibitor therapy within 14 days of initiating therapy, severe hypertension, severe coronary artery disease, hypersensitivity to pseudoephedrine, acrivastine (or other alkylamine antihistamines), or any component, renal impairment ($Cl_{cr}$ <48 mL/minute)

**Warnings/Precautions** Use with caution in patients >60 years of age; use with caution in patients with high blood pressure, ischemic heart disease, diabetes, increased intraocular pressure, GI or GU obstruction, asthma, thyroid disease, or prostatic hypertrophy; not recommended for use in children

**Pregnancy Risk Factor** B

**Pregnancy Implications** Enters breast milk/contraindicated

**Adverse Reactions**
>10%: Central nervous system: Drowsiness, headache
1% to 10%:
  Cardiovascular: Tachycardia, palpitations
(Continued)

## Acrivastine and Pseudoephedrine *(Continued)*

Central nervous system: Nervousness, dizziness, insomnia, vertigo, lightheadedness, fatigue

Gastrointestinal: Nausea, vomiting, xerostomia, diarrhea

Genitourinary: Dysuria

Neuromuscular & skeletal: Weakness

Respiratory: Pharyngitis, cough increase

Miscellaneous: Diaphoresis

<1%: Dysmenorrhea, dyspepsia

**Drug Interactions**

Decreased effect of guanethidine, reserpine, methyldopa, and beta-blockers

Increased toxicity with MAO inhibitors (hypertensive crisis), sympathomimetics, CNS depressants, alcohol (sedation)

**Duration** 12 hours

**Half-Life** 1.5 hours

**Special PA Issues**

**Patient Education:** Take as directed; do not exceed recommended dose. Avoid use of other depressants, alcohol, or sleep-inducing medications unless approved by prescriber. You may experience drowsiness or dizziness (use caution when driving or engaging in hazardous activity until response to medication is known); or dry mouth, nausea or vomiting (frequent small meals, frequent mouth care, chewing gum, or sucking hard candy may help). Report persistent dizziness, sedation, or agitation; chest pain, rapid heartbeat, or palpitations; difficulty breathing or increased cough; changes in urinary pattern; muscle weakness; or lack of improvement or worsening or condition.

- ◆ **ACT®** [OTC] *see* Fluoride *on page 383*
- ◆ **Actagen-C®** *see* Triprolidine, Pseudoephedrine, and Codeine *on page 941*
- ◆ **ActHIB®** *see* Haemophilus b Conjugate Vaccine *on page 432*
- ◆ **Acti-B₁₂®** *see* Hydroxocobalamin *on page 458*
- ◆ **Acticort 100®** *see* Hydrocortisone *on page 453*
- ◆ **Actidose-Aqua®** [OTC] *see* Charcoal *on page 184*
- ◆ **Actidose® With Sorbitol** [OTC] *see* Charcoal *on page 184*
- ◆ **Actifed® Allergy Tablet (Day)** [OTC] *see* Pseudoephedrine *on page 780*
- ◆ **Actigall™** *see* Ursodiol *on page 950*
- ◆ **Actinex® Topical** *see* Masoprocol *on page 558*
- ◆ **Actiprofen®** *see* Ibuprofen *on page 466*
- ◆ **Actiq®** *see* Fentanyl *on page 362*
- ◆ **Activase®** *see* Alteplase *on page 46*
- ◆ **Activated Carbon** *see* Charcoal *on page 184*
- ◆ **Activated Charcoal** *see* Charcoal *on page 184*
- ◆ **Activated Ergosterol** *see* Ergocalciferol *on page 326*
- ◆ **Actonel®** *see* Risedronate *on page 809*
- ◆ **Actron®** [OTC] *see* Ketoprofen *on page 507*
- ◆ **ACU-dyne®** [OTC] *see* Povidone-Iodine *on page 747*
- ◆ **Acular® Ophthalmic** *see* Ketorolac Tromethamine *on page 508*
- ◆ **Acutrim® 16 Hours** [OTC] *see* Phenylpropanolamine *on page 720*
- ◆ **Acutrim® II, Maximum Strength** [OTC] *see* Phenylpropanolamine *on page 720*
- ◆ **Acutrim® Late Day** [OTC] *see* Phenylpropanolamine *on page 720*
- ◆ **ACV** *see* Acyclovir *on this page*
- ◆ **Acycloguanosine** *see* Acyclovir *on this page*

## Acyclovir *(ay SYE kloe veer)*

**Pharmacologic Class** Antiviral Agent

**U.S. Brand Names** Zovirax®

**Mechanism of Action** Acyclovir is converted to acyclovir monophosphate by virus-specific thymidine kinase then further converted to acyclovir triphosphate by other cellular enzymes. Acyclovir triphosphate inhibits DNA synthesis and viral replication by competing with deoxyguanosine triphosphate for viral DNA polymerase and being incorporated into viral DNA.

**Use** Treatment of initial and prophylaxis of recurrent mucosal and cutaneous herpes simplex (HSV-1 and HSV-2) infections; herpes simplex encephalitis; herpes zoster; genital herpes infection; varicella-zoster infections in healthy, nonpregnant persons >13 years of age, children >12 months of age who have a chronic skin or lung disorder or are receiving long-term aspirin therapy, and immunocompromised patients; for herpes zoster, acyclovir should be started within 72 hours of the appearance of the rash to be effective; acyclovir will not prevent postherpetic neuralgias

**USUAL DOSAGE**

Dosing weight should be based on the smaller of lean body weight or total body weight

**Treatment of herpes simplex virus infections:** Children >12 years and Adults: I.V.:

Mucocutaneous HSV or severe initial herpes genitalis infection: 750 mg/m$^2$/day divided every 8 hours or 5 mg/kg/dose every 8 hours for 5-10 days

HSV encephalitis: 1500 mg/m$^2$/day divided every 8 hours or 10 mg/kg/dose for 10 days

**Treatment of genital herpes simplex virus infections:** Adults:

Oral: 200 mg every 4 hours while awake (5 times/day) for 10 days if initial episode; for 5 days if recurrence (begin at earliest signs of disease)

Topical: ½" ribbon of ointment for a 4" square surface area every 3 hours (6 times/day)

**Treatment of varicella-zoster virus (chickenpox) infections:**

Oral:

Children: 10-20 mg/kg/dose (up to 800 mg) 4 times/day for 5 days; begin treatment within the first 24 hours of rash onset

Adults: 600-800 mg/dose every 4 hours while awake (5 times/day) for 7-10 days or 1000 mg every 6 hours for 5 days

I.V.: Children and Adults: 1500 mg/m$^2$/day divided every 8 hours or 10 mg/kg/dose every 8 hours for 7 days

**Treatment of herpes zoster (shingles) infections:**

Oral:

Children (immunocompromised): 250-600 mg/m$^2$/dose 4-5 times/day for 7-10 days

Adults (immunocompromised): 800 mg every 4 hours (5 times/day) for 7-10 days

I.V.:

Children and Adults (immunocompromised): 10 mg/kg/dose or 500 mg/m$^2$/dose every 8 hours

Older Adults (immunocompromised): 7.5 mg/kg/dose every 8 hours

If nephrotoxicity occurs: 5 mg/kg/dose every 8 hours

**Prophylaxis in immunocompromised patients:**

Varicella zoster or herpes zoster in HIV-positive patients: Adults: Oral: 400 mg every 4 hours (5 times/day) for 7-10 days

Bone marrow transplant recipients: Children and Adults: I.V.:

Allogeneic patients who are HSV seropositive: 150 mg/m$^2$/dose (5 mg/kg) every 12 hours; with clinical symptoms of herpes simplex: 150 mg/m$^2$/dose every 8 hours

Allogeneic patients who are CMV seropositive: 500 mg/m$^2$/dose (10 mg/kg) every 8 hours; for clinically symptomatic CMV infection, consider replacing acyclovir with ganciclovir

**Chronic suppressive therapy for recurrent genital herpes simplex virus infections:** Adults: 200 mg 3-4 times/day or 400 mg twice daily for up to 12 months, followed by reevaluation

**Dosing adjustment in renal impairment:**

Oral: HSV/varicella-zoster:

Cl$_{cr}$ 10-25 mL/minute: Administer dose every 8 hours

Cl$_{cr}$ <10 mL/minute: Administer dose every 12 hours

I.V.:

Cl$_{cr}$ 25-50 mL/minute: 5-10 mg/kg/dose: Administer every 12 hours

Cl$_{cr}$ 10-25 mL/minute: 5-10 mg/kg/dose: Administer every 24 hours

Cl$_{cr}$ <10 mL/minute: 2.5-5 mg/kg/dose: Administer every 24 hours

Hemodialysis: Dialyzable (50% to 100%); administer dose postdialysis

Peritoneal dialysis: Dose as for Cl$_{cr}$ <10 mL/minute

Continuous arteriovenous or venovenous hemofiltration (CAVH/CAVHD) effects: Dose as for Cl$_{cr}$ <10 mL/minute

**Dosage Forms Cap:** 200 mg; **Powder for Inj:** 500 mg (10 mL); 1000 mg (20 mL); **Oint, top:** 5% [50 mg/g] (3 g, 15 g); **Susp, oral (banana flavor):** 200 mg/5 mL; **Tab:** 400 mg, 800 mg

**Contraindications** Hypersensitivity to acyclovir

**Warnings/Precautions** Use with caution in patients with pre-existing renal disease or in those receiving other nephrotoxic drugs concurrently; maintain adequate urine output during the first 2 hours after I.V. infusion; use with caution in patients with underlying neurologic abnormalities, serious hepatic or electrolyte abnormalities, or substantial hypoxia

**Pregnancy Risk Factor** C

**Adverse Reactions**

>10%: Local: Inflammation at injection site

1% to 10%:

Central nervous system: Lethargy, dizziness, seizures, confusion, agitation, coma, headache

Dermatologic: Rash

Gastrointestinal: Nausea, vomiting

Neuromuscular & skeletal: Tremor

Renal: Impaired renal function

<1%: Mental depression, insomnia, anorexia, LFT elevation, sore throat, hallucinations, leukopenia, thrombocytopenia, anemia

**Drug Interactions** Increased CNS side effects with zidovudine and probenecid

**Half-Life** 3 hours (normal renal function)

(Continued)

## Acyclovir *(Continued)*

**Special PA Issues**

**Patient Education:** This is not a cure for herpes (recurrences tend to appear within 3 months of original infection), nor will this medication reduce the risk of transmission to others when lesions are present. Take as directed for full course of therapy; do not discontinue even if feeling better. Maintain adequate hydration (2-3 L/day of fluids unless instructed to restrict fluid intake) to prevent renal complications. Avoid use of other topical creams, lotions, or ointments unless approved by prescriber. You may experience nausea or vomiting (small frequent meals or sucking on lozenges may help); lightheadedness or dizziness (use caution when driving or engaging in hazardous activities); headache, fever, muscle pain (an analgesic may be recommended). Report persistent lethargy, acute headache, severe nausea or vomiting, confusion or hallucinations, rash, or difficulty breathing.

**Monitoring Parameters:** Urinalysis, BUN, serum creatinine, liver enzymes, CBC

♦ **Adagen™** *see* Pegademase Bovine *on page 700*

♦ **Adalat®** *see* Nifedipine *on page 654*

♦ **Adalat® CC** *see* Nifedipine *on page 654*

♦ **Adalat® PA®** *see* Nifedipine *on page 654*

♦ **Adamantanamine Hydrochloride** *see* Amantadine *on page 48*

## Adapalene *(a DAP a leen)*

**Pharmacologic Class** Acne Products

**U.S. Brand Names** Differin®

**Mechanism of Action** Retinoid-like compound which is a modulator of cellular differentiation, keratinization and inflammatory processes, all of which represent important features in the pathology of acne vulgaris

**Use** Treatment of acne vulgaris

**USUAL DOSAGE** Children >12 years and Adults: Topical: Apply once daily at bedtime; therapeutic results should be noticed after 8-12 weeks of treatment

**Dosage Forms Gel, top (alcohol free):** 0.1% (15 g, 45 g)

**Contraindications** Hypersensitivity to adapalene or any of the components in the vehicle gel

**Warnings/Precautions** Use with caution in patients with eczema; avoid excessive exposure to sunlight and sunlamps; avoid contact with abraded skin, mucous membranes, eyes, mouth, angles of the nose

Certain cutaneous signs and symptoms such as erythema, dryness, scaling, burning or pruritus may occur during treatment; these are most likely to occur during the first 2-4 weeks and will usually lessen with continued use

**Pregnancy Risk Factor** C

**Pregnancy Implications**

Clinical effects on the fetus: No teratogenic effects were seen in rats at oral doses of adapalene 0.15 to 5 mg/kg/day

Breast feeding/lactation: There are no adequate and well controlled studies in pregnant women; it is not known whether adapalene is excreted in breast milk

**Adverse Reactions**

>10%: Dermatologic: Erythema, scaling, dryness, pruritus, burning, pruritus or burning immediately after application

≤1%: Skin irritation, stinging sunburn, acne flares

**Special PA Issues**

**Patient Education:** For external use only. Apply with gloves in thin film at night to thoroughly clean/dry skin; avoid area around eyes or mouth. Do not apply occlusive dressing. Results make take 8-12 weeks to appear. You may experience transient burning or stinging immediately after applying. Report worsening of condition or skin redness, dryness, peeling, or burning that persists between applications.

♦ **Adapin® Oral** *see* Doxepin *on page 304*

♦ **Adderall®** *see* Dextroamphetamine and Amphetamine *on page 269*

♦ **Adeflor®** *see* Vitamins, Multiple *on page 964*

♦ **Adenine Arabinoside** *see* Vidarabine *on page 961*

♦ **Adenocard®** *see* Adenosine *on this page*

## Adenosine *(a DEN oh seen)*

**Pharmacologic Class** Antiarrhythmic Agent, Class IV

**U.S. Brand Names** Adenocard®

**Mechanism of Action** Slows conduction time through the A-V node, interrupting the re-entry pathways through the A-V node, restoring normal sinus rhythm

**Use** Treatment of paroxysmal supraventricular tachycardia (PSVT) including that associated with accessory bypass tracts (Wolff-Parkinson-White syndrome); when clinically advisable, appropriate vagal maneuvers should be attempted prior to adenosine administration; not effective in atrial flutter, atrial fibrillation, or ventricular tachycardia; also used diagnostically as an adjunct to thallium-201 myocardial scintigraphy in patients unable to exercise adequately

**USUAL DOSAGE Rapid I.V. push (over 1-2 seconds) via peripheral line:**

Neonates: Initial dose: 0.05 mg/kg; if not effective within 2 minutes, increase dose by 0.05 mg/kg increments every 2 minutes to a maximum dose of 0.25 mg/kg or until termination of PSVT

Maximum single dose: 12 mg

Infants and Children: Pediatric advanced life support (PALS): Treatment of SVT: 0.1 mg/kg; if not effective, administer 0.2 mg/kg

Alternatively: Initial dose: 0.05 mg/kg; if not effective within 2 minutes, increase dose by 0.05 mg/kg increments every 2 minutes to a maximum dose of 0.25 mg/kg or until termination of PSVT; medium dose required: 0.15 mg/kg

Maximum single dose: 12 mg

Adults: 6 mg; if not effective within 1-2 minutes, 12 mg may be given; may repeat 12 mg bolus if needed

Maximum single dose: 12 mg

Hemodialysis: Significant drug removal is unlikely based on physiochemical characteristics

Peritoneal dialysis: Significant drug removal is unlikely based on physiochemical characteristics

**Note:** Patients who are receiving concomitant theophylline therapy may be less likely to respond to adenosine therapy

**Note:** Higher doses may be needed for administration via peripheral versus central vein

**Dosage Forms** Inj, preservative free: 3 mg/mL (2 mL)

**Contraindications** Known hypersensitivity to adenosine; second or third degree A-V block or sick-sinus syndrome (except in patients with a functioning artificial pacemaker), atrial flutter, atrial fibrillation, and ventricular tachycardia (the drug is not effective in converting these arrhythmias to sinus rhythm)

**Warnings/Precautions** Patients with pre-existing S-A nodal dysfunction may experience prolonged sinus pauses after adenosine; there have been reports of atrial fibrillation/flutter in patients with PSVT associated with accessory conduction pathways after adenosine; adenosine decreases conduction through the A-V node and may produce a short lasting first, second, or third degree heart block. Because of the very short half-life, the effects are generally self limiting. At the time of conversion to normal sinus rhythm, a variety of new rhythms may appear on the EKG.

A limited number of patients with asthma have received adenosine and have not experienced exacerbation of their asthma. Be alert to the possibility that adenosine could produce bronchoconstriction in patients with asthma.

**Pregnancy Risk Factor** C

**Pregnancy Implications** Excretion in breast milk unknown

Clinical effects on the fetus: Case reports (4) on administration during pregnancy have indicated no adverse effects on fetus or newborn attributable to adenosine

**Adverse Reactions**

>10%:

Cardiovascular: Facial flushing (18%), palpitations, chest pain, hypotension

Central nervous system: Headache

Respiratory: Shortness of breath/dyspnea (12%)

Miscellaneous: Diaphoresis

1% to 10%:

Central nervous system: Dizziness

Gastrointestinal: Nausea (3%)

Neuromuscular & skeletal: Paresthesia, numbness

Respiratory: Chest pressure (7%)

<1%: Lightheadedness, headache, dizziness, apprehension, intracranial pressure, metallic taste, tightness in throat, pressure in groin, neck and back pain, blurred vision, hyperventilation, burning sensation, heaviness in arms

**Drug Interactions**

Decreased effect: Methylxanthines antagonize effects

Increased effect: Dipyridamole potentiates effects of adenosine

Increased toxicity: Carbamazepine may increase heart block

**Onset** Clinical effects occur rapidly

**Duration** Very brief

**Half-Life** <10 seconds

**Special PA Issues**

Patient Education: Adenosine is administered in emergencies, patient education should be appropriate to the situation

**Monitoring Parameters:** EKG monitoring, heart rate, blood pressure

♦ **Adsorbocarpine® Ophthalmic** *see* Pilocarpine *on page 726*

♦ **Adsorbonac® Ophthalmic [OTC]** *see* Sodium Chloride *on page 839*

♦ **Advil® [OTC]** *see* Ibuprofen *on page 466*

♦ **AeroBid®-M Oral Aerosol Inhaler** *see* Flunisolide *on page 379*

♦ **AeroBid® Oral Aerosol Inhaler** *see* Flunisolide *on page 379*

♦ **Aerodine® [OTC]** *see* Povidone-Iodine *on page 747*

♦ **Aerolate®** *see* Theophylline Salts *on page 888*

♦ **Aerolate III®** *see* Theophylline Salts *on page 888*

♦ **Aerolate JR®** *see* Theophylline Salts *on page 888*

♦ **Aerolate SR®** *see* Theophylline Salts *on page 888*

♦ **Aerolone®** *see* Isoproterenol *on page 496*

♦ **Aeroseb-Dex®** *see* Dexamethasone *on page 264*

♦ **Aeroseb-HC®** *see* Hydrocortisone *on page 453*

♦ **A.F. Anacin®** *see* Acetaminophen *on page 21*

♦ **Afrin® Saline Mist [OTC]** *see* Sodium Chloride *on page 839*

♦ **Afrin® Tablet [OTC]** *see* Pseudoephedrine *on page 780*

♦ **Aftate® for Athlete's Foot [OTC]** *see* Tolnaftate *on page 915*

♦ **Aftate® for Jock Itch [OTC]** *see* Tolnaftate *on page 915*

♦ **Agenerase®** *see* Amprenavir *on page 67*

♦ **AgNO₃** *see* Silver Nitrate *on page 834*

♦ **Agrylin®** *see* Anagrelide *on page 68*

♦ **A-hydroCort®** *see* Hydrocortisone *on page 453*

♦ **Airet®** *see* Albuterol *on page 34*

♦ **Akarpine® Ophthalmic** *see* Pilocarpine *on page 726*

♦ **AKBeta®** *see* Levobunolol *on page 523*

♦ **AK-Chlor® Ophthalmic** *see* Chloramphenicol *on page 188*

♦ **AK-Cide® Ophthalmic** *see* Sulfacetamide Sodium and Prednisolone *on page 859*

♦ **AK-Con®** *see* Naphazoline *on page 635*

♦ **AK-Dex®** *see* Dexamethasone *on page 264*

♦ **AK-Dilate® Ophthalmic Solution** *see* Phenylephrine *on page 718*

♦ **AK-Fluor** *see* Fluorescein Sodium *on page 382*

♦ **AK-Homatropine® Ophthalmic** *see* Homatropine *on page 443*

♦ **AK-NaCl [OTC]** *see* Sodium Chloride *on page 839*

♦ **AK-Nefrin® Ophthalmic Solution** *see* Phenylephrine *on page 718*

♦ **AK-Neo-Dex® Ophthalmic** *see* Neomycin and Dexamethasone *on page 643*

♦ **AK-Pentolate®** *see* Cyclopentolate *on page 244*

♦ **AK-Poly-Bac® Ophthalmic** *see* Bacitracin and Polymyxin B *on page 97*

♦ **AK-Pred® Ophthalmic** *see* Prednisolone *on page 752*

♦ **AKPro® Ophthalmic** *see* Dipivefrin *on page 292*

♦ **AK-Spore H.C.® Ophthalmic Ointment** *see* Bacitracin, Neomycin, Polymyxin B, and Hydrocortisone *on page 97*

♦ **AK-Spore H.C.® Ophthalmic Suspension** *see* Neomycin, Polymyxin B, and Hydrocortisone *on page 645*

♦ **AK-Spore H.C.® Otic** *see* Neomycin, Polymyxin B, and Hydrocortisone *on page 645*

♦ **AK-Spore® Ophthalmic Ointment** *see* Bacitracin, Neomycin, and Polymyxin B *on page 97*

♦ **AK-Spore® Ophthalmic Solution** *see* Neomycin, Polymyxin B, and Gramicidin *on page 644*

♦ **AK-Sulf® Ophthalmic** *see* Sulfacetamide Sodium *on page 858*

♦ **AK-Taine®** *see* Proparacaine *on page 771*

♦ **AKTob® Ophthalmic** *see* Tobramycin *on page 907*

♦ **AK-Tracin® Ophthalmic** *see* Bacitracin *on page 96*

♦ **AK-Trol®** *see* Neomycin, Polymyxin B, and Dexamethasone *on page 644*

♦ **Ala-Cort®** *see* Hydrocortisone *on page 453*

♦ **Ala-Scalp®** *see* Hydrocortisone *on page 453*

♦ **Alatrovafloxacin Mesylate** *see* Trovafloxacin *on page 943*

♦ **Alba-Dex®** *see* Dexamethasone *on page 264*

♦ **Albalon® Liquifilm®** *see* Naphazoline *on page 635*

## Albendazole (al BEN da zole)

**Pharmacologic Class** Anthelmintic

**U.S. Brand Names** Albenza®

**Mechanism of Action** Active metabolite, albendazole, causes selective degeneration of cytoplasmic microtubules in intestinal and tegmental cells of intestinal helminths and larvae; glycogen is depleted, glucose uptake and cholinesterase secretion are impaired, and desecratory substances accumulate intracellulary. ATP production decreases causing energy depletion, immobilization, and worm death.

**Use** Treatment of parenchymal neurocysticercosis and cystic hydatid disease of the liver, lung, and peritoneum; albendazole has activity against *Ascaris lumbricoides* (roundworm), *Ancylostoma duodenal* and *Necator americanus* (hookworms), *Enterobius vermicularis* (pinworm), *Hymenolepis nana* and *Taenia* sp (tapeworms), *Opisthorchis sinensis* and *Opisthorchis viverrini* (liver flukes), *Strongyloides stercoralis* and *Trichuris trichiura* (whipworm); activity has also been shown against the liver fluke *Clonorchis sinensis*, *Giardia lamblia*, *Cysticercus cellulosae*, *Echinococcus granulosus*, *Echinococcus multilocularis*, and *Toxocara* sp.

**USUAL DOSAGE** Oral:
Neurocysticercosis:
<60 kg: 15 mg/kg/day in 2 divided doses (maximum: 800 mg/day) with meals for 8-30 days
≥60 kg: 400 mg twice daily for 8-30 days
Note: Give concurrent anticonvulsant and steroid therapy during first week
Hydatid:
<60 kg: 15 mg/kg/day in 2 divided doses with meals (maximum: 800 mg/day) for three 28-day cycles with 14-day drug-free interval in-between
≥60 kg: 400 mg twice daily for 3 cycles as above
Strongyloidiasis/tapeworm:
≤2 years: 200 mg/day for 3 days; may repeat in 3 weeks
>2 years and Adults: 400 mg/day for 3 days; may repeat in 3 weeks
Giardiasis: Adults: 400 mg/day for 3 days
Hookworm, pinworm, roundworm:
≤2 years: 200 mg as a single dose; may repeat in 3 weeks
>2 years and Adults: 400 mg as a single dose; may repeat in 3 weeks

**Dosage Forms** Tab: 200 mg

**Contraindications** Patients with hypersensitivity to albendazole or its components; pregnant women, if possible

**Warnings/Precautions** Discontinue therapy if LFT elevations are significant; may restart treatment when decreased to pretreatment values. Becoming pregnant within 1 month following therapy is not advised. Corticosteroids should be administered 1-2 days before albendazole therapy in patients with neurocysticercosis to minimize inflammatory reactions and steroid and anticonvulsant therapy should be used concurrently during the first week of therapy for neurocysticercosis to prevent cerebral hypertension. If retinal lesions exist in patients with neurocysticercosis, weigh risk of further retinal damage due to albendazole-induced changes to the retinal lesion vs benefit of disease treatment.

**Pregnancy Risk Factor** C

**Pregnancy Implications** Albendazole has been shown to be teratogenic in laboratory animals and should not be used during pregnancy, if at all possible

**Adverse Reactions** N = neurocysticercosis; H = hydatid disease
Central nervous system: Dizziness, vertigo, fever (≤1%); headache (11% - N; 1% - H); increased intracranial pressure
Dermatologic: Alopecia/rash/urticaria (<1%)
Gastrointestinal: Abdominal pain (6% - H, 0% - N); nausea/vomiting (3% to 6%)
Hematologic: Leukopenia (reversible) (<1%); granulocytopenia/agranulocytopenia/pancytopenia (rare)
Hepatic: Increased LFTs (~15% - H, <1% - N)
Miscellaneous: Allergic reactions (<1%)

**Drug Interactions** CYP1A enzyme inhibitor
Decreased effect: Carbamazepine may accelerate albendazole metabolism
Increased effect: Dexamethasone increases plasma levels of albendazole metabolites; praziquantel may increase plasma concentrations of albendazole by 50%; albendazole inhibits hepatic cytochrome P-450 1A and may consequently interact by increasing the concentrations of many drugs which are metabolized by this route; food (especially fatty meals) increases the oral bioavailability by 4-5 times

**Half-Life** 8-12 hours

**Special PA Issues**
Patient Education: Take according to prescribed dosage schedule with meals. You may experience loss of hair (reversible); dizziness or headaches (use caution when driving or engaging in tasks that require alertness). Report unusual fever, abdominal pain, unresolved vomiting, yellowing of skin or eyes, darkening of urine, or light colored stools.
Monitoring Parameters: Monitor fecal specimens for ova and parasites for 3 weeks after treatment; if positive, retreat; monitor LFTs, and clinical signs of hepatotoxicity; CBC at start of each 28-day cycle and every 2 weeks during therapy

# Albumin (al BYOO min)

**Pharmacologic Class** Blood Product Derivative; Plasma Volume Expander, Colloid

**U.S. Brand Names** Albuminar®; Albumisol®; Albunex®; Albutein®; Buminate®; Plasbumin®

**Mechanism of Action** Provides increase in intravascular oncotic pressure and causes mobilization of fluids from interstitial into intravascular space

**Use** Plasma volume expansion and maintenance of cardiac output in the treatment of certain types of shock or impending shock; may be useful for burn patients, ARDS, and cardiopulmonary bypass; other uses considered by some investigators (but not proven) are retroperitoneal surgery, peritonitis, and ascites; unless the condition responsible for hypoproteinemia can be corrected, albumin can provide only symptomatic relief or supportive treatment; nutritional supplementation is not an appropriate indication for albumin

**USUAL DOSAGE** I.V.:

**5%** should be used in hypovolemic patients or intravascularly-depleted patients

**25%** should be used in patients in whom fluid and sodium intake must be minimized

**Dose depends on condition of patient:**

Children:

Emergency initial dose: 25 g

Nonemergencies: 25% to 50% of the adult dose

Adults: Usual dose: 25 g; no more than 250 g should be administered within 48 hours

Hypoproteinemia: 0.5-1 g/kg/dose; repeat every 1-2 days as calculated to replace ongoing losses

Hypovolemia: 0.5-1 g/kg/dose; repeat as needed; maximum dose: 6 g/kg/day

**Dosage Forms Inj, as human:** 5% [50 mg/mL] (50 mL, 250 mL, 500 mL, 1000 mL); 25% [250 mg/mL] (10 mL, 20 mL, 50 mL, 100 mL)

**Contraindications** Patients with severe anemia or cardiac failure, known hypersensitivity to albumin; avoid 25% concentration in preterm infants due to risk of idiopathic ventricular hypertrophy

**Warnings/Precautions** Use with caution in patients with hepatic or renal failure because of added protein load; rapid infusion of albumin solutions may cause vascular overload. All patients should be observed for signs of hypervolemia such as pulmonary edema. Use with caution in those patients for whom sodium restriction is necessary. Rapid infusion may cause hypotension.

**Pregnancy Risk Factor** C

**Pregnancy Implications** Excretion in breast milk unknown/compatible

**Adverse Reactions** 1% to 10%:

Cardiovascular: Precipitation of congestive heart failure or hypotension, tachycardia, hypervolemia

Central nervous system: Fever, chills

Dermatologic: Rash

Gastrointestinal: Nausea, vomiting

Respiratory: Pulmonary edema

♦ **Albuminar®** see Albumin on this page

♦ **Albumin (Human)** see Albumin on this page

♦ **Albumisol®** see Albumin on this page

♦ **Albunex®** see Albumin on this page

♦ **Albutein®** see Albumin on this page

# Albuterol (al BYOO ter ole)

**Pharmacologic Class** Beta$_2$ Agonist

**U.S. Brand Names** Airet®; Proventil®; Proventil® HFA; Ventolin®; Ventolin® Rotocaps®; Volmax®

**Mechanism of Action** Relaxes bronchial smooth muscle by action on beta$_2$-receptors with little effect on heart rate

**Use** Bronchodilator in reversible airway obstruction due to asthma or COPD

**USUAL DOSAGE**

Oral:

Children:

2-6 years: 0.1-0.2 mg/kg/dose 3 times/day; maximum dose not to exceed 12 mg/day (divided doses)

6-12 years: 2 mg/dose 3-4 times/day; maximum dose not to exceed 24 mg/day (divided doses)

Children >12 years and Adults: 2-4 mg/dose 3-4 times/day; maximum dose not to exceed 32 mg/day (divided doses)

Elderly: 2 mg 3-4 times/day; maximum: 8 mg 4 times/day

Inhalation MDI: 90 mcg/spray:

Children <12 years: 1-2 inhalations 4 times/day using a tube spacer

Children ≥12 years and Adults: 1-2 inhalations every 4-6 hours; maximum: 12 inhalations/day

Exercise-induced bronchospasm: 2 inhalations 15 minutes before exercising

Inhalation: Nebulization: 0.01-0.05 mL/kg of 0.5% solution every 4-6 hours; intensive care patients may require more frequent administration; minimum dose: 0.1 mL; maximum dose: 1 mL diluted in 1-2 mL normal saline; continuous nebulized albuterol at 0.3 mg/kg/ hour has been used safely in the treatment of severe status asthmaticus in children; continuous nebulized doses of 3 mg/kg/hour ±2.2 mg/kg/hour in children whose mean age was 20.7 months resulted in no cardiac toxicity; the optimal dosage for continuous nebulization remains to be determined.

Hemodialysis: Not removed

Peritoneal dialysis: Significant drug removal is unlikely based on physiochemical characteristics

**Dosage Forms Aero:** 90 mcg/dose (17 g) [200 doses]; Proventil®, Ventolin®: 90 mcg/dose (17 g) [200 doses], Chlorofluorocarbon free (Proventil® HFA): 90 mcg/dose (17 g); **Cap for oral inhalation (Ventolin® Rotocaps®):** 200 mcg [to be used with Rotahaler® inhalation device]; **Sol, inhalation:** 0.083% (3 mL); 0.5% (20 mL), Airet®: 0.083%, Proventil®: 0.083% (3 mL); 0.5% (20 mL), Ventolin®: 0.5% (20 mL); **Syr, as sulfate:** 2 mg/5 mL (480 mL), Proventil®, Ventolin®: 2 mg/5 mL (480 mL); **Tab, as sulfate:** 2 mg, 4 mg, Proventil®, Ventolin®: 2 mg, 4 mg, extended release: Proventil® Repetabs®: 4 mg, Volmax®: 4 mg, 8 mg

**Contraindications** Hypersensitivity to albuterol, adrenergic amines or any ingredients

**Warnings/Precautions** Use with caution in patients with hyperthyroidism, diabetes mellitus, or sensitivity to sympathomimetic amines; cardiovascular disorders including coronary insufficiency or hypertension; excessive use may result in tolerance

Some adverse reactions may occur more frequently in children 2-5 years of age than in adults and older children

Because of its minimal effect on beta$_1$-receptors and its relatively long duration of action, albuterol is a rational choice in the elderly when a beta agonist is indicated. All patients should utilize a spacer device when using a metered dose inhaler. Oral use should be avoided in the elderly due to adverse effects.

**Pregnancy Risk Factor** C

**Pregnancy Implications**

Clinical effects on the fetus: Crosses the placenta. Tocolytic effects, fetal tachycardia, fetal hypoglycemia secondary to maternal hyperglycemia with oral or intravenous routes reported. Available evidence suggests safe use during pregnancy.

Breast-feeding/lactation: No data on crossing into breast milk or clinical effects on the infant

**Adverse Reactions**

>10%:

Cardiovascular: Tachycardia, palpitations, pounding heartbeat

Gastrointestinal: GI upset, nausea

1% to 10%:

Cardiovascular: Flushing of face, hypertension or hypotension

Central nervous system: Nervousness, CNS stimulation, hyperactivity, insomnia, dizziness, lightheadedness, drowsiness, headache

Gastrointestinal: Xerostomia, heartburn, vomiting, unusual taste

Genitourinary: Dysuria

Neuromuscular & skeletal: Muscle cramping, tremor, weakness

Respiratory: Coughing

Miscellaneous: Diaphoresis (increased)

<1%: Chest pain, unusual pallor, loss of appetite, paradoxical bronchospasm

**Drug Interactions**

Decreased effect: Beta-adrenergic blockers (eg, propranolol)

Increased therapeutic effect: Inhaled ipratropium may increase duration of bronchodilation, nifedipine may increase FEV-1

Increased toxicity: Cardiovascular effects are potentiated in patients also receiving MAO inhibitors, tricyclic antidepressants, sympathomimetic agents (eg, amphetamine, dopamine, dobutamine), inhaled anesthetics (eg, enflurane)

**Onset** Peak effect: Oral: 2-3 hours; Nebulization/oral inhalation: Within 0.5-2 hours

**Duration** Oral: 4-6 hours; Nebulization/oral inhalation: 3-4 hours

**Half-Life** Inhalation: 3.8 hours; Oral: 3.7-5 hours

**Special PA Issues**

**Patient Education:** Use exactly as directed (see Administration below). Do not use more often than recommended. Maintain adequate hydration (2-3 L/day of fluids unless instructed to restrict fluid intake). You may experience nervousness, dizziness, or fatigue (use caution when driving or engaging in hazardous activities until response to treatment is known); dry mouth, unpleasant taste, stomach upset (frequent small meals, frequent mouth care, chewing gum, or sucking hard candy may help); or difficulty urinating (always void before treatment). Report unresolved GI upset, dizziness or fatigue, vision changes, chest pain or palpitations, persistent inability to void, nervousness or insomnia, muscle cramping or tremor, or unusual cough.

**Administration**

Self-administered inhalation: Store canister upside down; do not freeze. Shake canister before using. Sit when using medication. Close eyes when administering albuterol to avoid spray getting into eyes. Exhale slowly and completely through nose; inhale deeply through mouth while administering aerosol. Hold breath for 1-3 seconds after

(Continued)

## Albuterol *(Continued)*

inhalation. Wait at least 1 full minute between inhalations. Wash mouthpiece between use. If more than one inhalation medication is used, use albuterol first and wait 5 minutes between medications.

Self-administered nebulizer: Wash hands before and after treatment. Wash and dry nebulizer after each treatment. Twist open the top of one unit dose vial and squeeze contents into nebulizer reservoir. Connect nebulizer reservoir to the mouthpiece or face-mask. Connect nebulizer to compressor. Sit in comfortable, upright position. Place mouthpiece in your mouth or put on face mask and turn on compressor. If face-mask is used, avoid leakage around the mask to avoid mist getting into eyes which may cause vision problems. Breath calmly and deeply until no more mist is formed in nebulizer (about 5 minutes). At this point treatment is finished.

**Monitoring Parameters:** Heart rate, CNS stimulation, asthma symptoms, arterial or capillary blood gases (if patients condition warrants)

♦ **Alcaine®** *see* Proparacaine *on page 771*

## Alclometasone *(al kloe MET a sone)*

**Pharmacologic Class** Corticosteroid, Topical

**U.S. Brand Names** Aclovate® Topical

**Mechanism of Action** Stimulates the synthesis of enzymes needed to decrease inflammation, suppress mitotic activity, and cause vasoconstriction

**Use** Treats inflammation of corticosteroid-responsive dermatosis (low potency topical corticosteroid)

**USUAL DOSAGE** Topical: Apply a thin film to the affected area 2-3 times/day

**Dosage Forms Crm:** 0.05% (15 g, 45 g, 60 g); **Oint, top:** 0.05% (15 g, 45 g, 60 g)

**Contraindications** Viral, fungal, or tubercular skin lesions, known hypersensitivity to alclometasone or any component

**Warnings/Precautions** Adverse systemic effects may occur when used on large areas of the body, denuded areas, for prolonged periods of time, with an occlusive dressing, and/or in infants or small children

**Pregnancy Risk Factor** C

**Adverse Reactions**

1% to 10%:

Dermatologic: Itching, erythema, dryness papular rashes

Local: Burning, irritation

<1%: Hypertrichosis, acneiform eruptions, hypopigmentation, perioral dermatitis, maceration of skin, skin atrophy, striae, miliaria

**Special PA Issues**

**Patient Education:** For external use only. Use exactly as directed; do not overuse. Do not apply to open wounds or weeping areas. Before using, wash and dry area gently. Apply a thin film to affected area and rub in gently If dressing is necessary, use a porous dressing. Avoid contact with eyes. Avoid exposing treated area to direct sunlight; sunburn can occur. Report increased swelling, redness, rash, itching, signs of infection, worsening of condition, or lack of healing.

♦ **Alclometasone Dipropionate** *see* Alclometasone *on this page*

♦ **Alconefrin® Nasal Solution [OTC]** *see* Phenylephrine *on page 718*

♦ **Aldactazide®** *see* Hydrochlorothiazide and Spironolactone *on page 448*

♦ **Aldactone®** *see* Spironolactone *on page 849*

♦ **Aldara™** *see* Imiquimod *on page 471*

## Aldesleukin *(al des LOO kin)*

**Pharmacologic Class** Biological Response Modulator

**U.S. Brand Names** Proleukin®

**Mechanism of Action** IL-2 promotes proliferation, differentiation, and recruitment of T and B cells, natural killer (NK) cells, and thymocytes; IL-2 also causes cytolytic activity in a subset of lymphocytes and subsequent interactions between the immune system and malignant cells; IL-2 can stimulate lymphokine-activated killer (LAK) cells and tumor-infiltrating lymphocytes (TIL) cells. LAK cells (which are derived from lymphocytes from a patient and incubated in IL-2) have the ability to lyse cells which are resistant to NK cells; TIL cells (which are derived from cancerous tissue from a patient and incubated in IL-2) have been shown to be 50% more effective than LAK cells in experimental studies.

**Use** Treatment of metastatic renal cell carcinoma; also, investigated in tumors known to have a response to immunotherapy, such as melanoma; has been used in conjunction with LAK cells, TIL cells, IL-1, and interferon

**USUAL DOSAGE** Refer to individual protocols; all orders must be written in million International units (million IU)

Adults: Metastatic renal cell carcinoma (RCC):

Treatment consists of two 5-day treatment cycles separated by a rest period. 600,000 units/kg (0.037 mg/kg)/dose administered every 8 hours by a 15-minute I.V. infusion for a total of 14 doses; following 9 days of rest, the schedule is repeated for another 14 doses, for a maximum of 28 doses per course

**Dose modification:** In high-dose therapy of RCC, see manufacturer's guidelines for holding and restarting therapy; hold or interrupt a dose - DO NOT DOSE REDUCE; or refer to specific protocol

**Retreatment:** Patients should be evaluated for response approximately 4 weeks after completion of a course of therapy and again immediately prior to the scheduled start of the next treatment course; additional courses of treatment may be given to patients only if there is some tumor shrinkage or stable disease following the last course and retreatment is not contraindicated. Each treatment course should be separated by a rest period of at least 7 weeks from the date of hospital discharge; tumors have continued to regress up to 12 months following the initiation of therapy

**Investigational regimen:** S.C.: 11 million Units (flat dose) daily x 4 days per week for 4 consecutive weeks; repeat every 6 weeks

**Dosage Forms** Powder for inj, lyophilized: $22 \times 10^6$ int. units [18 million int. units/mL = 1.1 mg/mL when reconstituted]

**Contraindications** Known history of hypersensitivity to interleukin-2 or any component; patients with an abnormal thallium stress test or pulmonary function test; patients who have had an organ allograft; retreatment in patients who have experienced sustained ventricular tachycardia ($\geq$5 beats); cardiac rhythm disturbances not controlled or unresponsive to management, recurrent chest pain with EKG changes (consistent with angina or myocardial infarction), intubation required >72 hours, pericardial tamponade; renal dysfunction requiring dialysis >72 hours, coma or toxic psychosis lasting >48 hours, repetitive or difficult to control seizures, bowel ischemia/perforation, GI bleeding requiring surgery

**Warnings/Precautions** High-dose IL-2 therapy has been associated with capillary leak syndrome (CLS); CLS results in hypotension and reduced organ perfusion which may be severe and can result in death; therapy should be restricted to patients with normal cardiac and pulmonary functions as defined by thallium stress and formal pulmonary function testing; extreme caution should be used in patients with normal thallium stress tests and pulmonary functions tests who have a history of prior cardiac or pulmonary disease. Postnephrectomy patients must have a serum creatinine of $\leq$1.5 mg/dL prior to treatment.

Intensive aldesleukin treatment is associated with impaired neutrophil function (reduced chemotaxis) and with an increased risk of disseminated infection, including sepsis and bacterial endocarditis, in treated patients. Consequently, pre-existing bacterial infections should be adequately treated prior to initiation of therapy. Additionally, all patients with indwelling central lines should receive antibiotic prophylaxis effective against *S. aureus*. Antibiotic prophylaxis which has been associated with a reduced incidence of staphylococcal infections in aldesleukin studies includes the use of oxacillin, nafcillin, ciprofloxacin, or vancomycin.

Standard prophylactic supportive care during high-dose IL-2 treatment includes acetaminophen to relieve constitutional symptoms and an $H_2$-antagonist to reduce the risk of GI ulceration and/or bleeding.

**Pregnancy Risk Factor** C

**Adverse Reactions**
>10%:
   Cardiovascular: Sensory dysfunction, sinus tachycardia, arrhythmias, pulmonary congestion; hypotension (dose-limiting toxicity) which may require vasopressor support and hemodynamic changes resembling those seen in septic shock can be seen within 2 hours of administration; angina, acute myocardial infarction, SVT with hypotension has been reported, edema
   Central nervous system: Dizziness, pain, fever, chills, cognitive changes, fatigue, malaise, disorientation, somnolence, paranoid delusion, and other behavioral changes; reversible and dose related; however, may continue to worsen for several days even after the infusion is stopped
   Dermatologic: Pruritus, erythema, rash, dry skin, exfoliative dermatitis, macular erythema
   Gastrointestinal: Nausea, vomiting, weight gain, diarrhea, stomatitis, anorexia, GI bleeding
   Hematologic: Anemia, thrombocytopenia, leukopenia, eosinophilia, coagulation disorders
   Hepatic: Elevated transaminase and alkaline phosphatase, jaundice
   Neuromuscular & skeletal: Weakness, rigors which can be decreased or ameliorated with acetaminophen or a nonsteroidal agent and meperidine
   Renal: Oliguria, anuria, proteinuria; renal failure (dose-limiting toxicity) manifested as oliguria noted within 24-48 hours of initiation of therapy; marked fluid retention, azotemia, and increased serum creatinine seen, which may return to baseline within 7 days of discontinuation of therapy; hypophosphatemia
   Respiratory: Dyspnea, pulmonary edema
1% to 10%: Cardiovascular: Increase in vascular permeability: Capillary-leak syndrome manifested by severe peripheral edema, ascites, pulmonary infiltration, and pleural effusion; occurs in 2% to 4% of patients and is resolved after therapy ends
<1%: Congestive heart failure, coma, seizure, alopecia, hypercalcemia, hypocalcemia, hypomagnesemia, hypothyroidism, increased plasma levels of stress-related hormones, acidosis, pancreatitis, polyuria, arthritis, muscle spasm, allergic reactions
(Continued)

## Aldesleukin *(Continued)*

**Drug Interactions**

Decreased toxicity: Corticosteroids have been shown to decrease toxicity of IL-2, but have not been used since there is concern that they may decrease the efficacy of the lympho-kine

Increased toxicity:

Aldesleukin may affect central nervous function; therefore, interactions could occur following concomitant administration of psychotropic drugs (eg, narcotics, analgesics, antiemetics, sedatives, tranquilizers)

Concomitant administration of drugs possessing nephrotoxic (eg, aminoglycosides, indo-methacin), myelotoxic (eg, cytotoxic chemotherapy), cardiotoxic (eg, doxorubicin), or hepatotoxic (eg, methotrexate, asparaginase) effects with aldesleukin may ↑ toxicity in these organ systems; the safety and efficacy of aldesleukin in combination with chemo-therapy agents has not been established

Beta-blockers and other antihypertensives may potentiate the hypotension seen with Proleukin®

Iodinated contrast media: Acute reactions including fever, chills, nausea, vomiting, pruritus, rash, diarrhea, hypotension, edema, and oliguria have occurred within hours of contrast infusion; this reaction may occur within 4 weeks or up to several months after IL-2 administration

**Half-Life** 20-120 minutes

**Special PA Issues**

**Patient Education:** This drug can only be administered by infusion. Avoid alcohol and all OTC or prescription drugs unless approved by your oncologist. You will be sensitive to sunlight; use of sunblock (15 SPF or greater), wear protective clothing, or avoid direct sun exposure. You will be susceptible to infection; avoid crowds or infected persons or persons with contagious diseases. Frequent mouth care and small frequent meals may help counteract any GI effects you may experience and will help maintain adequate nutrition and fluid intake. This drug may result in many side effects; you will be monitored and assessed closely during therapy, however, it is important that you report any changes or problems for evaluation. Report any changes in urination, unusual bruising or bleeding, chest pain or palpitations, acute dizziness, respiratory difficulty, fever or chills, changes in cognition, rash, feelings of pain or numbness in extremities, severe GI upset or diarrhea, vaginal discharge or mouth sores, yellowing of eyes or skin, or any changes in color of urine or stool.

**Monitoring Parameters:**

**The following clinical evaluations are recommended for all patients prior to begin-ning treatment and then daily during drug administration:**

Standard hematologic tests including CBC, differential, and platelet counts

Blood chemistries including electrolytes, renal and hepatic function tests

Chest x-rays

Daily monitoring during therapy should include vital signs (temperature, pulse, blood pressure, and respiration rate) and weight; in a patient with a decreased blood pressure, especially <90 mm Hg, constant cardiac monitoring for rhythm should be conducted. If an abnormal complex or rhythm is seen, an EKG should be performed; vital signs in these hypotension patients should be taken hourly and central venous pressure (CVP) checked.

During treatment, pulmonary function should be monitored on a regular basis by clinical examination, assessment of vital signs and pulse oximetry. Patients with dyspnea or clinical signs of respiratory impairment (tachypnea or rales) should be further assessed with arterial blood gas determination. These tests are to be repeated as often as clinically indicated.

Cardiac function is assessed daily by clinical examination and assessment of vital signs. Patients with signs or symptoms of chest pain, murmurs, gallops, irregular rhythm or palpitations should be further assessed with an EKG examination and CPK evaluation. If there is evidence of cardiac ischemia or congestive heart failure, a repeat thallium study should be done.

♦ **Aldoclor®** *see* Chlorothiazide and Methyldopa *on page 194*

♦ **Aldomet®** *see* Methyldopa *on page 590*

♦ **Aldoril®** *see* Methyldopa and Hydrochlorothiazide *on page 591*

## Alendronate *(a LEN droe nate)*

**Pharmacologic Class** Bisphosphonate Derivative

**U.S. Brand Names** Fosamax®

**Mechanism of Action** A bisphosphonate which inhibits bone resorption via actions on osteoclasts or on osteoclast precursors; decreases the rate of bone resorption direction, leading to an indirect decrease in bone formation

**Use** Osteoporosis in postmenopausal women; Paget's disease of the bone

**USUAL DOSAGE** Oral: Alendronate must be taken with plain water first thing in the morning and ≥30 minutes before the first food, beverage, or other medication of the day. Patients should be instructed to take alendronate with a full glass of water (6-8 oz) and not lie down for at least 30 minutes to improve alendronate absorption.

Adults: Patients with osteoporosis or Paget's disease should receive supplemental calcium and vitamin D if dietary intake is inadequate

**Osteoporosis in postmenopausal women:**
Prophylaxis: 5 mg once daily
Treatment: 10 mg once daily

**Paget's disease of bone:** 40 mg once daily for 6 months
Retreatment: Relapses during the 12 months following therapy occurred in 9% of patients who responded to treatment. Specific retreatment data are not available. Retreatment with alendronate may be considered, following a 6-month post-treatment evaluation period, in patients who have relapsed based on increases in serum alkaline phosphatase, which should be measured periodically. Retreatment may also be considered in those who failed to normalize their serum alkaline phosphatase.

Elderly: No dosage adjustment is necessary

**Dosage adjustment in renal impairment:**
$Cl_{cr}$ 30-60 mL/minute: None necessary
$Cl_{cr}$ <35 mL/minute: Alendronate is not recommended due to lack of experience

**Dosage adjustment in hepatic impairment:** None necessary

**Dosage Forms** Tab, as sodium: 5 mg, 10 mg, 40 mg

**Contraindications** Hypersensitivity to bisphosphonates or any component of the product; hypocalcemia; abnormalities of the esophagus which delay esophageal emptying such as stricture or achalasia; inability to stand or sit upright for at least 30 minutes

**Warnings/Precautions** Use caution in patients with renal impairment; concomitant hormone replacement therapy with alendronate for osteoporosis in postmenopausal women is not recommended; hypocalcemia must be corrected before therapy initiation with alendronate; ensure adequate calcium and vitamin D intake to provide for enhanced needs in patients with Paget's disease in whom the pretreatment rate of bone turnover may be greatly elevated.

**Pregnancy Risk Factor** C

**Adverse Reactions** Note: Incidence of adverse effects increases significantly in patients treated for Paget's disease at 40 mg/day, mostly GI adverse effects
1% to 10%:
Central nervous system: Headache (2.6%); pain (4.1%)
Gastrointestinal: Flatulence (2.6%); acid regurgitation (2%); esophagitis ulcer (1.5%); dysphagia, abdominal distention (1%)
<1%: Rash, erythema (rare), gastritis (0.5%)

**Half-Life** Estimated to exceed 10 years due to release of alendronate from the skeleton

**Special PA Issues**
**Patient Education:** Patients should be instructed that the expected benefits of alendronate may only be obtained when each tablet is taken with plain water the first thing in the morning and at least 30 minutes before the first food, beverage, or medication of the day. Also instruct them that waiting >30 minutes will improve alendronate absorption. Even dosing with orange juice or coffee markedly reduces the absorption of alendronate.

Instruct patients to take alendronate with a full glass of water (6-8 oz 180-240 mL) and not to lie down (stay fully upright sitting or standing) for at least 30 minutes following administration to facilitate delivery to the stomach and reduce the potential for esophageal irritation.

Patients should be instructed to take supplemental calcium and vitamin D if dietary intake is inadequate. Consider weight-bearing exercise along with the modification of certain behavioral factors, such as excessive cigarette smoking or alcohol consumption if these factors exist.

**Monitoring Parameters:** Alkaline phosphatase should be periodically measured; serum calcium, phosphorus, and possibly potassium due to its drug class; use of absorptiometry may assist in noting benefit in osteoporosis; monitor pain and fracture rate

**Reference Range:** Calcium (total): Adults: 9.0-11.0 mg/dL (2.05-2.54 mmol/L), may slightly decrease with aging; phosphorus: 2.5-4.5 mg/dL (0.81-1.45 mmol/L)

♦ **Alendronate Sodium** see Alendronate on previous page

♦ **Alesse™** see Ethinyl Estradiol and Levonorgestrel on page 347

♦ **Aleve® [OTC]** see Naproxen on page 636

♦ **Alfenta®** see Alfentanil on this page

# Alfentanil (al FEN ta nil)

**Pharmacologic Class** Analgesic, Narcotic

**U.S. Brand Names** Alfenta®

**Mechanism of Action** Binds with stereospecific receptors at many sites within the CNS, increases pain threshold, alters pain perception, inhibits ascending pain pathways; is an ultra short-acting narcotic

**Use** Analgesic adjunct given by continuous infusion or in incremental doses in maintenance of anesthesia with barbiturate or $N_2O$ or a primary anesthetic agent for the induction of
(Continued)

## Alfentanil (Continued)

anesthesia in patients undergoing general surgery in which endotracheal intubation and mechanical ventilation are required

**USUAL DOSAGE** Doses should be titrated to appropriate effects; wide range of doses is dependent upon desired degree of analgesia/anesthesia

Children <12 years: Dose not established
Adults: Dose should be based on ideal body weight; see table.

**Adult Dosing for Alfentanil**

| Indication | Approx Duration of Anesthesia (min) | Induction Period (Initial Dose) (mcg/kg) | Maintenance Period (Increments/ Infusion) | Total Dose (mcg/kg) | Effects |
|---|---|---|---|---|---|
| Incremental injection | ≤30 | 8-20 | 3-5 mcg/kg or 0.5-1 mcg/kg/ min | 8-40 | Spontaneously breathing or assisted ventilation when required. |
| | 30-60 | 20-50 | 5-15 mcg/kg | Up to 75 | Assisted or controlled ventilation required. Attenuation of response to laryngoscopy and intubation. |
| Continuous infusion | >45 | 50-75 | 0.5-3 mcg/kg/ min average infusion rate 1-1.5 mcg/kg/min | Dependent on duration of procedure | Assisted or controlled ventilation required. Some attenuation of response to intubation and incision, with intraoperative stability. |
| Anesthetic induction | >45 | 130-245 | 0.5-1.5 mcg/kg/ min or general anesthetic | Dependent on duration of procedure | Assisted or controlled ventilation required. Administer slowly (over 3 minutes). Concentration of inhalation agents reduced by 30% to 50% for initial hour. |

**Dosage Forms Inj, preservative free, as hydrochloride:** 500 mcg/mL (2 mL, 5 mL, 10 mL, 20 mL)

**Contraindications** Hypersensitivity to alfentanil hydrochloride or narcotics; increased intracranial pressure, severe respiratory depression

**Warnings/Precautions** Drug dependence, head injury, acute asthma and respiratory conditions; hypotension has occurred in neonates with respiratory distress syndrome; use caution when administering to patients with bradyarrhythmias; rapid I.V. infusion may result in skeletal muscle and chest wall rigidity → impaired ventilation → respiratory distress/arrest. Inject slowly over 3-5 minutes; nondepolarizing skeletal muscle relaxant may be required. Alfentanil may produce more hypotension compared to fentanyl, therefore, be sure to administer slowly and ensure patient has adequate hydration.

**Pregnancy Risk Factor** C

**Adverse Reactions**
>10%:
Cardiovascular: Bradycardia, peripheral vasodilation
Central nervous system: Drowsiness, sedation, increased intracranial pressure
Gastrointestinal: Nausea, vomiting, constipation
Endocrine & metabolic: Antidiuretic hormone release
Ocular: Miosis
1% to 10%:
Cardiovascular: Cardiac arrhythmias, orthostatic hypotension
Central nervous system: Confusion, CNS depression
Ocular: Blurred vision
<1%: Convulsions, mental depression, paradoxical CNS excitation or delirium, dizziness, dysesthesia, rash, urticaria, itching, biliary tract spasm, urinary tract spasm, respiratory depression, bronchospasm, laryngospasm, physical and psychological dependence with prolonged use, cold, clammy skin

**Drug Interactions** CYP3A3/4 enzyme substrate
Decreased effect: Phenothiazines may antagonize the analgesic effect of opiate agonists
Increased effect: Dextroamphetamine may enhance the analgesic effect of morphine and other opiate agonists
Increased toxicity: CNS depressants (eg, benzodiazepines, barbiturates, phenothiazines, tricyclic antidepressants), erythromycin, reserpine, beta-blockers

**Onset** Rapid

**Duration** 30-60 minutes (dose dependent)

**Half-Life**
Children: 40-60 minutes
Adults; 83-97 minutes

**Special PA Issues**
  **Monitoring Parameters:** Respiratory rate, blood pressure, heart rate
  **Reference Range:** 100-340 ng/mL (depending upon procedure)
**Related Information**
  Narcotic Agonists *on page 1023*

♦ **Alfentanil Hydrochloride** *see* Alfentanil *on page 39*

♦ **Alferon® N** *see* Interferon Alfa-n3 *on page 485*

# Alglucerase (al GLOO ser ase)

**Pharmacologic Class** Enzyme
**U.S. Brand Names** Ceredase®; Cerezyme®
**Mechanism of Action** Glucocerebrosidase is an enzyme prepared from human placental tissue. Gaucher's disease is an inherited metabolic disorder caused by the defective activity of beta-glucosidase and the resultant accumulation of glucosyl ceramide laden macrophages in the liver, bone, and spleen; acts by replacing the missing enzyme associated with Gaucher's disease.
**Use Orphan drug:** Treatment of Gaucher's disease
**USUAL DOSAGE** Usually administered as a 20-60 unit/kg I.V. infusion given with a frequency ranging from 3 times/week to once every 2 weeks
**Dosage Forms Inj:** 10 units/mL (5 mL), 80 units/mL (5 mL)
**Contraindications** Hypersensitivity to any component
**Warnings/Precautions** Prepared from pooled human placental tissue that may contain the causative agents of some viral diseases
**Pregnancy Risk Factor** C
**Pregnancy Implications** Excretion in breast milk unknown/use caution
**Adverse Reactions**
  >10%: Local: Discomfort, burning, and edema at the site of injection
  <1%: Fever, chills, abdominal discomfort, nausea, vomiting
**Special PA Issues**
  **Patient Education:** Treatment is required for life

# Alitretinoin (a li TRET i noyn)

**Pharmacologic Class** Antineoplastic Agent, Miscellaneous; Retinoic Acid Derivative
**U.S. Brand Names** Panretin®
**Mechanism of Action** Binds to retinoid receptors to inhibit growth of Kaposi's sarcoma
**Use** Topical treatment of cutaneous lesions in AIDS-related Kaposi's sarcoma; not indicated when systemic therapy for Kaposi's sarcoma is indicated
**USUAL DOSAGE** Topical: Apply gel twice daily to cutaneous Kaposi's sarcoma lesions
**Dosage Forms Gel:** 0.1%, 60 g tube
**Contraindications** Hypersensitivity to alitretinoin, other retinoids, or any component of the formulation
**Warnings/Precautions** May cause fetal harm if absorbed by a woman who is pregnant. Patients with cutaneous T cell lymphoma have a high incidence of treatment-limiting adverse reactions. May be photosensitizing (based on experience with other retinoids); minimize sun or other UV exposure of treated areas. Do not use concurrently with topical products containing DEET (increased toxicity may result). Safety in pediatric patients or geriatric patients has not been established. Occlusive dressing should not be used.
**Pregnancy Risk Factor** D
**Pregnancy Implications** Potentially teratogenic and/or embryotoxic; limb, craniofacial, or skeletal defects have been observed in animal models. If used during pregnancy or if the patient becomes pregnant while using alitretinoin, the woman should be advised of potential harm to the fetus. Women of childbearing potential should avoid becoming pregnant. Excretion in human breast milk is unknown; women are advised to discontinue breast-feeding prior to using this medication.
**Adverse Reactions**
  >10%:
    Central nervous system: Pain (0% to 34%)
    Dermatologic: Rash (25% to 77%), pruritus (8% to 11%)
    Neuromuscular & skeletal: Paresthesia (3% to 22%)
  5% to 10%:
    Cardiovascular: Edema (3% to 8%)
    Dermatologic: Exfoliative dermatitis (3% to 9%), skin disorder (0% to 8%)
**Drug Interactions** Increased toxicity of DEET may occur if products containing this compound are used concurrently with alitretinoin. Due to limited absorption after topical application, interaction with systemic medications is unlikely.
**Special PA Issues**
  **Patient Education:** For external use only; avoid UV light exposure (sun or sunlamps) of treated areas

♦ **Alka-Mints® [OTC]** *see* Calcium Carbonate *on page 139*

♦ **Alkeran®** *see* Melphalan *on page 565*

## Allopurinol (al oh PURE i nole)

**Pharmacologic Class** Xanthine Oxidase Inhibitor

**U.S. Brand Names** Zyloprim®

**Mechanism of Action** Allopurinol inhibits xanthine oxidase, the enzyme responsible for the conversion of hypoxanthine to xanthine to uric acid. Allopurinol is metabolized to oxypurinol which is also an inhibitor of xanthine oxidase; allopurinol acts on purine catabolism, reducing the production of uric acid without disrupting the biosynthesis of vital purines.

**Use** Prevention of attack of gouty arthritis and nephropathy; also used to treat secondary hyperuricemia which may occur during treatment of tumors or leukemia, and to prevent recurrent calcium oxalate calculi

**USUAL DOSAGE** Oral:

Children ≤10 years: 10 mg/kg/day in 2-3 divided doses **or** 200-300 mg/m²/day in 2-4 divided doses, maximum: 800 mg/24 hours

Alternative:

<6 years: 150 mg/day in 3 divided doses

6-10 years: 300 mg/day in 2-3 divided doses

Children >10 years and Adults: Daily doses >300 mg should be administered in divided doses

Myeloproliferative neoplastic disorders: 600-800 mg/day in 2-3 divided doses for prevention of acute uric acid nephropathy for 2-3 days starting 1-2 days before chemotherapy

Gout:

Mild: 200-300 mg/day

Severe: 400-600 mg/day

Elderly: Initial: 100 mg/day, increase until desired uric acid level is obtained

**Dosing adjustment in renal impairment:** Must be adjusted due to accumulation of allopurinol and metabolites; removed by hemodialysis. See table.

### Adult Maintenance Doses of Allopurinol*

| Creatinine Clearance (mL/min) | Maintenance Dose of Allopurinol (mg) |
|---|---|
| 140 | 400 qd |
| 120 | 350 qd |
| 100 | 300 qd |
| 80 | 250 qd |
| 60 | 200 qd |
| 40 | 150 qd |
| 20 | 100 qd |
| 10 | 100 q2d |
| 0 | 100 q3d |

*This table is based on a standard maintenance dose of 300 mg of allopurinol per day for a patient with a creatinine clearance of 100 mL/min.

Hemodialysis: Administer dose posthemodialysis or administer 50% supplemental dose

**Dosage Forms Tab:** 100 mg, 300 mg

**Contraindications** Not to be used in pregnancy or lactation, or in patients with a previous severe allergy reaction to allopurinol or any component

**Warnings/Precautions** Do not use to treat asymptomatic hyperuricemia. Discontinue at first signs of rash; reduce dosage in renal insufficiency, reinstate with caution in patients who have had a previous mild allergic reaction, use with caution in children; monitor liver function and complete blood counts before initiating therapy and periodically during therapy, use with caution in patients taking diuretics concurrently.

**Pregnancy Risk Factor** C

**Pregnancy Implications** Clinical effects on the fetus: There are few reports describing the use of allopurinol during pregnancy; no adverse fetal outcomes attributable to allopurinol have been reported in humans

**Adverse Reactions**

>10%: Dermatologic: Skin rash (usually maculopapular), exfoliative, urticarial or purpuric lesions, and Stevens-Johnson syndrome have been reported

1% to 10%:

Central nervous system: Drowsiness, chills, fever

Dermatologic: Alopecia

Gastrointestinal: Nausea, vomiting, diarrhea, abdominal pain, gastritis, dyspepsia

Hepatic: Increased alkaline phosphatase or AST/ALT, hepatomegaly, hyperbilirubinemia, and jaundice, hepatic necrosis has been reported

<1%: Vasculitis, headache, somnolence, toxic epidermal necrolysis, bone marrow suppression has been reported in patients receiving allopurinol with other myelosuppressive agents, thrombophlebitis, peripheral neuropathy, neuritis, paresthesia, cataracts, renal impairment, epistaxis, idiosyncratic reaction characterized by fever, chills, leukopenia, leukocytosis, eosinophilia, arthralgia, skin rash, pruritus, nausea, and vomiting

**Drug Interactions** Hepatic enzyme inhibitor

Decreased effect: Alcohol decreases effectiveness

Increased toxicity:

Inhibits metabolism of azathioprine and mercaptopurine

Use with ampicillin or amoxicillin may increase the incidence of skin rash

Urinary acidification with large amounts of vitamin C may increase kidney stone formation

Thiazide diuretics enhance toxicity, monitor renal function

Allopurinol prolongs half-life of oral anticoagulants; allopurinol increases serum half-life of theophylline; allopurinol may compete for excretion in renal tubule with chlorpropamide and increases chlorpropamide's serum half-life

**Onset** Decreases in serum uric acid occur in 1-2 days with nadir achieved in 1-2 weeks

**Half-Life** Parent drug: 1-3 hours; Oxypurinol: 18-30 hours; End-stage renal disease: Half-life prolonged

**Special PA Issues**

**Patient Education:** Take as directed. Maintain adequate hydration (2-3 L/day of fluids unless instructed to restrict fluid intake) to avoid possible adverse renal problems. While using this medication, do not use alcohol, other prescription or OTC medications, or vitamin substances without consulting prescriber. You may experience drowsiness (use caution when driving or engaging in hazardous tasks); nausea, vomiting, or heartburn (small frequent meals, good mouth care, chewing gum, or sucking on lozenges may help); hair loss (reversible). Report skin rash or lesions; painful urination or blood in urine or stool; unresolved nausea or vomiting; numbness of extremities; pain or irritation of the eyes; swelling of lips, mouth, or tongue; unusual fatigue; easy bruising or bleeding; yellowing of skin or eyes; or any change in color of urine or stool.

**Monitoring Parameters:** CBC, serum uric acid levels, I & O, hepatic and renal function, especially at start of therapy

**Reference Range:** Uric acid, serum: An increase occurs during childhood

Adults:

Male: 3.4-7 mg/dL or slightly more

Female: 2.4-6 mg/dL or slightly more

Values >7 mg/dL are sometimes arbitrarily regarded as hyperuricemia, but there is no sharp line between normals on the one hand, and the serum uric acid of those with clinical gout. Normal ranges cannot be adjusted for purine ingestion, but high purine diet increases uric acid. Uric acid may be increased with body size, exercise, and stress.

♦ **All-_trans_-Retinoic Acid** see Tretinoin, Oral on page 925

♦ **Almora® (Gluconate)** see Magnesium Salts (Other) on page 554

♦ **Alomide® Ophthalmic** see Lodoxamide Tromethamine on page 538

♦ **Alor® 5/500** see Hydrocodone and Aspirin on page 450

♦ **Alora® Transdermal** see Estradiol on page 332

♦ **Alpha-Baclofen®** see Baclofen on page 97

♦ **Alphagan®** see Brimonidine on page 120

♦ **Alphamin®** see Hydroxocobalamin on page 458

♦ **Alpha-Tamoxifen®** see Tamoxifen on page 871

♦ **Alphatrex®** see Betamethasone on page 111

# Alprazolam (al PRAY zoe lam)

**Pharmacologic Class** Benzodiazepine

**U.S. Brand Names** Alprazolam Intensol®; Xanax®

**Mechanism of Action** Binds at stereospecific receptors at several sites within the central nervous system, including the limbic system, reticular formation; effects may be mediated through GABA

**Use** Treatment of anxiety; adjunct in the treatment of depression; management of panic attacks

**USUAL DOSAGE** Oral:

Children <18 years: Safety and dose have not been established

(Continued)

## Alprazolam *(Continued)*

Adults:

Anxiety: Effective doses are 0.5-4 mg/day in divided doses; the manufacturer recommends starting at 0.25-0.5 mg 3 times/day; titrate dose upward; maximum: 4 mg/day

Depression: Average dose required: 2.5-3 mg/day in divided doses

Alcohol withdrawal: Usual dose: 2-2.5 mg/day in divided doses

Panic disorder: Many patients obtain relief at 2 mg/day, as much as 6 mg/day may be required

**Dosing adjustment in hepatic impairment**: Reduce dose by 50% to 60% or avoid in cirrhosis

**Note**: Treatment >4 months should be re-evaluated to determine the patient's need for the drug

**Dosage Forms Tab**: 0.25 mg, 0.5 mg, 1 mg, 2 mg

**Contraindications** Hypersensitivity to alprazolam or any component; there may be a cross-sensitivity with other benzodiazepines; severe uncontrolled pain, narrow-angle glaucoma, severe respiratory depression, pre-existing CNS depression; not to be used in pregnancy or lactation

**Warnings/Precautions** Withdrawal symptoms including seizures have occurred 18 hours to 3 days after abrupt discontinuation; when discontinuing therapy, decrease daily dose by no more than 0.5 mg every 3 days; reduce dose in patients with significant hepatic disease. Not intended for management of anxieties and minor distresses associated with everyday life.

**Pregnancy Risk Factor** D

**Pregnancy Implications** Enters breast milk/contraindicated

**Adverse Reactions**

>10%:

Cardiovascular: Tachycardia, chest pain

Central nervous system: Drowsiness, fatigue, ataxia, lightheadedness, memory impairment, insomnia, anxiety, depression, headache

Dermatologic: Rash

Endocrine & metabolic: Decreased libido

Gastrointestinal: Xerostomia, constipation, decreased salivation, nausea, vomiting, diarrhea, increased or decreased appetite

Neuromuscular & skeletal: Dysarthria

Ocular: Blurred vision

Miscellaneous: Diaphoresis

1% to 10%:

Cardiovascular: Syncope, hypotension

Central nervous system: Confusion, nervousness, dizziness, akathisia

Dermatologic: Dermatitis

Gastrointestinal: Weight gain or loss, increased salivation

Neuromuscular & skeletal: Rigidity, tremor, muscle cramps

Otic: Tinnitus

Respiratory: Nasal congestion, hyperventilation

**Drug Interactions** CYP3A3/4 enzyme substrate

Decreased therapeutic effect: Carbamazepine, disulfiram

Increased toxicity: Oral contraceptives, CNS depressants, cimetidine, lithium

**Onset** Within 1 hour

**Duration** Variable, 8-24 hours

**Half-Life** 12-15 hours

**Special PA Issues**

**Patient Education:** Take exactly as directed (do not increase dose or frequency); may cause physical and/or psychological dependence. Do not use excessive alcohol, or other prescription or OTC medications (especially pain medications, sedatives, antihistamines, or hypnotics) without consulting prescriber. Maintain adequate hydration (2-3 L/day of fluids unless instructed to restrict fluid intake). You may experience drowsiness, lightheadedness, impaired coordination, dizziness, or blurred vision (use caution when driving or engaging in hazardous tasks until response to medication is known); nausea, vomiting, or dry mouth (small frequent meals, good mouth care, chewing gum, or sucking lozenges may help); constipation (increased exercise, fluids, or dietary fruit and fiber may help); altered sexual drive or ability (reversible); photosensitivity (use sunscreen, protective clothing, and avoid extended exposure to direct sunlight). Report persistent CNS effects (eg, confusion, depression, increased sedation, excitation, headache, agitation, insomnia or nightmares, dizziness, fatigue, impaired coordination, changes in personality, or changes in cognition); changes in urinary pattern; muscle cramping, weakness, tremors, or rigidity; ringing in ears or visual disturbances; chest pain, palpitations, or rapid heartbeat; excessive perspiration; excessive GI symptoms (cramping, constipation, vomiting, anorexia); or worsening of condition.

**Dietary Considerations:** Alcohol: May have additive CNS effects, avoid use

**Monitoring Parameters:** Respiratory and cardiovascular status

♦ **Alprazolam Intensol®** *see Alprazolam on previous page*

## Alprostadil (al PROS ta dill)

**Pharmacologic Class** Prostaglandin

**U.S. Brand Names** Caverject® Injection; Edex™ Injection; Muse® Pellet; Prostin VR Pediatric® Injection

**Mechanism of Action** Causes vasodilation by means of direct effect on vascular and ductus arteriosus smooth muscle; relaxes trabecular smooth muscle by dilation of cavernosal arteries when injected along the penile shaft, allowing blood flow to and entrapment in the lacunar spaces of the penis (ie, corporeal veno-occlusive mechanism)

**Use** Temporary maintenance of patency of ductus arteriosus in neonates with ductal-dependent congenital heart disease until surgery can be performed. These defects include cyanotic (eg, pulmonary atresia, pulmonary stenosis, tricuspid atresia, Fallot's tetralogy, transposition of the great vessels) and acyanotic (eg, interruption of aortic arch, coarctation of aorta, hypoplastic left ventricle) heart disease; diagnosis and treatment of erectile dysfunction of vasculogenic, psychogenic, or neurogenic etiology; adjunct in the diagnosis of erectile dysfunction

**Investigational:** Treatment of pulmonary hypertension in infants and children with congenital heart defects with left-to-right shunts

### USUAL DOSAGE

**Patent ductus arteriosus** (Prostin VR Pediatric®):

I.V. continuous infusion into a large vein, or alternatively through an umbilical artery catheter placed at the ductal opening: 0.05-0.1 mcg/kg/minute with therapeutic response, rate is reduced to lowest effective dosage; with unsatisfactory response, rate is increased gradually; maintenance: 0.01-0.4 mcg/kg/minute

$PGE_1$ is usually given at an infusion rate of 0.1 mcg/kg/minute, but it is often possible to reduce the dosage to $1/2$ or even $1/10$ without losing the therapeutic effect. The mixing schedule is shown in the table.

**Alprostadil**

| Add 1 Ampul (500 mcg) to: | Concentration (mcg/mL) | Infusion Rate | |
|---|---|---|---|
| | | mL/min/kg Needed to Infuse 0.1 mcg/kg/min | mL/kg/24 h |
| 250 mL | 2 | 0.05 | 72 |
| 100 mL | 5 | 0.02 | 28.8 |
| 50 mL | 10 | 0.01 | 14.4 |
| 25 mL | 20 | 0.005 | 7.2 |

Therapeutic response is indicated by increased pH in those with acidosis or by an increase in oxygenation ($pO_2$) usually evident within 30 minutes

**Erectile dysfunction**

Caverject®, Edex®:

Vasculogenic, psychogenic, or mixed etiology: Individualize dose by careful titration; usual dose: 2.5-60 mcg (doses >60 mcg are not recommended); initiate dosage titration at 2.5 mcg, increasing by 2.5 mcg to a dose of 5 mcg and then in increments of 5-10 mcg depending on the erectile response until the dose produces an erection suitable for intercourse, not lasting >1 hour; if there is absolutely no response to initial 2.5 mcg dose, the second dose may increased to 7.5 mcg, followed by increments of 5-10 mcg

Neurogenic etiology (eg, spinal cord injury): Initiate dosage titration at 1.25 mcg, increasing to a doses of 2.5 mcg and then 5 mcg; increase further in increments 5 mcg until the dose is reached that produces an erection suitable for intercourse, not lasting >1 hour

**Note:** Patient must stay in the physician's office until complete detumescence occurs; if there is no response, then the next higher dose may be given within 1 hour; if there is still no response, a 1-day interval before giving the next dose is recommended; increasing the dose or concentration in the treatment of impotence results in increasing pain and discomfort

Muse® Pellet: Intraurethral: Administer as needed to achieve an erection; duration of action is about 30-60 minutes; use only two systems per 24-hour period

**Dosage Forms Inj:** Caverject®: 5 mcg, 10 mcg, 20 mcg, Edex®: 5 mcg, 10 mcg, 20 mcg, 40 mcg, Prostin VR Pediatric®: 500 mcg/mL (1 mL); **Pellet, urethral:** 125 mcg, 250 mcg, 500 mcg, 1000 mcg

**Contraindications** Hyaline membrane disease or persistent fetal circulation and when a dominant left-to-right shunt is present; respiratory distress syndrome; hypersensitivity to the drug or components; conditions predisposing patients to priapism (sickle cell anemia, multiple myeloma, leukemia); patients with anatomical deformation of the penis, penile implants; use in men for whom sexual activity is inadvisable or contraindicated; pregnancy

**Warnings/Precautions** Use cautiously in neonates with bleeding tendencies; apnea may occur in 10% to 12% of neonates with congenital heart defects, especially in those weighing <2 kg at birth; apnea usually appears during the first hour of drug infusion; priapism may (Continued)

## Alprostadil (Continued)

occur; treat immediately to avoid penile tissue damage and permanent loss of potency; discontinue therapy if signs of penile fibrosis develop (penile angulation, cavernosal fibrosis, or Peyronie's disease). When used in erectile dysfunction (Muse®), syncope occurring within 1 hour of administration, has been reported; the potential for drug-drug interactions may occur when Muse® is prescribed concomitantly with antihypertensives; some lowering of blood pressure may occur without symptoms, and swelling of leg veins, leg pain, perineal pain, and rapid pulse have been reported in <2% of patients during in-clinic titration and home treatment.

**Pregnancy Risk Factor** X

**Adverse Reactions**

>10%:
  Cardiovascular: Flushing
  Central nervous system: Fever
  Genitourinary: Penile pain
  Respiratory: Apnea

1% to 10%:
  Cardiovascular: Bradycardia, hypotension, hypertension, tachycardia, cardiac arrest, edema
  Central nervous system: Seizures, headache, dizziness
  Endocrine & metabolic: Hypokalemia
  Gastrointestinal: Diarrhea
  Genitourinary: Prolonged erection, penile fibrosis, penis disorder, penile rash, penile edema
  Hematologic: Disseminated intravascular coagulation
  Local: Injection site hematoma, injection site bruising
  Neuromuscular & skeletal: Back pain
  Respiratory: Upper respiratory infection, flu syndrome, sinusitis, nasal congestion, cough
  Miscellaneous: Sepsis, localized pain in structures other than the injection site

<1%: Cerebral bleeding, congestive heart failure, second degree heart block, shock, supraventricular tachycardia, ventricular fibrillation, hyperemia, hyperirritability, hypothermia, jitteriness, lethargy, hypoglycemia, hyperkalemia, gastric regurgitation, anuria, balanitis, urethral bleeding, penile numbness, yeast infection, penile pruritus and erythema, abnormal ejaculation, anemia, bleeding, thrombocytopenia, hyperbilirubinemia, hyperextension of neck, stiffness, hematuria, bradypnea, bronchial wheezing, peritonitis, leg pain, perineal pain

**Onset** Rapid

**Duration** <1 hour

**Half-Life** 5-10 minutes

**Special PA Issues**

  **Patient Education:** Use only as directed, no more than 3 times/week, allowing 24 hours between injections. Store in refrigerator and dilute with supplied diluent immediately before use. Use alternate sides of penis with each injection. Dispose of syringes and needle and single dose vials in a safe manner (do not share medication, syringes, or needles). Note that the risk of transmitting blood-borne disease is increased with use of alprostadil injections since a small amount of bleeding at injection site is possible. Stop using alprostadil and contact prescriber immediately if signs of priapism occur, erections last more than 4-6 hours, or you experience moderate to severe penile pain. Report penile problems (eg, nodules, new penile pain, rash, bruising, numbness, swelling, signs of infection, abnormal ejaculations); cardiac symptoms (hypo- or hypertension, chest pain, palpitations, irregular heartbeat); flushing, fever, flu-like symptoms; difficulty breathing, or wheezing; or other adverse reactions. Refer to prescriber every 3 months to ensure proper technique and for dosage evaluation.

  **Monitoring Parameters:** Arterial pressure, respiratory rate, heart rate, temperature, degree of penile pain, length of erection, signs of infection

♦ Alrex™ see Loteprednol on page 545
♦ Altace™ see Ramipril on page 793
♦ Altamisa see Feverfew on page 368

## Alteplase (AL te plase)

**Pharmacologic Class** Thrombolytic Agent

**U.S. Brand Names** Activase®

**Mechanism of Action** Initiates local fibrinolysis by binding to fibrin in a thrombus (clot) and converts entrapped plasminogen to plasmin

**Use** Management of acute myocardial infarction for the lysis of thrombi in coronary arteries; management of acute massive pulmonary embolism (PE) in adults

Acute myocardial infarction (AMI): Chest pain ≥20 minutes, ≤12-24 hours; S-T elevation ≥0.1 mV in at least two EKG leads

Acute pulmonary embolism (APE): Age ≤75 years: As soon as possible within 5 days of thrombotic event. Documented massive pulmonary embolism by pulmonary angiography or echocardiography or high probability lung scan with clinical shock.

Acute ischemic stroke (rule out hemorrhagic courses before administering)

## USUAL DOSAGE

Coronary artery thrombi: I.V.: Front loading dose: Total dose is 100 mg over 1.5 hours (for patients who weigh <65 kg, use 1.25 mg/kg/total dose). Add this dose to a 100 mL bag of 0.9% sodium chloride for a total volume of 200 mL. Infuse 15 mg (30 mL) over 1-2 minutes; infuse 50 mg (100 mL) over 30 minutes. Begin heparin 5000-10,000 unit bolus followed by continuous infusion of 1000 units/hour. Infuse 35 mg/hour (70 mL) for next 2 hours.

Acute pulmonary embolism: 100 mg over 2 hours

Acute ischemic stroke: Doses should be given within the first 3 hours of the onset of symptoms. Load with 0.09 mg/kg as a bolus, followed by 0.81 mg/kg as a continuous infusion over 60 minutes; maximum total dose should not exceed 90 mg

**Dosage Forms Powder for inj, lyophilized (recombinant):** 20 mg [11.6 million units] (20 mL), 50 mg [29 million units] (50 mL), 100 mg [58 million units] (100 mL)

**Contraindications** No central venous puncture (CVP line) or noncompressible arterial sticks. BP systolic ≥185, diastolic ≥110 unresponsive to nitrate or calcium antagonist; recent (within 1 month): cerebral-vascular accident, gastrointestinal bleeding, trauma or surgery, prolonged external cardiac massage; intracranial neoplasm, suspected aortic dissection, arteriovenous malformation or aneurysm, bleeding diathesis, hemostatic defects, seizure occurring at the time of stroke, suspicion of subarachnoid hemorrhage

**Warnings/Precautions** Doses >150 mg have been associated with an increase of intracranial hemorrhage; acute pericarditis, severe liver dysfunction, septic thrombophlebitis, patients receiving concurrent oral anticoagulants, advanced age

**Pregnancy Risk Factor** C

**Pregnancy Implications** Excretion in breast milk unknown

## Adverse Reactions

1% to 10%:
Cardiovascular: Hypotension
Central nervous system: Fever
Dermatologic: Bruising
Gastrointestinal: GI hemorrhage, nausea, vomiting
Genitourinary: GU hemorrhage

<1%: Retroperitoneal hemorrhage, gingival hemorrhage, intracranial hemorrhage, rapid lysis of coronary artery thrombi by thrombolytic agents may be associated with reperfusion-related atrial and/or ventricular arrhythmias; epistaxis

**Drug Interactions** Increased effect: Anticoagulants, aspirin, ticlopidine, dipyridamole, and heparin are at least additive

**Duration** >50% present in plasma is cleared within 5 minutes after the infusion has been terminated, and ~80% is cleared within 10 minutes

**Half-Life** Cleared rapidly by the liver; ~80% is cleared within 10 minutes after infusion is terminated

## Special PA Issues

**Patient Education:** This medication can only be administered I.V. You will have a tendency to bleed easily following this medication; use caution to prevent injury - use electric razor, soft toothbrush, and use caution with sharps. If bleeding occurs, apply pressure to bleeding spot until bleeding stops completely. Report unusual bruising or bleeding; blood in urine, stool, or vomitus; bleeding gums; changes in vision; difficulty breathing; or chest pain.

**Reference Range:** Not routinely measured; literature supports therapeutic levels of 0.52-1.8 µg/mL
Fibrinogen: 200-400 mg/dL
Activated partial thromboplastin time (APTT): 22.5-38.7 seconds
Prothrombin time (PT): 10.9-12.2 seconds

♦ **Alteplase, Recombinant** see Alteplase on previous page
♦ **Alteplase, Tissue Plasminogen Activator, Recombinant** see Alteplase on previous page
♦ **ALternaGEL® [OTC]** see Aluminum Hydroxide on this page
♦ **Alu-Cap® [OTC]** see Aluminum Hydroxide on this page

# Aluminum Acetate and Acetic Acid
(a LOO mi num AS e tate & a SEE tik AS id)
**Pharmacologic Class** Otic Agent, Anti-infective
**U.S. Brand Names** Otic Domeboro®
**Dosage Forms Soln, otic:** Aluminum acetate 10% and acetic acid 2% (60 mL)

# Aluminum Hydroxide (a LOO mi num hye DROKS ide)
**Pharmacologic Class** Antacid; Antidote
**U.S. Brand Names** ALternaGEL® [OTC]; Alu-Cap® [OTC]; Alu-Tab® [OTC]; Amphojel® [OTC]; Dialume® [OTC]; Nephrox Suspension [OTC]
(Continued)

## Aluminum Hydroxide *(Continued)*

**Use** Treatment of hyperacidity; hyperphosphatemia

**USUAL DOSAGE** Oral:

Peptic ulcer disease:

Children: 5-15 mL/dose every 3-6 hours or 1 and 3 hours after meals and at bedtime

Adults: 15-45 mL every 3-6 hours or 1 and 3 hours after meals and at bedtime

Prophylaxis against gastrointestinal bleeding:

Infants: 2-5 mL/dose every 1-2 hours

Children: 5-15 mL/dose every 1-2 hours

Adults: 30-60 mL/dose every hour

Titrate to maintain the gastric pH >5

Hyperphosphatemia:

Children: 50-150 mg/kg/24 hours in divided doses every 4-6 hours, titrate dosage to maintain serum phosphorus within normal range

Adults: 500-1800 mg, 3-6 times/day, between meals and at bedtime; best taken with a meal or within 20 minutes of a meal

Antacid: Adults: 30 mL 1 and 3 hours postprandial and at bedtime

**Dosage Forms Cap:** Alu-Cap®: 400 mg, Dialume®: 500 mg; **Liq:** 600 mg/5 mL, ALternaGEL®: 600 mg/5 mL; **Susp, oral:** 320 mg/5 mL, 450 mg/5 mL, 675 mg/5 mL, Amphojel®: 320 mg/5 mL; **Tab:** Amphojel®: 300 mg, 600 mg, Alu-Tab®: 500 mg

**Contraindications** Hypersensitivity to aluminum salts or drug components

**Warnings/Precautions** Hypophosphatemia may occur with prolonged administration or large doses; aluminum intoxication and osteomalacia may occur in patients with uremia. Use with caution in patients with congestive heart failure, renal failure, edema, cirrhosis, and low sodium diets, and patients who have recently suffered gastrointestinal hemorrhage; uremic patients not receiving dialysis may develop osteomalacia and osteoporosis due to phosphate depletion.

Elderly, due to disease and/or drug therapy, may be predisposed to constipation and fecal impaction. Careful evaluation of possible drug interactions must be done. When used as an antacid in ulcer treatment, consider buffer capacity (mEq/mL) to calculate dose; consider renal insufficiency as predisposition to aluminum toxicity.

**Pregnancy Risk Factor** C

**Pregnancy Implications** Excretion in breast milk unknown

Clinical effects on the fetus: No data available

**Adverse Reactions**

>10%: Gastrointestinal: Constipation, chalky taste, stomach cramps, fecal impaction

1% to 10%: Gastrointestinal: Nausea, vomiting, discoloration of feces (white speckles)

<1%: Hypophosphatemia, hypomagnesemia

**Drug Interactions** Decreased effect: Tetracyclines, digoxin, indomethacin, or iron salts, isoniazid, allopurinol, benzodiazepines, corticosteroids, penicillamine, phenothiazines, ranitidine, ketoconazole, itraconazole

**Special PA Issues**

**Patient Education:** Take as directed, preferably 2 hours before or 2 hours after meals and any other medications. Dilute liquid dose with water or juice and shake well. Do not increase sodium intake and maintain adequate hydration (2-3 L/day of fluids unless instructed to restrict fluid intake). Chew tablet thoroughly before swallowing with full glass of water. You may experience constipation (increased exercise or dietary fluids, fiber, and fruit may help). If unrelieved, see prescriber. Report unresolved nausea, malaise, muscle weakness, blood in stool, or abdominal pain.

**Monitoring Parameters:** Monitor phosphorous levels periodically when patient is on chronic therapy

- ◆ **Aluminum Sucrose Sulfate, Basic** *see* Sucralfate *on page 856*
- ◆ **Alupent®** *see* Metaproterenol *on page 575*
- ◆ **Alu-Tab® [OTC]** *see* Aluminum Hydroxide *on previous page*

## Amantadine *(a MAN ta deen)*

**Pharmacologic Class** Anti-Parkinson's Agent (Dopamine Agonist); Antiviral Agent

**U.S. Brand Names** Symadine®; Symmetrel®

**Mechanism of Action** As an antiviral, blocks the uncoating of influenza A virus preventing penetration of virus into host; antiparkinsonian activity may be due to its blocking the reuptake of dopamine into presynaptic neurons and causing direct stimulation of postsynaptic receptors

**Use** Symptomatic and adjunct treatment of parkinsonism; prophylaxis and treatment of influenza A viral infection; treatment of drug-induced extrapyramidal symptoms

**USUAL DOSAGE**

Children:

1-9 years: (<45 kg): 5-9 mg/kg/day in 1-2 divided doses to a maximum of 150 mg/day

10-12 years: 100-200 mg/day in 1-2 divided doses

Prophylaxis: Administer for 10-21 days following exposure if the vaccine is concurrently given or for 90 days following exposure if the vaccine is unavailable or contraindicated and re-exposure is possible

Adults:

Drug-induced extrapyramidal reactions: 100 mg twice daily; may increase to 300 mg/day, if needed

Parkinson's disease: 100 mg twice daily as sole therapy; may increase to 400 mg/day if needed with close monitoring; initial dose: 100 mg/day if with other serious illness or with high doses of other anti-Parkinson drugs

Influenza A viral infection: 200 mg/day in 1-2 divided doses

Prophylaxis: Minimum 10-day course of therapy following exposure if the vaccine is concurrently given or for 90 days following exposure if the vaccine is unavailable or contraindicated and re-exposure is possible

Elderly patients should take the drug in 2 daily doses rather than a single dose to avoid adverse neurologic reactions; see Warnings/Precautions

**Dosing interval in renal impairment:**

$Cl_{cr}$ 50-60 mL/minute: Administer 200 mg alternating with 100 mg/day

$Cl_{cr}$ 30-50 mL/minute: Administer 100 mg/day

$Cl_{cr}$ 20-30 mL/minute: Administer 200 mg twice weekly

$Cl_{cr}$ 10-20 mL/minute: Administer 100 mg 3 times/week

$Cl_{cr}$ <10 mL/minute: Administer 200 mg alternating with 100 mg every 7 days

Hemodialysis: Slightly hemodialyzable (5% to 20%); no supplemental dose is needed

Peritoneal dialysis: No supplemental dose is needed

Continuous arteriovenous or venovenous hemofiltration (CAVH/CAVHD): No supplemental dose is needed

**Dosage Forms Cap:** 100 mg; **Syr:** 50 mg/5 mL (480 mL)

**Contraindications** Hypersensitivity to amantadine hydrochloride or any component

**Warnings/Precautions** Use with caution in patients with liver disease, a history of recurrent and eczematoid dermatitis, uncontrolled psychosis or severe psychoneurosis, seizures and in those receiving CNS stimulant drugs; reduce dose in renal disease; when treating Parkinson's disease, do not discontinue abruptly. In many patients, the therapeutic benefits of amantadine are limited to a few months. Elderly patients may be more susceptible to the CNS effects (using 2 divided daily doses may minimize this effect).

**Pregnancy Risk Factor** C

**Adverse Reactions**

1% to 10%:

Cardiovascular: Orthostatic hypotension, peripheral edema

Central nervous system: Insomnia, depression, anxiety, irritability, dizziness, hallucinations, headache

Dermatologic: Livedo reticularis

Gastrointestinal: Nausea, anorexia, constipation, xerostomia

<1%: Congestive heart failure, slurred speech, confusion, fatigue, rash, decreased libido, urinary retention, vomiting, weakness, visual disturbances, dyspnea

**Drug Interactions**

Increased effect: Drugs with anticholinergic or CNS stimulant activity

Increased toxicity/levels: Hydrochlorothiazide plus triamterene, amiloride

**Onset** Onset of antidyskinetic action: Within 48 hours

**Half-Life** Normal renal function: 2-7 hours; End-stage renal disease: 7-10 days

**Special PA Issues**

**Patient Education:** Take as directed; do not increase dosage, take more often than prescribed, or discontinue without consulting prescriber. Maintain adequate hydration (2-3 L/day of fluids unless instructed to restrict fluid intake) and void before taking medication. Take last dose of day in the afternoon to reduce incidence of insomnia. Avoid alcohol, sedatives, or hypnotics unless consulting prescriber. You may experience decreased mental alertness or coordination (use caution when driving, climbing stairs, or engaging in tasks that require alertness); nausea, or dry mouth (small frequent meals, frequent mouth care, or sucking on lozenges may help). Report unusual swelling of extremities, difficulty breathing or shortness of breath, change in gait or increased tremors, or changes in mentation (depression, anxiety, irritability, hallucination, slurred speech).

**Monitoring Parameters:** Renal function, mental status, blood pressure

- ♦ **Amantadine Hydrochloride** see Amantadine on previous page
- ♦ **Amaphen®** see Butalbital Compound on page 131
- ♦ **Amaryl®** see Glimepiride on page 416
- ♦ **Ambenyl® Cough Syrup** see Bromodiphenhydramine and Codeine on page 123
- ♦ **Amber Touch-and-Feel** see St Johns Wort on page 852
- ♦ **Ambien™** see Zolpidem on page 977
- ♦ **Ambi® Skin Tone [OTC]** see Hydroquinone on page 457

## Amcinonide (am SIN oh nide)
**Pharmacologic Class** Corticosteroid, Topical
**U.S. Brand Names** Cyclocort®
**Mechanism of Action** Stimulates the synthesis of enzymes needed to decrease inflammation, suppress mitotic activity, and cause vasoconstriction
**Use** Relief of the inflammatory and pruritic manifestations of corticosteroid-responsive dermatoses (high potency corticosteroid)
**USUAL DOSAGE** Adults: Topical: Apply in a thin film 2-3 times/day
**Dosage Forms Crm:** 0.1% (15 g, 30 g, 60 g); **Lot:** 0.1% (20 mL, 60 mL); **Oint, top:** 0.1% (15 g, 30 g, 60 g)
**Contraindications** Hypersensitivity to amcinonide or any component; use on the face, groin, or axilla
**Warnings/Precautions** Adverse systemic effects may occur when used on large areas of the body, denuded areas, for prolonged periods of time, with an occlusive dressing, and/or in infants or small children; occlusive dressings should not be used in presence of infection or weeping lesions
**Pregnancy Risk Factor** C
**Adverse Reactions**
1% to 10%:
   Dermatologic: Itching, maceration of skin, skin atrophy, erythema, dryness, papular rashes
   Local: Burning, irritation
<1%: Hypertrichosis, acneiform eruptions, hypopigmentation, perioral dermatitis, striae, miliaria
**Special PA Issues**
   Patient Education: Before applying, gently wash area to reduce risk of infection; apply a thin film to cleansed area and rub in gently and thoroughly until medication vanishes; avoid exposure to sunlight, severe sunburn may occur

♦ **Amcort®** see Triamcinolone on page 928
♦ **Amen®** see Medroxyprogesterone Acetate on page 561
♦ **Amerge®** see Naratriptan on page 637
♦ **Americaine® [OTC]** see Benzocaine on page 105
♦ **A-methaPred® Injection** see Methylprednisolone on page 593
♦ **Amethocaine Hydrochloride** see Tetracaine on page 884
♦ **Amethopterin** see Methotrexate on page 585
♦ **Ametop™** see Tetracaine on page 884
♦ **Amfepramone** see Diethylpropion on page 277
♦ **Amgenal® Cough Syrup** see Bromodiphenhydramine and Codeine on page 123
♦ **Amicar®** see Aminocaproic Acid on page 52

## Amikacin (am i KAY sin)
**Pharmacologic Class** Antibiotic, Aminoglycoside
**U.S. Brand Names** Amikin® Injection
**Mechanism of Action** Inhibits protein synthesis in susceptible bacteria by binding to 30S ribosomal subunits
**Use** Treatment of serious infections due to organisms resistant to gentamicin and tobramycin including *Pseudomonas*, *Proteus*, *Serratia*, and other gram-positive bacilli (bone infections, respiratory tract infections, endocarditis, and septicemia); documented infection of mycobacterial organisms susceptible to amikacin
**USUAL DOSAGE** Individualization is critical because of the low therapeutic index
   **Use of ideal body weight (IBW) for determining the mg/kg/dose appears to be more accurate than dosing on the basis of total body weight (TBW)**
      In morbid obesity, dosage requirement may best be estimated using a dosing weight of IBW + 0.4 (TBW - IBW)
   Initial and periodic peak and trough plasma drug levels should be determined, particularly in critically ill patients with serious infections or in disease states known to significantly alter aminoglycoside pharmacokinetics (eg, cystic fibrosis, burns, or major surgery)
   Infants, Children, and Adults: I.M., I.V.: 5-7.5 mg/kg/dose every 8 hours
   Some clinicians suggest a daily dose of 15-20 mg/kg for all patients with normal renal function. This dose is at least as efficacious with similar, if not less, toxicity than conventional dosing.
   **Dosing interval in renal impairment:** Some patients may require larger or more frequent doses if serum levels document the need (ie, cystic fibrosis or febrile granulocytopenic patients)
      $Cl_{cr}$ ≥60 mL/minute: Administer every 8 hours
      $Cl_{cr}$ 40-60 mL/minute: Administer every 12 hours
      $Cl_{cr}$ 20-40 mL/minute: Administer every 24 hours
      $Cl_{cr}$ <20 mL/minute: Loading dose, then monitor levels
   Hemodialysis: Dialyzable (50% to 100%); administer dose postdialysis or administer 2/3 normal dose as a supplemental dose postdialysis and follow levels

Peritoneal dialysis: Dose as Cl$_{cr}$ <20 mL/minute: Follow levels
Continuous arteriovenous or venovenous hemodiafiltration (CAVH) effects: Dose as for Cl$_{cr}$ 20-40 mL/minute and follow levels

**Dosage Forms** Inj, as sulfate: 50 mg/mL (2 mL, 4 mL), 250 mg/mL (2 mL, 4 mL)

**Contraindications** Hypersensitivity to amikacin sulfate or any component; cross-sensitivity may exist with other aminoglycosides

**Warnings/Precautions** Dose and/or frequency of administration must be monitored and modified in patients with renal impairment; drug should be discontinued if signs of ototoxicity, nephrotoxicity, or hypersensitivity occur; ototoxicity is proportional to the amount of drug given and the duration of treatment; tinnitus or vertigo may be indications of vestibular injury and impending bilateral irreversible damage; renal damage is usually reversible

**Pregnancy Risk Factor** C

**Adverse Reactions**
1% to 10%:
Central nervous system: Neurotoxicity
Otic: Ototoxicity (auditory), ototoxicity (vestibular)
Renal: Nephrotoxicity
<1%: Hypotension, headache, drowsiness, drug fever, rash, nausea, vomiting, eosinophilia, paresthesia, tremor, arthralgia, weakness, dyspnea

**Drug Interactions**
Decreased effect of aminoglycoside: High concentrations of penicillins and/or cephalosporins (*in vitro* data)
Increased toxicity of aminoglycoside: Indomethacin I.V., amphotericin, loop diuretics, vancomycin, enflurane, methoxyflurane; increased toxicity of depolarizing and nondepolarizing neuromuscular blocking agents and polypeptide antibiotics with administration of aminoglycosides

**Half-Life** Dependent on renal function: Normal renal function: 1.4-2.3 hours; Anuria: End-stage renal disease: 28-86 hours

**Special PA Issues**
**Patient Education:** This drug can only be administered I.V. or I.M. It is important to maintain adequate hydration (2-3 L/day) unless informed by prescriber to restrict fluid intake. Report change in hearing acuity, ringing or roaring in ears, alteration in balance, vertigo, feeling of fullness in head; pain, tingling, or numbness of any body part; change in urinary pattern or decrease in urine; signs of opportunistic infection (eg, white plaques in mouth, vaginal discharge, unhealed sores, sore throat, unusual fever, chills); pain, redness, or swelling at injection site; or other adverse reactions.
**Monitoring Parameters:** Urinalysis, BUN, serum creatinine, appropriately timed peak and trough concentrations, vital signs, temperature, weight, I & O, hearing parameters
**Reference Range:**
Sample size: 0.5-2 mL blood (red top tube) or 0.1-1 mL serum (separated)
Therapeutic levels:
Peak:
Life-threatening infections: 25-30 µg/mL
Serious infections: 20-25 µg/mL
Urinary tract infections: 15-20 µg/mL
Trough:
Serious infections: 1-4 µg/mL
Life-threatening infections: 4-8 µg/mL
Toxic concentration: Peak: >35 µg/mL; Trough: >10 µg/mL
Timing of serum samples: Draw peak 30 minutes after completion of 30-minute infusion or at 1 hour following initiation of infusion or I.M. injection; draw trough within 30 minutes prior to next dose

♦ **Amikacin Sulfate** *see Amikacin on previous page*
♦ **Amikin®** *see Amikacin on previous page*
♦ **Amikin® Injection** *see Amikacin on previous page*

# Amiloride (a MIL oh ride)

**Pharmacologic Class** Diuretic, Potassium Sparing
**U.S. Brand Names** Midamor®
**Mechanism of Action** Interferes with potassium/sodium exchange (active transport) in the distal tubule, cortical collecting tubule and collecting duct by inhibiting sodium, potassium-ATPase; decreases calcium excretion; increases magnesium loss
**Use** Counteracts potassium loss induced by other diuretics in the treatment of hypertension or edematous conditions including CHF, hepatic cirrhosis, and hypoaldosteronism; usually used in conjunction with more potent diuretics such as thiazides or loop diuretics
**Investigational:** Cystic fibrosis
**USUAL DOSAGE** Oral:
Children: Although safety and efficacy have not been established by the FDA in children, a dosage of 0.625 mg/kg/day has been used in children weighing 6-20 kg
Adults: 5-10 mg/day (up to 20 mg)
Elderly: Initial: 5 mg once daily or every other day
(Continued)

## Amiloride *(Continued)*

**Dosing adjustment in renal impairment:**
Cl$_{cr}$ 10-50 mL/minute: Administer at 50% of normal dose
Cl$_{cr}$ <10 mL/minute: Avoid use

**Dosage Forms Tab, as hydrochloride:** 5 mg

**Contraindications** Hyperkalemia, potassium supplementation and impaired renal function or potassium-sparing diuretics, hypersensitivity to amiloride or any component

**Warnings/Precautions** Use cautiously in patients with severe hepatic insufficiency; may cause hyperkalemia (serum levels >5.5 mEq/L) which, if uncorrected, is potentially fatal; medication should be discontinued if potassium level are >6.5 mEq/L

**Pregnancy Risk Factor** B

**Adverse Reactions**

1% to 10%:
Central nervous system: Headache, fatigue, dizziness
Endocrine & metabolic: Hyperkalemia, hyperchloremic metabolic acidosis, dehydration, hyponatremia, gynecomastia
Gastrointestinal: Nausea, diarrhea, vomiting, abdominal pain, gas pain, appetite changes, constipation
Genitourinary: Impotence
Neuromuscular & skeletal: Muscle cramps, weakness
Respiratory: Cough, dyspnea
<1%: Angina pectoris, orthostatic hypotension, arrhythmias, palpitations, chest pain, vertigo, nervousness, insomnia, depression, rash or dryness, pruritus, alopecia, decreased libido, GI bleeding, heartburn, flatulence, dyspepsia, polyuria, bladder spasms, dysuria, jaundice, arthralgia, tremor, neck/shoulder pain, back pain, increased intraocular pressure, shortness of breath, thirst

**Drug Interactions**

Decreased effect of amiloride: Nonsteroidal anti-inflammatory agents
Increased risk of amiloride-associated hyperkalemia: Avoid use or use with extreme caution with triamterene, spironolactone, angiotensin-converting enzyme (ACE) inhibitors, potassium preparations, indomethacin
Increased toxicity of amantadine and lithium by reduction of renal excretion

**Onset** 2 hours

**Duration** 24 hours

**Half-Life** Normal renal function: 6-9 hours; End-stage renal disease: 8-144 hours

**Special PA Issues**

**Patient Education:** Take as directed, preferably early in day. Do not increase dietary intake of potassium unless instructed by prescriber (too much potassium can be as harmful as too little). You may experience dizziness or fatigue; use caution when driving or engaging in activities that require alertness. You may experience constipation (increased dietary fluid, fiber, or fruit may help), impotence (reversible), or loss of head hair (rare). Report muscle cramping or weakness, unresolved nausea or vomiting, palpitations, or difficulty breathing.

**Monitoring Parameters:** I & O, daily weights, blood pressure, serum electrolytes, renal function

**Related Information**

Heart Failure: Management of Patients with Left Ventricular Systolic Dysfunction *on page 1064*

## Amiloride and Hydrochlorothiazide

(a MIL oh ride & hye droe klor oh THYE a zide)

**Pharmacologic Class** Diuretic, Combination

**U.S. Brand Names** Moduretic®

**Dosage Forms Tab:** Amiloride hydrochloride 5 mg and hydrochlorothiazide 50 mg

♦ **Amiloride Hydrochloride** *see* Amiloride *on previous page*

♦ **2-Amino-6-Trifluoromethoxy-benzothiazole** *see* Riluzole *on page 806*

♦ **Aminobenzylpenicillin** *see* Ampicillin *on page 64*

## Aminocaproic Acid *(a mee noe ka PROE ik AS id)*

**Pharmacologic Class** Hemostatic Agent

**U.S. Brand Names** Amicar®

**Mechanism of Action** Competitively inhibits activation of plasminogen to plasmin, also, a lesser antiplasmin effect

**Use** Treatment of excessive bleeding from fibrinolysis

**USUAL DOSAGE** In the management of acute bleeding syndromes, oral dosage regimens are the same as the I.V. dosage regimens in adults and children

Chronic bleeding: Oral, I.V.: 5-30 g/day in divided doses at 3- to 6-hour intervals

Acute bleeding syndrome:

Children: Oral, I.V.: 100 mg/kg or 3 g/m² during the first hour, followed by continuous infusion at the rate of 33.3 mg/kg/hour or 1 g/m²/hour; total dosage should not exceed 18 g/m²/24 hours

Traumatic hyphema: Oral: 100 mg/kg/dose every 6-8 hours

Adults:

Oral: For elevated fibrinolytic activity, administer 5 g during first hour, followed by 1-1.25 g/hour for approximately 8 hours or until bleeding stops

I.V.: 4-5 g in 250 mL of diluent during first hour followed by continuous infusion at the rate of 1-1.25 g/hour in 50 mL of diluent, continue for 8 hours or until bleeding stops

Maximum daily dose: Oral, I.V.: 30 g

**Dosing adjustment in renal impairment:** Oliguria or ESRD: Reduce dose by 15% to 25%

**Dosage Forms Inj:** 250 mg/mL (20 mL, 96 mL, 100 mL); **Syr:** 1.25 g/5 mL (480 mL); **Tab:** 500 mg

**Contraindications** Disseminated intravascular coagulation, hematuria of upper urinary tract

**Warnings/Precautions** Rapid I.V. administration of the undiluted drug is not recommended; aminocaproic acid may accumulate in patients with decreased renal function; do not use in hematuria of upper urinary tract origin unless possible benefits outweigh risks; use with caution in patients with cardiac, renal or hepatic disease; do not administer without a definite diagnosis of laboratory findings indicative of hyperfibrinolysis; should not be used in nursing women

**Pregnancy Risk Factor** C

**Pregnancy Implications** Excretion in breast milk unknown

**Adverse Reactions**

1% to 10%:

Cardiovascular: Hypotension, bradycardia, arrhythmia

Central nervous system: Dizziness, headache, malaise, fatigue

Dermatologic: Rash

Gastrointestinal: GI irritation, nausea, cramps, diarrhea

Hematologic: Decreased platelet function, elevated serum enzymes

Neuromuscular & skeletal: Myopathy, weakness

Otic: Tinnitus

Respiratory: Nasal congestion

<1%: Convulsions, ejaculation problems, rhabdomyolysis, renal failure

**Drug Interactions** Increased toxic effect with oral contraceptives, estrogens

**Onset** Oral: Peak effect: Within 2 hours; Therapeutic effect: Within 1-72 hours after dose

**Half-Life** Oral: 1-2 hours

**Special PA Issues**

**Patient Education:** Take oral medication exactly as directed. This medication may cause dizziness and fatigue (use caution when driving or engaging in tasks that require alertness); hypotension (use caution when rising from a lying or sitting position or climbing stairs); menstrual irregularities, increased body hair, or sexual dysfunction (should reverse when treatment is completed); or nausea or vomiting (small frequent meals, frequent mouth care, or sucking on lozenges may help). Report immediately chest pain; dyspnea; swelling; nosebleed; warmth, swelling, pain, or redness in calves; skin rash; muscle pain or weakness; ringing in ears; or acute abdominal cramping.

**Monitoring Parameters:** Fibrinogen, fibrin split products, creatine phosphokinase (with long-term therapy)

**Reference Range:** Therapeutic concentration: >130 µg/mL (concentration necessary for inhibition of fibrinolysis)

♦ **Amino-Cerv™ Vaginal Cream** *see* Urea *on page 947*

# Aminoglutethimide (a mee noe gloo TETH i mide)

**Pharmacologic Class** Antineoplastic Agent, Miscellaneous

**U.S. Brand Names** Cytadren®

**Mechanism of Action** Blocks the enzymatic conversion of cholesterol to delta-5-pregnenolone, thereby reducing the synthesis of adrenal glucocorticoids, mineralocorticoids, estrogens, aldosterone, and androgens

**Use** Suppression of adrenal function in selected patients with Cushing's syndrome; also used successfully in postmenopausal patients with advanced breast carcinoma and in patients with metastatic prostate carcinoma as salvage (third-line hormonal agent)

**USUAL DOSAGE** Adults: Oral:

250 mg every 6 hours may be increased at 1- to 2-week intervals to a total of 2 g/day; administer in divided doses, 2-3 times/day to reduce incidence of nausea and vomiting. Follow adrenal cortical response by careful monitoring of plasma cortisol until the desired level of suppression is achieved.

Mineralocorticoid (fludrocortisone) replacement therapy may be necessary in up to 50% of patients. If glucocorticoid replacement therapy is necessary, 20-30 mg hydrocortisone orally in the morning will replace endogenous secretion.

**Dosing adjustment in renal impairment:** Dose reduction may be necessary

(Continued)

## Aminoglutethimide *(Continued)*

**Dosage Forms** Tab, scored: 250 mg

**Contraindications** Hypersensitivity to aminoglutethimide or any component and glutethimide

**Warnings/Precautions** Monitor blood pressure in all patients at appropriate intervals; hypothyroidism may occur; **mineralocorticoid replacement therapy may be necessary in up to 50% of patients** (ie, fludrocortisone); if glucocorticoid replacement therapy is necessary, 20-30 mg of hydrocortisone daily in the morning will replace endogenous secretion (steroid replacement regimen is controversial - high-dose versus low-dose)

**Pregnancy Risk Factor** D

**Pregnancy Implications** Suspected of causing virilization when given throughout pregnancy

**Adverse Reactions** Most adverse effects will diminish in incidence and severity after the first 2-6 weeks

>10%:

Central nervous system: Headache, dizziness, drowsiness, and lethargy are frequent at the start of therapy, clumsiness

Dermatologic: Skin rash

Gastrointestinal: Nausea, vomiting, anorexia

Hepatic: Cholestatic jaundice

Neuromuscular & skeletal: Myalgia

Renal: Nephrotoxicity

Respiratory: Pulmonary alveolar damage

Miscellaneous: Systemic lupus erythematosus

1% to 10%:

Cardiovascular: Hypotension and tachycardia, orthostatic hypotension

Dermatologic: Hirsutism in females

Endocrine & metabolic: Adrenocortical insufficiency

Hematologic: Rare cases of neutropenia, leukopenia, thrombocytopenia, pancytopenia, and agranulocytosis have been reported

<1%: Adrenal suppression, lipid abnormalities (hypercholesterolemia), hyperkalemia, hypothyroidism, goiter

**Drug Interactions** CYP 450 hepatic microsomal enzyme inducer

Decreased effect:

Dexamethasone: Reported to increase metabolism

Digitoxin: Increases clearance of digitoxin after 3-8 weeks of aminoglutethimide therapy

Theophylline: Aminoglutethimide increases metabolism of theophylline

Warfarin: Decreases anticoagulant response to warfarin

Increased toxicity: Propranolol: Case report of enhanced aminoglutethimide toxicity (rash and lethargy)

**Onset** 3-5 days

**Half-Life** 7-15 hours; shorter following multiple administrations than following single doses (induces hepatic enzymes increasing its own metabolism)

**Special PA Issues**

**Patient Education:** May be taken with food to reduce incidence of nausea. You may experience drowsiness or dizziness; avoid driving or use of hazardous machinery until response to medication is known. Small frequent meals may reduce incidence of nausea or vomiting. Masculinization may occur and is reversible when treatment is discontinued. Report rash, unresolved nausea, vomiting, lethargy, yellowing of skin or eyes, easy bruising or bleeding, change in color of urine or stool, increased growth of facial hair, thick tongue, severe mood swings, palpitations, or respiratory difficulty.

♦ **Amino-Opti-E® [OTC]** *see* Vitamin E *on page 963*

♦ **Aminophyllin™** *see* Theophylline Salts *on page 888*

♦ **Aminophylline** *see* Theophylline Salts *on page 888*

## Aminosalicylate Sodium *(a MEE noe sa LIS i late SOW dee um)*

**Pharmacologic Class** Salicylate

**U.S. Brand Names** Sodium P.A.S.

**Mechanism of Action** Aminosalicylic acid (PAS) is a highly specific bacteriostatic agent active against *M. tuberculosis*. Structurally related to para-aminobenzoic acid (PABA) and its mechanism of action is thought to be similar to the sulfonamides, a competitive antagonism with PABA; disrupts plate biosynthesis in sensitive organisms.

**Use** Adjunctive treatment of tuberculosis used in combination with other antitubercular agents; has also been used in Crohn's disease

**USUAL DOSAGE** Oral:

Children: 150 mg/kg/day in 3-4 equally divided doses

Adults: 150 mg/kg/day in 2-3 equally divided doses (usually 12-14 g/day)

**Dosing adjustment in renal impairment:**

$Cl_{cr}$ 10-50 mL/minute: Administer 50% to 75% of dose

$Cl_{cr}$ <10 mL/minute: Administer 50% of dose

Administer after hemodialysis

**Dosage Forms Tab:** 500 mg

**Contraindications** Hypersensitivity to aminosalicylate sodium

**Warnings/Precautions** Use with caution in patients with hepatic or renal dysfunction, patients with gastric ulcer, patients with CHF, and patients who are sodium restricted

**Pregnancy Risk Factor** C

**Adverse Reactions**

1% to 10%: Gastrointestinal: Nausea, vomiting, diarrhea, abdominal pain

<1%: Vasculitis, fever, skin eruptions, goiter with or without myxedema, leukopenia, agranulocytosis, thrombocytopenia, hemolytic anemia, jaundice, hepatitis

**Drug Interactions** Decreased levels of digoxin and vitamin $B_{12}$

**Special PA Issues**

**Patient Education:** May be taken with food. Do not take tablets that are discolored (brown or purple); see pharmacist for new prescription. Do not stop taking without consulting prescriber. Report persistent sore throat, fever, unusual bleeding or bruising, persistent nausea or vomiting, or abdominal pain.

♦ **5-Aminosalicylic Acid** *see* Mesalamine *on page 571*

# Amiodarone (a MEE oh da rone)

**Pharmacologic Class** Antiarrhythmic Agent, Class III

**U.S. Brand Names** Cordarone®; Pacerone®

**Mechanism of Action** Class III antiarrhythmic agent which inhibits adrenergic stimulation, prolongs the action potential and refractory period in myocardial tissue; decreases A-V conduction and sinus node function

**Use**

Oral: Management of life-threatening recurrent ventricular fibrillation (VF) or hemodynamically unstable ventricular tachycardia (VT)

I.V.: Initiation of treatment and prophylaxis of frequency recurring VF and unstable VT in patients refractory to other therapy. Also, for patients for whom oral amiodarone is indicated but who are unable to take oral medication.

**USUAL DOSAGE**

Oral:

Children (calculate doses for children <1 year on body surface area): Loading dose: 10-15 mg/kg/day or 600-800 mg/1.73 m²/day for 4-14 days or until adequate control of arrhythmia or prominent adverse effects occur (this loading dose may be given in 1-2 divided doses/day); dosage should then be reduced to 5 mg/kg/day or 200-400 mg/1.73 m²/day given once daily for several weeks; if arrhythmia does not recur, reduce to lowest effective dosage possible; usual daily minimal dose: 2.5 mg/kg/day; maintenance doses may be given for 5 of 7 days/week

Adults: Ventricular arrhythmias: 800-1600 mg/day in 1-2 doses for 1-3 weeks; then when adequate arrhythmia control is achieved decrease to 600-800 mg/day in 1-2 doses for 1 month; maintenance: 400 mg/day; lower doses are recommended for supraventricular arrhythmias

I.V.:

First 24 hours: 1000 mg according to following regimen

Step 1: 150 mg (10 mL) over first 10 minutes (mix 3 mL in 100 mL $D_5W$)

Step 2: 360 mg (200 mL) over next 6 hours (mix 18 mL in 500 mL $D_5W$)

Step 3: 540 mg (300 mL) over next 18 hours

After the first 24 hours: 0.5 mg/minute utilizing concentration of 1-6 mg/mL

Breakthrough VF or VT: 150 mg supplemental doses in 100 mL $D_5W$ over 10 minutes

**Note:** When switching from I.V. to oral therapy, use the following as a guide:

<1-week I.V. infusion → 800-1600 mg/day

1- to 3-week I.V. infusion → 600-800 mg/day

>3-week I.V. infusion → 400 mg/day

**Recommendations for conversion to intravenous amiodarone after oral administration:** During long-term amiodarone therapy (ie, ≥4 months), the mean plasma-elimination half-life of the active metabolite of amiodarone is 61 days; replacement therapy may not be necessary in such patients if oral therapy is discontinued for a period <2 weeks, since any changes in serum amiodarone concentrations during this period may **not** be clinically significant

**Dosing adjustment in hepatic impairment:** Probably necessary in substantial hepatic impairment

Hemodialysis: Not dialyzable (0% to 5%); supplemental dose is not necessary

Peritoneal dialysis effects: Not dialyzable (0% to 5%); supplemental dose is not necessary

**Dosage Forms Inj:** 50 mg/mL with benzyl alcohol (3 mL). **Tab**, scored: 200 mg

**Contraindications** Hypersensitivity to amiodarone; severe sinus node dysfunction, second and third degree A-V block, marked sinus bradycardia except if pacemaker is placed, pregnancy and lactation; administration with ritonavir or sparfloxacin

**Warnings/Precautions** Not considered first-line antiarrhythmic due to high incidence of significant and potentially fatal toxicity (ie, hypersensitivity pneumonitis or interstitial/alveolar pneumonitis, hepatic failure, heart block, bradycardia or exacerbated arrhythmias), especially with large doses; reserve for use in arrhythmias refractory to other therapy; hospitalize patients while loading dose is administered; use cautiously in elderly due to predisposition

(Continued)

## Amiodarone *(Continued)*

to toxicity; use very cautiously and with close monitoring in patients with thyroid or liver disease. Due to an extensive tissue distribution and prolonged elimination period, the time at which a life-threatening arrhythmia will recur following discontinued therapy or an interaction with subsequent treatment may occur is unpredictable; patients must be observed carefully and extreme caution taken when other antiarrhythmic agents are substituted after discontinuation of amiodarone.

**Pregnancy Risk Factor** D

**Pregnancy Implications** Enters breast milk/contraindicated

**Adverse Reactions** With large dosages (≥400 mg/day), adverse reactions occur in ~75% patients and require discontinuance in 5% to 20%

>10%:
  Cardiovascular: Hypotension (especially with I.V. form)
  Central nervous system: Ataxia, fatigue, malaise, dizziness, headache, insomnia, nightmares
  Dermatologic: Photosensitivity
  Gastrointestinal: Nausea, vomiting
  Neuromuscular & skeletal: Tremor, paresthesias, muscle weakness
  Respiratory: Pulmonary fibrosis (cough, fever, dyspnea, malaise), interstitial pneumonitis
  Miscellaneous: Alveolitis

1% to 10%:
  Cardiovascular: Congestive heart failure, cardiac arrhythmias (atropine-resistant bradycardia, heart block, sinus arrest, paroxysmal ventricular tachycardia), myocardial depression, flushing, edema
  Central nervous system: Fever, sleep disturbances
  Dermatologic: Solar dermatitis
  Endocrine & metabolic: Hypothyroidism or hyperthyroidism (less common), decreased libido
  Gastrointestinal: Constipation, anorexia, abdominal pain, abnormal salivation, abnormal taste (oral form)
  Hematologic: Coagulation abnormalities
  Hepatic: Abnormal LFTs
  Local: Phlebitis with concentrations >3 mg/mL
  Neuromuscular & skeletal: Paresthesia
  Ocular: Visual disturbances
  Miscellaneous: Abnormal smell (oral form)

<1%: Hypotension (with oral form), vasculitis, atrial fibrillation, increased Q-T interval, ventricular fibrillation, cardiogenic shock, pseudotumor cerebri, rash, alopecia, discoloration of skin (slate blue), Stevens-Johnson syndrome, hyperglycemia, hypertriglyceridemia, epididymitis, thrombocytopenia, cirrhosis, severe hepatotoxicity (potentially fatal hepatitis), increased ALT/AST, optic neuritis, corneal microdeposits, photophobia

**Drug Interactions** CYP3A3/4 enzyme substrate; CYP2C9, 2D6, and 3A3/4 enzyme inhibitor

Amiodarone appears to interfere with the hepatic metabolism of several drugs resulting in significantly increased plasma concentrations; see table.

**Onset** Onset of effect: 3 days to 3 weeks after starting therapy; Peak effect: 1 week to 5 months; onset of I.V. form may be more rapid

**Duration** Following discontinuation of therapy: 7-50 days

**Half-Life** Oral chronic therapy: 40-55 days (range: 26-107 days)

**Special PA Issues**
  **Patient Education:** Emergency use: Patient condition will determine amount of patient education. Oral: May be taken with food to reduce GI disturbance. Do not change dosage or discontinue drug without consulting prescriber. Regular blood work, ophthalmic exams, and cardiac assessment will be necessary while taking this medication on a long-term basis. You may experience dizziness, weakness, or insomnia (use caution when driving, climbing stairs, or engaging in hazardous tasks); hypotension (use caution changing position - rising from sitting or lying); nausea, vomiting, loss of appetite, or stomach discomfort, abnormal taste (small frequent meals, chewing gum, or sucking on lozenges may help); photosensitivity (use sunscreen, protective clothing, or avoid direct sunlight); or decreased libido (reversible). Report persistent dry cough or shortness of breath; chest pain, palpitations, irregular or slow heartbeat; unusual bruising or bleeding; blood in urine, feces, vomitus; pain, swelling, or warmth in calves; muscle tremor, weakness, numbness, or changes in gait; skin rash or irritation; or changes in urinary patterns.

  **Monitoring Parameters:** Monitor heart rate (EKG) and rhythm throughout therapy; assess patient for signs of thyroid dysfunction (thyroid function tests and liver enzymes), lethargy, edema of the hands, feet, weight loss, and pulmonary toxicity (baseline pulmonary function tests)

  **Reference Range:** Therapeutic: 0.5-2.5 mg/L (SI: 1-4 μmol/L) (parent); desethyl metabolite is active and is present in equal concentration to parent drug

## Amiodarone Common Drug Interactions

| Drug | Interaction |
|------|-------------|
| Anticoagulants, oral | The effects of the anticoagulant is increased due to inhibition of its metabolism. |
| β-adrenergic receptor antagonists | β-blocker effects are enhanced by amiodarone's inhibition of the β-blocker's hepatic metabolism. |
| Calcium channel antagonists | Additive effects of both drugs resulting in a reduction in cardiac sinus conduction, atrioventricular nodal conduction, and myocardial contractility. |
| Cholestyramine | Increased enterohepatic elimination of amiodarone may occur resulting in decreased serum levels and half-life. |
| Cimetidine | Increased amiodarone levels may result |
| Cyclosporine | Results in persistently elevated cyclosporine levels and elevated creatinine despite reduction in cyclosporine dosage. |
| Digoxin | Digoxin concentrations may be increased with resultant increases in activity and potential for toxicity. |
| Disopyramide | Q-T prolongation may occur in addition to arrhythmias. |
| Fentanyl | Concurrent use with amiodarone may result in hypotension, bradycardia, and decreased cardiac output. |
| Flecainide | Flecainide plasma concentrations are increased. |
| Methotrexate | Chronic use of amiodarone impairs MTX metabolism resulting in MTX toxicity. |
| Phenytoin | Phenytoin serum concentrations are increased due to reduction in phenytoin metabolism, with possible symptoms of phenytoin toxicity; amiodarone levels may be decreased. |
| Procainamide | Procainamide serum concentrations may be increased. |
| Quinidine | Quinidine serum concentrations may be increased and can potentially cause fatal cardiac dysrhythmias. |
| Ritonavir | Increased risk of amiodarone cardiotoxicity results. |
| Sparfloxacin | Risk of cardiotoxicity may be increased. |
| Theophylline | Increased theophylline levels and resultant toxicity may occur; effects may be delayed and may persist after amiodarone discontinuation |

- **Amiodarone Hydrochloride** *see* Amiodarone *on page 55*
- **Amitone® [OTC]** *see* Calcium Carbonate *on page 139*

# Amitriptyline (a mee TRIP ti leen)

**Pharmacologic Class** Antidepressant, Tricyclic (Tertiary Amine)

**U.S. Brand Names** Elavil®; Enovil®

**Mechanism of Action** Increases the synaptic concentration of serotonin and/or norepinephrine in the central nervous system by inhibition of their reuptake by the presynaptic neuronal membrane

**Use** Treatment of various forms of depression, often in conjunction with psychotherapy; analgesic for certain chronic and neuropathic pain, prophylaxis against migraine headaches

## USUAL DOSAGE

Children: Pain management: Oral: Initial: 0.1 mg/kg at bedtime, may advance as tolerated over 2-3 weeks to 0.5-2 mg/day at bedtime

Adolescents: Oral: Initial: 25-50 mg/day; may administer in divided doses; increase gradually to 100 mg/day in divided doses

Adults:

Oral: 30-100 mg/day single dose at bedtime or in divided doses; dose may be gradually increased up to 300 mg/day; once symptoms are controlled, decrease gradually to lowest effective dose

I.M.: 20-30 mg 4 times/day

**Dosing interval in hepatic impairment:** Use with caution and monitor plasma levels and patient response

Hemodialysis: Nondialyzable

**Dosage Forms Inj:** 10 mg/mL (10 mL); **Tab:** 10 mg, 25 mg, 50 mg, 75 mg, 100 mg, 150 mg

**Contraindications** Hypersensitivity to amitriptyline (cross-sensitivity with other tricyclics may occur); patients receiving MAO inhibitors within past 14 days; narrow-angle glaucoma; avoid use during pregnancy and lactation

## Warnings/Precautions

Amitriptyline should not be abruptly discontinued in patients receiving high doses for prolonged periods

Use with caution in patients with cardiac conduction disturbances; an EKG prior to initiation of therapy is advised; use with caution in patients with a history of hyperthyroidism, renal or hepatic impairment

(Continued)

## Amitriptyline *(Continued)*

The most anticholinergic and sedating of the antidepressants; pronounced effects on the cardiovascular system (hypotension), hence, many psychiatrists agree it is best to avoid in the elderly

**Pregnancy Risk Factor** D

**Pregnancy Implications** Enters breast milk/not recommended

**Adverse Reactions** Anticholinergic effects may be pronounced; moderate to marked sedation can occur (tolerance to these effects usually occurs)

>10%:
  Central nervous system: Dizziness, drowsiness, headache
  Gastrointestinal: Xerostomia, constipation, increased appetite, nausea, unpleasant taste, weight gain
  Neuromuscular & skeletal: Weakness

1% to 10%:
  Cardiovascular: Hypotension, postural hypotension, arrhythmias, tachycardia
  Central nervous system: Nervousness, restlessness, parkinsonian syndrome, insomnia, sedation, fatigue, anxiety, impaired cognitive function, seizures have occurred occasionally, extrapyramidal symptoms are possible
  Gastrointestinal: Diarrhea, heartburn
  Genitourinary: Sexual dysfunction, urinary retention
  Neuromuscular & skeletal: Tremor
  Ocular: Eye pain, blurred vision
  Miscellaneous: Diaphoresis (excessive)

<1%: Sudden death, alopecia, photosensitivity, breast enlargement, galactorrhea, rarely SIADH, trouble with gums, decreased lower esophageal sphincter tone may cause GE reflux, testicular edema, leukopenia, eosinophilia, rarely agranulocytosis, cholestatic jaundice, increased liver enzymes, increased intraocular pressure, tinnitus, allergic reactions

**Drug Interactions** CYP1A2, 2C9, 2C18, 2C19, 2D6, and 3A3/4 enzyme substrate

Decreased effect: Phenobarbital may increase the metabolism of amitriptyline; amitriptyline blocks the uptake of guanethidine and thus prevents the hypotensive effect of guanethidine

Increased toxicity: Clonidine → hypertensive crisis; amitriptyline may be additive with or may potentiate the action of other CNS depressants such as sedatives or hypnotics; with MAO inhibitors, hyperpyrexia, hypertension, tachycardia, confusion, seizures, and **deaths have been reported**; amitriptyline may increase the prothrombin time in patients stabilized on warfarin; amitriptyline potentiates the pressor and cardiac effects of sympathomimetic agents such as isoproterenol, epinephrine, etc; cimetidine and methylphenidate may decrease the metabolism of amitriptyline; additive anticholinergic effects seen with other anticholinergic agents

**Onset** Onset of therapeutic effect: 7-21 days

Desired therapeutic effect (for depression) may take as long as 3-4 weeks, at that point dosage should be reduced to lowest effective level.

When used for migraine headache prophylaxis, therapeutic effect may take as long as 6 weeks. A higher dosage may be required in a heavy smoker, because of increased metabolism.

**Half-Life** 9-25 hours (15-hour average)

**Special PA Issues**

  **Patient Education:** Take exactly as directed (do not increase dose or frequency); may take several weeks to achieve desired results; may cause physical and/or psychological dependence. Do not use alcohol, excess caffeine, and other prescription or OTC medications not approved by prescriber. Maintain adequate hydration (2-3 L/day of fluids unless instructed to restrict fluid intake). May turn urine blue-green (normal). You may experience drowsiness, lightheadedness, impaired coordination, dizziness, or blurred vision (use caution when driving or engaging in hazardous tasks until response to medication is known); constipation (increased exercise, fluids, or dietary fruit and fiber may help); urinary retention (void before taking medication); postural hypotension (use caution climbing stairs or when changing position from lying or sitting to standing); altered sexual drive or ability (reversible); or photosensitivity (use sunscreen, protective clothing, and avoid extended exposure to direct sunlight). Report persistent CNS effects (eg, nervousness, restlessness, insomnia, anxiety, excitation, headache, agitation, impaired coordination, changes in cognition); muscle cramping, weakness, tremors, or rigidity; ringing in ears or visual disturbances; chest pain, palpitations, or irregular heartbeat; blurred vision; or worsening of condition.

  **Dietary Considerations:** Alcohol: Additive CNS effects, avoid use

  **Monitoring Parameters:** Monitor blood pressure and pulse rate prior to and during initial therapy; evaluate mental status; monitor weight

  **Reference Range:** Therapeutic: Amitriptyline and nortriptyline 100-250 ng/mL (SI: 360-900 nmol/L); nortriptyline 50-150 ng/mL (SI: 190-570 nmol/L); Toxic: >0.5 µg/mL; plasma levels do not always correlate with clinical effectiveness

**Related Information**

Antidepressant Agents *on page 998*

## Amitriptyline and Chlordiazepoxide
(a mee TRIP ti leen & klor dye az e POKS ide)
**Pharmacologic Class** Antidepressant, Tricyclic (Tertiary Amine)
**U.S. Brand Names** Limbitrol® DS 10-25
**Dosage Forms Tab:** 5-12.5: Amitriptyline hydrochloride 12.5 mg and chlordiazepoxide 5 mg, 10-25: Amitriptyline hydrochloride 25 mg and chlordiazepoxide 10 mg

## Amitriptyline and Perphenazine (a mee TRIP ti leen & per FEN a zeen)
**Pharmacologic Class** Antidepressant, Tricyclic (Tertiary Amine)
**U.S. Brand Names** Etrafon®; Triavil®
**Dosage Forms Tab:** 2-10: Amitriptyline hydrochloride 10 mg and perphenazine 2 mg, 4-10: Amitriptyline hydrochloride 10 mg and perphenazine 4 mg, 2-25: Amitriptyline hydrochloride 25 mg and perphenazine 2 mg, 4-25: Amitriptyline hydrochloride 25 mg and perphenazine 4 mg, 4-50: Amitriptyline hydrochloride 50 mg and perphenazine 4 mg

♦ **Amitriptyline Hydrochloride** *see* Amitriptyline *on page 57*

## Amlexanox (am LEKS an oks)
**Pharmacologic Class** Anti-inflammatory, Locally Applied
**U.S. Brand Names** Aphthasol™
**Mechanism of Action** As a benzopyrano-bipyridine carboxylic acid derivative, amlexanox has anti-inflammatory and antiallergic properties; it inhibits chemical mediatory release of the slow-reacting substance of anaphylaxis (SRS-A) and may have antagonistic effect son interleukin-3
**Use** Treatment of aphthous ulcers (ie, canker sores); has been investigated in many allergic disorders
**USUAL DOSAGE** Administer (0.5 cm - ¼") directly on ulcers 4 times/day following oral hygiene, after meals, and at bedtime
**Dosage Forms Crm:** 5% (5 g)
**Contraindications** Hypersensitivity to amlexanox or components
**Warnings/Precautions** Discontinue therapy if rash or contact mucositis develops
**Pregnancy Risk Factor** B
**Pregnancy Implications** Due to lack of data, avoid use in pregnancy or lactation, if possible
**Adverse Reactions**
1% to 2%:
   Dermatologic: Allergic contact dermatitis
   Gastrointestinal: Oral irritation
<1%: Contact mucositis
**Special PA Issues**
   Patient Education: Apply as soon as possible and continue 4 times/day (after meals and at bedtime); wash hands after use; contact physician if no reduction in pain occurs within 10 days

## Amlodipine (am LOE di peen)
**Pharmacologic Class** Calcium Channel Blocker
**U.S. Brand Names** Norvasc®
**Mechanism of Action** Inhibits calcium ion from entering the "slow channels" or select voltage-sensitive areas of vascular smooth muscle and myocardium during depolarization, producing a relaxation of coronary vascular smooth muscle and coronary vasodilation; increases myocardial oxygen delivery in patients with vasospastic angina
**Use** Treatment of hypertension and angina (chronic stable or Prinzmetal's) with or without other blocking
**USUAL DOSAGE** Adults: Oral:
   Hypertension: Initial dose: 2.5-5 mg once daily; usual dose: 5 mg once daily; maximum dose: 10 mg once daily; in general, titrate in 2.5 mg increments over 7-14 days
   Angina: Usual dose: 10 mg; use lower doses for elderly or those with hepatic insufficiency (eg, 2.5-5 mg)
   Dialysis: Hemodialysis and peritoneal dialysis does not enhance elimination; supplemental dose is not necessary
   **Dosage adjustment in hepatic impairment:** 2.5 mg once daily
**Dosage Forms Tab:** 2.5 mg, 5 mg, 10 mg
**Contraindications** Hypersensitivity
**Warnings/Precautions** Use with caution and titrate dosages for patients with impaired renal or hepatic function; use caution when treating patients with congestive heart failure, sick-sinus syndrome, severe left ventricular dysfunction, hypertrophic cardiomyopathy (especially obstructive), concomitant therapy with beta-blockers or digoxin, edema, or increased intracranial pressure with cranial tumors; do not abruptly withdraw (may cause chest pain); elderly may experience hypotension and constipation more readily.
**Pregnancy Risk Factor** C
**Pregnancy Implications** Excretion in breast milk unknown/use caution
(Continued)

## Amlodipine *(Continued)*

Teratogenic and embryotoxic effects have been demonstrated in small animals. No well controlled studies have been conducted in pregnant women. Use in pregnancy only when clearly needed and when the benefits outweigh the potential hazard to the fetus.

Clinical effects on the fetus: No data on crossing the placenta

**Adverse Reactions**

>10%: Cardiovascular: Peripheral edema (1.8%-14.6% dose-related)

1% to 10%:

Cardiovascular: Flushing, palpitations

Central nervous system: Headache, fatigue, dizziness, somnolence (1% to 2%)

Dermatologic: Dermatitis, rash (1% to 2%); pruritus, urticaria (1% to 2%)

Endocrine & metabolic: Sexual dysfunction (1% to 2%)

Gastrointestinal: Nausea, abdominal pain (1% to 2%)

Respiratory: Shortness of breath (1% to 2%)

Neuromuscular & skeletal: Muscle cramps (1% to 2%)

<1%: Hypotension, bradycardia, arrhythmias, abnormal EKG, ventricular extrasystoles, syncope, tachycardia, nervousness, psychiatric disturbances, insomnia, malaise, alopecia, petechiae, weight gain, anorexia, diarrhea, constipation, vomiting, xerostomia, flatulence, micturition disorder, joint stiffness, weakness, paresthesia, tremor, tinnitus, nasal congestion, cough, epistaxis, diaphoresis

**Drug Interactions** CYP3A3/4 enzyme substrate

Increased effect:

Amlodipine and benazepril may increase hypotensive effect

Amlodipine and cyclosporine may increase cyclosporine levels

Beta-blockers in combination with calcium antagonists may result in increased cardiac depression

Severe hypotension or increased fluid volume requirements have occurred with fentanyl and calcium blockers

**Onset** 30-50 minutes; Peak effect: 6-12 hours

**Duration** 24 hours

**Half-Life** 30-50 hours

**Special PA Issues**

**Patient Education:** Take as prescribed; do not stop abruptly without consulting prescriber. You may experience headache (if unrelieved, consult prescriber), nausea or vomiting (frequent small meals may help), or constipation (increased dietary bulk and fluids may help). May cause drowsiness; use caution when driving or engaging in hazardous activities. Report unrelieved headache, vomiting, constipation, palpitations, peripheral or facial swelling, weight gain >5 lb/week, or respiratory changes.

**Related Information**

Calcium Channel Blocking Agents *on page 1004*

## Amlodipine and Benazepril *(am LOE di peen & ben AY ze pril)*

**Pharmacologic Class** Antihypertensive Agent, Combination

**U.S. Brand Names** Lotrel®

**Dosage Forms Cap:** Amlodipine 2.5 mg and benazepril hydrochloride 10 mg, Amlodipine 5 mg and benazepril hydrochloride 10 mg, Amlodipine 5 mg and benazepril hydrochloride 20 mg

♦ **Ammonapse** *see* Sodium Phenylbutyrate *on page 842*

♦ **AMO Vitrax®** *see* Sodium Hyaluronate *on page 841*

## Amoxapine *(a MOKS a peen)*

**Pharmacologic Class** Antidepressant, Tricyclic (Secondary Amine)

**U.S. Brand Names** Asendin®

**Mechanism of Action** Reduces the reuptake of serotonin and norepinephrine and blocks the response of dopamine receptors to dopamine

**Use** Treatment of neurotic and endogenous depression and mixed symptoms of anxiety and depression

**USUAL DOSAGE** Once symptoms are controlled, decrease gradually to lowest effective dose. Maintenance dose is usually given at bedtime to reduce daytime sedation. Oral:

Children: Not established in children <16 years of age

Adolescents: Initial: 25-50 mg/day; increase gradually to 100 mg/day; may administer as divided doses or as a single dose at bedtime

Adults: Initial: 25 mg 2-3 times/day, if tolerated, dosage may be increased to 100 mg 2-3 times/day; may be given in a single bedtime dose when dosage <300 mg/day

Elderly: Initial: 25 mg at bedtime increased by 25 mg weekly for outpatients and every 3 days for inpatients if tolerated; usual dose: 50-150 mg/day, but doses up to 300 mg may be necessary

Maximum daily dose:

Inpatient: 600 mg

Outpatient: 400 mg

**Dosage Forms Tab:** 25 mg, 50 mg, 100 mg, 150 mg

**Contraindications** Hypersensitivity to amoxapine; cross-sensitivity with other tricyclics may occur; narrow-angle glaucoma; patients receiving MAO inhibitors within past 14 days

**Warnings/Precautions** Use with caution in patients with seizures, cardiac conduction disturbances, cardiovascular diseases, urinary retention, hyperthyroidism, or those receiving thyroid replacement; do not discontinue abruptly in patients receiving high doses chronically; tolerance develops in 1-3 months in some patients, close medical follow-up is essential

**Pregnancy Risk Factor** C

**Pregnancy Implications** Enters breast milk/contraindicated

**Adverse Reactions**

>10%:

Central nervous system: Drowsiness

Gastrointestinal: Xerostomia, constipation, nausea, unpleasant taste, weight gain

1% to 10%:

Central nervous system: Dizziness, headache, confusion, nervousness, restlessness, insomnia, ataxia, excitement

Dermatologic: Edema, skin rash

Endocrine: Elevated prolactin levels

Gastrointestinal: Increased appetite

Neuromuscular & skeletal: Tremor, weakness

Ocular: Blurred vision

Miscellaneous: Diaphoresis

<1%: Hypotension, tachycardia, pallor, anxiety, seizures, neuroleptic malignant syndrome, tardive dyskinesia, photosensitivity, breast enlargement, galactorrhea, SIADH, increased or decreased libido, impotence, menstrual irregularity, painful ejaculation, epigastric distress, vomiting, flatulence, abdominal pain, abnormal taste, diarrhea, testicular edema, urinary retention, agranulocytosis, leukopenia, elevated liver enzymes, paresthesia, increased intraocular pressure, mydriasis, lacrimation, tinnitus, allergic reactions

**Drug Interactions**

Decreased effect of clonidine, guanethidine

Increased effect of CNS depressants, adrenergic agents, anticholinergic agents

Increased toxicity of MAO inhibitors (hyperpyrexia, tachycardia, hypertension, seizures and death may occur); similar interactions as with other tricyclics may occur

**Onset** Onset of antidepressant effect: Usually occurs after 1-2 weeks

**Half-Life** Parent drug: 11-16 hours; Active metabolite: 30 hours

**Special PA Issues**

**Patient Education:** Take exactly as directed (do not increase dose or frequency). Full effect may not occur for 3-5 weeks; may cause physical and/or psychological dependence. Do not use excessive alcohol or other prescription or OTC medications (especially pain medications, sedatives, antihistamines, or hypnotics) without consulting prescriber. Maintain adequate hydration (2-3 L/day of fluids unless instructed to restrict fluid intake). You may experience drowsiness, lightheadedness, impaired coordination, dizziness, or blurred vision (use caution when driving or engaging in hazardous tasks until response to medication is known); nausea, vomiting, increased appetite, or dry mouth (small frequent meals, good mouth care, chewing gum, or sucking lozenges may help); constipation (increased exercise, fluids, or dietary fruit and fiber may help); or altered sexual drive or ability (reversible). Report persistent CNS effects (confusion, restlessness, anxiety, insomnia, excitation, headache, dizziness, fatigue, impaired coordination); muscle cramping, weakness, tremors, or rigidity; visual disturbances; excessive GI symptoms (cramping, constipation, vomiting); or worsening of condition.

**Dietary Considerations:** Alcohol: Avoid use

**Monitoring Parameters:** Monitor blood pressure and pulse rate prior to and during initial therapy evaluate mental status; monitor weight

**Reference Range:** Therapeutic: Amoxapine: 20-100 ng/mL (SI: 64-319 nmol/L); 8-OH amoxapine: 150-400 ng/mL (SI: 478-1275 nmol/L); both: 200-500 ng/mL (SI: 637-1594 nmol/L)

**Related Information**

Antidepressant Agents *on page 998*

# Amoxicillin (a moks i SIL in)

**Pharmacologic Class** Antibiotic, Penicillin

**U.S. Brand Names** Amoxil®; Biomox®; Polymox®; Trimox®; Wymox®

**Mechanism of Action** Inhibits bacterial cell wall synthesis by binding to one or more of the penicillin binding proteins (PBPs); which in turn inhibits the final transpeptidation step of peptidoglycan synthesis in bacterial cell walls, thus inhibiting cell wall biosynthesis. Bacteria eventually lyse due to ongoing activity of cell wall autolytic enzymes (autolysins and murein hydrolases) while cell wall assembly is arrested.

**Use** Treatment of otitis media, sinusitis, and infections caused by susceptible organisms involving the respiratory tract, skin, and urinary tract; prophylaxis of bacterial endocarditis in patients undergoing surgical or dental procedures; approved in combination for eradication of *H. pylori*

(Continued)

## Amoxicillin *(Continued)*

**USUAL DOSAGE** Oral:
Children: 20-50 mg/kg/day in divided doses every 8 hours
  Subacute bacterial endocarditis prophylaxis: 50 mg/kg 1 hour before procedure
Adults: 250-500 mg every 8 hours or 500-875 mg twice daily; maximum dose: 2-3 g/day
  Endocarditis prophylaxis: 2 g 1 hour before procedure
*Helicobacter pylori:* 250-500 mg 3 times/day or 500-875 mg twice daily; clinically effective treatment regimens include triple therapy with amoxicillin or tetracycline, metronidazole, and bismuth subsalicylate; amoxicillin, metronidazole, and an $H_2$-receptor antagonist; amoxicillin, lansoprazole, and clarithromycin.

**Dosing interval in renal impairment:**
$Cl_{cr}$ 10-50 mL/minute: Administer every 12 hours
$Cl_{cr}$ <10 mL/minute: Administer every 24 hours
Dialysis: Moderately dialyzable (20% to 50%) by hemo- or peritoneal dialysis; approximately 50 mg of amoxicillin per liter of filtrate is removed by continuous arteriovenous or venovenous hemofiltration (CAVH); dose as per $Cl_{cr}$ <10 mL/minute guidelines

**Dosage Forms Cap, as trihydrate:** 250 mg, 500 mg; **Powder for oral susp, as trihydrate:** 125 mg/5 mL (5 mL, 80 mL, 100 mL, 150 mL, 200 mL), 250 mg/5 mL (5 mL, 80 mL, 100 mL, 150 mL, 200 mL); **Powder for oral susp, drops, as trihydrate:** 50 mg/mL (15 mL, 30 mL); **Tab, chewable, as trihydrate:** 125 mg, 250 mg; **Tab, film coated:** 500 mg, 875 mg

**Contraindications** Hypersensitivity to amoxicillin, penicillin, or any component

**Warnings/Precautions** In patients with renal impairment, doses and/or frequency of administration should be modified in response to the degree of renal impairment; a high percentage of patients with infectious mononucleosis have developed rash during therapy with amoxicillin; a low incidence of cross-allergy with other beta-lactams and cephalosporins exists

**Pregnancy Risk Factor** B

**Adverse Reactions**
1% to 10%:
  Central nervous system: Fever
  Dermatologic: Urticaria, rash
  Miscellaneous: Allergic reactions (includes serum sickness, rash, angioedema, bronchospasm, hypotension, etc)
<1%: Seizures, anxiety, confusion, hallucinations, depression (with large doses or patients with renal dysfunction), nausea, vomiting, leukopenia, neutropenia, thrombocytopenia, jaundice, interstitial nephritis

**Drug Interactions**
Decreased effect: Efficacy of oral contraceptives may be reduced
Increased effect: Disulfiram, probenecid may increase amoxicillin levels
Increased toxicity: Allopurinol theoretically has an additive potential for amoxicillin rash

**Half-Life** Adults with normal renal function: 0.7-1.4 hours; Patients with $Cl_{cr}$ <10 mL/minute. 7-21 hours

**Special PA Issues**
**Patient Education:** Take entire prescription, even if you are feeling better. Take at equal intervals around-the-clock; may be taken with milk, juice, or food. You may experience nausea or vomiting (small frequent meals, frequent mouth care, or sucking on lozenges may help). If diabetic, drug may cause false tests with Clinitest® urine glucose monitoring; use of glucose oxidase methods (Clinistix®) or serum glucose monitoring is preferable. This drug may interfere with oral contraceptives; an alternate form of birth control should be used. Report rash; unusual diarrhea; vaginal itching, burning, or pain; unresolved vomiting or constipation; fever or chills; unusual bruising or bleeding; or if condition being treated worsens or does not improve by the time prescription is completed.

**Dietary Considerations:** Food: May be taken with food

**Monitoring Parameters:** With prolonged therapy, monitor renal, hepatic, and hematologic function periodically; assess patient at beginning and throughout therapy for infection; monitor for signs of anaphylaxis during first dose

## Amoxicillin and Clavulanate Potassium

(a moks i SIL in & klav yoo LAN ate poe TASS ee um)
**Pharmacologic Class** Antibiotic, Penicillin
**U.S. Brand Names** Augmentin®

**Mechanism of Action** Clavulanic acid binds and inhibits beta-lactamases that inactivate amoxicillin resulting in amoxicillin having an expanded spectrum of activity. Amoxicillin inhibits bacterial cell wall synthesis by binding to one or more of the penicillin binding proteins (PBPs); which in turn inhibits the final transpeptidation step of peptidoglycan synthesis in bacterial cell walls, thus inhibiting cell wall biosynthesis. Bacteria eventually lyse due to ongoing activity of cell wall autolytic enzymes (autolysins and murein hydrolases) while cell wall assembly is arrested.

**Use** Treatment of otitis media, sinusitis, and infections caused by susceptible organisms involving the lower respiratory tract, skin and skin structure, and urinary tract; spectrum same as amoxicillin with additional coverage of beta-lactamase producing *B. catarrhalis, H. influenzae, N. gonorrhoeae,* and *S. aureus* (not MRSA).

**USUAL DOSAGE** Oral:

Children ≤40 kg: 20-40 mg (amoxicillin)/kg/day in divided doses every 8 hours or 45 mg/kg in divided doses every 12 hours

Children >40 kg and Adults: 250-500 mg every 8 hours or 875 mg every 12 hours

**Note:** Augmentin® 200 suspension or chewable tablets 200 mg dosed every 12 hours is considered equivalent to Augmentin® "125" dosed every 8 hours; Augmentin® 400 suspension and chewable tablets may be similarly dosed every 12 hours and are equivalent to Augmentin® "250" every 8 hours

**Dosing interval in renal impairment:**

Cl$_{cr}$ 10-30 mL/minute: Administer every 12 hours

Cl$_{cr}$ <10 mL/minute: Administer every 24 hours

Hemodialysis: Moderately dialyzable (20% to 50%)

Amoxicillin/clavulanic acid: Administer dose after dialysis

Peritoneal dialysis: Moderately dialyzable (20% to 50%)

Amoxicillin: Administer 250 mg every 12 hours

Clavulanic acid: Dose for Cl$_{cr}$ <10 mL/minute

Continuous arteriovenous or venovenous hemofiltration (CAVH) effects:

Amoxicillin: ~50 mg of amoxicillin/L of filtrate is removed

Clavulanic acid: Dose for Cl$_{cr}$ <10 mL/minute

**Dosage Forms Susp, oral:** 125 (banana flavor): Amoxicillin trihydrate 125 mg and clavulanate potassium 31.25 mg per 5 mL (75 mL, 150 mL), 200: Amoxicillin 200 mg and clavulanate potassium 28.5 mg per 5 mL (50 mL, 75 mL, 100 mL), 250 (orange flavor): Amoxicillin trihydrate 250 mg and clavulanate potassium 62.5 mg per 5 mL (75 mL, 150 mL), 400: Amoxicillin 400 mg and clavulanate potassium 57 mg per 5 mL (50 mL, 75 mL, 100 mL); **Tab:** 250: Amoxicillin trihydrate 250 mg and clavulanate potassium 125 mg, 500: Amoxicillin trihydrate 500 mg and clavulanate potassium 125 mg, 875: Amoxicillin trihydrate 875 mg and clavulanate potassium 125 mg; **Tab, chewable:** 125: Amoxicillin trihydrate 125 mg and clavulanate potassium 31.25 mg, 250: Amoxicillin trihydrate 250 mg and clavulanate potassium 62.5 mg

**Contraindications** Known hypersensitivity to amoxicillin, clavulanic acid, or penicillin; concomitant use of disulfiram

**Warnings/Precautions** In patients with renal impairment, doses and/or frequency of administration should be modified in response to the degree of renal impairment; high percentage of patients with infectious mononucleosis have developed rash during therapy; a low incidence of cross-allergy with cephalosporins exists; incidence of diarrhea is higher than with amoxicillin alone. Hepatic dysfunction, although rare, is more common in elderly and/or males, and occurs more frequently with prolonged treatment.

**Pregnancy Risk Factor** B

**Adverse Reactions**

1% to 10%:

Dermatologic: Rash, urticaria

Gastrointestinal: Nausea, vomiting, diarrhea

Genitourinary: Vaginitis

<1%: Headache, abdominal discomfort, flatulence

**Drug Interactions**

Decreased effect: Efficacy of oral contraceptives may be reduced

Increased effect: Disulfiram, probenecid may increase amoxicillin levels, increased effect of anticoagulants

Increased toxicity: Allopurinol theoretically has an additive potential for amoxicillin rash

**Half-Life** Adults with normal renal function: ~1 hour for both agents; Patients with Cl$_{cr}$ <10 mL/minute: 7-21 hours

**Special PA Issues**

**Patient Education:** Take entire prescription, even if you are feeling better. Take at equal intervals around-the-clock; may be taken with milk, juice, or food. You may experience nausea or vomiting (small frequent meals, frequent mouth care, or sucking on lozenges may help). If using oral contraceptives, use additional contraceptive measures; amoxicillin may reduce effectiveness of your oral contraceptive. Report rash; unusual diarrhea; vaginal itching, burning, or pain; unresolved vomiting or constipation; fever or chills; unusual bruising or bleeding; or if condition being treated worsens or does not improve by the time prescription is completed.

**Monitoring Parameters:** Assess patient at beginning and throughout therapy for infection; with prolonged therapy, monitor renal, hepatic, and hematologic function periodically; monitor for signs of anaphylaxis during first dose

♦ **Amoxicillin and Clavulanic Acid** *see* Amoxicillin and Clavulanate Potassium *on previous page*

♦ **Amoxicillin Trihydrate** *see* Amoxicillin *on page 61*

♦ **Amoxil®** *see* Amoxicillin *on page 61*

♦ **Amoxycillin** *see* Amoxicillin *on page 61*

## Amphetamine (am FET a meen)
**Pharmacologic Class** Stimulant

**Mechanism of Action** The amphetamines are noncatechol sympathomimetic amines with pharmacologic actions similar to ephedrine. They require breakdown by monoamine oxidase for inactivation; produce central nervous system and respiratory stimulation, a pressor response, mydriasis, bronchodilation, and contraction of the urinary sphincter; thought to have a direct effect on both alpha- and beta-receptor sites in the peripheral system, as well as release stores of norepinephrine in adrenergic nerve terminals. The central nervous system action is thought to occur in the cerebral cortex and reticular activating system. The anorexigenic effect is probably secondary to the CNS-stimulating effect; the site of action is probably the hypothalamic feeding center.

**Use** Treatment of narcolepsy; exogenous obesity; abnormal behavioral syndrome in children (minimal brain dysfunction); attention deficit/hyperactivity disorder (ADHD)

**USUAL DOSAGE** Oral:
Narcolepsy:
  Children:
    6-12 years: 5 mg/day, increase by 5 mg at weekly intervals
    >12 years: 10 mg/day, increase by 10 mg at weekly intervals
  Adults: 5-60 mg/day in 2-3 divided doses
Attention deficit/hyperactivity disorder: Children:
  3-5 years: 2.5 mg/day, increase by 2.5 mg at weekly intervals
  >6 years: 5 mg/day, increase by 5 mg at weekly intervals not to exceed 40 mg/day
Short-term adjunct to exogenous obesity: Children >12 years and Adults: 10 mg or 15 mg long-acting capsule daily, up to 30 mg/day; or 5-30 mg/day in divided doses (immediate release tablets only)

**Dosage Forms Tab, as sulfate:** 5 mg, 10 mg

**Contraindications** Patients with advanced arteriosclerosis, symptomatic cardiovascular disease, moderate to severe hypertension, hyperthyroidism, glaucoma, hypersensitivity, diabetes mellitus, agitated states, patients with a history of drug abuse, and during or within 14 days following MAO inhibitor therapy. Stimulant medications are contraindicated for use in children with attention deficit/hyperactivity disorders and concomitant Tourette's syndrome or tics.

**Warnings/Precautions** Cardiovascular disease, nephritis, angina pectoris, hypertension, glaucoma, patients with a history of drug abuse, known hypersensitivity to amphetamine

**Pregnancy Risk Factor** C

**Adverse Reactions**
>10%:
  Cardiovascular: Arrhythmia
  Central nervous system: False feeling of well being, nervousness, restlessness, insomnia
1% to 10%:
  Cardiovascular: Hypertension
  Central nervous system: Mood or mental changes, dizziness, lightheadedness, headache
  Endocrine & metabolic: Changes in libido
  Gastrointestinal: Diarrhea, nausea, vomiting, stomach cramps, constipation, anorexia, weight loss, xerostomia
  Ocular: Blurred vision
  Miscellaneous: Diaphoresis (increased)
<1%: Chest pain, CNS stimulation (severe), Tourette's syndrome, hyperthermia, seizures, paranoia, rash, urticaria, tolerance and withdrawal with prolonged use

**Drug Interactions** CYP2D6 enzyme substrate
  Increased toxicity of MAO inhibitors (hyperpyrexia, hypertension, arrhythmias, seizures, cerebral hemorrhage, and death has occurred)

**Onset** 1 hour

**Duration** 4-24 hours

**Special PA Issues**
  **Patient Education:** Take during day to avoid insomnia; do not discontinue abruptly, may cause physical and psychological dependence with prolonged use
  **Reference Range:** Therapeutic: 20-30 ng/mL; Toxic: >200 ng/mL

**Related Information**
  Hallucinogenic Drugs on page 1019

♦ **Amphetamine Sulfate** see Amphetamine on this page

♦ **Amphojel® [OTC]** see Aluminum Hydroxide on page 47

## Ampicillin (am pi SIL in)
**Pharmacologic Class** Antibiotic, Penicillin

**U.S. Brand Names** Marcillin®; Omnipen®; Omnipen®-N; Polycillin®; Polycillin-N®; Principen®; Totacillin®; Totacillin®-N

**Mechanism of Action** Inhibits bacterial cell wall synthesis by binding to one or more of the penicillin binding proteins (PBPs); which in turn inhibits the final transpeptidation step of peptidoglycan synthesis in bacterial cell walls, thus inhibiting cell wall biosynthesis. Bacteria eventually lyse due to ongoing activity of cell wall autolytic enzymes (autolysins and murein hydrolases) while cell wall assembly is arrested.

**Use** Treatment of susceptible bacterial infections (nonbeta-lactamase-producing organisms); susceptible bacterial infections caused by streptococci, pneumococci, nonpenicillinase-producing staphylococci, *Listeria*, meningococci; some strains of *H. influenzae*, *Salmonella*, *Shigella*, *E. coli*, *Enterobacter*, and *Klebsiella*

## USUAL DOSAGE
Neonates: I.M., I.V.:
  Postnatal age ≤7 days:
    ≤2000 g: Meningitis: 50 mg/kg/dose every 12 hours; other infections: 25 mg/kg/dose every 12 hours
    >2000 g: Meningitis: 50 mg/kg/dose every 8 hours; other infections: 25 mg/kg/dose every 8 hours
  Postnatal age >7 days:
    <1200 g: Meningitis: 50 mg/kg/dose every 12 hours; other infections: 25 mg/kg/dose every 12 hours
    1200-2000 g: Meningitis: 50 mg/kg/dose every 8 hours; other infections: 25 mg/kg/dose every 8 hours
    >2000 g: Meningitis: 50 mg/kg/dose every 6 hours; other infections: 25 mg/kg/dose every 6 hours
Infants and Children: I.M., I.V.: 100-400 mg/kg/day in doses divided every 4-6 hours
  Meningitis: 200 mg/kg/day in doses divided every 4-6 hours; maximum dose: 12 g/day
  Children: Oral: 50-100 mg/kg/day in doses divided every 6 hours; maximum dose: 2-3 g/day
Adults:
  Oral: 250-500 mg every 6 hours
  I.M.: 500 mg to 1.5 g every 4-6 hours
  I.V.: 500 mg to 3 g every 4-6 hours; maximum dose: 12 g/day
  Sepsis/meningitis: 150-250 mg/kg/24 hours divided every 3-4 hours
**Dosing interval in renal impairment:**
  $Cl_{cr}$ 30-50 mL/minute: Administer every 6-8 hours
  $Cl_{cr}$ 10-30 mL/minute: Administer every 8-12 hours
  $Cl_{cr}$ <10 mL/minute: Administer every 12 hours
  Hemodialysis: Moderately dialyzable (20% to 50%); administer dose after dialysis
  Peritoneal dialysis: Moderately dialyzable (20% to 50%)
    Administer 250 mg every 12 hours
  Continuous arteriovenous or venovenous hemofiltration (CAVH) effects: Dose as for $Cl_{cr}$ 10-50 mL/minute; ~50 mg of ampicillin per liter of filtrate is removed

**Dosage Forms Ampicillin anhydrous: Cap:** 250 mg, 500 mg; **Ampicillin sodium: Powder for inj:** 125 mg, 250 mg, 500 mg, 1 g, 2 g, 10 g; **Ampicillin trihydrate: Cap:** 250 mg, 500 mg; **Powder for oral susp:** 125 mg/5 mL (5 mL unit dose, 80 mL, 100 mL, 150 mL, 200 mL), 250 mg/5 mL (5 mL unit dose, 80 mL, 100 mL, 150 mL, 200 mL), 500 mg/5 mL (5 mL unit dose, 100 mL)
  Powder for oral susp, drops: 100 mg/mL (20 mL)

**Contraindications** Known hypersensitivity to ampicillin or other penicillins

**Warnings/Precautions** Dosage adjustment may be necessary in patients with renal impairment; a low incidence of cross-allergy with other beta-lactams exists; high percentage of patients with infectious mononucleosis have developed rash during therapy with ampicillin. Appearance of a rash should be carefully evaluated to differentiate a nonallergic ampicillin rash from a hypersensitivity reaction. Ampicillin rash occurs in 5% to 10% of children receiving ampicillin and is a generalized dull red, maculopapular rash, generally appearing 3-14 days after the start of therapy. It normally begins on the trunk and spreads over most of the body. It may be most intense at pressure areas, elbows, and knees.

**Pregnancy Risk Factor** B

**Adverse Reactions**
>10%: Local: Pain at injection site
1% to 10%:
  Dermatologic: Rash (appearance of a rash should be carefully evaluated to differentiate, if possible; nonallergic ampicillin rash from hypersensitivity reaction; incidence is higher in patients with viral infections, *Salmonella* infections, lymphocytic leukemia, or patients that have hyperuricemia)
  Gastrointestinal: Diarrhea, vomiting, oral candidiasis, abdominal cramps
  Miscellaneous: Allergic reaction (includes serum sickness, urticaria, angioedema, bronchospasm, hypotension, etc)
<1%: Penicillin encephalopathy, seizures (with large I.V. doses or patients with renal dysfunction), anemia, hemolytic anemia, thrombocytopenia, thrombocytopenic purpura, eosinophilia, leukopenia, granulocytopenia, decreased lymphocytes, interstitial nephritis (rare)

**Drug Interactions**
Decreased effect: Efficacy of oral contraceptives may be reduced
Increased effect: Disulfiram, probenecid may increase penicillin levels, increased effect of anticoagulants
Increased toxicity: Allopurinol theoretically has an additive potential for amoxicillin (ampicillin) rash
(Continued)

## Ampicillin *(Continued)*

**Half-Life** 1-1.8 hours; Anuria/end-stage renal disease: 7-20 hours
**Special PA Issues**
  **Patient Education:** Take entire prescription, even if you are feeling better. Take at equal intervals around-the-clock; preferably on an empty stomach with a full glass of water (1 hour before or 2 hours after meals). Maintain adequate hydration (2-3 L/day of fluids unless instructed to restrict fluid intake). You may experience nausea or vomiting (small frequent meals, frequent mouth care, or sucking on lozenges may help). If diabetic, drug may cause false tests with Clinitest® urine glucose monitoring; use of glucose oxidase methods (Clinistix®) or serum glucose monitoring is preferable. This drug may interfere with oral contraceptives; an alternate form of birth control should be used. Report rash; unusual diarrhea; unusual vaginal discharge, itching, burning, or pain; mouth sores; unresolved vomiting or constipation; fever or chills; unusual bruising or bleeding; or if condition being treated worsens or does not improve by the time prescription is completed.
  **Dietary Considerations:** Food: Decreases drug absorption rate; decreases drug serum concentration. Take on an empty stomach 1 hour before or 2 hours after meals.
  **Monitoring Parameters:** With prolonged therapy monitor renal, hepatic, and hematologic function periodically; observe signs and symptoms of anaphylaxis during first dose

## Ampicillin and Sulbactam *(am pi SIL in & SUL bak tam)*

**Pharmacologic Class** Antibiotic, Penicillin
**U.S. Brand Names** Unasyn®
**Mechanism of Action** The addition of sulbactam, a beta-lactamase inhibitor, to ampicillin extends the spectrum of ampicillin to include some beta-lactamase producing organisms; inhibits bacterial cell wall synthesis by binding to one or more of the penicillin binding proteins (PBPs); which in turn inhibits the final transpeptidation step of peptidoglycan synthesis in bacterial cell walls, thus inhibiting cell wall biosynthesis. Bacteria eventually lyse due to ongoing activity of cell wall autolytic enzymes (autolysins and murein hydrolases) while cell wall assembly is arrested.
**Use** Treatment of susceptible bacterial infections involved with skin and skin structure, intra-abdominal infections, gynecological infections; spectrum is that of ampicillin plus organisms producing beta-lactamases such as *S. aureus, H. influenzae, E. coli,* and anaerobes
**USUAL DOSAGE** Unasyn® (ampicillin/sulbactam) is a combination product. Each 3 g vial contains 2 g of ampicillin and 1 g of sulbactam. Sulbactam has very little antibacterial activity by itself, but effectively extends the spectrum of ampicillin to include beta-lactamase producing strains that are resistant to ampicillin alone. Therefore, dosage recommendations for Unasyn® are based on the ampicillin component.

  I.M., I.V.:
    Children (3 months to 12 years): 100-200 mg ampicillin/kg/day (150-300 mg Unasyn®) divided every 6 hours; maximum dose: 8 g ampicillin/day (12 g Unasyn®)
    Adults: 1-2 g ampicillin (1.5-3 g Unasyn®) every 6-8 hours; maximum dose: 8 g ampicillin/day (12 g Unasyn®)
  **Dosing interval in renal impairment:**
    Cl_cr 15-29 mL/minute: Administer every 12 hours
    Cl_cr 5-14 mL/minute: Administer every 24 hours
**Dosage Forms Powder for inj:** 1.5 g [ampicillin sodium 1 g and sulbactam sodium 0.5 g], 3 g [ampicillin sodium 2 g and sulbactam sodium 1 g]
**Contraindications** Hypersensitivity to ampicillin, sulbactam or any component, or penicillins
**Warnings/Precautions** Dosage adjustment may be necessary in patients with renal impairment; a low incidence of cross-allergy with other beta-lactams exists; high percentage of patients with infectious mononucleosis have developed rash during therapy with ampicillin. Appearance of a rash should be carefully evaluated to differentiate a nonallergic ampicillin rash from a hypersensitivity reaction. Ampicillin rash occurs in 5% to 10% of children receiving ampicillin and is a generalized dull red, maculopapular rash, generally appearing 3-14 days after the start of therapy. It normally begins on the trunk and spreads over most of the body. It may be most intense at pressure areas, elbows, and knees.
**Pregnancy Risk Factor** B
**Adverse Reactions**
  >10%: Local: Pain at injection site (I.M.)
  1% to 10%:
    Dermatologic: Rash
    Gastrointestinal: Diarrhea
    Local: Pain at injection site (I.V.)
    Miscellaneous: Allergic reaction (may include serum sickness, urticaria, bronchospasm, hypotension, etc)
  <1%: Chest pain, fatigue, malaise, headache, chills, penicillin encephalopathy, seizures (with large I.V. doses or patients with renal dysfunction), itching, nausea, vomiting, enterocolitis, pseudomembranous colitis, hairy tongue, dysuria, vaginitis, leukopenia, neutropenia, thrombocytopenia, decreased hemoglobin and hematocrit, increased liver enzymes, thrombophlebitis, increased BUN/creatinine, interstitial nephritis (rare)

**Drug Interactions**
Decreased effect: Efficacy of oral contraceptives may be reduced
Increased effect: Disulfiram, probenecid results in increased ampicillin levels
Increased toxicity: Allopurinol theoretically has an additive potential for ampicillin rash

**Half-Life** 1-1.8 hours

**Special PA Issues**
**Patient Education:** Take entire prescription, even if you are feeling better. Take at equal intervals around-the-clock; preferably on an empty stomach with a full glass of water (1 hour before or 2 hours after meals). Maintain adequate hydration (2-3 L/day of fluids unless instructed to restrict fluid intake). You may experience nausea or vomiting (small frequent meals, frequent mouth care, or sucking on lozenges may help). If diabetic, drug may cause false tests with Clinitest® urine glucose monitoring; use of glucose oxidase methods (Clinistix®) or serum glucose monitoring is preferable. This drug may interfere with oral contraceptives; an alternate form of birth control should be used. Report rash; unusual diarrhea; vaginal discharge, itching, burning, or pain; mouth sores; unresolved vomiting or constipation; fever or chills; unusual bruising or bleeding; or if condition being treated worsens or does not improve by the time prescription is completed.
**Monitoring Parameters:** With prolonged therapy, monitor hematologic, renal, and hepatic function; monitor for signs of anaphylaxis during first dose

♦ **Ampicillin Sodium** *see* Ampicillin *on page 64*
♦ **Ampicillin Trihydrate** *see* Ampicillin *on page 64*
♦ **Ampicin® Sodium** *see* Ampicillin *on page 64*

# Amprenavir (am PRE na veer)

**Pharmacologic Class** Antiretroviral Agent, Reverse Transcriptase Inhibitor (Non-Nucleoside); Protease Inhibitor

**U.S. Brand Names** Agenerase®

**Mechanism of Action** Binds to the protease activity site and inhibits the activity of the enzyme. HIV protease is required for the cleavage of viral polyprotein precursors into individual functional proteins found in infectious HIV. Inhibition prevents cleavage of these polyproteins, resulting in the formation of immature, noninfectious viral particles.

**Use** Treatment of HIV infections in combination with at least two other antiretroviral agents

**USUAL DOSAGE** Oral:
Capsules:
Children 4-12 years and older (<50 kg): 20 mg/kg twice daily or 15 mg/kg 3 times daily; maximum: 2400 mg/day
Children >13 years (>50 kg) and Adults: 1200 mg twice daily
Solution: Children 4-12 years or older (up to 18 years weighing <50 kg): 22 mg/kg twice daily or 17 mg/kg 3 times daily; maximum: 2400/day
**Dosage adjustment in hepatic impairment:**
Child-Pugh score between 5-8: 450 mg twice daily
Child-Pugh score between 9-12: 300 mg twice daily

**Dosage Forms Cap:** 50 mg, 150 mg, **Soln:** 15 mg/mL

**Contraindications** Hypersensitivity to amprenavir or any component; concurrent therapy with rifampin, astemizole, bepridil, cisapride, dihydroergotamine, ergotamine, midazolam, and triazolam; severe previous allergic reaction to sulfonamides

**Warnings/Precautions** Because of hepatic metabolism and effect on cytochrome P-450 enzymes, amprenavir should be used with caution in combination with other agents metabolized by this system (see Contraindications and Drug Interactions). Use with caution in patients with diabetes mellitus, sulfonamide allergy, hepatic impairment, or hemophilia. Redistribution of fat may occur (eg, buffalo hump, peripheral wasting, cushingoid appearance). Additional vitamin E supplements should be avoided. Concurrent use of sildenafil should be avoided.

**Pregnancy Risk Factor** Unknown

**Adverse Reactions** Protease inhibitors cause dyslipidemia which includes elevated cholesterol and triglycerides and a redistribution of body fat centrally to cause "protease paunch", buffalo hump, facial atrophy, and breast enlargement. These agents also cause hyperglycemia.
>10%:
Gastrointestinal: Nausea (38% to 73%), vomiting (20% to 29%), diarrhea (33% to 56%)
Dermatologic: Rash (28%)
Endocrine & metabolic: Hyperglycemia (37% to 41%), hypertriglyceridemia (38% to 27%)
Miscellaneous: Perioral tingling/numbness
1% to 10%:
Central nervous system: Depression (4% to 15%), headache, paresthesia, fatigue
Gastrointestinal: Taste disorders (1% to 10%)
Dermatologic: Stevens-Johnson syndrome (1% of total, 4% of patients who develop a rash)

**Drug Interactions** CYP3A4 inhibitor and substrate
Increased effect/toxicity: Abacavir, clarithromycin, indinavir, ketoconazole, and zidovudine increase the AUC of amprenavir. Nelfinavir had no effect on AUC, but increased the $C_{min}$
(Continued)

## Amprenavir *(Continued)*

of amprenavir. Amprenavir increased the AUC of ketoconazole, rifabutin, and zidovudine during concurrent therapy. Amprenavir may enhance the toxicity of astemizole, bepridil, cisapride, dihydroergotamine, ergotamine, midazolam, and triazolam - concurrent therapy with these drugs and amprenavir is contraindicated. May increase serum concentration of HMGCoA reductase inhibitors, diltiazem, nicardipine, nifedipine, nimodipine, alprazolam, clorazepate, diazepam, flurazepam, itraconazole, dapsone, erythromycin, loratadine, sildenafil, carbamazepine, and pimozide. May also increase the toxic effect of amiodarone, lidocaine, quinidine, warfarin, and tricyclic antidepressants. Serum concentration monitoring of these drugs is necessary.

**Additional Information** Capsules contain 109 Int. units of vitamin E per capsule; oral solution contains 46 Int. units of vitamin E per mL

**Special PA Issues**
**Patient Education:** Advise prescriber of any previous reactions to sulfonamides. Do not take this medication with antacids or high-fat meals. Do not take additional vitamin E supplements. Consult pharmacist or physician prior to taking any other medications, due to the potential for drug interactions. For women using oral contraceptives, an alternative method of contraception should be used.

## Amrinone *(AM ri none)*

**Pharmacologic Class** Phosphodiesterase Enzyme Inhibitor
**U.S. Brand Names** Inocor®
**Use** Congestive heart failure; adjunctive therapy of pulmonary hypertension; normally prescribed for patients who have not responded well to therapy with digitalis, diuretics, and vasodilators
**USUAL DOSAGE** Dosage is based on clinical response **(Note: Dose should not exceed 10 mg/kg/24 hours)**

Children and Adults: 0.75 mg/kg I.V. bolus over 2-3 minutes followed by maintenance infusion of 5-10 mcg/kg/minute; I.V. bolus may need to be repeated in 30 minutes
**Dosing adjustment in renal failure:** $Cl_{cr}$ <10 mL/minute: Administer 50% to 75% of dose
**Dosage Forms Inj, as lactate:** 5 mg/mL (20 mL)
**Contraindications** Hypersensitivity to amrinone lactate or sulfites (contains sodium metabisulfite)
**Pregnancy Risk Factor** C
**Pregnancy Implications** Excretion in breast milk unknown
**Onset** I.V.: Within 2-5 minutes
**Duration** Dose dependent (~30 minutes low dose, ~2 hours higher doses)
**Half-Life** Adults, normal: 3.6 hours; Adults with CHF: 5.8 hours
**Special PA Issues**
**Patient Education:** When used in emergency situations, patient instruction should be appropriate to situation. This medication can only be administered I.V. You will be monitored closely during infusion. Make any position changes slowly; ask for assistance and report any chest pain, palpitations, nausea, acute abdominal pain, or pain at infusion site.

♦ **Amrinone Lactate** *see* Amrinone *on this page*
♦ **Amvisc®** *see* Sodium Hyaluronate *on page 841*
♦ **Amvisc® Plus** *see* Sodium Hyaluronate *on page 841*
♦ **Anabolin® Injection** *see* Nandrolone *on page 634*
♦ **Anacin® [OTC]** *see* Aspirin *on page 80*
♦ **Anadrol®** *see* Oxymetholone *on page 688*
♦ **Anafranil®** *see* Clomipramine *on page 223*

## Anagrelide *(an AG gre lide)*

**Pharmacologic Class** Platelet Aggregation Inhibitor
**U.S. Brand Names** Agrylin®
**Mechanism of Action** Anagrelide appears to inhibit cyclic nucleotide phosphodiesterase and the release of arachidonic acid from phospholipase, possibly by inhibiting phospholipase A2. It also causes a dose-related reduction in platelet production, which results from decreased megakaryocyte hypermaturation. The drug disrupts the postmitotic phase of maturation.
**Use** Agent for essential thrombocythemia (ET); treatment of thrombocytopenia secondary to myeloproliferative disorders
**USUAL DOSAGE** Adults: Oral: 0.5 mg 4 times/day or 1 mg twice daily
Maintain for ≥1 week, then adjust to the lowest effective dose to reduce and maintain platelet count <600,000 µL ideally to the normal range; the dose must not be increased by >0.5 mg/day in any 1 week; maximum dose: 10 mg/day or 2.5 mg/dose
**Dosage Forms Cap, as hydrochloride:** 0.5 mg, 1 mg
**Contraindications** Hypersensitivity to anagrelide
**Warnings/Precautions** Use caution in patients with known or suspected heart disease, and only if the potential benefits of therapy outweigh the potential risks. Thrombocytopenia

appears to be the main dose-limiting side effect of anagrelide; palpitations, orthostatic hypotension, and headache have also been reported. Caution is warranted when anagrelide is used in patients with reduced renal function or hepatic dysfunction.

**Pregnancy Risk Factor** C

**Pregnancy Implications** Clinical effects on the fetus: The relative risks must be weighed carefully in relation to the potential benefits. Animal reproduction studies have shown an adverse effect on the fetus when anagrelide was administered during pregnancy. There are no adequate and well-controlled studies in humans; however, the potential benefits may warrant the use of this drug in pregnant women despite the potential risks.

**Adverse Reactions**

Cardiovascular: Palpitations (27.2%), chest pain (7.8%), tachycardia (7.3%), orthostatic hypotension, CHF, cardiomyopathy, myocardial infarction (rare), complete heart block, angina, and atrial fibrillation

Central nervous system: Headache (44%), dizziness (14.7%), bad dreams, impaired concentration ability

Hematologic: Anemia, thrombocytopenia, ecchymosis and lymphadenopathy have been reported rarely

**Drug Interactions** There is a single case report that suggests sucralfate may interfere with anagrelide absorption

**Duration** 6-24 hours

**Half-Life** 1.3 hours

**Special PA Issues**

**Patient Education:** Before using this drug, tell your physician your entire medical history, including any allergies (especially drug allergies), heart, kidney, or liver disease. Limit alcohol intake, as it may aggravate side effects. To avoid dizziness and lightheadedness when rising from a seated or lying position, get up slowly. This medication should be used only when clearly needed during pregnancy. Discuss the risks and benefits with your physician. It is not known whether this drug is excreted into breast milk. It is recommended to discontinue the drug or not to breast-feed, taking into account the risk to the infant. Tell your physician and pharmacist of all nonprescription and prescription medications you may use, especially sucralfate. Do not share this medication with others. Laboratory tests will be done to monitor the effectiveness and possible side effects of this drug.

**Dietary Considerations:** Food: No clinically significant effect on absorption

**Monitoring Parameters:** Anagrelide therapy requires close supervision of the patient. Because of the positive inotropic effects and side effects of anagrelide, a pretreatment cardiovascular examination is recommended along with careful monitoring during treatment; while the platelet count is being lowered (usually during the first 2 weeks of treatment), blood counts (hemoglobin, white blood cells), liver function test (AST, ALT) and renal function (serum creatinine, BUN) should be monitored.

**Reference Range:** Thrombocythemia: 60-300 ng/mL

♦ **Anagrelide Hydrochloride** see Anagrelide on previous page

♦ **Anandron®** see Nilutamide on page 656

♦ **Anapolon®** see Oxymetholone on page 688

♦ **Anaprox®** see Naproxen on page 636

♦ **Anaspaz®** see Hyoscyamine on page 463

# Anastrozole (an AS troe zole)

**Pharmacologic Class** Antineoplastic Agent, Miscellaneous

**U.S. Brand Names** Arimidex®

**Mechanism of Action** Potent and selective nonsteroidal aromatase inhibitor. It significantly lowers serum estradiol concentrations and has no detectable effect on formation of adrenal corticosteroids or aldosterone. In postmenopausal women, the principal source of circulating estrogen is conversion of adrenally generated androstenedione to estrone by aromatase in peripheral tissues.

**Use** Treatment of advanced breast cancer in postmenopausal women with disease progression following tamoxifen therapy. Patients with ER-negative disease and patients who did not respond to tamoxifen therapy rarely responded to anastrozole.

**USUAL DOSAGE** Breast cancer: Adults: Oral (refer to individual protocols): 1 mg once daily

**Dosage adjustment in renal impairment:** Because only about 10% is excreted unchanged in the urine, dosage adjustment in patients with renal insufficiency is not necessary

**Dosage adjustment in hepatic impairment:** Plasma concentrations in subjects with hepatic cirrhosis were within the range concentrations in normal subjects across all clinical trials; therefore, no dosage adjustment is needed

**Dosage Forms Tab:** 1 mg

**Contraindications** Hypersensitivity to any component

**Warnings/Precautions** Use with caution in patients with hyperlipidemias; mean serum total cholesterol and LDL cholesterol occurs in patients receiving anastrozole

**Pregnancy Risk Factor** C

(Continued)

## Anastrozole *(Continued)*

**Pregnancy Implications** Clinical effects on the fetus: Anastrozole can cause fetal harm when administered to a pregnant woman

**Adverse Reactions**
>5%:
  Cardiovascular: Flushing
  Gastrointestinal: Little to mild nausea (10%), vomiting
  Neuromuscular & skeletal: Increased bone and tumor pain
2% to 5%:
  Cardiovascular: Hypertension
  Central nervous system: Somnolence, confusion, insomnia, anxiety, nervousness, fever, malaise, accidental injury
  Dermatologic: Hair thinning, pruritus
  Endocrine & metabolic: Breast pain
  Gastrointestinal: Weight loss
  Genitourinary: Urinary tract infection
  Local: Thrombophlebitis
  Neuromuscular & skeletal: Myalgia, arthralgia, pathological fracture, neck pain
  Respiratory: Sinusitis, bronchitis, rhinitis
  Miscellaneous: Flu-like syndrome, infection

**Drug Interactions** CYP3A3/4 enzyme substrate; CYP1A2, 2C8, 2C9, and 3A3/4 enzyme inhibitor

Anastrozole inhibited *in vitro* metabolic reactions catalyzed by cytochromes P-450 1A2, 2C8/9, and 3A4, but only at relatively high concentrations. It is unlikely that coadministration of anastrozole with other drugs will result in clinically significant inhibition of cytochrome P-450-mediated metabolism of other drugs.

**Half-Life** 50 hours

**Special PA Issues**
  **Patient Education:** Take as prescribed. Maintain adequate hydration (2-3 L/day of fluids unless instructed to restrict fluid intake) and nutrition. If experiencing nausea, vomiting, or anorexia, small frequent meals, frequent mouth care, or sucking on lozenges may help or contact prescriber for relief. This medication may cause dizziness and fatigue (use caution when driving or engaging in tasks that require alertness); or increased bone pain (contact prescriber for analgesia). Report swelling of extremities, chest pain or palpitations, acute headache or dizziness, increased muscle pain or weakness, CNS changes (eg, confusion, insomnia, nervousness), breast or pelvic pain, unusual bruising or bleeding, flu-like symptoms, or respiratory difficulty.

♦ **Anbesol® [OTC]** *see* Benzocaine *on page 105*

♦ **Anbesol® Maximum Strength [OTC]** *see* Benzocaine *on page 105*

♦ **Ancef®** *see* Cefazolin *on page 161*

♦ **Ancobon®** *see* Flucytosine *on page 376*

♦ **Ancotil®** *see* Flucytosine *on page 376*

♦ **Androderm® Transdermal System** *see* Testosterone *on page 881*

♦ **Andro/Fem® Injection** *see* Estradiol and Testosterone *on page 334*

♦ **Android®** *see* Methyltestosterone *on page 595*

♦ **Andro-L.A.® Injection** *see* Testosterone *on page 881*

♦ **Androlone®-D Injection** *see* Nandrolone *on page 634*

♦ **Androlone® Injection** *see* Nandrolone *on page 634*

♦ **Andropository® Injection** *see* Testosterone *on page 881*

♦ **Anergan®** *see* Promethazine *on page 768*

♦ **Anestacon®** *see* Lidocaine *on page 531*

♦ **Aneurine Hydrochloride** *see* Thiamine *on page 894*

♦ **Anexate®** *see* Flumazenil *on page 378*

♦ **Anexsia®** *see* Hydrocodone and Acetaminophen *on page 449*

♦ **Animal and Human Bites** *see* Chart *on page 1118*

## Anisotropine *(an iss oh TROE peen)*

**Pharmacologic Class** Anticholinergic Agent

**U.S. Brand Names** Valpin® 50

**Mechanism of Action** Blocks the action of acetylcholine at parasympathetic sites in smooth muscle, secretory glands, and the CNS; increases cardiac output, dries secretions, antagonizes histamine and serotonin

**Use** Adjunctive treatment of peptic ulcer

**USUAL DOSAGE** Adults: Oral: 50 mg 3 times/day

**Dosage Forms** Tab, as methylbromide: 50 mg

**Contraindications** Narrow-angle glaucoma, obstructive GI tract or uropathy, severe ulcerative colitis, myasthenia gravis, intestinal atony, hepatic disease, hypersensitivity

**Warnings/Precautions** Drug-induced heatstroke can develop in hot or humid climates

**Pregnancy Risk Factor** C
**Adverse Reactions**
>10%:
Cardiovascular: Palpitations
Dermatologic: Dry skin
Gastrointestinal: Constipation, dry throat, xerostomia
Respiratory: Dry nose
Miscellaneous: Diaphoresis (decreased)
1% to 10%:
Endocrine & metabolic: Decreased flow of breast milk
Gastrointestinal: Decreased salivary secretion
<1%: Orthostatic hypotension, confusion, drowsiness, headache, loss of memory, fatigue, rash, bloated feeling, nausea, vomiting, decreased urination, weakness, increased intra-ocular pain, blurred vision, increased sensitivity to light
**Special PA Issues**
**Patient Education:** Dry mouth can be relieved by sugarless gum or hard candy; drink plenty of fluids
**Monitoring Parameters:** Monitor patient's vital signs and I & O

♦ **Anisotropine Methylbromide** *see* Anisotropine *on previous page*
♦ **Anisoylated Plasminogen Streptokinase Activator Complex** *see* Anistreplase *on this page*

# Anistreplase (a NISS tre plase)
**Pharmacologic Class** Thrombolytic Agent
**U.S. Brand Names** Eminase®
**Mechanism of Action** Activates the conversion of plasminogen to plasmin by forming a complex exposing plasminogen-activating site and cleavage of a peptide bond that converts plasminogen to plasmin; plasmin being capable of thrombolysis, by degrading fibrin, fibrinogen and other procoagulant proteins into soluble fragments, effective both outside and within the formed thrombus/embolus
**Use** Management of acute myocardial infarction (AMI) in adults; lysis of thrombi obstructing coronary arteries, reduction of infarct size; and reduction of mortality associated with AMI
**USUAL DOSAGE** Adults: I.V.: 30 units injected over 2-5 minutes as soon as possible after onset of symptoms
**Dosage Forms** Powder for inj, lyophilized: 30 units
**Contraindications** Active internal bleeding, history of CVA, intracranial neoplasma, known hypersensitivity to anistreplase or other kinases (streptokinase); history of cerebrovascular accident; recent intracranial surgery or trauma; arteriovenous malformation or aneurysm; severe uncontrolled hypertension
**Pregnancy Risk Factor** C
**Pregnancy Implications** Excretion in breast milk unknown
**Adverse Reactions**
>10%:
Cardiovascular: Arrhythmias, hypotension, perfusion arrhythmias
Hematologic: Bleeding or oozing from cuts
1% to 10%: Miscellaneous: Anaphylactic reaction
<1%: Headache, chills, rash, nausea, vomiting, anemia, eye hemorrhage, bronchospasm, epistaxis, diaphoresis
**Drug Interactions** Increased efficacy and bleeding potential: Anticoagulants (heparin, warfarin), antiplatelet agents (aspirin)
**Duration** Fibrinolytic effect persists for 4-6 hours following administration.
**Half-Life** 70-120 minutes
**Special PA Issues**
**Patient Education:** I.V. administration for cardiac emergencies: Patient instruction should be appropriate to situation. Following infusion, absolute bedrest is important; call for assistance changing position. You will have increased tendency to bleed; avoid razors, scissors or sharps, and use soft toothbrush or cotton swabs. Report back pain, abdominal pain, muscle cramping, acute onset headache, or chest pain.

♦ **Anodynos-DHC®** *see* Hydrocodone and Acetaminophen *on page 449*
♦ **Anoquan®** *see* Butalbital Compound *on page 131*
♦ **Ansaid® Oral** *see* Flurbiprofen *on page 391*
♦ **Ansamycin** *see* Rifabutin *on page 803*
♦ **Antabuse®** *see* Disulfiram *on page 297*
♦ **Antazone®** *see* Sulfinpyrazone *on page 863*
♦ **Anthra-Derm®** *see* Anthralin *on next page*
♦ **Anthraforte®** *see* Anthralin *on next page*

## Anthralin (AN thra lin)

**Pharmacologic Class** Antipsoriatic Agent; Keratolytic Agent

**U.S. Brand Names** Anthra-Derm®; Drithocreme®; Drithocreme® HP 1%; Dritho-Scalp®; Micanol® Cream

**Mechanism of Action** Reduction of the mitotic rate and proliferation of epidermal cells in psoriasis by inhibiting synthesis of nucleic protein from inhibition of DNA synthesis to affected areas

**Use** Treatment of psoriasis (quiescent or chronic psoriasis)

**USUAL DOSAGE Adults: Topical:** Generally, apply once a day or as directed. The irritant potential of anthralin is directly related to the strength being used and each patient's individual tolerance. Always commence treatment for at least one week using the lowest strength possible.

Skin application: Apply sparingly only to psoriatic lesions and rub gently and carefully into the skin until absorbed. Avoid applying an excessive quantity which may cause unnecessary soiling and staining of the clothing or bed linen.

Scalp application: Comb hair to remove scalar debris and, after suitably parting, rub cream well into the lesions, taking care to prevent the cream from spreading onto the forehead

Remove by washing or showering; optimal period of contact will vary according to the strength used and the patient's response to treatment. Continue treatment until the skin is entirely clear (ie, when there is nothing to feel with the fingers and the texture is normal)

**Dosage Forms Crm:** 0.1% (50 g, 65 g), 0.2% (65 g), 0.25% (50 g), 0.4% (65 g), 0.5% (50 g), 1% (50 g, 65 g); **Oint, top:** 0.1% (42.5 g), 0.25% (42.5 g), 0.4% (60 g), 0.5% (42.5 g), 1% (42.5 g)

**Contraindications** Hypersensitivity to anthralin or any component, acute psoriasis (acutely or actively inflamed psoriatic eruptions); use on the face

**Warnings/Precautions** If redness is observed, reduce frequency of dosage or discontinue application; avoid eye contact; should generally not be applied to intertriginous skin areas and high strengths should not be used on these sites; do not apply to face or genitalia; use caution in patients with renal disease and in those having extensive and prolonged applications; perform periodic urine tests for albuminuria.

**Pregnancy Risk Factor** C

**Adverse Reactions**

1% to 10%: Dermatologic: Transient primary irritation of uninvolved skin; temporary discoloration of hair and fingernails, may stain skin, hair, or fabrics

<1%: Rash, excessive irritation

**Drug Interactions** Increased toxicity: Long-term use of topical corticosteroids may destabilize psoriasis, and withdrawal may also give rise to a "rebound" phenomenon, allow an interval of at least 1 week between the discontinuance of topical corticosteroids and the commencement of therapy

**Special PA Issues**

**Patient Education:** For external use only. Use exactly as directed; do not overuse. Before using, wash and dry area gently. Wear gloves to apply a thin film to affected area and rub in gently. May discolor fabric, skin, or hair. If dressing is necessary, use a porous dressing. Avoid contact with eyes. Avoid exposing treated area to direct sunlight; sunburn can occur. Remove by washing; optimal period of contact will vary according to strength used and response to treatment. Report increased swelling, redness, rash, itching, signs of infection, worsening of condition, or lack of healing.

Scalp: Comb hair to remove scalar debris, part hair, and rub cream into lesions. Do not allow cream to spread to forehead or onto neck. Remove by washing hair.

## Antipyrine and Benzocaine (an tee PYE reen & BEN zoe kane)
**Pharmacologic Class** Otic Agent, Analgesic; Otic Agent, Cerumenolytic
**U.S. Brand Names** Allergan® Ear Drops; Auralgan®; Auroto®; Otocalm® Ear
**Dosage Forms Soln, otic:** Antipyrine 5.4% and benzocaine 1.4% (10 mL, 15 mL)

## Antirabies Serum (Equine) (an tee RAY beez SEER um EE kwine)
**Pharmacologic Class** Serum
**Mechanism of Action** Affords passive immunity against rabies
**Use** Rabies prophylaxis
**USUAL DOSAGE** 1000 units/55 lb in a single dose, infiltrate up to 50% of dose around the wound
**Dosage Forms Inj:** 125 units/mL (8 mL)
**Pregnancy Risk Factor** C
**Adverse Reactions** 1% to 10%:
  Central nervous system: Pain (local)
  Dermatologic: Urticaria
  Miscellaneous: Serum sickness

♦ **Antispas® Injection** see Dicyclomine on page 273
♦ **Antithymocyte Globulin (Equine)** see Lymphocyte Immune Globulin on page 550

## Antithymocyte Globulin (Rabbit) (ant i THYM o site GLOB yoo lin)
**Pharmacologic Class** Immunosuppressant Agent
**U.S. Brand Names** Thymoglobulin®
**Mechanism of Action** May involve elimination of antigen-reactive T-lymphocytes (killer cells) in peripheral blood or alteration of T-cell function
**Use** Treatment of renal transplant acute rejection in conjunction with concomitant immunosuppression
**USUAL DOSAGE** I.V.: 1.5 mg/kg/day for 7-14 days
**Dosage Forms Inj:** 25 mg vials (with diluent)
**Contraindications** Patients with history of allergy or anaphylaxis to rabbit proteins, or who have an acute viral illness
**Warnings/Precautions** Infusion may produce fever and chills. To minimize, the first dose should be infused over a minimum of 6 hours into a high-flow vein. Also, premedication with corticosteroids, acetaminophen, and/or an antihistamine and/or slowing the infusion rate may reduce reaction incidence and intensity.

Prolonged use or overdosage of Thymoglobulin® in association with other immunosuppressive agents may cause over-immunosuppression resulting in severe infections and may increase the incidence of lymphoma or post-transplant lymphoproliferative disease (PTLD) or other malignancies. Appropriate antiviral, antibacterial, antiprotozoal, and/or antifungal prophylaxis is recommended.

Thymoglobulin® should only be used by physicians experienced in immunosuppressive therapy for the treatment of renal transplant patients. Medical surveillance is required during the infusion. In rare circumstances, anaphylaxis has been reported with use. In such cases, the infusion should be terminated immediately. Medical personnel should be available to treat patients who experience anaphylaxis. Emergency treatment such as 0.3-0.5 mL aqueous epinephrine (1:1000 dilution) subcutaneously and other resuscitative measures including oxygen, intravenous fluids, antihistamines, corticosteroids, pressor amines, and airway management, as clinically indicated, should be provided. Thymoglobulin® or other rabbit immunoglobulins should not be administered again for such patients. Thrombocytopenia or neutropenia may result from cross-reactive antibodies and is reversible following dose adjustments.
**Pregnancy Risk Factor** C
**Adverse Reactions**
  >10%:
    Central nervous system: Fever, chills, headache
    Dermatologic: Rash
    Endocrine & metabolic: Hyperkalemia
    Gastrointestinal: Abdominal pain, diarrhea
    Hematologic: Leukopenia, thrombocytopenia
    Neuromuscular & skeletal: Weakness
    Respiratory: Dyspnea
    Miscellaneous: Systemic infection, pain
  1% to 10%:
    Gastrointestinal: Gastritis
    Respiratory: Pneumonia
    Miscellaneous: Sensitivity reactions: Anaphylaxis may be indicated by hypotension, respiratory distress, serum sickness, viral infection
**Special PA Issues**
  **Monitoring Parameters:** Lymphocyte profile, CBC with differential and platelet count, vital signs during administration

- **Antithymocyte Immunoglobulin** *see* Lymphocyte Immune Globulin *on page 550*
- **Antithymocyte Immunoglobulin** *see* Antithymocyte Globulin (Rabbit) *on previous page*
- **Anti-Tuss® Expectorant [OTC]** *see* Guaifenesin *on page 427*
- **Antivert®** *see* Meclizine *on page 559*
- **Antrizine®** *see* Meclizine *on page 559*
- **Anturan®** *see* Sulfinpyrazone *on page 863*
- **Anturane®** *see* Sulfinpyrazone *on page 863*
- **Anucort-HC® Suppository** *see* Hydrocortisone *on page 453*
- **Anuprep HC® Suppository** *see* Hydrocortisone *on page 453*
- **Anusol® HC-1 [OTC]** *see* Hydrocortisone *on page 453*
- **Anusol® HC-2.5% [OTC]** *see* Hydrocortisone *on page 453*
- **Anusol-HC® Suppository** *see* Hydrocortisone *on page 453*
- **Anxanil®** *see* Hydroxyzine *on page 462*
- **Anzemet®** *see* Dolasetron *on page 299*
- **Apacet® [OTC]** *see* Acetaminophen *on page 21*
- **APAP** *see* Acetaminophen *on page 21*
- **Aphthasol™** *see* Amlexanox *on page 59*
- **A.P.L.®** *see* Chorionic Gonadotropin *on page 205*
- **Aplisol®** *see* Tuberculin Tests *on page 945*
- **Aplitest®** *see* Tuberculin Tests *on page 945*
- **Aplonidine** *see* Apraclonidine *on page 76*
- **Apo®-Acetazolamide** *see* Acetazolamide *on page 23*
- **Apo®-Allopurinol** *see* Allopurinol *on page 42*
- **Apo®-Alpraz** *see* Alprazolam *on page 43*
- **Apo®-Amitriptyline** *see* Amitriptyline *on page 57*
- **Apo®-Amoxi** *see* Amoxicillin *on page 61*
- **Apo®-Ampi Trihydrate** *see* Ampicillin *on page 64*
- **Apo®-ASA** *see* Aspirin *on page 80*
- **Apo®-Atenol** *see* Atenolol *on page 84*
- **Apo® Bromocriptine** *see* Bromocriptine *on page 122*
- **Apo®-C** *see* Ascorbic Acid *on page 79*
- **Apo®-Cal** *see* Calcium Carbonate *on page 139*
- **Apo®-Capto** *see* Captopril *on page 146*
- **Apo®-Carbamazepine** *see* Carbamazepine *on page 148*
- **Apo®-Cefaclor** *see* Cefaclor *on page 158*
- **Apo®-Cephalex** *see* Cephalexin *on page 179*
- **Apo®-Chlordiazepoxide** *see* Chlordiazepoxide *on page 189*
- **Apo®-Chlorpromazine** *see* Chlorpromazine *on page 197*
- **Apo®-Chlorpropamide** *see* Chlorpropamide *on page 199*
- **Apo®-Chlorthalidone** *see* Chlorthalidone *on page 200*
- **Apo®-Cimetidine** *see* Cimetidine *on page 208*
- **Apo®-Clomipramine** *see* Clomipramine *on page 223*
- **Apo®-Clonidine** *see* Clonidine *on page 225*
- **Apo®-Clorazepate** *see* Clorazepate *on page 227*
- **Apo®-Cloxi** *see* Cloxacillin *on page 229*
- **Apo®-Diazepam** *see* Diazepam *on page 269*
- **Apo®-Diclo** *see* Diclofenac *on page 271*
- **Apo®-Diflunisal** *see* Diflunisal *on page 279*
- **Apo®-Diltiaz** *see* Diltiazem *on page 286*
- **Apo®-Dipyridamole FC** *see* Dipyridamole *on page 293*
- **Apo®-Dipyridamole SC** *see* Dipyridamole *on page 293*
- **Apo®-Doxepin** *see* Doxepin *on page 304*
- **Apo®-Doxy** *see* Doxycycline *on page 306*
- **Apo®-Doxy Tabs** *see* Doxycycline *on page 306*
- **Apo®-Enalapril** *see* Enalapril *on page 316*
- **Apo®-Erythro E-C** *see* Erythromycin *on page 329*
- **Apo®-Famotidine** *see* Famotidine *on page 358*
- **Apo®-Fluphenazine** *see* Fluphenazine *on page 388*
- **Apo®-Flurazepam** *see* Flurazepam *on page 390*
- **Apo®-Flurbiprofen** *see* Flurbiprofen *on page 391*
- **Apo®-Fluvoxamine** *see* Fluvoxamine *on page 395*
- **Apo®-Folic** *see* Folic Acid *on page 397*
- **Apo®-Furosemide** *see* Furosemide *on page 405*
- **Apo®-Gemfibrozil** *see* Gemfibrozil *on page 410*

- Apo®-Glyburide *see* Glyburide *on page 419*
- Apo®-Guanethidine *see* Guanethidine *on page 430*
- Apo®-Hydralazine *see* Hydralazine *on page 446*
- Apo®-Hydro *see* Hydrochlorothiazide *on page 447*
- Apo®-Hydroxyzine *see* Hydroxyzine *on page 462*
- Apo®-Ibuprofen *see* Ibuprofen *on page 466*
- Apo®-Imipramine *see* Imipramine *on page 469*
- Apo®-Indapadmide *see* Indapamide *on page 475*
- Apo®-Indomethacin *see* Indomethacin *on page 476*
- Apo®-ISDN *see* Isosorbide Dinitrate *on page 498*
- Apo®-Keto *see* Ketoprofen *on page 507*
- Apo®-Keto-E *see* Ketoprofen *on page 507*
- Apo®-Lisinopril *see* Lisinopril *on page 535*
- Apo®-Lorazepam *see* Lorazepam *on page 543*
- Apo®-Lovastatin *see* Lovastatin *on page 546*
- Apo®-Meprobamate *see* Meprobamate *on page 570*
- Apo®-Methyldopa *see* Methyldopa *on page 590*
- Apo®-Metoclop *see* Metoclopramide *on page 597*
- Apo®-Metoprolol (Type L) *see* Metoprolol *on page 599*
- Apo®-Metronidazole *see* Metronidazole *on page 601*
- Apo®-Minocycline *see* Minocycline *on page 610*
- Apo®-Nadol *see* Nadolol *on page 628*
- Apo®-Naproxen *see* Naproxen *on page 636*
- Apo®-Nifed *see* Nifedipine *on page 654*
- Apo®-Nitrofurantoin *see* Nitrofurantoin *on page 659*
- Apo®-Nizatidine *see* Nizatidine *on page 663*
- Apo®-Nortriptyline *see* Nortriptyline *on page 665*
- Apo®-Oxazepam *see* Oxazepam *on page 685*
- Apo®-Pentoxifylline SR *see* Pentoxifylline *on page 709*
- Apo®-Pen VK *see* Penicillin V Potassium *on page 706*
- Apo®-Perphenazine *see* Perphenazine *on page 713*
- Apo®-Pindol *see* Pindolol *on page 728*
- Apo®-Piroxicam *see* Piroxicam *on page 733*
- Apo®-Prazo *see* Prazosin *on page 750*
- Apo®-Prednisone *see* Prednisone *on page 754*
- Apo®-Primidone *see* Primidone *on page 756*
- Apo®-Procainamide *see* Procainamide *on page 759*
- Apo®-Propranolol *see* Propranolol *on page 775*
- Apo®-Ranitidine *see* Ranitidine Hydrochloride *on page 794*
- Apo®-Salvent *see* Albuterol *on page 34*
- Apo®-Selegiline *see* Selegiline *on page 826*
- Apo®-Sulfamethoxazole *see* Sulfamethoxazole *on page 861*
- Apo®-Sulfasalazine *see* Sulfasalazine *on page 862*
- Apo®-Sulfatrim *see* Co-Trimoxazole *on page 238*
- Apo®-Sulfinpyrazone *see* Sulfinpyrazone *on page 863*
- Apo®-Sulin *see* Sulindac *on page 865*
- Apo®-Tamox *see* Tamoxifen *on page 871*
- Apo®-Temazepam *see* Temazepam *on page 876*
- Apo®-Tetra *see* Tetracycline *on page 885*
- Apothecary/Metric Equivalents *see* Chart *on page 989*
- Apo®-Thioridazine *see* Thioridazine *on page 895*
- Apo®-Timol *see* Timolol *on page 905*
- Apo®-Timop *see* Timolol *on page 905*
- Apo®-Tolbutamide *see* Tolbutamide *on page 911*
- Apo®-Triazide *see* Hydrochlorothiazide and Triamterene *on page 449*
- Apo®-Triazo *see* Triazolam *on page 931*
- Apo®-Trihex *see* Trihexyphenidyl *on page 935*
- Apo®-Trimip *see* Trimipramine *on page 938*
- Apo®-Verap *see* Verapamil *on page 959*
- Apo®-Zidovudine *see* Zidovudine *on page 972*
- APPG *see* Penicillin G Procaine *on page 706*

## Apraclonidine (a pra KLOE ni deen)

**Pharmacologic Class** Alpha₂ Agonist, Ophthalmic

**U.S. Brand Names** Iopidine®

**Mechanism of Action** Apraclonidine is a potent alpha-adrenergic agent similar to clonidine; relatively selective for alpha₂-receptors but does retain some binding to alpha₁-receptors; appears to result in reduction of aqueous humor formation; its penetration through the blood-brain barrier is more polar than clonidine which reduces its penetration through the blood-brain barrier and suggests that its pharmacological profile is characterized by peripheral rather than central effects.

**Use** Prevention and treatment of postsurgical intraocular pressure elevation

**USUAL DOSAGE** Adults: Ophthalmic:

0.5%: Instill 1-2 drops in the affected eye(s) 3 times/day; since apraclonidine 0.5% will be used with other ocular glaucoma therapies, use an approximate 5-minute interval between instillation of each medication to prevent washout of the previous dose

1%: Instill 1 drop in operative eye 1 hour prior to anterior segment laser surgery, second drop in eye immediately upon completion of procedure

**Dosing adjustment in renal impairment:** Although the topical use of apraclonidine has not been studied in renal failure patients, structurally related clonidine undergoes a significant increase in half-life in patients with severe renal impairment; close monitoring of cardiovascular parameters in patients with impaired renal function is advised if they are candidates for topical apraclonidine therapy

**Dosing adjustment in hepatic impairment:** Close monitoring of cardiovascular parameters in patients with impaired liver function is advised because the systemic dosage form of clonidine is partially metabolized in the liver

**Dosage Forms Soln, ophth, as hydrochloride:** 0.5% (5 mL), 1% (0.1 mL, 0.25 mL)

**Contraindications** Known hypersensitivity to apraclonidine or clonidine

**Warnings/Precautions** Closely monitor patients who develop exaggerated reductions in intraocular pressure; use with caution in patients with cardiovascular disease and in patients with a history of vasovagal reactions

**Pregnancy Risk Factor** C

**Adverse Reactions**

1% to 10%:

Central nervous system: Lethargy

Gastrointestinal: Xerostomia

Ocular: Upper lid elevation, conjunctival blanching, mydriasis, burning and itching eyes, discomfort, conjunctival microhemorrhage, blurred vision

Respiratory: Dry nose

<1%: Allergic response, some systemic effects have also been reported including GI, CNS, and cardiovascular symptoms (arrhythmias)

**Drug Interactions** Increased effect: Topical beta-blockers, pilocarpine → additive ↓ intraocular pressure

**Onset** 1 hour

**Duration** 3-5 hours

**Special PA Issues**

**Monitoring Parameters:** Closely monitor patients who develop exaggerated reductions in intraocular pressure

♦ **Apraclonidine Hydrochloride** see Apraclonidine on this page

♦ **Apresazide®** see Hydralazine and Hydrochlorothiazide on page 447

♦ **Apresoline®** see Hydralazine on page 446

♦ **Aprodine® w/C** see Triprolidine, Pseudoephedrine, and Codeine on page 941

## Aprotinin (a proe TYE nin)

**Pharmacologic Class** Blood Product Derivative; Hemostatic Agent

**U.S. Brand Names** Trasylol®

**Mechanism of Action** Serine protease inhibitor; inhibits plasmin, kallikrein, and platelet activation producing antifibrinolytic effects; a weak inhibitor of plasma pseudocholinesterase. It also inhibits the contact phase activation of coagulation and preserves adhesive platelet glycoproteins making them resistant to damage from increased circulating plasmin or mechanical injury occurring during bypass

**Use** Reduction or prevention of blood loss in patients undergoing coronary artery bypass surgery when a high risk of excessive bleeding exists; this includes open heart reoperation, pre-existing coagulopathies, operations on the great vessels, and when a patient's beliefs prohibit blood transfusions

**USUAL DOSAGE**

Test dose: **All** patients should receive a 1 mL I.V. test dose at least 10 minutes prior to the loading dose to assess the potential for allergic reactions

Regimen A (standard dose):

2 million units (280 mg) loading dose I.V. over 20-30 minutes

2 million units (280 mg) into pump prime volume

500,000 units/hour (70 mg/hour) I.V. during operation

Regimen B (low dose):
1 million units (140 mg) loading dose I.V. over 20-30 minutes
1 million units (140 mg) into pump prime volume
250,000 units/hour (35 mg/hour) I.V. during operation

**Dosage Forms** Inj: 1.4 mg/mL [10,000 units/mL] (100 mL, 200 mL)

**Contraindications** Hypersensitivity to aprotinin or any component, patients with thrombo-embolic disease requiring anticoagulants or blood factor administration

**Warnings/Precautions** Patients with a previous exposure to aprotinin are at an increased risk of hypersensitivity reactions

**Pregnancy Risk Factor** B

**Pregnancy Implications** Excretion in breast milk unknown

**Adverse Reactions**
1% to 10%:
Cardiovascular: Atrial fibrillation, myocardial infarction, heart failure, atrial flutter, ventricular tachycardia, hypotension
Central nervous system: Fever, mental confusion
Local: Phlebitis
Renal: Increased potential for postoperative renal dysfunction
Respiratory: Dyspnea, bronchoconstriction
<1%: Cerebral embolism, cerebrovascular events, convulsions, hemolysis, liver damage, pulmonary edema, anaphylactic reactions have been reported in <0.5% of recipients, such reactions are more likely with repeated administration

**Drug Interactions**
Decreased effect: Fibrinolytic effects of streptokinase or anistreplase decrease effects of captopril
Increased effect: Heparin's whole blood clotting time may be prolonged; use with succinylcholine can produce prolonged or recurring apnea

**Half-Life** 150 minutes

**Special PA Issues**
**Patient Education:** You will be unaware of the effects of this drug, however, you will be closely monitored at all times
**Monitoring Parameters:** Bleeding times, prothrombin time, activated clotting time, platelet count, red blood cell counts, hematocrit, hemoglobin and fibrinogen degradation products; for toxicity also include renal function tests and blood pressure
**Reference Range:** Antiplasmin effects occur when plasma aprotinin concentrations are 125 KIU/mL and antikallikrein effects occur when plasma levels are 250-500 KIU/mL; it remains unknown if these plasma concentrations are required for clinical benefits to occur during cardiopulmonary bypass

♦ **APSAC** see Anistreplase on page 71
♦ **Aquacare® Topical [OTC]** see Urea on page 947
♦ **Aquachloral® Supprettes®** see Chloral Hydrate on page 186
♦ **AquaMEPHYTON® Injection** see Phytonadione on page 725
♦ **Aquaphyllin®** see Theophylline Salts on page 888
♦ **Aquasol A®** see Vitamin A on page 962
♦ **Aquasol E® [OTC]** see Vitamin E on page 963
♦ **Aquatag®** see Benzthiazide on page 107
♦ **Aqueous Procaine Penicillin G** see Penicillin G Procaine on page 706
♦ **Aqueous Testosterone** see Testosterone on page 881
♦ **Aquest®** see Estrone on page 338
♦ **Ara-A** see Vidarabine on page 961
♦ **Arabinofuranosyladenine** see Vidarabine on page 961
♦ **Aralen® Phosphate** see Chloroquine Phosphate on page 192
♦ **Aralen® Phosphate With Primaquine Phosphate** see Chloroquine and Primaquine on page 192
♦ **Arava™** see Leflunomide on page 517

# Ardeparin (ar dee PA rin)

**Pharmacologic Class** Low Molecular Weight Heparin

**U.S. Brand Names** Normiflo®

**Mechanism of Action** A low molecular weight heparin with antithrombotic properties; a partially depolymerized porcine mucosal heparin that has the same molecular subunits as heparin sodium, although its molecular weight is lower; acts at multiple sites in the normal coagulation system; binds to and accelerates the activity of antithrombin III, thereby inhibiting thrombosis by inactivating factor Xa and thrombin; inhibits thrombin by binding to heparin cofactor II

**Use** Prevention of deep vein thrombosis (DVT) which may lead to pulmonary embolism following knee replacement surgery

**USUAL DOSAGE** Adults: S.C.: 50 anti-Xa units/kg every 12 hours for DVT prophylaxis
(Continued)

## Ardeparin *(Continued)*

If the ardeparin formulation used contains 5000 anti-Xa units/0.5 mL (which is recommended for patients up to 100 kg or 220 lbs), the volume to be administered is calculated as follows:

Patient's weight (kg) x 0.005 mL/kg = volume (mL)

If the ardeparin formulation used contains 10,000 anti-Xa units/0.5 mL (which is recommended for patients >100 kg or 220 lbs), the volume to be administered is calculated as follows:

Patient's weight (kg) x 0.0025 mL/kg = volume (mL)

**Dosage adjustment in renal impairment:** No adjustment necessary

Not dialyzable

**Dosage Forms Inj, as sodium:** Anti-Xa units 5000 (0.5 mL), Anti-Xa units 10,000 (0.5 mL)

**Contraindications** Hypersensitivity to ardeparin, pork products, or other low-molecular weight heparins; cerebrovascular disease or other active hemorrhage; cerebral aneurysm; severe uncontrolled hypertension; thrombocytopenia associated with a positive *in vitro* test for antiplatelet antibodies in the presence of ardeparin

**Warnings/Precautions** Not intended for I.M. or I.V. use; use with extreme caution in patients with history of heparin-induced thrombocytopenia; may cause allergic-type reaction including anaphylactic symptoms and life-threatening or less severe asthmatic episodes in certain susceptible individuals; sulfite sensitivity more likely in asthmatics than nonasthmatics; use with extreme caution in patients with conditions having increased risk of hemorrhage (ie, bacterial endocarditis, congenital or acquired bleeding disorders, active ulcerative or angiodysplastic gastrointestinal disease, severe uncontrolled hypertension, hemorrhagic stroke, or shortly after brain, spinal, or ophthalmologic surgery) or in patients treated concomitantly with platelet inhibitors; use with caution in patients with hypersensitivity to methylparaben or propylparaben; use with caution in patients with bleeding diathesis, recent GI bleeding, thrombocytopenia or platelet defects, severe liver disease, hypertensive or diabetic retinopathy, or if undergoing invasive procedure especially if receiving other drugs known to interfere with hemostasis.

Patient should be observed closely for bleeding if ardeparin is administered during or immediately following diagnostic lumbar puncture, epidural anesthesia, or spinal anesthesia. If thromboembolism develops despite ardeparin prophylaxis, ardeparin should be discontinued and appropriate treatment should be initiated.

Carefully monitor patients receiving low molecular weight heparins or heparinoids. These drugs, when used concurrently with spinal or epidural anesthesia or spinal puncture, may cause bleeding or hematomas within the spinal column. Increased pressure on the spinal cord may result in permanent paralysis if not detected and treated immediately.

**Pregnancy Risk Factor** C

**Pregnancy Implications** Excretion in breast milk unknown/use caution

**Adverse Reactions** 1% to 10%:

Central nervous system: Fever (3%), confusion (<1%)

Dermatologic: Pruritus (2%), rash (2%), ecchymosis (2%)

Gastrointestinal: Nausea (3%), constipation (<1%), vomiting (1%)

Hematologic: Hemorrhage (5%), thrombocytopenia (2%), anemia (8%)

**Drug Interactions** Use with anticoagulants or platelet inhibitors, including aspirin and NSAIDs, may induce or augment bleeding

**Onset** Peak levels in 2-3 hours

**Duration** ~12 hours

**Half-Life** 3 hours (in plasma)

**Special PA Issues**

**Patient Education:** Inform prescriber of any over-the-counter or prescription medication you may take including aspirin, warfarin, NSAID (eg, ibuprofen, naproxen). Because this drug can alter the effects of certain laboratory tests, be sure to remind your prescriber that you are taking this medication when you are scheduled for any tests. This medication should not be mixed with, or added to, any other drug in the same syringe. Laboratory tests will be done periodically while taking this medication to monitor its effects and to prevent side effects. Use each dose at the scheduled time. If you miss a dose, use it as soon as remembered; do not use it if it is near the time for the next dose. Instead, skip the missed dose and resume your usual dosing schedule. Do not "double-up" the dose to catch up.

**Monitoring Parameters:** Monitor CBC including platelet counts, urinalysis, and occult blood in stool. Patients should be observed closely for bleeding if administered during or immediately following diagnostic lumbar puncture, epidural anesthesia, or spinal anesthesia. If thromboembolism develops despite ardeparin prophylaxis, ardeparin should be discontinued and appropriate treatment should be initiated. It is recommended during therapy to monitor complete blood counts including platelet counts, urinalysis, and occult blood in stools. Monitoring of coagulation parameters (APTT) during thromboprophylaxis with ardeparin is not required nor recommended.

♦ **Ardeparin Sodium** *see* Ardeparin *on previous page*

♦ **Aredia™** *see* Pamidronate *on page 693*

- **Argesic®-SA** *see* Salsalate *on page 820*
- **8-Arginine Vasopressin** *see* Vasopressin *on page 957*
- **Aricept®** *see* Donepezil *on page 301*
- **Arimidex®** *see* Anastrozole *on page 69*
- **Aristocort®** *see* Triamcinolone *on page 928*
- **Aristocort® A** *see* Triamcinolone *on page 928*
- **Aristocort® Forte** *see* Triamcinolone *on page 928*
- **Aristocort® Intralesional** *see* Triamcinolone *on page 928*
- **Aristospan® Intra-Articular** *see* Triamcinolone *on page 928*
- **Aristospan® Intralesional** *see* Triamcinolone *on page 928*
- **Arm-a-Med® Isoetharine** *see* Isoetharine *on page 493*
- **Arm-a-Med® Isoproterenol** *see* Isoproterenol *on page 496*
- **Arm-a-Med® Metaproterenol** *see* Metaproterenol *on page 575*
- **Armour® Thyroid** *see* Thyroid *on page 897*
- **Arrestin®** *see* Trimethobenzamide *on page 936*
- **ARS** *see* Antirabies Serum (Equine) *on page 73*
- **Artane®** *see* Trihexyphenidyl *on page 935*
- **Artha-G®** *see* Salsalate *on page 820*
- **Arthritis Foundation® Pain Reliever [OTC]** *see* Aspirin *on next page*
- **Arthritis Foundation® Pain Reliever, Aspirin Free [OTC]** *see* Acetaminophen *on page 21*
- **Arthropan® [OTC]** *see* Choline Salicylate *on page 204*
- **Arthrotec®** *see* Diclofenac and Misoprostol *on page 273*
- **Articulose-50® Injection** *see* Prednisolone *on page 752*
- **ASA** *see* Aspirin *on next page*
- **A.S.A. [OTC]** *see* Aspirin *on next page*
- **ASA®** *see* Aspirin *on next page*
- **5-ASA** *see* Mesalamine *on page 571*
- **Asacol® Oral** *see* Mesalamine *on page 571*
- **Asaphen** *see* Aspirin *on next page*
- **Ascorbic 500** *see* Ascorbic Acid *on this page*

## Ascorbic Acid (a SKOR bik AS id)

**Pharmacologic Class** Vitamin, Water Soluble

**U.S. Brand Names** Ascorbicap® [OTC]; C-Crystals® [OTC]; Cebid® Timecelles® [OTC]; Cecon® [OTC]; Cevalin® [OTC]; Cevi-Bid® [OTC]; Ce-Vi-Sol® [OTC]; Dull-C® [OTC]; Flavorcee® [OTC]; N'ice® Vitamin C Drops [OTC]; Vita-C® [OTC]

**Mechanism of Action** Not fully understood; necessary for collagen formation and tissue repair; involved in some oxidation-reduction reactions as well as other metabolic pathways, such as synthesis of carnitine, steroids, and catecholamines and conversion of folic acid to folinic acid

**Use** Prevention and treatment of scurvy and to acidify the urine

**Investigational:** In large doses to decrease the severity of "colds"; dietary supplementation; a 20-year study was recently completed involving 730 individuals which indicates a possible decreased risk of death by stroke when ascorbic acid at doses ≥45 mg/day was administered

**USUAL DOSAGE** Oral, I.M., I.V., S.C.:

Recommended daily allowance (RDA):
  <6 months: 30 mg
  6 months to 1 year: 35 mg
  1-3 years: 40 mg
  4-10 years: 45 mg
  11-14 years: 50 mg
  >14 years and Adults: 60 mg

Children:
  Scurvy: 100-300 mg/day in divided doses for at least 2 weeks
  Urinary acidification: 500 mg every 6-8 hours
  Dietary supplement: 35-100 mg/day

Adults:
  Scurvy: 100-250 mg 1-2 times/day for at least 2 weeks
  Urinary acidification: 4-12 g/day in 3-4 divided doses
  Prevention and treatment of colds: 1-3 g/day
  Dietary supplement: 50-200 mg/day

**Dosage Forms Cap, timed release:** 500 mg; **Crystals:** 4 g/teaspoonful (100 g, 500 g); 5 g/teaspoonful (180 g); **Inj:** 250 mg/mL (2 mL, 30 mL); 500 mg/mL (2 mL, 50 mL); **Liq, oral:** 35 mg/0.6 mL (50 mL); **Loz:** 60 mg; **Powder:** 4 g/teaspoonful (100 g, 500 g); **Soln, oral:** 100 mg/mL (50 mL); **Syr:** 500 mg/5 mL (5 mL, 10 mL, 120 mL, 480 mL); **Tab:** 25 mg, 50 mg, 100 mg, 250 mg, 500 mg, 1000 mg; **Tab, Chewable:** 100 mg, 250 mg, 500 mg; **Timed release:** 500 mg, 1000 mg, 1500 mg

(Continued)

## Ascorbic Acid *(Continued)*

**Contraindications** Large doses during pregnancy

**Warnings/Precautions** Diabetics and patients prone to recurrent renal calculi (eg, dialysis patients) should not take excessive doses for extended periods of time

**Pregnancy Risk Factor** A (C if used in doses above RDA recommendation)

**Pregnancy Implications** Enters breast milk/compatible

**Adverse Reactions**
1% to 10%: Renal: Hyperoxaluria with large doses
<1%: Flushing, faintness, dizziness, headache, fatigue, nausea, vomiting, heartburn, diarrhea, flank pain

**Drug Interactions**
Decreased effect:
Aspirin (decreases ascorbate levels, increases aspirin)
Fluphenazine (decreases fluphenazine levels)
Warfarin (decreased effect)
Increased effect:
Iron (absorption enhanced)
Oral contraceptives (increased contraceptive effect)

**Special PA Issues**
**Patient Education:** Take exactly as directed; do not take more than the recommended dose. Do not chew or crush extended release tablets. Take oral doses with 8 oz of water. Diabetics should use serum glucose monitoring method. Report pain on urination, faintness, or flank pain.
**Monitoring Parameters:** Monitor pH of urine when using as an acidifying agent

- **Ascorbicap® [OTC]** *see Ascorbic Acid on previous page*
- **Ascriptin® [OTC]** *see Aspirin on this page*
- **Asendin®** *see Amoxapine on page 60*
- **Asmalix®** *see Theophylline Salts on page 888*
- **A-Spas® S/L** *see Hyoscyamine on page 463*
- **Aspergum® [OTC]** *see Aspirin on this page*

## Aspirin *(AS pir in)*

**Pharmacologic Class** Salicylate

**U.S. Brand Names** Anacin® [OTC]; Arthritis Foundation® Pain Reliever [OTC]; A.S.A. [OTC]; Ascriptin® [OTC]; Aspergum® [OTC]; Asprimox® [OTC]; Bayer® Aspirin [OTC]; Bayer® Buffered Aspirin [OTC]; Bayer® Low Adult Strength [OTC]; Bufferin® [OTC]; Buffex® [OTC]; Cama® Arthritis Pain Reliever [OTC]; Easprin®; Ecotrin® [OTC]; Ecotrin® Low Adult Strength [OTC]; Empirin® [OTC]; Extra Strength Adprin-B® [OTC]; Extra Strength Bayer® Enteric 500 Aspirin [OTC]; Extra Strength Bayer® Plus [OTC]; Halfprin® 81® [OTC]; Regular Strength Bayer® Enteric 500 Aspirin [OTC]; St Joseph® Adult Chewable Aspirin [OTC]; ZORprin®

**Mechanism of Action** Inhibits prostaglandin synthesis, acts on the hypothalamus heat-regulating center to reduce fever; blocks prostaglandin synthetase action which prevents formation of the platelet-aggregating substance thromboxane $A_2$

**Use** Treatment of mild to moderate pain, inflammation, and fever; may be used as a prophylaxis of myocardial infarction and transient ischemic episodes; management of rheumatoid arthritis, rheumatic fever, osteoarthritis, and gout (high dose)

**USUAL DOSAGE**
Children:
Analgesic and antipyretic: Oral, rectal: 10-15 mg/kg/dose every 4-6 hours, up to a total of 60-80 mg/kg/24 hours
Anti-inflammatory: Oral: Initial: 60-90 mg/kg/day in divided doses; usual maintenance: 80-100 mg/kg/day divided every 6-8 hours, maximum dose: 3.6 g/day; monitor serum concentrations
Kawasaki disease: Oral: 80-100 mg/kg/day divided every 6 hours; after fever resolves: 8-10 mg/kg/day once daily; monitor serum concentrations
Antirheumatic: Oral: 60-100 mg/kg/day in divided doses every 4 hours
Adults:
Analgesic and antipyretic: Oral, rectal: 325-650 mg every 4-6 hours up to 4 g/day
Anti-inflammatory: Oral: Initial: 2.4-3.6 g/day in divided doses; usual maintenance: 3.6-5.4 g/day; monitor serum concentrations
TIA: Oral: 1.3 g/day in 2-4 divided doses
Myocardial infarction prophylaxis: 160-325 mg/day
**Dosing adjustment in renal impairment:** $Cl_{cr}$ <10 mL/minute: Avoid use
Hemodialysis: Dialyzable (50% to 100%)
**Dosing adjustment in hepatic disease:** Avoid use in severe liver disease
**Dosage Forms Cap:** 356.4 mg and caffeine 30 mg; **Supp, rectal:** 60 mg, 120 mg, 125 mg, 130 mg, 195 mg, 200 mg, 300 mg, 325 mg, 600 mg, 650 mg, 1.2 g; **Tab:** 65 mg, 75 mg, 81 mg, 325 mg, 500 mg, 400 mg and caffeine 32 mg; **Tab, buffered:** 325 mg and magnesium-aluminum hydroxide 150 mg, 325 mg, magnesium hydroxide 75 mg, aluminum hydroxide

75 mg, buffered with calcium carbonate, 325 mg and magnesium-aluminum hydroxide 75 mg; **Chewable:** 81 mg; **Controlled release:** 800 mg; **Delayed release:** 81 mg; **Enteric coated:** 81 mg, 325 mg, 500 mg, 650 mg, 975 mg; **Gum:** 227.5 mg; **Timed release:** 650 mg

**Contraindications** Bleeding disorders (factor VII or IX deficiencies), hypersensitivity to salicylates or other NSAIDs, tartrazine dye and asthma

**Warnings/Precautions** Use with caution in patients with platelet and bleeding disorders, renal dysfunction, erosive gastritis, or peptic ulcer disease, previous nonreaction does not guarantee future safe taking of medication; do not use aspirin in children <16 years of age for chickenpox or flu symptoms due to the association with Reye's syndrome

Otic: Discontinue use if dizziness, tinnitus, or impaired hearing occurs; surgical patients: avoid ASA if possible, for 1 week prior to surgery because of the possibility of postoperative bleeding; use with caution in impaired hepatic function

Elderly are a high-risk population for adverse effects from nonsteroidal anti-inflammatory agents. As much as 60% of elderly with GI complications to NSAIDs can develop peptic ulceration and/or hemorrhage asymptomatically. Also, concomitant disease and drug use contribute to the risk for GI adverse effects. Use lowest effective dose for shortest period possible. Consider renal function decline with age. Use of NSAIDs can compromise existing renal function especially when $Cl_{cr}$ is <30 mL/minute. Tinnitus may be a difficult and unreliable indication of toxicity due to age-related hearing loss or eighth cranial nerve damage. CNS adverse effects such as confusion, agitation, and hallucination are generally seen in overdose or high-dose situations, but elderly may demonstrate these adverse effects at lower doses than younger adults.

**Pregnancy Risk Factor** C (D if full-dose aspirin in 3rd trimester)

**Adverse Reactions**

>10%: Gastrointestinal: Nausea, vomiting, dyspepsia, epigastric discomfort, heartburn, stomach pains

1% to 10%:

Central nervous system: Fatigue
Dermatologic: Rash, urticaria
Gastrointestinal: Gastrointestinal ulceration
Hematologic: Hemolytic anemia
Neuromuscular & skeletal: Weakness
Respiratory: Dyspnea
Miscellaneous: Anaphylactic shock

<1%: Insomnia, nervousness, jitters, iron deficiency, occult bleeding, prolongation of bleeding time, leukopenia, thrombocytopenia, anemia, hepatotoxicity, impaired renal function, bronchospasm

**Drug Interactions**

Decreased effect: Possible decreased serum concentration of NSAIDs; aspirin may antagonize effects of probenecid

Increased toxicity: Aspirin may increase methotrexate serum levels and may displace valproic acid from binding sites which can result in toxicity; warfarin and aspirin may increase bleeding; NSAIDs and aspirin may increase GI adverse effects; buspirone increases free % *in vitro*; bleeding times may be additionally prolonged with verapamil

**Onset** Peak in 1-2 hours

**Duration** 4-6 hours

**Half-Life** Dose dependent; 3 hours at low dose, up to 10 hours at higher doses

**Special PA Issues**

**Patient Education:** If self-administered, use exactly as directed (do not increase dose or frequency); adverse reactions can occur with overuse. Take with food or milk. Do not use aspirin with strong vinegary odor. Do not crush or chew extended release products. While using this medication, avoid alcohol, excessive amounts of vitamin C, or salicylate-containing foods (curry powder, prunes, raisins, tea, or licorice), other prescription or OTC medications containing aspirin or salicylate, or other NSAIDs without consulting prescriber. Maintain adequate hydration (2-3 L/day of fluids unless instructed to restrict fluid intake). You may experience nausea, vomiting, gastric discomfort (frequent mouth care, small frequent meals, or sucking on lozenges may help). GI bleeding, ulceration, or perforation can occur with or without pain. Stop taking aspirin and report ringing in ears; persistent pain in stomach; unresolved nausea or vomiting; difficulty breathing or shortness of breath; unusual bruising or bleeding (mouth, urine, stool); or skin rash.

**Dietary Considerations:**

Alcohol: Combination causes GI irritation, possible bleeding; avoid or limit alcohol. Patients at increased risk include those prone to hypoprothrombinemia, vitamin K deficiency, thrombocytopenia, thrombotic thrombocytopenia purpura, severe hepatic impairment, and those receiving anticoagulants.

Food: May decrease the rate but not the extent of oral absorption. Drug may cause GI upset, bleeding, ulceration, perforation. Take with food or large volume of water or milk to minimize GI upset.

Folic acid: Hyperexcretion of folate; folic acid deficiency may result, leading to macrocytic anemia. Supplement with folic acid if necessary.

(Continued)

## Aspirin *(Continued)*

Iron: With chronic use and at doses of 3-4 g/day, iron deficiency anemia may result; supplement with iron if necessary

Sodium: Hypernatremia resulting from buffered aspirin solutions or sodium salicylate containing high sodium content. Avoid or use with caution in CHF or any condition where hypernatremia would be detrimental.

Curry powder, paprika, licorice, Benedictine liqueur, prunes, raisins, tea and gherkins: Potential salicylate accumulation. These foods contain 6 mg salicylate/100 g. An ordinarily American diet contains 10-200 mg/day of salicylate. Foods containing salicylates may contribute to aspirin hypersensitivity. Patients at greatest risk for aspirin hypersensitivity include those with asthma, nasal polyposis or chronic urticaria.

Fresh fruits containing vitamin C: Displaces drug from binding sites, resulting in increased urinary excretion of aspirin. Educate patients regarding the potential for a decreased analgesic effect of aspirin with consumption of foods high in vitamin C.

**Reference Range:** Timing of serum samples: Peak levels usually occur 2 hours after ingestion. Salicylate serum concentrations correlate with the pharmacological actions and adverse effects observed. See table.

### Serum Salicylate: Clinical Correlations

| Serum Salicylate Concentration (mcg/mL) | Desired Effects | Adverse Effects/Intoxication |
|---|---|---|
| ~100 | Antiplatelet Antipyresis Analgesia | GI intolerance and bleeding, hypersensitivity, hemostatic defects |
| 150-300 | Anti-inflammatory | Mild salicylism |
| 250-400 | Treatment of rheumatic fever | Nausea/vomiting, hyperventilation, salicylism, flushing, sweating, thirst, headache, diarrhea, and tachycardia |
| >400-500 | | Respiratory alkalosis, hemorrhage, excitement, confusion, asterixis, pulmonary edema, convulsions, tetany, metabolic acidosis, fever, coma, cardiovascular collapse, renal and respiratory failure |

## Aspirin and Codeine (AS pir in & KOE deen)

**Pharmacologic Class** Analgesic, Narcotic

**U.S. Brand Names** Empirin® With Codeine

**Mechanism of Action** Inhibits prostaglandin synthesis, acts on the hypothalamus heat-regulating center to reduce fever, blocks prostaglandin synthetase action which prevents formation of the platelet-aggregating substance thromboxane $A_2$; binds to opiate receptors in the CNS, causing inhibition of ascending pain pathways, altering the perception of and response to pain; causes cough supression by direct central action in the medulla; produces generalized CNS depression

**Use** Relief of mild to moderate pain

**USUAL DOSAGE** Oral:

Children:
Aspirin: 10 mg/kg/dose every 4 hours
Codeine: 0.5-1 mg/kg/dose every 4 hours
Adults: 1-2 tablets every 4-6 hours as needed for pain

**Dosing adjustment in renal impairment:**
$Cl_{cr}$ 10-50 mL/minute: Administer 75% of dose
$Cl_{cr}$ <10 mL/minute: Avoid use

**Dosing interval in hepatic disease:** Avoid use in severe liver disease

**Dosage Forms Tab:** #2: Aspirin 325 mg and codeine phosphate 15 mg, #3: Aspirin 325 mg and codeine phosphate 30 mg, #4: Aspirin 325 mg and codeine phosphate 60 mg

**Contraindications** Hypersensitivity to aspirin, codeine or any component; premature infants or during labor for delivery of a premature infant

**Warnings/Precautions** Use with caution in patients with impaired renal function, erosive gastritis, or peptic ulcer disease; children and teenagers should not use for chickenpox or flu symptoms before a physician is consulted about Reye's syndrome

**Pregnancy Risk Factor** D

**Adverse Reactions**

>10%:
Central nervous system: Lightheadedness, dizziness, sedation
Gastrointestinal: Nausea, heartburn, stomach pains, dyspepsia, epigastric discomfort, vomiting
Respiratory: Shortness of breath

1% to 10%:
  Central nervous system: Fatigue, euphoria, dysphoria
  Dermatologic: Rash, pruritus
  Gastrointestinal: Gastrointestinal ulceration, constipation
  Hematologic: Hemolytic anemia
  Neuromuscular & skeletal: Weakness
  Respiratory: Dyspnea
  Miscellaneous: Anaphylactic shock
<1%: Palpitations, hypotension, bradycardia, peripheral vasodilation, insomnia, nervousness, jitters, increased intracranial pressure, antidiuretic hormone release, iron deficiency, biliary tract spasm, urinary retention, occult bleeding, prolongation of bleeding time, leukopenia, thrombocytopenia, anemia, hepatotoxicity, miosis, impaired renal function, bronchospasm, respiratory depression, physical and psychological dependence

**Drug Interactions** Refer to individual monographs for Aspirin and Codeine
**Special PA Issues**
  **Dietary Considerations:** Alcohol: Additive CNS effects, avoid use
  **Monitoring Parameters:** Observe patient for excessive sedation, respiratory depression, pain relief, blood pressure, mental status

# Aspirin and Meprobamate (AS pir in & me proe BA mate)
**Pharmacologic Class** Antianxiety Agent, Miscellaneous
**U.S. Brand Names** Equagesic®
**Dosage Forms Tab:** Aspirin 325 mg and meprobamate 200 mg

- ♦ **Aspirin Free Anacin® Maximum Strength [OTC]** *see* Acetaminophen *on page 21*
- ♦ **Asprimox® [OTC]** *see* Aspirin *on page 80*
- ♦ **Astelin® Nasal Spray** *see* Azelastine *on page 92*

# Astemizole (a STEM mi zole)
**Pharmacologic Class** Antihistamine
**U.S. Brand Names** Hismanal®
**Mechanism of Action** Competes with histamine for $H_1$-receptor sites on effector cells in the gastrointestinal tract, blood vessels, and respiratory tract; binds to lung receptors significantly greater than it binds to cerebellar receptors, resulting in a reduced sedative potential
**Use** Perennial and seasonal allergic rhinitis and other allergic symptoms including urticaria
**USUAL DOSAGE** Oral:
  Children:
    <6 years: 0.2 mg/kg/day
    6-12 years: 5 mg/day (not to exceed 10 mg daily)
  Children >12 years and Adults: 10-30 mg/day; administer 30 mg on first day, 20 mg on second day, then 10 mg/day in a single dose
**Dosage Forms Tab:** 10 mg
**Contraindications** Hypersensitivity to astemizole or any component; concurrent use of erythromycin, quinine, ketoconazole, itraconazole, clarithromycin, troleandomycin, mibefradil dihydrochloride, or in patients with significant hepatic dysfunction
**Warnings/Precautions** Use with caution in patients receiving drugs which prolong QRS or rare cases of severe cardiovascular events (cardiac arrest, arrhythmias) have been reported. Safety and efficacy in children <12 years of age have not been established. Discontinue therapy immediately with signs of cardiotoxicity including syncope.

Concurrent use of fluoxetine, sertraline, fluvoxamine, nefazodone, paroxetine, ritonavir, indinavir, nelfinavir, saquinavir, zileuton, and other potent cytochrome P-450 3A4 inhibitors, including grapefruit juice is not recommended since these agents may inhibit astemizole clearance, thereby leading to increased astemizole serum concentrations and potential astemizole cardiotoxicity.

The recommended daily dose of astemizole should not be exceeded. Astemizole should not be used on an "as needed" (ie, prn) basis for immediate relief of symptoms. Patients should be advised that astemizole should not be taken with grapefruit juice because of the potential for grapefruit to influence the metabolism of astemizole.

**Pregnancy Risk Factor** C
**Pregnancy Implications** Excretion in breast milk unknown/not recommended
**Adverse Reactions**
  1% to 10%:
    Central nervous system: Drowsiness, headache, fatigue, nervousness, dizziness
    Gastrointestinal: Appetite increase, weight gain, nausea, diarrhea, abdominal pain, xerostomia
    Neuromuscular & skeletal: Arthralgia
    Respiratory: Pharyngitis
  <1%: Palpitations, edema, depression, angioedema, photosensitivity, rash, hepatitis, myalgia, paresthesia, bronchospasm, epistaxis, thickening of mucous
**Drug Interactions** CYP3A3/4 enzyme substrate
(Continued)

## Astemizole *(Continued)*

Increased toxicity: CNS depressants (sedation), triazole antifungals, macrolide antibiotics, mibefradil, and quinine may inhibit the metabolism of astemizole resulting in potentially life-threatening arrhythmias (torsade de pointes, etc); see Warnings and Contraindications

**Onset** <24 hours, but may take 2-3 days; Peak effect: 9-12 days

**Duration** Long-acting, with steady-state plasma levels seen within 4-8 weeks following initiation of chronic therapy

**Half-Life** 7-11 days

**Special PA Issues**

**Patient Education:** Notify prescriber if taking any cardiac medication. Take as directed; do not exceed recommended dose. Take on an empty stomach (1 hour before or 2 hours after meals). Avoid use of other depressants, alcohol, or sleep-inducing medications unless approved by prescriber. You may experience drowsiness or dizziness (use caution when driving or engaging in hazardous activity until response to medication is known); dry nasal membranes (use of humidifier may help); or dry mouth, abdominal pain, or nausea (frequent small meals, frequent mouth care, chewing gum, or sucking hard candy may help). Report persistent sedation, depression, or agitation; difficulty breathing or expectorating (thick secretions); tremors or loss of coordination; lack of improvement or worsening or condition.

♦ **Asthma Therapy Guidelines** *see Chart on page 1049*
♦ **Astramorph™ PF Injection** *see Morphine Sulfate on page 619*
♦ **Atacand™** *see Candesartan on page 144*
♦ **Atamet®** *see Levodopa and Carbidopa on page 525*
♦ **Atarax®** *see Hydroxyzine on page 462*
♦ **Atasol®** *see Acetaminophen on page 21*
♦ **Atasol® 8, 15, 30 With Caffeine** *see Acetaminophen and Codeine on page 22*

## Atenolol *(a TEN oh lole)*

**Pharmacologic Class** Beta Blocker, Beta$_1$ Selective

**U.S. Brand Names** Tenormin®

**Mechanism of Action** Competitively blocks response to beta-adrenergic stimulation, selectively blocks beta$_1$-receptors with little or no effect on beta$_2$-receptors except at high doses

**Use** Treatment of hypertension, alone or in combination with other agents; management of angina pectoris, postmyocardial infarction patients

**Unlabeled use:** Acute alcohol withdrawal, supraventricular and ventricular arrhythmias, and migraine headache prophylaxis

**USUAL DOSAGE**

Oral:

Children: 1-2 mg/kg/dose given daily

Adults:

Hypertension: 50 mg once daily, may increase to 100 mg/day; doses >100 mg are unlikely to produce any further benefit

Angina pectoris: 50 mg once daily, may increase to 100 mg/day; some patients may require 200 mg/day

Postmyocardial infarction: Follow I.V. dose with 100 mg/day or 50 mg twice daily for 6-9 days postmyocardial infarction

I.V.: Postmyocardial infarction: Early treatment: 5 mg slow I.V. over 5 minutes; may repeat in 10 minutes; if both doses are tolerated, may start oral atenolol 50 mg every 12 hours or 100 mg/day for 6-9 days postmyocardial infarction

**Dosing interval for oral atenolol in renal impairment:**

Cl$_{cr}$ 15-35 mL/minute: Administer 50 mg/day maximum

Cl$_{cr}$ <15 mL/minute: Administer 50 mg every other day maximum

Hemodialysis: Moderately dialyzable (20% to 50%) via hemodialysis; administer dose postdialysis or administer 25-50 mg supplemental dose

Peritoneal dialysis: Elimination is not enhanced; supplemental dose is not necessary

**Dosage Forms** Inj: 0.5 mg/mL (10 mL); Tab: 25 mg, 50 mg, 100 mg

**Contraindications** Hypersensitivity to beta-blocking agents, pulmonary edema, cardiogenic shock, bradycardia, heart block without a pacemaker, uncompensated congestive heart failure, sinus node dysfunction, A-V conduction abnormalities

**Warnings/Precautions** Safety and efficacy in children have not been established; administer with caution to patients (especially the elderly) with bronchospastic disease, CHF, renal dysfunction, severe peripheral vascular disease, myasthenia gravis, diabetes mellitus, hyperthyroidism. **Abrupt withdrawal of the drug should be avoided**, drug should be discontinued over 1-2 weeks; may potentiate hypoglycemia in a diabetic patient and mask signs and symptoms; modify dosage in patients with renal impairment.

**Pregnancy Risk Factor** C

**Pregnancy Implications** Enters breast milk/use caution

Clinical effects on the fetus: Crosses the placenta; persistent beta-blockade, bradycardia, IUGR; IUGR probably related to maternal hypertension. Available evidence suggest safe use during pregnancy and breast-feeding. Monitor breast-fed infant for symptoms of beta-blockade.

Clinical effects on the infant: Symptoms have been reported of beta-blockade including cyanosis, hypothermia, bradycardia

## Adverse Reactions
Cardiovascular: Persistent bradycardia, hypotension, chest pain, edema, heart failure, second or third degree A-V block, Raynaud's phenomenon

Central nervous system: Dizziness, fatigue, insomnia, lethargy, confusion, mental impairment, depression, headache, nightmares

Gastrointestinal: Constipation, diarrhea, nausea

Genitourinary: Impotence

Respiratory: Dyspnea (especially with large doses), wheezing

Miscellaneous: Cold extremities

## Drug Interactions
Decreased effect of some beta-blockers with aluminum salts, barbiturates, calcium salts, cholestyramine, colestipol, NSAIDs, penicillins (ampicillin), rifampin, salicylates, and sulfinpyrazone due to decreased bioavailability and plasma levels

Beta-blockers may decrease the effect of sulfonylureas

Increased effect/toxicity of beta-blockers with calcium blockers (diltiazem, felodipine, nicardipine), contraceptives, flecainide, hydralazine (metoprolol, propranolol), propafenone, quinidine (in extensive metabolizers), ciprofloxacin

Beta-blockers may increase the effect/toxicity of flecainide, hydralazine, clonidine (hypertensive crisis after or during withdrawal of either agent), epinephrine (initial hypertensive episode followed by bradycardia), nifedipine, verapamil, lidocaine, ergots, prazosin

Beta-blockers may affect the action or levels of ethanol, disopyramide, nondepolarizing muscle relaxants and theophylline although the effects are difficult to predict

**Onset** Peak concentrations in 1-2 hours with oral; more rapid with I.V.

**Duration** 12-24 hours in normal renal function

**Half-Life** Normal renal function: 6-9 hours, longer in those with renal impairment; End-stage renal disease: 15-35 hours

## Special PA Issues
**Patient Education:** Take exactly as directed. Do not increase, decrease, or adjust dosage without consulting prescriber. Take pulse daily, prior to medication and follow prescriber's instruction about holding medication. Do not take with antacids. Do not use alcohol or OTC medications (eg, cold remedies) without consulting prescriber. If diabetic, monitor serum sugars closely (may alter glucose tolerance or mask signs of hypoglycemia). May cause fatigue, dizziness, or postural hypotension; use caution when changing position from lying or sitting to standing, when driving, or when climbing stairs until response to medication is known. May cause alteration in sexual performance (reversible). Report unresolved swelling of extremities, difficulty breathing or new cough, unresolved fatigue, unusual weight gain, unresolved constipation, or unusual muscle weakness.

**Monitoring Parameters:** Monitor blood pressure, apical and radial pulses, fluid I & O, daily weight, respirations, and circulation in extremities before and during therapy

## Related Information
Beta-Blockers *on page 1002*

# Atenolol and Chlorthalidone (a TEN oh lole & klor THAL i done)
**Pharmacologic Class** Antihypertensive Agent, Combination

**U.S. Brand Names** Tenoretic®

**Dosage Forms** Tab: 50: Atenolol 50 mg and chlorthalidone 25 mg, 100: Atenolol 100 mg and chlorthalidone 25 mg

- ♦ **ATG** *see* Lymphocyte Immune Globulin *on page 550*
- ♦ **ATG** *see* Antithymocyte Globulin (Rabbit) *on page 73*
- ♦ **Atgam®** *see* Lymphocyte Immune Globulin *on page 550*
- ♦ **Ativan®** *see* Lorazepam *on page 543*
- ♦ **Atolone®** *see* Triamcinolone *on page 928*

# Atorvastatin (a TORE va sta tin)
**Pharmacologic Class** Antilipemic Agent (HMG-CoA Reductase Inhibitor)

**U.S. Brand Names** Lipitor®

**Mechanism of Action** Inhibitor of 3-hydroxy-3-methylglutaryl coenzyme A (HMG-CoA) reductase, the rate limiting enzyme in cholesterol synthesis (reduces the production of mevalonic acid from HMG-CoA); this then results in a compensatory increase in the expression of LDL receptors on hepatocyte membranes and a stimulation of LDL catabolism

**Use** Adjunct to diet for the reduction of elevated total and LDL-cholesterol levels in patients with hypercholesterolemia (Type IIa, IIb, and IIc); used in hypercholesterolemic patients without clinically evident heart disease to reduce the risk of myocardial infarction, to reduce the risk for revascularization, and reduce the risk of death due to cardiovascular causes

**USUAL DOSAGE** Adults: Oral: Initial: 10 mg once daily, titrate up to 80 mg/day if needed

**Dosing adjustment in renal impairment:** No dosage adjustment necessary

(Continued)

## Atorvastatin *(Continued)*

**Dosing adjustment in hepatic impairment:** Decrease dosage with severe disease (eg, chronic alcoholic liver disease)

**Dosage Forms** Tab: 10 mg, 20 mg, 40 mg

**Contraindications** Hypersensitivity to atorvastatin or its components; patients with active liver disease; pregnancy or lactation

**Warnings/Precautions** Discontinue therapy if symptoms of myopathy or renal failure due to rhabdomyolysis develop. Use with caution in patients with history of liver disease or who consume excessive amounts of alcohol. It is recommended that liver function tests (LFTs) be performed prior to and at 12 weeks following both the initiation of therapy and any elevation in dose, and periodically (eg, semiannually) thereafter.

**Pregnancy Risk Factor** X

**Adverse Reactions**

>1%:

Central nervous system: Headache
Gastrointestinal: Diarrhea, flatulence, abdominal pain (2% to 3%)
Neuromuscular & skeletal: Myalgia (1% to 5%)

<1%: Giddiness, euphoria, mild confusion, impaired short-term memory, mild LFT increases, pharyngitis, rhinitis

**Drug Interactions** CYP3A3/4 enzyme substrate

Increased toxicity: Gemfibrozil (musculoskeletal effects such as myopathy, myalgia and/or muscle weakness accompanied by markedly elevated CK concentrations, rash and/or pruritus), clofibrate, niacin (myopathy), erythromycin, cyclosporine, oral anticoagulants (elevated PT)

Increased effect/toxicity of levothyroxine

Concurrent use of erythromycin and atorvastatin may result in rhabdomyolysis

**Onset** Maximal reduction in plasma cholesterol and triglycerides in 2 weeks; initial changes in 3-5 days

**Half-Life** 14 hours (parent)

**Special PA Issues**

**Patient Education:** May take with meals at any time of day. Maintain adequate hydration (2-3 L/day of fluids unless instructed to restrict fluid intake). You will need laboratory evaluation during therapy. May cause headache (mild analgesic may help); diarrhea (yogurt or buttermilk may help); euphoria, giddiness, confusion (use caution when driving or engaging in tasks that require alertness until response to medication is known). Report unresolved diarrhea, excessive or acute muscle cramping or weakness, changes in mood or memory, yellowing of skin or eyes, easy bruising or bleeding, and unusual fatigue.

**Monitoring Parameters:** Lipid levels after 2-4 weeks; LFTs, CPK

It is recommended that liver function tests (LFTs) be performed prior to and at 12 weeks following both the initiation of therapy and any elevation in dose, and periodically (eg, semiannually) thereafter

**Related Information**

Lipid-Lowering Agents *on page 1022*

## Atovaquone *(a TOE va kwone)*

**Pharmacologic Class** Antiprotozoal

**U.S. Brand Names** Mepron™

**Mechanism of Action** Has not been fully elucidated; may inhibit electron transport in mitochondria inhibiting metabolic enzymes

**Use** Acute oral treatment of mild to moderate *Pneumocystis carinii* pneumonia (PCP) in patients who are intolerant to co-trimoxazole; prophylaxis of PCP in patients intolerant to co-trimoxazole; treatment/suppression of *Toxoplasma gondii* encephalitis, primary prophylaxis of HIV-infected persons at high risk for developing *Toxoplasma gondii* encephalitis

**USUAL DOSAGE** Adults: Oral: 750 mg twice daily with food for 21 days

**Dosage Forms** Susp, oral (citrus flavor): 750 mg/5 mL (210 mL)

**Contraindications** Life-threatening allergic reaction to the drug or formulation

**Warnings/Precautions** Has only been indicated in mild to moderate PCP; use with caution in elderly patients due to potentially impaired renal, hepatic, and cardiac function

**Pregnancy Risk Factor** C

**Adverse Reactions Note:** Adverse reaction statistics have been compiled from studies including patients with advanced HIV disease; consequently, it is difficult to distinguish reactions attributed to atovaquone from those caused by the underlying disease or a combination, thereof.

>10%:

Central nervous system: Headache, fever, insomnia, anxiety
Dermatologic: Rash
Gastrointestinal: Nausea, diarrhea, vomiting
Respiratory: Cough

1% to 10%:

Central nervous system: Dizziness

Dermatologic: Pruritus
Endocrine & metabolic: Hypoglycemia, hyponatremia
Gastrointestinal: Abdominal pain, constipation, anorexia, dyspepsia, increased amylase
Hematologic: Anemia, neutropenia, leukopenia
Hepatic: Elevated liver enzymes
Neuromuscular & skeletal: Weakness
Renal: Elevated BUN/creatinine
Miscellaneous: Oral moniliasis

**Drug Interactions**
Decreased effect: Rifamycins used concurrently decrease the steady-state plasma concentrations of atovaquone
**Note:** Possible increased toxicity with other highly protein bound drugs

**Half-Life** 2.9 days

**Special PA Issues**
Patient Education: Take as directed. Take with high-fat meals. You may experience dizziness or lightheadedness; use caution when driving or engaging in hazardous activity. Small meals may help reduce nausea. Report unresolved diarrhea, fever, mouth sores (use good mouth care), unresolved headache or vomiting.

- ♦ **Atozine®** *see* Hydroxyzine *on page 462*
- ♦ **ATRA** *see* Tretinoin, Oral *on page 925*
- ♦ **Atridox™** *see* Doxycycline *on page 306*
- ♦ **Atrohist® Plus** *see* Chlorpheniramine, Phenylephrine, Phenylpropanolamine, and Belladonna Alkaloids *on page 196*
- ♦ **Atromid-S®** *see* Clofibrate *on page 221*
- ♦ **Atropair® Ophthalmic** *see* Atropine *on this page*

# Atropine (A troe peen)

**Pharmacologic Class** Anticholinergic Agent; Anticholinergic Agent, Ophthalmic; Antidote; Antispasmodic Agent, Gastrointestinal; Ophthalmic Agent, Mydriatic
**U.S. Brand Names** Atropair® Ophthalmic; Atropine-Care® Ophthalmic; Atropisol® Ophthalmic; Isopto® Atropine Ophthalmic; I-Tropine® Ophthalmic; Ocu-Tropine® Ophthalmic
**Mechanism of Action** Blocks the action of acetylcholine at parasympathetic sites in smooth muscle, secretory glands and the CNS; increases cardiac output, dries secretions, antagonizes histamine and serotonin
**Use** Preoperative medication to inhibit salivation and secretions; treatment of sinus bradycardia; management of peptic ulcer; treat exercise-induced bronchospasm; antidote for organophosphate pesticide poisoning; produce mydriasis and cycloplegia for examination of the retina and optic disc and accurate measurement of refractive errors; uveitis
**USUAL DOSAGE Note:** Doses <0.1 mg have been associated with paradoxical bradycardia
Neonates, Infants, and Children:
Preanesthetic: Oral, I.M., I.V., S.C.:
<5 kg: 0.02 mg/kg/dose 30-60 minutes preop then every 4-6 hours as needed; use of a minimum dosage of 0.1 mg in neonates <5 kg will result in dosages >0.02 mg/kg; there is no documented minimum dosage in this age group
>5 kg: 0.01-0.02 mg/kg/dose to a maximum 0.4 mg/dose 30-60 minutes preop; minimum dose: 0.1 mg
Bradycardia: I.V., intratracheal: 0.02 mg/kg, minimum dose 0.1 mg, maximum single dose: 0.5 mg in children and 1 mg in adolescents; may repeat in 5-minute intervals to a maximum total dose of 1 mg in children or 2 mg in adolescents. (**Note:** For intratracheal administration, the dosage must be diluted with normal saline to a total volume of 1-2 mL); when treating bradycardia in neonates, reserve use for those patients unresponsive to improved oxygenation and epinephrine.
Children:
Bronchospasm: Inhalation: 0.03-0.05 mg/kg/dose 3-4 times/day
Preprocedure: Ophthalmic: 0.5% solution: Instill 1-2 drops twice daily for 1-3 days before the procedure
Uveitis: Ophthalmic: 0.5% solution: Instill 1-2 drops up to 3 times/day
Adults (doses <0.5 mg have been associated with paradoxical bradycardia):
Asystole: I.V.: 1 mg; may repeat every 3-5 minutes as needed
Preanesthetic: I.M., I.V., S.C.: 0.4-0.6 mg 30-60 minutes preop and repeat every 4-6 hours as needed
Bradycardia: I.V.: 0.5-1 mg every 5 minutes, not to exceed a total of 2 mg or 0.04 mg/kg; may give intratracheal in 1 mg/10 mL dilution only, intratracheal dose should be 2-2.5 times the I.V. dose
Neuromuscular blockade reversal: I.V.: 25-30 mcg/kg 30 seconds before neostigmine or 10 mcg/kg 30 seconds before edrophonium
Organophosphate or carbamate poisoning: I.V.: 1-2 mg/dose every 10-20 minutes until atropine effect (dry flushed skin, tachycardia, mydriasis, fever) is observed, then every 1-4 hours for at least 24 hours; up to 50 mg in first 24 hours and 2 g over several days may be given in cases of severe intoxication
(Continued)

## Atropine *(Continued)*

Bronchospasm: Inhalation: 0.025-0.05 mg/kg/dose every 4-6 hours as needed (maximum: 5 mg/dose)

Ophthalmic solution: 1%:
Preprocedure: Instill 1-2 drops 1 hour before the procedure
Uveitis: Instill 1-2 drops 4 times/day

Ophthalmic ointment: Apply a small amount in the conjunctival sac up to 3 times/day; compress the lacrimal sac by digital pressure for 1-3 minutes after instillation

**Dosage Forms Inj:** 0.1 mg/mL (5 mL, 10 mL), 0.3 mg/mL (1 mL, 30 mL), 0.4 mg/mL (1 mL, 20 mL, 30 mL), 0.5 mg/mL (1 mL, 5 mL, 30 mL), 0.8 mg/mL (0.5 mL, 1 mL), 1 mg/mL (1 mL, 10 mL); **Oint, ophth:** 0.5%, 1% (3.5 g); **Soln, ophth:** 0.5% (1 mL, 5 mL), 1% (1 mL, 2 mL, 5 mL, 15 mL), 2% (1 mL, 2 mL), 3% (5 mL); **Tab:** 0.4 mg

**Contraindications** Hypersensitivity to atropine sulfate or any component; narrow-angle glaucoma; tachycardia; thyrotoxicosis; obstructive disease of the GI tract; obstructive uropathy

**Warnings/Precautions** Use with caution in children with spastic paralysis; use with caution in elderly patients. Low doses cause a paradoxical decrease in heart rates. Some commercial products contain sodium metabisulfite, which can cause allergic-type reactions. May accumulate with multiple inhalational administration, particularly in the elderly. Heat prostration may occur in hot weather. Use with caution in patients with autonomic neuropathy, prostatic hypertrophy, hyperthyroidism, congestive heart failure, cardiac arrhythmias, chronic lung disease, biliary tract disease; anticholinergic agents are generally not well tolerated in the elderly and their use should be avoided when possible; atropine is rarely used except as a preoperative agent or in the acute treatment of bradyarrhythmias.

**Pregnancy Risk Factor** C

**Adverse Reactions**

>10%:
Dermatologic: Dry, hot skin
Gastrointestinal: Impaired GI motility, constipation, dry throat, xerostomia
Local: Irritation at injection site
Respiratory: Dry nose
Miscellaneous: Diaphoresis (decreased)

1% to 10%:
Dermatologic: Increased sensitivity to light
Endocrine & metabolic: Decreased flow of breast milk
Gastrointestinal: Dysphagia

<1%: Orthostatic hypotension, tachycardia, palpitations, ventricular fibrillation, confusion, drowsiness, ataxia, fatigue, delirium, headache, loss of memory, restlessness; the elderly may be at increased risk for confusion and hallucinations, rash, bloated feeling, nausea, vomiting, dysuria, tremor, weakness, increased intraocular pain, blurred vision, mydriasis

**Drug Interactions**

Decreased effect: Phenothiazines, levodopa, antihistamines with cholinergic mechanisms decrease anticholinergic effects of atropine

Increased toxicity: Amantadine increases anticholinergic effects, thiazides increase effect

**Onset** I.V.: Rapid onset

**Half-Life** 2-3 hours

**Special PA Issues**

**Patient Education:** Take exactly as directed, 30 minutes before meals. Maintain adequate hydration (2-3 L/day of fluids unless instructed to restrict fluid intake). Void before taking medication. You may experience dizziness, blurred vision, sensitivity to light (use caution when driving or engaging in hazardous activity until response to medication is known); dry mouth, nausea, or vomiting (small frequent meals or sucking on lozenges may help); orthostatic hypotension (use caution when climbing stairs and when rising from lying or sitting position); constipation (increased exercise, fluid, or dietary fiber may reduce constipation, if not effective consult prescriber); increased sensitivity to heat and decreased perspiration (avoid extremes of heat, reduce exercise in hot weather); decreased milk if breast-feeding. Report hot, dry, flushed skin; blurred vision or vision changes; difficulty swallowing; chest pain, palpitations, or rapid heartbeat; painful or difficult urination; increased confusion, depression, or loss of memory; rapid or difficult respirations; muscle weakness or tremors; or eye pain.

Ophthalmic: Instill as often as recommended. Wash hands before using. Sit or lie down, open eye, look at ceiling, and instill prescribed amount of solution. Do not blink for 30 seconds, close eye and roll eye in all directions, and apply gentle pressure to inner corner of eye for 1-2 minutes. Do not let tip of applicator touch eye or contaminate tip of applicator. Temporary stinging or blurred vision may occur.

**Monitoring Parameters:** Heart rate, blood pressure, pulse, mental status; intravenous administration requires a cardiac monitor

♦ **Atropine and Diphenoxylate** *see* Diphenoxylate and Atropine *on page 290*
♦ **Atropine-Care® Ophthalmic** *see* Atropine *on previous page*
♦ **Atropine Sulfate** *see* Atropine *on previous page*

- **Atropisol® Ophthalmic** *see Atropine on page 87*
- **Atrovent®** *see Ipratropium on page 490*
- **Augmentin®** *see Amoxicillin and Clavulanate Potassium on page 62*
- **Auralgan®** *see Antipyrine and Benzocaine on page 73*

# Auranofin (au RANE oh fin)

**Pharmacologic Class** Gold Compound

**U.S. Brand Names** Ridaura®

**Mechanism of Action** The exact mechanism of action of gold is unknown; gold is taken up by macrophages which results in inhibition of phagocytosis and lysosomal membrane stabilization; other actions observed are decreased serum rheumatoid factor and alterations in immunoglobulins. Additionally, complement activation is decreased, prostaglandin synthesis is inhibited, and lysosomal enzyme activity is decreased.

**Use** Management of active stage of classic or definite rheumatoid arthritis in patients that do not respond to or tolerate other agents; psoriatic arthritis; adjunctive or alternative therapy for pemphigus

**USUAL DOSAGE** Oral:

Children: Initial: 0.1 mg/kg/day divided daily; usual maintenance: 0.15 mg/kg/day in 1-2 divided doses; maximum: 0.2 mg/kg/day in 1-2 divided doses

Adults: 6 mg/day in 1-2 divided doses; after 3 months may be increased to 9 mg/day in 3 divided doses; if still no response after 3 months at 9 mg/day, discontinue drug

**Dosing adjustment in renal impairment:**

$Cl_{cr}$ 50-80 mL/minute: Reduce dose to 50%

$Cl_{cr}$ <50 mL/minute: Avoid use

**Dosage Forms Cap:** 3 mg [gold 29%]

**Contraindications** Renal disease, history of blood dyscrasias, congestive heart failure, exfoliative dermatitis, necrotizing enterocolitis, history of anaphylactic reactions

**Warnings/Precautions** NSAIDs and corticosteroids may be discontinued after starting gold therapy; therapy should be discontinued if platelet count falls to <100,000/mm³; WBC <4000, granulocytes <1500/mm³, explain possibility of adverse effects and their manifestations; use with caution in patients with renal or hepatic impairment

**Pregnancy Risk Factor** C

**Adverse Reactions**

>10%:

Dermatologic: Itching, rash

Gastrointestinal: Stomatitis

Ocular: Conjunctivitis

Renal: Proteinuria

1% to 10%:

Dermatologic: Urticaria, alopecia

Gastrointestinal: Glossitis

Hematologic: Eosinophilia, leukopenia, thrombocytopenia

Renal: Hematuria

<1%: Angioedema, ulcerative enterocolitis, GI hemorrhage, gingivitis, dysphagia, metallic taste, agranulocytosis, anemia, aplastic anemia, hepatotoxicity, peripheral neuropathy, interstitial pneumonitis

**Drug Interactions** Increased toxicity: Penicillamine, antimalarials, hydroxychloroquine, cytotoxic agents, immunosuppressants

**Onset** Delayed; may require as long as 3 months

**Duration** Prolonged

**Special PA Issues**

**Patient Education:** Take exactly as directed. Drug effects may not be seen for as long as 3 weeks to 3 months. You may experience metallic taste or mouth sores (frequent mouth care and lozenges may help); gray-blue color or irritation and reddening of skin (avoid excessive exposure to sunlight; use sunscreen, sunglasses, and protective clothing); nausea, bloating, or loss of appetite (small frequent meals, chewing gum, or sucking on lozenges may help); or loss of hair (reversible). Report unusual bruising; blood in mouth, urine, stool, vomitus; persistent fatigue; persistent metallic taste; abdominal cramping, vomiting, diarrhea; sores in mouth; skin rash or itching; or irritated or painful eyes.

**Monitoring Parameters:** Monitor urine for protein; CBC and platelets; monitor for mouth ulcers and skin reactions; may monitor auranofin serum levels

**Reference Range:** Gold: Normal: 0-0.1 µg/mL (SI: 0-0.0064 µmol/L); Therapeutic: 1-3 µg/mL (SI: 0.06-0.18 µmol/L); Urine: <0.1 µg/24 hours

- **Auro® Ear Drops [OTC]** *see Carbamide Peroxide on page 150*
- **Aurolate®** *see Gold Sodium Thiomalate on page 422*
- **Auroto®** *see Antipyrine and Benzocaine on page 73*
- **Avapro®** *see Irbesartan on page 491*
- **Avapro® HCT** *see Irbesartan and Hydrochlorothiazide on page 492*
- **AVC™ Cream** *see Sulfanilamide on page 862*
- **AVC™ Suppository** *see Sulfanilamide on page 862*

- **Aventyl® Hydrochloride** *see* Nortriptyline *on page 665*
- **Avirax™** *see* Acyclovir *on page 28*
- **Avita®** *see* Tretinoin, Topical *on page 927*
- **Avitene®** *see* Microfibrillar Collagen Hemostat *on page 605*
- **Avlosulfon®** *see* Dapsone *on page 256*
- **Avonex™** *see* Interferon Beta-1a *on page 486*
- **Awa** *see* Kava *on page 505*
- **Axid®** *see* Nizatidine *on page 663*
- **Axid® AR [OTC]** *see* Nizatidine *on page 663*
- **Axotal®** *see* Butalbital Compound *on page 131*
- **Ayercillin®** *see* Penicillin G Procaine *on page 706*
- **Ayr® Saline [OTC]** *see* Sodium Chloride *on page 839*
- **Azactam®** *see* Aztreonam *on page 94*

## Azatadine (a ZA ta deen)

**Pharmacologic Class** Antihistamine

**U.S. Brand Names** Optimine®

**Mechanism of Action** Azatadine is a piperidine-derivative antihistamine; has both anticholinergic and antiserotonin activity; has been demonstrated to inhibit mediator release from human mast cells *in vitro*; mechanism of this action is suggested to prevent calcium entry into the mast cell through voltage-dependent calcium channels

**Use** Treatment of perennial and seasonal allergic rhinitis and chronic urticaria

**USUAL DOSAGE** Children >12 years and Adults: Oral: 1-2 mg twice daily

**Dosage Forms** Tab, as maleate: 1 mg

**Contraindications** Hypersensitivity to azatadine or to other related antihistamines including cyproheptadine; patients taking monoamine oxidase inhibitors should not use azatadine

**Warnings/Precautions** Sedation and somnolence are the most commonly reported adverse effects

**Pregnancy Risk Factor** B

**Pregnancy Implications** Excretion in breast milk unknown/not recommended

**Adverse Reactions**

>10%:

Central nervous system: Slight to moderate drowsiness

Respiratory: Thickening of bronchial secretions

1% to 10%:

Central nervous system: Headache, fatigue, nervousness, dizziness

Gastrointestinal: Appetite increase, weight gain, nausea, diarrhea, abdominal pain, xerostomia

Neuromuscular & skeletal: Arthralgia

Respiratory: Pharyngitis

<1%: Palpitations, edema, depression, angioedema, photosensitivity, rash, hepatitis, myalgia, paresthesia, bronchospasm, epistaxis

**Drug Interactions** Increased effect/toxicity: Procarbazine, CNS depressants, tricyclic antidepressants, alcohol

**Onset** 1-2 hours

**Half-Life** ~8.7 hours

**Special PA Issues**

**Patient Education:** Take as directed; do not exceed recommended dose. Avoid use of other depressants, alcohol, or sleep-inducing medications unless approved by prescriber. You may experience drowsiness or dizziness (use caution when driving or engaging in hazardous activity until response to medication is known); or dry mouth, abdominal pain, or nausea (frequent small meals, frequent mouth care, chewing gum, or sucking hard candy may help). Report persistent sore throat, difficulty breathing, or expectorating (thick secretions); excessive sedation or mental stimulation; frequent nosebleeds; unusual joint or muscle pain; or lack of improvement or worsening or condition.

**Dietary Considerations:** Alcohol: Additive CNS effects, avoid use

## Azatadine and Pseudoephedrine (a ZA ta deen & soo doe e FED rin)

**Pharmacologic Class** Antihistamine/Decongestant Combination

**U.S. Brand Names** Trinalin®

**Dosage Forms** Tab: Azatadine maleate 1 mg and pseudoephedrine sulfate 120 mg

- **Azatadine Maleate** *see* Azatadine *on this page*

## Azathioprine (ay za THYE oh preen)

**Pharmacologic Class** Immunosuppressant Agent

**U.S. Brand Names** Imuran®

**Mechanism of Action** Antagonizes purine metabolism and may inhibit synthesis of DNA, RNA, and proteins; may also interfere with cellular metabolism and inhibit mitosis

**Use** Adjunct with other agents in prevention of rejection of solid organ transplants; also used in severe active rheumatoid arthritis unresponsive to other agents; other autoimmune diseases (ITP, SLE, MS, Crohn's Disease); **azathioprine is an imidazolyl derivative of 6-mercaptopurine**

**USUAL DOSAGE I.V. dose is equivalent to oral dose** (dosing should be based on ideal body weight):
Children and Adults: Solid organ transplantation: Oral, I.V.: 2-5 mg/kg/day to start, then 1-2 mg/kg/day maintenance
Adults: Rheumatoid arthritis: Oral: 1 mg/kg/day for 6-8 weeks; increase by 0.5 mg/kg every 4 weeks until response or up to 2.5 mg/kg/day

**Dosing adjustment in renal impairment:**
$Cl_{cr}$ 10-50 mL/minute: Administer 75% of normal dose daily
$Cl_{cr}$ <10 mL/minute: Administer 50% of normal dose daily
Hemodialysis: Slightly dialyzable (5% to 20%)
Administer dose posthemodialysis
CAPD effects: Unknown
CAVH effects: Unknown

**Dosage Forms Inj:** 100 mg (20 mL); **Tab (scored):** 50 mg

**Contraindications** Hypersensitivity to azathioprine or any component; pregnancy and lactation

**Warnings/Precautions** Chronic immunosuppression increases the risk of neoplasia; has mutagenic potential to both men and women and with possible hematologic toxicities; use with caution in patients with liver disease, renal impairment; monitor hematologic function closely

**Pregnancy Risk Factor** D

**Adverse Reactions** Dose reduction or temporary withdrawal allows reversal
>10%:
Central nervous system: Fever, chills
Gastrointestinal: Nausea, vomiting, anorexia, diarrhea
Hematologic: Thrombocytopenia, leukopenia, anemia
Miscellaneous: Secondary infection
1% to 10%:
Dermatologic: Rash
Hematologic: Pancytopenia
Hepatic: Hepatotoxicity
<1%: Hypotension, alopecia, maculopapular rash, aphthous stomatitis, arthralgias, which include myalgias, rigors, retinopathy, dyspnea, rare hypersensitivity reactions

**Drug Interactions** Increased toxicity: Allopurinol (decreases azathioprine dose to $\frac{1}{3}$ to $\frac{1}{4}$ of normal dose)

**Half-Life** Parent drug: 12 minutes; 6-mercaptopurine: 0.7-3 hours; End-stage renal disease: Slightly prolonged

**Special PA Issues**
**Patient Education:** Take as prescribed (may take in divided doses or with food if GI upset occurs).
Rheumatoid arthritis: Response may not occur for up to 3 months; do not discontinue without consulting prescriber.
Organ transplant: Azathioprine will usually be prescribed with other antirejection medications.
You will be susceptible to infection (avoid vaccinations unless approved by prescriber) and avoid crowds or infected persons or persons with contagious diseases. You may experience nausea, vomiting, loss of appetite (small frequent meals, chewing gum, or sucking on lozenges may help). Report abdominal pain and unresolved gastrointestinal upset (eg, persistent vomiting or diarrhea); unusual fever or chills, bleeding or bruising, sore throat, unhealed sores, or signs of infection; yellowing of skin or eyes; or change in color of urine or stool.
**Monitoring Parameters:** CBC, platelet counts, total bilirubin, alkaline phosphatase

♦ **Azathioprine Sodium** see Azathioprine on previous page
♦ **Azdone®** see Hydrocodone and Aspirin on page 450

# Azelaic Acid (a zeh LAY ik AS id)

**Pharmacologic Class** Topical Skin Product, Acne
**U.S. Brand Names** Azelex®
**Mechanism of Action** Exact mechanism is not known; in vitro, azelaic acid possesses antimicrobial activity against Propionibacterium acnes and Staphylococcus epidermidis; may decrease microcomedo formation
**Use** Acne vulgaris: Topical treatment of mild to moderate inflammatory acne vulgaris
**USUAL DOSAGE** Adults: Topical: After skin is thoroughly washed and patted dry, gently but thoroughly massage a thin film of azelaic acid cream into the affected areas twice daily, in the morning and evening. The duration of use can vary and depends on the severity of the acne. In the majority of patients with inflammatory lesions, improvement of the condition occurs within 4 weeks.
(Continued)

## Azelaic Acid *(Continued)*

**Dosage Forms** Crm: 20% (30 g)

**Contraindications** Known hypersensitivity to any of components

**Warnings/Precautions** For external use only; not for ophthalmic use; there have been isolated reports of hypopigmentation after use. If sensitivity or severe irritation develops, discontinue treatment and institute appropriate therapy.

**Pregnancy Risk Factor** B

**Pregnancy Implications** Breast-feeding/lactation: Since <4% of a topically applied dose is systemically absorbed, the uptake of azelaic acid into breast milk is not expected to cause a significant change from baseline azelaic acid levels in the milk. However, exercise caution when administering to a nursing mother.

**Adverse Reactions**
1% to 10%:
Dermatologic: Pruritus, stinging
Local: Burning
Neuromuscular & skeletal: Paresthesia
<1%: Erythema, dryness, rash, peeling, dermatitis, contact dermatitis, irritation

**Half-Life** Healthy subjects: 12 hours after topical dosing

**Special PA Issues**
Patient Education: Apply with gloves and wash hands following application. Use for the full prescribed treatment period. Avoid the use of occlusive dressings or wrappings. Keep away from the mouth, eyes and other mucous membranes. If it does come in contact with the eyes, wash eyes with large amounts of water and consult prescriber if eye irritation persists. Patients with dark complexion should report changes in skin color. Temporary skin irritation (eg, pruritus, burning or stinging) may occur when azelaic acid is applied to broken or inflamed skin, usually at the start of treatment. However, this irritation commonly subsides if treatment is continued. If it continues, apply only once a day, or stop the treatment until these effects have subsided. If irritation persists, discontinue use and consult prescriber.

## Azelastine (a ZEL as teen)

**Pharmacologic Class** Antihistamine

**U.S. Brand Names** Astelin® Nasal Spray

**Mechanism of Action** Competes with histamine for $H_1$-receptor sites on effector cells in the blood vessels and respiratory tract; reduces hyper-reactivity of the airways; increases the motility of bronchial epithelial cilia, improving mucociliary transport

**Use** Treatment of the symptoms of seasonal allergic rhinitis such as rhinorrhea, sneezing, and nasal pruritus in adults and children >12 years of age

**USUAL DOSAGE** Children ≥12 years and Adults: 2 sprays (137 mcg/spray) each nostril twice daily. Before initial use, the delivery system should be primed with 4 sprays or until a fine mist appears. If 3 or more days have elapsed since last use, the delivery system should be reprimed.

**Dosage Forms** Spray, nasal, as hydrochloride: 137 mcg/actuation [100 actuations/bottle]

**Contraindications** Hypersensitivity to azelastine or any component

**Warnings/Precautions** Use with caution in asthmatics; patients with hepatic or renal dysfunction may require lower doses

**Pregnancy Risk Factor** C

**Adverse Reactions**
>10%:
Central nervous system: Headache (14.8%), somnolence (11.5%)
Gastrointestinal: Bitter taste (19.7%)
2% to 10%:
Central nervous system: Dizziness (2%), fatigue (2.3%)
Gastrointestinal: Nausea (2.8%), weight increase (2%), dry mouth (2.8%)
Respiratory: Nasal burning (4.1%), pharyngitis (3.8%), paroxysmal sneezing (3.1%), rhinitis (2.3%), epistaxis (2%)
<2%:
Body as a whole: Allergic reactions, back pain, viral infections, malaise, extremity pain, abdominal pain
Cardiovascular: Flushing, hypertension, tachycardia
Central nervous system: Drowsiness, headache, somnolence, fatigue, vertigo, depression, nervousness, hypoesthesia
Dermatologic: Contact dermatitis, eczema, hair and follicle infection, furunculosis
Gastrointestinal: Constipation, gastroenteritis, glossitis, increased appetite, ulcerative stomatitis, vomiting, increased ALT, aphthous stomatitis
Genitourinary: Urinary frequency, hematuria, albuminuria, amenorrhea
Neuromuscular & skeletal: Myalgia, vertigo, temporomandibular dislocation, hypoesthesia, hyperkinesia
Ocular: Conjunctivitis, watery eyes, eye pain
Respiratory: Bronchospasm, coughing, throat burning, laryngitis

Psychological: Anxiety, depersonalization, depression, nervousness, sleep disorder, abnormal thinking

**Drug Interactions** May cause additive sedation when concomitantly administered with other CNS depressant medications; cimetidine can increase the AUC and $C_{max}$ of azelastine by as much as 65%

**Special PA Issues**

**Patient Education:** Causes drowsiness and may impair ability to perform hazardous activities requiring mental alertness or physical coordination; avoid spraying in eyes

♦ **Azelastine Hydrochloride** *see Azelastine on previous page*

♦ **Azelex®** *see Azelaic Acid on page 91*

♦ **Azidothymidine** *see Zidovudine on page 972*

# Azithromycin (az ith roe MYE sin)

**Pharmacologic Class** Antibiotic, Macrolide

**U.S. Brand Names** Zithromax™

**Mechanism of Action** Inhibits RNA-dependent protein synthesis at the chain elongation step; binds to the 50S ribosomal subunit resulting in blockage of transpeptidation

**Use**

Children: Treatment of acute otitis media due to *H. influenzae*, *M. catarrhalis*, or *S. pneumoniae*; pharyngitis/tonsillitis due to *S. pyogenes*

Adults:

Treatment of mild to moderate upper and lower respiratory tract infections, infections of the skin and skin structure, and sexually transmitted diseases due to susceptible strains of *C. trachomatis*, *M. catarrhalis*, *H. influenzae*, *S. aureus*, *S. pneumoniae*, *Mycoplasma pneumoniae*, and *C. psittaci*; community-acquired pneumonia, pelvic inflammatory disease (PID)

For preventing or delaying the onset of infection with *Mycobacterium avium* complex (MAC)

Prophylaxis of bacterial endocarditis in patients who are allergic to penicillin and undergoing surgical or dental procedures

**USUAL DOSAGE**

Oral:

Children ≥6 months: Otitis media and community-acquired pneumonia: 10 mg/kg on day 1 (maximum: 500 mg/day) followed by 5 mg/kg/day once daily on days 2-5 (maximum: 250 mg/day)

Children ≥2 years: Pharyngitis, tonsillitis: 12 mg/kg/day once daily for 5 days (maximum: 500 mg/day)

Children: *M. avium*-infected patients with acquired immunodeficiency syndrome: Not currently FDA approved for use; 10-20 mg/kg/day once daily (maximum: 40 mg/kg/day) has been used in clinical trials; prophylaxis for first episode of MAC: 5-12 mg/kg/day once daily (maximum: 500 mg/day)

Adolescents ≥16 years and Adults:

Respiratory tract, skin and soft tissue infections: 500 mg on day 1 followed by 250 mg/day on days 2-5 (maximum: 500 mg/day)

Uncomplicated chlamydial urethritis/cervicitis or chancroid: Single 1 g dose

Gonococcal urethritis/cervicitis: Single 2 g dose

Prophylaxis of disseminated *M. avium* complex disease in patient with advanced HIV infection: 1200 mg once weekly (may be combined with rifabutin)

Prophylaxis for bacterial endocarditis: 500 mg 1 hour prior to the procedure

I.V.: Adults:

Community-acquired pneumonia: 500 mg as a single dose for at least 2 days, follow I.V. therapy by the oral route with a single daily dose of 500 mg to complete a 7-10 day course of therapy

Pelvic inflammatory disease (PID): 500 mg as a single dose for 1-2 days, follow I.V. therapy by the oral route with a single daily dose of 250 mg to complete a 7 day course of therapy

**Dosage Forms Cap:** 250 mg; **Cap, (Z-PAK™):** 6 capsules per package: 250 mg; **Powder for oral susp:** 100 mg/5 mL (15 mL), 200 mg/5 mL (15 mL, 22.5 mL), 1 g (single-dose packet); **Tab:** 250 mg, 600 mg

**Contraindications** Hepatic impairment, known hypersensitivity to azithromycin, other macrolide antibiotics, or any azithromycin components; use with pimozide

**Warnings/Precautions** Use with caution in patients with hepatic dysfunction; hepatic impairment with or without jaundice has occurred chiefly in older children and adults; it may be accompanied by malaise, nausea, vomiting, abdominal colic, and fever; discontinue use if these occur; may mask or delay symptoms of incubating gonorrhea or syphilis, so appropriate culture and susceptibility tests should be performed prior to initiating azithromycin; pseudomembranous colitis has been reported with use of macrolide antibiotics; safety and efficacy have not been established in children <6 months of age with acute otitis media and in children <2 years of age with pharyngitis/tonsillitis

**Pregnancy Risk Factor** B

(Continued)

## Azithromycin *(Continued)*

### Adverse Reactions
1% to 10%: Gastrointestinal: Diarrhea, nausea, abdominal pain, cramping, vomiting (especially with high single-dose regimens)

<1%: Ventricular arrhythmias, fever, headache, dizziness, rash, angioedema, hypertrophic pyloric stenosis, vaginitis, eosinophilia, elevated LFTs, cholestatic jaundice, thrombophlebitis, ototoxicity, nephritis, allergic reactions

### Drug Interactions CYP3A3/4 enzyme inhibitor
Decreased peak serum levels: Aluminum- and magnesium-containing antacids by 24% but not total absorption

Increased effect/toxicity: Azithromycin may increase levels of tacrolimus, phenytoin, ergot alkaloids, alfentanil, astemizole, terfenadine, bromocriptine, carbamazepine, cyclosporine, digoxin, disopyramide, and triazolam; azithromycin did not affect the response to warfarin or theophylline although caution is advised when administered together

Avoid use with pimozide due to significant risk of cardiotoxicity

### Half-Life 68 hours

### Special PA Issues
**Patient Education:** Take as directed. Take all of prescribed medication. Do not discontinue until prescription is completed. Take 1 hour before or 2 hours after meals. Do not take with aluminum- or magnesium-containing antacids. May cause transient abdominal distress, diarrhea, headache. Report signs of additional infections (eg, sores in mouth or vagina, vaginal discharge, unresolved fever, severe vomiting, or diarrhea).

**Dietary Considerations:** Food: Rate and extent of GI absorption decreased; take on an empty stomach

Azithromycin suspension, not tablet form, has significantly decreased absorption (46%) with food

**Monitoring Parameters:** Liver function tests, CBC with differential

♦ **Azithromycin Dihydrate** *see* Azithromycin *on previous page*

♦ **Azmacort™** *see* Triamcinolone *on page 928*

♦ **Azopt™** *see* Brinzolamide *on page 121*

♦ **Azo-Standard® [OTC]** *see* Phenazopyridine *on page 714*

♦ **Azo-Sulfisoxazole** *see* Sulfisoxazole and Phenazopyridine *on page 865*

♦ **AZT** *see* Zidovudine *on page 972*

♦ **AZT + 3TC** *see* Zidovudine and Lamivudine *on page 973*

♦ **Aztreonam** *see* Aztreonam *on this page*

## Aztreonam *(AZ tree oh nam)*

**Pharmacologic Class** Antibiotic, Miscellaneous

**U.S. Brand Names** Azactam®

**Mechanism of Action** Inhibits bacterial cell wall synthesis by binding to one or more of the penicillin binding proteins (PBPs), which in turn inhibits the final transpeptidation step of peptidoglycan synthesis in bacterial cell walls, thus inhibiting cell wall biosynthesis. Bacteria eventually lyse due to ongoing activity of cell wall autolytic enzymes (autolysins and murein hydrolases) while cell wall assembly is arrested. Monobactam structure makes cross-allergenicity with beta-lactams unlikely.

**Use** Treatment of patients with urinary tract infections, lower respiratory tract infections, septicemia, skin/skin structure infections, intra-abdominal infections, and gynecological infections caused by susceptible gram-negative bacilli; often useful in patients with allergies to penicillins or cephalosporins

### USUAL DOSAGE
Neonates: I.M., I.V.:
    Postnatal age ≤7 days:
        <2000 g: 30 mg/kg/dose every 12 hours
        >2000 g: 30 mg/kg/dose every 8 hours
    Postnatal age >7 days:
        <1200 g: 30 mg/kg/dose every 12 hours
        1200-2000 g: 30 mg/kg/dose every 8 hours
        >2000 g: 30 mg/kg/dose every 6 hours
Children >1 month: I.M., I.V.: 90-120 mg/kg/day divided every 6-8 hours
    Cystic fibrosis: 50 mg/kg/dose every 6-8 hours (ie, up to 200 mg/kg/day); maximum: 6-8 g/day
Adults:
    Urinary tract infection: I.M., I.V.: 500 mg to 1 g every 8-12 hours
    Moderately severe systemic infections: 1 g I.V. or I.M. or 2 g I.V. every 8-12 hours
    Severe systemic or life-threatening infections (especially caused by *Pseudomonas aeruginosa*): I.V.: 2 g every 6-8 hours; maximum: 8 g/day

**Dosing adjustment in renal impairment:** Adults:
    $Cl_{cr}$ >50 mL/minute: 500 mg to 1 g every 6-8 hours
    $Cl_{cr}$ 10-50 mL/minute: 50% to 75% of usual dose given at the usual interval
    $Cl_{cr}$ <10 mL/minute: 25% of usual dosage given at the usual interval

Hemodialysis: Moderately dialyzable (20% to 50%); administer dose postdialysis or supplemental dose of 500 mg after dialysis

Peritoneal dialysis: Administer as for $Cl_{cr}$ <10 mL/minute

Continuous arteriovenous or venovenous hemofiltration (CAVH/CAVHD): Dose as for $Cl_{cr}$ 10-50 mL/minute

**Dosage Forms Powder for inj:** 500 mg (15 mL, 100 mL), 1 g (15 mL, 100 mL), 2 g (15 mL, 100 mL)

**Contraindications** Hypersensitivity to aztreonam or any component

**Warnings/Precautions** Rare cross-allergenicity to penicillins and cephalosporins; requires dosing adjustment in renal impairment

**Pregnancy Risk Factor** B

**Adverse Reactions**
1% to 10%:
Dermatologic: Rash
Gastrointestinal: Diarrhea, nausea, vomiting
Local: Thrombophlebitis, pain at injection site

<1%: Hypotension, seizures, confusion, headache, vertigo, insomnia, dizziness, fever, breast tenderness, pseudomembranous colitis, aphthous ulcer, abnormal taste, halitosis, numb tongue, vaginitis, hepatitis, jaundice, elevated liver enzymes, thrombocytopenia, eosinophilia, leukopenia, neutropenia, myalgia, weakness, diplopia, tinnitus, sneezing, anaphylaxis

**Half-Life** Normal renal function: 1.7-2.9 hours; End-stage renal disease: 6-8 hours

**Special PA Issues**
**Patient Education:** This medication can only be administered I.M. or I.V. You may experience nausea or GI distress. Frequent mouth care and frequent small meals, or sucking on lozenges may help relieve these symptoms. May cause false readings with urine glucose testing. Diabetics should use alternate means of monitoring glucose. Report any unrelieved diarrhea or vomiting, pain at injection sites, unresolved fever, unhealed or new sores in mouth or vagina, vaginal discharge, or acute onset of respiratory difficulty.

**Monitoring Parameters:** Periodic liver function test; monitor for signs of anaphylaxis during first dose

♦ **Azulfidine®** see Sulfasalazine on page 862
♦ **Azulfidine® EN-tabs®** see Sulfasalazine on page 862
♦ **Babee® Teething® [OTC]** see Benzocaine on page 105
♦ **B-A-C®** see Butalbital Compound on page 131

# Bacampicillin (ba kam pi SIL in)

**Pharmacologic Class** Antibiotic, Penicillin

**U.S. Brand Names** Spectrobid®

**Mechanism of Action** Interferes with bacterial cell wall synthesis during active multiplication causing cell wall death and resultant bactericidal activity against susceptible bacteria

**Use** Treatment of susceptible bacterial infections involving the urinary tract, skin structure, upper and lower respiratory tract; activity is identical to that of ampicillin

**USUAL DOSAGE** Oral:
Children <25 kg: 25-50 mg/kg/day in divided doses every 12 hours
Children >25 kg and Adults: 400-800 mg every 12 hours
**Dosing interval in renal impairment:**
$Cl_{cr}$ 10-30 mL/minute: Administer every 24 hours
$Cl_{cr}$ <10 mL/minute: Administer every 36 hours

**Dosage Forms Powder for oral susp:** 125 mg/5 mL [chemically equivalent to ampicillin 87.5 mg per 5 mL] (70 mL); **Tab:** 400 mg [chemically equivalent to ampicillin 280 mg]

**Contraindications** Hypersensitivity to bacampicillin or any component or penicillins

**Warnings/Precautions** Use with caution in patients allergic to cephalosporins; modify dosage in patients with renal impairment; high percentage of patients with infectious mononucleosis develop a rash during amoxicillin therapy

**Pregnancy Risk Factor** B

**Adverse Reactions**
1% to 10%: Gastrointestinal: Gastric upset, diarrhea, nausea
<1%: Rash, pseudomembranous colitis, agranulocytosis, mildly increased AST, hypersensitivity reactions

**Drug Interactions**
Decreased effect of oral contraceptives
Increased levels with probenecid; allopurinol theoretically has has an additive potential for amoxicillin/ampicillin rash

**Special PA Issues**
**Patient Education:** Take oral suspension 1 hour before or 2 hours after a meal; report diarrhea promptly; entire course of medication (10-14 days) should be taken to ensure eradication of organism; should be taken in equal intervals around-the-clock to maintain adequate blood levels; may interfere with oral contraceptives, females should report symptoms of vaginitis
(Continued)

## Bacampicillin *(Continued)*

**Monitoring Parameters:** Renal, hepatic, and hematologic function tests

♦ **Bacampicillin Hydrochloride** *see Bacampicillin on previous page*
♦ **Bachelor's Buttons** *see Feverfew on page 368*
♦ **Bacid® [OTC]** *see Lactobacillus acidophilus and Lactobacillus bulgaricus on page 512*
♦ **Baciguent® Topical [OTC]** *see Bacitracin on this page*
♦ **Bacigvent** *see Bacitracin on this page*
♦ **Baci-IM® Injection** *see Bacitracin on this page*
♦ **Bacitin** *see Bacitracin on this page*

## Bacitracin *(bas i TRAY sin)*

**Pharmacologic Class** Antibiotic, Ophthalmic; Antibiotic, Topical; Antibiotic, Miscellaneous

**U.S. Brand Names** AK-Tracin® Ophthalmic; Baciguent® Topical [OTC]; Baci-IM® Injection

**Mechanism of Action** Inhibits bacterial cell wall synthesis by preventing transfer of mucopeptides into the growing cell wall

**Use** Treatment of susceptible bacterial infections mainly has activity against gram-positive bacilli; due to toxicity risks, systemic and irrigant uses of bacitracin should be limited to situations where less toxic alternatives would not be effective; oral administration has been successful in antibiotic-associated colitis and has been used for enteric eradication of vancomycin-resistant enterococci (VRE)

**USUAL DOSAGE** Children and Adults (**do not administer I.V.**):

Infants: I.M.:
≤2.5 kg: 900 units/kg/day in 2-3 divided doses
>2.5 kg: 1000 units/kg/day in 2-3 divided doses

Children: I.M.: 800-1200 units/kg/day divided every 8 hours

Adults: Antibiotic-associated colitis: Oral: 25,000 units 4 times/day for 7-10 days

Topical: Apply 1-5 times/day

Ophthalmic, ointment: Instill ¼" to ½" ribbon every 3-4 hours into conjunctival sac for acute infections, or 2-3 times/day for mild to moderate infections for 7-10 days

Irrigation, solution: 50-100 units/mL in normal saline, lactated Ringer's, or sterile water for irrigation; soak sponges in solution for topical compresses 1-5 times/day or as needed during surgical procedures

**Dosage Forms Inj:** 50,000 units; **Oint: Ophth:** 500 units/g (3.5 g, 3.75 g), AK-Tracin®: 500 units/g (3.5 g); **Top:** 500 units/g (1.5 g, 3.75 g, 15 g, 30 g, 120 g, 454 g)

**Contraindications** Hypersensitivity to bacitracin or any component; I.M. use is contraindicated in patients with renal impairment

**Warnings/Precautions** Prolonged use may result in overgrowth of nonsusceptible organisms; I.M. use may cause renal failure due to tubular and glomerular necrosis; **do not administer intravenously** because severe thrombophlebitis occurs

**Pregnancy Risk Factor** C

**Adverse Reactions** 1% to 10%:
Cardiovascular: Hypotension, edema of the face/lips, tightness of chest
Central nervous system: Pain
Dermatologic: Rash, itching
Gastrointestinal: Anorexia, nausea, vomiting, diarrhea, rectal itching
Hematologic: Blood dyscrasias
Miscellaneous: Diaphoresis

**Drug Interactions** Increased toxicity: Nephrotoxic drugs, neuromuscular blocking agents, and anesthetics (↑ neuromuscular blockade)

**Duration** 6-8 hours

**Special PA Issues**
**Patient Education:**
Oral, I.M.: Maintain adequate hydration (2-3 L/day of fluids unless instructed to restrict fluid intake). Report rash, redness, or itching; change in urinary pattern; acute dizziness; swelling of face or lips; chest pain or tightness; acute nausea or vomiting; or loss of appetite (small frequent meals or frequent mouth care may help).

Ophthalmic: Instill as many times per day as directed. Wash hands before using. Gently pull lower eyelid forward, instill prescribed amount of ointment into lower eyelid. Close eye and roll eyeball in all directions. May cause blurred vision; use caution when driving or engaging in tasks that require clear vision. Report any adverse reactions such as rash or itching, swelling of face or lips, burning or pain in eye, worsening of condition, or if condition does not improve.

Topical: Apply a thin film as many times as day as prescribed to the affected area. May cover with porous sterile bandage (avoid occlusive dressings). Do not use longer than 1 week unless advised by healthcare provider.

**Monitoring Parameters:** I.M.: Urinalysis, renal function tests

# Bacitracin and Polymyxin B (bas i TRAY sin & pol i MIKS in bee)

**Pharmacologic Class** Antibiotic, Ophthalmic; Antibiotic, Topical

**U.S. Brand Names** AK-Poly-Bac® Ophthalmic; Betadine® First Aid Antibiotics + Moisturizer [OTC]; Polysporin® Ophthalmic; Polysporin® Topical

**Dosage Forms** Oint, **Ophth:** Bacitracin 500 units and polymyxin B sulfate 10,000 units per g (3.5 g), Top: Bacitracin 500 units and polymyxin B sulfate 10,000 units per g in white petrolatum (15 g, 30 g); **Powder:** Bacitracin 500 units and polymyxin B sulfate 10,000 units per g (10 g)

# Bacitracin, Neomycin, and Polymyxin B
(bas i TRAY sin, nee oh MYE sin & pol i MIKS in bee)

**Pharmacologic Class** Antibiotic, Ophthalmic; Antibiotic, Topical

**U.S. Brand Names** AK-Spore® Ophthalmic Ointment; Medi-Quick® Topical Ointment [OTC]; Mycitracin® Topical [OTC]; Neomixin® Topical [OTC]; Neosporin® Ophthalmic Ointment; Neosporin® Topical Ointment [OTC]; Ocutricin® Topical Ointment; Septa® Topical Ointment [OTC]; Triple Antibiotic® Topical

**Dosage Forms** Oint: **Ophth:** Bacitracin 400 units, neomycin sulfate 3.5 mg, and polymyxin B sulfate 10,000 units and per g; **Top:** Bacitracin 400 units, neomycin sulfate 3.5 mg, and polymyxin B sulfate 5000 units per g

# Bacitracin, Neomycin, Polymyxin B, and Hydrocortisone
(bas i TRAY sin, nee oh MYE sin, pol i MIKS in bee & hye droe KOR ti sone)

**Pharmacologic Class** Antibiotic, Ophthalmic; Antibiotic, Otic; Antibiotic, Topical; Corticosteroid, Ophthalmic; Corticosteroid, Otic; Corticosteroid, Topical

**U.S. Brand Names** AK-Spore H.C.® Ophthalmic Ointment; Cortisporin® Ophthalmic Ointment; Cortisporin® Topical Ointment; Neotricin HC® Ophthalmic Ointment

**Dosage Forms** Oint: **Ophth:** Bacitracin 400 units, neomycin sulfate 3.5 mg, polymyxin B sulfate 10,000 units, and hydrocortisone 10 mg per g (3.5 g), Top: Bacitracin 400 units, neomycin sulfate 3.5 mg, polymyxin B sulfate 10,000 units, and hydrocortisone 10 mg per g (15 g)

# Baclofen (BAK loe fen)

**Pharmacologic Class** Skeletal Muscle Relaxant

**U.S. Brand Names** Lioresal®

**Mechanism of Action** Inhibits the transmission of both monosynaptic and polysynaptic reflexes at the spinal cord level, possibly by hyperpolarization of primary afferent fiber terminals, with resultant relief of muscle spasticity

**Use** Treatment of reversible spasticity associated with multiple sclerosis or spinal cord lesions

**Unlabeled use:** Intractable hiccups, intractable pain relief, and bladder spasticity

**USUAL DOSAGE**

Oral (avoid abrupt withdrawal of drug):

Children:

2-7 years: Initial: 10-15 mg/24 hours divided every 8 hours; titrate dose every 3 days in increments of 5-15 mg/day to a maximum of 40 mg/day

≥8 years: Maximum: 60 mg/day in 3 divided doses

Adults: 5 mg 3 times/day, may increase 5 mg/dose every 3 days to a maximum of 80 mg/day

Hiccups: Adults: Usual effective dose: 10-20 mg 2-3 times/day

Intrathecal:

Test dose: 50-100 mcg, doses >50 mcg should be given in 25 mcg increments, separated by 24 hours

Maintenance: After positive response to test dose, a maintenance intrathecal infusion can be administered via an implanted intrathecal pump. Initial dose via pump: Infusion at a 24-hour rate dosed at twice the test dose.

**Dosing adjustment in renal impairment:** It is necessary to reduce dosage in renal impairment but there are no specific guidelines available

Hemodialysis: Poor water solubility allows for accumulation during chronic hemodialysis. Low-dose therapy is recommended. There have been several case reports of accumulation of baclofen resulting in toxicity symptoms (organic brain syndrome, myoclonia, deceleration and steep potentials in EEG) in patients with renal failure who have received normal doses of baclofen.

**Dosage Forms** Inj, intrathecal, preservative free: 500 mcg/mL (20 mL), 2000 mcg/mL (5 mL); **Tab:** 10 mg, 20 mg

**Contraindications** Hypersensitivity to baclofen or any component

**Warnings/Precautions** Use with caution in patients with seizure disorder, impaired renal function; avoid abrupt withdrawal of the drug; elderly are more sensitive to the effects of baclofen and are more likely to experience adverse CNS effects at higher doses.

**Pregnancy Risk Factor** C

(Continued)

## Baclofen *(Continued)*

### Adverse Reactions
>10%:
  Central nervous system: Drowsiness, vertigo, psychiatric disturbances, insomnia, slurred speech, ataxia, hypotonia
  Neuromuscular & skeletal: Weakness
1% to 10%:
  Cardiovascular: Hypotension
  Central nervous system: Fatigue, confusion, headache
  Dermatologic: Rash
  Gastrointestinal: Nausea, constipation
  Genitourinary: Polyuria
<1%: Palpitations, chest pain, syncope, euphoria, excitement, depression, hallucinations, xerostomia, anorexia, abnormal taste, abdominal pain, vomiting, diarrhea, enuresis, urinary retention, dysuria, impotence, inability to ejaculate, nocturia, paresthesia, hematuria, dyspnea

### Drug Interactions
Increased effect: Opiate analgesics, benzodiazepines, hypertensive agents
Increased toxicity: CNS depressants and alcohol (sedation), tricyclic antidepressants (short-term memory loss), clindamycin (neuromuscular blockade), guanabenz (sedation), MAO inhibitors (decrease blood pressure, CNS, and respiratory effects)

**Onset** Muscle relaxation effect requires 3-4 days; Peak effect: Maximal clinical effect is not seen for 5-10 days

**Half-Life** 3.5 hours

### Special PA Issues
**Patient Education:** Take this drug as prescribed. Do not discontinue without consulting prescriber (abrupt discontinuation may cause hallucinations). Do not take any prescription or OTC sleep-inducing drugs, sedatives, antispasmodics without consulting prescriber. Avoid alcohol use. You may experience transient drowsiness, lethargy, or dizziness; use caution when driving or engaging in hazardous activities. Frequent small meals or lozenges may reduce GI upset. Report unresolved insomnia, painful urination, change in urinary patterns, constipation, or persistent confusion.

- ◆ **Bacticort® Otic** *see* Neomycin, Polymyxin B, and Hydrocortisone *on page 645*
- ◆ **Bactocill®** *see* Oxacillin *on page 682*
- ◆ **BactoShield® Topical [OTC]** *see* Chlorhexidine Gluconate *on page 190*
- ◆ **Bactrim™** *see* Co-Trimoxazole *on page 238*
- ◆ **Bactrim™ DS** *see* Co-Trimoxazole *on page 238*
- ◆ **Bactroban®** *see* Mupirocin *on page 622*
- ◆ **Bactroban® Nasal** *see* Mupirocin *on page 622*
- ◆ **Baking Soda** *see* Sodium Bicarbonate *on page 838*
- ◆ **Baldex®** *see* Dexamethasone *on page 264*
- ◆ **Balminil® Decongestant** *see* Pseudoephedrine *on page 780*
- ◆ **Balminil® Expectorant** *see* Guaifenesin *on page 427*
- ◆ **Bancap®** *see* Butalbital Compound *on page 131*
- ◆ **Bancap HC®** *see* Hydrocodone and Acetaminophen *on page 449*
- ◆ **Banophen® Oral [OTC]** *see* Diphenhydramine *on page 289*
- ◆ **Bapadin®** *see* Bepridil *on page 109*
- ◆ **Barbidonna®** *see* Hyoscyamine, Atropine, Scopolamine, and Phenobarbital *on page 464*
- ◆ **Barc™ Liquid [OTC]** *see* Pyrethrins *on page 783*
- ◆ **Baridium® [OTC]** *see* Phenazopyridine *on page 714*
- ◆ **Barophen®** *see* Hyoscyamine, Atropine, Scopolamine, and Phenobarbital *on page 464*

## Basiliximab *(ba si LIKS i mab)*
**Pharmacologic Class** Immunosuppressant Agent; Monoclonal Antibody
**U.S. Brand Names** Simulect®
**Mechanism of Action** Chimeric (murine/human) monoclonal antibody which blocks the alpha-chain of the interleukin-2 (IL-2) receptor complex; this receptor is expressed on activated T lymphocytes and is a critical pathway for activating cell-mediated allograft rejection
**Use** Prophylaxis of acute organ rejection in renal transplantation
**USUAL DOSAGE** I.V.:
  Children 2-15 years of age: 12 mg/m² (maximum: 20 mg) within 2 hours prior to transplant surgery, followed by a second dose of 12 mg/m² (maximum: 20 mg/dose) 4 days after transplantation
  Adults: 20 mg within 2 hours prior to transplant surgery, followed by a second 20 mg dose 4 days after transplantation
  **Dosing adjustment/comments in renal or hepatic impairment**: No specific dosing adjustment recommended

**Dosage Forms** Powder for inj: 20 mg

**Contraindications** Known hypersensitivity to murine proteins or any component of this product

**Warnings/Precautions** To be used as a component of immunosuppressive regimen which includes cyclosporine and corticosteroids. Only physicians experienced in transplantation and immunosuppression should prescribe, and patients should receive the drug in a facility with adequate equipment and staff capable of providing the laboratory and medical support required for transplantation.

The incidence of lymphoproliferative disorders and/or opportunistic infections may be increased by immunosuppressive therapy. Hypersensitivity reactions have not been observed in clinical trials. However, similar medications have been associated with reactions including urticaria, dyspnea, and hypotension. Discontinue the drug if a reaction occurs. Medications for the treatment of hypersensitivity reactions should be available for immediate use. Effects of readministration have not been evaluated in humans. Treatment may result in the development of human antimurine antibodies (HAMA); however, limited evidence suggesting the use of muromonab-CD3 or other murine products is not precluded.

**Pregnancy Risk Factor** B

**Pregnancy Implications** IL-2 receptors play an important role in the development of the immune system. Use in pregnant women only when benefit exceeds potential risk to the fetus. Women of childbearing potential should use effective contraceptive measures before beginning treatment and for 2 months after completion of therapy with this agent.

It is not known whether basiliximab is excreted in human milk. Because many immunoglobulins are secreted in milk and the potential for serious adverse reactions exists, a decision should be made whether to discontinue nursing or discontinue the drug, taking into account the importance of the drug to the mother.

**Adverse Reactions** Administration of basiliximab did not appear to increase the incidence or severity of adverse effects in clinical trials. Adverse events were reported in 99% of both the placebo and basiliximab groups.

>10%:
Cardiovascular: Edema, peripheral edema, hypertension
Central nervous system: Fever, headache, dizziness, insomnia
Dermatologic: Wound complications, acne
Endocrine and metabolic: Hypokalemia, hyperkalemia, hyperglycemia, hyperuricemia, hypophosphatemia, hypocalcemia, hypercholesterolemia, acidosis
Gastrointestinal: Constipation, nausea, diarrhea, abdominal pain, vomiting, dyspepsia, moniliasis, weight gain
Genitourinary: Dysuria, urinary tract infection
Hematologic: Anemia
Neuromuscular and skeletal: Leg pain, back pain, tremor
Respiratory: Dyspnea, infection (upper respiratory), coughing, rhinitis, pharyngitis
Miscellaneous: Viral infection, asthenia

3% to 10%:
Cardiovascular: Chest pain, cardiac failure, hypotension, arrhythmia, tachycardia, vascular disorder, generalized edema
Central nervous system: Hypoesthesia, neuropathy, agitation, anxiety, depression, malaise, fatigue, rigors
Dermatologic: Cyst, herpes infection, hypertrichosis, pruritus, rash, skin disorder, skin ulceration
Endocrine and metabolic: Dehydration, diabetes mellitus, fluid overload, hypercalcemia, hyperlipidemia, hypoglycemia, hypomagnesemia
Gastrointestinal: Flatulence, gastroenteritis, GI hemorrhage, gingival hyperplasia, melena, esophagitis, stomatitis
Genitourinary: Impotence, genital edema, albuminuria, bladder disorder, hematuria, urinary frequency, oliguria, abnormal renal function, renal tubular necrosis, ureteral disorder, urinary retention
Hematologic: Hematoma, hemorrhage, purpura, thrombocytopenia, thrombosis, polycythemia
Neuromuscular and skeletal: Arthralgia, arthropathy, cramps, fracture, hernia, myalgia, paresthesia
Ocular: Cataract, conjunctivitis, abnormal vision
Renal: Increased BUN
Respiratory: Bronchitis, bronchospasm, pneumonia, pulmonary edema, sinusitis
Miscellaneous: Accidental trauma, facial edema, sepsis, infection, increased glucocorticoids

**Drug Interactions** Basiliximab is an immunoglobulin; specific drug interactions have not been evaluated, but are not anticipated

**Duration** Mean: 36 days (determined by IL-2R alpha saturation)

**Half-Life** Mean: 7.2 days

**Special PA Issues**
    **Patient Education:** This medication, which may help to reduce transplant rejection, can only be given by infusion. You will be monitored and assessed closely during infusion and
(Continued)

## Basiliximab (Continued)

thereafter, however, it is important that you report any changes or problems for evaluation. You will be susceptible to infection; avoid crowds or infected persons or persons with contagious diseases. Frequent mouth care and small frequent meals may help counteract any GI effects you may experience and will help maintain adequate nutrition and fluid intake. Report any changes in urination; unusual bruising or bleeding; chest pain or palpitations; acute dizziness; respiratory difficulty; fever or chills; changes in cognition; rash; feelings of pain or numbness in extremities; severe GI upset or diarrhea; unusual back or leg pain or muscle tremors; vision changes; or any sign of infection (chills, fever, sore throat, easy bruising or bleeding, mouth sores, unhealed sores, vaginal discharge).

**Monitoring Parameters:** Signs and symptoms of acute rejection

- ♦ **Baycol™** see Cerivastatin on page 182
- ♦ **Bayer® Aspirin [OTC]** see Aspirin on page 80
- ♦ **Bayer® Buffered Aspirin [OTC]** see Aspirin on page 80
- ♦ **Bayer® Low Adult Strength [OTC]** see Aspirin on page 80
- ♦ **BAY W6228** see Cerivastatin on page 182
- ♦ **B Complex** see Vitamins, Multiple on page 964
- ♦ **B Complex With C** see Vitamins, Multiple on page 964

## Becaplermin (be KAP ler min)

**Pharmacologic Class** Growth Factor, Platelet-derived; Topical Skin Product

**U.S. Brand Names** Regranex®

**Mechanism of Action** Recombinant B-isoform homodimer of human platelet-derived growth factor (rPDGF-BB) which enhances formation of new granulation tissue, induces fibroblast proliferation, and differentiation to promote wound healing

**Use** Debridement adjunct for the treatment of diabetic ulcers that occur on the lower limbs and feet

**USUAL DOSAGE** Adults: Topical:

Diabetic ulcers: Apply appropriate amount of gel once daily with a cotton swab or similar tool, as a coating over the ulcer

The amount of becaplermin to be applied will vary depending on the size of the ulcer area. To calculate the length of gel to apply to the ulcer, measure the greatest length of the ulcer by the greatest width of the ulcer in inches. Refer to following table to calculate the length of gel to administer.

### Formula to Calculate Length of Gel in Inches to be Applied Daily

| Tube Size | Formula |
| --- | --- |
| 15 or 7.5 g tube | length x width x 0.6 |
| 2 g tube | length x width x 1.3 |

**Note:** If the ulcer does not decrease in size by ~30% after 10 weeks of treatment or complete healing has not occurred in 20 weeks, continued treatment with becaplermin gel should be reassessed.

**Dosage Forms Gel, top:** 0.01%

**Contraindications** Hypersensitivity to becaplermin or any component of its formulation; known neoplasm(s) at the site(s) of application; active infection at ulcer site

**Warnings/Precautions** Concurrent use of corticosteroids, cancer chemotherapy, or other immunosuppressive agents; ulcer wounds related to arterial or venous insufficiency. Thermal, electrical, or radiation burns at wound site. Malignancy (potential for tumor proliferation, although unproven; topical absorption is minimal). Should not be used in wounds that close by primary intention. For external use only.

**Pregnancy Risk Factor** C

**Adverse Reactions** <1%: Erythema with purulent discharge, ulcer infection, tunneling of ulcer, exuberant granulation tissue, local pain, skin ulceration

**Special PA Issues**

**Patient Education:**

Hands should be washed thoroughly before applying. The tip of the tube should not come into contact with the ulcer or any other surface; the tube should be recapped tightly after each use. A cotton swab, tongue depressor, or other application aid should be used to apply gel.

Step-by-step instructions for application:

Squeeze the calculated length of gel on to a clean, firm, nonabsorbable surface (wax paper)

With a clean cotton swab, tongue depressor, or similar application aid, spread the measured gel over the ulcer area to obtain an even layer

Cover with a saline-moistened gauze dressing. After ~12 hours, the ulcer should be gently rinsed with saline or water to remove residual gel and covered with a saline-moistened gauze dressing (**without** gel).

**Monitoring Parameters:** Ulcer volume (pressure ulcers); wound area; evidence of closure; drainage (diabetic ulcers); signs/symptoms of toxicity (erythema, local infections)

♦ **Beclodisk®** *see* Beclomethasone *on this page*

♦ **Becloforte®** *see* Beclomethasone *on this page*

# Beclomethasone (be kloe METH a sone)

**Pharmacologic Class** Corticosteroid, Oral Inhaler; Corticosteroid, Nasal

**U.S. Brand Names** Beclovent® Oral Inhaler; Beconase AQ® Nasal Inhaler; Beconase® Nasal Inhaler; Vancenase® AQ Inhaler; Vancenase® Nasal Inhaler; Vanceril® Oral Inhaler

**Mechanism of Action** Controls the rate of protein synthesis, depresses the migration of polymorphonuclear leukocytes, fibroblasts, reverses capillary permeability, and lysosomal stabilization at the cellular level to prevent or control inflammation

**Use**

Oral inhalation: Treatment of bronchial asthma in patients who require chronic administration of corticosteroids

Nasal aerosol: Symptomatic treatment of seasonal or perennial rhinitis and nasal polyposis

**USUAL DOSAGE** Nasal inhalation and oral inhalation dosage forms are not to be used interchangeably

Aqueous inhalation, nasal:

Vancenase® AQ, Beconase® AQ: Children ≥6 years and Adults: 1-2 inhalations each nostril twice daily

Vancenase® AQ 84 mcg: Children ≥6 years and Adults: 1-2 inhalations in each nostril once daily

Intranasal (Vancenase®, Beconase®):

Children 6-12 years: 1 inhalation in each nostril 3 times/day

Children ≥12 years and Adults: 1 inhalation in each nostril 2-4 times/day or 2 inhalations each nostril twice daily; usual maximum maintenance: 1 inhalation in each nostril 3 times/day

Oral inhalation (doses should be titrated to the lowest effective dose once asthma is controlled):

Beclovent®, Vanceril®:

Children 6-12 years: 1-2 inhalations 3-4 times/day (alternatively: 2-4 inhalations twice daily); maximum dose: 10 inhalations/day

Children ≥12 years and Adults: 2 inhalations 3-4 times/day (alternatively: 4 inhalations twice daily); maximum dose: 20 inhalations/day; patients with severe asthma: Initial: 12-16 inhalations/day (divided 3-4 times/day); dose should be adjusted downward according to patient's response

Vanceril® 84 mcg double strength:

Children 6-12 years: 2 inhalations twice daily; maximum dose: 5 inhalations/day

Children ≥12 years and Adults: 2 inhalations twice daily; maximum dose: 10 inhalations/day; patients with severe asthma: Initial: 6-8 inhalations/day (divided twice daily); dose should be adjusted downward according to patient's response

NIH Guidelines (NIH, 1997) (give in divided doses):

Children:

"Low" dose: 84-336 mcg/day (42 mcg/puff: 2-8 puffs/day or 84 mcg/puff: 1-4 puffs/day)

"Medium" dose: 336-672 mcg/day (42 mcg/puff: 8-16 puffs/day or 84 mcg/puff: 4-8 puffs/day)

"High" dose: >672 mcg/day (42 mcg/puff: >16 puffs/day or 84 mcg/puff >8 puffs/day)

Adults:

"Low" dose: 168-504 mcg/day (42 mcg/puff: 4-12 puffs/day or 84 mcg/puff: 2-6 puffs/day)

"Medium" dose: 504-840 mcg/day (42 mcg/puff: 12-20 puffs/day or 84 mcg/puff: 6-10 puffs/day)

"High" dose: >840 mcg/day (42 mcg/puff: >20 puffs/day or 84 mcg/puff: >10 puffs/day)

**Dosage Forms Beclomethasone dipropionate: Nasal: Inhalation:** (Beconase®, Vancenase®): 42 mcg/inhalation [200 metered doses] (16.8 g), **Spray, (Vancenase® AQ Nasal):** 0.084% [120 actuations] (19 g) **Spray, aqueous, nasal, (Beconase® AQ, Vancenase® AQ):** 42 mcg/inhalation [≥200 metered doses] (25 g), 84 mcg/inhalation [≥200 metered doses] (25 g); **Oral: Inhalation:** Beclovent®, Vanceril®: 42 mcg/inhalation [200 metered doses] (16.8 g), Vanceril® Double Strength: 84 mcg/inhalation (5.4 g - 40 metered doses, 12.2 g - 120 metered doses)

**Contraindications** Status asthmaticus; hypersensitivity to the drug or fluorocarbons, oleic acid in the formulation, systemic fungal infections

**Warnings/Precautions** Not to be used in status asthmaticus; safety and efficacy in children <6 years of age have not been established; avoid using higher than recommended dosages since suppression of hypothalamic, pituitary, or adrenal function may occur
(Continued)

# Beclomethasone *(Continued)*

Controlled clinical studies have shown that inhaled and intranasal corticosteroids may cause a reduction in growth velocity in pediatric patients. Growth velocity provides a means of comparing the rate of growth among children of the same age.

In studies involving inhaled corticosteroids, the average reduction in growth velocity was approximately 1 cm (about 1/3 of an inch) per year. It appears that the reduction is related to dose and how long the child takes the drug.

FDA's Pulmonary and Allergy Drugs and Metabolic and Endocrine Drugs advisory committees discussed this issue at a July 1998 meeting. They recommended that the agency develop class-wide labeling to inform healthcare providers so they would understand this potential side effect and monitor growth routinely in pediatric patients who are treated with inhaled corticosteroids, intranasal corticosteroids or both.

Long-term effects of this reduction in growth velocity on final adult height are unknown. Likewise, it also has not yet been determined whether patients' growth will "catch up" if treatment in discontinued. Drug manufacturers will continue to monitor these drugs to learn more about long-term effects. Children are prescribed inhaled corticosteroids to treat asthma. Intranasal corticosteroids are generally used to prevent and treat allergy-related nasal symptoms.

Patients are advised not to stop using their inhaled or intranasal corticosteroids without first speaking to their healthcare providers about the benefits of these drugs compared to their risks.

**Pregnancy Risk Factor** C

**Pregnancy Implications** Data does not support an association between drug and congenital defects in humans

Clinical effects on fetus: No data on crossing the placenta or effects on the fetus

Breast-feeding/lactation: No data on crossing into breast milk or effects on the infant

**Adverse Reactions**
>10%:
Local: Growth of *Candida* in the mouth, irritation and burning of the nasal mucosa
Respiratory: Cough, hoarseness
1% to 10%:
Gastrointestinal: Xerostomia
Local: Nasal ulceration
Respiratory: Epistaxis
<1%: Headache, rash, dysphagia, bronchospasm, rhinorrhea, nasal congestion, sneezing, nasal septal perforations

**Onset** Therapeutic effect: Within 1-4 weeks of use

**Half-Life** Oral: Initial: 3 hours; Terminal: 15 hours

**Special PA Issues**
**Patient Education:** Use as directed; do not increase dosage or discontinue abruptly without consulting prescriber. It may take 1-4 weeks for you to realize full effects of treatment. Review use of inhaler or spray with prescriber or follow package insert for directions. Keep oral inhaler clean and unobstructed. Always rinse mouth and throat after use of inhaler to prevent opportunistic infection. If you are also using an inhaled bronchodilator, wait 10 minutes before using this steroid aerosol. Report adverse effects such as skin redness, rash, or irritation; pain or burning of nasal mucosa; white plaques in mouth or fuzzy tongue; unresolved headache; or worsening of condition or lack of improvement.

**Related Information**
Asthma Therapy Guidelines *on page 1049*

- ♦ **Beclomethasone Dipropionate** *see Beclomethasone on previous page*
- ♦ **Beclovent® Oral Inhaler** *see Beclomethasone on previous page*
- ♦ **Beconase AQ® Nasal Inhaler** *see Beclomethasone on previous page*
- ♦ **Beconase® Nasal Inhaler** *see Beclomethasone on previous page*
- ♦ **Becotin® Pulvules®** *see Vitamins, Multiple on page 964*
- ♦ **Beepen-VK®** *see Penicillin V Potassium on page 706*
- ♦ **Belix® Oral [OTC]** *see Diphenhydramine on page 289*

# Belladonna and Opium *(bel a DON a & OH pee um)*

**Pharmacologic Class** Analgesic, Narcotic

**U.S. Brand Names** B&O Supprettes®

**Mechanism of Action** Anticholinergic alkaloids act primarily by competitive inhibition of the muscarinic actions of acetylcholine on structures innervated by postganglionic cholinergic neurons and on smooth muscle; resulting effects include antisecretory activity on exocrine glands and intestinal mucosa and smooth muscle relaxation. Contains many narcotic alkaloids including morphine; its mechanism for gastric motility inhibition is primarily due to this morphine content; it results in a decrease in digestive secretions, an increase in GI muscle tone, and therefore a reduction in GI propulsion.

**Use** Relief of moderate to severe pain associated with rectal or bladder tenesmus that may occur in postoperative states and neoplastic situations; pain associated with ureteral spasms not responsive to non-narcotic analgesics and to space intervals between injections of opiates

**USUAL DOSAGE** Adults: Rectal: 1 suppository 1-2 times/day, up to 4 doses/day

**Dosage Forms** Supp: #15 A: Belladonna extract 15 mg and opium 30 mg, #16 A: Belladonna extract 15 mg and opium 60 mg

**Contraindications** Glaucoma, severe renal or hepatic disease, bronchial asthma, respiratory depression, convulsive disorders, acute alcoholism, premature labor

**Warnings/Precautions** Usual precautions of opiate agonist therapy should be observed; infants <3 months of age are more susceptible to respiratory depression, use with caution and generally in reduced doses in this age group

**Pregnancy Risk Factor** C

**Adverse Reactions**
>10%:
Dermatologic: Dry skin
Gastrointestinal: Constipation, dry throat, xerostomia
Local: Irritation at injection site
Respiratory: Dry nose
Miscellaneous: Diaphoresis (decreased)

1% to 10%:
Dermatologic: Increased sensitivity to light
Endocrine & metabolic: Decreased flow of breast milk
Gastrointestinal: Dysphagia

<1%: Orthostatic hypotension, ventricular fibrillation, tachycardia, palpitations, confusion, drowsiness, headache, loss of memory, fatigue, ataxia, CNS depression, rash, antidiuretic hormone release, bloated feeling, nausea, vomiting, constipation, biliary tract spasm, dysuria, urinary retention, urinary tract spasm, increased intraocular pain, blurred vision, weakness, respiratory depression, histamine release, physical and psychological dependence, diaphoresis

**Drug Interactions**
Decreased effect: Phenothiazines
Increased effect/toxicity: CNS depressants, tricyclic antidepressants

**Onset** Belladonna: 1-2 hours; Opium: Within 30 minutes

**Special PA Issues**
**Patient Education:** If self-administered, use exactly as directed (do not increase dose or frequency); may cause physical and/or psychological dependence. Take with food or milk. While using this medication, do not use alcohol and other prescription or OTC medications (especially sedatives, tranquilizers, antihistamines, or pain medications) without consulting prescriber. Maintain adequate hydration (2-3 L/day of fluids unless instructed to restrict fluid intake). May cause hypotension, dizziness, or drowsiness (use caution when driving, climbing stairs, or changing position (rising from sitting or lying to standing) or when engaging in hazardous activities until response to medication is known); dry mouth or throat (frequent mouth care, frequent sips of fluids, chewing gum, or sucking on lozenges may help); constipation (increased exercise, fluids, or dietary fruit and fiber may help - if constipation remains an unresolved problem, consult prescriber about use of stool softeners); photosensitivity (wear protective clothing and eye wear, use sunscreen, and avoid extensive exposure to direct sunlight); decreased perspiration (avoid extremes in temperature or excessive activity in hot environments). Report chest pain or palpitations; persistent dizziness; changes in mentation; changes in gait; blurred vision; shortness of breath or difficulty breathing.

## Belladonna, Phenobarbital, and Ergotamine Tartrate
(bel AY DON a, fee noe BAR bi tal, & er GOT a meen TAR trate)
**Pharmacologic Class** Ergot Derivative
**U.S. Brand Names** Bellergal-S®; Bel-Phen-Ergot S®; Phenerbel-S®
**Dosage Forms** Tab, sustained release: l-alkaloids of belladonna 0.2 mg, phenobarbital 40 mg, and ergotamine tartrate 0.6 mg
**Half-Life** Ergotamine: 21 hours

♦ **Bellergal-S®** see Belladonna, Phenobarbital, and Ergotamine Tartrate on this page
♦ **Bel-Phen-Ergot S®** see Belladonna, Phenobarbital, and Ergotamine Tartrate on this page
♦ **Benadryl® Injection** see Diphenhydramine on page 289
♦ **Benadryl® Oral [OTC]** see Diphenhydramine on page 289
♦ **Benadryl® Topical** see Diphenhydramine on page 289
♦ **Ben-Allergin-50® Injection** see Diphenhydramine on page 289

## Benazepril (ben AY ze pril)
**Pharmacologic Class** Angiotensin-Converting Enzyme (ACE) Inhibitors
**U.S. Brand Names** Lotensin®
**Mechanism of Action** Competitive inhibition of angiotensin I being converted to angiotensin II, a potent vasoconstrictor, through the angiotensin I-converting enzyme (ACE)
(Continued)

## Benazepril *(Continued)*

activity, with resultant lower levels of angiotensin II which causes an increase in plasma renin activity and a reduction in aldosterone secretion

**Use** Treatment of hypertension, either alone or in combination with other antihypertensive agents

**USUAL DOSAGE** Adults: Oral: 20-40 mg/day as a single dose or 2 divided doses; base dosage adjustments on peak (2-6 hours after dosing) and trough responses

**Dosing interval in renal impairment:** $Cl_{cr}$ <30 mL/minute: Administer 5 mg/day initially; maximum daily dose: 40 mg

Hemodialysis: Moderately dialyzable (20% to 50%); administer dose postdialysis or administer 25% to 35% supplemental dose

Peritoneal dialysis: Supplemental dose is not necessary

**Dosage Forms** Tab, as hydrochloride: 5 mg, 10 mg, 20 mg, 40 mg

**Contraindications** Hypersensitivity to benazepril or any component or other ACE inhibitors

**Warnings/Precautions** Use with caution in patients with collagen vascular disease, hypovolemia, valvular stenosis, hyperkalemia, recent anesthesia; modify dosage in patients with renal impairment (especially renal artery stenosis), severe congestive heart failure, or with coadministered diuretic therapy; experience in children is limited; severe hypotension may occur in patients who are sodium and/or volume depleted; initiate lower doses and monitor closely when starting therapy in these patients

**Pregnancy Risk Factor** C (1st trimester); D (2nd & 3rd trimester)

**Pregnancy Implications** Enters breast milk/compatible

Clinical effects on the fetus: No data available on crossing the placenta. Cranial defects, hypocalvaria/acalvaria, oligohydramnios, persistent anuria following delivery, hypotension, renal defects, renal dysgenesis/dysplasia, renal failure, pulmonary hypoplasia, limb contractures secondary to oligohydramnios and stillbirth reported. ACE inhibitors should be avoided during pregnancy.

**Adverse Reactions**

1% to 10%:

Central nervous system: Headache, dizziness, fatigue

Gastrointestinal: Nausea (1% to 2%)

Respiratory: Transient cough

<1%: Hypotension, tachycardia, anxiety, insomnia, nervousness, rash, photosensitivity, angioedema, hyperkalemia, constipation, gastritis, vomiting, melena, impotence, urinary tract infection, hypertonia, paresthesia, arthralgia, arthritis, myalgia, weakness, asthma, bronchitis, dyspnea, sinusitis, diaphoresis

**Drug Interactions** See Drug-Drug Interactions With ACEIs table *on page 997*

**Onset**

Reduction in plasma angiotensin-converting enzyme activity: Oral: Peak effect: 1-2 hours after administration of 2-20 mg dose

Reduction in blood pressure: Peak effect after single oral dose: 2-6 hours; Maximum response with continuous therapy: 2 weeks

**Duration** >90% inhibition for 24 hours has been observed after 5-20 mg dose

**Half-Life** Parent drug: 0.6 hour; Metabolite elimination: 22 hours (from 24 hours after dosing onward); Metabolite: 1.5-2 hours after fasting or 2-4 hours after a meal

**Special PA Issues**

**Patient Education:** Take exactly as directed; do not discontinue without consulting prescriber. May cause dizziness, fainting, lightheadedness (use caution when driving or engaging in hazardous tasks); postural hypotension (use caution when rising from lying or sitting position or climbing stairs); nausea, dry cough, or transient loss of appetite (small frequent meals, frequent mouth care, or sucking on lozenges may help - report if these persist). Report mouth sores; fever or chills; swelling of extremities, face and mouth, or tongue; or difficulty in breathing.

**Related Information**

ACE Inhibitors *on page 995*

Drug-Drug Interactions With ACEIs *on page 997*

## Benazepril and Hydrochlorothiazide

(ben AY ze pril & hye droe klor oh THYE a zide)

**Pharmacologic Class** Antihypertensive Agent, Combination

**U.S. Brand Names** Lotensin® HCT

**Dosage Forms** Tab: Benazepril 5 mg and hydrochlorothiazide 6.25 mg, Benazepril 10 mg and hydrochlorothiazide 12.5 mg, Benazepril 20 mg and hydrochlorothiazide 12.5 mg, Benazepril 20 mg and hydrochlorothiazide 25 mg

♦ **Benazepril Hydrochloride** *see* Benazepril *on previous page*

♦ **Benemid®** *see* Probenecid *on page 758*

## Bentoquatam (ben to KWA tam)

**Pharmacologic Class** Topical Skin Product

**U.S. Brand Names** IvyBlock®

**Mechanism of Action** An organoclay substance which is capable of absorbing or binding to urushiol, the active principle in poison oak, ivy, and sumac. Bentoquatam serves as a barrier, blocking urushiol skin contact/absorption.

**Use** Skin protectant for the prevention of allergic contact dermatitis to poison oak, ivy, and sumac

**USUAL DOSAGE** Children >6 years and Adults: Topical: Apply to skin 15 minutes prior to potential exposure to poison ivy, poison oak, or poison sumac, and reapply every 4 hours

**Dosage Forms Lot:** 5% (120 mL)

**Contraindications** Hypersensitivity to bentoquatam

**Warnings/Precautions** Use with caution in patients with history of allergic-type responses to medications (especially topical formulations); open wounds, psoriatic lesions, or other cutaneous conditions. Use with caution in patients who are postexposure to poison oak, ivy, or sumac (lack of efficacy).

**Adverse Reactions** <1%: Erythema

**Special PA Issues**

**Patient Education:** Do not use this medication if you have had an allergic reaction to bentoquatam. Do not use this medication on children <6 years of age, unless ordered by your child's physician. Do not use this medication to treat a rash caused by poison ivy, oak, or sumac.

Use this medication on your skin only. Read and follow the instructions on the medicine label. The medication must be used at least 15 minutes **before** you are exposed to poison ivy, poison oak, or poison sumac. Shake the bottle well before each use. Rub a thin layer of the lotion on your skin to form a smooth wet layer. When the lotion dries, you will see a clay-like coating on the protected parts of your skin. You will need to apply more lotion on your skin at least every 4 hours or sooner if the medication rubs off. Do not use the medication in or near your eyes. If you do get the medication in your eyes, rinse them well with cool water for at least 20 minutes. Tell your physician if you have eye redness or eye pain that does not go away.

**Monitoring Parameters:** Signs and symptoms of exposure to poison oak, ivy, or sumac (rash, swelling, blisters)

- ◆ **Bentyl® Hydrochloride Injection** *see* Dicyclomine *on page 273*
- ◆ **Bentyl® Hydrochloride Oral** *see* Dicyclomine *on page 273*
- ◆ **Bentylol®** *see* Dicyclomine *on page 273*
- ◆ **Benuryl™** *see* Probenecid *on page 758*
- ◆ **Benylin® Cough Syrup [OTC]** *see* Diphenhydramine *on page 289*
- ◆ **Benylin® Expectorant [OTC]** *see* Guaifenesin and Dextromethorphan *on page 428*
- ◆ **Benzamycin®** *see* Erythromycin and Benzoyl Peroxide *on page 330*
- ◆ **Benzathine Benzylpenicillin** *see* Penicillin G Benzathine, Parenteral *on page 704*
- ◆ **Benzathine Penicillin G** *see* Penicillin G Benzathine, Parenteral *on page 704*
- ◆ **Benzazoline Hydrochloride** *see* Tolazoline *on page 911*
- ◆ **Benzene Hexachloride** *see* Lindane *on page 534*
- ◆ **Benzhexol Hydrochloride** *see* Trihexyphenidyl *on page 935*

# Benzocaine (BEN zoe kane)

**Pharmacologic Class** Local Anesthetic

**U.S. Brand Names** Americaine® [OTC]; Anbesol® [OTC]; Anbesol® Maximum Strength [OTC]; Babee® Teething® [OTC]; Benzocol® [OTC]; Benzodent® [OTC]; Chigger-Tox® [OTC]; Cylex® [OTC]; Dermoplast® [OTC]; Foille® [OTC]; Foille® Medicated First Aid [OTC]; Hurricaine®; Lanacane® [OTC]; Maximum Strength Anbesol® [OTC]; Maximum Strength Orajel® [OTC]; Mycinettes® [OTC]; Numzitdent® [OTC]; Numzit Teething® [OTC]; Orabase®-B [OTC]; Orabase®-O [OTC]; Orajel® Brace-Aid Oral Anesthetic [OTC]; Orajel® Maximum Strength [OTC]; Orajel® Mouth-Aid [OTC]; Orasept® [OTC]; Orasol® [OTC]; Oratect™ [OTC]; Rhulicaine® [OTC]; Rid-A-Pain® [OTC]; Slim-Mint® [OTC]; Solarcaine® [OTC]; Spec-T® [OTC]; Tanac® [OTC]; Trocaine® [OTC]; Unguentine® [OTC]; Vicks® Children's Chloraseptic® [OTC]; Vicks® Chloraseptic® Sore Throat [OTC]; Zilactin-B® Medicated [OTC]

**Mechanism of Action** Ester local anesthetic blocks both the initiation and conduction of nerve impulses by decreasing the neuronal membrane's permeability to sodium ions, which results in inhibition of depolarization with resultant blockade of conduction

**Use** Temporary relief of pain associated with local anesthetic for pruritic dermatosis, pruritus, minor burns, acute congestive and serous otitis media, swimmer's ear, otitis externa, toothache, minor sore throat pain, canker sores, hemorrhoids, rectal fissures, anesthetic lubricant for passage of catheters and endoscopic tubes; nonprescription diet aide

**USUAL DOSAGE**

Children and Adults:

Mucous membranes: Dosage varies depending on area to be anesthetized and vascularity of tissues

Oral mouth/throat preparations: Do not administer for >2 days or in children <2 years of age, unless directed by a physician; refer to specific package labeling

Topical: Apply to affected area as needed

(Continued)

# Benzocaine *(Continued)*

Adults: Nonprescription diet aid: 6-15 mg just prior to food consumption, not to exceed 45 mg/day

**Dosage Forms** Topical for mucous membranes: **Gel:** 6% (7.5 g), 20% (2.5 g, 3.75 g, 7.5 g, 30 g]; **Liq:** 20% (3.75 mL, 9 mL, 13.3 mL, 30 mL);

Topical for skin disorders: **Aero, external use:** 5% (92 mL, 105 g), 20% (82.5 mL, 90 mL, 92 mL, 150 mL); **Crm:** (30 g, 60 g), 5% (30 g, 1 lb), 6% (28.4 g); **Lot:** (120 mL), 8% (90 mL); **Oint:** 5% (3.5 g, 28 g); **Spray:** 5% (97.5 mL), 20% (20 g, 60 g, 120 g, 13.3 mL, 120 mL)

Mouth/throat preparations: **Crm:** 5% (10 g); **Gel:** 6.3% (7.5 g), 7.5% (7.2 g, 9.45 g, 14.1 g), 10% (6 g, 9.45 g, 10 g, 15 g), 15% (10.5 g), 20% (9.45 g, 14.1 g); **Liq:** 20% (3.7 mL), 5% (8.8 mL), 6.3% (9 mL, 22 mL, 14.79 mL), 10% (13 mL), 20% (13.3 mL); **Lot:** 0.2% (15 mL), 2.5% (15 mL); **Loz:** 5 mg, 6 mg, 10 mg, 15 mg; **Oint:** 20% (30 g); **Paste:** 20% (5 g, 15 g);

Nonprescription diet aid: **Candy:** 6 mg; **Gum:** 6 mg

**Contraindications** Children <1 year of age; secondary bacterial infection of area; ophthalmic use; known hypersensitivity to benzocaine or other ester type local anesthetics

**Warnings/Precautions** Not intended for use when infections are present

**Pregnancy Risk Factor** C

**Adverse Reactions** Dose-related and may result in high plasma levels

1% to 10%:
 Dermatologic: Angioedema, contact dermatitis
 Local: Burning, stinging
<1%: Edema, urticaria, urethritis, methemoglobinemia in infants, tenderness

**Special PA Issues**

**Patient Education:** Use as directed; do not overuse. Do not apply when infections are present and do not apply to large areas of broken skin. Do not eat or drink for 1 hour following oral application. Discontinue application and report if swelling of mouth, lips, tongue, or throat occurs; or if skin irritation occurs at application site.

# Benzocaine, Butyl Aminobenzoate, Tetracaine, and Benzalkonium Chloride

(BEN zoe kane, BYOO til a meen oh BENZ oh ate, TET ra kane, & benz al KOE nee um KLOR ide)

**Pharmacologic Class** Local Anesthetic

**U.S. Brand Names** Cetacaine®

**Dosage Forms Aero:** Benzocaine 14%, butyl aminobenzoate 2%, tetracaine 2%, and benzalkonium chloride 0.5% (56 g)

♦ **Benzocol®** [OTC] *see Benzocaine on previous page*

♦ **Benzodent®** [OTC] *see Benzocaine on previous page*

# Benzonatate *(ben ZOE na tate)*

**Pharmacologic Class** Antitussive

**U.S. Brand Names** Tessalon® Perles

**Mechanism of Action** Tetracaine congener with antitussive properties; suppresses cough by topical anesthetic action on the respiratory stretch receptors

**Use** Symptomatic relief of nonproductive cough

**USUAL DOSAGE** Children >10 years and Adults: Oral: 100 mg 3 times/day or every 4 hours up to 600 mg/day

**Dosage Forms Cap:** 100 mg

**Contraindications** Known hypersensitivity to benzonatate or related compounds (such as tetracaine)

**Pregnancy Risk Factor** C

**Adverse Reactions** 1% to 10%:
 Central nervous system: Sedation, headache, dizziness
 Dermatologic: Rash
 Gastrointestinal: GI upset
 Neuromuscular & skeletal: Numbness in chest
 Ocular: Burning sensation in eyes
 Respiratory: Nasal congestion

**Onset** Therapeutic: Within 15-20 minutes

**Duration** 3-8 hours

**Special PA Issues**

**Patient Education:** Take only as prescribed; do not exceed prescribed dose or frequency. Do not break or chew tablet. Maintain adequate hydration (2-3 L/day of fluids unless instructed to restrict fluid intake). Avoid use of other depressants, alcohol, or sleep-inducing medications unless approved by prescriber. You may experience drowsiness, impaired coordination, blurred vision, or increased anxiety (use caution when driving or engaging in hazardous tasks until response to therapy is known); or upset stomach or nausea (frequent small meals, frequent mouth care, chewing gum, or sucking hard candy may help). Report persistent CNS changes (dizziness, sedation, tremor, or agitation), numbness in chest or feeling of chill, visual changes or burning in eyes, numbness of mouth or difficulty swallowing, or lack of improvement or worsening or condition.

**Monitoring Parameters:** Monitor patient's chest sounds and respiratory pattern

# Benzoyl Peroxide and Hydrocortisone
(BEN zoe il peer OKS ide & hye droe KOR ti sone)
**Pharmacologic Class** Acne Products
**U.S. Brand Names** Vanoxide-HC®
**Dosage Forms Lot:** Benzoyl peroxide 5% and hydrocortisone alcohol 0.5% (25 mL)

# Benzthiazide (benz THYE a zide)
**Pharmacologic Class** Diuretic, Thiazide
**U.S. Brand Names** Aquatag®; Exna®; Hydrex®; Marazide®; Proaqua®
**Use** Management of mild to moderate hypertension; treatment of edema in congestive heart failure and hepatic cirrhosis, corticosteroid and estrogen therapy, and renal dysfunction
  **Unlabeled use:** Calcium nephrolithiasis, osteoporosis, diabetes insipidus
**USUAL DOSAGE** Adults: Oral:
  Edema: 50-200 mg/day; maintenance: 50-150 mg/day; use divided doses after morning and evening meal if total dose exceeds 100 mg
  Hypertension: 50-100 mg/day; maintenance: individualize dose (maximum effective dose: 200 mg/day)
**Dosage Forms Tab:** 50 mg
**Contraindications** Anuria, renal decompensation, hypersensitivity to benzthiazide or any component, cross-sensitivity with other thiazides and sulfonamide derivatives
**Warnings/Precautions** Hypokalemia, renal disease, hepatic disease, gout, lupus erythematosus, diabetes mellitus; use with caution in severe renal diseases
**Pregnancy Risk Factor** C
**Pregnancy Implications** Excretion in breast milk unknown/use caution
**Adverse Reactions**
  1% to 10%:
    Cardiovascular: Orthostatic hypotension
    Endocrine & metabolic: Hyponatremia, hypokalemia
    Gastrointestinal: Anorexia, upset stomach, diarrhea
  <1%: Drowsiness, hyperuricemia, nausea, vomiting, polyuria, aplastic anemia, hemolytic anemia, leukopenia, agranulocytosis, thrombocytopenia, hepatitis, hepatic function impairment, paresthesia, uremia, allergic reactions
**Drug Interactions**
  Decreased effect of oral hypoglycemics; decreased absorption with cholestyramine and colestipol
  Increased effect with furosemide and other loop diuretics
  Increased toxicity/levels of lithium
**Onset** Within 2 hours
**Duration** 12 hours
**Special PA Issues**
  **Patient Education:** Take early in the day and take last dose in early evening to avoid frequent night urination. Take with food to reduce GI upset. Weigh yourself on a regular basis (same time, same clothes). Report unresolved weight gain (more than 3-5 pounds in 3 days). You may experience dizziness or drowsiness; change positions slowly and use caution when driving or engaging in hazardous tasks. May cause photosensitivity; avoid excessive sunlight, use sunblock, wear protective clothing and glasses. You may experience decreased sexual function; this will resolve when medication is discontinued. Report increased swelling of ankles, fingers, dizziness or trembling, cramps, or muscle pain.
  **Monitoring Parameters:** Assess weight, I & O reports daily to determine fluid loss; blood pressure, serum electrolytes, BUN, creatinine

# Benztropine (BENZ troe peen)
**Pharmacologic Class** Anticholinergic Agent; Anti-Parkinson's Agent (Anticholinergic)
**U.S. Brand Names** Cogentin®
**Mechanism of Action** Thought to partially block striatal cholinergic receptors to help balance cholinergic and dopaminergic activity
**Use** Adjunctive treatment of Parkinson's disease; also used in treatment of drug-induced extrapyramidal effects (except tardive dyskinesia) and acute dystonic reactions
**USUAL DOSAGE** Use in children <3 years of age should be reserved for life-threatening emergencies

Drug-induced extrapyramidal reaction: Oral, I.M., I.V.:
  Children >3 years: 0.02-0.05 mg/kg/dose 1-2 times/day
  Adults: 1-4 mg/dose 1-2 times/day
Acute dystonia: Adults: I.M., I.V.: 1-2 mg
(Continued)

## Benztropine *(Continued)*

Parkinsonism: Oral:
Adults: 0.5-6 mg/day in 1-2 divided doses; if one dose is greater, administer at bedtime; titrate dose in 0.5 mg increments at 5- to 6-day intervals
Elderly: Initial: 0.5 mg once or twice daily; increase by 0.5 mg as needed at 5-6 days; maximum: 6 mg/day

**Dosage Forms** Benztropine mesylate: **Inj:** 1 mg/mL (2 mL); **Tab:** 0.5 mg, 1 mg, 2 mg

**Contraindications** Children <3 years of age, use with caution in older children (dosage not established); patients with narrow-angle glaucoma; hypersensitivity to any component; pyloric or duodenal obstruction, stenosing peptic ulcers; bladder neck obstructions; achalasia; myasthenia gravis

**Warnings/Precautions** Use with caution in hot weather or during exercise. Elderly patients frequently develop increased sensitivity and require strict dosage regulation - side effects may be more severe in elderly patients with atherosclerotic changes. Use with caution in patients with tachycardia, cardiac arrhythmias, hypertension, hypotension, prostatic hypertrophy (especially in the elderly) or any tendency toward urinary retention, liver or kidney disorders and obstructive disease of the GI or GU tract. When given in large doses or to susceptible patients, may cause weakness and inability to move particular muscle groups.

**Pregnancy Risk Factor** C

**Pregnancy Implications** Excretion in breast milk unknown

**Adverse Reactions**
>10%:
Dermatologic: Dry skin
Gastrointestinal: Constipation, dry throat, xerostomia
Respiratory: Dry nose
Miscellaneous: Diaphoresis (decreased)
1% to 10%:
Dermatologic: Increased sensitivity to light
Endocrine & metabolic: Decreased flow of breast milk
Gastrointestinal: Dysphagia
<1%: Tachycardia, orthostatic hypotension, ventricular fibrillation, palpitations, coma, drowsiness, nervousness, hallucinations; the elderly may be at increased risk for confusion and hallucinations; headache, loss of memory, fatigue, ataxia, rash, nausea, vomiting, bloated feeling, dysuria, blurred vision, mydriasis, increased intraocular pain, weakness

**Drug Interactions**
Decreased effect: May increase gastric degradation of levodopa and decrease the amount of levodopa absorbed by delaying gastric emptying - the opposite may be true for digoxin
Increased toxicity: Central anticholinergic syndrome can occur when administered with narcotic analgesics, phenothiazines and other antipsychotics, tricyclic antidepressants, quinidine and some other antiarrhythmics, and antihistamines

**Onset** Oral: Within 1 hour; Parenteral: Within 15 minutes

**Duration** 6-48 hours (wide range)

**Special PA Issues**
Patient Education: Take exactly as directed; do not increase, decrease, or discontinue without consulting prescriber. Take at same time each day. Do not use alcohol and all prescription or OTC sedatives or CNS depressants without consulting prescriber. You may experience drowsiness, dizziness, confusion, and blurred vision (use caution when driving, climbing stairs, or engaging in hazardous tasks); increased susceptibility to heat stroke, decreased perspiration (use caution in hot weather - maintain adequate fluids and reduce exercise activity); constipation (increased exercise, fluids, or dietary fruit and fiber may help). Report unresolved nausea, vomiting, or gastric disturbances; rapid or pounding heartbeat, chest pain or palpitation; difficulty breathing; CNS changes (hallucination, loss of memory, nervousness, etc); eye pain; prolonged fever; painful or difficult urination; unresolved constipation; increased muscle spasticity or rigidity; skin rash; or significant worsening of condition.
Dietary Considerations: Alcohol: Additive CNS effects, avoid use

◆ **Benztropine Mesylate** *see Benztropine on previous page*
◆ **Benzylpenicillin Benzathine** *see Penicillin G Benzathine, Parenteral on page 704*
◆ **Benzylpenicillin Potassium** *see Penicillin G, Parenteral, Aqueous on page 705*
◆ **Benzylpenicillin Sodium** *see Penicillin G, Parenteral, Aqueous on page 705*

## Benzylpenicilloyl-polylysine (BEN zil pen i SIL oyl pol i LIE seen)

**Pharmacologic Class** Diagnostic Agent, Penicillin Allergy Skin Test

**U.S. Brand Names** Pre-Pen®

**Mechanism of Action** Elicits IgE antibodies which produce type I accelerate urticarial reactions to penicillins

**Use** Adjunct in assessing the risk of administering penicillin (penicillin or benzylpenicillin) in adults with a history of clinical penicillin hypersensitivity

**USUAL DOSAGE** PPL is administered by a scratch technique or by intradermal injection. For initial testing, PPL should always be applied via the scratch technique. **Do not administer intradermally to patients who have positive reactions to a scratch test.** PPL test alone does not identify those patients who react to a minor antigenic determinant and does not appear to predict reliably the occurrence of late reactions.

**Scratch test:** Use scratch technique with a 20-gauge needle to make 3-5 mm nonbleeding scratch on epidermis, apply a small drop of solution to scratch, rub in gently with applicator or toothpick. A positive reaction consists of a pale wheal surrounding the scratch site which develops within 10 minutes and ranges from 5-15 mm or more in diameter.

**Intradermal test:** Use intradermal test with a tuberculin syringe with a 26- to 30-gauge short bevel needle; a dose of 0.01-0.02 mL is injected intradermally. A control of 0.9% sodium chloride should be injected at least 1.5" from the PPL test site. Most skin responses to the intradermal test will develop within 5-15 minutes.

**Interpretation:**

(-) Negative: No reaction

(±) Ambiguous: Wheal only slightly larger than original bleb with or without erythematous flare and larger than control site

(+) Positive: Itching and marked increase in size of original bleb

Control site should be reactionless

**Dosage Forms Soln:** 0.25 mL

**Contraindications** Patients known to be extremely hypersensitive to penicillin

**Warnings/Precautions** PPL test alone does not identify those patients who react to a minor antigenic determinant and does not appear to predict reliably the occurrence of late reactions. A negative skin test is associated with an incidence of allergic reactions <5% after penicillin administration and a positive skin test is associated with a >20% incidence of allergic reaction after penicillin administration; have epinephrine 1:1000 available.

**Pregnancy Risk Factor** C

**Adverse Reactions**

1% to 10%: Local: Intense local inflammatory response at skin test site

<1%: Edema, pruritus, erythema, urticaria, wheal (locally), systemic allergic reactions occur rarely

**Drug Interactions**

Decreased effect: Corticosteroids and other immunosuppressive agents may inhibit the immune response to the skin test

# Bepridil (BE pri dil)

**Pharmacologic Class** Calcium Channel Blocker

**U.S. Brand Names** Vascor®

**Mechanism of Action** Bepridil, a type 4 calcium antagonist, possesses characteristics of the traditional calcium antagonists, inhibiting calcium ion from entering the "slow channels" or select voltage-sensitive areas of vascular smooth muscle and myocardium during depolarization and producing a relaxation of coronary vascular smooth muscle and coronary vasodilation. However, bepridil may also inhibit fast sodium channels (inward) which may account for some of its side effects (eg, arrhythmias); a direct bradycardia effect of bepridil has been postulated via direct action on the S-A node.

**Use** Treatment of chronic stable angina; due to side effect profile, reserve for patients who have been intolerant of other antianginal therapy; bepridil may be used alone or in combination with nitrates or beta-blockers

**USUAL DOSAGE** Adults: Oral: Initial: 200 mg/day, then adjust dose at 10-day intervals until optimal response is achieved; usual dose: 300 mg/day; maximum daily dose: 400 mg

**Dosage Forms Tab, as hydrochloride:** 200 mg, 300 mg, 400 mg

**Contraindications** History of serious ventricular or atrial arrhythmias (especially tachycardia or those associated with accessory conduction pathways), uncompensated cardiac insufficiency, congenital Q-T interval prolongation, patients taking other drugs that prolong the Q-T interval, history of hypersensitivity to bepridil or any component, calcium channel blockers, or adenosine; concurrent administration with ritonavir or sparfloxacin

**Warnings/Precautions** Use with great caution in patients with history of IHSS, second or third degree A-V block, cardiogenic shock; reserve for patients in whom other antianginals have failed. Carefully titrate dosages for patients with impaired renal or hepatic function; use caution when treating patients with congestive heart failure, significant hypotension, severe left ventricular dysfunction, hypertrophic cardiomyopathy (especially obstructive), concomitant therapy with beta-blockers or digoxin, edema, or increased intracranial pressure with cranial tumors; do not abruptly withdraw (may cause chest pain); elderly may experience hypotension and constipation more readily.

If dosage reduction does not maintain the Q-T within a safe range (not to exceed 0.52 seconds during therapy), discontinue the medication; has class I antiarrhythmic properties and can induce new arrhythmias, including VT/VF; it can also cause torsade de pointes type ventricular tachycardia due to its ability to prolong the Q-T interval; avoid use in patients in the immediate period postinfarction.

**Pregnancy Risk Factor** C

**Pregnancy Implications** Enters breast milk/compatible

(Continued)

# Bepridil (Continued)

## Adverse Reactions

>10%:
Central nervous system: Dizziness
Gastrointestinal: Nausea, dyspepsia
Neuromuscular & skeletal: Weakness

1% to 10%:
Cardiovascular: Bradycardia, edema, palpitations
Central nervous system: Nervousness, headache (7% to 13%), drowsiness, psychiatric disturbances (<2%), insomnia (2% to 3%)
Dermatologic: Rash (≤2%)
Endocrine & metabolic: Sexual dysfunction
Gastrointestinal: Diarrhea, anorexia, xerostomia, constipation, abdominal pain, dyspepsia, flatulence
Neuromuscular & skeletal: Weakness (6.5% to 14%), tremor (<9%), paresthesia (2.5%)
Ocular: Blurred vision
Otic: Tinnitus
Respiratory: Rhinitis, dyspnea (≤8.7%), cough (≤2%)
Miscellaneous (≤2%): Flu syndrome, diaphoresis

<1%: Ventricular premature contractions, hypertension, syncope, prolonged Q-T intervals, fever, altered behavior, akathisia, abnormal taste, arthritis, pharyngitis

## Drug Interactions CYP3A3/4 enzyme substrate

Increased toxicity/effect/levels:
Bepridil and cyclosporine may increase cyclosporine levels (other calcium channel blockers have been shown to interact)
Bepridil and digitalis glycoside may increase digitalis glycoside levels
Use with ritonavir may increase risk of bepridil and sparfloxacin toxicity, especially its cardiotoxicity
Coadministration with beta-blocking agents may result in increased depressant effects on myocardial contractility or A-V conduction
Severe hypotension or increased fluid volume requirements may occur with concomitant fentanyl

## Onset 1 hour

## Half-Life 24 hours

## Special PA Issues

**Patient Education:** Take as directed (may be taken with food to reduce gastric side effects). Do not discontinue without consulting prescriber. Regular EKGs and follow-up with prescriber may be required. If taking potassium supplements or potassium-sparing diuretics, serum potassium monitoring will be required. May cause dizziness, shakiness, visual disturbances, or headache; use caution when driving or engaging in hazardous tasks. Report irregular or pounding heartbeat, respiratory difficulty, swelling of hands or feet, unresolved headache, dizziness, constipation, or any unusual bleeding or bruising.

**Monitoring Parameters:** EKG and serum electrolytes, blood pressure, signs and symptoms of congestive heart failure; elderly may need very close monitoring due to underlying cardiac and organ system defects

**Reference Range:** 1-2 ng/mL

### Related Information

Calcium Channel Blocking Agents *on page 1004*

♦ **Bepridil Hydrochloride** *see* Bepridil *on previous page*

# Beractant (ber AKT ant)

## Pharmacologic Class Lung Surfactant

## U.S. Brand Names Survanta®

## Mechanism of Action Replaces deficient or ineffective endogenous lung surfactant in neonates with respiratory distress syndrome (RDS) or in neonates at risk of developing RDS. Surfactant prevents the alveoli from collapsing during expiration by lowering surface tension between air and alveolar surfaces.

## Use Prevention and treatment of respiratory distress syndrome (RDS) in premature infants

Prophylactic therapy: Body weight <1250 g in infants at risk for developing or with evidence of surfactant deficiency
Rescue therapy: Treatment of infants with RDS confirmed by x-ray and requiring mechanical ventilation (administer as soon as possible - within 8 hours of age)

## USUAL DOSAGE

Prophylactic treatment: Administer 100 mg phospholipids (4 mL/kg) intratracheal as soon as possible; as many as 4 doses may be administered during the first 48 hours of life, no more frequently than 6 hours apart. The need for additional doses is determined by evidence of continuing respiratory distress; if the infant is still intubated and requiring at least 30% inspired oxygen to maintain a PaO$_2$ ≤80 torr.
Rescue treatment: Administer 100 mg phospholipids (4 mL/kg) as soon as the diagnosis of RDS is made; may repeat if needed, no more frequently than every 6 hours to a maximum of 4 doses

**Dosage Forms Susp:** 200 mg (8 mL)

**Warnings/Precautions** Rapidly affects oxygenation and lung compliance and should be restricted to a highly supervised use in a clinical setting with immediate availability of clinicians experienced with intubation and ventilatory management of premature infants. If transient episodes of bradycardia and decreased oxygen saturation occur, discontinue the dosing procedure and initiate measures to alleviate the condition; produces rapid improvements in lung oxygenation and compliance that may require immediate reductions in ventilator settings and $FiO_2$.

**Adverse Reactions** During the dosing procedure:

Cardiovascular: Transient bradycardia, vasoconstriction, hypotension, hypertension, pallor

Respiratory: Oxygen desaturation, endotracheal tube blockage, hypocarbia, hypercarbia, apnea, pulmonary air leaks, pulmonary interstitial emphysema

Miscellaneous: Increased probability of post-treatment nosocomial sepsis

**Special PA Issues**

**Monitoring Parameters:** Continuous EKG and transcutaneous $O_2$ saturation should be monitored during administration; frequent arterial blood gases are necessary to prevent postdosing hyperoxia and hypocarbia

- **Berocca®** *see* Vitamin B Complex With Vitamin C and Folic Acid *on page 963*
- **Berubigen®** *see* Cyanocobalamin *on page 242*
- **Beta-2®** *see* Isoetharine *on page 493*
- **Beta-Blockers** *see* Chart *on page 1002*

## Beta-Carotene (BAY tah KARE oh teen)

**Pharmacologic Class** Vitamin, Fat Soluble

**U.S. Brand Names** Solatene®

**Mechanism of Action** The exact mechanism of action in erythropoietic protoporphyria has not as yet been elucidated; although patient must become carotenemic before effects are observed, there appears to be more than a simple internal light screen responsible for the drug's action. A protective effect was achieved when beta-carotene was added to blood samples. The concentrations of solutions used were similar to those achieved in treated patients. Topically applied beta-carotene is considerably less effective than systemic therapy.

**Use** Reduces severity of photosensitivity reactions in patients with erythropoietic protoporphyria (EPP)

**Unlabeled use:** Prophylaxis and treatment of polymorphous light eruption and prophylaxis against photosensitivity reactions in erythropoietic protoporphyria

**USUAL DOSAGE** Oral:

Children <14 years: 30-150 mg/day

Adults: 30-300 mg/day

**Dosage Forms Cap:** 15 mg, 30 mg

**Contraindications** Hypersensitivity to beta-carotene

**Warnings/Precautions** Use with caution in patients with renal or hepatic impairment; not proven effective as a sunscreen

**Pregnancy Risk Factor** C

**Pregnancy Implications** Excretion in breast milk unknown/use caution

**Adverse Reactions**

>10%: Dermatologic: Carotenodermia (yellowing of palms, hands, or soles of feet, and to a lesser extent the face)

<1%: Dizziness, bruising, diarrhea, arthralgia

**Drug Interactions** Fulfills vitamin A requirements, do not prescribe additional vitamin A

**Special PA Issues**

**Patient Education:** Take exactly as directed; do not take more than the recommended dose. Take with meals. Skin may appear slightly yellow-orange. Not a proven sunblock.

- **Betachron E-R®** *see* Propranolol *on page 775*
- **Betadine® [OTC]** *see* Povidone-Iodine *on page 747*
- **Betadine® First Aid Antibiotics + Moisturizer [OTC]** *see* Bacitracin and Polymyxin B *on page 97*
- **9-Beta-D-ribofuranosyladenine** *see* Adenosine *on page 30*
- **Betagan® [OTC]** *see* Povidone-Iodine *on page 747*
- **Betagan® Liquifilm®** *see* Levobunolol *on page 523*
- **Betaloc®** *see* Metoprolol *on page 599*
- **Betaloc® Durules®** *see* Metoprolol *on page 599*

## Betamethasone (bay ta METH a sone)

**Pharmacologic Class** Corticosteroid, Oral; Corticosteroid, Parenteral; Corticosteroid, Topical

**U.S. Brand Names** Alphatrex®; Betatrex®; Beta-Val®; Celestone®; Celestone® Soluspan®; Cel-U-Jec®; Diprolene®; Diprolene® AF; Diprosone®; Luxiq™; Maxivate®; Psorion® Cream; Teladar®; Valisone®

(Continued)

# Betamethasone (Continued)

**Mechanism of Action** Controls the rate of protein synthesis, depresses the migration of polymorphonuclear leukocytes, fibroblasts, reverses capillary permeability, and lysosomal stabilization at the cellular level to prevent or control inflammation

**Use** Inflammatory dermatoses such as seborrheic or atopic dermatitis, neurodermatitis, anogenital pruritus, psoriasis, inflammatory phase of xerosis

**USUAL DOSAGE** Base dosage on severity of disease and patient response

Children: Use lowest dose listed as initial dose for adrenocortical insufficiency (physiologic replacement)

I.M.: 0.0175-0.125 mg base/kg/day divided every 6-12 hours **or** 0.5-7.5 mg base/m$^2$/day divided every 6-12 hours

Oral: 0.0175-0.25 mg/kg/day divided every 6-8 hours **or** 0.5-7.5 mg/m$^2$/day divided every 6-8 hours

Adolescents and Adults:

Oral: 2.4-4.8 mg/day in 2-4 doses; range: 0.6-7.2 mg/day

I.M.: Betamethasone sodium phosphate and betamethasone acetate: 0.6-9 mg/day (generally, $^1/_3$ to $^1/_2$ of oral dose) divided every 12-24 hours

Foam: Apply twice daily, once in the morning and once at night

**Dosing adjustment in hepatic impairment:** Adjustments may be necessary in patients with liver failure because betamethasone is extensively metabolized in the liver

Intrabursal, intra-articular, intradermal: 0.25-2 mL

Intralesional: Rheumatoid arthritis/osteoarthritis:

Very large joints: 1-2 mL

Large joints: 1 mL

Medium joints: 0.5-1 mL

Small joints: 0.25-0.5 mL

Topical: Apply thin film 2-4 times/day

**Dosage Forms** Betamethasone base (Celestone®), Oral: **Syr:** 0.6 mg/5 mL (118 mL); **Tab:** 0.6 mg

Betamethasone dipropionate (Diprosone®): **Aero:** 0.1% (85 g); **Crm:** 0.05% (15 g, 45 g); **Lot:** 0.05% (20 mL, 30 mL, 60 mL); **Oint:** 0.05% (15 g, 45 g)

Betamethasone dipropionate augmented (Diprolene®) **Crm:** 0.05% (15 g, 45 g); **Gel:** 0.05% (15 g, 45 g); **Lot:** 0.05% (30 mL, 60 mL); **Oint, top:** 0.05% (15 g, 45 g)

Betamethasone valerate (Betatrex®, Valisone®) **Crm:** 0.01% (15 g, 60 g), 0.1% (15 g, 45 g, 110 g, 430 g); **Lot:** 0.1% (20 mL, 60 mL); **Oint:** 0.1% (15 g, 45 g); (Beta-Val®): **Crm:** 0.01% (15 g, 60 g), 0.1% (15 g, 45 g, 110 g, 430 g); Lot: 0.1% (20 mL, 60 mL); (Luxiq™): **Foam:** 100 g aluminum can (box of 1)

**Inj: Sodium phosphate (Celestone® Phosphate, Cel-U-Jec®):** 4 mg betamethasone phosphate/mL (equivalent to 3 mg betamethasone/mL) (5 mL); **Inj, susp:** Sodium phosphate and acetate (Celestone® Soluspan®): 6 mg/mL (3 mg of betamethasone sodium phosphate and 3 mg of betamethasone acetate per mL) (5 mL)

**Contraindications** Systemic fungal infections; hypersensitivity to betamethasone or any component

**Warnings/Precautions** Fatalities have occurred due to adrenal insufficiency in asthmatic patients during and after transfer from systemic corticosteroids to aerosol steroids; several months may be required for recovery of this syndrome; during this period, aerosol steroids do **not** provide the systemic steroid needed to treat patients having trauma, surgery, or infections; use with caution in patients with hypothyroidism, cirrhosis, ulcerative colitis; do not use occlusive dressings on weeping or exudative lesions and general caution with occlusive dressings should be observed; discontinue if skin irritation or contact dermatitis should occur; do not use in patients with decreased skin circulation

**Pregnancy Risk Factor** C

**Pregnancy Implications** Clinical effects on the fetus: There are no reports linking the use of betamethasone with congenital defects in the literature; betamethasone is often used in patients with premature labor [26-34 weeks gestation] to stimulate fetal lung maturation

**Adverse Reactions**

>10%:

Central nervous system: Insomnia

Gastrointestinal: Increased appetite, indigestion

Ocular: Temporary mild blurred vision

1% to 10%:

Dermatologic: Erythema, itching

Endocrine & metabolic: Diabetes mellitus

Local: Dryness, irritation, papular rashes, burning

Ocular: Cataracts

<1%: Hypertension, convulsions, vertigo, confusion, headache, thin fragile skin, hyperpigmentation or hypertrichosis, hypopigmentation, impaired wound healing, acneiform eruptions, perioral dermatitis, maceration of skin, skin atrophy, striae, miliaria, cushingoid state, sodium retention, peptic ulcer, sterile abscess, myalgia, osteoporosis, glaucoma, sudden blindness

**Drug Interactions** CYP3A enzyme substrate

Decreased effect (corticosteroid) by barbiturates, phenytoin, rifampin

**Half-Life** 6.5 hours

**Special PA Issues**

**Patient Education:** Take exactly as directed; do not increase dose or discontinue abruptly, consult prescriber. Take oral medication with or after meals. Limit intake of caffeine or stimulants. Prescriber may recommend increased dietary vitamins, minerals, or iron. Diabetics should monitor glucose levels closely (antidiabetic medication may need to be adjusted). Inform prescriber if you are experiencing greater than normal levels of stress (medication may need adjustment). Some forms of this medication may cause GI upset (oral medication may be taken with meals to reduce GI upset; small frequent meals and frequent mouth care may reduce GI upset). You may be more susceptible to infection (avoid crowds and persons with contagious or infective conditions). Report promptly excessive nervousness or sleep disturbances; signs of infection (sore throat, unhealed injuries); excessive growth of body hair or loss of skin color; changes in vision; excessive or sudden weight gain (>3 lb/week); swelling of face or extremities; difficulty breathing; muscle weakness; change in color of stools (tarry) or persistent abdominal pain; or worsening of condition or failure to improve.

Topical: For external use only, Not for eyes or mucous membranes or open wounds. Apply in a thin layer (may rub in lightly). Apply light dressing (if necessary) to area being treated. Do not use occlusive dressing unless so advised by prescriber. Avoid prolonged or excessive use around sensitive tissues, genital, or rectal areas. Inform prescriber if condition worsens (redness, swelling, irritation, open sores) or fails to improve.

**Related Information**

Corticosteroids *on page 1007*

# Betamethasone and Clotrimazole (bay ta METH a sone & kloe TRIM a zole)

**Pharmacologic Class** Antifungal/Corticosteroid

**U.S. Brand Names** Lotrisone®

**Dosage Forms Crm:** Betamethasone dipropionate 0.05% and clotrimazole 1% (15 g, 45 g)

- ♦ **Betamethasone Dipropionate** *see Betamethasone on page 111*
- ♦ **Betamethasone Dipropionate, Augmented** *see Betamethasone on page 111*
- ♦ **Betamethasone Sodium Phosphate** *see Betamethasone on page 111*
- ♦ **Betamethasone Valerate** *see Betamethasone on page 111*
- ♦ **Betapace®** *see Sotalol on page 845*
- ♦ **Betapen®-VK** *see Penicillin V Potassium on page 706*
- ♦ **Betasept® [OTC]** *see Chlorhexidine Gluconate on page 190*
- ♦ **Betaseron®** *see Interferon Beta-1b on page 486*
- ♦ **Betatrex®** *see Betamethasone on page 111*
- ♦ **Beta-Val®** *see Betamethasone on page 111*
- ♦ **Betaxin®** *see Thiamine on page 894*

# Betaxolol (be TAKS oh lol)

**Pharmacologic Class** Beta Blocker, Beta$_1$ Selective; Ophthalmic Agent, Antiglaucoma

**U.S. Brand Names** Betoptic® Ophthalmic; Betoptic® S Ophthalmic; Kerlone® Oral

**Mechanism of Action** Competitively blocks beta$_1$-receptors, with little or no effect on beta$_2$-receptors; ophthalmic reduces intraocular pressure by reducing the production of aqueous humor

**Use** Treatment of chronic open-angle glaucoma and ocular hypertension; management of hypertension

**USUAL DOSAGE** Adults:

Ophthalmic: Instill 1 drop twice daily

Oral: 10 mg/day; may increase dose to 20 mg/day after 7-14 days if desired response is not achieved; initial dose in elderly patients: 5 mg/day

**Dosage Forms Soln, ophth, (Betoptic®):** 0.5% (2.5 mL, 5 mL, 10 mL); **Susp, ophth, (Betoptic® S):** 0.25% (2.5 mL, 10 mL, 15 mL); **Tab, (Kerlone®):** 10 mg, 20 mg

**Contraindications** Bronchial asthma, sinus bradycardia, second and third degree A-V block, cardiac failure (unless a functioning pacemaker present), cardiogenic shock, hypersensitivity to betaxolol or any component

**Warnings/Precautions** Some products contain sulfites which can cause allergic reactions; diminished response occurs over time; use with caution in patients with decreased renal or hepatic function (dosage adjustment required); patients with a history of asthma, congestive heart failure, diabetes mellitus, or bradycardia appear to be at a higher risk for adverse effects

**Pregnancy Risk Factor** C

**Adverse Reactions**

1% to 10%:

Cardiovascular: Bradycardia, palpitations, edema, congestive heart failure

Central nervous system: Dizziness, fatigue, lethargy, headache

Dermatologic: Erythema, itching

Ocular: Mild ocular stinging and discomfort, tearing, photophobia, decreased corneal sensitivity, keratitis

(Continued)

## Betaxolol *(Continued)*

Miscellaneous: Cold extremities

<1%: Chest pain, nervousness, depression, hallucinations, thrombocytopenia

**Drug Interactions** CYP1A2 and 2D6 enzyme substrate

Decreased effect of some beta-blockers with aluminum salts, barbiturates, calcium salts, cholestyramine, colestipol, NSAIDs, penicillins (ampicillin), rifampin, salicylates and sulfinpyrazone due to decreased bioavailability and plasma levels

Beta-blockers may decrease the effect of sulfonylureas

Increased effect/toxicity of beta-blockers with calcium blockers (diltiazem, felodipine, nicardipine), contraceptives, flecainide, hydralazine (metoprolol, propranolol), propafenone, quinidine (in extensive metabolizers), ciprofloxacin

Beta-blockers may increase the effect/toxicity of flecainide, hydralazine, clonidine (hypertensive crisis after or during withdrawal of either agent), epinephrine (initial hypertensive episode followed by bradycardia), nifedipine, verapamil, lidocaine, ergots, prazosin

Beta-blockers may affect the action or levels of ethanol, disopyramide, nondepolarizing muscle relaxants and theophylline although the effects are difficult to predict

**Onset** Ophthalmic: 30 minutes; Oral: 1-1.5 hours

**Duration** Ophthalmic: 12 hours

**Half-Life** Oral: 12-22 hours

**Special PA Issues**

**Patient Education:**

Oral: Use as directed; do not increase dose unless directed by prescriber. You may experience dizziness or blurred vision (use caution when driving or engaging in hazardous activities); nausea or vomiting (small frequent meals, frequent mouth care, or sucking lozenges may help). Report persistent GI response (nausea, vomiting, diarrhea, or constipation); chest pain or palpitations; unusual cough, difficulty breathing, swelling or coolness of extremities; or unusual mental depression.

Ophthalmic: Shake well before using. Tilt head back and instill in eye. Keep eye open; do not blink for 30 seconds. Apply gentle pressure to corner of eye for 1 minute. Wipe away excess from skin. Do not touch applicator to eyes or contaminate tip of applicator. Report if condition does not improve or if you experience eye pain, vision disturbances, or other adverse eye response.

**Monitoring Parameters:** Ophthalmic: Intraocular pressure. Systemic: Blood pressure, pulse

**Related Information**

Beta-Blockers *on page 1002*

♦ **Betaxolol Hydrochloride** *see* Betaxolol *on previous page*

## Bethanechol *(be THAN e kole)*

**Pharmacologic Class** Cholinergic Agonist

**U.S. Brand Names** Duvoid®; Myotonachol™; Urabeth®; Urecholine®

**Mechanism of Action** Stimulates cholinergic receptors in the smooth muscle of the urinary bladder and gastrointestinal tract resulting in increased peristalsis, increased GI and pancreatic secretions, bladder muscle contraction, and increased ureteral peristaltic waves

**Use** Nonobstructive urinary retention and retention due to neurogenic bladder; treatment and prevention of bladder dysfunction caused by phenothiazines; diagnosis of flaccid or atonic neurogenic bladder; gastroesophageal reflux

**USUAL DOSAGE**

Children:

Oral:

Abdominal distention or urinary retention: 0.6 mg/kg/day divided 3-4 times/day

Gastroesophageal reflux: 0.1-0.2 mg/kg/dose given 30 minutes to 1 hour before each meal to a maximum of 4 times/day

S.C.: 0.15-0.2 mg/kg/day divided 3-4 times/day

Adults:

Oral: 10-50 mg 2-4 times/day

S.C.: 2.5-5 mg 3-4 times/day, up to 7.5-10 mg every 4 hours for neurogenic bladder

**Dosage Forms Inj:** 5 mg/mL (1 mL); **Tab:** 5 mg, 10 mg, 25 mg, 50 mg

**Contraindications** Hypersensitivity to bethanechol; do not use in patients with mechanical obstruction of the GI or GU tract or when the strength or integrity of the GI or bladder wall is in question. It is also contraindicated in patients with hyperthyroidism, peptic ulcer disease, epilepsy, obstructive pulmonary disease, bradycardia, vasomotor instability, atrioventricular conduction defects, hypotension, or parkinsonism; **contraindicated for I.M. or I.V. use due to a likely severe cholinergic reaction**

**Warnings/Precautions** Potential for reflux infection if the sphincter fails to relax as bethanechol contracts the bladder; use with caution when administering to nursing women, as it is unknown if the drug is excreted in breast milk; safety and efficacy in children <5 years of age have not been established; syringe containing atropine should be readily available for treatment of serious side effects; for S.C. injection only; do not administer I.M. or I.V.

**Pregnancy Risk Factor** C

**Adverse Reactions**
Oral: <1%: Hypotension, cardiac arrest, flushed skin, abdominal cramps, diarrhea, nausea, vomiting, salivation, bronchial constriction, diaphoresis, vasomotor response
Subcutaneous: 1% to 10%:
Cardiovascular: Hypotension, cardiac arrest, flushed skin
Gastrointestinal: Abdominal cramps, diarrhea, nausea, vomiting, salivation
Respiratory: Bronchial constriction
Miscellaneous: Diaphoresis, vasomotor response

**Drug Interactions**
Decreased effect: Procainamide, quinidine
Increased toxicity: Bethanechol and ganglionic blockers → critical fall in blood pressure; cholinergic drugs or anticholinesterase agents

**Onset** Oral: 30-90 minutes; S.C.: 5-15 minutes

**Duration** Oral: Up to 6 hours; S.C.: 2 hours

**Special PA Issues**
**Patient Education:** Oral: Take as directed, on an empty stomach to avoid nausea or vomiting. Do not discontinue without consulting prescriber. Maintain adequate hydration (2-3 L/day of fluids unless instructed to restrict fluid intake). May cause dizziness or hypotension (rise slowly from sitting or lying position and use caution when driving or climbing stairs); vomiting or loss of appetite (frequent small meals, frequent mouth care, or sucking lozenges may help). Report persistent abdominal discomfort; significantly increased salivation, sweating, tearing, or urination; flushed skin; chest pain or palpitations; acute headache; unresolved diarrhea; excessive fatigue, insomnia, dizziness, or depression; increased muscle, joint, or body pain; vision changes or blurred vision; or respiratory difficulty or wheezing.
**Monitoring Parameters:** Observe closely for side effects

- **Bethanechol Chloride** see Bethanechol on previous page
- **Betimol® Ophthalmic** see Timolol on page 905
- **Betnesol® [Disodium Phosphate]** see Betamethasone on page 111
- **Betoptic® Ophthalmic** see Betaxolol on page 113
- **Betoptic® S Ophthalmic** see Betaxolol on page 113
- **Bewon®** see Thiamine on page 894
- **Bexophene®** see Propoxyphene and Aspirin on page 774
- **Biaxin™** see Clarithromycin on page 215

# Bicalutamide (bye ka LOO ta mide)

**Pharmacologic Class** Androgen

**U.S. Brand Names** Casodex®

**Mechanism of Action** Pure nonsteroidal antiandrogen that binds to androgen receptors; specifically a competitive inhibitor for the binding of dihydrotestosterone and testosterone; prevents testosterone stimulation of cell growth in prostate cancer

**Use** In combination therapy with LHRH agonist analogues in treatment of advanced prostatic carcinoma

**USUAL DOSAGE** Adults: Oral: 1 tablet once daily (morning or evening), with or without food. It is recommended that bicalutamide be taken at the same time each day; start treatment with bicalutamide at the same time as treatment with an LHRH analog.
**Dosage adjustment in renal impairment:** None necessary as renal impairment has no significant effect on elimination
**Dosage adjustment in liver impairment:** Limited data in subjects with severe hepatic impairment suggest that excretion of bicalutamide may be delayed and could lead to further accumulation. Use with caution in patients with moderate to severe hepatic impairment.

**Dosage Forms** Tab: 50 mg

**Contraindications** Known hypersensitivity to drug or any components of the product; pregnancy

**Pregnancy Risk Factor** X

**Adverse Reactions**
>10%: Endocrine & metabolic: Hot flashes (49%)
≥2% to <5%:
Cardiovascular: Angina pectoris, congestive heart failure, edema
Central nervous system: Anxiety, depression, confusion, somnolence, nervousness, fever, chills
Dermatologic: Dry skin, pruritus, alopecia
Endocrine & metabolic: Breast pain, diabetes mellitus, decreased libido, dehydration, gout
Gastrointestinal: Anorexia, dyspepsia, rectal hemorrhage, xerostomia, melena, weight gain
Genitourinary: Polyuria, urinary impairment, dysuria, urinary retention, urinary urgency
Hepatic: Alkaline phosphatase increased
Neuromuscular & skeletal: Myasthenia, arthritis, myalgia, leg cramps, pathological fracture, neck pain, hypertonia, neuropathy
(Continued)

## Bicalutamide *(Continued)*

Renal: Creatinine increased
Respiratory: Cough increased, pharyngitis, bronchitis, pneumonia, rhinitis, lung disorder
Miscellaneous: Sepsis, neoplasma
<1%: Diarrhea (0.5%)

**Half-Life** Active enantiomer is 5.8 days

**Special PA Issues**

**Patient Education:** Bicalutamide and the drug used for medical castration (LHRH analog) are administered concomitantly. Do not interrupt or stop taking medication without consulting prescriber. Take at same time each day with or without food. May cause dizziness, confusion, or drowsiness; use caution when driving or engaging in hazardous activities until response to drug is known. May cause nausea; small frequent meals may help. Increased exercise and increased dietary fluids, fruit, or fiber may reduce constipation. Report yellowing of skin or eyes, change in color of urine or stool, easy bruising or bleeding, unusual fatigue, chest pain, swelling of feet or ankles, unresolved anxiety or depression, or other unusual signs of adverse reactions.

**Monitoring Parameters:** Serum prostate-specific antigen, alkaline phosphatase, acid phosphatase, or prostatic acid phosphatase; prostate gland dimensions; skeletal survey; liver scans; chest x-rays; physical exam every 3 months; bone scan every 3-6 months; CBC, LFTs, EKG, echocardiograms, and serum testosterone and luteinizing hormone (periodically)

- **Bicillin® C-R** *see* Penicillin G Benzathine and Procaine Combined *on page 703*
- **Bicillin® C-R 900/300** *see* Penicillin G Benzathine and Procaine Combined *on page 703*
- **Bicillin® L-A** *see* Penicillin G Benzathine, Parenteral *on page 704*
- **Bicitra®** *see* Sodium Citrate and Citric Acid *on page 840*
- **Biltricide®** *see* Praziquantel *on page 749*
- **Biocef** *see* Cephalexin *on page 179*
- **Bioderm®** *see* Bacitracin and Polymyxin B *on page 97*
- **Biodine [OTC]** *see* Povidone-Iodine *on page 747*
- **Biohist-LA®** *see* Carbinoxamine and Pseudoephedrine *on page 152*
- **Biomox®** *see* Amoxicillin *on page 61*
- **Bio-Tab® Oral** *see* Doxycycline *on page 306*
- **Biozyme-C®** *see* Collagenase *on page 235*
- **Bismatrol® [OTC]** *see* Bismuth *on this page*

## Bismuth *(BIZ muth)*

**Pharmacologic Class** Antidiarrheal

**U.S. Brand Names** Bismatrol® [OTC]; Devrom® [OTC]; Pepto-Bismol® [OTC]; Pink Bismuth® [OTC]

**Mechanism of Action** Bismuth subsalicylate exhibits both antisecretory and antimicrobial action. This agent may provide some anti-inflammatory action as well. The salicylate moiety provides antisecretory effect and the bismuth exhibits antimicrobial directly against bacterial and viral gastrointestinal pathogens. Bismuth has some antacid properties.

**Use** Symptomatic treatment of mild, nonspecific diarrhea; indigestion, nausea, control of traveler's diarrhea (enterotoxigenic *Escherichia coli*); an adjunct with other agents such as metronidazole, tetracycline, and an $H_2$-antagonist in the treatment of *Helicobacter pylori*-associated duodenal ulcer disease

**USUAL DOSAGE** Oral:

Nonspecific diarrhea: Subsalicylate:

Children: Up to 8 doses/24 hours:

3-6 years: $^1/_3$ tablet or 5 mL every 30 minutes to 1 hour as needed
6-9 years: $^2/_3$ tablet or 10 mL every 30 minutes to 1 hour as needed
9-12 years: 1 tablet or 15 mL every 30 minutes to 1 hour as needed

Adults: 2 tablets or 30 mL every 30 minutes to 1 hour as needed up to 8 doses/24 hours

Prevention of traveler's diarrhea: 2.1 g/day or 2 tablets 4 times/day before meals and at bedtime

Subgallate: 1-2 tablets 3 times/day with meals

*Helicobacter pylori*: Chew 2 tablets 4 times/day with meals and at bedtime with other agents in selected regiment (eg, an $H_2$-antagonist, tetracycline and metronidazole) for 14 days

**Dosing adjustment in renal impairment:** Should probably be avoided in patients with renal failure

**Dosage Forms** Liq, as subsalicylate (Pepto-Bismol®, Bismatrol®): 262 mg/15 mL (120 mL, 240 mL, 360 mL, 480 mL), 524 mg/15 mL (120 mL, 240 mL, 360 mL); **Tab:** Chewable, as subsalicylate (Pepto-Bismol®, Bismatrol®): 262 mg, Chewable, as subgallate (Devrom®): 200 mg

**Contraindications** Do not use subsalicylate in patients with influenza or chickenpox because of risk of Reye's syndrome; do not use in patients with known hypersensitivity to salicylates; history of severe GI bleeding; history of coagulopathy

**Warnings/Precautions** Subsalicylate should be used with caution if patient is taking aspirin; use with caution in children, especially those <3 years of age and those with viral illness; may be neurotoxic with very large doses

**Pregnancy Risk Factor** C (D in 3rd trimester)

**Adverse Reactions**
>10%: Gastrointestinal: Discoloration of the tongue (darkening), grayish black stools
<1%: Anxiety, confusion, slurred speech, headache, mental depression, impaction may occur in infants and debilitated patients, muscle spasms, weakness, hearing loss, tinnitus

**Drug Interactions**
Decreased effect: Tetracyclines and uricosurics
Increased toxicity: Aspirin, warfarin, hypoglycemics

**Special PA Issues**
**Patient Education:** Chew tablet well or shake suspension well before using; may darken stools; if diarrhea persists for more than 2 days, consult a physician; can turn tongue black; tinnitus may indicate toxicity and use should be discontinued

- ♦ **Bismuth Subgallate** *see Bismuth on previous page*
- ♦ **Bismuth Subsalicylate** *see Bismuth on previous page*

# Bismuth Subsalicylate, Metronidazole, and Tetracycline
(BIZ muth sub sa LIS i late, me troe NI da zole, & tet ra SYE kleen)
**Pharmacologic Class** Antidiarrheal
**U.S. Brand Names** Helidac™
**Dosage Forms Cap:** Tetracycline: 500 mg; **Tab:** Bismuth subsalicylate: Chewable: 262.4 mg, Metronidazole: 250 mg

## Bisoprolol (bis OH proe lol)
**Pharmacologic Class** Beta Blocker, Beta₁ Selective
**U.S. Brand Names** Zebeta®
**Mechanism of Action** Selective inhibitor of beta$_1$-adrenergic receptors; competitively blocks beta$_1$-receptors, with little or no effect on beta$_2$-receptors at doses <10 mg
**Use** Treatment of hypertension, alone or in combination with other agents
**Unlabeled use:** Angina pectoris, supraventricular arrhythmias, PVCs
**USUAL DOSAGE** Oral:
Adults: 5 mg once daily, may be increased to 10 mg, and then up to 20 mg once daily, if necessary
Elderly: Initial dose: 2.5 mg/day; may be increased by 2.5-5 mg/day; maximum recommended dose: 20 mg/day
**Dosing adjustment in renal/hepatic impairment:** Cl$_{cr}$ <40 mL/minute: Initial: 2.5 mg/day; increase cautiously
Hemodialysis: Not dialyzable
**Dosage Forms Tab, as fumarate:** 5 mg, 10 mg
**Contraindications** Hypersensitivity to beta-blocking agents, uncompensated congestive heart failure; cardiogenic shock; bradycardia or heart block; sinus node dysfunction; A-V conduction abnormalities. Although bisoprolol primarily blocks beta$_1$-receptors, high doses can result in beta$_2$-receptor blockage. Therefore, use with caution in patients (especially elderly) with bronchospastic lung disease and renal dysfunction.
**Warnings/Precautions** Use with caution in patients with inadequate myocardial function, bronchospastic disease, hyperthyroidism, undergoing anesthesia; and in those with impaired hepatic function; acute withdrawal may exacerbate symptoms (gradually taper over a 2-week period)
**Pregnancy Risk Factor** C
**Pregnancy Implications** Enters breast milk/use caution
**Adverse Reactions**
>10%: Central nervous system: Fatigue, lethargy
1% to 10%:
Cardiovascular: Hypotension, chest pain, heart failure, Raynaud's phenomenon, heart block, edema, bradycardia
Central nervous system: Headache, dizziness, insomnia, confusion, depression, abnormal dreams
Dermatologic: Rash
Gastrointestinal: Constipation, diarrhea, dyspepsia, nausea, flatulence, anorexia
Genitourinary: Polyuria, impotence, urinary retention
Hepatic: Increased LFTs
Neuromuscular & skeletal: Arthralgia, myalgia
Ocular: Abnormal vision
Respiratory: Dyspnea, rhinitis, cough
**Drug Interactions** CYP2D6 enzyme substrate
Decreased effect of some beta-blockers with aluminum salts, barbiturates, calcium salts, cholestyramine, colestipol, NSAIDs, penicillins (ampicillin), rifampin, salicylates, and sulfinpyrazone due to decreased bioavailability and plasma levels
Beta-blockers may decrease the effect of sulfonylureas
(Continued)

## Bisoprolol (Continued)

Increased effect/toxicity of beta-blockers with calcium blockers (diltiazem, felodipine, nicardipine), contraceptives, flecainide, hydralazine (metoprolol, propranolol), propafenone, quinidine (in extensive metabolizers), ciprofloxacin,

Beta-blockers may increase the effect/toxicity of flecainide, hydralazine, clonidine (hypertensive crisis after or during withdrawal of either agent), epinephrine (initial hypertensive episode followed by bradycardia), nifedipine, verapamil, lidocaine, ergots, prazosin

Beta-blockers may affect the action or levels of ethanol, disopyramide, nondepolarizing muscle relaxants and theophylline although the effects are difficult to predict

**Onset** 1-2 hours

**Half-Life** 9-12 hours

**Special PA Issues**

**Patient Education:** Take exactly as directed. Do not increase, decrease, or adjust dosage without consulting prescriber. Do not take with antacids and do not use alcohol or OTC medications (eg, cold remedies) without consulting prescriber. If diabetic, monitor serum sugars closely (may alter glucose tolerance or mask signs of hypoglycemia). May cause fatigue, dizziness, or postural hypotension; use caution when changing position from lying or sitting to standing, or when driving or climbing stairs until response to medication is known. May cause alteration in sexual performance (reversible). Report palpitations, unresolved swelling of extremities, difficulty breathing or new cough, unresolved fatigue, unusual weight gain, unresolved constipation, or unusual muscle weakness.

**Monitoring Parameters:** Blood pressure, EKG, neurologic status

**Related Information**

Beta-Blockers on page 1002

## Bisoprolol and Hydrochlorothiazide

(bis OH proe lol & hye droe klor oh THYE a zide)

**Pharmacologic Class** Antihypertensive Agent, Combination

**U.S. Brand Names** Ziac™

**Dosage Forms Tab:** Bisoprolol fumarate 2.5 mg and hydrochlorothiazide 6.25 mg, Bisoprolol fumarate 5 mg and hydrochlorothiazide 6.25 mg, Bisoprolol fumarate 10 mg and hydrochlorothiazide 6.25 mg

♦ **Bisoprolol Fumarate** see Bisoprolol on previous page

♦ **Bistropamide** see Tropicamide on page 943

## Bitolterol (bye TOLE ter ole)

**Pharmacologic Class** Beta$_2$ Agonist

**U.S. Brand Names** Tornalate®

**Mechanism of Action** Selectively stimulates beta$_2$-adrenergic receptors in the lungs producing bronchial smooth muscle relaxation; minor beta$_1$ activity

**Use** Prevention and treatment of bronchial asthma and bronchospasm

**USUAL DOSAGE** Children >12 years and Adults:

Bronchospasm: 2 inhalations at an interval of at least 1-3 minutes, followed by a third inhalation if needed

Prevention of bronchospasm: 2 inhalations every 8 hours; do not exceed 3 inhalations every 6 hours or 2 inhalations every 4 hours

**Dosage Forms Aero, oral:** 0.8% [370 mcg/metered spray, 300 inhalations] (15 mL); **Soln, inh:** 0.2% (10 mL, 30 mL, 60 mL)

**Contraindications** Known hypersensitivity to bitolterol

**Warnings/Precautions** Use with caution in patients with unstable vasomotor symptoms, diabetes, hyperthyroidism, prostatic hypertrophy or a history of seizures; also use caution in the elderly and those patients with cardiovascular disorders such as coronary artery disease, arrhythmias, and hypertension; excessive use may result in cardiac arrest and death; do not use concurrently with other sympathomimetic bronchodilators

**Pregnancy Risk Factor** C

**Adverse Reactions**

>10%: Neuromuscular & skeletal: Trembling

1% to 10%:

Cardiovascular: Flushing of face, hypertension, pounding heartbeat

Central nervous system: Dizziness, lightheadedness, nervousness

Gastrointestinal: Xerostomia, nausea, unpleasant taste

Respiratory: Bronchial irritation, coughing

<1%: Chest pain, arrhythmias, tachycardia, insomnia, paradoxical bronchospasm

**Drug Interactions**

Decreased effect: Beta-adrenergic blockers (eg, propranolol)

Increased effect: Inhaled ipratropium may increase duration of bronchodilation, nifedipine may increase FEV-1

Increased toxicity: MAO inhibitors, tricyclic antidepressants, sympathomimetic agents (eg, amphetamine, dopamine, dobutamine), inhaled anesthetics (eg, enflurane)

**Onset** Rapid

**Duration** 4-8 hours

**Half-Life** 3 hours

**Special PA Issues**

**Patient Education:** Use exactly as directed (see Administration below). Do not use more often than recommended. Maintain adequate hydration (2-3 L/day of fluids unless instructed to restrict fluid intake). You may experience nervousness, dizziness, or fatigue (use caution when driving or engaging in hazardous activities until response to treatment is known); or dry mouth, stomach upset (frequent small meals, frequent mouth care, chewing gum, or sucking hard candy may help). Report unresolved GI upset; dizziness or fatigue; vision changes; chest pain, rapid heartbeat, or palpitations; nervousness or insomnia; muscle cramping or tremor; or unusual cough.

**Administration:** Self-administered inhalation: Store canister upside down; do not freeze. Shake canister before using. Sit when using medication. Close eyes when administering bitolterol to avoid spray getting into eyes. Exhale slowly and completely through nose; inhale deeply through mouth while administering aerosol. Hold breath for 1-3 seconds after inhalation. Wait at least 1 full minute between inhalations. Wash mouthpiece between use. If more than one inhalation medication is used, use bitolterol first and wait 5 minutes between medications.

Self-administered nebulizer: Wash hands before and after treatment. Wash and dry nebulizer after each treatment. Twist open the top of one unit dose vial and squeeze contents into nebulizer reservoir. Connect nebulizer reservoir to the mouthpiece or face-mask. Connect nebulizer to compressor. Sit in comfortable, upright position. Place mouthpiece in your mouth or put on face-mask and turn on compressor. If face-mask is used, avoid leakage around the mask to avoid mist getting into eyes which may cause vision problems. Breath calmly and deeply until no more mist is formed in nebulizer (about 5 minutes). At this point treatment is finished.

**Monitoring Parameters:** Assess lung sounds, pulse, and blood pressure before administration and during peak of medication; observe patient for wheezing after administration

♦ **Bitolterol Mesylate** *see Bitolterol on previous page*

♦ **Black Susans** *see Echinacea on page 310*

♦ **Bleph®-10 Ophthalmic** *see Sulfacetamide Sodium on page 858*

♦ **Blephamide® Ophthalmic** *see Sulfacetamide Sodium and Prednisolone on page 859*

♦ **Blis-To-Sol® [OTC]** *see Tolnaftate on page 915*

♦ **Blocadren® Oral** *see Timolol on page 905*

♦ **Body Mass Index Chart** *see Chart on page 988*

♦ **Body Surface Area of Adults and Children** *see Chart on page 986*

♦ **Bonine® [OTC]** *see Meclizine on page 559*

♦ **B&O Supprettes®** *see Belladonna and Opium on page 102*

♦ **Botox®** *see Botulinum Toxin Type A on this page*

# Botulinum Toxin Type A (BOT yoo lin num TOKS in type aye)

**Pharmacologic Class** Ophthalmic Agent, Toxin

**U.S. Brand Names** Botox®

**Mechanism of Action** Botulinum A toxin is a neurotoxin produced by *Clostridium botulinum*, spore-forming anaerobic bacillus, which appears to affect only the presynaptic membrane of the neuromuscular junction in humans, where it prevents calcium-dependent release of acetylcholine and produces a state of denervation. Muscle inactivation persists until new fibrils grow from the nerve and form junction plates on new areas of the muscle-cell walls. The antagonist muscle shortens simultaneously ("contracture"), taking up the slack created by agonist paralysis; following several weeks of paralysis, alignment of the eye is measurably changed, despite return of innervation to the injected muscle.

**Use** Treatment of strabismus and blepharospasm associated with dystonia (including benign essential blepharospasm or VII nerve disorders in patients ≥12 years of age)

**Unlabeled use:** Treatment of hemifacial spasms, spasmodic torticollis (ie, cervical dystonia, clonic twisting of the head), oromandibular dystonia, spasmodic dysphonia (laryngeal dystonia) and other dystonias (ie, writer's cramp, focal task-specific dystonias)

**Orphan drug:** Treatment of dynamic muscle contracture in pediatric cerebral palsy patients

**USUAL DOSAGE**

Strabismus: 1.25-5 units (0.05-0.15 mL) injected into any one muscle

Subsequent doses for residual/recurrent strabismus: Re-examine patients 7-14 days after each injection to assess the effect of that dose. Subsequent doses for patients experiencing incomplete paralysis of the target may be increased up to two fold the previously administered dose. Maximum recommended dose as a single injection for any one muscle is 25 units.

Blepharospasm: 1.25-2.5 units (0.05-0.10 mL) injected into the orbicularis oculi muscle

Subsequent doses: Each treatment lasts approximately 3 months. At repeat treatment sessions, the dose may be increased up to twofold if the response from the initial treatment is considered insufficient (usually defined as an effect that does not last >2 months). There appears to be little benefit obtainable from injecting >5 units per site.

(Continued)

## Botulinum Toxin Type A *(Continued)*

Some tolerance may be found if treatments are given any more frequently than every 3 months.

The cumulative dose should not exceed 200 units in a 30-day period

**Dosage Forms** Inj: 100 units *Clostridium botulinum* toxin type A

**Contraindications** Hypersensitivity to botulinum A toxin; relative contraindications to botulinum toxin therapy include diseases of neuromuscular transmission and coagulopathy, including anticoagulant therapy; injections into the central area of the upper eyelid (rapid diffusion of toxin into the levator can occur resulting in a marked ptosis).

**Warnings/Precautions** Use with caution in patients taking aminoglycosides or any other antibiotic or other drugs that interfere with neuromuscular transmission; do not exceed recommended dose

**Pregnancy Risk Factor** C

**Adverse Reactions**

>10%: Ocular: Dry eyes, lagophthalmos, ptosis, photophobia, vertical deviation

1% to 10%:
  Dermatologic: Diffuse rash
  Ocular: Eyelid edema, blepharospasm

<1%: Ectropion, keratitis, diplopia, entropion

**Drug Interactions** Increased effect: Botulinum toxin may be potentiated by aminoglycosides

**Special PA Issues**

  **Patient Education:** Patients with blepharospasm may have been extremely sedentary for a long time; caution these patients to resume activity slowly and carefully following administration

- **Bovine Lung Surfactant** *see* Beractant *on page 110*
- **Breast-Feeding and Drugs** *see* Chart *on page 1120*
- **Breathe Free® [OTC]** *see* Sodium Chloride *on page 839*
- **Breezee® Mist Antifungal [OTC]** *see* Tolnaftate *on page 915*
- **Breezee® Mist Antifungal [OTC]** *see* Miconazole *on page 604*
- **Breonesin® [OTC]** *see* Guaifenesin *on page 427*
- **Brethaire® Inhalation Aerosol** *see* Terbutaline *on page 879*
- **Brethine® Injection** *see* Terbutaline *on page 879*
- **Brethine® Oral** *see* Terbutaline *on page 879*
- **Brevicon®** *see* Ethinyl Estradiol and Norethindrone *on page 348*
- **Bricanyl® Injection** *see* Terbutaline *on page 879*
- **Bricanyl® Oral** *see* Terbutaline *on page 879*

## Brimonidine *(bri MOE ni deen)*

**Pharmacologic Class** Alpha$_2$ Agonist, Ophthalmic; Ophthalmic Agent, Antiglaucoma

**U.S. Brand Names** Alphagan®

**Mechanism of Action** Selective for alpha$_2$-receptors; appears to result in reduction of aqueous humor formation and increase uveoscleral outflow

**Use** Lowering of intraocular pressure in patients with open-angle glaucoma or ocular hypertension

**USUAL DOSAGE** Adults: Ophthalmic: Instill 1 drop in affected eye(s) 3 times/day (approximately every 8 hours)

**Dosage Forms** Soln, ophth, as tartrate: 0.2% (5 mL, 10 mL)

**Contraindications** Known hypersensitivity to brimonidine tartrate or any component of this medication; patients receiving monoamine oxidase (MAO) inhibitor therapy

**Warnings/Precautions** Exercise caution in treating patients with severe cardiovascular disease. Use with caution in patients with depression, cerebral or coronary insufficiency, Raynaud's phenomenon, orthostatic hypotension or thromboangiitis obliterans

The preservative in brimonidine tartrate, benzalkonium chloride, may be absorbed by soft contact lenses; instruct patients wearing soft contact lenses to wait at least 15 minutes after instilling brimonidine tartrate to insert soft contact lenses

Use with caution in patients with hepatic or renal impairment

Loss of effect in some patients may occur. The IOP-lowering efficacy observed with brimonidine tartrate during the first of month of therapy may not always reflect the long term level of IOP reduction. Routinely monitor IOP.

**Pregnancy Risk Factor** B

**Adverse Reactions**

>10%:
  Central nervous system: Headache, fatigue/drowsiness
  Gastrointestinal: Xerostomia
  Ocular: Ocular hyperemia, burning and stinging, blurring, foreign body sensation, conjunctival follicles, ocular allergic reactions and ocular pruritus

1% to 10%:
  Central nervous system: Dizziness

Ocular: Corneal staining/erosion, photophobia, eyelid erythema, ocular ache/pain, ocular dryness, tearing, eyelid edema, conjunctival edema, blepharitis, ocular irritation, conjunctival blanching, abnormal vision, lid crusting, conjunctival hemorrhage, abnormal taste, conjunctival discharge

Respiratory: Upper respiratory symptoms

<1%: Allergic response, some systemic effects have also been reported including GI, CNS, and cardiovascular symptoms (arrhythmias)

**Drug Interactions**

Increased effect:

CNS depressants (eg, alcohol, barbiturates, opiates, sedatives, anesthetics): Additive or potentiating effect

Topical beta-blockers, pilocarpine → additive decreased intraocular pressure, antihypertensives, cardiac glycosides

Decreased effect: Tricyclic antidepressants can affect the metabolism and uptake of circulating amines

**Onset** 1-4 hours

**Duration** 12 hours

**Special PA Issues**

**Patient Education:** For ophthalmic use only. Store in refrigerator. If you wear soft contact lenses, remove before using medication and wait at least 15 minutes before replacing. Apply prescribed amount as often as directed. Wash hands before using and do not let tip of applicator touch eye or contaminate tip of applicator. Tilt head back and look upward. Gently pull down lower lid and put drop(s) in inner corner of eye. Close eye and roll eyeball in all directions. Do not blink for $^1/_2$ minute. Apply gentle pressure to inner corner of eye for 30 seconds. Wipe away excess from skin around eye. Do not use any other eye preparation for at least 10 minutes. Do not touch tip of applicator to eye or contaminate tip of applicator. Do not share medication with anyone else. Temporary stinging or blurred vision may occur. May cause tiredness or dizziness (use caution when driving or engaging in tasks that require alertness). Inform prescriber if you experience persistent eye pain, redness, burning, watering, dryness, double vision, puffiness around eye, vision disturbances, or other adverse eye response; worsening of condition or lack of improvement.

**Monitoring Parameters:** Closely monitor patients who develop fatigue or drowsiness

♦ **Brimonidine Tartrate** see Brimonidine on previous page

# Brinzolamide (brin ZOH la mide)

**Pharmacologic Class** Carbonic Anhydrase Inhibitor; Ophthalmic Agent, Antiglaucoma

**U.S. Brand Names** Azopt™

**Mechanism of Action** Inhibition of carbonic anhydrase decreases aqueous humor secretion. This results in a reduction of intraocular pressure.

**Use** Lowers intraocular pressure to treat glaucoma in patients with ocular hypertension or open-angle glaucoma

**USUAL DOSAGE** Adults: Ophthalmic: Instill 1 drop in affected eye(s) 3 times/day

**Dosage Forms** Susp, ophth: 1% (2.5 mL, 5 mL, 10 mL, 15 mL)

**Contraindications** Hypersensitivity to brinzolamide or any component

**Warnings/Precautions** Effects of prolonged use on corneal epithelial cells have not been evaluated; has not been studied in acute angle-closure glaucoma; renal impairment (parent and metabolite may accumulate). Patients with allergy to sulfonamides (brinzolamide is a sulfonamide); systemic absorption may cause serious hypersensitivity reactions to recur.

**Pregnancy Risk Factor** C

**Adverse Reactions**

1% to 10%:

Dermatologic: Dermatitis (1% to 5%)

Gastrointestinal: Taste disturbances (5% to 10%)

Ocular: Blurred vision (5% to 10%), blepharitis (1% to 5%), dry eye (1% to 5%), foreign body sensation (1% to 5%), eye discharge (1% to 5%), eye pain (1% to 5%), itching of eye (1% to 5%)

Respiratory: Rhinitis

<1%: Dizziness, headache, urticaria, alopecia, diarrhea, nausea, xerostomia, diplopia, eye fatigue, lid crusting, dyspnea, pharyngitis, allergic reactions

**Drug Interactions**

Concurrent use of oral carbonic anhydrase inhibitors (CAIs) - additive effects and toxicity

High-dose salicylates may result in toxicity from CAIs

**Onset** Peak: 2 hours

**Duration** 8-12 hours

**Special PA Issues**

**Patient Education:** If using other ophthalmic preparations, administer 10 minutes apart. Avoid excessive use of aspirin or aspirin-containing medications (may cause toxicity). May cause taste changes; runny nose; or vision disturbances (blurred vision, dry eye, foreign body sensation, eye discharge, temporary sensitivity to bright light, blurring or

(Continued)

## Brinzolamide *(Continued)*

stinging, altered distance perception, reduced night vision acuity). Report persistent dizziness or headache, skin rash, loss of hair, unresolved gastrointestinal disturbance, difficulty breathing, or persistent sore throat.

**Administration:** Tilt head back, place medication in conjunctival sac, and close eyes. Apply finger pressure at corner of eye for 1 minute following application. Do not allow tip of applicator to touch eye or any contaminated surface.

**Monitoring Parameters:** Intraocular pressure

♦ **Bromanate® DC** *see* Brompheniramine, Phenylpropanolamine, and Codeine *on next page*

♦ **Bromanyl® Cough Syrup** *see* Bromodiphenhydramine and Codeine *on next page*

## Bromocriptine (broe moe KRIP teen)

**Pharmacologic Class** Anti-Parkinson's Agent (Dopamine Agonist); Ergot Derivative

**U.S. Brand Names** Parlodel®

**Mechanism of Action** Semisynthetic ergot alkaloid derivative with dopaminergic properties; inhibits prolactin secretion and can improve symptoms of Parkinson's disease by directly stimulating dopamine receptors in the corpus stratum

**Use**

Usually used with levodopa or levodopa/carbidopa to treat Parkinson's disease - treatment of parkinsonism in patients unresponsive or allergic to levodopa

Prolactin-secreting pituitary adenomas

Acromegaly

Amenorrhea/galactorrhea secondary to hyperprolactinemia in the absence of primary tumor

**The indication for prevention of postpartum lactation has been withdrawn** voluntarily by Sandoz Pharmaceuticals Corporation

**USUAL DOSAGE** Adults: Oral:

Parkinsonism: 1.25 mg 2 times/day, increased by 2.5 mg/day in 2- to 4-week intervals (usual dose range is 30-90 mg/day in 3 divided doses), though elderly patients can usually be managed on lower doses

Hyperprolactinemia: 2.5 mg 2-3 times/day

Acromegaly: Initial: 1.25-2.5 mg increasing as necessary every 3-7 days; usual dose: 20-30 mg/day

**Dosing adjustment in hepatic impairment:** No guidelines are available, however, may be necessary

**Dosage Forms** Bromocriptine mesylate: **Cap:** 5 mg; **Tab:** 2.5 mg

**Contraindications** Hypersensitivity to bromocriptine or any component, severe ischemic heart disease or peripheral vascular disorders, pregnancy

**Warnings/Precautions** Use with caution in patients with impaired renal or hepatic function

**Pregnancy Risk Factor** C (See Contraindications)

**Pregnancy Implications** Enters breast milk/contraindicated

**Adverse Reactions** Incidence of adverse effects is high, especially at beginning of treatment and with dosages >20 mg/day

1% to 10%:
Cardiovascular: Hypotension, Raynaud's phenomenon
Central nervous system: Mental depression, confusion, hallucinations
Gastrointestinal: Nausea, constipation, anorexia
Neuromuscular & skeletal: Leg cramps
Respiratory: Nasal congestion
<1%: Hypertension, myocardial infarction, syncope, dizziness, drowsiness, fatigue, insomnia, headache, seizures, vomiting, abdominal cramps

**Drug Interactions** CYP3A3/4 enzyme substrate

Decreased effect: Amitriptyline, butyrophenones, imipramine, methyldopa, phenothiazines, reserpine, may decrease bromocriptine's efficacy at reducing prolactin

Increased toxicity: Ergot alkaloids (increased cardiovascular toxicity)

**Onset** Peak serum concentrations: 1-2 hours

**Half-Life** Half-life (biphasic): Initial: 6-8 hours; Terminal: 50 hours

**Special PA Issues**

**Patient Education:** Take exactly as directed (may be prescribed in conjunction with levodopa/carbidopa); do not change dosage or discontinue without consulting prescriber. Therapeutic effects may take several weeks or months to achieve and you may need frequent monitoring during first weeks of therapy. Take with meals if GI upset occurs, before meals if dry mouth occurs, after eating if drooling or if nausea occurs. Take at same time each day. Maintain adequate hydration (2-3 L/day of fluids unless instructed to restrict fluid intake); void before taking medication. Do not use alcohol and prescription or OTC sedatives or CNS depressants without consulting prescriber. Urine or perspiration may appear darker. You may experience drowsiness, dizziness, confusion, or vision changes (use caution when driving, climbing stairs, or engaging in hazardous tasks); orthostatic hypotension (use caution when changing position - rising to standing from sitting or lying); constipation (increased exercise, fluids, or dietary fruit and fiber may help); nasal congestion (consult prescriber for appropriate relief); nausea, vomiting, loss of appetite, or stomach discomfort (small frequent meals, chewing gum, or sucking on lozenges may help). Report unresolved constipation or vomiting; chest pain or irregular heartbeat; acute headache or dizziness; CNS changes (hallucination, loss of memory, seizures, acute headache, nervousness, etc); painful or difficult urination; increased muscle spasticity, rigidity, or involuntary movements; skin rash; or significant worsening of condition.

**Monitoring Parameters:** Monitor blood pressure closely as well as hepatic, hematopoietic, and cardiovascular function

♦ **Bromocriptine Mesylate** see Bromocriptine on previous page

# Bromodiphenhydramine and Codeine
(brome oh dye fen HYE dra meen & KOE deen)

**Pharmacologic Class** Antihistamine/Antitussive

**U.S. Brand Names** Ambenyl® Cough Syrup; Amgenal® Cough Syrup; Bromanyl® Cough Syrup; Bromotuss® w/Codeine Cough Syrup

**Dosage Forms Liq:** Bromodiphenhydramine hydrochloride 12.5 mg and codeine phosphate 10 mg per 5 mL

♦ **Bromotuss® w/Codeine Cough Syrup** see Bromodiphenhydramine and Codeine on this page

♦ **Bromphen® DC w/Codeine** see Brompheniramine, Phenylpropanolamine, and Codeine on this page

# Brompheniramine, Phenylpropanolamine, and Codeine
(brome fen IR a meen, fen il proe pa NOLE a meen, & KOE deen)

**Pharmacologic Class** Antihistamine/Decongestant/Antitussive

**U.S. Brand Names** Bromanate® DC; Bromphen® DC w/Codeine; Dimetane®-DC; Myphetane DC®; Poly-Histine CS®

**Dosage Forms Liq:** Brompheniramine maleate 2 mg, phenylpropanolamine hydrochloride 12.5 mg, and codeine phosphate 10 mg per 5 mL with alcohol 0.95% (480 mL)

♦ **Bronalide®** see Flunisolide on page 379
♦ **Bronchial®** see Theophylline and Guaifenesin on page 888
♦ **Bronkodyl®** see Theophylline Salts on page 888
♦ **Bronkometer®** see Isoetharine on page 493
♦ **Bronkosol®** see Isoetharine on page 493
♦ **Brontex® Liquid** see Guaifenesin and Codeine on page 428
♦ **Brontex® Tablet** see Guaifenesin and Codeine on page 428
♦ **Bucladin®-S Softab®** see Buclizine on this page

# Buclizine (BYOO kli zeen)

**Pharmacologic Class** Antihistamine

**U.S. Brand Names** Bucladin®-S Softab®; Vibazine®

**Mechanism of Action** Buclizine acts centrally to suppress nausea and vomiting. It is a piperazine antihistamine closely related to cyclizine and meclizine. It also has CNS depressant, anticholinergic, antispasmodic, and local anesthetic effects, and suppresses labyrinthine activity and conduction in vestibular-cerebellar nerve pathways.

**Use** Prevention and treatment of motion sickness; symptomatic treatment of vertigo

**USUAL DOSAGE** Adults: Oral:

Motion sickness (prophylaxis): 50 mg 30 minutes prior to traveling; may repeat 50 mg after 4-6 hours

Vertigo: 50 mg twice daily, up to 150 mg/day

**Dosage Forms Tab, chewable, as hydrochloride:** 50 mg

**Contraindications** Known hypersensitivity to buclizine

**Warnings/Precautions** Product contains tartrazine; use with caution in patients with angle-closure glaucoma, peptic ulcer, urinary tract obstruction, hyperthyroidism; some preparations contain sodium bisulfite; syrup contains alcohol

**Pregnancy Risk Factor** C

**Pregnancy Implications** Excretion in breast milk unknown/contraindicated

**Adverse Reactions**

>10%: Central nervous system: Drowsiness

<1%: Hypotension, palpitations, sedation, dizziness, paradoxical excitement, fatigue, insomnia, nausea, vomiting, urinary retention, tremor, blurred vision

**Drug Interactions** Increased toxicity: CNS depressants, MAO inhibitors, tricyclic antidepressants

**Special PA Issues**

**Patient Education:** Take as directed. Do not increase dose or take more often than recommended. May cause drowsiness; use caution when driving or engaging in hazardous activities. May cause dry mouth; lozenges, gum, or liquids may help. May cause headache or feelings of jitteriness or anxiety; these will go away when drug is discontinued.

♦ **Buclizine Hydrochloride** *see* Buclizine *on previous page*

# Budesonide (byoo DES oh nide)

**Pharmacologic Class** Corticosteroid, Oral Inhaler; Corticosteroid, Nasal; Corticosteroid, Topical

**U.S. Brand Names** Pulmicort Turbuhaler®; Rhinocort®

**Mechanism of Action** Controls the rate of protein synthesis, depresses the migration of polymorphonuclear leukocytes, fibroblasts, reverses capillary permeability, and lysosomal stabilization at the cellular level to prevent or control inflammation

**Use**
Intranasal: Children and Adults: Management of symptoms of seasonal or perennial rhinitis
Oral inhalation: Maintenance and prophylactic treatment of asthma; includes patients who require corticosteroids and those who may benefit from systemic dose reduction/elimination

## USUAL DOSAGE
Children <6 years: Not recommended
Aerosol inhalation: Children ≥6 years and Adults: Nasal: Initial: 8 sprays (4 sprays/nostril) per day (256 mcg/day), given as either 2 sprays in each nostril in the morning and evening or as 4 sprays in each nostril in the morning; after symptoms decrease (usually by 3-7 days), reduce dose slowly every 2-4 weeks to the smallest amount needed to control symptoms
Oral inhalation:
Children ≥6 years:
Previous therapy of bronchodilators alone: 200 mcg twice initially which may be increased up to 400 mcg twice daily
Previous therapy of inhaled corticosteroids: 200 mcg twice initially which may be increased up to 400 mcg twice daily
Previous therapy of oral corticosteroids: The highest recommended dose in children is 400 mcg twice daily
Adults:
Previous therapy of bronchodilators alone: 200-400 mcg twice initially which may be increased up to 400 mcg twice daily
Previous therapy of inhaled corticosteroids: 200-400 mcg twice initially which may be increased up to 800 mcg twice daily
Previous therapy of oral corticosteroids: 400-800 mcg twice daily which may be increased up to 800 mcg twice daily
NIH Guidelines (NIH, 1997) (give in divided doses twice daily):
Children:
"Low" dose: 100-200 mcg/day
"Medium" dose: 200-400 mcg/day (1-2 inhalations/day)
"High" dose: >400 mcg/day (>2 inhalation/day)
Adults:
"Low" dose: 200-400 mcg/day (1-2 inhalations/day)
"Medium" dose: 400-600 mcg/day (2-3 inhalations/day)
"High" dose: >600 mcg/day (>3 inhalation/day)

**Dosage Forms Aero, nasal:** 32 mcg per actuation (7 g); **Powder (dry) for inhalation:** 200 mcg per metered dose

**Warnings/Precautions** Controlled clinical studies have shown that inhaled and intranasal corticosteroids may cause a reduction in growth velocity in pediatric patients. Growth velocity provides a means of comparing the rate of growth among children of the same age.

In studies involving inhaled corticosteroids, the average reduction in growth velocity was approximately 1 cm (about ⅓ of an inch) per year. It appears that the reduction is related to dose and how long the child takes the drug.

FDA's Pulmonary and Allergy Drugs and Metabolic and Endocrine Drugs advisory committees discussed this issue at a July 1998 meeting. They recommended that the agency develop class-wide labeling to inform healthcare providers so they would understand this potential side effect and monitor growth routinely in pediatric patients who are treated with inhaled corticosteroids, intranasal corticosteroids or both.

Long-term effects of this reduction in growth velocity on final adult height are unknown. Likewise, it also has not yet been determined whether patients' growth will "catch up" if treatment is discontinued. Drug manufacturers will continue to monitor these drugs to learn more about long-term effects. Children are prescribed inhaled corticosteroids to treat asthma. Intranasal corticosteroids are generally used to prevent and treat allergy-related nasal symptoms.

Patients are advised not to stop using their inhaled or intranasal corticosteroids without first speaking to their healthcare providers about the benefits of these drugs compared to their risks.

**Adverse Reactions**
>10%:
Cardiovascular: Pounding heartbeat
Central nervous system: Nervousness, headache, dizziness

Dermatologic: Itching, rash
Gastrointestinal: GI irritation, bitter taste, oral candidiasis
Respiratory: Coughing, upper respiratory tract infection, bronchitis, hoarseness
Miscellaneous: Increased susceptibility to infections, diaphoresis
1% to 10%:
Central nervous system: Insomnia, psychic changes
Dermatologic: Acne, urticaria
Endocrine & metabolic: Menstrual problems
Gastrointestinal: Anorexia, increase in appetite, xerostomia, dry throat, loss of taste perception
Ocular: Cataracts
Respiratory: Epistaxis
Miscellaneous: Loss of smell
<1%: Abdominal fullness, bronchospasm, shortness of breath

**Drug Interactions** CYP3A3/4 enzyme substrate
Although there have been no reported drug interactions to date, one would expect budesonide could potentially interact with drugs known to interact with other corticosteroids

**Special PA Issues**
**Patient Education:** Use as directed; do not increase dosage or discontinue abruptly without consulting prescriber. It may take several days for you to realize full effects of treatment. If you are also using an inhaled bronchodilator, wait 10 minutes before using this steroid aerosol. You may experience dizziness, anxiety, or blurred vision (rise slowly from sitting or lying position and use caution when driving or engaging in hazardous tasks until response to drug is known); or taste disturbance or aftertaste (frequent mouth care and mouth rinses may help). Report pounding heartbeat or chest pain; acute nervousness or inability to sleep; severe sneezing or nosebleed; difficulty breathing, sore throat, hoarseness, or bronchitis; respiratory difficulty or bronchospasms; disturbed menstrual pattern; vision changes; loss of taste or smell perception; or worsening of condition or lack of improvement.

**Administration:** Take 3-5 deep breaths. Use inhaler on inspiration. Allow 1 full minute between inhalations. Rinse mouth with water after use to reduce aftertaste and incidence of candidiasis.

**Related Information**
Asthma Therapy Guidelines *on page 1049*

♦ **Bufferin® [OTC]** *see* Aspirin *on page 80*
♦ **Buffex® [OTC]** *see* Aspirin *on page 80*

# Bumetanide (byoo MET a nide)
**Pharmacologic Class** Diuretic, Loop
**U.S. Brand Names** Bumex®
**Mechanism of Action** Inhibits reabsorption of sodium and chloride in the ascending loop of Henle and proximal renal tubule, interfering with the chloride-binding cotransport system, thus causing increased excretion of water, sodium, chloride, magnesium, phosphate and calcium; it does not appear to act on the distal tubule
**Use** Management of edema secondary to congestive heart failure or hepatic or renal disease including nephrotic syndrome; may be used alone or in combination with antihypertensives in the treatment of hypertension; can be used in furosemide-allergic patients; (1 mg = 40 mg furosemide)
**USUAL DOSAGE**
Children (not FDA-approved for use in children <18 years of age):
<6 months: Dose not established
>6 months:
Oral: Initial: 0.015 mg/kg/dose once daily or every other day; maximum dose: 0.1 mg/kg/day
I.M., I.V.: Dose not established
Adults:
Oral: 0.5-2 mg/dose 1-2 times/day; maximum: 10 mg/day
I.M., I.V.: 0.5-1 mg/dose; maximum: 10 mg/day
Continuous I.V. infusions of 0.9-1 mg/hour may be more effective than bolus dosing
**Dosage Forms** Inj: 0.25 mg/mL (2 mL, 4 mL, 10 mL); **Tab:** 0.5 mg, 1 mg, 2 mg
**Contraindications** Hypersensitivity to bumetanide or any component; in anuria or increasing azotemia
**Warnings/Precautions** Profound diuresis with fluid and electrolyte loss is possible; close medical supervision and dose evaluation is required; use caution when dosing in patients with hepatic failure
**Pregnancy Risk Factor** D
**Pregnancy Implications** Excretion in breast milk unknown/use caution
**Adverse Reactions**
>10%:
Endocrine & metabolic: Hyperuricemia, hypochloremia, hypokalemia
Renal: Azotemia
(Continued)

## Bumetanide *(Continued)*

1% to 10%:
Central nervous system: Dizziness, encephalopathy, headache
Endocrine & metabolic: Hyponatremia
Neuromuscular & skeletal: Muscle cramps, weakness
<1%: Hypotension, rash, pruritus, hyperglycemia, hyperuricemia, cramps, nausea, vomiting, altered LFTs, hearing loss, increased serum creatinine

**Drug Interactions**
Decreased effect: Indomethacin and other NSAIDs, probenecid
Increased effect: Other antihypertensive agents; lithium's excretion may be decreased

**Onset** Oral, I.M.: 0.5-1 hour I.V.: 2-3 minutes

**Duration** 6 hours

**Half-Life** Adults: 1-1.5 hours

**Special PA Issues**
**Patient Education:** May be taken with food to reduce GI effects. Take single dose early in day (single dose) or last dose early in afternoon (twice daily) to prevent sleep interruptions. Include orange juice or bananas (or other sources of potassium-rich foods) in your daily diet but do not take supplemental potassium without consulting prescriber. You may experience dizziness, hypotension, lightheadedness, or weakness; use caution when changing position (rising from sitting or lying position), when driving, exercising, climbing stairs, or performing hazardous tasks, and avoid excessive exercise in hot weather. Report swelling of ankles or feet, weight increase or decrease more than 3 pounds in any one day, increased fatigue, muscle cramps or trembling, and any changes in hearing.
**Monitoring Parameters:** Blood pressure, serum electrolytes, renal function

**Related Information**
Heart Failure: Management of Patients with Left Ventricular Systolic Dysfunction *on page 1064*

♦ **Bumex®** *see* Bumetanide *on previous page*
♦ **Buminate®** *see* Albumin *on page 34*
♦ **Buphenyl®** *see* Sodium Phenylbutyrate *on page 842*

## Bupivacaine *(byoo PIV a kane)*

**Pharmacologic Class** Local Anesthetic

**U.S. Brand Names** Marcaine®; Sensorcaine®; Sensorcaine®-MPF

**Mechanism of Action** Blocks both the initiation and conduction of nerve impulses by decreasing the neuronal membrane's permeability to sodium ions, which results in inhibition of depolarization with resultant blockade of conduction

**Use** Local anesthetic (injectable) for peripheral nerve block, infiltration, sympathetic block, caudal or epidural block, retrobulbar block

**USUAL DOSAGE** Dose varies with procedure, depth of anesthesia, vascularity of tissues, duration of anesthesia and condition of patient. Metabisulfites (in epinephrine-containing injection); do not use solutions containing preservatives for caudal or epidural block.

Caudal block (with or without epinephrine):
Children: 1-3.7 mg/kg
Adults: 15-30 mL of 0.25% or 0.5%
Epidural block (other than caudal block):
Children: 1.25 mg/kg/dose
Adults: 10-20 mL of 0.25% or 0.5%
Peripheral nerve block: 5 mL dose of 0.25% or 0.5% (12.5-25 mg); maximum: 2.5 mg/kg (plain); 3 mg/kg (with epinephrine); up to a maximum of 400 mg/day
Sympathetic nerve block: 20-50 mL of 0.25% (no epinephrine) solution

**Dosage Forms** Inj, as hydrochloride: 0.25% (10 mL, 20 mL, 30 mL, 50 mL), 0.5% (10 mL, 20 mL, 30 mL, 50 mL), 0.75% (2 mL, 10 mL, 20 mL, 30 mL); **Inj, as hydrochloride, with epinephrine (1:200,000):** 0.25% (10 mL, 30 mL, 50 mL), 0.5% (1.8 mL, 3 mL, 5 mL, 10 mL, 30 mL), 0.75% (30 mL)

**Contraindications** Hypersensitivity to bupivacaine hydrochloride or any component, para-aminobenzoic acid or parabens

**Warnings/Precautions** Use with caution in patients with liver disease. Some commercially available formulations contain sodium metabisulfite, which may cause allergic-type reactions. Pending further data, should not be used in children <12 years of age and the solution for spinal anesthesia should not be used in children <18 years of age. **Do not use solutions containing preservatives for caudal or epidural block**; convulsions due to systemic toxicity leading to cardiac arrest have been reported, presumably following unintentional intravascular injection. 0.75% is **not** recommended for obstetrical anesthesia.

**Pregnancy Risk Factor** C

**Adverse Reactions** 1% to 10% (dose related):
Cardiovascular: Cardiac arrest, hypotension, bradycardia, palpitations
Central nervous system: Seizures, restlessness, anxiety, dizziness
Gastrointestinal: Nausea, vomiting
Neuromuscular & skeletal: Weakness

Ocular: Blurred vision
Otic: Tinnitus
Respiratory: Apnea

**Drug Interactions**
Increased effect: Hyaluronidase
Increased toxicity: Beta-blockers, ergot-type oxytocics, MAO inhibitors, TCAs, phenothiazines, vasopressors

**Onset** Onset of anesthesia (dependent on route administered): Within 4-10 minutes generally

**Duration** 1.5-8.5 hours

**Half-Life** 1.5-5.5 hours

**Special PA Issues**
**Patient Education:** This medication is given to reduce sensation in the injected area. You will experience decreased sensation to pain, heat, or cold in the area and/or decreased muscle strength (depending on area of application) until the effects wear off; use necessary caution to reduce incidence of possible injury until full sensation returns. If used in mouth, do not eat or drink until full sensation returns. Immediately report chest pain or palpitations; increased restlessness, anxiety, or dizziness; skeletal or muscle weakness; difficulty breathing; ringing in ears; or changes in vision.

**Monitoring Parameters:** Monitor fetal heart rate during paracervical anesthesia

♦ **Bupivacaine Hydrochloride** see Bupivacaine on previous page

♦ **Buprenex®** see Buprenorphine on this page

# Buprenorphine (byoo pre NOR feen)

**Pharmacologic Class** Analgesic, Narcotic

**U.S. Brand Names** Buprenex®

**Mechanism of Action** Opiate agonist/antagonist that produces analgesia by binding to kappa and mu opiate receptors in the CNS

**Use** Management of moderate to severe pain

**USUAL DOSAGE** I.M., slow I.V.:
Children ≥13 years and Adults: 0.3-0.6 mg every 6 hours as needed
Elderly: 0.15 mg every 6 hours; elderly patients are more likely to suffer from confusion and drowsiness compared to younger patients
Long-term use is not recommended

**Dosage Forms** Inj, as hydrochloride: 0.3 mg/mL (1 mL)

**Contraindications** Hypersensitivity to buprenorphine or any component

**Warnings/Precautions** Use with caution in patients with hepatic dysfunction or possible neurologic injury; may precipitate abstinence syndrome in narcotic-dependent patients; tolerance or drug dependence may result from extended use

**Pregnancy Risk Factor** C

**Adverse Reactions**
>10%: Central nervous system: Drowsiness
1% to 10%:
Cardiovascular: Hypotension
Central nervous system: Respiratory depression, dizziness, headache
Gastrointestinal: Vomiting, nausea
<1%: Euphoria, slurred speech, malaise, allergic dermatitis, urinary retention, paresthesia, blurred vision

**Drug Interactions** Increased toxicity: Barbiturates, benzodiazepines (increase CNS and respiratory depression)

**Onset** Onset of analgesia: Within 10-30 minutes

**Duration** 6-8 hours

**Half-Life** 2.2-3 hours (range: 1.2-7.2 hours)

**Special PA Issues**
**Patient Education:** If self-administered, use exactly as directed (do not increase dose or frequency). While using this medication, do not use alcohol and other prescription or OTC medications (especially sedatives, tranquilizers, antihistamines, or pain medications) without consulting prescriber. May cause dizziness, drowsiness, confusion, or blurred vision (use caution when driving, climbing stairs, or changing position - rising from sitting or lying to standing, or when engaging in hazardous activities until response to medication is known). You may experience nausea or vomiting (frequent mouth care, small frequent meals, or sucking on lozenges may help). Report unresolved nausea or vomiting; difficulty breathing or shortness of breath; excessive sedation or unusual weakness; rapid heartbeat or palpitations.

**Monitoring Parameters:** Pain relief, respiratory and mental status, CNS depression, blood pressure

**Related Information**
Narcotic Agonists on page 1023

♦ **Buprenorphine Hydrochloride** see Buprenorphine on this page

# Bupropion (byoo PROE pee on)

**Pharmacologic Class** Antidepressant, Dopamine-Reuptake Inhibitor

**U.S. Brand Names** Wellbutrin®; Wellbutrin® SR; Zyban™

**Mechanism of Action** Antidepressant structurally different from all other previously marketed antidepressants; like other antidepressants the mechanism of bupropion's activity is not fully understood; weak blocker of serotonin and norepinephrine re-uptake, inhibits neuronal dopamine re-uptake and is **not** a monoamine oxidase A or B inhibitor

**Use** Treatment of depression; adjunct in smoking cessation

**USUAL DOSAGE** Oral:

Adults:

Depression: 100 mg 3 times/day; begin at 100 mg twice daily; may increase to a maximum dose of 450 mg/day

Smoking cessation: Initiate with 150 mg once daily for 3 days; increase to 150 mg twice daily; treatment should continue for 7-12 weeks

Elderly: Depression: 50-100 mg/day, increase by 50-100 mg every 3-4 days as tolerated; there is evidence that the elderly respond at 150 mg/day in divided doses, but some may require a higher dose

**Dosing adjustment/comments in renal or hepatic impairment:** Patients with renal or hepatic failure should receive a reduced dosage initially and be closely monitored

**Dosage Forms Tab:** 75 mg, 100 mg; **Tab:** sustained release: 100 mg, 150 mg; **Tab:** sustained release (Zyban™): 150 mg

**Contraindications** Seizure disorder, prior diagnosis of bulimia or anorexia nervosa, known hypersensitivity to bupropion, concurrent use of a monoamine oxidase (MAO) inhibitor

**Warnings/Precautions** The estimated seizure potential is increased many fold in doses in the 450-600 mg/day range; giving a single dose <150 mg will lessen the seizure potential; use in patients with renal or hepatic impairment increases possible toxic effects

**Pregnancy Risk Factor** B

**Pregnancy Implications** Enters breast milk/not recommended

**Adverse Reactions**

>10%:

Central nervous system: Agitation, insomnia, fever, headache, psychosis, confusion, anxiety, restlessness, dizziness, seizures, chills, akathisia

Gastrointestinal: Nausea, vomiting, xerostomia, constipation, weight loss

Genitourinary: Impotence

Neuromuscular & skeletal: Tremor

1% to 10%:

Central nervous system: Hallucinations, fatigue

Dermatologic: Rash

Ocular: Blurred vision

<1%: Syncope, drowsiness

**Drug Interactions** CYP2B6 and 2D6 enzyme substrate, CYP3A3/4 enzyme substrate (minor)

Decreased effects: Increased clearance: Carbamazepine, phenytoin, cimetidine, phenobarbital

Increased effects: Levodopa, MAO inhibitors

**Onset** >2 weeks to therapeutic effect

**Half-Life** 14 hours

**Special PA Issues**

**Patient Education:**

Depression: Take as directed, in equally divided doses, do not take in larger dose or more often than recommended. Do not discontinue without consulting prescriber. Do not use excessive alcohol or OTC medications not approved by prescriber. May cause drowsiness, clouded sensorium, restlessness, or agitation (use caution when driving or engaging in tasks that require clear judgment); nausea, vomiting, or dry mouth (small frequent meals, good mouth care, chewing gum, or sucking lozenges may help); constipation (increased exercise, fluids, or dietary fruit and fiber may help); or impotence (reversible). Report persistent CNS effects (agitation, confusion, anxiety, restlessness, insomnia, psychosis, hallucinations, seizures); muscle weakness or tremor; skin rash or irritation; chest pain or palpitations, abdominal pain or blood in stools; yellowing of skin or eyes; difficulty breathing, bronchitis, or unusual cough.

Smoking cessation: Use as directed, do not take extra doses. Do not combine narcotic patches with use of Zyban™ unless approved by prescriber. May cause dry mouth and insomnia (these may resolve with continued use). Report any difficulty breathing, unusual cough, dizziness, or muscle tremors.

**Dietary Considerations:** Alcohol: Additive CNS effects, avoid use

**Monitoring Parameters:** Monitor body weight

**Reference Range:** Therapeutic levels (trough, 12 hours after last dose): 50-100 ng/mL

**Related Information**

Antidepressant Agents on page 998

♦ **Burinex®** see Bumetanide on page 125

♦ **BuSpar®** see Buspirone on next page

# Buspirone (byoo SPYE rone)

**Pharmacologic Class** Antianxiety Agent, Miscellaneous

**U.S. Brand Names** BuSpar®

**Mechanism of Action** The mechanism of action of buspirone is unknown; it differs from typical benzodiazepine anxiolytics in that it does not exert anticonvulsant or muscle relaxant effects; it also lacks the prominent sedative effect that is associated with more typical anxiolytics; in vitro preclinical studies have shown that buspirone has a high affinity for serotonin (5-HT$_{1A}$) receptors; buspirone has no significant affinity for benzodiazepine receptors and does not affect GABA binding in vitro or in vivo when tested in preclinical models; buspirone has moderate affinity for brain D$_2$-dopamine receptors; some studies do suggest that buspirone may have indirect effects on other neurotransmitter systems

**Use** Management of anxiety; has shown little potential for abuse

**USUAL DOSAGE** Adults: Oral: 15 mg/day (5 mg 3 times/day); may increase in increments of 5 mg/day every 2-4 days to a maximum of 60 mg/day

**Note:** The safety and efficacy profile of buspirone in elderly patients has been demonstrated to be similar to those in younger patients; there were no effects of age on its pharmacokinetics

**Dosing adjustment in renal or hepatic impairment:** Dosage should be decreased in patients with severe hepatic insufficiency; in anuric patients, doses should be reduced by 25% to 50% of usual dose

**Dosage Forms Tab, as hydrochloride:** 5 mg, 10 mg

**Contraindications** Hypersensitivity to buspirone or any component

**Warnings/Precautions** Safety and efficacy not established in children <18 years of age; use in hepatic or renal impairment is not recommended; does not prevent or treat withdrawal from benzodiazepines

**Pregnancy Risk Factor** B

**Pregnancy Implications** Excretion in breast milk unknown/not recommended

**Adverse Reactions**

>10%:
Central nervous system: Dizziness, lightheadedness, headache, restlessness
Gastrointestinal: Nausea
1% to 10%: Central nervous system: Drowsiness
<1%: Chest pain, tachycardia, confusion, insomnia, nightmares, sedation, disorientation, excitement, fever, ataxia, rash, urticaria, xerostomia, vomiting, diarrhea, flatulence, leukopenia, eosinophilia, muscle weakness, blurred vision, tinnitus

**Drug Interactions** CYP3A3/4 enzyme substrate
Increased effects/toxicity: MAO inhibitors, phenothiazines, CNS depressants; increased toxicity of digoxin and haloperidol; coadministration of buspirone with cimetidine was found to increase the maximal concentrations of buspirone, but to have no effects on the AUC

**Onset** Peak serum concentration: Within 1 hour

**Half-Life** 2-3 hours

**Special PA Issues**

**Patient Education:** Take only as directed; do not increase dose or take more often than prescribed. May take 2-3 weeks to see full effect; do not discontinue without consulting prescriber. Do not use excessive alcohol or other prescription or OTC medications (especially pain medications, sedatives, antihistamines, or hypnotics) without consulting prescriber. Maintain adequate hydration (2-3 L/day of fluids unless instructed to restrict fluid intake). You may experience drowsiness, lightheadedness, impaired coordination, dizziness, or blurred vision (use caution when driving or engaging in hazardous tasks until response to medication is known); or upset stomach, nausea (small frequent meals, good mouth care, chewing gum, or sucking lozenges may help). Report persistent vomiting, chest pain or rapid heartbeat, persistent CNS effects (eg, confusion, restlessness, anxiety, insomnia, excitation, headache, dizziness, fatigue, impaired coordination), or worsening of condition.

**Monitoring Parameters:** Mental status, symptoms of anxiety; monitor for benzodiazepine withdrawal

♦ **Buspirone Hydrochloride** see Buspirone on this page

# Busulfan (byoo SUL fan)

**Pharmacologic Class** Antineoplastic Agent, Alkylating Agent

**U.S. Brand Names** Myleran®

**Mechanism of Action** Reacts with N-7 position of guanosine and interferes with DNA replication and transcription of RNA. Busulfan has a more marked effect on myeloid cells (and is, therefore, useful in the treatment of CML) than on lymphoid cells. The drug is also very toxic to hematopoietic stem cells (thus its usefulness in high doses in BMT preparative regimens). Busulfan exhibits little immunosuppressive activity. Interferes with the normal function of DNA by alkylation and cross-linking the strands of DNA.

**Use**

Oral: Chronic myelogenous leukemia and bone marrow disorders, such as polycythemia vera and myeloid metaplasia, conditioning regimens for bone marrow transplantation
(Continued)

## Busulfan *(Continued)*

I.V.: Combination therapy with cyclophosphamide as a conditioning regimen prior to alloge-neic hematopoietic progenitor cell transplantation for chronic myelogenous leukemia

**USUAL DOSAGE** Busulfan should be based on adjusted ideal body weight because actual body weight, ideal body weight, or other factors can produce significant differences in busulfan clearance among lean, normal, and obese patients

Oral (refer to individual protocols):

Children:

For remission induction of CML: 0.06-0.12 mg/kg/day **OR** 1.8-4.6 mg/m$^2$/day; titrate dosage to maintain leukocyte count above 40,000/mm$^3$; reduce dosage by 50% if the leukocyte count reaches 30,000-40,000/mm$^3$; discontinue drug if counts fall to ≤20,000/mm$^3$

BMT marrow-ablative conditioning regimen: 1 mg/kg/dose (ideal body weight) every 6 hours for 16 doses

Adults:

BMT marrow-ablative conditioning regimen: 1 mg/kg/dose (ideal body weight) every 6 hours for 16 doses

Remission: Induction of CML: 4-8 mg/day (may be as high as 12 mg/day); Maintenance doses: Controversial, range from 1-4 mg/day to 2 mg/week; treatment is continued until WBC reaches 10,000-20,000 cells/mm$^3$ at which time drug is discontinued; when WBC reaches 50,000/mm$^3$, maintenance dose is resumed

**Unapproved uses:**

Polycythemia vera: 2-6 mg/day

Thrombocytosis: 4-6 mg/day

I.V.: 0.8 mg/kg (ideal body weight or actual body weight, whichever is lower) every 6 hours for 4 days (a total of 16 doses)

I.V. dosing in morbidly obese patients: Dosing should be based on adjusted ideal body weight (AIBW) which should be calculated as ideal body weight (IBW) + 0.25 times (actual weight minus ideal body weight)

AIBW = IBW + 0.25 x (AW - IBW)

Cyclophosphamide, in combination with busulfan, is given on each of two days as a 1-hour infusion at a dose of 160 mg/m$^2$ beginning on day 3, 6 hours following the 16th dose of busulfan

**Dosage Forms** Inj: 60 mg/10 mL ampuls; **Tab:** 2 mg

**Contraindications** Failure to respond to previous courses; should not be used in pregnancy or lactation; hypersensitivity to busulfan or any component

**Warnings/Precautions** The U.S. Food and Drug Administration (FDA) currently recommends that procedures for proper handling and disposal of antineoplastic agents be considered. May induce severe bone marrow hypoplasia; reduce or discontinue dosage at first sign, as reflected by an abnormal decrease in any of the formed elements of the blood; use with caution in patients recently given other myelosuppressive drugs or radiation treatment. If white blood count is high, hydration and allopurinol should be employed to prevent hyperuricemia.

**Pregnancy Risk Factor** D

**Adverse Reactions**

>10%:

Cardiovascular: Endocardial fibrosis

Dermatologic: Skin hyperpigmentation (busulfan tan), urticaria, erythema, alopecia

Endocrine & metabolic: Ovarian suppression, amenorrhea, sterility

Genitourinary: Azospermia, testicular atrophy; malignant tumors have been reported in patients on busulfan therapy

Hematologic: Severe pancytopenia, leukopenia, thrombocytopenia, anemia, and bone marrow suppression are common and patients should be monitored closely while on therapy; since this is a delayed effect (busulfan affects the stem cells), the drug should be discontinued temporarily at the first sign of a large or rapid fall in any blood element; some patients may develop bone marrow fibrosis or chronic aplasia which is probably due to the busulfan toxicity; in large doses, busulfan is myeloablative and is used for this reason in BMT

Myelosuppressive:

WBC: Moderate

Platelets: Moderate

Onset (days): 7-10

Nadir (days): 14-21

Recovery (days): 28

1% to 10%:

Dermatologic: Hyperpigmentation

Endocrine & metabolic: Amenorrhea

Gastrointestinal: Nausea, vomiting, diarrhea; drug has little effect on the GI mucosal lining

Emetic potential: Low (<10%)

Hepatic: Elevated LFTs

Neuromuscular & skeletal: Weakness

Ocular: Cataracts

<1%: Generalized or myoclonic seizures and loss of consciousness have been associated with high-dose busulfan (4 mg/kg/day), adrenal suppression, gynecomastia, hyperuricemia, isolated cases of hemorrhagic cystitis have been reported, hepatic dysfunction, cataracts, blurred vision; after long-term or high-dose therapy, a syndrome known as busulfan lung may occur; this syndrome is manifested by a diffuse interstitial pulmonary fibrosis and persistent cough, fever, rales, and dyspnea. May be relieved by corticosteroids

**Drug Interactions** CYP3A3/4 enzyme substrate

**Duration** 28 days

**Half-Life** After first dose: 3.4 hours; After last dose: 2.3 hours

**Special PA Issues**

**Patient Education:** Take oral medication as directed with chilled liquids. Maintain adequate hydration (2-3 L/day of fluids unless instructed to restrict fluid intake) to help prevent kidney complications. Avoid alcohol, acidic or spicy foods, aspirin or OTC medications unless approved by prescriber. Brush teeth with soft toothbrush or cotton swab. You may lose head hair or experience darkening of skin color (reversible when medication is discontinued), amenorrhea, sterility, or skin rash. You may experience nausea, vomiting, anorexia, or constipation (small frequent meals, increased exercise, and increased dietary fruit or fiber may help). You will be more susceptible to infection (avoid crowds or contagious persons, and do not receive any vaccinations unless approved by prescriber). Report palpitations or chest pain, excessive dizziness, confusion, respiratory difficulty, numbness or tingling of extremities, unusual bruising or bleeding, pain or changes in urination, or other adverse effects.

**Monitoring Parameters:** CBC with differential and platelet count, hemoglobin, liver function tests

♦ **Butace®** see Butalbital Compound on this page

## Butalbital Compound (byoo TAL bi tal KOM pound)

**Pharmacologic Class** Barbiturate

**U.S. Brand Names** Amaphen®; Anoquan®; Axotal®; B-A-C®; Bancap®; Butace®; Endolor®; Esgic®; Femcet®; Fiorgen PF®; Fioricet®; Fiorinal®; G-1®; Isollyl® Improved; Lanorinal®; Marnal®; Medigesic®; Phrenilin®; Phrenilin® Forte; Repan®; Sedapap-10®; Triapin®; Two-Dyne®

**Mechanism of Action** Butalbital, like other barbiturates, has a generalized depressant effect on the central nervous system (CNS). Barbiturates have little effect on peripheral nerves or muscle at usual therapeutic doses. However, at toxic doses serious effects on the cardiovascular system and other peripheral systems may be observed. These effects may result in hypotension or skeletal muscle weakness. While all areas of the central nervous system are acted on by barbiturates, the mesencephalic reticular activating system is extremely sensitive to their effects. Barbiturates act at synapses where gamma-aminobenzoic acid is a neurotransmitter, but they may act in other areas as well.

**Use** Relief of symptomatic complex of tension or muscle contraction headache

**USUAL DOSAGE** Adults: Oral: 1-2 tablets or capsules every 4 hours; not to exceed 6/day

**Dosing interval in renal or hepatic impairment:** Should be reduced

**Dosage Forms Cap, with acetaminophen:** Amaphen®, Anoquan®, Butace®, Endolor®, Esgic®, Femcet®, G-1®, Medigesic®, Repan®, Two-Dyne®: Butalbital 50 mg, caffeine 40 mg, and acetaminophen 325 mg, **Bancap®, Triapin®:** Butalbital 50 mg and acetaminophen 325 mg, **Phrenilin® Forte:** Butalbital 50 mg and acetaminophen 650 mg; **Cap, with aspirin: (Fiorgen PF®, Fiorinal®, Isollyl® Improved, Lanorinal®, Marnal®):** Butalbital 50 mg, caffeine 40 mg, and aspirin 325 mg; **Tab, with acetaminophen: Esgic®, Fioricet®, Repan®:** Butalbital 50 mg, caffeine 40 mg, and acetaminophen 325 mg, **Phrenilin®:** Butalbital 50 mg and acetaminophen 325 mg, **Sedapap-10®:** Butalbital 50 mg and acetaminophen 650 mg; **Tab, with aspirin: Axotal®:** Butalbital 50 mg and aspirin 650 mg, **B-A-C®:** Butalbital 50 mg, caffeine 40 mg, and aspirin 650 mg, **Fiorinal®, Isollyl® Improved, Lanorinal®, Marnal®:** Butalbital 50 mg, caffeine 40 mg, and aspirin 325 mg

**Contraindications** Patients with porphyria, known hypersensitivity to butalbital or any component

**Warnings/Precautions** Children and teenagers should not use for chickenpox or flu symptoms before a physician is consulted about Reye's syndrome (Fiorinal®)

**Pregnancy Risk Factor** D

**Adverse Reactions**

>10%:

Central nervous system: Dizziness, lightheadedness, drowsiness, "hangover" effect

Gastrointestinal: Nausea, heartburn, stomach pains, dyspepsia, epigastric discomfort

1% to 10%:

Central nervous system: Confusion, mental depression, unusual excitement, nervousness, faint feeling, headache, insomnia, nightmares, fatigue

Dermatologic: Rash

Gastrointestinal: Constipation, vomiting, gastrointestinal ulceration

Hematologic: Hemolytic anemia

(Continued)

## Butalbital Compound *(Continued)*

Neuromuscular & skeletal: Weakness
Respiratory: Dyspnea
Miscellaneous: Anaphylactic shock
<1%: Hypotension, hallucinations, jitters, exfoliative dermatitis, Stevens-Johnson syndrome, agranulocytosis, megaloblastic anemia, occult bleeding, prolongation of bleeding time, leukopenia, thrombocytopenia, iron deficiency anemia, hepatotoxicity, thrombophlebitis, impaired renal function, respiratory depression, bronchospasm

**Drug Interactions**
Decreased effect: Phenothiazines, haloperidol, quinidine, cyclosporine, TCAs, corticosteroids, theophylline, ethosuximide, warfarin, oral contraceptives, chloramphenicol, griseofulvin, doxycycline, beta-blockers
Increased effect/toxicity: Propoxyphene, benzodiazepines, CNS depressants, valproic acid, methylphenidate, chloramphenicol

**Special PA Issues**
**Patient Education:** Children and teenagers should not use this product; may cause drowsiness, avoid alcohol or other CNS depressants, may impair judgment and coordination; may cause physical and psychological dependence with prolonged use; do not exceed recommended dose
**Dietary Considerations:** Alcohol: Additive CNS effects, avoid use

## Butenafine *(byoo TEN a fine)*
**Pharmacologic Class** Antifungal Agent, Topical
**U.S. Brand Names** Mentax®
**Mechanism of Action** Butenafine exerts antifungal activity by blocking squalene epoxidation, resulting in inhibition of ergosterol synthesis (antidermatophyte and *Sporothrix schenckii* activity). In higher concentrations, the drug disrupts fungal cell membranes (anticandidal activity).
**Use** Topical treatment of tinea pedis (athlete's foot) and tinea cruris (jock itch)
**USUAL DOSAGE** Children >12 years and Adults: Topical: Apply once daily for 4 weeks to the affected area and surrounding skin
**Dosage Forms Crm, as hydrochloride:** 1% (2 g, 15 g, 30 g)
**Contraindications** Hypersensitivity to butenafine or components
**Warnings/Precautions** Only for topical use (not ophthalmic, vaginal, or internal routes); patients sensitive to other allylamine antifungals may cross-react with butenafine
**Pregnancy Risk Factor** B
**Adverse Reactions**
>1%: Dermatologic: Burning, stinging, irritation, erythema, pruritus (2%)
<1%: Contact dermatitis
**Special PA Issues**
**Patient Education:** Report any signs of rash or allergy to your physician immediately; do not apply other topical medications on the same area as butenafine unless directed by your physician
**Monitoring Parameters:** Culture and KOH exam, clinical signs of tinea pedis
**Related Information**
Antifungal Agents, Topical *on page 1000*

♦ **Butenafine Hydrochloride** *see* Butenafine *on this page*

## Butoconazole *(byoo toe KOE na zole)*
**Pharmacologic Class** Antifungal Agent, Vaginal
**U.S. Brand Names** Femstat®
**Mechanism of Action** Increases cell membrane permeability in susceptible fungi (*Candida*)
**Use** Local treatment of vulvovaginal candidiasis
**USUAL DOSAGE** Adults:
Nonpregnant: Insert 1 applicatorful (~5 g) intravaginally at bedtime as a single dose; therapy may extend for up to 6 days, if necessary, as directed by physician
Pregnant: **Use only during 2nd or 3rd trimester**
**Dosage Forms Crm, vaginal, as nitrate:** 2% with applicator (28 g)
**Contraindications** Known hypersensitivity to butoconazole
**Warnings/Precautions** In pregnancy, use only during 2nd or 3rd trimesters; if irritation or sensitization occurs, discontinue use
**Pregnancy Risk Factor** C (For use only in 2nd or 3rd trimester)
**Adverse Reactions**
1% to 10%: Genitourinary: Vulvar/vaginal burning
<1%: Vulvar itching, soreness, edema, or discharge; polyuria
**Special PA Issues**
**Patient Education:** May cause burning or stinging on application; if symptoms of vaginitis persist, contact physician

♦ **Butoconazole Nitrate** *see* Butoconazole *on this page*

# Butorphanol (byoo TOR fa nole)

**Pharmacologic Class** Analgesic, Narcotic

**U.S. Brand Names** Stadol®; Stadol® NS

**Mechanism of Action** Mixed narcotic agonist-antagonist with central analgesic actions; binds to opiate receptors in the CNS, causing inhibition of ascending pain pathways, altering the perception of and response to pain; produces generalized CNS depression

**Use** Management of moderate to severe pain

**USUAL DOSAGE** Adults:

I.M.: 1-4 mg every 3-4 hours as needed

I.V.: 0.5-2 mg every 3-4 hours as needed

Nasal spray: Headache: 1 spray in 1 nostril; if adequate pain relief is not achieved within 60-90 minutes, an additional 1 spray in 1 nostril may be given (each spray gives ~1 mg of butorphanol); may repeat in 3-4 hours after the last dose as needed

**Dosing adjustment in renal impairment:**

$Cl_{cr}$ 10-50 mL/minute: Administer 75% of dose

$Cl_{cr}$ <10 mL/minute: Administer 50% of dose

**Dosage Forms Inj:** 1 mg/mL (1 mL), 2 mg/mL (1 mL, 2 mL, 10 mL); **Spray, nasal:** 10 mg/mL [14-15 doses] (2.5 mL)

**Contraindications** Hypersensitivity to butorphanol or any component; avoid use in opiate-dependent patients who have not been detoxified, may precipitate opiate withdrawal

**Warnings/Precautions** Use with caution in patients with hepatic/renal dysfunction, may elevate CSF pressure, may increase cardiac workload; tolerance of drug dependence may result from extended use

**Pregnancy Risk Factor** B (D if used for prolonged periods or in high doses at term)

**Adverse Reactions**

>10%: Central nervous system: Drowsiness

1% to 10%:

Cardiovascular: Flushing of the face, hypotension

Central nervous system: Dizziness, lightheadedness, headache

Gastrointestinal: Anorexia, nausea, vomiting

Genitourinary: Decreased urination

Miscellaneous: Diaphoresis (increased)

<1%: Bradycardia or tachycardia, hypertension, paradoxical CNS stimulation, confusion, hallucinations, mental depression, false sense of well being, malaise, restlessness, nightmares, CNS depression, rash, stomach cramps, constipation, xerostomia, painful urination, blurred vision, tinnitus, weakness, shortness of breath, dyspnea, respiratory depression, dependence with prolonged use

**Drug Interactions** Increased toxicity: CNS depressants, phenothiazines, barbiturates, skeletal muscle relaxants, alfentanil, guanabenz, MAO inhibitors

**Onset** I.M.: 5-10 minutes; I.V.: <10 minutes; Nasal: Within 15 minutes

**Duration** I.M./I.V.: 3-4 hours; Nasal: 4-5 hours

**Half-Life** 2.5-4 hours

**Special PA Issues**

**Patient Education:** If self-administered, use exactly as directed (do not increase dose or frequency); may cause physical and/or psychological dependence. While using this medication, do not use alcohol and other prescription or OTC medications (especially sedatives, tranquilizers, antihistamines, or pain medications) without consulting prescriber. May cause dizziness, drowsiness, confusion, or blurred vision (use caution when driving, climbing stairs, or changing position - rising from sitting or lying to standing, or when engaging in hazardous activities until response to medication is known); nausea or vomiting, or loss of appetite (frequent mouth care, small frequent meals, or sucking on lozenges may help). Report unresolved nausea or vomiting; difficulty breathing or shortness of breath; restlessness, insomnia, euphoria, or nightmares; excessive sedation or unusual weakness; facial flushing, rapid heartbeat, or palpitations; urinary difficulty; or vision changes.

**Dietary Considerations:** Alcohol: Additive CNS effects, avoid or limit use; watch for sedation

**Monitoring Parameters:** Pain relief, respiratory and mental status, blood pressure

**Reference Range:** 0.7-1.5 ng/mL

**Related Information**

Narcotic Agonists *on page 1023*

♦ **Butorphanol Tartrate** *see* Butorphanol *on this page*

♦ **BW-430C** *see* Lamotrigine *on page 514*

♦ **Byclomine® Injection** *see* Dicyclomine *on page 273*

♦ **Bydramine® Cough Syrup [OTC]** *see* Diphenhydramine *on page 289*

# Cabergoline (ca BER go leen)

**Pharmacologic Class** Ergot Derivative

**U.S. Brand Names** Dostinex®

(Continued)

## Cabergoline *(Continued)*

**Mechanism of Action** Cabergoline is a long-acting dopamine receptor agonist with a high affinity for $D_2$ receptors; prolactin secretion by the anterior pituitary is predominantly under hypothalamic inhibitory control exerted through the release of dopamine

**Use** Treatment of hyperprolactinemic disorders, either idiopathic or due to pituitary adenomas

**Unlabeled use:** Adjunct for the treatment of Parkinson's disease

**USUAL DOSAGE** Initial dose: Oral: 0.25 mg twice weekly; the dose may be increased by 0.25 mg twice weekly up to a maximum of 1 mg twice weekly according to the patient's serum prolactin level. Dosage increases should not occur more rapidly than every 4 weeks. Once a normal serum prolactin level is maintained for 6 months, the dose may be discontinued and prolactin levels monitored to determine if cabergoline is still required. The durability of efficacy beyond 24 months of therapy has not been established.

**Dosage Forms Tab:** 0.5 mg

**Contraindications** Patients with uncontrolled hypertension or hypersensitivity to ergot derivatives

**Warnings/Precautions** Initial doses >1 mg may cause orthostatic hypotension. Use caution when patients are receiving other medications which may reduce blood pressure. Not indicated for the inhibition or suppression of physiologic lactation since it has been associated with cases of hypertension, stroke, and seizures. Because cabergoline is extensively metabolized by the liver, careful monitoring in patients with hepatic impairment is warranted. Female patients should instruct the physician if they are pregnant, become pregnant, or intend to become pregnant. Should not be used in patients with pregnancy-induced hypertension unless benefit outweighs potential risk. Do not give to postpartum women who are breast-feeding or planning to breast-feed. In all patients, prolactin concentrations should be monitored monthly until normalized.

**Pregnancy Risk Factor** B

**Adverse Reactions**
>10%:
  Central nervous system: Headache (26%), dizziness (17%)
  Gastrointestinal: Nausea (29%)
1% to 10%:
  Body as whole: Asthenia (6%), fatigue (5%), syncope (1%), influenza-like symptoms (1%), malaise (1%), periorbital edema (1%), peripheral edema (1%)
  Cardiovascular: Hot flashes (3%), hypotension (1%), dependent edema (1%), palpitations (1%)
  Central nervous system: Vertigo (4%), depression (3%), somnolence (2%), anxiety (1%), insomnia (1%), impaired concentration (1%), nervousness (1%)
  Dermatologic: Acne (1%), pruritus (1%)
  Endocrine: Breast pain (2%), dysmenorrhea (1%)
  Gastrointestinal: Constipation (7%), abdominal pain (5%), dyspepsia (5%), vomiting (4%), xerostomia (2%), diarrhea (2%), flatulence (2%), throat irritation (1%), toothache (1%), anorexia (1%)
  Neuromuscular & skeletal: Pain (2%), arthralgia (1%), paresthesias (2%)
  Ocular: Abnormal vision (1%)
  Respiratory: Rhinitis (1%)

**Drug Interactions**
Additive hypotensive effects may occur when cabergoline is administered with antihypertensive medications; dosage adjustment of the antihypertensive medication may be required
Decreased effect: Dopamine antagonists (eg, phenothiazines, butyrophenones, thioxanthenes, or metoclopramide) may reduce the therapeutic effects of cabergoline and should not be used concomitantly

**Special PA Issues**
**Patient Education:** Patient should be instructed to notify physician if she suspects she is pregnant, becomes pregnant, or intends to become pregnant during therapy with cabergoline. A pregnancy test should be done if there is any suspicion of pregnancy and continuation of treatment should be discussed with physician.

♦ **Cafatine®** *see* Ergotamine *on page 328*
♦ **Cafatine-PB®** *see* Ergotamine *on page 328*
♦ **Cafergot®** *see* Ergotamine *on page 328*
♦ **Cafetrate®** *see* Ergotamine *on page 328*

## Caffeine and Sodium Benzoate (KAF een & SOW dee um BEN zoe ate)

**Pharmacologic Class** Diuretic, Miscellaneous

**Dosage Forms Inj:** Caffeine 125 mg and sodium benzoate 125 mg per mL (2 mL)

♦ **Calan®** *see* Verapamil *on page 959*
♦ **Calan® SR** *see* Verapamil *on page 959*
♦ **Cal Carb-HD® [OTC]** *see* Calcium Carbonate *on page 139*
♦ **Calci-Chew™ [OTC]** *see* Calcium Carbonate *on page 139*
♦ **Calciday-667® [OTC]** *see* Calcium Carbonate *on page 139*

## Calcifediol (kal si fe DYE ole)

**Pharmacologic Class** Vitamin D Analog

**U.S. Brand Names** Calderol®

**Mechanism of Action** Vitamin D analog that (along with calcitonin and parathyroid hormone) regulates serum calcium homeostasis by promoting absorption of calcium and phosphorus in the small intestine; promotes renal tubule resorption of phosphate; increases rate of accretion and resorption in bone minerals

**Use** Treatment and management of metabolic bone disease associated with chronic renal failure or hypocalcemia in patients on chronic renal dialysis

**USUAL DOSAGE** Oral: Hepatic osteodystrophy:

Infants: 5-7 mcg/kg/day

Children and Adults: Usual dose: 20-100 mcg/day or 20-200 mcg every other day; titrate to obtain normal serum calcium/phosphate levels; increase dose at 4-week intervals; initial dose: 300-350 mcg/week, administered daily or on alternate days

**Dosage Forms Cap:** 20 mcg, 50 mcg

**Contraindications** Hypercalcemia; known hypersensitivity to calcifediol; malabsorption syndrome; hypervitaminosis D; significantly decreased renal function

**Warnings/Precautions** Adequate (supplemental) dietary calcium is necessary for clinical response to vitamin D; calcium-phosphate product (serum calcium times phosphorus) must not exceed 70; avoid hypercalcemia

**Pregnancy Risk Factor** C

**Pregnancy Implications** Enters breast milk/compatible

**Adverse Reactions**

Cardiovascular: Hypotension, cardiac arrhythmias, hypertension

Central nervous system: Irritability, headache, somnolence, seizures (rare)

Dermatologic: Pruritus

Endocrine & metabolic: Hypercalcemia, polydipsia, hypermagnesemia

Gastrointestinal: Nausea, vomiting, constipation, anorexia, pancreatitis, metallic taste, xerostomia

Genitourinary: Polyuria

Hepatic: Elevated LFTs

Neuromuscular & skeletal: Myalgia, bone pain

Ocular: Conjunctivitis, photophobia

**Drug Interactions**

Decreased effect: Cholestyramine, colestipol

Increased effect: Thiazide diuretics

Additive effect: Antacids (magnesium)

**Onset** Time to peak serum concentration: 4 hours

**Half-Life** 12-22 days

**Special PA Issues**

**Patient Education:** Take exact dose as prescribed; do not increase dose. Maintain recommended diet and calcium supplementation. Avoid taking magnesium-containing antacids. You may experience nausea, vomiting, or metallic taste (frequent small meals, frequent mouth care, or sucking on lozenges may help) or hypotension (use caution when rising from sitting or lying position or when climbing stairs or bending over). Report chest pain or palpitations, acute headache, skin rash, change in vision or eye irritation, CNS changes, weakness or lethargy.

♦ **Calciferol™ Injection** see Ergocalciferol on page 326

♦ **Calciferol™ Oral** see Ergocalciferol on page 326

♦ **Calcijex™** see Calcitriol on page 137

♦ **Calcimar® Injection** see Calcitonin on next page

♦ **Calci-Mix™ [OTC]** see Calcium Carbonate on page 139

## Calcipotriene (kal si POE try een)

**Pharmacologic Class** Topical Skin Product; Vitamin, Fat Soluble

**U.S. Brand Names** Dovonex®

**Mechanism of Action** Synthetic vitamin $D_3$ analog which regulates skin cell production and proliferation

**Use** Treatment of moderate plaque psoriasis

**USUAL DOSAGE** Adults: Topical: Apply in a thin film to the affected skin twice daily and rub in gently and completely

**Dosage Forms Crm:** 0.005% (30 g, 60 g, 100 g); **Oint, top:** 0.005% (30 g, 60 g, 100 g); **Soln, top:** 0.005%

**Contraindications** Hypersensitivity to any components of the preparation; patients with demonstrated hypercalcemia or evidence of vitamin D toxicity; use on the face

**Warnings/Precautions** Use may cause irritations of lesions and surrounding uninvolved skin. If irritation develops, discontinue use. Transient, rapidly reversible elevation of serum calcium has occurred during use. If elevation in serum calcium occurs above the normal range, discontinue treatment until calcium levels are normal. For external use only; not for ophthalmic, oral or intravaginal use.

(Continued)

## Calcipotriene *(Continued)*

**Pregnancy Risk Factor** C

**Adverse Reactions**

>10%: Dermatologic: Burning, itching, skin irritation, erythema, dry skin, peeling, rash, worsening of psoriasis

1% to 10%: Dermatologic: Dermatitis

<1%: Skin atrophy, hyperpigmentation, folliculitis, hypercalcemia

**Special PA Issues**

Patient Education: For external use only. Use exactly as directed; do not overuse. Before using, wash and dry area gently. Wear gloves to apply a thin film to affected area and rub in gently. If dressing is necessary, use a porous dressing. Avoid contact with eyes. Avoid exposing treated area to direct sunlight; sunburn can occur. Report increased swelling, redness, rash, itching, signs of infection, worsening of condition, or lack of healing.

♦ **Calcite-500** *see* Calcium Carbonate *on page 139*

## Calcitonin *(kal si TOE nin)*

**Pharmacologic Class** Antidote

**U.S. Brand Names** Calcimar® Injection; Cibacalcin® Injection; Miacalcin® Injection; Miacalcin® Nasal Spray; Osteocalcin® Injection; Salmonine® Injection

**Mechanism of Action** Structurally similar to human calcitonin; it directly inhibits osteoclastic bone resorption; promotes the renal excretion of calcium, phosphate, sodium, magnesium and potassium by decreasing tubular reabsorption; increases the jejunal secretion of water, sodium, potassium, and chloride

**Use**

Calcitonin (salmon): Treatment of Paget's disease of bone and as adjunctive therapy for hypercalcemia; also used in postmenopausal osteoporosis and osteogenesis imperfecta

Calcitonin (human): Treatment of Paget's disease of bone

**USUAL DOSAGE**

Children: Dosage not established

Adults:

Paget's disease:

Salmon calcitonin: I.M., S.C.: 100 units/day to start, 50 units/day or 50-100 units every 1-3 days maintenance dose

Human calcitonin: S.C.: Initial: 0.5 mg/day (maximum: 0.5 mg twice daily); maintenance: 0.5 mg 2-3 times/week or 0.25 mg/day

Hypercalcemia: Initial: Salmon calcitonin: I.M., S.C.: 4 units/kg every 12 hours; may increase up to 8 units/kg every 12 hours to a maximum of every 6 hours

Osteogenesis imperfecta: Salmon calcitonin: I.M., S.C.: 2 units/kg 3 times/week

Postmenopausal osteoporosis: Salmon calcitonin:

I.M., S.C.: 100 units/day

Intranasal: 200 units (1 spray)/day

**Dosage Forms** Inj: Human (Cibacalcin®): 0.5 mg/vial, Salmon: 200 units/mL (2 mL); **Spray, nasal:** 200 units/activation (0.09 mL/dose) (2 mL glass bottle with pump)

**Contraindications** Hypersensitivity to salmon protein or gelatin diluent

**Warnings/Precautions** A skin test should be performed prior to initiating therapy of calcitonin salmon; have epinephrine immediately available for a possible hypersensitivity reaction

**Pregnancy Risk Factor** C

**Adverse Reactions**

>10%:

Cardiovascular: Facial flushing

Gastrointestinal: Nausea, diarrhea, anorexia

Local: Edema at injection site

1% to 10%: Genitourinary: Polyuria

<1%: Edema, chills, headache, dizziness, rash, urticaria, paresthesia, weakness, shortness of breath, nasal congestion

**Onset** Hypercalcemia: Onset of reduction in calcium: 2 hours

**Duration** Hypercalcemia: 6-8 hours

**Half-Life** S.C.: 1.2 hours

**Special PA Issues**

Patient Education: When this drug is given subcutaneously or I.M. it will be necessary for you or a significant other to learn to prepare and give the injections (keep drug vials in a refrigerator - do not freeze). Report significant nasal irritation if using calcitonin nasal spray. Follow directions exactly. Increased warmth and flushing may be experienced with this drug and should only last about 1 hour after administration (taking drug in the evening may minimize these discomforts). Immediately report twitching, muscle spasm, dark colored urine, hives, significant skin rash, palpitations, or difficulty breathing.

Monitoring Parameters: Serum electrolytes and calcium; alkaline phosphatase and 24-hour urine collection for hydroxyproline excretion (Paget's disease); serum calcium

**Reference Range:** Therapeutic: <19 pg/mL (SI: 19 ng/L) basal, depending on the assay

♦ **Calcitonin (Human)** see Calcitonin on previous page
♦ **Calcitonin (Salmon)** see Calcitonin on previous page

# Calcitriol (kal si TRYE ole)

**Pharmacologic Class** Vitamin D Analog

**U.S. Brand Names** Calcijex™; Rocaltrol®

**Mechanism of Action** Promotes absorption of calcium in the intestines and retention at the kidneys thereby increasing calcium levels in the serum; decreases excessive serum phosphatase levels, parathyroid hormone levels, and decreases bone resorption; increases renal tubule phosphate resorption

**Use** Management of hypocalcemia in patients on chronic renal dialysis; reduce elevated parathyroid hormone levels

    **Unlabeled use:** Decrease severity of psoriatic lesions in psoriatic vulgaris; vitamin D resistant rickets

**USUAL DOSAGE** Individualize dosage to maintain calcium levels of 9-10 mg/dL

  Renal failure:
    Children:
      Oral: 0.25-2 mcg/day have been used (with hemodialysis); 0.014-0.041 mcg/kg/day (not receiving hemodialysis); increases should be made at 4- to 8-week intervals
      I.V.: 0.01-0.05 mcg/kg 3 times/week if undergoing hemodialysis
    Adults:
      Oral: 0.25 mcg/day or every other day (may require 0.5-1 mcg/day); increases should be made at 4- to 8-week intervals
      I.V.: 0.5 mcg/day 3 times/week (may require from 0.5-3 mcg/day given 3 times/week) if undergoing hemodialysis
  Hypoparathyroidism/pseudohypoparathyroidism: Oral (evaluate dosage at 2- to 4-week intervals):
    Children:
      <1 year: 0.04-0.08 mcg/kg once daily
      1-5 years: 0.25-0.75 mcg once daily
    Children >6 years and Adults: 0.5-2 mcg once daily
  Vitamin D-dependent rickets: Children and Adults: Oral: 1 mcg once daily
  Vitamin D-resistant rickets (familial hypophosphatemia): Children and Adults: Oral: Initial: 0.015-0.02 mcg/kg once daily; maintenance: 0.03-0.06 mcg/kg once daily; maximum dose: 2 mcg once daily
  Hypocalcemia in premature infants: Oral: 1 mcg once daily for 5 days
  Hypocalcemic tetany in premature infants: I.V.: 0.05 mcg/kg once daily for 5-12 days

**Dosage Forms Cap:** 0.25 mcg, 0.5 mcg; **Inj:** 1 mcg/mL (1 mL); 2 mcg/mL (1 mL); **Soln, oral:** 1 mcg/mL

**Contraindications** Hypercalcemia; vitamin D toxicity; abnormal sensitivity to the effects of vitamin D; malabsorption syndrome

**Warnings/Precautions** Adequate dietary (supplemental) calcium is necessary for clinical response to vitamin D; maintain adequate fluid intake; calcium-phosphate product (serum calcium times phosphorus) must not exceed 70; avoid hypercalcemia or use with renal function impairment and secondary hyperparathyroidism

**Pregnancy Risk Factor** C

**Pregnancy Implications** Enters breast milk/compatible

**Adverse Reactions**
  Cardiovascular: Hypotension, cardiac arrhythmias, hypertension
  Central nervous system: Irritability, headache, somnolence, seizures (rare)
  Dermatologic: Pruritus
  Endocrine & metabolic: Hypercalcemia, polydipsia, hypermagnesemia
  Gastrointestinal: Nausea, vomiting, constipation, anorexia, pancreatitis, metallic taste, xerostomia
  Genitourinary: Polyuria
  Hepatic: Elevated LFTs
  Neuromuscular & skeletal: Myalgia, bone pain
  Ocular: Conjunctivitis, photophobia

**Drug Interactions**
  Decreased effect/absorption: Cholestyramine, colestipol
  Increased effect: Thiazide diuretics
  Additive effect: Magnesium-containing antacids

**Onset** ~2-6 hours

**Duration** 3-5 days

**Half-Life** 3-8 hours

**Special PA Issues**
  **Patient Education:** Take exact dose as prescribed; do not increase dose. Maintain recommended diet and calcium supplementation. Avoid taking magnesium-containing antacids. You may experience nausea, vomiting, loss of appetite, or metallic taste
  (Continued)

## Calcitriol *(Continued)*

(frequent small meals, frequent mouth care, or sucking on lozenges may help); or hypotension (use caution when rising from sitting or lying position or when climbing stairs or bending over). Report chest pain or palpitations; acute headache; skin rash; change in vision or eye irritation; CNS changes; unusual weakness or fatigue; persistent nausea, vomiting, cramps, or diarrhea; or muscle or bone pain.

**Monitoring Parameters:** Monitor symptoms of hypercalcemia (weakness, fatigue, somnolence, headache, anorexia, dry mouth, metallic taste, nausea, vomiting, cramps, diarrhea, muscle pain, bone pain and irritability)

**Reference Range:** Calcium (serum) 9-10 mg/dL (4.5-5 mEq/L) but do not include the I.V. dosages; phosphate: 2.5-5 mg/dL

## Calcium Acetate (KAL see um AS e tate)

**Pharmacologic Class** Antidote; Calcium Salt; Electrolyte Supplement, Oral

**U.S. Brand Names** Calphron®; PhosLo®

**Mechanism of Action** Combines with dietary phosphate to form insoluble calcium phosphate which is excreted in feces

**Use** Control of hyperphosphatemia in end-stage renal failure; calcium acetate binds phosphorus in the GI tract better than other calcium salts due to its lower solubility and subsequent reduced absorption and increased formation of calcium phosphate; calcium acetate does not promote aluminum absorption

**USUAL DOSAGE**

Oral: Adults, on dialysis: Initial: 2 tablets with each meal, can be increased gradually to 3-4 tablets with each meal to bring the serum phosphate value <6 mg/dL as long as hypercalcemia does not develop

I.V.: Dose is dependent on the requirements of the individual patient; in central venous total parental nutrition (TPN), calcium is administered at a concentration of 5 mEq (10 mL)/L of TPN solution; the additive maintenance dose in neonatal TPN is 0.5 mEq calcium/kg/day (1.0 mL/kg/day)

Neonates: 70-200 mg/kg/day

Infants and Children: 70-150 mg/kg/day

Adolescents: 18-35 mg/kg/day

**Dosage Forms** Elemental calcium listed in brackets **Cap (Phos-Ex® 125):** 500 mg [125 mg]; **Tab:** Calphron®: 667 mg [169 mg], PhosLo®: 667 mg [169 mg]

**Contraindications** Hypercalcemia, renal calculi, hypophosphatemia

**Warnings/Precautions** Calcium absorption is impaired in achlorhydria (common in elderly - try alternate salt, administer with food); administration is followed by increased gastric acid secretion within 2 hours of administration; while hypercalcemia and hypercalciuria may result when therapeutic replacement amounts are given for prolonged periods, they are most likely to occur in hypoparathyroid patients receiving high doses of vitamin D

**Pregnancy Risk Factor** C

**Adverse Reactions**

Mild hypercalcemia (calcium: >10.5 mg/dL) may be asymptomatic or manifest itself as constipation, anorexia, nausea, and vomiting

More severe hypercalcemia (calcium: >12 mg/dL) is associated with confusion, delirium, stupor, and coma

<1%: Headache, hypophosphatemia, hypercalcemia, nausea, anorexia, vomiting, abdominal pain, constipation, thirst

**Drug Interactions**

Decreased effect:

Calcium acetate may significantly decrease the bioavailability of tetracyclines

Large intakes of dietary fiber may decrease calcium absorption due to a decreased GI transit time and the formation of fiber-calcium complexes

Increased effect: Calcium acetate may increase the effects of quinidine

**Special PA Issues**

**Patient Education:** Take as directed, with a full glass of water or juice 2 hours before or after other medications. Do not take with fiber-rich meals, whole grain cereals, or food high in oxalates (eg spinach, rhubarb). Avoid antacids, excess alcohol, caffeine containing beverages, or additional calcium supplements unless approved by prescriber. Increasing exercise or dietary fluid, fiber, or fruits may help reduce incidence of constipation. Report severe, unresolved GI disturbances and unusual emotional lability (mood swings).

**Reference Range:**

Serum calcium: 8.4-10.2 mg/dL

Due to a poor correlation between the serum ionized calcium (free) and total serum calcium, particularly in states of low albumin or acid/base imbalances, direct measurement of ionized calcium is recommended

In low albumin states, the corrected **total** serum calcium may be estimated by this equation (assuming a normal albumin of 4 g/dL)

Corrected total calcium = total serum calcium + 0.8 (4.0 - measured serum albumin)

**or**

Corrected calcium = measured calcium - measured albumin + 4.0

# Calcium Carbonate (KAL see um KAR bun ate)

**Pharmacologic Class** Antacid; Antidote; Calcium Salt; Electrolyte Supplement, Oral

**U.S. Brand Names** Alka-Mints® [OTC]; Amitone® [OTC]; Cal Carb-HD® [OTC]; Calci-Chew™ [OTC]; Calciday-667® [OTC]; Calci-Mix™ [OTC]; Cal-Plus® [OTC]; Caltrate® 600 [OTC]; Caltrate, Jr.® [OTC]; Chooz® [OTC]; Dicarbosil® [OTC]; Equilet® [OTC]; Florical® [OTC]; Gencalc® 600 [OTC]; Mallamint® [OTC]; Nephro-Calci® [OTC]; Os-Cal® 500 [OTC]; Oyst-Cal 500 [OTC]; Oystercal® 500; Rolaids® Calcium Rich [OTC]; Tums® [OTC]; Tums® E-X Extra Strength Tablet [OTC]; Tums® Extra Strength Liquid [OTC]

**Mechanism of Action** As dietary supplements to prevent or treat negative calcium balance (eg, osteoporosis), the calcium in calcium salts moderates nerve and muscle performance and allows normal cardiac function; also used to treat hyperphosphatemia in patients with advanced renal insufficiency by combining with dietary phosphate to form insoluble calcium phosphate, which is excreted in feces; calcium salts as antacids neutralize gastric acidity resulting in increased gastric an duodenal bulb pH; they additionally inhibit proteolytic activity of peptic if the pH is increased >4 and increase lower esophageal sphincter tone.

**Use** As an antacid, and treatment and prevention of calcium deficiency or hyperphosphatemia (eg, osteoporosis, osteomalacia, mild/moderate renal insufficiency, hypoparathyroidism, postmenopausal osteoporosis, rickets); has been used to bind phosphate

**USUAL DOSAGE** Oral (dosage is in terms of elemental calcium):

**Adequate intakes:**
  0-6 months: 210 mg/day
  7-12 months: 270 mg/day
  1-3 years: 500 mg/day
  4-8 years: 800 mg/day
  Adults, male/female:
    9-18 years: 1300 mg/day
    19-50 years: 1000 mg/day
    >51 years: 1200 mg/day
  Female: Pregnancy:
    ≤18 years: 1300 mg/day
    >19 years: 1000 mg/day
  Female: Lactating:
    ≤18 years: 1300 mg/day
    >19 years: 1000 mg/day
  Hypocalcemia (dose depends on clinical condition and serum calcium level): Dose expressed in mg of **elemental calcium**
    Neonates: 50-150 mg/kg/day in 4-6 divided doses; not to exceed 1 g/day
    Children: 45-65 mg/kg/day in 4 divided doses
    Adults: 1-2 g or more/day in 3-4 divided doses
  Adults:
    Dietary supplementation: 500 mg to 2 g divided 2-4 times/day
    Antacid: 2 tablets or 10 mL every 2 hours, up to 12 times/day
  Adults >51 years of age: Osteoporosis: 1200 mg/day
  **Dosing adjustment in renal impairment:** Cl$_{cr}$ <25 mL/minute: Dosage adjustments may be necessary depending on the serum calcium levels

**Dosage Forms** Elemental calcium listed in brackets **Cap:** 1500 mg [600 mg], Calci-Mix™: 1250 mg [500 mg], Florical®: 364 mg [145.6 mg] with sodium fluoride 8.3 mg; **Liq (Tums® Extra Strength):** 1000 mg/5 mL (360 mL); **Loz (Mylanta® Soothing Antacids):** 600 mg [240 mg]; **Powder (Cal Carb-HD®):** 6.5 g/packet [2.6 g]; **Susp, oral:** 1250 mg/5 mL [500 mg]; **Tab:** 650 mg [260 mg], 1500 mg [600 mg], Calciday-667®: 667 mg [267 mg], Os-Cal® 500, Oyst-Cal 500, Oystercal® 500: 1250 mg [500 mg], Cal-Plus®, Caltrate® 600, Gencalc® 600, Nephro-Calci®: 1500 mg [600 mg]; **Chewable:** Alka-Mints®: 850 mg [340 mg], Amitone®: 350 mg [140 mg], Caltrate, Jr.®: 750 mg [300 mg], Calci-Chew™, Os-Cal®: 750 mg [300 mg], Chooz®, Dicarbosil®, Equilet®, Tums®: 500 mg [200 mg], Mallamint®: 420 mg [168 mg], Rolaids® Calcium Rich: 550 mg [220 mg], Tums® E-X Extra Strength: 750 mg [300 mg], Tums® Ultra®: 1000 mg [400 mg], Florical®: 364 mg [145.6 mg]with sodium fluoride 8.3 mg

**Contraindications** Hypercalcemia, renal calculi, hypophosphatemia

**Warnings/Precautions** Calcium carbonate absorption is impaired in achlorhydria (common in elderly - use alternate salt, administer with food); administration is followed by increased gastric acid secretion within 2 hours of administration; while hypercalcemia and hypercalciuria may result when therapeutic replacement amounts are given for prolonged periods, they are most likely to occur in hypoparathyroid patients receiving high doses of vitamin D

**Pregnancy Risk Factor** C

**Pregnancy Implications**
  Clinical effects on the fetus: No data available; available evidence suggests safe use during pregnancy and breast-feeding
  Breast-feeding/lactation: No data available

**Adverse Reactions** Well tolerated
  Central nervous system: Headache
  (Continued)

## Calcium Carbonate (Continued)

Endocrine & metabolic: Hypophosphatemia, hypercalcemia

Gastrointestinal: Constipation, laxative effect, acid rebound, nausea, vomiting, anorexia, abdominal pain, xerostomia, flatulence

Miscellaneous: Milk alkali syndrome with very high, chronic dosing and/or renal failure (headache, nausea, irritability, and weakness or alkalosis, hypercalcemia, renal impairment)

**Drug Interactions** Decreased effect:

May significantly decrease the bioavailability of tetracyclines and fluoroquinolones, iron salts, and salicylates

Large intakes of dietary fiber may decrease calcium absorption due to a decreased GI transit time and the formation of fiber-calcium complexes

**Special PA Issues**

**Patient Education:** Follow instructions for dosing. Take with a full glass of water or juice, 1-3 hours after meals and other medications and 1-2 hours before any iron supplements. Avoid alcohol, other antacids, caffeine, or other calcium supplements unless approved by prescriber. You may experience constipation (increasing exercise or dietary fluid, fiber, or fruits may help). Report severe, unresolved GI disturbances and unusual emotional lability (mood swings).

**Reference Range:**

Serum calcium: 8.4-10.2 mg/dL: Monitor plasma calcium levels if using calcium salts as electrolyte supplements for deficiency

Due to a poor correlation between the serum ionized calcium (free) and total serum calcium, particularly in states of low albumin or acid/base imbalances, direct measurement of ionized calcium is recommended

In low albumin states, the corrected **total** serum calcium may be estimated by: Corrected total calcium = total serum calcium + 0.8 (4.0 - measured serum albumin)

## Calcium Carbonate and Magnesium Carbonate

(KAL see um KAR bun ate & mag NEE zhum KAR bun ate)

**Pharmacologic Class** Antacid

**U.S. Brand Names** Mylanta® Gelcaps®

**Dosage Forms Cap:** Calcium carbonate 311 mg and magnesium carbonate 232 mg

♦ **Calcium Channel Blocking Agents** see Chart on page 1004

## Calcium Chloride (KAL see um KLOR ide)

**Pharmacologic Class** Calcium Salt; Electrolyte Supplement, Parenteral

**Mechanism of Action** Moderates nerve and muscle performance via action potential excitation threshold regulation

**Use** Cardiac resuscitation when epinephrine fails to improve myocardial contractions, cardiac disturbances of hyperkalemia, hypocalcemia, or calcium channel blocking agent toxicity; emergent treatment of hypocalcemic tetany, treatment of hypermagnesemia

**USUAL DOSAGE Note:** Calcium chloride is 3 times as potent as calcium gluconate

Cardiac arrest in the presence of hyperkalemia or hypocalcemia, magnesium toxicity, or calcium antagonist toxicity: I.V.:

Infants and Children: 20 mg/kg; may repeat in 10 minutes if necessary

Adults: 2-4 mg/kg (10% solution), repeated every 10 minutes if necessary

Hypocalcemia: I.V.:

Infants and Children: 10-20 mg/kg/dose (infants <1 mEq; children 1-7 mEq), repeat every 4-6 hours if needed

Adults: 500 mg to 1 g (7-14 mEq)/dose repeated every 4-6 hours if needed

Hypocalcemic tetany: I.V.:

Infants and Children: 10 mg/kg (0.5-0.7 mEq/kg) over 5-10 minutes; may repeat after 6-8 hours or follow with an infusion with a maximum dose of 200 mg/kg/day

Adults: 1 g over 10-30 minutes; may repeat after 6 hours

Hypocalcemia secondary to citrated blood transfusion: I.V.:

Neonates: Give 0.45 mEq **elemental** calcium for each 100 mL citrated blood infused

Adults: 1.35 mEq calcium with each 100 mL of citrated blood infused

**Dosing adjustment in renal impairment:** $Cl_{cr}$ <25 mL/minute: Dosage adjustments may be necessary depending on the serum calcium levels

**Dosage Forms** Elemental calcium listed in brackets **Inj:** 10% = 100 mg/mL [27.2 mg/mL] (10 mL)

**Contraindications** In ventricular fibrillation during cardiac resuscitation, hypercalcemia, and in patients with risk of digitalis toxicity, renal or cardiac disease

**Warnings/Precautions** Avoid too rapid I.V. administration (<1 mL/minute) and extravasation; use with caution in digitalized patients, respiratory failure, or acidosis; hypercalcemia may occur in patients with renal failure, and frequent determination of serum calcium is necessary; avoid metabolic acidosis (ie, administer only 2-3 days then change to another calcium salt)

**Pregnancy Risk Factor** C

**Adverse Reactions** <1%: Vasodilation, hypotension, bradycardia, cardiac arrhythmias, ventricular fibrillation, syncope, lethargy, coma, mania, erythema, decreased serum magnesium, hypercalcemia, elevated serum amylase, tissue necrosis, muscle weakness, hypercalciuria

**Drug Interactions**

Decreased effect: Calcium may antagonize the effects of calcium channel blockers, atenolol, and sodium polystyrene sulfonate

Increased toxicity: Administer cautiously to a digitalized patient, may precipitate arrhythmias; hypercalcemia induced by thiazides may be increased with calcium administration

**Special PA Issues**

**Patient Education:** This medication can only be given I.V. Do not make rapid postural changes while calcium is infusing. Report any feelings of excitation, chest pain, irregular or pounding heartbeat, vomiting, acute headache, or dizziness.

**Reference Range:**

Serum calcium: 8.4-10.2 mg/dL

Due to a poor correlation between the serum ionized calcium (free) and total serum calcium, particularly in states of low albumin or acid/base imbalances, direct measurement of ionized calcium is recommended

In low albumin states, the corrected **total** serum calcium may be estimated by this equation (assuming a normal albumin of 4 g/dL)

Corrected total calcium = total serum calcium + 0.8 (4.0 - measured serum albumin)

**or**

Corrected calcium = measured calcium - measured albumin + 4.0

Serum/plasma chloride: 95-108 mEq/L

# Calcium Glubionate (KAL see um gloo BYE oh nate)

**Pharmacologic Class** Calcium Salt

**U.S. Brand Names** Neo-Calglucon® [OTC]

**Mechanism of Action** As dietary supplements, to prevent or treat negative calcium balance (eg, osteoporosis), the calcium in calcium salts moderates nerve and muscle performance and allows normal cardiac function

**Use** Adjunct in treatment and prevention of postmenopausal osteoporosis; treatment and prevention of calcium depletion or hyperphosphatemia (eg, osteoporosis, osteomalacia, mild/moderate renal insufficiency, hypoparathyroidism, rickets)

**USUAL DOSAGE** Dosage is in terms of **elemental** calcium

**Adequate intakes:**

0-6 months: 210 mg/day

7-12 months: 270 mg/day

1-3 years: 500 mg/day

4-8 years: 800 mg/day

Adults, male/female:

9-18 years: 1300 mg/day

19-50 years: 1000 mg/day

>51 years: 1200 mg/day

Female: Pregnancy:

≤18 years: 1300 mg/day

>19 years: 1000 mg/day

Female: Lactating:

≤18 years: 1300 mg/day

>19 years: 1000 mg/day

Syrup is a hyperosmolar solution; dosage is in terms of calcium glubionate, elemental calcium is in parentheses

Neonatal hypocalcemia: 1200 mg (77 mg $Ca^{++}$)/kg/day in 4-6 divided doses

Maintenance: Infants and Children: 600-2000 mg (38-128 mg $Ca^{++}$)/kg/day in 4 divided doses up to a maximum of 9 g (575 mg $Ca^{++}$)/day

Adults: 6-18 g (~0.5-1 g $Ca^{++}$)/day in divided doses

**Dosing adjustment in renal impairment:** $Cl_{cr}$ <25 mL/minute: Dosage adjustments may be necessary depending on the serum calcium levels

**Dosage Forms** Elemental calcium listed in brackets **Syr:** 1.8 g/5 mL [115 mg/5 mL] (480 mL)

**Contraindications** Hypercalcemia, renal calculi, ventricular fibrillation

**Warnings/Precautions** Calcium absorption is impaired in achlorhydria (common in elderly - try alternate salt, administer with food); administration is followed by increased gastric acid secretion within 2 hours of administration; while hypercalcemia and hypercalciuria may result when therapeutic replacement amounts are given for prolonged periods, they are most likely to occur in hypoparathyroid patients receiving high doses of vitamin D

**Pregnancy Risk Factor** C

**Adverse Reactions**

Mild hypercalcemia (calcium: >10.5 mg/dL) may be asymptomatic or manifest itself as constipation, anorexia, nausea, and vomiting

More severe hypercalcemia (calcium: >12 mg/dL) is associated with confusion, delirium, stupor, and coma

(Continued)

## Calcium Glubionate *(Continued)*

<1%: Headache, hypophosphatemia, hypercalcemia, nausea, anorexia, vomiting, abdominal pain, constipation, thirst

**Drug Interactions**
Decreased effect:
Calcium glubionate may significantly decrease the bioavailability of tetracyclines
Large intakes of dietary fiber may decrease calcium absorption due to a decreased GI transit time and the formation of fiber-calcium complexes
Increased effect: Calcium glubionate may increase the effects of quinidine

**Special PA Issues**
**Patient Education:** Follow instructions for dosing. Take with a full glass of water or juice, 1-3 hours after meals and other medications and 1-2 hours before any iron supplements. Avoid alcohol, other antacids, caffeine, or other calcium supplements unless approved by prescriber. You may experience constipation (increasing exercise or dietary fluid, fiber, or fruits may help). Report severe, unresolved GI disturbances and unusual emotional lability (mood swings).

**Reference Range:**
Serum calcium: 8.4-10.2 mg/dL: Monitor plasma calcium levels if using calcium salts as electrolyte supplements for deficiency
Due to a poor correlation between the serum ionized calcium (free) and total serum calcium, particularly in states of low albumin or acid/base imbalances, direct measurement of ionized calcium is recommended
In low albumin states, the corrected **total** serum calcium may be estimated by: Corrected total calcium = total serum calcium + 0.8 (4.0 - measured serum albumin)

## Calcium Gluceptate *(KAL see um gloo SEP tate)*

**Pharmacologic Class** Calcium Salt; Electrolyte Supplement, Parenteral

**Mechanism of Action** Moderates nerve and muscle performance via action potential excitation threshold regulation

**Use** Treatment of cardiac disturbances of hyperkalemia, hypocalcemia, or calcium channel blocker toxicity; cardiac resuscitation when epinephrine fails to improve myocardial contractions; treatment of hypermagnesemia and hypocalcemia

**USUAL DOSAGE** Dose expressed in mg of calcium gluceptate (elemental calcium is in parentheses)
Cardiac resuscitation in the presence of hypocalcemia, hyperkalemia, magnesium toxicity, or calcium channel blocker toxicity: I.V.:
Children: 110 mg (9 mg Ca⁺⁺)/kg/dose
Adults: 1.1-1.5 g (90-123 mg Ca⁺⁺)
Hypocalcemia:
I.M.:
Children: 200-500 mg (16.4-41 mg Ca⁺⁺)/kg/day divided every 6 hours
Adults: 500 mg to 1.1 g/dose as needed
I.V.: Adults: 1.1-4.4 g (90-360 mg Ca⁺⁺) administered slowly as needed (≤2 mL/minute)
After citrated blood administration: Children and Adults: I.V.: 0.45 mEq Ca⁺⁺/100 mL blood infused

**Dosing adjustment in renal impairment:** $Cl_{cr}$ <25 mL/minute: Dosage adjustments may be necessary depending on the serum calcium levels

**Dosage Forms** Elemental calcium listed in brackets **Inj:** 220 mg/mL [18 mg/mL] (5 mL, 50 mL)

**Contraindications** In ventricular fibrillation during cardiac resuscitation; patients with risk of digitalis toxicity, renal or cardiac disease; hypercalcemia

**Warnings/Precautions** Avoid too rapid I.V. administration; avoid extravasation; use with caution in digitalized patients, respiratory failure or acidosis; metabolic acidosis (administer for only 2-3 days then change to another calcium salt)

**Pregnancy Risk Factor** C

**Adverse Reactions** <1%: Vasodilation, hypotension, bradycardia, cardiac arrhythmias, ventricular fibrillation, syncope, lethargy, mania, coma, erythema, hypomagnesemia, hypercalcemia, elevated serum amylase, tissue necrosis, muscle weakness, hypercalciuria

**Drug Interactions**
Decreased effect: Calcium may antagonize the effects of calcium channel blockers, atenolol, and sodium polystyrene sulfonate
Increased toxicity: Administer cautiously to a digitalized patient, may precipitate arrhythmias; hypercalcemia induced by thiazides may be increased with calcium administration

**Special PA Issues**
**Reference Range:**
Serum calcium: 8.4-10.2 mg/dL
Due to a poor correlation between the serum ionized calcium (free) and total serum calcium, particularly in states of low albumin or acid/base imbalances, direct measurement of ionized calcium is recommended
In low albumin states, the corrected **total** serum calcium may be estimated by this equation (assuming a normal albumin of 4 g/dL)

Corrected total calcium = total serum calcium + 0.8 (4.0 - measured serum albumin)
or
Corrected calcium = measured calcium - measured albumin + 4.0

# Calcium Gluconate (KAL see um GLOO koe nate)

**Pharmacologic Class** Calcium Salt; Electrolyte Supplement, Oral; Electrolyte Supplement, Parenteral

**U.S. Brand Names** Kalcinate®

**Mechanism of Action** When used to prevent or treat negative calcium balance (eg, osteoporosis), the calcium in calcium salts moderates nerve and muscle performance and allows normal cardiac function

**Use** Treatment and prevention of hypocalcemia; treatment of tetany, cardiac disturbances of hyperkalemia, cardiac resuscitation when epinephrine fails to improve myocardial contractions, hypocalcemia, or calcium channel blocker toxicity; calcium supplementation

**USUAL DOSAGE** Dosage is in terms of **elemental** calcium

**Adequate intakes:**

0-6 months: 210 mg/day
7-12 months: 270 mg/day
1-3 years: 500 mg/day
4-8 years: 800 mg/day
Adults, male/female:
9-18 years: 1300 mg/day
19-50 years: 1000 mg/day
>51 years: 1200 mg/day
Female: Pregnancy:
≤18 years: 1300 mg/day
>19 years: 1000 mg/day
Female: Lactating:
≤18 years: 1300 mg/day
>19 years: 1000 mg/day

Dosage expressed in terms of **calcium gluconate**

Hypocalcemia: I.V.:
Neonates: 200-800 mg/kg/day as a continuous infusion or in 4 divided doses
Infants and Children: 200-500 mg/kg/day as a continuous infusion or in 4 divided doses
Adults: 2-15 g/24 hours as a continuous infusion or in divided doses

Hypocalcemia: Oral:
Children: 200-500 mg/kg/day divided every 6 hours
Adults: 500 mg to 2 g 2-4 times/day
Osteoporosis/bone loss: Oral: 1000-1500 mg in divided doses/day

Hypocalcemia secondary to citrated blood infusion: I.V.: Give 0.45 mEq **elemental** calcium for each 100 mL citrated blood infused

Hypocalcemic tetany: I.V.:
Neonates: 100-200 mg/kg/dose, may follow with 500 mg/kg/day in 3-4 divided doses or as an infusion
Infants and Children: 100-200 mg/kg/dose (0.5-0.7 mEq/kg/dose) over 5-10 minutes; may repeat every 6-8 hours **or** follow with an infusion of 500 mg/kg/day
Adults: 1-3 g (4.5-16 mEq) may be administered until therapeutic response occurs

Calcium antagonist toxicity, magnesium intoxication or cardiac arrest in the presence of hyperkalemia or hypocalcemia: Calcium chloride is recommended calcium salt: I.V.:
Infants and Children: 100 mg/kg/dose (maximum: 3 g/dose)
Adults: 500-800 mg; maximum: 3 g/dose

Maintenance electrolyte requirements for total parenteral nutrition: I.V.: Daily requirements:
Adults: 8-16 mEq/1000 kcal/24 hours

**Dosing adjustment in renal impairment:** $Cl_{cr}$ <25 mL/minute: Dosage adjustments may be necessary depending on the serum calcium levels

**Dosage Forms** Elemental calcium listed in brackets **Inj:** 10% = 100 mg/mL [9 mg/mL] (10 mL, 50 mL, 100 mL, 200 mL); **Tab:** 500 mg [45 mg], 650 mg [58.5 mg], 975 mg [87.75 mg], 1 g [90 mg]

**Contraindications** In ventricular fibrillation during cardiac resuscitation; patients with risk of digitalis toxicity, renal or cardiac disease, hypercalcemia, renal calculi, hypophosphatemia

**Warnings/Precautions** Avoid too rapid I.V. administration (1.5-3.3 mL/minute); use with caution in digitalized patients, severe hyperphosphatemia, respiratory failure or acidosis; avoid extravasation; may produce cardiac arrest; hypercalcemia may occur in patients with renal failure and frequent determination of serum calcium is necessary; the serum calcium level should be monitored twice weekly during the early dose adjustment period

**Pregnancy Risk Factor** C

**Adverse Reactions** <1%: Vasodilation, hypotension, bradycardia, cardiac arrhythmias, ventricular fibrillation, syncope, lethargy, mania, coma, erythema, decrease serum magnesium, hypercalcemia, elevated serum amylase, constipation, nausea, vomiting, abdominal pain, tissue necrosis, muscle weakness, hypercalciuria
(Continued)

## Calcium Gluconate *(Continued)*

### Drug Interactions
Decreased effect:

Calcium may decrease the bioavailability of tetracyclines, fluoroquinolones, iron salts and salicylates, atenolol, and sodium polystyrene sulfonate

I.V. calcium may antagonize the effects of verapamil; large intakes of dietary fiber may decrease calcium absorption due to a decreased GI transit time and the formation of fiber-calcium complexes

Increased effect: I.V. calcium may increase the effects of quinidine and digitalis

### Special PA Issues

**Patient Education:**

I.V.: Do not make rapid postural changes while calcium is infusing. Report any feelings of excitation, chest pain, irregular or pounding heartbeat, vomiting, acute headache, or dizziness.

Oral: Take as directed, with a full glass of water or juice 2 hours before or after other medications. Do not take with fiber rich meals, whole grain cereals, or food high in oxalates (eg, spinach, rhubarb). Avoid antacids, excess alcohol, caffeine-containing beverages, or additional calcium supplements unless approved by prescriber. Increasing exercise or dietary fluid, fiber, or fruits may help reduce incidence of constipation. Report severe, unresolved GI disturbances and unusual emotional lability (mood swings).

**Reference Range:**

Serum calcium: 8.4-10.2 mg/dL: Monitor plasma calcium levels if using calcium salts as electrolyte supplements for deficiency

Due to a poor correlation between the serum ionized calcium (free) and total serum calcium, particularly in states of low albumin or acid/base imbalances, direct measurement of ionized calcium is recommended

In low albumin states, the corrected **total** serum calcium may be estimated by: Corrected total calcium = total serum calcium + 0.8 (4.0 - measured serum albumin)

- ♦ **Calcium Leucovorin** *see* Leucovorin *on page 520*
- ♦ **CaldeCORT®** *see* Hydrocortisone *on page 453*
- ♦ **CaldeCORT® Anti-Itch Spray** *see* Hydrocortisone *on page 453*
- ♦ **Calderol®** *see* Calcifediol *on page 135*
- ♦ **Calmylin Expectorant** *see* Guaifenesin *on page 427*
- ♦ **Calphron®** *see* Calcium Acetate *on page 138*
- ♦ **Cal-Plus® [OTC]** *see* Calcium Carbonate *on page 139*
- ♦ **Calsan®** *see* Calcium Carbonate *on page 139*
- ♦ **Caltine®** *see* Calcitonin *on page 136*
- ♦ **Caltrate® 600 [OTC]** *see* Calcium Carbonate *on page 139*
- ♦ **Caltrate, Jr.® [OTC]** *see* Calcium Carbonate *on page 139*
- ♦ **Cama® Arthritis Pain Reliever [OTC]** *see* Aspirin *on page 80*
- ♦ **Camphorated Tincture of Opium** *see* Paregoric *on page 697*

## Candesartan *(kan de SAR tan)*

**Pharmacologic Class** Angiotensin II Antagonists

**U.S. Brand Names** Atacand™

**Mechanism of Action** Candesartan is an angiotensin receptor antagonist. Angiotensin II acts as a vasoconstrictor. In addition to causing direct vasoconstriction, angiotensin II also stimulates the release of aldosterone. Once aldosterone is released, sodium as well as water are reabsorbed. The end result is an elevation in blood pressure. Candesartan binds to the AT1 angiotensin II receptor. This binding prevents angiotensin II from binding to the receptor thereby blocking the vasoconstriction and the aldosterone secreting effects of angiotensin II.

**Use** Alone or in combination with other antihypertensive agents in treating essential hypertension; may have an advantage over losartan due to minimal metabolism requirements and consequent use in mild to moderate hepatic impairment

**USUAL DOSAGE** Adults: Oral: Usual dose is 4-32 mg once daily; dosage must be individualized; blood pressure response is dose-related over the range of 2-32 mg; the usual recommended starting dose of 16 mg once daily when it is used as monotherapy in patients who are not volume depleted; it can be administered once or twice daily with total daily doses ranging from 8-32 mg; larger doses do not appear to have a greater effect and there is relatively little experience with such doses

No initial dosage adjustment is necessary for elderly patients (although higher concentrations ($C_{max}$) and AUC were observed in these populations), for patients with mildly impaired renal function, or for patients with mildly impaired hepatic function.

**Dosage Forms Tab, as cilexetil:** 4 mg, 8 mg, 16 mg, 32 mg

**Contraindications** Hypersensitivity to candesartan or any component; sensitivity to other A-II receptor antagonists; pregnancy; hyperaldosteronism (primary); renal artery stenosis (bilateral)

**Warnings/Precautions** Avoid use or use smaller dose in volume-depleted patients. Drugs which alter renin-angiotensin system have been associated with deterioration in renal function, including oliguria, acute renal failure and progressive azotemia. Use with caution in patients with renal artery stenosis (unilateral or bilateral) to avoid decrease in renal function; use caution in patients with pre-existing renal insufficiency (may decrease renal perfusion).

**Pregnancy Risk Factor** C (1st trimester); D (2nd and 3rd trimester)

**Pregnancy Implications** Enters breast milk/contraindicated

Drugs which act directly on renin-angiotensin can cause fetal and neonatal morbidity and death

**Adverse Reactions**

1% to 10%:

Cardiovascular: Flushing, chest pain, peripheral edema

Central nervous system: Dizziness, lightheadedness, drowsiness, fatigue, headache

Dermatologic: Rash

Gastrointestinal: Nausea, diarrhea, vomiting

Neuromuscular & skeletal: Back pain, arthralgia

Respiratory: Upper respiratory tract infection, pharyngitis, rhinitis, bronchitis, cough, sinusitis

<1%: Tachycardia, palpitations, angina, myocardial infarction, vertigo, anxiety, depression, somnolence, fever, angioedema, rash, hyperglycemia, hypertriglyceridemia, hyperuricemia, dyspepsia, gastroenteritis, paresthesias, increased CPK, myalgia, weakness, hematuria, epistaxis, dyspnea, diaphoresis (increased)

**Drug Interactions** Potassium salts/supplements; candesartan is not metabolized by cytochrome P-450

**Onset** 2-3 hours; peak effect: 6-8 hours

**Duration** >24 hours

**Half-Life** Dose-dependent: 5-9 hours

**Special PA Issues**

**Patient Education:** Take exactly as directed; do not miss doses, alter dosage, or discontinue without consulting prescriber. Do not alter salt or potassium intake without consulting prescriber. Change position slowly when rising from sitting or lying or when climbing stairs. May cause transient drowsiness, dizziness, or headache; avoid driving or engaging in tasks that require alertness until response to drug is known. Small frequent meals may help reduce any nausea or vomiting. Report unusual weight gain or swelling of ankles and hands; persistent fatigue; unusual flu or cold symptoms or dry cough; difficulty breathing; chest pain or palpitations; swelling of eyes, face, or lips; skin rash; muscle pain or weakness; unusual bleeding (in urine, stool, or gums); or excessive sweating.

**Dietary Considerations:** Food reduces the time to maximal concentration and increases the $C_{max}$

**Monitoring Parameters:** Supine blood pressure, electrolytes, serum creatinine, BUN, urinalysis, symptomatic hypotension, and tachycardia

♦ **Candesartan Cilexetil** see Candesartan on previous page

♦ **C. angustifolia** see Senna on page 828

♦ **Capastat® Sulfate** see Capreomycin on this page

♦ **Capital® and Codeine** see Acetaminophen and Codeine on page 22

♦ **Capoten®** see Captopril on next page

♦ **Capozide®** see Captopril and Hydrochlorothiazide on page 147

# Capreomycin (kap ree oh MYE sin)

**Pharmacologic Class** Antibiotic, Miscellaneous; Antitubercular Agent

**U.S. Brand Names** Capastat® Sulfate

**Mechanism of Action** Capreomycin is a cyclic polypeptide antimicrobial. It is administered as a mixture of capreomycin IA and capreomycin IB. The mechanism of action of capreomycin is not well understood. Mycobacterial species that have become resistant to other agents are usually still sensitive to the action of capreomycin. However, significant cross-resistance with viomycin, kanamycin, and neomycin occurs.

**Use** Treatment of tuberculosis in conjunction with at least one other antituberculosis agent

**USUAL DOSAGE** I.M.:

Infants and Children: 15 mg/kg/day, up to 1 g/day maximum

Adults: 15-20 mg/kg/day up to 1 g/day for 60-120 days, followed by 1 g 2-3 times/week

Dosing interval in renal impairment: Adults:

$Cl_{cr}$ >100 mL/minute: Administer 13-15 mg/kg every 24 hours

$Cl_{cr}$ 80-100 mL/minute: Administer 10-13 mg/kg every 24 hours

$Cl_{cr}$ 60-80 mL/minute: Administer 7-10 mg/kg every 24 hours

$Cl_{cr}$ 40-60 mL/minute: Administer 11-14 mg/kg every 48 hours

$Cl_{cr}$ 20-40 mL/minute: Administer 10-14 mg/kg every 72 hours

$Cl_{cr}$ <20 mL/minute: Administer 4-7 mg/kg every 72 hours

**Dosage Forms** Inj, as sulfate: 100 mg/mL (10 mL)

**Contraindications** Known hypersensitivity to capreomycin sulfate

(Continued)

145

## Capreomycin *(Continued)*

**Warnings/Precautions** Use in patients with renal insufficiency or pre-existing auditory impairment must be undertaken with great caution, and the risk of additional eighth nerve impairment or renal injury should be weighed against the benefits to be derived from therapy. Since other parenteral antituberculous agents (eg, streptomycin) also have similar and sometimes irreversible toxic effects, particularly on eighth cranial nerve and renal function, simultaneous administration of these agents with capreomycin is not recommended. Use with nonantituberculous drugs (ie, aminoglycoside antibiotics) having ototoxic or nephrotoxic potential should be undertaken only with great caution.

**Pregnancy Risk Factor** C

**Adverse Reactions**

>10%:

Otic: Ototoxicity [subclinical hearing loss (11%), clinical loss (3%)], tinnitus

Renal: Nephrotoxicity (36%, increased BUN)

1% to 10%: Hematologic: Eosinophilia (dose-related, mild)

<1%: Vertigo, hypokalemia, leukocytosis, thrombocytopenia (rare); pain, induration, and bleeding at injection site; hypersensitivity (urticaria, rash, fever)

**Drug Interactions**

Increased effect/duration of nondepolarizing neuromuscular blocking agents

Additive toxicity (nephro- and ototoxicity, respiratory paralysis): Aminoglycosides (eg, streptomycin)

**Half-Life** Dependent upon renal function and varies with creatinine clearance; 4-6 hours

**Special PA Issues**

**Patient Education:** Take as prescribed; do not discontinue without consulting prescriber. Maintain adequate hydration (2-3 L/day of fluids unless instructed to restrict fluid intake) to reduce incidence of nephrotoxicity. While taking this medication, routine blood tests and auditory tests will be necessary. Report any hearing loss, dizziness or vertigo, persistent nausea or vomiting, loss of appetite, or increased frequency of urination.

**Reference Range:** 10 µg/mL

♦ **Capreomycin Sulfate** *see Capreomycin on previous page*

## Captopril *(KAP toe pril)*

**Pharmacologic Class** Angiotensin-Converting Enzyme (ACE) Inhibitors

**U.S. Brand Names** Capoten®

**Mechanism of Action** Competitive inhibitor of angiotensin-converting enzyme (ACE); prevents conversion of angiotensin I to angiotensin II, a potent vasoconstrictor; results in lower levels of angiotensin II which causes an increase in plasma renin activity and a reduction in aldosterone secretion

**Use** Management of hypertension and treatment of congestive heart failure; left ventricular dysfunction after myocardial infarction (MI), diabetic nephropathy

**Unlabeled use:** Hypertensive crisis, rheumatoid arthritis, diagnosis of anatomic renal artery stenosis, hypertension secondary to scleroderma renal crisis, diagnosis of aldosteronism, idiopathic edema, Bartter's syndrome, increase circulation in Raynaud's phenomenon

**USUAL DOSAGE Note:** Dosage must be titrated according to patient's response; use lowest effective dose. Oral:

Infants: Initial: 0.15-0.3 mg/kg/dose; titrate dose upward to maximum of 6 mg/kg/day in 1-4 divided doses; usual required dose: 2.5-6 mg/kg/day

Children: Initial: 0.5 mg/kg/dose; titrate upward to maximum of 6 mg/kg/day in 2-4 divided doses

Older Children: Initial: 6.25-12.5 mg/dose every 12-24 hours; titrate upward to maximum of 6 mg/kg/day

Adolescents: Initial: 12.5-25 mg/dose given every 8-12 hours; increase by 25 mg/dose to maximum of 450 mg/day

Adults:

Hypertension:

Initial dose: 12.5-25 mg 2-3 times/day; may increase by 12.5-25 mg/dose at 1- to 2-week intervals up to 50 mg 3 times/day; add diuretic before further dosage increases

Maximum dose: 150 mg 3 times/day

Congestive heart failure:

Initial dose: 6.25-12.5 mg 3 times/day in conjunction with cardiac glycoside and diuretic therapy; initial dose depends upon patient's fluid/electrolyte status

Target dose: 50 mg 3 times/day

Maximum dose: 150 mg 3 times/day

LVD after MI: Initial dose: 6.25 mg followed by 12.5 mg 3 times/day; then increase to 25 mg 3 times/day during next several days and then over next several weeks to target dose of 50 mg 3 times/day

Diabetic nephropathy: 25 mg 3 times/day; other antihypertensives often given concurrently

**Dosing adjustment in renal impairment:**

$Cl_{cr}$ 10-50 mL/minute: Administer at 75% of normal dose

$Cl_{cr}$ <10 mL/minute: Administer at 50% of normal dose

**Note:** Smaller dosages given every 8-12 hours are indicated in patients with renal dysfunction; renal function and leukocyte count should be carefully monitored during therapy

Hemodialysis: Moderately dialyzable (20% to 50%); administer dose postdialysis or administer 25% to 35% supplemental dose

Peritoneal dialysis: Supplemental dose is not necessary

**Dosage Forms** Tab: 12.5 mg, 25 mg, 50 mg, 100 mg

**Contraindications** Hypersensitivity to captopril, other ACE inhibitors, or any component

**Warnings/Precautions** Use with caution and decrease dosage in patients with renal impairment (especially renal artery stenosis), severe congestive heart failure, or with coadministered diuretic therapy; experience in children is limited. Severe hypotension may occur in patients who are sodium and/or volume depleted, initiate lower doses and monitor closely when starting therapy in these patients; ACE inhibitors may be preferred agents in elderly patients with congestive heart failure and diabetes mellitus (diabetic proteinuria is reduced, minimal CNS effects, and enhanced insulin sensitivity); however due to decreased renal function, tolerance must be carefully monitored.

**Pregnancy Risk Factor** C (1st trimester); D (2nd and 3rd trimesters)

**Pregnancy Implications** Enters breast milk/compatible

Clinical effects on the fetus: No data available on crossing the placenta. Cranial defects, hypocalvaria/acalvaria, oligohydramnios, persistent anuria following delivery, hypotension, renal defects, renal dysgenesis/dysplasia, renal failure, pulmonary hypoplasia, limb contractures secondary to oligohydramnios and stillbirth reported. ACE inhibitors should be avoided during pregnancy.

**Adverse Reactions**

>1%:

Cardiovascular: Tachycardia, chest pain, palpitations

Central nervous system: Insomnia, headache, dizziness, fatigue, malaise

Dermatologic: Rash (4% to 7%), pruritus, alopecia

Gastrointestinal: Abdominal pain, vomiting, nausea, diarrhea, anorexia, constipation, abnormal taste (2% to 4%), xerostomia

Neuromuscular & skeletal: Paresthesias

Renal: Oliguria

Respiratory: Transient cough (0.5% to 2%)

<1%: Hypotension, angioedema, hyperkalemia, neutropenia, agranulocytosis, proteinuria, increased BUN/serum creatinine

**Drug Interactions** CYP2D6 enzyme substrate

Increased toxicity: See Drug-Drug Interactions With ACEIs table *on page 997*

**Onset** Maximal decrease in blood pressure 1-1.5 hours after dose

**Duration** Dose related, may require several weeks of therapy before full hypotensive effect is seen

**Half-Life** Dependent upon renal and cardiac function: Adults, normal: 1.9 hours; Congestive heart failure: 2.06 hours; Anuria: 20-40 hours

**Special PA Issues**

**Patient Education:** Take as directed, preferably on an empty stomach (1 hour before or 2 hours after meals). Do not change dosage or stop taking without consulting prescriber. Follow prescribed diet. You may experience dizziness, fainting, or lightheadedness (use caution when driving or performing hazardous tasks and use caution when rising from sitting or lying position, climbing stairs, or bending over until response to medication is known). Report loss of taste; sore throat, fever, or chills; rash; swelling of hands, feet, or legs; respiratory difficulty; chest pains or irregular heartbeat; unusual cough; or persistent vomiting, diarrhea, or perspiration.

**Monitoring Parameters:** BUN, serum creatinine, urine dipstick for protein, complete leukocyte count, and blood pressure

**Related Information**

ACE Inhibitors *on page 995*

Heart Failure: Management of Patients with Left Ventricular Systolic Dysfunction *on page 1064*

Drug-Drug Interactions With ACEIs *on page 997*

# Captopril and Hydrochlorothiazide

(KAP toe pril & hye droe klor oh THYE a zide)

**Pharmacologic Class** Antihypertensive Agent, Combination

**U.S. Brand Names** Capozide®

**Dosage Forms** Tab: 25/15: Captopril 25 mg and hydrochlorothiazide 15 mg, 25/25: Captopril 25 mg and hydrochlorothiazide 25 mg, 50/15: Captopril 50 mg and hydrochlorothiazide 15 mg, 50/25: Captopril 50 mg and hydrochlorothiazide 25 mg

♦ **Carafate®** *see* Sucralfate *on page 856*

## Caramiphen and Phenylpropanolamine
(kar AM i fen & fen il proe pa NOLE a meen)
**Pharmacologic Class** Antihistamine
**U.S. Brand Names** Ordrine AT® Extended Release Capsule; Rescaps-D® S.R. Capsule; Tuss-Allergine® Modified T.D. Capsule; Tussogest® Extended Release Capsule
**Dosage Forms Cap, timed release:** Caramiphen edisylate 40 mg and phenylpropanolamine hydrochloride 75 mg; **Liq:** Caramiphen edisylate 6.7 mg and phenylpropanolamine hydrochloride 12.5 mg per 5 mL

♦ **Carampicillin Hydrochloride** see Bacampicillin on page 95

## Carbachol (KAR ba kole)
**Pharmacologic Class** Cholinergic Agonist; Ophthalmic Agent, Antiglaucoma; Ophthalmic Agent, Miotic
**U.S. Brand Names** Carbastat® Ophthalmic; Carboptic® Ophthalmic; Isopto® Carbachol Ophthalmic; Miostat® Intraocular
**Mechanism of Action** Synthetic direct-acting cholinergic agent that causes miosis by stimulating muscarinic receptors in the eye
**Use** Lowers intraocular pressure in the treatment of glaucoma; cause miosis during surgery
**USUAL DOSAGE** Adults:
Ophthalmic: Instill 1-2 drops up to 3 times/day
Intraocular: 0.5 mL instilled into anterior chamber before or after securing sutures
**Dosage Forms Soln:** Intraocular (Carbastat®, Miostat®): 0.01% (1.5 mL); **Top, ophth:** Carboptic®: 3% (15 mL), Isopto® Carbachol: 0.75% (15 mL, 30 mL), 1.5% (15 mL, 30 mL), 2.25% (15 mL), 3% (15 mL, 30 mL)
**Contraindications** Acute iritis, acute inflammatory disease of the anterior chamber, hypersensitivity to carbachol or any component
**Warnings/Precautions** Use with caution in patients undergoing general anesthesia and in presence of corneal abrasion
**Pregnancy Risk Factor** C
**Adverse Reactions**
1% to 10%: Ocular: Blurred vision, eye pain
<1%: Transient fall in blood pressure, headache, stomach cramps, diarrhea, ciliary spasm with temporary decrease of visual acuity, corneal clouding, persistent bullous keratopathy, postoperative keratitis, retinal detachment, transient ciliary and conjunctival injection, asthma, increased peristalsis
**Onset** Ophthalmic instillation: Onset of miosis: 10-20 minutes; Intraocular administration: Onset of miosis: Within 2-5 minutes
**Duration** Ophthalmic instillation: Duration of reduction in intraocular pressure: 4-8 hours; Intraocular administration: 24 hours
**Special PA Issues**
**Patient Education:** For ophthalmic use only. Store at room temperature, away from light. Do not use discolored solution. Apply prescribed amount as often as directed. Wash hands before using and do not let tip of applicator touch eye or contaminate tip of applicator. Tilt head back and look upward. Gently pull down lower lid and put drop(s) in inner corner of eye. Close eye and roll eyeball in all directions. Do not blink for ½ minute. Apply gentle pressure to inner corner of eye for 30 seconds. Wipe away excess from skin around eye. Do not use any other eye preparation for at least 10 minutes. Do not touch tip of applicator to eye or contaminate tip of applicator. Do not share medication with anyone else. Temporary stinging or blurred vision may occur. May cause altered distance vision or decreased night vision (use caution when driving or in areas that are poorly lit). Report persistent eye pain; redness, burning, watering, dryness, or double vision; puffiness around eye; vision disturbances or other adverse eye response; worsening of condition or lack of improvement.

♦ **Carbacholine** see Carbachol on this page

## Carbamazepine (kar ba MAZ e peen)
**Pharmacologic Class** Anticonvulsant, Miscellaneous
**U.S. Brand Names** Carbatrol®; Epitol®; Tegretol®; Tegretol®-XR
**Mechanism of Action** In addition to anticonvulsant effects, carbamazepine has anticholinergic, antineuralgic, antidiuretic, muscle relaxant and antiarrhythmic properties; may depress activity in the nucleus ventralis of the thalamus or decrease synaptic transmission or decrease summation of temporal stimulation leading to neural discharge by limiting influx of sodium ions across cell membrane or other unknown mechanisms; stimulates the release of ADH and potentiates its action in promoting reabsorption of water; chemically related to tricyclic antidepressants
**Use** Prophylaxis of generalized tonic-clonic, partial (especially complex partial), and mixed partial or generalized seizure disorder; pain relief of trigeminal neuralgia
**Unlabeled use:** Treat bipolar disorders and other affective disorders; resistant schizophrenia, alcohol withdrawal, restless leg syndrome, and psychotic behavior associated with dementia

**USUAL DOSAGE** Oral (adjust dose according to patient's response and serum concentrations):

Children:

&lt;6 years: Initial: 5 mg/kg/day; dosage may be increased every 5-7 days to 10 mg/kg/day; then up to 20 mg/kg/day if necessary; administer in 2-4 divided doses/day

6-12 years: Initial: 100 mg twice daily or 10 mg/kg/day in 2 divided doses; increase by 100 mg/day at weekly intervals depending upon response; usual maintenance: 20-30 mg/kg/day in 2-4 divided doses/day; maximum dose: 1000 mg/day

Children &gt;12 years and Adults: 200 mg twice daily to start, increase by 200 mg/day at weekly intervals until therapeutic levels achieved; usual dose: 800-1200 mg/day in 3-4 divided doses; some patients have required up to 1.6-2.4 g/day

Trigeminal or glossopharyngeal neuralgia: Initial: 100 mg twice daily with food, gradually increasing in increments of 100 mg twice daily as needed; usual maintenance: 400-800 mg/day in 2 divided doses

**Dosing adjustment in renal impairment:** $Cl_{cr}$ &lt;10 mL/minute: Administer 75% of dose

**Dosage Forms Susp, oral (citrus-vanilla flavor):** 100 mg/5 mL (450 mL); **Tab:** 200 mg; **Tab, chewable:** 100 mg; **Tab, extended release:** 100 mg, 200 mg, 400 mg

**Contraindications** Hypersensitivity to carbamazepine or any component; **may have cross-sensitivity with tricyclic antidepressants**; should not be used in any patient with bone marrow suppression, MAO inhibitor use; the oral suspension should not be administered simultaneously with other liquid medicinal agents or diluents

**Warnings/Precautions** MAO inhibitors should be discontinued for a minimum of 14 days before carbamazepine is begun; administer with caution to patients with history of cardiac damage or hepatic disease; potentially fatal blood cell abnormalities have been reported following treatment; early detection of hematologic change is important; advise patients of early signs and symptoms including fever, sore throat, mouth ulcers, infections, easy bruising, petechial or purpuric hemorrhage; carbamazepine is not effective in absence, myoclonic or akinetic seizures; exacerbation of certain seizure types have been seen after initiation of carbamazepine therapy in children with mixed seizure disorders. Elderly may have increased risk of SIADH-like syndrome.

**Pregnancy Risk Factor** D

**Pregnancy Implications** Enters breast milk/compatible

Clinical effects on the fetus: Crosses the placenta. Dysmorphic facial features, cranial defects, cardiac defects, spina bifida, IUGR, and multiple other malformations reported. Epilepsy itself, number of medications, genetic factors, or a combination of these probably influence the teratogenicity of anticonvulsant therapy. Benefit:risk ratio usually favors continued use during pregnancy and breast-feeding.

**Adverse Reactions**

Dermatologic: Rash; but does not necessarily mean the drug should not be stopped

&gt;10%:

Central nervous system: Sedation, dizziness, fatigue, ataxia, confusion

Gastrointestinal: Nausea, vomiting

Ocular: Blurred vision, nystagmus

1% to 10%:

Dermatologic: Stevens-Johnson syndrome, toxic epidermal necrolysis

Endocrine & metabolic: Hyponatremia, SIADH

Gastrointestinal: Diarrhea

Miscellaneous: Diaphoresis

&lt;1%: Edema, congestive heart failure, syncope, bradycardia, hypertension or hypotension, A-V block, arrhythmias, slurred speech, mental depression, hypocalcemia, hyponatremia, urinary retention, sexual problems in males, neutropenia (can be transient), aplastic anemia, agranulocytosis, eosinophilia, leukopenia, pancytopenia, thrombocytopenia, bone marrow suppression, hepatitis, peripheral neuritis, diplopia, swollen glands, hypersensitivity

**Drug Interactions** CYP2C8 and CYP3A3/4 enzyme substrate; CYP1A2, 2C, 2C9, 2C18, 2C19, 2D6, and 3A3/4 inducer

Decreased effect: Carbamazepine may induce the metabolism of warfarin, cyclosporine, doxycycline, oral contraceptives, phenytoin, theophylline, benzodiazepines, ethosuximide, valproic acid, corticosteroids, and thyroid hormones

Increased toxicity: Erythromycin, isoniazid, propoxyphene, verapamil, danazol, diltiazem, and cimetidine may inhibit hepatic metabolism of carbamazepine with resultant increase of carbamazepine serum concentrations and toxicity

Carbamazepine suspension is **incompatible** with chlorpromazine solution and thioridazine liquid; a number of patients have found rubbery orange mass to indicate a decreased bioavailability. Schedule carbamazepine suspension at least 1-2 hours apart from other liquid medicinals.

**Onset** Requires several days to reach steady-state concentrations; absorption is erratic and slow

**Half-Life** Initial: 18-55 hours; Multiple dosing: 12-17 hours

**Special PA Issues**

**Patient Education:** Take exactly as directed (do not increase dose or frequency or discontinue without consulting prescriber). While using this medication, do not use (Continued)

## Carbamazepine *(Continued)*

alcohol and other prescription or OTC medications (especially pain medications, sedatives, antihistamines, or hypnotics) without consulting prescriber. Maintain adequate
hydration (2-3 L/day of fluids unless instructed to restrict fluid intake). You may experience drowsiness, dizziness, or blurred vision (use caution when driving or engaging in
hazardous tasks); nausea, vomiting, loss of appetite, or dry mouth (small frequent meals,
good mouth care, chewing gum, or sucking on lozenges may help). Wear identification of
epileptic status and medications. Report CNS changes, mentation changes, or changes
in cognition; muscle cramping, weakness, tremors, changes in gait; persistent GI symptoms (cramping, constipation, vomiting, anorexia); rash or skin irritations; unusual
bruising or bleeding (mouth, urine, stool); worsening of seizure activity, or loss of seizure
control.

**Dietary Considerations:**
Food: Drug may cause GI upset, take with large amount of water or food to decrease GI
upset. May need to split doses to avoid GI upset.
Sodium: SIADH and water intoxication; monitor fluid status; may need to restrict fluid

**Reference Range:**
Timing of serum samples: Absorption is slow, peak levels occur 6-8 hours after ingestion
of the first dose; the half-life ranges from 8-60 hours, therefore, steady-state is
achieved in 2-5 days
Therapeutic levels: 6-12 µg/mL (SI: 25-51 µmol/L)
Toxic concentration: >15 µg/mL; patients who require higher levels of 8-12 µg/mL (SI: 34-
51 µmol/L) should be watched closely. Side effects including CNS effects occur
commonly at higher dosage levels. If other anticonvulsants are given therapeutic range
is 4-8 µg/mL.

♦ **Carbamide** *see Urea on page 947*

## Carbamide Peroxide (KAR ba mide per OKS ide)

**Pharmacologic Class** Otic Agent, Cerumenolytic
**U.S. Brand Names** Auro® Ear Drops [OTC]; Debrox® Otic [OTC]; E•R•O Ear [OTC]; Gly-
Oxide® Oral [OTC]; Mollifene® Ear Wax Removing Formula [OTC]; Murine® Ear Drops
[OTC]; Orajel® Perioseptic® [OTC]; Proxigel® Oral [OTC]
**Mechanism of Action** Carbamide peroxide releases hydrogen peroxide which serves as a
source of nascent oxygen upon contact with catalase; deodorant action is probably due to
inhibition of odor-causing bacteria; softens impacted cerumen due to its foaming action
**Use** Relief of minor inflammation of gums, oral mucosal surfaces and lips including canker
sores and dental irritation; emulsify and disperse ear wax
**USUAL DOSAGE** Children and Adults:
Gel: Gently massage on affected area 4 times/day; do not drink or rinse mouth for 5 minutes
after use
Oral solution (should not be used for >7 days): Oral preparation should not be used in
children <3 years of age; apply several drops undiluted on affected area 4 times/day after
meals and at bedtime; expectorate after 2-3 minutes or place 10 drops onto tongue, mix
with saliva, swish for several minutes, expectorate
Otic:
Children <12 years: Tilt head sideways and individualize the dose according to patient
size; 3 drops (range: 1-5 drops) twice daily for up to 4 days, tip of applicator should not
enter ear canal; keep drops in ear for several minutes by keeping head tilted and
placing cotton in ear
Children ≥12 years and Adults: Tilt head sideways and instill 5-10 drops twice daily up to
4 days, tip of applicator should not enter ear canal; keep drops in ear for several
minutes by keeping head tilted and placing cotton in ear
**Dosage Forms Gel, oral (Proxigel®):** 10% (34 g); **Soln: Oral:** Gly-Oxide®: 10% in glycerin
(15 mL, 60 mL), Orajel® Perioseptic®: 15% in glycerin (13.3 mL); **Otic (Auro® Ear Drops,
Debrox®, Mollifene® Ear Wax Removing, Murine® Ear Drops):** 6.5% in glycerin (15 mL,
30 mL)
**Contraindications** Otic preparation should not be used in patients with a perforated
tympanic membrane; ear drainage, ear pain or rash in the ear; do not use in the eye; do not
use otic preparation longer than 4 days; oral preparation should not be used in children <3
years
**Warnings/Precautions**
Oral: With prolonged use of oral carbamide peroxide, there is a potential for overgrowth of
opportunistic organisms; damage to periodontal tissues; delayed wound healing; should
not be used for longer than 7 days
Otic: Do not use if ear drainage or discharge, ear pain, irritation, or rash in ear; should not
be used for longer than 4 days
**Pregnancy Risk Factor** C
**Adverse Reactions** 1% to 10%:
Dermatologic: Rash
Local: Irritation, redness
Miscellaneous: Superinfections

**Special PA Issues**
**Patient Education:** Contact physician if dizziness or otic redness, rash, irritation, tenderness, pain, drainage, or discharge develop; do not drink or rinse mouth for 5 minutes after oral use of gel

♦ **Carbamylcholine Chloride** *see Carbachol on page 148*
♦ **Carbastat® Ophthalmic** *see Carbachol on page 148*
♦ **Carbatrol®** *see Carbamazepine on page 148*

# Carbenicillin (kar ben i SIL in)
**Pharmacologic Class** Antibiotic, Penicillin
**U.S. Brand Names** Geocillin®
**Mechanism of Action** Inhibits bacterial cell wall synthesis by binding to one or more of the penicillin binding proteins (PBPs); which in turn inhibits the final transpeptidation step of peptidoglycan synthesis in bacterial cell walls, thus inhibiting cell wall biosynthesis. Bacteria eventually lyse due to ongoing activity of cell wall autolytic enzymes (autolysins and murein hydrolases) while cell wall assembly is arrested.
**Use** Treatment of serious urinary tract infections and prostatitis caused by susceptible gram-negative aerobic bacilli
**USUAL DOSAGE** Oral:
Children: 30-50 mg/kg/day divided every 6 hours; maximum dose: 2-3 g/day
Adults: 1-2 tablets every 6 hours for urinary tract infections or 2 tablets every 6 hours for prostatitis
**Dosing interval in renal impairment:** Adults:
$Cl_{cr}$ 10-50 mL/minute: Administer 382-764 mg every 12-24 hours
$Cl_{cr}$ <10 mL/minute: Administer 382-764 mg every 24-48 hours
Moderately dialyzable (20% to 50%)
**Dosage Forms** Tab, film coated, as indanyl sodium ester: 382 mg [base]
**Contraindications** Hypersensitivity to carbenicillin or any component or penicillins
**Warnings/Precautions** Do not use in patients with severe renal impairment ($Cl_{cr}$ <10 mL/minute); dosage modification required in patients with impaired renal and/or hepatic function; oral carbenicillin should be limited to treatment of urinary tract infections. Use with caution in patients with history of hypersensitivity to cephalosporins.
**Pregnancy Risk Factor** B
**Adverse Reactions**
>10%: Gastrointestinal: Diarrhea
1% to 10%: Gastrointestinal: Nausea, bad taste, vomiting, flatulence, glossitis
<1%: Headache, skin rash, urticaria, anemia, thrombocytopenia, leukopenia, neutropenia, eosinophilia, hyperthermia, itchy eyes, vaginitis, hypokalemia, hematuria, thrombophlebitis
**Drug Interactions**
Decreased effect with administration of aminoglycosides within 1 hour; may inactivate both drugs
Increased duration of half-life with probenecid
**Half-Life** 1-1.5 hours, prolonged to 10-20 hours with renal insufficiency
**Special PA Issues**
**Patient Education:** Take as prescribed, at equal intervals around-the-clock, with a full glass of water, and preferably on an empty stomach (1 hour before or 2 hours after meals). Do not skip doses and take full course of treatment even if feeling better. Frequent mouth care will help relieve dry mouth and bitter aftertaste. Report swelling, respiratory difficulty, easy bruising or bleeding, or signs of opportunistic infection (eg, sore throat, fever, chills, fatigue, thrush, vaginal discharge, diarrhea). If diabetic, drug may cause false tests with Clinitest® urine glucose monitoring; use of glucose oxidase methods (Clinistix®) or serum glucose monitoring is preferable.
**Monitoring Parameters:** Renal, hepatic, and hematologic function tests
**Reference Range:** Therapeutic: Not established; Toxic: >250 µg/mL (SI: >660 µmol/L)

# Carbidopa (kar bi DOE pa)
**Pharmacologic Class** Anti-Parkinson's Agent (Dopamine Agonist)
**U.S. Brand Names** Lodosyn®
**Mechanism of Action** Carbidopa is a peripheral decarboxylase inhibitor with little or no pharmacological activity when given alone in usual doses. It inhibits the peripheral decarboxylation of levodopa to dopamine; and as it does not cross the blood-brain barrier, unlike levodopa, effective brain concentrations of dopamine are produced with lower doses of levodopa. At the same time, reduced peripheral formation of dopamine reduces peripheral side-effects, notably nausea and vomiting, and cardiac arrhythmias, although the dyskinesias and adverse mental effects associated with levodopa therapy tend to develop earlier.
**Use** Given with levodopa in the treatment of parkinsonism to enable a lower dosage of levodopa to be used and a more rapid response to be obtained and to decrease side-effects; for details of administration and dosage, see Levodopa; has no effect without levodopa
**USUAL DOSAGE** Adults: Oral: 70-100 mg/day; maximum daily dose: 200 mg
(Continued)

## Carbidopa *(Continued)*

**Dosage Forms Tab:** 25 mg

**Contraindications** Hypersensitivity to carbidopa or levodopa

**Pregnancy Risk Factor** C

**Adverse Reactions** Adverse reactions are associated with concomitant administration with levodopa

>10%: Central nervous system: Anxiety, confusion, nervousness, mental depression

1% to 10%:

Cardiovascular: Orthostatic hypotension, palpitations, cardiac arrhythmias

Central nervous system: Memory loss, nervousness, insomnia, fatigue, hallucinations, ataxia, dystonic movements

Gastrointestinal: Nausea, vomiting, GI bleeding

Ocular: Blurred vision

<1%: Hypertension, duodenal ulcer, hemolytic anemia

**Drug Interactions** Increased toxicity: Tricyclic antidepressant → hypertensive reactions and dyskinesia

**Special PA Issues**

**Patient Education:** Can take with food to prevent GI upset, do not stop taking this drug even if you do not think it is working; dizziness, lightheadedness, fainting may occur when getting up from a sitting or lying position

♦ **Carbidopa and Levodopa** *see* Levodopa and Carbidopa *on page 525*

## Carbinoxamine and Pseudoephedrine

(kar bi NOKS a meen & soo doe e FED rin)

**Pharmacologic Class** Adrenergic Agonist Agent; Antihistamine, $H_1$ Blocker; Decongestant

**U.S. Brand Names** Biohist-LA®; Carbiset® Tablet; Carbiset-TR® Tablet; Carbodec® Syrup; Carbodec® Tablet; Carbodec® TR Tablet; Cardec-S® Syrup; Rondec® Drops; Rondec® Filmtab®; Rondec® Syrup; Rondec-TR®

**Mechanism of Action** Carbinoxamine competes with histamine for $H_1$-receptor sites on effector cells in the gastrointestinal tract, blood vessels, and respiratory tract

**Use** Temporary relief of nasal congestion, running nose, sneezing, itching of nose or throat, and itchy, watery eyes due to the common cold, hay fever, or other respiratory allergies

**USUAL DOSAGE** Oral:

Children:

Drops: 1-18 months: 0.25-1 mL 4 times/day

Syrup:

18 months to 6 years: 2.5 mL 3-4 times/day

>6 years: 5 mL 2-4 times/day

Adults:

Liquid: 5 mL 4 times/day

Tablets: 1 tablet 4 times/day

**Dosage Forms Drops:** Carbinoxamine maleate 2 mg and pseudoephedrine hydrochloride 25 mg per mL (30 mL with dropper); **Syr:** Carbinoxamine maleate 4 mg and pseudoephedrine hydrochloride 60 mg per 5 mL (120 mL, 480 mL); **Tab: Film-coated:** Carbinoxamine maleate 4 mg and pseudoephedrine hydrochloride 60 mg; **Sustained release:** Carbinoxamine maleate 8 mg and pseudoephedrine hydrochloride 120 mg

**Contraindications** Hypersensitivity to carbinoxamine or pseudoephedrine or any component; severe hypertension or coronary artery disease, MAO inhibitor therapy, GI or GU obstruction, narrow-angle glaucoma; avoid use in premature or term infants due to a possible association with SIDS

**Warnings/Precautions** Narrow-angle glaucoma, bladder neck obstruction, symptomatic prostatic hypertrophy, asthmatic attack, and stenosing peptic ulcer

**Pregnancy Risk Factor** C

**Pregnancy Implications** Excretion in breast milk unknown/contraindicated

**Adverse Reactions**

>10%:

Central nervous system: Slight to moderate drowsiness

Respiratory: Thickening of bronchial secretions

1% to 10%:

Central nervous system: Headache, fatigue, nervousness, dizziness

Gastrointestinal: Appetite increase, weight gain, nausea, diarrhea, abdominal pain, xerostomia

Neuromuscular & skeletal: Arthralgia

Respiratory: Pharyngitis

<1%: Edema, palpitations, depression, angioedema, photosensitivity, rash, hepatitis, myalgia, paresthesia, bronchospasm, epistaxis

**Drug Interactions** Increased toxicity: Barbiturates, TCAs, MAO inhibitors, ethanolamine antihistamines

### Special PA Issues
**Patient Education:** Take as directed; do not exceed recommended dose. Maintain adequate hydration (2-3 L/day of fluids unless instructed to restrict fluid intake). Avoid use of other depressants, alcohol, or sleep-inducing medications unless approved by prescriber. You may experience drowsiness, impaired coordination, blurred vision, or increased anxiety (use caution when driving or engaging in hazardous tasks until response to therapy is known); or dry mouth or nausea (frequent small meals, frequent mouth care, chewing gum, or sucking hard candy may help). Report persistent dizziness, sedation, or agitation; difficulty breathing or increased cough; changes in urinary pattern; muscle weakness; or lack of improvement or worsening or condition.

# Carbinoxamine, Pseudoephedrine, and Dextromethorphan
(kar bi NOKS a meen, soo doe e FED rin, & deks troe meth OR fan)

**Pharmacologic Class** Antihistamine/Decongestant/Antitussive

**U.S. Brand Names** Carbodec DM®; Cardec DM®; Pseudo-Car® DM; Rondamine-DM® Drops; Rondec®-DM; Tussafed® Drops

**Dosage Forms Drops:** Carbinoxamine maleate 2 mg, pseudoephedrine hydrochloride 25 mg, and dextromethorphan hydrobromide 4 mg per mL (30 mL); **Syr:** Carbinoxamine maleate 4 mg, pseudoephedrine hydrochloride 60 mg, and dextromethorphan hydrobromide 15 mg per 5 mL (120 mL, 480 mL, 4000 mL)

♦ **Carbiset® Tablet** see Carbinoxamine and Pseudoephedrine on previous page

♦ **Carbiset-TR® Tablet** see Carbinoxamine and Pseudoephedrine on previous page

♦ **Carbocaine®** see Mepivacaine on page 569

♦ **Carbodec DM®** see Carbinoxamine, Pseudoephedrine, and Dextromethorphan on this page

♦ **Carbodec® Syrup** see Carbinoxamine and Pseudoephedrine on previous page

♦ **Carbodec® Tablet** see Carbinoxamine and Pseudoephedrine on previous page

♦ **Carbodec® TR Tablet** see Carbinoxamine and Pseudoephedrine on previous page

# Carboprost Tromethamine (KAR boe prost tro METH a meen)

**Pharmacologic Class** Abortifacient; Prostaglandin

**U.S. Brand Names** Hemabate™

**Mechanism of Action** Carboprost tromethamine is a prostaglandin similar to prostaglandin $F_2$ alpha (dinoprost) except for the addition of a methyl group at the C-15 position. This substitution produces longer duration of activity than dinoprost; carboprost stimulates uterine contractility which usually results in expulsion of the products of conception and is used to induce abortion between 13-20 weeks of pregnancy. Hemostasis at the placentation site is achieved through the myometrial contractions produced by carboprost.

**Use** Termination of pregnancy and refractory postpartum uterine bleeding
**Investigational:** Hemorrhagic cystitis

**USUAL DOSAGE** Adults: I.M.:
Abortion: Initial: 250 mcg, then 250 mcg at $1^1/_2$-hour to $3^1/_2$-hour intervals depending on uterine response; a 500 mcg dose may be given if uterine response is not adequate after several 250 mcg doses; do not exceed 12 mg total dose or continuous administration for >2 days

Refractory postpartum uterine bleeding: Initial: 250 mcg; may repeat at 15- to 90-minute intervals to a total dose of 2 mg

Bladder irrigation for hemorrhagic cystitis (refer to individual protocols): [0.4-1.0 mg/dL as solution] 50 mL instilled into bladder 4 times/day for 1 hour

**Dosage Forms Inj:** Carboprost 250 mcg and tromethamine 83 mcg per mL (1 mL)

**Contraindications** Hypersensitivity to carboprost tromethamine or any component; acute pelvic inflammatory disease; pregnancy

**Warnings/Precautions** Use with caution in patients with history of asthma, hypotension or hypertension, cardiovascular, adrenal, renal or hepatic disease, anemia, jaundice, diabetes, epilepsy or compromised uteri

**Pregnancy Risk Factor** X

**Adverse Reactions**
>10%: Gastrointestinal: Nausea (33%)
1% to 10%: Cardiovascular: Flushing (7%)
<1%: Hypertension, hypotension, drowsiness, vertigo, nervousness, fever, headache, dystonia, vasovagal syndrome, breast tenderness, xerostomia, vomiting, diarrhea, hematemesis, abnormal taste, bladder spasms, myalgia, blurred vision, coughing, asthma, respiratory distress, septic shock, hiccups

**Drug Interactions** Increased toxicity: Oxytocic agents

**Special PA Issues**
**Patient Education:** This medication is used to stimulate expulsion of uterine contents (fetal tissue) or stimulate uterine contractions to reduce uterine bleeding. Report increased blood loss, acute abdominal cramping, persistent elevation of temperature, foul-smelling vaginal discharge. Increased temperature (elevated temperature) may occur 1-16 hours after therapy and last for several hours.

- **Carboptic® Ophthalmic** *see* Carbachol *on page 148*
- **Cardec DM®** *see* Carbinoxamine, Pseudoephedrine, and Dextromethorphan *on previous page*
- **Cardec-S® Syrup** *see* Carbinoxamine and Pseudoephedrine *on page 152*
- **Cardene®** *see* Nicardipine *on page 651*
- **Cardene® I.V.** *see* Nicardipine *on page 651*
- **Cardene® SR** *see* Nicardipine *on page 651*
- **Cardioquin®** *see* Quinidine *on page 789*
- **Cardizem® CD** *see* Diltiazem *on page 286*
- **Cardizem® Injectable** *see* Diltiazem *on page 286*
- **Cardizem® SR** *see* Diltiazem *on page 286*
- **Cardizem® Tablet** *see* Diltiazem *on page 286*
- **Cardura®** *see* Doxazosin *on page 304*
- **Carindacillin** *see* Carbenicillin *on page 151*
- **Carisoprodate** *see* Carisoprodol *on this page*

# Carisoprodol (kar i soe PROE dole)

**Pharmacologic Class** Skeletal Muscle Relaxant
**U.S. Brand Names** Rela®; Sodol®; Soma®; Soprodol®; Soridol®
**Mechanism of Action** Precise mechanism is not yet clear, but many effects have been ascribed to its central depressant actions
**Use** Skeletal muscle relaxant
**USUAL DOSAGE** Adults: Oral: 350 mg 3-4 times/day; take last dose at bedtime; compound: 1-2 tablets 4 times/day
**Dosage Forms Tab:** 350 mg
**Contraindications** Acute intermittent porphyria, hypersensitivity to carisoprodol, meprobamate or any component
**Warnings/Precautions** Use with caution in renal and hepatic dysfunction
**Pregnancy Risk Factor** C
**Adverse Reactions**
>10%: Central nervous system: Drowsiness
1% to 10%:
  Cardiovascular: Tachycardia, tightness in chest, flushing of face, syncope
  Central nervous system: Mental depression, allergic fever, dizziness, lightheadedness, headache, paradoxical CNS stimulation
  Dermatologic: Angioedema
  Gastrointestinal: Nausea, vomiting, stomach cramps
  Neuromuscular & skeletal: Trembling
  Ocular: Burning eyes
  Respiratory: Shortness of breath
  Miscellaneous: Hiccups
<1%: Ataxia, rash, urticaria, erythema multiforme, aplastic anemia, leukopenia, eosinophilia, blurred vision
**Drug Interactions** CYP2C19 enzyme substrate
  Increased toxicity: Alcohol, CNS depressants, phenothiazines
**Onset** Within 30 minutes
**Duration** 4-6 hours
**Half-Life** 8 hours
**Special PA Issues**
  **Patient Education:** Take exactly as directed with food. Do not increase dose or discontinue without consulting prescriber. Do not use alcohol, prescriptive or OTC antidepressants, sedatives, and pain medications without consulting prescriber. You may experience drowsiness, dizziness, lightheadedness (avoid driving or engaging in tasks that require alertness until response to therapy is known); nausea, vomiting, or cramping (small, frequent meals, frequent mouth care, or sucking hard candy may help); or postural hypotension (change position slowly when rising from sitting or lying or when climbing stairs). Report excessive drowsiness or mental agitation; palpitations, rapid heartbeat, or chest pain; skin rash; muscle cramping or tremors; or respiratory difficulty.
  **Dietary Considerations:** Alcohol: Additive CNS effects, avoid use
  **Monitoring Parameters:** Look for relief of pain and/or muscle spasm and avoid excessive drowsiness

# Carisoprodol and Aspirin (kar i soe PROE dole & AS pir in)

**Pharmacologic Class** Skeletal Muscle Relaxant
**U.S. Brand Names** Soma® Compound
**Dosage Forms Tab:** Carisoprodol 200 mg and aspirin 325 mg

# Carisoprodol, Aspirin, and Codeine

(kar i soe PROE dole, AS pir in, and KOE deen)
**Pharmacologic Class** Skeletal Muscle Relaxant
**U.S. Brand Names** Soma® Compound w/Codeine

**Dosage Forms Tab:** Carisoprodol 200 mg, aspirin 325 mg, and codeine phosphate 16 mg

♦ **Carmol-HC® Topical** see Urea and Hydrocortisone on page 948
♦ **Carmol® Topical [OTC]** see Urea on page 947

# Carteolol (KAR tee oh lole)

**Pharmacologic Class** Beta Blocker (with Intrinsic Sympathomimetic Activity); Ophthalmic Agent, Antiglaucoma

**U.S. Brand Names** Cartrol® Oral; Ocupress® Ophthalmic

**Mechanism of Action** Blocks both $beta_1$- and $beta_2$-receptors and has mild intrinsic sympathomimetic activity; has negative inotropic and chronotropic effects and can significantly slow A-V nodal conduction

**Use** Management of hypertension; treatment of chronic open-angle glaucoma and intraocular hypertension

**USUAL DOSAGE** Adults:

Oral: 2.5 mg as a single daily dose, with a maintenance dose normally 2.5-5 mg once daily; doses >10 mg do not increase response and may in fact decrease effect

Ophthalmic: Instill 1 drop in affected eye(s) twice daily

**Dosing interval in renal impairment:**

$Cl_{cr}$ >60 mL/minute/1.73 $m^2$: Administer every 24 hours

$Cl_{cr}$ 20-60 mL/minute/1.73 $m^2$: Administer every 48 hours

$Cl_{cr}$ <20 mL/minute/1.73 $m^2$: Administer every 72 hours

**Dosage Forms Soln, ophth (Ocupress®):** 1% (5 mL, 10 mL); **Tab (Cartrol®):** 2.5 mg, 5 mg

**Contraindications** Bronchial asthma, sinus bradycardia, second and third degree A-V block, cardiac failure (unless a functioning pacemaker present), cardiogenic shock, hypersensitivity to betaxolol or any component

**Warnings/Precautions** Some products contain sulfites which can cause allergic reactions; diminished response over time; may increase muscle weaknesses; use with a miotic in angle-closure glaucoma; use with caution in patients with decreased renal or hepatic function (dosage adjustment required) or patients with a history of asthma, congestive heart failure, or bradycardia; severe CNS, cardiovascular, and respiratory adverse effects have been seen following ophthalmic use

**Pregnancy Risk Factor** C

**Pregnancy Implications** Excretion in breast milk unknown/use caution

**Adverse Reactions**

1% to 10%:

Cardiovascular: Congestive heart failure, arrhythmia

Central nervous system: Mental depression, headache, dizziness

Neuromuscular & skeletal: Back pain, arthralgia

<1%: Bradycardia, chest pain, mesenteric arterial thrombosis, A-V block, persistent bradycardia, hypotension, edema, Raynaud's phenomenon, fatigue, insomnia, lethargy, nightmares, confusion, purpura, hyperglycemia, ischemic colitis, constipation, nausea, diarrhea, impotence, thrombocytopenia, bronchospasm, cold extremities

**Drug Interactions**

Decreased effect of beta-blockers with aluminum salts, barbiturates, calcium salts, cholestyramine, colestipol, NSAIDs, penicillins (ampicillin), rifampin, salicylates, and sulfinpyrazone due to decreased bioavailability and plasma levels

Beta-blockers may decrease the effect of sulfonylureas

Increased effect/toxicity of beta-blockers with calcium blockers (diltiazem, felodipine, nicardipine), contraceptives, flecainide, haloperidol (propranolol, hypotensive effects), $H_2$-antagonists (metoprolol, propranolol only by cimetidine, possibly ranitidine), hydralazine (metoprolol, propranolol), loop diuretics (propranolol, not atenolol), MAO inhibitors (metoprolol, nadolol, bradycardia), phenothiazines (propranolol), propafenone (metoprolol, propranolol), quinidine (in extensive metabolizers), ciprofloxacin, thyroid hormones (metoprolol, propranolol, when hypothyroid patient is converted to euthyroid state)

Beta-blockers may increase the effect/toxicity of flecainide, haloperidol (hypotensive effects), hydralazine, phenothiazines, acetaminophen, anticoagulants (propranolol, warfarin), benzodiazepines (not atenolol), clonidine (hypertensive crisis after or during withdrawal of either agent), epinephrine (initial hypertensive episode followed by bradycardia), nifedipine and verapamil lidocaine, ergots (peripheral ischemia), prazosin (postural hypotension)

Beta-blockers may affect the action or levels of ethanol, disopyramide, nondepolarizing muscle relaxants and theophylline although the effects are difficult to predict

**Onset** Onset of effect: Oral: 1-1.5 hours; Peak effect: 2 hours

**Duration** 12 hours

**Half-Life** 6 hours

**Special PA Issues**

**Patient Education:**

Oral: Take exactly as directed. Do not increase, decrease, or adjust dosage without consulting prescriber. Take pulse daily, prior to medication; follow prescriber's instruction about holding medication. Do not take with antacids and avoid alcohol or OTC medications (eg, cold remedies) without consulting prescriber. If diabetic, monitor

(Continued)

## Carteolol *(Continued)*

serum blood glucose closely (may alter glucose tolerance or mask signs of hypogly-cemia). May cause fatigue, dizziness, or postural hypotension; use caution when changing position from lying or sitting to standing, when driving, or climbing stairs until response to medication is known. May cause alteration in sexual performance (revers-ible). Report unresolved swelling of extremities, difficulty breathing or new cough, unresolved fatigue, unusual weight gain, unresolved constipation, or unusual muscle weakness.

Ophthalmic: Wash hands before instilling. Sit or lie down to instill. Open eye, look at ceiling, and instill prescribed amount of medication. Close eye and apply gentle pres-sure to inner corner of eye. Do not let tip of applicator touch eye or contaminate tip of applicator. Temporary stinging or burning may occur. Report persistent pain, burning, vision disturbances, swelling, itching, or worsening of condition.

**Monitoring Parameters:** Ophthalmic: Intraocular pressure; Systemic: Blood pressure, pulse, CNS status

**Related Information**

Beta-Blockers *on page 1002*

♦ **Carteolol Hydrochloride** *see* Carteolol *on previous page*

♦ **Cartia XT®** *see* Diltiazem *on page 286*

♦ **Cartrol® Oral** *see* Carteolol *on previous page*

## Carvedilol *(KAR ve dil ole)*

**Pharmacologic Class** Alpha-/Beta- Blocker

**U.S. Brand Names** Coreg®

**Mechanism of Action** As a racemic mixture, carvedilol has nonselective beta-adrenore-ceptor and alpha-adrenergic blocking activity at equal potency. No intrinsic sympathomi-metic activity has been documented. Associated effects include reduction of cardiac output, exercise- or beta agonist-induced tachycardia, reduction of reflex orthostatic tachycardia, vasodilation, decreased peripheral vascular resistance (especially in standing position), decreased renal vascular resistance, reduced plasma renin activity, and increased levels of atrial natriuretic peptide.

**Use** Management of hypertension; can be used alone or in combination with other agents, especially thiazide-type diuretics; treatment of mild or moderate congestive heart failure of ischemia or cardiomyopathic origin in conjunction with digitalis, diuretics, and ACE inhibitors to reduce the progression of disease as evidenced by cardiovascular death, cardiovascular hospitalizations, or the need to adjust other heart failure medications

**Unlabeled use:** Appears to be effective in the treatment of angina and idiopathic cardiomy-opathy

**USUAL DOSAGE** Adults: Oral:

Hypertension: 6.25 mg twice daily; if tolerated, dose should be maintained for 1-2 weeks, then increased to 12.5 mg twice daily; dosage may be increased to a maximum of 25 mg twice daily after 1-2 weeks; reduce dosage if heart rate drops to <55 beats/minute

Congestive heart failure: 3.125 mg twice daily for 2 weeks; if this dose is tolerated, may increase to 6.25 mg twice daily. Double the dose every 2 weeks to the highest dose tolerated by patient. (Prior to initiating therapy, other heart failure medications should be stabilized.)

Maximum recommended dose:

<85 kg: 25 mg twice daily

>85 kg: 50 mg twice daily

Angina pectoris (unlabeled use): 25-50 mg twice daily

Idiopathic cardiomyopathy (unlabeled use): 6.25-25 mg twice daily

**Dosing adjustment in renal impairment:** None necessary

**Dosing adjustment in hepatic impairment:** Use is contraindicated in liver dysfunction

**Dosage Forms Tab:** 3.125 mg, 6.25 mg, 12.5 mg, 25 mg

**Contraindications** Uncompensated congestive heart failure (NYHA Class IV), asthma or bronchospastic disease (status asthmaticus may result), cardiogenic shock, severe brady-cardia or second or third degree heart block, and symptomatic hepatic disease; hypersensi-tivity to any component

**Warnings/Precautions** Use with caution in patients with congestive heart failure treated with digitalis, diuretic, or ACE inhibitor since A-V conduction may be slowed; discontinue therapy if any evidence of liver injury occurs; use caution in patients with peripheral vascular disease, those undergoing anesthesia, in hyperthyroidism and diabetes mellitus. If no other antihypertensive is tolerated, very small doses may be cautiously used in patients with bronchospastic disease. Abrupt withdrawal of the drug should be avoided, drug should be discontinued over 1-2 weeks; do not use in pregnant or nursing women; may potentiate hypoglycemia in a diabetic patient and mask signs and symptoms; safety and efficacy in children have not been established.

**Pregnancy Risk Factor** C

**Pregnancy Implications** Excretion in breast milk unknown/contraindicated

Clinical effects on the fetus: Use during pregnancy only if the potential benefit justifies the risk

**Adverse Reactions**
>1%:
Cardiovascular: Bradycardia, postural hypotension, edema
Central nervous system: Dizziness, somnolence, insomnia, fatigue
Gastrointestinal: Diarrhea, abdominal pain
Neuromuscular & skeletal: Back pain
Respiratory: Rhinitis, pharyngitis, dyspnea
<1%: A-V block, extrasystoles, hypertension, hypotension, palpitations, peripheral ischemia, syncope, ataxia, vertigo, depression, nervousness, malaise, pruritus, rash, decreased male libido, hypercholesterolemia, hyperglycemia, hyperuricemia, constipation, flatulence, xerostomia, impotence, anemia, leukopenia, hyperbilirubinemia, increased LFTs, paresthesia, myalgia, weakness, abnormal vision, tinnitus, asthma, cough, diaphoresis (increased)

**Drug Interactions** CYP2C, 2C9, and 2D6 enzyme substrate
Decreased effect: Rifampin may reduce the plasma concentration of carvedilol by up to 70%; decreased effect of other beta-blockers has also occurred with aluminum salts, barbiturates, calcium salts, cholestyramine, colestipol, NSAIDs, penicillins (ampicillin), salicylates, and sulfinpyrazone due to decreased bioavailability and plasma levels; beta-blockers may decrease the effect of sulfonylureas
Increased effect: Carvedilol may enhance the action of antidiabetic agents, calcium channel blockers, digoxin; clonidine and carvedilol may result in augmented blood pressure and heart rate lowering effects; cimetidine increases the effect and AUC of carvedilol. Other drugs likely to increase carvedilol's levels and effects include quinidine, fluoxetine, paroxetine, and propafenone since these drugs inhibit CYP2D6.
Increased effect/toxicity of other beta-blockers occurs with contraceptives, flecainide, epinephrine (initial hypertensive episode followed by bradycardia), lidocaine, ergots (peripheral ischemia), and prazosin (postural hypotension)

**Onset** Within 1-2 hours
**Half-Life** 7-10 hours
**Special PA Issues**
Patient Education: Take exactly as directed. Do not increase, decrease, or adjust dosage without consulting prescriber. Take pulse daily, prior to medication; follow prescriber's instruction about holding medication. Do not take with antacids and avoid alcohol or OTC medications (eg, cold remedies) without consulting prescriber. If diabetic, monitor serum glucose closely (may alter glucose tolerance or mask signs of hypoglycemia). May cause fatigue, dizziness, or postural hypotension; use caution when changing position from lying or sitting to standing, when driving, or climbing stairs until response to medication is known. May cause alteration in sexual performance (reversible). Report unresolved swelling of extremities, difficulty breathing or new cough, unresolved fatigue, unusual weight gain, unresolved constipation, or unusual muscle weakness.
Monitoring Parameters: Heart rate, blood pressure (base need for dosage increase on trough blood pressure measurements and for tolerance on standing systolic pressure 1 hour after dosing)
**Related Information**
Beta-Blockers *on page 1002*

## Cascara Sagrada (kas KAR a sah GRAH dah)

**Pharmacologic Class** Laxative, Stimulant
**Mechanism of Action** Direct chemical irritation of the intestinal mucosa resulting in an increased rate of colonic motility and change in fluid and electrolyte secretion
**Use** Temporary relief of constipation; sometimes used with milk of magnesia ("black and white" mixture)
**USUAL DOSAGE Note:** Cascara sagrada fluid extract is 5 times more potent than cascara sagrada aromatic fluid extract

Oral (aromatic fluid extract):
Infants: 1.25 mL/day (range: 0.5-1.5 mL) as needed
Children 2-11 years: 2.5 mL/day (range: 1-3 mL) as needed
Children ≥12 years and Adults: 5 mL/day (range: 2-6 mL) as needed at bedtime (1 tablet as needed at bedtime)
**Dosage Forms Aromatic fluid extract:** 120 mL, 473 mL; **Tab:** 325 mg
**Contraindications** Nausea, vomiting, abdominal pain, fecal impaction, intestinal obstruction, GI bleeding, appendicitis, congestive heart failure
**Warnings/Precautions** Excessive use can lead to electrolyte imbalance, fluid imbalance, vitamin deficiency, steatorrhea, osteomalacia, cathartic colon, and dependence; should be avoided during nursing because it may have a laxative effect on the infant
**Pregnancy Risk Factor** C
**Pregnancy Implications** Enters breast milk/use caution
**Adverse Reactions** 1% to 10%:
Central nervous system: Faintness
Endocrine & metabolic: Electrolyte and fluid imbalance
(Continued)

## Cascara Sagrada *(Continued)*

Gastrointestinal: Abdominal cramps, nausea, diarrhea
Genitourinary: Discoloration of urine (reddish pink or brown)
**Drug Interactions** Decreased effect of oral anticoagulants
**Onset** 6-10 hours
**Special PA Issues**
**Patient Education:** Take with water on an empty stomach for better absorption. Do not take within 1 hour of antacids, milk, or cimetidine. Evacuation will usually occur 6-12 hours after taking. Cascara should not be used regularly for more than 1 week. A regular toileting routine, adequate fluids, regular exercise, and a diet that includes roughage and bulk will help to prevent constipation. Urine and feces may become yellowish or reddish-brown in color.

- ♦ **Casodex®** *see Bicalutamide on page 115*
- ♦ *Cassia acutifolia see Senna on page 828*
- ♦ **Cataflam® Oral** *see Diclofenac on page 271*
- ♦ **Catapres® Oral** *see Clonidine on page 225*
- ♦ **Catapres-TTS® Transdermal** *see Clonidine on page 225*
- ♦ **Caverject® Injection** *see Alprostadil on page 45*
- ♦ **CCNU** *see Lomustine on page 539*
- ♦ **C-Crystals® [OTC]** *see Ascorbic Acid on page 79*
- ♦ **2-CdA** *see Cladribine on page 214*
- ♦ **Cebid® Timecelles® [OTC]** *see Ascorbic Acid on page 79*
- ♦ **Ceclor®** *see Cefaclor on this page*
- ♦ **Ceclor® CD** *see Cefaclor on this page*
- ♦ **Cecon® [OTC]** *see Ascorbic Acid on page 79*
- ♦ **Cedax®** *see Ceftibuten on page 173*
- ♦ **Cedocard®-SR** *see Isosorbide Dinitrate on page 498*
- ♦ **CeeNU®** *see Lomustine on page 539*

## Cefaclor *(SEF a klor)*

**Pharmacologic Class** Antibiotic, Cephalosporin (Second Generation)
**U.S. Brand Names** Ceclor®; Ceclor® CD
**Mechanism of Action** Inhibits bacterial cell wall synthesis by binding to one or more of the penicillin-binding proteins (PBPs) which in turn inhibits the final transpeptidation step of peptidoglycan synthesis in bacterial cell walls, thus inhibiting cell wall biosynthesis. Bacteria eventually lyse due to ongoing activity of cell wall autolytic enzymes (autolysins and murein hydrolases) while cell wall assembly is arrested.
**Use** Infections caused by susceptible organisms including *Staphylococcus aureus* and *H influenzae*; treatment of otitis media, sinusitis, and infections involving the respiratory tract, skin and skin structure, bone and joint, and urinary tract
**USUAL DOSAGE** Oral:
Children >1 month: 20-40 mg/kg/day divided every 8-12 hours; maximum dose: 2 g/day (total daily dose may be divided into two doses for treatment of otitis media or pharyngitis)
Adults: 250-500 mg every 8 hours
Extended release tablets: 500 mg every 12 hours for 7 days for acute bacterial exacerbations of or secondary infections with chronic bronchitis or 375 mg every 12 hour for 10 days for pharyngitis or tonsillitis or for uncomplicated skin and skin structure infections
**Dosing adjustment in renal impairment:** $Cl_{cr}$ <50 mL/minute: Administer 50% of dose
Hemodialysis: Moderately dialyzable (20% to 50%)
**Dosage Forms** Cap: 250 mg, 500 mg; **Powder for oral susp (strawberry flavor):** 125 mg/5 mL (75 mL, 150 mL), 187 mg/5 mL (50 mL, 100 mL), 250 mg/5 mL (75 mL, 150 mL), 375 mg/5 mL (50 mL, 100 mL); **Tab, extended release:** 375 mg, 500 mg
**Contraindications** Hypersensitivity to cefaclor, any component, or cephalosporins
**Warnings/Precautions** Modify dosage in patients with severe renal impairment; prolonged use may result in superinfection; a low incidence of cross-hypersensitivity to penicillins exists
**Pregnancy Risk Factor** B
**Adverse Reactions**
1% to 10%:
Gastrointestinal: Diarrhea (1.5%)
Hematologic: Eosinophilia (2%)
Hepatic: Elevated transaminases (2.5%)
Dermatologic: Rash (maculopapular, erythematous, or morbilliform) (1% to 1.5%)
<1%: Anaphylaxis, urticaria, pruritus, angioedema, serum-sickness, arthralgia, hepatitis, cholestatic jaundice, Stevens-Johnson syndrome, nausea, vomiting, pseudomembranous colitis, vaginitis, hemolytic anemia, neutropenia, interstitial nephritis, CNS irritability, hyperactivity, agitation, nervousness, insomnia, confusion, dizziness, hallucinations, somnolence, seizures, prolonged PT

Reactions reported with other cephalosporins include fever, abdominal pain, superinfection, renal dysfunction, toxic nephropathy, hemorrhage, cholestasis

**Drug Interactions**
Increased effect: Probenecid may decrease cephalosporin elimination
Increased toxicity: Furosemide, aminoglycosides may be a possible additive to nephrotoxicity

**Half-Life** 0.5-1 hour, prolonged with renal impairment

**Special PA Issues**
**Patient Education:** Take as directed, at regular intervals around-the-clock (with or without food). Chilling oral suspension improves flavor (do not freeze). Do not chew or crush extended release tablets. Complete full course of medication, even if you feel better. Drink 2-3 L fluid/day. Small frequent meals, frequent mouth care, or sucking on lozenges may reduce nausea or vomiting. If diarrhea occurs, yogurt or buttermilk may help. May cause false-positive test with Clinitest®; use another form of testing. May interfere with oral contraceptives; additional contraceptive measures are necessary. Report severe, unresolved diarrhea; vaginal itching or drainage; sores in mouth; blood, pus, or mucus in stool or urine; easy bleeding or bruising; unusual fever or chills; rash; or respiratory difficulty.
**Monitoring Parameters:** Assess patient at beginning and throughout therapy for infection; monitor for signs of anaphylaxis during first dose

## Cefadroxil (sef a DROKS il)

**Pharmacologic Class** Antibiotic, Cephalosporin (First Generation)

**U.S. Brand Names** Duricef®; Ultracef®

**Mechanism of Action** Inhibits bacterial cell wall synthesis by binding to one or more of the penicillin-binding proteins (PBPs) which in turn inhibits the final transpeptidation step of peptidoglycan synthesis in bacterial cell walls, thus inhibiting cell wall biosynthesis. Bacteria eventually lyse due to ongoing activity of cell wall autolytic enzymes (autolysins and murein hydrolases) while cell wall assembly is arrested.

**Use** Treatment of susceptible gram-positive bacilli and cocci (not enterococcus); some gram-negative bacilli including *E. coli*, *Proteus*, and *Klebsiella* may be susceptible

**USUAL DOSAGE** Oral:
Children: 30 mg/kg/day divided twice daily up to a maximum of 2 g/day
Adults: 1-2 g/day in 2 divided doses
Prophylaxis against bacterial endocarditis: 2 g 1 hour prior to the procedure
**Dosing interval in renal impairment:**
Cl$_{cr}$ 10-25 mL/minute: Administer every 24 hours
Cl$_{cr}$ <10 mL/minute: Administer every 36 hours

**Dosage Forms Cap:** 500 mg; **Susp, oral:** 125 mg/5 mL, 250 mg/5 mL, 500 mg/5 mL (50 mL, 100 mL); **Tab:** 1 g

**Contraindications** Hypersensitivity to cefadroxil or other cephalosporins

**Warnings/Precautions** Modify dosage in patients with severe renal impairment; prolonged use may result in superinfection; use with caution in patients with a history of penicillin allergy especially IgE-mediated reactions (eg, anaphylaxis, urticaria); may cause antibiotic-associated colitis or colitis secondary to *C. difficile*

**Pregnancy Risk Factor** B

**Adverse Reactions**
1% to 10%: Gastrointestinal: Diarrhea
<1%: Anaphylaxis, rash (maculopapular and erythematous), erythema multiforme, Stevens-Johnson syndrome, serum sickness, arthralgia, urticaria, pruritus, angioedema, pseudomembranous colitis, abdominal pain, dyspepsia, nausea, vomiting, elevated transaminases, cholestasis, vaginitis, neutropenia, agranulocytosis, thrombocytopenia, fever

Reactions reported with other cephalosporins include toxic epidermal necrolysis, abdominal pain, superinfection. renal dysfunction, toxic nephropathy, aplastic anemia, hemolytic anemia, hemorrhage, prolonged prothrombin time, increased BUN, increased creatinine, eosinophilia, pancytopenia, seizures

**Drug Interactions**
Increased effect: Probenecid may decrease cephalosporin elimination
Increased toxicity: Furosemide, aminoglycosides may be a possible additive to nephrotoxicity

**Half-Life** 1-2 hours; 20-24 hours in renal failure

**Special PA Issues**
**Patient Education:** Take as directed, at regular intervals around-the-clock (with or without food). Chilling oral suspension improves flavor (do not freeze). Complete full course of medication, even if you feel better. Drink 2-3 L fluid/day. If diarrhea occurs, yogurt or buttermilk may help. May cause false-positive test with Clinitest®; use another form of testing. May interfere with oral contraceptives; additional contraceptive measures are necessary. Report severe, unresolved diarrhea; vaginal itching or drainage; sores in mouth; blood, pus, or mucus in stool or urine; easy bleeding or bruising; unusual fever or chills; rash; or respiratory difficulty.

(Continued)

## Cefadroxil *(Continued)*

**Monitoring Parameters:** Observe for signs and symptoms of anaphylaxis during first dose

♦ **Cefadroxil Monohydrate** *see Cefadroxil on previous page*
♦ **Cefadyl®** *see Cephapirin on page 180*

## Cefamandole (sef a MAN dole)

**Pharmacologic Class** Antibiotic, Cephalosporin (Second Generation)
**U.S. Brand Names** Mandol®
**Mechanism of Action** Inhibits bacterial cell wall synthesis by binding to one or more of the penicillin-binding proteins (PBPs) which in turn inhibits the final transpeptidation step of peptidoglycan synthesis in bacterial cell walls, thus inhibiting cell wall biosynthesis. Bacteria eventually lyse due to ongoing activity of cell wall autolytic enzymes (autolysins and murein hydrolases) while cell wall assembly is arrested.
**Use** Treatment of susceptible bacterial infection; mainly respiratory tract, skin and skin structure, bone and joint, urinary tract and gynecologic, septicemia; surgical prophylaxis. Active against methicillin-sensitive staphylococci, many streptococci, and various gram-negative bacilli including *E. coli*, some *Klebsiella*, *P. mirabilis*, *H. influenzae*, and *Moraxella*.
**USUAL DOSAGE** I.M., I.V.:
Children: 50-150 mg/kg/day in divided doses every 4-8 hours
Adults: Usual dose: 500-1000 mg every 4-8 hours; in life-threatening infections: 2 g every 4 hours may be needed
**Dosing interval in renal impairment:**
$Cl_{cr}$ 25-50 mL/minute: 1-2 g every 8 hours
$Cl_{cr}$ 10-25 mL/minute: 1 g every 8 hours
$Cl_{cr}$ <10 mL/minute: 1 g every 12 hours
Hemodialysis: Moderately dialyzable (20% to 50%)
**Dosage Forms** Powder for inj, as nafate: 500 mg (10 mL), 1 g (10 mL, 100 mL), 2 g (20 mL, 100 mL), 10 g (100 mL)
**Contraindications** Hypersensitivity to cefamandole nafate, any component, or cephalosporins
**Warnings/Precautions** Modify dosage in patients with severe renal impairment; prolonged use may result in superinfection; although rare, cefamandole may interfere with hemostasis via destruction of vitamin K producing intestinal bacteria, prevention of activation of prothrombin by the attachment of a methyltetrazolethiol side chain, and by an immune-mediated thrombocytopenia. Use with caution in patients with a history of penicillin allergy especially IgE-mediated reactions (eg, anaphylaxis, urticaria); may cause antibiotic-associated colitis or colitis secondary to *C. difficile*.
**Pregnancy Risk Factor** B
**Adverse Reactions** Contains MTT side chain which may lead to increased risk of hypoprothrombinemia and bleeding.

1% to 10%:
Gastrointestinal: Diarrhea
Local: Thrombophlebitis
<1%: Anaphylaxis, rash (maculopapular and erythematous), urticaria, pseudomembranous colitis, nausea, vomiting, elevated transaminases, cholestasis, eosinophilia, neutropenia, thrombocytopenia, increased BUN, increased creatinine, fever, prolonged PT

Reactions reported with other cephalosporins include toxic epidermal necrolysis, Stevens-Johnson syndrome, abdominal pain, superinfection, renal dysfunction, toxic nephropathy, aplastic anemia, hemolytic anemia, hemorrhage, pancytopenia, vaginitis, seizures
**Drug Interactions**
Disulfiram-like reaction has been reported when taken within 72 hours of alcohol consumption
Increased cefamandole plasma levels: Probenecid
Increased nephrotoxicity: Aminoglycosides, furosemide
Hypoprothrombinemic effect increased: Warfarin and heparin
**Half-Life** 30-60 minutes; prolonged in renal impairment
**Special PA Issues**
**Patient Education:** This medication is administered I.M. or I.V. Drink 2-3 L fluid/day. Avoid alcohol during therapy and for 72 hours after last dose (may cause severe disulfiram-like reactions). If diarrhea occurs, yogurt or buttermilk may help. May cause false-positive test with Clinitest®; use another form of testing. May interfere with oral contraceptives; additional contraceptive measures are necessary. Report severe, unresolved diarrhea; vaginal itching or drainage; sores in mouth; blood, pus, or mucus in stool or urine; easy bleeding or bruising; unusual fever or chills; rash; or respiratory difficulty.
**Monitoring Parameters:** Monitor for signs of bruising or bleeding; observe for signs and symptoms of anaphylaxis during first dose

♦ **Cefamandole Nafate** *see Cefamandole on this page*

# Cefazolin (sef A zoe lin)

**Pharmacologic Class** Antibiotic, Cephalosporin (First Generation)

**U.S. Brand Names** Ancef®; Kefzol®; Zolicef®

**Mechanism of Action** Inhibits bacterial cell wall synthesis by binding to one or more of the penicillin-binding proteins (PBPs) which in turn inhibits the final transpeptidation step of peptidoglycan synthesis in bacterial cell walls, thus inhibiting cell wall biosynthesis. Bacteria eventually lyse due to ongoing activity of cell wall autolytic enzymes (autolysins and murein hydrolases) while cell wall assembly is arrested.

**Use** Treatment of gram-positive bacilli and cocci (except enterococcus); some gram-negative bacilli including *E. coli*, *Proteus*, and *Klebsiella* may be susceptible

**USUAL DOSAGE** I.M., I.V.:

Children >1 month: 25-100 mg/kg/day divided every 6-8 hours; maximum: 6 g/day

Adults: 250 mg to 2 g every 6-12 (usually 8) hours, depending on severity of infection; maximum dose: 12 g/day

**Dosing adjustment in renal impairment:**

$Cl_{cr}$ 10-30 mL/minute: Administer every 12 hours

$Cl_{cr}$ <10 mL/minute: Administer every 24 hours

Hemodialysis: Moderately dialyzable (20% to 50%); administer dose postdialysis or administer supplemental dose of 0.5-1 g after dialysis

Peritoneal dialysis: Administer 0.5 g every 12 hours

Continuous arteriovenous or venovenous hemofiltration (CAVH/CAVHD): Dose as for $Cl_{cr}$ 10-30 mL/minute; removes 30 mg of cefazolin per liter of filtrate per day

**Dosage Forms** Inf, premixed in $D_5W$ (frozen) (Ancef®): 500 mg (50 mL), 1 g (50 mL); **Inj** (Kefzol®): 500 mg, 1 g; **Powder for inj** (Ancef®, Zolicef®): 250 mg, 500 mg, 1 g, 5 g, 10 g, 20 g

**Contraindications** Hypersensitivity to cefazolin sodium, any component, or cephalosporins

**Warnings/Precautions** Modify dosage in patients with severe renal impairment; prolonged use may result in superinfection; use with caution in patients with a history of penicillin allergy especially IgE-mediated reactions (eg, anaphylaxis, urticaria); may cause antibiotic-associated colitis or colitis secondary to *C. difficile*

**Pregnancy Risk Factor** B

**Adverse Reactions**

1% to 10%:

Gastrointestinal: Diarrhea

Local: Pain at injection site

<1%: Anaphylaxis, rash, pruritus, Stevens-Johnson syndrome, oral candidiasis, nausea, vomiting, abdominal cramps, anorexia, pseudomembranous colitis, eosinophilia, neutropenia, leukopenia, thrombocytopenia, thrombocytosis, elevated transaminases, phlebitis, vaginitis, fever, seizures

Other reactions with cephalosporins include toxic epidermal necrolysis, abdominal pain, cholestasis, superinfection, renal dysfunction, toxic nephropathy, aplastic anemia, hemolytic anemia, hemorrhage, prolonged prothrombin time, pancytopenia

**Drug Interactions**

Increased effect: High-dose probenecid decreases clearance

Increased toxicity: Aminoglycosides increase nephrotoxic potential

**Half-Life** 90-150 minutes (prolonged with renal impairment); End-stage renal disease: 40-70 hours

**Special PA Issues**

**Patient Education:** This drug is administered I.V. or I.M. Drink 2-3 L fluid/day. If diarrhea occurs, yogurt or buttermilk may help. May cause false-positive test with Clinitest®; use another form of testing. May interfere with oral contraceptives; additional contraceptive measures are necessary. Report severe, unresolved diarrhea; vaginal itching or drainage; sores in mouth; blood, pus, or mucus in stool or urine; easy bleeding or bruising; unusual fever or chills; rash; or respiratory difficulty.

**Monitoring Parameters:** Renal function periodically when used in combination with other nephrotoxic drugs, hepatic function tests, CBC; monitor for signs of anaphylaxis during first dose

♦ **Cefazolin Sodium** see Cefazolin on this page

# Cefdinir (SEF di ner)

**Pharmacologic Class** Antibiotic, Cephalosporin (Third Generation)

**U.S. Brand Names** Omnicef®

**Mechanism of Action** Inhibits bacterial cell wall synthesis by binding to one or more of the penicillin-binding proteins (PBPs) which in turn inhibits the final transpeptidation step of peptidoglycan synthesis in bacterial cell walls, thus inhibiting cell wall biosynthesis. Bacteria eventually lyse due to ongoing activity of cell wall autolytic enzymes (autolysins and murein hydrolases) while cell wall assembly is arrested.

**Use** Treatment of community-acquired pneumonia, acute exacerbations of chronic bronchitis, acute bacterial otitis media, acute maxillary sinusitis, pharyngitis/tonsillitis, and uncomplicated skin and skin structure infections.

(Continued)

## Cefdinir *(Continued)*

**USUAL DOSAGE** Oral:
  Children: 7 mg/kg/dose twice daily or 14 mg/kg/dose once daily for 10 days (maximum: 600 mg/day)
  Adolescents and Adults: 300 mg twice daily or 600 mg once daily for 10 days
  **Dosing adjustment in renal impairment:** $Cl_{cr}$ <30 mL/minute: 300 mg once daily
  Hemodialysis removes cefdinir; recommended initial dose: 300 mg (or 7 mg/kg/dose) every other day. At the conclusion of each hemodialysis session, 300 mg (or 7 mg/kg/dose) should be given. Subsequent doses (300 mg or 7 mg/kg/dose) should be administered every other day.

**Dosage Forms Cap:** 300 mg; **Susp, oral:** 125 mg/5 mL (60 mL, 100 mL)

**Contraindications** Hypersensitivity to cephalosporins or related antibiotics

**Warnings/Precautions** Administer cautiously to penicillin-sensitive patients. There is evidence of partial cross-allergenicity and cephalosporins cannot be assumed to be an absolutely safe alternative to penicillin in the penicillin-allergic patient. Serum sickness-like reactions have been reported. Signs and symptoms occur after a few days of therapy and resolve a few days after drug discontinuation with no serious sequelae. Pseudomembranous colitis occurs; consider its diagnosis in patients who develop diarrhea with antibiotic use.

**Pregnancy Risk Factor** B

**Adverse Reactions**
  >1%: Gastrointestinal: Diarrhea
  <1%: Seizures (with high doses and renal dysfunction), headache, nervousness, rash, urticaria, pruritus, Stevens-Johnson syndrome, nausea, vomiting, pseudomembranous colitis, eosinophilia, hemolytic anemia, neutropenia, positive Coombs' test, thrombocytopenia, cholestatic jaundice, slightly increased AST/ALT, arthralgia, nephrotoxicity with transient elevations of BUN/creatinine, interstitial nephritis, serum sickness, candidiasis

**Drug Interactions**
  Decreased effect: Coadministration with iron or antacids reduces the rate and extent of cefdinir absorption
  Increased effect: Probenecid increases the effects of cephalosporins by decreasing the renal elimination in those which are secreted by tubular secretion
  Increased toxicity: Anticoagulant effects may be increased when administered with cephalosporins

**Half-Life** 2-4 hours

**Special PA Issues**
  **Monitoring Parameters:** Observe for signs and symptoms of anaphylaxis during first dose

## Cefepime *(SEF e pim)*

**Pharmacologic Class** Antibiotic, Cephalosporin (Fourth Generation)

**U.S. Brand Names** Maxipime®

**Mechanism of Action** Inhibits bacterial cell wall synthesis by binding to one or more of the penicillin-binding proteins (PBPs) which in turn inhibits the final transpeptidation step of peptidoglycan synthesis in bacterial cell walls, thus inhibiting cell wall biosynthesis. Bacterial eventually lyse due to ongoing activity of cell wall autolytic enzymes (autolysis and murein hydrolases) while cell wall assembly is arrested.

**Use** Treatment of uncomplicated and complicated urinary tract infections, including pyelonephritis caused by typical urinary tract pathogens; monotherapy for febrile neutropenia; uncomplicated skin and skin structure infections caused by *Streptococcus pyogenes*; moderate to severe pneumonia caused by pneumococcus, *Pseudomonas aeruginosa*, and other gram-negative organisms; complicated intra-abdominal infections (in combination with metronidazole). Also active against methicillin-susceptible staphylococci, *Enterobacter* sp, and many other gram-negative bacilli.

  Pediatrics (2 months to 16 years of age): Empiric therapy of febrile neutropenia patients, uncomplicated skin/soft tissue infections, pneumonia, and uncomplicated/complicated urinary tract infections.

**USUAL DOSAGE** I.V.:
  Children:
    Febrile neutropenia: 50 mg/kg every 8 hours for 7-10 days
    Uncomplicated skin/soft tissue infections, pneumonia, and complicated/uncomplicated UTI: 50 mg/kg twice daily
  Adults:
    Most infections: 1-2 g every 12 hours for 5-10 days; higher doses or more frequent administration may be required in pseudomonal infections
    Urinary tract infections, uncomplicated: 500 mg every 12 hours
    Monotherapy for febrile neutropenic patients: 2 g every 8 hours for 7 days or until the neutropenia resolves

**Dosing adjustment in renal impairment:**

| Creatinine Clearance (mL/minute) | Recommended Maintenance Schedule | | |
|---|---|---|---|
| >60<br>Normal recommended dosing schedule | 500 mg every 12 hours | 1 g every 12 hours | 2 g every 12 hours |
| 30-60 | 500 mg every 24 hours | 1 g every 24 hours | 1 g every 24 hours |
| 11-29 | 500 mg every 24 hours | 500 mg every 24 hours | 1 g every 24 hours |
| <10 | 250 mg every 24 hours | 250 mg every 24 hours | 500 mg every 24 hours |

Hemodialysis: Removed by dialysis; administer supplemental dose of 250 mg after each dialysis session

Peritoneal dialysis: Removed to a lesser extent than hemodialysis; administer 250 mg every 48 hours

Continuous arteriovenous or venovenous hemofiltration (CAVH/CAVHD): Dose as normal $Cl_{cr}$ (eg, >30 mL/minute)

**Dosage Forms** Powder for inj, as hydrochloride: 500 mg, 1 g, 2 g

**Contraindications** Hypersensitivity to cefepime or its components, or other cephalosporins

**Warnings/Precautions** Modify dosage in patients with severe renal impairment; prolonged use may result in superinfection; use with caution in patients with a history of penicillin or cephalosporin allergy, especially IgE-mediated reactions (eg, anaphylaxis, urticaria); may cause antibiotic-associated colitis or colitis secondary to *C. difficile*

**Pregnancy Risk Factor** B

**Adverse Reactions**
>10%: Hematologic: Positive Coombs' test without hemolysis
1% to 10%:
　Dermatologic: Rash, pruritus
　Gastrointestinal: : Diarrhea, nausea, vomiting
　Central nervous system: Fever (1%), headache (1%)
　Local: Pain, erythema at injection site
<1%: Leukopenia, neutropenia, agranulocytosis, thrombocytopenia, myoclonus, seizures, encephalopathy, neuromuscular excitability

Other reactions with cephalosporins include toxic epidermal necrolysis, Stevens-Johnson syndrome, erythema multiforme, renal dysfunction, toxic nephropathy, aplastic anemia, hemolytic anemia, hemorrhage, prolonged PT, pancytopenia, vaginitis, superinfection

**Drug Interactions**
Increased effect: High-dose probenecid decreases clearance
Increased toxicity: Aminoglycosides increase nephrotoxic potential

**Half-Life** 2 hours; prolonged in renal impairment

**Special PA Issues**
　**Patient Education:** This drug is administered I.V. or I.M. Drink 2-3 L fluid/day. If diarrhea occurs, yogurt or buttermilk may help. May cause false-positive test with Clinitest®; use another form of testing. May interfere with oral contraceptives; additional contraceptive measures are necessary. Report severe, unresolved diarrhea; vaginal itching or drainage; sores in mouth; blood, pus, or mucus in stool or urine; easy bleeding or bruising; unusual fever or chills; rash; or respiratory difficulty.
　**Monitoring Parameters:** Obtain specimen for culture and sensitivity prior to the first dose; monitor for signs of anaphylaxis during first dose

# Cefixime (sef IKS eem)

**Pharmacologic Class** Antibiotic, Cephalosporin (Third Generation)

**U.S. Brand Names** Suprax®

**Mechanism of Action** Inhibits bacterial cell wall synthesis by binding to one or more of the penicillin binding proteins (PBPs); which in turn inhibits the final transpeptidation step of peptidoglycan synthesis in bacterial cell walls, thus inhibiting cell wall biosynthesis. Bacteria eventually lyse due to ongoing activity of cell wall autolytic enzymes (autolysins and murein hydrolases) while cell wall assembly is arrested.

**Use** Treatment of urinary tract infections, otitis media, respiratory infections due to susceptible organisms including *S. pneumoniae* and *S. pyogenes*, *H. influenzae* and many Enterobacteriaceae; documented poor compliance with other oral antimicrobials; outpatient therapy of serious soft tissue or skeletal infections due to susceptible organisms; single-dose oral treatment of uncomplicated cervical/urethral gonorrhea due to *N. gonorrhoeae*

**USUAL DOSAGE** Oral:
Children: 8 mg/kg/day divided every 12-24 hours
Adolescents and Adults: 400 mg/day divided every 12-24 hours
　Uncomplicated cervical/urethral gonorrhea due to *N. gonorrhoeae*: 400 mg as a single dose
(Continued)

## Cefixime *(Continued)*

For *S. pyogenes* infections, treat for 10 days; use suspension for otitis media due to increased peak serum levels as compared to tablet form

**Dosing adjustment in renal impairment:**

Cl$_{cr}$ 21-60 mL/minute or with renal hemodialysis: Administer 75% of the standard dose

Cl$_{cr}$ <20 mL/minute or with CAPD: Administer 50% of the standard dose

Moderately dialyzable (10%)

**Dosage Forms Powder for oral susp (strawberry flavor):** 100 mg/5 mL (50 mL, 100 mL); **Tab, film coated:** 200 mg, 400 mg

**Contraindications** Hypersensitivity to cefixime or cephalosporins

**Warnings/Precautions** Prolonged use may result in superinfection; modify dosage in patients with renal impairment; use with caution in patients with a history of penicillin allergy especially IgE-mediated reactions (eg, anaphylaxis, urticaria); may cause antibiotic-associated colitis or colitis secondary to *C. difficile*

**Pregnancy Risk Factor** B

**Adverse Reactions**

>10%: Gastrointestinal: Diarrhea (16%)

1% to 10%: Gastrointestinal: Abdominal pain, nausea, dyspepsia, flatulence

<1%: Rash, urticaria, pruritus, erythema multiforme, Stevens-Johnson syndrome, serum sickness -like reaction, fever, vomiting, pseudomembranous colitis, transaminase elevations, increased BUN, increased creatinine, headache, dizziness, thrombocytopenia, leukopenia, eosinophilia, prolonged PT, vaginitis, candidiasis

Other reactions with cephalosporins include anaphylaxis, seizures, toxic epidermal necrolysis, renal dysfunction, toxic nephropathy, interstitial nephritis, cholestasis, aplastic anemia, hemolytic anemia, hemorrhage, pancytopenia, neutropenia, agranulocytosis, colitis, superinfection

**Drug Interactions**

Increased effect: Probenecid may decrease cephalosporin elimination

Increased toxicity: Furosemide, aminoglycosides may be a possible additive to nephrotoxicity

**Half-Life** Normal renal function: 3-4 hours; Renal failure: Up to 11.5 hours

**Special PA Issues**

**Patient Education:** Take as directed, at regular intervals around-the-clock (with or without food). Chilling oral suspension improves flavor (do not freeze). Complete full course of medication, even if you feel better. Drink 2-3 L fluid/day. If diarrhea occurs, yogurt or buttermilk may help. May cause false-positive test with Clinitest®; use another form of testing. May interfere with oral contraceptives; additional contraceptive measures are necessary. Report severe, unresolved diarrhea; vaginal itching or drainage; sores in mouth; blood, pus, or mucus in stool or urine; easy bleeding or bruising; unusual fever or chills,; rash; or respiratory difficulty.

**Monitoring Parameters:** With prolonged therapy, monitor renal and hepatic function periodically, observe for signs and symptoms of anaphylaxis during first dose

♦ **Cefizox®** *see* Ceftizoxime *on page 174*

## Cefmetazole *(sef MET a zole)*

**Pharmacologic Class** Antibiotic, Cephalosporin (Second Generation)

**U.S. Brand Names** Zefazone®

**Mechanism of Action** Inhibits bacterial cell wall synthesis by binding to one or more of the penicillin-binding proteins (PBPs) which in turn inhibits the final transpeptidation step of peptidoglycan synthesis in bacterial cell walls, thus inhibiting cell wall biosynthesis. Bacteria eventually lyse due to ongoing activity of cell wall autolytic enzymes (autolysins and murein hydrolases) while cell wall assembly is arrested.

**Use** Second generation cephalosporin, useful for susceptible aerobic and anaerobic grampositive and gram-negative bacteria; surgical prophylaxis, specifically colorectal and OB-GYN

**USUAL DOSAGE** Adults: I.V.:

Infections: 2 g every 6-12 hours for 5-14 days

Prophylaxis: 2 g 30-90 minutes before surgery **or** 1 g 30-90 minutes before surgery; repeat 8 and 16 hours later

**Dosing interval in renal impairment:**

Cl$_{cr}$ 50-90 mL/minute: Administer every 12 hours

Cl$_{cr}$ 10-50 mL/minute: Administer every 16-24 hours

Cl$_{cr}$ <10 mL/minute: Administer every 48 hours

**Dosage Forms Powder for inj, as sodium:** 1 g, 2 g

**Contraindications** Hypersensitivity to cefmetazole or any component or cephalosporins

**Warnings/Precautions** Modify dosage in patients with severe renal impairment; prolonged use may result in superinfection; use with caution in patients with a history of penicillin allergy especially IgE-mediated reactions (eg, anaphylaxis, urticaria); may cause antibiotic-associated colitis or colitis secondary to *C. difficile*

**Pregnancy Risk Factor** B

**Adverse Reactions** Contains MTT side chain which may lead to increased risk of hypoprothrombinemia and bleeding.

1% to 10%:
Dermatologic: Rash
Gastrointestinal: Diarrhea

<1%: Pain at injection site, phlebitis, pseudomembranous colitis, epigastric pain, candidiasis, bleeding, shock, hypotension, headache, hot flashes, dyspnea, epistaxis, respiratory distress, fever, vaginitis

Other reactions with cephalosporins include anaphylaxis, seizures, toxic epidermal necrolysis, erythema multiforme, Stevens-Johnson syndrome, renal dysfunction, interstitial nephritis, toxic nephropathy, cholestasis, aplastic anemia, hemolytic anemia, hemorrhage, pancytopenia, neutropenia, agranulocytosis, colitis, superinfection

**Drug Interactions**
Increased effect: Probenecid may decrease cephalosporin elimination
Increased toxicity: Furosemide, aminoglycosides may be a possible additive to nephrotoxicity

**Half-Life** 72 minutes; prolonged in renal impairment

**Special PA Issues**
**Patient Education:** This drug is administered I.V. or I.M. Drink 2-3 L fluid/day. Avoid alcohol during therapy and for 72 hours after last dose (may cause severe disulfiram-like reactions). If diarrhea occurs, yogurt or buttermilk may help. May cause false-positive test with Clinitest®; use another form of testing. May interfere with oral contraceptives; additional contraceptive measures are necessary. Report severe, unresolved diarrhea; vaginal itching or drainage; sores in mouth; blood, pus, or mucus in stool or urine; easy bleeding or bruising; unusual fever or chills; rash; or respiratory difficulty.

**Monitoring Parameters:** Monitor prothrombin times; observe for signs and symptoms of anaphylaxis during first dose

♦ **Cefmetazole Sodium** *see* Cefmetazole *on previous page*
♦ **Cefobid®** *see* Cefoperazone *on next page*
♦ **Cefol® Filmtab®** *see* Vitamins, Multiple *on page 964*

## Cefonicid (se FON i sid)
**Pharmacologic Class** Antibiotic, Cephalosporin (Second Generation)
**U.S. Brand Names** Monocid®
**Mechanism of Action** Inhibits bacterial cell wall synthesis by binding to one or more of the penicillin-binding proteins (PBPs) which in turn inhibits the final transpeptidation step of peptidoglycan synthesis in bacterial cell walls, thus inhibiting cell wall biosynthesis. Bacteria eventually lyse due to ongoing activity of cell wall autolytic enzymes (autolysins and murein hydrolases) while cell wall assembly is arrested.
**Use** Treatment of susceptible bacterial infection; mainly respiratory tract, skin and skin structure, bone and joint, urinary tract and gynecologic, septicemia; active against methicillin-sensitive staphylococci, many streptococci, and various gram-negative bacilli including *E. coli*, some *Klebsiella*, *P. mirabilis*, *H. influenzae*, and *Moraxella*.
**USUAL DOSAGE** Adults: I.M., I.V.: 0.5-2 g every 24 hours
Prophylaxis: Preop: 1 g/hour
**Dosing interval in renal impairment:** See table.

### Cefonicid Sodium

| Cl$_{cr}$ (mL/min/1.73 m$^2$) | Dose (mg/kg) for Each Dosing Interval |
|---|---|
| 60-79 | 10-24 q24h |
| 40-59 | 8-20 q24h |
| 20-39 | 4-15 q24h |
| 10-19 | 4-15 q48h |
| 5-9 | 4-15 q3-5d |
| <5 | 3-4 q3-5d |

**Dosage Forms** Powder for inj, as sodium: 500 mg, 1 g, 10 g
**Contraindications** Hypersensitivity to cefonicid sodium, any component, or cephalosporins
**Warnings/Precautions** Modify dosage in patients with severe renal impairment; prolonged use may result in superinfection; use with caution in patients with a history of penicillin allergy especially IgE-mediated reactions (eg, anaphylaxis, urticaria); may cause antibiotic-associated colitis or colitis secondary to *C. difficile*
**Pregnancy Risk Factor** B
**Adverse Reactions**
1% to 10%:
Hematologic: Increased eosinophils (2.9%), increased platelets (1.7%)
(Continued)

## Cefonicid *(Continued)*

Hepatic: Altered liver function tests (increased transaminases, LDH, alkaline phosphatase) (1.6%)

Local: Pain, burning at injection site (5.7%)

<1%: Fever, rash, pruritus, erythema, anaphylactoid reactions, diarrhea, pseudomembranous colitis, abdominal pain, increased transaminases, increased BUN, increased creatinine, interstitial nephritis, neutropenia, decreased WBC, thrombocytopenia

Other reactions with cephalosporins include anaphylaxis, seizures, Stevens-Johnson syndrome, toxic epidermal necrolysis, renal dysfunction, toxic nephropathy, cholestasis, aplastic anemia, hemolytic anemia, hemorrhage, pancytopenia, agranulocytosis, colitis, superinfection

**Drug Interactions**

Increased effect: Probenecid may decrease cephalosporin elimination

Increased toxicity: Furosemide, aminoglycosides may be a possible additive to nephrotoxicity

**Half-Life** 6-7 hours; prolonged in renal impairment

**Special PA Issues**

**Patient Education:** This medication is administered I.M. or I.V. Drink 2-3 L fluid/day. If diarrhea occurs, yogurt or buttermilk may help. May cause false-positive test with Clinitest®; use another form of testing. May interfere with oral contraceptives; additional contraceptive measures are necessary. Report severe, unresolved diarrhea; vaginal itching or drainage; sores in mouth; blood, pus, or mucus in stool or urine; easy bleeding or bruising; unusual fever or chills; rash; or respiratory difficulty.

**Monitoring Parameters:** Observe for signs and symptoms of anaphylaxis during first dose

♦ **Cefonicid Sodium** *see* Cefonicid *on previous page*

## Cefoperazone (sef oh PER a zone)

**Pharmacologic Class** Antibiotic, Cephalosporin (Third Generation)

**U.S. Brand Names** Cefobid®

**Mechanism of Action** Inhibits bacterial cell wall synthesis by binding to one or more of the penicillin-binding proteins (PBPs) which in turn inhibits the final transpeptidation step of peptidoglycan synthesis in bacterial cell walls, thus inhibiting cell wall biosynthesis. Bacteria eventually lyse due to ongoing activity of cell wall autolytic enzymes (autolysins and murein hydrolases) while cell wall assembly is arrested.

**Use** Treatment of susceptible bacterial infection; mainly respiratory tract, skin and skin structure, bone and joint, urinary tract and gynecologic as well as septicemia. Active against a variety of gram-negative bacilli, some gram-positive cocci, and has some activity against *Pseudomonas aeruginosa*.

**USUAL DOSAGE** I.M., I.V.:

Children (not approved): 100-150 mg/kg/day divided every 8-12 hours; up to 12 g/day

Adults: 2-4 g/day in divided doses every 12 hours; up to 12 g/day

**Dosing adjustment in hepatic impairment:** Reduce dose 50% in patients with advanced liver cirrhosis; maximum daily dose: 4 g

**Dosage Forms Inj, premixed (frozen):** 1 g (50 mL); 2 g (50 mL); **Powder for inj:** 1 g, 2 g

**Contraindications** Hypersensitivity to cefoperazone or any component or cephalosporins

**Warnings/Precautions** Modify dosage in patients with severe renal or hepatic impairment; prolonged use may result in superinfection; although rare, cefoperazone may interfere with hemostasis via destruction of vitamin K-producing intestinal bacteria, prevention of activation of prothrombin by the attachment of a methyltetrazolethiol side chain, and by an immune-mediated thrombocytopenia; use with caution in patients with a history of penicillin allergy especially IgE-mediated reactions (eg, anaphylaxis, urticaria); may cause antibiotic-associated colitis or colitis secondary to *C. difficile*

**Pregnancy Risk Factor** B

**Adverse Reactions** Contains MTT side chain which may lead to increased risk of hypoprothrombinemia and bleeding.

1% to 10%:

Dermatologic: Rash (maculopapular or erythematous) (2%)

Gastrointestinal: Diarrhea (3%)

Hematologic: Decreased neutrophils (2%), decreased hemoglobin or hematocrit (5%), eosinophilia (10%)

Hepatic: Increased transaminases (5% to 10%)

<1%: Hypoprothrombinemia, bleeding, pseudomembranous colitis, nausea, vomiting, elevated BUN, elevated creatinine, pain at injection site, induration at injection site, phlebitis, drug fever

Other reactions with cephalosporins include anaphylaxis, seizures, Stevens-Johnson syndrome, toxic epidermal necrolysis, renal dysfunction, toxic nephropathy, cholestasis, aplastic anemia, hemolytic anemia, pancytopenia, agranulocytosis, colitis, superinfection

### Drug Interactions

Disulfiram-like reaction has been reported when taken within 72 hours of alcohol consumption

Increased nephrotoxicity: Aminoglycosides, furosemide

**Half-Life** 2 hours, higher with hepatic disease or biliary obstruction

### Special PA Issues

**Patient Education:** This drug is administered I.M. or I.V. Drink 2-3 L fluid/day. Avoid alcohol during therapy and for 72 hours after last dose (may cause severe disulfiram-like reactions). If diarrhea occurs, yogurt or buttermilk may help. May cause false-positive test with Clinitest®; use another form of testing. May interfere with oral contraceptives; additional contraceptive measures are necessary. Report severe, unresolved diarrhea; vaginal itching or drainage; sores in mouth; blood, pus, or mucus in stool or urine; easy bleeding or bruising; unusual fever or chills; rash; or respiratory difficulty.

**Monitoring Parameters:** Monitor for coagulation abnormalities and diarrhea; observe for signs and symptoms of anaphylaxis during first dose

♦ **Cefoperazone Sodium** *see* Cefoperazone *on previous page*

♦ **Cefotan®** *see* Cefotetan *on next page*

## Cefotaxime (sef oh TAKS eem)

**Pharmacologic Class** Antibiotic, Cephalosporin (Third Generation)

**U.S. Brand Names** Claforan®

**Mechanism of Action** Inhibits bacterial cell wall synthesis by binding to one or more of the penicillin-binding proteins (PBPs) which in turn inhibits the final transpeptidation step of peptidoglycan synthesis in bacterial cell walls, thus inhibiting cell wall biosynthesis. Bacteria eventually lyse due to ongoing activity of cell wall autolytic enzymes (autolysins and murein hydrolases) while cell wall assembly is arrested.

**Use** Treatment of susceptible infection in respiratory tract, skin and skin structure, bone and joint, urinary tract, gynecologic as well as septicemia, and documented or suspected meningitis. Active against most gram-negative bacilli (not *Pseudomonas*) and gram-positive cocci (not enterococcus). Active against many penicillin-resistant pneumococci.

### USUAL DOSAGE

Neonates: I.V.:
  0-1 week: 50 mg/kg every 12 hours
  1-4 weeks: 50 mg/kg every 8 hours
Infants and Children 1 month to 12 years: I.M., I.V.: <50 kg: 50-180 mg/kg/day in divided doses every 4-6 hours
  Meningitis: 200 mg/kg/day in divided doses every 6 hours
Children >12 years and Adults:
  Gonorrhea: I.M.: 1 g as a single dose
  Uncomplicated infections: I.M., I.V.: 1 g every 12 hours
  Moderate/severe infections: I.M., I.V.: 1-2 g every 8 hours
  Infections commonly needing higher doses (eg, septicemia): I.V.: 2 g every 6-8 hours
  Life-threatening infections: I.V.: 2 g every 4 hours
  Preop: I.M., I.V.: 1 g 30-90 minutes before surgery
  C-section: 1 g as soon as the umbilical cord is clamped, then 1 g I.M., I.V. at 6- and 12-hours intervals
**Dosing interval in renal impairment:**
  Cl_cr 10-50 mL/minute: Administer every 8-12 hours
  Cl_cr <10 mL/minute: Administer every 24 hours
Hemodialysis: Moderately dialyzable
**Dosing adjustment in hepatic impairment:** Moderate dosage reduction is recommended in severe liver disease
Continuous arteriovenous or venovenous hemodiafiltration (CAVH) effects: Administer 1 g every 12 hour

**Dosage Forms Inf, premixed in D₅W** (frozen): 1 g (50 mL); 2 g (50 mL); **Powder for inj:** 500 mg, 1 g, 2 g, 10 g

**Contraindications** Hypersensitivity to cefotaxime, any component, or cephalosporins

**Warnings/Precautions** Modify dosage in patients with severe renal impairment; prolonged use may result in superinfection; a potentially life-threatening arrhythmia has been reported in patients who received a rapid bolus injection via central line. Use caution in patients with colitis; minimize tissue inflammation by changing infusion sites when needed. Use with caution in patients with a history of penicillin allergy especially IgE-mediated reactions (eg, anaphylaxis, urticaria); may cause antibiotic-associated colitis or colitis secondary to *C. difficile.*

### Pregnancy Risk Factor B

### Adverse Reactions

1% to 10%:
  Dermatologic: Rash, pruritus
  Gastrointestinal: Diarrhea, nausea, vomiting, colitis
  Local: Pain at injection site
(Continued)

## Cefotaxime *(Continued)*

<1%: Anaphylaxis, urticaria, arrhythmias (after rapid IV injection via central catheter), pseu-domembranous colitis, neutropenia, thrombocytopenia, eosinophilia, headache, fever, transaminase elevations, interstitial nephritis, increased BUN, increased creatinine, increased transaminases, phlebitis, candidiasis, vaginitis,

Other reactions with cephalosporins include seizures, Stevens-Johnson syndrome, toxic epidermal necrolysis, renal dysfunction, toxic nephropathy, cholestasis, aplastic anemia, hemolytic anemia, hemorrhage, pancytopenia, agranulocytosis, colitis, superinfection

**Drug Interactions**
Increased effect: Probenecid may decrease cephalosporin elimination
Increased toxicity: Furosemide, aminoglycosides may be a possible additive to nephrotox-icity

**Half-Life**
Cefotaxime: 1-1.5 hours (prolonged with renal and/or hepatic impairment)
Desacetylcefotaxime: 1.5-1.9 hours (prolonged with renal impairment)

**Special PA Issues**
**Patient Education:** This medication is administered I.M. or I.V. Drink 2-3 L fluid/day. If diarrhea occurs, yogurt or buttermilk may help. May cause false-positive test with Clin-itest®; use another form of testing. May interfere with oral contraceptives; additional contraceptive measures are necessary. Report severe, unresolved diarrhea; vaginal itching or drainage; sores in mouth; blood, pus, or mucus in stool or urine; easy bleeding or bruising; unusual fever or chills; rash; or respiratory difficulty.
**Monitoring Parameters:** Observe for signs and symptoms of anaphylaxis during first dose; CBC with differential (especially with long courses)

♦ **Cefotaxime Sodium** *see* Cefotaxime *on previous page*

## Cefotetan *(SEF oh tee tan)*
**Pharmacologic Class** Antibiotic, Cephalosporin (Second Generation)
**U.S. Brand Names** Cefotan®
**Mechanism of Action** Inhibits bacterial cell wall synthesis by binding to one or more of the penicillin-binding proteins (PBPs) which in turn inhibits the final transpeptidation step of peptidoglycan synthesis in bacterial cell walls, thus inhibiting cell wall biosynthesis. Bacteria eventually lyse due to ongoing activity of cell wall autolytic enzymes (autolysins and murein hydrolases) while cell wall assembly is arrested.
**Use** Less active against staphylococci and streptococci than first generation cephalosporins, but active against anaerobes including *Bacteroides fragilis*; active against gram-negative enteric bacilli including *E. coli*, *Klebsiella*, and *Proteus*; used predominantly for respiratory tract, skin and skin structure, bone and joint, urinary tract and gynecologic as well as septicemia; surgical prophylaxis; intra-abdominal infections and other mixed infections

**USUAL DOSAGE** I.M., I.V.:
Children: 20-40 mg/kg/dose every 12 hours
Adults: 1-6 g/day in divided doses every 12 hours; usual dose: 1-2 g every 12 hours for 5-10 days; 1-2 g may be given every 24 hours for urinary tract infection
**Dosing interval in renal impairment:**
Cl$_{cr}$ 10-30 mL/minute: Administer every 24 hours
Cl$_{cr}$ <10 mL/minute: Administer every 48 hours
Hemodialysis: Slightly dialyzable (5% to 20%)
Continuous arteriovenous or venovenous hemodiafiltration (CAVH) effects: Administer 750 mg every 12 hours
**Dosage Forms Powder for inj, as disodium:** 1 g (10 mL, 100 mL), 2 g (20 mL, 100 mL), 10 g (100 mL)
**Contraindications** Hypersensitivity to cefotetan, any component, or cephalosporins
**Warnings/Precautions** Modify dosage in patients with severe renal impairment; prolonged use may result in superinfection; although cefotetan contains the methyltetrazolethial side chain, bleeding has not been a significant problem; use with caution in patients with a history of penicillin allergy especially IgE-mediated reactions (eg, anaphylaxis, urticaria); may cause antibiotic-associated colitis or colitis secondary to *C. difficile*
**Pregnancy Risk Factor** B
**Adverse Reactions** Contains MTT side chain which may lead to increased risk of hypopro-thrombinemia and bleeding.
1% to 10%:
Gastrointestinal: Diarrhea (1.3%)
Hepatic: Increased transaminases (1.2%)
Miscellaneous: Hypersensitivity reactions (1.2%)
<1%: Anaphylaxis, urticaria, rash, pruritus, pseudomembranous colitis, nausea, vomiting, eosinophilia, thrombocytosis, agranulocytosis, hemolytic anemia, leukopenia, thrombocy-topenia, prolonged PT, bleeding, elevated BUN, elevated creatinine, nephrotoxicity, phle-bitis, fever

Other reactions with cephalosporins include: Seizures, Stevens-Johnson syndrome, toxic epidermal necrolysis, renal dysfunction, toxic nephropathy, cholestasis, aplastic anemia, hemolytic anemia, hemorrhage, pancytopenia, agranulocytosis, colitis, superinfection

**Drug Interactions**

Disulfiram-like reaction has been reported when taken within 72 hours of alcohol consumption

Increased cefamandole plasma levels: Probenecid

Increased nephrotoxicity: Aminoglycosides, furosemide

**Half-Life** 1.5-3 hours; prolonged in severe renal impairment

**Special PA Issues**

**Patient Education:** This medication is administered I.V. or I.M. Drink 2-3 L fluid/day. Avoid alcohol during therapy and for 72 hours after last dose (may cause severe disulfiram-like reactions). If diarrhea occurs, yogurt or buttermilk may help. May cause false-positive test with Clinitest®; use another form of testing. May interfere with oral contraceptives; additional contraceptive measures are necessary. Report severe, unresolved diarrhea; vaginal itching or drainage; sores in mouth; blood, pus, or mucus in stool or urine; easy bleeding or bruising; unusual fever or chills; rash; or respiratory difficulty.

**Monitoring Parameters:** Observe for signs and symptoms of anaphylaxis during first dose

♦ **Cefotetan Disodium** *see* Cefotetan *on previous page*

# Cefoxitin (se FOKS i tin)

**Pharmacologic Class** Antibiotic, Cephalosporin (Second Generation)

**U.S. Brand Names** Mefoxin®

**Mechanism of Action** Inhibits bacterial cell wall synthesis by binding to one or more of the penicillin-binding proteins (PBPs) which in turn inhibits the final transpeptidation step of peptidoglycan synthesis in bacterial cell walls, thus inhibiting cell wall biosynthesis. Bacteria eventually lyse due to ongoing activity of cell wall autolytic enzymes (autolysins and murein hydrolases) while cell wall assembly is arrested.

**Use** Less active against staphylococci and streptococci than first generation cephalosporins, but active against anaerobes including *Bacteroides fragilis*; active against gram-negative enteric bacilli including *E. coli*, *Klebsiella*, and *Proteus*; used predominantly for respiratory tract, skin and skin structure, bone and joint, urinary tract and gynecologic as well as septicemia; surgical prophylaxis; intra-abdominal infections and other mixed infections

**USUAL DOSAGE** I.M., I.V.:

Infants >3 months and Children:
  Mild to moderate infection: 80-100 mg/kg/day in divided doses every 4-6 hours
  Severe infection: 100-160 mg/kg/day in divided doses every 4-6 hours
  Maximum dose: 12 g/day

Adults: 1-2 g every 6-8 hours (I.M. injection is painful); up to 12 g/day

**Dosing interval in renal impairment:**
  $Cl_{cr}$ 30-50 mL/minute: Administer every 8-12 hours
  $Cl_{cr}$ 10-30 mL/minute: Administer every 12-24 hours
  $Cl_{cr}$ <10 mL/minute: Administer every 24-48 hours

Hemodialysis: Moderately dializable (20% to 50%)

Continuous arteriovenous or venovenous hemodiafiltration (CAVH) effects: Dose as for $Cl_{cr}$ 10-30 mL/minute

**Dosage Forms Inf,** premixed in D₅W (frozen): 1 g (50 mL); 2 g (50 mL); **Powder for inj:** 1 g, 2 g, 10 g

**Contraindications** Hypersensitivity to cefoxitin, any component, or cephalosporins

**Warnings/Precautions** Use with caution in patients with history of colitis; cefoxitin may increase resistance of organisms by inducing beta-lactamase; modify dosage in patients with severe renal impairment; prolonged use may result in superinfection; use with caution in patients with a history of penicillin allergy especially IgE-mediated reactions (eg, anaphylaxis, urticaria); may cause antibiotic-associated colitis or colitis secondary to *C. difficile*

**Pregnancy Risk Factor** B

**Adverse Reactions**

1% to 10%: Gastrointestinal: Diarrhea

<1%: Anaphylaxis, dyspnea, fever, rash, exfoliative dermatitis, toxic epidermal necrolysis, pruritus, angioedema, nausea, hypotension, vomiting, dyspnea, pseudomembranous colitis, phlebitis, interstitial nephritis, increased BUN, increased creatinine, leukopenia, thrombocytopenia, hemolytic anemia, bone marrow suppression, eosinophilia, increased transaminases, jaundice, thrombophlebitis, increased nephrotoxicity (with aminoglycosides), exacerbation of myasthenia gravis, prolonged PT

Other reactions with cephalosporins include: Seizures, Stevens-Johnson syndrome, toxic epidermal necrolysis, erythema multiforme, urticaria, serum-sickness reactions, renal dysfunction, toxic nephropathy, cholestasis, aplastic anemia, hemolytic anemia, hemorrhage, pancytopenia, agranulocytosis, colitis, vaginitis, superinfection

**Drug Interactions**

Increased effect: Probenecid may decrease cephalosporin elimination
(Continued)

## Cefoxitin *(Continued)*

Increased toxicity: Furosemide, aminoglycosides may be a possible additive to nephrotoxicity

**Half-Life** 45-60 minutes, increases significantly with renal insufficiency

### Special PA Issues

**Patient Education:** This medication is administered I.M. or I.V. Drink 2-3 L fluid/day. If diarrhea occurs, yogurt or buttermilk may help. May cause false-positive test with Clinitest®; use another form of testing. May interfere with oral contraceptives; additional contraceptive measures are necessary. Report severe, unresolved diarrhea; vaginal itching or drainage; sores in mouth; blood, pus, or mucus in stool or urine; easy bleeding or bruising; unusual fever or chills; rash; or respiratory difficulty.

**Monitoring Parameters:** Monitor renal function periodically when used in combination with other nephrotoxic drugs; observe for signs and symptoms of anaphylaxis during first dose

◆ **Cefoxitin Sodium** *see* Cefoxitin *on previous page*

## Cefpodoxime *(sef pode OKS eem)*

**Pharmacologic Class** Antibiotic, Cephalosporin (Second Generation)

**U.S. Brand Names** Vantin®

**Mechanism of Action** Inhibits bacterial cell wall synthesis by binding to one or more of the penicillin-binding proteins (PBPs) which in turn inhibits the final transpeptidation step of peptidoglycan synthesis in bacterial cell walls, thus inhibiting cell wall biosynthesis. Bacteria eventually lyse due to ongoing activity of cell wall autolytic enzymes (autolysins and murein hydrolases) while cell wall assembly is arrested.

**Use** Treatment of susceptible acute, community-acquired pneumonia caused by *S. pneumoniae* or nonbeta-lactamase producing *H. influenzae*; acute uncomplicated gonorrhea caused by *N. gonorrhoeae*; uncomplicated skin and skin structure infections caused by *S. aureus* or *S. pyogenes*; acute otitis media caused by *S. pneumoniae, H. influenzae*, or *M. catarrhalis*; pharyngitis or tonsillitis; and uncomplicated urinary tract infections caused by *E. coli, Klebsiella*, and *Proteus*

**USUAL DOSAGE** Oral:

Children >5 months to 12 years:

Acute otitis media: 10 mg/kg/day as a single dose or divided every 12 hours (400 mg/day)

Pharyngitis/tonsillitis: 10 mg/kg/day in 2 divided doses (maximum: 200 mg/day)

Children ≥13 years and Adults:

Acute community-acquired pneumonia and bacterial exacerbations of chronic bronchitis: 200 mg every 12 hours for 14 days and 10 days, respectively

Skin and skin structure: 400 mg every 12 hours for 7-14 days

Uncomplicated gonorrhea (male and female) and rectal gonococcal infections (female): 200 mg as a single dose

Pharyngitis/tonsillitis: 100 mg every 12 hours for 10 days

Uncomplicated urinary tract infection: 100 mg every 12 hours for 7 days

**Dosing adjustment in renal impairment:** Cl$_{cr}$ <30 mL/minute: Administer every 24 hours

**Dosage Forms** Granules for oral susp **(lemon creme flavor):** 50 mg/5 mL (100 mL), 100 mg/5 mL (100 mL); **Tab, film coated:** 100 mg, 200 mg

**Contraindications** Hypersensitivity to cefpodoxime or cephalosporins

**Warnings/Precautions** Modify dosage in patients with severe renal impairment; prolonged use may result in superinfection; a low incidence of cross-hypersensitivity to penicillins exists

**Pregnancy Risk Factor** B

### Adverse Reactions

>10%:

Dermatologic: Diaper rash (12.1%)

Gastrointestinal: Diarrhea in infants and toddlers (15.4%)

1% to 10%:

Central nervous system: Headache (1.1%)

Dermatologic: Rash (1.4%)

Gastrointestinal: Diarrhea (7.2%), nausea (3.8%), abdominal pain (1.6%), vomiting (1.1% to 2.1%)

Genitourinary: Vaginal infections (3.1%)

<1%: Anaphylaxis, chest pain, hypotension, fungal skin infection, pseudomembranous colitis, vaginal candidiasis, pruritus, flatulence, decreased salivation, malaise, fever, decreased appetite, cough, epistaxis, dizziness, fatigue, anxiety, insomnia, flushing, weakness, nightmares, taste alteration, eye itching, tinnitus, purpuric nephritis

Other reactions with cephalosporins include seizures, Stevens-Johnson syndrome, toxic epidermal necrolysis, erythema multiforme, urticaria, serum-sickness reactions, renal dysfunction, interstitial nephritis toxic nephropathy, cholestasis, aplastic anemia, hemolytic anemia, hemorrhage, pancytopenia, agranulocytosis, colitis, vaginitis, superinfection

### Drug Interactions

Decreased effect: Antacids and $H_2$-receptor antagonists (reduce absorption and serum concentration of cefpodoxime)

Increased effect: Probenecid may decrease cephalosporin elimination

Increased toxicity: Furosemide, aminoglycosides may be a possible additive to nephrotoxicity

**Half-Life** 2.2 hours (prolonged with renal impairment)

### Special PA Issues

**Patient Education:** Take as directed, at regular intervals around-the-clock (with or without food). Chilling oral suspension improves flavor (do not freeze). Complete full course of medication, even if you feel better. Drink 2-3 L fluid/day. If diarrhea occurs, yogurt or buttermilk may help. May cause false-positive test with Clinitest®; use another form of testing. May interfere with oral contraceptives; additional contraceptive measures are necessary. Report severe, unresolved diarrhea; vaginal itching or drainage; sores in mouth; blood, pus, or mucus in stool or urine; easy bleeding or bruising; unusual fever or chills; rash; or respiratory difficulty.

**Monitoring Parameters:** Observe for signs and symptoms of anaphylaxis during first dose

♦ **Cefpodoxime Proxetil** *see* Cefpodoxime *on previous page*

# Cefprozil (sef PROE zil)

**Pharmacologic Class** Antibiotic, Cephalosporin (Second Generation)

**U.S. Brand Names** Cefzil®

**Mechanism of Action** Inhibits bacterial cell wall synthesis by binding to one or more of the penicillin-binding proteins (PBPs) which in turn inhibits the final transpeptidation step of peptidoglycan synthesis in bacterial cell walls, thus inhibiting cell wall biosynthesis. Bacteria eventually lyse due to ongoing activity of cell wall autolytic enzymes (autolysins and murein hydrolases) while cell wall assembly is arrested.

**Use** Treatment of otitis media and infections involving the respiratory tract and skin and skin structure; Active against methicillin-sensitive staphylococci, many streptococci, and various gram-negative bacilli including *E. coli*, some *Klebsiella*, *P. mirabilis*, *H. influenzae*, and *Moraxella*.

### USUAL DOSAGE Oral:

Infants and Children >6 months to 12 years: Otitis media: 15 mg/kg every 12 hours for 10 days

Pharyngitis/tonsillitis:

Children 2-12 years: 7.5 -15 mg/kg/day divided every 12 hours for 10 days (administer for >10 days if due to *S. pyogenes*); maximum: 1 g/day

Children >13 years and Adults: 500 mg every 24 hours for 10 days

Uncomplicated skin and skin structure infections:

Children 2-12 years: 20 mg/kg every 24 hours for 10 days; maximum: 1 g/day

Children >13 years and Adults: 250 mg every 12 hours, or 500 mg every 12-24 hours for 10 days

Secondary bacterial infection of acute bronchitis or acute bacterial exacerbation of chronic bronchitis: 500 mg every 12 hours for 10 days

**Dosing adjustment in renal impairment:** $Cl_{cr}$ <30 mL/minute: Reduce dose by 50%

Hemodialysis: Reduced by hemodialysis; administer dose after the completion of hemodialysis

**Dosage Forms** Powder for oral susp, as anhydrous: 125 mg/5 mL (50 mL, 75 mL, 100 mL), 250 mg/5 mL (50 mL, 75 mL, 100 mL); Tab, as anhydrous: 250 mg, 500 mg

**Contraindications** Hypersensitivity to cefprozil or any component or cephalosporins

**Warnings/Precautions** Modify dosage in patients with severe renal impairment; prolonged use may result in superinfection; use with caution in patients with a history of penicillin allergy especially IgE-mediated reactions (eg, anaphylaxis, urticaria); may cause antibiotic-associated colitis or colitis secondary to *C. difficile*

**Pregnancy Risk Factor** B

### Adverse Reactions

1% to 10%:

Central nervous system: Dizziness (1%)

Dermatologic: Diaper rash (1.5%)

Gastrointestinal: Diarrhea (2.9%), nausea (3.5%), vomiting (1%), abdominal pain (1%)

Genitourinary: Vaginitis, genital pruritus (1.6%)

Hepatic: Increased transaminases (2%)

Miscellaneous: Superinfection

<1%: Anaphylaxis, angioedema, pseudomembranous colitis, rash, urticaria, erythema multiforme, serum sickness, Stevens-Johnson syndrome, hyperactivity, headache, insomnia, confusion, somnolence, leukopenia, eosinophilia, thrombocytopenia, elevated BUN, elevated creatinine, arthralgia, cholestatic jaundice, fever

Other reactions with cephalosporins include: Seizures, toxic epidermal necrolysis, renal dysfunction, interstitial nephritis, toxic nephropathy, aplastic anemia, hemolytic anemia, hemorrhage, pancytopenia, agranulocytosis, colitis, vaginitis, superinfection

(Continued)

## Cefprozil *(Continued)*

### Drug Interactions

Increased effect: Probenecid may decrease cephalosporin elimination

Increased toxicity: Furosemide, aminoglycosides may be a possible additive to nephrotoxicity

**Half-Life** 1.3 hours (normal renal function)

### Special PA Issues

**Patient Education:** Take as directed, at regular intervals around-the-clock (with or without food). Chilling oral suspension improves flavor (do not freeze). Complete full course of medication, even if you feel better. Drink 2-3 L fluid/day. If diarrhea occurs, yogurt or buttermilk may help. May cause false-positive test with Clinitest®; use another form of testing. May interfere with oral contraceptives; additional contraceptive measures are necessary. Report severe, unresolved diarrhea; vaginal itching or drainage; sores in mouth; blood, pus, or mucus in stool or urine; easy bleeding or bruising; unusual fever or chills; rash; or respiratory difficulty.

**Monitoring Parameters:** Assess patient at beginning and throughout therapy for infection; monitor for signs of anaphylaxis during first dose

## Ceftazidime (SEF tay zi deem)

**Pharmacologic Class** Antibiotic, Cephalosporin (Third Generation)

**U.S. Brand Names** Ceptaz™; Fortaz®; Tazicef®; Tazidime®

**Mechanism of Action** Inhibits bacterial cell wall synthesis by binding to one or more of the penicillin-binding proteins (PBPs) which in turn inhibits the final transpeptidation step of peptidoglycan synthesis in bacterial cell walls, thus inhibiting cell wall biosynthesis. Bacteria eventually lyse due to ongoing activity of cell wall autolytic enzymes (autolysins and murein hydrolases) while cell wall assembly is arrested.

**Use** Treatment of documented susceptible *Pseudomonas aeruginosa* infection and infections due to other susceptible aerobic gram-negative organisms; empiric therapy of a febrile, granulocytopenic patient

### USUAL DOSAGE

Neonates 0-4 weeks: I.V.: 30 mg/kg every 12 hours

Infants and Children 1 month to 12 years: I.V.: 30-50 mg/kg/dose every 8 hours; maximum dose: 6 g/day

Adults: I.M., I.V.: 500 mg to 2 g every 8-12 hours

Urinary tract infections: 250-500 mg every 12 hours

**Dosing interval in renal impairment:**

$Cl_{cr}$ 30-50 mL/minute: Administer every 12 hours

$Cl_{cr}$ 10-30 mL/minute: Administer every 24 hours

$Cl_{cr}$ <10 mL/minute: Administer every 48-72 hours

Hemodialysis: Dialyzable (50% to 100%)

Continuous arteriovenous or venovenous hemodiafiltration (CAVH) effects: Dose as for $Cl_{cr}$ 30-50 mL/minute

**Dosage Forms Inj, premixed (frozen) (Fortaz®):** 1 g (50 mL), 2 g (50 mL); **Powder for inj:** 500 mg, 1 g, 2 g, 6 g

**Contraindications** Hypersensitivity to ceftazidime, any component, or cephalosporins

**Warnings/Precautions** Modify dosage in patients with severe renal impairment; prolonged use may result in superinfection; use with caution in patients with a history of penicillin allergy especially IgE-mediated reactions (eg, anaphylaxis, urticaria); may cause antibiotic-associated colitis or colitis secondary to *C. difficile*

**Pregnancy Risk Factor** B

### Adverse Reactions

1% to 10%:

Gastrointestinal: Diarrhea (1.3%)

Local: Pain at injection site (1.4%)

Miscellaneous: Hypersensitivity reactions (2%)

<1%: Anaphylaxis, fever, headache, dizziness, paresthesia, pruritus, rash, Stevens-Johnson syndrome, toxic epidermal necrolysis, erythema multiforme, angioedema, nausea, vomiting, pseudomembranous colitis, eosinophilia, thrombocytosis, leukopenia, hemolytic anemia, elevated transaminases, increased BUN, increased creatinine, phlebitis, candidiasis, vaginitis, encephalopathy, asterixis, neuromuscular excitability

Other reactions with cephalosporins include: seizures, urticaria, serum-sickness reactions, renal dysfunction, interstitial nephritis, toxic nephropathy, elevated BUN, elevated creatinine, cholestasis, aplastic anemia, hemolytic anemia, pancytopenia, agranulocytosis, colitis, prolonged PT, hemorrhage, superinfection

### Drug Interactions

Increased effect: Probenecid may decrease cephalosporin elimination; aminoglycosides: *in vitro* studies indicate additive or synergistic effect against some strains of Enterobacteriaceae and *Pseudomonas aeruginosa*

Increased toxicity: Furosemide, aminoglycosides may be a possible additive to nephrotoxicity

**Half-Life** 1-2 hours (prolonged with renal impairment)

### Special PA Issues

**Patient Education:** This medication is administered I.M. or I.V. Drink 2-3 L fluid/day. If diarrhea occurs, yogurt or buttermilk may help. May cause false-positive test with Clinitest®; use another form of testing. May interfere with oral contraceptives; additional contraceptive measures are necessary. Report severe, unresolved diarrhea; vaginal itching or drainage; sores in mouth; blood, pus, or mucus in stool or urine; easy bleeding or bruising; unusual fever or chills; rash; or respiratory difficulty.

**Monitoring Parameters:** Observe for signs and symptoms of anaphylaxis during first dose

## Ceftibuten (sef TYE byoo ten)

**Pharmacologic Class** Antibiotic, Cephalosporin (Third Generation)

**U.S. Brand Names** Cedax®

**Mechanism of Action** Inhibits bacterial cell wall synthesis by binding to one or more of the penicillin-binding proteins (PBPs) which in turn inhibits the final transpeptidation step of peptidoglycan synthesis in bacterial cell walls, thus inhibiting cell wall biosynthesis. Bacteria eventually lyse due to ongoing activity of cell wall autolytic enzymes (autolysins and murein hydrolases) while cell wall assembly is arrested.

**Use** Oral cephalosporin for bronchitis, otitis media, and pharyngitis/tonsillitis due to *H. influenzae* and *M. catarrhalis*, both beta-lactamase-producing and nonproducing strains, as well as *S. pneumoniae* (weak) and *S. pyogenes*

**USUAL DOSAGE** Oral:

Children <12 years: 9 mg/kg/day for 10 days; maximum daily dose: 400 mg

Children ≥12 years and Adults: 400 mg once daily for 10 days; maximum: 400 mg

**Dosage adjustment in renal impairment:**

$Cl_{cr}$ 30-49 mL/minute: Administer 4.5 mg/kg or 200 mg every 24 hours

$Cl_{cr}$ <29 mL/minute: Administer 2.25 mg/kg or 100 mg every 24 hours

**Dosage Forms Cap:** 400 mg; **Powder for oral susp (cherry flavor):** 90 mg/5 mL (30 mL, 60 mL, 120 mL), 180 mg/5 mL (30 mL, 60 mL, 120 mL)

**Contraindications** In patients with known allergy to the cephalosporin group of antibiotics

**Warnings/Precautions** Modify dosage in patients with severe renal impairment, prolonged use may result in superinfection; use with caution in patients with a history of penicillin allergy, especially IgE-mediated reactions (eg, anaphylaxis, urticaria); may cause antibiotic-associated colitis or colitis secondary to *C. difficile*

**Pregnancy Risk Factor** B

**Adverse Reactions**

1% to 10%:

Central nervous system: Headache (3%), dizziness (1%)

Gastrointestinal: Nausea (4%), diarrhea (3%), dyspepsia (2%), vomiting (1%), abdominal pain (1%)

Hematologic: Increased eosinophils (3%), decreased hemoglobin (2%), thrombocytosis

Hepatic: Increased ALT (1%), increased bilirubin (1%)

Renal: Increased BUN (4%)

<1%: Anorexia, agitation, constipation, diaper rash, dry mouth, dyspnea, dysuria, fatigue, candidiasis, rash, urticaria, irritability, paresthesia, nasal congestion, insomnia, rigors, increased transaminases, increased creatinine, leukopenia

Other reactions with cephalosporins include anaphylaxis, fever, paresthesia, pruritus, Stevens-Johnson syndrome, toxic epidermal necrolysis, erythema multiforme, angioedema, pseudomembranous colitis, hemolytic anemia, candidiasis, vaginitis, encephalopathy, asterixis, neuromuscular excitability, seizures, serum-sickness reactions, renal dysfunction, interstitial nephritis, toxic nephropathy, cholestasis, aplastic anemia, hemolytic anemia, pancytopenia, agranulocytosis, colitis, prolonged PT, hemorrhage, superinfection

**Drug Interactions**

Increased effect: High-dose probenecid decreases clearance

Increased toxicity: Aminoglycosides increase nephrotoxic potential

**Half-Life** 2 hours

### Special PA Issues

**Patient Education:** Take as directed, at regular intervals around-the-clock (with or without food). Chilling oral suspension improves flavor (do not freeze). Complete full course of medication, even if you feel better. Drink 2-3 L fluid/day. If diarrhea occurs, yogurt or buttermilk may help. May cause false-positive test with Clinitest®; use another form of testing. May interfere with oral contraceptives; additional contraceptive measures are necessary. Report severe, unresolved diarrhea; vaginal itching or drainage; sores in mouth; blood, pus, or mucus in stool or urine; easy bleeding or bruising; unusual fever or chills; rash; or respiratory difficulty.

**Monitoring Parameters:** Observe for signs and symptoms of anaphylaxis during first dose; with prolonged therapy, monitor renal, hepatic, and hematologic function periodically

♦ **Ceftin® Oral** *see* Cefuroxime *on page 176*

# Ceftizoxime (sef ti ZOKS eem)

**Pharmacologic Class** Antibiotic, Cephalosporin (Third Generation)

**U.S. Brand Names** Cefizox®

**Mechanism of Action** Inhibits bacterial cell wall synthesis by binding to one or more of the penicillin-binding proteins (PBPs) which in turn inhibits the final transpeptidation step of peptidoglycan synthesis in bacterial cell walls, thus inhibiting cell wall biosynthesis. Bacteria eventually lyse due to ongoing activity of cell wall autolytic enzymes (autolysins and murein hydrolases) while cell wall assembly is arrested.

**Use** Treatment of susceptible bacterial infection, mainly respiratory tract, skin and skin structure, bone and joint, urinary tract and gynecologic, as well as septicemia; active against many gram-negative bacilli (not *Pseudomonas*), some gram-positive cocci (not *Enterococcus*), and some anaerobes

**USUAL DOSAGE** I.M., I.V.:

Children ≥6 months: 150-200 mg/kg/day divided every 6-8 hours (maximum of 12 g/24 hours)

Adults: 1-2 g every 8-12 hours, up to 2 g every 4 hours or 4 g every 8 hours for life-threatening infections

**Dosing adjustment in renal impairment:** Adults:

$Cl_{cr}$ 10-30 mL/minute: Administer 1 g every 12 hours

$Cl_{cr}$ <10 mL/minute: Administer 1 g every 24 hours

Moderately dialyzable (20% to 50%)

Continuous arteriovenous or venovenous hemodiafiltration (CAVH) effects: Dose as for $Cl_{cr}$ 10-30 mL/minute

**Dosage Forms** Inj in $D_5W$ (frozen): 1 g (50 mL); 2 g (50 mL); **Powder for inj:** 500 mg, 1 g, 2 g, 10 g

**Contraindications** Hypersensitivity to ceftizoxime, any component, or cephalosporins

**Warnings/Precautions** Modify dosage in patients with severe renal impairment, prolonged use may result in superinfection; use with caution in patients with a history of penicillin allergy, especially IgE-mediated reactions (eg, anaphylaxis, urticaria); may cause antibiotic-associated colitis or colitis secondary to *C. difficile*

**Pregnancy Risk Factor** B

**Adverse Reactions**

1% to 10%:

Central nervous system: Fever

Dermatologic: Rash, pruritus

Hematologic: Eosinophilia, thrombocytosis

Hepatic: Elevated transaminases, alkaline phosphatase

Local: Pain, burning at injection site

<1%: Anaphylaxis, diarrhea, nausea, vomiting, injection site reactions, phlebitis, paresthesia, numbness, increased bilirubin, increased BUN, increased creatinine, anemia, leukopenia, neutropenia, thrombocytopenia, vaginitis

Other reactions reported with cephalosporins include Stevens-Johnson syndrome, toxic epidermal necrolysis, erythema multiforme, pseudomembranous colitis, angioedema, hemolytic anemia, candidiasis, encephalopathy, asterixis, neuromuscular excitability, seizures, serum-sickness reactions, renal dysfunction, interstitial nephritis, toxic nephropathy, cholestasis, aplastic anemia, hemolytic anemia, pancytopenia, agranulocytosis, colitis, prolonged PT, hemorrhage, superinfection

**Drug Interactions**

Increased effect: Probenecid may decrease cephalosporin elimination

Increased toxicity: Furosemide, aminoglycosides may be a possible additive to nephrotoxicity

**Half-Life** 1.6 hours, increases to 25 hours when $Cl_{cr}$ falls to <10 mL/minute

**Special PA Issues**

**Patient Education:** This medication is administered I.M. or I.V. Drink 2-3 L fluid/day. If diarrhea occurs, yogurt or buttermilk may help. May cause false-positive test with Clinitest®; use another form of testing. May interfere with oral contraceptives; additional contraceptive measures are necessary. Report severe, unresolved diarrhea; vaginal itching or drainage; sores in mouth; blood, pus, or mucus in stool or urine; easy bleeding or bruising; unusual fever or chills; rash; or respiratory difficulty.

**Monitoring Parameters:** Observe for signs and symptoms of anaphylaxis during first dose

♦ **Ceftizoxime Sodium** *see* Ceftizoxime *on this page*

# Ceftriaxone (sef trye AKS one)

**Pharmacologic Class** Antibiotic, Cephalosporin (Third Generation)

**U.S. Brand Names** Rocephin®

**Mechanism of Action** Inhibits bacterial cell wall synthesis by binding to one or more of the penicillin-binding proteins (PBPs) which in turn inhibits the final transpeptidation step of peptidoglycan synthesis in bacterial cell walls, thus inhibiting cell wall biosynthesis. Bacteria eventually lyse due to ongoing activity of cell wall autolytic enzymes (autolysins and murein hydrolases) while cell wall assembly is arrested.

**Use** Treatment of lower respiratory tract infections, skin and skin structure infections, bone and joint infections, intra-abdominal and urinary tract infections, sepsis and meningitis due to susceptible organisms; documented or suspected infection due to susceptible organisms in home care patients and patients without I.V. line access; treatment of documented or suspected gonococcal infection or chancroid; emergency room management of patients at high risk for bacteremia, periorbital or buccal cellulitis, salmonellosis or shigellosis, and pneumonia of unestablished etiology (<5 years of age); treatment of Lyme disease, depends on the stage of the disease (used in Stage II and Stage III, but not stage I; doxycycline is the drug of choice for Stage I)

## USUAL DOSAGE I.M., I.V.:

Neonates:

Postnatal age ≤7 days: 50 mg/kg/day given every 24 hours

Postnatal age >7 days:

≤2000 g: 50 mg/kg/day given every 24 hours

>2000 g: 50-75 mg/kg/day given every 24 hours

Gonococcal prophylaxis: 25-50 mg/kg as a single dose (dose not to exceed 125 mg)

Gonococcal infection: 25-50 mg/kg/day (maximum dose: 125 mg) given every 24 hours for 10-14 days

Infants and Children: 50-75 mg/kg/day in 1-2 divided doses every 12-24 hours; maximum: 2 g/24 hours

Meningitis: 100 mg/kg/day divided every 12-24 hours, up to a maximum of 4 g/24 hours; loading dose of 75 mg/kg/dose may be given at start of therapy

Otitis media: Single I.M. injection

Uncomplicated gonococcal infections, sexual assault, and STD prophylaxis: I.M.: 125 mg as a single dose plus doxycycline

Complicated gonococcal infections:

Infants: I.M., I.V.: 25-50 mg/kg/day in a single dose (maximum: 125 mg/dose); treat for 7 days for disseminated infection and 7-14 days for documented meningitis

<45 kg: 50 mg/kg/day once daily; maximum: 1 g/day; for ophthalmia, peritonitis, arthritis, or bacteremia: 50-100 mg/kg/day divided every 12-24 hours; maximum: 2 g/day for meningitis or endocarditis

>45 kg: 1 g/day once daily for disseminated gonococcal infections; 1-2 g dose every 12 hours for meningitis or endocarditis

Acute epididymitis: I.M.: 250 mg in a single dose

Adults: 1-2 g every 12-24 hours (depending on the type and severity of infection); maximum dose: 2 g every 12 hours for treatment of meningitis

Uncomplicated gonorrhea: I.M.: 250 mg as a single dose

Surgical prophylaxis: 1 g 30 minutes to 2 hours before surgery

**Dosing adjustment in renal or hepatic impairment:** No change necessary

Hemodialysis: Not dialyzable (0% to 5%); administer dose postdialysis

Peritoneal dialysis: Administer 750 mg every 12 hours

Continuous arteriovenous or venovenous hemofiltration (CAVH/CAVHD): Removes 10 mg of ceftriaxone per liter of filtrate per day

**Dosage Forms** Inf, premixed (frozen): 1 g in $D_{3.8}W$ (50 mL), 2 g in $D_{2.4}W$ (50 mL); **Powder for inj:** 250 mg, 500 mg, 1 g, 2 g, 10 g

**Contraindications** Hypersensitivity to ceftriaxone sodium, any component, or cephalosporins; **do not use in hyperbilirubinemic neonates**, particularly those who are premature since ceftriaxone is reported to displace bilirubin from albumin binding sites

**Warnings/Precautions** Modify dosage in patients with severe renal impairment, prolonged use may result in superinfection; use with caution in patients with a history of penicillin allergy, especially IgE-mediated reactions (eg, anaphylaxis, urticaria); may cause antibiotic-associated colitis or colitis secondary to *C. difficile*

**Pregnancy Risk Factor** B

**Adverse Reactions**

1% to 10%:

Dermatologic: Rash (1.7%)

Gastrointestinal: Diarrhea (2.7%)

Hematologic: Eosinophilia (6%), thrombocytosis (5.1%), leukopenia (2.1%)

Hepatic: Elevated transaminases (3.1% to 3.3%)

Local: Pain, induration at injection site (1%)

Renal: Increased BUN (1.2%)

<1%: Phlebitis, pruritus, fever, chills, anemia, hemolytic anemia, neutropenia, lymphopenia, thrombocytopenia, prolonged PT, nausea, vomiting, dysgeusia, increased alkaline phosphatase, increased bilirubin, increased creatinine, urinary casts, headache, dizziness, candidiasis, vaginitis, diaphoresis, flushing

Other reactions with cephalosporins include anaphylaxis, paresthesia, Stevens-Johnson syndrome, toxic epidermal necrolysis, erythema multiforme, angioedema, pseudomembranous colitis, hemolytic anemia, encephalopathy, asterixis, neuromuscular excitability, (Continued)

## Ceftriaxone (Continued)

seizures, serum-sickness reactions, renal dysfunction, interstitial nephritis, toxic nephropathy, cholestasis, aplastic anemia, hemolytic anemia, pancytopenia, agranulocytosis, colitis, hemorrhage, superinfection

**Drug Interactions**
Increased effect:
Aminoglycosides may result in synergistic antibacterial activity
High-dose probenecid decreases clearance
Increased toxicity: Aminoglycosides increase nephrotoxic potential

**Half-Life** Normal renal and hepatic function: 5-9 hours

**Special PA Issues**
**Patient Education:** This medication is administered I.M. or I.V. Drink 2-3 L fluid/day. If diarrhea occurs, yogurt or buttermilk may help. May cause false-positive test with Clinitest®; use another form of testing. May interfere with oral contraceptives; additional contraceptive measures are necessary. Report severe, unresolved diarrhea; vaginal itching or drainage; sores in mouth; blood, pus, or mucus in stool or urine; easy bleeding or bruising; unusual fever or chills; rash; or respiratory difficulty.

**Monitoring Parameters:** Observe for signs and symptoms of anaphylaxis

♦ **Ceftriaxone Sodium** see Ceftriaxone on page 174

## Cefuroxime (se fyoor OKS eem)

**Pharmacologic Class** Antibiotic, Cephalosporin (Second Generation)

**U.S. Brand Names** Ceftin® Oral; Kefurox® Injection; Zinacef® Injection

**Mechanism of Action** Inhibits bacterial cell wall synthesis by binding to one or more of the penicillin-binding proteins (PBPs) which in turn inhibits the final transpeptidation step of peptidoglycan synthesis in bacterial cell walls, thus inhibiting cell wall biosynthesis. Bacteria eventually lyse due to ongoing activity of cell wall autolytic enzymes (autolysins and murein hydrolases) while cell wall assembly is arrested.

**Use** Treatment of infections caused by staphylococci, group B streptococci, H. influenzae (type A and B), E. coli, Enterobacter, Salmonella, and Klebsiella; treatment of susceptible infections of the lower respiratory tract, otitis media, urinary tract, skin and soft tissue, bone and joint, sepsis and gonorrhea

**USUAL DOSAGE**
Children:
Pharyngitis, tonsillitis: Oral:
Suspension: 20 mg/kg/day (maximum: 500 mg/day) in 2 divided doses
Tablet: 125 mg every 12 hours
Acute otitis media, impetigo: Oral:
Suspension: 30 mg/kg/day (maximum: 1 g/day) in 2 divided doses
Tablet: 250 mg every 12 hours
I.M., I.V.: 75-150 mg/kg/day divided every 8 hours; maximum dose: 6 g/day
Meningitis: Not recommended (doses of 200-240 mg/kg/day divided every 6-8 hours have been used); maximum dose: 9 g/day
Adults:
Oral: 250-500 mg twice daily; uncomplicated urinary tract infection: 125-250 mg every 12 hours
I.M., I.V.: 750 mg to 1.5 g/dose every 8 hours or 100-150 mg/kg/day in divided doses every 6-8 hours; maximum: 6 g/24 hours
**Dosing adjustment in renal impairment:**
Cl_cr 10-20 mL/minute: Administer every 12 hours
Cl_cr <10 mL/minute: Administer every 24 hours
Hemodialysis: Dialyzable (25%)
**Note:** Cefuroxime axetil film-coated tablets and oral suspension are not bioequivalent and are not substitutable on a mg/mg basis
Continuous arteriovenous or venovenous hemodiafiltration (CAVH) effects: Dose as for Cl_cr 10-20 mL/minute

**Dosage Forms** Cefuroxime sodium: **Inf, premixed (frozen) (Zinacef®):** 750 mg (50 mL), 1.5 g (50 mL); **Powder for inj:** 750 mg, 1.5 g, 7.5 g, Powder for inj (Kefurox®, Zinacef®): 750 mg, 1.5 g, 7.5 g
Cefuroxime axetil: **Powder for oral susp (tutti-frutti flavor) (Ceftin®):** 125 mg/5 mL (50 mL, 100 mL, 200 mL); **Tab (Ceftin®):** 125 mg, 250 mg, 500 mg

**Contraindications** Hypersensitivity to cefuroxime, any component, or cephalosporins

**Warnings/Precautions** Modify dosage in patients with severe renal impairment, prolonged use may result in superinfection; use with caution in patients with a history of penicillin allergy, especially IgE-mediated reactions (eg, anaphylaxis, urticaria); may cause antibiotic-associated colitis or colitis secondary to C. difficile

**Pregnancy Risk Factor** B

**Adverse Reactions**
1% to 10%:
Hematologic: Eosinophilia (7%), decreased hemoglobin and hematocrit (10%)
Hepatic: Increased transaminases (4%), increased alkaline phosphatase (2%)

Local: Thrombophlebitis (1.7%)

<1%: Anaphylaxis, erythema multiforme, toxic epidermal necrolysis, Stevens-Johnson syndrome, interstitial nephritis, dizziness, fever, headache, rash, nausea, vomiting, diarrhea, stomach cramps, GI bleeding, colitis, neutropenia, leukopenia, increased creatinine, increased BUN, pain at injection site, vaginitis, seizures, angioedema, pseudomembranous colitis

Other reactions with cephalosporins include toxic nephropathy, cholestasis, agranulocytosis, colitis, pancytopenia, aplastic anemia, hemolytic anemia, hemorrhage, prolonged PT, encephalopathy, asterixis, neuromuscular excitability, serum-sickness reactions, superinfection

**Drug Interactions**
Increased effect: High-dose probenecid decreases clearance
Increased toxicity: Aminoglycosides increase nephrotoxic potential

**Half-Life** 1-2 hours (prolonged in renal impairment)

**Special PA Issues**
**Patient Education:** Take as directed, at regular intervals around-the-clock (with or without food). Chilling oral suspension improves flavor (do not freeze). Complete full course of medication, even if you feel better. Drink 2-3 L fluid/day. If diarrhea occurs, yogurt or buttermilk may help. May cause false-positive test with Clinitest®; use another form of testing. May interfere with oral contraceptives; additional contraceptive measures are necessary. Report severe, unresolved diarrhea; vaginal itching or drainage; sores in mouth; blood, pus, or mucus in stool or urine; easy bleeding or bruising; unusual fever or chills; rash; or respiratory difficulty.

**Monitoring Parameters:** Observe for signs and symptoms of anaphylaxis during first dose; with prolonged therapy, monitor renal, hepatic, and hematologic function periodically

♦ **Cefuroxime Axetil** *see* Cefuroxime *on previous page*
♦ **Cefuroxime Sodium** *see* Cefuroxime *on previous page*
♦ **Cefzil®** *see* Cefprozil *on page 171*
♦ **Celebrex®** *see* Celecoxib *on this page*

## Celecoxib (ce le COX ib)

**Pharmacologic Class** Sedative, Miscellaneous

**U.S. Brand Names** Celebrex®

**Mechanism of Action** Inhibits prostaglandin synthesis by decreasing the activity of the enzyme, cyclo-oxygenase-2 (COX-2), which results in decreased formation of prostaglandin precursors. Celecoxib does not inhibit cyclo-oxygenase-1 (COX-1) at therapeutic concentrations.

**Use** Relief of the signs and symptoms of osteoarthritis; relief of the signs and symptoms of rheumatoid arthritis in adults

**USUAL DOSAGE** Adults: Oral:
Osteoarthritis: 200 mg/day as a single dose or in divided dose twice daily
Rheumatoid arthritis: 100-200 mg twice daily
**Dosing adjustment in renal impairment:** No specific dosage adjustment is recommended
**Dosing adjustment in hepatic impairment:** Reduced dosage is recommended (AUC may be increased by 40% to 180%)
Dosing adjustment for elderly: No specific adjustment is recommended. However, the AUC in elderly patients may be increased by 50% as compared to younger subjects. Use the lowest recommended dose in patients weighing <50 kg.

**Dosage Forms Cap:** 100 mg, 200 mg

**Contraindications** Hypersensitivity to celecoxib or any component, sulfonamides, aspirin, or other nonsteroidal anti-inflammatory drugs (NSAIDs)

**Warnings/Precautions** Gastrointestinal irritation, ulceration, bleeding, and perforation may occur with NSAIDs (it is unclear whether celecoxib is associated with rates of these events which are similar to nonselective NSAIDs). Use with caution in patients with a history of GI disease (bleeding or ulcers), decreased renal function, hepatic disease, congestive heart failure, hypertension, or asthma. Anaphylactoid reactions may occur, even with no prior exposure to celecoxib. Use caution in patients with known or suspected deficiency of cytochrome P-450 isoenzyme 2C9.

**Pregnancy Risk Factor** C (D after 34 weeks gestation or close to delivery)

**Pregnancy Implications** In late pregnancy may cause premature closure of the ductus arteriosus. In animal studies, celecoxib has been found to be excreted in milk; it is not known whether celecoxib is excreted in human milk. Because many drugs are excreted in milk, and the potential for serious adverse reactions exists, a decision should be made whether to discontinue nursing or discontinue the drug, taking into account the importance of the drug to the mother.

**Adverse Reactions**
>10%: Central nervous system: Headache (15.8%)
2% to 10%:
Cardiovascular: Peripheral edema (2.1%)
Central nervous system: Insomnia (2.3%), dizziness (2%)
(Continued)

177

## Celecoxib *(Continued)*

Dermatologic: Skin rash (2.2%)

Gastrointestinal: Dyspepsia (8.8%), diarrhea (5.6%), abdominal pain (4.1%), nausea (3.5%), flatulence (2.2%)

Neuromuscular & skeletal: Back pain (2.8%)

Respiratory: Upper respiratory tract infection (8.1%), sinusitis (5%), pharyngitis (2.3%), rhinitis (2%)

Miscellaneous: Accidental injury (2.9%)

0.1% to 2%:

Cardiovascular: Hypertension (aggravated), chest pain, myocardial infarction, palpitation, tachycardia, facial edema, peripheral edema

Central nervous system: Migraine, vertigo, hypoesthesia, fatigue, fever, pain, hypotonia, anxiety, depression, nervousness, somnolence

Dermatologic: Alopecia, dermatitis, photosensitivity, pruritus, rash (maculopapular), rash (erythematous), dry skin, urticaria

Endocrine & metabolic: Hot flashes, diabetes mellitus, hyperglycemia, hypercholesterolemia, breast pain, dysmenorrhea, menstrual disturbances, hypokalemia

Gastrointestinal: Constipation, tenesmus, diverticulitis, eructation, esophagitis, gastroenteritis, vomiting, gastroesophageal reflux, hemorrhoids, hiatal hernia, melena, stomatitis, anorexia, increased appetite, taste disturbance, dry mouth, tooth disorder, weight gain

Genitourinary: Prostate disorder, vaginal bleeding, vaginitis, monilial vaginitis, dysuria, cystitis, urinary frequency, incontinence, urinary tract infection,

Hepatic: Elevated transaminases, increased alkaline phosphatase

Hematologic: Anemia, thrombocytopenia, ecchymosis

Neuromuscular & skeletal: Leg cramps, increased CPK, neck stiffness, arthralgia, myalgia, bone disorder, fracture, synovitis, tendonitis, neuralgia, paresthesia, neuropathy, weakness

Ocular: Glaucoma, blurred vision, cataract, conjunctivitis, eye pain

Otic: Deafness, tinnitus, earache, otitis media

Renal: Increased BUN, increased creatinine, albuminuria, hematuria, renal calculi

Respiratory: Bronchitis, bronchospasm, cough, dyspnea, laryngitis, pneumonia, epistaxis

Miscellaneous: Allergic reactions, flu-like syndrome, breast cancer, herpes infection, bacterial infection, moniliasis, viral infection, increased diaphoresis

<0.1% (limited to severe): Congestive heart failure, ventricular fibrillation, pulmonary embolism, syncope, cerebrovascular accident, gangrene, thrombophlebitis, thrombocytopenia, ataxia, acute renal failure, intestinal obstruction, pancreatitis, intestinal perforation, gastrointestinal bleeding, colitis, esophageal perforation, sepsis, sudden death

**Drug Interactions** Celecoxib may be a cytochrome oxidase P-450 isoenzyme 2C9 substrate and an inhibitor of isoenzyme 2D6

Decreased effect: Efficacy of thiazide diuretics, loop diuretics (furosemide), or ACE inhibitors may be diminished by celecoxib; aluminum and magnesium-containing antacids may decrease AUC and $C_{max}$ of celecoxib 10% and 37% respectively

Increased effect: Inhibitors of isoenzyme 2C9 may result in significant increases in celecoxib concentrations. Coadministration of drugs by 2D6 may result in increased serum concentrations of these agents. Fluconazole increases celecoxib concentrations two-fold. Lithium concentrations may be increased by celecoxib. Celecoxib may be used with low-dose aspirin, however rates of gastrointestinal bleeding may be increased with coadministration. Celecoxib has not been shown to alter warfarin effects, although bleeding complications may be increased.

**Half-Life** 11 hours

**Special PA Issues**

Patient Education: Do not take more than recommended dose. May be taken with food to reduce GI upset. Do not take with antacids. Avoid alcohol, aspirin, and OTC medication unless approved by prescriber. You may experience dizziness, confusion, or blurred vision (avoid driving or engaging in tasks that require alertness until response to drug is known); anorexia, nausea, vomiting, taste disturbance, gastric distress (small frequent meals, frequent mouth care, or sucking lozenges may help). GI bleeding, ulceration, or perforation can occur with or without pain; it is unclear whether celecoxib has rates of these events which are similar to nonselective NSAIDs. Stop taking medication and report immediately stomach pain or cramping, unusual bleeding or bruising, or blood in vomitus, stool, or urine. Report persistent insomnia; skin rash; unusual fatigue or easy bruising or bleeding; muscle pain, tremors, or weakness; sudden weight gain; changes in hearing (ringing in ears); changes in vision; changes in urination pattern; or respiratory difficulty.

Dietary Considerations: Peak concentrations are delayed and AUC is increased by 10% to 20% when taken with a high-fat meal; celecoxib may be taken without regard to meals

**Monitoring Parameters:** Periodic LFTs

♦ **Celestone®** *see* Betamethasone *on page 111*
♦ **Celestone® Soluspan®** *see* Betamethasone *on page 111*
♦ **Celexa®** *see* Citalopram *on page 213*
♦ **CellCept®** *see* Mycophenolate *on page 624*

- **Cel-U-Jec®** *see* Betamethasone *on page 111*
- **Cenafed® [OTC]** *see* Pseudoephedrine *on page 780*
- **Cena-K®** *see* Potassium Chloride *on page 742*
- **Cenolate®** *see* Sodium Ascorbate *on page 838*

# Cephalexin (sef a LEKS in)

**Pharmacologic Class** Antibiotic, Cephalosporin (First Generation)

**U.S. Brand Names** Biocef; Keflex®; Keftab®

**Mechanism of Action** Inhibits bacterial cell wall synthesis by binding to one or more of the penicillin-binding proteins (PBPs) which in turn inhibits the final transpeptidation step of peptidoglycan synthesis in bacterial cell walls, thus inhibiting cell wall biosynthesis. Bacteria eventually lyse due to ongoing activity of cell wall autolytic enzymes (autolysins and murein hydrolases) while cell wall assembly is arrested.

**Use** Treatment of susceptible bacterial infections, including those caused by group A beta-hemolytic *Streptococcus, Staphylococcus, Klebsiella pneumoniae, E. coli, Proteus mirabilis,* and *Shigella*; predominantly used for lower respiratory tract, urinary tract, skin and soft tissue, and bone and joint; prophylaxis against bacterial endocarditis in high-risk patients undergoing surgical or dental procedures who are allergic to penicillin

**USUAL DOSAGE** Oral:

Children: 25-50 mg/kg/day every 6 hours; severe infections: 50-100 mg/kg/day in divided doses every 6 hours; maximum: 3 g/24 hours

Adults: 250-1000 mg every 6 hours; maximum: 4 g/day

Prophylaxis of bacterial endocarditis: 2 g 1 hour prior to the procedure

**Dosing adjustment in renal impairment:** Adults:

$Cl_{cr}$ 10-40 mL/minute: 250-500 mg every 8-12 hours

$Cl_{cr}$ <10 mL/minute: 250 mg every 12-24 hours

Hemodialysis: Moderately dialyzable (20% to 50%)

**Dosage Forms**

Cephalexin monohydrate: **Cap:** 250 mg, 500 mg; **Powder, for oral susp:** 125 mg/5 mL (5 mL unit dose, 60 mL, 100 mL, 200 mL), 250 mg/5 mL (5 mL unit dose, 100 mL, 200 mL);

**Susp, oral, pediatric:** 100 mg/mL [5 mg/drop] (10 mL); **Tab:** 250 mg, 500 mg, 1 g;

Cephalexin hydrochloride: **Tab:** 500 mg

**Contraindications** Hypersensitivity to cephalexin, any component, or cephalosporins

**Warnings/Precautions** Modify dosage in patients with severe renal impairment; prolonged use may result in superinfection; use with caution in patients with a history of penicillin allergy, especially IgE-mediated reactions (eg, anaphylaxis, urticaria); may cause antibiotic-associated colitis or colitis secondary to *C. difficile*

**Pregnancy Risk Factor** B

**Adverse Reactions**

1% to 10%: Gastrointestinal: Diarrhea

<1%: Dizziness, fatigue, headache, rash, urticaria, angioedema, anaphylaxis, erythema multiforme, toxic epidermal necrolysis, Stevens-Johnson syndrome, serum-sickness reaction, nausea, vomiting, dyspepsia, gastritis, abdominal pain, pseudomembranous colitis, interstitial nephritis, agitation, hallucinations, confusion, arthralgia, eosinophilia, neutropenia, thrombocytopenia, anemia, increased transaminases, hepatitis, cholestasis

Other reactions with cephalosporins include anaphylaxis, vomiting, agranulocytosis, colitis, pancytopenia, aplastic anemia, hemolytic anemia, hemorrhage, prolonged PT, encephalopathy, asterixis, neuromuscular excitability, seizures, superinfection

**Drug Interactions**

Increased effect: High-dose probenecid decreases clearance

Increased toxicity: Aminoglycosides increase nephrotoxic potential

**Half-Life** 0.5-1.2 hours (prolonged with renal impairment)

**Special PA Issues**

**Patient Education:** Take as directed, at regular intervals around-the-clock (with or without food). Chilling oral suspension improves flavor (do not freeze). Complete full course of medication, even if you feel better. Drink 2-3 L fluid/day. If diarrhea occurs, yogurt or buttermilk may help. May cause false-positive test with Clinitest®; use another form of testing. May interfere with oral contraceptives; additional contraceptive measures are necessary. Report severe, unresolved diarrhea; vaginal itching or drainage; sores in mouth; blood, pus, or mucus in stool or urine; easy bleeding or bruising; unusual fever or chills; rash; or respiratory difficulty.

**Dietary Considerations:** Food: Peak antibiotic serum concentration is lowered and delayed, but total drug absorbed is not affected; take on an empty stomach. If GI distress, take with food.

**Monitoring Parameters:** With prolonged therapy monitor renal, hepatic, and hematologic function periodically; monitor for signs of anaphylaxis during first dose

- **Cephalexin Hydrochloride** *see* Cephalexin *on this page*
- **Cephalexin Monohydrate** *see* Cephalexin *on this page*

# Cephalothin (sef A loe thin)

**Pharmacologic Class** Antibiotic, Cephalosporin (First Generation)

**Mechanism of Action** Inhibits bacterial cell wall synthesis by binding to one or more of the penicillin-binding proteins (PBPs) which in turn inhibits the final transpeptidation step of peptidoglycan synthesis in bacterial cell walls, thus inhibiting cell wall biosynthesis. Bacteria eventually lyse due to ongoing activity of cell wall autolytic enzymes (autolysins and murein hydrolases) while cell wall assembly is arrested.

**Use** Treatment of infections when caused by susceptible strains in respiratory, genitourinary, gastrointestinal, skin and soft tissue, bone and joint infections; septicemia; treatment of susceptible gram-positive bacilli and cocci (never enterococcus); some gram-negative bacilli including *E. coli*, *Proteus*, and *Klebsiella* may be susceptible

**USUAL DOSAGE** I.M., I.V.:

Neonates:

Postnatal age <7 days:

<2000 g: 20 mg every 12 hours

>2000 g: 20 mg every 8 hours

Postnatal age >7 days:

<2000 g: 20 mg every 8 hours

>2000 g: 20 mg every 6 hours

Children: 75-125 mg/kg/day divided every 4-6 hours; maximum dose: 10 g in a 24-hour period

Adults: 500 mg to 2 g every 4-6 hours

**Dosing interval in renal impairment:**

$Cl_{cr}$ 10-50 mL/minute: Administer every 6-8 hours

$Cl_{cr}$ <10 mL/minute: Administer every 12 hours

Continuous arteriovenous or venovenous hemodiafiltration (CAVH) effects: Administer 1 g every 8 hours

**Dosage Forms** Inf, in $D_5W$ (frozen): 1 g (50 mL), 2 g (50 mL); **Powder for inj:** 1 g, 2 g, 20 g

**Contraindications** Hypersensitivity to cephalothin or cephalosporins

**Warnings/Precautions** Modify dosage in patients with severe renal impairment, prolonged use may result in superinfection; use with caution in patients with a history of penicillin allergy, especially IgE-mediated reactions (eg, anaphylaxis, urticaria); may cause antibiotic-associated colitis or colitis secondary to *C. difficile*

**Pregnancy Risk Factor** B

**Adverse Reactions**

1% to 10%: Gastrointestinal: Diarrhea, nausea, vomiting

<1%: Maculopapular and erythematous rash, dyspepsia, pseudomembranous colitis, bleeding, pain and induration at injection site

Other reactions with cephalosporins include anaphylaxis, erythema multiforme, toxic epidermal necrolysis, Stevens-Johnson syndrome, dizziness, fever, headache, CNS irritability, seizures, decreased hemoglobin, neutropenia, leukopenia, agranulocytosis, pancytopenia, aplastic anemia, hemolytic anemia, interstitial nephritis, toxic nephropathy, vaginitis, angioedema, cholestasis, hemorrhage, prolonged PT, serum-sickness reactions, superinfection

**Half-Life** 30-60 minutes; prolonged in renal impairment

**Special PA Issues**

**Monitoring Parameters:** Observe for signs and symptoms of anaphylaxis during first dose

♦ **Cephalothin Sodium** *see* Cephalothin *on this page*

# Cephapirin (sef a PYE rin)

**Pharmacologic Class** Antibiotic, Cephalosporin (First Generation)

**U.S. Brand Names** Cefadyl®

**Mechanism of Action** Inhibits bacterial cell wall synthesis by binding to one or more of the penicillin-binding proteins (PBPs) which in turn inhibits the final transpeptidation step of peptidoglycan synthesis in bacterial cell walls, thus inhibiting cell wall biosynthesis. Bacteria eventually lyse due to ongoing activity of cell wall autolytic enzymes (autolysins and murein hydrolases) while cell wall assembly is arrested.

**Use** Treatment of infections when caused by susceptible strains in respiratory, genitourinary, gastrointestinal, skin and soft tissue, bone and joint infections; septicemia; treatment of susceptible gram-positive bacilli and cocci (never enterococcus); some gram-negative bacilli including *E. coli*, *Proteus*, and *Klebsiella* may be susceptible

**USUAL DOSAGE** I.M., I.V.:

Children: 10-20 mg/kg/dose every 6 hours up to 4 g/24 hours

Adults: 500 mg to 1 g every 6 hours up to 12 g/day

Perioperative prophylaxis: 1-2 g 30 minutes to 1 hour prior to surgery and every 6 hours as needed for 24 hours following

**Dosing interval in renal impairment:**

$Cl_{cr}$ 10-50 mL/minute: Administer every 6-8 hours

$Cl_{cr}$ <10 mL/minute: Administer every 12 hours

Continuous arteriovenous or venovenous hemodiafiltration (CAVH) effects: Administer 1 g every 8 hours

**Dosage Forms** Powder for inj, as sodium: 500 mg, 1 g, 2 g, 4 g, 20 g

**Contraindications** Hypersensitivity to cephapirin sodium, any component, or cephalosporins

**Warnings/Precautions** Modify dosage in patients with severe renal impairment, prolonged use may result in superinfection; use with caution in patients with a history of penicillin allergy, especially IgE-mediated reactions (eg, anaphylaxis, urticaria); may cause antibiotic-associated colitis or colitis secondary to *C. difficile*

**Pregnancy Risk Factor** B

**Adverse Reactions**

1% to 10%: Gastrointestinal: Diarrhea

<1%: CNS irritation, seizures, fever, rash, urticaria, leukopenia, thrombocytopenia, increased transaminases

Other reactions with cephalosporins include anaphylaxis, erythema multiforme, toxic epidermal necrolysis, Stevens-Johnson syndrome, dizziness, fever, headache, encephalopathy, asterixis, neuromuscular excitability, seizures, nausea, vomiting, pseudomembranous colitis, decreased hemoglobin, agranulocytosis, pancytopenia, aplastic anemia, hemolytic anemia, interstitial nephritis, toxic nephropathy, pain at injection site, vaginitis, angioedema, cholestasis, hemorrhage, prolonged PT, serum-sickness reactions, superinfection

**Drug Interactions**

Increased effect: High-dose probenecid decreases clearance

Increased toxicity: Aminoglycosides increase nephrotoxic potential

**Half-Life** 36-60 minutes; prolonged in renal impairment

**Special PA Issues**

Patient Education: This drug is administered I.M. or I.V. Drink 2-3 L fluid/day. If diarrhea occurs, yogurt or buttermilk may help. May cause false-positive test with Clinitest®; use another form of testing. May interfere with oral contraceptives; additional contraceptive measures are necessary. Report severe, unresolved diarrhea; vaginal itching or drainage; sores in mouth; blood, pus, or mucus in stool or urine; easy bleeding or bruising; unusual fever or chills; rash; or respiratory difficulty.

Monitoring Parameters: Observe for signs and symptoms of anaphylaxis during first dose

♦ **Cephapirin Sodium** *see* Cephapirin *on previous page*

# Cephradine (SEF ra deen)

**Pharmacologic Class** Antibiotic, Cephalosporin (First Generation)

**U.S. Brand Names** Velosef®

**Mechanism of Action** Inhibits bacterial cell wall synthesis by binding to one or more of the penicillin-binding proteins (PBPs) which in turn inhibits the final transpeptidation step of peptidoglycan synthesis in bacterial cell walls, thus inhibiting cell wall biosynthesis. Bacteria eventually lyse due to ongoing activity of cell wall autolytic enzymes (autolysins and murein hydrolases) while cell wall assembly is arrested.

**Use** Treatment of infections when caused by susceptible strains in respiratory, genitourinary, gastrointestinal, skin and soft tissue, bone and joint infections; treatment of susceptible gram-positive bacilli and cocci (never enterococcus); some gram-negative bacilli including *E. coli*, *Proteus*, and *Klebsiella* may be susceptible

**USUAL DOSAGE** Oral:

Children ≥9 months: 25-50 mg/kg/day in divided doses every 6 hours

Adults: 250-500 mg every 6-12 hours

Dosing adjustment in renal impairment: Adults:

$Cl_{cr}$ 10-50 mL/minute: 250 mg every 6 hours

$Cl_{cr}$ <10 mL/minute: 125 mg every 6 hours

**Dosage Forms** Cap: 250 mg, 500 mg; **Powder for inj:** 250 mg, 500 mg, 1 g, 2 g (in ready to use infusion bottles); **Powder for oral susp:** 125 mg/5 mL (5 mL, 100 mL, 200 mL), 250 mg/5 mL (5 mL, 100 mL, 200 mL)

**Contraindications** Hypersensitivity to cephradine, any component, or cephalosporins

**Warnings/Precautions** Modify dosage in patients with severe renal impairment, prolonged use may result in superinfection; use with caution in patients with a history of penicillin allergy, especially IgE-mediated reactions (eg, anaphylaxis, urticaria); may cause antibiotic-associated colitis or colitis secondary to *C. difficile*

**Pregnancy Risk Factor** B

**Adverse Reactions**

1% to 10%: Gastrointestinal: Diarrhea

<1%: Rash, nausea, vomiting, pseudomembranous colitis, increased BUN, increased creatinine

(Continued)

## Cephradine (Continued)

Other reactions with cephalosporins include anaphylaxis, erythema multiforme, toxic epidermal necrolysis, Stevens-Johnson syndrome, dizziness, fever, headache, encephalopathy, asterixis, neuromuscular excitability, seizures, neutropenia, leukopenia, agranulocytosis, pancytopenia, aplastic anemia, hemolytic anemia, interstitial nephritis, toxic nephropathy, vaginitis, angioedema, cholestasis, hemorrhage, prolonged PT, serum-sickness reactions, superinfection

**Drug Interactions**
Increased effect: High-dose probenecid decreases clearance
Increased toxicity: Aminoglycosides increase nephrotoxic potential

**Half-Life** 1-2 hours; prolonged in renal impairment

**Special PA Issues**
**Patient Education:** Oral: Take as directed, at regular intervals around-the-clock (with or without food). Chilling oral suspension improves flavor (do not freeze). Complete full course of medication, even if you feel better. Drink 2-3 L fluid/day. If diarrhea occurs, yogurt or buttermilk may help. May cause false-positive test with Clinitest®; use another form of testing. May interfere with oral contraceptives; additional contraceptive measures are necessary. Report severe, unresolved diarrhea; vaginal itching or drainage; sores in mouth; blood, pus, or mucus in stool or urine; easy bleeding or bruising; unusual fever or chills; rash; or respiratory difficulty.

**Monitoring Parameters:** Observe for signs and symptoms of anaphylaxis during first dose

♦ **Cephulac®** see Lactulose on page 512

♦ **Ceptaz™** see Ceftazidime on page 172

♦ **Ceptaz™** see Ceftazidime on page 172

♦ **Ceredase®** see Alglucerase on page 41

♦ **Cerezyme®** see Alglucerase on page 41

## Cerivastatin (se ree va STAT in)

**Pharmacologic Class** Antilipemic Agent (HMG-CoA Reductase Inhibitor)

**U.S. Brand Names** Baycol™

**Mechanism of Action** As an HMG-CoA reductase inhibitor, cerivastatin competitively inhibits 3-hydroxyl-3-methylglutaryl coenzyme A (HMG-CoA) reductase, the enzyme that catalyzes the rate-limiting step in cholesterol biosynthesis

**Use** Adjunct to dietary therapy to for the reduction of elevated total and LDL cholesterol levels in patients with primary hypercholesterolemia and mixed dyslipidemia when the response to dietary restriction of saturated fat and cholesterol and other nonpharmacological measures alone has been inadequate

**USUAL DOSAGE** Adults: Oral: 0.3 mg once daily in the evening; may be taken with or without food

**Dosing adjustment with renal impairment:** Moderate to severe impairment (<60 mL/minute): Starting dose: 0.2 mg

**Dosing adjustment in hepatic impairment:** Avoidance suggested; no guidelines for dosage reduction available

**Dosage Forms Tab, as sodium:** 0.2 mg, 0.3 mg

**Contraindications** Hypersensitivity or severe adverse reactions to cerivastatin or other statins; active hepatic disease, pregnancy

**Warnings/Precautions** Use with caution in patients with history of liver disease, those who are breast-feeding, and those predisposed to renal failure

**Pregnancy Risk Factor** X

**Pregnancy Implications** Enters breast milk/contraindicated

**Adverse Reactions**
1% to 10%:
Cardiovascular: Chest pain, peripheral edema (2%)
Central nervous system: Headache, dizziness, insomnia, asthenia (2%)
Gastrointestinal: Pain (3%), diarrhea (4%), dyspepsia (6%), nausea (3%), constipation (2%)
Neuromuscular & skeletal: Myalgia (3%), arthralgia (7%), leg pain (2%)
<1%: Increased LFTs, myopathy, possible rhabdomyolysis with renal failure, sinusitis, rhinitis, cough

**Drug Interactions** CYP3A3/4 enzyme substrate
Concurrent therapy with cyclosporine, fibric acid derivative, erythromycin, azole antifungals, and niacin may increase risk of myopathy/rhabdomyolysis with renal failure
Decreased effect of cerivastatin with cholestyramine
Increased cerivastatin with erythromycin

**Onset** Maximal reductions in ~2 weeks

**Half-Life** 2-3 hours

**Special PA Issues**
**Patient Education:** Take prescribed dose in the evening (with or without food). You will need laboratory evaluation during therapy. Maintain adequate hydration (2-3 L/day of fluids unless instructed to restrict fluid intake). May cause headache (mild analgesic may help); drowsiness, dizziness, or blurred vision (use caution when driving or engaging in tasks that require alertness until response to medication is known). Report chest pain; swelling of extremities; weight gain (>5 lb/week); respiratory difficulty; persistent vomiting or abdominal pain; muscle weakness or pain; persistent cough; swelling of mouth, lips, or face; unusual bruising or bleeding; or skin rash.
**Monitoring Parameters:** Serum total cholesterol, LDL, HDL, triglycerides, apolipoprotein B, diet, weight, LFTs
**Related Information**
Lipid-Lowering Agents *on page 1022*

♦ **Cerivastatin Sodium** *see* Cerivastatin *on previous page*
♦ **Cerumenex® Otic** *see* Triethanolamine Polypeptide Oleate-Condensate *on page 933*
♦ **Cervidil® Vaginal Insert** *see* Dinoprostone *on page 288*
♦ **C.E.S.™** *see* Estrogens, Conjugated *on page 335*
♦ **C.E.S.** *see* Estrogens, Conjugated *on page 335*
♦ **Cetacaine®** *see* Benzocaine, Butyl Aminobenzoate, Tetracaine, and Benzalkonium Chloride *on page 106*
♦ **Cetacort®** *see* Hydrocortisone *on page 453*
♦ **Cetamide® Ophthalmic** *see* Sulfacetamide Sodium *on page 858*
♦ **Cetapred® Ophthalmic** *see* Sulfacetamide Sodium and Prednisolone *on page 859*

## Cetirizine (se TI ra zeen)
**Pharmacologic Class** Antihistamine
**U.S. Brand Names** Zyrtec®
**Mechanism of Action** Competes with histamine for $H_1$-receptor sites on effector cells in the gastrointestinal tract, blood vessels, and respiratory tract
**Use** Perennial and seasonal allergic rhinitis and other allergic symptoms including urticaria
**USUAL DOSAGE** Children ≥6 years and Adults: Oral: 5-10 mg once daily, depending upon symptom severity
**Dosing interval in renal/hepatic impairment:** $Cl_{cr}$ ≤31 mL/minute: Administer 5 mg once daily
**Dosage Forms** Cetirizine hydrochloride: **Syr:** 5 mg/5 mL (120 mL); **Tab:** 5 mg, 10 mg
**Contraindications** Hypersensitivity to cetirizine, hydroxyzine, or any component
**Warnings/Precautions** Cetirizine should be used cautiously in patients with hepatic or renal dysfunction, the elderly and in nursing mothers. Doses >10 mg/day may cause significant drowsiness
**Pregnancy Risk Factor** B
**Pregnancy Implications** Enters breast milk/not recommended
**Adverse Reactions**
>10%: Central nervous system: Headache has been reported to occur in 10% to 12% of patients, drowsiness has been reported in as much as 26% of patients on high doses
1% to 10%:
Central nervous system: Somnolence, fatigue, dizziness
Gastrointestinal: Xerostomia
<1%: Depression
**Drug Interactions** Increased toxicity: CNS depressants, anticholinergics
**Onset** Within 15-30 minutes
**Half-Life** 8-11 hours
**Special PA Issues**
**Patient Education:** Take as directed; do not exceed recommended dose. Avoid use of other depressants, alcohol, or sleep-inducing medications unless approved by prescriber. You may experience drowsiness or dizziness (use caution when driving or engaging in hazardous activity until response to medication is known); or dry mouth, (frequent small meals, frequent mouth care, chewing gum, or sucking hard candy may help). Report persistent sedation, confusion, or agitation; persistent nausea or vomiting; changes in urinary pattern; blurred vision; chest pain or palpitations; or lack of improvement or worsening or condition.
**Monitoring Parameters:** Relief of symptoms, sedation and anticholinergic effects

♦ **Cetirizine Hydrochloride** *see* Cetirizine *on this page*
♦ **Cevalin® [OTC]** *see* Ascorbic Acid *on page 79*
♦ **Cevi-Bid® [OTC]** *see* Ascorbic Acid *on page 79*
♦ **Ce-Vi-Sol® [OTC]** *see* Ascorbic Acid *on page 79*
♦ **CFDN** *see* Cefdinir *on page 161*
♦ **CG** *see* Chorionic Gonadotropin *on page 205*

## Chamomile

**Mechanism of Action** Pharmacologic activities include antispasmodic, anti-inflammatory, antiulcer, and antibacterial effects; a sedative effect has also been documented

**Use** Has been used for indigestion and its hypnotic properties; topical anti-inflammatory agent; used for hemorrhoids, irritable bowel, eczema, mastitis and leg ulcers; used to flavor cigarette tobacco

**USUAL DOSAGE**

Tea: ±150 mL $H_2O$ poured over heaping tablespoon (±3 g) of chamomile, covered and steeped 5-10 minutes; tea used 3-4 times/day for G.I. upset

Liquid extract: 1-4 mL 3 times/day

**Contraindications** Known hypersensitivity to *Asteraceae/Compositae* family

**Warnings/Precautions** Use with caution in asthmatics; cross sensitivity may occur in individuals allergic to ragweed pollens, asters, or chrysanthemums

**Pregnancy Implications** Excessive use should be avoided due to potential teratogenicity

**Adverse Reactions**

Dermatologic: Contact dermatitis, immunologic contact urticaria

Gastrointestinal: Emesis (from dried flowering heads)

Miscellaneous: Anaphylaxis

While the toxicity of its main chemical constituent (Bisabolol) is low, the tea is essentially prepared from various allergens (ie, pollen-laden flower heads) which can cause hypersensitivity reactions especially in atopic individuals; contains various flavonoids (apigenin, herniarin)

**Drug Interactions** May increase effect of coumarin-type anticoagulants at high dosages

♦ **Charcoaid® [OTC]** *see* Charcoal *on this page*

## Charcoal (CHAR kole)

**Pharmacologic Class** Antidiarrheal; Antidote; Antiflatulent

**U.S. Brand Names** Actidose-Aqua® [OTC]; Actidose® With Sorbitol [OTC]; Charcoaid® [OTC]; Charcocaps® [OTC]; Insta-Char® [OTC]; Liqui-Char® [OTC]

**Mechanism of Action** Adsorbs toxic substances or irritants, thus inhibiting GI absorption; adsorbs intestinal gas; the addition of sorbitol results in hyperosmotic laxative action causing catharsis

**Use** Emergency treatment in poisoning by drugs and chemicals; repetitive doses for gastric dialysis in uremia to adsorb various waste products, and repetitive doses have proven useful to enhance the elimination of certain drugs (eg, theophylline, phenobarbital, and aspirin)

**USUAL DOSAGE** Oral:

Acute poisoning:

Charcoal with sorbitol: Single-dose:

Children 1-12 years: 1-2 g/kg/dose or 15-30 g or approximately 5-10 times the weight of the ingested poison; 1 g adsorbs 100-1000 mg of poison; the use of repeat oral charcoal with sorbitol doses is not recommended. In young children, sorbitol should be repeated no more than 1-2 times/day.

Adults: 30-100 g

Charcoal in water:

Single-dose:

Infants <1 year: 1 g/kg

Children 1-12 years: 15-30 g or 1-2 g/kg

Adults: 30-100 g or 1-2 g/kg

Multiple-dose:

Infants <1 year: 0.5 g/kg every 4-6 hours

Children 1-12 years: 20-60 g or 0.5-1 g/kg every 2-6 hours until clinical observations, serum drug concentration have returned to a subtherapeutic range, or charcoal stool apparent

Adults: 20-60 g or 0.5-1 g/kg every 2-6 hours

Gastric dialysis: Adults: 20-50 g every 6 hours for 1-2 days

Intestinal gas, diarrhea, GI distress: Adults: 520-975 mg after meals or at first sign of discomfort; repeat as needed to a maximum dose of 4.16 g/day

**Dosage Forms Cap (Charcocaps®):** 260 mg; **Liq, activated:** Actidose-Aqua®: 12.5 g (60 mL), 25 g (120 mL), Liqui-Char®: 12.5 g (60 mL), 15 g (75 mL), 25 g (120 mL), 30 g (120 mL), 50 g (240 mL), SuperChar®: 30 g (240 mL); **Liq, activated, with propylene glycol:** 12.5 g (60 mL), 25 g (120 mL); **Liq, activated, with sorbitol:** Actidose® With Sorbitol: 25 g (120 mL); 50 g (240 mL), Charcoaid®: 30 g (150 mL); **Powder for susp, activated:** 15 g, 30 g, 40 g, 120 g, 240 g

**Contraindications** Not effective for cyanide, mineral acids, caustic alkalis, organic solvents, iron, ethanol, methanol poisoning, lithium; do not use charcoal with sorbitol in patients with fructose intolerance; charcoal with sorbitol is not recommended in children <1 year.

**Warnings/Precautions** When using ipecac with charcoal, induce vomiting with ipecac before administering activated charcoal since charcoal adsorbs ipecac syrup; charcoal may cause vomiting which is hazardous in petroleum distillate and caustic ingestions; if charcoal in sorbitol is administered, doses should be limited to prevent excessive fluid and electrolyte losses; do not mix charcoal with milk, ice cream, or sherbet

**Pregnancy Risk Factor** C

**Pregnancy Implications** Does not enter breast milk/compatible

**Adverse Reactions**

>10%:
Gastrointestinal: Vomiting, diarrhea with sorbitol, constipation
Miscellaneous: Stools will turn black

<1%: Swelling of abdomen

**Drug Interactions** Do not administer concomitantly with syrup of ipecac; do not mix with milk, ice cream, or sherbet

**Special PA Issues**

Patient Education: Charcoal will cause your stools to turn black. Do not self-administer as an antidote before calling the poison control center, hospital emergency room, or physician for instructions (charcoal is not the antidote for all poisons).

♦ **Charcocaps® [OTC]** see Charcoal on previous page
♦ **Chealamide®** see Edetate Disodium on page 312
♦ **Chelated Manganese® [OTC]** see Manganese on page 556
♦ **Chenix®** see Chenodiol on this page
♦ **Chenodeoxycholic Acid** see Chenodiol on this page

# Chenodiol (kee noe DYE ole)

**Pharmacologic Class** Bile Acid

**U.S. Brand Names** Chenix®

**Mechanism of Action** Chenodiol is a primary acid excreted into bile, normally constituting one-third of the total biliary bile acids. Synthesis of chenodiol is regulated by the relative composition and flux of cholesterol and bile acids through the hepatocyte by a negative feedback effect on the rate-limiting enzymes for synthesis of cholesterol (HMG CoA reductase) and bile acids (cholesterol 7 alpha-hydroxyl).

**Use** Oral dissolution of cholesterol gallstones in selected patients

**USUAL DOSAGE** Adults: Oral: 13-16 mg/kg/day in 2 divided doses, starting with 250 mg twice daily the first 2 weeks and increasing by 250 mg/day each week thereafter until the recommended or maximum tolerated dose is achieved

Dosing comments in hepatic impairment: Contraindicated for use in presence of known hepatocyte dysfunction or bile ductal abnormalities

**Dosage Forms** Tab, film coated: 250 mg

**Contraindications** Presence of known hepatocyte dysfunction or bile ductal abnormalities; a gallbladder confirmed as nonvisualizing after two consecutive single doses of dye; radiopaque stones; gallstone complications or compelling reasons for gallbladder surgery; inflammatory bowel disease or active gastric or duodenal ulcer; pregnancy

**Warnings/Precautions** Chenodiol is hepatotoxic in animal models including subhuman Primates; chenodiol should be discontinued if aminotransferases exceed 3 times the upper normal limit; chenodiol may contribute to colon cancer in otherwise susceptible individuals

**Pregnancy Risk Factor** X

**Pregnancy Implications** Excretion in breast milk unknown/not recommended

**Adverse Reactions**

>10%:
Gastrointestinal: Diarrhea (mild), biliary pain
Miscellaneous: Aminotransferase increases

1% to 10%:
Endocrine & metabolic: Increases in cholesterol and LDL cholesterol
Gastrointestinal: Dyspepsia

<1%: Diarrhea (severe), cramps, nausea, vomiting, flatulence, constipation, leukopenia, intrahepatic cholestasis, higher cholecystectomy rates

**Drug Interactions** Decreased effect: Antacids, cholestyramine, colestipol, oral contraceptives

**Special PA Issues**

Patient Education: Take as directed, for entire length of therapy. Medication may need to be taken for 24 months before dissolution will occur. Avoid aluminum-based antacids during entire course of therapy. Blood studies and x-rays studies will be necessary during therapy. Report persistent diarrhea and gallstone attacks (abdominal pain, nausea and vomiting, yellowing of skin or eyes).

Monitoring Parameters: Oral cholecystograms and/or ultrasonograms should be used to monitor response; dissolutions of stones should be confirmed 1-3 months later

♦ **Cheracol®** see Guaifenesin and Codeine on page 428
♦ **Cheracol® D [OTC]** see Guaifenesin and Dextromethorphan on page 428
♦ **Chibroxin™ Ophthalmic** see Norfloxacin on page 664
♦ **Chigger-Tox® [OTC]** see Benzocaine on page 105
♦ **Children's Advil® Oral Suspension [OTC]** see Ibuprofen on page 466

- **Children's Motrin® Oral Suspension [OTC]** *see* Ibuprofen *on page 466*
- **Children's Silapap® [OTC]** *see* Acetaminophen *on page 21*
- **Children's Silfedrine® [OTC]** *see* Pseudoephedrine *on page 780*
- **Children's Vitamins** *see* Vitamins, Multiple *on page 964*
- **Chloral** *see* Chloral Hydrate *on this page*

## Chloral Hydrate (KLOR al HYE drate)

**Pharmacologic Class** Hypnotic, Miscellaneous

**U.S. Brand Names** Aquachloral® Supprettes®

**Mechanism of Action** Central nervous system depressant effects are due to its active metabolite trichloroethanol, mechanism unknown

**Use** Short-term sedative and hypnotic (<2 weeks), sedative/hypnotic for dental and diagnostic procedures; sedative prior to EEG evaluations

**USUAL DOSAGE**

Children:

Sedation, anxiety: Oral, rectal: 5-15 mg/kg/dose every 8 hours, maximum: 500 mg/dose

Prior to EEG: Oral, rectal: 20-25 mg/kg/dose, 30-60 minutes prior to EEG; may repeat in 30 minutes to maximum of 100 mg/kg or 2 g total

Hypnotic: Oral, rectal: 20-40 mg/kg/dose up to a maximum of 50 mg/kg/24 hours or 1 g/dose or 2 g/24 hours

Sedation, nonpainful procedure: Oral: 50-75 mg/kg/dose 30-60 minutes prior to procedure; may repeat 30 minutes after initial dose if needed, to a total maximum dose of 120 mg/kg or 1 g total

Adults: Oral, rectal:

Sedation, anxiety: 250 mg 3 times/day

Hypnotic: 500-1000 mg at bedtime or 30 minutes prior to procedure, not to exceed 2 g/24 hours

**Dosing adjustment/comments in renal impairment:** $Cl_{cr}$ <50 mL/minute: Avoid use

Hemodialysis: Dialyzable (50% to 100%); supplemental dose is not necessary

**Dosing adjustment/comments in hepatic impairment:** Avoid use in patients with severe hepatic impairment

**Dosage Forms Supp, rectal:** 324 mg, 500 mg, 648 mg; **Syr:** 250 mg/5 mL (10 mL), 500 mg/5 mL (5 mL, 10 mL, 480 mL)

**Contraindications** Hypersensitivity to chloral hydrate or any component; hepatic or renal impairment; gastritis or ulcers; severe cardiac disease

**Warnings/Precautions** Use with caution in patients with porphyria; use with caution in neonates, drug may accumulate with repeated use, prolonged use in neonates associated with hyperbilirubinemia; tolerance to hypnotic effect develops, therefore, not recommended for use >2 weeks; taper dosage to avoid withdrawal with prolonged use; trichloroethanol (TCE), a metabolite of chloral hydrate, is a carcinogen in mice; there is no data in humans. Chloral hydrate is considered a second line hypnotic agent in the elderly. Recent interpretive guidelines from the Health Care Financing Administration (HCFA) discourage the use of chloral hydrate in residents of long-term care facilities.

**Pregnancy Risk Factor** C

**Adverse Reactions**

>10%: Gastrointestinal: Gastric irritation, nausea, vomiting, diarrhea

1% to 10%:

Central nervous system: Ataxia, hallucinations, drowsiness, "hangover" effect

Dermatologic: Rash, urticaria

<1%: Disorientation, sedation, ataxia, excitement (paradoxical), dizziness, fever, headache, confusion, flatulence, leukopenia, eosinophilia, physical and psychological dependence may occur with prolonged use of large doses

**Drug Interactions** Increased toxicity: May potentiate effects of warfarin, central nervous system depressants, alcohol; vasodilation reaction (flushing, tachycardia, etc) may occur with concurrent use of alcohol; concomitant use of furosemide (I.V.) may result in flushing, diaphoresis, and blood pressure changes

**Duration** 4-8 hours

**Half-Life** Active metabolite: 8-11 hours

**Special PA Issues**

**Patient Education:** Use exactly as directed (do not increase dose or frequency or discontinue without consulting prescriber); may cause physical and/or psychological dependence. While using this medication, do not use alcohol and other prescription or OTC medications (especially, pain medications, sedatives, antihistamines, or hypnotics) without consulting prescriber. Maintain adequate hydration (2-3 L/day of fluids unless instructed to restrict fluid intake). You may experience drowsiness, dizziness, or blurred vision (use caution when driving or engaging in hazardous tasks); nausea, vomiting, unpleasant taste (small frequent meals, good mouth care, chewing gum, or sucking lozenges may help); diarrhea (buttermilk, boiled milk, yogurt may help). Report skin rash or irritation, CNS changes (confusion, depression, increased sedation, excitation, headache, insomnia, or nightmares), unresolved gastrointestinal distress, chest pain or palpitations, or ineffectiveness of medication.

**Dietary Considerations:** Alcohol: Additive CNS effects, avoid use
**Monitoring Parameters:** Vital signs, $O_2$ saturation and blood pressure with doses used for conscious sedation

# Chlorambucil (klor AM byoo sil)
**Pharmacologic Class** Antineoplastic Agent, Alkylating Agent
**U.S. Brand Names** Leukeran®
**Mechanism of Action** Interferes with DNA replication and RNA transcription by alkylation and cross-linking the strands of DNA
**Use** Management of chronic lymphocytic leukemia, Hodgkin's and non-Hodgkin's lymphoma; breast and ovarian carcinoma; Waldenström's macroglobulinemia, testicular carcinoma, thrombocythemia, choriocarcinoma
**USUAL DOSAGE** Oral (refer to individual protocols):
Children:
General short courses: 0.1-0.2 mg/kg/day OR 4.5 mg/m²/day for 3-6 weeks for remission induction (usual: 4-10 mg/day); maintenance therapy: 0.03-0.1 mg/kg/day (usual: 2-4 mg/day)
Nephrotic syndrome: 0.1-0.2 mg/kg/day every day for 5-15 weeks with low-dose prednisone
Chronic lymphocytic leukemia (CLL):
Biweekly regimen: Initial: 0.4 mg/kg/dose every 2 weeks; increase dose by 0.1 mg/kg every 2 weeks until a response occurs and/or myelosuppression occurs
Monthly regimen: Initial: 0.4 mg/kg, increase dose by 0.2 mg/kg every 4 weeks until a response occurs and/or myelosuppression occurs
Malignant lymphomas:
Non-Hodgkin's lymphoma: 0.1 mg/kg/day
Hodgkin's lymphoma: 0.2 mg/kg/day
Adults: 0.1-0.2 mg/kg/day OR 3-6 mg/m²/day for 3-6 weeks, then adjust dose on basis of blood counts. Pulse dosing has been used in CLL as intermittent, biweekly, or monthly doses of 0.4 mg/kg and increased by 0.1 mg/kg until the disease is under control or toxicity ensues. An alternate regimen is 14 mg/m²/day for 5 days, repeated every 21-28 days.
Hemodialysis: Supplemental dosing is not necessary
Peritoneal dialysis: Supplemental dosing is not necessary
**Dosage Forms** Tab, sugar coated: 2 mg
**Contraindications** Previous resistance; hypersensitivity to chlorambucil or any component or other alkylating agents
**Warnings/Precautions** The U.S. Food and Drug Administration (FDA) currently recommends that procedures for proper handling and disposal of antineoplastic agents be considered. Use with caution in patients with seizure disorder and bone marrow suppression; reduce initial dosage if patient has received radiation therapy, myelosuppressive drugs or has a depressed baseline leukocyte or platelet count within the previous 4 weeks. Can severely suppress bone marrow function; affects human fertility; carcinogenic in humans and probably mutagenic and teratogenic as well; chromosomal damage has been documented; secondary AML may be associated with chronic therapy.
**Pregnancy Risk Factor** D
**Pregnancy Implications** Clinical effects on the fetus: Carcinogenic and mutagenic in humans
**Adverse Reactions**
>10%:
Hematologic: Myelosuppressive: Use with caution when receiving radiation; bone marrow suppression frequently occurs and occasionally bone marrow failure has occurred; blood counts should be monitored closely while undergoing treatment; leukopenia, thrombocytopenia, anemia
WBC: Moderate
Platelets: Moderate
Onset (days): 7
Nadir (days): 10-14
Recovery (days): 28
1% to 10%:
Dermatologic: Skin rashes
Endocrine & metabolic: Hyperuricemia, menstrual changes
Gastrointestinal: Nausea, vomiting, diarrhea, oral ulceration are all infrequent
Emetic potential: Low (<10%)
<1%: Confusion, agitation, drug fever, ataxia, hallucination; rarely generalized or focal seizures, rash, fertility impairment: Has caused chromosomal damage in men, both reversible and permanent sterility have occurred in both sexes; can produce amenorrhea in females, oral ulceration, oligospermia, hepatotoxicity, hepatic necrosis, weakness, tremors, muscular twitching, peripheral neuropathy, pulmonary fibrosis, secondary malignancies; Increased incidence of AML; skin hypersensitivity
**Duration** ~4 weeks
**Half-Life** 90 minutes to 2 hours
(Continued)

# Chlorambucil *(Continued)*

## Special PA Issues

**Patient Education:** Take exactly as directed (may be taken with chilled liquids). Maintain adequate hydration (2-3 L/day of fluids unless instructed to restrict fluid intake). Avoid alcohol, acidic, spicy, or hot foods, aspirin, or OTC medications unless approved by prescriber. Hair may be lost during treatment (reversible). You may experience menstrual irregularities and/or sterility. You will be more susceptible to infection; avoid crowds and exposure to infection. Frequent mouth care with soft toothbrush or cotton swab may reduce occurrence of mouth sores. Report easy bruising or bleeding; fever or chills; numbness, pain, or tingling of extremities; muscle cramping or weakness; unusual swelling of extremities; menstrual irregularities; or any difficulty breathing.

**Monitoring Parameters:** Liver function tests, CBC, leukocyte counts, platelets, serum uric acid

# Chloramphenicol *(klor am FEN i kole)*

**Pharmacologic Class** Antibiotic, Ophthalmic; Antibiotic, Otic; Antibiotic, Miscellaneous

**U.S. Brand Names** AK-Chlor® Ophthalmic; Chloromycetin®; Chloroptic® Ophthalmic

**Mechanism of Action** Reversibly binds to 50S ribosomal subunits of susceptible organisms preventing amino acids from being transferred to growing peptide chains thus inhibiting protein synthesis

**Use** Treatment of serious infections due to organisms resistant to other less toxic antibiotics or when its penetrability into the site of infection is clinically superior to other antibiotics to which the organism is sensitive; useful in infections caused by *Bacteroides*, *H. influenzae*, *Neisseria meningitidis*, *Salmonella*, and *Rickettsia*; active against many vancomycin-resistant enterococci

## USUAL DOSAGE

Meningitis: I.V.: Infants >30 days and Children: 50-100 mg/kg/day divided every 6 hours

Other infections: I.V.:

Infants >30 days and Children: 50-75 mg/kg/day divided every 6 hours; maximum daily dose: 4 g/day

Adults: 50-100 mg/kg/day in divided doses every 6 hours; maximum daily dose: 4 g/day

Ophthalmic: Children and Adults: Instill 1-2 drops or 1.25 cm (½" of ointment every 3-4 hours); increase interval between applications after 48 hours to 2-3 times/day

Otic solution: Instill 2-3 drops into ear 3 times/day

Topical: Gently rub into the affected area 1-4 times/day

**Dosing adjustment/comments in hepatic impairment:** Avoid use in severe liver impairment as increased toxicity may occur

Hemodialysis: Slightly dialyzable (5% to 20%) via hemo- and peritoneal dialysis; no supplemental doses needed in dialysis or continuous arteriovenous or veno-venous hemofiltration (CAVH/CAVHD)

**Dosage Forms Cap:** 250 mg, **Oint, ophth:** 1% [10 mg/g] (3.5 g), AK-Chlor®, Chloromycetin®, Chloroptic® S.O.P.®: 1% [10 mg/g] (3.5 g); **Powder for inj, as sodium succinate:** 1 g; **Powder for ophth soln (Chloromycetin®):** 25 mg/vial (15 mL); **Soln:** 0.5% [5 mg/mL] (7.5 mL, 15 mL), **Ophth (AK-Chlor®, Chloroptic®):** 0.5% [5 mg/mL] (2.5 mL, 7.5 mL, 15 mL), **Otic (Chloromycetin®):** 0.5% (15 mL)

**Contraindications** Hypersensitivity to chloramphenicol or any component

**Warnings/Precautions** Use with caution in patients with impaired renal or hepatic function and in neonates; reduce dose with impaired liver function; use with care in patients with glucose 6-phosphate dehydrogenase deficiency. Serious and fatal blood dyscrasias have occurred after both short-term and prolonged therapy; should not be used when less potentially toxic agents are effective; prolonged use may result in superinfection.

**Pregnancy Risk Factor** C

**Adverse Reactions** <1%: Nightmares, headache, rash, diarrhea, stomatitis, enterocolitis, nausea, vomiting, bone marrow suppression, aplastic anemia, peripheral neuropathy, optic neuritis, gray syndrome

### Three (3) major toxicities associated with chloramphenicol include:

Aplastic anemia, an idiosyncratic reaction which can occur with any route of administration; usually occurs 3 weeks to 12 months after initial exposure to chloramphenicol

Bone marrow suppression is thought to be dose-related with serum concentrations >25 µg/mL and reversible once chloramphenicol is discontinued; anemia and neutropenia may occur during the first week of therapy

Gray syndrome is characterized by circulatory collapse, cyanosis, acidosis, abdominal distention, myocardial depression, coma, and death; reaction appears to be associated with serum levels ≥50 µg/mL; may result from drug accumulation in patients with impaired hepatic or renal function

**Drug Interactions** CYP2C9 enzyme inhibitor

Decreased effect: Phenobarbital and rifampin may decrease concentration of chloramphenicol

Increased toxicity: Chloramphenicol inhibits the metabolism of chlorpropamide, phenytoin, oral anticoagulants

**Half-Life** Prolonged with markedly reduced liver function or combined liver/kidney dysfunction; Normal renal function: 1.6-3.3 hours; End-stage renal disease: 3-7 hours; Cirrhosis: 10-12 hours

**Special PA Issues**

**Patient Education:**

Oral: Take as directed, at regular intervals around-the-clock, with a large glass of water. Maintain adequate hydration (2-3 L/day of fluids unless instructed to restrict fluid intake). During I.V. administration, a bitter taste may occur; this will pass. Diabetics: Drug may cause false-positive test with Clinitest® glucose monitoring; use alternative glucose monitoring. This drug may interfere with effectiveness of oral contraceptives. You may experience nausea, vomiting (frequent small meals, frequent mouth care, or sucking on lozenges may help). Report persistent rash, diarrhea; pain, burning, or numbness of extremities; petechiae; sore throat; fatigue; unusual bleeding or bruising; vaginal itching or discharge; mouth sores; yellowing of skin or eyes; dark urine or pale stool; CNS disturbances (nightmares acute headache); or lack or improvement or worsening of condition.

Ophthalmic: Wash hands before instilling. Sit or lie down to instill. Open eye, look at ceiling, and instill prescribed amount of medication. Close eye and apply gentle pressure to inner corner of eye. Do not let tip of applicator touch eye or contaminate tip of applicator. Temporary stinging or burning may occur. Report persistent pain, burning, vision disturbances, swelling, itching, rash, or worsening of condition.

Otic: Wash hands before instilling. Tilt head with affected ear upward. Gently grasp ear lobe and lift back and upward. Instill prescribed drops into ear canal. Do not push dropper into ear. Remain with head tilted for 2 minutes. Report ringing in ears, discharge, or worsening of condition.

Topical: Wash hands before applying or wear gloves. Apply thin film to affected area. May apply porous dressing. Report persistent burning, swelling, itching, or worsening of condition.

**Dietary Considerations:** Folic acid, iron salts, vitamin $B_{12}$: May decrease intestinal absorption of vitamin $B_{12}$; may have increased dietary need for riboflavin, pyridoxine, and vitamin $B_{12}$; monitor hematological status

**Monitoring Parameters:** CBC with reticulocyte and platelet counts, periodic liver and renal function tests, serum drug concentration

**Reference Range:**
Therapeutic levels: 15-20 µg/mL; Toxic concentration: >40 µg/mL; Trough: 5-10 µg/mL
Timing of serum samples: Draw levels 1.5 hours and 3 hours after completion of I.V. or oral dose; trough levels may be preferred; should be drawn ≤1 hour prior to dose

# Chloramphenicol and Prednisolone (klor am FEN i kole & pred NIS oh lone)
**Pharmacologic Class** Antibiotic/Corticosteroid, Ophthalmic
**U.S. Brand Names** Chloroptic-P® Ophthalmic
**Dosage Forms Oint, ophth:** Chloramphenicol 1% and prednisolone 0.5% (3.5 g)

# Chloramphenicol, Polymyxin B, and Hydrocortisone (klor am FEN i kole, pol i MIKS in bee, & hye droe KOR ti sone)
**Pharmacologic Class** Antibiotic/Corticosteroid, Ophthalmic
**Dosage Forms Soln, ophth:** Chloramphenicol 1%, polymyxin B sulfate 10,000 units, and hydrocortisone acetate 0.5% per g (3.75 g)

# Chlordiazepoxide (klor dye az e POKS ide)
**Pharmacologic Class** Benzodiazepine
**U.S. Brand Names** Libritabs®; Librium®; Mitran® Oral; Reposans-10® Oral
**Use** Approved for anxiety, may be useful for acute alcohol withdrawal symptoms
**USUAL DOSAGE**

Children:
<6 years: Not recommended
>6 years: Anxiety: Oral, I.M.: 0.5 mg/kg/24 hours divided every 6-8 hours

Adults:
Anxiety:
Oral: 15-100 mg divided 3-4 times/day
I.M., I.V.: Initial: 50-100 mg followed by 25-50 mg 3-4 times/day as needed
Preoperative anxiety: I.M.: 50-100 mg prior to surgery
Alcohol withdrawal symptoms: Oral, I.V.: 50-100 mg to start, dose may be repeated in 2-4 hours as necessary to a maximum of 300 mg/24 hours

**Dosing adjustment in renal impairment:** $Cl_{cr}$ <10 mL/minute: Administer 50% of dose
Hemodialysis: Not dialyzable (0% to 5%)
**Dosing adjustment/comments in hepatic impairment:** Avoid use
**Dosage Forms Cap:** 5 mg, 10 mg, 25 mg; **Powder for inj:** 100 mg; **Tab:** 5 mg, 10 mg, 25 mg
**Contraindications** Hypersensitivity to chlordiazepoxide or any component, pre-existing CNS depression, severe uncontrolled pain
(Continued)

## Chlordiazepoxide *(Continued)*

**Warnings/Precautions** Use with caution in patients with respiratory depression, CNS impairment, liver dysfunction, or a history of drug dependence

**Pregnancy Risk Factor** D

**Adverse Reactions**

>10%:
  Cardiovascular: Chest pain
  Central nervous system: Drowsiness, fatigue, ataxia, lightheadedness, memory impairment, insomnia, anxiety, depression, headache
  Dermatologic: Skin eruptions, rash
  Endocrine & metabolic: Decreased libido
  Gastrointestinal: Nausea, constipation, vomiting, diarrhea, xerostomia, increased or decreased appetite, decreased salivation
  Neuromuscular & skeletal: Dysarthria
  Ocular: Blurred vision
  Miscellaneous: Diaphoresis

1% to 10%:
  Cardiovascular: Hypotension, tachycardia, edema, syncope
  Central nervous system: Ataxia, confusion, mental impairment, nervousness, dizziness, akathisia
  Dermatologic: Dermatitis
  Gastrointestinal: Weight gain or loss, increased salivation
  Neuromuscular & skeletal: Rigidity, tremor, muscle cramps
  Otic: Tinnitus
  Respiratory: Nasal congestion, hyperventilation

<1%: Menstrual irregularities, blood dyscrasias, depressed reflexes, drug dependence

**Drug Interactions** Increased toxicity (CNS depression): Oral anticoagulants, alcohol, tricyclic antidepressants, sedative-hypnotics, MAO inhibitors

**Onset** Peak concentrations in ~2 hours

**Duration** 48 hours to 1 week

**Half-Life** 6.6-25 hours; End-stage renal disease: 5-30 hours; Cirrhosis: 30-63 hours

**Special PA Issues**

**Patient Education:** Oral: Take exactly as directed (do not increase dose or frequency); may cause physical and/or psychological dependence. Do not use excessive alcohol or other prescription or OTC medications (especially pain medications, sedatives, antihistamines, or hypnotics) without consulting prescriber. Maintain adequate hydration (2-3 L/day of fluids unless instructed to restrict fluid intake). You may experience drowsiness, lightheadedness, impaired coordination, dizziness, or blurred vision (use caution when driving or engaging in hazardous tasks until response to medication is known); nausea or dry mouth (small frequent meals, good mouth care, chewing gum, or sucking lozenges may help); constipation (increased exercise, fluids, or dietary fruit and fiber may help); or altered sexual drive or ability (reversible). Report persistent CNS effects (eg, euphoria, confusion, increased sedation, depression); chest pain, palpitations, or rapid heartbeat; muscle cramping, weakness, tremors, rigidity, or altered gait; or worsening of condition.

**Dietary Considerations:** Alcohol: Additive CNS effects, avoid use

**Monitoring Parameters:** Respiratory and cardiovascular status, mental status, check for orthostasis

**Reference Range:** Therapeutic: 0.1-3 µg/mL (SI: 0-10 µmol/L); Toxic: >23 µg/mL (SI: >77 µmol/L)


## Chlorhexidine Gluconate *(klor HEKS i deen GLOO koe nate)*

**Pharmacologic Class** Antibacterial, Oral Rinse; Mouthwash

**U.S. Brand Names** BactoShield® Topical [OTC]; Betasept® [OTC]; Dyna-Hex® Topical [OTC]; Exidine® Scrub [OTC]; Hibiclens® Topical [OTC]; Hibistat® Topical [OTC]; Peridex® Oral Rinse; PerioChip®; PerioGard®

**Mechanism of Action** The bactericidal effect of chlorhexidine is a result of the binding of this cationic molecule to negatively charged bacterial cell walls and extramicrobial complexes. At low concentrations, this causes an alteration of bacterial cell osmotic equilibrium and leakage of potassium and phosphorous resulting in a bacteriostatic effect. At high concentrations of chlorhexidine, the cytoplasmic contents of the bacterial cell precipitate and result in cell death.

**Use** Skin cleanser for surgical scrub, cleanser for skin wounds, germicidal hand rinse, and as antibacterial dental rinse. Chlorhexidine is active against gram-positive and gram-negative organisms, facultative anaerobes, aerobes, and yeast.

**USUAL DOSAGE** Adults: Oral rinse (Peridex®):

Precede use of solution by flossing and brushing teeth; completely rinse toothpaste from mouth. Swish 15 mL undiluted oral rinse around in mouth for 30 seconds, then expectorate. Caution patient not to swallow the medicine. Avoid eating for 2-3 hours after treatment. (The cap on bottle of oral rinse is a measure for 15 mL.)

When used as a treatment of gingivitis, the regimen begins with oral prophylaxis. Patient treats mouth with 15 mL chlorhexidine, swishes for 30 seconds, then expectorates. This is repeated twice daily (morning and evening). Patient should have a re-evaluation followed by a dental prophylaxis every 6 months.

Cleanser:

Surgical scrub: Scrub 3 minutes and rinse thoroughly, wash for an additional 3 minutes

Hand wash: Wash for 15 seconds and rinse

Hand rinse: Rub 15 seconds and rinse

**Dosage Forms Chip, for periodontal pocket insertion (PerioChip®):** 2.5 mg; **Foam, top, with isopropyl alcohol 4% (BactoShield®):** 4% (180 mL); **Liq, top, with isopropyl alcohol 4%:** Dyna-Hex® Skin Cleanser: 2% (120 mL, 240 mL, 480 mL, 960 mL, 4000 mL), 4% (120 mL, 240 mL, 480 mL, 4000 mL), BactoShield® 2: 2% (960 mL), BactoShield®, Betasept®, Exidine® Skin Cleanser, Hibiclens® Skin Cleanser: 4% (15 mL, 120 mL, 240 mL, 480 mL, 960 mL, 4000 mL); **Rinse: Oral (mint flavor) (Peridex®, PerioGard®):** 0.12% with alcohol 11.6% (480 mL); **Top (Hibistat® Hand Rinse):** 0.5% with isopropyl alcohol 70% (120 mL, 240 mL); **Sponge/Brush (Hibiclens®):** 4% with isopropyl alcohol 4% (22 mL); **Wipes (Hibistat®):** 0.5% (50s)

**Contraindications** Known hypersensitivity to chlorhexidine gluconate

**Warnings/Precautions** Staining of oral surfaces, tooth restorations, and dorsum of tongue may occur; keep out of eyes and ears; for topical use only; there have been case reports of anaphylaxis following chlorhexidine disinfection

**Pregnancy Risk Factor** B

**Adverse Reactions**

>10%: Oral: Increase of tartar on teeth, changes in taste. Staining of oral surfaces (mucosa, teeth, dorsum of tongue) may be visible as soon as 1 week after therapy begins and is more pronounced when there is a heavy accumulation of unremoved plaque and when teeth fillings have rough surfaces. Stain does not have a clinically adverse effect but because removal may not be possible, patient with frontal restoration should be advised of the potential permanency of the stain.

1% to 10%: Gastrointestinal: Tongue irritation, oral irritation

<1%: Facial edema, nasal congestion, shortness of breath

**Special PA Issues**

**Patient Education:**

Oral rinse: Do not swallow, do not rinse after use; may cause reduced taste perception which is reversible; may cause discoloration of teeth

Topical administration is for external use only

♦ **2-Chlorodeoxyadenosine** see Cladribine on page 214

♦ **Chloromycetin®** see Chloramphenicol on page 188

# Chloroprocaine (klor oh PROE kane)

**Pharmacologic Class** Local Anesthetic

**U.S. Brand Names** Nesacaine®; Nesacaine®-MPF

**Mechanism of Action** Chloroprocaine HCl is benzoic acid, 4-amino-2-chloro-2-(diethylamino) ethyl ester monohydrochloride. Chloroprocaine is an ester-type local anesthetic, which stabilizes the neuronal membranes and prevents initiation and transmission of nerve impulses thereby affecting local anesthetic actions. Local anesthetics including chloroprocaine, reversibly prevent generation and conduction of electrical impulses in neurons by decreasing the transient increase in permeability to sodium. The differential sensitivity generally depends on the size of the fiber; small fibers are more sensitive than larger fibers and require a longer period for recovery. Sensory pain fibers are usually blocked first, followed by fibers that transmit sensations of temperature, touch, and deep pressure. High concentrations block sympathetic somatic sensory and somatic motor fibers. The spread of anesthesia depends upon the distribution of the solution. This is primarily dependent on the volume of drug injected.

**Use** Infiltration anesthesia and peripheral and epidural anesthesia

**USUAL DOSAGE** Dosage varies with anesthetic procedure, the area to be anesthetized, the vascularity of the tissues, depth of anesthesia required, degree of muscle relaxation required, and duration of anesthesia; range: 1.5-25 mL of 2% to 3% solution; single adult dose should not exceed 800 mg

Infiltration and peripheral nerve block: 1% to 2%

Infiltration, peripheral and central nerve block, including caudal and epidural block: 2% to 3%, without preservatives

**Dosage Forms Inj, as hydrochloride: Preservative free (Nesacaine®-MPF):** 2% (30 mL), 3% (30 mL); **With preservative (Nesacaine®):** 1% (30 mL), 2% (30 mL)

**Contraindications** Known hypersensitivity to chloroprocaine, or other ester type anesthetics; myasthenia gravis; concurrent use of bupivacaine; do not use for subarachnoid administration

**Warnings/Precautions** Use with caution in patients with cardiac disease, renal disease, and hyperthyroidism; convulsions and cardiac arrest have been reported presumably due to intravascular injection

**Pregnancy Risk Factor** C

**Adverse Reactions** <1%: Myocardial depression, hypotension, bradycardia, cardiovascular collapse, edema, anxiety, restlessness, disorientation, confusion, seizures, drowsiness, (Continued)

## Chloroprocaine *(Continued)*

unconsciousness, chills, urticaria, nausea, vomiting, transient stinging or burning at injection site, tremor, blurred vision, tinnitus, respiratory arrest, anaphylactoid reactions, shivering

**Onset** 6-12 minutes

**Duration** 30-60 minutes

**Special PA Issues**

**Patient Education:** This medication is given to reduce sensation in the injected area. You will experience decreased sensation to pain, heat, or cold in the area and/or decreased muscle strength (depending on area of application) until the effects wear off; use necessary caution to reduce incidence of possible injury until full sensation returns. Immediately report chest pain or palpitations; increased restlessness, confusion, anxiety, or dizziness; difficulty breathing; chills, shivering, or tremors; ringing in ears; or changes in vision.

♦ **Chloroprocaine Hydrochloride** *see Chloroprocaine on previous page*

♦ **Chloroptic® Ophthalmic** *see Chloramphenicol on page 188*

♦ **Chloroptic-P® Ophthalmic** *see Chloramphenicol and Prednisolone on page 189*

## Chloroquine and Primaquine (KLOR oh kwin & PRIM a kween)

**Pharmacologic Class** Antimalarial Agent

**U.S. Brand Names** Aralen® Phosphate With Primaquine Phosphate

**Mechanism of Action** Chloroquine concentrates within parasite acid vesicles and raises internal pH resulting in inhibition of parasite growth; may involve aggregates of ferriprotoporphyrin IX acting as chloroquine receptors causing membrane damage; may also interfere with nucleoprotein synthesis. Primaquine eliminates the primary tissue exoerythrocytic forms of *P. falciparum*; disrupts mitochondria and binds to DNA.

**Use** Prophylaxis of malaria, regardless of species, in all areas where the disease is endemic

**USUAL DOSAGE** Oral: Start at least 1 day before entering the endemic area; continue for 8 weeks after leaving the endemic area

Children: For suggested weekly dosage (based on body weight), see table:

| Weight | | Chloroquine Base (mg) | Primaquine Base (mg) | Dose* (mL) |
| lb | kg | | | |
|---|---|---|---|---|
| 10-15 | 4.5-6.8 | 20 | 3 | 2.5 |
| 16-25 | 7.3-11.4 | 40 | 6 | 5 |
| 26-35 | 11.8-15.9 | 60 | 9 | 7.5 |
| 36-45 | 16.4-20.5 | 80 | 12 | 10 |
| 46-55 | 20.9-25 | 100 | 15 | 12.5 |
| 56-100 | 25.4-45.4 | 160 | 22.5 | ½ tablet |
| 100+ | >45.4 | 300 | 45 | 1 tablet |

*Dose based on liquid containing approximately 40 mg of chloroquine base and 6 mg primaquine base per 5 mL, prepared from chloroquine phosphate with primaquine phosphate tablets.

Adults: 1 tablet/week on the same day each week

**Dosage Forms Tab:** Chloroquine phosphate 500 mg [base 300 mg] and primaquine phosphate 79 mg [base 45 mg]

**Contraindications** Retinal or visual field changes, known hypersensitivity to chloroquine or primaquine

**Warnings/Precautions** Use with caution in patients with psoriasis, porphyria, hepatic dysfunction, G-6-PD deficiency

**Pregnancy Risk Factor** C

**Adverse Reactions**

1% to 10%: Gastrointestinal: Diarrhea, nausea

<1%: Hypotension, EKG changes, fatigue, personality changes, headache, pruritus, hair bleaching, anorexia, vomiting, stomatitis, blood dyscrasias, retinopathy, blurred vision

**Drug Interactions**

Decreased absorption if administered concomitantly with kaolin and magnesium trisilicate

Increased toxicity/levels with cimetidine

**Special PA Issues**

**Monitoring Parameters:** Periodic CBC, examination for muscular weakness, and ophthalmologic examination in patients receiving prolonged therapy

## Chloroquine Phosphate (KLOR oh kwin FOS fate)

**Pharmacologic Class** Aminoquinoline (Antimalarial)

**U.S. Brand Names** Aralen® Phosphate

**Mechanism of Action** Binds to and inhibits DNA and RNA polymerase; interferes with metabolism and hemoglobin utilization by parasites; inhibits prostaglandin effects; chloroquine concentrates within parasite acid vesicles and raises internal pH resulting in inhibition of parasite growth; may involve aggregates of ferriprotoporphyrin IX acting as chloroquine receptors causing membrane damage; may also interfere with nucleoprotein synthesis

**Use** Suppression or chemoprophylaxis of malaria; treatment of uncomplicated or mild to moderate malaria; extraintestinal amebiasis

**Unlabeled use:** Rheumatoid arthritis; discoid lupus erythematosus, scleroderma, pemphigus

**USUAL DOSAGE** Oral (**dosage expressed in terms of mg of base**):

Suppression or prophylaxis of malaria:

Children: Administer 5 mg base/kg/week on the same day each week (not to exceed 300 mg base/dose); begin 1-2 weeks prior to exposure; continue for 4-6 weeks after leaving endemic area; if suppressive therapy is not begun prior to exposure, double the initial loading dose to 10 mg base/kg and administer in 2 divided doses 6 hours apart, followed by the usual dosage regimen

Adults: 300 mg/week (base) on the same day each week; begin 1-2 weeks prior to exposure; continue for 4-6 weeks after leaving endemic area; if suppressive therapy is not begun prior to exposure, double the initial loading dose to 600 mg base and administer in 2 divided doses 6 hours apart, followed by the usual dosage regimen

Acute attack:

Oral:

Children: 10 mg/kg on day 1, followed by 5 mg/kg 6 hours later and 5 mg/kg on days 2 and 3

Adults: 600 mg on day 1, followed by 300 mg 6 hours later, followed by 300 mg on days 2 and 3

I.M. (as hydrochloride):

Children: 5 mg/kg, repeat in 6 hours

Adults: Initial: 160-200 mg, repeat in 6 hours if needed; maximum: 800 mg first 24 hours; begin oral dosage as soon as possible and continue for 3 days until 1.5 g has been given

Extraintestinal amebiasis:

Children: Oral: 10 mg/kg once daily for 2-3 weeks (up to 300 mg base/day)

Adults:

Oral: 600 mg base/day for 2 days followed by 300 mg base/day for at least 2-3 weeks

I.M., as hydrochloride: 160-200 mg/day for 10 days; resume oral therapy as soon as possible

**Dosing adjustment in renal impairment:** $Cl_{cr}$ <10 mL/minute: Administer 50% of dose

Hemodialysis: Minimally removed by hemodialysis

**Dosage Forms Tab:** 250 mg [150 mg base], 500 mg [300 mg base]

**Contraindications** Retinal or visual field changes; patients with psoriasis; known hypersensitivity to chloroquine

**Warnings/Precautions** Use with caution in patients with liver disease, G-6-PD deficiency, alcoholism or in conjunction with hepatotoxic drugs, psoriasis, porphyria may be exacerbated; retinopathy (irreversible) has occurred with long or high-dose therapy; discontinue drug if any abnormality in the visual field or if muscular weakness develops during treatment

**Pregnancy Risk Factor** C

**Adverse Reactions**

>1%: Gastrointestinal: Nausea, diarrhea

<1%: Hypotension, EKG changes, fatigue, personality changes, headache, pruritus, hair bleaching, anorexia, vomiting, stomatitis, blood dyscrasias, retinopathy, blurred vision

**Drug Interactions**

Chloroquine and other 4-aminoquinolones may be decreased due to GI binding with kaolin or magnesium trisilicate

Increased effect: Cimetidine increases levels of chloroquine and probably other 4-aminoquinolones

**Half-Life** 3-5 days

**Special PA Issues**

**Patient Education:** It is important to complete full course of therapy which may take up to 6 months for full effect. May be taken with meals to decrease GI upset and bitter aftertaste. Avoid alcohol. You should have regular ophthalmic exams (every 4-6 months) if using this medication over extended periods. You may experience skin discoloration (blue/black), hair bleaching, or skin rash. If you have psoriasis, you may experience exacerbation. May turn urine red/brown (normal). You may experience nausea, vomiting, or loss of appetite (small frequent meals, frequent mouth care, or sucking lozenges may help) or increased sensitivity to sunlight (wear dark glasses and protective clothing, use sunblock, and avoid direct exposure to sunlight). Report vision changes, rash or itching, persistent diarrhea or GI disturbances, change in hearing acuity or ringing in the ears, chest pain or palpitation, CNS changes, unusual fatigue, easy bruising or bleeding, or any other persistent adverse reactions.

**Monitoring Parameters:** Periodic CBC, examination for muscular weakness, and ophthalmologic examination in patients receiving prolonged therapy

# Chlorothiazide (klor oh THYE a zide)

**Pharmacologic Class** Diuretic, Thiazide

**U.S. Brand Names** Diurigen®; Diuril®

**Mechanism of Action** Inhibits sodium reabsorption in the distal tubules causing increased excretion of sodium and water as well as potassium and hydrogen ions, magnesium, phosphate, calcium

**Use** Management of mild to moderate hypertension, or edema associated with congestive heart failure, pregnancy, or nephrotic syndrome in patients unable to take oral hydrochloro-thiazide, when a thiazide is the diuretic of choice

**USUAL DOSAGE**

Infants <6 months:
  Oral: 20-40 mg/kg/day in 2 divided doses
  I.V.: 2-8 mg/kg/day in 2 divided doses

Infants >6 months and Children:
  Oral: 20 mg/kg/day in 2 divided doses
  I.V.: 4 mg/kg/day

Adults:
  Oral: 500 mg to 2 g/day divided in 1-2 doses
  I.V.: 100-500 mg/day (for edema only)

Elderly: Oral: 500 mg once daily **or** 1 g 3 times/week

**Dosage Forms Powder for inj, lyophilized, as sodium:** 500 mg; **Susp, oral:** 250 mg/5 mL (237 mL); **Tab:** 250 mg, 500 mg

**Contraindications** Hypersensitivity to chlorothiazide or any component; cross-sensitivity with other thiazides or sulfonamides; do not use in anuric patients.

**Warnings/Precautions** Injection must not be administered S.C. or I.M.; may cause hyper-bilirubinemia, hypokalemia, hypokalemia, alkalosis, hyperglycemia, hyperuricemia; chlorothiazide is mini-mally effective in patients with a Cl$_{cr}$ <40 mL/minute; this may limit the usefulness of chlorothiazide in the elderly; use the I.V. form only when oral therapy is prohibitive or in an emergency, do not use in children if possible; avoid coadministration with blood

**Pregnancy Risk Factor** B

**Pregnancy Implications**

Clinical effects on the fetus: Crosses the placenta. Hypoglycemia, thrombocytopenia, hemolytic anemia, electrolyte disturbances reported. May exhibit a tocolytic effect. Gener-ally, use of diuretics during pregnancy is avoided due to risk of decreased placental perfusion.

Breast-feeding/lactation: Crosses into breast milk; may suppress lactation with high doses. American Academy of Pediatrics considers **compatible** with breast-feeding.

**Adverse Reactions**

1% to 10%: Endocrine & metabolic: Hypokalemia, hyponatremia

<1%: Arrhythmia, weak pulse, orthostatic hypotension, dizziness, vertigo, headache, fever, rash, photosensitivity, hypochloremic alkalosis, hyperglycemia, hyperlipidemia, hyperuri-cemia, rarely blood dyscrasias, leukopenia, agranulocytosis, aplastic anemia, paresthe-sias, prerenal azotemia

**Drug Interactions**

Decreased effect:
  Thiazides may decrease the effect of anticoagulants, antigout agents, sulfonylureas
  Bile acid sequestrants, methenamine, and NSAIDs may decrease the effect of the thia-zides

Increased effect: Thiazides may increase the toxicity of allopurinol, anesthetics, antine-oplastics, calcium salts, diazoxide, digitalis, lithium, loop diuretics, methyldopa, nondepo-larizing muscle relaxants, vitamin D; amphotericin B and anticholinergics may increase the toxicity of thiazides

**Onset** Onset of diuresis: Oral: 2 hours

**Duration** Oral: 6-12 hours; I.V.: ~2 hours

**Half-Life** 1-2 hours

**Special PA Issues**

**Patient Education:** Take once daily dose of chlorothiazide in morning or last of daily doses in early evening to avoid night-time disturbances. Additional potassium may be recommended; follow dietary suggestions of prescriber. You will be more sensitive to sunlight; use sunblock, wear protective clothing, or avoid direct sunlight. You may experi-ence dizziness, weakness, or drowsiness; use caution when driving or engaging in tasks that require alertness until response to drug is known. You may experience postural hypotension; use caution when rising from sitting or lying position or when climbing stairs. Report muscle twitching or cramps; acute loss of appetite; GI distress; severe rash, redness, or itching of skin; sexual dysfunction; palpitations; or respiratory difficulty.

**Monitoring Parameters:** Serum electrolytes, renal function, blood pressure; assess weight, I & O reports daily to determine fluid loss

# Chlorothiazide and Methyldopa (klor oh THYE a zide & meth il DOE pa)

**Pharmacologic Class** Antihypertensive Agent, Combination

**U.S. Brand Names** Aldoclor®

**Dosage Forms Tab:** 150: Chlorothiazide 150 mg and methyldopa 250 mg, 250: Chlorothiazide 250 mg and methyldopa 250 mg

# Chlorothiazide and Reserpine (klor oh THYE a zide & re SER peen)
**Pharmacologic Class** Antihypertensive Agent, Combination
**Dosage Forms Tab:** 250: Chlorothiazide 250 mg and reserpine 0.125 mg, 500: Chlorothiazide 500 mg and reserpine 0.125 mg

# Chlorotrianisene (klor oh trye AN i seen)
**Pharmacologic Class** Estrogen Derivative
**U.S. Brand Names** TACE®
**Mechanism of Action** Diethylstilbestrol derivative with similar estrogenic actions
**Use** Treat inoperable prostatic cancer; management of atrophic vaginitis, female hypogonadism, vasomotor symptoms of menopause
**USUAL DOSAGE** Adults: Oral:
Atrophic vaginitis: 12-25 mg/day in 28-day cycles (21 days on and 7 days off)
Female hypogonadism: 12-25 mg cyclically for 21 days. May be followed by I.M. progesterone 100 mg or 5 days of oral progestin; next course may begin on day 5 of induced uterine bleeding.
Postpartum breast engorgement: 12 mg 4 times/day for 7 days or 50 mg every 6 hours for 6 doses; administer first dose within 8 hours after delivery
Vasomotor symptoms associated with menopause: 12-25 mg cyclically for 30 days; one or more courses may be prescribed
Prostatic cancer (inoperable/progressing): 12-25 mg/day
**Dosage Forms Cap:** 12 mg, 25 mg
**Contraindications** Thrombophlebitis, breast cancer, undiagnosed abnormal vaginal bleeding, known or suspected pregnancy
**Warnings/Precautions** Estrogens have been reported to increase the risk of endometrial carcinoma; do not use estrogens during pregnancy
**Pregnancy Risk Factor** X
**Adverse Reactions**
>10%:
Cardiovascular: Peripheral edema
Endocrine & metabolic: Enlargement of breasts (female and male), breast tenderness
Gastrointestinal: Nausea, anorexia, bloating
1% to 10%:
Central nervous system: Headache
Endocrine & metabolic: Increased libido (female), decreased libido (male)
Gastrointestinal: Vomiting, diarrhea
<1%: Hypertension, thromboembolism, myocardial infarction, edema, depression, dizziness, anxiety, stroke, chloasma, melasma, rash, amenorrhea, alterations in frequency and flow of menses, decreased glucose tolerance, increased triglycerides and LDL, nausea, GI distress, cholestatic jaundice, intolerance to contact lenses, increased susceptibility to *Candida* infection, breast tumors
**Onset** Commonly occurs within 14 days of therapy
**Special PA Issues**
Patient Education: Take as directed. May cause enlargement of breast (male/female), menstrual irregularity, increased libido (female), decreased libido (male), nausea or vomiting (small frequent meals, frequent mouth care may help), or acute headache (mild analgesic may help). Report persistent diarrhea; swelling of feet, hands, or legs; sudden severe headache; disturbance of speech or vision; warmth, swelling, or pain in calves; severe abdominal pain; rash; emotional lability; chest pain or palpitations; or signs of vaginal infection.

# Chlorpheniramine and Phenylephrine (klor fen IR a meen & fen il EF rin)
**Pharmacologic Class** Antihistamine/Decongestant Combination
**U.S. Brand Names** Dallergy-D® Syrup; Ed A-Hist® Liquid; Histatab® Plus Tablet [OTC]; Histor-D® Syrup; Rolatuss® Plain Liquid; Ru-Tuss® Liquid
**Dosage Forms Cap, sustained release:** Chlorpheniramine maleate 8 mg and phenylephrine hydrochloride 20 mg; **Liq:** Dallergy-D®, Histor-D®, Rolatuss® Plain, Ru-Tuss®: Chlorpheniramine maleate 2 mg and phenylephrine hydrochloride 5 mg per 5 mL, Ed A-Hist® Liquid: Chlorpheniramine maleate 4 mg and phenylephrine hydrochloride 10 mg per 5 mL; **Tab (Histatab® Plus):** Chlorpheniramine maleate 2 mg and phenylephrine hydrochloride 5 mg

# Chlorpheniramine, Ephedrine, Phenylephrine, and Carbetapentane
(klor fen IR a meen, e FED rin, fen il EF rin, & kar bay ta PEN tane)
**Pharmacologic Class** Antihistamine/Decongestant/Antitussive
**U.S. Brand Names** Rentamine®; Rynatuss® Pediatric Suspension; Tri-Tannate Plus® (Continued)

195

## Chlorpheniramine, Ephedrine, Phenylephrine, and Carbetapentane *(Continued)*

**Dosage Forms Liq:** Carbetapentane tannate 30 mg, ephedrine tannate 5 mg, phenylephrine tannate 5 mg, and chlorpheniramine tannate 4 mg per 5 mL

## Chlorpheniramine, Phenindamine, and Phenylpropanolamine
(klor fen IR a meen, fen IN dah meen, & fen il proe pa NOLE a meen)
**Pharmacologic Class** Antihistamine/Decongestant Combination
**U.S. Brand Names** Nolamine®
**Dosage Forms Tab, timed release:** Chlorpheniramine maleate 4 mg, phenindamine tartrate 24 mg, and phenylpropanolamine hydrochloride 50 mg

## Chlorpheniramine, Phenylephrine, and Codeine
(klor fen IR a meen, fen il EF rin, & KOE deen)
**Pharmacologic Class** Antihistamine/Decongestant/Antitussive
**U.S. Brand Names** Pediacof®; Pedituss®
**Dosage Forms Liq:** Chlorpheniramine maleate 0.75 mg, phenylephrine hydrochloride 2.5 mg, and codeine phosphate 5 mg with potassium iodide 75 mg per 5 mL

## Chlorpheniramine, Phenylephrine, and Methscopolamine
(klor fen IR a meen, fen il EF rin, & meth skoe POL a meen)
**Pharmacologic Class** Antihistamine/Decongestant/Anticholinergic
**U.S. Brand Names** D.A.II® Tablet; Dallergy®; Dura-Vent/DA®; Extendryl® SR; Histor-D® Timecelles®
**Dosage Forms Cap, sustained release:** Chlorpheniramine maleate 8 mg, phenylephrine hydrochloride 20 mg, and methscopolamine nitrate 2.5 mg, Chlorpheniramine maleate 8 mg, phenylephrine hydrochloride 10 mg, and methscopolamine nitrate 2.5 mg; **Syr:** Chlorpheniramine maleate 2 mg, phenylephrine hydrochloride 10 mg, and methscopolamine nitrate 0.625 mg per 5 mL; **Tab:** Chlorpheniramine maleate 4 mg, phenylephrine hydrochloride 10 mg, and methscopolamine nitrate 1.25 mg

## Chlorpheniramine, Phenylephrine, and Phenylpropanolamine
(klor fen IR a meen, fen il EF rin, & fen il proe pa NOLE a meen)
**Pharmacologic Class** Antihistamine/Decongestant Combination
**U.S. Brand Names** Hista-Vadrin® Tablet
**Dosage Forms Tab:** Chlorpheniramine maleate 6 mg, phenylephrine hydrochloride 5 mg, and phenylpropanolamine hydrochloride 40 mg

## Chlorpheniramine, Phenylephrine, and Phenyltoloxamine
(klor fen IR a meen, fen il EF rin, & fen il tole LOKS a meen)
**Pharmacologic Class** Antihistamine/Decongestant Combination
**U.S. Brand Names** Comhist®; Comhist® LA
**Dosage Forms Cap, sustained release (Comhist® LA):** Chlorpheniramine maleate 4 mg, phenylephrine hydrochloride 20 mg, and phenyltoloxamine citrate 50 mg; **Tab (Comhist®):** Chlorpheniramine maleate 2 mg, phenylephrine hydrochloride 10 mg, and phenyltoloxamine citrate 25 mg

## Chlorpheniramine, Phenylephrine, Phenylpropanolamine, and Belladonna Alkaloids
(klor fen IR a meen, fen il EF rin, fen il proe pa NOLE a meen, & bel a DON a AL ka loydz)
**Pharmacologic Class** Cold Preparation
**U.S. Brand Names** Atrohist® Plus; Phenahist-TR®; Phenchlor® S.H.A.; Ru-Tuss®; Stahist®
**Dosage Forms Tab, sustained release:** Chlorpheniramine 8 mg, phenylephrine 25 mg, phenylpropanolamine 50 mg, hyoscyamine 0.19 mg, atropine 0.04 mg, and scopolamine 0.01 mg

## Chlorpheniramine, Phenyltoloxamine, Phenylpropanolamine, and Phenylephrine
(klor fen IR a meen, fen il tole LOKS a meen, fen il proe pa NOLE a meen & fen il EF rin)
**Pharmacologic Class** Antihistamine/Decongestant Combination
**U.S. Brand Names** Naldecon®; Naldelate®; Nalgest®; Nalspan®; New Decongestant®; Par Decon®; Tri-Phen-Chlor®; Uni-Decon®
**Dosage Forms Drops, pediatric:** Chlorpheniramine maleate 0.5 mg, phenyltoloxamine citrate 2 mg, phenylpropanolamine hydrochloride 5 mg, and phenylephrine hydrochloride 1.25 mg per mL; **Syr:** Chlorpheniramine maleate 2.5 mg, phenyltoloxamine citrate 7.5 mg, phenylpropanolamine hydrochloride 20 mg, and phenylephrine hydrochloride 5 mg per 5 mL; **Syr, pediatric:** Chlorpheniramine maleate 0.5 mg, phenyltoloxamine citrate 2 mg, phenylpropanolamine hydrochloride 5 mg, and phenylephrine hydrochloride 1.25 mg per 5

mL; **Tab, sustained release:** Chlorpheniramine maleate 5 mg, phenyltoloxamine citrate 15 mg, phenylpropanolamine hydrochloride 40 mg, and phenylephrine hydrochloride 10 mg

# Chlorpheniramine, Pseudoephedrine, and Codeine
(klor fen IR a meen, soo doe e FED rin, & KOE deen)

**Pharmacologic Class** Antihistamine/Decongestant/Antitussive

**U.S. Brand Names** Codehist® DH; Decohistine® DH; Dihistine® DH; Ryna-C® Liquid

**Dosage Forms Liq:** Chlorpheniramine maleate 2 mg, pseudoephedrine hydrochloride 30 mg, and codeine phosphate 10 mg (120 mL, 480 mL)

# Chlorpheniramine, Pyrilamine, and Phenylephrine
(klor fen IR a meen, pye RIL a meen, & fen il EF rin)

**Pharmacologic Class** Antihistamine/Decongestant Combination

**U.S. Brand Names** Rhinatate® Tablet; R-Tannamine® Tablet; R-Tannate® Tablet; Rynatan® Pediatric Suspension; Rynatan® Tablet; Tanoral® Tablet; Triotann® Tablet; Tri-Tannate® Tablet

**Dosage Forms Liq:** Chlorpheniramine tannate 2 mg, pyrilamine tannate 12.5 mg, and phenylephrine tannate 5 mg per 5 mL; **Tab:** Chlorpheniramine tannate 8 mg, pyrilamine maleate 12.5 mg, and phenylephrine tannate 25 mg

# Chlorpheniramine, Pyrilamine, Phenylephrine, and Phenylpropanolamine
(klor fen IR a meen, pye RIL a meen, fen il EF rin, & fen il proe pa NOLE a meen)

**Pharmacologic Class** Antihistamine/Decongestant Combination

**U.S. Brand Names** Histalet Forte® Tablet

**Dosage Forms Tab:** Chlorpheniramine maleate 4 mg, pyrilamine maleate 25 mg, phenylephrine hydrochloride 10 mg, and phenylpropanolamine hydrochloride 50 mg

♦ **Chlorprom®** see Chlorpromazine on this page
♦ **Chlorpromanyl®** see Chlorpromazine on this page

# Chlorpromazine (klor PROE ma zeen)

**Pharmacologic Class** Antipsychotic Agent, Phenothiazine, Aliphatic

**U.S. Brand Names** Ormazine; Thorazine®

**Mechanism of Action** Blocks postsynaptic mesolimbic dopaminergic receptors in the brain; exhibits a strong alpha-adrenergic blocking effect and depresses the release of hypothalamic and hypophyseal hormones; believed to depress the reticular activating system, thus affecting basal metabolism, body temperature, wakefulness, vasomotor tone, and emesis

**Use** Treatment of nausea and vomiting; psychoses; Tourette's syndrome; mania; intractable hiccups (adults); behavioral problems (children)

**USUAL DOSAGE**

Children >6 months:
  Psychosis:
    Oral: 0.5-1 mg/kg/dose every 4-6 hours; older children may require 200 mg/day or higher
    I.M., I.V.: 0.5-1 mg/kg/dose every 6-8 hours; maximum dose for <5 years (22.7 kg): 40 mg/day; maximum for 5-12 years (22.7-45.5 kg): 75 mg/day
  Nausea and vomiting:
    Oral: 0.5-1 mg/kg/dose every 4-6 hours as needed
    I.M., I.V.: 0.5-1 mg/kg/dose every 6-8 hours; maximum dose for <5 years (22.7 kg): 40 mg/day; maximum for 5-12 years (22.7-45.5 kg): 75 mg/day
    Rectal: 1 mg/kg/dose every 6-8 hours as needed
Adults:
  Psychosis:
    Oral: Range: 30-800 mg/day in 1-4 divided doses, initiate at lower doses and titrate as needed; usual dose: 200 mg/day; some patients may require 1-2 g/day
    I.M., I.V.: Initial: 25 mg, may repeat (25-50 mg) in 1-4 hours, gradually increase to a maximum of 400 mg/dose every 4-6 hours until patient is controlled; usual dose: 300-800 mg/day
  Intractable hiccups: Oral, I.M.: 25-50 mg 3-4 times/day
  Nausea and vomiting:
    Oral: 10-25 mg every 4-6 hours
    I.M., I.V.: 25-50 mg every 4-6 hours
    Rectal: 50-100 mg every 6-8 hours
Elderly (nonpsychotic patient; dementia behavior): Initial: 10-25 mg 1-2 times/day; increase at 4- to 7-day intervals by 10-25 mg/day. Increase dose intervals (bid, tid, etc) as necessary to control behavior response or side effects; maximum daily dose: 800 mg; gradual increases (titration) may prevent some side effects or decrease their severity.
Hemodialysis: Not dialyzable (0% to 5%)
**Dosing adjustment/comments in hepatic impairment:** Avoid use in severe hepatic dysfunction
(Continued)

# Chlorpromazine *(Continued)*

**Dosage Forms** Chlorpromazine hydrochloride: **Cap, sustained action:** 30 mg, 75 mg, 150 mg, 200 mg, 300 mg; **Conc, oral:** 30 mg/mL (120 mL); 100 mg/mL (60 mL, 240 mL); **Inj:** 25 mg/mL (1 mL, 2 mL, 10 mL); **Syr:** 10 mg/5 mL (120 mL); **Tab:** 10 mg, 25 mg, 50 mg, 100 mg, 200 mg

**Supp, rectal, as base:** 25 mg, 100 mg

**Contraindications** Hypersensitivity to chlorpromazine hydrochloride or any component; cross-sensitivity with other phenothiazines may exist; avoid use in patients with narrow-angle glaucoma

**Warnings/Precautions** Safety in children <6 months of age has not been established; use with caution in patients with seizures, bone marrow suppression, or severe liver disease

Significant hypotension may occur, especially when the drug is administered parenterally; injection contains benzyl alcohol; injection also contains sulfites which may cause allergic reaction

Tardive dyskinesia: Prevalence rate may be 40% in elderly; development of the syndrome and the irreversible nature are proportional to duration and total cumulative dose over time. May be reversible if diagnosed early in therapy.

Extrapyramidal reactions are more common in elderly with up to 50% developing these reactions after 60 years of age. Drug-induced **Parkinson's syndrome** occurs often. **Akathisia** is the most common extrapyramidal reaction in elderly.

Increased confusion, memory loss, psychotic behavior, and agitation frequently occur as a consequence of anticholinergic effects

Orthostatic hypotension is due to alpha-receptor blockade, the elderly are at greater risk for orthostatic hypotension

Antipsychotic associated sedation in nonpsychotic patients is extremely unpleasant due to feelings of depersonalization, derealization, and dysphoria

Life-threatening arrhythmias have occurred at therapeutic doses of antipsychotics

**Pregnancy Risk Factor** C

**Adverse Reactions**

>10%:

Cardiovascular: Hypotension (especially with I.V. use), tachycardia, arrhythmias, orthostatic hypotension

Central nervous system: Pseudoparkinsonism, akathisia, dystonias, tardive dyskinesia (persistent), dizziness

Gastrointestinal: Constipation

Ocular: Pigmentary retinopathy

Respiratory: Nasal congestion

Miscellaneous: Diaphoresis (decreased)

1% to 10%:

Dermatologic: Pruritus, rash, increased sensitivity to sun

Endocrine & metabolic: Amenorrhea, galactorrhea, gynecomastia, changes in libido, pain in breasts

Gastrointestinal: GI upset, nausea, vomiting, stomach pain, weight gain, xerostomia

Genitourinary: Dysuria, ejaculatory disturbances, urinary retention

Neuromuscular & skeletal: Trembling of fingers

Ocular: Blurred vision

<1%: Sedation, drowsiness, restlessness, anxiety, extrapyramidal reactions, seizures, altered central temperature regulation, lowering of seizures threshold, neuroleptic malignant syndrome (NMS), discoloration of skin (blue-gray), photosensitivity, galactorrhea, priapism, agranulocytosis (more often in women between 4th and 10th weeks of therapy), leukopenia (usually in patients with large doses for prolonged periods), cholestatic jaundice, hepatotoxicity, cornea and lens changes, anaphylactoid reactions

**Drug Interactions** CYP1A2, 2D6, and 3A3/4 enzyme substrate; CYP2D6 enzyme inhibitor

Increased toxicity: Additive effects with other CNS-depressants; epinephrine (hypotension); may increase valproic acid serum concentrations

**Onset** Peak concentration after oral dose: 1-2 hours

**Half-Life** Half-life, biphasic: Initial: 2 hours; Terminal: 30 hours

**Special PA Issues**

**Patient Education:** Use exactly as directed (do not increase dose or frequency); may cause physical and/or psychological dependence. Do not discontinue without consulting prescriber. Tablets/capsules may be taken with food. Mix oral solution with 2-4 oz of liquid (eg, juice, milk, water). Do not take within 2 hours of any antacid. Store away from light. Avoid excess alcohol or caffeine and other prescription or OTC medications not approved by prescriber. Maintain adequate hydration (2-3 L/day of fluids unless instructed to restrict fluid intake). May turn urine red-brown (normal). You may experience excess drowsiness, lightheadedness, dizziness, or blurred vision (use caution driving or when engaging in hazardous tasks until response to medication is known); dry mouth, upset stomach, nausea, vomiting, anorexia (small frequent meals, frequent mouth care, or sucking lozenges may help); constipation (increased exercise, fluids, or dietary fruit and fiber may help); postural hypotension (use caution climbing stairs or when changing position from lying or sitting to standing); urinary retention (void before taking medication); ejaculatory dysfunction (reversible); decreased perspiration (avoid strenuous exercise in hot environments); or photosensitivity (use sunscreen, protective clothing, and avoid prolonged exposure to direct sunlight). Report persistent CNS effects (trembling fingers, altered gait or balance, excessive sedation, seizures, unusual movements, anxiety, abnormal thoughts, confusion, personality changes); chest pain, palpitations, rapid heartbeat, or severe dizziness; unresolved urinary retention or changes in urinary pattern; altered menstrual pattern, change in libido, swelling or pain in breasts (male or female); vision changes, skin rash, irritation, or changes in color of skin (gray-blue); or worsening of condition.

**Dietary Considerations:** Alcohol: Additive CNS effects, avoid use

**Monitoring Parameters:** Orthostatic blood pressures; tremors, gait changes, abnormal movement in trunk, neck, buccal area, or extremities; monitor target behaviors for which the agent is given; watch for hypotension when administering I.M. or I.V.

**Reference Range:** Therapeutic: 50-300 ng/mL (SI: 157-942 nmol/L); Toxic: >750 ng/mL (SI: >2355 nmol/L); serum concentrations poorly correlate with expected response

**Related Information**
Antipsychotic Agents on page 1001

♦ **Chlorpromazine Hydrochloride** see Chlorpromazine on page 197

# Chlorpropamide (klor PROE pa mide)

**Pharmacologic Class** Antidiabetic Agent (Sulfonylurea)

**U.S. Brand Names** Diabinese®

**Mechanism of Action** Stimulates insulin release from the pancreatic beta cells; reduces glucose output from the liver; insulin sensitivity is increased at peripheral target sites

**Use** Control blood sugar in adult onset, noninsulin-dependent diabetes (type II)

**Unlabeled use:** Neurogenic diabetes insipidus

**USUAL DOSAGE** Oral: The dosage of chlorpropamide is variable and should be individualized based upon the patient's response

Initial dose:
  Adults: 250 mg/day in mild to moderate diabetes in middle-aged, stable diabetic
  Elderly: 100-125 mg/day in older patients
Subsequent dosages may be increased or decreased by 50-125 mg/day at 3- to 5-day intervals
Maintenance dose: 100-250 mg/day; severe diabetics may require 500 mg/day; avoid doses >750 mg/day

**Dosing adjustment/comments in renal impairment:** $Cl_{cr}$ <50 mL/minute: Avoid use
Hemodialysis: Removed with hemoperfusion
Peritoneal dialysis: Supplemental dose is not necessary

**Dosing adjustment in hepatic impairment:** Dosage reduction is recommended. Conservative initial and maintenance doses are recommended in patients with liver impairment because chlorpropamide undergoes extensive hepatic metabolism.

**Dosage Forms Tab:** 100 mg, 250 mg

**Contraindications** Cross-sensitivity may exist with other hypoglycemics or sulfonamides; do not use with type I diabetes or with severe renal, hepatic, thyroid, or other endocrine disease

**Warnings/Precautions**
Patients should be properly instructed in the early detection and treatment of hypoglycemia; long half-life may complicate recovery from excess effects
Because of chlorpropamide's long half-life, duration of action, and the increased risk for hypoglycemia, it is not considered a hypoglycemic agent of choice in the elderly

**Pregnancy Risk Factor** D

**Pregnancy Implications**
Clinical effects on the fetus: Crosses the placenta. Hypoglucemia; ear defects reported; other malformations reported but may have been secondary to poor maternal glucose control/diabetes. Insulin is the drug of choice for the control of diabetes mellitus during pregnancy.
Breast-feeding/lactation: Crosses into breast milk

**Adverse Reactions**
>10%:
  Central nervous system: Headache, dizziness
  Gastrointestinal: Anorexia, constipation, heartburn, epigastric fullness, nausea, vomiting, diarrhea
1% to 10%: Dermatologic: Skin rash, urticaria, photosensitivity
<1%: Edema, hypoglycemia, hyponatremia, SIADH, blood dyscrasias, aplastic anemia, hemolytic anemia, bone marrow suppression, thrombocytopenia, agranulocytosis, cholestatic jaundice

**Drug Interactions**
Decreased effect: Thiazides and hydantoins (eg, phenytoin) decrease chlorpropamide effectiveness may increase blood glucose
Increased toxicity:
  Increases alcohol-associated disulfiram reactions
(Continued)

# Chlorpropamide *(Continued)*

Increases oral anticoagulant effects

Salicylates may increase chlorpropamide effects may decrease blood glucose

Sulfonamides may decrease sulfonylureas clearance

**Onset** Oral: Within 6-8 hours

**Half-Life** 30-42 hours; prolonged in the elderly or with renal disease; End-stage renal disease: 50-200 hours

**Special PA Issues**

**Patient Education:** Take at the same time each day (usually before breakfast). Avoid hypoglycemia, eat regularly, do not skip meals. Carry a quick source of sugar. Avoid alcohol. Alcohol will cause "disulfiram"-type reaction consisting of flushing, headache, nausea, and in some patients, vomiting and chest and/or abdominal pain. Use sunblock to reduce photosensitivity reactions. This medication is used to control, not to cure diabetes. Other components of treatment plan are also important. Follow prescribed diet, medication, and exercise regimen as directed.

**Dietary Considerations:**

Alcohol: A disulfiram-like reaction characterized by flushing, headache, nausea, vomiting, sweating or tachycardia; avoid use. Inform patient of chlorpropamide-alcohol flush (facial reddening and an increase in facial temperature).

Food: Chlorpropamide may cause GI upset; take with food. Take at the same time each day; eat regularly and do not skip meals.

Glucose: Decreases blood glucose concentration; hypoglycemia may occur. Educate patients how to detect and treat hypoglycemia. Monitor for signs and symptoms of hypoglycemia. Administer glucose if necessary. Evaluate patient's diet and exercise regimen. May need to decrease or discontinue dose of sulfonylurea.

Sodium: Reports of hyponatremia and SIADH. Those at increased risk include patients on medications or who have medical conditions that predispose them to hyponatremia. Monitor sodium serum concentration and fluid status. May need to restrict water intake.

**Monitoring Parameters:** Fasting blood glucose, normal Hgb $A_{1c}$ or fructosamine levels; monitor for signs and symptoms of hypoglycemia, (fatigue, sweating, numbness of extremities); monitor urine for glucose and ketones

**Reference Range:** Target range: Adults: Fasting blood glucose: <120 mg/dL; Glycosylated hemoglobin: <7%

**Related Information**

Hypoglycemic Drugs *on page 1020*

# Chlorthalidone *(klor THAL i done)*

**Pharmacologic Class** Diuretic, Thiazide

**U.S. Brand Names** Hygroton®; Thalitone®

**Mechanism of Action** Sulfonamide-derived diuretic that inhibits sodium and chloride reabsorption in the cortical-diluting segment of the ascending loop of Henle

**Use** Management of mild to moderate hypertension, used alone or in combination with other agents; treatment of edema associated with congestive heart failure, nephrotic syndrome, or pregnancy. Recent studies have found chlorthalidone effective in the treatment of isolated systolic hypertension in the elderly.

**USUAL DOSAGE** Oral:

Children (nonapproved): 2 mg/kg/dose 3 times/week or 1-2 mg/kg/day

Adults:

Edema: 50-100 mg/day or 100 mg every other day; may increase to 200 mg but greater doses do not usually result in increased response

Hypertension: Initial: 25 mg/day, increase slowly to 100 mg/day or add additional antihypertensives

Elderly: Initial: 12.5-25 mg/day or every other day; there is little advantage to using doses >25 mg/day

**Note:** Thalidone 30 mg = chlorthalidone 25 mg

**Dosing interval in renal impairment:** $Cl_{cr}$ <10 mL/minute: Administer every 48 hours

**Dosage Forms Tab:** 25 mg, 50 mg, 100 mg, Hygroton®: 25 mg, 50 mg, 100 mg, Thalitone®: 15 mg, 25 mg

**Contraindications** Hypersensitivity to chlorthalidone or any component, cross-sensitivity with other thiazides or sulfonamides; do not use in anuric patients

**Warnings/Precautions** Use with caution in patients with hypokalemia, renal disease, hepatic disease, gout, lupus erythematosus, diabetes mellitus; use with caution in severe renal diseases

**Pregnancy Risk Factor** B

**Adverse Reactions**

1% to 10%: Endocrine & metabolic: Hypokalemia

<1%: Hypotension, photosensitivity, fluid and electrolyte imbalances (hypocalcemia, hypomagnesemia, hyponatremia), hyperglycemia, rarely blood dyscrasias, prerenal azotemia

**Drug Interactions**
Decreased effect: NSAIDs + chlorthalidone → decreased antihypertensive effect; decreased absorption of thiazides with cholestyramine resins; chlorthalidone causes a decreased effect of oral hypoglycemics
Increased toxicity: Digitalis glycosides, lithium (decreased clearance), probenecid
Increased effect: Furosemide and other loop diuretics

**Onset** Peak effect: 2-6 hours

**Half-Life** 35-55 hours; may be prolonged with renal impairment, with anuria: 81 hours

**Special PA Issues**
**Patient Education:** Take prescribed dose with food early in the day. Include orange juice or bananas in your diet, but do not take potassium supplements without consulting prescriber. You may experience postural hypotension (use caution when rising from lying or sitting position, when climbing stairs, or when driving); photosensitivity (use sunblock, wear protective clothing and eyewear, or avoid direct sunlight); decreased accommodation to heat (avoid excessive exercise in hot weather). Report muscle weakness, tremors, or cramping; persistent nausea or vomiting; swelling of extremities; significant increase in weight; respiratory difficulty; rash; unusual weakness or fatigue; or easy bruising or bleeding.
**Monitoring Parameters:** Assess weight, I & O records daily to determine fluid loss; blood pressure, serum electrolytes, renal function

**Related Information**
Heart Failure: Management of Patients with Left Ventricular Systolic Dysfunction *on page 1064*

## Chlorzoxazone (klor ZOKS a zone)
**Pharmacologic Class** Skeletal Muscle Relaxant
**U.S. Brand Names** Flexaphen®; Paraflex®; Parafon Forte™ DSC
**Mechanism of Action** Acts on the spinal cord and subcortical levels by depressing polysynaptic reflexes
**Use** Symptomatic treatment of muscle spasm and pain associated with acute musculoskeletal conditions
**USUAL DOSAGE** Oral:
Children: 20 mg/kg/day or 600 mg/m²/day in 3-4 divided doses
Adults: 250-500 mg 3-4 times/day up to 750 mg 3-4 times/day
**Dosage Forms Caplet (Parafon Forte™ DSC):** 500 mg; **Cap (Flexaphen®, Mus-Lax®):** 250 mg with acetaminophen 300 mg; **Tab:** Paraflex®: 250 mg
**Contraindications** Known hypersensitivity to chlorzoxazone; impaired liver function
**Pregnancy Risk Factor** C
**Adverse Reactions**
>10%: Central nervous system: Drowsiness
1% to 10%:
Cardiovascular: Tachycardia, tightness in chest, flushing of face, syncope
Central nervous system: Mental depression, allergic fever, dizziness, lightheadedness, headache, paradoxical stimulation
Dermatologic: Angioedema
Gastrointestinal: Nausea, vomiting, stomach cramps
Neuromuscular & skeletal: Trembling
Ocular: Burning of eyes
Respiratory: Shortness of breath
Miscellaneous: Hiccups
<1%: Ataxia, rash, urticaria, erythema multiforme, aplastic anemia, leukopenia, eosinophilia, blurred vision
**Drug Interactions** CYP2E1 enzyme substrate
Increased effect/toxicity: Alcohol, CNS depressants
**Onset** Within 1 hour
**Duration** 6-12 hours
**Special PA Issues**
**Patient Education:** Take exactly as directed, with food. Do not increase dose or discontinue without consulting prescriber. Do not use alcohol, prescriptive or OTC antidepressants, sedatives, or pain medications without consulting prescriber. May turn urine orange or red (normal). You may experience drowsiness, dizziness, lightheadedness (avoid driving or engaging in tasks that require alertness until response to therapy is known); nausea, vomiting, or cramping (small, frequent meals, frequent mouth care, or sucking hard candy may help); postural hypotension (change position slowly when rising from sitting or lying or when climbing stairs); or constipation (increased dietary fluids and fibers or increased exercise may help). Report excessive drowsiness or mental agitation; palpitations, rapid heartbeat, or chest pain; skin rash or swelling of mouth or face; persistent diarrhea or constipation; or unusual weakness or bleeding.
**Dietary Considerations:** Alcohol: Additive CNS effects, avoid use
**Monitoring Parameters:** Periodic liver functions tests

♦ **Chlorzoxazone with Acetaminophen** *see* Chlorzoxazone *on this page*

♦ **Cholac®** *see* Lactulose *on page 512*
♦ **Choledyl®** *see* Theophylline Salts *on page 888*

# Cholestyramine Resin (koe LES tir a meen REZ in)

**Pharmacologic Class** Antilipemic Agent (Bile Acid Seqestrant)

**U.S. Brand Names** Prevalite®; Questran®; Questran® Light

**Mechanism of Action** Forms a nonabsorbable complex with bile acids in the intestine, releasing chloride ions in the process; inhibits enterohepatic reuptake of intestinal bile salts and thereby increases the fecal loss of bile salt-bound low density lipoprotein cholesterol

**Use** Adjunct in the management of primary hypercholesterolemia; pruritus associated with elevated levels of bile acids; diarrhea associated with excess fecal bile acids; binding toxicologic agents; pseudomembraneous colitis

**USUAL DOSAGE** Oral (dosages are expressed in terms of anhydrous resin):
Powder:
Children: 240 mg/kg/day in 3 divided doses; need to titrate dose depending on indication
Adults: 4 g 1-2 times/day to a maximum of 24 g/day and 6 doses/day
Tablet: Adults: Initial: 4 g once or twice daily; maintenance: 8-16 g/day in 2 divided doses
Dialysis: Not removed by hemo- or peritoneal dialysis; supplemental doses not necessary with dialysis or continuous arteriovenous or venovenous hemofiltration effects

**Dosage Forms Powder:** 4 g of resin/9 g of powder (9 g, 378 g), For oral susp: With aspartame: 4 g of resin/5 g of powder (5 g, 210 g), With phenylalanine: 4 g of resin/5.5 g of powder (60s)

**Contraindications** Avoid using in complete biliary obstruction; hypersensitive to cholestyramine or any component; hypolipoproteinemia types III, IV, V

**Warnings/Precautions** Use with caution in patients with constipation (GI dysfunction); caution patients with phenylketonuria (Questran® Light contains aspartame); overdose may result in GI obstruction

**Pregnancy Risk Factor** C

**Adverse Reactions**
1% to 10%: Gastrointestinal: Constipation
<1%: Rash, irritation of perianal area or skin, hyperchloremic acidosis, nausea, vomiting, abdominal distention and pain, malabsorption of fat-soluble vitamins, intestinal obstruction, steatorrhea, tongue irritation, hypoprothrombinemia (secondary to vitamin K deficiency), increased urinary calcium excretion

**Drug Interactions** Decreased effect: Decreased absorption (oral) of digitalis glycosides, warfarin, thyroid hormones, valproic acid, thiazide diuretics, propranolol, phenobarbital, amiodarone, methotrexate, NSAIDs, fat-soluble vitamins, aspirin, clofibrate, furosemide, glipizide, hydrocortisone, imipramine, methyldopa, niacin, penicillin G, phenytoin, phosphate, tetracyclines, tolbutamide, and other drugs by binding to the drug in the intestine

**Onset** Peak effect: 21 days

**Special PA Issues**
**Patient Education:** Take once or twice a day as directed. Do not take the powder in its dry form; mix with fluid, applesauce, pudding, or jello. Chew bars thoroughly. Take other medications 2 hours before or 4 hours after cholestyramine. Ongoing medical follow-up and laboratory tests may be required. You may experience GI effects (these should resolve after continued use); nausea and vomiting (small frequent meals, frequent oral care, and sucking on lozenges may help); constipation (increased exercise, dietary fluid, fiber, or fruit may help - consult prescriber about use of stool softener or laxative). Report unusual stomach cramping, pain or blood in stool; unresolved nausea, vomiting, or constipation.

# Choline Magnesium Trisalicylate
(KOE leen mag NEE zhum trye sa LIS i late)

**Pharmacologic Class** Salicylate

**U.S. Brand Names** Tricosal®; Trilisate®

**Mechanism of Action** Inhibits prostaglandin synthesis; acts on the hypothalamus heat-regulating center to reduce fever; blocks the generation of pain impulses

**Use** Management of osteoarthritis, rheumatoid arthritis, and other arthritis; salicylate salts may not inhibit platelet aggregation and, therefore, should not be substituted for aspirin in the prophylaxis of thrombosis

**USUAL DOSAGE** Oral (based on total salicylate content):
Children <37 kg: 50 mg/kg/day given in 2 divided doses
Adults: 500 mg to 1.5 g 2-3 times/day; usual maintenance dose: 1-4.5 g/day
**Dosing adjustment/comments in renal impairment:** Avoid use in severe renal impairment

**Dosage Forms Liq:** 500 mg/5 mL [choline salicylate 293 mg and magnesium salicylate 362 mg per 5 mL] (237 mL); **Tab:** 500 mg: Choline salicylate 293 mg and magnesium salicylate 362 mg, 750 mg: Choline salicylate 440 mg and magnesium salicylate 544 mg, 1000 mg: Choline salicylate 587 mg and magnesium salicylate 725 mg

**Contraindications** Bleeding disorders; hypersensitivity to salicylates or other nonacetylated salicylates or other NSAIDs; tartrazine dye hypersensitivity, asthma

**Warnings/Precautions** Use with caution in patients with impaired renal function, erosive gastritis, or peptic ulcer; avoid use in patients with suspected varicella or influenza (salicylates have been associated with Reye's syndrome in children <16 years of age when used to treat symptoms of chickenpox or the flu). Tinnitus or impaired hearing may indicate toxicity; discontinue use 1 week prior to surgical procedures.

Elderly are a high-risk population for adverse effects from nonsteroidal anti-inflammatory agents. As much as 60% of elderly can develop peptic ulceration and/or hemorrhage asymptomatically. Use lowest effective dose for shortest period possible. Tinnitus may be a difficult and unreliable indication of toxicity due to age-related hearing loss or eighth cranial nerve damage. CNS adverse effects may be observed in the elderly at lower doses than younger adults.

**Pregnancy Risk Factor** C

**Adverse Reactions**
>10%: Gastrointestinal: Nausea, heartburn, stomach pains, dyspepsia, epigastric discomfort

1% to 10%:
  Central nervous system: Fatigue
  Dermatologic: Rash
  Gastrointestinal: Gastrointestinal ulceration
  Hematologic: Hemolytic anemia
  Neuromuscular & skeletal: Weakness
  Respiratory: Dyspnea
  Miscellaneous: Anaphylactic shock

<1%: Insomnia, nervousness, jitters, occult bleeding, prolongation of bleeding time, leukopenia, thrombocytopenia, iron deficiency anemia, hepatotoxicity, impaired renal function, bronchospasm, increased uric acid

**Drug Interactions**
Decreased effect: Antacids + Trilisate® may decrease salicylate concentration
Increased toxicity: Warfarin + Trilisate® may possibly increase hypoprothrombinemic effect

**Onset** Peak concentrations in ~2 hours after oral dose

**Half-Life** Dose-dependent ranging from 2-3 hours at low doses to 30 hours at high doses

**Special PA Issues**
Patient Education: If self-administered, use exactly as directed (do not increase dose or frequency); adverse reactions can occur with overuse. Take with food or milk. While using this medication, do not use alcohol, excessive amounts of vitamin C, or salicylate-containing foods (curry powder, prunes, raisins, tea, or licorice), other prescription or OTC medications containing aspirin or salicylate, or other NSAIDs without consulting prescriber. Maintain adequate hydration (2-3 L/day of fluids unless instructed to restrict fluid intake). You may experience nausea, vomiting, gastric discomfort (frequent mouth care, small frequent meals, or sucking on lozenges may help). GI bleeding, ulceration, or perforation can occur with or without pain. Stop taking medication and report ringing in ears; persistent pain in stomach; unresolved nausea or vomiting; difficulty breathing or shortness of breath; unusual bruising or bleeding (mouth, urine, stool); or skin rash.

**Dietary Considerations:**
Alcohol: Combination causes GI irritation, possible bleeding; avoid or limit alcohol. Patients at increased risk include those prone to hypoprothrombinemia, vitamin K deficiency, thrombocytopenia, thrombotic thrombocytopenia purpura, severe hepatic impairment, and those receiving anticoagulants.

Food: May decrease the rate but not the extent of oral absorption. Drug may cause GI upset, bleeding, ulceration, perforation. Take with food or or large volume of water or milk to minimize GI upset.

Folic acid: Hyperexcretion of folate; folic acid deficiency may result, leading to macrocytic anemia. Supplement with folic acid if necessary.

Iron: With chronic use and at doses of 3-4 g/day, iron deficiency anemia may result; supplement with iron if necessary

Magnesium: Hypermagnesemia resulting from magnesium salicylate; avoid or use with caution in renal insufficiency

Sodium: Hypernatremia resulting from buffered aspirin solutions or sodium salicylate containing high sodium content. Avoid or use with caution in CHF or any condition where hypernatremia would be detrimental.

Curry powder, paprika, licorice, Benedictine liqueur, prunes, raisins, tea and gherkins: Potential salicylate accumulation. These foods contain 6 mg salicylate/100 g. An ordinary American diet contains 10-200 mg/day of salicylate. Foods containing salicylates may contribute to aspirin hypersensitivity. Patients at greatest risk for aspirin hypersensitivity include those with asthma, nasal polyposis, or chronic urticaria.

**Monitoring Parameters:** Serum magnesium with high dose therapy or in patients with impaired renal function; serum salicylate levels, renal function, hearing changes or tinnitus, abnormal bruising, weight gain and response (ie, pain)

**Reference Range:** Salicylate blood levels for anti-inflammatory effect: 150-300 μg/mL; analgesia and antipyretic effect: 30-50 μg/mL

## Choline Salicylate (KOE leen sa LIS i late)

**Pharmacologic Class** Nonsteroidal Anti-Inflammatory Agent (NSAID); Salicylate

**U.S. Brand Names** Arthropan® [OTC]

**Mechanism of Action** Inhibits prostaglandin synthesis; acts on the hypothalamus heat-regulating center to reduce fever; blocks the generation of pain impulses

**Use** Temporary relief of pain of rheumatoid arthritis, rheumatic fever, osteoarthritis, and other conditions for which oral salicylates are recommended; useful in patients in which there is difficulty in administering doses in a tablet or capsule dosage form, because of the liquid dosage form

**USUAL DOSAGE**
Children >12 years and Adults: Oral: 5 mL (870 mg) every 3-4 hours, if necessary, but not more than 6 doses in 24 hours
Rheumatoid arthritis: 870-1740 mg (5-10 mL) up to 4 times/day
**Dosing adjustment/comments in renal impairment:** Avoid use in severe renal impairment

**Dosage Forms Liq** (mint flavor): 870 mg/5 mL (240 mL, 480 mL)

**Contraindications** Hypersensitivity to salicylates or any component or other nonacetylated salicylates

**Warnings/Precautions** Use with caution in patients with impaired renal function, erosive gastritis, or peptic ulcer; avoid use in patients with suspected varicella or influenza (salicylates have been associated with Reye's syndrome in children <16 years of age when used to treat symptoms of chickenpox or the flu)

**Pregnancy Risk Factor** C

**Adverse Reactions**
>10%: Gastrointestinal: Nausea, heartburn, stomach pains, dyspepsia, epigastric discomfort
1% to 10%:
Central nervous system: Fatigue
Dermatologic: Rash
Gastrointestinal: Gastrointestinal ulceration
Hematologic: Hemolytic anemia
Neuromuscular & skeletal: Weakness
Respiratory: Dyspnea
Miscellaneous: Anaphylactic shock
<1%: Insomnia, nervousness, jitters, occult bleeding, prolongation of bleeding time, leukopenia, thrombocytopenia, iron deficiency anemia, hepatotoxicity, impaired renal function, bronchospasm

**Drug Interactions**
Decreased effect with antacids
Increased effect of warfarin

**Onset** Peak concentration: 2 hours

**Half-Life** 2-30 hours

**Special PA Issues**
**Patient Education:** Take with food; do not take with antacids; watch for bleeding gums or any signs of GI bleeding; take with food or milk to minimize GI distress, notify physician if ringing in ears or persistent GI pain occurs

♦ **Choline Theophyllinate** *see* Theophylline Salts *on page 888*

## Chondroitin Sulfate-Sodium Hyaluronate
(kon DROY tin SUL fate-SOW de um hye a loo ROE nate)

**Pharmacologic Class** Ophthalmic Agent, Viscoelastic

**U.S. Brand Names** Duovisc® With Kit; Viscoat®

**Mechanism of Action** Functions as a tissue lubricant and is thought to play an important role in modulating the interactions between adjacent tissues

**Use** Surgical aid in anterior segment procedures, protects corneal endothelium and coats intraocular lens thus protecting it

**USUAL DOSAGE** Carefully introduce (using a 27-gauge needle or cannula) into anterior chamber after thoroughly cleaning the chamber with a balanced salt solution

**Dosage Forms Soln:** Sodium chondroitin 40 mg and sodium hyaluronate 30 mg (0.25 mL, 0.5 mL)

**Contraindications** Hypersensitivity to hyaluronate

**Warnings/Precautions** Product is extracted from avian tissues and contains minute amounts of protein, potential risks of hypersensitivity may exist. Intraocular pressure may be elevated as a result of pre-existing glaucoma, compromised outflow and by operative procedures and sequelae, including coma, compromised outflow and by operative procedures and sequelae, including enzymatic zonulysis, absence of an iridectomy, trauma to filtration structures and by blood and lenticular remnants in the anterior chamber. Monitor IOP, especially during the immediate postoperative period.

**Pregnancy Risk Factor** C

**Adverse Reactions** 1% to 10%: Ocular: Increased intraocular pressure

♦ **Chooz®** [OTC] *see* Calcium Carbonate *on page 139*

♦ **Chorex®** *see* Chorionic Gonadotropin *on this page*

# Chorionic Gonadotropin (kor ee ON ik goe NAD oh troe pin)

**Pharmacologic Class** Ovulation Stimulator

**U.S. Brand Names** A.P.L.®; Chorex®; Choron®; Follutein®; Glukor®; Gonic®; Pregnyl®; Profasi® HP

**Mechanism of Action** Stimulates production of gonadal steroid hormones by causing production of androgen by the testis; as a substitute for luteinizing hormone (LH) to stimulate ovulation

**Use** Induces ovulation and pregnancy in anovulatory, infertile females; treatment of hypogonadotropic hypogonadism, prepubertal cryptorchidism

**USUAL DOSAGE** I.M.:

Children:

Prepubertal cryptorchidism: 1000-2000 units/m$^2$/dose 3 times/week for 3 weeks **OR** 4000 units 3 times/week for 3 weeks **OR** 5000 units every second day for 4 injections **OR** 500 units 3 times/week for 4-6 weeks

Hypogonadotropic hypogonadism: 500-1000 units 3 times/week for 3 weeks, followed by the same dose twice weekly for 3 weeks **OR** 1000-2000 units 3 times/week **OR** 4000 units 3 times/week for 6-9 months; reduce dosage to 2000 units 3 times/week for additional 3 months

Adults: Induction of ovulation: 5000-10,000 units one day following last dose of menotropins

**Dosage Forms Powder for inj:** 200 units/mL (10 mL, 25 mL), 500 units/mL (10 mL), 1000 units/mL (10 mL), 2000 units/mL (10 mL)

**Contraindications** Hypersensitivity to chorionic gonadotropin or any component; precocious puberty, prostatic carcinoma or similar neoplasms

**Warnings/Precautions** Use with caution in asthma, seizure disorders, migraine, cardiac or renal disease; **not** effective in the treatment of obesity

**Pregnancy Risk Factor** C

**Adverse Reactions**

1% to 10%:

Central nervous system: Mental depression, fatigue

Endocrine & metabolic: Pelvic pain, ovarian cysts, enlargement of breasts, precocious puberty

Local: Pain at the injection site

Neuromuscular & skeletal: Premature closure of epiphyses

<1%: Peripheral edema, irritability, restlessness, headache, ovarian hyperstimulation syndrome, gynecomastia

**Half-Life** Half-life, biphasic: Initial: 11 hours; Terminal: 23 hours

**Special PA Issues**

**Patient Education:** Discontinue immediately if possibility of pregnancy

**Reference Range:** Depends on application and methodology; <3 mIU/mL (SI: <3 units/L) usually normal (nonpregnant)

♦ **Choron®** *see* Chorionic Gonadotropin *on this page*

♦ **Chromagen® OB** [OTC] *see* Vitamins, Multiple *on page 964*

# Chromium

**Mechanism of Action** Chromium picolinate is the only active form of chromium. It appears that chromium, in its trivalent form, increases insulin sensitivity and improves glucose transport into cells. The mechanism by which this happens could include one or more of the following:

Increase the number of insulin receptors

Enhance insulin binding to target tissues

Promote activation of insulin-receptor tyrosine kinase activity

Enhance beta cell sensitivity in the pancreas

**Use** Improves glycemic control; increases lean body mass; reduces obesity; improves lipid profile by decreasing total cholesterol and triglycerides, increasing HDL

**USUAL DOSAGE** 50-600 mcg/day

**Adverse Reactions** Gastrointestinal: Nausea, loose stools, flatulence, changes in appetite Isolated reports of anemia, cognitive impairment, renal failure

**Drug Interactions** Any medications that may also affect blood sugars; (eg, beta-blockers, thiazides, any medications prescribed to treat diabetes); discuss chromium use prior to initiating

♦ **Chronulac®** *see* Lactulose *on page 512*

♦ **Cibacalcin® Injection** *see* Calcitonin *on page 136*

# Ciclopirox (sye kloe PEER oks)

**Pharmacologic Class** Antifungal Agent, Topical

**U.S. Brand Names** Loprox®

*(Continued)*

## Ciclopirox *(Continued)*

**Mechanism of Action** Inhibiting transport of essential elements in the fungal cell causing problems in synthesis of DNA, RNA, and protein

**Use** Treatment of tinea pedis (athlete's foot), tinea cruris (jock itch), tinea corporis (ringworm), cutaneous candidiasis, and tinea versicolor (pityriasis)

**USUAL DOSAGE** Children >10 years and Adults: Apply twice daily, gently massage into affected areas; if no improvement after 4 weeks of treatment, re-evaluate the diagnosis

**Dosage Forms Crm, top:** 1% (15 g, 30 g, 90 g); **Gel:** 1%; **Lot:** 1% (30 mL)

**Contraindications** Known hypersensitivity to ciclopirox or any of its components; avoid occlusive wrappings or dressings

**Warnings/Precautions** For external use only; avoid contact with eyes

**Pregnancy Risk Factor** B

**Adverse Reactions** 1% to 10%:
Dermatologic: Pruritus
Local: Irritation, redness, burning, or pain

**Special PA Issues**
**Patient Education:** Avoid contact with eyes; if sensitivity or irritation occurs, discontinue use

**Related Information**
Antifungal Agents, Topical *on page 1000*

♦ **Ciclopirox Olamine** *see* Ciclopirox *on previous page*

## Cidofovir (si DOF o veer)

**Pharmacologic Class** Antiviral Agent

**U.S. Brand Names** Vistide®

**Mechanism of Action** Cidofovir is converted to cidofovir diphosphate which is the active intracellular metabolite; cidofovir diphosphate suppresses CMV replication by selective inhibition of viral DNA synthesis. Incorporation of cidofovir into growing viral DNA chain results in reductions in the rate of viral DNA synthesis.

**Use** Treatment of cytomegalovirus (CMV) retinitis in patients with acquired immunodeficiency syndrome (AIDS). **Note:** Should be administered with probenecid.

**USUAL DOSAGE**
Induction: 5 mg/kg I.V. over 1 hour once weekly for 2 consecutive weeks
Maintenance: 5 mg/kg over 1 hour once every other week
**Administer with probenecid - 2 g orally 3 hours prior to each cidofovir dose and 1 g at 2 and 8 hours after completion of the infusion (total: 4 g)**
Hydrate with 1 L of 0.9% NS I.V. prior to cidofovir infusion; a second liter may be administered over a 1- to 3-hour period immediately following infusion, if tolerated
**Dosing adjustment in renal impairment:**
$Cl_{cr}$ 41-55 mL/minute: 2 mg/kg
$Cl_{cr}$ 30-40 mL/minute: 1.5 mg/kg
$Cl_{cr}$ 20-29 mL/minute: 1 mg/kg
$Cl_{cr}$ <19 mL/minute: 0.5 mg/kg
If the creatinine increases by 0.3-0.4 mg/dL, reduce the cidofovir dose to 3 mg/kg; discontinue therapy for increases ≥0.5 mg/dL or development of ≥3+ proteinuria

**Dosage Forms Inj:** 75 mg/mL (5 mL)

**Contraindications** Patients with hypersensitivity to cidofovir and in patients with a history of clinically severe hypersensitivity to probenecid or other sulfa-containing medications

**Warnings/Precautions** Dose-dependent nephrotoxicity requires dose adjustment or discontinuation if changes in renal function occur during therapy (eg, proteinuria, glycosuria, decreased serum phosphate, uric acid or bicarbonate, and elevated creatinine); avoid use in patients with creatinine >1.5 mg/dL; $Cl_{cr}$ <55 mL/minute; use great caution with elderly patients; neutropenia and ocular hypotony have also occurred; safety and efficacy have not been established in children; administration must be accompanied by oral probenecid and intravenous saline prehydration; prepare admixtures in a class two laminar flow hood, wearing protective gear; dispose of cidofovir as directed

**Pregnancy Risk Factor** C

**Pregnancy Implications**
Clinical effect on the fetus: Although studies are inconclusive, adenocarcinomas have occurred in animal studies with cidofovir; use during pregnancy only if the potential benefit justifies the potential risk to the fetus
Breast-feeding/lactation: Excretion of cidofovir into breast milk is unknown

**Adverse Reactions**
>10%:
Central nervous system: Infection, chills, fever, headache, amnesia, anxiety, confusion, seizures, insomnia
Dermatologic: Alopecia, rash, acne, skin discoloration
Gastrointestinal: Nausea, vomiting, diarrhea, anorexia, abdominal pain, constipation, dyspepsia, gastritis
Hematologic: Thrombocytopenia, neutropenia, anemia

Neuromuscular & skeletal: Weakness, paresthesia
Ocular: Amblyopia, conjunctivitis, ocular hypotony
Renal: Tubular damage, proteinuria, elevated creatinine
Respiratory: Asthma, bronchitis, coughing, dyspnea, pharyngitis
1% to 10%:
Cardiovascular: Hypotension, pallor, syncope, tachycardia
Central nervous system: Dizziness, hallucinations, depression, somnolence, malaise
Dermatologic: Pruritus, urticaria
Endocrine & metabolic: Hyperglycemia, hyperlipidemia, hypocalcemia, hypokalemia, dehydration
Gastrointestinal: Abnormal taste, stomatitis
Genitourinary: Glycosuria, urinary incontinence, urinary tract infections
Neuromuscular & skeletal: Skeletal pain
Ocular: Retinal detachment, iritis, uveitis, abnormal vision
Renal: Hematuria
Respiratory: Pneumonia, rhinitis, sinusitis
Miscellaneous: Diaphoresis, allergic reactions

**Drug Interactions** Increased effect/toxicity: Drugs with nephrotoxic potential (eg, amphotericin B, aminoglycosides, foscarnet, and I.V. pentamidine) should be avoided during cidofovir therapy

**Half-Life** ~2.6 hours (when administered with probenecid)

**Special PA Issues**
**Patient Education:** This drug can only be administered I.V. You may experience hair loss (reversible). You may be more susceptible to infection; avoid crowds and infectious situations. You may experience headache, anxiety, confusion; use caution when driving or engaging in tasks requiring alertness. You may experience GI upset (buttermilk or yogurt may help relieve diarrhea); frequent small meals, frequent mouth care, or sucking on lozenges may relieve nausea, heartburn, or vomiting; and increased exercise and increased dietary fruit, fluids, or fiber may reduce constipation. You may experience postural hypotension; use caution changing from lying to sitting or standing position and when climbing stairs. Report severe unresolved vomiting, constipation or diarrhea, chills, fever, signs of infection, difficulty breathing or coughing, palpitations, chest pain, syncope, CNS changes (eg, hallucinations, depression, excessive sedation, amnesia, seizures, insomnia), or other severe side effects.

**Monitoring Parameters:** Renal function (Cr, BUN, UAs), LFTs, WBCs, intraocular pressure and visual acuity

# Cilostazol (sil OH sta zol)

**Pharmacologic Class** Platelet Aggregation Inhibitor
**U.S. Brand Names** Pletal®

**Mechanism of Action** Cilostazol and its metabolites are inhibitors of phosphodiesterase III. As a result cyclic AMP is increased leading to inhibition of platelet aggregation and vasodilation. Other effects of phosphodiesterase III inhibition include increased cardiac contractility, accelerated AV nodal conduction, increased ventricular automaticity, heart rate, and coronary blood flow.

**Use** Symptomatic management of peripheral vascular disease, primarily intermittent claudication; currently being investigated for the treatment of acute coronary syndromes

**USUAL DOSAGE** Adults: Oral: 100 mg twice daily taken at least one-half hour before or 2 hours after breakfast and dinner; dosage should be reduced to 50 mg twice daily during concurrent therapy with inhibitors of CYP3A4 or CYP2C19 (see Drug Interactions)

**Dosage Forms** Tab: 50 mg, 100 mg

**Contraindications** Hypersensitivity to cilostazol or any component of the formulation; heart failure (of any severity)

**Warnings/Precautions** Use with caution in patients receiving platelet aggregation inhibitors (effects are unknown), hepatic impairment (not studied). Use with caution in patients receiving inhibitors of CYP3A4 (such as ketoconazole or erythromycin) or inhibitors of CYP2C19 (such as omeprazole); use with caution in severe underlying heart disease; use is not recommended in nursing mothers

**Pregnancy Risk Factor** C

**Pregnancy Implications** In animal studies, abnormalities of the skeletal, renal and cardiovascular system were increased. In addition, the incidence of stillbirth and decreased birth weights were increased. It is not known whether cilostazol is excreted in human milk. Because of the potential risk to nursing infants, a decision to discontinue the drug or discontinue nursing should be made.

**Adverse Reactions**
>10%:
Central nervous system: Headache (27% to 34%)
Gastrointestinal: Abnormal stools (12% to 15%), diarrhea (12% to 19%)
Miscellaneous: Infection (10% to 14%)
2% to 10%:
Cardiovascular: Peripheral edema (7% to 9%), palpitation (5% to 10%), tachycardia (4%)
Central nervous system: Dizziness (9% to 10%)

(Continued)

## Cilostazol *(Continued)*

Gastrointestinal: Dyspepsia (6%), nausea (6% to 7%), abdominal pain (4% to 5%), flatulence (2% to 3%)

Neuromuscular & skeletal: Back pain (6% to 7%), myalgia (2% to 3%)

Respiratory: Rhinitis (7% to 12%), pharyngitis (7% to 10%), cough (3% to 4%)

<2%: Chills, facial edema, fever, edema, malaise, nuchal rigidity, pelvic pain, retroperitoneal hemorrhage, cerebral infarction/ischemia, congestive heart failure, cardiac arrest, hemorrhage, hypotension, myocardial infarction/ischemia, postural hypotension, ventricular arrhythmia, supraventricular arrhythmia, syncope, anorexia, cholelithiasis, colitis, duodenitis, peptic ulcer, duodenal ulcer, esophagitis, esophageal hemorrhage, gastritis, hematemesis, melena, tongue edema, diabetes mellitus, anemia, ecchymosis, polycythemia, purpura, increased creatinine, gout, hyperlipidemia, hyperuricemia, arthralgia, bone pain, bursitis, anxiety, insomnia, neuralgia, dry skin, urticaria, amblyopia, blindness, conjunctivitis, diplopia, retinal hemorrhage, cystitis, albuminuria, vaginitis, vaginal hemorrhage, urinary frequency

**Drug Interactions** CYP3A4 and CYP2C19 cytochrome enzyme substrate

Increased effect/toxicity: Increased concentrations of cilostazol have been observed during concurrent therapy with omeprazole, an inhibitor of CYP2C19 and during concurrent therapy with inhibitors of CYP3A4 such as clarithromycin, erythromycin, itraconazole, fluconazole, miconazole, fluvoxamine, fluoxetine, nefazodone, sertraline, and diltiazem. Platelet aggregation with aspirin is further inhibited when coadministered with cilostazol, it remains unclear whether concurrent oral anticoagulants or other antiplatelet drugs can increase cilostazol toxicity.

**Onset** 2-4 weeks

**Special PA Issues**

**Dietary Considerations:** Avoid concurrent ingestion of grapefruit juice due to the potential to inhibit CYP3A4. Avoid administration with meals. Taking cilostazol with a high-fat meal increases the AUC by 25% and the peak concentration may be increased by 90%; it is best to take cilostazol 30 minutes before or 2 hours after meals.

♦ **Ciloxan™ Ophthalmic** *see Ciprofloxacin on next page*

## Cimetidine *(sye MET i deen)*

**Pharmacologic Class** Histamine H$_2$ Antagonist

**U.S. Brand Names** Tagamet®; Tagamet® HB [OTC]

**Mechanism of Action** Competitive inhibition of histamine at H$_2$-receptors of the gastric parietal cells resulting in reduced gastric acid secretion, gastric volume and hydrogen ion concentration reduced

**Use** Short-term treatment of active duodenal ulcers and benign gastric ulcers; long-term prophylaxis of duodenal ulcer; gastric hypersecretory states; gastroesophageal reflux; prevention of upper GI bleeding in critically ill patients.

**USUAL DOSAGE**

Children: Oral, I.M., I.V.: 20-40 mg/kg/day in divided doses every 4 hours

Adults: Short-term treatment of active ulcers:

Oral: 300 mg 4 times/day or 800 mg at bedtime or 400 mg twice daily for up to 8 weeks

I.M., I.V.: 300 mg every 6 hours or 37.5 mg/hour by continuous infusion; I.V. dosage should be adjusted to maintain an intragastric pH ≥5

Patients with an active bleed: Administer cimetidine as a continuous infusion (see above)

Duodenal ulcer prophylaxis: Oral: 400-800 mg at bedtime

Gastric hypersecretory conditions: Oral, I.M., I.V.: 300-600 mg every 6 hours; dosage not to exceed 2.4 g/day

**Dosing adjustment/interval in renal impairment:** Children and Adults:

Cl$_{cr}$ 20-40 mL/minute: Administer every 8 hours or 75% of normal dose

Cl$_{cr}$ 0-20 mL/minute: Administer every 12 hours or 50% of normal dose

Hemodialysis: Slightly dialyzable (5% to 20%)

**Dosing adjustment/comments in hepatic impairment:** Usual dose is safe in mild liver disease but use with caution and in reduced dosage in severe liver disease; increased risk of CNS toxicity in cirrhosis suggested by enhanced penetration of CNS

**Dosage Forms Inf, as hydrochloride, in NS:** 300 mg (50 mL); **Inj, as hydrochloride:** 150 mg/mL (2 mL, 8 mL); **Liq, oral, as hydrochloride (mint-peach flavor):** 300 mg/5 mL with alcohol 2.8% (5 mL, 240 mL); **Tab:** 200 mg, 300 mg, 400 mg, 800 mg

**Contraindications** Hypersensitivity to cimetidine, other component, or other H$_2$-antagonists

**Warnings/Precautions** Adjust dosages in renal/hepatic impairment or patients receiving drugs metabolized through the P-450 system

**Pregnancy Risk Factor** B

**Adverse Reactions**

1% to 10%:

Central nervous system: Dizziness, agitation, headache, drowsiness

Gastrointestinal: Diarrhea, nausea, vomiting

<1%: Bradycardia, hypotension, tachycardia, confusion, fever, rash, gynecomastia, edema of the breasts, decreased sexual ability, neutropenia, agranulocytosis, thrombocytopenia, increased AST/ALT, myalgia, elevated creatinine

**Drug Interactions** CYP3A3/4 enzyme substrate; CYP1A2, 2C9, 2C18, 2C19, 2D6, and 3A3/4 enzyme inhibitor

Increased toxicity: Decreased elimination of lidocaine, theophylline, phenytoin, metronidazole, triamterene, procainamide, quinidine, and propranolol

Inhibition of warfarin metabolism, tricyclic antidepressant metabolism, diazepam elimination and cyclosporine elimination

**Onset** 1 hour; peak serum concentrations ~1 hour after oral dose

**Duration** 6 hours

**Half-Life** Normal renal function: 2 hours

**Special PA Issues**

**Patient Education:** Take with meals. Limit xanthine-containing foods and beverages which may decrease iron absorption. To be effective, continue to take for the prescribed time (possibly 4-8 weeks) even though symptoms may have improved. Smoking decreases the effectiveness of cimetidine; stop smoking if possible. Avoid use of caffeine or aspirin products. Report diarrhea, black tarry stools, coffee ground like emesis, dizziness, confusion, rash, unusual bleeding or bruising, sore throat, and fever.

**Dietary Considerations:** Alcohol: Additive CNS effects, avoid or limit use

**Monitoring Parameters:** Blood pressure with I.V. push administration, CBC, gastric pH, signs and symptoms of peptic ulcer disease, occult blood with GI bleeding, monitor renal function to correct dose; monitor for side effects

♦ **Cinobac® Pulvules®** *see* Cinoxacin *on this page*

# Cinoxacin (sin OKS a sin)

**Pharmacologic Class** Antibiotic, Quinolone

**U.S. Brand Names** Cinobac® Pulvules®

**Mechanism of Action** Inhibits microbial synthesis of DNA with resultant inhibition of protein synthesis

**Use** Treatment of urinary tract infections

**USUAL DOSAGE** Children >12 years and Adults: Oral: 1 g/day in 2-4 doses for 7-14 days

**Dosing interval in renal impairment:**

$Cl_{cr}$ 20-50 mL/minute: 250 mg twice daily

$Cl_{cr}$ <20 mL/minute: 250 mg/day

**Dosage Forms Cap:** 250 mg, 500 mg

**Contraindications** History of convulsive disorders, hypersensitivity to cinoxacin or any component or other quinolones

**Warnings/Precautions** CNS stimulation may occur (tremor, restlessness, confusion, and very rarely hallucinations or seizures). Use with caution in patients with known or suspected CNS disorders or renal impairment. Not recommended in children <18 years of age, ciprofloxacin (a related compound), has caused a transient arthropathy in children; prolonged use may result in superinfection; modify dosage in patients with renal impairment.

**Pregnancy Risk Factor** B

**Adverse Reactions** Generally well tolerated

1% to 10%:

Central nervous system: Headache, dizziness

Gastrointestinal: Heartburn, abdominal pain, GI bleeding, belching, flatulence, anorexia, nausea

<1%: Insomnia, confusion, seizures (rare), diarrhea, thrombocytopenia, photophobia, tinnitus

**Drug Interactions**

Decreased effect: Decreased urine levels with probenecid; decreased absorption with aluminum-, magnesium-, calcium-containing antacids

Increased serum levels: Probenecid

**Half-Life** 1.5 hours, prolonged in renal impairment

**Special PA Issues**

**Patient Education:** Take prescribed dose with food. Maintain adequate hydration (2-3 L/day of fluids unless instructed to restrict fluid intake). Avoid antacid use. May cause dizziness; avoid driving or hazardous activity until response to drug is known. Small frequent meals, frequent mouth care, or sucking on lozenges may reduce nausea or vomiting. Report skin rash, itching, redness, or swelling; pain, inflammation, or rupture of tendon; pain or burning on urination; or persistent diarrhea or vomiting.

♦ **Cipro™** *see* Ciprofloxacin *on this page*

# Ciprofloxacin (sip roe FLOKS a sin)

**Pharmacologic Class** Antibiotic, Ophthalmic; Antibiotic, Quinolone

**U.S. Brand Names** Ciloxan™ Ophthalmic; Cipro™; Cipro™ I.V.

**Mechanism of Action** Inhibits DNA-gyrase in susceptible organisms; inhibits relaxation of supercoiled DNA and promotes breakage of double-stranded DNA

**Use** Treatment of documented or suspected infections of the lower respiratory tract, sinuses, skin and skin structure, bone/joints, and urinary tract including prostatitis, due to susceptible
(Continued)

## Ciprofloxacin *(Continued)*

bacterial strains; especially indicated for *Pseudomonal* infections and those due to multi-drug resistant gram-negative organisms, chronic bacterial prostatitis, infectious diarrhea, complicated gram-negative and anaerobic intra-abdominal infections (with metronidazole) due to *E. coli* (enteropathic strains),*B. fragilis, P. mirabilis, K. pneumoniae, P. aeruginosa, Campylobacter jejuni* or *Shigella*; approved for acute sinusitis caused by *H. influenzae* or *M. catarrhalis*; also used to treat typhoid fever due to *Salmonella typhi* (although eradication of the chronic typhoid carrier state has not been proven), osteomyelitis when parenteral therapy is not feasible, and sexually transmitted diseases such as uncomplicated cervical and urethral gonorrhea due to *Neisseria gonorrhoeae*; used ophthalmologically for superficial ocular infections (corneal ulcers, conjunctivitis) due to susceptible strains

### USUAL DOSAGE

Children (see Warnings/Precautions):
Oral: 20-30 mg/kg/day in 2 divided doses; maximum: 1.5 g/day
Cystic fibrosis: 20-40 mg/kg/day divided every 12 hours
I.V.: 15-20 mg/kg/day divided every 12 hours
Cystic fibrosis: 15-30 mg/kg/day divided every 8-12 hours
Adults: Oral:
Urinary tract infection: 250-500 mg every 12 hours for 7-10 days, depending on severity of infection and susceptibility; (3 investigations (n=975) indicate the minimum effective dose for women with acute, uncomplicated urinary tract infection may be 100 mg twice daily for 3 days)
Lower respiratory tract, skin/skin structure infections: 500-750 mg twice daily for 7-14 days depending on severity and susceptibility
Bone/joint infections: 500-750 mg twice daily for 4-6 weeks, depending on severity and susceptibility
Infectious diarrhea: 500 mg every 12 hours for 5-7 days
Typhoid fever: 500 mg every 12 hours for 10 days
Urethral/cervical gonococcal infections: 250-500 mg as a single dose (CDC recommends concomitant doxycycline or azithromycin due to developing resistance; avoid use in Asian or Western Pacific travelers)
Disseminated gonococcal infection: 500 mg twice daily to complete 7 days of therapy (initial treatment with ceftriaxone 1 g I.M./I.V. daily for 24-48 hours after improvement begins)
Chancroid: 500 mg twice daily for 3 days
Mild to moderate sinusitis: 500 mg every 12 hours for 10 days
Adults: I.V.
Urinary tract infection: 200-400 mg every 12 hours for 7-10 days
Lower respiratory tract, skin/skin structure infection (mild to moderate): 400 mg every 12 hours for 7-14 days
Ophthalmic: Instill 1-2 drops in eye(s) every 2 hours while awake for 2 days and 1-2 drops every 4 hours while awake for the next 5 days
**Dosing adjustment in renal impairment:**
$Cl_{cr}$ >30 mL/minute:
250 mg every 12 hours or
500 mg every 12 hours or
750 mg every 12 hours
$Cl_{cr}$ <30 mL/minute:
500 mg every 24 hours or
750 mg every 24 hours
Dialysis: Only small amounts of ciprofloxacin are removed by hemo- or peritoneal dialysis (<10%); usual dose: 250-500 mg every 24 hours following dialysis
Continuous arteriovenous or venovenous hemodiafiltration (CAVH) effects: Administer 200-400 mg I.V. every 12 hours

**Dosage Forms Inf in D₅W:** 400 mg (200 mL); **Inf in NS or D₅W:** 200 mg (100 mL); **Inj:** 200 mg (20 mL), 400 mg (40 mL); **Soln, ophth:** 3.5 mg/mL (2.5 mL, 5 mL); **Susp, oral:** 250 mg/5 mL x 100 mL, 500 mg/5 mL x 100 mL; **Tab:** 100 mg, 250 mg, 500 mg, 750 mg

**Contraindications** Hypersensitivity to ciprofloxacin, any component or other quinolones

**Warnings/Precautions** Not recommended in children <18 years of age; has caused transient arthropathy in children; CNS stimulation may occur (tremor, restlessness, confusion, and very rarely hallucinations or seizures); use with caution in patients with known or suspected CNS disorder; green discoloration of teeth in newborns has been reported; prolonged use may result in superinfection; may rarely cause inflamed or ruptured tendons (discontinue use immediately with signs of inflammation or tendon pain)

**Pregnancy Risk Factor** C

### Adverse Reactions

1% to 10%:
Central nervous system: Headache, restlessness
Gastrointestinal: Nausea, diarrhea, vomiting, abdominal pain
Dermatologic: Rash
<1%: Dizziness, confusion, seizures, anemia, increased liver enzymes, tremor, arthralgia, ruptured tendons, acute renal failure

**Drug Interactions** CYP1A2 enzyme inhibitor

Decreased effect:

Enteral feedings may decrease plasma concentrations of ciprofloxacin probably by >30% inhibition of absorption. Ciprofloxacin should not be administered with enteral feedings. The feeding would need to be discontinued for 1-2 hours prior to and after ciprofloxacin administration. Nasogastric administration produces a greater loss of ciprofloxacin bioavailability than does nasoduodenal administration.

Aluminum/magnesium products, didanosine, and sucralfate may decrease absorption of ciprofloxacin by ≥90% if administered concurrently

RECOMMENDATION: Administer ciprofloxacin 2 hours before dose OR administer ciprofloxacin at least 4 hours and preferably 6 hours after the dose of these agents OR change to an $H_2$-antagonist or omeprazole

Calcium, iron, zinc, and multivitamins with minerals products may decrease absorption of ciprofloxacin significantly if administered concurrently

RECOMMENDATION: Administer ciprofloxacin 2 hours before dose OR administer ciprofloxacin at least 2 hours after the dose of these agents

Increased toxicity:

Caffeine and theophylline → CNS stimulation when concurrent with ciprofloxacin

Cyclosporine may increase serum creatinine levels

**Half-Life** Adults with normal renal function: 3-5 hours

**Special PA Issues**

**Patient Education:** May be taken with nondairy food. Do not consume dairy products, antacids, or other medications 2 hours prior to or 2 hours after taking ciprofloxacin. Avoid excessive use of caffeine or chocolate. Maintain adequate hydration (2-3 L/day of fluids unless instructed to restrict fluid intake) to avoid concentrated urine and crystal formation. May cause dizziness, drowsiness, or lightheadedness (avoid driving or hazardous activity until response to drug is known); nausea or vomiting (small frequent meals, frequent mouth care, or sucking on lozenges may help); photosensitivity (use sunscreen, wear protective clothing and eyewear, or avoid extended exposure to direct sunlight). Report unresolved diarrhea or abdominal pain; rash, itching, or redness; fever; chills; vaginal itching or discharge; white places in mouth; CNS disturbance (agitation, confusion, hallucinations, tremors); join swelling or pain; pain, inflammation, or rupture of tendon; or respiratory difficulty.

Ophthalmic: Wash hands before instilling. Sit or lie down to instill. Open eye, look at ceiling, and instill prescribed amount of medication. Close eye and apply gentle pressure to inner corner of eye. Do not let tip of applicator touch eye or contaminate tip of applicator. Temporary stinging or burning may occur. Report persistent pain, burning, vision disturbances, swelling, itching, foreign body sensation, rash, or worsening of condition.

**Dietary Considerations:**

Food: Decreases rate, but not extent, of absorption. Drug may cause GI upset; take without regard to meals (manufacturer prefers that drug is taken 2 hours after meals)

Dairy products, oral multivitamins, and mineral supplements: Absorption decreased by divalent and trivalent cations. These cations bind to and form insoluble complexes with quinolones. Avoid taking these substrates with ciprofloxacin. The manufacturer states that the usual dietary intake of calcium has not been shown to interfere with ciprofloxacin absorption.

Caffeine: Possible exaggerated or prolonged effects of caffeine. Ciprofloxacin reduces total body clearance of caffeine. Patients consuming regular large quantities of caffeinated beverages may need to restrict caffeine intake if excessive cardiac or CNS stimulation occurs.

**Monitoring Parameters:** Patients receiving concurrent ciprofloxacin, theophylline, or cyclosporine should have serum levels monitored

**Reference Range:** Therapeutic: 2.6-3 µg/mL; Toxic: >5 µg/mL

# Ciprofloxacin and Hydrocortisone

(sip roe FLOKS a sin & hye droe KOR ti sone)

**Pharmacologic Class** Antibiotic/Corticosteroid, Otic

**U.S. Brand Names** Cipro™ HC Otic

**Dosage Forms Susp, otic:** Ciprofloxacin hydrochloride 0.2% and hydrocortisone 1%

♦ **Ciprofloxacin Hydrochloride** *see* Ciprofloxacin *on page 209*

♦ **Cipro™ HC Otic** *see* Ciprofloxacin and Hydrocortisone *on this page*

♦ **Cipro™ I.V.** *see* Ciprofloxacin *on page 209*

# Cisapride (SIS a pride)

**Pharmacologic Class** Gastrointestinal Agent, Prokinetic

**U.S. Brand Names** Propulsid®

**Mechanism of Action** Enhances the release of acetylcholine at the myenteric plexus. *In vitro* studies have shown cisapride to have serotonin-4 receptor agonistic properties which may increase gastrointestinal motility and cardiac rate; increases lower esophageal

(Continued)

## Cisapride *(Continued)*

sphincter pressure and lower esophageal peristalsis; accelerates gastric emptying of both liquids and solids.

**Use** Treatment of nocturnal symptoms of gastroesophageal reflux disease (GERD), also demonstrated effectiveness for gastroparesis, refractory constipation, and nonulcer dyspepsia

**USUAL DOSAGE** Oral:

Children: 0.15-0.3 mg/kg/dose 3-4 times/day; maximum: 10 mg/dose

Adults: Initial: 10 mg 4 times/day at least 15 minutes before meals and at bedtime; in some patients the dosage will need to be increased to 20 mg to obtain a satisfactory result

**Dosage Forms Susp, oral (cherry cream flavor):** 1 mg/mL (450 mL); **Tab, scored:** 10 mg, 20 mg

### Contraindications

Hypersensitivity to cisapride or any of its components; GI hemorrhage, mechanical obstruction, GI perforation, or other situations when GI motility stimulation is dangerous

Serious cardiac arrhythmias including ventricular tachycardia, ventricular fibrillation, torsade de pointes, and QT prolongation have been reported in patients taking cisapride with other drugs that inhibit CYP3A4. Some of these events have been fatal. Concomitant oral or intravenous administration of the following drugs with cisapride may lead to elevated cisapride blood levels and is contraindicated:

Antibiotics: Oral or I.V. erythromycin, clarithromycin, troleandomycin

Antidepressants: Nefazodone

Antifungals: Oral or I.V. fluconazole, itraconazole, miconazole, oral ketoconazole

Protease inhibitors: Indinavir, ritonavir

Cisapride is also contraindicated for patients with history of prolonged electrocardiographic QT intervals, renal failure, history of ventricular arrhythmias, ischemic heart disease, and congestive heart failure; uncorrected electrolyte disorders (hypokalemia, hypomagnesemia); respiratory failure; and concomitant medications known to prolong the QT interval and increase the risk of arrhythmia, such as certain antiarrhythmics, certain antipsychotics, certain antidepressants, astemizole, bepridil, sparfloxacin, and terodiline. The preceding lists of drugs are not comprehensive. Cisapride should not be used in patients with uncorrected hypokalemia or hypomagnesemia or who might experience rapid reduction of plasma potassium such as those administered potassium-wasting diuretics and/or insulin in acute settings.

**Warnings/Precautions Serious cardiac arrhythmias including ventricular tachycardia, ventricular fibrillation, torsade de pointes, and QT prolongation have been reported in patients taking this drug.** Many of these patients also took drugs expected to increase cisapride blood levels by inhibiting the cytochrome P-450 3A4 enzymes that metabolize cisapride. These drugs include clarithromycin, erythromycin, troleandomycin, nefazodone, fluconazole, itraconazole, ketoconazole, indinavir and ritonavir. Some of these events have been fatal. Cisapride is contraindicated in patients taking any of these drugs. **QT prolongation, torsade de pointes (sometimes with syncope), cardiac arrest and sudden death have been reported in patients taking cisapride without the above mentioned contraindicated drugs.** Most patients had disorders that may have predisposed them to arrhythmias with cisapride. Cisapride is contraindicated for those patients with: history of prolonged electrocardiographic QT intervals; renal failure; history of ventricular arrhythmias, ischemic heart disease, and congestive heart failure; uncorrected electrolyte disorders (hypokalemia, hypomagnesemia); respiratory failure; and concomitant medications known to prolong the QT interval and increase the risk of arrhythmia, such as certain antiarrhythmics, including those of Class 1A (such as quinidine and procainamide) and Class III (such as sotalol); tricyclic antidepressants (such as amitriptyline); certain tetracyclic antidepressants (such as maprotiline); certain antipsychotic medications (such as certain phenothiazines and sertindole), astemizole, bepridil, sparfloxacin and terodiline. (The preceding lists of drugs are not comprehensive.) Recommended doses of cisapride should not be exceeded.

Potential benefits should be weighed against risks prior administration of cisapride to patients who have or may develop prolongation of cardiac conduction intervals, particularly QTc. These include patients with conditions that could predispose them to the development of serious arrhythmias, such as multiple organ failure, COPD, apnea and advanced cancer. Cisapride should not be used in patients with uncorrected hypokalemia or hypomagnesemia, such as those with severe dehydration, vomiting or malnutrition, or those taking potassium-wasting diuretics. Cisapride should not be used in patients who might experience rapid reduction of plasma potassium, such as those administered potassium-wasting diuretics and/or insulin in acute settings.

**Pregnancy Risk Factor** C

### Adverse Reactions

>5%:

Central nervous system: Headache

Dermatologic: Rash

Gastrointestinal: Diarrhea, GI cramping, dyspepsia, flatulence, nausea, xerostomia

Respiratory: Rhinitis

&lt;5%:
Cardiovascular: Tachycardia
Central nervous system: Extrapyramidal effects, somnolence, fatigue, seizures, insomnia, anxiety
Hematologic: Thrombocytopenia, increased LFTs, pancytopenia, leukopenia, granulocytopenia, aplastic anemia
Respiratory: Sinusitis, coughing, upper respiratory tract infection, increased incidence of viral infection

**Drug Interactions** CYP3A3/4 enzyme substrate
Decreased effect: Atropine, digoxin
Increased toxicity: Warfarin, diazepam increased levels, cimetidine, and ranitidine, CNS depressants; erythromycin and other macrolides and the azole-derivative antifungal agents such as ketoconazole, miconazole, itraconazole, and fluconazole have increased cisapride levels, which has been associated with prolonged Q-T intervals and the potential for torsade de pointes

**Onset** 0.5-1 hour

**Half-Life** 6-12 hours

**Special PA Issues**
Patient Education: Take before meals. Avoid alcohol and other CNS depressants. May cause increased sedation. Report severe abdominal pain, prolonged diarrhea, weight loss, or extreme fatigue.

♦ **13-*cis*-Retinoic Acid** *see* Isotretinoin *on page 499*

# Citalopram (sye TAL oh pram)

**Pharmacologic Class** Antidepressant, Selective Serotonin Reuptake Inhibitor

**U.S. Brand Names** Celexa®

**Mechanism of Action** Inhibits CNS neuronal reuptake of serotonin, which enhances serotonergic activity. Activity as an antidepressant has been presumed to be associated with this effect. Has limited or no affinity for histamine, dopamine, acetylcholine (muscarinic), GABA, benzodiazepine, and adrenergic (alpha- and beta-) receptors. Antagonism of these receptors is believed to be associated with sedative, anticholinergic and cardiovascular adverse effects of tricyclic antidepressants.

**Use** Treatment of depression; currently being evaluated for use in the treatment of dementia, smoking cessation, alcohol abuse, obsessive-compulsive disorder, and diabetic neuropathy

**USUAL DOSAGE** Oral: 20 mg once daily, in the morning or evening. Dose is generally increased to 40 mg once daily. Doses should be increased by 20 mg at intervals of not less than 1 week. Doses >40 mg/day are not generally recommended, although some patients may respond to doses up to 60 mg/day.

Elderly or hepatically impaired patients: Initial dose of 20 mg is recommended; increase dose to 40 mg/day only in nonresponders
Maintenance: Generally, patients are maintained on the dose required for acute stabilization. If side effects are bothersome, dose reduction by 20 mg/day may be considered.
Dosing adjustment in renal impairment: None necessary in mild to moderate renal impairment; best avoided in severely impaired renal function (Cl$_{cr}$ <20 mL/minute)

**Dosage Forms** Tab, as hydrobromide: 20 mg, 40 mg, 60 mg

**Contraindications** Known hypersensitivity to citalopram; hypersensitivity or other adverse sequelae during therapy with other SSRIs; concomitant use with MAO inhibitors or within 2 weeks of discontinuing MAO inhibitors. Potential for severe reaction when used with MAO inhibitors - serotonin syndrome (hyperthermia, muscular rigidity, mental status changes/agitation, autonomic instability) may occur, possibly resulting in death. Do not use citalopram and MAO inhibitors within 14 days of each other.

**Warnings/Precautions** As with all antidepressants, use with caution in patients with a history of mania (may activate hypomania/mania). Use with caution in patients with a history of seizures and patients at high risk of suicide. Has potential to impair cognitive/motor performance - should use caution operating hazardous machinery. Elderly and patients with hepatic insufficiency should receive lower dosages. Use with caution in renal insufficiency and other concomitant illness (due to limited drug experience). May cause hyponatremia/SIADH.

**Pregnancy Risk Factor** C

**Pregnancy Implications** Animal reproductive studies have revealed adverse effects on fetal and postnatal development (at doses higher than human therapeutic doses). Should be used in pregnancy only if potential benefit justifies potential risk. Citalopram is excreted in human milk; a decision should be made whether to continue or discontinue nursing or discontinue the drug.

**Adverse Reactions**
>10%:
Central nervous system: Somnolence (18%), insomnia (15%)
Gastrointestinal: Nausea (21%), dry mouth (20%)
Miscellaneous: Increased diaphoresis (11%)
(Continued)

## Citalopram *(Continued)*

1% to 10%:
   Central nervous system: Fatigue (5%), anxiety (4%), agitation (3%), yawning (2%), fever (2%)
   Endocrine/metabolic: Dysmenorrhea (3%), decreased libido (males 3.8%, females 1.3%), anorgasmia (females 1.1%)
   Gastrointestinal: Diarrhea (8%), dyspepsia (5%), vomiting (4%), anorexia (4%), abdominal pain (3%)
   Genitourinary: Ejaculation disorder (6%), impotence (3%)
   Neuromuscular/skeletal: Tremor (8%), arthralgia (2%), myalgia (2%)
   Respiratory: Upper respiratory tract infection (5%), rhinitis (5%), sinusitis (3%)

The following events had an incidence >2% in clinical trials but the incidence on placebo was greater than or equal to the incidence on citalopram: Headache, asthenia, dizziness, constipation, palpitation, abnormal vision, sleep disorder, nervousness, pharyngitis, micturition disorder, back pain

The following treatment emergent effects were also noted at a frequency ≥1% in premarketing trials: Migraine, impaired concentration, confusion, hypotension, postural hypotension, tachycardia, suicide attempt, rash, pruritus, weight gain or loss, abnormal taste, increased appetite, amenorrhea, paresthesia, abnormal accommodation, cough

Several cases of hyponatremia and SIADH have been reported with citalopram. As with other antidepressants, hypomania/mania may be activated in a small proportion of patients with major affective disorders.

**Drug Interactions Extensive metabolism via CYP450 isoenzymes 3A4 and 2C19.** Decreases in citalopram clearance are possible when used with inhibitors of these isoenzymes (including ketoconazole, itraconazole, fluconazole, and erythromycin). Citalopram is also a weak inhibitor of CYP450 isoenzymes 1A2, 2D6, and 2C19.

Caution when use with other CNS active agents. See Contraindications and Warnings regarding the use of MAO inhibitors. Cimetidine increases AUC by 43%, lithium may enhance serotonergic effects, and carbamazepine may increase clearance of citalopram via enzyme induction. Citalopram may increase the serum concentration of metoprolol. Serum concentrations of imipramine metabolite (desipramine) may be increased.

**Onset** Usually >2 weeks

**Half-Life** 24-48 hours (average 35 hours - doubled in patients with hepatic impairment)

**Special PA Issues**

   **Patient Education:** The effects of this medication may take up to 3 weeks. Take as directed; do not alter dose or frequency without consulting prescriber. Avoid alcohol, caffeine, and CNS stimulants. You may experience sexual dysfunction (reversible). May cause dizziness, anxiety, or blurred vision (rise slowly from sitting or lying position and use caution when driving or engaging in hazardous tasks until response to drug is known); nausea or dry mouth (frequent small meals, chewing gum, or sucking on lozenges may help). Report confusion or impaired concentration, severe headache, palpitations, rash, insomnia or nightmares, changes in personality, muscle weakness or tremors, altered gait pattern, signs and symptoms of respiratory infection, or excessive perspiration.

   **Monitoring Parameters:** Monitor patient periodically for symptom resolution, heart rate, blood pressure, liver function tests, and CBC with continued therapy

   **Related Information**
      Antidepressant Agents *on page 998*

♦ **Citrate of Magnesia** *see* Magnesium Citrate *on page 552*
♦ **Citrovorum Factor** *see* Leucovorin *on page 520*
♦ **CI-719** *see* Gemfibrozil *on page 410*
♦ **Cla** *see* Clarithromycin *on next page*

## Cladribine *(KLA dri been)*

**Pharmacologic Class** Antineoplastic Agent, Antimetabolite

**U.S. Brand Names** Leustatin™

**Mechanism of Action** A purine nucleoside analogue; prodrug which is activated via phosphorylation by deoxycytidine kinase to a 5'-triphosphate derivative. This active form incorporates into susceptible cells and into DNA to result in the breakage of DNA strand and shutdown of DNA synthesis. This also results in a depletion of nicotinamide adenine dinucleotide and adenosine triphosphate (ATP). The induction of strand breaks results in a drop in the cofactor nicotinamide adenine dinucleotide and disruption of cell metabolism. ATP is depleted to deprive cells of an important source of energy. Cladribine effectively kills resting as well as dividing cells.

**Use** Treatment of hairy cell leukemia (HCL) and chronic lymphocytic leukemias

**USUAL DOSAGE** I.V.:

Children:
   Acute leukemia: The safety and effectiveness of cladribine in children have not been established; in a phase I study involving patients 1-21 years of age with relapsed acute

leukemia, cladribine was administered by CIV at doses ranging from 3-10.7 mg/m²/day for 5 days (0.5-2 times the dose recommended in HCL). Investigators reported beneficial responses in this study; the dose-limiting toxicity was severe myelosuppression with profound neutropenia and thrombocytopenia.

CIV: 15-18 mg/m²/day for 5 days

Adults:

Hairy cell leukemia:

CIV: 0.09-0.1 mg/kg/day continuous infusion for 7 consecutive days

CIV: 4 mg/m²/day for 7 days

Non-Hodgkin's lymphoma: CIV: 0.1 mg/kg/day for 7 days

**Dosage Forms Inj, preservative free:** 1 mg/mL (10 mL)

**Contraindications** Patients with a prior history of hypersensitivity to cladribine

**Warnings/Precautions** The U.S. Food and Drug Administration (FDA) currently recommends that procedures for proper handling and disposal of antineoplastic agents be considered. Because of its myelosuppressive properties, cladribine should be used with caution in patients with pre-existing hematologic or immunologic abnormalities; prophylactic administration of allopurinol should be considered in patients receiving cladribine because of the potential for hyperuricemia secondary to tumor lysis; appropriate antibiotic therapy should be administered promptly in patients exhibiting signs and symptoms of neutropenia and infection.

**Pregnancy Risk Factor** D

**Adverse Reactions**

>10%:

Bone marrow suppression: Commonly observed in patients treated with cladribine, especially at high doses; at the initiation of treatment, however, most patients in clinical studies had hematologic impairment as a result of HCL. During the first 2 weeks after treatment initiation, mean platelet counts decline and subsequently increased with normalization of mean counts by day 12. Absolute neutrophil counts and hemoglobin declined and subsequently increased with normalization of mean counts by week 5 and week 6. CD4 counts nadir at approximately 270, 4-6 months after treatments. Mean CD4 counts after 15 months were <500/mm³. Patients should be considered immunosuppressed for up to one year after cladribine therapy.

Central nervous system: Fatigue, headache

Fever: Temperature ≥101°F has been associated with the use of cladribine in approximately 66% of patients in the first month of therapy. Although 69% of patients developed fevers, <33% of febrile events were associated with documented infection.

Dermatologic: Rash

Gastrointestinal: Nausea and vomiting are not severe with cladribine at any dose level. Most cases of nausea were mild, not accompanied by vomiting and did not require treatment with antiemetics. In patients requiring antiemetics, nausea was easily controlled most often by chlorpromazine.

Local: Injection site reactions

1% to 10%:

Cardiovascular: Edema, tachycardia

Central nervous system: Dizziness, insomnia, pain, chills, malaise

Dermatologic: Pruritus, erythema

Gastrointestinal: Constipation, abdominal pain

Neuromuscular & skeletal: Myalgia, arthralgia, weakness

Miscellaneous: Diaphoresis, trunk pain

**Half-Life** Half-life: Biphasic: Alpha: 25 minutes; Beta: 6.7 hours; Terminal, mean (normal renal function): 5.4 hours

**Special PA Issues**

Patient Education: This drug can only be administered by infusion. Do not use alcohol, aspirin-containing products, and OTC medications without consulting prescriber. It is important to maintain adequate hydration (2-3 L/day of fluids unless instructed to restrict fluid intake) and nutrition during therapy; frequent small meals may help. You may experience nausea or vomiting (frequent small meals, frequent mouth care, and sucking on lozenges may help). You will be more susceptible to infection (avoid crowds and exposure to infection). You may experience muscle weakness or pain (mild analgesics may help). Frequent mouth care with soft toothbrush or cotton swabs and frequent mouth rinses may help relieve mouth sores. Report rash; fever; chills; unusual bruising or bleeding; signs of infection; excessive fatigue; yellowing of eyes or skin; change in color of urine or stool; swelling, warmth, or pain in extremities; or difficult respirations.

♦ **Claforan®** see Cefotaxime on page 167
♦ **Claripex®** see Clofibrate on page 221

# Clarithromycin (kla RITH roe mye sin)

**Pharmacologic Class** Antibiotic, Macrolide

**U.S. Brand Names** Biaxin™

(Continued)

## Clarithromycin *(Continued)*

**Mechanism of Action** Exerts its antibacterial action by binding to 50S ribosomal subunit resulting in inhibition of protein synthesis. The 14-OH metabolite of clarithromycin is twice as active as the parent compound against certain organisms.

**Use** In adults, for treatment of pharyngitis/tonsillitis, acute maxillary sinusitis, acute exacerbation of chronic bronchitis, pneumonia, uncomplicated skin/skin structure infections due to susceptible *S. pyogenes*, *S. pneumoniae*, *S. agalactiae*, viridans *Streptococcus*, *M. catarrhalis*, *C. trachomatis*, *Legionella* sp, *Mycoplasma pneumoniae*,*S. aureus*, *H. influenzae*; has activity against *M. avium* and *M. intracellulare* infection and is indicated for treatment of and prevention of disseminated mycobacterial infections due to *M. avium* complex disease (eg, patients with advanced HIV infection); indicated for the treatment of duodenal ulcer disease due to *H. pylori* in regimens with other drugs including amoxicillin and lansoprazole or omeprazole, ranitidine, bismuth citrate, bismuth subsalicylate, tetracycline and/or an H$_2$-antagonist; also indicated for prophylaxis of bacterial endocarditis in patients who are allergic to penicillin and undergoing surgical or dental procedures

In children, for treatment of pharyngitis/tonsillitis, acute maxillary sinusitis, acute otitis media, uncomplicated skin/skin structure infections due to the above organisms; treatment of and prevention of disseminated mycobacterial infections due to *M. avium* complex disease (eg, patients with advanced HIV infection)

Exhibits the same spectrum of *in vitro* activity as erythromycin, but with significantly increased potency against those organisms

**USUAL DOSAGE** Safe use in children has not been established

Children ≥6 months: 15 mg/kg/day divided every 12 hours; dosages of 7.5 mg/kg twice daily up to 500 mg twice daily children with AIDS and disseminated MAC infection

Adults: Oral: Usual dose: 250-500 mg every 12 hours for 7-14 days

Upper respiratory tract: 250-500 mg every 12 hours for 10-14 days

Pharyngitis/tonsillitis: 250 mg every 12 hours for 10 days

Acute maxillary sinusitis: 500 mg every 12 hours for 14 days

Lower respiratory tract: 250-500 mg every 12 hours for 7-14 days

Acute exacerbation of chronic bronchitis due to:

M. catarrhalis and S. pneumoniae: 250 mg every 12 hours for 7-14 days

H. influenzae: 500 mg every 12 hours for 7-14 days

Pneumonia due to *M. pneumoniae* and *S. pneumoniae*: 250 mg every 12 hours for 7-14 days

Mycobacterial infection (prevention and treatment): 500 mg twice daily (use with other antimycobacterial drugs, eg, ethambutol, clofazimine, or rifampin)

Prophylaxis of bacterial endocarditis: 500 mg 1 hour prior to procedure

Uncomplicated skin and skin structure: 250 mg every 12 hours for 7-14 days

*Helicobacter pylori*: In combination regimen with bismuth subsalicylate, tetracycline, and an H$_2$-receptor antagonist; or in combination with omeprazole (and possibly metronidazole or amoxicillin) or ranitidine bismuth citrate (Tritec®) (and possibly tetracycline or amoxicillin or lansoprazole and amoxicillin); 250 mg twice daily to 500 mg 3 times/day (for first 2 weeks only of regimen with Tritec® or omeprazole)

**Dosing adjustment in renal impairment:** Adults: Oral:

Cl$_{cr}$ <30 mL/minute: 500 mg loading dose, then 250 mg once or twice daily

**Dosing adjustment in severe renal impairment:** Decreased doses or prolonged dosing intervals are recommended

**Dosage Forms Granules for oral susp:** 125 mg/5 mL (50 mL, 100 mL), 250 mg/5 mL (50 mL, 100 mL); **Tab, film coated:** 250 mg, 500 mg

**Contraindications** Hypersensitivity to clarithromycin, erythromycin, or any macrolide antibiotic; use with pimozide, astemizole, cisapride, terfenadine

**Warnings/Precautions** In presence of severe renal impairment with or without coexisting hepatic impairment, decreased dosage or prolonged dosing interval may be appropriate; antibiotic-associated colitis has been reported with use of clarithromycin; elderly patients have experienced increased incidents of adverse effects due to known age-related decreases in renal function

**Pregnancy Risk Factor** C

**Adverse Reactions**

1% to 10%:

Central nervous system: Headache

Gastrointestinal: Diarrhea, nausea, abnormal taste, dyspepsia, abdominal pain

<1%: Ventricular tachycardia, manic behavior, tremor, hypoglycemia, torsade de pointes, neutropenia, leukopenia, prolonged PT, increased AST, alkaline phosphatase, and bilirubin; elevated BUN/serum creatinine

**Drug Interactions** CYP3A3/4 enzyme substrate; CYP1A2 and 3A3/4 enzyme inhibitor

Increased levels:

Clarithromycin increases serum theophylline levels by as much as 20%

Increased concentration of HMG CoA-reductase inhibitors (lovastatin and simvastatin)

Significantly increases carbamazepine levels and those of cyclosporine, digoxin, ergot alkaloid, tacrolimus, omeprazole and triazolam

Peak levels (but not AUC) of zidovudine are often increased; terfenadine and astemizole should be avoided with use of clarithromycin since plasma levels may be increased by >3 times; serious arrhythmias have occurred with cisapride and other drugs which inhibit cytochrome P-450 3A4 (eg, clarithromycin)

Fluconazole increases clarithromycin levels and AUC by ~25%; death has been reported with administration of pimozide and clarithromycin

**Note:** While other drug interactions (bromocriptine, disopyramide, lovastatin, phenytoin, and valproate) known to occur with erythromycin have not been reported in clinical trials with clarithromycin, concurrent use of these drugs should be monitored closely

**Half-Life** 5-7 hours

**Special PA Issues**

**Patient Education:** Take full course of therapy; do not discontinue without consulting prescriber. Do not refrigerate oral suspension, more palatable when taken at room temperature. Maintain adequate hydration (2-3 L/day of fluids unless instructed to restrict fluid intake). You may experience nausea (small frequent meals, or sucking on lozenges may help); abnormal taste (frequent mouth care or chewing gum may help); diarrhea, headache, or abdominal cramps (medication may be ordered). Report persistent fever or chills, easy bruising or bleeding, or joint pain. Report severe persistent diarrhea, skin rash, sores in mouth, foul-smelling urine, rapid heartbeat or palpitations, or difficulty breathing.

♦ **Claritin®** *see* Loratadine *on page 542*

♦ **Claritin-D®** *see* Loratadine and Pseudoephedrine *on page 542*

♦ **Claritin-D® 24-Hour** *see* Loratadine and Pseudoephedrine *on page 542*

♦ **Clavulin®** *see* Amoxicillin and Clavulanate Potassium *on page 62*

♦ **Clear Eyes® [OTC]** *see* Naphazoline *on page 635*

♦ **Clear Tussin® 30** *see* Guaifenesin and Dextromethorphan *on page 428*

## Clemastine (KLEM as teen)

**Pharmacologic Class** Antihistamine

**U.S. Brand Names** Antihist-1® [OTC]; Tavist®; Tavist®-1 [OTC]

**Mechanism of Action** Competes with histamine for $H_1$-receptor sites on effector cells in the gastrointestinal tract, blood vessels, and respiratory tract

**Use** Perennial and seasonal allergic rhinitis and other allergic symptoms including urticaria

**USUAL DOSAGE** Oral:

Children: <12 years: 0.4-1 mg twice daily

Children >12 years and Adults: 1.34 mg twice daily to 2.68 mg 3 times/day; do not exceed 8.04 mg/day; lower doses should be considered in patients >60 years

**Dosage Forms** Clemastine fumarate: **Syr (citrus flavor):** 0.67 mg/5 mL with alcohol 5.5% (120 mL); **Tab:** 1.34 mg, 2.68 mg

**Contraindications** Narrow-angle glaucoma, hypersensitivity to clemastine or any component

**Warnings/Precautions** Safety and efficacy have not been established in children <6 years of age; bladder neck obstruction, symptomatic prostate hypertrophy, asthmatic attacks, and stenosing peptic ulcer

**Pregnancy Risk Factor** C

**Adverse Reactions**

>10%:

Central nervous system: Slight to moderate drowsiness

Respiratory: Thickening of bronchial secretions

1% to 10%:

Central nervous system: Headache, fatigue, nervousness, increased dizziness

Gastrointestinal: Appetite increase, weight gain, nausea, diarrhea, abdominal pain, xerostomia

Neuromuscular & skeletal: Arthralgia

Respiratory: Pharyngitis

<1%: Edema, palpitations, depression, angioedema, photosensitivity, rash, hepatitis, myalgia, paresthesia, bronchospasm, epistaxis

**Drug Interactions** Increased toxicity (CNS depression): CNS depressants, MAO inhibitors, tricyclic antidepressants, phenothiazines

**Onset** Peak concentrations in 1-2 hours

**Duration** 8-16 hours

**Special PA Issues**

**Patient Education:** Avoid alcohol; may cause drowsiness, may impair coordination or judgment

**Dietary Considerations:** Alcohol: Additive CNS effects, avoid use

**Monitoring Parameters:** Look for a reduction of rhinitis, urticaria, eczema, pruritus, or other allergic symptoms

## Clemastine and Phenylpropanolamine
(KLEM as teen & fen il proe pa NOLE a meen)
**Pharmacologic Class** Antihistamine/Decongestant Combination
**U.S. Brand Names** Antihist-D®; Tavist-D®
**Dosage Forms Tab:** Clemastine fumarate 1.34 mg and phenylpropanolamine hydrochloride 75 mg

♦ **Clemastine Fumarate** see Clemastine on previous page
♦ **Cleocin HCl®** see Clindamycin on this page
♦ **Cleocin Pediatric®** see Clindamycin on this page
♦ **Cleocin Phosphate®** see Clindamycin on this page
♦ **Cleocin T®** see Clindamycin on this page

## Clidinium and Chlordiazepoxide (kli DI nee um & klor dye az e POKS ide)
**Pharmacologic Class** Antispasmodic Agent, Gastrointestinal
**U.S. Brand Names** Clindex®; Librax®
**Dosage Forms Cap:** Clidinium bromide 2.5 mg and chlordiazepoxide hydrochloride 5 mg

♦ **Climara® Transdermal** see Estradiol on page 332
♦ **Clinda-Derm® Topical Solution** see Clindamycin on this page

## Clindamycin (klin da MYE sin)
**Pharmacologic Class** Antibiotic, Miscellaneous
**U.S. Brand Names** Cleocin HCl®; Cleocin Pediatric®; Cleocin Phosphate®; Cleocin T®; Clinda-Derm® Topical Solution; C/T/S® Topical Solution
**Mechanism of Action** Reversibly binds to 50S ribosomal subunits preventing peptide bond formation thus inhibiting bacterial protein synthesis; bacteriostatic or bactericidal depending on drug concentration, infection site, and organism
**Use** Treatment against aerobic and anaerobic streptococci (except enterococci), most staphylococci, *Bacteroides* sp and *Actinomyces*; used topically in treatment of severe acne, vaginally for *Gardnerella vaginalis*, alternate treatment for toxoplasmosis; prophylaxis in the prevention of bacterial endocarditis in high-risk patients undergoing surgical or dental procedures in patients allergic to penicillin; may be useful in PCP
**USUAL DOSAGE** Avoid in neonates (contains benzyl alcohol)
Infants and Children:
Oral: 8-20 mg/kg/day as hydrochloride; 8-25 mg/kg/day as palmitate in 3-4 divided doses; minimum dose of palmitate: 37.5 mg 3 times/day
I.M., I.V.:
<1 month: 15-20 mg/kg/day
>1 month: 20-40 mg/kg/day in 3-4 divided doses
Children and Adults: Topical: Apply a thin film twice daily
Adults:
Oral: 150-450 mg/dose every 6-8 hours; maximum dose: 1.8 g/day
I.M., I.V.: 1.2-1.8 g/day in 2-4 divided doses; maximum dose: 4.8 g/day
Bacterial endocarditis prophylaxis: 600 mg 1 hour prior to the procedure
Pelvic inflammatory disease: I.V.: 900 mg every 8 hours with gentamicin 2 mg/kg, then 1.5 mg/kg every 8 hours; continue after discharge with doxycycline 100 mg twice daily or oral clindamycin 450 mg 5 times/day for 10-14 days
*Pneumocystis carinii* pneumonia:
Oral: 300-450 mg 4 times/day with primaquine
I.M., I.V.: 1200-2400 mg/day with pyrimethamine
I.V.: 600 mg 4 times/day with primaquine
Vaginal: One full applicator (100 mg) inserted intravaginally once daily before bedtime for 3 or 7 consecutive days
**Dosing adjustment in hepatic impairment:** Adjustment recommended in patients with severe hepatic disease
**Dosage Forms** Clindamycin hydrochloride: **Cap:** 75 mg, 150 mg, 300 mg
Clindamycin palmitate: **Granules for oral soln:** 75 mg/5 mL (100 mL)
Clindamycin phosphate: **Crm, vaginal:** 2% (40 g), **Gel, top:** 1% [10 mg/g] (7.5 g, 30 g), **Inf in D₅W:** 300 mg (50 mL); 600 mg (50 mL), **Inj:** 150 mg/mL (2 mL, 4 mL, 6 mL, 50 mL, 60 mL), **Soln, top:** 1% [10 mg/mL] (30 mL, 60 mL, 480 mL), **Lot, top:** 1% [10 mg/mL] (60 mL)
**Contraindications** Hypersensitivity to clindamycin or any component; previous pseudomembranous colitis, hepatic impairment
**Warnings/Precautions** Dosage adjustment may be necessary in patients with severe hepatic dysfunction; can cause severe and possibly fatal colitis; use with caution in patients with a history of pseudomembranous colitis; discontinue drug if significant diarrhea, abdominal cramps, or passage of blood and mucus occurs
**Pregnancy Risk Factor** B
**Adverse Reactions**
>10%: Gastrointestinal: Diarrhea

1% to 10%:
Dermatologic: Rashes
Gastrointestinal: Pseudomembranous colitis (more common with oral form), nausea, vomiting
<1%: Hypotension, urticaria, Stevens-Johnson syndrome, eosinophilia, neutropenia, granulocytopenia, thrombocytopenia, elevated liver enzymes, thrombophlebitis, sterile abscess at I.M. injection site, polyarthritis, rare renal dysfunction
**Drug Interactions** CYP3A3/4 enzyme substrate
Increased duration of neuromuscular blockade from tubocurarine, pancuronium
**Half-Life** 1.6-5.3 hours, average: 2-3 hours
**Special PA Issues**
**Patient Education:**
Oral: Take each dose with a full glass of water. Complete full prescription, even if feeling better. You may experience nausea or vomiting (small frequent meals, frequent mouth care, or sucking on lozenges may help). Report dizziness; persistent gastrointestinal effects (pain, diarrhea, vomiting); skin redness, rash, or burning; fever; chills; unusual bruising or bleeding; signs of infection; excessive fatigue; yellowing of eyes or skin; change in color of urine or stool; swelling, warmth, or pain in extremities; difficult respirations; bloody or fatty stool (do not take antidiarrheal without consulting prescriber); or lack or improvement or worsening of condition.
Topical: Wash hands before applying or wear gloves. Apply thin film of gel, lotion, or solution to affected area. May apply porous dressing. Report persistent burning, swelling, itching, or worsening of condition.
Vaginal: Wash hands before using. At bedtime, gently insert full applicator into vagina and expel cream. Wash applicator with soap and water following use. Remain lying down for 30 minutes following administration. Avoid intercourse during 7 days of therapy. Report adverse reactions (dizziness, nausea, vomiting, stomach cramps, or headache) or lack of improvement or worsening of condition.
**Monitoring Parameters:** Observe for changes in bowel frequency, monitor for colitis and resolution of symptoms; during prolonged therapy monitor CBC, liver and renal function tests periodically

- **Clindamycin Hydrochloride** see Clindamycin on previous page
- **Clindamycin Phosphate** see Clindamycin on previous page
- **Clindex®** see Clidinium and Chlordiazepoxide on previous page
- **Clinoril®** see Sulindac on page 865

# Clioquinol (klye oh KWIN ole)
**Pharmacologic Class** Antifungal Agent, Topical
**U.S. Brand Names** Vioform® [OTC]
**Mechanism of Action** Chelates bacterial surface and trace metals needed for bacterial growth
**Use** Topically in the treatment of tinea pedis, tinea cruris, and skin infections caused by dermatophytic fungi (ringworm)
**USUAL DOSAGE** Children and Adults: Topical: Apply 2-3 times/day; do not use for longer than 7 days
**Dosage Forms Crm:** 3% (30 g); **Oint, top:** 3% (30 g)
**Contraindications** Not effective in the treatment of scalp or nail fungal infections; children <2 years of age, hypersensitivity to any component
**Warnings/Precautions** May irritate sensitized skin; topical application poses a potential risk of toxicity to infants and children; known to cause serious and irreversible optic atrophy and peripheral neuropathy with muscular weakness, sensory loss, spastic paraparesis, and blindness; use with caution in patients with iodine intolerance
**Pregnancy Risk Factor** C
**Adverse Reactions** 1% to 10%:
Dermatologic: Skin irritation, rash
Neuromuscular & skeletal: Peripheral neuropathy
Ocular: Optic atrophy
**Special PA Issues**
**Patient Education:** Cleanse affected area before application; can stain skin and fabrics; for external use only; avoid contact with eyes and mucous membranes
**Related Information**
Antifungal Agents, Topical on page 1000

# Clioquinol and Hydrocortisone (klye oh KWIN ole & hye droe KOR ti sone)
**Pharmacologic Class** Antifungal/Corticosteroid
**U.S. Brand Names** Corque® Topical; Pedi-Cort V® Creme
**Dosage Forms Crm:** Clioquinol 3% and hydrocortisone 1% (20 g)

# Clobetasol (kloe BAY ta sol)
**Pharmacologic Class** Corticosteroid, Topical
**U.S. Brand Names** Embeline E® Emollient Cream; Temovate® Topical
(Continued)

## Clobetasol *(Continued)*

**Mechanism of Action** Stimulates the synthesis of enzymes needed to decrease inflammation, suppress mitotic activity, and cause vasoconstriction

**Use Short-term** relief of inflammation of moderate to severe corticosteroid-responsive dermatosis (very high potency topical corticosteroid)

**USUAL DOSAGE** Adults: Topical: Apply twice daily for up to 2 weeks with no more than 50 g/week

**Dosage Forms Crm:** 0.05% (15 g, 30 g, 45 g), **Crm in emollient base:** 0.05% (15 g, 30 g, 60 g), **Gel:** 0.05% (15 g, 30 g, 45 g), **Oint, top:** 0.05% (15 g, 30 g, 45 g), **Scalp application:** 0.05% (25 mL, 50 mL)

**Contraindications** Known hypersensitivity to clobetasol; viral, fungal, or tubercular skin lesions

**Warnings/Precautions** Adrenal suppression can occur if used for >14 days

**Pregnancy Risk Factor** C

**Adverse Reactions**
1% to 10%:
Dermatologic: Itching, erythema
Local: Burning, dryness, irritation, papular rashes
<1%: Hypertrichosis, acneiform eruptions, maceration of skin, skin atrophy, striae, hypopigmentation, perioral dermatitis, miliaria

**Special PA Issues**
Patient Education: For external use only. Use exactly as directed; do not overuse. Do not apply to open wounds or weeping areas. Before using, wash and dry area gently. Apply a thin film to affected area and rub in gently. If dressing is necessary, use a porous dressing. Avoid contact with eyes. Avoid exposing treated area to direct sunlight; sunburn can occur. Report increased swelling, redness, rash, itching, signs of infection, worsening of condition, or lack of healing.

♦ **Clobetasol Propionate** *see Clobetasol on previous page*
♦ **Clocort® Maximum Strength** *see Hydrocortisone on page 453*

## Clocortolone *(kloe KOR toe lone)*

**Pharmacologic Class** Corticosteroid, Topical

**U.S. Brand Names** Cloderm® Topical

**Mechanism of Action** Stimulates the synthesis of enzymes needed to decrease inflammation, suppress mitotic activity, and cause vasoconstriction

**Use** Inflammation of corticosteroid-responsive dermatoses (medium potency topical corticosteroid)

**USUAL DOSAGE** Adults: Apply sparingly and gently; rub into affected area from 1-4 times/day

**Dosage Forms Crm, as pivalate:** 0.1% (15 g, 45 g)

**Contraindications** Known hypersensitivity to clocortolone; viral, fungal, or tubercular skin lesions

**Warnings/Precautions** Adrenal suppression can occur if used for >14 days

**Pregnancy Risk Factor** C

**Adverse Reactions**
1% to 10%:
Dermatologic: Itching, erythema
Local: Burning, dryness, irritation, papular rashes
<1%: Hypertrichosis, acneiform eruptions, maceration of skin, skin atrophy, striae, hypopigmentation, perioral dermatitis, miliaria

**Special PA Issues**
Patient Education: For external use only. Use exactly as directed; do not overuse. Do not apply to open wounds or weeping areas. Before using, wash and dry area gently. Apply a thin film to affected area and rub in gently. If dressing is necessary, use a porous dressing. Avoid contact with eyes. Avoid exposing treated area to direct sunlight; sunburn can occur. Report increased swelling, redness, rash, itching, signs of infection, worsening of condition, or lack of healing.

♦ **Clocortolone Pivalate** *see Clocortolone on this page*
♦ **Cloderm® Topical** *see Clocortolone on this page*

## Clofazimine *(kloe FA zi meen)*

**Pharmacologic Class** Leprostatic Agent

**U.S. Brand Names** Lamprene®

**Mechanism of Action** Binds preferentially to mycobacterial DNA to inhibit mycobacterial growth; also has some anti-inflammatory activity through an unknown mechanism

**Use Orphan drug:** Treatment of dapsone-resistant leprosy; multibacillary dapsone-sensitive leprosy; erythema nodosum leprosum; *Mycobacterium avium-intracellulare* (MAI) infections

**USUAL DOSAGE** Oral:
Children: Leprosy: 1 mg/kg/day every 24 hours in combination with dapsone and rifampin

Adults:

Dapsone-resistant leprosy: 100 mg/day in combination with one or more antileprosy drugs for 3 years; then alone 100 mg/day

Dapsone-sensitive multibacillary leprosy: 100 mg/day in combination with two or more antileprosy drugs for at least 2 years and continue until negative skin smears are obtained, then institute single drug therapy with appropriate agent

Erythema nodosum leprosum: 100-200 mg/day for up to 3 months or longer then taper dose to 100 mg/day when possible

Pyoderma gangrenosum: 300-400 mg/day for up to 12 months

**Dosing adjustment in hepatic impairment:** Should be considered in severe hepatic dysfunction

**Dosage Forms** Cap, as palmitate: 50 mg

**Contraindications** Hypersensitivity to clofazimine or any component

**Warnings/Precautions** Use with caution in patients with GI problems; dosages >100 mg/day should be used for as short a duration as possible; skin discoloration may lead to depression

**Pregnancy Risk Factor** C

**Adverse Reactions**

>10%:

Dermatologic: Dry skin

Gastrointestinal: Abdominal pain, nausea, vomiting, diarrhea

Miscellaneous: Pink to brownish-black discoloration of the skin and conjunctiva

1% to 10%:

Dermatologic: Rash, pruritus

Endocrine & metabolic: Elevated blood sugar

Gastrointestinal: Fecal discoloration

Genitourinary: Discoloration of urine

Ocular: Irritation of the eyes

Miscellaneous: Discoloration of sputum, sweat

<1%: Edema, vascular pain, dizziness, drowsiness, fatigue, headache, giddiness, taste disorder, fever, erythroderma, acneiform eruptions, monilial cheilosis, phototoxicity, hypokalemia, bowel obstruction, GI bleeding, anorexia, constipation, weight loss, eosinophilic enteritis, cystitis, eosinophilia, anemia, hepatitis, jaundice, enlarged liver; increased albumin, serum bilirubin, and AST; bone pain, neuralgia, diminished vision, lymphadenopathy

**Drug Interactions** Decreased effect with dapsone (unconfirmed)

**Half-Life** Terminal: 8 days; Tissue: 70 days

**Special PA Issues**

**Patient Education:** May be taken with meals. Drug may cause a pink to brownish-black discoloration of the skin, conjunctiva, tears, sweat, urine, feces, and nasal secretions. Although reversible, it may take months to years for skin discoloration to disappear after therapy is complete. Report promptly bone or joint pain, GI disturbance, or vision disturbances.

♦ **Clofazimine Palmitate** *see* Clofazimine *on previous page*

# Clofibrate (kloe FYE brate)

**Pharmacologic Class** Antilipemic Agent (Fibric Acid)

**U.S. Brand Names** Atromid-S®

**Mechanism of Action** Mechanism is unclear but thought to reduce cholesterol synthesis and triglyceride hepatic-vascular transference

**Use** Adjunct to dietary therapy in the management of hyperlipidemias associated with high triglyceride levels (types III, IV, V); primarily lowers triglycerides and very low density lipoprotein

**USUAL DOSAGE** Adults: Oral: 500 mg 4 times/day; some patients may respond to lower doses

**Dosing interval in renal impairment:**

$Cl_{cr}$ >50 mL/minute: Administer every 6-12 hours

$Cl_{cr}$ 10-50 mL/minute: Administer every 12-18 hours

$Cl_{cr}$ <10 mL/minute: Avoid use

Hemodialysis: Elimination is not enhanced via hemodialysis; supplemental dose is not necessary

**Dosage Forms** Cap: 500 mg

**Contraindications** Hypersensitivity to clofibrate or any component, severe hepatic or renal impairment, primary biliary cirrhosis

**Warnings/Precautions** Clofibrate has been shown to be tumorigenic in animal studies; increased risk of cholelithiasis, cholecystitis; discontinue if lipid response is not obtained; no evidence substantiates a beneficial effect on cardiovascular mortality

**Pregnancy Risk Factor** C

**Adverse Reactions**

Cardiovascular: Angina, cardiac arrhythmias

Central nervous system: Headache, dizziness, fatigue

(Continued)

## Clofibrate (Continued)

Dermatologic: Rash, urticaria, pruritus, alopecia

Gastrointestinal: Nausea, diarrhea, vomiting, dyspepsia, flatulence, abdominal distress, gallstones

Genitourinary: Impotence

Hematologic: Leukopenia, anemia, eosinophilia, agranulocytosis

Hepatic: Increased LFTs

Neuromuscular & skeletal: Muscle cramping, aching, weakness, myalgia

Renal: Renal toxicity, rhabdomyolysis-induced renal failure

Miscellaneous: Dry, brittle hair

**Drug Interactions**

Decreased effect: Oral contraceptives may increase elimination of clofibrate

Increased effect: Effects of warfarin, insulin, dantrolene, furosemide, and sulfonylureas may be increased

Increased toxicity/levels: Clofibrate's levels may be increased with probenecid

**Half-Life** 6-24 hours, increases significantly with reduced renal function; with anuria: 110 hours

**Special PA Issues**

**Patient Education:** This drug will have to be taken long-term and ongoing follow-up is essential. Adherence to a cardiac risk reduction program, including adherence to prescribed diet, is of major importance. This drug may cause stomach upset; if this occurs, take medication with food or milk. Report chest pain, shortness of breath, irregular heartbeat, palpitations, severe stomach pain with nausea and vomiting, persistent fever, sore throat, or unusual bleeding or bruising.

**Monitoring Parameters:** Serum lipids, cholesterol and triglycerides, LFTs, CBC

♦ **Clomid®** see Clomiphene on this page

## Clomiphene (KLOE mi feen)

**Pharmacologic Class** Ovulation Stimulator

**U.S. Brand Names** Clomid®; Milophene®; Serophene®

**Mechanism of Action** Induces ovulation by stimulating the release of pituitary gonadotropins

**Use** Treatment of ovulatory failure in patients desiring pregnancy

**Unlabeled use:** Male infertility

**USUAL DOSAGE** Adults: Oral:

Male (infertility): 25 mg/day for 25 days with 5 days rest, or 100 mg every Monday, Wednesday, Friday

Female (ovulatory failure): 50 mg/day for 5 days (first course); start the regimen on or about the fifth day of cycle. The dose should be increased only in those patients who do not ovulate in response to cyclic 50 mg Clomid®. A low dosage or duration of treatment course is particularly recommended if unusual sensitivity to pituitary gonadotropin is suspected, such as in patients with polycystic ovary syndrome.

If ovulation does not appear to occur after the first course of therapy, a second course of 100 mg/day (two 50 mg tablets given as a single daily dose) for 5 days should be given. This course may be started as early as 30 days after the previous one after precautions are taken to exclude the presence of pregnancy. Increasing the dosage or duration of therapy beyond 100 mg/day for 5 days is not recommended. The majority of patients who are going to ovulate will do so after the first course of therapy. If ovulation does not occur after 3 courses of therapy, further treatment is not recommended and the patient should be re-evaluated. If 3 ovulatory responses occur, but pregnancy has not been achieved, further treatment is not recommended. If menses does not occur after an ovulatory response, the patient should be re-evaluated. Long-term cyclic therapy is not recommended beyond a total of about 6 cycles.

**Dosage Forms Tab, as citrate:** 50 mg

**Contraindications** Hypersensitivity or allergy to clomiphene citrate or any of its components; liver disease, abnormal uterine bleeding, suspected pregnancy, enlargement or development of ovarian cyst, uncontrolled thyroid or adrenal dysfunction in the presence of an organic intracranial lesion such as pituitary tumor

**Warnings/Precautions** Patients unusually sensitive to pituitary gonadotropins (eg, polycystic ovary disease); multiple pregnancies, blurring or other visual symptoms can occur, ovarian hyperstimulation syndrome, and abdominal pain

**Pregnancy Risk Factor** X

**Adverse Reactions**

>10%: Endocrine & metabolic: Hot flashes, ovarian enlargement

1% to 10%:

Cardiovascular: Thromboembolism

Central nervous system: Mental depression, headache

Endocrine & metabolic: Breast enlargement (males), breast discomfort (females), abnormal menstrual flow

Gastrointestinal: Distention, bloating, nausea, vomiting, hepatotoxicity

Ocular: Blurring of vision, diplopia, floaters, after-images, phosphenes, photophobia
<1%: Insomnia, fatigue, alopecia (reversible), weight gain, polyuria

**Half-Life** 5-7 days

**Special PA Issues**
**Patient Education:** Follow recommended schedule of dosing. You may experience hot flashes (cool clothes and cool environment may help). Report acute sudden headache; difficulty breathing; warmth, pain, redness, or swelling in calves; breast enlargement (male) or breast discomfort (female); abnormal menstrual bleeding; vision changes (blurring, diplopia, photophobia, floaters); acute abdominal discomfort; or fever.

**Reference Range:** FSH and LH are expected to peak 5-9 days after completing clomiphene; ovulation assessed by basal body temperature or serum progesterone 2 weeks after last clomiphene dose

♦ **Clomiphene Citrate** *see Clomiphene on previous page*

# Clomipramine (kloe MI pra meen)

**Pharmacologic Class** Antidepressant, Tricyclic (Tertiary Amine)

**U.S. Brand Names** Anafranil®

**Mechanism of Action** Clomipramine appears to affect serotonin uptake while its active metabolite, desmethylclomipramine, affects norepinephrine uptake

**Use** Treatment of obsessive-compulsive disorder (OCD); may also relieve depression, panic attacks, and chronic pain

**USUAL DOSAGE** Oral: Initial:
Children >10 years of age: 25 mg/day and gradually increase, as tolerated, to a maximum of 3 mg/kg/day or 200 mg/day, whichever is smaller
The safety and efficacy of clomipramine in pediatric patients <10 years of age have not been established and, therefore, dosing recommendations cannot be made
Adults: 25 mg/day and gradually increase, as tolerated, to 100 mg/day the first 2 weeks, may then be increased to a total of 250 mg/day maximum

**Dosage Forms** Cap, as hydrochloride: 25 mg, 50 mg, 75 mg

**Contraindications** Patients in acute recovery stage of recent myocardial infarction; not to be used within 14 days of MAO inhibitors

**Warnings/Precautions** Seizures are likely and are dose-related; can be additive when coadministered with other drugs that can lower the seizure threshold; use with caution in patients with asthma, bladder outlet destruction, narrow-angle glaucoma

**Pregnancy Risk Factor** C

**Adverse Reactions**
>10%:
Central nervous system: Dizziness, drowsiness, headache
Gastrointestinal: Xerostomia, constipation, increased appetite, nausea, unpleasant taste, weight gain
Neuromuscular & skeletal: Weakness
1% to 10%:
Cardiovascular: Arrhythmias, hypotension
Central nervous system: Confusion, delirium, hallucinations, nervousness, restlessness, parkinsonian syndrome, insomnia
Gastrointestinal: Diarrhea, heartburn
Genitourinary: Dysuria, sexual dysfunction
Neuromuscular & skeletal: Fine muscle tremors
Ocular: Blurred vision, eye pain
Miscellaneous: Diaphoresis (excessive)
<1%: Anxiety, seizures, alopecia, photosensitivity, breast enlargement, galactorrhea, SIADH, trouble with gums, decreased lower esophageal sphincter tone may cause GE reflux, testicular edema, agranulocytosis, leukopenia, eosinophilia, cholestatic jaundice, increased liver enzymes, increased intraocular pressure, tinnitus, allergic reactions

**Drug Interactions** CYP1A2, 2C9, 2C18, 2C19, 2D6, and 3A3/4 enzyme substrate; CYP2D6 enzyme inhibitor

Decreased effect with barbiturates, carbamazepine, phenytoin
Increased effect of alcohol, CNS depressants, anticholinergics, sympathomimetics
Increased toxicity: MAO inhibitors (increase temperature, seizures, coma, and death)

**Onset** Usually >2 weeks to therapeutic effect

**Half-Life** 20-30 hours

**Special PA Issues**
**Patient Education:** Take multiple dose medication with meals to reduce side effects. Take single daily dose at bedtime to reduce daytime sedation. The effect of this drug may take several weeks to appear. Do not use excessive alcohol, caffeine, and other prescriptive or OTC medications without consulting prescriber. May cause dizziness, drowsiness, headache, or seizures (use caution when driving or engaging in tasks that require alertness until response to drug is known); dry mouth or unpleasant aftertaste (sucking lozenges and frequent mouth care may help); constipation (increased fluids, dietary fiber and fruits, or exercise may help); or orthostatic hypotension (use caution when rising from
(Continued)

## Clomipramine (Continued)

lying or sitting to standing position or when climbing stairs). Report unresolved constipation or GI upset, unusual muscle weakness, palpitations, or persistent CNS disturbances (hallucinations, delirium, insomnia, or impaired gait).

**Related Information**

Antidepressant Agents on page 998

♦ **Clomipramine Hydrochloride** see Clomipramine on previous page

## Clonazepam (kloe NA ze pam)

**Pharmacologic Class** Benzodiazepine

**U.S. Brand Names** Klonopin™

**Mechanism of Action** Suppresses the spike-and-wave discharge in absence seizures by depressing nerve transmission in the motor cortex

**Use** Prophylaxis of petit mal, petit mal variant (Lennox-Gastaut), akinetic, and myoclonic seizures

**Unlabeled use:** Restless legs syndrome, neuralgia, multifocal tic disorder, parkinsonian dysarthria, acute manic episodes, and adjunct therapy for schizophrenia

**USUAL DOSAGE** Oral:

Children <10 years or 30 kg:

Initial daily dose: 0.01-0.03 mg/kg/day (maximum: 0.05 mg/kg/day) given in 2-3 divided doses; increase by no more than 0.5 mg every third day until seizures are controlled or adverse effects seen

Usual maintenance dose: 0.1-0.2 mg/kg/day divided 3 times/day; not to exceed 0.2 mg/kg/day

Adults:

Initial daily dose not to exceed 1.5 mg given in 3 divided doses; may increase by 0.5-1 mg every third day until seizures are controlled or adverse effects seen

Usual maintenance dose: 0.05-0.2 mg/kg; do not exceed 20 mg/day

Hemodialysis: Supplemental dose is not necessary

**Dosage Forms** Tab: 0.5 mg, 1 mg, 2 mg

**Contraindications** Hypersensitivity to clonazepam, any component, or other benzodiazepines; severe liver disease; acute narrow-angle glaucoma

**Warnings/Precautions** Use with caution in patients with chronic respiratory disease or impaired renal function; abrupt discontinuance may precipitate withdrawal symptoms, status epilepticus or seizures, in patients with a history of substance abuse; clonazepam-induced behavioral disturbances may be more frequent in mentally handicapped patients

**Pregnancy Risk Factor** C

**Pregnancy Implications**

Clinical effects on the fetus: Two reports of cardiac defects; respiratory depression, lethargy, hypotonia may be observed in newborns exposed near time of delivery. Epilepsy itself, number of medications, genetic factors, or a combination of these probably influence the teratogenicity of anticonvulsant therapy. Benefit:risk ratio usually favors continued use during pregnancy and breast-feeding.

Breast-feeding/lactation: Crosses into breast milk

Clinical effects on the infant: CNS depression, respiratory depression reported. No recommendation from the American Academy of Pediatrics.

**Adverse Reactions**

\>10%:

Cardiovascular: Tachycardia, chest pain

Central nervous system: Drowsiness, fatigue, ataxia, lightheadedness, memory impairment, insomnia, anxiety, depression, headache

Dermatologic: Rash

Endocrine & metabolic: Decreased libido

Gastrointestinal: Xerostomia, constipation, diarrhea, nausea, increased or decreased appetite, vomiting, decreased salivation

Neuromuscular & skeletal: Dysarthria

Ocular: Blurred vision

Miscellaneous: Diaphoresis

1% to 10%:

Cardiovascular: Syncope, hypotension

Central nervous system: Confusion, nervousness, dizziness, akathisia

Dermatologic: Dermatitis

Gastrointestinal: Weight gain or loss, increased salivation

Neuromuscular & skeletal: Rigidity, tremor, muscle cramps

Otic: Tinnitus

Respiratory: Nasal congestion, hyperventilation

<1%: Menstrual irregularities, blood dyscrasias, reflex slowing, drug dependence

**Drug Interactions** CYP3A3/4 enzyme substrate

Decreased effect: Phenytoin, barbiturates may increase clonazepam clearance

Increased toxicity: CNS depressants may increase sedation

**Onset** 20-60 minutes

**Duration** Up to 12 hours

**Half-Life** 19-50 hours

**Special PA Issues**

**Patient Education:** Take exactly as directed (do not increase dose or frequency); may cause physical and/or psychological dependence. While using this medication, do not use alcohol and other prescription or OTC medications (especially pain medications, sedatives, antihistamines, or hypnotics) without consulting prescriber. Maintain adequate hydration (2-3 L/day of fluids unless instructed to restrict fluid intake). You may experience drowsiness, dizziness, or blurred vision (use caution when driving or engaging in hazardous tasks); nausea, vomiting, loss of appetite, or dry mouth (small frequent meals, good mouth care, chewing gum, or sucking on lozenges may help); constipation (increased exercise, fluids, or dietary fruit and fiber may help). If medication is used to control seizures, wear identification that you are taking an antiepileptic medication. Report excessive drowsiness, dizziness, fatigue, or impaired coordination; CNS changes (confusion, depression, increased sedation, excitation, headache, agitation, insomnia, or nightmares) or changes in cognition; difficulty breathing or shortness of breath; changes in urinary pattern, changes in sexual activity; muscle cramping, weakness, tremors, or rigidity; ringing in ears or visual disturbances, excessive perspiration, or excessive GI symptoms (cramping, constipation, vomiting, anorexia); worsening of seizure activity, or loss of seizure control.

**Dietary Considerations:** Alcohol: Additive CNS depression has been reported with benzodiazepines; avoid or limit alcohol

**Reference Range:** Relationship between serum concentration and seizure control is not well established

Timing of serum samples: Peak serum levels occur 1-3 hours after oral ingestion; the half-life is 20-40 hours; therefore, steady-state occurs in 5-7 days

Therapeutic levels: 20-80 ng/mL; Toxic concentration: >80 ng/mL

# Clonidine (KLOE ni deen)

**Pharmacologic Class** Alpha$_2$ Agonist

**U.S. Brand Names** Catapres® Oral; Catapres-TTS® Transdermal; Duraclon® Injection

**Mechanism of Action** Stimulates alpha$_2$-adrenoceptors in the brain stem, thus activating an inhibitory neuron, resulting in reduced sympathetic outflow, producing a decrease in vasomotor tone and heart rate; epidural clonidine may produce pain relief at spinal presynaptic and postjunctional alpha$_2$-adrenoceptors by preventing pain signal transmission; pain relief occurs only for the body regions innervated by the spinal segments where analgesic concentrations of clonidine exist

**Use** Management of mild to moderate hypertension; either used alone or in combination with other antihypertensives; not recommended for first-line therapy for hypertension; as a second-line agent for decreasing heroin or nicotine withdrawal symptoms in patients with severe symptoms; indicated by the epidural route, in combination with opiates, for treatment of severe pain in refractory cancer patients (most effective in patients with neuropathic pain); other uses may include prophylaxis of migraines, glaucoma, and diabetes-associated diarrhea

## USUAL DOSAGE

Oral:

Children: Initial: 5-10 mcg/kg/day in divided doses every 8-12 hours; increase gradually at 5- to 7-day intervals to 25 mcg/kg/day in divided doses every 6 hours; maximum: 0.9 mg/day

Clonidine tolerance test (test of growth hormone release from pituitary): 0.15 mg/m$^2$ or 4 mcg/kg as single dose

Adults: Initial dose: 0.1 mg twice daily, usual maintenance dose: 0.2-1.2 mg/day in 2-4 divided doses; maximum recommended dose: 2.4 mg/day

Nicotine withdrawal symptoms: 0.1 mg twice daily to maximum of 0.4 mg/day for 3-4 weeks

Elderly: Initial: 0.1 mg once daily at bedtime, increase gradually as needed

Transdermal: Apply once every 7 days; for initial therapy start with 0.1 mg and increase by 0.1 mg at 1- to 2-week intervals; dosages >0.6 mg do not improve efficacy

Epidural infusion: Starting dose: 30 mcg/hour; titrate as required for relief of pain or presence of side effects; minimal experience with doses >40 mcg/hour; should be considered an adjunct to intraspinal opiate therapy

**Dosing adjustment in renal impairment:** Cl$_{cr}$ <10 mL/minute: Administer 50% to 75% of normal dose initially

Dialysis: Not dialyzable (0% to 5%) via hemo- or peritoneal dialysis; supplemental dose not necessary

**Dosage Forms** Clonidine hydrochloride: **Inj, preservative free:** 100 mcg/mL (10 mL), **Patch, transdermal:** 1, 2, and 3 (0.1, 0.2, 0.3 mg/day, 7-day duration), **Tab:** 0.1 mg, 0.2 mg, 0.3 mg

**Contraindications** Hypersensitivity to clonidine hydrochloride or any component

**Warnings/Precautions** Use with caution in cerebrovascular disease, coronary insufficiency, renal impairment, sinus node dysfunction; do not abruptly discontinue as rapid increase in blood pressure and symptoms of sympathetic overactivity (ie, increased heart (Continued)

## Clonidine *(Continued)*

rate, tremor, agitation, anxiety, insomnia, sweating, palpitations) may occur; **if need to discontinue, taper dose gradually over 1 week or more (2-4 days with epidural product)**; adjust dosage in patients with renal dysfunction (especially the elderly); not recommended for obstetrical, postpartum or perioperative pain management or in those with severe hemodynamic instability due to unacceptable risk of hypotension and bradycardia; clonidine injection should be administered via a continuous epidural infusion device

**Pregnancy Risk Factor** C

**Pregnancy Implications**

Clinical effects on the fetus: Crosses the placenta. Caution should be used with this drug due to the potential of rebound hypertension with abrupt discontinuation.

Breast-feeding/lactation: Crosses into breast milk. American Academy of Pediatrics has NO RECOMMENDATION.

**Adverse Reactions**

>10%:

Cardiovascular: Orthostatic hypotension (especially with epidural route), rebound hypertension, bradycardia

Central nervous system: Drowsiness, dizziness, confusion, anxiety

Gastrointestinal: Xerostomia, constipation, nausea

1% to 10%:

Central nervous system: Mental depression, headache, fatigue, hyperaesthesia, pain

Dermatologic: Rash, skin ulcer

Respiratory: Dyspnea, hypoventilation

Cardiovascular: Chest pain

Endocrine & metabolic: Decreased sexual activity, loss of libido

Gastrointestinal: vomiting, constipation

Genitourinary: Nocturia, impotence

Hepatic: Abnormal LFTs

Neuromuscular & skeletal: Weakness

Otic: Tinnitus

<1%: Palpitations, tachycardia, Raynaud's phenomenon, congestive heart failure, insomnia, vivid dreams, delirium, fever, pruritus, urticaria, alopecia, gynecomastia, weight gain, urinary retention, dysuria, infection possible, burning eyes, blurred vision

**Drug Interactions**

Decreased effect: Tricyclic antidepressants antagonize hypotensive effects of clonidine

Increased toxicity: Beta-blockers may potentiate bradycardia in patients receiving clonidine and may increase the rebound hypertension of withdrawal; discontinue beta-blocker several days before clonidine is tapered; tricyclic antidepressants may enhance the hypertensive response associated with abrupt clonidine withdrawal; narcotic analgesics may potentiate hypotensive effects of clonidine; alcohol and barbiturates may increase the CNS depression; epidural clonidine may prolong the sensory and motor blockade of local anesthetics

**Onset** Oral: 0.5-1 hour; $T_{max}$: 2-4 hours

**Duration** >24 hours

**Half-Life** Normal renal function: 6-20 hours; Renal impairment: 18-41 hours

**Special PA Issues**

**Patient Education:** Take as directed, at bedtime. Do not skip doses or discontinue without consulting prescriber. If using patch, check daily for correct placement. Follow recommended diet and exercise program. Do not use OTC medications which may affect blood pressure (eg, cough or cold remedies, diet pills, stay-awake medications) without consulting prescriber. This medication may cause drowsiness, dizziness, or impaired judgment (use caution when driving or engaging in tasks that require alertness until response is known); decreased libido or sexual function (will resolve when drug is discontinued); postural hypotension (use caution when rising from sitting or lying position or when climbing stairs); or dry mouth or nausea (frequent mouth care or sucking lozenges may help). Report difficulty, pain, or burning on urination; increased nervousness or depression; sudden weight gain (weigh yourself in the same clothes at same time of day once a week); unusual or persistent swelling of ankles, feet, or extremities; wet cough or respiratory difficulty; chest pain or palpitations; muscle weakness, fatigue, or pain; or other persistent side effects.

**Monitoring Parameters:** Blood pressure, standing and sitting/supine, respiratory rate and depth, pain relief, mental status, heart rate (bradycardia may be treated with atropine)

**Reference Range:** Therapeutic: 1-2 ng/mL (SI: 4.4-8.7 nmol/L)

## Clonidine and Chlorthalidone *(KLOE ni deen & klor THAL i done)*

**Pharmacologic Class** Antihypertensive Agent, Combination

**U.S. Brand Names** Combipres®

**Dosage Forms Tab:** 0.1: Clonidine 0.1 mg and chlorthalidone 15 mg, 0.2: Clonidine 0.2 mg and chlorthalidone 15 mg, 0.3: Clonidine 0.3 mg and chlorthalidone 15 mg

♦ **Clonidine Hydrochloride** *see* Clonidine *on previous page*

# Clopidogrel (kloh PID oh grel)

**Pharmacologic Class** Antiplatelet Agent

**U.S. Brand Names** Plavix®

**Mechanism of Action** Blocks the ADP receptors, which prevent fibrinogen binding at that site and thereby reduce the possibility of platelet adhesion and aggregation

**Use** The reduction of atherosclerotic events (myocardial infarction, stroke, vascular deaths) in patients with atherosclerosis documented by recent myocardial infarctions, recent stroke or established peripheral arterial disease

**USUAL DOSAGE** Adults: Oral: 75 mg once daily

**Dosing adjustment in renal impairment and elderly:** None necessary

**Dosage Forms** Tab, as bisulfate: 75 mg

**Contraindications** In patients with active bleeding (eg, peptic ulcer disease, intracranial hemorrhage), patients with coagulation disorders, or patients who have demonstrated hypersensitivity to the drug or any components of the drug product

**Warnings/Precautions** Patients receiving anticoagulants or other antiplatelet drugs concurrently, liver disease, patients having a previous hypersensitivity or other untoward effects related to ticlopidine, hypertension, renal impairment, history of bleeding or hemostatic disorders or drug-related hematologic disorders, and consider discontinuing in patients scheduled for major surgery, 7 days prior to that surgery

**Pregnancy Risk Factor** B

**Adverse Reactions**

>10%: Gastrointestinal: Indigestion, nausea, vomiting (15%)

1% to 10%:

Dermatologic: Rash (4.2%), pruritus (3.3%)

Gastrointestinal: Diarrhea (4.5%), GI hemorrhage (2%)

Hepatic: Hepatotoxicity (≤3%)

<1%: Neutropenia (0.1%), prolonged bleeding time, intracranial bleeding (0.35%)

**Drug Interactions** Increased effect/toxicity: When used with other drugs that can increase bleeding risk such as heparins, warfarins, NSAIDs and other antiplatelet drugs

**Half-Life** 7-8 hours

**Special PA Issues**

Patient Education: Take as directed. May cause headache or dizziness; use caution when driving or engaging in hazardous activities. Small frequent meals, frequent mouth care, or sucking on lozenges may reduce nausea or vomiting. Mild analgesics may reduce arthralgia or back pain. Report immediately unusual or acute chest pain or respiratory difficulties, skin rash, unresolved diarrhea or gastrointestinal distress, nosebleed, or acute headache.

Dietary Considerations: Food: May be taken without regard to meals

Monitoring Parameters: Signs of bleeding

♦ **Clopidogrel Bisulfate** see Clopidogrel on this page

♦ **Clopra®** see Metoclopramide on page 597

# Clorazepate (klor AZ e pate)

**Pharmacologic Class** Benzodiazepine

**U.S. Brand Names** Gen-XENE®; Tranxene®

**Mechanism of Action** Facilitates gamma aminobutyric acid (GABA)-mediated transmission inhibitory neurotransmitter action, depresses subcortical levels of CNS

**Use** Treatment of generalized anxiety and panic disorders; management of alcohol withdrawal; adjunct anticonvulsant in management of partial seizures

**USUAL DOSAGE** Oral:

Children 9-12 years: Anticonvulsant: Initial: 3.75-7.5 mg/dose twice daily; increase dose by 3.75 mg at weekly intervals, not to exceed 60 mg/day in 2-3 divided doses

Children >12 years and Adults: Anticonvulsant: Initial: Up to 7.5 mg/dose 2-3 times/day; increase dose by 7.5 mg at weekly intervals; not to exceed 90 mg/day

Adults:

Anxiety: 7.5-15 mg 2-4 times/day, or given as single dose of 11.25 or 22.5 mg at bedtime

Alcohol withdrawal: Initial: 30 mg, then 15 mg 2-4 times/day on first day; maximum daily dose: 90 mg; gradually decrease dose over subsequent days

**Dosage Forms** Clorazepate dipotassium: **Cap:** 3.75 mg, 7.5 mg, 15 mg; **Tab:** 3.75 mg, 7.5 mg, 15 mg; **Tab, single dose:** 11.25 mg, 22.5 mg

**Contraindications** Hypersensitivity to clorazepate dipotassium or any component; cross-sensitivity with other benzodiazepines may exist; avoid using in patients with pre-existing CNS depression, severe uncontrolled pain, or narrow-angle glaucoma

**Warnings/Precautions** Use with caution in patients with hepatic or renal disease; abrupt discontinuation may cause withdrawal symptoms or seizures

**Pregnancy Risk Factor** D

**Adverse Reactions**

>10%:

Cardiovascular: Tachycardia, chest pain

(Continued)

## Clorazepate *(Continued)*

Central nervous system: Drowsiness, fatigue, ataxia, lightheadedness, memory impairment, insomnia, anxiety, headache, depression
Dermatologic: Rash
Endocrine & metabolic: Decreased libido
Gastrointestinal: Xerostomia, constipation, diarrhea, decreased salivation, nausea, vomiting, increased or decreased appetite
Neuromuscular & skeletal: Dysarthria
Ocular: Blurred vision
Miscellaneous: Diaphoresis
1% to 10%:
Cardiovascular: Syncope, hypotension
Central nervous system: Confusion, nervousness, dizziness, akathisia
Dermatologic: Dermatitis
Gastrointestinal: Nausea, increased salivation, weight gain or loss
Neuromuscular & skeletal: Rigidity, tremor, muscle cramps
Otic: Tinnitus
Respiratory: Nasal congestion, hyperventilation
<1%: Menstrual irregularities, blood dyscrasias, reflex slowing, drug dependence, long-term use may also be associated with renal or hepatic injury and reduced hematocrit
**Drug Interactions** Increased effect: Cimetidine, CNS depressants, alcohol
**Onset** ~1 hour
**Duration** Variable, 8-24 hours
**Half-Life** Desmethyldiazepam: 48-96 hours; Oxazepam: 6-8 hours
**Special PA Issues**
**Patient Education:** Take exactly as directed (do not increase dose or frequency); may cause physical and/or psychological dependence. Do not use excessive alcohol and other prescription or OTC medications (especially pain medications, sedatives, antihistamines, or hypnotics) without consulting prescriber. Maintain adequate hydration (2-3 L/day of fluids unless instructed to restrict fluid intake). You may experience drowsiness, lightheadedness, impaired coordination, dizziness, or blurred vision (use caution when driving or engaging in hazardous tasks until response to medication is known); nausea, vomiting, or dry mouth (small frequent meals, good mouth care, chewing gum, or sucking lozenges may help); constipation (increased exercise, fluids, or dietary fruit and fiber may help); altered sexual drive or ability (reversible); or photosensitivity (use sunscreen, protective clothing, and avoid extended exposure to direct sunlight). Report persistent CNS effects (eg, confusion, depression, increased sedation, excitation, headache, agitation, insomnia or nightmares, dizziness, fatigue, impaired coordination, changes in personality, or changes in cognition); changes in urinary pattern; muscle cramping, weakness, tremors, or rigidity; ringing in ears or visual disturbances; chest pain, palpitations, or rapid heartbeat; excessive perspiration; excessive GI symptoms (cramping, constipation, vomiting, anorexia); or worsening of condition.
**Dietary Considerations:** Alcohol: Additive CNS effects, avoid use
**Monitoring Parameters:** Respiratory and cardiovascular status, excess CNS depression
**Reference Range:** Therapeutic: 0.12-1 µg/mL (SI: 0.36-3.01 µmol/L)

♦ **Clorazepate Dipotassium** *see* Clorazepate *on previous page*

## Clotrimazole *(kloe TRIM a zole)*

**Pharmacologic Class** Antifungal Agent, Oral Nonabsorbed; Antifungal Agent, Topical; Antifungal Agent, Vaginal
**U.S. Brand Names** Femizole-7® [OTC]; Fungoid® Solution; Gyne-Lotrimin® [OTC]; Gynix® Vaginal Tablets; Lotrimin®; Lotrimin® AF Cream [OTC]; Lotrimin® AF Lotion [OTC]; Lotrimin® AF Solution [OTC]; Mycelex®; Mycelex®-7; Mycelex®-G
**Mechanism of Action** Binds to phospholipids in the fungal cell membrane altering cell wall permeability resulting in loss of essential intracellular elements
**Use** Treatment of susceptible fungal infections, including oropharyngeal, candidiasis, dermatophytoses, superficial mycoses, and cutaneous candidiasis, as well as vulvovaginal candidiasis; limited data suggest that clotrimazole troches may be effective for prophylaxis against oropharyngeal candidiasis in neutropenic patients
**USUAL DOSAGE**
Children >3 years and Adults:
Oral:
Prophylaxis: 10 mg troche dissolved 3 times/day for the duration of chemotherapy or until steroids are reduced to maintenance levels
Treatment: 10 mg troche dissolved slowly 5 times/day for 14 consecutive days
Topical: Apply twice daily; if no improvement occurs after 4 weeks of therapy, re-evaluate diagnosis
Children >12 years and Adults:
Vaginal:
Cream: Insert 1 applicatorful of 1% vaginal cream daily (preferably at bedtime) for 7 consecutive days

Tablet: Insert 100 mg/day for 7 days or 500 mg single dose

Topical: Apply to affected area twice daily (morning and evening) for 7 consecutive days

**Dosage Forms Combination pack (Mycelex-7®):** Vaginal tab 100 mg (7's) and vaginal cream 1% (7 g); **Crm:** Topical (Lotrimin®, Lotrimin® AF, Mycelex®, Mycelex® OTC): 1% (15 g, 30 g, 45 g, 90 g), Vaginal (Femizole-7®, Gyne-Lotrimin®, Mycelex®-G): 1% (45 g, 90 g); **Lot (Lotrimin®):** 1% (30 mL); **Soln, top (Fungoid®, Lotrimin®, Lotrimin® AF, Mycelex®, Mycelex® OTC):** 1% (10 mL, 30 mL); **Tab, vaginal (Gyne-Lotrimin®, Gynix®; Mycelex®-G):** 100 mg (7s), 500 mg (1s); **Troche (Mycelex®):** 10 mg; **Twin pack (Mycelex®):** Vaginal tab 500 mg (1's) and vaginal cream 1% (7 g)

**Contraindications** Hypersensitivity to clotrimazole or any component

**Warnings/Precautions** Clotrimazole should not be used for treatment of systemic fungal infection; safety and effectiveness of clotrimazole lozenges (troches) in children <3 years of age have not been established

**Pregnancy Risk Factor** B; C (oral)

**Adverse Reactions**
>10%: Hepatic: Abnormal LFTs, causal relationship between troches and elevated LFTs not clearly established

1% to 10%:
Gastrointestinal: Nausea and vomiting may occur in patients on clotrimazole troches
Local: Mild burning, irritation, stinging to skin or vaginal area

**Drug Interactions** CYP3A3/4 and 3A5-7 enzyme inhibitor

**Special PA Issues**
Patient Education:
Oral: Do not swallow oral medication whole; allow to dissolve slowly in mouth. You may experience nausea or vomiting (small frequent meals, frequent mouth care, or sucking on lozenges may help). Report signs of opportunistic infection (eg, white plaques in mouth, fever, chills, perianal itching or vaginal discharge, fatigue, unhealed wounds or sores).
Topical: Wash hands before applying or wear gloves. Apply thin film of gel, lotion, or solution to affected area. May apply porous dressing. Report persistent burning, swelling, itching, worsening of condition, or lack of response to therapy.
Vaginal: Wash hands before using. Insert full applicator into vagina gently and expel cream, or insert tablet into vagina, at bedtime. Wash applicator with soap and water following use. Remain lying down for 30 minutes following administration. Avoid intercourse during therapy (sexual partner may experience penile burning or itching). Report adverse reactions (eg, vulvular itching, frequent urination), worsening of condition, or lack of response to therapy.
**Monitoring Parameters:** Periodic liver function tests during oral therapy with clotrimazole lozenges

# Cloxacillin (kloks a SIL in)

**Pharmacologic Class** Antibiotic, Penicillin

**U.S. Brand Names** Cloxapen®; Tegopen®

**Mechanism of Action** Inhibits bacterial cell wall synthesis by binding to one or more of the penicillin-binding proteins (PBPs) which in turn inhibits the final transpeptidation step of peptidoglycan synthesis in bacterial cell walls, thus inhibiting cell wall biosynthesis. Bacteria eventually lyse due to ongoing activity of cell wall autolytic enzymes (autolysins and murein hydrolases) while cell wall assembly is arrested.

**Use** Treatment of susceptible bacterial infections, notably penicillinase-producing staphylococci causing respiratory tract, skin and skin structure, bone and joint, urinary tract infections

**USUAL DOSAGE** Oral:
Children >1 month (<20 kg): 50-100 mg/kg/day in divided doses every 6 hours; up to a maximum of 4 g/day
Children (>20 kg) and Adults: 250-500 mg every 6 hours
Hemodialysis: Not dialyzable (0% to 5%)

**Dosage Forms Cap:** 250 mg, 500 mg; **Powder for oral susp:** 125 mg/5 mL (100 mL, 200 mL)

**Contraindications** Hypersensitivity to cloxacillin or any component, or penicillins

**Warnings/Precautions** Monitor PT if patient concurrently on warfarin, elimination of drug is slow in renally impaired; use with caution in patients allergic to cephalosporins due to a low incidence of cross-hypersensitivity

**Pregnancy Risk Factor** B

**Adverse Reactions**
1% to 10%: Gastrointestinal: Nausea, diarrhea, abdominal pain
<1%: Fever, seizures with extremely high doses and/or renal failure, rash (maculopapular to exfoliative), vomiting, pseudomembranous colitis, vaginitis, eosinophilia, leukopenia, neutropenia, thrombocytopenia, agranulocytosis, anemia, hemolytic anemia, prolonged PT, hepatotoxicity, transient elevated LFTs, hematuria, interstitial nephritis, increased BUN/creatinine, serum sickness-like reactions, hypersensitivity

**Drug Interactions**
Decreased effect: Efficacy of oral contraceptives may be reduced
(Continued)

## Cloxacillin (Continued)

Increased effect: Disulfiram, probenecid may increase penicillin levels, increased effect of anticoagulants

**Half-Life** 0.5-1.5 hours (prolonged with renal impairment and in neonates)

**Special PA Issues**

**Patient Education:** Take 1 hour before or 2 hours after meals with water. Finish all medication; do not skip doses. Take around-the-clock. If diabetic, drug may cause false tests with Clinitest® urine glucose monitoring; use of glucose oxidase methods (Clinistix®) or serum glucose monitoring is preferable. This drug may interfere with oral contraceptives; an alternate form of birth control should be used. Immediately report any signs or symptoms of anaphylactic reactions (eg, chills, fever, wheezing, tightness in chest), excessive GI side effects, or signs or symptoms of opportunistic infection (eg, white spots or sores in mouth, vaginal discharge or sores, fever, fatigue, unhealed sores or wounds).

**Monitoring Parameters:** Observe for signs and symptoms of anaphylaxis during first dose

♦ **Cloxacillin Sodium** see Cloxacillin on previous page

♦ **Cloxapen®** see Cloxacillin on previous page

## Clozapine (KLOE za peen)

**Pharmacologic Class** Antipsychotic Agent, Dibenzodiazepine

**U.S. Brand Names** Clozaril®

**Mechanism of Action** Clozapine is a weak dopamine$_1$ and dopamine$_2$ receptor blocker; in addition, it blocks the serotonin$_2$, alpha-adrenergic, and histamine H$_1$ central nervous system receptors

**Use** Management of schizophrenic patients

**USUAL DOSAGE** Adults: Oral: 25 mg once or twice daily initially and increased, as tolerated to a target dose of 300-450 mg/day after 2 weeks, but may require doses as high as 600-900 mg/day

**Dosage Forms Tab:** 25 mg, 100 mg

**Contraindications** In patients with WBC ≤3500 cells/mm$^3$ before therapy; if WBC falls to <3000 cells/mm$^3$ during therapy the drug should be withheld until signs and symptoms of infection disappear and WBC rises to >3000 cells/mm$^3$

**Warnings/Precautions** Medication should not be stopped abruptly; taper off over 1-2 weeks. WBC testing should occur weekly for the first 6 months of therapy; thereafter, if acceptable WBC counts are maintained (WBC ≥3000/mm$^3$, ANC ≥1500/mm$^3$) then WBC counts can be monitored every other week. WBCs must be monitored weekly for the first 4 weeks after therapy discontinuation. Significant risk of agranulocytosis, potentially life-threatening. Use with caution in patients receiving other marrow suppressive agents.

**Pregnancy Risk Factor** B

**Adverse Reactions**

>10%:
Cardiovascular: Tachycardia, hypotension, orthostatic hypotension
Central nervous system: Fever, headache, drowsiness
Gastrointestinal: Constipation, nausea, vomiting, unusual weight gain

1% to 10%:
Cardiovascular: EKG changes, hypertension
Central nervous system: Agitation, akathisia
Gastrointestinal: Abdominal discomfort, heartburn, xerostomia
Ocular: Blurred vision
Miscellaneous: Diaphoresis (increased)

<1%: Insomnia, seizures, tardive dyskinesia, neuroleptic malignant syndrome, dysuria, impotence, agranulocytosis, eosinophilia, granulocytopenia, leukopenia, thrombocytopenia, rigidity, tremor

**Drug Interactions** CYP1A2, 2C, 2E1, 3A3/4 enzyme substrate, CYP2D6 enzyme substrate (minor)
Decreased effect of epinephrine; decreased effect with phenytoin
Increased effect of CNS depressants, guanabenz, anticholinergics
Increased toxicity with cimetidine, MAO inhibitors, neuroleptics, TCAs

**Half-Life** Mean half-life: 12 hours (range: 4-66 hours)

**Special PA Issues**

**Patient Education:** Use exactly as directed (do not increase dose or frequency); may cause physical and/or psychological dependence. Do not discontinue without consulting prescriber. Avoid excess alcohol or caffeine and other prescription or OTC medications not approved by prescriber. Maintain adequate hydration (2-3 L/day of fluids unless instructed to restrict fluid intake). You may experience headache, excess drowsiness, dizziness, or blurred vision (use caution driving or when engaging in hazardous tasks until response to medication is known); dry mouth, nausea, vomiting (small frequent meals, frequent mouth care, or sucking lozenges may help); or postural hypotension (use caution climbing stairs or when changing position from lying or sitting to standing). Report persistent CNS effects (insomnia, depression, altered consciousness); palpitations, rapid heartbeat, severe dizziness; vision changes; hypersalivation, tearing, sweating; difficulty breathing; or worsening of condition.

**Related Information**
Antipsychotic Agents *on page 1001*

♦ **Clozaril®** *see* Clozapine *on previous page*
♦ **CMV-IGIV** *see* Cytomegalovirus Immune Globulin (Intravenous-Human) *on page 249*
♦ **Cobex®** *see* Cyanocobalamin *on page 242*

## Cocaine (koe KANE)
**Pharmacologic Class** Local Anesthetic
**Mechanism of Action** Ester local anesthetic blocks both the initiation and conduction of nerve impulses by decreasing the neuronal membrane's permeability to sodium ions, which results in inhibition of depolarization with resultant blockade of conduction; interferes with the uptake of norepinephrine by adrenergic nerve terminals producing vasoconstriction
**Use** Topical anesthesia (ester derivative) for mucous membranes
**USUAL DOSAGE** Dosage depends on the area to be anesthetized, tissue vascularity, technique of anesthesia, and individual patient tolerance; use the lowest dose necessary to produce adequate anesthesia should be used, not to exceed 1 mg/kg. Use reduced dosages for children, elderly, or debilitated patients.

Topical application (ear, nose, throat, bronchoscopy): Concentrations of 1% to 4% are used; concentrations >4% are not recommended because of potential for increased incidence and severity of systemic toxic reactions
**Dosage Forms Powder:** 5 g, 25 g; **Soln, top:** 4% [40 mg/mL] (2 mL, 4 mL, 10 mL), 10% [100 mg/mL] (4 mL, 10 mL); **Soln, top, viscous:** 4% [40 mg/mL] (4 mL, 10 mL), 10% [100 mg/mL] (4 mL, 10 mL); **Tab, soluble, for top soln:** 135 mg
**Contraindications** Systemic use, hypersensitivity to cocaine or any component; pregnancy if nonmedicinal use
**Warnings/Precautions** Use with caution in patients with hypertension, severe cardiovascular disease, or thyrotoxicosis; use with caution in patients with severely traumatized mucosa and sepsis in the region of intended application. Repeated topical application can result in psychic dependence and tolerance. May cause cornea to become clouded or pitted, therefore, normal saline should be used to irrigate and protect cornea during surgery; not for injection.
**Pregnancy Risk Factor** C (X if nonmedicinal use)
**Adverse Reactions**
>10%:
Central nervous system: CNS stimulation
Gastrointestinal: Loss of taste perception
Respiratory: Chronic rhinitis, nasal congestion
Miscellaneous: Loss of smell
1% to 10%:
Cardiovascular: Decreased heart rate with low doses, increased heart rate with moderate doses, hypertension, tachycardia, cardiac arrhythmias
Central nervous system: Nervousness, restlessness, euphoria, excitement, hallucination, seizures
Gastrointestinal: Vomiting
Neuromuscular & skeletal: Tremors and clonic-tonic reactions
Ocular: Sloughing of the corneal epithelium, ulceration of the cornea
Respiratory: Tachypnea, respiratory failure
**Drug Interactions** CYP3A3/4 enzyme substrate
Increased toxicity: MAO inhibitors
**Onset** Onset of action: Within 1 minute; Peak action: Within 5 minutes
**Duration** ≥30 minutes, depending on dosage administered
**Half-Life** Following topical administration to mucosa: 75 minutes
**Special PA Issues**
**Patient Education:** When used orally, do not take anything by mouth until full sensation returns. Ocular: Use caution when driving or engaging in tasks that require alert vision (mydriasis may last for several hours). At time of use or immediately thereafter, report any unusual cardiovascular, CNS, or respiratory symptoms immediately. Following use, report skin irritation or eruption; alterations in vision, eye pain or irritation; persistent gastrointestinal effects; muscle or skeletal tremors, numbness, or rigidity; urinary or genital problems; or persistent fatigue. When used orally, do not take anything by mouth until full sensation returns.
**Monitoring Parameters:** Vital signs
**Reference Range:** Therapeutic: 100-500 ng/mL (SI: 330 nmol/L); Toxic: >1000 ng/mL (SI: >3300 nmol/L)
**Related Information**
Hallucinogenic Drugs *on page 1019*

♦ **Cocaine Hydrochloride** *see* Cocaine *on this page*
♦ **Codafed® Expectorant** *see* Guaifenesin, Pseudoephedrine, and Codeine *on page 429*

♦ **Codamine®** *see* Hydrocodone and Phenylpropanolamine *on page 453*
♦ **Codamine® Pediatric** *see* Hydrocodone and Phenylpropanolamine *on page 453*
♦ **Codehist® DH** *see* Chlorpheniramine, Pseudoephedrine, and Codeine *on page 197*

# Codeine (KOE deen)

**Pharmacologic Class** Analgesic, Narcotic; Antitussive

**Mechanism of Action** Binds to opiate receptors in the CNS, causing inhibition of ascending pain pathways, altering the perception of and response to pain; causes cough supression by direct central action in the medulla; produces generalized CNS depression

**Use** Treatment of mild to moderate pain; antitussive in lower doses; dextromethorphan has equivalent antitussive activity but has much lower toxicity in accidental overdose

**USUAL DOSAGE** Doses should be titrated to appropriate analgesic effect; when changing routes of administration, note that oral dose is $^2/_3$ as effective as parenteral dose

Analgesic:
  Children: Oral, I.M., S.C.: 0.5-1 mg/kg/dose every 4-6 hours as needed; maximum: 60 mg/dose
  Adults: Oral, I.M., I.V., S.C.: 30 mg/dose; range: 15-60 mg every 4-6 hours as needed; maximum: 360 mg/24 hours
Antitussive: Oral (for nonproductive cough):
  Children: 1-1.5 mg/kg/day in divided doses every 4-6 hours as needed: Alternative dose according to age:
    2-6 years: 2.5-5 mg every 4-6 hours as needed; maximum: 30 mg/day
    6-12 years: 5-10 mg every 4-6 hours as needed; maximum: 60 mg/day
  Adults: 10-20 mg/dose every 4-6 hours as needed; maximum: 120 mg/day
**Dosing adjustment in renal impairment:**
  Cl$_{cr}$ 10-50 mL/minute: Administer 75% of dose
  Cl$_{cr}$ <10 mL/minute: Administer 50% of dose
**Dosing adjustment in hepatic impairment:** Probably necessary in hepatic insufficiency

**Dosage Forms** Codeine phosphate: **Inj:** 30 mg (1 mL, 2 mL); 60 mg (1 mL, 2 mL); **Tab, soluble:** 30 mg, 60 mg
  Codeine sulfate: **Tab:** 15 mg, 30 mg, 60 mg; **Tab, soluble:** 15 mg, 30 mg, 60 mg

**Contraindications** Hypersensitivity to codeine or any component

**Warnings/Precautions** Use with caution in patients with hypersensitivity reactions to other phenanthrene derivative opioid agonists (morphine, hydrocodone, hydromorphone, levorphanol, oxycodone, oxymorphone); respiratory diseases including asthma, emphysema, COPD, or severe liver or renal insufficiency; some preparations contain sulfites which may cause allergic reactions; tolerance or drug dependence may result from extended use

Not recommended for use for cough control in patients with a productive cough; not recommended as an antitussive for children <2 years of age; the elderly may be particularly susceptible to the CNS depressant and confusion as well as constipating effects of narcotics

**Pregnancy Risk Factor** C (D if used for prolonged periods or in high doses at term)

**Adverse Reactions**
Percentage unknown: Increased AST, ALT
>10%:
  Central nervous system: Drowsiness
  Gastrointestinal: Constipation
1% to 10%:
  Cardiovascular: Tachycardia or bradycardia, hypotension
  Central nervous system: Dizziness, lightheadedness, false feeling of well being, malaise, headache, restlessness, paradoxical CNS stimulation, confusion
  Dermatologic: Rash, urticaria
  Gastrointestinal: Xerostomia, anorexia, nausea, vomiting,
  Genitourinary: Decreased urination, ureteral spasm
  Hepatic: Increased LFTs
  Local: Burning at injection site
  Ocular: Blurred vision
  Neuromuscular & skeletal: Weakness
  Respiratory: Shortness of breath, dyspnea
  Miscellaneous: Histamine release
<1%: Convulsions, hallucinations, mental depression, nightmares, insomnia, paralytic ileus, biliary spasm, stomach cramps, muscle rigidity, trembling

**Drug Interactions** CYP2D6 and 3A3/4 enzyme substrate; CYP2D6 enzyme inhibitor
  Decreased effect with cigarette smoking
  Increased toxicity: CNS depressants, TCAs, other narcotic analgesics, guanabenz, MAO inhibitors, neuromuscular blockers

**Onset**
  Onset of action: Oral: 0.5-1 hour; I.M.: 10-30 minutes
  Peak action: Oral: 1-1.5 hours; I.M.: 0.5-1 hour

**Duration** 4-6 hours

**Half-Life** 2.5-3.5 hours

**Special PA Issues**

**Patient Education:** If self-administered, use exactly as directed (do not increase dose or frequency); may cause physical and/or psychological dependence. While using this medication, do not use alcohol and other prescription or OTC medications (especially sedatives, tranquilizers, antihistamines, or pain medications) without consulting prescriber. Maintain adequate hydration (2-3 L/day of fluids unless instructed to restrict fluid intake). May cause dizziness, drowsiness, confusion, agitation, impaired coordination, or blurred vision (use caution when driving, climbing stairs, or changing position - rising from sitting or lying to standing, or when engaging in hazardous activities until response to medication is known); nausea or vomiting, or loss of appetite (frequent mouth care, small frequent meals, or sucking on lozenges may help); constipation (increased exercise, fluids, or dietary fruit and fiber may help - if constipation remains an unresolved problem, consult prescriber about use of stool softeners). Report confusion, insomnia, excessive nervousness, excessive sedation or drowsiness, or shakiness; acute GI upset; difficulty breathing or shortness of breath; facial flushing, rapid heartbeat or palpitations; urinary difficulty; unusual muscle weakness; or vision changes.

**Dietary Considerations:**

Alcohol: Additive CNS effects, avoid or limit alcohol; watch for sedation

Food: Glucose may cause hyperglycemia; monitor blood glucose concentrations

**Monitoring Parameters:** Pain relief, respiratory and mental status, blood pressure, heart rate

**Reference Range:** Therapeutic: Not established; Toxic: >1.1 µg/mL

**Related Information**

Narcotic Agonists on page 1023

♦ **Codeine and Acetaminophen** see Acetaminophen and Codeine on page 22

♦ **Codeine and Aspirin** see Aspirin and Codeine on page 82

♦ **Codeine and Guaifenesin** see Guaifenesin and Codeine on page 428

♦ **Codeine Contin®** see Codeine on previous page

♦ **Codeine Phosphate** see Codeine on previous page

♦ **Codeine Sulfate** see Codeine on previous page

♦ **Codiclear® DH** see Hydrocodone and Guaifenesin on page 451

♦ **Codoxy®** see Oxycodone and Aspirin on page 688

♦ **Codroxomin®** see Hydroxocobalamin on page 458

♦ **Cogentin®** see Benztropine on page 107

♦ **Co-Gesic®** see Hydrocodone and Acetaminophen on page 449

♦ **Cognex®** see Tacrine on page 868

♦ **Colace® [OTC]** see Docusate on page 298

♦ **Colax-C®** see Docusate on page 298

## Colchicine (KOL chi seen)

**Pharmacologic Class** Colchicine

**Mechanism of Action** Decreases leukocyte motility, decreases phagocytosis in joints and lactic acid production, thereby reducing the deposition of urate crystals that perpetuates the inflammatory response

**Use** Treat acute gouty arthritis attacks and prevent recurrences of such attacks, management of familial Mediterranean fever

**USUAL DOSAGE**

Prophylaxis of familial Mediterranean fever: Oral:

Children:

≤5 years: 0.5 mg/day

>5 years: 1-1.5 mg/day in 2-3 divided doses

Adults: 1-2 mg/day in 2-3 divided doses

Gouty arthritis, acute attacks: Adults:

Oral: Initial: 0.5-1.2 mg, then 0.5-0.6 mg every 1-2 hours or 1-1.2 mg every 2 hours until relief or GI side effects (nausea, vomiting, or diarrhea) occur to a maximum total dose of 8 mg; wait 3 days before initiating another course of therapy

I.V.: Initial: 1-3 mg, then 0.5 mg every 6 hours until response, not to exceed 4 mg/day; if pain recurs, it may be necessary to administer a daily dose of 1-2 mg for several days, however, do not administer more colchicine by any route for at least 7 days after a full course of I.V. therapy (4 mg), transfer to oral colchicine in a dose similar to that being given I.V.

Gouty arthritis, prophylaxis of recurrent attacks: Adults: Oral: 0.5-0.6 mg/day or every other day

**Dosing adjustment in renal impairment:**

Cl$_{cr}$ <50 mL/minute: Avoid chronic use or administration

Cl$_{cr}$ <10 mL/minute: Decrease dose by 50% for treatment of acute attacks

Hemodialysis: Not dialyzable (0% to 5%); supplemental dose is not necessary

Peritoneal dialysis: Supplemental dose is not necessary

(Continued)

## Colchicine *(Continued)*

**Dosage Forms Inj:** 0.5 mg/mL (2 mL); **Tab:** 0.5 mg, 0.6 mg

**Contraindications** Hypersensitivity to colchicine or any component; serious renal, gastrointestinal, hepatic, or cardiac disorders; blood dyscrasias

**Warnings/Precautions** Severe local irritation can occur following S.C. or I.M. administration; use with caution in debilitated patients or elderly patients or patients with severe GI, renal, or liver disease

**Pregnancy Risk Factor** C (oral)/D (parenteral)

**Adverse Reactions**
>10%: Gastrointestinal: Nausea, vomiting, diarrhea, abdominal pain
1% to 10%:
  Dermatologic: Alopecia
  Gastrointestinal: Anorexia
<1%: Rash, azoospermia, agranulocytosis, aplastic anemia, bone marrow suppression, hepatotoxicity, myopathy, peripheral neuritis

**Drug Interactions**
Decreased effect: Vitamin $B_{12}$ absorption may be decreased
Increased toxicity:
  Sympathomimetic agents
  CNS depressant effects are enhanced

**Onset** Oral: Relief of pain and inflammation occurs after 24-48 hours; I.V.: 6-12 hours

**Half-Life** 12-30 minutes; End-stage renal disease: 45 minutes

**Special PA Issues**
**Patient Education:** Take as directed; do not exceed recommended dosage. Consult prescriber about a low-purine diet. Maintain adequate hydration (2-3 L/day of fluids unless instructed to restrict fluid intake). Do not use alcohol or aspirin-containing medication without consulting prescriber. You may experience nausea, vomiting, or anorexia (small frequent meals, frequent mouth care, or sucking on lozenges may help); hair loss (reversible). Stop medication and report to prescriber if severe vomiting, watery or bloody diarrhea, or abdominal pain occurs. Report muscle tremors or weakness; fatigue; easy bruising or bleeding; yellowing of eyes or skin; or pale stool or dark urine.
**Dietary Considerations:**
Alcohol: Avoid use
Food: Cyanocobalamin (Vitamin $B_{12}$): Malabsorption of the substrate. May result in macrocytic anemia or neurologic dysfunction. May need to supplement with Vitamin $B_{12}$.
**Monitoring Parameters:** CBC and renal function test

## Colchicine and Probenecid *(KOL chi seen & proe BEN e sid)*

**Pharmacologic Class** Antigout Agent

**Dosage Forms Tab:** Colchicine 0.5 mg and probenecid 0.5 g

♦ **Colestid®** *see* Colestipol *on this page*

## Colestipol *(koe LES ti pole)*

**Pharmacologic Class** Antilipemic Agent (Bile Acid Seqestrant)

**U.S. Brand Names** Colestid®

**Mechanism of Action** Binds with bile acids to form an insoluble complex that is eliminated in feces; it thereby increases the fecal loss of bile acid-bound low density lipoprotein cholesterol

**Use** Adjunct in management of primary hypercholesterolemia; regression of arterioloscle-rosis; relief of pruritus associated with elevated levels of bile acids; possibly used to decrease plasma half-life of digoxin in toxicity

**USUAL DOSAGE** Adults: Oral:
Granules: 5-30 g/day given once or in divided doses 2-4 times/day; initial dose: 5 g 1-2 times/day; increase by 5 g at 1- to 2-month intervals
Tablets: 2-16 g/day; initial dose: 2 g 1-2 times/day; increase by 2 g at 1- to 2-month intervals

**Dosage Forms** Colestipol hydrochloride: **Granules:** 5 g packet, 300 g, 500 g; **Tab:** 1 g

**Contraindications** Hypersensitivity to colestipol or any component; avoid using in complete biliary obstruction

**Warnings/Precautions** Avoid in patients with high triglycerides, GI dysfunction (constipation); may be associated with increased bleeding tendency as a result of hypothrombinemia secondary to vitamin K deficiency; may cause depletion of vitamins A, D, E

**Pregnancy Risk Factor** C

**Adverse Reactions**
>10%: Gastrointestinal: Constipation
1% to 10%: Gastrointestinal: Abdominal pain and distention, belching, flatulence, nausea, vomiting, diarrhea
<1%: Headache, dizziness, anxiety, vertigo, drowsiness, fatigue, dermatitis, urticaria, peptic ulceration, GI irritation and bleeding, anorexia, cholelithiasis, cholecystitis, arthralgia,

arthritis, weakness, shortness of breath, increased serum phosphorous and chloride with decrease of sodium and potassium

**Drug Interactions** Decreased absorption of tetracycline, penicillin G, vitamins A, D, E and K, digitalis glycosides, warfarin, thyroid hormones, thiazide diuretics, propranolol, phenobarbital, amiodarone, methotrexate, NSAIDs, gemfibrozil, ursodiol, aspirin, clindamycin, clofibrate, furosemide, glipizide, hydrocortisone, imipramine, methyldopa, niacin, phenytoin, phosphate, tolbutamide, and other drugs by binding to the drug in the intestine

**Special PA Issues**
**Patient Education:** Take with 38-45 oz of water or fruit juice. Rinse glass with small amount of water to ensure full dose is taken. Other medications should be taken 2 hours before or 2 hours after colestipol. You may experience constipation (increased exercise, increased dietary fluids, fruit, fiber, or stool softener may help) or drowsiness or dizziness (use caution when driving or engaging in tasks that require alertness until response is known). Report acute gastric pain, tarry stools, or difficulty breathing.

**Related Information**
Lipid-Lowering Agents *on page 1022*

♦ **Colestipol Hydrochloride** *see* Colestipol *on previous page*

# Colfosceril Palmitate (kole FOS er il PALM i tate)

**Pharmacologic Class** Lung Surfactant
**U.S. Brand Names** Exosurf® Neonatal
**Mechanism of Action** Replaces deficient or ineffective endogenous lung surfactant in neonates with respiratory distress syndrome (RDS) or in neonates at risk of developing RDS; reduces surface tension and stabilizes the alveoli from collapsing
**Use** Neonatal respiratory distress syndrome:
Prophylactic therapy: Body weight <1350 g in infants at risk for developing RDS; body weight >1350 g in infants with evidence of pulmonary immaturity
Rescue therapy: Treatment of infants with RDS based on respiratory distress not attributable to any other causes and chest radiographic findings consistent with RDS
**USUAL DOSAGE** For intratracheal use only. Neonates:
Prophylactic treatment: Administer 5 mL/kg (as two 2.5 mL/kg half-doses) as soon as possible; the second and third doses should be administered at 12 and 24 hours later to those infants remaining on ventilators
Rescue treatment: Administer 5 mL/kg (as two 2.5 mL/kg half-doses) as soon as the diagnosis of RDS is made; the second 5 mL/kg (as two 2.5 mL/kg half-doses) dose should be administered 12 hours later
**Dosage Forms Powder for inj, lyophilized:** 108 mg (10 mL)
**Warnings/Precautions** Pulmonary hemorrhaging may occur especially in infants <700 g. Mucous plugs may have formed in the endotracheal tube in those infants whose ventilation was markedly impaired during or shortly after dosing. If chest expansion improves substantially, the ventilator PIP setting should be reduced immediately. Hyperoxia and hypocarbia (hypocarbia can decrease blood flow to the brain) may occur requiring appropriate ventilator adjustments.
**Adverse Reactions** 1% to 10%: Respiratory: Pulmonary hemorrhage, apnea, mucous plugging, decrease in transcutaneous $O_2$ of >20%
**Special PA Issues**
**Monitoring Parameters:** Continuous EKG and transcutaneous $O_2$ saturation should be monitored during administration; frequent ABG sampling is necessary to prevent postdosing hyperoxia and hypocarbia

# Colistin, Neomycin, and Hydrocortisone
(koe LIS tin, nee oh MYE sin & hye droe KOR ti sone)
**Pharmacologic Class** Antibiotic/Corticosteroid, Otic
**U.S. Brand Names** Coly-Mycin® S Otic Drops; Cortisporin-TC® Otic
**Dosage Forms Susp, otic:** Colistin sulfate 0.3%, neomycin sulfate 0.47%, and hydrocortisone acetate 1% (5 mL, 10 mL)

♦ **Collagen** *see* Microfibrillar Collagen Hemostat *on page 605*

# Collagenase (KOL la je nase)

**Pharmacologic Class** Enzyme, Topical Debridement
**U.S. Brand Names** Biozyme-C®; Santyl®
**Mechanism of Action** Collagenase is an enzyme derived from the fermentation of *Clostridium histolyticum* and differs from other proteolytic enzymes in that its enzymatic action has a high specificity for native and denatured collagen. Collagenase will not attack collagen in healthy tissue or newly formed granulation tissue. In addition, it does not act on fat, fibrin, keratin, or muscle.
**Use** Promotes debridement of necrotic tissue in dermal ulcers and severe burns
**USUAL DOSAGE** Topical: Apply once daily (or more frequently if the dressing becomes soiled)
(Continued)

## Collagenase *(Continued)*

**Dosage Forms Oint, top:** 250 units/g (15 g, 30 g)

**Contraindications** Known hypersensitivity to collagenase

**Warnings/Precautions** For external use only; avoid contact with eyes; monitor debilitated patients for systemic bacterial infections because debriding enzymes may increase the risk of bacteremia

**Pregnancy Risk Factor** C

**Adverse Reactions**

1% to 10%: Local: Irritation

<1%: Pain and burning may occur at site of application

**Drug Interactions** Decreased effect: Enzymatic activity is inhibited by detergents, benzalkonium chloride, hexachlorophene, nitrofurazone, tincture of iodine, and heavy metal ions (silver and mercury)

**Special PA Issues**

**Patient Education:** Use exactly as directed; do not overuse. Wear gloves to apply a thin film to affected area. If dressing is necessary, use a porous dressing. Avoid contact with eyes. Report increased swelling, redness, rash, itching, signs of infection, worsening of condition, or lack of healing.

♦ **Colovage®** *see* Polyethylene Glycol-Electrolyte Solution *on page 736*
♦ **Coly-Mycin® S Otic Drops** *see* Colistin, Neomycin, and Hydrocortisone *on previous page*
♦ **Colyte®** *see* Polyethylene Glycol-Electrolyte Solution *on page 736*
♦ **Comb Flower** *see* Echinacea *on page 310*
♦ **Combipres®** *see* Clonidine and Chlorthalidone *on page 226*
♦ **Combivent®** *see* Ipratropium and Albuterol *on page 491*
♦ **Combivir®** *see* Zidovudine and Lamivudine *on page 973*
♦ **Comfort® [OTC]** *see* Naphazoline *on page 635*
♦ **Comhist®** *see* Chlorpheniramine, Phenylephrine, and Phenyltoloxamine *on page 196*
♦ **Comhist® LA** *see* Chlorpheniramine, Phenylephrine, and Phenyltoloxamine *on page 196*
♦ **Community Acquired Pneumonia in Adults** *see* Chart *on page 1057*
♦ **Compazine®** *see* Prochlorperazine *on page 763*
♦ **Comphor of the Poor** *see* Garlic *on page 410*
♦ **Compound E** *see* Cortisone Acetate *on next page*
♦ **Compound F** *see* Hydrocortisone *on page 453*
♦ **Compound S** *see* Zidovudine *on page 972*
♦ **Compoz® Gel Caps [OTC]** *see* Diphenhydramine *on page 289*
♦ **Compoz® Nighttime Sleep Aid [OTC]** *see* Diphenhydramine *on page 289*
♦ **Comvax™** *see* Haemophilus b Conjugate and Hepatitis b Vaccine *on page 431*
♦ **Congest** *see* Estrogens, Conjugated *on page 335*
♦ **Constant-T®** *see* Theophylline Salts *on page 888*
♦ **Constilac®** *see* Lactulose *on page 512*
♦ **Constipation, Treatment Options** *see* Chart *on page 1124*
♦ **Constulose®** *see* Lactulose *on page 512*
♦ **Contac® Cough Formula Liquid [OTC]** *see* Guaifenesin and Dextromethorphan *on page 428*
♦ **Control® [OTC]** *see* Phenylpropanolamine *on page 720*
♦ **Copaxone®** *see* Glatiramer Acetate *on page 415*
♦ **Cophene XP®** *see* Hydrocodone, Pseudoephedrine, and Guaifenesin *on page 453*
♦ **Copolymer-1** *see* Glatiramer Acetate *on page 415*
♦ **Coptin®** *see* Sulfadiazine *on page 859*
♦ **Coradur®** *see* Isosorbide Dinitrate *on page 498*
♦ **Corax®** *see* Chlordiazepoxide *on page 189*
♦ **Cordarone®** *see* Amiodarone *on page 55*
♦ **Cordran®** *see* Flurandrenolide *on page 390*
♦ **Cordran® SP** *see* Flurandrenolide *on page 390*
♦ **Coreg®** *see* Carvedilol *on page 156*
♦ **Corgard®** *see* Nadolol *on page 628*
♦ **Corque® Topical** *see* Clioquinol and Hydrocortisone *on page 219*
♦ **CortaGel® [OTC]** *see* Hydrocortisone *on page 453*
♦ **Cortaid® Maximum Strength [OTC]** *see* Hydrocortisone *on page 453*
♦ **Cortaid® With Aloe [OTC]** *see* Hydrocortisone *on page 453*
♦ **Cortatrigen® Otic** *see* Neomycin, Polymyxin B, and Hydrocortisone *on page 645*
♦ **Cort-Dome®** *see* Hydrocortisone *on page 453*
♦ **Cortef®** *see* Hydrocortisone *on page 453*
♦ **Cortef® Feminine Itch** *see* Hydrocortisone *on page 453*
♦ **Cortenema®** *see* Hydrocortisone *on page 453*

♦ **Corticaine®** **Topical** *see* Dibucaine and Hydrocortisone *on page 271*
♦ **Corticosteroids** *see* Chart *on page 1007*
♦ **Cortifoam®** *see* Hydrocortisone *on page 453*
♦ **Cortisol** *see* Hydrocortisone *on page 453*

# Cortisone Acetate (KOR ti sone AS e tate)

**Pharmacologic Class** Corticosteroid, Oral; Corticosteroid, Parenteral
**U.S. Brand Names** Cortone® Acetate
**Mechanism of Action** Decreases inflammation by suppression of migration of polymorpho-nuclear leukocytes and reversal of increased capillary permeability
**Use** Management of adrenocortical insufficiency
**USUAL DOSAGE** If possible, administer glucocorticoids before 9 AM to minimize adreno-cortical suppression; dosing depends upon the condition being treated and the response of the patient; supplemental doses may be warranted during times of stress in the course of withdrawing therapy

Children:
 Anti-inflammatory or immunosuppressive: Oral: 2.5-10 mg/kg/day **or** 20-300 mg/m²/day in divided doses every 6-8 hours
 Physiologic replacement: Oral: 0.5-0.75 mg/kg/day **or** 20-25 mg/m²/day in divided doses every 8 hours
Adults: Oral: 25-300 mg/day in divided doses every 12-24 hours
Hemodialysis: Supplemental dose is not necessary
Peritoneal dialysis: Supplemental dose is not necessary
**Dosage Forms Inj:** 50 mg/mL (10 mL); **Tab:** 5 mg, 10 mg, 25 mg
**Contraindications** Serious infections, except septic shock or tuberculous meningitis; administration of live virus vaccines
**Warnings/Precautions** Use with caution in patients with hypothyroidism, cirrhosis, hyper-tension, congestive heart failure, ulcerative colitis, thromboembolic disorders, osteoporosis, convulsive disorders, peptic ulcer, diabetes mellitus, myasthenia gravis; prolonged therapy (>5 days) of pharmacologic doses of corticosteroids may lead to hypothalamic-pituitary-adrenal suppression, the degree of adrenal suppression varies with the degree and duration of glucocorticoid therapy; this must be taken into consideration when taking patients off steroids
**Pregnancy Risk Factor** D
**Adverse Reactions**
>10%:
 Central nervous system: Insomnia, nervousness
 Gastrointestinal: Increased appetite, indigestion
1% to 10%:
 Dermatologic: Hirsutism
 Endocrine & metabolic: Diabetes mellitus
 Neuromuscular & skeletal: Arthralgia
 Ocular: Cataracts, glaucoma
 Respiratory: Epistaxis
<1%: Edema, hypertension, vertigo, seizures, headache, psychoses, pseudotumor cerebri, mood swings, delirium, hallucinations, euphoria, acne, skin atrophy, bruising, hyperpig-mentation, Cushing's syndrome, pituitary-adrenal axis suppression, growth suppression, glucose intolerance, hypokalemia, alkalosis, amenorrhea, sodium and water retention, hyperglycemia, peptic ulcer, nausea, vomiting, abdominal distention, ulcerative esopha-gitis, pancreatitis, myalgia, osteoporosis, fractures, muscle wasting, hypersensitivity reac-tions
**Drug Interactions** CYP3A3/4 enzyme substrate
Decreased effect:
 Barbiturates, phenytoin, rifampin may decrease cortisone effects
 Live virus vaccines, diuretics (potassium depleting)
 Anticholinesterase agents may decrease effect
 Cortisone may decrease warfarin effects
 Cortisone may decrease effects of salicylates
Increased effect: Estrogens (increase cortisone effects)
Increased toxicity:
 Cortisone + NSAIDs may increase ulcerogenic potential
 Cortisone may increase potassium deletion due to diuretics
**Onset** Peak effect: Oral: Within 2 hours; I.M.: Within 20-48 hours
**Half-Life** 30 minutes to 2 hours; End-stage renal disease: 3.5 hours
**Special PA Issues**
 **Patient Education:** Take oral formulation as directed, with food or milk in the morning. Do not take more than prescribed or discontinue without consulting prescriber. Maintain adequate nutritional intake; consult prescriber for possibility of special dietary instructions. If diabetic, monitor serum glucose closely and notify prescriber of any changes; this medication can alter hypoglycemic requirements. Inform prescriber if you are experi-encing unusual stress; dosage may need to be adjusted. You will be susceptible to
(Continued)

## Cortisone Acetate *(Continued)*

infection; avoid crowds or infected persons or persons with contagious diseases. You may experience insomnia or nervousness; use caution when driving or engaging in tasks requiring alertness until response to medication is known. Report excessive or sudden weight gain, swelling of extremities, difficulty breathing, muscle pain or weakness, change in menstrual pattern, vision changes, signs of hyperglycemia, signs of infection (eg, fever, chills, mouth sores, perianal itching, vaginal discharge), other persistent side effects, or worsening of condition.

**Related Information**
Corticosteroids *on page 1007*

♦ **Cortisporin® Ophthalmic Ointment** *see* Bacitracin, Neomycin, Polymyxin B, and Hydrocortisone *on page 97*

♦ **Cortisporin® Ophthalmic Suspension** *see* Neomycin, Polymyxin B, and Hydrocortisone *on page 645*

♦ **Cortisporin® Otic** *see* Neomycin, Polymyxin B, and Hydrocortisone *on page 645*

♦ **Cortisporin-TC® Otic** *see* Colistin, Neomycin, and Hydrocortisone *on page 235*

♦ **Cortisporin® Topical Cream** *see* Neomycin, Polymyxin B, and Hydrocortisone *on page 645*

♦ **Cortisporin® Topical Ointment** *see* Bacitracin, Neomycin, Polymyxin B, and Hydrocortisone *on page 97*

♦ **Cortizone®-5 [OTC]** *see* Hydrocortisone *on page 453*

♦ **Cortizone®-10 [OTC]** *see* Hydrocortisone *on page 453*

♦ **Cortone® Acetate** *see* Cortisone Acetate *on previous page*

♦ **Cortrosyn®** *see* Cosyntropin *on this page*

♦ **Corvert®** *see* Ibutilide *on page 467*

♦ **Coryphen® Codeine** *see* Aspirin and Codeine *on page 82*

## Cosyntropin *(koe sin TROE pin)*

**Pharmacologic Class** Diagnostic Agent, Adrenocortical Insufficiency

**U.S. Brand Names** Cortrosyn®

**Mechanism of Action** Stimulates the adrenal cortex to secrete adrenal steroids (including hydrocortisone, cortisone), androgenic substances, and a small amount of aldosterone

**Use** Diagnostic test to differentiate primary adrenal from secondary (pituitary) adrenocortical insufficiency

**USUAL DOSAGE**
Adrenocortical insufficiency: I.M., I.V. (over 2 minutes): Peak plasma cortisol concentrations usually occur 45-60 minutes after cosyntropin administration
Neonates: 0.015 mg/kg/dose
Children <2 years: 0.125 mg
Children >2 years and Adults: 0.25-0.75 mg
When greater cortisol stimulation is needed, an I.V. infusion may be used:
Children >2 years and Adults: 0.25 mg administered at 0.04 mg/hour over 6 hours
Congenital adrenal hyperplasia evaluation: 1 mg/m²/dose up to a maximum of 1 mg

**Dosage Forms** Powder for inj: 0.25 mg

**Contraindications** Known hypersensitivity to cosyntropin

**Warnings/Precautions** Use with caution in patients with pre-existing allergic disease or a history of allergic reactions to corticotropin

**Pregnancy Risk Factor** C

**Adverse Reactions**
1% to 10%:
Cardiovascular: Flushing
Central nervous system: Mild fever
Dermatologic: Pruritus
Gastrointestinal: Chronic pancreatitis
<1%: Hypersensitivity reactions

**Special PA Issues**
**Reference Range:** Normal baseline cortisol; increase in serum cortisol after cosyntropin injection of >7 µg/dL or peak response >18 µg/dL; plasma cortisol concentrations should be measured immediately before and exactly 30 minutes after a dose

♦ **Cotazym®** *see* Pancrelipase *on page 694*

♦ **Cotazym-S®** *see* Pancrelipase *on page 694*

♦ **Cotrim®** *see* Co-Trimoxazole *on this page*

♦ **Cotrim® DS** *see* Co-Trimoxazole *on this page*

## Co-Trimoxazole *(koe trye MOKS a zole)*

**Pharmacologic Class** Antibiotic, Sulfonamide Derivative

**U.S. Brand Names** Bactrim™; Bactrim™ DS; Cotrim®; Cotrim® DS; Septra®; Septra® DS; Sulfatrim®

**Mechanism of Action** Sulfamethoxazole interferes with bacterial folic acid synthesis and growth via inhibition of dihydrofolic acid formation from para-aminobenzoic acid; trimethoprim inhibits dihydrofolic acid reduction to tetrahydrofolate resulting in sequential inhibition of enzymes of the folic acid pathway

**Use**

Oral treatment of urinary tract infections due to *E. coli*, *Klebsiella* and *Enterobacter* sp, *M. morganii*, *P. mirabilis* and *P. vulgaris*; acute otitis media in children and acute exacerbations of chronic bronchitis in adults due to susceptible strains of *H. influenzae* or *S. pneumoniae*; prophylaxis of *Pneumocystis carinii* pneumonitis (PCP), traveler's diarrhea due to enterotoxigenic *E. coli* or *Cyclospora*

I.V. treatment or severe or complicated infections when oral therapy is not feasible, for documented PCP, empiric treatment of PCP in immune compromised patients; treatment of documented or suspected shigellosis, typhoid fever, *Nocardia asteroides* infection, or other infections caused by susceptible bacteria

**Unlabeled use:** Cholera and salmonella-type infections and nocardiosis; chronic prostatitis; as prophylaxis in neutropenic patients with *P. carinii* infections, in leukemics, and in patients following renal transplantation, to decrease incidence of gram-negative rod infections

**USUAL DOSAGE** Dosage recommendations are based on the trimethoprim component

Children >2 months:

Mild to moderate infections: Oral, I.V.: 8 mg TMP/kg/day in divided doses every 12 hours

Serious infection/*Pneumocystis*: I.V.: 20 mg TMP/kg/day in divided doses every 6 hours

Urinary tract infection prophylaxis: Oral: 2 mg TMP/kg/dose daily

Prophylaxis of *Pneumocystis*: Oral, I.V.: 10 mg TMP/kg/day or 150 mg TMP/m²/day in divided doses every 12 hours for 3 days/week; dose should not exceed 320 mg trimethoprim and 1600 mg sulfamethoxazole 3 days/week

Adults:

Urinary tract infection/chronic bronchitis: Oral: 1 double strength tablet every 12 hours for 10-14 days

Sepsis: I.V.: 20 TMP/kg/day divided every 6 hours

*Pneumocystis carinii*:

Prophylaxis: Oral: 1 double strength tablet daily or 3 times/week

Treatment: Oral, I.V.: 15-20 mg TMP/kg/day in 3-4 divided doses

**Dosing adjustment in renal impairment:** Adults:

I.V.:

$Cl_{cr}$ 15-30 mL/minute: Administer 2.5-5 mg/kg every 12 hours

$Cl_{cr}$ <15 mL/minute: Administer 2.5-5 mg/kg every 24 hours

Oral:

$Cl_{cr}$ 15-30 mL/minute: Administer 1 double strength tablet every 24 hours or 1 single strength tablet every 12 hours

$Cl_{cr}$ <15 mL/minute: Not recommended

**Dosage Forms** The 5:1 ratio (SMX to TMP) remains constant in all dosage forms: **Inj:** Sulfamethoxazole 80 mg and trimethoprim 16 mg per mL (5 mL, 10 mL, 20 mL, 30 mL, 50 mL); **Susp, oral:** Sulfamethoxazole 200 mg and trimethoprim 40 mg per 5 mL (20 mL, 100 mL, 150 mL, 200 mL, 480 mL); **Tab:** Sulfamethoxazole 400 mg and trimethoprim 80 mg, **Double strength:** Sulfamethoxazole 800 mg and trimethoprim 160 mg

**Contraindications** Hypersensitivity to any sulfa drug or any component; porphyria; megaloblastic anemia due to folate deficiency; infants <2 months of age; marked hepatic damage

**Warnings/Precautions** Use with caution in patients with G-6-PD deficiency, impaired renal or hepatic function; maintain adequate hydration to prevent crystalluria; adjust dosage in patients with renal impairment. Injection vehicle contains benzyl alcohol and sodium metabisulfite. Fatalities associated with severe reactions including Stevens-Johnson syndrome, toxic epidermal necrolysis, hepatic necrosis, agranulocytosis, aplastic anemia and other blood dyscrasias; discontinue use at first sign of rash. Elderly patients appear at greater risk for more severe adverse reactions. May cause hypoglycemia, particularly in malnourished, or patients with renal or hepatic impairment. Use with caution in patients with porphyria or thyroid dysfunction. Slow acetylators may be more prone to adverse reactions.

**Pregnancy Risk Factor** C

**Pregnancy Implications** Do not use at term to avoid kernicterus in the newborn and use during pregnancy only if risks outweigh the benefits since folic acid metabolism may be affected

**Adverse Reactions**

>10%:

Dermatologic: Allergic skin reactions including rashes and urticaria, photosensitivity

Gastrointestinal: Nausea, vomiting, anorexia

1% to 10%:

Dermatologic: Stevens-Johnson syndrome, toxic epidermal necrolysis (rare)

Hematologic: Blood dyscrasias

Hepatic: Hepatitis

(Continued)

239

## Co-Trimoxazole *(Continued)*

<1%: Confusion, depression, hallucinations, seizures, fever, ataxia, kernicterus in neonates, erythema multiforme, stomatitis, diarrhea, pseudomembranous colitis, pancytopenia, pancreatitis, rhabdomyolysis, thrombocytopenia, megaloblastic anemia, granulocytopenia, aplastic anemia, hemolysis (with G-6-PD deficiency), cholestatic jaundice, interstitial nephritis, serum sickness

**Drug Interactions** CYP2C9 enzyme inhibitor

Decreased effect: Cyclosporines

Increased effect/toxicity: Phenytoin, cyclosporines (nephrotoxicity), methotrexate (displaced from binding sites), dapsone, sulfonylureas, and oral anticoagulants; may compete for renal secretion of methotrexate; digoxin concentrations increased

**Half-Life** SMX: 9 hours; TMP: 6-17 hours, both are prolonged in renal failure

**Special PA Issues**

**Patient Education:** Take oral medication with 8 oz of water on an empty stomach (1 hour before or 2 hours after meals) for best absorption. Finish all medication; do not skip doses. You may experience increased sensitivity to sunlight; use sunblock, wear protective clothing and dark glasses, or avoid direct exposure to sunlight. Small frequent meals, frequent mouth care, or sucking on lozenges may reduce nausea or vomiting. Report skin rash, sore throat, or unusual bruising or bleeding immediately.

## Cromolyn Sodium *(KROE moe lin SOW dee um)*

**Pharmacologic Class** Antihistamine, Inhalation; Mast Cell Stabilizer

**U.S. Brand Names** Crolom® Ophthalmic Solution; Gastrocrom® Oral; Intal® Nebulizer Solution; Intal® Oral Inhaler; Nasalcrom® Nasal Solution

**Mechanism of Action** Prevents the mast cell release of histamine, leukotrienes and slow-reacting substance of anaphylaxis by inhibiting degranulation after contact with antigens

**Use** Adjunct in the prophylaxis of allergic disorders, including rhinitis, giant papillary conjunctivitis, and asthma; inhalation product may be used for prevention of exercise-induced bronchospasm; systemic mastocytosis, food allergy, and treatment of inflammatory bowel disease; **cromolyn is a prophylactic drug with no benefit for acute situations**

**USUAL DOSAGE**

Oral:

Systemic mastocytosis:

Neonates and preterm Infants: Not recommended

Infants and Children <2 years: 20 mg/kg/day in 4 divided doses; may increase in patients 6 months to 2 years of age if benefits not seen after 2-3 weeks; do not exceed 30 mg/kg/day

Children 2-12 years: 100 mg 4 times/day; not to exceed 40 mg/kg/day

Children >12 years and Adults: 200 mg 4 times/day

Food allergy and inflammatory bowel disease:

Children <2 years: Not recommended

Children 2-12 years: Initial dose: 100 mg 4 times/day; may double the dose if effect is not satisfactory within 2-3 weeks; not to exceed 40 mg/kg/day

Children >12 years and Adults: Initial dose: 200 mg 4 times/day; may double the dose if effect is not satisfactory within 2-3 weeks; up to 400 mg 4 times/day

Once desired effect is achieved, dose may be tapered to lowest effective dose

Inhalation:

For chronic control of asthma, taper frequency to the lowest effective dose (ie, 4 times/day to 3 times/day to twice daily):

Nebulization solution: Children >2 years and Adults: Initial: 20 mg 4 times/day; usual dose: 20 mg 3-4 times/day

Metered spray:
- Children 5-12 years: Initial: 2 inhalations 4 times/day; usual dose: 1-2 inhalations 3-4 times/day
- Children ≥12 years and Adults: Initial: 2 inhalations 4 times/day; usual dose: 2-4 inhalations 3-4 times/day

Prevention of allergen- or exercise-induced bronchospasm: Administer 10-15 minutes prior to exercise or allergen exposure but no longer than 1 hour before:
- Nebulization solution: Children >2 years and Adults: Single dose of 20 mg
- Metered spray: Children >5 years and Adults: Single dose of 2 inhalations

**Dosage Forms Inh, oral (Intal®):** 800 mcg/spray (8.1 g); **Soln:** For nebulization: 10 mg/mL (2 mL), Intal®: 10 mg/mL (2 mL); **Soln, as sodium, oral (Gastrocrom®):** 100 mg/5 mL; **Nasal (Nasalcrom®):** 40 mg/mL (13 mL); **Ophth (Crolom®):** 4% (2.5 mL, 10 mL)

**Contraindications** Hypersensitivity to cromolyn or any component; acute asthma attacks

**Warnings/Precautions** Severe anaphylactic reactions may occur rarely; cromolyn is a prophylactic drug with no benefit for acute situations; do not use in patients with severe renal or hepatic impairment; caution should be used when withdrawing the drug or tapering the dose as symptoms may reoccur; use with caution in patients with a history of cardiac arrhythmias

**Pregnancy Risk Factor** B

**Pregnancy Implications**
Clinical effects on the fetus: No data on whether cromolyn crosses the placenta or clinical effects on the fetus. Available evidence suggests safe use during pregnancy.

Breast-feeding/lactation: No data on whether cromolyn crosses into breast milk or clinical effects on the infant

**Adverse Reactions**
>10%:
- Gastrointestinal: Unpleasant taste (inhalation aerosol)
- Respiratory: Hoarseness, coughing

1% to 10%:
- Dermatologic: Angioedema
- Gastrointestinal: Xerostomia
- Genitourinary: Dysuria
- Respiratory: Sneezing, nasal congestion

<1%: Dizziness, headache, rash, urticaria, nausea, vomiting, diarrhea, arthralgia, ocular stinging, lacrimation, wheezing, throat irritation, eosinophilic pneumonia, pulmonary infiltrates, nasal burning, anaphylactic reactions

**Half-Life** 80-90 minutes

**Special PA Issues**
Patient Education: Oral: Use as directed; do not increase dosage or discontinue abruptly without consulting prescriber. You may experience dizziness or nervousness (use caution when driving or engaging in hazardous tasks until response to medication is known); diarrhea (boiled milk, yogurt, or buttermilk may help); or headache or muscle pain (mild analgesic may offer relief). Report persistent insomnia; skin rash or irritation; abdominal pain or difficulty swallowing; unusual cough, bronchospasm, or difficulty breathing; decreased urination; or if condition worsens or fails to improve.

Nebulizer: Store nebulizer solution away from light. Prepare nebulizer according to package instructions. Clear as much mucus as possible before use. Rinse mouth following each use to prevent opportunistic infection and reduce unpleasant aftertaste. Report if symptoms worsen or condition fails to improve.

Nasal: Instill 1 spray into each nostril 3-4 times a day. You may experience unpleasant taste (rinsing mouth and frequent oral care may help); or headache (mild analgesic may help). Report increased sneezing, burning, stinging, or irritation inside of nose; sore throat, hoarseness, nosebleed; anaphylactic reaction (skin rash, fever, chills, backache, difficulty breathing, chest pain); or worsening of condition or lack of improvement.

Ophthalmic: For ophthalmic use only. Wash hands before using. Tilt head back and look upward. Put drops of suspension or apply thin ribbon of ointment inside lower eyelid. Close eye and roll eyeball in all directions. Do not blink for 30 seconds. Apply gentle pressure to inner corner of eye for 30 seconds. Do not use any other eye preparation for at least 10 minutes. Do not let tip of applicator touch eye or contaminate tip of applicator. Do not share medication with anyone else. Temporary stinging or blurred vision may occur. Inform prescriber if condition worsens or fails to improve or if you experience eye pain, redness, burning, watering, dryness, double vision, puffiness around eye, vision disturbances, or other adverse eye response; or worsening of condition or lack of improvement.

Monitoring Parameters: Periodic pulmonary function tests

# Crotamiton (kroe TAM i tonn)
**Pharmacologic Class** Scabicidal Agent
**U.S. Brand Names** Eurax® Topical
**Mechanism of Action** Crotamiton has scabicidal activity against *Sarcoptes scabiei*; mechanism of action unknown
(Continued)

# Crotamiton (Continued)

**Use** Treatment of scabies (*Sarcoptes scabiei*) and symptomatic treatment of pruritus
**USUAL DOSAGE** Topical:
Scabicide: Children and Adults: Wash thoroughly and scrub away loose scales, then towel dry; apply a thin layer and massage drug onto skin of the entire body from the neck to the toes (with special attention to skin folds, creases, and interdigital spaces). Repeat application in 24 hours. Take a cleansing bath 48 hours after the final application. Treatment may be repeated after 7-10 days if live mites are still present.
Pruritus: Massage into affected areas until medication is completely absorbed; repeat as necessary
**Dosage Forms Cream:** 10% (60 g); **Lotion:** 10% (60 mL, 454 mL)
**Contraindications** Hypersensitivity to crotamiton or other components; patients who manifest a primary irritation response to topical medications
**Warnings/Precautions** Avoid contact with face, eyes, mucous membranes, and urethral meatus; do not apply to acutely inflamed or raw skin; for external use only
**Pregnancy Risk Factor** C
**Adverse Reactions** <1%: Local irritation, pruritus, contact dermatitis, warm sensation
**Special PA Issues**
Patient Education: For topical use only. Apply lotion to whole body from the chin down being sure to cover all skin folds and creases. Apply a second application 24 hours later. Avoid eyes. Take a bath 48 hours after application. All contaminated clothing and bed linen should be washed to avoid reinfestation. If cure is not achieved after 2 doses, use alternative therapy.

- ◆ **Crystalline Penicillin** *see* Penicillin G, Parenteral, Aqueous *on page 705*
- ◆ **Crystal Violet** *see* Gentian Violet *on page 413*
- ◆ **Crystamine®** *see* Cyanocobalamin *on this page*
- ◆ **Crysti 1000®** *see* Cyanocobalamin *on this page*
- ◆ **Crysticillin® A.S.** *see* Penicillin G Procaine *on page 706*
- ◆ **Crystodigin®** *see* Digitoxin *on page 280*
- ◆ **CsA** *see* Cyclosporine *on page 245*
- ◆ **C/T/S® Topical Solution** *see* Clindamycin *on page 218*
- ◆ **Cuprimine®** *see* Penicillamine *on page 702*
- ◆ **Curretab®** *see* Medroxyprogesterone Acetate *on page 561*
- ◆ **Cutivate™** *see* Fluticasone *on page 393*
- ◆ **CyA** *see* Cyclosporine *on page 245*

# Cyanocobalamin (sye an oh koe BAL a min)

**Pharmacologic Class** Vitamin, Water Soluble
**U.S. Brand Names** Berubigen®; Cobex®; Crystamine®; Crysti 1000®; Cyanoject®; Cyomin®; Ener-B® [OTC]; Kaybovite-1000®; Nascobal®; Redisol®; Rubramin-PC®; Sytobex®
**Mechanism of Action** Coenzyme for various metabolic functions, including fat and carbohydrate metabolism and protein synthesis, used in cell replication and hematopoiesis
**Use** Treatment of pernicious anemia; vitamin $B_{12}$ deficiency; increased $B_{12}$ requirements due to pregnancy, thyrotoxicosis, hemorrhage, malignancy, liver or kidney disease
**USUAL DOSAGE**
Recommended daily allowance (RDA):
Children: 0.3-2 mcg
Adults: 2 mcg
Nutritional deficiency: Oral: 25-250 mcg/day
Anemias: I.M. or deep S.C. (oral is not generally recommended due to poor absorption and I.V. is not recommended due to more rapid elimination):
Pernicious anemia, congenital (if evidence of neurologic involvement): 1000 mcg/day for at least 2 weeks; maintenance: 50-100 mcg/month or 100 mcg for 6-7 days; if there is clinical improvement, give 100 mcg every other day for 7 doses, then every 3-4 days for 2-3 weeks; follow with 100 mcg/month for life. Administer with folic acid if needed.
Children: 30-50 mcg/day for 2 or more weeks (to a total dose of 1000-5000 mcg), then follow with 100 mcg/month as maintenance dosage
Adults: 100 mcg/day for 6-7 days; if improvement, administer same dose on alternate days for 7 doses; then every 3-4 days for 2-3 weeks; once hematologic values have returned to normal, maintenance dosage: 100 mcg/month. **Note:** Use only parenteral therapy as oral therapy is not dependable.
Vitamin $B_{12}$ deficiency:
Children:
Neurologic signs: 100 mcg/day for 10-15 days (total dose of 1-1.5 mg), then once or twice weekly for several months; may taper to 60 mcg every month
Hematologic signs: 10-50 mcg/day for 5-10 days, followed by 100-250 mcg/dose every 2-4 weeks
Adults: Initial: 30 mcg/day for 5-10 days; maintenance: 100-200 mcg/month
Schilling test: I.M.: 1000 mcg

**Dosage Forms Gel, nasal:** Ener-B®: 400 mcg/0.1 mL, Nascobal®: 500 mcg/0.1 mL (5 mL);
**Inj:** 30 mcg/mL (30 mL), 100 mcg/mL (1 mL, 10 mL, 30 mL), 1000 mcg/mL (1 mL, 10 mL, 30 mL); **Tab [OTC]:** 25 mcg, 50 mcg, 100 mcg, 250 mcg, 500 mcg, 1000 mcg

**Contraindications** Hypersensitivity to cyanocobalamin or any component, cobalt; patients with hereditary optic nerve atrophy

**Warnings/Precautions** I.M. route used to treat pernicious anemia; vitamin $B_{12}$ deficiency for >3 months results in irreversible degenerative CNS lesions; treatment of vitamin $B_{12}$ megaloblastic anemia may result in severe hypokalemia, sometimes, fatal, when anemia corrects due to cellular potassium requirements. $B_{12}$ deficiency masks signs of polycythemia vera; vegetarian diets may result in $B_{12}$ deficiency; pernicious anemia occurs more often in gastric carcinoma than in general population.

**Pregnancy Risk Factor** A (C if dose exceeds RDA recommendation)

**Adverse Reactions**
1% to 10%:
  Dermatologic: Itching
  Gastrointestinal: Diarrhea
<1%: Peripheral vascular thrombosis, urticaria, anaphylaxis

**Special PA Issues**
  **Patient Education:** Use exactly as directed. Pernicious anemia may require monthly injections for life. Report skin rash; swelling, pain, or redness of extremities; or acute persistent diarrhea.
  **Monitoring Parameters:** Serum potassium, erythrocyte and reticulocyte count, hemoglobin, hematocrit
  **Reference Range:** Normal range of serum $B_{12}$ is 150-750 pg/mL; this represents 0.1% of total body content. Metabolic requirements are 2-5 μg/day; years of deficiency required before hematologic and neurologic signs and symptoms are seen. Occasional patients with significant neuropsychiatric abnormalities may have no hematologic abnormalities and normal serum cobalamin levels, 200 pg/mL (SI: >150 pmol/L), or more commonly between 100-200 pg/mL (SI: 75-150 pmol/L). There exists evidence that people, particularly elderly whose serum cobalamin concentrations <300 pg/mL, should receive replacement parenteral therapy; this recommendation is based upon neuropsychiatric disorders and cardiovascular disorders associated with lower sodium cobalamin concentrations.

♦ **Cyanoject®** see Cyanocobalamin *on previous page*
♦ **Cyclen®** see Ethinyl Estradiol and Norgestimate *on page 350*

# Cyclobenzaprine (sye kloe BEN za preen)

**Pharmacologic Class** Skeletal Muscle Relaxant
**U.S. Brand Names** Flexeril®
**Mechanism of Action** Centrally acting skeletal muscle relaxant pharmacologically related to tricyclic antidepressants; reduces tonic somatic motor activity influencing both alpha and gamma motor neurons
**Use** Treatment of muscle spasm associated with acute painful musculoskeletal conditions; supportive therapy in tetanus
**USUAL DOSAGE** Oral: **Note:** Do not use longer than 2-3 weeks
  Children: Dosage has not been established
  Adults: 20-40 mg/day in 2-4 divided doses; maximum dose: 60 mg/day
**Dosage Forms Tab, as hydrochloride:** 10 mg
**Contraindications** Hypersensitivity to cyclobenzaprine or any component; do not use concomitantly or within 14 days of MAO inhibitors; hyperthyroidism, congestive heart failure, arrhythmias
**Warnings/Precautions** Cyclobenzaprine shares the toxic potentials of the tricyclic antidepressants and the usual precautions of tricyclic antidepressant therapy should be observed; use with caution in patients with urinary hesitancy or angle-closure glaucoma
**Pregnancy Risk Factor** B
**Adverse Reactions**
>10%:
  Central nervous system: Drowsiness, dizziness, lightheadedness
  Gastrointestinal: Xerostomia
1% to 10%:
  Cardiovascular: Edema of the face/lips, syncope
  Gastrointestinal: Bloated feeling
  Genitourinary: Problems in urinating, polyuria
  Hepatic: Hepatitis
  Neuromuscular & skeletal: Problems in speaking, muscle weakness
  Ocular: Blurred vision
  Otic: Tinnitus
<1%: Tachycardia, hypotension, arrhythmia, headache, fatigue, nervousness, confusion, ataxia, rash, dermatitis, dyspepsia, nausea, constipation, stomach cramps, unpleasant taste
**Drug Interactions** CYP1A2, 2D6 and 3A3/4 enzyme substrate
(Continued)

## Cyclobenzaprine *(Continued)*

Increased toxicity:

Do not use concomitantly or within 14 days after MAO inhibitors

Because of similarities to the tricyclic antidepressants, may have additive toxicities

Anticholinergics: Because of cyclobenzaprine's anticholinergic action, use with caution in patients receiving these agents

Alcohol, barbiturates, and other CNS depressants: Effects may be enhanced by cyclobenzaprine

**Onset** Commonly occurs within 1 hour

**Duration** 8 to >24 hours

**Half-Life** 1-3 days

**Special PA Issues**

**Patient Education:** Take exactly as directed. Do not increase dose or discontinue without consulting prescriber. Do not use alcohol, prescriptive or OTC antidepressants, sedatives, or pain medications without consulting prescriber. You may experience drowsiness, dizziness, lightheadedness (avoid driving or engaging in tasks that require alertness until response to therapy is known); or urinary retention (void before taking medication). Report excessive drowsiness or mental agitation, chest pain, skin rash, swelling of mouth/face, difficulty speaking, ringing in ears, or blurred vision.

- ♦ **Cyclobenzaprine Hydrochloride** *see* Cyclobenzaprine *on previous page*
- ♦ **Cyclocort®** *see* Amcinonide *on page 50*
- ♦ **Cyclogyl®** *see* Cyclopentolate *on this page*
- ♦ **Cyclomen®** *see* Danazol *on page 253*
- ♦ **Cyclomydril® Ophthalmic** *see* Cyclopentolate and Phenylephrine *on this page*

## Cyclopentolate *(sye kloe PEN toe late)*

**Pharmacologic Class** Anticholinergic Agent, Ophthalmic; Ophthalmic Agent, Mydriatic

**U.S. Brand Names** AK-Pentolate®; Cyclogyl®; I-Pentolate®

**Mechanism of Action** Prevents the muscle of the ciliary body and the sphincter muscle of the iris from responding to cholinergic stimulation, causing mydriasis and cycloplegia

**Use** Diagnostic procedures requiring mydriasis and cycloplegia

**USUAL DOSAGE**

Infants: Instill 1 drop of 0.5% into each eye 5-10 minutes before examination

Children: Instill 1 drop of 0.5%, 1%, or 2% in eye followed by 1 drop of 0.5% or 1% in 5 minutes, if necessary

Adults: Instill 1 drop of 1% followed by another drop in 5 minutes; 2% solution in heavily pigmented iris

**Dosage Forms Soln, ophth, as hydrochloride:** 0.5% (2 mL, 5 mL, 15 mL), 1% (2 mL, 5 mL, 15 mL), 2% (2 mL, 5 mL, 15 mL)

**Contraindications** Narrow-angle glaucoma, known hypersensitivity to drug

**Warnings/Precautions** 2% solution may result in psychotic reactions and behavioral disturbances in children, usually occurring approximately 30-45 minutes after instillation; use with caution in elderly patients and other patients who may be predisposed to increased intraocular pressure

**Pregnancy Risk Factor** C

**Adverse Reactions** 1% to 10%:

Cardiovascular: Tachycardia

Central nervous system: Restlessness, hallucinations, psychosis, hyperactivity, seizures, incoherent speech, ataxia

Dermatologic: Burning sensation

Ocular: Increase in intraocular pressure, loss of visual accommodation

Miscellaneous: Allergic reaction

**Drug Interactions** Decreased effect of carbachol, cholinesterase inhibitors

**Special PA Issues**

**Patient Education:** May cause blurred vision and increased sensitivity to light

## Cyclopentolate and Phenylephrine *(sye kloe PEN toe late & fen il EF rin)*

**Pharmacologic Class** Anticholinergic/Adrenergic Agonist

**U.S. Brand Names** Cyclomydril® Ophthalmic

**Dosage Forms Soln, ophth:** Cyclopentolate hydrochloride 0.2% and phenylephrine hydrochloride 1% (2 mL, 5 mL)

- ♦ **Cyclopentolate Hydrochloride** *see* Cyclopentolate *on this page*

## Cycloserine *(sye kloe SER een)*

**Pharmacologic Class** Antibiotic, Miscellaneous; Antitubercular Agent

**U.S. Brand Names** Seromycin® Pulvules®

**Mechanism of Action** Inhibits bacterial cell wall synthesis by competing with amino acid (D-alanine) for incorporation into the bacterial cell wall; bacteriostatic or bactericidal

**Use** Adjunctive treatment in pulmonary or extrapulmonary tuberculosis; has been studied for use in Gaucher's disease

**USUAL DOSAGE** Some of the neurotoxic effects may be relieved or prevented by the concomitant administration of pyridoxine

Tuberculosis: Oral:
Children: 10-20 mg/kg/day in 2 divided doses up to 1000 mg/day for 18-24 months
Adults: Initial: 250 mg every 12 hours for 14 days, then administer 500 mg to 1 g/day in 2 divided doses for 18-24 months (maximum daily dose: 1 g)

**Dosing interval in renal impairment:**
$Cl_{cr}$ 10-50 mL/minute: Administer every 24 hours
$Cl_{cr}$ <10 mL/minute: Administer every 36-48 hours

**Dosage Forms Capsule:** 250 mg

**Contraindications** Known hypersensitivity to cycloserine

**Warnings/Precautions** Epilepsy, depression, severe anxiety, psychosis, severe renal insufficiency, chronic alcoholism

**Pregnancy Risk Factor** C

**Adverse Reactions** Percentage unknown: Cardiac arrhythmias, drowsiness, headache, dizziness, vertigo, seizures, confusion, psychosis, paresis, coma, rash, folate deficiency, elevated liver enzymes, tremor, vitamin $B_{12}$ deficiency

**Drug Interactions** Increased toxicity: Alcohol, isoniazid, ethionamide increase toxicity of cycloserine; cycloserine inhibits the hepatic metabolism of phenytoin

**Half-Life** 10 hours in patients with normal renal function

**Special PA Issues**
**Patient Education:** Take as directed (may be taken with food); do not skip doses. Avoid alcohol and maintain adequate hydration (2-3 L/day of fluids unless instructed to restrict fluid intake). Dietary requirements for vitamin $B_{12}$ and folic acid may be increased; consult prescriber. May cause drowsiness; use caution with tasks that require alertness. Report skin rash, acute headache, tremors, changes in mentation (acute confusion or suicidal ideation), changes in behavior, respiratory difficulty, or unusual swelling of extremities.
**Monitoring Parameters:** Periodic renal, hepatic, hematological tests, and plasma cyclo-serine concentrations
**Reference Range:** Toxicity is greatly increased at levels >30 µg/mL

♦ **Cyclosporin A** see Cyclosporine on this page

# Cyclosporine (SYE kloe spor een)

**Pharmacologic Class** Immunosuppressant Agent

**U.S. Brand Names** Neoral® Oral; Sandimmune® Injection; Sandimmune® Oral; Sang® CyA

**Mechanism of Action** Inhibition of production and release of interleukin II and inhibits interleukin II-induced activation of resting T-lymphocytes

**Use** Immunosuppressant which may be used with azathioprine and/or corticosteroids to prolong organ and patient survival in kidney, liver, heart, and bone marrow transplants; severe psoriasis; also used in some cases of severe autoimmune disease that are resistant to corticosteroids and other therapy.

**USUAL DOSAGE** Children and Adults (oral dosage is ~3 times the I.V. dosage); dosage should be based on ideal body weight:

I.V.:
Initial: 5-6 mg/kg/day beginning 4-12 hours prior to organ transplantation; patients should be switched to oral cyclosporine as soon as possible; dose should be infused over 2-24 hours
Maintenance: 2-10 mg/kg/day in divided doses every 8-12 hours; dose should be adjusted to maintain whole blood FPIA trough concentrations in the reference range
Oral: Solution or soft gelatin capsule (Sandimmune®):
Initial: 14-18 mg/kg/day, beginning 4-12 hours prior to organ transplantation

### Cyclosporine

| Condition | Cyclosporine |
| --- | --- |
| Switch from I.V. to oral therapy | Threefold increase in dose |
| T-tube clamping | Decrease dose; increase availability of bile facilitates absorption of CsA |
| Pediatric patients | About 2-3 times higher dose compared to adults |
| Liver dysfunction | Decrease I.V. dose; increase oral dose |
| Renal dysfunction | Decrease dose to decrease levels if renal dysfunction is related to the drug |
| Dialysis | Not removed |
| Inhibitors of hepatic metabolism | Decrease dose |
| Inducers of hepatic metabolism | Monitor drug level; may need to increase dose |

(Continued)

# Cyclosporine (Continued)

Maintenance: 5-15 mg/kg/day divided every 12-24 hours; maintenance dose is usually tapered to 3-10 mg/kg/day

Focal segmental glomerulosclerosis: Initial: 3 mg/kg/day divided every 12 hours

Autoimmune diseases: 1-3 mg/kg/day

Dosing considerations of cyclosporine, see table.

Oral: **Solution or soft gelatin capsule in a microemulsion (Neoral®):** Based on the organ transplant population:

Initial: Same as the initial dose for solution or soft gelatin capsule (listed above) **or**

Renal: 9 mg/kg/day (range: 6-12 mg/kg/day)

Liver: 8 mg/kg/day (range: 4-12 mg/kg/day)

Heart: 7 mg/kg/day (range: 4-10 mg/kg/day)

**Note:** A 1:1 ratio conversion from Sandimmune® to Neoral® has been recommended initially; however, lower doses of Neoral® may be required after conversion to prevent overdose. Total daily doses should be adjusted based on the cyclosporine trough blood concentration and clinical assessment of organ rejection. CsA blood trough levels should be determined prior to conversion. After conversion to Neoral®, CsA trough levels should be monitored every 4-7 days. **Neoral® and Sandimmune® are not bioequivalent and cannot be used interchangeably.**

Hemodialysis: Supplemental dose is not necessary

Peritoneal dialysis: Supplemental dose is not necessary

**Dosing adjustment in hepatic impairment:** Probably necessary, monitor levels closely

**Dosing adjustment recommendations for renal impairment during cyclosporine therapy for severe psoriasis:**

**Serum creatinine levels ≥25% above pretreatment levels:** Take another sample within 2 weeks. If the level remains ≥25% above pretreatment levels, decrease dosage of cyclosporine microemulsion by 25% to 50%. If 2 dosage adjustments do not reverse the increase in serum creatinine levels, treatment should be discontinued.

**Serum creatinine ≥50% above pretreatment levels:** Decrease cyclosporine dosage by 25% to 50%. If 2 dosage adjustments do not reverse the increase in serum creatinine levels, treatment should be discontinued.

**Note:** Increase the frequency of blood pressure monitoring after each alteration in dosage of cyclosporine. Cyclosporine dosage should be decreased by 25% to 50% in patients with no history of hypertension who develop sustained hypertension during therapy and, if hypertension persists, treatment with cyclosporine should be discontinued.

**Dosage Forms Cap (Sandimmune®):** 25 mg, 100 mg, **Soft gel (Sandimmune®):** 50 mg, **Soft gel for microemulsion (Neoral®):** 25 mg, 100 mg; **Inj (Sandimmune®):** 50 mg/mL (5 mL); **Soln: Oral (Sandimmune®):** 100 mg/mL (50 mL), **Oral for microemulsion (Neoral®):** 100 mg/mL (50 mL)

## Contraindications

Hypersensitivity to cyclosporine, Cremaphor EL® (I.V. solution), or any other I.V. component (ie, polyoxyl 35 castor oil is an ingredient of the parenteral formulation and polyoxyl 40 hydrogenated castor oil is an ingredient of the cyclosporine capsules and solution for microemulsion)

Use in severe psoriasis therapy: Concomitant treatment of cyclosporine with other psoriasis treatments such as psoralens + ultraviolet A (UVA) light PUVA, UVB therapy, other radiation therapy or other immunosuppressive agents may result in excessive immuno-suppression and increased risk of malignancies. Concomitant treatment of cyclosporine with methotrexate or coal tar. The risk of skin malignancies is increased in patients who have previously been treated with these other psoriasis therapies prior to cyclosporine therapy.

**Warnings/Precautions** Infection and possible development of lymphoma may result. Make dose adjustments to avoid toxicity or possible organ rejection using cyclosporine blood levels because absorption is erratic and elimination is highly variable. Adjustment of dose should only be made under the direct supervision of an experienced physician; reserve the use of I.V. for use only in patients who cannot take oral; adequate airway and other supportive measures and agents for treating anaphylaxis should be present when I.V. drug is given. Nephrotoxic, if possible avoid concomitant use of other potentially nephrotoxic drugs (eg, acyclovir, aminoglycoside antibiotics, amphotericin B, ciprofloxacin). Can cause systemic hypertension or nephrotoxicity when used with other psoriasis therapies.

**Pregnancy Risk Factor** C

**Pregnancy Implications** Clinical effects on the fetus: Based on small numbers of patients, the use of cyclosporine during pregnancy apparently does not pose a major risk to the fetus

**Adverse Reactions**

>10%:

Cardiovascular: Hypertension

Dermatologic: Hirsutism

Gastrointestinal: Gingival hypertrophy

Neuromuscular & skeletal: Tremor

Renal: Nephrotoxicity

1% to 10%:
    Central nervous system: Seizure, headache
    Dermatologic: Acne
    Gastrointestinal: Abdominal discomfort, nausea, vomiting
    Neuromuscular & skeletal: Leg cramps
<1%: Hypotension, tachycardia, warmth, flushing, hyperkalemia, hypomagnesemia, hyper-uricemia, pancreatitis, hepatotoxicity, myositis, paresthesias, respiratory distress, sinus-itis, anaphylaxis, increased susceptibility to infection, and sensitivity to temperature extremes

**Drug Interactions** CYP3A3/4 enzyme substrate
    Decreased effect: Drugs that decrease cyclosporine concentrations: Carbamazepine, phenobarbital, phenytoin, rifampin, isoniazid
    Increased toxicity:
        Drugs that increase cyclosporine concentrations: Azithromycin, clarithromycin, diltiazem, erythromycin, fluconazole, itraconazole, ketoconazole, nicardipine, verapamil, grape-fruit juice
        Drugs that enhance nephrotoxicity of cyclosporine: Aminoglycosides, amphotericin B, acyclovir
        Lovastatin - myositis, myalgias, rhabdomyolysis, acute renal failure
        Nifedipine - increases risk of gingival hyperplasia

**Half-Life**
    Solution or soft gelatin capsule (Sandimmune®): Biphasic, alpha phase: 1.4 hours and terminal phase 6-24 hours
    Solution or soft gelatin capsule in a microemulsion (Neoral®): 8.4 hours

**Special PA Issues**
    **Patient Education:** Use glass container for liquid solution (do not use plastic or styrofoam cup). Mixing with milk, chocolate milk, or orange juice at room temperature improves flavor. Mix thoroughly and drink at once. Take dose at same time each day. You will be susceptible to infection; avoid crowds and exposure to any infectious diseases. Do not have any vaccinations without consulting prescriber. Practice good oral hygiene to reduce gum inflammation; see dentist regularly during treatment. Report acute headache; unusual hair growth or deepening of voice; mouth sores or swollen gums; persistent nausea, vomiting, or abdominal pain; muscle pain or cramping; unusual swelling of extremities, weight gain, or change in urination; or chest pain or rapid heartbeat.

    **Monitoring Parameters:**
    Cyclosporine trough levels, serum electrolytes, renal function, hepatic function, blood pressure, serum cholesterol
    Psoriasis therapy: Biweekly monitoring of blood pressure, complete blood count, and levels of BUN, uric acid, potassium, lipids and magnesium during the first three months of treatment for psoriasis. Monthly monitoring is recommended after this initial period.

    **Reference Range:** Reference ranges are method dependent and specimen dependent; use the same analytical method consistently; trough levels should be obtained immedi-ately prior to next dose
    **Method-dependent and specimen-dependent**
    Trough levels should be obtained:
        Oral: 12-18 hours after dose (chronic usage)
        I.V.: 12 hours after dose **or** immediately prior to next dose
    **Therapeutic range: Not absolutely defined, dependent on organ transplanted, time after transplant, organ function and CsA toxicity**
    General range of 100-400 ng/mL
    Toxic level: Not well defined, nephrotoxicity may occur at any level

♦ **Cycofed® Pediatric** see Guaifenesin, Pseudoephedrine, and Codeine on page 429
♦ **Cycrin®** see Medroxyprogesterone Acetate on page 561
♦ **Cylert®** see Pemoline on page 701
♦ **Cylex® [OTC]** see Benzocaine on page 105
♦ **Cyomin®** see Cyanocobalamin on page 242

# Cyproheptadine (si proe HEP ta deen)

**Pharmacologic Class** Antihistamine
**U.S. Brand Names** Periactin®
**Mechanism of Action** A potent antihistamine and serotonin antagonist, competes with histamine for $H_1$-receptor sites on effector cells in the gastrointestinal tract, blood vessels, and respiratory tract
**Use** Perennial and seasonal allergic rhinitis and other allergic symptoms including urticaria
    **Unlabeled use:** Appetite stimulation, blepharospasm, cluster headaches, migraine head-aches, Nelson's syndrome, pruritus, schizophrenia, spinal cord damage associated spas-ticity, and tardive dyskinesia
**USUAL DOSAGE** Oral:
    Children: 0.25 mg/kg/day in 2-3 divided doses or 8 mg/m²/day in 2-3 divided doses
        2-6 years: 2 mg every 8-12 hours (not to exceed 12 mg/day)
        7-14 years: 4 mg every 8-12 hours (not to exceed 16 mg/day)
(Continued)

## Cyproheptadine *(Continued)*

Adults: 4-20 mg/day divided every 8 hours (not to exceed 0.5 mg/kg/day)

**Dosing adjustment in hepatic impairment:** Dosage should be reduced in patients with significant hepatic dysfunction

**Dosage Forms** Cyproheptadine hydrochloride: **Syr:** 2 mg/5 mL with alcohol 5% (473 mL); **Tab:** 4 mg

**Contraindications** Hypersensitivity to cyproheptadine or any component; narrow-angle glaucoma, bladder neck obstruction, acute asthmatic attack, stenosing peptic ulcer, GI tract obstruction, those on MAO inhibitors; avoid use in premature and term newborns due to potential association with SIDS

**Warnings/Precautions** Do not use in neonates, safety and efficacy have not been established in children <2 years of age; symptomatic prostate hypertrophy; antihistamines are more likely to cause dizziness, excessive sedation, syncope, toxic confusion states, and hypotension in the elderly. In case reports, cyproheptadine has promoted weight gain in anorexic adults, though it has not been specifically studied in the elderly. All cases of weight loss or decreased appetite should be adequately assessed.

**Pregnancy Risk Factor** B

**Adverse Reactions**

>10%:
Central nervous system: Slight to moderate drowsiness
Respiratory: Thickening of bronchial secretions

1% to 10%:
Central nervous system: Headache, fatigue, nervousness, dizziness
Gastrointestinal: Appetite stimulation, nausea, diarrhea, abdominal pain, xerostomia
Neuromuscular & skeletal: Arthralgia
Respiratory: Pharyngitis

<1%: Tachycardia, palpitations, edema, sedation, CNS stimulation, seizures, depression, photosensitivity, rash, angioedema, hemolytic anemia, leukopenia, thrombocytopenia, hepatitis, myalgia, paresthesia, bronchospasm, epistaxis, allergic reactions

**Drug Interactions** Increased toxicity: MAO inhibitors → hallucinations

**Special PA Issues**

**Patient Education:** Take as directed; do not exceed recommended dose. Avoid use of other depressants, alcohol, or sleep-inducing medications unless approved by prescriber. You may experience drowsiness or dizziness (use caution when driving or engaging in hazardous activity until response to medication is known); or dry mouth, nausea, or abdominal pain (frequent small meals, frequent mouth care, chewing gum, or sucking hard candy may help). Report persistent sedation, confusion, or agitation; changes in urinary pattern; blurred vision; chest pain or palpitations; sore throat difficulty breathing or expectorating (thick secretions); or lack of improvement or worsening of condition.

**Dietary Considerations:** Alcohol: Additive CNS effects, avoid use

♦ **Cyproheptadine Hydrochloride** *see* Cyproheptadine *on previous page*

♦ **Cystagon®** *see* Cysteamine *on this page*

## Cysteamine *(sis TEE a meen)*

**Pharmacologic Class** Anticystine Agent; Urinary Tract Product

**U.S. Brand Names** Cystagon®

**Mechanism of Action** Reacts with cystine in the lysosome to convert it to cysteine and to a cysteine-cysteamine mixed disulfide, both of which can then exit the lysosome in patients with cystinosis, an inherited defect of lysosomal transport

**Use Orphan drug:** Management of nephropathic cystinosis

**USUAL DOSAGE** Initiate therapy with $1/4$ to $1/8$ of maintenance dose; titrate slowly upward over 4-6 weeks

Children <12 years: Oral: Maintenance: 1.3 g/m²/day divided into 4 doses
Children >12 years and Adults (>110 lbs): 2 g/day in 4 divided doses; dosage may be increased to 1.95 g/m²/day if cystine levels are <1 nmol/$1/2$ cystine/mg protein, although intolerance and incidence of adverse events may be increased

**Dosage Forms Cap, as bitartrate:** 50 mg, 150 mg

**Contraindications** Hypersensitivity to cysteamine or penicillamine

**Warnings/Precautions** Withhold cysteamine if a mild rash develops; restart at a lower dose and titrate to therapeutic dose; adjust cysteamine dose if CNS symptoms due to the drug develop, rather than the disease; adjust cysteamine dose downward if severe GI symptoms develop (most common during initiation of therapy)

**Pregnancy Risk Factor** C

**Pregnancy Implications**

Clinical effects on the fetus: Use only when the potential benefits outweigh the potential hazards to the fetus; in animal studies, cysteamine reduced the fertility of rats and offspring survival at very large doses

Breast-feeding/lactation: It is unknown whether cysteamine is excreted in breast milk; discontinue nursing or discontinue drug during lactation

**Adverse Reactions**
>5%:
Gastrointestinal: Vomiting (35%), anorexia (31%), diarrhea (16%)
Central nervous system: Fever, lethargy (11%)
Dermatologic: Rash (7%)
<5%:
Cardiovascular: Hypertension
Central nervous system: Somnolence, encephalopathy, headache, seizures, ataxia, confusion, dizziness, jitteriness, nervousness, impaired cognition, emotional changes, hallucinations, nightmares
Dermatologic: Urticaria
Endocrine & metabolic: Dehydration
Gastrointestinal: Bad breath, abdominal pain, dyspepsia, constipation, gastroenteritis, duodenitis, duodenal ulceration
Hematologic: Anemia, leukopenia
Hepatic: Abnormal LFTs
Neuromuscular & skeletal: Tremor, hyperkinesia
Otic: Decreased hearing

**Special PA Issues**
**Patient Education:** Take as directed. Maintain adequate hydration (2-3 L/day of fluids unless instructed to restrict fluid intake). It may be necessary to include other medication in treatment regimen. Periodic blood tests will need to be performed. You may experience dizziness, confusion, or lethargy; use caution with tasks that require alertness until response to drug is known. Report fever, gastric disturbances, or rash.
**Monitoring Parameters:** Blood counts and LFTs during therapy; monitor leukocyte cystine measurements every 3 months to determine adequate dosage and compliance (measure 5-6 hours after administration); monitor more frequently when switching salt forms
**Reference Range:** Leukocyte cystine: <1 nmol/$\frac{1}{2}$ cystine/mg protein

- ◆ **Cysteamine Bitartrate** *see* Cysteamine *on previous page*
- ◆ **Cystospaz®** *see* Hyoscyamine *on page 463*
- ◆ **Cystospaz-M®** *see* Hyoscyamine *on page 463*
- ◆ **Cytadren®** *see* Aminoglutethimide *on page 53*
- ◆ **Cytochrome P-450 and Drug Interactions** *see* Chart *on page 1009*
- ◆ **CytoGam™** *see* Cytomegalovirus Immune Globulin (Intravenous-Human) *on this page*

# Cytomegalovirus Immune Globulin (Intravenous-Human)
(sye toe meg a low VYE rus i MYUN GLOB yoo lin in tra VEE nus HYU man)
**Pharmacologic Class** Immune Globulin
**U.S. Brand Names** CytoGam™
**Mechanism of Action** CMV-IGIV is a preparation of immunoglobulin G derived from pooled healthy blood donors with a high titer of CMV antibodies; administration provides a passive source of antibodies against cytomegalovirus
**Use** Attenuation of primary CMV disease associated with immunosuppressed recipients of kidney transplantation; especially indicated for CMV-negative recipients of CMV-positive donor; has been used as adjunct therapy in the treatment of CMV disease in immunocompromised patients
**USUAL DOSAGE** I.V.:
Dosing schedule:
Initial dose (within 72 hours after transplant): 150 mg/kg/dose
2, 4, 6, 8 weeks after transplant: 100 mg/kg/dose
12 and 16 weeks after transplant: 50 mg/kg/dose
Severe CMV pneumonia: Regimens of 400 mg/kg on days 1, 2, 7 or 8, followed by 200 mg/kg have been used

Administration rate: Administer at 15 mg/kg/hour initially, then increase to 30 mg/kg/hour after 30 minutes if no untoward reactions, then increase to 60 mg/kg/hour after another 30 minutes; volume not to exceed 75 mL/hour
**Dosage Forms** Powder for inj, lyophilized, detergent treated: 2500 mg ±250 mg (50 mL)
**Contraindications** Hypersensitivity to any component, patients with selective immunoglobulin A deficiency (↑ potential for anaphylaxis); persons with IgA deficiency
**Warnings/Precautions** Studies indicate that product carries little or no risk for transmission of HIV; give with caution to patients with prior allergic reactions to human immunoglobulin preparations; do not perform skin testing
**Pregnancy Risk Factor** C
**Adverse Reactions**
1% to 10%:
Cardiovascular: Flushing of face
Gastrointestinal: Nausea, vomiting
Neuromuscular & skeletal: Muscle cramps, back pain
Respiratory: Wheezing
(Continued)

## Cytomegalovirus Immune Globulin (Intravenous-Human)
### (Continued)

Miscellaneous: Diaphoresis

<1%: Tightness in the chest, dizziness, fever, headache, chills, aseptic meningitis syndrome, hypersensitivity reactions

**Drug Interactions** May inactivate live virus vaccines (eg, measles, mumps, rubella); if IGIV administration within 3 months of vaccination with live virus products, revaccinate

**Special PA Issues**

**Patient Education:** This medication can only be administered by infusion. You will be monitored closely during the infusion. If you experience nausea ask for assistance, do not get up alone. Do not have any vaccination for the next 3 months without consulting prescriber. Immediately report chills, muscle cramping, low back pain, chest pain or tightness, or difficulty breathing.

♦ **Cytotec®** *see* Misoprostol *on page 612*
♦ **Cytovene®** *see* Ganciclovir *on page 408*
♦ **D-3-Mercaptovaline** *see* Penicillamine *on page 702*
♦ **d4T** *see* Stavudine *on page 851*

## Dacliximab (da KLIK si mab)

**Pharmacologic Class** Immunosuppressant Agent

**U.S. Brand Names** Zenapax®

**Mechanism of Action** Inhibits the binding of IL-2 to the high affinity IL-2 receptor, thus suppressing T cell activity against allografts. Its active ingredient, dacliximab, a humanized monoclonal antibody, binds to the alpha subunit of the high affinity interleukin-2 receptor (IL-2R) which is expressed on activated T cells.

**Use** Prophylaxis of acute organ rejection in patients receiving renal transplants; used as part of an immunosuppressive regimen that includes cyclosporine and corticosteroids

**USUAL DOSAGE** Children and Adults: IVPB: 1 mg/kg, used as part of an immunosuppressive regimen that includes cyclosporine and corticosteroids for a total of 5 doses; give the first dose ≤24 hours before transplantation. The 4 remaining doses should be administered at intervals of 14 days.

**Dosing adjustment in renal impairment:** None necessary

**Dosage Forms Inj:** 5 mg/mL (5 mL)

**Contraindications** Hypersensitivity to any component of the product

**Warnings/Precautions** Only physicians experienced in immunosuppressive therapy and management of organ transplant patients should prescribe dacliximab. Manage patients receiving the drug in facilities equipped and staffed with adequate laboratory and supportive medical resources. Readministration of dacliximab after an initial course of therapy has not been studied in humans. The potential risks of such readministration, specifically those associated with immunosuppression or the occurrence of anaphylaxis/anaphylactoid reactions, are not known.

**Adverse Reactions**

>10%: Endocrine & metabolic: Hyperglycemia (32%)

1% to 10%:

Cardiovascular: Peripheral edema, hypertension, hypotension, aggravated hypertension, tachycardia, thrombosis, bleeding, chest pain

Central nervous system: Headache, dizziness, prickly sensation, depression, anxiety, fever, fatigue, insomnia, shivering, generalized weakness

Dermatologic: Impaired wound healing without infection, acne, pruritus, hirsutism, rash

Endocrine & metabolic: Fluid overload, diabetes mellitus, dehydration, edema

Gastrointestinal: Constipation, nausea, diarrhea, vomiting, abdominal pain, pyrosis, dyspepsia, abdominal distention, epigastric pain (not food-related), flatulence, gastritis, hemorrhoids

Genitourinary: Dysuria, urinary tract disorder, urinary retention

Hematologic: Urinary tract bleeding

Local: Injection site pain

Neuromuscular & skeletal: Tremor, musculoskeletal pain, back pain, arthralgia, leg cramps, myalgia, pain

Ocular: Blurred vision

Renal: Oliguria, renal tubular necrosis, renal damage, hydronephrosis, renal insufficiency

Respiratory: Dyspnea, pulmonary edema, coughing, atelectasis, congestion, rhinitis, pharyngitis, hypoxia, rales, abnormal breath sounds, pleural effusion

Miscellaneous: Increased diaphoresis, night sweats, post-traumatic pain

♦ **D.A.II® Tablet** *see* Chlorpheniramine, Phenylephrine, and Methscopolamine *on page 196*
♦ **Dakin's Solution** *see* Sodium Hypochlorite Solution *on page 842*
♦ **Dalacin® C [Hydrochloride]** *see* Clindamycin *on page 218*
♦ **Dalalone L.A.®** *see* Dexamethasone *on page 264*
♦ **Dallergy®** *see* Chlorpheniramine, Phenylephrine, and Methscopolamine *on page 196*
♦ **Dallergy-D® Syrup** *see* Chlorpheniramine and Phenylephrine *on page 195*

♦ **Dalmane®** *see* Flurazepam *on page 390*

♦ **d-Alpha Tocopherol** *see* Vitamin E *on page 963*

# Dalteparin (dal TE pa rin)

**Pharmacologic Class** Low Molecular Weight Heparin

**U.S. Brand Names** Fragmin®

**Mechanism of Action** Low molecular weight heparin analog with a molecular weight of 4000-6000 daltons; the commercial product contains 3% to 15% heparin with a molecular weight <3000 daltons, 65% to 78% with a molecular weight of 3000-8000 daltons and 14% to 26% with a molecular weight >8000 daltons; while dalteparin has been shown to inhibit both factor Xa and factor IIa (thrombin), the antithrombotic effect of dalteparin is characterized by a higher ratio of antifactor Xa to antifactor IIa activity (ratio = 4)

**Use** Prevention of deep vein thrombosis which may lead to pulmonary embolism, in patients requiring hip arthroplasty or abdominal surgery who are at risk for thromboembolism complications (ie, patients >40 years of age, obese, patients with malignancy, history of deep vein thrombosis or pulmonary embolism, and surgical procedures requiring general anesthesia and lasting longer than 30 minutes)

**USUAL DOSAGE** Adults: S.C.:

Low-moderate risk patients undergoing abdominal surgery: 2500 units 1-2 hours prior to surgery, then once daily for 5-10 days postoperatively

High risk patients undergoing abdominal surgery: 5000 units 1-2 hours prior to surgery and then once daily for 5-10 days postoperatively

Patients undergoing total hip surgery: 2500 units 1-2 hours prior to surgery, then 2500 units 6 hours after surgery (evening of the day of surgery), followed by 5000 units once daily for 7-10 days

**Dosage Forms Inj:** Prefilled syringe: 2500 units (16 mg) in 0.2 mL

**Contraindications** Hypersensitivity to dalteparin or other low-molecular weight heparins; cerebrovascular disease or other active hemorrhage; cerebral aneurysm; severe uncontrolled hypertension

**Warnings/Precautions** Use with caution in patients with pre-existing thrombocytopenia, recent childbirth, subacute bacterial endocarditis, peptic ulcer disease, pericarditis or pericardial effusion, liver or renal function impairment, recent lumbar puncture, vasculitis, concurrent use of aspirin (increased bleeding risk), previous hypersensitivity to heparin, heparin-associated thrombocytopenia. Patients should be observed closely for bleeding if dalteparin is administered during or immediately following diagnostic lumbar puncture, epidural anesthesia, or spinal anesthesia. If thromboembolism develops despite dalteparin prophylaxis, dalteparin should be discontinued and appropriate treatment should be initiated.

**Pregnancy Risk Factor** B

**Adverse Reactions** 1% to 10%:

Central nervous system: Allergic fever

Dermatologic: Pruritus, rash, bullous eruption, skin necrosis

Hematologic: Bleeding, thrombocytopenia, wound hematoma

Local: Pain at injection site, injection site hematoma, injection site reactions

Miscellaneous: Anaphylactoid reactions, allergic reactions

**Drug Interactions** Increased toxicity: Caution should be used when using aspirin, other platelet inhibitors, and oral anticoagulants in combination with dalteparin due to an increased risk of bleeding

**Onset** 1-2 hours

**Duration** >12 hours

**Special PA Issues**

**Patient Education:** To avoid injury while on this drug, brush teeth with soft brush and floss with waxed floss, use electric razor, and avoid scissors and sharp knives or potentially harmful activities. Report any unusual bleeding or bruising, bleeding gums, nosebleed, blood in urine, black or tarry stools, petechiae, back pain, or severe head pain.

**Monitoring Parameters:** Periodic CBC including platelet count; stool occult blood tests; monitoring of PT and PTT is not necessary

♦ **Damason-P®** *see* Hydrocodone and Aspirin *on page 450*

# Danaparoid (da NAP a roid)

**Pharmacologic Class** Anticoagulant

**U.S. Brand Names** Orgaran®

**Use** Prevention of postoperative deep vein thrombosis following elective hip replacement surgery

**Unlabeled use:** System anticoagulation for patients with heparin-induced thrombocytopenia: Factor Xa inhibition is used to monitor degree of anticoagulation if necessary

**USUAL DOSAGE** S.C.:

Children: Safety and effectiveness have not been established

Adults: 750 anti-Xa units twice daily; beginning 1-4 hours before surgery and then not sooner than 2 hours after surgery and every 12 hours until the risk of DVT has diminished, the average duration of therapy is 7-10 days

(Continued)

# Danaparoid *(Continued)*

Treatment: See table.

### Adult Danaparoid Treatment Dosing Regimens

| | Body Weight (kg) | I.V. Bolus aFXaU | Long–Term Infusion aFXaU | Level of aFXaU/mL | Monitoring |
|---|---|---|---|---|---|
| Deep Vein Thrombosis OR Acute Pulmonary Embolism | <55 | 1250 | 400 units/h over 4 h then 300 units/h over 4 h, then 150-200 units/h maintenance dose | 0.5-0.8 | Days 1-3 daily, then every alternate day |
| | 55-90 | 2500 | | | |
| | >90 | 3750 | | | |
| Deep Vein Thrombosis OR Pulmonary Embolism >5 d old | <90 | 1250 | S.C.: 3 x 750/d | <0.5 | Not necessary |
| | >90 | 1250 | S.C.: 3 x 1250/d | | |
| Embolectomy | <90 | 2500 preoperatively | S.C.: 2 x 1250/d postoperatively | <0.4 | Not necessary |
| | >90 and high risk | 2500 preoperatively | 750 units/20 mL NaCl perioperatively, arterial irrigation if necessary | 0.5-0.8 | Days 1-3 daily, then every alternate day |
| Peripheral Arterial Bypass | | 2500 preoperatively | 150-200 units/h | 0.5-0.8 | Days 1-3 daily, then every alternate day |
| Cardiac Catheter | <90 | 2500 preoperatively | | | |
| | >90 | 3750 preoperatively | | | |
| Surgery (excluding vascular) | | | S.C.: 750, 1-4 h preoperatively | <0.35 | Not necessary |
| | | | S.C.: 750, 2-5 h postoperatively, then 2 x 750/d | | |

**Dosing adjustment in elderly and severe renal impairment:** Adjustment may be necessary; patients with serum creatinine levels ≥2.0 mg/dL should be carefully monitored
Hemodialysis: See table

### Haemodialysis With Danaparoid Sodium

| Dialysis on alternate days | Dosage prior to dialysis in aFXaU (dosage for body wt <55 kg) | |
|---|---|---|
| First dialysis | 3750 (2500) | |
| Second dialysis | 3750 (2000) | |
| **Further dialysis:** | | |
| aFXa level before dialysis (eg, day 5) | Bolus before next dialysis, aFXaU (eg, day 7) | aFXa level during dialysis |
| <0.3 | 3000 (<55 kg 2000) | 0.5-0.8 |
| 0.3-0.35 | 2500 (2000) | |
| 0.35-0.4 | 2000 (1500) | |
| >0.4 | 0 | |
| | if fibrin strands occur, 1500 aFXaU I.V. | |
| Monitoring: 30 minutes before dialysis and after 4 hours of dialysis | | |
| **Daily Dialysis** | | |
| First dialysis | 3750 (2500) | |
| Second dialysis | 2500 (2000) | |
| Further dialyses | See above | |
| As with "dialysis on alternate days", always take the aFXa activity preceding the previous dialysis as a basis for the current dosage. | | |

**Dosage Forms** Inj, as sodium: 750 anti-Xa units/0.6 mL

**Contraindications** Patients with severe hemorrhagic diathesis including active major bleeding, hemorrhagic stroke in the acute phase, hemophilia and idiopathic thrombocytopenic purpura; type II thrombocytopenia associated with a positive *in vitro* test for antiplatelet antibody in the presence of danaparoid, hypersensitivity to danaparoid or known hypersensitivity to pork products

**Warnings/Precautions** Do not administer intramuscularly; use with extreme caution in patients with a history of bacterial endocarditis, hemorrhagic stroke, recent CNS or ophthalmological surgery, bleeding diathesis, uncontrolled arterial hypertension, or a history of recent gastrointestinal ulceration and hemorrhage. Danaparoid shows a low cross-sensitivity with antiplatelet antibodies in individuals with type II heparin-induced thrombocytopenia. This product contains sodium sulfite which may cause allergic-type reactions, including anaphylactic symptoms and life-threatening asthmatic episodes in susceptible people; this is seen more frequently in asthmatics.

Carefully monitor patients receiving low molecular weight heparins or heparinoids. These drugs, when used concurrently with spinal or epidural anesthesia or spinal puncture, may cause bleeding or hematomas within the spinal column. Increased pressure on the spinal cord may result in permanent paralysis if not detected and treated immediately.

**Note:** Danaparoid is **not** effectively antagonized by protamine sulfate. No other antidote is available, so extreme caution is needed in monitoring dose given and resulting Xa inhibition effect.

**Pregnancy Risk Factor** B

**Adverse Reactions** 1% to 10%:

Cardiovascular: Peripheral edema, generalized edema

Central nervous system: Fever, insomnia, headache, dizziness

Dermatologic: Rash, pruritus

Gastrointestinal: Nausea, constipation, vomiting

Genitourinary: Urinary tract infections, urinary retention

Hematologic: Anemia, hemorrhage, hematoma

Local: Injection site pain

Neuromuscular & skeletal: Joint disorder, weakness

**Drug Interactions** Increased toxicity with oral anticoagulants, platelet inhibitors

**Onset** Maximum antifactor Xa and antithrombin (antifactor IIa) activities occur 2-5 hours after S.C. administration

**Half-Life** Plasma: Mean terminal half-life: ~24 hours

**Special PA Issues**

**Patient Education:** This medication is given to reduce formation of unwanted venous thrombi. Use caution shaving (use safety razor), with needles or scissors (use blunt end scissors). Brush teeth with soft toothbrush and use precautions against injury. Report bleeding gums; blood in urine or stool; severe abdominal cramping; swelling of extremities; rash, itching, or burning in peri area or with urination; pain, cramping, or unusual weakness in joints or muscles; severe nausea or vomiting or diarrhea; heat, pain, or pain in calves or respiratory difficulty.

**Monitoring Parameters:** Platelets, occult blood, and anti-Xa activity, if available; the monitoring of PT and/or PTT is not necessary

♦ **Danaparoid Sodium** *see* Danaparoid *on page 251*

# Danazol (DA na zole)

**Pharmacologic Class** Androgen

**U.S. Brand Names** Danocrine®

**Mechanism of Action** Suppresses pituitary output of follicle-stimulating hormone and luteinizing hormone that causes regression and atrophy of normal and ectopic endometrial tissue; decreases rate of growth of abnormal breast tissue; reduces attacks associated with hereditary angioedema by increasing levels of C4 component of complement

**Use** Treatment of endometriosis, fibrocystic breast disease, and hereditary angioedema

**USUAL DOSAGE** Adults: Oral:

Female: Endometriosis: Initial: 200-400 mg/day in 2 divided doses for mild disease; individualize dosage. Usual maintenance dose: 800 mg/day in 2 divided doses to achieve amenorrhea and rapid response to painful symptoms. Continue therapy uninterrupted for 3-6 months (up to 9 months).

Female: Fibrocystic breast disease: Range: 10-400 mg/day in 2 divided doses

Male/Female: Hereditary angioedema: Initial: 200 mg 2-3 times/day; after favorable response, decrease the dosage by 50% or less at intervals of 1-3 months or longer if the frequency of attacks dictates. If an attack occurs, increase the dosage by up to 200 mg/day.

**Dosage Forms** Cap: 50 mg, 100 mg, 200 mg

**Contraindications** Undiagnosed genital bleeding, hypersensitivity to danazol or any component; pregnancy

(Continued)

## Danazol *(Continued)*

**Warnings/Precautions** Use with caution in patients with seizure disorders, migraine, or conditions influenced by edema; impaired hepatic, renal, or cardiac disease, pregnancy, lactation

**Pregnancy Risk Factor** X

**Adverse Reactions**

>10%:
  Cardiovascular: Edema
  Dermatologic: Oily skin, acne, hirsutism
  Endocrine & metabolic: Fluid retention, breakthrough bleeding, irregular menstrual periods, decreased breast size
  Gastrointestinal: Weight gain
  Hepatic: Hepatic impairment
  Miscellaneous: Voice deepening

1% to 10%:
  Endocrine & metabolic: Virilization, androgenic effects, amenorrhea, hypoestrogenism
  Neuromuscular & skeletal: Weakness

<1%: Benign intracranial hypertension, dizziness, headache, skin rashes, photosensitivity, pancreatitis, bleeding gums, monilial vaginitis, testicular atrophy, enlarged clitoris, cholestatic jaundice, carpal tunnel syndrome

**Drug Interactions** CYP3A3/4 enzyme inhibitor

Increased toxicity: Decreased insulin requirements; warfarin may increase anticoagulant effects

**Onset** Within 4 weeks following daily doses

**Half-Life** 4.5 hours (variable)

**Special PA Issues**

Patient Education: Take as directed; do not stop without consulting prescriber. Therapy for endometriosis usually requires 3-6 months and may exceed 9 months. Relief of pain and tenderness in fibrocystic breast disease usually occurs within 1 month and is eliminated in 2-3 months. Elimination of nodules usually takes 4-6 months.

Hereditary angioedema: Initial response may require 1-3 months and dosage may be decreased at 1-3 month intervals. Amenorrhea is expected with higher doses; menstruation should resume within 2-3 months after therapy is completed. Female: Report menstrual irregularities or masculinity (ie, facial hair, deepening of voice). Male: Report persistent penile erections. All patients should report persistent GI distress, diarrhea, jaundice, fever, and easy bruising. Male/female: Perform self breast exam regularly during therapy and report any changes or nodules in breast.

♦ **Danocrine®** *see Danazol on previous page*
♦ **Dantrium®** *see Dantrolene on this page*

## Dantrolene *(DAN troe leen)*

**Pharmacologic Class** Skeletal Muscle Relaxant

**U.S. Brand Names** Dantrium®

**Mechanism of Action** Acts directly on skeletal muscle by interfering with release of calcium ion from the sarcoplasmic reticulum; prevents or reduces the increase in myoplasmic calcium ion concentration that activates the acute catabolic processes associated with malignant hyperthermia

**Use** Treatment of spasticity associated with spinal cord injury, stroke, cerebral palsy, or multiple sclerosis; also used as treatment of malignant hyperthermia

**USUAL DOSAGE**

Spasticity: Oral:
  Children: Initial: 0.5 mg/kg/dose twice daily, increase frequency to 3-4 times/day at 4- to 7-day intervals, then increase dose by 0.5 mg/kg to a maximum of 3 mg/kg/dose 2-4 times/day up to 400 mg/day
  Adults: 25 mg/day to start, increase frequency to 2-4 times/day, then increase dose by 25 mg every 4-7 days to a maximum of 100 mg 2-4 times/day or 400 mg/day

Malignant hyperthermia: Children and Adults:
  Oral: 4-8 mg/kg/day in 4 divided doses
    Preoperative prophylaxis: Begin 1-2 days prior to surgery with last dose 3-4 hours prior to surgery
  I.V.: 1 mg/kg; may repeat dose up to cumulative dose of 10 mg/kg (mean effective dose is 2.5 mg/kg), then switch to oral dosage
    Preoperative: 2.5 mg/kg ~1¼ hours prior to anesthesia and infused over 1 hour with additional doses as needed and individualized

**Dosage Forms Cap:** 25 mg, 50 mg, 100 mg; **Powder for Inj:** 20 mg

**Contraindications** Active hepatic disease; should not be used where spasticity is used to maintain posture or balance

**Warnings/Precautions** Use with caution in patients with impaired cardiac function or impaired pulmonary function; has potential for hepatotoxicity; overt hepatitis has been most frequently observed between the third and twelfth month of therapy; hepatic injury appears to be greater in females and in patients >35 years of age

**Pregnancy Risk Factor** C

**Adverse Reactions**

>10%:

Central nervous system: Drowsiness, dizziness, lightheadedness, fatigue

Dermatologic: Rash

Gastrointestinal: Diarrhea (mild), nausea, vomiting

Neuromuscular & skeletal: Muscle weakness

1% to 10%:

Cardiovascular: Pleural effusion with pericarditis

Central nervous system: Chills, fever, headache, insomnia, nervousness, mental depression

Gastrointestinal: Diarrhea (severe), constipation, anorexia, stomach cramps

Ocular: Blurred vision

Respiratory: Respiratory depression

<1%: Seizures, confusion, hepatitis

**Drug Interactions** Increased toxicity: Estrogens (hepatotoxicity), CNS depressants (sedation), MAO inhibitors, phenothiazines, clindamycin (increased neuromuscular blockade), verapamil (hyperkalemia and cardiac depression), warfarin, clofibrate and tolbutamide

**Half-Life** 8.7 hours

**Special PA Issues**

**Patient Education:** Take exactly as directed. Do not increase dose or discontinue without consulting prescriber. Do not use alcohol, prescriptive or OTC antidepressants, sedatives, or pain medications without consulting prescriber. You may experience drowsiness, dizziness, lightheadedness (avoid driving or engaging in tasks that require alertness until response to therapy is known); nausea or vomiting (small, frequent meals, frequent mouth care, or sucking hard candy may help); or diarrhea (buttermilk, boiled milk, or yogurt may help). Report excessive confusion; drowsiness or mental agitation; chest pain, palpitations, or difficulty breathing; skin rash; or vision disturbances.

**Dietary Considerations:** Alcohol: Additive CNS effects, avoid use

**Monitoring Parameters:** Motor performance should be monitored for therapeutic outcomes; nausea, vomiting, and liver function tests should be monitored for potential hepatotoxicity; intravenous administration requires cardiac monitor and blood pressure monitor

♦ **Dantrolene Sodium** see Dantrolene on previous page

# Dapiprazole (DA pi pray zole)

**Pharmacologic Class** Alpha₁ Blocker, Ophthalmic

**U.S. Brand Names** Rēv-Eyes™

**Mechanism of Action** Dapiprazole is a selective alpha-adrenergic blocking agent, exerting effects primarily on alpha₁-adrenoceptors. It induces miosis via relaxation of the smooth dilator (radial) muscle of the iris, which causes pupillary constriction. It is devoid of cholinergic effects. Dapiprazole also partially reverses the cycloplegia induced with parasympatholytic agents such as tropicamide. Although the drug has no significant effect on the ciliary muscle per se, it may increase accommodative amplitude, therefore relieving the symptoms of paralysis of accommodation.

**Use** Reverse dilation due to drugs (adrenergic or parasympathomimetic) after eye exams

**USUAL DOSAGE** Adults: Administer 2 drops followed 5 minutes later by an additional 2 drops applied to the conjunctiva of each eye; should not be used more frequently than once a week in the same patient

**Dosage Forms** Powder, lyophilized, as hydrochloride: 25 mg [0.5% solution when mixed with supplied diluent]

**Contraindications** Contraindicated in the presence of conditions where miosis is unacceptable, such as acute iritis and in patients with a history of hypersensitivity to any component of the formulation

**Warnings/Precautions** For ophthalmic use only

**Pregnancy Risk Factor** B

**Adverse Reactions**

>10%:

Central nervous system: Headache

Ocular: Conjunctival injection, burning and itching eyes, lid edema, ptosis, lid erythema, chemosis, punctate keratitis, corneal edema, photophobia

1% to 10%: Ocular: Dry eyes, blurring of vision, tearing of eye

**Special PA Issues**

**Patient Education:** May still be sensitive to sunlight and sensitivity may return in 2 or more hours; exercise caution when driving at night or performing other activities in poor illumination. To avoid contamination, do not touch tip of container to any surface.

♦ **Dapiprazole Hydrochloride** see Dapiprazole on this page

# Dapsone (DAP sone)

**Pharmacologic Class** Antibiotic, Miscellaneous

**U.S. Brand Names** Avlosulfon®

**Mechanism of Action** Competitive antagonists of para-aminobenzoic acid (PABA) and prevent normal bacterial utilization of PABA for the synthesis of folic acid.

**Use** Treatment of leprosy and dermatitis herpetiformis (infections caused by *Mycobacterium leprae*)

Prophylaxis of toxoplasmosis in severely immunocompromised patients; alternative agent for *Pneumocystis carinii* pneumonia prophylaxis (given alone) and treatment (given with trimethoprim)

May be useful in relapsing polychondritis, prophylaxis of malaria, inflammatory bowel disorders, *Leishmaniasis*, rheumatic/connective tissue disorders, brown recluse spider bites

**USUAL DOSAGE** Oral:

Leprosy:

Children: 1-2 mg/kg/24 hours, up to a maximum of 100 mg/day

Adults: 50-100 mg/day for 3-10 years

Dermatitis herpetiformis: Adults: Start at 50 mg/day, increase to 300 mg/day, or higher to achieve full control, reduce dosage to minimum level as soon as possible

Prophylaxis of *Pneumocystis carinii* pneumonia:

Children >1 month: 1 mg/kg/day; maximum: 100 mg

Adults: 100 mg/day

Treatment of *Pneumocystis carinii* pneumonia: Adults: 100 mg/day in combination with trimethoprim (15-20 mg/kg/day) for 21 days

**Dosing in renal impairment:** No specific guidelines are available

**Dosage Forms Tab:** 25 mg, 100 mg

**Contraindications** Hypersensitivity to dapsone or any component

**Warnings/Precautions** Use with caution in patients with severe anemia, G-6-PD, methemoglobin reductase or hemoglobin M deficiency; hypersensitivity to other sulfonamides; aplastic anemia, agranulocytosis and other severe blood dyscrasias have resulted in death; monitor carefully; treat severe anemia prior to therapy; serious dermatologic reactions (including toxic epidermal necrolysis) are rare but potential occurrences; sulfone reactions may also occur as potentially fatal hypersensitivity reactions; these, but not leprosy reactional states, require drug discontinuation; dapsone is carcinogenic in small animals

**Pregnancy Risk Factor** C

**Adverse Reactions**

1% to 10%: Hematologic: Hemolysis, methemoglobinemia

<1%: Reactional states (ie, abrupt changes in clinical activity occurring during any leprosy treatment; classified as reversal of erythema nodosum leprosum reactions); insomnia, headache, exfoliative dermatitis, photosensitivity, nausea, vomiting, anemia, leukopenia, agranulocytosis, hepatitis, cholestatic jaundice, peripheral neuropathy (usually in nonleprosy patients), blurred vision, tinnitus, SLE

**Drug Interactions** CYP2C9, 2E1, and 3A3/4 enzyme substrate

Decreased effect/levels: Para-aminobenzoic acid, didanosine, and rifampin decrease dapsone effects

Increased toxicity: Folic acid antagonists may increase the risk of hematologic reactions of dapsone; probenecid decreases dapsone excretion; trimethoprim with dapsone may increase toxic effects of both drugs

**Half-Life** 30 hours (range: 10-50 hours)

**Special PA Issues**

Patient Education: Take as directed, for full term of therapy (treatment for leprosy may take 3-10 years). Do not take with antacids, alkaline foods, or drugs (may decrease dapsone absorption). Frequent blood tests may be required during therapy. Discontinue if rash develops and notify prescriber. Report persistent sore throat, fever, chills; constant fatigue; yellowing of skin or eyes; or easy bruising or bleeding.

Monitoring Parameters: Monitor patient for signs of jaundice and hemolysis; CBC weekly for first month, monthly for 6 months, and semiannually thereafter

- **Debrisan®** [OTC] *see* Dextranomer *on page 267*
- **Debrox® Otic** [OTC] *see* Carbamide Peroxide *on page 150*
- **Decaderm®** *see* Dexamethasone *on page 264*
- **Decadron®** *see* Dexamethasone *on page 264*
- **Decadron®-LA** *see* Dexamethasone *on page 264*
- **Decadron® Turbinaire®** *see* Dexamethasone *on page 264*
- **Deca-Durabolin® Injection** *see* Nandrolone *on page 634*
- **Decaject-L.A.®** *see* Dexamethasone *on page 264*
- **Decaspray®** *see* Dexamethasone *on page 264*
- **Declomycin®** *see* Demeclocycline *on page 259*
- **Decofed® Syrup** [OTC] *see* Pseudoephedrine *on page 780*
- **Decohistine® DH** *see* Chlorpheniramine, Pseudoephedrine, and Codeine *on page 197*
- **Decohistine® Expectorant** *see* Guaifenesin, Pseudoephedrine, and Codeine *on page 429*
- **Deconsal® Sprinkle®** *see* Guaifenesin and Phenylephrine *on page 429*
- **Degest® 2** [OTC] *see* Naphazoline *on page 635*
- **Dehydral™** *see* Methenamine *on page 582*
- **Dekasol-L.A.®** *see* Dexamethasone *on page 264*
- **Deladumone® Injection** *see* Estradiol and Testosterone *on page 334*
- **Delatest® Injection** *see* Testosterone *on page 881*
- **Delatestryl® Injection** *see* Testosterone *on page 881*

## Delavirdine (de la VIR deen)

**Pharmacologic Class** Antiretroviral Agent, Reverse Transcriptase Inhibitor (Non-Nucleoside)

**U.S. Brand Names** Rescriptor®

**Mechanism of Action** Delavirdine binds directly to reverse transcriptase, blocking RNA-dependent and DNA-dependent DNA polymerase activities

**Use** Treatment of HIV-1 infection in combination with at least two additional antiretroviral agents

**USUAL DOSAGE** Adults: Oral: 400 mg 3 times/day

**Dosage Forms** Tab: 100 mg

**Contraindications** Known hypersensitivity to delavirdine or any components

**Warnings/Precautions** Avoid use with terfenadine, astemizole, benzodiazepines, clarithromycin, dapsone, cisapride, rifabutin, rifampin; use with caution in patients with hepatic or renal dysfunction; due to rapid emergence of resistance, delavirdine should not be used as monotherapy; cross-resistance may be conferred to other non-nucleoside reverse transcriptase inhibitors, although potential for cross-resistance with protease inhibitors is low. Long-term effects of delavirdine are not known. Safety and efficacy have not been established in children. Rash, which occurs frequently, may require discontinuation of therapy; usually occurs within 1-3 weeks and lasts <2 weeks. Most patients may resume therapy following a treatment interruption.

**Pregnancy Risk Factor** C

**Pregnancy Implications**
Clinical effects on the fetus: Administer during pregnancy only if benefits to mother outweigh risks to the fetus
Breast-feeding/lactation: HIV-infected mothers are discouraged from breast-feeding to decrease potential transmission of HIV

**Adverse Reactions** >2%:
Central nervous system: Headache, fatigue
Dermatologic: Rash, pruritus
Gastrointestinal: Nausea, diarrhea, vomiting
Metabolic: Increased ALT/AST

**Drug Interactions** CYP2D6 and 3A3/4 enzyme substrate; CYP2D6 and 3A3/4 enzyme inhibitor
Increased plasma concentrations of delavirdine: Clarithromycin, ketoconazole, fluoxetine
Decreased plasma concentrations of delavirdine: Carbamazepine, phenobarbital, phenytoin, rifabutin, rifampin, didanosine, saquinavir
Decreased absorption of delavirdine: Antacids, histamine-2 receptor antagonists, didanosine
Delavirdine increases plasma concentrations of: Indinavir, saquinavir, terfenadine, astemizole, clarithromycin, dapsone, rifabutin, ergot derivatives, alprazolam, midazolam, triazolam, dihydropyridines, cisapride, quinidine, warfarin
Delavirdine decreases plasma concentrations of: Didanosine

**Half-Life** 2-11 hours

**Special PA Issues**
Patient Education: Delavirdine is not a cure for HIV nor has it been found to reduce transmission of HIV. Take as directed, with food. Do not take antacids within 1 hour of delavirdine. Mix 4 tablets in 3-5 oz of water, allow to stand a few minutes, and stir; drink immediately. You may experience nausea or vomiting (small frequent meals or sucking
(Continued)

## Delavirdine *(Continued)*

on lozenges may help - consult prescriber if nausea or vomiting persists). Report mouth sores; skin rash or irritation; muscle weakness or tremors; easy bruising or bleeding, fever or chills; CNS changes (eg, hallucinations, confusion, dizziness, altered coordination); swelling of face, lips, or tongue; yellowing of eyes or skin; or dark urine or pale stools.

**Dietary Considerations:** Delavirdine may be taken without regard to food

**Monitoring Parameters:** Liver function tests if administered with saquinavir

♦ **Delaxin®** *see* Methocarbamol *on page 585*

♦ **Delcort®** *see* Hydrocortisone *on page 453*

♦ **Delestrogen® Injection** *see* Estradiol *on page 332*

♦ **Delta-Cortef® Oral** *see* Prednisolone *on page 752*

♦ **Deltacortisone** *see* Prednisone *on page 754*

♦ **Deltadehydrocortisone** *see* Prednisone *on page 754*

♦ **Deltahydrocortisone** *see* Prednisolone *on page 752*

♦ **Deltasone®** *see* Prednisone *on page 754*

♦ **Delta-Tritex®** *see* Triamcinolone *on page 928*

♦ **Del-Vi-A®** *see* Vitamin A *on page 962*

♦ **Demadex®** *see* Torsemide *on page 918*

## Demecarium *(dem e KARE ee um)*

**Pharmacologic Class** Cholinergic Agonist; Ophthalmic Agent, Antiglaucoma; Ophthalmic Agent, Miotic

**U.S. Brand Names** Humorsol® Ophthalmic

**Mechanism of Action** Cholinesterase inhibitor (anticholinesterase) which causes acetylcholine to accumulate at cholinergic receptor sites and produces effects equivalent to excessive stimulation of cholinergic receptors. Demecarium mainly acts by inhibiting true (erythrocyte) cholinesterase and causes a reduction in intraocular pressure due to facilitation of outflow of aqueous humor; the reduction is likely to be particularly marked in eyes in which the pressure is elevated.

**Use** Management of chronic simple glaucoma, chronic and acute angle-closure glaucoma; strabismus

**USUAL DOSAGE** Children/Adults: Ophthalmic:

Glaucoma: Instill 1 drop into eyes twice weekly to a maximum dosage of 1 or 2 drops twice daily for up to 4 months

Strabismus:

Diagnosis: Instill 1 drop daily for 2 weeks, then 1 drop every 2 days for 2-3 weeks. If eyes become straighter, an accommodative factor is demonstrated.

Therapy: Instill not more than 1 drop at a time in both eyes every day for 2-3 weeks. Then reduce dosage to 1 drop every other day for 3-4 weeks and re-evaluate. Continue at 1 drop every 2 days to 1 drop twice a week and evaluate the patient's condition every 4-12 weeks. If improvement continues, reduce dose to 1 drop once a week and eventually off of medication. Discontinue therapy after 4 months if control of the condition still requires 1 drop every 2 days.

**Dosage Forms Soln, ophth, as bromide:** 0.125% (5 mL), 0.25% (5 mL)

**Contraindications** Hypersensitivity to demecarium or any component, acute inflammatory disease of anterior chamber; pregnancy

**Pregnancy Risk Factor** C

**Pregnancy Implications** Although there are no reports of use in pregnancy, demecarium is an ophthalmic medication and transplacental passage in significant amounts would not be expected

**Adverse Reactions**

1% to 10%: Ocular: Stinging, burning eyes, myopia, visual blurring

<1%: Bradycardia, hypotension, flushing, nausea, vomiting, diarrhea, muscle weakness, retinal detachment, miosis, twitching eyelids, watering eyes, dyspnea, diaphoresis

**Special PA Issues**

**Patient Education:** For ophthalmic use only. Apply prescribed amount as often as directed. Wash hands before using and do not touch tip of applicator to eye or contaminate tip of applicator. Tilt head back and look upward. Gently pull down lower lid and put drop(s) inside lower eyelid at inner corner. Close eye and roll eyeball in all directions. Do not blink for ½ minute. Apply gentle pressure to inner corner of eye for 30 seconds. Wipe away excess from skin around eye. Do not use any other eye preparation for at least 10 minutes. Do not share medication with anyone else. Temporary stinging or blurred vision may occur. Immediately report any adverse cardiac or CNS effects (usually signifies overdose). Report persistent eye pain, redness, burning, watering, dryness, double vision, puffiness around eye, vision disturbances, other adverse eye response, worsening of condition or lack of improvement.

♦ **Demecarium Bromide** *see* Demecarium *on this page*

## Demeclocycline (dem e kloe SYE kleen)

**Pharmacologic Class** Antibiotic, Tetracycline Derivative

**U.S. Brand Names** Declomycin®

**Mechanism of Action** Inhibits protein synthesis by binding with the 30S and possibly the 50S ribosomal subunit(s) of susceptible bacteria; may also cause alterations in the cytoplasmic membrane; inhibits the action of ADH in patients with chronic SIADH

**Use** Treatment of susceptible bacterial infections (acne, gonorrhea, pertussis and urinary tract infections) caused by both gram-negative and gram-positive organisms; used when penicillin is contraindicated (other agents are preferred); treatment of chronic syndrome of inappropriate secretion of antidiuretic hormone (SIADH)

**USUAL DOSAGE** Oral:

Children ≥8 years: 8-12 mg/kg/day divided every 6-12 hours

Adults: 150 mg 4 times/day or 300 mg twice daily

Uncomplicated gonorrhea (penicillin sensitive): 600 mg stat, 300 mg every 12 hours for 4 days (3 g total)

SIADH: 900-1200 mg/day or 13-15 mg/kg/day divided every 6-8 hours initially, then decrease to 600-900 mg/day

**Dosing adjustment/comments in renal/hepatic impairment:** Should be avoided in patients with renal/hepatic dysfunction

**Dosage Forms Cap:** 150 mg; **Tab:** 150 mg, 300 mg

**Contraindications** Hypersensitivity to demeclocycline, tetracyclines, or any component

**Warnings/Precautions** Do not administer to children <9 years of age; photosensitivity reactions occur frequently with this drug, avoid prolonged exposure to sunlight, do not use tanning equipment

**Pregnancy Risk Factor** D

**Adverse Reactions**

1% to 10%:

Dermatologic: Photosensitivity

Gastrointestinal: Nausea, diarrhea

<1%: Pericarditis, increased intracranial pressure, bulging fontanels in infants, dermatologic effects, pruritus, exfoliative dermatitis, diabetes insipidus syndrome, vomiting, esophagitis, anorexia, abdominal cramps, paresthesia, acute renal failure, azotemia, superinfections, anaphylaxis, pigmentation of nails

**Drug Interactions**

Decreased effect with antacids (aluminum, calcium, zinc, or magnesium), bismuth salts, sodium bicarbonate, barbiturates, carbamazepine, hydantoins

Decreased effect of oral contraceptives

Increased effect of warfarin

**Onset** Onset of action for diuresis in SIADH: Several days

**Half-Life** Reduced renal function: 10-17 hours

**Special PA Issues**

**Patient Education:** Preferable to take on an empty stomach (1 hour before or 2 hours after meals). Take at regularly scheduled times around-the-clock. Avoid antacids, iron, or dairy products within 2 hours of taking demeclocycline. You may experience photosensitivity (use sunblock, wear protective clothing, or avoid exposure to direct sunlight); dizziness or lightheadedness (use caution when driving or engaging in hazardous tasks); nausea/vomiting (frequent small meals, frequent mouth care, sucking on lozenges may help); or diarrhea (buttermilk, yogurt, or boiled milk may help). If diabetic, drug may cause false tests with Clinitest® urine glucose monitoring; use of glucose oxidase methods (Clinistix®) or serum glucose monitoring is preferable. Report rash or intense itching; yellowing of skin or eyes; change in color of urine or stools; fever or chills; dark urine or pale stools; vaginal itching or discharge; foul-smelling stools; excessive thirst or urination; acute headache; unresolved diarrhea; or difficulty breathing.

**Monitoring Parameters:** CBC, renal and hepatic function

- **Depogen® Injection** *see* Estradiol *on page 332*
- **Depoject® Injection** *see* Methylprednisolone *on page 593*
- **Depo-Medrol® Injection** *see* Methylprednisolone *on page 593*
- **Deponit® Patch** *see* Nitroglycerin *on page 660*
- **Depopred® Injection** *see* Methylprednisolone *on page 593*
- **Depo-Provera® Injection** *see* Medroxyprogesterone Acetate *on page 561*
- **Depo-Testadiol® Injection** *see* Estradiol and Testosterone *on page 334*
- **Depotest® Injection** *see* Testosterone *on page 881*
- **Depotestogen® Injection** *see* Estradiol and Testosterone *on page 334*
- **Depo®-Testosterone Injection** *see* Testosterone *on page 881*
- **Deprenyl** *see* Selegiline *on page 826*
- **Deproic** *see* Valproic Acid and Derivatives *on page 952*
- **Deproist® Expectorant With Codeine** *see* Guaifenesin, Pseudoephedrine, and Codeine *on page 429*
- **Dermacort®** *see* Hydrocortisone *on page 453*
- **Dermaflex® Gel** *see* Lidocaine *on page 531*
- **Dermarest Dricort®** *see* Hydrocortisone *on page 453*
- **Derma-Smoothe/FS®** *see* Fluocinolone *on page 381*
- **Dermasone** *see* Clobetasol *on page 219*
- **Dermatop®** *see* Prednicarbate *on page 751*
- **Dermazin™** *see* Silver Sulfadiazine *on page 835*
- **DermiCort®** *see* Hydrocortisone *on page 453*
- **Dermolate® [OTC]** *see* Hydrocortisone *on page 453*
- **Dermoplast® [OTC]** *see* Benzocaine *on page 105*
- **Dermovate®** *see* Clobetasol *on page 219*
- **Dermtex® HC With Aloe** *see* Hydrocortisone *on page 453*
- **DES** *see* Diethylstilbestrol *on page 277*
- **Desiccated Thyroid** *see* Thyroid *on page 897*

## Desipramine (des IP ra meen)

**Pharmacologic Class** Antidepressant, Tricyclic (Secondary Amine)

**U.S. Brand Names** Norpramin®

**Mechanism of Action** Traditionally believed to increase the synaptic concentration of norepinephrine in the central nervous system by inhibition of its reuptake by the presynaptic neuronal membrane. However, additional receptor effects have been found including desensitization of adenyl cyclase, down regulation of beta-adrenergic receptors, and down regulation of serotonin receptors.

**Use** Treatment of various forms of depression, often in conjunction with psychotherapy; analgesic adjunct in chronic pain

**Unlabeled use:** Peripheral neuropathies

**USUAL DOSAGE** Oral:

Children 6-12 years: 10-30 mg/day or 1-5 mg/kg/day in divided doses; do not exceed 5 mg/kg/day

Adolescents: Initial: 25-50 mg/day; gradually increase to 100 mg/day in single or divided doses; maximum: 150 mg/day

Adults: Initial: 75 mg/day in divided doses; increase gradually to 150-200 mg/day in divided or single dose; maximum: 300 mg/day

Elderly: Initial dose: 10-25 mg/day; increase by 10-25 mg every 3 days for inpatients and every week for outpatients if tolerated; usual maintenance dose: 75-100 mg/day, but doses up to 150 mg/day may be necessary

Hemodialysis/peritoneal dialysis: Supplemental dose is not necessary

**Dosage Forms** Tab, as hydrochloride: 10 mg, 25 mg, 50 mg, 75 mg, 100 mg, 150 mg

**Contraindications** Hypersensitivity to desipramine (cross-sensitivity with other tricyclic antidepressants may occur); patients receiving MAO inhibitors within past 14 days; narrow-angle glaucoma; use immediately postmyocardial infarction

**Warnings/Precautions** Use with caution in patients with cardiovascular disease, conduction disturbances, urinary retention, seizure disorders, hyperthyroidism or those receiving thyroid replacement; do not discontinue abruptly in patients receiving long-term high-dose therapy

**Pregnancy Risk Factor** C

**Adverse Reactions**

>10%:

Central nervous system: Dizziness, drowsiness, headache

Gastrointestinal: Xerostomia, constipation, increased appetite, nausea, unpleasant taste, weight gain

Neuromuscular & skeletal: Weakness

1% to 10%:

Cardiovascular: Arrhythmias, hypotension

Central nervous system: Confusion, delirium, hallucinations, nervousness, restlessness, parkinsonian syndrome, insomnia

Gastrointestinal: Diarrhea, heartburn

Genitourinary: Dysuria, sexual dysfunction

Neuromuscular & skeletal: Fine muscle tremors

Ocular: Blurred vision, eye pain

Miscellaneous: Diaphoresis (excessive)

<1%: Anxiety, seizures, alopecia, photosensitivity, breast enlargement, galactorrhea, SIADH, trouble with gums, decreased lower esophageal sphincter tone may cause GE reflux, testicular edema, agranulocytosis, leukopenia, eosinophilia, cholestatic jaundice, increased liver enzymes, increased intraocular pressure, tinnitus, allergic reactions

**Drug Interactions** CYP1A2 and 2D6 enzyme substrate; CYP2D6 inhibitor

Decreased effects of guanethidine, clonidine; decreased effect of desipramine with barbiturates, carbamazepine, phenytoin

Increased effects: Sympathomimetics, benzodiazepines

Increased toxicity: Anticholinergics; increased toxicity with MAO inhibitors (hyperpyrexia, tachycardia, hypertension, seizures, and death may occur), alcohol, CNS depressants, cimetidine

**Onset** 1-3 weeks (maximum antidepressant effects: after >2 weeks)

**Half-Life** 7-60 hours

**Special PA Issues**

**Patient Education:** Take exactly as directed (do not increase dose or frequency); may take several weeks to achieve desired results; may cause physical and/or psychological dependence. Avoid excessive alcohol, excess caffeine, and other prescription or OTC medications not approved by prescriber. Maintain adequate hydration (2-3 L/day of fluids unless instructed to restrict fluid intake). You may experience drowsiness, lightheadedness, impaired coordination, dizziness, or blurred vision (use caution when driving or engaging in hazardous tasks until response to medication is known); constipation (increased exercise, fluids, or dietary fruit and fiber may help); urinary retention (void before taking medication); postural hypotension (use caution climbing stairs or when changing position from lying or sitting to standing); altered sexual drive or ability (reversible); or photosensitivity (use sunscreen, protective clothing, and avoid extended exposure to direct sunlight). Report persistent CNS effects (eg, nervousness, restlessness, insomnia, anxiety, excitation, headache, agitation, impaired coordination, changes in cognition); muscle cramping, weakness, tremors, or rigidity; chest pain, palpitations, or irregular heartbeat; blurred vision or eye pain; yellowing of skin or eyes; or worsening of condition.

**Dietary Considerations:** Alcohol: Additive CNS effects, avoid use

**Monitoring Parameters:** Monitor blood pressure and pulse rate prior to and during initial therapy; evaluate mental status; monitor weight

**Reference Range: Plasma levels do not always correlate with clinical effectiveness**
Timing of serum samples: Draw trough just before next dose

Therapeutic: 50-300 ng/mL

In elderly patients the response rate is greatest with steady-state plasma concentrations >115 ng/mL

Possible toxicity: >300 ng/mL

Toxic: >1000 ng/mL

**Related Information**
Antidepressant Agents on page 998

♦ **Desipramine Hydrochloride** see Desipramine on previous page

♦ **Desmethylimipramine Hydrochloride** see Desipramine on previous page

# Desmopressin Acetate (des moe PRES in AS e tate)

**Pharmacologic Class** Vasopressin Analog, Synthetic

**U.S. Brand Names** DDAVP® Nasal Spray; Stimate® Nasal

**Mechanism of Action** Enhances reabsorption of water in the kidneys by increasing cellular permeability of the collecting ducts; possibly causes smooth muscle constriction with resultant vasoconstriction; raises plasma levels of von Willebrand factor and factor VIII

**Use** Treatment of diabetes insipidus and controlling bleeding in mild hemophilia, von Willebrand disease, and thrombocytopenia (eg, uremia), nocturnal enuresis

**USUAL DOSAGE**

Children:

Diabetes insipidus: 3 months to 12 years: Intranasal (using 100 mcg/mL nasal solution): Initial: 5 mcg/day (0.05 mL/day) divided 1-2 times/day; range: 5-30 mcg/day (0.05-0.3 mL/day) divided 1-2 times/day; adjust morning and evening doses separately for an adequate diurnal rhythm of water turnover

Hemophilia: >3 months: I.V. 0.3 mcg/kg; may repeat dose if needed; begin 30 minutes before procedure; dilute I.V. dose in 50 mL 0.9% sodium chloride and infuse over 15-30 minutes

(Continued)

## Desmopressin Acetate *(Continued)*

Nocturnal enuresis: ≥6 years: Intranasal (using 100 mcg/mL nasal solution): Initial: 20 mcg (0.2 mL) at bedtime; range: 10-40 mcg; it is recommended that ¹/₂ of the dose be given in each nostril

Children 12 years and Adults:

Diabetes insipidus:

I.V., S.C.: 2-4 mcg/day in 2 divided doses or ¹/₁₀ of the maintenance intranasal dose; dilute I.V. dose in 50 mL 0.9% sodium chloride and infuse over 15-30 minutes

Intranasal (using 100 mcg/mL nasal solution): 5-40 mcg/day (0.05-0.4 mL) divided 1-3 times/day; adjust morning and evening doses separately for an adequate diurnal rhythm of water turnover. **Note:** The nasal spray pump can only deliver doses of 10 mcg (0.1 mL) or multiples of 10 mcg (0.1 mL), if doses other than this are needed, the rhinal tube delivery system is preferred.

Hemophilia/uremic bleeding:

I.V.: 0.3 mcg/kg by slow infusion, begin 30 minutes before procedure; dilute I.V. dose in 50 mL 0.9% sodium chloride and infuse over 15-30 minutes

Nasal spray: Using high concentration spray: <50 kg: 150 mcg (1 spray); >50 kg: 300 mcg (1 spray each nostril); repeat use is determined by the patient's clinical condition and laboratory work; if using preoperatively, administer 2 hours before surgery

Oral: Begin therapy 12 hours after the last intranasal dose for patients previously on intranasal therapy

Children: Initial: 0.05 mg; fluid restrictions are required in children to prevent hyponatremia and water intoxication

Adults: 0.05 mg twice daily; adjust individually to optimal therapeutic dose. Total daily dose should be increased or decreased (range: 0.1-1.2 mg divided 2-3 times/day) as needed to obtain adequate antidiuresis.

**Dosage Forms Inj (DDAVP®):** 4 mcg/mL (1 mL); **Soln, nasal:** DDAVP®: 100 mcg/mL (2.5 mL, 5 mL), Stimate®: 1.5 mg/mL (2.5 mL); **Tab (DDAVP®):** 0.1 mg, 0.2 mg

**Contraindications** Hypersensitivity to desmopressin or any component; avoid using in patients with type IIB or platelet-type von Willebrand disease, patients with <5% factor VIII activity level

**Warnings/Precautions** Avoid overhydration especially when drug is used for its hemostatic effect

**Pregnancy Risk Factor** B

**Adverse Reactions**

1% to 10%:

Cardiovascular: Facial flushing

Central nervous system: Headache, dizziness

Gastrointestinal: Nausea, abdominal cramps

Genitourinary: Vulval pain

Local: Pain at the injection site

Respiratory: Nasal congestion

<1%: Increase in blood pressure, hyponatremia, water intoxication

**Drug Interactions**

Decreased effect: Demeclocycline, lithium may decrease ADH effects

Increased effect: Chlorpropamide, fludrocortisone may increase ADH response

**Onset**

Intranasal administration: Onset of ADH effects: Within 1 hour; Peak effect: Within 1-5 hours

I.V. infusion: Onset of increased factor VIII activity: Within 15-30 minutes; Peak effect: 90 minutes to 3 hours

**Duration** Intranasal administration: 5-21 hours

**Half-Life** I.V. infusion: Elimination (terminal): 75 minutes

**Special PA Issues**

**Patient Education:** Use specific product as directed. Diabetes insipidus: Avoid overhydration. Weigh yourself daily at same time in the same clothes. Report increased weight or swelling of extremities. If using intranasal product, inspect nasal membranes regularly. Report swelling or increased nasal congestion. All uses: Report unresolved headache, difficulty breathing, acute heartburn or nausea, abdominal cramping, or vulval pain.

**Monitoring Parameters:** Blood pressure and pulse should be monitored during I.V. infusion

Diabetes insipidus: Fluid intake, urine volume, specific gravity, plasma and urine osmolality, serum electrolytes

Hemophilia: Factor VIII antigen levels, APTT, bleeding time (for von Willebrand disease and thrombocytopathies)

♦ **Desocort®** *see* Desonide *on this page*

♦ **Desogen®** *see* Ethinyl Estradiol and Desogestrel *on page 345*

## Desonide *(DES oh nide)*

**Pharmacologic Class** Corticosteroid, Topical

**U.S. Brand Names** DesOwen® Topical; Tridesilon® Topical

**Mechanism of Action** Stimulates the synthesis of enzymes needed to decrease inflammation, suppress mitotic activity, and cause vasoconstriction

**Use** Adjunctive therapy for inflammation in acute and chronic corticosteroid responsive dermatosis (low potency corticosteroid)

**USUAL DOSAGE** Children and Adults: Topical: Apply 2-4 times/day sparingly

**Dosage Forms Crm, top:** 0.05% (15 g, 60 g); **Lot:** 0.05% (60 mL, 120 mL); **Oint, top:** 0.05% (15 g, 60 g)

**Contraindications** Known hypersensitivity to desonide, fungal infections, tuberculosis of skin, herpes simplex

**Warnings/Precautions** Use with caution in patients with impaired circulation, skin infections

**Pregnancy Risk Factor** C

**Adverse Reactions** <1%: Itching, dry skin, folliculitis, hypertrichosis, acneiform eruptions, hypopigmentation, perioral dermatitis, allergic contact dermatitis, skin maceration, skin atrophy, striae; local burning, irritation, miliaria; secondary infection

**Onset** Commonly noted within 7 days of continued therapy

**Special PA Issues**

**Patient Education:** For external use only. Use exactly as directed; do not overuse. Do not apply to open wounds or weeping areas. Before using, wash and dry area gently. Apply a thin film to affected area and rub in gently. If dressing is necessary, use a porous dressing. Avoid contact with eyes. Avoid exposing treated area to direct sunlight; sunburn can occur. Report increased swelling, redness, rash, itching, signs of infection, worsening of condition, or lack of healing.

♦ **DesOwen® Topical** see Desonide on previous page

## Desoximetasone (des oks i MET a sone)

**Pharmacologic Class** Corticosteroid, Topical

**U.S. Brand Names** Topicort®; Topicort®-LP

**Mechanism of Action** Stimulates the synthesis of enzymes needed to decrease inflammation, suppress mitotic activity, and cause vasoconstriction; high potency, fluorinated topical corticosteroid

**Use** Relieves inflammation and pruritic symptoms of corticosteroid-responsive dermatosis [medium to high potency topical corticosteroid]

**USUAL DOSAGE** Desoximetasone is a potent fluorinated topical corticosteroid. All of the preparations are considered high potency.

Children: Apply sparingly in a very thin film to affected area 1-2 times/day

Adults: Apply sparingly in a thin film twice daily

**Dosage Forms Crm, top:** Topicort®: 0.25% (15 g, 60 g, 120 g), Topicort®-LP: 0.05% (15 g, 60 g); **Gel, top:** 0.05% (15 g, 60 g); **Oint, top (Topicort®):** 0.25% (15 g, 60 g)

**Contraindications** Known hypersensitivity to desoximetasone, topical fungal infections, tuberculosis of skin herpes simplex

**Warnings/Precautions** Use with caution in patients with impaired circulation; skin infections

**Pregnancy Risk Factor** C

**Adverse Reactions** <1%: Itching, dry skin, folliculitis, hypertrichosis, acneiform eruptions, allergic contact dermatitis, skin maceration, skin atrophy, striae, perioral dermatitis, hypopigmentation; local burning, irritation, miliaria; secondary infection

**Special PA Issues**

**Patient Education:** For external use only. Use exactly as directed; do not overuse. Do not apply to open wounds or weeping areas. Before using, wash and dry area gently. Apply a thin film to affected area and rub in gently. If dressing is necessary, use a porous dressing. Avoid contact with eyes. Avoid exposing treated area to direct sunlight; sunburn can occur. Report increased swelling, redness, rash, itching, signs of infection, worsening of condition, or lack of healing.

♦ **Desoxyephedrine Hydrochloride** see Methamphetamine on page 581

♦ **Desoxyn®** see Methamphetamine on page 581

♦ **Desoxyn Gradumet®** see Methamphetamine on page 581

♦ **Desoxyphenobarbital** see Primidone on page 756

♦ **Desyrel®** see Trazodone on page 924

♦ **Detensol®** see Propranolol on page 775

♦ **Detrol™** see Tolterodine on page 915

♦ **Detussin® Expectorant** see Hydrocodone, Pseudoephedrine, and Guaifenesin on page 453

♦ **Detussin® Liquid** see Hydrocodone and Pseudoephedrine on page 453

♦ **Devrom® [OTC]** see Bismuth on page 116

♦ **Dexacidin®** see Neomycin, Polymyxin B, and Dexamethasone on page 644

♦ **Dexair®** see Dexamethasone on next page

# Dexamethasone (deks a METH a sone)

**Pharmacologic Class** Corticosteroid, Oral; Corticosteroid, Oral Inhaler; Corticosteroid, Nasal; Corticosteroid, Ophthalmic; Corticosteroid, Parenteral; Corticosteroid, Topical

**U.S. Brand Names** Aeroseb-Dex®; AK-Dex®; Alba-Dex®; Baldex®; Dalalone L.A.®; Decadern®; Decadron®; Decadron®-LA; Decadron® Turbinaire®; Decaject-LA.®; Decaspray®; Dekasol-L.A.®; Dexair®; Dexasone L.A.®; Dexone®; Dexone L.A.®; Dezone®; Hexadrol®; I-Methasone®; Maxidex®; Ocu-Dex®; Solurex L.A.®

**Mechanism of Action** Decreases inflammation by suppression of migration of polymorphonuclear leukocytes and reversal of increased capillary permeability; suppresses normal immune response

**Use** Systemically and locally for chronic inflammation, allergic, hematologic, neoplastic, and autoimmune diseases; may be used in management of cerebral edema, septic shock, as a diagnostic agent, antiemetic

## USUAL DOSAGE

Neonates:

Airway edema or extubation: I.V.: Usual: 0.25 mg/kg/dose given 4 hours prior to scheduled extubation and then every 8 hours for 3 doses total; range: 0.25-1 mg/kg/dose for 1-3 doses; maximum dose: 1 mg/kg/day. **Note:** A longer duration of therapy may be needed with more severe cases.

Bronchopulmonary dysplasia (to facilitate ventilator weaning): Oral:, I.V.: Numerous dosing schedules have been proposed; range: 0.5-0.6 mg/kg/day given in divided doses every 12 hours for 3-7 days, then taper over 1-6 weeks

Children:

Antiemetic (prior to chemotherapy): I.V. (should be given as sodium phosphate): 10 mg/$m^2$/dose (maximum: 20 mg) for first dose then 5 mg/$m^2$/dose every 6 hours as needed

Anti-inflammatory immunosuppressant: Oral, I.M., I.V. (injections should be given as sodium phosphate): 0.08-0.3 mg/kg/day **or** 2.5-10 mg/$m^2$/day in divided doses every 6-12 hours

Extubation or airway edema: Oral, I.M., I.V. (injections should be given as sodium phosphate): 0.5-2 mg/kg/day in divided doses every 6 hours beginning 24 hours prior to extubation and continuing for 4-6 doses afterwards

Cerebral edema: I.V. (should be given as sodium phosphate): Loading dose: 1-2 mg/kg/dose as a single dose; maintenance: 1-1.5 mg/kg/day (maximum: 16 mg/day) in divided doses every 4-6 hours for 5 days then taper for 5 days, then discontinue

Bacterial meningitis in infants and children >2 months: I.V. (should be given as sodium phosphate): 0.6 mg/kg/day in 4 divided doses every 6 hours for the first 4 days of antibiotic treatment; start dexamethasone at the time of the first dose of antibiotic

Physiologic replacement: Oral, I.M., I.V.: 0.03-0.15 mg/kg/day or 0.6-0.75 mg/$m^2$/day in divided doses every 6-12 hours

Adults:

Acute nonlymphoblastic leukemia (ANLL) protocol: I.V.: 2 mg/$m^2$/dose every 8 hours for 12 doses

Antiemetic (prior to chemotherapy): Oral/I.V. (should be given as sodium phosphate): 10 mg/$m^2$/dose (usually 20 mg) for first dose then 5 mg/$m^2$/dose every 6 hours as needed

Anti-inflammatory:

Oral, I.M., I.V. (injections should be given as sodium phosphate): 0.75-9 mg/day in divided doses every 6-12 hours

I.M. (as acetate): 8-16 mg; may repeat in 1-3 weeks

Intralesional (as acetate): 0.8-1.6 mg

Intra-articular/soft tissue (as acetate): 4-16 mg; may repeat in 1-3 weeks

Intra-articular, intralesional, or soft tissue (as sodium phosphate): 0.4-6 mg/day

Cerebral edema: I.V. 10 mg stat, 4 mg I.M./I.V. (should be given as sodium phosphate) every 6 hours until response is maximized, then switch to oral regimen, then taper off if appropriate; dosage may be reduced after 24 days and gradually discontinued over 5-7 days

Diagnosis for Cushing's syndrome: Oral: 1 mg at 11 PM, draw blood at 8 AM the following day for plasma cortisol determination

Physiological replacement: Oral, I.M., I.V. (should be given as sodium phosphate): 0.03-0.15 mg/kg/day OR 0.6-0.75 mg/$m^2$/day in divided doses every 6-12 hours

Shock therapy:

Addisonian crisis/shock (ie, adrenal insufficiency/responsive to steroid therapy): I.V. (given as sodium phosphate): 4-10 mg as a single dose, which may be repeated if necessary

Unresponsive shock (ie, unresponsive to steroid therapy): I.V. (given as sodium phosphate): 1-6 mg/kg as a single I.V. dose or up to 40 mg initially followed by repeat doses every 2-6 hours while shock persists

Hemodialysis: Supplemental dose is not necessary

Peritoneal dialysis: Supplemental dose is not necessary

Ophthalmic:

Ointment: Apply thin coating into conjunctival sac 3-4 times/day; gradually taper dose to discontinue

Suspension: Instill 2 drops into conjunctival sac every hour during the day and every other hour during the night; gradually reduce dose to every 3-4 hours, then to 3-4 times/day
Topical: Apply 1-4 times/day

**Dosage Forms** Dexamethasone acetate: **Inj:** Dalalone L.A.®, Decadron®-LA, Decaject-LA®, Dexasone® L.A., Dexone® LA, Solurex L.A.®: 8 mg/mL (1 mL, 5 mL), Dalalone D.P.®: 16 mg/mL (1 mL, 5 mL)

Dexamethasone base: **Aero, top:** Aeroseb-Dex®: 0.01% (58 g); **Elix (Decadron®, Hexadrol®):** 0.5 mg/5 mL (5 mL, 20 mL, 100 mL, 120 mL, 240 mL, 500 mL); **Soln, oral:** 0.5 mg/5 mL (5 mL, 20 mL, 500 mL); **Soln, oral concentrate:** 0.5 mg/0.5 mL (30 mL); **Susp, ophth:** 0.1% (5 mL), Maxidex®: 0.1% (5 mL, 15 mL); **Tab (Decadron®, Dexone®, Hexadrol®):** 0.25 mg, 0.5 mg, 0.75 mg, 1 mg, 1.5 mg, 2 mg, 4 mg, 6 mg; **Therapeutic pack:** Six 1.5 mg tabs and eight 0.75 mg tabs

Dexamethasone sodium phosphate: **Aero, nasal (Dexacort®):** 84 mcg/activation [170 metered doses] (12.6 g); **Aero, oral (Dexacort®):** 84 mcg/activation [170 metered doses] (12.6 g); **Crm (Decadron® Phosphate):** 0.1% (15 g, 30 g); **Inj:** Dalalone®, Decadron® Phosphate, Decaject®, Dexasone®, Hexadrol® Phosphate, Solurex®: 4 mg/mL (1 mL, 2 mL, 2.5 mL, 5 mL, 10 mL, 30 mL), Hexadrol® Phosphate: 10 mg/mL (1 mL, 10 mL); 20 mg/mL (5 mL) Decadron® Phosphate: 24 mg/mL (5 mL, 10 mL); **Oint, ophth:** 0.05% (3.5 g), AK-Dex®, Baldex®, Decadron® Phosphate, Maxidex®: 0.05% (3.5 g); **Soln, ophth (AK-Dex®, Baldex®, Decadron® Phosphate, Dexotic®):** 0.1% (5 mL)

**Contraindications** Active untreated infections; use in ophthalmic viral, fungal, or tuberculosis diseases of the eye

**Warnings/Precautions** Fatalities have occurred due to adrenal insufficiency in asthmatic patients during and after transfer from systemic corticosteroids to aerosol steroids; aerosol steroids do **not** provide the systemic steroid needed to treat patients having trauma, surgery, or infections; use with caution in patients with hypothyroidism, cirrhosis, hypertension, congestive heart failure, ulcerative colitis, thromboembolic disorders. Because of the risk of adverse effects, systemic corticosteroids should be used cautiously in the elderly in the smallest possible dose and for the shortest possible time.

Controlled clinical studies have shown that inhaled and intranasal corticosteroids may cause a reduction in growth velocity in pediatric patients. Growth velocity provides a means of comparing the rate of growth among children of the same age.

In studies involving inhaled corticosteroids, the average reduction in growth velocity was approximately 1 cm (about ⅓ of an inch) per year. It appears that the reduction is related to dose and how long the child takes the drug.

FDA's Pulmonary and Allergy Drugs and Metabolic and Endocrine Drugs advisory committees discussed this issue at a July 1998 meeting. They recommended that the agency develop class-wide labeling to inform health care providers so they would understand this potential side effect and monitor growth routinely in pediatric patients who are treated with inhaled corticosteroids, intranasal corticosteroids or both.

Long-term effects of this reduction in growth velocity on final adult height are unknown. Likewise, it also has not yet been determined whether patients' growth will "catch up" if treatment is discontinued. Drug manufacturers will continue to monitor these drugs to learn more about long-term effects. Children are prescribed inhaled corticosteroids to treat asthma. Intranasal corticosteroids are generally used to prevent and treat allergy-related nasal symptoms.

Patients are advised not to stop using their inhaled or intranasal corticosteroids without first speaking to their health care providers about the benefits of these drugs compared to their risks.

**Pregnancy Risk Factor** C

**Pregnancy Implications** Dexamethasone has been used in patients with premature labor (26-34 weeks gestation) to stimulate fetal lung maturation

Clinical effects on the fetus: Crosses the placenta; transient leukocytosis reported. Available evidence suggests safe use during pregnancy
Breast-feeding/lactation: No data on crossing into breast milk or effects on the infant

**Adverse Reactions**
**Systemic:**
>10%:
Central nervous system: Insomnia, nervousness
Gastrointestinal: Increased appetite, indigestion
1% to 10%:
Dermatologic: Hirsutism
Endocrine & metabolic: Diabetes mellitus
Neuromuscular & skeletal: Arthralgia
Ocular: Cataracts
Respiratory: Epistaxis
<1%: Seizures, mood swings, headache, delirium, hallucinations, euphoria, skin atrophy, bruising, hyperpigmentation, acne, amenorrhea, sodium and water retention, Cushing's
(Continued)

## Dexamethasone (Continued)

syndrome, hyperglycemia, bone growth suppression, abdominal distention, ulcerative esophagitis, pancreatitis, muscle wasting, hypersensitivity reactions

**Topical:** <1%: Itching, dryness, folliculitis, hypertrichosis, acneiform eruptions, hypopigmentation, perioral dermatitis, allergic contact dermatitis, skin maceration, skin atrophy, striae; miliaria, local burning, irritation; secondary infection

**Drug Interactions** CYP3A3/4 enzyme substrate; CYP3A3/4 enzyme inducer; CYP3A3/4 enzyme inhibitor

Decreased effect: Barbiturates, phenytoin, rifampin may decrease dexamethasone effects; dexamethasone decreases effect of salicylates, vaccines, toxoids

**Duration** Duration of metabolic effect: Can last for 72 hours; acetate is a long-acting repository preparation with a prompt onset of action.

**Half-Life** Normal renal function: 1.8-3.5 hours; Biological half-life: 36-54 hours

**Special PA Issues**

**Patient Education:** Take exactly as directed; do not increase dose or discontinue abruptly without consulting prescriber. Take oral medication with or after meals. Limit intake of caffeine or stimulants. Prescriber may recommend increased dietary vitamins, minerals, or iron. Diabetics should monitor glucose levels closely (antidiabetic medication may need to be adjusted). Inform prescriber if you are experiencing greater than normal levels of stress (medication may need adjustment). Some forms of this medication may cause GI upset (oral medication may be taken with meals to reduce GI upset; small frequent meals and frequent mouth care may reduce GI upset). You may be more susceptible to infection (avoid crowds and persons with contagious or infective conditions). Report promptly excessive nervousness or sleep disturbances; any signs of infection (sore throat, unhealed injuries); excessive growth of body hair or loss of skin color; changes in vision; excessive or sudden weight gain (>3 lb/week); swelling of face or extremities; difficulty breathing; muscle weakness; change in color of stools (tarry) or persistent abdominal pain; or worsening of condition or failure to improve.

Ophthalmic: For ophthalmic use only. Wash hands before using. Tilt head back and look upward. Put drops of suspension or apply thin ribbon of ointment inside lower eyelid. Close eye and roll eyeball in all directions. Do not blink for 30 seconds. Apply gentle pressure to inner corner of eye for 30 seconds. Do not use any other eye preparation for at least 10 minutes. Do not touch tip of applicator to eye or contaminate tip of applicator. Do not share medication with anyone else. Wear sunglasses when in sunlight; you may be more sensitive to bright light. Inform prescriber if condition worsens or fails to improve or if you experience eye pain, disturbances of vision, or other adverse eye response.

Topical: For external use only. Not for eyes or mucous membranes or open wounds. Apply in very thin layer to occlusive dressing. Apply dressing to area being treated. Avoid prolonged or excessive use around sensitive tissues, genital, or rectal areas. Inform prescriber if condition worsens (swelling, redness, irritation, pain, open sores) or fails to improve.

Aerosol: Not for use during acute asthmatic attack. Follow directions that accompany product. Rinse mouth and throat after use to prevent candidiasis. Do not use intranasal product if you have a nasal infection, nasal injury, or recent nasal surgery. If using two products, consult prescriber in which order to use the two products. Inform prescriber if condition worsens or does not improve.

**Monitoring Parameters:** Hemoglobin, occult blood loss, serum potassium, and glucose

**Reference Range:** Dexamethasone suppression test, overnight: 8 AM cortisol <6 µg/100 mL (dexamethasone 1 mg); plasma cortisol determination should be made on the day after giving dose

**Related Information**

Corticosteroids on page 1007

♦ **Dexamethasone Acetate** see Dexamethasone on page 264
♦ **Dexamethasone and Tobramycin** see Tobramycin and Dexamethasone on page 909
♦ **Dexamethasone Sodium Phosphate** see Dexamethasone on page 264
♦ **Dexasone L.A.®** see Dexamethasone on page 264
♦ **Dexasporin®** see Neomycin, Polymyxin B, and Dexamethasone on page 644
♦ **Dexatrim® Pre-Meal [OTC]** see Phenylpropanolamine on page 720
♦ **Dexchlor®** see Dexchlorpheniramine on this page

## Dexchlorpheniramine (deks klor fen EER a meen)

**Pharmacologic Class** Antihistamine

**U.S. Brand Names** Dexchlor®; Poladex®; Polaramine®

**Use** Perennial and seasonal allergic rhinitis and other allergic symptoms including urticaria

**USUAL DOSAGE** Oral:

Children:

2-5 years: 0.5 mg every 4-6 hours (do not use timed release)

6-11 years: 1 mg every 4-6 hours or 4 mg timed release at bedtime

Adults: 2 mg every 4-6 hours or 4-6 mg timed release at bedtime or every 8-10 hours

**Dosage Forms** Dexchlorpheniramine maleate: **Syr (orange flavor):** 2 mg/5 mL with alcohol 6% (480 mL); **Tab:** 2 mg; **Tab, sustained action:** 4 mg, 6 mg

**Contraindications** Narrow-angle glaucoma, hypersensitivity to dexchlorpheniramine or any component

**Pregnancy Risk Factor** B

**Onset** ~1 hour

**Duration** 3-6 hours

**Special PA Issues**
  **Patient Education:** Take as directed; do not exceed recommended dose. Do not chew or crush sustained release tablet. Avoid use of other depressants, alcohol, or sleep-inducing medications unless approved by prescriber. You may experience drowsiness or dizziness (use caution when driving or engaging in hazardous activity until response to medication is known); or dry mouth, nausea, or abdominal pain (frequent small meals, frequent mouth care, chewing gum, or sucking hard candy may help). Report persistent sedation, confusion, or agitation; changes in urinary pattern; blurred vision; sore throat, difficulty breathing or expectorating (thick secretions); or lack of improvement or worsening or condition.

- **Dexchlorpheniramine Maleate** see Dexchlorpheniramine on previous page
- **Dexedrine®** see Dextroamphetamine on next page
- **Dexferrum®** see Iron Dextran Complex on page 492
- **Dexone®** see Dexamethasone on page 264
- **Dexone L.A.®** see Dexamethasone on page 264

## Dexpanthenol (deks PAN the nole)
**Pharmacologic Class** Gastrointestinal Agent, Stimulant
**U.S. Brand Names** Ilopan®; Ilopan-Choline®; Panthoderm® [OTC]
**Use** Prophylactic use to minimize paralytic ileus, treatment of postoperative distention
**USUAL DOSAGE**
  Children and Adults: Relief of itching and aid in skin healing: Topical: Apply to affected area 1-2 times/day
  Adults:
    Relief of gas retention: Oral: 2-3 tablets 3 times/day
    Prevention of postoperative ileus: I.M.: 250-500 mg stat, repeat in 2 hours, followed by doses every 6 hours until danger passes
    Paralyzed ileus: I.M.: 500 mg stat, repeat in 2 hours, followed by doses every 6 hours, if needed
**Dosage Forms Crm:** 2% (30 g, 60 g); **Inj (Ilopan®):** 250 mg/mL (2 mL, 10 mL, 30 mL); **Tab (Ilopan-Choline®):** 50 mg with choline bitartrate 25 mg
**Contraindications** Hemophilia; mechanical obstruction of ileus
**Pregnancy Risk Factor** C

## Dextranomer (deks TRAN oh mer)
**Pharmacologic Class** Topical Skin Product
**U.S. Brand Names** Debrisan® [OTC]
**Mechanism of Action** Dextranomer is a network of dextran-sucrose beads possessing a great many exposed hydroxy groups; when this network is applied to an exudative wound surface, the exudate is drawn by capillary forces generated by the swelling of the beads, with vacuum forces producing an upward flow of exudate into the network
**Use** Clean exudative ulcers and wounds such as venous stasis ulcers, decubitus ulcers, and infected traumatic and surgical wounds; no controlled studies have found dextranomer to be more effective than conventional therapy
**USUAL DOSAGE** Debride and clean wound prior to application; apply to affected area once or twice daily in a ¼" layer; apply a dressing and seal on all four sides; removal should be done by irrigation
**Dosage Forms Beads:** 4 g, 25 g, 60 g, 120 g; **Paste:** 10 g foil packets
**Contraindications** Deep fistulas, sinus tracts, hypersensitivity to any component
**Warnings/Precautions** Do not use in deep fistulas or any area where complete removal is not assured; do not use on dry wounds (ineffective); avoid contact with eyes
**Pregnancy Risk Factor** C
**Adverse Reactions** 1% to 10%:
  Local: Transitory pain, blistering
  Dermatologic: Maceration may occur, erythema
  Hematologic: Bleeding
**Special PA Issues**
  **Patient Education:** Use exactly as directed; do not overuse. Clean wound as directed. Sprinkle beads into or apply paste to ¼" thickness. Change dressing 1-4 times/day before dressing is completely dry to facilitate removal. Wash hands carefully following application. Avoid contact with eyes or other nonulcerous tissue. Report increased swelling, redness, rash, itching, signs of infection, worsening of condition, or lack of healing.

# Dextroamphetamine (deks troe am FET a meen)

**Pharmacologic Class** Stimulant

**U.S. Brand Names** Dexedrine®; Oxydess® II; Spancap® No. 1

**Mechanism of Action** Blocks reuptake of dopamine and norepinephrine from the synapse, thus increases the amount of circulating dopamine and norepinephrine in cerebral cortex to reticular activating system; inhibits the action of monoamine oxidase and causes catecholamines to be released

**Use** Narcolepsy, exogenous obesity, abnormal behavioral syndrome in children (minimal brain dysfunction), attention deficit/hyperactivity disorder (ADHD)

**USUAL DOSAGE** Oral:

Children:

Narcolepsy: 6-12 years: Initial: 5 mg/day, may increase at 5 mg increments in weekly intervals until side effects appear; maximum dose: 60 mg/day

Attention deficit/hyperactivity disorder:

3-5 years: Initial: 2.5 mg/day given every morning; increase by 2.5 mg/day in weekly intervals until optimal response is obtained, usual range: 0.1-0.5 mg/kg/dose every morning with maximum of 40 mg/day

≥6 years: 5 mg once or twice daily; increase in increments of 5 mg/day at weekly intervals until optimal response is reached, usual range: 0.1-0.5 mg/kg/dose every morning (5-20 mg/day) with maximum of 40 mg/day

Children >12 years and Adults:

Narcolepsy: Initial: 10 mg/day, may increase at 10 mg increments in weekly intervals until side effects appear; maximum: 60 mg/day

Exogenous obesity: 5-30 mg/day in divided doses of 5-10 mg 30-60 minutes before meals

**Dosage Forms Cap, sustained release:** 5 mg, 10 mg, 15 mg; **Tab:** 5 mg, 10 mg (5 mg tabs contain tartrazine)

**Contraindications** Hypersensitivity to dextroamphetamine or any component; advanced arteriosclerosis, hypertension, hyperthyroidism, glaucoma, MAO inhibitors

**Warnings/Precautions** Use with caution in patients with psychopathic personalities, cardiovascular disease, HTN, angina, and glaucoma; has high potential for abuse; use in weight reduction programs only when alternative therapy has been ineffective; prolonged administration may lead to drug dependence

**Pregnancy Risk Factor** C

**Adverse Reactions**

>10%:

Cardiovascular: Arrhythmia

Central nervous system: False feeling of well being, nervousness, restlessness, insomnia

1% to 10%:

Cardiovascular: Hypertension

Central nervous system: Mood or mental changes, dizziness, lightheadedness, headache

Endocrine & metabolic: Changes in libido

Gastrointestinal: Diarrhea, nausea, vomiting, stomach cramps, constipation, anorexia, weight loss, xerostomia

Ocular: Blurred vision

Miscellaneous: Diaphoresis (increased)

<1%: Chest pain, CNS stimulation (severe), Tourette's syndrome, hyperthermia, seizures, paranoia, rash, urticaria, tolerance and withdrawal with prolonged use

**Drug Interactions**

Decreased effect: Methyldopa decreased antihypertensive efficacy; ethosuximide; decreased effect with acidifiers, psychotropics

Increased toxicity: May precipitate hypertensive crisis in patients receiving MAO inhibitors and arrhythmias in patients receiving general anesthetics

Increased effect/toxicity of TCAs, phenytoin, phenobarbital, propoxyphene, norepinephrine and meperidine

**Onset** 1-1.5 hours

**Half-Life** 34 hours (urine pH dependent)

**Special PA Issues**

**Patient Education:** Take exactly as directed (do not increase dose or frequency without consulting prescriber); may cause physical and/or psychological dependence. Take early in day to avoid sleep disturbance, 30 minutes before meals. Avoid alcohol, caffeine, or OTC medications that act as stimulants. You may experience restlessness, false sense of euphoria, or impaired judgment (use caution when driving or engaging in hazardous activities); dry mouth (frequent mouth care, sucking on lozenges, or chewing gum may help); nausea or vomiting (small frequent meals, frequent mouth care may help); constipation (increased exercise, dietary fiber, fruit, or fluid may help); diarrhea (buttermilk, boiled milk, or yogurt may help); or altered libido (reversible). Diabetics need to monitor serum glucose closely (may alter antidiabetic medication requirements). Report chest pain, palpitations, or irregular heartbeat; extreme fatigue or depression; CNS changes (aggressiveness, restlessness, euphoria, sleep disturbances); severe unremitting abdominal distress or cramping; changes in sexual activity; or blurred vision.

**Monitoring Parameters:** Growth in children and CNS activity in all

# Dextroamphetamine and Amphetamine
(deks troe am FET a meen & am FET a meen)

**Pharmacologic Class** Stimulant

**U.S. Brand Names** Adderall®

**Dosage Forms Tab:** 10 mg [dextroamphetamine sulfate 2.5 mg, dextroamphetamine saccharate 2.5 mg and amphetamine aspartate 2.5 mg, amphetamine sulfate 2.5 mg], 30 mg [dextroamphetamine sulfate 7.5 mg, dextroamphetamine saccharate 7.5 mg and amphetamine aspartate 7.55 mg, amphetamine sulfate 7.5 mg]

♦ **Dextroamphetamine Sulfate** *see* Dextroamphetamine *on previous page*
♦ **Dextromethorphan and Guaifenesin** *see* Guaifenesin and Dextromethorphan *on page 428*
♦ **Dextropropoxyphene** *see* Propoxyphene *on page 773*
♦ **Dey-Dose® Isoproterenol** *see* Isoproterenol *on page 496*
♦ **Dey-Dose® Metaproterenol** *see* Metaproterenol *on page 575*
♦ **Dey-Drop® Ophthalmic Solution** *see* Silver Nitrate *on page 834*
♦ **Dey-Lute® Isoetharine** *see* Isoetharine *on page 493*
♦ **Dezone®** *see* Dexamethasone *on page 264*
♦ **DFMO** *see* Eflornithine *on page 315*
♦ **DFP** *see* Isoflurophate *on page 494*
♦ **DHC Plus®** *see* Dihydrocodeine Compound *on page 284*
♦ **D.H.E. 45® Injection** *see* Dihydroergotamine *on page 285*
♦ **DHPG Sodium** *see* Ganciclovir *on page 408*
♦ **DHT™** *see* Dihydrotachysterol *on page 285*
♦ **Diaβeta®** *see* Glyburide *on page 419*
♦ **Diabetes Mellitus Treatment** *see* Chart *on page 1063*
♦ **Diabetic Tussin DM® [OTC]** *see* Guaifenesin and Dextromethorphan *on page 428*
♦ **Diabetic Tussin EX® [OTC]** *see* Guaifenesin *on page 427*
♦ **Diabinese®** *see* Chlorpropamide *on page 199*
♦ **Dialose® [OTC]** *see* Docusate *on page 298*
♦ **Dialume® [OTC]** *see* Aluminum Hydroxide *on page 47*
♦ **Diaminodiphenylsulfone** *see* Dapsone *on page 256*
♦ **Diamox®** *see* Acetazolamide *on page 23*
♦ **Diamox Sequels®** *see* Acetazolamide *on page 23*
♦ **Diapid® Nasal Spray** *see* Lypressin *on page 551*
♦ **Diar-aid® [OTC]** *see* Loperamide *on page 540*
♦ **Diastat® Rectal Delivery System** *see* Diazepam *on this page*
♦ **Diazemuls®** *see* Diazepam *on this page*
♦ **Diazemuls® Injection** *see* Diazepam *on this page*

# Diazepam (dye AZ e pam)

**Pharmacologic Class** Benzodiazepine

**U.S. Brand Names** Diastat® Rectal Delivery System; Diazemuls® Injection; Diazepam Intensol®; Dizac® Injectable Emulsion; Valium® Injection; Valium® Oral

**Mechanism of Action** Depresses all levels of the CNS, including the limbic and reticular formation, probably through the increased action of gamma-aminobutyric acid (GABA), which is a major inhibitory neurotransmitter in the brain

**Use** Management of general anxiety disorders, panic disorders, and provide preoperative sedation, light anesthesia, and amnesia; treatment of status epilepticus, alcohol withdrawal symptoms; used as a skeletal muscle relaxant

**USUAL DOSAGE Oral absorption is more reliable than I.M.**

Children:

Conscious sedation for procedures: Oral: 0.2-0.3 mg/kg (maximum: 10 mg) 45-60 minutes prior to procedure

Sedation or muscle relaxation or anxiety:

Oral: 0.12-0.8 mg/kg/day in divided doses every 6-8 hours

I.M., I.V.: 0.04-0.3 mg/kg/dose every 2-4 hours to a maximum of 0.6 mg/kg within an 8-hour period if needed

Status epilepticus:

Infants 30 days to 5 years: I.V.: 0.05-0.3 mg/kg/dose given over 2-3 minutes, every 15-30 minutes to a maximum total dose of 5 mg; repeat in 2-4 hours as needed **or** 0.2-0.5 mg/dose every 2-5 minutes to a maximum total dose of 5 mg

>5 years: I.V.: 0.05-0.3 mg/kg/dose given over 2-3 minutes every 15-30 minutes to a maximum total dose of 10 mg; repeat in 2-4 hours as needed **or** 1 mg/dose given over 2-3 minutes, every 2-5 minutes to a maximum total dose of 10 mg

Rectal: 0.5 mg/kg, then 0.25 mg/kg in 10 minutes if needed

(Continued)

## Diazepam *(Continued)*

Adolescents: Conscious sedation for procedures:
  Oral: 10 mg
  I.V.: 5 mg, may repeat with ½ dose if needed
Adults:
  Anxiety/sedation/skeletal muscle relaxation:
    Oral: 2-10 mg 2-4 times/day
    I.M., I.V.: 2-10 mg, may repeat in 3-4 hours if needed
    Status epilepticus: I.V.: 5-10 mg every 10-20 minutes, up to 30 mg in an 8-hour period; may repeat in 2-4 hours if necessary
Elderly: Oral: Initial:
    Anxiety: 1-2 mg 1-2 times/day; increase gradually as needed, rarely need to use >10 mg/ day
    Skeletal muscle relaxant: 2-5 mg 2-4 times/day
Hemodialysis: Not dialyzable (0% to 5%); supplemental dose is not necessary
**Dosing adjustment in hepatic impairment:** Reduce dose by 50% in cirrhosis and avoid in severe/acute liver disease

**Dosage Forms Gel, rectal:** Adult: 10 mg, 15 mg, 20 mg, Pediatric: 2.5 mg, 5 mg, 10 mg; **Inj:** 5 mg/mL (1 mL, 2 mL, 5 mL, 10 mL); **Inj, emulsified (Dizac®):** 5 mg/mL (3 mL); **Soln, oral (wintergreen-spice flavor):** 5 mg/5 mL (5 mL, 10 mL, 500 mL); **Soln, oral concentrate:** 5 mg/mL (30 mL); **Tab:** 2 mg, 5 mg, 10 mg

**Contraindications** Hypersensitivity to diazepam or any component; there may be a cross-sensitivity with other benzodiazepines; do not use in a comatose patient, in those with pre-existing CNS depression, respiratory depression, narrow-angle glaucoma, or severe uncontrolled pain; do not use in pregnant women

**Warnings/Precautions** Use with caution in patients receiving other CNS depressants, patients with low albumin, hepatic dysfunction, and in the elderly and young infants. Due to its long-acting metabolite, diazepam is not considered a drug of choice in the elderly; long-acting benzodiazepines have been associated with falls in the elderly.

**Pregnancy Risk Factor** D

**Pregnancy Implications**

Clinical effects on the fetus: Crosses the placenta. Oral clefts reported, however, more recent data does not support an association between drug and oral clefts; inguinal hernia, cardiac defects, spina bifida, dysmorphic facial features, skeletal defects, multiple other malformations reported; hypotonia and withdrawal symptoms reported following use near time of delivery

Breast-feeding/lactation: Crosses into breast milk

Clinical effects on the infant: Sedation; American Academy of Pediatrics reports that USE MAY BE OF CONCERN.

**Adverse Reactions**

>10%:
  Cardiovascular: Cardiac arrest, hypotension, bradycardia, cardiovascular collapse, tachycardia, chest pain
  Central nervous system: Drowsiness, ataxia, amnesia, slurred speech, paradoxical excitement or rage, fatigue, lightheadedness, insomnia, memory impairment, headache, anxiety, depression
  Dermatologic: Rash
  Endocrine & metabolic: Decreased libido
  Gastrointestinal: Xerostomia, changes in salivation, constipation, nausea, vomiting, diarrhea, increased or decreased appetite
  Local: Phlebitis, pain with injection
  Neuromuscular & skeletal: Dysarthria
  Ocular: Blurred vision, diplopia
  Respiratory: Decrease in respiratory rate, apnea, laryngospasm
  Miscellaneous: Diaphoresis
1% to 10%:
  Cardiovascular: Syncope, hypotension
  Central nervous system: Confusion, nervousness, dizziness, akathisia
  Dermatologic: Dermatitis
  Gastrointestinal: Weight gain or loss
  Neuromuscular & skeletal: Rigidity, tremor, muscle cramps
  Otic: Tinnitus
  Respiratory: Nasal congestion, hyperventilation
  Miscellaneous: Hiccups
<1%: Menstrual irregularities, blood dyscrasias, reflex slowing, physical and psychological dependence with prolonged use

**Drug Interactions** CYP1A2, 2C8, and 2C9 enzyme substrate, CYP3A3/4 enzyme substrate (minor), and diazepam and desmethyldiazepam are CYP2C19 enzyme substrates

Decreased effect: Enzyme inducers may increase the metabolism of diazepam
Increased toxicity: CNS depressants (alcohol, barbiturates, opioids) may enhance sedation and respiratory depression; cimetidine may decrease the metabolism of diazepam;

cisapride can significantly increase diazepam levels; valproic acid may displace diazepam from binding sites which may result in an increase in sedative effects; selective serotonin reuptake inhibitors (eg, fluoxetine, sertraline, paroxetine) have greatly increased diazepam levels by altering its clearance

**Onset** I.V. for status epilepticus: Almost immediate

**Duration** I.V. for status epilepticus: Short, 20-30 minutes

**Half-Life**

Parent drug: 20-50 hours; increased half-life in the elderly and those with severe hepatic disorders

Active major metabolite (desmethyldiazepam): 50-100 hours

**Special PA Issues**

**Patient Education:** Take exactly as directed (do not increase dose or frequency); may cause physical and/or psychological dependence. While using this medication, do not use alcohol and other prescription or OTC medications (especially pain medications, sedatives, antihistamines, or hypnotics) without consulting prescriber. Maintain adequate hydration (2-3 L/day of fluids unless instructed to restrict fluid intake). You may experience drowsiness, dizziness, or blurred vision (use caution when driving or engaging in hazardous tasks); nausea, vomiting, loss of appetite, or dry mouth (small frequent meals, good mouth care, chewing gum, or sucking on lozenges may help); constipation (increased exercise, fluids, or dietary fruit and fiber may help). If medication is used to control seizures, wear identification that you are taking an antiepileptic medication. Report CNS changes (confusion, depression, increased sedation, excitation, headache, agitation, insomnia or nightmares, dizziness, fatigue, or impaired coordination) or changes in cognition; difficulty breathing or shortness of breath; changes in urinary pattern; changes in sexual activity; muscle cramping, weakness, tremors, or rigidity; ringing in ears or visual disturbances, excessive perspiration, or excessive GI symptoms (cramping, constipation, vomiting, anorexia); worsening of seizure activity, or loss of seizure control.

**Dietary Considerations:** Alcohol: Additive CNS depression has been reported with benzodiazepines; avoid or limit alcohol

**Monitoring Parameters:** Respiratory rate, heart rate, blood pressure with I.V. use

**Reference Range:** Therapeutic: Diazepam: 0.2-1.5 µg/mL (SI: 0.7-5.3 µmol/L); N-desmethyldiazepam (nordiazepam): 0.1-0.5 µg/mL (SI: 0.35-1.8 µmol/L)

♦ **Diazepam Intensol®** *see* Diazepam *on page 269*

♦ **Dibent® Injection** *see* Dicyclomine *on page 273*

# Dibucaine and Hydrocortisone (DYE byoo kane & hye droe KOR ti sone)

**Pharmacologic Class** Anesthetic/Corticosteroid

**U.S. Brand Names** Corticaine® Topical

**Dosage Forms Crm:** Dibucaine 5% and hydrocortisone 5%

♦ **Dicarbosil® [OTC]** *see* Calcium Carbonate *on page 139*

# Dichlorodifluoromethane and Trichloromonofluoromethane

(dye klor oh dye flor oh METH ane & tri klor oh mon oh flor oh METH ane)

**Pharmacologic Class** Analgesic, Topical

**U.S. Brand Names** Fluori-Methane® Topical Spray

**Dosage Forms Spray, top:** Dichlorodifluoromethane 15% and trichloromonofluoromethane 85%

♦ **Dichysterol** *see* Dihydrotachysterol *on page 285*

# Diclofenac (dye KLOE fen ak)

**Pharmacologic Class** Nonsteroidal Anti-Inflammatory Agent (NSAID)

**U.S. Brand Names** Cataflam® Oral; Voltaren® Ophthalmic; Voltaren® Oral; Voltaren-XR® Oral

**Mechanism of Action** Inhibits prostaglandin synthesis by decreasing the activity of the enzyme, cyclo-oxygenase, which results in decreased formation of prostaglandin precursors

**Use** Acute treatment of mild to moderate pain; acute and chronic treatment of rheumatoid arthritis, ankylosing spondylitis, and osteoarthritis; used for juvenile rheumatoid arthritis, gout, dysmenorrhea; ophthalmic solution for postoperative inflammation after cataract extraction

**USUAL DOSAGE** Adults:

Oral:

Analgesia: Starting dose: 50 mg 3 times/day

Rheumatoid arthritis: 150-200 mg/day in 2-4 divided doses (100 mg/day of sustained release product)

Osteoarthritis: 100-150 mg/day in 2-3 divided doses (100-200 mg/day of sustained release product)

Ankylosing spondylitis: 100-125 mg/day in 4-5 divided doses

(Continued)

## Diclofenac (Continued)

Ophthalmic: Instill 1 drop into affected eye 4 times/day beginning 24 hours after cataract surgery and continuing for 2 weeks

**Dosage Forms** Diclofenac sodium: **Soln, ophth (Voltaren®):** 0.1% (2.5 mL, 5 mL); **Tab, delayed release (Voltaren®):** 25 mg, 50 mg, 75 mg; **Tab, extended release, as sodium (Voltaren-XR®):** 100 mg

Diclofenac potassium: **Tab (Cataflam®):** 50 mg

**Contraindications** Known hypersensitivity to diclofenac, any component, aspirin or other nonsteroidal anti-inflammatory drugs (NSAIDs); porphyria

**Warnings/Precautions** Use with caution in patients with congestive heart failure, hypertension, decreased renal or hepatic function, history of GI disease, or those receiving anticoagulants

**Pregnancy Risk Factor** B

**Adverse Reactions**

>10%:

Dermatologic: Rash

Gastrointestinal: Abdominal cramps, heartburn, indigestion, nausea

1% to 10%:

Cardiovascular: Angina pectoris, arrhythmias

Central nervous system: Dizziness, nervousness

Dermatologic: Itching

Gastrointestinal: GI ulceration, vomiting

Genitourinary: Vaginal bleeding

Otic: Tinnitus

<1%: Chest pain, congestive heart failure, hypertension, tachycardia, convulsions, forgetfulness, mental depression, drowsiness, insomnia, urticaria, exfoliative dermatitis, erythema multiforme, Stevens-Johnson syndrome, angioedema, stomatitis, cystitis, agranulocytosis, anemia, pancytopenia, leukopenia, thrombocytopenia, hepatitis, peripheral neuropathy, trembling, weakness, blurred vision, change in vision, decreased hearing, interstitial nephritis, nephrotic syndrome, renal impairment, wheezing, laryngeal edema, shortness of breath, epistaxis, anaphylaxis, diaphoresis (increased)

**Drug Interactions** CYP2C8 and 2C9 enzyme substrate; CYP2C9 enzyme inhibitor

Decreased effect with aspirin; decreased effect of thiazides, furosemide

Increased toxicity of digoxin, methotrexate, cyclosporine, lithium, insulin, sulfonylureas, potassium-sparing diuretics, aspirin, warfarin

**Onset** Cataflam® has a more rapid onset of action than does the sodium salt (Voltaren®), because it is absorbed in the stomach instead of the duodenum.

**Half-Life** 2 hours

**Special PA Issues**

**Patient Education:**

Oral: Take this medication exactly as directed; do not increase dose without consulting prescriber. Do not crush or chew tablets. Take with 8 oz of water, along with food or milk products to reduce GI distress. Maintain adequate fluid intake (2-3 L/day). Avoid excessive alcohol, aspirin and aspirin-containing medication, and all other anti-inflammatory medications unless consulting prescriber. You may experience dizziness, nervousness, or headache (use caution when driving or performing hazardous tasks); nausea, vomiting, dry mouth, or heartburn (frequent small meals, frequent oral care, sucking lozenges, or chewing gum may help); or constipation (increased exercise, fluids, or dietary fruit and fiber may help). GI bleeding, ulceration, or perforation can occur with or without pain; discontinue medication and contact prescriber if persistent abdominal pain or cramping, or blood in stool occurs. Report chest pain or palpitations; breathlessness or difficulty breathing; unusual bruising/bleeding or blood in urine, stool, mouth, or vomitus; unusual fatigue; skin rash or itching; unusual weight gain or swelling of extremities; change in urinary pattern; change in vision or hearing; or ringing in ears.

Ophthalmic: For ophthalmic use only. Apply prescribed amount as often as directed. Wash hands before using and do not let tip of applicator touch eye or contaminate tip of applicator. Tilt head back and look upward. Gently pull down lower lid and put drop(s) in inner corner of eye. Close eye and roll eyeball in all directions. Do not blink for ½ minute. Apply gentle pressure to inner corner of eye for 30 seconds. Wipe away excess from skin around eye. Do not use any other eye preparation for at least 10 minutes. Do not touch tip of applicator to eye or contaminate tip of applicator. Do not share medication with anyone else. May cause sensitivity to bright light (dark glasses may help); temporary stinging or blurred vision may occur. Inform prescriber if you experience eye pain, redness, burning, watering, dryness, double vision, puffiness around eye, vision disturbances, or other adverse eye response; worsening of condition or lack of improvement. Consult prescriber if pregnant or breast-feeding.

**Monitoring Parameters:** Monitor CBC, liver enzymes; monitor urine output and BUN/serum creatinine in patients receiving diuretics; occult blood loss

**Related Information**

Nonsteroidal Anti-Inflammatory Agents on page 1026

## Diclofenac and Misoprostol (dye KLOE fen ak & mye soe PROST ole)

**Pharmacologic Class** Nonsteroidal Anti-Inflammatory Agent (NSAID); Prostaglandin

**U.S. Brand Names** Arthrotec®

**Dosage Forms Tab:** Diclofenac 50 mg and misoprostol 200 mcg, diclofenac 75 mg and misoprostol 200 mcg

♦ **Diclofenac Potassium** see Diclofenac on page 271

♦ **Diclofenac Sodium** see Diclofenac on page 271

## Dicloxacillin (dye kloks a SIL in)

**Pharmacologic Class** Antibiotic, Penicillin

**U.S. Brand Names** Dycill®; Dynapen®; Pathocil®

**Mechanism of Action** Inhibits bacterial cell wall synthesis by binding to one or more of the penicillin binding proteins (PBPs); which in turn inhibits the final transpeptidation step of peptidoglycan synthesis in bacterial cell walls, thus inhibiting cell wall biosynthesis. Bacteria eventually lyse due to ongoing activity of cell wall autolytic enzymes (autolysins and murein hydrolases) while cell wall assembly is arrested.

**Use** Treatment of systemic infections such as pneumonia, skin and soft tissue infections, and osteomyelitis caused by penicillinase-producing staphylococci

**USUAL DOSAGE** Oral:

Use in newborns not recommended

Children <40 kg: 12.5-25 mg/kg/day divided every 6 hours; doses of 50-100 mg/kg/day in divided doses every 6 hours have been used for therapy of osteomyelitis

Children >40 kg and Adults: 125-250 mg every 6 hours

**Dosage adjustment in renal impairment:** Not necessary

Hemodialysis: Not dialyzable (0% to 5%); supplemental dosage not necessary

Peritoneal dialysis: Supplemental dosage not necessary

Continuous arteriovenous or venovenous hemofiltration (CAVH/CAVHD): Supplemental dosage not necessary

**Dosage Forms Cap:** 125 mg, 250 mg, 500 mg; **Powder for oral susp:** 62.5 mg/5 mL (80 mL, 100 mL, 200 mL)

**Contraindications** Known hypersensitivity to dicloxacillin, penicillin, or any components

**Warnings/Precautions** Monitor PT if patient concurrently on warfarin; elimination of drug is slow in neonates; use with caution in patients allergic to cephalosporins; bad taste of suspension may make compliance difficult

**Pregnancy Risk Factor** B

**Adverse Reactions**

1% to 10%: Gastrointestinal: Nausea, diarrhea, abdominal pain

<1%: Fever, seizures with extremely high doses and/or renal failure, rash (maculopapular to exfoliative), vomiting, pseudomembranous colitis, vaginitis, eosinophilia, leukopenia, neutropenia, thrombocytopenia, agranulocytosis, anemia, hemolytic anemia, prolonged PT, hepatotoxicity, transient elevated LFTs, hematuria, interstitial nephritis, increased BUN/creatinine, serum sickness-like reactions, hypersensitivity

**Drug Interactions**

Decreased effect: Efficacy of oral contraceptives may be reduced; decreased effect of warfarin

Increased effect: Disulfiram, probenecid may increase penicillin levels

**Half-Life** 0.6-0.8 hours; slightly prolonged in patients with renal impairment

**Special PA Issues**

**Patient Education:** Take medication as directed, with a large glass of water 1 hour before or 2 hours after meals. Take at regular intervals around-the-clock and take for length of time prescribed. You may experience some gastric distress (small frequent meals may help) and diarrhea (if this persists, consult prescriber). If diabetic, drug may cause false tests with Clinitest® urine glucose monitoring; use of glucose oxidase methods (Clinistix®) or serum glucose monitoring is preferable. This drug may interfere with oral contraceptives; an alternate form of birth control should be used. Report fever, vaginal itching, sores in the mouth, loose foul-smelling stools, yellowing of skin or eyes, and change in color of urine or stool.

**Dietary Considerations:** Food: Decreases drug absorption rate; decreases drug serum concentration. Administer on an empty stomach 1 hour before or 2 hours after meals.

**Monitoring Parameters:** Monitor prothrombin time if patient concurrently on warfarin; monitor for signs of anaphylaxis during first dose

♦ **Dicloxacillin Sodium** see Dicloxacillin on this page

## Dicyclomine (dye SYE kloe meen)

**Pharmacologic Class** Anticholinergic Agent

**U.S. Brand Names** Antispas® Injection; Bentyl® Hydrochloride Injection; Bentyl® Hydrochloride Oral; Byclomine® Injection; Dibent® Injection; Dilomine® Injection; Di-Spaz® Injection; Di-Spaz® Oral; Or-Tyl® Injection

**Mechanism of Action** Blocks the action of acetylcholine at parasympathetic sites in smooth muscle, secretory glands and the CNS

(Continued)

## Dicyclomine *(Continued)*

**Use** Treatment of functional disturbances of GI motility such as irritable bowel syndrome
  **Unlabeled use:** Urinary incontinence

**USUAL DOSAGE**

Oral:

  Infants >6 months: 5 mg/dose 3-4 times/day

  Children: 10 mg/dose 3-4 times/day

  Adults: Begin with 80 mg/day in 4 equally divided doses, then increase up to 160 mg/day

I.M. **(should not be used I.V.):** Adults: 80 mg/day in 4 divided doses (20 mg/dose)

**Dosage Forms Cap:** 10 mg, 20 mg; **Inj:** 10 mg/mL (2 mL, 10 mL); **Syr:** 10 mg/5 mL (118 mL, 473 mL, 946 mL); **Tab:** 20 mg

**Contraindications** Hypersensitivity to any anticholinergic drug; narrow-angle glaucoma, myasthenia gravis; should not be used in infants <6 months of age; nursing mothers

**Warnings/Precautions** Use with caution in patients with hepatic or renal disease, ulcerative colitis, hyperthyroidism, cardiovascular disease, hypertension, tachycardia, GI obstruction, obstruction of the urinary tract. The elderly are at increased risk for anticholinergic effects, confusion and hallucinations.

**Pregnancy Risk Factor** B

**Adverse Reactions** Adverse reactions are included here that have been reported for pharmacologically similar drugs with anticholinergic/antispasmodic action

Cardiovascular: Syncope, tachycardia, palpitations

Central nervous system: Dizziness, lightheadedness, tingling, headache, drowsiness, nervousness, numbness, mental confusion and/or excitement, dyskinesia, lethargy, speech disturbance, insomnia

Dermatologic: Rash, urticaria, itching, and other dermal manifestations; severe allergic reaction or drug idiosyncrasies including anaphylaxis

Endocrine & metabolic: Suppression of lactation

Gastrointestinal: Xerostomia, nausea, vomiting, constipation, bloated feeling, abdominal pain, taste loss, anorexia

Genitourinary: Urinary hesitancy, urinary retention, impotence

Neuromuscular & skeletal: Weakness

Ocular: Blurred vision, diplopia, mydriasis, cycloplegia, increased ocular tension

Respiratory: Dyspnea, apnea, asphyxia, nasal stuffiness or congestion, sneezing, throat congestion

Miscellaneous: Decreased diaphoresis

**Drug Interactions**

Decreased effect: Phenothiazines, anti-Parkinson's drugs, haloperidol, sustained release dosage forms; decreased effect with antacids

Increased toxicity: Anticholinergics, amantadine, narcotic analgesics, type I antiarrhythmics, antihistamines, phenothiazines, TCAs

**Onset** 1-2 hours

**Duration** Up to 4 hours

**Half-Life** Initial phase: 1.8 hours; Terminal phase: 9-10 hours

**Special PA Issues**

  **Patient Education:** Take prescribed dose 1 hour before meals. Void before taking medication. You may experience constipation (frequent exercise, increased dietary fruit, fiber, and fluid may help); dry mouth (sucking on lozenges, frequent mouth care, or chewing gum may help); drowsiness, impaired judgment (use caution when driving or engaging in hazardous tasks); impotence (reversible); or difficulty urinating (void before taking medication, maintain adequate hydration). Report respiratory difficulty, skin rash or redness, soreness at injection site, increased sweating, sensitivity to light, difficulty swallowing, blurred vision, or other unusual adverse reactions.

  **Dietary Considerations:** Alcohol: Additive CNS effects, avoid use

  **Monitoring Parameters:** Pulse, anticholinergic effect, urinary output, GI symptoms

♦ **Dicyclomine Hydrochloride** *see* Dicyclomine *on previous page*

♦ **Dicycloverine Hydrochloride** *see* Dicyclomine *on previous page*

## Didanosine *(dye DAN oh seen)*

**Pharmacologic Class** Antiretroviral Agent, Reverse Transcriptase Inhibitor (Nucleoside)

**U.S. Brand Names** Videx®

**Mechanism of Action** Didanosine, a purine nucleoside analogue and the deamination product of dideoxyadenosine (ddA), inhibits HIV replication *in vitro* in both T cells and monocytes. Didanosine is converted within the cell to the mono-, di-, and triphosphates of ddA. These ddA triphosphates act as substrate and inhibitor of HIV reverse transcriptase substrate and inhibitor of HIV reverse transcriptase thereby blocking viral DNA synthesis and suppressing HIV replication.

**Use** Treatment of HIV infection; always to be used in combination with at least two other antiretroviral agents

**USUAL DOSAGE** Oral (administer on an empty stomach):

Children: 180 mg/m$^2$/day divided every 12 hours **or** dosing is based on body surface area (m$^2$): See table.

### Didanosine — Pediatric Dosing

| Body Surface Area (m$^2$) | Dosing (Tablets) (mg bid) |
|---|---|
| ≤0.4 | 25 |
| 0.5-0.7 | 50 |
| 0.8-1 | 75 |
| 1.1-1.4 | 100 |

Adults: Dosing is based on patient weight: See table.

### Didanosine — Adult Dosing

| Patient Weight (kg) | Dosing (Tablets) (mg bid) |
|---|---|
| 35-49 | 125 |
| 50-74 | 200 |
| ≥75 | 300 |

**Note:** Children >1 year and Adults should receive 2 tablets per dose and children <1 year should receive 1 tablet per dose for adequate buffering and absorption; tablets should be chewed; didanosine has also been used as 300 mg once daily

**Dosing adjustment in renal impairment:**

### Recommended Dose (mg) of Didanosine by Body Weight

| Creatinine Clearance (mL/min) | ≥60 kg | | <60 kg | | Interval (hours) |
|---|---|---|---|---|---|
| | Tablet[a] | Solution[b] | Tablet[a] | Solution[b] | |
| ≥60 | 200 | 250 | 125 | 167 | 12 |
| 30-59 | 100 | 100 | 75 | 100 | 12 |
| 10-29 | 150 | 167 | 100 | 100 | 24 |
| <10 | 100 | 100 | 75 | 100 | 24 |

[a] Chewable/dispersible buffered tablet; 2 tablets must be taken with each dose; different strengths of tablets may be combined to yield the recommended dose.

[b] Buffered powder for oral solution

Hemodialysis: Removed by hemodialysis (40% to 60%)

**Dosing adjustment in hepatic impairment:** Should be considered

**Dosage Forms Powder for oral soln: Buffered (single dose packet):** 100 mg, 167 mg, 250 mg, 375 mg, **Pediatric:** 2 g, 4 g; **Tab, buffered, chewable (mint flavor):** 25 mg, 50 mg, 100 mg, 150 mg

**Contraindications** Hypersensitivity to any component

**Warnings/Precautions** Peripheral neuropathy occurs in ~35% of patients receiving the drug; pancreatitis (sometimes fatal) occurs in ~9%; risk factors for developing pancreatitis include a previous history of the condition, concurrent cytomegalovirus or *Mycobacterium avium-intracellulare* infection, and concomitant use of pentamidine or co-trimoxazole; discontinue didanosine if clinical signs of pancreatitis occur. Didanosine may cause retinal depigmentation in children receiving doses >300 mg/m$^2$/day. Patients should undergo retinal examination every 6-12 months. Use with caution in patients with decreased renal or hepatic function, phenylketonuria, sodium-restricted diets, or with edema, congestive heart failure or hyperuricemia; in high concentrations, didanosine is mutagenic. Lactic acidosis and severe hepatomegaly have occurred with antiretroviral nucleoside analogues.

**Pregnancy Risk Factor** B

**Pregnancy Implications**

Clinical effects on the fetus: Administer during pregnancy only if benefits to mother outweigh risks to the fetus

Breast-feeding/lactation: HIV-infected mothers are discouraged from breast-feeding to decrease potential transmission of HIV

**Adverse Reactions**

>10%:

Central nervous system: Anxiety, headache, irritability, insomnia, restlessness

Gastrointestinal: Abdominal pain, nausea, diarrhea

Neuromuscular & skeletal: Peripheral neuropathy

1% to 10%:

Central nervous system: Depression

Dermatologic: Rash, pruritus

(Continued)

## Didanosine (Continued)

Gastrointestinal: Pancreatitis (2% to 3%)

<1%: Seizures, anemia, granulocytopenia, leukopenia, thrombocytopenia, hepatitis, lactic acidosis/hepatomegaly, alopecia, anaphylactoid reaction, diabetes mellitus, optic neuritis, retinal depigmentation, renal impairment, hypersensitivity

**Drug Interactions** Drugs whose absorption depends on the level of acidity in the stomach such as ketoconazole, itraconazole, and dapsone should be administered at least 2 hours prior to didanosine

Decreased effect: Didanosine may decrease absorption of quinolones or tetracyclines, didanosine should be held during PCP treatment with pentamidine; didanosine may decrease levels of indinavir

Increased toxicity: Concomitant administration of other drugs which have the potential to cause peripheral neuropathy or pancreatitis may increase the risk of these toxicities

**Half-Life**

Normal renal function: 1.5 hours; however, its active metabolite ddATP has an intracellular half-life >12 hours in vitro. This permits the drug to be dosed at 12-hour intervals; total body clearance averages 800 mL/minute.

Impaired renal function: Half-life is increased, with values ranging from 2.5-5 hours.

**Special PA Issues**

**Patient Education:** Take as directed, 1 hour before or 2 hours after eating. Chew tablets thoroughly and/or dissolve in water. Pour powder into 4 oz of liquid, stir, and drink immediately. Do not mix with fruit juice or other acid-containing liquids. You may experience dizziness; use caution when driving or engaging in hazardous tasks until response to therapy is known. You will be susceptible to infection; avoid crowds. Report numbness or tingling of fingers, toes, or feet; abdominal pain; or persistent nausea or vomiting. Should have a retinal exam every 6-12 months.

**Monitoring Parameters:** Serum potassium, uric acid, creatinine; hemoglobin, CBC with neutrophil and platelet count, CD4 cells; viral load; liver function tests, amylase; weight gain; perform dilated retinal exam every 6 months

♦ **Dideoxycytidine** see Zalcitabine on page 971

♦ **Didronel®** see Etidronate Disodium on page 354

## Dienestrol (dye en ES trole)

**Pharmacologic Class** Estrogen Derivative

**U.S. Brand Names** DV® Vaginal Cream; Ortho® Dienestrol Vaginal

**Mechanism of Action** Increases the synthesis of DNA, RNA, and various proteins in target tissues; reduces the release of gonadotropin-releasing hormone from the hypothalamus; reduces FSH and LH release from the pituitary

**Use** Symptomatic management of atrophic vaginitis or kraurosis vulvae in postmenopausal women

**USUAL DOSAGE** Adults: Vaginal: Insert 1 applicatorful once or twice daily for 1-2 weeks and then 1/2 of that dose for 1-2 weeks; maintenance dose: 1 applicatorful 1-3 times/week for 3-6 months

**Dosage Forms Crm, vaginal:** 0.01% (30 g, 78 g)

**Contraindications** Pregnancy; should not be used during lactation or undiagnosed vaginal bleeding

**Warnings/Precautions** Use with caution in patients with a history of thromboembolism, stroke, myocardial infarction (especially age >40 who smoke), liver tumor, hypertension, cardiac, renal or hepatic insufficiency

**Pregnancy Risk Factor** X

**Adverse Reactions**

1% to 10%:

Cardiovascular: Peripheral edema

Endocrine & metabolic: Breast tenderness, breast enlargement

Gastrointestinal: Anorexia, abdominal cramping

<1%: Hypertension, thromboembolism, myocardial infarction, stroke, migraine, dizziness, anxiety, depression, headache, chloasma, melasma, rash, decreased glucose tolerance, alterations in frequency and flow of menses, breast tenderness or enlargement, increased triglycerides and LDL, nausea, GI distress, cholestatic jaundice, increased susceptibility to Candida infection

**Special PA Issues**

**Patient Education:** Use as directed. Insert cream high in vagina. Remain lying down for 30 minutes following insertion. Use of sanitary napkin following administration will protect clothing; do not use a tampon. May cause breast tenderness or enlargement (consult prescriber for relief). Discontinue use and report promptly any pain, redness, warmth, or swelling in calves; sudden onset difficulty breathing; headache; loss of vision; difficulty speaking; sharp or sudden chest pain; severe abdominal pain; or unusual bleeding.

## Diethylpropion (dye eth il PROE pee on)

**Pharmacologic Class** Anorexiant

**U.S. Brand Names** Tenuate®; Tenuate® Dospan®

**Mechanism of Action** Diethylpropion is used as an anorexiant agent possessing pharmacological and chemical properties similar to those of amphetamines. The mechanism of action of diethylpropion in reducing appetite appears to be secondary to CNS effects, specifically stimulation of the hypothalamus to release catecholamines into the central nervous system; anorexiant effects are mediated via norepinephrine and dopamine metabolism. An increase in physical activity and metabolic effects (inhibition of lipogenesis and enhancement of lipolysis) may also contribute to weight loss.

**Use** Short-term adjunct in exogenous obesity

**USUAL DOSAGE** Adults: Oral:

Tablet: 25 mg 3 times/day before meals or food

Tablet, controlled release: 75 mg at midmorning

**Dosage Forms** Diethylpropion hydrochloride: **Tab:** 25 mg; **Tab, controlled release:** 75 mg

**Contraindications** Known hypersensitivity to diethylpropion; during or within 14 days following administration of MAO inhibitors (hypertensive crises may result)

**Warnings/Precautions** Prolonged administration may lead to dependence; use with caution in patients with mental illness or diabetes mellitus, advanced arteriosclerosis, cardiovascular disease, nephritis, angina pectoris, hypertension, glaucoma, and patients with a history of drug abuse

**Pregnancy Risk Factor** B

**Adverse Reactions**

>10%:

Cardiovascular: Hypertension

Central nervous system: Euphoria, nervousness, insomnia

1% to 10%:

Central nervous system: Confusion, mental depression

Endocrine & metabolic: Changes in libido

Gastrointestinal: Nausea, vomiting, restlessness, constipation

Hematologic: Blood dyscrasias

Neuromuscular & skeletal: Tremor

Ocular: Blurred vision

<1%: Tachycardia, arrhythmias, depression, headache, alopecia, diarrhea, abdominal cramps, dysuria, polyuria, myalgia, tremor, dyspnea, diaphoresis (increased)

**Drug Interactions**

Decreased effect of guanethidine; decreased effect with phenothiazines

Increased effect/toxicity with MAO inhibitors (hypertensive crisis), CNS depressants, general anesthetics (arrhythmias), sympathomimetics

**Onset** 1 hour

**Duration** 12-24 hours

**Special PA Issues**

**Patient Education:** Take exactly as directed (do not increase dose or frequency without consulting prescriber); may cause physical and/or psychological dependence. Do not crush or chew extended release tablets. Take early in day to avoid sleep disturbance, 1 hour before meals. Avoid alcohol, caffeine, or OTC medications that act as stimulants. You may experience restlessness, false sense of euphoria, or impaired judgment (use caution when driving or engaging in hazardous activities); dry mouth (frequent mouth care, sucking on lozenges, or chewing gum may help); nausea or vomiting (small frequent meals, frequent mouth care may help); constipation (increased exercise, dietary fiber, fruit, or fluid may help); diarrhea (buttermilk, boiled milk, or yogurt may help); or altered libido (reversible). Diabetics need to monitor serum glucose closely (may alter antidiabetic medication requirements). Report chest pain, palpitations, or irregular heartbeat; muscle weakness or tremors; extreme fatigue or depression; CNS changes (aggressiveness, restlessness, euphoria, sleep disturbances); severe unremitting abdominal distress or cramping; changes in sexual activity; changes in urinary pattern; or blurred vision.

**Dietary Considerations:** Alcohol: Avoid use

**Monitoring Parameters:** Monitor CNS

♦ **Diethylpropion Hydrochloride** see Diethylpropion on this page

## Diethylstilbestrol (dye eth il stil BES trole)

**Pharmacologic Class** Estrogen Derivative

**U.S. Brand Names** Stilphostrol®

**Mechanism of Action** Competes with estrogenic and androgenic compounds for binding onto tumor cells and thereby inhibits their effects on tumor growth

**Use** Palliative treatment of inoperable metastatic prostatic carcinoma and postmenopausal inoperable, progressing breast cancer

**USUAL DOSAGE** Adults:

Male:

Prostate carcinoma (inoperable, progressing): Oral: 1-3 mg/day

(Continued)

## Diethylstilbestrol *(Continued)*

Diphosphate: (inoperable, progressing): Oral: 50 mg 3 times/day; increase up to 200 mg or more 3 times/day; maximum daily dose: 1 g

I.V.: Administer 0.5 g, dissolved in 250 mL of saline or $D_5W$, administer slowly the first 10-15 minutes then adjust rate so that the entire amount is given in 1 hour; repeat for ≥5 days depending on patient response, then repeat 0.25-0.5 g 1-2 times for one week or change to oral therapy

Female: Postmenopausal (inoperable, progressing) breast carcinoma: Oral: 15 mg/day

**Dosage Forms** Diethylstilbestrol base: **Tab:** 1 mg, 2.5 mg, 5 mg

Diethylstilbestrol diphosphate sodium: **Inj (Stilphostrol®):** 0.25 g (5 mL); **Tab (Stilphostrol®):** 50 mg

**Contraindications** Undiagnosed vaginal bleeding, during pregnancy; breast cancer except in select patients with metastatic disease

**Warnings/Precautions** Use with caution in patients with a history of thromboembolism, stroke, myocardial infarction (especially >40 years of age who smoke), liver tumor, hypertension, cardiac, renal or hepatic insufficiency; estrogens have been reported to increase the risk of endometrial carcinoma; do not use estrogens during pregnancy

**Pregnancy Risk Factor** X

**Adverse Reactions**

>10%:

Cardiovascular: Peripheral edema

Endocrine & metabolic: Enlargement of breasts (female and male), breast tenderness

Gastrointestinal: Nausea, anorexia, bloating

1% to 10%:

Central nervous system: Headache

Endocrine & metabolic: Increased libido (female), decreased libido (male)

Gastrointestinal: Vomiting, diarrhea

<1%: Hypertension, thromboembolism, myocardial infarction, edema, stroke, depression, dizziness, anxiety, chloasma, melasma, rash, amenorrhea, alterations in frequency and flow of menses, increased triglycerides, nausea, GI distress, increased LDL, cholestatic jaundice, intolerance to contact lenses, decreased glucose tolerance, increased susceptibility to *Candida* infection, breast tumors

**Special PA Issues**

**Patient Education:** Use as directed with or after meals (sustained release may be taken at midmorning - do not crush or chew). May cause breast tenderness or enlargement (consult prescriber for relief). You may be more sensitive to sunlight; use sunblock, wear protective clothing and dark glasses, or avoid direct exposure to sunlight. If you are diabetic, monitor serum glucose closely; antidiabetic agent may need to be adjusted. Discontinue use and report promptly any pain, redness, warmth, or swelling in calves; sudden onset difficulty breathing; headache; loss of vision; difficulty speaking; sharp or sudden chest pain; severe abdominal pain; or unusual bleeding or speech.

♦ **Diethylstilbestrol Diphosphate Sodium** *see Diethylstilbestrol on previous page*

## Difenoxin and Atropine *(dye fen OKS in & A troe peen)*

**Pharmacologic Class** Antidiarrheal

**U.S. Brand Names** Motofen®

**Dosage Forms Tab:** Difenoxin hydrochloride 1 mg and atropine sulfate 0.025 mg

♦ **Differin®** *see Adapalene on page 30*

## Diflorasone *(dye FLOR a sone)*

**Pharmacologic Class** Corticosteroid, Topical

**U.S. Brand Names** Florone®; Florone E®; Maxiflor®; Psorcon™

**Mechanism of Action** Decreases inflammation by suppression of migration of polymorphonuclear leukocytes and reversal of increased capillary permeability

**Use** Relieves inflammation and pruritic symptoms of corticosteroid-responsive dermatosis (high to very high potency topical corticosteroid)

Maxiflor®: High potency topical corticosteroid

Psorcon™: Very high potency topical corticosteroid

**USUAL DOSAGE** Topical: Apply ointment sparingly 1-3 times/day; apply cream sparingly 2-4 times/day

**Dosage Forms Crm:** 0.05% (15 g, 30 g, 60 g); **Oint, top:** 0.05% (15 g, 30 g, 60 g)

**Contraindications** Known hypersensitivity to diflorasone

**Warnings/Precautions** Use with caution in patients with impaired circulation; skin infections

**Pregnancy Risk Factor** C

**Adverse Reactions** <1%: Itching, folliculitis, maceration, burning, dryness, muscle atrophy, arthralgia, secondary infection

**Special PA Issues**
  **Patient Education:** For external use only. Use exactly as directed; do not overuse. Do not apply to open wounds or weeping areas. Before using, wash and dry area gently. Apply a thin film to affected area and rub in gently. If dressing is necessary, use a porous dressing. Avoid contact with eyes. Avoid exposing treated area to direct sunlight; sunburn can occur. Report increased swelling, redness, rash, itching, signs of infection, worsening of condition, or lack of healing.

♦ **Diflorasone Diacetate** see Diflorasone on previous page
♦ **Diflucan®** see Fluconazole on page 375

# Diflunisal (dye FLOO ni sal)
**Pharmacologic Class** Nonsteroidal Anti-Inflammatory Agent (NSAID)
**U.S. Brand Names** Dolobid®
**Mechanism of Action** Inhibits prostaglandin synthesis by decreasing the activity of the enzyme, cyclo-oxygenase, which results in decreased formation of prostaglandin precursors
**Use** Management of inflammatory disorders usually including rheumatoid arthritis and osteoarthritis; can be used as an analgesic for treatment of mild to moderate pain
**USUAL DOSAGE** Adults: Oral:
  Pain: Initial: 500-1000 mg followed by 250-500 mg every 8-12 hours; maximum daily dose: 1.5 g
  Inflammatory condition: 500-1000 mg/day in 2 divided doses; maximum daily dose: 1.5 g
  **Dosing adjustment in renal impairment:** $Cl_{cr}$ <50 mL/minute: Administer 50% of normal dose
**Dosage Forms Tab:** 250 mg, 500 mg
**Contraindications** Hypersensitivity to diflunisal or any component, may be a cross-sensitivity with other nonsteroidal anti-inflammatory agents including aspirin; should not be used in patients with active GI bleeding
**Warnings/Precautions** Peptic ulceration and GI bleeding have been reported; platelet function and bleeding time are inhibited; ophthalmologic effects; impaired renal function, use lower dosage; peripheral edema; possibility of Reye's syndrome; elevation in liver tests
**Pregnancy Risk Factor** C (D if used in the 3rd trimester)
**Adverse Reactions**
  >10%:
    Central nervous system: Headache
    Endocrine & metabolic: Fluid retention
  1% to 10%:
    Cardiovascular: Angina pectoris, arrhythmias
    Central nervous system: Dizziness
    Dermatologic: Rash
    Gastrointestinal: GI ulceration
    Genitourinary: Vaginal bleeding
    Otic: Tinnitus
  <1%: Chest pain, vasculitis, tachycardia, convulsions, hallucinations, mental depression, drowsiness, nervousness, insomnia, toxic epidermal necrolysis, urticaria, exfoliative dermatitis, itching, erythema multiforme, Stevens-Johnson syndrome, angioedema, stomatitis, esophagitis or gastritis, cystitis, hemolytic anemia, agranulocytosis, thrombocytopenia, hepatitis, peripheral neuropathy, trembling, weakness, blurred vision, change in vision, decreased hearing, interstitial nephritis, nephrotic syndrome, renal impairment, wheezing, shortness of breath, anaphylaxis, diaphoresis (increased)
**Drug Interactions**
  Decreased effect with antacids
  Increased effect/toxicity of digoxin, methotrexate, anticoagulants, phenytoin, sulfonylureas, sulfonamides, lithium, indomethacin, hydrochlorothiazide, acetaminophen (levels)
**Onset** Onset of analgesia: Within 1 hour
**Duration** 8-12 hours
**Half-Life** 8-12 hours; prolonged with renal impairment
**Special PA Issues**
  **Patient Education:** If self-administered, use exactly as directed (do not increase dose or frequency); adverse reactions can occur with overuse. Do not take longer than 3 days for fever, or 10 days for pain without consulting medical advisor. Take with food or milk. While using this medication, do not use alcohol, excessive amounts of vitamin C, or salicylate-containing foods (curry powder, prunes, raisins, tea, or licorice), other prescription or OTC medications containing aspirin or salicylate, or other NSAIDs without consulting prescriber. Maintain adequate hydration (2-3 L/day of fluids unless instructed to restrict fluid intake). You may experience nausea, vomiting, gastric discomfort (frequent mouth care, small frequent meals, or sucking on lozenges may help). GI bleeding, ulceration, or perforation can occur with or without pain. Stop taking medication and report ringing in ears; persistent pain in stomach; unresolved nausea or vomiting; difficulty breathing or shortness of breath; unusual bruising or bleeding (mouth, urine, stool); skin rash; unusual swelling of extremities; chest pain; or palpitations.

♦ **Digibind®** *see* Digoxin Immune Fab *on page 283*

# Digitoxin (di ji TOKS in)

**Pharmacologic Class** Antiarrhythmic Agent, Miscellaneous; Cardiac Glycoside

**U.S. Brand Names** Crystodigin®

**Mechanism of Action** Digitalis binds to and inhibits magnesium and adenosine triphosphate dependent sodium and potassium ATPase thereby increasing the influx of calcium ions, from extracellular to intracellular cytoplasm due to the inhibition of sodium and potassium ion movement across the myocardial membranes; this increase in calcium ions results in a potentiation of the activity of the contractile heart muscle fibers and an increase in the force of myocardial contraction (positive inotropic effect); digitalis may also increase intracellular entry of calcium via slow calcium channel influx; stimulates release and blocks reuptake of norepinephrine; decreases conduction through the S-A and A-V nodes

**Use** Treatment of congestive heart failure, atrial fibrillation, atrial flutter, paroxysmal atrial tachycardia, and cardiogenic shock

## USUAL DOSAGE Oral:

Children: Doses are very individualized; **when recommended**, digitalizing dose is as follows:

<1 year: 0.045 mg/kg

1-2 years: 0.04 mg/kg

>2 years: 0.03 mg/kg which is equivalent to 0.75 mg/m$^2$

Maintenance: Approximately $^1/_{10}$ of the digitalizing dose

Adults: Oral:

Rapid loading dose: Initial: 0.6 mg followed by 0.4 mg and then 0.2 mg at intervals of 4-6 hours

Slow loading dose: 0.2 mg twice daily for a period of 4 days followed by a maintenance dose

Maintenance: 0.05-0.3 mg/day

Most common dose: 0.15 mg/day

**Dosing adjustment in renal impairment:** $Cl_{cr}$ <10 mL/minute: Administer 50% to 75% of normal dose

Hemodialysis: Not dialyzable (0% to 5%)

**Dosing adjustment in hepatic impairment:** Dosage reduction is necessary in severe liver disease

**Dosage Forms** Tab: 0.1 mg, 0.2 mg

**Contraindications** Hypersensitivity to digitoxin or any component (rare); digitalis toxicity, beriberi heart disease, A-V block, idiopathic hypertrophic subaortic stenosis, constrictive pericarditis, ventricular fibrillation, or tachycardia

**Warnings/Precautions** Use with caution in patients with hypoxia, hypothyroidism, acute myocarditis,; do not use to treat obesity; patients with incomplete A-V block (Stokes-Adams attack) may progress to complete block with digitalis drug administration; use with caution in patients with acute myocardial infarction, severe pulmonary disease, advanced heart failure, idiopathic hypertrophic subaortic stenosis, Wolff-Parkinson-White syndrome, sick-sinus syndrome (bradyarrhythmias), amyloid heart disease, and constrictive cardiomyopathies; adjust dose with renal or hepatic impairment and aged patients; elderly may develop exaggerated serum/tissue concentrations due to decreased lean body mass, total body water, and age-related reduction in renal/hepatic function; exercise will reduce serum concentrations of digoxin due to increased skeletal muscle uptake

**Pregnancy Risk Factor** C

## Adverse Reactions

1% to 10%: Gastrointestinal: Anorexia, nausea, vomiting

<1%: Sinus bradycardia, A-V block, S-A block, atrial or nodal ectopic beats, ventricular arrhythmias, bigeminy, trigeminy, atrial tachycardia with A-V block, drowsiness, headache, fatigue, lethargy, vertigo, disorientation, hyperkalemia with acute toxicity, feeding intolerance, abdominal pain, diarrhea, neuralgia, blurred vision, halos, yellow or green vision, diplopia, photophobia, flashing lights

**Drug Interactions** CYP3A4 enzyme substrate

Decreased effect/levels of digoxin: Antacids (magnesium, aluminum)•, penicillamine•, dietary bran fiber•, radiotherapy+, antineoplastic drugs+, sucralfate+, sulfasalazine+, thiazide and loop diuretics+, aminosalicylic acid+, neomycin••, phenytoin••, cholestyramine/colestipol/kaolin-pectin••, aminoglutethimide••

Decreased effect/levels of digitoxin: Antacids (magnesium, aluminum)•, phenylbutazone••, phenobarbital••, phenytoin••, cholestyramine••, aminoglutethimide••, rifampin++

Increased effect/toxicity/levels of digoxin: Diltiazem•, spironolactone/triamterene•, ibuprofen•, cimetidine•, omeprazole•, flecainide+, acetylsalicylic acid+, indomethacin+, benzodiazepines+, bepridil••, reserpine••, amphotericin B••, erythromycin••, quinine sulfate••, tetracycline••, cyclosporine••, amiodarone++, propafenone++, quinidine++, verapamil++, calcium preparations++, itraconazole++

Increased effect/toxicity/levels of digitoxin: Diltiazem•, spironolactone•, amphotericin B••, quinidine++, calcium preparations++

**Note:**

• = improbable clinical importance

\* = uncertain clinical significance

•• = interaction proven needing monitoring for possible dosage adjustments

♦♦ = important interaction needing monitoring, dosage adjustments are likely

**Special PA Issues**

**Patient Education:** Do not discontinue medication without physician's advice; instruct patients to notify physician if they suffer loss of appetite, visual changes, nausea, vomiting, weakness, drowsiness, headache, confusion, or depression

**Reference Range:** Therapeutic: 20-35 ng/mL; Toxic: >45 ng/mL

# Digoxin (di JOKS in)

**Pharmacologic Class** Antiarrhythmic Agent, Class IV; Cardiac Glycoside

**U.S. Brand Names** Lanoxicaps®; Lanoxin®

**Mechanism of Action**

Congestive heart failure: Inhibition of the sodium/potassium ATPase pump which acts to increase the intracellular sodium-calcium exchange to increase intracellular calcium leading to increased contractility

Supraventricular arrhythmias: Direct suppression of the A-V node conduction to increase effective refractory period and decrease conduction velocity - positive inotropic effect, enhanced vagal tone, and decreased ventricular rate to fast atrial arrhythmias. Atrial fibrillation may decrease sensitivity and increase tolerance to higher serum digoxin concentrations.

**Use** Treatment of congestive heart failure and to slow the ventricular rate in tachyarrhythmias such as atrial fibrillation, atrial flutter, and supraventricular tachycardia (paroxysmal atrial tachycardia); cardiogenic shock; may not slow progression of heart failure or affect survival but proven to relieve signs and symptoms of heart failure.

**USUAL DOSAGE** When changing from oral (tablets or liquid) or I.M. to I.V. therapy, dosage should be reduced by 20% to 25%. See table.

### Dosage Recommendations for Digoxin

| Age | Total Digitalizing Dose† (mcg/kg*) | | Daily Maintenance Dose‡ (mcg/kg*) | |
|---|---|---|---|---|
| | P.O. | I.V. or I.M. | P.O. | I.V. or I.M. |
| Preterm infant* | 20-30 | 15-25 | 5-7.5 | 4-6 |
| Full-term infant* | 25-35 | 20-30 | 6-10 | 5-8 |
| 1 mo - 2 y* | 35-60 | 30-50 | 10-15 | 7.5-12 |
| 2-5 y* | 30-40 | 25-35 | 7.5-10 | 6-9 |
| 5-10 y* | 20-35 | 15-30 | 5-10 | 4-8 |
| >10 y* | 10-15 | 8-12 | 2.5-5 | 2-3 |
| Adults | 0.75-1.5 mg | 0.5-1 mg | 0.125-0.5 mg | 0.1-0.4 mg |

*Based on lean body weight and normal renal function for age. Decrease dose in patients with ↓ renal function; digitalizing dose often not recommended in infants and children.

†Give one-half of the total digitalizing dose (TDD) in the initial dose, then give one-quarter of the TDD in each of two subsequent doses at 8- to 12-hour intervals. Obtain EKG 6 hours after each dose to assess potential toxicity.

‡Divided every 12 hours in infants and children <10 years of age. Given once daily to children >10 years of age and adults.

**Dosing adjustment/interval in renal impairment:**

$Cl_{cr}$ 10-50 mL/minute: Administer 25% to 75% of dose or every 36 hours

$Cl_{cr}$ <10 mL/minute: Administer 10% to 25% of dose or every 48 hours

Reduce loading dose by 50% in ESRD

Hemodialysis: Not dialyzable (0% to 5%)

**Dosage Forms Cap:** 50 mcg, 100 mcg, 200 mcg; **Elix:** 50 mcg/mL with alcohol 10% (60 mL); **Inj:** 250 mcg/mL (1 mL, 2 mL); **Inj, pediatric:** 100 mcg/mL (1 mL); **Tab:** 125 mcg, 250 mcg, 500 mcg

**Contraindications** Hypersensitivity to digoxin or any component; A-V block, idiopathic hypertrophic subaortic stenosis, or constrictive pericarditis

**Warnings/Precautions** Use with caution in patients with hypoxia, myxedema, hypothyroidism, acute myocarditis; patients with incomplete A-V block (Stokes-Adams attack) may progress to complete block with digitalis drug administration; use with caution in patients with acute myocardial infarction, severe pulmonary disease, advanced heart failure, idiopathic hypertrophic subaortic stenosis, Wolff-Parkinson-White syndrome, sick-sinus syndrome (bradyarrhythmias), amyloid heart disease, and constrictive cardiomyopathies; adjust dose with renal impairment; elderly and neonates may develop exaggerated serum/tissue concentrations due to age-related alterations in clearance and pharmacodynamic differences; exercise will reduce serum concentrations of digoxin due to increased skeletal muscle uptake; recent studies indicate photopsia, chromatopsia and decreased visual acuity may occur even with therapeutic serum drug levels

**Pregnancy Risk Factor** C

(Continued)

## Digoxin *(Continued)*

### Adverse Reactions

1% to 10%: Gastrointestinal: Anorexia, nausea, vomiting

<1%: Sinus bradycardia, A-V block, S-A block, atrial or nodal ectopic beats, ventricular arrhythmias, bigeminy, trigeminy, atrial tachycardia with A-V block, drowsiness, headache, fatigue, lethargy, vertigo, disorientation, hyperkalemia with acute toxicity, feeding intolerance, abdominal pain, diarrhea, neuralgia, blurred vision, halos, yellow or green vision, diplopia, photophobia, flashing lights

### Drug Interactions

Decreased effect/levels of digoxin: Antacids (magnesium, aluminum)•, penicillamine•, dietary bran fiber•, radiotherapy⁺, antineoplastic drugs⁺, sucralfate⁺, sulfasalazine⁺, thiazide and loop diuretics⁺, aminosalicylic acid⁺, neomycin••, phenytoin••, cholestyramine/colestipol/kaolin-pectin••, aminoglutethimide••

Decreased effect/levels of digitoxin: Antacids (magnesium, aluminum)•, phenylbutazone••, phenobarbital••, phenytoin••, cholestyramine••, aminoglutethimide••, rifampin⁺⁺

Increased effect/toxicity/levels of digoxin: Diltiazem•, spironolactone/triamterene•, ibuprofen•, cimetidine•, omeprazole•, flecainide⁺, acetylsalicylic acid⁺, indomethacin⁺, benzodiazepines⁺, bepridil••, reserpine••, amphotericin B••, erythromycin••, clarithromycin, quinine sulfate••, tetracycline••, nefazodone, cyclosporin••, amiodarone⁺⁺, propafenone⁺⁺, quinidine⁺⁺, verapamil⁺⁺, calcium preparations⁺⁺, itraconazole⁺⁺

Increased effect/toxicity/levels of digitoxin: diltiazem•, spironolactone•, amphotericin B••, quinidine⁺⁺, calcium preparations⁺⁺

### Note:

• = improbable clinical importance

⁺ = uncertain clinical significance

•• = interaction proven needing monitoring for possible dosage adjustments

⁺⁺ important interaction needing monitoring, dosage adjustments are likely

**Onset** Oral: 1-2 hours; I.V.: 5-30 minutes; Peak effect: Oral: 2-8 hours; I.V.: 1-4 hours

**Duration** 3-4 days both forms

### Half-Life

Dependent upon age, renal and cardiac function: Adults: 38-48 hours; Adults, anephric: 4-6 days

Half-life: Parent drug: 38 hours; Metabolites: Digoxigenin: 4 hours; Monodigitoxoside: 3-12 hours

### Special PA Issues

**Patient Education:** Take as directed; do not discontinue without consulting prescriber. Maintain adequate dietary intake of potassium (do not increase without consulting prescriber). Adequate dietary potassium will reduce risk of digoxin toxicity. Take pulse at same time each day; follow prescriber instructions for holding medication if pulse is below 50. Notify prescriber of acute changes in pulse. Report loss of appetite, nausea, vomiting, persistent diarrhea, swelling of extremities, palpitations, "yellowing" or blurred vision, mental confusion or depression, or unusual fatigue.

### Monitoring Parameters

When to draw serum digoxin concentrations: Digoxin serum concentrations are monitored because digoxin possesses a narrow therapeutic serum range; the therapeutic endpoint is difficult to quantify and digoxin toxicity may be life-threatening. Digoxin serum levels should be drawn **at least 4 hours after an intravenous dose** and **at least 6 hours after an oral dose (optimally 12-24 hours after a dose).**

Initiation of therapy:

**If a loading dose is given:** Digoxin serum concentration may be drawn within 12-24 hours after the initial loading dose administration. Levels drawn this early may confirm the relationship of digoxin plasma levels and response but are of little value in determining maintenance doses.

**If a loading dose is not given:** Digoxin serum concentration should be obtained after 3-5 days of therapy

Maintenance therapy:

**Trough** concentrations should be followed just prior to the next dose or at a minimum of 4 hours after an I.V. dose and at least 6 hours after an oral dose

Digoxin serum concentrations should be obtained within 5-7 days (approximate time to steady-state) after any dosage changes. Continue to obtain digoxin serum concentrations 7-14 days after any change in maintenance dose. **Note:** In patients with end-stage renal disease, it may take 15-20 days to reach steady-state.

Additionally, patients who are receiving potassium-depleting medications such as diuretics, should be monitored for potassium, magnesium, and calcium levels

Digoxin serum concentrations should be obtained whenever any of the following conditions occur:

Questionable patient compliance or to evaluate clinical deterioration following an initial good response

Changing renal function

Suspected digoxin toxicity

Initiation or discontinuation of therapy with drugs (amiodarone, quinidine, verapamil) which potentially interact with digoxin; if quinidine therapy is started; digoxin levels should be drawn within the first 24 hours after starting quinidine therapy, then 7-14 days later or empirically skip one day's digoxin dose and decrease the daily dose by 50%

Any disease changes (hypothyroidism)

Heart rate and rhythm should be monitored along with periodic EKGs to assess both desired effects and signs of toxicity

Follow closely (especially in patients receiving diuretics or amphotericin) for decreased serum potassium and magnesium or increased calcium, all of which predispose to digoxin toxicity

Assess renal function

Be aware of drug interactions

## Reference Range:
### Digoxin therapeutic serum concentrations:
Congestive heart failure: 0.8-2 ng/mL
Arrhythmias: 1.5-2.5 ng/mL

Adults: <0.5 ng/mL; probably indicates underdigitalization unless there are special circumstances

Toxic: >2.5 ng/mL; tachyarrhythmias commonly require levels >2 ng/mL

Digoxin-like immunoreactive substance (DLIS) may cross-react with digoxin immunoassay. DLIS has been found in patients with renal and liver disease, congestive heart failure, neonates, and pregnant women (3rd trimester).

## Related Information
Heart Failure: Management of Patients with Left Ventricular Systolic Dysfunction *on page 1064*

# Digoxin Immune Fab (di JOKS in i MYUN fab)
**Pharmacologic Class** Antidote
**U.S. Brand Names** Digibind®
**Mechanism of Action** Binds with molecules of digoxin or digitoxin and then is excreted by the kidneys and removed from the body
**Use** Digoxin immune Fab are specific antibodies for the treatment of digitalis intoxication in carefully selected patients; use in life-threatening ventricular arrhythmias secondary to digoxin, acute digoxin ingestion (ie, >10 mg in adults or >4 mg in children), hyperkalemia (serum potassium >5 mEq/L) in the setting of digoxin toxicity
**USUAL DOSAGE** Each vial of Digibind® 40 mg will bind ~0.6 mg of digoxin or digitoxin

Estimation of the dose is based on the body burden of digitalis. This may be calculated if the amount ingested is known or the postdistribution serum drug level is known.

| Tablets Ingested (0.25 mg) | Fab Dose (mg) | (vials) |
|---|---|---|
| 5 | 68 | 1.7 |
| 10 | 136 | 3.4 |
| 25 | 340 | 8.5 |
| 50 | 680 | 17 |
| 75 | 1000 | 25 |
| 100 | 1360 | 34 |
| 150 | 2000 | 50 |

**Fab dose based on serum drug level postdistribution:**
Digoxin:
No. of vials = level (ng/mL) x body weight (kg) divided by 100
Digitoxin:
No. of vials = digitoxin (ng/mL) x body weight (kg) divided by 1000
If neither amount ingested nor drug level are known, dose empirically with 10 and 5 vials for acute and chronic toxicity, respectively

**Dosage Forms Powder for inj, lyophilized:** 38 mg
**Contraindications** Hypersensitivity to sheep products
**Warnings/Precautions** Use with caution in renal or cardiac failure; allergic reactions possible (sheep product)-skin testing not routinely recommended; epinephrine should be immediately available, Fab fragments may be eliminated more slowly in patients with renal failure, heart failure may be exacerbated as digoxin level is reduced; total serum digoxin concentration may rise precipitously following administration of Digibind®, but this will be almost entirely bound to the Fab fragment and not able to react with receptors in the body; Digibind® will interfere with digitalis immunoassay measurements - this will result in clinically misleading serum digoxin concentrations until the Fab fragment is eliminated from the body (several days to >1 week after Digibind® administration). Hypokalemia has been reported to occur following reversal of digitalis intoxication as has exacerbation of underlying heart failure. Serum digoxin levels drawn prior to therapy may be difficult to evaluate if 6-8 hours have not elapsed after the last dose of digoxin (time to equilibration between serum and (Continued)

## Digoxin Immune Fab *(Continued)*

tissue); redigitalization should not be initiated until Fab fragments have been eliminated from the body, which may occur over several days or greater than a week in patients with impaired renal function.

**Pregnancy Risk Factor** C

**Adverse Reactions** <1%: Worsening of low cardiac output or congestive heart failure, rapid ventricular response in patients with atrial fibrillation as digoxin is withdrawn, facial edema and redness, hypokalemia, urticarial rash, allergic reactions

**Onset** I.V.: Improvement in signs or symptoms occur within 2-30 minutes

**Half-Life** 15-20 hours; prolonged in patients with renal impairment

**Special PA Issues**

**Patient Education:** Patient education and instruction will be determined by patient condition and ability to understand. Immediately report dizziness, palpitations, cramping, or difficulty breathing.

**Monitoring Parameters:** Serum potassium, serum digoxin concentration prior to first dose of digoxin immune Fab; **digoxin levels will greatly increase with Digibind® use and are not an accurate determination of body stores**

♦ **Dihistine® DH** *see* Chlorpheniramine, Pseudoephedrine, and Codeine *on page 197*

♦ **Dihistine® Expectorant** *see* Guaifenesin, Pseudoephedrine, and Codeine *on page 429*

♦ **Dihydrex® Injection** *see* Diphenhydramine *on page 289*

## Dihydrocodeine Compound *(dye hye droe KOE deen KOM pound)*

**Pharmacologic Class** Analgesic, Narcotic

**U.S. Brand Names** DHC Plus®; Synalgos®-DC

**Mechanism of Action** Binds to opiate receptors in the CNS, causing inhibition of ascending pain pathways, altering the perception of and response to pain; causes cough suppression by direct central action in the medulla; produces generalized CNS depression

**Use** Management of mild to moderate pain that requires relaxation

**USUAL DOSAGE** Adults: Oral: 1-2 capsules every 4-6 hours as needed for pain

**Dosage Forms Cap:** DHC Plus®: Dihydrocodeine bitartrate 16 mg, acetaminophen 356.4 mg, and caffeine 30 mg, Synalgos®-DC: Dihydrocodeine bitartrate 16 mg, aspirin 356.4 mg, and caffeine 30 mg

**Contraindications** Hypersensitivity to dihydrocodeine or any component

**Warnings/Precautions** Use with caution in patients with hypersensitivity reactions to other phenanthrene derivative opioid agonists (morphine, hydrocodone, hydromorphone, levorphanol, oxycodone, oxymorphone); respiratory diseases including asthma, emphysema, COPD, or severe liver or renal insufficiency; some preparations contain sulfites which may cause allergic reactions; dextromethorphan has equivalent antitussive activity but has much lower toxicity in accidental overdose; tolerance of drug dependence may result from extended use

**Pregnancy Risk Factor** B (D if used for prolonged periods or in high doses at term)

**Adverse Reactions**

>10%:

Central nervous system: Lightheadedness, dizziness, drowsiness, sedation

Dermatologic: Pruritus, skin reactions

Gastrointestinal: Nausea, vomiting, constipation

1% to 10%:

Cardiovascular: Hypotension, palpitations, bradycardia, peripheral vasodilation

Central nervous system: Increased intracranial pressure

Endocrine & metabolic: Antidiuretic hormone release

Gastrointestinal: Biliary tract spasm

Genitourinary: Urinary tract spasm

Ocular: Miosis

Respiratory: Respiratory depression

Miscellaneous: Histamine release, physical and psychological dependence with prolonged use

**Drug Interactions** CYP2D6 enzyme substrate

Increased toxicity: MAO inhibitors may increase adverse symptoms

**Onset** 4-5 hours

**Half-Life** 3.5-4.5 hours

**Special PA Issues**

**Patient Education:** If self-administered, use exactly as directed (do not increase dose or frequency); may cause physical and/or psychological dependence. While using this medication, do not use alcohol and other prescription or OTC medications (especially sedatives, tranquilizers, antihistamines, or pain medications) without consulting prescriber. Maintain adequate hydration (2-3 L/day of fluids unless instructed to restrict fluid intake). May cause dizziness, drowsiness, impaired coordination, or blurred vision (use caution when driving, climbing stairs, or changing position - rising from sitting or lying to standing or when engaging in hazardous activities until response to medication is known); nausea or vomiting (frequent mouth care, small frequent meals, or sucking on lozenges may help); constipation (increased exercise, fluids, or dietary fruit and fiber may help - if constipation remains an unresolved problem, consult prescriber about use of stool softeners). Report chest pain or rapid heartbeat; acute headache; swelling of extremities or unusual weight gain; changes in urinary elimination; acute headache; back or flank pain or spasms; or other adverse reactions.

**Dietary Considerations:** Alcohol: Additive CNS effects, avoid use

# Dihydroergotamine (dye hye droe er GOT a meen)

**Pharmacologic Class** Ergot Derivative

**U.S. Brand Names** D.H.E. 45® Injection; Migranal® Nasal Spray

**Mechanism of Action** Ergot alkaloid alpha-adrenergic blocker directly stimulates vascular smooth muscle to vasoconstrict peripheral and cerebral vessels; also has effects on serotonin receptors

**Use** Aborts or prevents vascular headaches; also as an adjunct for DVT prophylaxis for hip surgery, for orthostatic hypotension, xerostomia secondary to antidepressant use, and pelvic congestion with pain

**USUAL DOSAGE** Adults:

I.M.: 1 mg at first sign of headache; repeat hourly to a maximum dose of 3 mg total
I.V.: Up to 2 mg maximum dose for faster effects; maximum dose: 6 mg/week
Intranasal: 1 spray (0.5 mg) of nasal spray should be administered into each nostril; repeat as needed within 15 minutes, up to a total of 6 sprays in any 24-hour period and no more than 8 sprays in a week

**Dosing adjustment in hepatic impairment:** Dosage reductions are probably necessary but specific guidelines are not available

**Dosage Forms** Dihydroergotamine mesylate: **Inj:** 1 mg/mL (1 mL); **Spray, nasal:** 4 mg/mL [0.5 mg/spray] (1 mL)

**Contraindications** High-dose aspirin therapy, hypersensitivity to dihydroergotamine or any component. DHE should not be used within 24 hours of sumatriptan, zolmitriptan, other serotonin agonists or ergot-like agents. DHE should be avoided during or within 2 weeks of discontinuing MAO inhibitors. Pregnancy is contraindicated.

**Warnings/Precautions** Use with caution in hypertension, angina, peripheral vascular disease, impaired renal or hepatic function; avoid pregnancy

**Pregnancy Risk Factor** X

**Adverse Reactions**

>10%:
Cardiovascular: Localized edema, peripheral vascular effects (numbness and tingling of fingers and toes)
Central nervous system: Drowsiness, dizziness
Gastrointestinal: Xerostomia, diarrhea, nausea, vomiting
1% to 10%:
Cardiovascular: Precordial distress and pain, transient tachycardia or bradycardia
Neuromuscular & skeletal: Muscle pain in the extremities, weakness in the legs

**Drug Interactions**
Increased effect of heparin
Increased toxicity with erythromycin, clarithromycin, nitroglycerin, propranolol, troleandomycin

**Onset** Within 15-30 minutes

**Duration** 3-4 hours

**Half-Life** 1.3-3.9 hours

**Special PA Issues**

**Patient Education:** Take this drug as rapidly as possible when first symptoms occur. Rare feelings of numbness or tingling of fingers, toes, or face may occur; use caution and avoid injury. May cause drowsiness; avoid activities requiring alertness until effects of medication are known. Report heart palpitations, severe nausea or vomiting, or severe numbness of fingers or toes.

**Reference Range:** Minimum concentration for vasoconstriction is reportedly 0.06 ng/mL

♦ **Dihydroergotamine Mesylate** see Dihydroergotamine on this page

♦ **Dihydroergotoxine** see Ergoloid Mesylates on page 327

♦ **Dihydrogenated Ergot Alkaloids** see Ergoloid Mesylates on page 327

♦ **Dihydrohydroxycodeinone** see Oxycodone on page 687

♦ **Dihydromorphinone** see Hydromorphone on page 456

# Dihydrotachysterol (dye hye droe tak IS ter ole)

**Pharmacologic Class** Vitamin D Analog

**U.S. Brand Names** DHT™; Hytakerol®

**Mechanism of Action** Synthetic analogue of vitamin D with a faster onset of action; stimulates calcium and phosphate absorption from the small intestine, promotes secretion of calcium from bone to blood; promotes renal tubule resorption of phosphate

**Use** Treatment of hypocalcemia associated with hypoparathyroidism; prophylaxis of hypocalcemic tetany following thyroid surgery
(Continued)

## Dihydrotachysterol *(Continued)*

**USUAL DOSAGE** Oral
Hypoparathyroidism:
Infants and young Children: Initial: 1-5 mg/day for 4 days, then 0.1-0.5 mg/day
Older Children and Adults: Initial: 0.8-2.4 mg/day for several days followed by maintenance doses of 0.2-1 mg/day
Nutritional rickets: 0.5 mg as a single dose or 13-50 mcg/day until healing occurs
Renal osteodystrophy: Maintenance: 0.25-0.6 mg/24 hours adjusted as necessary to achieve normal serum calcium levels and promote bone healing

**Dosage Forms Cap (Hytakerol®):** 0.125 mg; **Soln: Oral Concentrate (DHT™):** 0.2 mg/mL (30 mL), **Oral, in oil (Hytakerol®):** 0.25 mg/mL (15 mL); **Tab (DHT™):** 0.125 mg, 0.2 mg, 0.4 mg

**Contraindications** Hypercalcemia, known hypersensitivity to dihydrotachysterol

**Warnings/Precautions** Calcium-phosphate product (serum calcium and phosphorus) must not exceed 70; avoid hypercalcemia; use with caution in coronary artery disease, decreased renal function (especially with secondary hyperparathyroidism), renal stones, and elderly

**Pregnancy Risk Factor** A (D if used in doses above the recommended daily allowance)

**Adverse Reactions**
>10%:
Endocrine & metabolic: Hypercalcemia
Renal: Elevated serum creatinine, hypercalciuria
<1%: Convulsions, polydipsia, nausea, vomiting, anorexia, weight loss, polyuria, anemia, weakness, metastatic calcification, renal damage

**Drug Interactions**
Decreased effect/levels of vitamin D: Cholestyramine, colestipol, mineral oil; phenytoin and phenobarbital may inhibit activation may decrease effectiveness
Increased toxicity: Thiazide diuretics increase calcium

**Onset** Peak hypercalcemic effect: Within 2-4 weeks

**Duration** Can be as long as 9 weeks

**Special PA Issues**
**Patient Education:** Take exact dose prescribed; do not take more than recommended. Your prescriber may recommend a special diet. Do not increase calcium intake without consulting prescriber. Avoid magnesium supplements or magnesium-containing antacids. You may experience nausea, vomiting, or metallic taste (frequent small meals, frequent mouth care, or sucking hard candy may help); hypotension (use caution when rising from sitting or lying position or when climbing stairs or bending over). Report chest pain or palpitations; acute headache, dizziness, or feeling of weakness; unresolved nausea or vomiting; persistent metallic taste; unrelieved muscle or bone pain; or CNS irritability.
**Monitoring Parameters:** Monitor renal function, serum calcium, and phosphate concentrations; if hypercalcemia is encountered, discontinue agent until serum calcium returns to normal
**Reference Range:** Calcium (serum): 9-10 mg/dL (4.5-5 mEq/L)

♦ **1,25 Dihydroxycholecalciferol** *see* Calcitriol *on page 137*
♦ **Diiodohydroxyquin** *see* Iodoquinol *on page 487*
♦ **Diisopropyl Fluorophosphate** *see* Isoflurophate *on page 494*
♦ **Dilacor™ XR** *see* Diltiazem *on this page*
♦ **Dilantin®** *see* Phenytoin *on page 721*
♦ **Dilatrate®-SR** *see* Isosorbide Dinitrate *on page 498*
♦ **Dilaudid®** *see* Hydromorphone *on page 456*
♦ **Dilaudid-5®** *see* Hydromorphone *on page 456*
♦ **Dilaudid-HP®** *see* Hydromorphone *on page 456*
♦ **Dilocaine®** *see* Lidocaine *on page 531*
♦ **Dilomine® Injection** *see* Dicyclomine *on page 273*

## Diloxanide Furoate *(eye LOKS ah nide FYOOR oh ate)*
**Pharmacologic Class** Amebicide
**U.S. Brand Names** Furamide®
**Use** Treatment of amebiasis (asymptomatic cyst passers)

## Diltiazem *(dil TYE a zem)*
**Pharmacologic Class** Calcium Channel Blocker
**U.S. Brand Names** Cardizem® CD; Cardizem® Injectable; Cardizem® SR; Cardizem® Tablet; Cartia XT®; Dilacor™ XR; Tiamate®; Tiazac™
**Mechanism of Action** Inhibits calcium ion from entering the "slow channels" or select voltage-sensitive areas of vascular smooth muscle and myocardium during depolarization, producing a relaxation of coronary vascular smooth muscle and coronary vasodilation; increases myocardial oxygen delivery in patients with vasospastic angina

**Use**

Capsule: Essential hypertension (alone or in combination) - sustained release only; chronic stable angina or angina from coronary artery spasm

Injection: Atrial fibrillation or atrial flutter; paroxysmal supraventricular tachycardia (PSVT)

**Unlabeled use:** Prevention of reinfarction of non-Q-wave myocardial infarction, dyskinesia, and Raynaud's syndrome

**USUAL DOSAGE** Adults:

Angina: Oral: Usual starting dose: 30 mg 4 times/day; sustained release: 120-180 mg once daily; dosage should be increased gradually at 1- to 2-day intervals until optimum response is obtained. Doses up to 360 mg/day have been effectively used. Hypertension is controllable with single daily doses of sustained release products, or divided daily doses of regular release products, in the range of 240-360 mg/day

Sustained-release capsules:

**Cardizem® SR:** Initial: 60-120 mg twice daily; adjust to maximum antihypertensive effect (usually within 14 days); usual range: 240-360 mg/day

**Cardizem® CD, Tiazac™:** Hypertension: Total daily dose of short-acting administered once daily or initially 180 or 240 mg once daily; adjust to maximum effect (usually within 14 days); maximum: 480 mg/day; usual range: 240-360 mg/day

**Cardizem® CD:** Angina: Initial: 120-180 mg once daily; maximum: 480 mg once/day

**Dilacor™ XR:**

Hypertension: 180-240 mg once daily; maximum: 540 mg/day; usual range: 180-480 mg/day; use lower dose in elderly

Angina: Initial: 120 mg/day; titrate slowly over 7-14 days up to 480 mg/day, as needed

I.V. (requires an infusion pump): See table.

### Diltiazem — I.V. Dosage and Administration

| Initial Bolus Dose | 0.25 mg/kg actual body weight over 2 min (average adult dose: 20 mg) |
|---|---|
| **Repeat Bolus Dose**<br>May be administered after 15 min if the response is inadequate. | 0.35 mg/kg actual body weight over 2 min (average adult dose: 25 mg) |
| **Continuous Infusion**<br>Infusions >24 h or infusion rates >15 mg/h are not recommended. | Initial infusion rate of 10 mg/h; rate may be increased in 5 mg/h increments up to 15 mg/h as needed; some patients may respond to an initial rate of 5 mg/h. |

If Cardizem® injectable is administered by continuous infusion for >24 hours, the possibility of decreased diltiazem clearance, prolonged elimination half-life, and increased diltiazem and/or diltiazem metabolite plasma concentrations should be considered

**Conversion from I.V. diltiazem to oral diltiazem:** Start oral approximately 3 hours after bolus dose

**Oral dose (mg/day) is approximately equal to [rate (mg/hour) x 3 + 3] x 10**

3 mg/hour = 120 mg/day
5 mg/hour = 180 mg/day
7 mg/hour = 240 mg/day
11 mg/hour = 360 mg/day

**Dosing comments in renal/hepatic impairment:** Use with caution as extensively metabolized by the liver and excreted in the kidneys and bile

Dialysis: Not removed by hemo- or peritoneal dialysis; supplemental dose is not necessary

**Dosage Forms Cap, sustained release, as hydrochloride:** Cardizem® CD: 120 mg, 180 mg, 240 mg, 300 mg, Cardizem® SR: 60 mg, 90 mg, 120 mg, Dilacor™ XR: 180 mg, 240 mg, Tiazac™: 120 mg, 180 mg, 240 mg, 300 mg, 360 mg; **Inj, as hydrochloride:** 5 mg/mL (5 mL, 10 mL), Cardizem®: 5 mg/mL (5 mL, 10 mL); **Tab, as hydrochloride (Cardizem®):** 30 mg, 60 mg, 90 mg, 120 mg; **Tab, extended release, as hydrochloride (Tiamate®):** 120 mg, 180 mg, 240 mg

**Contraindications** Severe hypotension (<90 mm Hg systolic) or second and third degree heart block except with a functioning pacemaker; hypersensitivity to diltiazem; sick sinus syndrome, acute myocardial infarction, and pulmonary congestion

**Warnings/Precautions** Use with caution and titrate dosages for patients with hypotension or patients taking antihypertensives, impaired renal or hepatic function, or when treating patients with congestive heart failure. Use caution with concomitant therapy with beta-blockers or digoxin. Monitor LFTs during therapy since these enzymes may rarely be increased and symptoms of hepatic injury may occur; usually reverses with drug discontinuation; avoid abrupt withdrawal of calcium blockers since rebound angina is theoretically possible.

**Pregnancy Risk Factor** C

**Pregnancy Implications**

Clinical effects on the fetus: Teratogenic and embryotoxic effects have been demonstrated in small animals given doses 5-10 times the adult dose (mg/kg)

Breast-feeding/lactation: Freely diffuses into breast milk; however, the American Academy of Pediatrics considers diltiazem to be **compatible** with breast-feeding. Available evidence suggest safe use during breast-feeding.

(Continued)

## Diltiazem *(Continued)*

### Adverse Reactions
1% to 10% (generally well tolerated):
Cardiovascular: Bradycardia, A-V block (0.6% to 7.6%), EKG abnormality, peripheral edema, flushing
Central nervous system: Dizziness, headache
Gastrointestinal: Nausea
Neuromuscular & skeletal: Weakness
<1%: Congestive heart failure, tachycardia, angina, hypotension, palpitations, sleep disturbances, psychiatric disturbances, insomnia, nervousness, somnolence, urticaria, photosensitivity, alopecia, rash, petechiae, ecchymosis, anorexia, constipation, diarrhea, abnormal taste, dyspepsia, vomiting, abdominal cramps, xerostomia, micturition disorder, sexual difficulties, leukopenia, paresthesia, tremor, joint stiffness, amblyopia, retinopathy, tinnitus, nasal or chest congestion, shortness of breath

### Drug Interactions
CYP3A3/4 enzyme substrate; CYP1A2, 2D6, and 3A3/4 enzyme inhibitor
Decreased effect: Moricizine has decreased diltiazem concentrations and decreased its half-life
Increased toxicity:
Diltiazem has increased peak plasma moricizine levels and decreased oral clearance; side effect frequency increases
Diltiazem and amiodarone may cause increased bradycardia and decreased cardiac output
Diltiazem and cimetidine may cause increased bioavailability of diltiazem
Severe hypotension possible with concurrent administration with fentanyl
Both increased and decreased lithium levels have occurred with diltiazem; use caution with coadministration
Diltiazem and cyclosporine may cause increased cyclosporine levels and subsequent renal toxicity
Diltiazem and digoxin may cause increased digoxin levels and additive effects
Diltiazem and beta-blockers may result in increased cardiac depression
Theophylline effects possibly enhanced with diltiazem
Diltiazem with carbamazepine may result in increased carbamazepine levels and possible toxic effects

### Onset
Oral: 30-60 minutes (including sustained release)

### Half-Life
4-6 hours, may increase with renal impairment; 5-7 hours with sustained release

### Special PA Issues
Patient Education: Oral: Take as directed; do not alter dosage or discontinue therapy without consulting prescriber. Do not crush or chew extended release form. Avoid (or limit) alcohol and caffeine. You may experience dizziness or lightheadedness (use caution when driving or engaging in tasks that require alertness); nausea or vomiting (small frequent meals, frequent mouth care, or sucking on lozenges may help); constipation (increased exercise, dietary fiber, fruit, or fluid may help); diarrhea (buttermilk, boiled milk, or yogurt may help). Report chest pain, palpitations, irregular heartbeat, unusual cough, difficulty breathing, swelling of extremities, muscle tremors or weakness, confusion or acute lethargy, or skin rash.
Dietary Considerations: Alcohol: Avoid use
Monitoring Parameters: Liver function tests, blood pressure, EKG

### Related Information
Calcium Channel Blocking Agents *on page 1004*

- ◆ **Diltiazem Hydrochloride** *see* Diltiazem *on page 286*
- ◆ **Dimetane®-DC** *see* Brompheniramine, Phenylpropanolamine, and Codeine *on page 123*
- ◆ **Dimethoxyphenyl Penicillin Sodium** *see* Methicillin *on page 583*
- ◆ **β,β-Dimethylcysteine** *see* Penicillamine *on page 702*

## Dinoprostone *(dye noe PROST one)*

Pharmacologic Class Abortifacient; Prostaglandin
U.S. Brand Names Cervidil® Vaginal Insert; Prepidil® Vaginal Gel; Prostin E$_2$® Vaginal Suppository
Mechanism of Action A synthetic prostaglandin E$_2$ abortifacient that stimulates uterine contractions similar to those seen during natural labor

### Use
Gel: Promote cervical ripening prior to labor induction; usage for gel include any patient undergoing induction of labor with an unripe cervix, most commonly for pre-eclampsia, eclampsia, postdates, diabetes, intrauterine growth retardation, and chronic hypertension
Suppositories: Terminate pregnancy from 12th through 28th week of gestation; evacuate uterus in cases of missed abortion or intrauterine fetal death; manage benign hydatidiform mole

### USUAL DOSAGE
Abortifacient: Insert 1 suppository high in vagina, repeat at 3- to 5-hour intervals until abortion occurs up to 240 mg (maximum dose); continued administration for longer than 2 days is not advisable

Cervical ripening:
Gel:
Intracervical: 0.25-1 mg
Intravaginal: 2.5 mg
Suppositories: Intracervical: 2-3 mg

**Dosage Forms** Insert, vaginal (Cervidil®): 10 mg; Gel, vaginal: 0.5 mg in 3 g syringes [each package contains a 10-mm and 20-mm shielded catheter]; Supp, vaginal: 20 mg

**Contraindications**
Gel: Hypersensitivity to prostaglandins or any constituents of the cervical gel, history of asthma, contracted pelvis, malpresentation of the fetus
Gel: The following are "relative" contraindications and should only be considered by the physician under these circumstances: Patients in whom vaginal delivery is not indicated (ie, herpes genitalia with a lesion at the time of delivery), prior uterine surgery, breech presentation, multiple gestation, polyhydramnios, premature rupture of membranes
Suppository: Known hypersensitivity to dinoprostone, acute pelvic inflammatory disease, uterine fibroids, cervical stenosis

**Warnings/Precautions** Dinoprostone should be used only by medically trained personnel in a hospital; caution in patients with cervicitis, infected endocervical lesions, acute vaginitis, compromised (scarred) uterus or history of asthma, hypertension or hypotension, epilepsy, diabetes mellitus, anemia, jaundice, or cardiovascular, renal, or hepatic disease. Oxytocin should not be used simultaneously with Prepidil® (>6 hours of the last dose of Prepidil®).

**Pregnancy Risk Factor** X

**Adverse Reactions**
>10%:
Central nervous system: Headache
Gastrointestinal: Vomiting, diarrhea, nausea
1% to 10%:
Cardiovascular: Bradycardia
Central nervous system: Fever
Neuromuscular & skeletal: Back pain
<1%: Hypotension, cardiac arrhythmias, syncope, flushing, tightness of the chest, vasomotor and vasovagal reactions, dizziness, chills, pain, hot flashes, wheezing, dyspnea, coughing, bronchospasm, shivering

**Drug Interactions** Increased effect of oxytocics

**Onset** Onset of effect (uterine contractions): Within 10 minutes

**Duration** Up to 2-3 hours

**Special PA Issues**
**Patient Education:** Nausea and vomiting, cramping or uterine pain, or fever may occur. Report acute pain, respiratory difficulty, or skin rash. Closely monitor for vaginal discharge for several days. Report vaginal bleeding, itching, malodorous or bloody discharge, or severe cramping.

♦ **Diochloram** see Chloramphenicol on page 188
♦ **Diocto®** [OTC] see Docusate on page 298
♦ **Diocto-K®** [OTC] see Docusate on page 298
♦ **Dioctyl Calcium Sulfosuccinate** see Docusate on page 298
♦ **Dioctyl Potassium Sulfosuccinate** see Docusate on page 298
♦ **Dioctyl Sodium Sulfosuccinate** see Docusate on page 298
♦ **Diodoquin®** see Iodoquinol on page 487
♦ **Dioeze®** [OTC] see Docusate on page 298
♦ **Diomycin** see Erythromycin on page 329
♦ **Dionephrine** see Phenylephrine on page 718
♦ **Dioval® Injection** see Estradiol on page 332
♦ **Diovan™** see Valsartan on page 953
♦ **Diovan™ HCT** see Valsartan and Hydrochlorothiazide on page 954
♦ **Dipalmitoylphosphatidylcholine** see Colfosceril Palmitate on page 235
♦ **Dipentum®** see Olsalazine on page 674
♦ **Diphenacen-50® Injection** see Diphenhydramine on this page
♦ **Diphen® Cough** [OTC] see Diphenhydramine on this page
♦ **Diphenhist** [OTC] see Diphenhydramine on this page

# Diphenhydramine (dye fen HYE dra meen)

**Pharmacologic Class** Antihistamine

**U.S. Brand Names** AllerMax® Oral [OTC]; Banophen® Oral [OTC]; Belix® Oral [OTC]; Benadryl® Injection; Benadryl® Oral [OTC]; Benadryl® Topical; Ben-Allergin-50® Injection; Benylin® Cough Syrup [OTC]; Bydramine® Cough Syrup [OTC]; Compoz® Gel Caps [OTC]; Compoz® Nighttime Sleep Aid [OTC]; Dihydrex® Injection; Diphenacen-50® Injection; Diphen® Cough [OTC]; Diphenhist [OTC]; Dormarex® 2 Oral [OTC]; Dormin® Oral [OTC]; Genahist® Oral; Hydramyn® Syrup [OTC]; Hyrexin-50® Injection; Maximum Strength Nytol® [OTC]; Miles Nervine® Caplets [OTC]; Nordryl® Injection; Nordryl® Oral; Nytol® Oral [OTC]; (Continued)

## Diphenhydramine (Continued)

Phendry® Oral [OTC]; Siladryl® Oral [OTC]; Silphen® Cough [OTC]; Sleep-eze 3® Oral [OTC]; Sleepinal® [OTC]; Sleepwell 2-nite® [OTC]; Sominex® Oral [OTC]; Tusstat® Syrup; Twilite® Oral [OTC]; Uni-Bent® Cough Syrup; 40 Winks® [OTC]

**Mechanism of Action** Competes with histamine for $H_1$-receptor sites on effector cells in the gastrointestinal tract, blood vessels, and respiratory tract

**Use** Symptomatic relief of allergic symptoms caused by histamine release which include nasal allergies and allergic dermatosis; can be used for mild nighttime sedation; prevention of motion sickness and as an antitussive; has antinauseant and topical anesthetic properties; treatment of phenothiazine-induced dystonic reactions

### USUAL DOSAGE

Children:

Oral: (>10 kg): 12.5-25 mg 3-4 times/day; maximum daily dose: 300 mg

I.M., I.V.: 5 mg/kg/day or 150 mg/m²/day in divided doses every 6-8 hours, not to exceed 300 mg/day

Adults:

Oral: 25-50 mg every 6-8 hours

Nighttime sleep aid: 50 mg at bedtime

I.M., I.V.: 10-50 mg in a single dose every 2-4 hours, not to exceed 400 mg/day

Topical: For external application, not longer than 7 days

**Dosage Forms** Diphenhydramine hydrochloride: **Cap:** 25 mg, 50 mg; **Crm:** 1%, 2%; **Elix:** 12.5 mg/5 mL (5 mL, 10 mL, 20 mL, 120 mL, 480 mL, 3780 mL); **Inj:** 10 mg/mL (10 mL, 30 mL); 50 mg/mL (1 mL, 10 mL); **Lot:** 1% (75 mL); **Soln, top spray:** 1% (60 mL); **Syr:** 12.5 mg/5 mL (5 mL, 120 mL, 240 mL, 480 mL, 3780 mL); **Tab:** 25 mg, 50 mg

**Contraindications** Hypersensitivity to diphenhydramine or any component; should not be used in acute attacks of asthma

**Warnings/Precautions** Use with caution in patients with angle-closure glaucoma, peptic ulcer, urinary tract obstruction, hyperthyroidism; some preparations contain sodium bisulfite; syrup contains alcohol; diphenhydramine has high sedative and anticholinergic properties, so it may not be considered the antihistamine of choice for prolonged use in the elderly

**Pregnancy Risk Factor** C

### Adverse Reactions

>10%:

Central nervous system: Slight to moderate drowsiness

Respiratory: Thickening of bronchial secretions

1% to 10%:

Central nervous system: Headache, fatigue, nervousness

Gastrointestinal: Nausea, vomiting, diarrhea, abdominal pain, xerostomia, appetite increase, weight gain, dry mucous membranes

Neuromuscular & skeletal: Arthralgia

Respiratory: Pharyngitis

<1%: Hypotension, palpitations, edema, sedation, dizziness, paradoxical excitement, insomnia, depression, photosensitivity, rash, angioedema, urinary retention, hepatitis, myalgia, paresthesia, tremor, blurred vision, bronchospasm, epistaxis

**Drug Interactions** CYP2D6 enzyme substrate

Increased toxicity: CNS depressants worsens CNS and respiratory depression, monoamine oxidase inhibitors may increase anticholinergic effects; syrup should not be given to patients taking drugs that can cause disulfiram reactions (ie, metronidazole, chlorpropamide) due to high alcohol content

**Onset** Maximum sedative effect: 1-3 hours; I.V. more rapid

**Duration** 4-7 hours

**Half-Life** 2-8 hours; elderly: 13.5 hours

### Special PA Issues

**Patient Education:** Take as directed; do not exceed recommended dose. Avoid use of other depressants, alcohol, or sleep-inducing medications unless approved by prescriber. You may experience drowsiness or dizziness (use caution when driving or engaging in hazardous activity until response to medication is known); or dry mouth, nausea, or vomiting (frequent small meals, frequent mouth care, chewing gum, or sucking hard candy may help). Report persistent sedation, confusion, or agitation; changes in urinary pattern; blurred vision; sore throat, difficulty breathing, or expectorating (thick secretions); or lack of improvement or worsening or condition.

**Dietary Considerations:** Alcohol: Additive CNS effects, avoid use

**Reference Range:** Antihistamine effects at levels >25 ng/mL; drowsiness at levels 30-40 ng/mL; mental impairment at levels >60 ng/mL

Therapeutic: Not established; Toxic: >0.1 µg/mL

♦ **Diphenhydramine Hydrochloride** see Diphenhydramine on previous page

## Diphenoxylate and Atropine (dye fen OKS i late & A troe peen)

**Pharmacologic Class** Antidiarrheal

**U.S. Brand Names** Lofene®; Logen®; Lomanate®; Lomodix®; Lomotil®; Lonox®; Low-Quel®

**Mechanism of Action** Diphenoxylate inhibits excessive GI motility and GI propulsion; commercial preparations contain a subtherapeutic amount of atropine to discourage abuse

**Use** Treatment of diarrhea

**USUAL DOSAGE** Oral:

Children (use with caution in young children due to variable responses): Liquid: 0.3-0.4 mg of diphenoxylate/kg/day in 2-4 divided doses **or**

<2 years: Not recommended

2-5 years: 2 mg of diphenoxylate 3 times/day

5-8 years: 2 mg of diphenoxylate 4 times/day

8-12 years: 2 mg of diphenoxylate 5 times/day

Adults: 15-20 mg/day of diphenoxylate in 3-4 divided doses; maintenance: 5-15 mg/day in 2-3 divided doses

**Dosage Forms Soln, oral:** Diphenoxylate hydrochloride 2.5 mg and atropine sulfate 0.025 mg per 5 mL (4 mL, 10 mL, 60 mL); **Tab:** Diphenoxylate hydrochloride 2.5 mg and atropine sulfate 0.025 mg

**Contraindications** Hypersensitivity to diphenoxylate, atropine or any component; severe liver disease, jaundice, dehydrated patient, and narrow-angle glaucoma; it should not be used for children <2 years of age

**Warnings/Precautions** High doses may cause physical and psychological dependence with prolonged use; use with caution in patients with ulcerative colitis, dehydration, and hepatic dysfunction; reduction of intestinal motility may be deleterious in diarrhea resulting from *Shigella*, *Salmonella*, toxigenic strains of *E. coli*, and from pseudomembranous enterocolitis associated with broad spectrum antibiotics; children may develop signs of atropinism (dryness of skin and mucous membranes, thirst, hyperthermia, tachycardia, urinary retention, flushing) even at the recommended dosages; if there is no response with 48 hours, the drug is unlikely to be effective and should be discontinued; if chronic diarrhea is not improved symptomatically within 10 days at maximum dosage of 20 mg/day, control is unlikely with further use.

**Pregnancy Risk Factor** C

**Adverse Reactions**

1% to 10%:

Central nervous system: Nervousness, restlessness, dizziness, drowsiness, headache, mental depression

Gastrointestinal: Paralytic ileus, xerostomia

Genitourinary: Urinary retention and dysuria

Ocular: Blurred vision

Respiratory: Respiratory depression

<1%: Tachycardia, sedation, euphoria, hyperthermia Pruritus, urticaria, nausea, vomiting, abdominal discomfort, pancreatitis, stomach cramps, muscle cramps, weakness, diaphoresis (increased)

**Drug Interactions** Increased toxicity: MAO inhibitors (hypertensive crisis), CNS depressants, antimuscarinics (paralytic ileus); may prolong half-life of drugs metabolized in liver

**Onset** Onset of action: Within 45-60 minutes; Peak effect: Within 2 hours

**Duration** 3-4 hours

**Half-Life** Diphenoxylate: 2.5 hours

**Special PA Issues**

**Patient Education:** Take as directed; do not exceed recommended dosage. If no response within 48 hours, notify prescriber. Avoid alcohol or other prescriptive or OTC sedatives or depressants. You may experience drowsiness, blurred vision, impaired coordination; use caution when driving or performing hazardous tasks. Sucking on lozenges or chewing gum may reduce dry mouth. Report difficulty urinating, persistent diarrhea, respiratory difficulties, fever, or palpitations.

**Dietary Considerations:** Alcohol: Additive CNS effects, avoid use

**Monitoring Parameters:** Watch for signs of atropinism (dryness of skin and mucous membranes, tachycardia, thirst, flushing); monitor number and consistency of stools; observe for signs of toxicity, fluid and electrolyte loss, hypotension, and respiratory depression

♦ **Diphenylan Sodium®** *see* Phenytoin *on page 721*

♦ **Diphenylhydantoin** *see* Phenytoin *on page 721*

# Diphtheria and Tetanus Toxoid (dif THEER ee a & TET a nus TOKS oyd)

**Pharmacologic Class** Toxoid

**Use** Active immunity against diphtheria and tetanus when pertussis vaccine is contraindicated; tetanus prophylaxis in wound management

DT: Infants and children through 6 years of age

Td: Children and adults ≥7 years of age

**USUAL DOSAGE** I.M.:

Infants and Children (DT):

6 weeks to 1 year: Three 0.5 mL doses at least 4 weeks apart; administer a reinforcing dose 6-12 months after the third injection

(Continued)

## Diphtheria and Tetanus Toxoid *(Continued)*

1-6 years: Two 0.5 mL doses at least 4 weeks apart; reinforcing dose 6-12 months after second injection; if final dose is given after seventh birthday, use adult preparation

4-6 years (booster immunization): 0.5 mL; not necessary if all 4 doses were given after fourth birthday - routinely administer booster doses at 10-year intervals with the adult preparation

Children >7 years and Adults: Should receive Td; 2 primary doses of 0.5 mL each, given at an interval of 4-6 weeks; third (reinforcing) dose of 0.5 mL 6-12 months later; boosters every 10 years

### Tetanus Prophylaxis in Wound Management

| Number of Prior Tetanus Toxoid Doses | Clean, Minor Wounds | | All Other Wounds | |
|---|---|---|---|---|
| | Td* | TIG† | Td* | TIG† |
| Unknown or <3 | Yes | No | Yes | Yes |
| ≥3‡ | No# | No | No¶ | No |

*Adult tetanus and diphtheria toxoids; use pediatric preparations (DT or DTP) if the patient is <7 years old.

†Tetanus immune globulin.

‡If only three doses of fluid tetanus toxoid have been received, a fourth dose of toxoid, preferably an adsorbed toxoid, should be given.

#Yes, if >10 years since last dose.

¶Yes, if >5 years since last dose.

Adapted from Report of the Committee on Infectious Diseases, American Academy of Pediatrics, Elk Grove Village, IL: American Academy of Pediatrics, 1986.

**Dosage Forms Inj: Pediatric use:** Diphtheria 6.6 Lf units and tetanus 5 Lf units per 0.5 mL (5 mL); Diphtheria 10 Lf units and tetanus 5 Lf units per 0.5 mL (0.5 mL, 5 mL); Diphtheria 12.5 Lf units and tetanus 5 Lf units per 0.5 mL (5 mL); Diphtheria 15 Lf units and tetanus 10 Lf units per 0.5 mL (5 mL)

**Adult use:** Diphtheria 1.5 Lf units and tetanus 5 Lf units per 0.5 mL (0.5 mL, 5 mL); Diphtheria 2 Lf units and tetanus 5 Lf units per 0.5 mL (5 mL); Diphtheria 2 Lf units and tetanus 10 Lf units per 0.5 mL (5 mL)

**Contraindications** Patients receiving immunosuppressive agents, prior anaphylactic, allergic, or systemic reactions; hypersensitivity to diphtheria and tetanus toxoid or any component; acute respiratory infection or other active infection

**Warnings/Precautions** History of a neurologic reaction or immediate hypersensitivity reaction following a previous dose. History of severe local reaction (Arthus-type) following previous dose (such individuals should not be given further routine or emergency doses of tetanus and diphtheria toxoids for 10 years). Do not confuse pediatric DT with adult diphtheria and tetanus toxoid (Td); absorbed (Td) is used in patients >7 years of age; primary immunization should be postponed until the second year of life due to possibility of CNS damage or convulsion; have epinephrine 1:1000 available.

**Pregnancy Risk Factor** C

**Pregnancy Implications** Clinical effects on the fetus: Td and T vaccines are not known to cause special problems for pregnant women or their unborn babies. While physicians do not usually recommend giving any drugs or vaccines to pregnant women, a pregnant woman who needs Td vaccine should get it; wait until 2nd trimester if possible.

**Adverse Reactions** Severe adverse reactions must be reported to the FDA

>10%: Central nervous system: Fretfulness, drowsiness

1% to 10%:

Central nervous system: Persistent crying

Gastrointestinal: Anorexia, vomiting

<1%: Tachycardia, hypotension, edema, convulsions (rarely), pain, redness, urticaria, pruritus, tenderness, Arthus-type hypersensitivity reactions, transient fever

**Drug Interactions** Decreased effect with immunosuppressive agents, immunoglobulins if given within 1 month (eg, concomitant administration with tetanus immune globulin decreased the immune response to Td)

**Special PA Issues**

**Patient Education:** DT, Td and T vaccines cause few problems (mild fever or soreness, swelling, and redness/knot at the injection site); these problems usually last 1-2 days, but this does not happen nearly as often as with DTP vaccine

♦ **Diphtheria CRM₁₉₇ Protein Conjugate** *see Haemophilus* b Conjugate Vaccine *on page 432*

♦ **Diphtheria Toxoid Conjugate** *see Haemophilus* b Conjugate Vaccine *on page 432*

♦ **Dipivalyl Epinephrine** *see Dipivefrin on this page*

## Dipivefrin *(dye PI ve frin)*

**Pharmacologic Class** Alpha/Beta Agonist; Ophthalmic Agent, Antiglaucoma; Ophthalmic Agent, Vasoconstrictor

**U.S. Brand Names** AKPro® Ophthalmic; Propine® Ophthalmic

**Mechanism of Action** Dipivefrin is a prodrug of epinephrine which is the active agent that stimulates alpha- and/or beta-adrenergic receptors increasing aqueous humor outflow

**Use** Reduces elevated intraocular pressure in chronic open-angle glaucoma; also used to treat ocular hypertension, low tension, and secondary glaucomas

**USUAL DOSAGE** Adults: Ophthalmic: Instill 1 drop every 12 hours into the eyes

**Dosage Forms** Soln, ophth, as hydrochloride: 0.1% (5 mL, 10 mL, 15 mL)

**Contraindications** Hypersensitivity to dipivefrin, ingredients in the formulation, or epinephrine; contraindicated in patients with angle-closure glaucoma

**Warnings/Precautions** Use with caution in patients with vascular hypertension or cardiac disorders and in aphakic patients; contains sodium metabisulfite

**Pregnancy Risk Factor** B

**Adverse Reactions**

1% to 10%:
  Central nervous system: Headache
  Local: Burning, stinging
  Ocular: Ocular congestion, photophobia, mydriasis, blurred vision, ocular pain, bulbar conjunctival follicles, blepharoconjunctivitis, cystoid macular edema
<1%: Arrhythmias, hypertension

**Drug Interactions** Increased or synergistic effect when used with other agents to lower intraocular pressure

**Onset** Ocular pressure effect: Within 30 minutes; Mydriasis: May occur within 30 minutes

**Duration** Ocular pressure effect: ≥12 hours; Mydriasis: Several hours

**Special PA Issues**

**Patient Education:** For ophthalmic use only. Store away from light. Do not use discolored solution. Apply prescribed amount as often as directed. Wash hands before using and do not let tip of applicator touch eye or contaminate tip of applicator. Tilt head back and look upward. Gently pull down lower lid and put drop(s) in inner corner of eye. Close eye and roll eyeball in all directions. Do not blink for ½ minute. Apply gentle pressure to inner corner of eye for 30 seconds. Wipe away excess from skin around eye. Do not use any other eye preparation for at least 10 minutes. Do not touch tip of applicator to eye or contaminate tip of applicator. Do not share medication with anyone else. Temporary stinging or blurred vision may occur. May cause sensitivity to sunlight (wearing dark glasses may help). Report persistent eye pain, redness, burning, watering, dryness, double vision, puffiness around eye, vision disturbances, or other adverse eye response; worsening of condition or lack of improvement.

- **Dipivefrin Hydrochloride** see Dipivefrin on previous page
- **Diprivan®** see Propofol on page 772
- **Diprolene®** see Betamethasone on page 111
- **Diprolene® AF** see Betamethasone on page 111
- **Diprolene® Glycol [Dipropionate]** see Betamethasone on page 111
- **Dipropylacetic Acid** see Valproic Acid and Derivatives on page 952
- **Diprosone®** see Betamethasone on page 111

## Dipyridamole (dye peer ID a mole)

**Pharmacologic Class** Antiplatelet Agent; Vasodilator

**U.S. Brand Names** Persantine®

**Mechanism of Action** Inhibits the activity of adenosine deaminase and phosphodiesterase, which causes an accumulation of adenosine, adenine nucleotides, and cyclic AMP; these mediators then inhibit platelet aggregation and may cause vasodilation; may also stimulate release of prostacyclin or $PGD_2$; causes coronary vasodilation

**Use** Maintains patency after surgical grafting procedures including coronary artery bypass; used with warfarin to decrease thrombosis in patients after artificial heart valve replacement; used with aspirin to prevent coronary artery thrombosis; in combination with aspirin or warfarin to prevent other thromboembolic disorders. Dipyridamole may also be given 2 days prior to open heart surgery to prevent platelet activation by extracorporeal bypass pump and as a diagnostic agent in CAD; also approved as an alternative to exercise during Thallium myocardial perfusion imaging for the evaluation of coronary artery disease in patients who cannot exercise adequately

**USUAL DOSAGE**

Children: Oral: 3-6 mg/kg/day in 3 divided doses
  Doses of 4-10 mg/kg/day have been used investigationally to treat proteinuria in pediatric renal disease
  Mechanical prosthetic heart valves: Oral: 2-5 mg/kg/day (used in combination with an oral anticoagulant in children who have systemic embolism despite adequate oral anticoagulant therapy, and used in combination with low-dose oral anticoagulation (INR 2-3) plus aspirin in children in whom full-dose oral anticoagulation is contraindicated)
Adults:
  Oral: 75-400 mg/day in 3-4 divided doses
(Continued)

## Dipyridamole *(Continued)*

Evaluation of coronary artery disease: I.V.: 0.14 mg/kg/minute for 4 minutes; maximum dose: 60 mg

Hemodialysis: Significant drug removal is unlikely based on physiochemical characteristics

**Dosage Forms Inj:** 10 mg/2 mL; **Tab:** 25 mg, 50 mg, 75 mg

**Contraindications** Hypersensitivity to dipyridamole or any component

**Warnings/Precautions** Safety and effectiveness in children <12 years of age have not been established; may further decrease blood pressure in patients with hypotension due to peripheral vasodilation; use with caution in patients taking other drugs which affect platelet function or coagulation and in patients with hemostatic defects. Since evidence suggests that clinically used doses are ineffective for prevention of platelet aggregation, consideration for low-dose aspirin (81-325 mg/day) alone may be necessary; this will decrease cost as well as inconvenience.

**Pregnancy Risk Factor** B

**Adverse Reactions**

>10%:
Cardiovascular: Exacerbation of angina pectoris (I.V.), headache (I.V.)
Central nervous system: Dizziness

1% to 10%:
Cardiovascular: Hypotension, hypertension, tachycardia
Central nervous system: Headache
Dermatologic: Rash
Gastrointestinal: Abdominal distress
Respiratory: Dyspnea

<1%: Vasodilatation, flushing, syncope, edema, angina, migraine, diarrhea, vomiting, hepatic dysfunction, weakness, hypertonia, rhinitis, hyperventilation, allergic reaction, pleural pain

**Drug Interactions**

Increased toxicity: Heparin may increase anticoagulation
Decreased hypotensive effect (I.V.): Theophylline

**Half-Life** 10-12 hours

**Special PA Issues**

Patient Education: Oral: Take exactly as directed, with or without food. You may experience mild headache, transient diarrhea, or temporary dizziness (sit or lie down when taking medication). You may have a tendency to bleed easy; use caution with sharps, needles, or razors. Report chest pain, redness around mouth, acute abdominal cramping or severe diarrhea, acute and persistent headache or dizziness, rash, difficulty breathing, or swelling of extremities.

## Dirithromycin (dye RITH roe mye sin)

**Pharmacologic Class** Antibiotic, Macrolide

**U.S. Brand Names** Dynabac®

**Mechanism of Action** After being converted during intestinal absorption to its active form, erythromycylamine, dirithromycin inhibits protein synthesis by binding to the 50S ribosomal subunits of susceptible microorganisms

**Use** Treatment of mild to moderate upper and lower respiratory tract infections due to *Moraxella catarrhalis*, *Streptococcus pneumoniae*, *Legionella pneumophila*, or *S. pyogenes* ie, acute exacerbation of chronic bronchitis, secondary bacterial infection of acute bronchitis, community-acquired pneumonia, pharyngitis/tonsillitis, and uncomplicated infections of the skin and skin structure due to *Staphylococcus aureus*

**USUAL DOSAGE** Adults: Oral: 500 mg once daily for 5-14 days (14 days required for treatment of community-acquired pneumonia due to *Legionella*, *Mycoplasma*, or *S. pneumoniae*; 10 days is recommended for treatment of *S. pyogenes* pharyngitis/tonsillitis)

Dosing adjustment in renal impairment: None necessary
Dosing adjustment in hepatic impairment: None needed in mild dysfunction; not studied in moderate to severe dysfunction

**Dosage Forms Tab, enteric coated:** 250 mg

**Contraindications** Hypersensitivity to any macrolide or component of dirithromycin; use with pimozide

**Warnings/Precautions** Contrary to potential serious consequences with other macrolides (eg, cardiac arrhythmias), the combination of terfenadine and dirithromycin has not shown alteration of terfenadine metabolism; however, caution should be taken during coadministration of dirithromycin and terfenadine; pseudomembranous colitis has been reported and should be considered in patients presenting with diarrhea subsequent to therapy with dirithromycin

**Pregnancy Risk Factor** C

**Pregnancy Implications**

Clinical effects on the fetus: Animal studies indicate the use of dirithromycin during pregnancy should be avoided if possible
Breast-feeding/lactation: Use caution when administering to nursing women

## Adverse Reactions

1% to 10%:
Central nervous system: Headache, dizziness, vertigo, insomnia
Dermatologic: Rash, pruritus, urticaria
Endocrine & metabolic: Hyperkalemia
Gastrointestinal: Abdominal pain, nausea, diarrhea, vomiting, dyspepsia, flatulence
Hematologic: Thrombocytosis, eosinophilia, segmented neutrophils
Neuromuscular & skeletal: Weakness, pain, increased CPK
Respiratory: Increased cough, dyspnea

<1%: Palpitations, vasodilation, syncope, edema, anxiety, depression, somnolence, fever, malaise, dysmenorrhea, hypochloremia, hypophosphatemia, increased uric acid, dehydration, abnormal stools, anorexia, gastritis, constipation, abnormal taste, xerostomia, abdominal pain, mouth ulceration, polyuria, vaginitis, neutropenia, thrombocytopenia, decreased hemoglobin/hematocrit; increased alkaline phosphatase, bands, basophils; leukocytosis, monocytosis, Increased ALT/AST, GGT; hyperbilirubinemia, paresthesia, tremor, myalgia, amblyopia, tinnitus, increased creatinine, phosphorus, epistaxis, hemoptysis, hyperventilation, hypoalbuminemia, flu-like syndrome, diaphoresis, thirst

**Drug Interactions** CYP3A3/4 enzyme inhibitor
Increased effect: Absorption of dirithromycin is slightly enhanced with concomitant antacids and $H_2$-antagonists; dirithromycin may, like erythromycin, increase the effect of alfentanil, anticoagulants, bromocriptine, carbamazepine, cyclosporine, digoxin, disopyramide, ergots, methylprednisolone, cisapride, astemizole
Increased toxicity: Avoid use with pimozide (due to risk of significant cardiotoxicity) and triazolam
**Note:** Interactions with nonsedating antihistamines (eg, terfenadine, astemizole), cisapride, and theophylline are not known to occur, however, caution is advised with coadministration.

**Half-Life** 8 hours (range: 2-36 hours)

## Special PA Issues

**Patient Education:** Take with food or after meals around-the-clock. Do not chew, cut, or crush tablets. Take complete prescription even if you are feeling better. You may experience dizziness or drowsiness (use caution when driving or engaging in hazardous activities); nausea or vomiting (small frequent meals, frequent mouth care may help); constipation (increased exercise, dietary fiber, fruit, or fluid may help); or diarrhea (buttermilk, boiled milk, or yogurt may help). Report skin rash or itching, easy bruising or bleeding, unhealed sores of mouth, itching or vaginal discharge, fever or chills, unusual cough, muscle cramping or weakness, or palpitations or chest pain.

**Monitoring Parameters:** Temperature, CBC

- ♦ **Disalcid®** see Salsalate on page 820
- ♦ **Disalicylic Acid** see Salsalate on page 820
- ♦ **Discoloration of Feces and Urine Due to Drugs** see Chart on page 1126
- ♦ **Disodium Cromoglycate** see Cromolyn Sodium on page 240
- ♦ **d-Isoephedrine Hydrochloride** see Pseudoephedrine on page 780
- ♦ **Disonate®** [OTC] see Docusate on page 298

# Disopyramide (dye soe PEER a mide)

**Pharmacologic Class** Antiarrhythmic Agent, Class I-A

**U.S. Brand Names** Norpace®

**Mechanism of Action** Class IA antiarrhythmic: Decreases myocardial excitability and conduction velocity; reduces disparity in refractory between normal and infarcted myocardium; possesses anticholinergic, peripheral vasoconstrictive, and negative inotropic effects

**Use** Suppression and prevention of unifocal and multifocal premature, ventricular premature complexes, coupled ventricular tachycardia; effective in the conversion of atrial fibrillation, atrial flutter, and paroxysmal atrial tachycardia to normal sinus rhythm and prevention of the reoccurrence of these arrhythmias after conversion by other methods

**USUAL DOSAGE** Oral:
Children:
<1 year: 10-30 mg/kg/24 hours in 4 divided doses
1-4 years: 10-20 mg/kg/24 hours in 4 divided doses
4-12 years: 10-15 mg/kg/24 hours in 4 divided doses
12-18 years: 6-15 mg/kg/24 hours in 4 divided doses
Adults:
<50 kg: 100 mg every 6 hours or 200 mg every 12 hours (controlled release)
>50 kg: 150 mg every 6 hours or 300 mg every 12 hours (controlled release); if no response, may increase to 200 mg every 6 hours; maximum dose required for patients with severe refractory ventricular tachycardia is 400 mg every 6 hours

**Dosing adjustment in renal impairment:** 100 mg (nonsustained release) given at the following intervals: See table.
or alter the dose as follows:
$Cl_{cr}$ 30-<40 mL/minute: Reduce dose 50%
$Cl_{cr}$ 15-30 mL/minute: Reduce dose 75%
(Continued)

# Disopyramide *(Continued)*

### Disopyramide Phosphate

| Creatinine Clearance (mL/min) | Dosage Interval |
|---|---|
| 30-40 | q8h |
| 15-30 | q12h |
| <15 | q24h |

Dialysis: Not dialyzable (0% to 5%) by hemo- or peritoneal methods; supplemental dose not necessary

**Dosing interval in hepatic impairment:** 100 mg every 6 hours or 200 mg every 12 hours (controlled release)

**Dosage Forms** Disopyramide phosphate: **Cap:** 100 mg, 150 mg; **Cap, sustained action:** 100 mg, 150 mg

**Contraindications** Pre-existing second or third degree A-V block, cardiogenic shock, or known hypersensitivity to the drug; coadministration with sparfloxacin

**Warnings/Precautions** Pre-existing urinary retention, family history, or existing angle-closure glaucoma, myasthenia gravis, hypotension during initiation of therapy, congestive heart failure unless caused by an arrhythmias, widening of QRS complex during therapy or Q-T interval (>25% to 50% of baseline QRS complex or Q-T interval), sick-sinus syndrome or WPW, renal or hepatic impairment require decrease in dosage; disopyramide ineffective in hypokalemia and potentially toxic with hyperkalemia. Due to changes in total clearance (decreased) in elderly, monitor closely; the anticholinergic action may be intolerable and require discontinuation.

**Pregnancy Risk Factor** C

**Adverse Reactions**
>10%: Genitourinary: Urinary retention/hesitancy
1% to 10%:
Cardiovascular: Chest pains, congestive heart failure, hypotension
Endocrine & metabolic: Hypokalemia
Gastrointestinal: Stomach pain, bloating, xerostomia
Neuromuscular & skeletal: Muscle weakness
Ocular: Blurred vision
<1%: Syncope and conduction disturbances including A-V block, widening QRS complex and lengthening of Q-T interval, fatigue, malaise, nervousness, acute psychosis, depression, dizziness, headache, pain, generalized rashes, hypoglycemia, may initiate contractions of pregnant uterus, hyperkalemia may enhance toxicities, increased cholesterol and triglycerides, constipation, nausea, vomiting, diarrhea, flatulence, anorexia, weight gain, dry throat, hepatic cholestasis, elevated liver enzymes, dry eyes, dyspnea, dry nose

**Drug Interactions** CYP3A3/4 enzyme substrate
Decreased effect with hepatic microsomal enzyme-inducing agents (ie, phenytoin, phenobarbital, rifampin)
Increased effect/levels/toxicity with sparfloxacin; increased levels of digoxin
Increased effect/levels/toxicity with erythromycin; disopyramide levels when administered with erythromycin resulting in excessive QRS complex widening and/or prolongation of the Q-T interval

**Onset** 0.5-3.5 hours

**Duration** 1.5-8.5 hours

**Half-Life** 4-10 hours, increased half-life with hepatic or renal disease

**Special PA Issues**
**Patient Education:** Take as directed, at regular intervals around-the-clock. Do not alter dosage or discontinue therapy without consulting prescriber. Do not crush or chew extended release form. Avoid (or limit) alcohol and caffeine. You may experience dizziness or blurred vision (use caution when driving or engaging in tasks that require alertness); or dry mouth (frequent mouth care or sucking on lozenges may help). Report any change in urinary pattern or difficulty urinating; chest pain, palpitations, irregular heartbeat; unusual cough, difficulty breathing, swelling of extremities; muscle tremors or weakness; confusion or acute lethargy; or skin rash.
**Monitoring Parameters:** EKG, blood pressure, disopyramide drug level, urinary retention, CNS anticholinergic effects (confusion, agitation, hallucinations, etc)
**Reference Range:**
Therapeutic concentration: Atrial arrhythmias: 2.8-3.2 µg/mL; Ventricular arrhythmias 3.3-7.5 µg/mL
Toxic concentration: >7 µg/mL

♦ **Disopyramide Phosphate** *see* Disopyramide *on previous page*

♦ **Disotate®** *see* Edetate Disodium *on page 312*

♦ **Di-Spaz® Injection** *see* Dicyclomine *on page 273*

♦ **Di-Spaz® Oral** *see* Dicyclomine *on page 273*

♦ **Dispos-a-Med® Isoproterenol** *see Isoproterenol on page 496*

# Disulfiram (dye SUL fi ram)

**Pharmacologic Class** Aldehyde Dehydrogenase Inhibitor

**U.S. Brand Names** Antabuse®

**Mechanism of Action** Disulfiram is a thiuram derivative which interferes with aldehyde dehydrogenase. When taken concomitantly with alcohol, there is an increase in serum acetaldehyde levels. High acetaldehyde causes uncomfortable symptoms including flushing, nausea, thirst, palpitations, chest pain, vertigo, and hypotension. This reaction is the basis for disulfiram use in postwithdrawal long-term care of alcoholism.

**Use** Management of chronic alcoholism

**USUAL DOSAGE** Adults: Oral: Do not administer until the patient has abstained from alcohol for at least 12 hours

Initial: 500 mg/day as a single dose for 1-2 weeks; maximum daily dose is 500 mg

Average maintenance dose: 250 mg/day; range: 125-500 mg; duration of therapy is to continue until the patient is fully recovered socially and a basis for permanent self control has been established; maintenance therapy may be required for months or even years

**Dosage Forms Tab:** 250 mg, 500 mg

**Contraindications** Severe myocardial disease and coronary occlusion, hypersensitivity to disulfiram or any component, patient receiving alcohol, paraldehyde, alcohol-containing preparations like cough syrup or tonics

**Warnings/Precautions** Use with caution in patients with diabetes, hypothyroidism, seizure disorders, hepatic cirrhosis, or insufficiency; should never be administered to a patient when he/she is in a state of alcohol intoxication, or without his/her knowledge

**Pregnancy Risk Factor** C

**Adverse Reactions**

>10%: Central nervous system: Drowsiness

1% to 10%:

Central nervous system: Headache, fatigue, mood changes, neurotoxicity

Dermatologic: Rash

Gastrointestinal: Metallic or garlic-like aftertaste

Genitourinary: Impotence

<1%: Encephalopathy, hepatitis

**Disulfiram reaction with alcohol:** Flushing, diaphoresis, cardiovascular collapse, myocardial infarction, vertigo, seizures, headache, nausea, vomiting, dyspnea, chest pain, death

**Drug Interactions** CYP2C9 and 2E1 enzyme inhibitor, both disulfiram and diethyldithiocarbamate (disulfiram metabolite) are CYP3A3/4 enzyme inhibitors

Increased effect: Diazepam, chlordiazepoxide

Increased toxicity:

Alcohol and disulfiram: Antabuse® reaction

Tricyclic antidepressants, metronidazole, isoniazid: Encephalopathy

Phenytoin may increase serum levels and toxicity

Warfarin may increase prothrombin time

**Onset** Full effect: 12 hours

**Duration** May persist for 1-2 weeks after last dose

**Special PA Issues**

**Patient Education:** Tablets can be crushed or mixed with water or juice. Metallic aftertaste may occur; this will go away. Do not drink any alcohol, including products containing alcohol (cough and cold syrups), or use alcohol-containing skin products for at least 3 days and preferably 14 days after stopping this medication or while taking this medication. Drowsiness, tiredness, or visual changes may occur. Use care when driving or engaging in hazardous activity. Report yellow color in eyes or skin and any respiratory difficulty.

**Dietary Considerations:** Alcohol: Avoid use, including alcohol-containing products

♦ **Ditropan®** *see Oxybutynin on page 686*
♦ **Ditropan XL®** *see Oxybutynin on page 686*
♦ **Diuchlor®** *see Hydrochlorothiazide on page 447*
♦ **Diurigen®** *see Chlorothiazide on page 194*
♦ **Diuril®** *see Chlorothiazide on page 194*
♦ **Divalproex Sodium** *see Valproic Acid and Derivatives on page 952*
♦ **Dixarit®** *see Clonidine on page 225*
♦ **Dizac® Injectable Emulsion** *see Diazepam on page 269*
♦ **Dizmiss® [OTC]** *see Meclizine on page 559*
♦ **dl-Alpha Tocopherol** *see Vitamin E on page 963*
♦ **dl-Norephedrine Hydrochloride** *see Phenylpropanolamine on page 720*
♦ **D-Mannitol** *see Mannitol on page 557*
♦ **D-Med® Injection** *see Methylprednisolone on page 593*

## Dobutamine (doe BYOO ta meen)

**Pharmacologic Class** Adrenergic Agonist Agent; Sympathomimetic

**U.S. Brand Names** Dobutrex® Injection

**Mechanism of Action** Stimulates beta$_1$-adrenergic receptors, causing increased contractility and heart rate, with little effect on beta$_2$- or alpha-receptors

**Use** Short-term management of patients with cardiac decompensation

**USUAL DOSAGE** Administration requires the use of an infusion pump; I.V. infusion: See table.

### Infusion Rates of Various Dilutions of Dobutamine

| Desired Delivery Rate (mcg/kg/min) | Infusion Rate (mL/kg/min) | |
|---|---|---|
| | 250 mg/500 mL diluent (500 mcg/mL) | 500 mg/500 mL diluent (1 mg/mL) |
| 2.5 | 0.005 | 0.0025 |
| 5 | 0.01 | 0.005 |
| 7.5 | 0.015 | 0.0075 |
| 10 | 0.02 | 0.01 |
| 12.5 | 0.025 | 0.0125 |
| 15 | 0.03 | 0.015 |
| 20 | 0.04 | 0.02 |

Neonates: 2-15 mcg/kg/minute, titrate to desired response

Children and Adults: 2.5-20 mcg/kg/minute; maximum: 40 mcg/kg/minute, titrate to desired response

**Dosage Forms Inf, as hydrochloride:** 12.5 mg/mL (20 mL)

**Contraindications** Hypersensitivity to sulfites (commercial preparation contains sodium bisulfite); patients with idiopathic hypertrophic subaortic stenosis, atrial fibrillation or atrial flutter

**Warnings/Precautions** Hypovolemia should be corrected prior to use; infiltration causes local inflammatory changes, extravasation may cause dermal necrosis; use with extreme caution following myocardial infarction; potent drug, must be diluted prior to use

**Pregnancy Risk Factor** C

**Adverse Reactions**

>10%: Cardiovascular: Ectopic heartbeats, increased heart rate, chest pain, angina, palpitations, elevated blood pressure; in higher doses ventricular tachycardia or arrhythmias may be seen; patients with atrial fibrillation or flutter are at risk of developing a rapid ventricular response

1% to 10%:
Cardiovascular: Premature ventricular beats
Central nervous system: Headache
Gastrointestinal: Nausea, vomiting
Neuromuscular & skeletal: Mild leg cramps, paresthesia
Respiratory: Dyspnea, shortness of breath

**Drug Interactions**

Decreased effect: Beta-adrenergic blockers (increased peripheral resistance)

Increased toxicity: General anesthetics (ie, halothane or cyclopropane) and usual doses of dobutamine have resulted in ventricular arrhythmias in animals

**Onset** I.V.: 1-10 minutes; Peak effect: Within 10-20 minutes

**Half-Life** 2 minutes

**Special PA Issues**

**Patient Education:** When administered in emergencies, patient education should be appropriate to the situation. If patient is aware, instruct to promptly report chest pain, palpitations, rapid heartbeat, headache, nervousness, or restlessness, nausea or vomiting, or difficulty breathing.

**Monitoring Parameters:** Blood pressure, EKG, heart rate, CVP, RAP, MAP, urine output; if pulmonary artery catheter is in place, monitor CI, PCWP, and SVR; also monitor serum potassium

♦ **Dobutamine Hydrochloride** see Dobutamine on this page

♦ **Dobutrex® Injection** see Dobutamine on this page

## Docusate (DOK yoo sate)

**Pharmacologic Class** Stool Softener

**U.S. Brand Names** Colace® [OTC]; DC 240® Softgels® [OTC]; Dialose® [OTC]; Diocto® [OTC]; Diocto-K® [OTC]; Dioeze® [OTC]; Disonate® [OTC]; DOK® [OTC]; DOS® Softgel® [OTC]; D-S-S® [OTC]; Kasof® [OTC]; Modane® Soft [OTC]; Pro-Cal-Sof® [OTC]; Regulax SS® [OTC]; Sulfalax® [OTC]; Surfak® [OTC]

**Mechanism of Action** Reduces surface tension of the oil-water interface of the stool resulting in enhanced incorporation of water and fat allowing for stool softening

**Use** Stool softener in patients who should avoid straining during defecation and constipation associated with hard, dry stools; prophylaxis for straining (Valsalva) following myocardial infarction. A safe agent to be used in elderly; some evidence that doses <200 mg are ineffective; stool softeners are unnecessary if stool is well hydrated or "mushy" and soft; shown to be ineffective used long-term.

**USUAL DOSAGE** Docusate salts are interchangeable; the amount of sodium, calcium, or potassium per dosage unit is clinically insignificant

Infants and Children <3 years: Oral: 10-40 mg/day in 1-4 divided doses
Children: Oral:
   3-6 years: 20-60 mg/day in 1-4 divided doses
   6-12 years: 40-150 mg/day in 1-4 divided doses
Adolescents and Adults: Oral: 50-500 mg/day in 1-4 divided doses
Older Children and Adults: Rectal: Add 50-100 mg of docusate liquid to enema fluid (saline or water); administer as retention or flushing enema

**Dosage Forms Cap:** As calcium: DC 240® Softgels®, Pro-Cal-Sof®, Sulfalax®: 240 mg, Surfak®: 50 mg, 240 mg; **As potassium:** Diocto-K®: 100 mg, Kasof®: 240 mg; **As sodium:** Colace®: 50 mg, 100 mg, Dioeze®: 250 mg, Disonate®: 100 mg, 240 mg, DOK®: 100 mg, 250 mg, DOS® Softgel®: 100 mg, 250 mg, D-S-S®: 100 mg, Modane® Soft: 100 mg, Regulax SS®: 100 mg, 250 mg; **Liq, as sodium** (Diocto®, Colace®, Disonate®, DOK®): 150 mg/15 mL (30 mL, 60 mL, 480 mL); **Soln, oral, as sodium** (Doxinate®): 50 mg/mL with alcohol 5% (60 mL, 3780 mL); **Syr, as sodium:** 50 mg/15 mL (15 mL, 30 mL), Colace®, Diocto®, Disonate®, DOK®: 60 mg/15 mL (240 mL, 480 mL, 3780 mL); **Tab, as sodium** (Dialose®): 100 mg

**Contraindications** Concomitant use of mineral oil; intestinal obstruction, acute abdominal pain, nausea, vomiting; hypersensitivity to docusate or any component

**Warnings/Precautions** Prolonged, frequent or excessive use may result in dependence or electrolyte imbalance

**Pregnancy Risk Factor** C

**Adverse Reactions** 1% to 10%:
Gastrointestinal: Intestinal obstruction, diarrhea, abdominal cramping
Miscellaneous: Throat irritation

**Drug Interactions**
Decreased effect of Coumadin® with high doses of docusate
Increased toxicity with mineral oil, phenolphthalein

**Onset** 12-72 hours

**Special PA Issues**
Patient Education: Docusate should be taken with a full glass of water, milk, or fruit juice. Do not use if abdominal pain, nausea, or vomiting are present. Laxative use should be used for a short period of time (<1 week). Prolonged use may result in abuse, dependence, as well as fluid and electrolyte loss. Report bleeding or if constipation occurs.

♦ **Docusate Calcium** see Docusate on previous page
♦ **Docusate Potassium** see Docusate on previous page
♦ **Docusate Sodium** see Docusate on previous page
♦ **DOK® [OTC]** see Docusate on previous page
♦ **Doktors® Nasal Solution [OTC]** see Phenylephrine on page 718
♦ **Dolacet®** see Hydrocodone and Acetaminophen on page 449

# Dolasetron (dol A se tron)

**Pharmacologic Class** Selective 5-HT₃ Receptor Antagonist

**U.S. Brand Names** Anzemet®

**Mechanism of Action** Dolasetron is a pseudopelletierine-derived serotonin antagonist. Serotonin antagonists block the serotonin receptors in the chemoreceptor trigger zone and in the gastrointestinal tract. Once the receptor site is blocked, antagonism of vomiting occurs.

**Use** Prevention of nausea and vomiting associated with emetogenic cancer chemotherapy, including initial and repeat courses; prevention of postoperative nausea and vomiting and treatment of postoperative nausea and vomiting (injectable form only)

Agents with high emetogenic potential (>90%) (dose/m²):
   Amifostine
   Azacitidine
   Carmustine ≥200 mg/m²
   Cisplatin ≥50 mg/m²
   Cyclophosphamide ≥1 g/m²
   Cytarabine ≥1500 mg/m²
   Dacarbazine ≥500 mg/m²
   Dactinomycin
   Doxorubicin ≥60 mg/m²
   Lomustine ≥60 mg/m²
   Mechlorethamine
   Melphalan ≥100 mg/m²
(Continued)

## Dolasetron *(Continued)*

Streptozocin
Thiotepa ≥100 mg/m$^2$
**or** two agents classified as having high or moderately high emetogenic potential as listed:

Agents with moderately high emetogenic potential (60% to 90%) (dose/m$^2$):
Carboplatin 200-400 mg/m$^2$
Carmustine <200 mg/m$^2$
Cisplatin <50 mg/m$^2$
Cyclophosphamide 600-999 mg/m$^2$
Dacarbazine <500 mg/m$^2$
Doxorubicin 21-59 mg/m$^2$
Hexamethyl melamine
Ifosfamide ≥5000 mg/m$^2$
Lomustine <60 mg/m$^2$
Methotrexate ≥250 mg/m$^2$
Pentostatin
Procarbazine

### USUAL DOSAGE

Children <2 years: Not recommended for use
Nausea and vomiting associated with chemotherapy (including initial and repeat courses):
Children 2-16 years:
Oral: 1.8 mg/kg within 1 hour before chemotherapy; maximum: 100 mg/dose
I.V.: 1.8 mg/kg ~30 minutes before chemotherapy; maximum: 100 mg/dose
Adults:
Oral: 100 mg within 1 hour before chemotherapy
I.V.: 1.8 mg/kg ~30 minutes before chemotherapy or may give 100 mg
Prevention of postoperative nausea and vomiting:
Children 2-16 years:
Oral: 1.2 mg within 2 hours before surgery; maximum: 100 mg/dose
I.V.: 0.35 mg/kg (maximum: 12.5 mg) ~15 minutes before stopping anesthesia
Adults:
Oral: 100 mg within 2 hours before surgery
I.V.: 12.5 mg ~15 minutes before stopping anesthesia
Treatment of postoperative nausea and vomiting: I.V. only:
Children 2-16 years: 0.35 mg/kg as soon as needed
Adults: 12.5 mg as soon as needed
**Dosing adjustment for elderly, renal/hepatic impairment:** No dosage adjustment is recommended

**Dosage Forms** Dolasetron mesylate: **Inj:** 20 mg/mL; **Tab:** 50 mg, 100 mg

**Contraindications** Patients known to have hypersensitivity to the drug

**Warnings/Precautions** Dolasetron should be administered with caution in patients who have or may develop prolongation of cardiac conduction intervals, particularly QTc intervals. These include patients with hypokalemia or hypomagnesemia, patients taking diuretics with potential for inducing electrolyte abnormalities, patients with congenital Q-T syndrome, patients taking antiarrhythmic drugs or other drugs which lead to Q-T prolongation, and cumulative high-dose anthracycline therapy.

**Pregnancy Risk Factor** B

**Adverse Reactions** Dolasetron can cause electrocardiographic interval changes, which are related in frequency and magnitude to blood levels of the metabolite, hydrodolasetron

>2%:
Cardiovascular: Hypertension
Central nervous system: Headache, fatigue, dizziness, fever, chills and shivering
Gastrointestinal: Diarrhea, abdominal pain
Genitourinary: Urinary retention
Hepatic: Transient increases in liver enzymes

**Drug Interactions** CYP2D6 and 3A3/4 enzyme substrate
Blood levels of the active metabolite are increased when dolasetron is coadministered with cimetidine, decreased with rifampin. Clearance of hydrodolasetron decreases when dolasetron is given with atenolol.

**Half-Life** Dolasetron: <10 minutes; hydrodolasetron 7.3 hours

**Special PA Issues**
**Patient Education:** This drug is given to reduce the incidence of nausea and vomiting. You may experience headache or dizziness; request assistance when getting up or changing position. Report immediately unusual pain, chills, or fever; chest pain, palpitations, or tightness; swelling of throat or feeling of tightness in throat; or difficulty urinating.
**Monitoring Parameters:** Liver function tests, blood pressure and pulse, and EKG in patients with cardiovascular disease

♦ **Dolasetron Mesylate** *see* Dolasetron *on previous page*
♦ **Dolene®** *see* Propoxyphene *on page 773*
♦ **Dolobid®** *see* Diflunisal *on page 279*

♦ **Dolophine®** *see* Methadone *on page 579*

♦ **Dome Paste Bandage** *see* Zinc Gelatin *on page 975*

## Donepezil (don EH pa zil)

**Pharmacologic Class** Acetylcholinesterase Inhibitor (Central)

**U.S. Brand Names** Aricept®

**Mechanism of Action** Alzheimer's disease is characterized by cholinergic deficiency in the cortex and basal forebrain, which contributes to cognitive deficits. Donepezil reversibly and noncompetitively inhibits centrally-active acetylcholinesterase, the enzyme responsible for hydrolysis of acetylcholine. This appears to result in increased concentrations of acetylcholine available for synaptic transmission in the central nervous system.

**Use** Treatment of mild to moderate dementia of the Alzheimer's type

**USUAL DOSAGE** Adults: Initial: 5 mg/day at bedtime; may increase to 10 mg/day at bedtime after 4-6 weeks

**Dosage Forms Tab:** 5 mg, 10 mg

**Contraindications** Patients who are hypersensitive to donepezil or piperidine derivatives

**Warnings/Precautions** Use with caution in patients with sick sinus syndrome or other supraventricular cardiac conduction abnormalities, in patients with seizures or asthma; avoid use in nursing mothers

**Pregnancy Risk Factor** C

**Adverse Reactions**

>10%:

Central nervous system: Headache

Gastrointestinal: Nausea, diarrhea

1% to 10%:

Cardiovascular: Syncope, chest pain

Central nervous system: Fatigue, insomnia, dizziness, depression, abnormal dreams, somnolence

Dermatologic: Bruising

Gastrointestinal: Anorexia, vomiting, weight loss

Genitourinary: Polyuria

Neuromuscular & skeletal: Muscle cramps, arthritis, body pain

**Drug Interactions** CYP2D6 and 3A3/4 enzyme substrate

Increased effects of succinylcholine, cholinesterase inhibitors, or cholinergic agonists (bethanechol). Concomitant NSAIDs may increase the risk of gastrointestinal bleeding.

**Onset** May require extended treatment

**Duration** May be prolonged, particularly in older patients

**Half-Life** 70 hours

**Special PA Issues**

**Patient Education:** This medication will not cure the disease, but may help reduce symptoms. Use as directed; do not increase dose or discontinue without consulting prescriber. Maintain adequate hydration (2-3 L/day of fluids unless instructed to restrict fluid intake). May cause dizziness, sedation, or hypotension (rise slowly from sitting or lying position and use caution when driving or climbing stairs); vomiting or loss of appetite (frequent small meals, frequent mouth care, or sucking lozenges may help); or diarrhea (boiled milk, yogurt, or buttermilk may help). Report persistent abdominal discomfort; significantly increased salivation, sweating, tearing, or urination; flushed skin; chest pain or palpitations; acute headache; unresolved diarrhea; excessive fatigue, insomnia, dizziness, or depression; increased muscle, joint, or body pain; vision changes or blurred vision; or shortness of breath or wheezing.

♦ **Donnamar®** *see* Hyoscyamine *on page 463*

♦ **Donnapectolin-PG®** *see* Hyoscyamine, Atropine, Scopolamine, Kaolin, Pectin, and Opium *on page 465*

♦ **Donnapine®** *see* Hyoscyamine, Atropine, Scopolamine, and Phenobarbital *on page 464*

♦ **Donna-Sed®** *see* Hyoscyamine, Atropine, Scopolamine, and Phenobarbital *on page 464*

♦ **Donnatal®** *see* Hyoscyamine, Atropine, Scopolamine, and Phenobarbital *on page 464*

♦ **Dopamet®** *see* Methyldopa *on page 590*

## Dopamine (DOE pa meen)

**Pharmacologic Class** Adrenergic Agonist Agent; Sympathomimetic

**U.S. Brand Names** Intropin® Injection

**Mechanism of Action** Stimulates both adrenergic and dopaminergic receptors, lower doses are mainly dopaminergic stimulating and produce renal and mesenteric vasodilation, higher doses also are both dopaminergic and beta₁-adrenergic stimulating and produce cardiac stimulation and renal vasodilation; large doses stimulate alpha-adrenergic receptors

**Use** Adjunct in the treatment of shock which persists after adequate fluid volume replacement

**USUAL DOSAGE** I.V. infusion (administration requires the use of an infusion pump):

Neonates: 1-20 mcg/kg/minute continuous infusion, titrate to desired response

Children: 1-20 mcg/kg/minute, maximum: 50 mcg/kg/minute continuous infusion, titrate to desired response

(Continued)

## Dopamine *(Continued)*

> Adults: 1-5 mcg/kg/minute up to 50 mcg/kg/minute, titrate to desired response; infusion may be increased by 1-4 mcg/kg/minute at 10- to 30-minute intervals until optimal response is obtained
>
> If dosages >20-30 mcg/kg/minute are needed, a more direct-acting pressor may be more beneficial (ie, epinephrine, norepinephrine)
>
> **The hemodynamic effects of dopamine are dose-dependent:**
>> Low-dose: 1-3 mcg/kg/minute, increased renal blood flow and urine output
>>
>> Intermediate-dose: 3-10 mcg/kg/minute, increased renal blood flow, heart rate, cardiac contractility, and cardiac output
>>
>> High-dose: >10 mcg/kg/minute, alpha-adrenergic effects begin to predominate, vasoconstriction, increased blood pressure

**Dosage Forms Inf in D₅W:** 0.8 mg/mL (250 mL, 500 mL), 1.6 mg/mL (250 mL, 500 mL), 3.2 mg/mL (250 mL, 500 mL); **Inj:** 40 mg/mL (5 mL, 10 mL, 20 mL), 80 mg/mL (5 mL, 20 mL), 160 mg/mL (5 mL)

**Contraindications** Hypersensitivity to sulfites (commercial preparation contains sodium bisulfite); pheochromocytoma or ventricular fibrillation

**Warnings/Precautions** Safety in children has not been established; hypovolemia should be corrected by appropriate plasma volume expanders before administration; extravasation may cause tissue necrosis; potent drug, must be diluted prior to use; patient's hemodynamic status should be monitored; use with caution in patients with cardiovascular disease or cardiac arrhythmias or patients with occlusive vascular disease

**Pregnancy Risk Factor** C

**Adverse Reactions**
> >10%:
>> Cardiovascular: Ectopic heartbeats, tachycardia, vasoconstriction, hypotension, cardiac conduction abnormalities, widened QRS complex, ventricular arrhythmias
>>
>> Central nervous system: Headache
>>
>> Gastrointestinal: Nausea, vomiting
>>
>> Respiratory: Dyspnea
>
> 1% to 10%: Cardiovascular: Bradycardia, hypertension, gangrene of the extremities
>
> <1%: Vasoconstriction, anxiety, piloerection, azotemia, decreased urine output

**Drug Interactions** Increased effect: Dopamine's effects are prolonged and intensified by MAO inhibitors, alpha- and beta-adrenergic blockers, general anesthetics, phenytoin

**Onset** 5 minutes

**Duration** <10 minutes

**Half-Life** 2 minutes

**Special PA Issues**
> **Patient Education:** When administered in emergencies, patient education should be appropriate to the situation. If patient is aware, instruct to promptly report chest pain, palpitations, rapid heartbeat, headache, nervousness or restlessness, nausea or vomiting, or difficulty breathing.
>
> **Monitoring Parameters:** Blood pressure, EKG, heart rate, CVP, RAP, MAP, urine output; if pulmonary artery catheter is in place, monitor CI, PCWP, SVR, and PVR

- ◆ **Dopamine Hydrochloride** *see Dopamine on previous page*
- ◆ **Dopar®** *see Levodopa on page 524*
- ◆ **Dopram® Injection** *see Doxapram on next page*
- ◆ **Dormarex® 2 Oral [OTC]** *see Diphenhydramine on page 289*
- ◆ **Dormin® Oral [OTC]** *see Diphenhydramine on page 289*
- ◆ **Doryx®** *see Doxycycline on page 306*

## Dorzolamide *(dor ZOLE a mide)*

**Pharmacologic Class** Carbonic Anhydrase Inhibitor; Ophthalmic Agent, Antiglaucoma

**U.S. Brand Names** Trusopt®

**Mechanism of Action** Reversible inhibition of the enzyme carbonic anhydrase resulting in reduction of hydrogen ion secretion at renal tubule and an increased renal excretion of sodium, potassium, bicarbonate, and water to decrease production of aqueous humor; also inhibits carbonic anhydrase in central nervous system to retard abnormal and excessive discharge from CNS neurons

**Use** Lowers intraocular pressure to treat glaucoma in patients with ocular hypertension or open-angle glaucoma

**USUAL DOSAGE** Adults: Glaucoma: Instill 1 drop in the affected eye(s) 3 times/day

**Dosage Forms Soln, ophth, as hydrochloride:** 2%

**Contraindications** Hypersensitivity to any component of the product; contains benzalkonium chloride as a preservative

**Warnings/Precautions**
> Although administered topically, systemic absorption occurs. Same types of adverse reactions attributed to sulfonamides may occur with topical administration.

Because dorzolamide and its metabolite are excreted predominantly by the kidney, it is not recommended for use in patients with severe renal impairment ($Cl_{cr}$ <30 mL/minute); use with caution in patients with hepatic impairment

Local ocular adverse effects (conjunctivitis and lid reactions) were reported with chronic administration. Many resolved with discontinuation of drug therapy. If such reactions occur, discontinue dorzolamide.

There is a potential for an additive effect in patients receiving an oral carbonic anhydrase inhibitor and dorzolamide. The concomitant administration of dorzolamide and oral carbonic anhydrase inhibitors is not recommended.

Benzalkonium chloride is the preservative in dorzolamide which may be absorbed by soft contact lenses. Dorzolamide should not be administered while wearing soft contact lenses.

**Pregnancy Risk Factor** C

**Adverse Reactions**
>10%:
Gastrointestinal: Bitter taste following administration (25%)
Ocular: Burning, stinging or discomfort immediately following administration (33%); superficial punctate keratitis (10% to 15%); signs and symptoms of ocular allergic reaction (10%)
5% to 10% Ocular: Blurred vision, tearing, dryness, photophobia
<1%: Headache, fatigue, rashes, nausea, urolithiasis, weakness, iridocyclitis

**Drug Interactions** Increased toxicity: Salicylates use may result in carbonic anhydrase inhibitor accumulation and toxicity including CNS depression and metabolic acidosis

**Onset** Peak effect: 2 hours

**Duration** 8-12 hours

**Half-Life** Terminal RBC half-life of 147 days

**Special PA Issues**
**Patient Education:** For ophthalmic use only. Store at room temperature, do not use discolored solution. If you wear soft contact lenses, remove before using medication and wait at least 15 minutes before replacing. Apply prescribed amount as often as directed. Wash hands before using and do not touch tip of applicator to eye or contaminate tip of applicator. Tilt head back and look upward. Gently pull down lower lid and put drop(s) inside lower eyelid at inner corner. Close eye and roll eyeball in all directions. Do not blink for 1/2 minute. Apply gentle pressure to inner corner of eye for 30 seconds. Wipe away excess from skin around eye. Do not use any other eye preparation for at least 10 minutes. Do not share medication with anyone else. Temporary stinging or blurred vision may occur. May cause sensitivity to sunlight (wearing dark glasses may help). Report persistent eye pain, redness, burning, watering, dryness, double vision, puffiness around eye, vision disturbances, or other adverse eye response; worsening of condition or lack of improvement.

**Monitoring Parameters:** Monitor serum electrolyte levels (potassium) and blood pH levels; Ophthalmic exams and IOP periodically

♦ **Dorzolamide Hydrochloride** see Dorzolamide on previous page
♦ **DOSS** see Docusate on page 298
♦ **DOS® Softgel® [OTC]** see Docusate on page 298
♦ **Dostinex®** see Cabergoline on page 133
♦ **Dovonex®** see Calcipotriene on page 135

# Doxapram (DOKS a pram)

**Pharmacologic Class** Respiratory Stimulant; Stimulant

**U.S. Brand Names** Dopram® Injection

**Use** Respiratory and CNS stimulant; stimulates respiration in patients with drug-induced CNS depression or postanesthesia respiratory depression; in hospitalized patients with COPD associated with acute hypercapnia

**USUAL DOSAGE** Not for use in newborns since doxapram contains a significant amount of benzyl alcohol (0.9%)

Neonatal apnea (apnea of prematurity): I.V.:
Initial: 1-1.5 mg/kg/hour
Maintenance: 0.5-2.5 mg/kg/hour, titrated to the lowest rate at which apnea is controlled
Adults: Respiratory depression following anesthesia: I.V.:
Initial: 0.5-1 mg/kg; may repeat at 5-minute intervals; maximum total dose: 2 mg/kg
I.V. infusion: Initial: 5 mg/minute until adequate response or adverse effects seen; decrease to 1-3 mg/minute; usual total dose: 0.5-4 mg/kg; maximum: 300 mg
Hemodialysis: Not dialyzable

**Dosage Forms Inj, as hydrochloride:** 20 mg/mL (20 mL)

**Contraindications** Hypersensitivity to doxapram or any component; epilepsy, cerebral edema, head injury, severe pulmonary disease, pheochromocytoma, cardiovascular disease, hypertension, hyperthyroidism

**Pregnancy Risk Factor** B
(Continued)

## Doxapram *(Continued)*

**Onset** Respiratory stimulation begins: I.V.: Within 20-40 seconds; Peak effect: Within 1-2 minutes

**Duration** 5-12 minutes

**Half-Life** 3.4 hours (mean half-life)

**Special PA Issues**

**Patient Education:** This drug is generally used in an emergency. Teaching should be appropriate to patient education. Someone will be observing response at all times.

♦ **Doxapram Hydrochloride** *see* Doxapram *on previous page*

## Doxazosin (doks AYE zoe sin)

**Pharmacologic Class** Alpha₁ Blockers

**U.S. Brand Names** Cardura®

**Mechanism of Action** Competitively inhibits postsynaptic alpha-adrenergic receptors which results in vasodilation of veins and arterioles and a decrease in total peripheral resistance and blood pressure; approximately 50% as potent on a weight by weight basis as prazosin

**Use** Treatment of hypertension alone or in conjunction with diuretics, cardiac glycosides, ACE inhibitors or calcium antagonists (particularly appropriate for those with hypertension and other cardiovascular risk factors such as hypercholesterolemia and diabetes mellitus); treatment of urinary outflow obstruction and/or obstructive and irritative symptoms associated with benign prostatic hyperplasia (particularly useful in patients with troublesome symptoms who are unable or unwilling to undergo invasive procedures, but who require rapid symptomatic relief)

**USUAL DOSAGE** Oral:

Adults: 1 mg once daily in morning or evening; may be increased to 2 mg once daily; thereafter titrate upwards, if needed, over several weeks, balancing therapeutic benefit with doxazosin-induced postural hypotension; maximum dose for hypertension: 16 mg/day, for BPH: 8 mg/day

Elderly: Initial: 0.5 mg once daily

**Dosage Forms** Tab: 1 mg, 2 mg, 4 mg, 8 mg

**Contraindications** Hypersensitivity to doxazosin or any component

**Warnings/Precautions** Use with caution in patients with renal impairment. Can cause marked hypotension and syncope with sudden loss of consciousness with the first dose. Anticipate a similar effect if therapy is interrupted for a few days, if dosage is increased rapidly, or if another antihypertensive drug is introduced.

**Pregnancy Risk Factor** B

**Adverse Reactions**

>10%: Central nervous system: Dizziness

1% to 10%:

Cardiovascular: Palpitations, arrhythmia

Central nervous system: Vertigo, nervousness, somnolence, anxiety

Endocrine & metabolic: Decreased libido

Gastrointestinal: Nausea, vomiting, xerostomia, diarrhea, constipation

Neuromuscular & skeletal: Shoulder, neck, back pain

Ocular: Abnormal vision

Respiratory: Rhinitis

<1%: Hypotension, tachycardia, depression, abdominal discomfort, flatulence, incontinence, polyuria, conjunctivitis, tinnitus, dyspnea, sinusitis, epistaxis

**Drug Interactions**

Decreased effect with NSAIDs

Increased effect with diuretics and antihypertensive medications (especially beta-blockers)

**Onset** Peak serum concentration: 1-2 hours

**Duration** >24 hours

**Special PA Issues**

**Patient Education:** Take as directed, at bedtime. Do not skip dose or discontinue without consulting prescriber. Follow recommended diet and exercise program. Do not use OTC medications which may affect blood pressure (eg, cough or cold remedies, diet pills, stay-awake medications) without consulting prescriber. This medication may cause drowsiness, dizziness, or impaired judgment (use caution when driving or engaging in tasks that require alertness until response is known); postural hypotension (use caution when rising from sitting or lying position or when climbing stairs); or dry mouth or nausea (frequent mouth care or sucking lozenges may help). Report increased nervousness or depression; sudden weight gain (weigh yourself in the same clothes at same time of day once a week); unusual or persistent swelling of ankles, feet, or extremities; palpitations or rapid heartbeat; muscle weakness, fatigue, or pain; or other persistent side effects.

**Monitoring Parameters:** Blood pressure, standing and sitting/supine

## Doxepin (DOKS e pin)

**Pharmacologic Class** Antidepressant, Tricyclic (Tertiary Amine); Topical Skin Product

**U.S. Brand Names** Adapin® Oral; Sinequan® Oral; Zonalon® Topical Cream

**Mechanism of Action** Increases the synaptic concentration of serotonin and/or norepinephrine in the central nervous system by inhibition of their reuptake by the presynaptic neuronal membrane

**Use**

Oral: Treatment of various forms of depression, usually in conjunction with psychotherapy; treatment of anxiety disorders

**Unlabeled use:** Analgesic for certain chronic and neuropathic pain

Topical: Short-term (<8 days) management of moderate pruritus in adults with atopic dermatitis or lichen simplex chronicus

**USUAL DOSAGE**

Oral (entire daily dose may be given at bedtime):

Adolescents: Initial: 25-50 mg/day in single or divided doses; gradually increase to 100 mg/day

Adults: Initial: 30-150 mg/day at bedtime or in 2-3 divided doses; may gradually increase up to 300 mg/day; single dose should not exceed 150 mg; select patients may respond to 25-50 mg/day

**Dosing adjustment in hepatic impairment:** Use a lower dose and adjust gradually

Topical: Adults: Apply a thin film 4 times/day with at least 3- to 4-hour interval between applications

**Dosage Forms** Doxepin hydrochloride: **Cap:** 10 mg, 25 mg, 50 mg, 75 mg, 100 mg, 150 mg; **Conc, oral:** 10 mg/mL (120 mL); **Crm (Zonalon®):** 5% (30 g)

**Contraindications** Hypersensitivity to doxepin or any component (cross-sensitivity with other tricyclic antidepressants may occur); narrow-angle glaucoma

**Warnings/Precautions** Use with caution in patients with cardiovascular disease, conduction disturbances, seizure disorders, urinary retention, hyperthyroidism, or those receiving thyroid replacement; avoid use during lactation; use with caution in pregnancy; do not discontinue abruptly in patients receiving chronic high-dose therapy

**Pregnancy Risk Factor** C

**Adverse Reactions**

>10%:

Central nervous system: Sedation, drowsiness, dizziness, headache

Gastrointestinal: Xerostomia, constipation, increased appetite, nausea, unpleasant taste, weight gain

Neuromuscular & skeletal: Weakness

1% to 10%:

Cardiovascular: Hypotension, arrhythmias

Central nervous system: Confusion, delirium, hallucinations, nervousness, restlessness, parkinsonian syndrome, insomnia

Gastrointestinal: Diarrhea, heartburn

Genitourinary: Sexual dysfunction, dysuria

Neuromuscular & skeletal: Fine muscle tremors

Ocular: Blurred vision, eye pain

Miscellaneous: Diaphoresis (excessive)

<1%: Anxiety, seizures, alopecia, photosensitivity, breast enlargement, galactorrhea, SIADH, trouble with gums, decreased lower esophageal sphincter tone may cause GE reflux, urinary retention, testicular edema, agranulocytosis, leukopenia, eosinophilia, hepatitis, cholestatic jaundice and increased liver enzymes, increased intraocular pressure, tinnitus, allergic reactions

**Drug Interactions** CYP2D6 enzyme substrate

Decreased effect of bretylium, guanethidine, clonidine, levodopa; decreased effect with ascorbic acid, cholestyramine

Increased effect/toxicity of carbamazepine, amphetamines, thyroid preparations, sympathomimetics

Increased toxicity with fluoxetine (seizures), thyroid preparations, MAO inhibitors, albuterol, CNS depressants (ie, benzodiazepines, opiate analgesics, phenothiazines, alcohol), anticholinergics, cimetidine

**Onset** Peak antidepressant effect: Usually more than 2 weeks; anxiolytic effects may occur sooner

**Half-Life** 6-8 hours

**Special PA Issues**

**Patient Education:**

Oral: Take exactly as directed (do not increase dose or frequency); may take several weeks to achieve desired results; may cause physical and/or psychological dependence. Avoid excessive alcohol, caffeine, and other prescription or OTC medications not approved by prescriber. Maintain adequate hydration (2-3 L/day of fluids unless instructed to restrict fluid intake). You may experience drowsiness, lightheadedness, impaired coordination, dizziness, or blurred vision (use caution when driving or engaging in hazardous tasks until response to medication is known); constipation (increased exercise, fluids, or dietary fruit and fiber may help); urinary retention (void before taking medication); postural hypotension (use caution climbing stairs or when changing position from lying or sitting to standing); altered sexual drive or ability (reversible); or photosensitivity (use sunscreen, protective clothing, and avoid extended

(Continued)

## Doxepin *(Continued)*

exposure to direct sunlight). Report persistent CNS effects (eg, nervousness, restlessness, insomnia, anxiety, excitation, headache, agitation, impaired coordination, changes in cognition); muscle cramping, weakness, tremors, or rigidity; chest pain, palpitations, or irregular heartbeat; blurred vision or eye pain; yellowing of skin or eyes; or worsening of condition.

Topical: Use as directed. Apply in thin layer; do not overuse. Report increased skin irritation, worsening of condition or lack of improvement.

**Dietary Considerations:** Alcohol: Additive CNS effect, avoid use

**Monitoring Parameters:** Monitor blood pressure and pulse rate prior to and during initial therapy; monitor mental status, weight

**Reference Range:** Therapeutic: 30-150 ng/mL; Toxic: >500 ng/mL; utility of serum level monitoring is controversial

**Related Information**

Antidepressant Agents *on page 998*

- ◆ **Doxepin Hydrochloride** *see Doxepin on page 304*
- ◆ **Doxy**® *see Doxycycline on this page*
- ◆ **Doxychel**® *see Doxycycline on this page*
- ◆ **Doxycin** *see Doxycycline on this page*

## Doxycycline (doks i SYE kleen)

**Pharmacologic Class** Antibiotic, Tetracycline Derivative

**U.S. Brand Names** Atridox™; Bio-Tab® Oral; Doryx®; Doxy®; Doxychel®; Periostat™; Vibramycin®; Vibramycin® IV; Vibra-Tabs®

**Mechanism of Action** Inhibits protein synthesis by binding with the 30S and possibly the 50S ribosomal subunit(s) of susceptible bacteria; may also cause alterations in the cytoplasmic membrane

**Use** Principally in the treatment of infections caused by susceptible *Rickettsia*, *Chlamydia*, and *Mycoplasma* along with uncommon susceptible gram-negative and gram-positive organisms; alternative to mefloquine for malaria prophylaxis; treatment for syphilis in penicillin-allergic patients; often active against vancomycin-resistant enterococci; used for community-acquired pneumonia and other common infections due to susceptible organisms; sclerosing agent for pleural effusions

**USUAL DOSAGE** Oral, I.V.:

Children ≥8 years (<45 kg): 2-5 mg/kg/day in 1-2 divided doses, not to exceed 200 mg/day

Children >8 years (>45 kg) and Adults: 100-200 mg/day in 1-2 divided doses

Acute gonococcal infection: 200 mg immediately, then 100 mg at bedtime on the first day followed by 100 mg twice daily for 3 days **OR** 300 mg immediately followed by 300 mg in 1 hour

Primary and secondary syphilis: 300 mg/day in divided doses for ≥10 days

Uncomplicated chlamydial infections: 100 mg twice daily for ≥7 days

Endometritis, salpingitis, parametritis, or peritonitis: 100 mg I.V. twice daily with cefoxitin 2 g every 6 hours for 4 days and for ≥48 hours after patient improves; then continue with oral therapy 100 mg twice daily to complete a 10- to 14-day course of therapy

Sclerosing agent for pleural effusion injection: 500 mg as a single dose in 30-50 mL of NS or SWI

**Dosing adjustment in renal impairment:** Cl$_{cr}$ <10 mL/minute: 100 mg every 24 hours

Dialysis: Not dialyzable; 0% to 5% by hemo- and peritoneal methods or by continuous arteriovenous or venovenous hemofiltration (CAVH/CAVHD); no supplemental dosage necessary

**Dosage Forms**

Doxycycline calcium: **Syr (raspberry-apple flavor) (Vibramycin®):** 50 mg/5 mL (30 mL, 473 mL)

Doxycycline hyclate; **Cap:** (Periostat™): 20 mg, (Doxychel®, Vibramycin®): 50 mg, (Doxy®, Doxychel®, Vibramycin®): 100 mg; **Cap, coated pellets (Doryx®):** 100 mg; **Gel, for subgingival application** (Atridox™): 50 mg in each 500 mg of blended formulation; 2-syringe system contains doxycycline syringe (50 mg) and delivery system syringe (450 mg) along with a blunt cannula; **Powder for inj (Doxy®, Doxychel®, Vibramycin® IV):** 100 mg, 200 mg; **Tab:** (Doxychel®): 50 mg, (Bio-Tab®, Doxychel®, Vibra-Tabs®): 100 mg

Doxycycline monohydrate **Cap (Monodox®):** 50 mg, 100 mg; **Powder for oral susp (raspberry flavor) (Vibramycin®):** 25 mg/5 mL (60 mL)

**Contraindications** Hypersensitivity to doxycycline, tetracycline or any component; children <8 years of age; severe hepatic dysfunction

**Warnings/Precautions** Use of tetracyclines during tooth development may cause permanent discoloration of the teeth and enamel hypoplasia; prolonged use may result in superinfection; photosensitivity reaction may occur with this drug; avoid prolonged exposure to sunlight or tanning equipment. Do not administer to children ≤8 years of age.

**Pregnancy Risk Factor** D

**Adverse Reactions**

>10%: Miscellaneous: Discoloration of teeth in children

1% to 10%: Gastrointestinal: Esophagitis

<1%: Increased intracranial pressure, bulging fontanels in infants, rash, photosensitivity, nausea, diarrhea, neutropenia, eosinophilia, hepatotoxicity, phlebitis

**Drug Interactions** CYP3A3/4 enzyme substrate

Decreased effect with antacids containing aluminum, calcium, or magnesium

Iron and bismuth subsalicylate may decrease doxycycline bioavailability

Barbiturates, phenytoin, and carbamazepine decrease doxycycline's half-life

Increased effect of warfarin

**Half-Life** 12-15 hours (usually increases to 22-24 hours with multiple dosing); End-stage renal disease: 18-25 hours

**Special PA Issues**

**Patient Education:** Take as directed, for the entire prescription, even if you are feeling better. Avoid alcohol and maintain adequate hydration (2-3 L/day of fluids unless instructed to restrict fluid intake). You may be very sensitive to sunlight; use sunblock, wear protective clothing and eyewear, or avoid exposure to direct sunlight. You may experience lightheadedness, dizziness, or drowsiness (use caution when driving or engaging in hazardous activities); nausea or vomiting (small frequent meals, frequent mouth care may help); or diarrhea (buttermilk, boiled milk, or yogurt may help). If diabetic, drug may cause false tests with Clinitest® urine glucose monitoring; use of glucose oxidase methods (Clinistix®) or serum glucose monitoring is preferable. Report skin rash or itching, easy bruising or bleeding, yellowing of skin or eyes, pale stool or dark urine, unhealed sores of mouth, itching or vaginal discharge, fever or chills, or unusual cough.

# Dronabinol (droe NAB i nol)

**Pharmacologic Class** Antiemetic

**U.S. Brand Names** Marinol®

**Mechanism of Action** Not well defined, probably inhibits the vomiting center in the medulla oblongata

**Use** When conventional antiemetics fail to relieve the nausea and vomiting associated with cancer chemotherapy, AIDS-related anorexia

**USUAL DOSAGE** Oral:

Children: NCI protocol recommends 5 mg/m$^2$ starting 6-8 hours before chemotherapy and every 4-6 hours after to be continued for 12 hours after chemotherapy is discontinued

Adults: 5 mg/m$^2$ 1-3 hours before chemotherapy, then administer 5 mg/m$^2$/dose every 2-4 hours after chemotherapy for a total of 4-6 doses/day; dose may be increased up to a maximum of 15 mg/m$^2$/dose if needed (dosage may be increased by 2.5 mg/m$^2$ increments)

Appetite stimulant (AIDS-related): Initial: 2.5 mg twice daily (before lunch and dinner); titrate up to a maximum of 20 mg/day

**Dosage Forms Cap:** 2.5 mg, 5 mg, 10 mg

**Contraindications** Use only for cancer chemotherapy-induced nausea; should not be used in patients with a history of schizophrenia or in patients with known hypersensitivity to dronabinol or any component

**Warnings/Precautions** Use with caution in patients with heart disease, hepatic disease, or seizure disorders; reduce dosage in patients with severe hepatic impairment

**Pregnancy Risk Factor** B

**Adverse Reactions**

>10%: Central nervous system: Drowsiness, dizziness, detachment, anxiety, difficulty concentrating, mood change

1% to 10%:

Cardiovascular: Orthostatic hypotension, tachycardia

Central nervous system: Ataxia, depression, headache, vertigo, hallucinations, memory lapse

(Continued)

## Dronabinol *(Continued)*

Gastrointestinal: Xerostomia
Neuromuscular & skeletal: Paresthesia, weakness
<1%: Syncope, nightmares, speech difficulties, diarrhea, myalgia, tinnitus, diaphoresis

**Drug Interactions** CYP2C18 and 3A3/4 enzyme substrate
Increased toxicity (drowsiness) with alcohol, barbiturates, benzodiazepines

**Onset** Within 1 hour

**Half-Life** 19-24 hours

**Special PA Issues**

**Patient Education:** Take exactly as directed; do not increase dose or take more often than prescribed. Avoid all alcohol intake and any other CNS depressants. This drug may induce severe psychotic reactions and impair coordination and judgment; do not drive or engage in any activities which require alertness and motor coordination. You may experience mood changes (eg, euphoria, anxiety, depression, memory lapse), weakness or faintness, or dizziness or drowsiness (change position slowly). Report excessive bizarre thought patterns, inability to control behavior or thoughts, fainting, respiratory difficulties, or rapid heartbeat.

**Dietary Considerations:** Alcohol: Additive CNS effect, avoid use

**Monitoring Parameters:** CNS effects, heart rate, blood pressure

**Reference Range:** Antinauseant effects: 5-10 ng/mL

## Droperidol *(droe PER i dole)*

**Pharmacologic Class** Antiemetic

**U.S. Brand Names** Inapsine®

**Mechanism of Action** Alters the action of dopamine in the CNS, at subcortical levels, to produce sedation; reduces emesis by blocking dopamine stimulation of the chemotrigger zone

**Use** Tranquilizer and antiemetic in surgical and diagnostic procedures; antiemetic for cancer chemotherapy; preoperative medication; has good antiemetic effect as well as sedative and antianxiety effects

**USUAL DOSAGE** Titrate carefully to desired effect

Children 2-12 years:
Premedication: I.M.: 0.1-0.15 mg/kg; smaller doses may be sufficient for control of nausea or vomiting
Adjunct to general anesthesia: I.V. induction: 0.088-0.165 mg/kg
Nausea and vomiting: I.M., I.V.: 0.05-0.06 mg/kg/dose every 4-6 hours as needed

Adults:
Premedication: I.M.: 2.5-10 mg 30 minutes to 1 hour preoperatively
Adjunct to general anesthesia: I.V. induction: 0.22-0.275 mg/kg; maintenance: 1.25-2.5 mg/dose
Alone in diagnostic procedures: I.M.: Initial: 2.5-10 mg 30 minutes to 1 hour before; then 1.25-2.5 mg if needed
Nausea and vomiting: I.M., I.V.: 2.5-5 mg/dose every 3-4 hours as needed

**Dosage Forms Inj:** 2.5 mg/mL (1 mL, 2 mL, 5 mL, 10 mL)

**Contraindications** Hypersensitivity to droperidol or any component

**Warnings/Precautions** Safety in children <6 months of age has not been established; use with caution in patients with seizures, bone marrow suppression, or severe liver disease

Significant hypotension may occur, especially when the drug is administered parenterally; injection contains benzyl alcohol; injection also contains sulfites which may cause allergic reaction

Tardive dyskinesia: Prevalence rate may be 40% in elderly; development of the syndrome and the irreversible nature are proportional to duration and total cumulative dose over time. May be reversible if diagnosed early in therapy.

Extrapyramidal reactions are more common in elderly with up to 50% developing these reactions after 60 years of age. Drug-induced **Parkinson's syndrome** occurs often. **Akathisia** is the most common extrapyramidal reaction in elderly.

Increased confusion, memory loss, psychotic behavior, and agitation frequently occur as a consequence of anticholinergic effects

Orthostatic hypotension is due to alpha-receptor blockade, the elderly are at greater risk for orthostatic hypotension

Antipsychotic associated sedation in nonpsychotic patients is extremely unpleasant due to feelings of depersonalization, derealization, and dysphoria

Life-threatening arrhythmias have occurred at therapeutic doses of antipsychotics

**Pregnancy Risk Factor** C

**Pregnancy Implications**
Clinical effects on the fetus: Crosses the placenta
Breast-feeding/lactation: No data available

**Adverse Reactions**
>10%:
Cardiovascular: Mild to moderate hypotension, tachycardia
Central nervous system: Postoperative drowsiness

**1% to 10%:**
Cardiovascular: Hypertension
Central nervous system: Extrapyramidal reactions
Respiratory: Respiratory depression
<1%: Dizziness, chills, postoperative hallucinations, laryngospasm, bronchospasm, shivering

**Drug Interactions** Increased toxicity: CNS depressants, fentanyl and other analgesics increased blood pressure; conduction anesthesia decreased blood pressure; epinephrine decreased blood pressure; atropine, lithium

**Onset** Following parenteral administration: Peak effect: Within 30 minutes

**Duration** Following parenteral administration: 2-4 hours, may extend to 12 hours

**Half-Life** 2.3 hours

**Special PA Issues**
**Patient Education:** This drug may cause you to feel very sleepy; do not attempt to get up without assistance. Immediately report any difficulty breathing, confusion, loss of thought processes, or palpitations.
**Monitoring Parameters:** Blood pressure, heart rate, respiratory rate; observe for dystonias, extrapyramidal side effects, and temperature changes

# Droperidol and Fentanyl (droe PER i dole & FEN ta nil)
**Pharmacologic Class** Analgesic, Narcotic
**U.S. Brand Names** Innovar®
**Dosage Forms** Inj: Droperidol 2.5 mg and fentanyl 50 mcg per mL (2 mL, 5 mL)

- **Drotic® Otic** see Neomycin, Polymyxin B, and Hydrocortisone on page 645
- **Droxia™** see Hydroxyurea on page 460
- **Dr Scholl's Athlete's Foot [OTC]** see Tolnaftate on page 915
- **Dr Scholl's® Cracked Heel Relief Cream [OTC]** see Lidocaine on page 531
- **Dr Scholl's Maximum Strength Tritin [OTC]** see Tolnaftate on page 915
- **Drug-Drug Interactions With ACEIs** see Chart on page 997
- **Drugs in Pregnancy** see Chart on page 1127
- **DSCG** see Cromolyn Sodium on page 240
- **D-S-S® [OTC]** see Docusate on page 298
- **DSS** see Docusate on page 298
- **DT** see Diphtheria and Tetanus Toxoid on page 291
- **DTO** see Opium Tincture on page 677
- **Dull-C® [OTC]** see Ascorbic Acid on page 79
- **DuoCet™** see Hydrocodone and Acetaminophen on page 449
- **Duo-Cyp® Injection** see Estradiol and Testosterone on page 334
- **Duofilm® Solution** see Salicylic Acid and Lactic Acid on page 819
- **Duo-Medihaler® Aerosol** see Isoproterenol and Phenylephrine on page 497
- **Duo-Trach® see Lidocaine** on page 531
- **Duovisc® With Kit** see Chondroitin Sulfate-Sodium Hyaluronate on page 204
- **DuP 753** see Losartan on page 544
- **Duphalac®** see Lactulose on page 512
- **Durabolin® Injection** see Nandrolone on page 634
- **Duraclon® Injection** see Clonidine on page 225
- **Duradyne DHC®** see Hydrocodone and Acetaminophen on page 449
- **Dura-Estrin® Injection** see Estradiol on page 332
- **Durafuss-G®** see Guaifenesin on page 427
- **Duragen® Injection** see Estradiol on page 332
- **Duragesic® Transdermal** see Fentanyl on page 362
- **Duralone® Injection** see Methylprednisolone on page 593
- **Duramorph® Injection** see Morphine Sulfate on page 619
- **Duranest®** see Etidocaine on page 353
- **Duraphyl™** see Theophylline Salts on page 888
- **Duratest® Injection** see Testosterone on page 881
- **Duratestrin® Injection** see Estradiol and Testosterone on page 334
- **Durathate® Injection** see Testosterone on page 881
- **Dura-Vent/DA®** see Chlorpheniramine, Phenylephrine, and Methscopolamine on page 196
- **Duricef®** see Cefadroxil on page 159
- **Durrax®** see Hydroxyzine on page 462
- **Duvoid®** see Bethanechol on page 114
- **DV® Vaginal Cream** see Dienestrol on page 276
- **Dyazide®** see Hydrochlorothiazide and Triamterene on page 449
- **Dycill®** see Dicloxacillin on page 273
- **Dyclone®** see Dyclonine on next page

## Dyclonine (DYE kloe neen)

**Pharmacologic Class** Local Anesthetic; Local Anesthetic, Oral

**U.S. Brand Names** Dyclone®; Sucrets® [OTC]

**Mechanism of Action** Blocks impulses at peripheral nerve endings in skin and mucous membranes by altering cell membrane permeability to ionic transfer

**Use** Local anesthetic prior to laryngoscopy, bronchoscopy, or endotracheal intubation; use topically for temporary relief of pain associated with oral mucosa or anogenital lesions

**USUAL DOSAGE** Use the lowest dose needed to provide effective anesthesia

Children and Adults: Topical solution:

Mouth sores: 5-10 mL of 0.5% or 1% to oral mucosa (swab or swish and then spit) 3-4 times/day as needed; maximum single dose: 200 mg (40 mL of 0.5% solution or 20 mL of 1% solution)

Bronchoscopy: Use 2 mL of the 1% solution or 4 mL of the 0.5% solution sprayed onto the larynx and trachea every 5 minutes until the reflex has been abolished

**Dosage Forms Lozenges, as hydrochloride:** 1.2 mg, 3 mg; **Soln, top, as hydrochloride:** 0.5% (30 mL), 1% (30 mL)

**Contraindications** Contraindicated in patients allergic to chlorobutanol (preservative used in dyclonine) or dyclonine

**Warnings/Precautions** Use with caution in patients with sepsis or traumatized mucosa in the area of application to avoid rapid systemic absorption; may impair swallowing and enhance the danger of aspiration; use with caution in patients with shock or heart block; resuscitative equipment, oxygen, and resuscitative drugs should be immediately available when dyclonine topical solution is administered to mucous membranes; **not for injection or ophthalmic use**

**Pregnancy Risk Factor** C

**Adverse Reactions** <1%: Hypotension, bradycardia, respiratory arrest, cardiac arrest, excitation, drowsiness, nervousness, dizziness, seizures, slight irritation and stinging may occur when applied, blurred vision, allergic reactions

**Onset** Onset of local anesthesia: 2-10 minutes

**Duration** 30-60 minutes

**Special PA Issues**

**Patient Education:** This medication is given to reduce sensation in the injected area. When used in mouth or throat; do not eat or drink anything for at least 1 hour following treatment. Take small sips of water at first to ensure that you can swallow without difficulty. Your tongue and mouth may be numb - use caution to avoid biting yourself. Immediately report swelling of face, lips, tongue; chest pain or palpitations; increased restlessness, confusion, anxiety, or dizziness.

♦ **Dyclonine Hydrochloride** see Dyclonine on this page
♦ **Dyflos** see Isoflurophate on page 494
♦ **Dynabac®** see Dirithromycin on page 294
♦ **Dynacin® Oral** see Minocycline on page 610
♦ **DynaCirc®** see Isradipine on page 500
♦ **Dyna-Hex® Topical [OTC]** see Chlorhexidine Gluconate on page 190
♦ **Dynapen®** see Dicloxacillin on page 273
♦ **Dyrenium®** see Triamterene on page 930
♦ **E2020** see Donepezil on page 301
♦ **Ear-Eze® Otic** see Neomycin, Polymyxin B, and Hydrocortisone on page 645
♦ **Easprin®** see Aspirin on page 80
♦ **E-Base®** see Erythromycin on page 329

## Echinacea

**Mechanism of Action** Contains a caffeic acid glycoside named echinacoside (0.1% concentration) which is bactericidal. Other caffeic acid glycosides and isolutylamides associated with the plant can cause immune stimulation by increasing leukocyte phagocytosis and promoting T-cell activation. Also has an antihyaluronidase and anti-inflammatory activity; constituents have been associated with antitumor, antispasmodic effects

**Use** Prophylaxis and treatment of cold and flu; also used as an immunostimulant in herbal medicine; used to treat minor upper respiratory tract infections, urinary tract infections, wound/skin infections, arthritis, vaginal yeast infections

**USUAL DOSAGE** Continuous use should not exceed 8 weeks

Per Commission E: Expressed juice (of fresh herb): 6-9 mL/day
Capsule/tablet or tea form: 500 mg to 2 g 3 times/day
Liquid extract: 0.25-1 mL 3 times/day
Tincture: 1-2 mL 3 times/day
May be applied topically

**Contraindications** Autoimmune diseases, such as collagen vascular disease (Lupus, RA), multiple sclerosis; allergy to sunflowers, daisies, ragweed; tuberculosis, HIV, AIDS, pregnancy, breast-feeding; parenteral administration only contraindicated per Commission E; oral use of Echinacea not contraindicated during pregnancy by Commission E

**Warnings/Precautions** May alter immunosuppression; persons allergic to sunflowers may display cross-allergy potential

**Adverse Reactions** May become immunosuppressive with continuous use over 6-8 weeks
Gastrointestinal: Tingling sensation of tongue
Miscellaneous: Allergic reactions (rarely)
Per Commission E: None known for oral and external use

**Drug Interactions** Theoretically may alter response to immunosuppressive therapy

♦ **Echinacea angustifolia** see Echinacea on previous page

## Echothiophate Iodide (ek oh THYE oh fate EYE oh dide)

**Pharmacologic Class** Ophthalmic Agent, Antiglaucoma;  Ophthalmic Agent, Miotic

**U.S. Brand Names** Phospholine Iodide® Ophthalmic

**Mechanism of Action** Produces miosis and changes in accommodation by inhibiting cholinesterase, thereby preventing the breakdown of acetylcholine; acetylcholine is, therefore, allowed to continuously stimulate the iris and ciliary muscles of the eye

**Use** Reverse toxic CNS effects caused by anticholinergic drugs; used as miotic in treatment of open-angle glaucoma; may be useful in specific case of narrow-angle glaucoma; accommodative esotropia

**USUAL DOSAGE** Adults:
Ophthalmic: Glaucoma: Instill 1 drop twice daily into eyes with 1 dose just prior to bedtime; some patients have been treated with 1 dose daily or every other day
Accommodative esotropia:
Diagnosis: Instill 1 drop of 0.125% once daily into both eyes at bedtime for 2-3 weeks
Treatment: Use lowest concentration and frequency which gives satisfactory response, with a maximum dose of 0.125% once daily, although more intensive therapy may be used for short periods of time

**Dosage Forms Powder for reconstitution, ophth:** 1.5 mg [0.03%] (5 mL), 3 mg [0.06%] (5 mL), 6.25 mg [0.125%] (5 mL), 12.5 mg [0.25%] (5 mL)

**Contraindications** Hypersensitivity to echothiophate or any component; most cases of angle-closure glaucoma; active uveal inflammation or any inflammatory disease of the iris or ciliary body, glaucoma associated with iridocyclitis

**Warnings/Precautions** Tolerance may develop after prolonged use; a rest period restores response to the drug

**Pregnancy Risk Factor** C

**Adverse Reactions**
1% to 10%: Ocular: Stinging, burning eyes, myopia, visual blurring
<1%: Bradycardia, hypotension, flushing, nausea, vomiting, diarrhea, muscle weakness, retinal detachment, diaphoresis, browache, miosis, twitching eyelids, watering eyes, dyspnea

**Drug Interactions** Increased toxicity: Carbamate or organophosphate insecticides and pesticides; succinylcholine; systemic acetylcholinesterases may increase neuromuscular effects

**Onset** Miosis: 10-30 minutes; Intraocular pressure decrease: 4-8 hours; Peak intraocular pressure decrease: 24 hours

**Duration** Up to 1-4 weeks

**Special PA Issues**
Patient Education: For ophthalmic use only. Keep refrigerated, do not use discolored solution. Apply prescribed amount as often as directed. Wash hands before using and do not touch tip of applicator to eye or contaminate tip of applicator. Tilt head back and look upward. Gently pull down lower lid and put drop(s) inside lower eyelid at inner corner. Close eye and roll eyeball in all directions. Do not blink for ½ minute. Apply gentle pressure to inner corner of eye for 30 seconds. Wipe away excess from skin around eye. Do not use any other eye preparation for at least 10 minutes. Do not share medication with anyone else. Temporary stinging or blurred vision may occur (this should resolve in 5-7 days). Report systemic response (abdominal cramping or diarrhea, increased anxiety, or excess perspiration or salivation) or persistent eye pain, redness, burning, watering, dryness, double vision, puffiness around eye, vision disturbances or other adverse eye response, or worsening of ophthalmic condition or lack of improvement. If the benefits of this medication appear to wear off after time, contact prescriber; tolerance could develop which may necessitate a brief vacation from this medication.

♦ **E-Complex-600® [OTC]** see Vitamin E on page 963

## Econazole (e KONE a zole)

**Pharmacologic Class** Antifungal Agent, Topical

**U.S. Brand Names** Spectazole™ Topical

**Mechanism of Action** Alters fungal cell wall membrane permeability; may interfere with RNA and protein synthesis, and lipid metabolism

**Use** Topical treatment of tinea pedis (athlete's foot), tinea cruris (jock itch), tinea corporis (ringworm), tinea versicolor, and cutaneous candidiasis

**USUAL DOSAGE** Children and Adults: Topical:
(Continued)

## Econazole (Continued)

Tinea pedis, tinea cruris, tinea corporis, tinea versicolor: Apply sufficient amount to cover affected areas once daily

Cutaneous candidiasis: Apply sufficient quantity twice daily (morning and evening)

Duration of treatment: Candidal infections and tinea cruris, versicolor, and corporis should be treated for 2 weeks and tinea pedis for 1 month; occasionally, longer treatment periods may be required

**Dosage Forms Crm, as nitrate:** 1% (15 g, 30 g, 85 g)

**Contraindications** Known hypersensitivity to econazole or any component

**Warnings/Precautions** Discontinue drug if sensitivity or chemical irritation occurs; not for ophthalmic or intravaginal use

**Pregnancy Risk Factor** C

**Pregnancy Implications** Clinical effect on the fetus: Do not use during the 1st trimester of pregnancy, unless essential to a patient's welfare; use during the second and third trimesters only if clearly needed

**Adverse Reactions** 1% to 10%:

Dermatologic: Pruritus, erythema

Local: Burning, stinging

**Special PA Issues**

**Patient Education:** For external use only. Apply exactly as directed and for the length of time prescribed. Report if conditions worsens or persists or if infection occurs.

- ◆ **Econazole Nitrate** see Econazole on previous page
- ◆ **Econopred® Ophthalmic** see Prednisolone on page 752
- ◆ **Econopred® Plus Ophthalmic** see Prednisolone on page 752
- ◆ **Ecostatin®** see Econazole on previous page
- ◆ **Ecostigmine Iodide** see Echothiophate Iodide on previous page
- ◆ **Ecotrin® [OTC]** see Aspirin on page 80
- ◆ **Ecotrin® Low Adult Strength [OTC]** see Aspirin on page 80
- ◆ **Ed A-Hist® Liquid** see Chlorpheniramine and Phenylephrine on page 195
- ◆ **Edathamil Disodium** see Edetate Disodium on this page
- ◆ **Edecrin®** see Ethacrynic Acid on page 341

## Edetate Disodium (ED e tate dye SOW dee um)

**Pharmacologic Class** Antidote; Chelating Agent

**U.S. Brand Names** Chealamide®; Disotate®; Endrate®

**Mechanism of Action** Chelates with divalent or trivalent metals to form a soluble complex that is then eliminated in urine

**Use** Emergency treatment of hypercalcemia; control digitalis-induced cardiac dysrhythmias (ventricular arrhythmias)

**USUAL DOSAGE** Hypercalcemia: I.V.:

Children: 40-70 mg/kg/day slow infusion over 3-4 hours or more to a maximum of 3 g/24 hours; administer for 5 days and allow 5 days between courses of therapy

Adults: 50 mg/kg/day over 3 or more hours to a maximum of 3 g/24 hours; a suggested regimen of 5 days followed by 2 days without drug and repeated courses up to 15 total doses

**Dosage Forms Inj:** 150 mg/mL (20 mL)

**Contraindications** Severe renal failure or anuria

**Warnings/Precautions** Use of this drug is recommended only when the severity of the clinical condition justifies the aggressive measures associated with this type of therapy; use with caution in patients with renal dysfunction, intracranial lesions, seizure disorders, coronary or peripheral vascular disease

**Pregnancy Risk Factor** C

**Adverse Reactions**

Rapid I.V. administration or excessive doses may cause a sudden drop in serum calcium concentration which may lead to hypocalcemic tetany, seizures, arrhythmias, and death from respiratory arrest. Do not exceed recommended dosage and rate of administration.

1% to 10%: Gastrointestinal: Nausea, vomiting, abdominal cramps, diarrhea

<1%: Arrhythmias, transient hypotension, acute tubular necrosis, seizures, fever, headache, tetany, chills, eruptions, dermatologic lesions, hypomagnesemia, hypokalemia, anemia, thrombophlebitis, pain at the site of injection, paresthesia may occur, back pain, muscle cramps, nephrotoxicity, death from respiratory arrest

**Drug Interactions** Increased effect of insulin (edetate disodium may decrease blood glucose concentrations and reduce insulin requirements in diabetic patients treated with insulin)

**Half-Life** 20-60 minutes

**Special PA Issues**

**Patient Education:** Patient education and instruction will be determined by patient condition and ability to understand. You will require frequent blood tests and monitoring during this infusion. You must remain supine during infusion and for a period of time following treatment; change position slowly and ask for assistance if you must get up. Immediately report any difficulty breathing, chest pain, or irregular heartbeat; headache, abdominal cramps, chills, back pain, or muscle rigidity or cramping; or pain at injection/infusion site.

**Monitoring Parameters:** Cardiac function (EKG monitoring); blood pressure during infusion; renal function should be assessed before and during therapy; monitor calcium, magnesium, and potassium levels; cardiac monitor required

♦ **Edex™ Injection** *see* Alprostadil *on page 45*

# Edrophonium (ed roe FOE nee um)

**Pharmacologic Class** Antidote; Cholinergic Agonist; Diagnostic Agent, Myasthenia Gravis

**U.S. Brand Names** Enlon® Injection; Reversol® Injection; Tensilon® Injection

**Mechanism of Action** Inhibits destruction of acetylcholine by acetylcholinesterase. This facilitates transmission of impulses across myoneural junction and results in increased cholinergic responses such as miosis, increased tonus of intestinal and skeletal muscles, bronchial and ureteral constriction, bradycardia, and increased salivary and sweat gland secretions.

**Use** Diagnosis of myasthenia gravis; differentiation of cholinergic crises from myasthenia crises; reversal of nondepolarizing neuromuscular blockers; treatment of paroxysmal atrial tachycardia

**USUAL DOSAGE** Usually administered I.V., however, if not possible, I.M. or S.C. may be used:

Infants:

  I.M.: 0.5-1 mg

  I.V.: Initial: 0.1 mg, followed by 0.4 mg if no response; total dose = 0.5 mg

Children:

  Diagnosis: Initial: 0.04 mg/kg over 1 minute followed by 0.16 mg/kg if no response, to a maximum total dose of 5 mg for children <34 kg, or 10 mg for children >34 kg

  I.M.:

    <34 kg: 1 mg

    >34 kg: 5 mg

  Titration of oral anticholinesterase therapy: 0.04 mg/kg once given 1 hour after oral intake of the drug being used in treatment; if strength improves, an increase in neostigmine or pyridostigmine dose is indicated

Adults:

  Diagnosis:

    I.V.: 2 mg test dose administered over 15-30 seconds; 8 mg given 45 seconds later if no response is seen; test dose may be repeated after 30 minutes

    I.M.: Initial: 10 mg; if no cholinergic reaction occurs, administer 2 mg 30 minutes later to rule out false-negative reaction

  Titration of oral anticholinesterase therapy: 1-2 mg given 1 hour after oral dose of anticholinesterase; if strength improves, an increase in neostigmine or pyridostigmine dose is indicated

  Reversal of nondepolarizing neuromuscular blocking agents (neostigmine with atropine usually preferred): I.V.: 10 mg over 30-45 seconds; may repeat every 5-10 minutes up to 40 mg

  Termination of paroxysmal atrial tachycardia: I.V. rapid injection: 5-10 mg

  Differentiation of cholinergic from myasthenic crisis: I.V.: 1 mg; may repeat after 1 minute. **Note:** Intubation and controlled ventilation may be required if patient has cholinergic crisis

**Dosing adjustment in renal impairment:** Dose may need to be reduced in patients with chronic renal failure

**Dosage Forms Inj, as chloride:** 10 mg/mL (1 mL, 10 mL, 15 mL)

**Contraindications** Hypersensitivity to edrophonium or any component, GI or GU obstruction, hypersensitivity to sulfite agents

**Warnings/Precautions** Use with caution in patients with bronchial asthma and those receiving a cardiac glycoside; atropine sulfate should always be readily available as an antagonist. Overdosage can cause cholinergic crisis which may be fatal. I.V. atropine should be readily available for treatment of cholinergic reactions.

**Pregnancy Risk Factor** C

**Adverse Reactions**

  >10%:

    Gastrointestinal: Nausea, vomiting, diarrhea, excessive salivation, stomach cramps

    Miscellaneous: Diaphoresis (increased)

  1% to 10%:

    Genitourinary: Polyuria

    Ocular: Small pupils, lacrimation

    Respiratory: Increased bronchial secretions

  <1%: Bradycardia, A-V block, seizures, headache, drowsiness, dysphoria, weakness, muscle cramps, muscle spasms, thrombophlebitis, diplopia, miosis, laryngospasm, bronchospasm, respiratory paralysis, hypersensitivity, hyper-reactive cholinergic responses

(Continued)

## Edrophonium *(Continued)*

### Drug Interactions

Decreased effect: Atropine, nondepolarizing muscle relaxants, procainamide, quinidine

Increased effect: Succinylcholine, digoxin, I.V. acetazolamide, neostigmine, physostigmine

**Onset** I.M.: Within 2-10 minutes; I.V.: Within 30-60 seconds

**Duration** I.M.: 5-30 minutes; I.V.: 10 minutes

**Half-Life** 1.8 hours

♦ **Edrophonium Chloride** *see Edrophonium on previous page*

♦ **ED-SPAZ®** *see Hyoscyamine on page 463*

♦ **EDTA** *see Edetate Disodium on page 312*

♦ **E.E.S.®** *see Erythromycin on page 329*

## Efavirenz *(e FAV e renz)*

**Pharmacologic Class** Antiretroviral Agent, Reverse Transcriptase Inhibitor (Non-Nucleoside)

**U.S. Brand Names** Sustiva™

**Mechanism of Action** As a non-nucleoside reverse transcriptase inhibitor, efavirenz has activity against HIV-1 by binding to reverse transcriptase. It consequently blocks the RNA-dependent and DNA-dependent DNA polymerase activities including HIV-1 replication. It does not require intracellular phosphorylation for antiviral activity.

**Use** Treatment of HIV-1 infections in combination with at least two other antiretroviral agents. Also has some activity against hepatitis B virus and herpes viruses.

**USUAL DOSAGE** Oral: Dosing at bedtime is recommended to limit central nervous system effects; should not be used as single-agent therapy

Children: Dosage is based on body weight

10 kg to <15 kg: 200 mg once daily

15 kg to <20 kg: 250 mg once daily

20 kg to <25 kg: 300 mg once daily

25 kg to <32.5 kg: 350 mg once daily

32.5 kg to <40 kg: 400 mg once daily

≥40 kg: 600 mg once daily

Adults: 600 mg once daily

**Dosing adjustment in renal impairment:** None recommended

**Dosing comments in hepatic impairment:** Limited clinical experience, use with caution

**Dosage Forms Cap:** 50 mg, 100 mg, 200 mg

**Contraindications** Clinically significant hypersensitivity to any component of the formulation

**Warnings/Precautions** Do not use as single-agent therapy; avoid pregnancy; women of childbearing potential should undergo pregnancy testing prior to initiation of therapy; do not administer with other agents metabolized by cytochrome P-450 isoenzyme 3A4 including astemizole, cisapride, midazolam, triazolam or ergot alkaloids (potential for life-threatening adverse effects); history of mental illness/drug abuse (predisposition to psychological reactions); may cause depression and/or other psychiatric symptoms including impaired concentration, dizziness or drowsiness (avoid potentially hazardous tasks such as driving or operating machinery if these effects are noted); discontinue if severe rash (involving blistering, desquamation, mucosal involvement or fever) develops. Caution in patients with known or suspected hepatitis B or C infection (monitoring of liver function is recommended); hepatic impairment. Persistent elevations of serum transaminases >5 times the upper limit of normal should prompt evaluation - benefit of continued therapy should be weighed against possible risk of hepatotoxicity. Children are more susceptible to development of rash - prophylactic antihistamines may be used.

**Pregnancy Risk Factor** C

**Pregnancy Implications** Teratogenic effects have been observed in Primates receiving efavirenz. Pregnancy should be avoided. Women of childbearing potential should undergo pregnancy testing prior to initiation of efavirenz. Barrier contraception should be used in combination with other (hormonal) methods of contraception.

### Adverse Reactions

2% to 10%:

Central nervous system: Dizziness (2% to 10%), inability to concentrate (0% to 9%), insomnia (0% to 7%), headache (5% to 6%) abnormal dreams (0% to 4%), somnolence (0% to 3%), depression (0% to 2%), anorexia (0% to 5%), nervousness (0% to 2%), fatigue (2% to 7%), hypoesthesia (1% to 2%)

Dermatologic: Rash (5% to 20%), pruritus (0% to 2%)

Gastrointestinal: Nausea (0% to 12%), vomiting (0% to 7%), diarrhea (2% to 12%), dyspepsia (0% to 4%), elevated transaminases (2% to 3%), abdominal pain (0% to 3%)

Miscellaneous: Increased sweating (0% to 2%)

<2%: Edema (peripheral), syncope, flushing, palpitations, tachycardia, fever, pain, malaise, ataxia, depression, seizures, hallucinations, psychosis, depersonalization, amnesia, anxiety, apathy, emotional lability, agitation, confusion, euphoria, impaired coordination, migraine, speech disorder, vertigo, alopecia, eczema, folliculitis, skin exfoliation, urticaria,

increased cholesterol and triglycerides, hot flashes, pancreatitis, dry mouth, taste disturbance, flatulence, renal calculus, hematuria, hepatitis, thrombophlebitis, asthenia, neuralgia, paresthesia, peripheral neuropathy, tremor, arthralgia, myalgia, abnormal vision, diplopia, tinnitus, asthma, alcohol intolerance, allergic reaction, parosmia

Pediatric patients: Rash (40%), diarrhea (39%), fever (26%), cough (25%), nausea/vomiting (16%), central nervous system reactions (9%)

**Drug Interactions**

Increased effect: CYP3A4, 2C9, 2C19 inhibitor; CYP3A4 inducer; coadministration with medications metabolized by these enzymes may lead to increased concentration-related effects. Astemizole, cisapride, midazolam, triazolam and ergot alkaloids may result in life-threatening toxicities. The AUC of nelfinavir is increased (20%); AUC of both ritonavir and efavirenz are increased by 20% during concurrent therapy. The AUC of ethinyl estradiol is increased 37% by efavirenz (clinical significance unknown). May increase effect of warfarin.

Decreased effect: Other inducers of this enzyme (including phenobarbital, rifampin and rifabutin) may decrease serum concentrations of efavirenz. Concentrations of indinavir may be reduced; dosage increase to 1000 mg 3 times/day is recommended. Concentrations of saquinavir may be decreased (use as sole protease inhibitor is not recommended). Plasma concentrations of clarithromycin are decreased (clinical significance unknown). May decrease effect of warfarin.

**Half-Life** Single dose: 52-76 hours; after multiple doses: 40-55 hours

**Special PA Issues**

**Patient Education:** Efavirenz is not a cure for HIV, nor will it reduce transmission of HIV. Take as directed (usually at bedtime to reduce CNS effects), with or without food. Do not alter dose or discontinue without consulting prescriber. Avoid high fat meals when taking this medication. Maintain adequate hydration (2-3 L/day of fluids unless instructed to restrict fluid intake). Avoid excessive alcohol (severe reaction), prescription, and OTC sedatives unless consulting prescriber. You may experience dry mouth, taste disturbances, nausea, or vomiting (small frequent meals or sucking hard candy may help - consult prescriber if nausea or vomiting persists); diarrhea (buttermilk, boiled milk, or yogurt may help); or dizziness, anxiety, tremor, impaired coordination (use caution when driving or engaging in hazardous tasks until response to drug is known). Report CNS changes (acute headache, abnormal dreams, sleepiness or fatigue, seizures, hallucinations, amnesia, emotional lability, confusion); sense of fullness or ringing in ears; vision changes or double vision; muscle pain, weakness, tremors, numbness, spasticity, or change in gait; skin rash or irritation; chest pain or palpitations; or other unusual effects related to this medication.

**Dietary Considerations:** May be taken with or without food. Avoid high-fat meals when taking this medication. High-fat meals increase the absorption of efavirenz.

**Monitoring Parameters:** Serum transaminases (discontinuation of treatment should be considered for persistent elevations greater than five times the upper limit of normal), cholesterol, triglycerides, signs and symptoms of infection

♦ **Effer-K™** see Potassium Bicarbonate and Potassium Citrate, Effervescent on page 741

♦ **Effer-Syllium® [OTC]** see Psyllium on page 781

♦ **Effexor®** see Venlafaxine on page 958

♦ **Effexor® XR** see Venlafaxine on page 958

♦ **Efidac/24® [OTC]** see Pseudoephedrine on page 780

# Eflornithine (ee FLOR ni theen)

**Pharmacologic Class** Antiprotozoal

**U.S. Brand Names** Ornidyl®

**Mechanism of Action** Eflornithine exerts antitumor and antiprotozoal effects through specific, irreversible ("suicide") inhibition of the enzyme ornithine decarboxylase (ODC). ODC is the rate-limiting enzyme in the biosynthesis of putrescine, spermine, and spermidine, the major polyamines in nucleated cells. Polyamines are necessary for the synthesis of DNA, RNA, and proteins and are, therefore, necessary for cell growth and differentiation. Although many microorganisms and higher plants are able to produce polyamines from alternate biochemical pathways, all mammalian cells depend on ornithine decarboxylase to produce polyamines. Eflornithine inhibits ODC and rapidly depletes animal cells of putrescine and spermidine; the concentration of spermine remains the same or may even increase. Rapidly dividing cells appear to most susceptible to the effects of eflornithine.

**Use** Treatment of meningoencephalitic stage of *Trypanosoma brucei gambiense* infection (sleeping sickness)

**USUAL DOSAGE** Adults: I.V. infusion: 100 mg/kg/dose given every 6 hours (over at least 45 minutes) for 14 days

**Dosing adjustment in renal impairment:** Dose should be adjusted although no specific guidelines are available

**Dosage Forms Inj, as hydrochloride:** 200 mg/mL (100 mL)

**Contraindications** Hypersensitivity to eflornithine or any component

(Continued)

## Eflornithine *(Continued)*

**Warnings/Precautions** Must be diluted before use; frequent monitoring for myelosuppression should be done; use with caution in patients with a history of seizures and in patients with renal impairment; serial audiograms should be obtained; due to the potential for relapse, patients should be followed up for at least 24 months

**Pregnancy Risk Factor** C

**Adverse Reactions**

>10%: Hematologic (reversible): Anemia (55%), leukopenia (37%), thrombocytopenia (14%)

1% to 10%:

Central nervous system: Seizures (may be due to the disease) (8%), dizziness

Dermatologic: Alopecia

Gastrointestinal: Vomiting, diarrhea

Hematologic: Eosinophilia

Otic: Hearing impairment

<1%: Facial edema, headache, abdominal pain, anorexia, weakness

**Special PA Issues**

**Patient Education:** Report any persistent or unusual fever, sore throat, fatigue, bleeding, or bruising; frequent blood tests are needed during therapy

**Monitoring Parameters:** CBC with platelet counts

- **Eflornithine Hydrochloride** *see Eflornithine on previous page*
- **Efodine®** [OTC] *see Povidone-Iodine on page 747*
- **Efudex® Topical** *see Fluorouracil on page 384*
- **EHDP** *see Etidronate Disodium on page 354*
- **Elase-Chloromycetin® Topical** *see Fibrinolysin and Desoxyribonuclease on page 369*
- **Elase® Topical** *see Fibrinolysin and Desoxyribonuclease on page 369*
- **Elavil®** *see Amitriptyline on page 57*
- **Eldecort®** *see Hydrocortisone on page 453*
- **Eldepryl®** *see Selegiline on page 826*
- **Eldercaps® [OTC]** *see Vitamins, Multiple on page 964*
- **Eldopaque® [OTC]** *see Hydroquinone on page 457*
- **Eldopaque Forte®** *see Hydroquinone on page 457*
- **Eldoquin® [OTC]** *see Hydroquinone on page 457*
- **Eldoquin® Forte®** *see Hydroquinone on page 457*
- **Electrolyte Lavage Solution** *see Polyethylene Glycol-Electrolyte Solution on page 736*
- **Elimite™ Cream** *see Permethrin on page 712*
- **Elixophyllin®** *see Theophylline Salts on page 888*
- **Elixophyllin® SR** *see Theophylline Salts on page 888*
- **Elocom** *see Mometasone Furoate on page 617*
- **Elocon® Topical** *see Mometasone Furoate on page 617*
- **Eltor®** *see Pseudoephedrine on page 780*
- **Eltroxin®** *see Levothyroxine on page 529*
- **Embeline E® Emollient Cream** *see Clobetasol on page 219*
- **Emcyt®** *see Estramustine on page 334*
- **Eminase®** *see Anistreplase on page 71*
- **EMLA®** *see Lidocaine and Prilocaine on page 533*
- **Empirin® [OTC]** *see Aspirin on page 80*
- **Empirin® With Codeine** *see Aspirin and Codeine on page 82*
- **Empracet® 30, 60** *see Acetaminophen and Codeine on page 22*
- **Emtec-30®** *see Acetaminophen and Codeine on page 22*
- **E-Mycin®** *see Erythromycin on page 329*

## Enalapril *(e NAL a pril)*

**Pharmacologic Class** Angiotensin-Converting Enzyme (ACE) Inhibitors

**U.S. Brand Names** Vasotec®; Vasotec® I.V.

**Mechanism of Action** Competitive inhibitor of angiotensin-converting enzyme (ACE); prevents conversion of angiotensin I to angiotensin II, a potent vasoconstrictor; results in lower levels of angiotensin II which causes an increase in plasma renin activity and a reduction in aldosterone secretion

**Use** Management of mild to severe hypertension and congestive heart failure; believed to prolong survival in heart failure

**Unlabeled use:** Hypertensive crisis, diabetic nephropathy, rheumatoid arthritis, diagnosis of anatomic renal artery stenosis, hypertension secondary to scleroderma renal crisis, diagnosis of aldosteronism, idiopathic edema, Bartter's syndrome, postmyocardial infarction for prevention of ventricular failure

**USUAL DOSAGE** Use lower listed initial dose in patients with hyponatremia, hypovolemia, severe congestive heart failure, decreased renal function, or in those receiving diuretics

Infants and Children:

Investigational initial oral doses of **enalapril**: 0.1 mg/kg/day increasing as needed over 2 weeks to 0.5 mg/kg/day have been used to treat severe congestive heart failure in infants

Investigational I.V. doses of **enalaprilat**: 5-10 mcg/kg/dose administered every 8-24 hours have been used for the treatment of neonatal hypertension; monitor patients carefully; select patients may require higher doses

Adults:

Oral: **Enalapril**

Hypertension: 2.5-5 mg/day then increase as required, usual therapeutic dose for hypertension: 10-40 mg/day in 1-2 divided doses. **Note:** Initiate with 2.5 mg if patient taking diuretic which cannot be discontinued; may add a diuretic if blood pressure cannot be controlled with enalapril alone

Heart failure: As adjunct with diuretics and digitalis, initiate with 2.5 mg once or twice daily (usual range: 5-20 mg/day in 2 divided doses; maximum: 40 mg)

Asymptomatic left ventricular dysfunction: 2.5 mg twice daily, titrated as tolerated to 20 mg/day

I.V.: **Enalaprilat**

Hypertension: 1.25 mg/dose, given over 5 minutes every 6 hours; doses as high as 5 mg/dose every 6 hours have been tolerated for up to 36 hours. **Note:** If patients are concomitantly receiving diuretic therapy, begin with 0.625 mg I.V. over 5 minutes; if the effect is not adequate after 1 hour, repeat the dose and administer 1.25 mg at 6-hour intervals thereafter; if adequate, administer 0.625 mg I.V. every 6 hours

Conversion from I.V. to oral therapy if not concurrently on diuretics: 5 mg once daily; subsequent titration as needed; if concurrently receiving diuretics and responding to 0.625 mg I.V. every 6 hours, initiate with 2.5 mg/day

**Dosing adjustment in renal impairment:**

Oral: Enalapril:

$Cl_{cr}$ 30-80 mL/minute: Administer 5 mg/day titrated upwards to maximum of 40 mg

$Cl_{cr}$ <30 mL/minute: Administer 2.5 mg day; titrated upward until blood pressure is controlled

For heart failure patients with sodium <130 mEq/L or serum creatinine >1.6 mg/dL, initiate dosage with 2.5 mg/day, increasing to twice daily as needed; increase further in increments of 2.5 mg/dose at >4-day intervals to a maximum daily dose of 40 mg

I.V.: Enalaprilat:

$Cl_{cr}$ >30 mL/minute: Initiate with 1.25 mg every 6 hours and increase dose based on response

$Cl_{cr}$ <30 mL/minute: Initiate with 0.625 mg every 6 hours and increase dose based on response

Hemodialysis: Moderately dialyzable (20% to 50%); administer dose postdialysis (eg, 0.625 mg I.V. every 6 hours) or administer 20% to 25% supplemental dose following dialysis; Clearance: 62 mL/minute

Peritoneal dialysis: Supplemental dose is not necessary, although some removal of drug occurs

**Dosing adjustment in hepatic impairment:** Hydrolysis of enalapril to enalaprilat may be delayed and/or impaired in patients with severe hepatic impairment, but the pharmacodynamic effects of the drug do not appear to be significantly altered; no dosage adjustment

**Dosage Forms Enalaprilat: Inj:** 1.25 mg/mL (1 mL, 2 mL); **Enalapril maleate: Tab:** 2.5 mg, 5 mg, 10 mg, 20 mg

**Contraindications** Hypersensitivity to enalapril, enalaprilat, other ACE inhibitors, or any component

**Warnings/Precautions** Use with caution and modify dosage in patients with renal impairment (especially renal artery stenosis), severe congestive heart failure, or with coadministered diuretic therapy, valvular stenosis, hyperkalemia (>5.7 mEq/L); experience in children is limited. Severe hypotension may occur in patients who are sodium and/or volume depleted; initiate lower doses and monitor closely when starting therapy in these patients.

**Pregnancy Risk Factor** C (1st trimester); D (2nd and 3rd trimester)

**Pregnancy Implications**

Clinical effects on the fetus: No data available on crossing the placenta. Cranial defects, hypocalvaria/acalvaria, oligohydramnios, persistent anuria following delivery, hypotension, renal defects, renal dysgenesis/dysplasia, renal failure, pulmonary hypoplasia, limb contractures secondary to oligohydramnios and stillbirth reported. ACE inhibitors should be avoided during pregnancy.

Breast-feeding/lactation: Crosses into breast milk. Detectable levels but appears clinically insignificant. American Academy of Pediatrics considers **compatible** with breast-feeding.

**Adverse Reactions**

1% to 10%:

Cardiovascular: Chest pain (2%), syncope (2%), hypotension (6.7%)

Central nervous system: Headache (2% to 5%), dizziness (4% to 8%), fatigue (2% to 3%)

Dermatologic: Rash (1.5%)

Gastrointestinal: Abnormal taste, abdominal pain, vomiting, nausea, diarrhea, anorexia, constipation

Neuromuscular & skeletal: Weakness

(Continued)

## Enalapril *(Continued)*

Respiratory (1% to 2%): Bronchitis, cough, dyspnea

<1%: Angina pectoris, pulmonary edema, palpitations, arrest, CVA, myocardial infarction, orthostatic hypotension, rhythm, insomnia, ataxia, drowsiness, confusion, depression, nervousness, vertigo, alopecia, erythema multiforme, pruritus, Stevens-Johnson syndrome, urticaria, angioedema, pemphigus, hypoglycemia, hyperkalemia, gynecomastia, stomatitis, xerostomia, dyspepsia, glossitis, pancreatitis, ileus, urinary tract infection, impotence, agranulocytosis, neutropenia, anemia, hemolysis with G-6-PD, jaundice, hepatitis, paresthesia, blurred vision, conjunctivitis, tinnitus, oliguria, renal dysfunction, asthma, bronchospasm, URI, diaphoresis

**Drug Interactions** CYP3A3/4 enzyme substrate

See Drug-Drug Interactions With ACEIs *on page 997*

**Onset** Oral: ~1 hour

**Duration** Oral: 12-24 hours

**Half-Life**

Enalapril: Healthy: 2 hours; With congestive heart failure: 3.4-5.8 hours
Enalaprilat: 35-38 hours

**Special PA Issues**

**Patient Education:** Take as directed. Do not stop taking medication without consulting prescriber. Limit use of salt substitutes or potassium-containing foods (eg, bananas, nuts, oranges). You may experience GI upset, loss of appetite, or mouth sores (frequent small meals, frequent mouth care, and sucking on lozenges may help); or dizziness or weakness for a few days (use caution driving until these disappear). Report signs of dehydration (eg, excessive sweating, diarrhea or vomiting, excessively dry skin or mouth); swelling of face or mouth; irregular heartbeat or chest pains; or difficulty breathing.

**Monitoring Parameters:** Blood pressure, renal function, WBC, serum potassium; blood pressure monitor required during intravenous administration

**Related Information**

ACE Inhibitors *on page 995*

Heart Failure: Management of Patients with Left Ventricular Systolic Dysfunction *on page 1064*

Drug-Drug Interactions With ACEIs *on page 997*

## Enalapril and Diltiazem (e NAL a pril & dil TYE a zem)

**Pharmacologic Class** Antihypertensive Agent, Combination

**U.S. Brand Names** Teczem®

**Dosage Forms Tab, extended release:** Enalapril maleate 5 mg and diltiazem maleate 180 mg

## Enalapril and Felodipine (e NAL a pril & fe LOE di peen)

**Pharmacologic Class** Antihypertensive Agent, Combination

**U.S. Brand Names** Lexxel™

**Dosage Forms Tab, extended release:** Enalapril maleate 5 mg and felodipine 5 mg

## Enalapril and Hydrochlorothiazide

(e NAL a pril & hye droe klor oh THYE a zide)

**Pharmacologic Class** Antihypertensive Agent, Combination

**U.S. Brand Names** Vaseretic® 10-25

**Dosage Forms Tab:** Enalapril maleate 5 mg and hydrochlorothiazide 12.5 mg, Enalapril maleate 10 mg and hydrochlorothiazide 25 mg

- ◆ **Enalaprilat** *see* Enalapril *on page 316*
- ◆ **Enalapril Maleate** *see* Enalapril *on page 316*
- ◆ **Enbrel®** *see* Etanercept *on page 340*
- ◆ **Endal®** *see* Guaifenesin and Phenylephrine *on page 429*
- ◆ **Endantadine®** *see* Amantadine *on page 48*
- ◆ **End Lice® Liquid [OTC]** *see* Pyrethrins *on page 783*
- ◆ **Endocet®** *see* Oxycodone and Acetaminophen *on page 688*
- ◆ **Endodan®** *see* Oxycodone and Aspirin *on page 688*
- ◆ **Endolor®** *see* Butalbital Compound *on page 131*
- ◆ **Endrate®** *see* Edetate Disodium *on page 312*
- ◆ **Ener-B® [OTC]** *see* Cyanocobalamin *on page 242*
- ◆ **English Hawthorn** *see* Hawthorn *on page 438*
- ◆ **Enlon® Injection** *see* Edrophonium *on page 313*
- ◆ **Enovil®** *see* Amitriptyline *on page 57*

## Enoxacin (en OKS a sin)

**Pharmacologic Class** Antibiotic, Quinolone

**U.S. Brand Names** Penetrex™

**Mechanism of Action** Inhibits DNA-gyrase in susceptible organisms; inhibits relaxation of supercoiled DNA and promotes breakage of double-stranded DNA

**Use** Treatment of complicated and uncomplicated urinary tract infections caused by susceptible gram-negative and gram-positive bacteria and uncomplicated urethral or cervical gonorrhea due to *N. gonorrhoeae*

**USUAL DOSAGE** Adults: Oral:

Complicated urinary tract infection: 400 mg twice daily for 14 days

Cystitis: 200 mg twice daily for 7 days

Uncomplicated gonorrhea: 400 mg as single dose

**Dosing adjustment in renal impairment:** $Cl_{cr}$ <50 mL/minute: Administer 50% of dose

**Dosage Forms Tab:** 200 mg, 400 mg

**Contraindications** Hypersensitivity to enoxacin, any component, or other quinolones

**Warnings/Precautions** Use with caution in patients with a history of convulsions or epilepsy, renal dysfunction, psychosis, elevated intracranial pressure, prepubertal children, and pregnancy; nalidixic acid and ciprofloxacin (related compounds) have been associated with erosions of the cartilage in weight-bearing joints and other signs of arthropathy in immature animals and children; similar precautions are advised for enoxacin although no data is available; has rarely caused ruptured tendons (discontinue immediately with signs of inflammation or tendon pain)

**Pregnancy Risk Factor** C

**Adverse Reactions**

1% to 10%:

Central nervous system: Dizziness (<3%), headache (<2%), vertigo (3%)

Gastrointestinal: Nausea (2.9%), vomiting (6% to 9%), abdominal pain (1% to 2%), diarrhea (1% to 2%)

<1%: Palpitations, syncope, edema, restlessness, confusion, seizures, fatigue, drowsiness, depression, insomnia, confusion, chills, fever, rash, photosensitivity, pruritus, exfoliative dermatitis, hypo/hyperkalemia, GI bleeding, dyspepsia, xerostomia, constipation, flatulence, anorexia, vaginitis, anemia, leukopenia, eosinophilia, leukocytosis, increased liver enzymes, tremor, arthralgia, ruptured tendons, paresthesias, visual disturbances, increased serum creatinine/BUN, acute renal failure, proteinuria

**Drug Interactions** CYP1A2 enzyme inhibitor

Decreased effect of enoxacin with antacids (magnesium, aluminum), iron and zinc salts, sucralfate, bismuth salts, antineoplastics

Increased toxicity/levels of warfarin, cyclosporine, digoxin, caffeine, and theophylline with enoxacin

Increased levels of enoxacin with cimetidine, probenecid

**Half-Life** 3-6 hours (average)

**Special PA Issues**

**Patient Education:** Take as prescribed and for as long as directed. Take on an empty stomach (1 hour prior to or after meals). Do not use antacids within 2 hours of medication. Maintain adequate hydration (2-3 L/day of fluids unless instructed to restrict fluid intake). You may experience stomach discomfort (eat small, frequent meals) and dizziness or blurred vision (use caution when driving). May cause photosensitivity (wear protective clothing, sunscreen, and eyewear). Report skin rash; visual changes; severe gastric upset; weakness; pain, inflammation, or rupture of tendon; or signs or symptoms of opportunistic infection (eg, white spots or sores in mouth or perineal area, itching or vaginal discharge, unhealed sores, fever).

# Enoxaparin (ee noks a PA rin)

**Pharmacologic Class** Anticoagulant

**U.S. Brand Names** Lovenox® Injection

**Mechanism of Action** Standard heparin consists of components with molecular weights ranging from 4000 to 30,000 daltons with a mean of 16,000 daltons. Heparin acts as an anticoagulant by enhancing the inhibition rate of clotting proteases by antithrombin III impairing normal hemostasis and inhibition of factor Xa. Low molecular weight heparins have a small effect on the activated partial thromboplastin time and strongly inhibit factor Xa. Enoxaparin is derived from porcine heparin that undergoes benzylation followed by alkaline depolymerization. The average molecular weight of enoxaparin is 4500 daltons which is distributed as (≤20%) 2000 daltons, (≥68%) 2000-8000 daltons, and (≤15%) >8000 daltons. Enoxaparin has a higher ratio of antifactor Xa to antifactor IIa activity than unfractionated heparin.

**Use**

Prophylaxis of thromboembolic disorders (deep vein thrombosis) which may lead to pulmonary embolism following hip replacement therapy or total knee replacement

Prophylaxis of thromboembolic disorders (deep vein thrombosis) which may lead to pulmonary embolism in high-risk patients who are undergoing abdominal surgery. High-risk patients include those with one or more of the following risk factors: >40 years of age, obese, general anesthesia lasting >30 minutes, malignancy, history of deep vein thrombosis or pulmonary embolism.

Prevention of ischemic complications of unstable angina and non-Q-wave myocardial infarction when concurrently administered with aspirin

(Continued)

## Enoxaparin *(Continued)*

Treatment of thromboembolic disorders (deep vein thrombosis with or without pulmonary embolism)

**USUAL DOSAGE** S.C.:

Prophylaxis of DVT following abdominal, hip replacement or knee replacement surgery:

Children: Safety and effectiveness have not been established

Adults:

DVT prophylaxis in hip replacement:

30 mg twice daily: First dose within 12-24 hours after surgery and every 12 hours until risk of deep vein thrombosis has diminished or the patient is adequately anticoagulated on warfarin. Average duration of therapy: 7-10 days

40 mg once daily: First dose within 9-15 hours before surgery and daily until risk of deep vein thrombosis has diminished or the patient is adequately anticoagulated on warfarin. Average duration of therapy: 7-10 days unless warfarin is not given concurrently, then 40 mg S.C. once daily should be continued for 3 more weeks (4 weeks total)

DVT prophylaxis in knee replacement:

30 mg twice daily: First dose within 12-24 hours after surgery and every 12 hours until risk of deep vein thrombosis has diminished. Average duration of therapy: 7-10 days; maximum course: 14 days

Patients who weigh <100 lbs or are >65 years of age: Some clinicians recommend 0.5 mg/kg/dose every 12 hours to reduce the risk of bleeding

DVT prophylaxis in high-risk patients undergoing abdominal surgery: 40 mg once daily, with initial dose given 2 hours prior to surgery; usual duration: 7-10 days and up to 12 days has been tolerated in clinical trials

Treatment of acute proximal DVT: Start warfarin within 72 hours and continue enoxaparin until INR is between 2.0 and 3.0 (usually 7 days)

Inpatient treatment of DVT with or without pulmonary embolism: Adults: S.C. 1 mg/kg/dose every 12 hours or 1.5 mg/kg once daily

Outpatient treatment of DCT without pulmonary embolism: Adults: S.C.: 1 mg/kg/dose every 12 hours

Prevention of ischemic complications with unstable angina or non-Q-wave myocardial infarction: S.C.: 1 mg/kg twice daily in conjunction with oral aspirin therapy (100-325 mg once daily); treatment should be continued for a minimum of 2 days and continued until clinical stabilization (usually 2-8 days)

**Dosing adjustment in renal impairment:** Total clearance is lower and elimination is delayed in patients with renal failure; adjustment may be necessary in elderly and patients with severe renal impairment

Hemodialysis: Supplemental dose is not necessary

Peritoneal dialysis: Significant drug removal is unlikely based on physiochemical characteristics

**Dosage Forms** Inj, as sodium, preservative free: 30 mg/0.3 mL, 40 mg/0.4 mL; **Grad prefilled syringe:** 60 mg/0.6 mL, 80 mg/0.8 mL, 100 mg/1.0 mL; **Ampul:** 30 mg/0.3 mL

**Contraindications** Patients with active major bleeding, thrombocytopenia associated with a positive *in vitro* test for antiplatelet antibody or enoxaparin-induced platelet aggregation, hypersensitivity to enoxaparin, known hypersensitivity to heparin or pork products

**Warnings/Precautions** Do not administer intramuscularly; use with extreme caution in patients with a history of heparin-induced thrombocytopenia; bacterial endocarditis, hemorrhagic stroke, recent CNS or ophthalmological surgery, bleeding diathesis, uncontrolled arterial hypertension, or a history of recent gastrointestinal ulceration and hemorrhage. Elderly and patients with renal insufficiency may show delayed elimination of enoxaparin; avoid use in lactation. Patients should be observed closely for bleeding if enoxaparin is administered during or immediately following diagnostic lumbar puncture, epidural anesthesia, or spinal anesthesia. If thromboembolism develops despite enoxaparin prophylaxis, enoxaparin should be discontinued and appropriate treatment should be initiated.

Carefully monitor patients receiving low molecular weight heparins or heparinoids. These drugs, when used concurrently with spinal or epidural anesthesia or spinal puncture, may cause bleeding or hematomas within the spinal column. Increased pressure on the spinal cord may result in permanent paralysis if not detected and treated immediately.

**Pregnancy Risk Factor** B

**Adverse Reactions** 1% to 10%:

Central nervous system: Fever, confusion, pain

Dermatologic: Erythema, bruising

Gastrointestinal: Nausea

Hematologic: Hemorrhage, thrombocytopenia, hypochromic anemia, hematoma

Local: Irritation

At the recommended doses, single injections of enoxaparin do not significantly influence platelet aggregation or affect global clotting time (ie, PT or APTT)

**Drug Interactions** Increased toxicity with oral anticoagulants, platelet inhibitors

**Onset** Maximum antifactor Xa and antithrombin (antifactor IIa) activities occur 3-5 hours after S.C. administration.

**Duration** Following a 40 mg dose, significant antifactor Xa activity persists in plasma for ~12 hours.

**Half-Life** Half-life, plasma: Low molecular weight heparin is 2-4 times longer than standard heparin independent of the dose.

**Special PA Issues**

**Patient Education:** Use soft toothbrush, electric razor, and avoid injury potential activities. Report any signs of bleeding gums, blood in urine or tarry stools, nosebleeds, excessive bruising, or acute headache or backache.

**Monitoring Parameters:** Platelets, occult blood, and anti-Xa activity, if available; the monitoring of PT and/or PTT is not necessary

♦ **Enoxaparin Sodium** see Enoxaparin on page 319

♦ **Entocort®** see Budesonide on page 124

♦ **Entrophen®** see Aspirin on page 80

♦ **Entuss-D® Liquid** see Hydrocodone and Pseudoephedrine on page 453

♦ **Enulose®** see Lactulose on page 512

♦ **Enzone®** see Pramoxine and Hydrocortisone on page 748

♦ **E Pam®** see Diazepam on page 269

## Ephedrine (e FED rin)

**Pharmacologic Class** Alpha/Beta Agonist

**U.S. Brand Names** Kondon's Nasal® [OTC]; Pretz-D® [OTC]

**Mechanism of Action** Releases tissue stores of epinephrine and thereby produces an alpha- and beta-adrenergic stimulation; longer-acting and less potent than epinephrine

**Use** Treatment of bronchial asthma, nasal congestion, acute bronchospasm, idiopathic orthostatic hypotension

**USUAL DOSAGE**

Children:

Oral, S.C.: 3 mg/kg/day or 25-100 mg/m$^2$/day in 4-6 divided doses every 4-6 hours

I.M., slow I.V. push: 0.2-0.3 mg/kg/dose every 4-6 hours

Adults:

Oral: 25-50 mg every 3-4 hours as needed

I.M., S.C.: 25-50 mg, parenteral adult dose should not exceed 150 mg in 24 hours

I.V.: 5-25 mg/dose slow I.V. push repeated after 5-10 minutes as needed, then every 3-4 hours not to exceed 150 mg/24 hours

**Dosage Forms Inj:** 25 mg/mL (1 mL); 50 mg/mL (1 mL, 10 mL); **Jelly (Kondon's Nasal®):** 1% (20 g); **Spray (Pretz-D®):** 0.25% (15 mL)

**Contraindications** Hypersensitivity to ephedrine or any component, cardiac arrhythmias, angle-closure glaucoma, patients on other sympathomimetic agents

**Warnings/Precautions** Blood volume depletion should be corrected before ephedrine therapy is instituted; use caution in patients with unstable vasomotor symptoms, diabetes, hyperthyroidism, prostatic hypertrophy, or a history of seizures; also use caution in the elderly and those patients with cardiovascular disorders such as coronary artery disease, arrhythmias, and hypertension. Ephedrine may cause hypertension resulting in intracranial hemorrhage. Long-term use may cause anxiety and symptoms of paranoid schizophrenia. Avoid as a bronchodilator; generally not used as a bronchodilator since new beta$_2$ agents are less toxic. Use with caution in the elderly, since it crosses the blood-brain barrier and may cause confusion.

**Pregnancy Risk Factor** C

**Adverse Reactions**

>10%: Central nervous system: CNS stimulating effects, nervousness, anxiety, apprehension, fear, tension, agitation, excitation, restlessness, irritability, insomnia, hyperactivity

1% to 10%:

Cardiovascular: Hypertension, tachycardia, palpitations, elevation or depression of blood pressure, unusual pallor

Central nervous system: Dizziness, headache

Gastrointestinal: Xerostomia, nausea, anorexia, GI upset, vomiting

Genitourinary: Painful urination

Neuromuscular & skeletal: Trembling, tremor (more common in the elderly), weakness

Miscellaneous: Diaphoresis (increased)

<1%: Chest pain, arrhythmias, dyspnea

**Drug Interactions**

Decreased effect: Alpha- and beta-adrenergic blocking agents decrease ephedrine vasopressor effects

Increased toxicity: Additive cardiostimulation with other sympathomimetic agents; theophylline → cardiostimulation; MAO inhibitors or atropine may increase blood pressure; cardiac glycosides or general anesthetics may increase cardiac stimulation

**Onset** Oral: Onset of bronchodilation: Within 0.25-1 hour

**Duration** Oral: 3-6 hours

**Half-Life** 2.5-3.6 hours

(Continued)

## Ephedrine *(Continued)*

### Special PA Issues

**Patient Education:** Use this medication exactly as directed; do not take more than recommended dosage. Avoid other stimulant prescriptive or OTC medications to avoid serious overdose reactions. Store this medication away from light. You may experience dizziness, blurred vision, restlessness (use caution when driving or engaging in hazardous activities); or difficulty urinating (empty bladder immediately before taking this medication). Report excessive nervousness or excitation, inability to sleep, facial flushing, pounding heartbeat, muscle tremors or weakness, chest pain or palpitations, bronchial irritation or coughing, or increased sweating.

**Monitoring Parameters:** Blood pressure, pulse, urinary output, mental status; cardiac monitor and blood pressure monitor required

- ◆ **Ephedrine Sulfate** *see* Ephedrine *on previous page*
- ◆ **E-Pilo-x® Ophthalmic** *see* Pilocarpine and Epinephrine *on page 727*
- ◆ **Epimorph®** *see* Morphine Sulfate *on page 619*
- ◆ **Epitol®** *see* Carbamazepine *on page 148*
- ◆ **Epivir®** *see* Lamivudine *on page 513*
- ◆ **Epivir® HBV** *see* Lamivudine *on page 513*
- ◆ **EPO** *see* Epoetin Alfa *on this page*

## Epoetin Alfa *(e POE e tin AL fa)*

**Pharmacologic Class** Colony Stimulating Factor

**U.S. Brand Names** Epogen®; Procrit®

**Mechanism of Action** Induces erythropoiesis by stimulating the division and differentiation of committed erythroid progenitor cells; induces the release of reticulocytes from the bone marrow into the bloodstream, where they mature to erythrocytes. There is a dose response relationship with this effect. This results in an increase in reticulocyte counts followed by a rise in hematocrit and hemoglobin levels.

### Use

Treatment of anemia associated with chronic renal failure, including patients on dialysis (end-stage renal disease) and patients not on dialysis

Treatment of anemia related to zidovudine therapy in HIV-infected patients; in patients when the endogenous erythropoietin level is ≤500 mIU/mL and the dose of zidovudine is ≤4200 mg/week

Treatment of anemia in cancer patients on chemotherapy; in patients with nonmyeloid malignancies where anemia is caused by the effect of the concomitantly administered chemotherapy; to decrease the need for transfusions in patients who will be receiving chemotherapy for a minimum of 2 months

Reduction of allogeneic block transfusion in surgery patients scheduled to undergo elective, noncardiac, nonvascular surgery

### USUAL DOSAGE

Chronic renal failure patients: I.V., S.C.:

Initial dose: 50-100 units/kg 3 times/week

Reduce dose by 25 units/kg when

1) hematocrit approaches 36% **or**

2) when hematocrit increases >4 points in any 2-week period

Increase dose if hematocrit does not increase by 5-6 points after 8 weeks of therapy and hematocrit is below suggested target range

Suggested target hematocrit range: 30% to 36%

Maintenance dose: Individualize to target range

Dialysis patients: Median dose: 75 units/kg 3 times/week

Nondialysis patients: Doses of 75-150 units/kg

Zidovudine-treated, HIV-infected patients: Patients with erythropoietin levels >500 mIU/mL are **unlikely** to respond

Initial dose: I.V., S.C.: 100 units/kg 3 times/week for 8 weeks

Increase dose by 50-100 units/kg 3 times/week if response is not satisfactory in terms of reducing transfusion requirements or increasing hematocrit after 8 weeks of therapy

Evaluate response every 4-8 weeks thereafter and adjust the dose accordingly by 50-100 units/kg increments 3 times/week

If patients have not responded satisfactorily to a 300 unit/kg dose 3 times/week, it is unlikely that they will respond to higher doses

Stop dose if hematocrit exceeds 40% and resume treatment at a 25% dose reduction when hematocrit drops to 36%

Cancer patients on chemotherapy: Treatment of patients with erythropoietin levels >200 mU/mL is **not recommended**

Initial dose: S.C.: 150 units/kg 3 times/week

Dose adjustment: If response is not satisfactory in terms of reducing transfusion requirement or increasing hematocrit after 8 weeks of therapy, the dose may be increased up to 300 units/kg 3 times/week. If patients do not respond, it is unlikely that they will respond to higher doses.

If hematocrit exceeds 40%, hold the dose until it falls to 36% and reduce the dose by 25% when treatment is resumed

Surgery patients: Prior to initiating treatment, obtain a hemoglobin to establish that is is >10 mg/dL or ≤13 mg/dL

Initial dose: S.C.: 300 units/kg/day for 10 days before surgery, on the day of surgery, and for 4 days after surgery

Alternative dose: S.C.: 600 units/kg in once-weekly doses (21, 14, and 7 days before surgery) plus a fourth dose on the day of surgery

**Dosage Forms 1 mL single-dose vials: Preservative-free soln** 2000 units/mL, 3000 units/mL, 4000 units/mL, 10,000 units/mL; **2 mL multidose vials: Preserved soln:** 10,000 units/mL

**Contraindications** Known hypersensitivity to albumin (human) or mammalian cell-derived products; uncontrolled hypertension

**Warnings/Precautions** Use with caution in patients with porphyria, hypertension, or a history of seizures; prior to and during therapy, iron stores must be evaluated. It is recommended that the epoetin dose be decreased if the hematocrit increase exceeds 4 points in any 2-week period.

**Pretherapy parameters:**

Serum ferritin >100 ng/dL

Transferrin saturation (serum iron/iron binding capacity x 100) of 20% to 30%

Iron supplementation (usual oral dosing of 325 mg 2-3 times/day) should be given during therapy to provide for increased requirements during expansion of the red cell mass secondary to marrow stimulation by EPO unless iron stores are already in excess

For patients with endogenous serum EPO levels which are inappropriately low for hemoglobin level, documentation of the serum EPO level will indicate which patients may benefit from EPO therapy. Serum EPO levels can be ordered routinely from Clinical Chemistry (red-top serum separator tube). Refer to "Reference Range" for information on interpretation of EPO levels.

See table:

### Factors Limiting Response to Epoetin Alfa

| Factor | Mechanism |
|---|---|
| Iron deficiency | Limits hemoglobin synthesis |
| Blood loss/hemolysis | Counteracts epoetin alfa-stimulated erythropoiesis |
| Infection/inflammation | Inhibits iron transfer from storage to bone marrow |
| | Suppresses erythropoiesis through activated macrophages |
| Aluminum overload | Inhibits iron incorporation into heme protein |
| Bone marrow replacement Hyperparathyroidsm Metastatic, neoplastic | Limits bone marrow volume |
| Folic acid/vitamin $B_{12}$ deficiency | Limits hemoglobin synthesis |
| Patient compliance | Self-administered epoetin alfa or iron therapy |

Increased mortality has occurred when aggressive dosing is used in CHF or anginal patients undergoing hemodialysis. An Amgen-funded study determined that when patients were targeted for a hematocrit of 42% versus a less aggressive 30%, mortality was higher (35% versus 29%).

**Pregnancy Risk Factor** C

**Pregnancy Implications** Clinical effect on the fetus: Epoetin alfa has been shown to have adverse effects in rats when given in doses 5X the human dose. There are no adequate and well-controlled studies in pregnant women. Epoetin alfa should be used only if potential benefit justifies the potential risk to the fetus.

**Adverse Reactions**

>10%:

Cardiovascular: Hypertension

Central nervous system: Fatigue, headache, fever

1% to 10%:

Cardiovascular: Edema, chest pain

Gastrointestinal: Nausea, vomiting, diarrhea

Hematologic: Clotted access

Neuromuscular & skeletal: Arthralgias, asthenia

<1%: Myocardial infarction, CVA/TIA, rash, hypersensitivity reactions

**Onset** Several days; Peak effect: 2-3 weeks

**Half-Life** Circulating: 4-13 hours in patients with chronic renal failure; 20% shorter in patients with normal renal function

(Continued)

## Epoetin Alfa *(Continued)*

### Special PA Issues

**Patient Education:** You will require frequent blood tests to determine appropriate dosage. Do not take other medications, vitamin or iron supplements, or make significant changes in your diet without consulting prescriber. Report signs or symptoms of edema (eg, swollen extremities, difficulty breathing, rapid weight gain), onset of severe headache, acute back pain, chest pain, or muscular tremors or seizure activity.

### Monitoring Parameters:

Careful monitoring of blood pressure is indicated; problems with hypertension have been noted especially in renal failure patients treated with rHuEPO. Other patients are less likely to develop this complication.

See table.

| Test | Initial Phase Frequency | Maintenance Phase Frequency |
|------|------------------------|----------------------------|
| Hematocrit/hemoglobin | 2 x/week | 2-4 x/month |
| Blood pressure | 3 x/week | 3 x/week |
| Serum ferritin | Monthly | Quarterly |
| Transferrin saturation | Monthly | Quarterly |
| Serum chemistries including CBC with differential, creatinine, blood urea nitrogen, potassium, phosphorous | Regularly per routine | Regularly per routine |

Hematocrit should be determined twice weekly until stabilization within the target range (30% to 36%), and twice weekly for at least 2 to 6 weeks after a dose increase

**Reference Range:** Guidelines should be based on the following figure or published literature

Guidelines for estimating appropriateness of endogenous EPO levels for varying levels of anemia via the EIA assay method: See figure. The reference range for erythropoietin in serum, for subjects with normal hemoglobin and hematocrit, is 4.1-22.2 mIU/mL by the EIA method. Erythropoietin levels are typically inversely related to hemoglobin (and hematocrit) levels in anemias not attributed to impaired erythropoietin production.

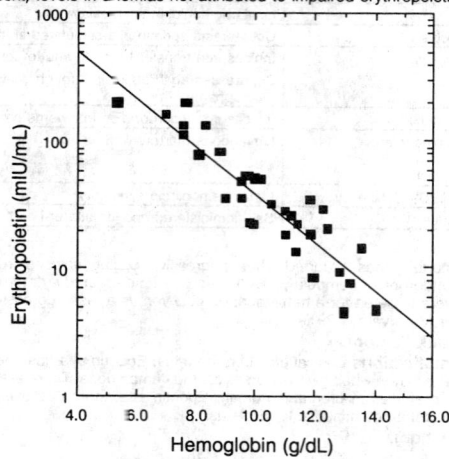

Zidovudine-treated HIV patients: Available evidence indicates patients with endogenous serum erythropoietin levels >500 mIU/mL are unlikely to respond

Cancer chemotherapy patients: Treatment of patients with endogenous serum erythropoietin levels >200 mIU/mL is not recommended

♦ **Epogen®** *see* Epoetin Alfa *on page 322*

## Epoprostenol *(e poe PROST en ole)*

**Pharmacologic Class** Plasma Volume Expander, Colloid; Prostaglandin

**U.S. Brand Names** Flolan® Injection

**Mechanism of Action** Epoprostenol is also known as prostacyclin and $PGI_2$. It is a strong vasodilator of all vascular beds. In addition, it is a potent endogenous inhibitor of platelet aggregation. The reduction in platelet aggregation results from epoprostenol's activation of intracellular adenylate cyclase and the resultant increase in cyclic adenosine monophosphate concentrations within the platelets. Additionally, it is capable of decreasing thrombogenesis and platelet clumping in the lungs by inhibiting platelet aggregation.

**Use** Treatment of primary pulmonary hypertension in NYHA Class III and IV patients

    **Off-label uses:** Other potential uses include pulmonary hypertension associated with ARDS, SLE, or CHF, neonatal pulmonary hypertension, cardiopulmonary bypass surgery, hemodialysis, atherosclerosis, peripheral vascular disorders, and neonatal purpura fulminans

**USUAL DOSAGE** I.V.: The drug is administered by continuous intravenous infusion via a central venous catheter using an ambulatory infusion pump; during dose ranging it may be administered peripherally

    **Acute dose ranging:** The initial infusion rate should be 2 ng/kg/minute by continuous I.V. and increased in increments of 2 ng/kg/minute every 15 minutes or longer until dose-limiting effects are elicited (such as chest pain, anxiety, dizziness, changes in heart rate, dyspnea, nausea, vomiting, headache, hypotension and/or flushing)

    **Continuous chronic infusion:** Initial: 4 ng/kg/minute **less** than the maximum-tolerated infusion rate determined during acute dose ranging

    If maximum-tolerated infusion rate is <5 ng/kg/minute, the chronic infusion rate should be ½ the maximum-tolerated acute infusion rate

    **Dosage adjustments:** Dose adjustments in the chronic infusion rate should be based on persistence, recurrence, or worsening of patient symptoms of pulmonary hypertension

    If symptoms persist or recur after improving, the infusion rate should be increased by 1-2 ng/kg/minute increments, every 15 minutes or greater; following establishment of a new chronic infusion rate, the patient should be observed and vital signs monitored.

**Preparation of Infusion**

| To make 100 mL of solution with concentration: | Directions |
| --- | --- |
| 3000 ng/mL | Dissolve one 0.5 mg vial with 5 mL supplied diluent, withdraw 3 mL, and add to sufficient diluent to make a total of 100 mL. |
| 5000 ng/mL | Dissolve one 0.5 mg vial with 5 mL supplied diluent, withdraw entire vial contents, and add a sufficient volume of diluent to make a total of 100 mL. |
| 10,000 ng/mL | Dissolve two 0.5 mg vials each with 5 mL supplied diluent, withdraw entire vial contents, and add a sufficient volume of diluent to make a total of 100 mL. |
| 15,000 ng/mL | Dissolve one 1.5 mg vial with 5 mL supplied diluent, withdraw entire vial contents, and add a sufficient volume of diluent to make a total of 100 mL. |

**Dosage Forms Inj, as sodium:** 0.5 mg/vial and 1.5 mg/vial, each supplied with 50 mL of sterile diluent

**Contraindications** Chronic use in patients with CHF due to severe left ventricular systolic dysfunction; hypersensitivity to epoprostenol or to structurally-related compounds

**Warnings/Precautions** Abrupt interruptions or large sudden reductions in dosage may result in rebound pulmonary hypertension; some patients with primary pulmonary hypertension have developed pulmonary edema during dose ranging, which may be associated with pulmonary veno-occlusive disease; during chronic use, unless contraindicated, anticoagulants should be coadministered to reduce the risk of thromboembolism

**Pregnancy Risk Factor** B

**Adverse Reactions**

  >10%:

    Cardiovascular: Flushing, tachycardia, shock, syncope, heart failure

    Central nervous system: Fever, chills, anxiety, nervousness, dizziness, headache, hyperesthesia, pain

    Gastrointestinal: Diarrhea, nausea, vomiting

    Neuromuscular & skeletal: Jaw pain, myalgia, tremor, paresthesia

    Respiratory: Hypoxia

    Miscellaneous: Sepsis, flu-like symptoms

  1% to 10%:

    Cardiovascular: Bradycardia, hypotension, angina pectoris, edema, arrhythmias, pallor, cyanosis, palpitations, cerebrovascular accident, myocardial ischemia, chest pain

    Central nervous system: Seizures, confusion, depression, insomnia

    Dermatologic: Pruritus, rash

    Endocrine & metabolic: Hypokalemia, weight change

    Gastrointestinal: Abdominal pain, anorexia, constipation

    Hematologic: Hemorrhage

    Hepatic: Ascites

    Neuromuscular & skeletal: Arthralgias, bone pain, weakness

    Hematologic: Disseminated intravascular coagulation

(Continued)

## Epoprostenol *(Continued)*

Ocular: Amblyopia
Respiratory: Cough increase, dyspnea, epistaxis, pleural effusion
Miscellaneous: Diaphoresis

**Drug Interactions** Increased toxicity: The hypotensive effects of epoprostenol may be exacerbated by other vasodilators, diuretics, or by using acetate in dialysis fluids. Patients treated with anticoagulants and epoprostenol should be monitored for increased bleeding risk because of shared effects on platelet aggregation.

**Half-Life** 2.7-6 minute; steady-state levels are reached in about 15 minutes with continuous infusions

**Special PA Issues**

**Patient Education:** You will be on this medication through a portable continuous infusion pump and you will be instructed on the proper care and operation of the pump and preparation of all solutions. You may experience mild headache, nausea or vomiting, and some muscular pains (use of a mild analgesia may be recommended by your prescriber). Report immediately any signs or symptoms of pump problems, acute or severe headache, back pain, increased difficult breathing, flushing, fever or chills, any unusual bleeding or bruising, or any onset of unresolved diarrhea.

**Monitoring Parameters:** Monitor for improvements in pulmonary function, decreased exertional dyspnea, fatigue, syncope and chest pain, pulmonary vascular resistance, pulmonary arterial pressure and quality of life. In addition, the pump device and catheters should be monitored frequently to avoid "system" related failure.

- ◆ **Epoprostenol Sodium** *see* Epoprostenol *on page 324*
- ◆ **Epsom Salts** *see* Magnesium Sulfate *on page 555*
- ◆ **Equagesic®** *see* Aspirin and Meprobamate *on page 83*
- ◆ **Equanil®** *see* Meprobamate *on page 570*
- ◆ **Equilet® [OTC]** *see* Calcium Carbonate *on page 139*
- ◆ **Eramycin®** *see* Erythromycin *on page 329*
- ◆ **Ercaf®** *see* Ergotamine *on page 328*
- ◆ **Ergamisol®** *see* Levamisole *on page 522*

## Ergocalciferol *(er goe kal SIF e role)*

**Pharmacologic Class** Vitamin D Analog

**U.S. Brand Names** Calciferol™ Injection; Calciferol™ Oral; Drisdol® Oral

**Mechanism of Action** Stimulates calcium and phosphate absorption from the small intestine, promotes secretion of calcium from bone to blood; promotes renal tubule phosphate resorption

**Use** Treatment of refractory rickets, hypophosphatemia, hypoparathyroidism

**USUAL DOSAGE** Oral dosing is preferred; I.M. therapy required with GI, liver, or biliary disease associated with malabsorption

Dietary supplementation (each mcg = 40 USP units):
  Premature infants: 10-20 mcg/day (400-800 units), up to 750 mcg/day (30,000 units)
  Infants and healthy Children: 10 mcg/day (400 units)
  Adults: 10 mcg/day (400 units)
Renal failure:
  Children: 100-1000 mcg/day (4000-40,000 units)
  Adults: 500 mcg/day (20,000 units)
Hypoparathyroidism:
  Children: 1.25-5 mg/day (50,000-200,000 units) and calcium supplements
  Adults: 625 mcg to 5 mg/day (25,000-200,000 units) and calcium supplements
Vitamin D-dependent rickets:
  Children: 75-125 mcg/day (3000-5000 units); maximum: 1500 mcg/day
  Adults: 250 mcg to 1.5 mg/day (10,000-60,000 units)
Nutritional rickets and osteomalacia:
  Children and Adults (with normal absorption): 25-125 mcg/day (1000-5000 units)
  Children with malabsorption: 250-625 mcg/day (10,000-25,000 units)
  Adults with malabsorption: 250-7500 mcg (10,000-300,000 units)
Vitamin D-resistant rickets:
  Children: Initial: 1000-2000 mcg/day (40,000-80,000 units) with phosphate supplements; daily dosage is increased at 3- to 4-month intervals in 250-500 mcg (10,000-20,000 units) increments
  Adults: 250-1500 mcg/day (10,000-60,000 units) with phosphate supplements
Familial hypophosphatemia: 10,000-80,000 units daily plus 1-2 g/day elemental phosphorus
Osteoporosis prophylaxis: Adults:
  51-70 years of age: 400 units/day
  >70 years of age: 600 units/day
  Maximum daily dose: 2000 units/day

**Dosage Forms Cap (Drisdol®):** 50,000 units [1.25 mg]; **Inj (Calciferol™):** 500,000 units/mL [12.5 mg/mL] (1 mL); **Liq (Calciferol™, Drisdol®):** 8000 units/mL [200 mcg/mL] (60 mL); **Tab (Calciferol™):** 50,000 units [1.25 mg]

**Contraindications** Hypercalcemia, hypersensitivity to ergocalciferol or any component; malabsorption syndrome; evidence of vitamin D toxicity

**Warnings/Precautions** Administer with extreme caution in patients with impaired renal function, heart disease, renal stones, or arteriosclerosis; must administer concomitant calcium supplementation; maintain adequate fluid intake; avoid hypercalcemia; renal function impairment with secondary hyperparathyroidism

**Pregnancy Risk Factor** A (C if dose exceeds RDA recommendation)

**Adverse Reactions** Generally well tolerated

Cardiovascular: Cardiac arrhythmias, hypertension (late)

Central nervous system: Irritability, headache, psychosis (rare), somnolence, hyperthermia (late)

Dermatologic: Pruritus

Endocrine & metabolic: Decreased libido (late), hypercholesterolemia, mild acidosis (late), polydipsia (late)

Gastrointestinal: Nausea, vomiting, anorexia, pancreatitis, metallic taste, weight loss (rare), xerostomia, constipation

Genitourinary: Polyuria (late), increased BUN (late)

Hepatic: Increased LFTs (late)

Neuromuscular & skeletal: Bone pain, myalgia, weakness

Ocular: Conjunctivitis, photophobia (late)

Miscellaneous: Vascular/nephrocalcinosis (rare)

**Drug Interactions**

Decreased effect: Cholestyramine, colestipol, mineral oil may decrease oral absorption

Increased effect: Thiazide diuretics may increase vitamin D effects

Increased toxicity: Cardiac glycosides may increase toxicity

**Onset** Peak effect: ~1 month following daily doses

**Special PA Issues**

Patient Education: Take exact dose prescribed; do not take more than recommended. Your prescriber may recommend a special diet; do not increase calcium intake without consulting prescriber. Avoid magnesium supplements or magnesium-containing antacids. You may experience nausea, vomiting, or metallic taste (frequent small meals, frequent mouth care, or sucking hard candy may help); hypotension (use caution when rising from sitting or lying position or when climbing stairs or bending over). Report chest pain or palpitations; acute headache, dizziness, or feeling of weakness; unresolved nausea or vomiting; persistent metallic taste; unrelieved muscle or bone pain; or CNS irritability.

Monitoring Parameters: Measure serum calcium, BUN, and phosphorus every 1-2 weeks; x-ray bones monthly until stabilized

Reference Range: Serum calcium times phosphorus should not exceed 70 mg/dL to avoid ectopic calcification; ergocalciferol levels: 10-60 ng/mL; serum calcium: 9-10 mg/dL, phosphorus: 2.5-5 mg/dL

# Ergoloid Mesylates (ER goe loid MES i lates)

**Pharmacologic Class** Ergot Derivative

**U.S. Brand Names** Germinal®; Hydergine®; Hydergine® LC

**Use** Treatment of cerebrovascular insufficiency in primary progressive dementia, Alzheimer's dementia, and senile onset

**USUAL DOSAGE** Adults: Oral: 1 mg 3 times/day up to 4.5-12 mg/day; up to 6 months of therapy may be necessary

**Dosage Forms Cap, liq (Hydergine® LC):** 1 mg; **Liq (Hydergine®):** 1 mg/mL (100 mL); **Tab: Oral:** 0.5 mg, Gerimal®, Hydergine®: 1 mg, **Sublingual:** Gerimal®, Hydergine®: 0.5 mg, 1 mg

**Contraindications** Acute or chronic psychosis, hypersensitivity to ergot or any component

**Pregnancy Risk Factor** C

♦ **Ergomar®** *see* Ergotamine *on next page*

♦ **Ergometrine Maleate** *see* Ergonovine *on this page*

# Ergonovine (er goe NOE veen)

**Pharmacologic Class** Ergot Derivative

**U.S. Brand Names** Ergotrate® Maleate

**Mechanism of Action** Ergot alkaloid alpha-adrenergic agonist directly stimulates vascular smooth muscle to vasoconstrict peripheral and cerebral vessels; may also have antagonist effects on serotonin

**Use** Prevention and treatment of postpartum and postabortion hemorrhage caused by uterine atony or subinvolution

Unlabeled use: Migraine headaches, diagnostically to identify Prinzmetal's angina

**USUAL DOSAGE** Adults: I.M., I.V. (I.V. should be reserved for emergency use only): 0.2 mg, repeat dose in 2-4 hours as needed

**Dosage Forms Inj, as maleate:** 0.2 mg/mL (1 mL)

**Contraindications** Induction of labor, threatened spontaneous abortion, hypersensitivity to ergonovine or any component

(Continued)

## Ergonovine *(Continued)*

**Warnings/Precautions** Use with caution in patients with sepsis, heart disease, hypertension, or with hepatic or renal impairment; restore uterine responsiveness in calcium-deficient patients who do not respond to ergonovine by I.V. calcium administration; avoid prolonged use; discontinue if ergotism develops

**Pregnancy Risk Factor** X

**Adverse Reactions**

1% to 10%: Gastrointestinal: Nausea, vomiting

<1%: Palpitations, bradycardia, transient chest pain, hypertension (sometimes extreme - treat with I.V. chlorpromazine), cerebrovascular accidents, shock, myocardial infarction, ergotism, seizures, dizziness, headache, thrombophlebitis, tinnitus, dyspnea, diaphoresis

**Onset** Oral: Within 5-15 minutes; I.M.: Within 2-5 minutes

**Duration** Uterine effects persist for 3 hours, except when given I.V., then effects persist for ~45 minutes.

**Special PA Issues**

**Patient Education:** For angina diagnosis cardiologist will instruct patient about what to expect. For postpartum hemorrhage (an emergency situation) patient needs to know why the drug is being given and what side effects she might experience (eg, mild nausea and vomiting, dizziness, headache, ringing ears) and instructed to report difficulty breathing, acute headache, or numbness and cold feeling in extremities, or severe abdominal cramping.

♦ **Ergonovine Maleate** *see* Ergonovine *on previous page*

## Ergotamine (er GOT a meen)

**Pharmacologic Class** Ergot Derivative

**U.S. Brand Names** Cafatine®; Cafatine-PB®; Cafergot®; Cafetrate®; Ercaf®; Ergomar®; Wigraine®

**Mechanism of Action** Has partial agonist and/or antagonist activity against tryptaminergic, dopaminergic and alpha-adrenergic receptors depending upon their site; is a highly active uterine stimulant; it causes constriction of peripheral and cranial blood vessels and produces depression of central vasomotor centers

**Use** Abort or prevent vascular headaches, such as migraine or cluster

**USUAL DOSAGE** Adults:

Oral:

Cafergot®: 2 tablets at onset of attack; then 1 tablet every 30 minutes as needed; maximum: 6 tablets per attack; do not exceed 10 tablets/week

Ergostat®: 1 tablet under tongue at first sign, then 1 tablet every 30 minutes, 3 tablets/24 hours, 5 tablets/week

Rectal (Cafergot® suppositories, Wigraine® suppositories, Cafatine® suppositories): 1 at first sign of an attack; follow with second dose after 1 hour, if needed; maximum dose: 2 per attack; do not exceed 5/week

**Dosage Forms Supp, rectal (Cafatine®, Cafergot®, Cafetrate®, Wigraine®):** Ergotamine tartrate 2 mg and caffeine 100 mg (12s); **Tab (Ercaf®, Wigraine®):** Ergotamine tartrate 1 mg and caffeine 100 mg; **Sublingual (Ergomar®):** Ergotamine tartrate 2 mg

**Contraindications** Hypersensitivity to ergotamine, caffeine, or any component; peripheral vascular disease, hepatic or renal disease, hypertension, peptic ulcer disease, sepsis; avoid during pregnancy

**Warnings/Precautions** Avoid prolonged administration or excessive dosage because of the danger of ergotism and gangrene; patients who take ergotamine for extended periods of time may become dependent on it. May be harmful due to reduction in cerebral blood flow; may precipitate angina, myocardial infarction, or aggravate intermittent claudication; therefore, not considered a drug of choice in the elderly.

**Pregnancy Risk Factor** X

**Adverse Reactions**

>10%:

Cardiovascular: Tachycardia, bradycardia, arterial spasm, claudication and vasoconstriction; rebound headache may occur with sudden withdrawal of the drug in patients on prolonged therapy; localized edema, peripheral vascular effects (numbness and tingling of fingers and toes)

Central nervous system: Drowsiness, dizziness

Gastrointestinal: Nausea, vomiting, diarrhea, xerostomia

1% to 10%:

Cardiovascular: Transient tachycardia or bradycardia, precordial distress and pain

Neuromuscular & skeletal: Weakness in the legs, abdominal or muscle pain, muscle pains in the extremities, paresthesia

**Drug Interactions** Increased toxicity:

Propranolol: One case of severe vasoconstriction with pain and cyanosis has been reported

Erythromycin, troleandomycin and other macrolide antibiotics: Monitor for signs of ergot toxicity

**Special PA Issues**
**Patient Education:** Take this drug as directed; do not increase dose or use more often than prescribed. If relief is not obtained, contact your prescriber. Avoid caffeine-containing products (eg, tea, coffee, colas, cocoa); caffeine increases GI absorption of ergotamines. May cause drowsiness (avoid activities requiring alertness until effects of medication are known). You may experience mild nausea/vomiting (you may have an antiemetic prescribed), mild weakness or numbness of extremities (avoid injury). Inspect your extremities for coldness, numbness, or injury. Report immediately extreme numbness, pain, tingling or weakness in extremities (toes, fingers), severe unresolved nausea or vomiting, difficulty breathing or irregular heartbeat.
Inhaler: Follow directions for use on package insert. If more than one inhalation is necessary, wait 5 minutes between inhalations (maximum dose of 6 inhalations/24 hours or 15 inhalations/week)

♦ **Ergotamine Tartrate** see Ergotamine on previous page
♦ **Ergotamine Tartrate and Caffeine** see Ergotamine on previous page
♦ **Ergotrate® Maleate** see Ergonovine on page 327
♦ **E•R•O Ear [OTC]** see Carbamide Peroxide on page 150
♦ **Erybid™** see Erythromycin on this page
♦ **Eryc®** see Erythromycin on this page
♦ **EryPed®** see Erythromycin on this page
♦ **Ery-Tab®** see Erythromycin on this page
♦ **Erythro-Base®** see Erythromycin on this page
♦ **Erythrocin®** see Erythromycin on this page

# Erythromycin (er ith roe MYE sin)
**Pharmacologic Class** Antibiotic, Macrolide
**U.S. Brand Names** E-Base®; E.E.S.®; E-Mycin®; Eramycin®; Eryc®; EryPed®; Ery-Tab®; Erythrocin®; Ilosone®; PCE®
**Mechanism of Action** Inhibits RNA-dependent protein synthesis at the chain elongation step; binds to the 50S ribosomal subunit resulting in blockage of transpeptidation
**Use** Treatment of susceptible bacterial infections including *S. pyogenes*, some *S. pneumoniae*, some *S. aureus*, *M. pneumoniae*, *Legionella pneumophila*, diphtheria, pertussis, chancroid, *Chlamydia*, erythrasma, *N. gonorrhoeae*, *E. histolytica*, syphilis and nongonococcal urethritis, and *Campylobacter* gastroenteritis; used in conjunction with neomycin for decontaminating the bowel; treatment of gastroparesis

**USUAL DOSAGE**
Infants and Children (Note: 400 mg ethylsuccinate = 250 mg base, stearate, or estolate salts):
Oral: 30-50 mg/kg/day divided every 6-8 hours; may double doses in severe infections
Preop bowel preparation: 20 mg/kg erythromycin base at 1, 2, and 11 PM on the day before surgery combined with mechanical cleansing of the large intestine and oral neomycin
I.V.: Lactobionate: 20-40 mg/kg/day divided every 6 hours
Adults:
Oral:
Base: 250-500 mg every 6-12 hours
Ethylsuccinate: 400-800 mg every 6-12 hours
Preop bowel preparation: Oral: 1 g erythromycin base at 1, 2, and 11 PM on the day before surgery combined with mechanical cleansing of the large intestine and oral neomycin
I.V.: Lactobionate: 15-20 mg/kg/day divided every 6 hours or 500 mg to 1 g every 6 hours, or given as a continuous infusion over 24 hours (maximum: 4 g/24 hours)
Children and Adults: Ophthalmic: Instill ½" (1.25 cm) 2-8 times/day depending on the severity of the infection
Dialysis: Slightly dialyzable (5% to 20%); no supplemental dosage necessary in hemo or peritoneal dialysis or in continuous arteriovenous or venovenous hemofiltration (CAVH/CAVHD)
Erythromycin has been used as a prokinetic agent to improve gastric emptying time and intestinal motility. In adults, 200 mg was infused I.V. initially followed by 250 mg orally 3 times/day 30 minutes before meals. In children, erythromycin 3 mg/kg I.V. has been infused over 60 minutes initially followed by 20 mg/kg/day orally in 3-4 divided doses before meals or before meals and at bedtime
**Dosage Forms** Erythromycin base: **Cap: Delayed release:** 250 mg, **Delayed release, enteric coated pellets (Eryc®):** 250 mg; **Tab: Delayed release:** 333 mg, **Enteric coated (E-Mycin®, Ery-Tab®, E-Base®):** 250 mg, 333 mg, 500 mg, **Film coated:** 250 mg, 500 mg, **Polymer coated particles (PCE®):** 333 mg, 500 mg
Erythromycin estolate: **Cap (Ilosone® Pulvules®):** 250 mg; **Susp, oral (Ilosone®):** 125 mg/5 mL (480 mL), 250 mg/5 mL (480 mL); **Tab (Ilosone®):** 500 mg
Erythromycin ethylsuccinate: **Granules for oral susp (EryPed®):** 400 mg/5 mL (60 mL, 100 mL, 200 mL); **Powder for oral susp (E.E.S.®):** 200 mg/5 mL (100 mL, 200 mL); **Susp: Oral (E.E.S.®, EryPed®):** 200 mg/5 mL (5 mL, 100 mL, 200 mL, 480 mL), 400 mg/5 mL (5 (Continued)

## Erythromycin *(Continued)*

mL, 60 mL, 100 mL, 200 mL, 480 mL), **Oral [drops] (EryPed®):** 100 mg/2.5 mL (50 mL);
**Tab (E.E.S.®):** 400 mg, **Tab, chewable (EryPed®):** 200 mg

Erythromycin gluceptate: **Inj:** 1000 mg (30 mL)

Erythromycin lactobionate: **Powder for inj:** 500 mg, 1000 mg

Erythromycin stearate: **Tab, film coated (Eramycin®, Erythrocin®):** 250 mg, 500 mg

**Contraindications** Hepatic impairment, known hypersensitivity to erythromycin or its components; pre-existing liver disease (erythromycin estolate); concomitant use with pimozide, terfenadine, astemizole, or cisapride

**Warnings/Precautions** Hepatic impairment with or without jaundice has occurred, it may be accompanied by malaise, nausea, vomiting, abdominal colic, and fever; discontinue use if these occur; avoid using erythromycin lactobionate in neonates since formulations may contain benzyl alcohol which is associated with toxicity in neonates; observe for superinfections

**Pregnancy Risk Factor** B

**Adverse Reactions**

>10%: Gastrointestinal: Abdominal pain, cramping, nausea, vomiting

1% to 10%:

Gastrointestinal: Oral candidiasis

Hepatic: Cholestatic jaundice

Local: Phlebitis at the injection site

Miscellaneous: Hypersensitivity reactions

<1%: Ventricular arrhythmias, fever, rash, hypertrophic pyloric stenosis, diarrhea, pseudomembranous colitis, eosinophilia, cholestatic jaundice (most common with estolate), thrombophlebitis, allergic reactions

**Drug Interactions** CYP3A3/4 enzyme substrate; CYP1A2 and 3A3/4 enzyme inhibitor

Increased toxicity:

Erythromycin decreases clearance of carbamazepine, cyclosporine, and triazolam, alfentanil, bromocriptine, digoxin (~10% of patients), disopyramide, ergot alkaloids, methylprednisolone; may decrease clearance of protease inhibitors

Erythromycin may decrease theophylline clearance and increase theophylline's half-life by up to 60% (patients on high-dose theophylline and erythromycin or who have received erythromycin for >5 days may be at higher risk)

Decreases metabolism of terfenadine, cisapride, and astemizole resulting in an increase in Q-T interval and potential heart failure

Inhibits felodipine (and other dihydropyridine calcium antagonist) metabolism in the liver resulting in a twofold increase in levels and consequent toxicity

Death has been reported by potentiation of pimozide's cardiotoxicity when given concurrently with erythromycin

May potentiate anticoagulant effect of warfarin and decrease metabolism of vinblastine

Concurrent use of erythromycin and lovastatin and simvastatin may result in significantly increased levels and rhabdomyolysis

**Half-Life** 1.5-2 hours (peak); End-stage renal disease: 5-6 hours

**Special PA Issues**

**Patient Education:** Take as directed, around-the-clock, with a full glass of water (not juice or milk), preferably on an empty stomach (1 hour before or 2 hours after meals). Take complete prescription even if you are feeling better. You may experience nausea, vomiting, or mouth sores (small frequent meals, frequent mouth care may help). Report skin rash or itching; easy bruising or bleeding; unhealed sores of mouth; itching or vaginal discharge; watery or bloody diarrhea; unresolved vomiting; yellowing of skin or eyes; easy fatigue; pale stool or dark urine; skin rash or itching; white plaques, sores, or fuzziness in mouth; or any change in hearing.

Ophthalmic: Wash hands before applying. Pull down lower eyelid gently, instill thin ribbon of ointment into lower lid, close eye, roll eyeball in all directions. Blurred vision and stinging is temporary. Report persistent pain, burning, vision disturbances, swelling, itching, or worsening of condition.

**Dietary Considerations:** Food: Increased drug absorption with meals. Drug may cause GI upset; may take with food.

## Erythromycin and Benzoyl Peroxide

(er ith roe MYE sin & BEN zoe il per OKS ide)

**Pharmacologic Class** Acne Products

**U.S. Brand Names** Benzamycin®

**Dosage Forms Gel:** Erythromycin 30 mg and benzoyl peroxide 50 mg per g

## Erythromycin and Sulfisoxazole (er ith roe MYE sin & sul fi SOKS a zole)

**Pharmacologic Class** Antibiotic, Macrolide; Antibiotic, Sulfonamide Derivative

**U.S. Brand Names** Eryzole®; Pediazole®

**Mechanism of Action** Erythromycin inhibits bacterial protein synthesis; sulfisoxazole competitively inhibits bacterial synthesis of folic acid from para-aminobenzoic acid

**Use** Treatment of susceptible bacterial infections of the upper and lower respiratory tract, otitis media in children caused by susceptible strains of *Haemophilus influenzae*, and many other infections in patients allergic to penicillin

**USUAL DOSAGE** Oral (dosage recommendation is based on the product's erythromycin content):

Children ≥2 months: 50 mg/kg/day erythromycin and 150 mg/kg/day sulfisoxazole in divided doses every 6 hours; not to exceed 2 g erythromycin/day or 6 g sulfisoxazole/day for 10 days

Adults >45 kg: 400 mg erythromycin and 1200 mg sulfisoxazole every 6 hours

**Dosing adjustment in renal impairment** (sulfisoxazole must be adjusted in renal impairment):

$Cl_{cr}$ 10-50 mL/minute: Administer every 8-12 hours

$Cl_{cr}$ <10 mL/minute: Administer every 12-24 hours

**Dosage Forms Susp, oral:** Erythromycin ethylsuccinate 200 mg and sulfisoxazole acetyl 600 mg per 5 mL (100 mL, 150 mL, 200 mL, 250 mL)

**Contraindications** Hepatic dysfunction, known hypersensitivity to erythromycin or sulfonamides; infants <2 months of age (sulfas compete with bilirubin for binding sites); patients with porphyria; concurrent use with pimozide, terfenadine, astemizole, or cisapride

**Warnings/Precautions** Use with caution in patients with impaired renal or hepatic function, G-6-PD deficiency (hemolysis may occur)

**Pregnancy Risk Factor** C

**Adverse Reactions**

>10%: Gastrointestinal: Abdominal pain, cramping, nausea, vomiting

1% to 10%:

Gastrointestinal: Oral candidiasis

Local: Phlebitis at the injection site

Miscellaneous: Hypersensitivity reactions

<1%: Ventricular arrhythmias, fever, headache, rash, Stevens-Johnson syndrome, toxic epidermal necrolysis, hypertrophic pyloric stenosis, diarrhea, pseudomembranous colitis, crystalluria, eosinophilia, agranulocytosis, aplastic anemia, hepatic necrosis, cholestatic jaundice, thrombophlebitis, toxic nephrosis

**Drug Interactions**

Increased effect/toxicity/levels with erythromycin/sulfisoxazole on alfentanil, astemizole, terfenadine (resulting in potentially life-threatening prolonged Q-T interval), bromocriptine, carbamazepine, cyclosporine, digoxin, disopyramide, theophylline, triazolam, lovastatin/simvastatin, ergots, methylprednisolone, cisapride, pimozide, felodipine, phenytoin, barbiturate anesthetics, methotrexate, sulfonylureas, uricosuric agents, and warfarin; may inhibit metabolism of protease inhibitors

Increased toxicity of sulfonamides occurs with concurrent diuretics, indomethacin, methenamine, probenecid, and salicylates

**Special PA Issues**

**Monitoring Parameters:** CBC and periodic liver function test

# Estazolam (es TA zoe lam)

**Pharmacologic Class** Benzodiazepine

**U.S. Brand Names** ProSom™

**Mechanism of Action** Benzodiazepines may exert their pharmacologic effect through potentiation of the inhibitory activity of GABA. Benzodiazepines do not alter the synthesis, release, reuptake, or enzymatic degradation of GABA.

(Continued)

## Estazolam *(Continued)*

**Use** Short-term management of insomnia; there has been little experience with this drug in the elderly, but because of its lack of active metabolites, it is a reasonable choice when a benzodiazepine hypnotic is indicated

**USUAL DOSAGE** Adults: Oral: 1 mg at bedtime, some patients may require 2 mg; start at doses of 0.5 mg in debilitated or small elderly patients

**Dosing adjustment in hepatic impairment:** May be necessary

**Dosage Forms Tab:** 1 mg, 2 mg

**Contraindications** Pregnancy; hypersensitivity to estazolam, cross-sensitivity with other benzodiazepines may occur, pre-existing CNS depression, sleep apnea, narrow-angle glaucoma

**Warnings/Precautions** Abrupt discontinuance may precipitate withdrawal or rebound insomnia; use with caution in patients receiving other CNS depressants, patients with low albumin, hepatic dysfunction, and in the elderly; do not use in pregnant women; may cause drug dependency; safety and efficacy have not been established in children <15 years of age, not recommended in nursing mothers

**Pregnancy Risk Factor** X

**Adverse Reactions**

>10%:

Cardiovascular: Tachycardia, chest pain

Central nervous system: Drowsiness, fatigue, ataxia, lightheadedness, memory impairment, insomnia, anxiety, depression, headache

Dermatologic: Rash

Endocrine & metabolic: Decreased libido

Gastrointestinal: Xerostomia, constipation, decreased salivation, nausea, vomiting, diarrhea, increased or decreased appetite

Neuromuscular & skeletal: Dysarthria

Ocular: Blurred vision

Miscellaneous: Diaphoresis

1% to 10%:

Cardiovascular: Syncope, hypotension

Central nervous system: Confusion, nervousness, dizziness, akathisia

Dermatologic: Dermatitis

Gastrointestinal: Weight gain or loss, increased salivation

Neuromuscular & skeletal: Rigidity, tremor, muscle cramps

Otic: Tinnitus

Respiratory: Nasal congestion, hyperventilation

<1%: Menstrual irregularities, blood dyscrasias, reflex slowing, drug dependence

**Drug Interactions**

Decreased effect: Enzyme inducers may increase the metabolism of estazolam

Increased toxicity: CNS depressants may increase CNS adverse effects; cimetidine may decrease metabolism of estazolam

**Onset** Within 1 hour

**Duration** Variable

**Special PA Issues**

**Patient Education:** Use exactly as directed (do not increase dose or frequency or discontinue without consulting prescriber); may cause physical and/or psychological dependence. While using this medication, do not use alcohol or other prescription or OTC medications (especially, pain medications, sedatives, antihistamines, or hypnotics) without consulting prescriber. Maintain adequate hydration (2-3 L/day of fluids unless instructed to restrict fluid intake). You may experience drowsiness, dizziness, or blurred vision (use caution when driving or engaging in hazardous tasks); GI upset (take with water or milk). Report CNS changes (confusion, depression, increased sedation, excitation, headache, abnormal thinking, insomnia, or nightmares), altered voiding patterns or blood in urine, difficulty breathing, chest pain or palpitations, altered gait pattern, or ineffectiveness of medication.

**Dietary Considerations:** Alcohol: Additive CNS effect, avoid use

**Monitoring Parameters:** Respiratory and cardiovascular status

♦ **Estinyl®** *see* Ethinyl Estradiol *on page 344*

♦ **Estivin® II [OTC]** *see* Naphazoline *on page 635*

♦ **Estrace® Oral** *see* Estradiol *on this page*

♦ **Estraderm® Transdermal** *see* Estradiol *on this page*

♦ **Estra-D® Injection** *see* Estradiol *on this page*

## Estradiol *(es tra DYE ole)*

**Pharmacologic Class** Estrogen Derivative

**U.S. Brand Names** Alora® Transdermal; Climara® Transdermal; Delestrogen® Injection; depGynogen® Injection; Depo®-Estradiol Injection; Depogen® Injection; Dioval® Injection; Dura-Estrin® Injection; Duragen® Injection; Esclim® Transdermal; Estrace® Oral;

Estraderm® Transdermal; Estra-D® Injection; Estra-L® Injection; Estring®; Estro-Cyp® Injection; Estroject-L.A.® Injection; FemPatch® Transdermal; Gynogen L.A.® Injection; Valergen® Injection; Vivelle® Transdermal

**Mechanism of Action** Increases the synthesis of DNA, RNA, and various proteins in target tissues; reduces the release of gonadotropin-releasing hormone from the hypothalamus; reduces FSH and LH release from the pituitary

**Use** Treatment of atrophic vaginitis, atrophic dystrophy of vulva, menopausal symptoms, female hypogonadism, ovariectomy, primary ovarian failure, inoperable breast cancer, inoperable prostatic cancer, mild to severe vasomotor symptoms associated with menopause

**USUAL DOSAGE** Adults (all dosage needs to be adjusted based upon the patient's response):

Male:

Prostate cancer: Valerate: I.M.: ≥30 mg or more every 1-2 weeks

Prostate cancer (androgen-dependent, inoperable, progressing): Oral: 10 mg 3 times/day for at least 3 months

Female:

Breast cancer (inoperable, progressing): Oral: 10 mg 3 times/day for at least 3 months

Osteoporosis prevention: Oral: 0.5 mg/day in a cyclic regimen (3 weeks on and 1 week off of drug)

Hypogonadism, moderate to severe vasomotor symptoms:

Oral: 1-2 mg/day in a cyclic regimen for 3 weeks on drug, then 1 week off drug

I.M.: Valerate: 10-20 mg every 4 weeks given cyclically

Moderate to severe vasomotor symptoms:

Oral: 1-2 mg/day; adjust to control presenting symptoms and titrate to the minimal effective dose for maintenance therapy. Use the lowest dose and regimen that will control symptoms and discontinue medication as soon as possible. Attempt to discontinue or taper medication at 3- to 6-month intervals.

I.M.: Cypionate: 1-5 mg every 3-4 weeks; attempt to discontinue or taper medication at 3- to 6-month intervals

I.M.: Valerate: 10-20 mg every 4 weeks

Postpartum breast engorgement: I.M.: Valerate: 10-25 mg at end of first stage of labor

Transdermal: Apply 0.05 mg patch initially (titrate dosage to response) applied twice weekly (once weekly for Climara® Transdermal) in a cyclic regimen, for 3 weeks on drug and 1 week off drug in patients with an intact uterus and continuously in patients without a uterus

Atrophic vaginitis, kraurosis vulvae: Vaginal: Insert 2-4 g/day for 2 weeks then gradually reduce to 1/2 the initial dose for 2 weeks followed by a maintenance dose of 1 g 1-3 times/week

**Dosing adjustment in hepatic impairment:**

Mild to moderate liver impairment: Dosage reduction of estrogens is recommended

Severe liver impairment: **Not recommended**

**Dosage Forms** Estradiol base: **Crm, vaginal (Estrace®):** 0.1 mg/g (42.5 g); **Tab, micronized (Estrace®):** 1 mg, 2 mg; **Transdermal system:** Alora®: 0.05 mg/24 hours [18 cm²], total estradiol 1.5 mg; 0.075 mg/24 hours [27 cm²], total estradiol 2.3 mg; 0.1 mg/24 hours [36 cm²], total estradiol 3 mg; Climara®: 0.05 mg/24 hours [12.5 cm²], total estradiol 3.9 mg; 0.1 mg/24 hours [25 cm²], total estradiol 7.8 mg; Esclim®: 0.025 mg/24 hours; 0.0375 mg/24 hours; 0.05 mg/24 hours; 0.075 mg/24 hours; Estraderm®: 0.05 mg/24 hours [10 cm²], total estradiol 4 mg; 0.1 mg/24 hours [20 cm²], total estradiol 8 mg; Vivelle®: 0.0375 mg/day, 0.05 mg/day, 0.075 mg/day; **Vaginal ring (Estring®):** 2 mg gradually released over 90 days; **Estradiol cypionate: Inj (depGynogen®, Depo®-Estradiol, Depogen®, Dura-Estrin®, Estra-D®, Estro-Cyp®, Estroject-L.A.®):** 5 mg/mL (5 mL, 10 mL); **Estradiol valerate: Inj:** Valergen®: 10 mg/mL (5 mL, 10 mL), 20 mg/mL (1 mL, 5 mL, 10 mL), 40 mg/mL (5 mL, 10 mL), Dioval®, Duragen®, Estra-L®, Gynogen L.A.®: 20 mg/mL (10 mL); 40 mg/mL (10 mL)

**Contraindications** Known or suspected pregnancy, undiagnosed genital bleeding, carcinoma of the breast (except in patients treated for metastatic disease), estrogen-dependent tumors, history of thrombophlebitis, thrombosis, or thromboembolic disorders associated with estrogen use

**Warnings/Precautions** Use with caution in patients with renal or hepatic insufficiency; estrogens may cause premature closure of epiphyses in young individuals; in patients with a history of thromboembolism, stroke, myocardial infarction (especially >40 years of age who smoke), liver tumor, hypertension.

Estrogens have been reported to increase the risk of endometrial carcinoma; do not use estrogens during pregnancy. Before prescribing estrogen therapy to postmenopausal women, the risks and benefits must be weighed for each patient. Women should be informed of these risks and benefits, as well as possible side effects and the return of menstrual bleeding (when cycled with a progestin), and be involved in the decision to prescribe. Oral therapy may be more convenient for vaginal atrophy and stress incontinence.

**Pregnancy Risk Factor** X

(Continued)

## Estradiol *(Continued)*

### Adverse Reactions

>10%:

Cardiovascular: Peripheral edema

Endocrine & metabolic: Enlargement of breasts (female and male), breast tenderness

Gastrointestinal: Nausea, anorexia, bloating

1% to 10%:

Central nervous system: Headache

Endocrine & metabolic: Increased libido (female), decreased libido (male)

Gastrointestinal: Vomiting, diarrhea

<1%: Increase in blood pressure, edema, thromboembolic disorders, myocardial infarction, depression, dizziness, anxiety, stroke, chloasma, melasma, rash, hypercalcemia, folate deficiency, change in menstrual flow, breast tumors, amenorrhea, decreased glucose tolerance, increased triglycerides and LDL, GI distress, cholestatic jaundice, pain at injection site, intolerance to contact lenses, increased susceptibility to *Candida* infection

**Drug Interactions** CYP1A2 and 3A3/4 enzyme substrate

Decreased effect: Rifampin decreases estrogen serum concentrations

Increased toxicity: Hydrocortisone increases corticosteroid toxic potential; increased potential for thromboembolic events with anticoagulants

**Half-Life** 50-60 minutes

### Special PA Issues

**Patient Education:** Use this drug in cycles or term as prescribed. Periodic gynecologic exam and breast exams are important. You may experience nausea or vomiting (small frequent meals may help); dizziness or mental depression (use caution when driving); photosensitivity (avoid direct sun, use sunblock or wear protective clothing); rash; loss of scalp hair; enlargement/tenderness of breasts; increased/decreased libido. Report sudden acute pain in legs or calves, chest, or abdomen; shortness of breath; severe headache or vomiting; weakness or numbness of arms or legs; unusual vaginal bleeding; yellowing of skin or eyes; change in color of urine or stool; or easy bruising or bleeding.

Transdermal patch: Apply to clean dry skin. Do not apply transdermal patch to breasts. Apply to trunk of body (preferably abdomen). Rotate application sites. Aerosol topical corticosteroids may reduce allergic skin reaction; report persistent skin reaction.

Intravaginal cream: Insert high in vagina. Wash hands and applicator before and after use.

**Reference Range:**

Children: <10 pg/mL (SI: <37 pmol/L)

Male: 10-50 pg/mL (SI: 37-184 pmol/L)

Female: Premenopausal: 30-400 pg/mL (SI: 110-1468 pmol/L); Postmenopausal: 0-30 pg/mL (SI: 0-110 pmol/L)

## Estradiol and Testosterone (es tra DYE ole & tes TOS ter one)

**Pharmacologic Class** Estrogen Derivative

**U.S. Brand Names** Andro/Fem® Injection; Deladumone® Injection; depAndrogyn® Injection; Depo-Testadiol® Injection; Depotestogen® Injection; Duo-Cyp® Injection; Duratestrin® Injection; Valertest No.1® Injection

**Dosage Forms Inj:** Andro/Fem®, depAndrogyn®, Depo-Testadiol®, Depotestogen®, Duo-Cyp®, Duratestrin®: Estradiol cypionate 2 mg and testosterone cypionate 50 mg per mL in cottonseed oil (1 mL, 10 mL), Androgyn L.A.®, Deladumone®, Estra-Testrin®, Valertest No.1®: Estradiol valerate 4 mg and testosterone enanthate 90 mg per mL in sesame oil (5 mL, 10 mL)

♦ **Estradiol Cypionate** *see Estradiol on page 332*

♦ **Estradiol Transdermal** *see Estradiol on page 332*

♦ **Estradiol Valerate** *see Estradiol on page 332*

♦ **Estra-L® Injection** *see Estradiol on page 332*

## Estramustine (es tra MUS teen)

**Pharmacologic Class** Antineoplastic Agent, Alkylating Agent

**U.S. Brand Names** Emcyt®

**Mechanism of Action** Mechanism is not completely clear, thought to act as an alkylating agent and as estrogen

**Use** Palliative treatment of prostatic carcinoma (progressive or metastatic)

**USUAL DOSAGE** Adults: Oral: 14 mg/kg/day (range: 10-16 mg/kg/day) in 3-4 divided doses for 30-90 days; some patients have been maintained for >3 years on therapy

**Dosage Forms Cap, as phosphate sodium:** 140 mg

**Contraindications** Active thrombophlebitis or thromboembolic disorders, hypersensitivity to estramustine or any component, estradiol or nitrogen mustard

**Warnings/Precautions** The U.S. Food and Drug Administration (FDA) currently recommends that procedures for proper handling and disposal of antineoplastic agents be considered. Glucose tolerance may be decreased; elevated blood pressure may occur;

exacerbation of peripheral edema or congestive heart disease may occur; use with caution in patients with impaired liver function, renal insufficiency, or metabolic bone diseases.

**Pregnancy Risk Factor** C

**Adverse Reactions**

>10%:
  Cardiovascular: Edema
  Gastrointestinal: Diarrhea, nausea, mild increases in AST (SGOT) or LDH
  Endocrine & metabolic: Decreased libido, breast tenderness, breast enlargement
  Respiratory: Dyspnea

1% to 10%:
  Cardiovascular: Myocardial infarction
  Central nervous system: Insomnia, lethargy
  Gastrointestinal: Anorexia, flatulence
  Hematologic: Leukopenia
  Local: Thrombophlebitis
  Neuromuscular & skeletal: Leg cramps
  Respiratory: Pulmonary embolism

<1%: Cardiac arrest, depression, pigment changes, hypercalcemia, hot flashes, tinnitus, night sweats

**Drug Interactions** Decreased effect: Milk products and calcium-rich foods/drugs may impair the oral absorption of estramustine phosphate sodium

**Half-Life** 20 hours

**Special PA Issues**

**Patient Education:** It may take several weeks to manifest effects of this medication. Store capsules in refrigerator. Do not take with milk or milk products. Preferable to take on empty stomach (1 hour before or 2 hours after meals). Small frequent meals, frequent mouth care may reduce incidence of nausea or vomiting. You may experience flatulence, diarrhea, decreased libido (reversible), breast tenderness or enlargement. Report sudden acute pain or cramping in legs or calves, chest pain, shortness of breath, weakness or numbness of arms or legs, difficulty breathing, or edema (increased weight, swelling of legs or feet).

♦ **Estramustine Phosphate Sodium** see Estramustine *on previous page*

♦ **Estratab®** see Estrogens, Esterified *on page 337*

♦ **Estratest®** see Estrogens and Methyltestosterone *on this page*

♦ **Estratest® H.S.** see Estrogens and Methyltestosterone *on this page*

♦ **Estring®** see Estradiol *on page 332*

♦ **Estro-Cyp® Injection** see Estradiol *on page 332*

♦ **Estrogenic Substance Aqueous** see Estrone *on page 338*

♦ **Estrogenic Substances, Conjugated** see Estrogens, Conjugated *on this page*

## Estrogens and Medroxyprogesterone
(ES troe jenz & me DROKS ee proe JES te rone)

**Pharmacologic Class** Estrogen Derivative

**U.S. Brand Names** Premphase™; Prempro™

**Dosage Forms Premphase™: Two separate tabs in therapy pack:** Conjugated estrogens 0.625 mg [Premarin®] (28s) taken orally for 28 days and medroxyprogesterone acetate [Cycrin®] 5 mg (14s) which are taken orally with a Premarin® tab on days 15 through 28, **Prempro™:** Conjugated estrogens 0.625 mg and medroxyprogesterone acetate 2.5 mg (14s)

## Estrogens and Methyltestosterone (ES troe jenz & meth il tes TOS te rone)

**Pharmacologic Class** Estrogen Derivative

**U.S. Brand Names** Estratest®; Estratest® H.S.; Premarin® With Methyltestosterone

**Dosage Forms Tab:** Estratest®, Menogen®: Esterified estrogen 1.25 mg and methyltestosterone 2.5 mg, Estratest® H.S., Menogen H.S.®: Esterified estrogen 0.625 mg and methyltestosterone 1.25 mg, Premarin® With Methyltestosterone: Conjugated estrogen 0.625 mg and methyltestosterone 5 mg; conjugated estrogen 1.25 mg and methyltestosterone 10 mg

## Estrogens, Conjugated (ES troe jenz KON joo gate ed)

**Pharmacologic Class** Estrogen Derivative

**U.S. Brand Names** Premarin®

**Mechanism of Action** Increases the synthesis of DNA, RNA, and various proteins in target tissues; reduces the release of gonadotropin-releasing hormone from the hypothalamus; reduces FSH and LH release from the pituitary

**Use** Atrophic vaginitis; hypogonadism; primary ovarian failure; vasomotor symptoms of menopause; prostatic carcinoma; osteoporosis prophylactic

**USUAL DOSAGE** Adolescents and Adults:

Male: Prostate cancer: Oral: 1.25-2.5 mg 3 times/day

(Continued)

## Estrogens, Conjugated *(Continued)*

Female:

Osteoporosis in postmenopausal women: Oral: 0.625 mg/day, cyclically (3 weeks on, 1 week off)

Dysfunctional uterine bleeding:

Stable hematocrit: Oral: 1.25 mg twice daily for 21 days; if bleeding persists after 48 hours, increase to 2.5 mg twice daily; if bleeding persists after 48 more hours, increase to 2.5 mg 4 times/day; some recommend starting at 2.5 mg 4 times/day. **(Note:** Medroxyprogesterone acetate 10 mg/day is also given on days 17-21.)

Unstable hematocrit: Oral: I.V.: 5 mg 2-4 times/day; if bleeding is profuse, 20-40 mg every 4 hours up to 24 hours may be used. **Note:** A progestational-weighted contraception pill should also be given (eg, Ovral® 2 tablets stat and 1 tablet 4 times/day or medroxyprogesterone acetate 5-10 mg 4 times/day)

Alternatively: I.V.: 25 mg every 6-12 hours until bleeding stops

Hypogonadism: Oral: 2.5-7.5 mg/day for 20 days, off 10 days and repeat until menses occur. If bleeding does not occur by the end of this period, repeat dosage schedule. If bleeding occurs before the end of the 10-day period, begin a 20-day estrogen-progestin cyclic regimen with 2.5-7.5 mg estrogen daily in divided doses for 1-20 days. During the last 5 days of estrogen therapy, give an oral progestin. If bleeding occurs before this regimen is concluded, discontinue therapy and resume on day 5 of bleeding.

Moderate to severe vasomotor symptoms: Oral: 1.25 mg/day if patient has not menstruated in ≥2 months, start cyclic administration arbitrarily. If patient is menstruating, begin administration on day 5 of bleeding.

Postpartum breast engorgement: Oral: 3.75 mg every 4 hours for 5 doses, then 1.25 mg every 4 hours for 5 days

Atrophic vaginitis, kraurosis vulvae:

Oral: 0.3-1.25 mg or more daily depending on tissue response of the patient; administer cyclically (3 weeks of daily estrogen and 1 week off)

Vaginal: 2-4 g instilled/day 3 weeks on and 1 week off

Female castration and primary ovarian failure: Oral: 1.25 mg/day cyclically (3 weeks on, 1 week off). Adjust according to severity of symptoms and patient response. For maintenance, adjust to the lowest effective dose.

Male/Female: Uremic bleeding: I.V.: 0.6 mg/kg/dose daily for 5 days

**Dosing adjustment in hepatic impairment:**

Mild to moderate liver impairment: Dosage reduction of estrogens is recommended

Severe liver impairment: **Not recommended**

**Dosage Forms Crm, vaginal:** 0.625 mg/g (42.5 g); **Inj:** 25 mg (5 mL); **Tab:** 0.3 mg, 0.625 mg, 0.9 mg, 1.25 mg, 2.5 mg

**Contraindications** Undiagnosed vaginal bleeding; hypersensitivity to estrogens or any component; thrombophlebitis, liver disease, known or suspected pregnancy, carcinoma of the breast, estrogen dependent tumor

**Warnings/Precautions** Use with caution in patients with asthma, epilepsy, migraine, diabetes, cardiac or renal dysfunction; estrogens may cause premature closure of the epiphyses in young individuals; safety and efficacy in children have not been established; estrogens have been reported to increase the risk of endometrial carcinoma; do not use estrogens during pregnancy

**Pregnancy Risk Factor** X

**Adverse Reactions**

>10%:

Cardiovascular: Peripheral edema

Endocrine & metabolic: Breast tenderness, hypercalcemia, enlargement of breasts

Gastrointestinal: Nausea, anorexia, bloating

1% to 10%:

Central nervous system: Headache

Endocrine & metabolic: Increased libido

Gastrointestinal: Vomiting, diarrhea

Local: Pain at injection site

<1%: Increase in blood pressure, edema, thromboembolic disorder, myocardial infarction, hypertension, depression, dizziness, anxiety, stroke, chloasma, melasma, rash, breast tumors, amenorrhea, alterations in frequency and flow of menses, decreased glucose tolerance, increased triglycerides and LDL, GI distress, cholestatic jaundice, intolerance to contact lenses, increased susceptibility to *Candida* infection

**Drug Interactions** CYP1A2 enzyme inducer

Decreased effect: Rifampin decreases estrogen serum concentrations

Increased toxicity:

Hydrocortisone increases corticosteroid toxic potential

Increased potential for thromboembolic events with anticoagulants

**Special PA Issues**

**Patient Education:** Follow prescribed schedule and dose. Periodic gynecologic exam and breast exams are important with long-term use. Consult prescriber for specific dietary recommendations. You may experience nausea or vomiting (small frequent meals may help); dizziness or mental depression (use caution when driving); photosensitivity (avoid direct sun exposure, wear sunscreen or protective clothing); rash, loss of scalp hair (reversible); enlargement/tenderness of breasts (both male and female); increased (female)/decreased (male) libido; or headache (use of mild analgesic may help). Report swelling of extremities or unusual weight gain; chest pain or palpitations; sudden acute pain, warmth, or weakness in legs or calves; shortness of breath; severe headache or vomiting; or unusual vaginal bleeding, amenorrhea, or alterations in frequency and flow of menses.

Intravaginal cream: Insert high in vagina; wash hands and applicator before and after application.

**Reference Range:**
Children: <10 µg/24 hours (SI: <35 µmol/day) (values at Mayo Medical Laboratories)
Adults:
  Male: 15-40 µg/24 hours (SI: 52-139 µmol/day)
  Female: Menstruating: 15-80 µg/24 hours (SI: 52-277 µmol/day); Postmenopausal: <20 µg/24 hours (SI: <69 µmol/day)

# Estrogens, Esterified (ES troe jenz, es TER i fied)

**Pharmacologic Class** Estrogen Derivative

**U.S. Brand Names** Estratab®; Menest®

**Mechanism of Action** Primary effects on the interphase DNA-protein complex (chromatin) by binding to a receptor (usually located in the cytoplasm of a target cell) and initiating translocation of the hormone-receptor complex to the nucleus

**Use** Atrophic vaginitis; hypogonadism; primary ovarian failure; vasomotor symptoms of menopause; prostatic carcinoma; osteoporosis prophylactic

**USUAL DOSAGE** Adults: Oral:

Male: Prostate cancer (inoperable, progressing): 1.25-2.5 mg 3 times/day
Female:

Hypogonadism: 2.5-7.5 mg of estrogen daily for 20 days followed by a 10-day rest period. Administer cyclically (3 weeks on and 1 week off). If bleeding does not occur by the end of the 10-day period, begin an estrogen-progestin cyclic regimen of 2.5-7.5 mg/day in divided doses for 20 days. During the last days of estrogen therapy, give an oral progestin. If bleeding occurs before this regimen is concluded, discontinue therapy and resume on the fifth day of bleeding.

Moderate to severe vasomotor symptoms: 1.25 mg/day administered cyclically (3 weeks on and 1 week off). If patient has not menstruated within the last 2 months or more, cyclic administration is started arbitrary. If the patient is menstruating, cyclical administration is started on day 5 of the bleeding. For short-term use only and should be discontinued as soon as possible. Re-evaluate at 3- to 6-month intervals for tapering or discontinuation of therapy.

Atopic vaginitis and kraurosis vulvae: 0.3 to ≥1.25 mg/day, depending on the tissue response of the individual patient. Administer cyclically. For short-term use only and should be discontinued as soon as possible. Re-evaluate at 3- to 6-month intervals for tapering or discontinuation of therapy.

Breast cancer (inoperable, progressing): 10 mg 3 times/day for at least 3 months
Osteoporosis, in postmenopausal women: Initial: 0.3 mg/day and increase to a maximum daily dose of 1.25 mg/day; initiate therapy as soon as possible after menopause; cyclical therapy is recommended

Female castration and primary ovarian failure: 1.25 mg/day, cyclically. Adjust dosage up- or downward according to the severity of symptoms and patient response. For maintenance, adjust dosage to lowest level that will provide effective control.

**Dosing adjustment in hepatic impairment:**
Mild to moderate liver impairment: Dosage reduction of estrogens is recommended
Severe liver impairment: **Not recommended**

**Dosage Forms Tab:** 0.3 mg, 0.625 mg, 1.25 mg, 2.5 mg

**Contraindications** Known or suspected cancer of the breast, except in appropriately selected patients being treated for metastatic disease; known or suspected estrogen-dependent neoplasia; known or suspected pregnancy; undiagnosed abnormal genital bleeding; active thrombophlebitis or thromboembolic disorders; past history of thrombophlebitis, thrombosis, or thromboembolic disorders associated with previous estrogen use except when used in the treatment of breast or prostatic malignancy

**Warnings/Precautions** Use with caution in patients with asthma, epilepsy, migraine, diabetes, cardiac or renal dysfunction; estrogens may cause premature closure of the epiphyses in young individuals; safety and efficacy in children have not been established; estrogens have been reported to increase the risk of endometrial carcinoma; do not use estrogens during pregnancy

**Pregnancy Risk Factor** X

**Adverse Reactions**
>10%:
  Cardiovascular: Peripheral edema
  Endocrine & metabolic: Enlargement of breasts, breast tenderness
  Gastrointestinal: Nausea, anorexia, bloating
(Continued)

## Estrogens, Esterified (Continued)

1% to 10%:
Central nervous system: Headache
Endocrine & metabolic: Increased libido
Gastrointestinal: Vomiting, diarrhea

<1%: Hypertension, thromboembolism, myocardial infarction, edema, stroke, depression, dizziness, anxiety, chloasma, melasma, rash, amenorrhea, alterations in frequency and flow of menses, decreased glucose tolerance, increased triglycerides and LDL, GI distress, cholestatic jaundice, intolerance to contact lenses, increased susceptibility to *Candida* infection, breast tumors

### Drug Interactions

Decreased effect: Rifampin decreases estrogen serum concentrations
Increased toxicity:
Hydrocortisone increases corticosteroid toxic potential
Anticoagulants: Increases potential for thromboembolic events with anticoagulants
Carbamazepine, tricyclic antidepressants, and corticosteroids; increased thromboembolic potential with oral anticoagulants

### Special PA Issues

**Patient Education:** Use this drug in cycles or term as prescribed. Take each day at the same time with food. Periodic gynecologic exam and breast exams are important. You may experience nausea or vomiting (small frequent meals may help); dizziness or mental depression (use caution when driving); rash; loss of scalp hair; enlargement/tenderness of breasts; or increased/decreased libido. Report significant swelling of extremities, sudden acute pain in legs or calves, chest, or abdomen; shortness of breath; severe headache or vomiting; weakness or numbness of arms or legs; or unusual vaginal bleeding.

♦ **Estroject-L.A.® Injection** *see* Estradiol *on page 332*

## Estrone (ES trone)

**Pharmacologic Class** Estrogen Derivative

**U.S. Brand Names** Aquest®; Kestrone®

**Mechanism of Action** Estrone is a natural ovarian estrogenic hormone that is available as an aqueous mixture of water insoluble estrone and water soluble estrone potassium sulfate; all estrogens, including estrone, act in a similar manner; there is no evidence that there are biological differences among various estrogen preparations other than their ability to bind to cellular receptors inside the target cells

**Use** Hypogonadism; primary ovarian failure; vasomotor symptoms of menopause; prostatic carcinoma; inoperable breast cancer, kraurosis vulvae, abnormal uterine bleeding due to hormone imbalance

**USUAL DOSAGE** Adults: I.M.:

Male: Prostatic carcinoma: 2-4 mg 2-3 times/week

Female:
Senile vaginitis and kraurosis vulvae: 0.1-0.5 mg 2-3 times/week; cyclical (3 weeks on and 1 week off)
Breast cancer (inoperable, progressing): 5 mg 3 or more times/week
Primary ovarian failure, hypogonadism: 0.1-1 mg/week, up to 2 mg/week in single or divided doses; cyclical (3 weeks on and 1 week off)
Abnormal uterine bleeding: Brief courses of intensive therapy: 2-5 mg/day for several days

**Dosing adjustment in hepatic impairment:**
Mild to moderate liver impairment: Dosage reduction of estrogens is recommended
Severe liver impairment: **Not recommended**

**Dosage Forms Inj:** 2 mg/mL (10 mL, 30 mL), 5 mg/mL (10 mL)

**Contraindications** Thrombophlebitis, undiagnosed vaginal bleeding, hypersensitivity to estrogens or any component, pregnancy

**Warnings/Precautions** Use with caution in patients with asthma, epilepsy, migraine, diabetes, cardiac or renal dysfunction; estrogens may cause premature closure of the epiphyses in young individuals; safety and efficacy in children have not been established; estrogens have been reported to increase the risk of endometrial carcinoma, do not use estrogens during pregnancy

**Pregnancy Risk Factor** X

**Adverse Reactions**

>10%:
Cardiovascular: Peripheral edema
Endocrine & metabolic: Enlargement of breasts, breast tenderness
Gastrointestinal: Nausea, anorexia, bloating

1% to 10%:
Central nervous system: Headache
Endocrine & metabolic: Increased libido
Gastrointestinal: Vomiting, diarrhea

&lt;1%: Hypertension, thromboembolism, myocardial infarction, edema, stroke, depression, dizziness, anxiety, chloasma, melasma, rash, amenorrhea, alterations in frequency and flow of menses, decreased glucose tolerance, increased triglycerides and LDL, GI distress, cholestatic jaundice, intolerance to contact lenses, increased susceptibility to *Candida* infection, breast tumors

**Drug Interactions**
Decreased effect: Rifampin decreases estrogen serum concentrations
Increased toxicity:
  Hydrocortisone increases corticosteroid toxic potential
  Anticoagulants: Increases potential for thromboembolic events with anticoagulants
  Carbamazepine, tricyclic antidepressants, and corticosteroids; increased thromboembolic potential with oral anticoagulants

**Special PA Issues**
**Patient Education:** This drug can only be given I.M. It is important to maintain schedule of drug days and drug-free days. Periodic gynecologic exam and breast exams are important. You may experience nausea or vomiting (small frequent meals may help); dizziness or mental depression (use caution when driving); rash; loss of scalp hair; enlargement/tenderness of breasts; or increased/decreased libido. Report significant swelling of extremities, sudden acute pain in legs or calves, chest, or abdomen; shortness of breath; severe headache or vomiting; weakness or numbness of arms or legs; or unusual vaginal bleeding.

# Estropipate (ES troe pih pate)

**Pharmacologic Class** Estrogen Derivative
**U.S. Brand Names** Ogen® Oral; Ogen® Vaginal; Ortho-Est® Oral
**Mechanism of Action** Crystalline estrone that has been solubilized as the sulfate and stabilized with piperazine. Primary effects on the interphase DNA-protein complex (chromatin) by binding to a receptor (usually located in the cytoplasm of a target cell) and initiating translocation of the hormone receptor complex to the nucleus.
**Use** Atrophic vaginitis; hypogonadism; primary ovarian failure; vasomotor symptoms of menopause; osteoporosis prophylactic

**USUAL DOSAGE** Adults: Female:
Moderate to severe vasomotor symptoms: Oral: Usual dosage range: 0.75-6 mg estropipate daily. Use the lowest dose and regimen that will control symptoms, and discontinue as soon as possible. Attempt to discontinue or taper medication at 3- to 6-month intervals. If a patient with vasomotor symptoms has not menstruated within the last ≥2 months, start the cyclic administration arbitrarily. If the patient has menstruated, start cyclic administration on day 5 of bleeding.
Hypogonadism or primary ovarian failure: Oral: 1.5-9 mg/day for the first 3 weeks, followed by a rest period of 8-10 days. Repeat if bleeding does not occur by the end of the rest period. The duration of therapy necessary to product the withdrawal bleeding will vary according to the responsiveness of the endometrium. If satisfactory withdrawal bleeding does not occur, give an oral progestin in addition to estrogen during the third week of the cycle.
Osteoporosis prevention: Oral: 0.625 mg/day for 25 days of a 31-day cycle
Atrophic vaginitis or kraurosis vulvae: Vaginal: Instill 2-4 g/day 3 weeks on and 1 week off
**Dosing adjustment in hepatic impairment:**
Mild to moderate liver impairment: Dosage reduction of estrogens is recommended
Severe liver impairment: **Not recommended**

**Dosage Forms Crm, vaginal:** 0.15% [estropipate 1.5 mg/g] (42.5 g tube); **Tab:** 0.625 mg [estropipate 0.75 mg], 1.25 mg [estropipate 1.5 mg], 2.5 mg [estropipate 3 mg], 5 mg [estropipate 6 mg]
**Contraindications** Thrombophlebitis, undiagnosed vaginal bleeding, hypersensitivity to estrogens or any component; pregnancy
**Warnings/Precautions** Use with caution in patients with asthma, epilepsy, migraine, diabetes, cardiac or renal dysfunction; estrogens may cause premature closure of the epiphyses in young individuals; safety and efficacy in children have not been established; estrogens have been reported to increase the risk of endometrial carcinoma, do not use estrogens during pregnancy
**Pregnancy Risk Factor** X
**Adverse Reactions**
&gt;10%:
  Cardiovascular: Peripheral edema
  Endocrine & metabolic: Enlargement of breasts, breast tenderness
  Gastrointestinal: Nausea, anorexia, bloating
1% to 10%:
  Central nervous system: Headache
  Endocrine & metabolic: Increased libido
  Gastrointestinal: Vomiting, diarrhea
&lt;1%: Hypertension, thromboembolism, myocardial infarction, edema, stroke, depression, dizziness, anxiety, chloasma, melasma, rash, amenorrhea, alterations in frequency and flow of menses, decreased glucose tolerance, increased triglycerides and LDL, GI
(Continued)

## Estropipate *(Continued)*

distress, cholestatic jaundice, intolerance to contact lenses, increased susceptibility to *Candida* infection, breast tumors

**Drug Interactions**

Decreased effect: Rifampin decreases estrogen serum concentrations

Increased toxicity:

Hydrocortisone increases corticosteroid toxic potential

Anticoagulants: Increases potential for thromboembolic events with anticoagulants

Carbamazepine, tricyclic antidepressants, and corticosteroids; increased thromboembolic potential with oral anticoagulants

**Special PA Issues**

**Patient Education:** It is important to maintain schedule of drug days and drug-free days. Periodic gynecologic exam and breast exams are important. You may experience nausea or vomiting (small frequent meals may help); dizziness or mental depression (use caution when driving); rash; loss of scalp hair; enlargement/tenderness of breasts; or increased/decreased libido. Report significant swelling of extremities, sudden acute pain in legs or calves, chest or abdomen; shortness of breath; severe headache or vomiting; weakness or numbness of arms or legs; or unusual vaginal bleeding.

Intravaginal cream: Insert high in vagina, wash hands and applicator before and after application.

- ♦ **Estrostep® 21** *see* Ethinyl Estradiol and Norethindrone *on page 348*
- ♦ **Estrostep® Fe** *see* Ethinyl Estradiol and Norethindrone *on page 348*
- ♦ **Estrouis®** *see* Estropipate *on previous page*

## Etanercept (et a NER cept)

**Pharmacologic Class** Antirheumatic, Disease Modifying

**U.S. Brand Names** Enbrel®

**Mechanism of Action** Etanercept is a recombinant DNA-derived protein composed of tumor necrosis factor receptor (TNFR) linked to the Fc portion of human IgG1. Etanercept binds tumor necrosis factor (TNF) and blocks its interaction with cell surface receptors. TNF plays an important role in the inflammatory processes of rheumatoid arthritis (RA) and the resulting joint pathology.

**Use** Reduction in signs and symptoms of moderately to severely active rheumatoid arthritis in patients who have had an inadequate response to one or more disease-modifying antirheumatic drugs (DMARDs).

**USUAL DOSAGE** S.C.:

Children: 0.4 mg/kg (maximum: 25 mg dose)

Adult: 25 mg given twice weekly; if the physician determines that it is appropriate, patients may self-inject after proper training in injection technique

Elderly: Although greater sensitivity of some elderly patients cannot be ruled out, no overall differences in safety or effectiveness were observed

**Dosage Forms Powder for inj:** 25 mg

**Contraindications** Etanercept should not be administered to patients with sepsis (mortality may be increased). Do not administer to patients with known hypersensitivity to etanercept or any of its components.

**Warnings/Precautions** Etanercept may affect defenses against infections and malignancies. Safety and efficacy in patients with immunosuppression or chronic infections have not been evaluated. Discontinue administration if patient develops a serious infection. Impact on the development and course of malignancies is not fully defined. Treatment may result in the formation of autoimmune antibodies; cases of autoimmune disease have not been described. Non-neutralizing antibodies to etanercept may also be formed. No correlation of antibody development to clinical response or adverse events has been observed. The long-term immunogenicity, carcinogenic potential, or effect on fertility are unknown. No evidence of mutagenic activity has been observed *in vitro* or *in vivo*. The safety of etanercept has not been studied in children <4 years of age.

Allergic reactions may occur (<0.5%), but anaphylaxis has not been observed. If an anaphylactic reaction or other serious allergic reaction occurs, administration of etanercept should be discontinued immediately and appropriate therapy initiated.

Patients should be brought up to date with all immunizations before initiating therapy. No data are available concerning the effects of etanercept on vaccination. Live vaccines should not be given concurrently. No data are available concerning secondary transmission of live vaccines in patients receiving etanercept. Patients with a significant exposure to varicella virus should temporarily discontinue etanercept. Treatment with varicella zoster immune globulin should be considered.

**Pregnancy Risk Factor** B

**Pregnancy Implications** Developmental toxicity studies performed in animals have revealed no evidence of harm to the fetus. There are no studies in pregnant women; this drug should be used during pregnancy only if clearly needed.

It is not known whether etanercept is excreted in human milk or absorbed systemically after ingestion. Because many immunoglobulins are excreted in human milk, and because of the potential for serious adverse reactions in nursing infants from etanercept, a decision should be made whether to discontinue nursing or to discontinue the drug.

**Adverse Reactions** Events reported include those >3% with incidence higher than placebo

>10%:
Central nervous system: Headache (17%)
Local: Injection site reaction (37%)
Respiratory: Respiratory tract infection (38%), upper respiratory tract infection (29%), rhinitis (12%)
Miscellaneous: Infection (35%), positive ANA (11%), positive anti-double stranded DNA antibodies (15% by RIA, 3% by *Crithidia lucilae* assay)

>3% to 10%:
Central nervous system: Dizziness (7%)
Dermatologic: Rash (5%)
Gastrointestinal: Abdominal pain (5%), dyspepsia (4%)
Neuromuscular and skeletal: Weakness (5%)
Respiratory: Pharyngitis (7%), respiratory disorder (5%), sinusitis (3%)

<3%: Malignancies, serious infection, heart failure, myocardial infarction, myocardial ischemia, cerebral ischemia, hypertension, hypotension, cholecystitis, pancreatitis, gastrointestinal hemorrhage, bursitis, depression, dyspnea

Pediatric patients (JRA): The percentages of patients reporting abdominal pain (17%) and vomiting (14.5%) was higher than in adult RA. Two patients developed varicella infection associated with aseptic meningitis which resolved without complications (see Warnings/Precautions).

**Drug Interactions** Specific drug interaction studies have not been conducted with etanercept

**Onset** Within 2-3 weeks

**Half-Life** 115 hours (98-300 hours)

**Special PA Issues**
Patient Education: If self-injecting, follow instructions for injection and disposal of needles exactly. If redness, swelling, or irritation appears at the injection site, contact prescriber. Do not have any vaccinations while using this medication without consulting prescriber first. You may experience headache or dizziness (use caution when driving or engaging in hazardous tasks until response to medication is known). If stomach pain or cramping, unusual bleeding or bruising, blood in vomitus, stool, or urine occurs, stop taking medication and contact prescriber. Report skin rash, unusual muscle or bone weakness, or signs of respiratory flu or other infection (eg, chills, fever, sore throat, easy bruising or bleeding, mouth sores, unhealed sores).

♦ **Ethacrynate Sodium** *see* Ethacrynic Acid *on this page*

# Ethacrynic Acid (eth a KRIN ik AS id)

**Pharmacologic Class** Diuretic, Loop

**U.S. Brand Names** Edecrin®

**Mechanism of Action** Inhibits reabsorption of sodium and chloride in the ascending loop of Henle and distal renal tubule, interfering with the chloride-binding cotransport system, thus causing increased excretion of water, sodium, chloride, magnesium, and calcium

**Use** Management of edema associated with congestive heart failure; hepatic cirrhosis or renal disease; short-term management of ascites due to malignancy, idiopathic edema, and lymphedema

**USUAL DOSAGE** I.V. formulation should be diluted in D₅W or NS (1 mg/mL) and infused over several minutes

Children: Oral: 1 mg/kg/dose once daily; increase at intervals of 2-3 days as needed, to a maximum of 3 mg/kg/day
Adults:
Oral: 50-200 mg/day in 1-2 divided doses; may increase in increments of 25-50 mg at intervals of several days; doses up to 200 mg twice daily may be required with severe, refractory edema
I.V.: 0.5-1 mg/kg/dose (maximum: 100 mg/dose); repeat doses not routinely recommended; however, if indicated, repeat doses every 8-12 hours

Dosing adjustment/comments in renal impairment: Cl$_{cr}$ <10 mL/minute: Avoid use
Dialysis: Not removed by hemo- or peritoneal dialysis; supplemental dose is not necessary

**Dosage Forms** Powder for inj, as ethacrynate sodium: 50 mg (50 mL); **Tab:** 25 mg, 50 mg

**Contraindications** Hypersensitivity to ethacrynic acid or any component; anuria, hypotension, dehydration with low serum sodium concentrations; metabolic alkalosis with hypokalemia, or history of severe, watery diarrhea from ethacrynic acid

**Warnings/Precautions** Use with caution in patients with advanced hepatic cirrhosis, diabetes mellitus, hypotension, dehydration, history of watery diarrhea from ethacrynic acid, hearing impairment; ototoxicity occurs more frequently than with other loop diuretics; safety and efficacy in infants have not been established
(Continued)

## Ethacrynic Acid *(Continued)*

**Pregnancy Risk Factor** B

**Pregnancy Implications**

Clinical effects on the fetus: No data available. Generally, use of diuretics during pregnancy is avoided due to risk of decreased placental perfusion.

Breast-feeding/lactation: No data available

### Adverse Reactions

>10%: Gastrointestinal: Diarrhea

1% to 10%:

Cardiovascular: Orthostatic hypotension

Central nervous system: Headache

Endocrine & metabolic: Hyponatremia, hypochloremic alkalosis, hypokalemia

Gastrointestinal: Loss of appetite, nausea, vomiting

Ocular: Blurred vision

<1%: Nervousness, confusion, fatigue, malaise, fever, chills, rash, hyperuricemia, gout, GI bleeding, pancreatitis, stomach cramps, dysphagia, hepatic dysfunction, abnormal LFTs, jaundice, leukopenia, agranulocytosis, thrombocytopenia, irritation, ototoxicity (irreversible), renal injury, hematuria

### Drug Interactions

Increased toxicity:

Thiazide diuretics may synergistically result in profound diuresis and serious electrolyte disturbances

Hypotensive agents → additive decreased blood pressure

Drugs affected by or causing potassium depletion → additive decreased potassium

Increased ototoxicity potential with aminoglycosides, cisplatin

Ethacrynic acid increases digoxin's cardiotoxic potential → arrhythmias

Increased warfarin anticoagulant effects; increased lithium levels

Decreased effect:

Probenecid, NSAIDs, salicylates decrease diuretic effects

Decreased effectiveness of antidiabetic agents

### Onset

Onset of diuretic effect: Oral: Within 30 minutes; I.V.: 5 minutes

Peak effect: Oral: 2 hours; I.V.: 30 minutes

**Duration** Oral: 12 hours; I.V.: 2 hours

**Half-Life** Normal renal function: 2-4 hours

### Special PA Issues

**Patient Education:** Take prescribed dose with food early in day. Include orange juice or bananas (or other potassium-rich foods) in your diet, but do not take potassium supplements without consulting prescriber. You may experience postural hypotension (use caution when rising from lying or sitting position, when climbing stairs, or when driving); lightheadedness, dizziness, or drowsiness (use caution driving or when engaging in hazardous activities); diarrhea (buttermilk, boiled milk, or yogurt may help); or decreased accommodation to heat (avoid excessive exercise in hot weather). Diabetics should monitor serum glucose closely (this medication may interfere with antidiabetic medications). Report changes in hearing or ringing in ears, persistent headache, unusual confusion or nervousness, abdominal pain or blood stool, palpitations, chest pain, rapid heartbeat, joint or muscle soreness or weakness, flu-like symptoms, skin rash or itching, or blurred vision. Report swelling of ankles or feet, weight changes of more than 3 lb/day, increased fatigue, or muscle cramping or trembling.

**Monitoring Parameters:** Blood pressure, renal function, serum electrolytes, and fluid status closely, including weight and I & O daily; hearing

### Related Information

Heart Failure: Management of Patients with Left Ventricular Systolic Dysfunction *on page 1064*

## Ethambutol *(e THAM byoo tole)*

**Pharmacologic Class** Antitubercular Agent

**U.S. Brand Names** Myambutol®

**Mechanism of Action** Suppresses mycobacteria multiplication by interfering with RNA synthesis

**Use** Treatment of tuberculosis and other mycobacterial diseases in conjunction with other antituberculosis agents

**USUAL DOSAGE** Oral:

Ethambutol is generally not recommended in children whose visual acuity cannot be monitored (<6 years of age). However, ethambutol should be considered for all children with organisms resistant to other drugs, when susceptibility to ethambutol has been demonstrated, or susceptibility is likely.

**Note:** A four-drug regimen (isoniazid, rifampin, pyrazinamide, and either streptomycin or ethambutol) is preferred for the initial, empiric treatment of TB. When the drug susceptibility results are available, the regimen should be altered as appropriate.

Children (>6 years) and Adults:
Daily therapy: 15-25 mg/kg/day (maximum: 2.5 g/day)
Directly observed therapy (DOT): Twice weekly: 50 mg/kg (maximum: 2.5 g)
DOT: 3 times/week: 25-30 mg/kg (maximum: 2.5 g)
**Dosing interval in renal impairment:**
$Cl_{cr}$ 10-50 mL/minute: Administer every 24-36 hours
$Cl_{cr}$ <10 mL/minute: Administer every 48 hours
Hemodialysis: Slightly dialyzable (5% to 20%); Administer dose postdialysis
Peritoneal dialysis: Dose for $Cl_{cr}$ <10 mL/minute
Continuous arteriovenous or venovenous hemofiltration: Administer every 24-36 hours
**Dosage Forms Tab, as hydrochloride:** 100 mg, 400 mg
**Contraindications** Hypersensitivity to ethambutol or any component; optic neuritis
**Warnings/Precautions** Use only in children whose visual acuity can accurately be determined and monitored (not recommended for use in children <13 years of age); dosage modification required in patients with renal insufficiency
**Pregnancy Risk Factor** B
**Adverse Reactions**
1% to 10%:
Central nervous system: Headache, confusion, disorientation
Endocrine & metabolic: Acute gout or hyperuricemia
Gastrointestinal: Abdominal pain, anorexia, nausea, vomiting
<1%: Malaise, mental confusion, fever, rash, pruritus, abnormal LFTs, peripheral neuritis, optic neuritis, anaphylaxis
**Drug Interactions** Decreased absorption with aluminum salts
**Half-Life** 2.5-3.6 hours; End-stage renal disease: 7-15 hours
**Special PA Issues**
**Patient Education:** Take as scheduled, with meals. Avoid missing doses and do not discontinue without consulting prescriber. You may experience GI distress (frequent small meals and good oral care may help), dizziness, disorientation, drowsiness (avoid driving or engaging in hazardous tasks until response is known). You will need to have frequent ophthalmic exams and periodic medical check-ups to evaluate drug effects. Report changes in vision, numbness or tingling of extremities, or persistent loss of appetite.
**Monitoring Parameters:** Periodic visual testing in patients receiving more than 15 mg/kg/day; periodic renal, hepatic, and hematopoietic tests

♦ **Ethambutol Hydrochloride** see Ethambutol on previous page
♦ **Ethamolin®** see Ethanolamine Oleate on this page
♦ **Ethanoic Acid** see Acetic Acid on page 25

# Ethanolamine Oleate (ETH a nol a meen OH lee ate)
**Pharmacologic Class** Sclerosing Agent
**U.S. Brand Names** Ethamolin®
**Mechanism of Action** Derived from oleic acid and similar in physical properties to sodium morrhuate; however, the exact mechanism of the hemostatic effect used in endoscopic injection sclerotherapy is not known. Intravenously injected ethanolamine oleate produces a sterile inflammatory response resulting in fibrosis and occlusion of the vein; a dose-related extravascular inflammatory reaction occurs when the drug diffuses through the venous wall. Autopsy results indicate that variceal obliteration occurs secondary to mural necrosis and fibrosis. Thrombosis appears to be a transient reaction.
**Use** Mild sclerosing agent for bleeding esophageal varices
**USUAL DOSAGE** Adults: 1.5-5 mL per varix, up to 20 mL total or 0.4 mL/kg for a 50 kg patient; doses should be decreased in patients with severe hepatic dysfunction and should receive less than recommended maximum dose
**Dosage Forms Inj:** 5% [50 mg/mL] (2 mL)
**Contraindications** Hypersensitivity to agent or oleic acid
**Warnings/Precautions** Fatal anaphylactic shock has been reported following administration; use with caution and decrease doses in patients with significant liver dysfunction (child class C), with concomitant cardiorespiratory disease, or in the elderly or critically ill
**Pregnancy Risk Factor** C
**Adverse Reactions**
1% to 10%:
Central nervous system: Pyrexia (1.8%)
Gastrointestinal: Esophageal ulcer (2%), esophageal stricture (1.3%)
Respiratory: Pleural effusion (2%), pneumonia (1.2%)
Miscellaneous: Retrosternal pain (1.6%)
<1%: Esophagitis, perforation, injection necrosis, acute renal failure, anaphylaxis

# Ethchlorvynol (eth klor VI nole)
**Pharmacologic Class** Hypnotic, Miscellaneous
**U.S. Brand Names** Placidyl®
**Mechanism of Action** Causes nonspecific depression of the reticular activating system
**Use** Short-term management of insomnia
(Continued)

## Ethchlorvynol *(Continued)*

**USUAL DOSAGE** Adults: Oral: 500-1000 mg at bedtime

**Dosing adjustment in renal impairment:** $Cl_{cr}$ <50 mL/minute: Avoid use

**Dosage Forms Cap:** 200 mg, 500 mg, 750 mg

**Contraindications** Porphyria, hypersensitivity to ethchlorvynol or any component

**Warnings/Precautions** Administer with caution to depressed or suicidal patients or to patients with a history of drug abuse; intoxication symptoms may appear with prolonged daily doses of as little as 1 g; withdrawal symptoms may be seen upon abrupt discontinuation; use with caution in the elderly and in patients with hepatic or renal dysfunction; use with caution in patients who have a history of paradoxical restlessness to barbiturates or alcohol; some products may contain tartrazine

**Pregnancy Risk Factor** C

**Adverse Reactions**

>10%:

Central nervous system: Dizziness

Gastrointestinal: Indigestion, nausea, stomach pain, unpleasant aftertaste

Neuromuscular & skeletal: Weakness

Ocular: Blurred vision

1% to 10%:

Central nervous system: Nervousness, excitement, ataxia, confusion, drowsiness (daytime)

Dermatologic: Rash

<1%: Bradycardia, hyperthermia, slurred speech, cholestatic jaundice, trembling, weakness (severe), shortness of breath

**Drug Interactions**

Decreased effect of oral anticoagulants

Increased toxicity (CNS depression) with alcohol, CNS depressants, MAO inhibitors, TCAs (delirium)

**Onset** 15-60 minutes

**Duration** 5 hours

**Half-Life** 10-20 hours

**Special PA Issues**

**Patient Education:** Use exactly as directed (do not increase dose or frequency or discontinue without consulting prescriber); may cause physical and/or psychological dependence. While using this medication, do not use alcohol or other prescription or OTC medications (especially, pain medications, sedatives, antihistamines, or hypnotics) without consulting prescriber. Maintain adequate hydration (2-3 L/day of fluids unless instructed to restrict fluid intake). You may experience drowsiness, dizziness, or blurred vision (use caution when driving or engaging in hazardous tasks); or nausea, vomiting, unpleasant taste (small frequent meals, good mouth care, chewing gum, or sucking lozenges may help). Report rash or skin irritation, CNS changes (confusion, depression, increased sedation, excitation, headache, abnormal thinking, insomnia, or nightmares), muscle pain or weakness, difficulty breathing, chest pain or palpitations, yellow skin or change in color of urine or stool, or ineffectiveness of medication.

**Dietary Considerations:** Alcohol: Additive CNS effect, avoid use

**Monitoring Parameters:** Cardiac and respiratory function and abuse potential

**Reference Range:** Therapeutic: 2-9 µg/mL; Toxic: >20 µg/mL

## Ethinyl Estradiol *(ETH in il es tra DYE ole)*

**Pharmacologic Class** Estrogen Derivative

**U.S. Brand Names** Estinyl®

**Mechanism of Action** Increases the synthesis of DNA, RNA, and various proteins in target tissues; reduces the release of gonadotropin-releasing hormone from the hypothalamus; reduces FSH and LH release from the pituitary

**Use** Hypogonadism; primary ovarian failure; vasomotor symptoms of menopause; prostatic carcinoma; breast cancer

**USUAL DOSAGE** Adults: Oral:

Male: Prostatic cancer (inoperable, progressing): 0.15-2 mg/day for palliation

Female:

Hypogonadism: 0.05 mg 1-3 times/day during the first 2 weeks of a theoretical menstrual cycle. Follow with a progesterone during the last half of the arbitrary cycle. Continue for 3-6 months. The patient should not be treated for the following 2 months.

Vasomotor symptoms: Usual dosage range: 0.02-0.05 mg/day; give cyclically for short-term use only and use the lowest dose that will control symptoms. Discontinue as soon as possible and administer cyclically (3 weeks on and 1 week off). Attempt to discontinue or taper medication at 3- to 6-month intervals.

Breast cancer (inoperable, progressing): 1 mg 3 times/day for palliation

**Dosing adjustment in hepatic impairment:**

Mild to moderate liver impairment: Dosage reduction of estrogens is recommended

Severe liver impairment: **Not recommended**

**Dosage Forms** Tab: 0.02 mg, 0.05 mg, 0.5 mg

**Contraindications** Thrombophlebitis, undiagnosed vaginal bleeding, hypersensitivity to ethinyl estradiol or any component, pregnancy, estrogen-dependent neoplasia

**Warnings/Precautions** Use with caution in patients with asthma, seizure disorders, migraine, cardiac, renal or hepatic impairment, cerebrovascular disorders or history of breast cancer, past or present thromboembolic disease, smokers >35 years of age

**Pregnancy Risk Factor** X

**Adverse Reactions**
>10%:
  Cardiovascular: Peripheral edema
  Endocrine & metabolic: Enlargement of breasts, breast tenderness, bloating
  Gastrointestinal: Nausea, anorexia
1% to 10%:
  Central nervous system: Headache
  Endocrine & metabolic: Increased libido
  Gastrointestinal: Vomiting, diarrhea
<1%: Hypertension, thromboembolism, myocardial infarction, edema, stroke, depression, dizziness, anxiety, chloasma, melasma, rash, breast tumors, amenorrhea, alterations in frequency and flow of menses, decreased glucose tolerance, increased triglycerides and LDL, GI distress, cholestatic jaundice, intolerance to contact lenses, increased susceptibility to *Candida* infection

**Drug Interactions** CYP3A3/4 and 3A5-7 enzyme substrate; CYP1A2 enzyme inhibitor
Increased toxicity:
  Carbamazepine, tricyclic antidepressants, and corticosteroids
Increased thromboembolic potential with oral anticoagulants

**Special PA Issues**
  **Patient Education:** Take according to recommended schedule. It is important to maintain schedule of drug days and drug-free days. Periodic gynecologic exam and breast exams for females are important. You may experience nausea or vomiting (small frequent meals may help); dizziness or mental depression (use caution when driving); rash; loss of scalp hair; enlargement/tenderness of breasts; or increased/decreased libido. Report significant swelling in extremities, sudden acute pain in legs or calves, chest, or abdomen; shortness of breath; severe headache or vomiting; weakness or numbness of arms or legs; or unusual vaginal bleeding.

# Ethinyl Estradiol and Desogestrel
(ETH in il es tra DYE ole & des oh JES trel)

**Pharmacologic Class** Contraceptive, Oral

**U.S. Brand Names** Desogen®; Ortho-Cept®

**Dosage Forms** Tab: Ethinyl estradiol 0.03 mg and desogestrel 0.15 mg (21s, 28s)

# Ethinyl Estradiol and Ethynodiol Diacetate
(ETH in il es tra DYE ole & e thye noe DYE ole dye AS e tate)

**Pharmacologic Class** Contraceptive, Oral (Intermediate Potency Estrogen, Intermediate Potency Progestin); Contraceptive, Oral (Low Potency Estrogen, Intermediate Potency Progestin); Contraceptive, Oral (Monophasic); Estrogen Derivative, Oral; Progestin

**U.S. Brand Names** Demulen®; Zovia®

**Mechanism of Action** Combination oral contraceptives inhibit ovulation via a negative feedback mechanism on the hypothalamus, which alters the normal pattern of gonadotropin secretion of a follicle-stimulating hormone (FSH) and luteinizing hormone by the anterior pituitary. The follicular phase FSH and midcycle surge of gonadotropins are inhibited. In addition, oral contraceptives produce alterations in the genital tract, including changes in the cervical mucus, rendering it unfavorable for sperm penetration even if ovulation occurs. Changes in the endometrium may also occur, producing an unfavorable environment for nidation. Oral contraceptive drugs may alter the tubal transport of the ova through the fallopian tubes. Progestational agents may also alter sperm fertility.

**Use** Prevention of pregnancy; treatment of hypermenorrhea, endometriosis, female hypogonadism

**USUAL DOSAGE** Adults: Female: Oral:
  For 21-tablet cycle packs, with 21 active tablets (28-day packs have 21 active tablets and 7 inert tablets): Take 1 tablet daily starting on the fifth day of menstrual cycle, with day 1 being the first day of menstruation; begin taking a new cycle pack on the eighth day after taking the last tablet from the previous pack
  With 28-tablet packages, dosage is 1 tablet daily without interruption; extra tablets are placebos or contain iron. If next menstrual period does not begin on schedule, rule out pregnancy before starting new dosing cycle. If menstrual period begins, start new dosing cycle 7 days after last tablet was taken. If all doses have been taken on schedule and one menstrual period is missed, continue dosing cycle. If two consecutive menstrual periods are missed, pregnancy test is required before new dosing cycle is started.
  One dose missed: Take as soon as remembered or take 2 tablets next day
  Two doses missed: Take 2 tablets as soon as remembered or 2 tablets next 2 days
  Three doses missed: Begin new compact of tablets starting on day 1 of next cycle
(Continued)

345

## Ethinyl Estradiol and Ethynodiol Diacetate *(Continued)*

**Dosage Forms Tab:** 1/35: Ethinyl estradiol 0.035 mg and ethynodiol diacetate 1 mg (21s, 28s), 1/50: Ethinyl estradiol 0.05 mg and ethynodiol diacetate 1 mg (21s, 28s)

**Contraindications** Known or suspected pregnancy, undiagnosed genital bleeding, carcinoma of the breast, estrogen-dependent tumor

**Warnings/Precautions** In patients with a history of thromboembolism, stroke, myocardial infarction (especially >40 years of age who smoke), liver tumor, hypertension, cardiac, renal or hepatic insufficiency; use of any progestin during the first 4 months of pregnancy is not recommended; risk of cardiovascular side effects increases in those women who smoke cigarettes and in women >35 years of age

**Pregnancy Risk Factor** X

**Adverse Reactions**

>10%:

Cardiovascular: Peripheral edema

Endocrine & metabolic: Enlargement of breasts, breast tenderness

Gastrointestinal: Nausea, anorexia, bloating

1% to 10%:

Central nervous system: Headache

Endocrine & metabolic: Increased libido

Gastrointestinal: Vomiting, diarrhea

<1%: Hypertension, thromboembolism, stroke, myocardial infarction, edema, depression, dizziness, anxiety, chloasma, melasma, rash, decreased glucose tolerance, amenorrhea, alterations in frequency and flow of menses, increased triglycerides and LDL, GI distress, cholestatic jaundice, intolerance to contact lenses, increased susceptibility to *Candida* infection, breast tumors

See tables.

### Achieving Proper Hormonal Balance in an Oral Contraceptive

| Estrogen | | Progestin | |
|---|---|---|---|
| **Excess** | **Deficiency** | **Excess** | **Deficiency** |
| Nausea, bloating | Early or midcycle | Increased appetite | Late breakthrough |
| Cervical mucorrhea, | breakthrough | Weight gain | bleeding |
| polyposis | bleeding | Tiredness, fatigue | Amenorrhea |
| Melasma | Increased spotting | Hypomenorrhea | Hypermenorrhea |
| Migraine headache | Hypomenorrhea | Acne, oily scalp* | |
| Breast fullness or | | Hair loss, hirsutism* | |
| tenderness | | Depression | |
| Edema | | Monilial vaginitis | |
| Hypertension | | Breast regression | |

*Result of androgenic activity of progestins.

### Pharmacological Effects of Progestins Used in Oral Contraceptives

| | Progestin | Estrogen | Antiestrogen | Androgen |
|---|---|---|---|---|
| Norgestrel/levonorgestrel | +++ | 0 | ++ | +++ |
| Ethynodiol diacetate | ++ | +* | +* | + |
| Norethindrone acetate | + | + | +++ | + |
| Norethindrone | + | +* | +* | + |
| Norethynodrel | + | +++ | 0 | 0 |

*Has estrogenic effect at low doses; may have antiestrogenic effect at higher doses.

+++ = pronounced effect

++ = moderate effect

+ = slight effect

0 = no effect

**Drug Interactions** Ethinyl estradiol is a CYP3A3/4 and 3A5-7 enzyme substrate; CYP1A2 enzyme inhibitor

Decreased effect of oral contraceptives with barbiturates, hydantoins - phenytoin, rifampin, antibiotics - penicillins, tetracyclines, griseofulvin

Increased toxicity of acetaminophen, anticoagulants, benzodiazepines, caffeine, corticosteroids, metoprolol, theophylline, tricyclic antidepressants

**Special PA Issues**

**Patient Education:** Photosensitivity may occur

Inform your physician if signs or symptoms of any of the following occur: Thromboembolic or thrombotic disorders including sudden severe headache or vomiting, disturbance of vision or speech, loss of vision, numbness or weakness in an extremity, sharp or crushing chest pain, calf pain, shortness of breath, severe abdominal pain or mass, mental depression or unusual bleeding.

If any doses are missed, alternative contraceptive methods should be used for the next 2 days or until 2 days into the new cycle

Discontinue taking the medication if you suspect you are pregnant or become pregnant

# Ethinyl Estradiol and Levonorgestrel
(ETH in il es tra DYE ole & LEE voe nor jes trel)

**Pharmacologic Class** Contraceptive, Oral (Low Potency Estrogen, Intermediate Potency Progestin); Contraceptive, Oral (Low Potency Estrogen, Low Potency Progestin); Contraceptive, Oral (Monophasic); Contraceptive, Oral (Triphasic); Estrogen Derivative, Oral; Progestin

**U.S. Brand Names** Alesse™; Levlen®; Levlite®; Levora®; Nordette®; Tri-Levlen®; Triphasil®

**Mechanism of Action** Combination oral contraceptives inhibit ovulation via a negative feedback mechanism on the hypothalamus, which alters the normal pattern of gonadotropin secretion of a follicle-stimulating hormone (FSH) and luteinizing hormone by the anterior pituitary. The follicular phase FSH and midcycle surge of gonadotropins are inhibited. In addition, oral contraceptives produce alterations in the genital tract, including changes in the cervical mucus, rendering it unfavorable for sperm penetration even if ovulation occurs. Changes in the endometrium may also occur, producing an unfavorable environment for nidation. Oral contraceptive drugs may alter the tubal transport of the ova through the fallopian tubes. Progestational agents may also alter sperm fertility.

**Use** Prevention of pregnancy; treatment of hypermenorrhea, endometriosis, female hypogonadism

**USUAL DOSAGE** Adults: Female: Oral:

Contraception: 1 tablet daily, beginning on day 5 of menstrual cycle (first day of menstrual flow is day 1). With 20-tablet and 21-tablet packages, new dosing cycle begins 7 days after last tablet taken. With 28-tablet packages, dosage is 1 tablet daily without interruption; extra tablets are placebos or contain iron. If next menstrual period does not begin on schedule, rule out pregnancy before starting new dosing cycle. If menstrual period begins, start new dosing cycle 7 days after last tablet was taken. If all doses have been taken on schedule and one menstrual period is missed, continue dosing cycle. If two consecutive menstrual periods are missed, pregnancy test is required before new dosing cycle is started.

One dose missed: Take as soon as remembered or take 2 tablets next day

Two doses missed: Take 2 tablets as soon as remembered or 2 tablets next 2 days

Three doses missed: Begin new compact of tablets starting on day 1 of next cycle

Triphasic oral contraceptive (Tri-Levlen®, Triphasil®): 1 tablet/day in the sequence specified by the manufacturer

**Dosage Forms** Tab: Alesse™, Levlite®: Ethinyl estradiol 0.02 mg and levonorgestrel 0.1 mg (21s, 28s), Levlen®, Levora®, Nordette®: Ethinyl estradiol 0.03 mg and levonorgestrel 0.15 mg (21s, 28s), Tri-Levlen®, Triphasil®: Phase 1 (6 brown tabs): Ethinyl estradiol 0.03 mg and levonorgestrel 0.05 mg, Phase 2 (5 white tabs): Ethinyl estradiol 0.04 mg and levonorgestrel 0.075 mg, Phase 3 (10 yellow tabs): Ethinyl estradiol 0.03 mg and levonorgestrel 0.125 mg (21s, 28s)

**Contraindications** Thrombophlebitis, undiagnosed vaginal bleeding, hypersensitivity to ethinyl estradiol or any component, known or suspected pregnancy, carcinoma of the breast, estrogen-dependent tumor

**Warnings/Precautions** Use of any progestin during the first 4 months of pregnancy is not recommended; use with caution in patients with asthma, seizure disorders, migraine, cardiac, renal or hepatic impairment, cerebrovascular disorders or history of breast cancer, past and present thromboembolic disease, smokers >35 years of age

**Pregnancy Risk Factor** X

**Adverse Reactions**

>10%:

Cardiovascular: Peripheral edema

Endocrine & metabolic: Enlargement of breasts, breast tenderness

Gastrointestinal: Nausea, anorexia, bloating

1% to 10%:

Central nervous system: Headache

Endocrine & metabolic: Increased libido

Gastrointestinal: Vomiting, diarrhea

<1%: Hypertension, thromboembolism, stroke, myocardial infarction, edema, depression, dizziness, anxiety, chloasma, melasma, rash, decreased glucose tolerance, amenorrhea, alterations in frequency and flow of menses, increased triglycerides and LDL, GI distress, cholestatic jaundice, intolerance to contact lenses, increased susceptibility to *Candida* infection, breast tumors

See tables.

**Drug Interactions** Ethinyl estradiol is a CYP3A3/4 and 3A5-7 enzyme substrate; CYP1A2 enzyme inhibitor

Decreased effect of oral contraceptives with barbiturates, hydantoins - phenytoin, rifampin, antibiotics - penicillins, tetracyclines, griseofulvin

(Continued)

# Ethinyl Estradiol and Levonorgestrel *(Continued)*

Increased toxicity of acetaminophen, anticoagulants, benzodiazepines, caffeine, corticosteroids, metoprolol, theophylline, tricyclic antidepressants

### Achieving Proper Hormonal Balance in an Oral Contraceptive

| Estrogen | | Progestin | |
|---|---|---|---|
| **Excess** | **Deficiency** | **Excess** | **Deficiency** |
| Nausea, bloating | Early or midcycle | Increased appetite | Late breakthrough |
| Cervical mucorrhea, | breakthrough | Weight gain | bleeding |
| polyposis | bleeding | Tiredness, fatigue | Amenorrhea |
| Melasma | Increased spotting | Hypomenorrhea | Hypermenorrhea |
| Migraine headache | Hypomenorrhea | Acne, oily scalp* | |
| Breast fullness or | | Hair loss, hirsutism* | |
| tenderness | | Depression | |
| Edema | | Monilial vaginitis | |
| Hypertension | | Breast regression | |

*Result of androgenic activity of progestins.

### Pharmacological Effects of Progestins Used in Oral Contraceptives

| | Progestin | Estrogen | Antiestrogen | Androgen |
|---|---|---|---|---|
| Norgestrel/levonorgestrel | +++ | 0 | ++ | +++ |
| Ethynodiol diacetate | ++ | +* | +* | + |
| Norethindrone acetate | + | + | +++ | + |
| Norethindrone | + | +* | +* | + |
| Norethynodrel | + | +++ | 0 | 0 |

*Has estrogenic effect at low doses; may have antiestrogenic effect at higher doses.

+++ = pronounced effect

++ = moderate effect

+ = slight effect

0 = no effect

## Special PA Issues
### Patient Education:
Inform your physician if signs or symptoms of any of the following occur: Thromboembolic or thrombotic disorders including sudden severe headache or vomiting, disturbance of vision or speech, loss of vision, numbness or weakness in an extremity, sharp or crushing chest pain, calf pain, shortness of breath, severe abdominal pain or mass, mental depression or unusual bleeding

If any doses are missed, alternative contraceptive methods should be used for the next 2 days or until 2 days into the new cycle

Discontinue taking the medication if you suspect you are pregnant or become pregnant

# Ethinyl Estradiol and Norethindrone
(ETH in il es tra DYE ole & nor eth IN drone)

**Pharmacologic Class** Contraceptive, Oral (Biphasic); Contraceptive, Oral (Intermediate Potency Estrogen, Intermediate Potency Progestin); Contraceptive, Oral (Intermediate Potency Estrogen, Low Potency Progestin); Contraceptive, Oral (Low Potency Estrogen, Low Potency Progestin); Contraceptive, Oral (Monophasic); Contraceptive, Oral (Triphasic); Estrogen Derivative, Oral; Progestin

**U.S. Brand Names** Brevicon®; Estrostep® 21; Estrostep® Fe; Genora® 0.5/35; Genora® 1/35; Jenest-28™; Loestrin®; Modicon™; N.E.E.® 1/35; Nelova™ 0.5/35E; Nelova™ 10/11; Norethin™ 1/35E; Norinyl® 1+35; Ortho-Novum® 1/35; Ortho-Novum® 7/7/7; Ortho-Novum® 10/11; Ovcon® 35; Ovcon® 50; Tri-Norinyl®

**Mechanism of Action** Combination oral contraceptives inhibit ovulation via a negative feedback mechanism on the hypothalamus, which alters the normal pattern of gonadotropin secretion of a follicle-stimulating hormone (FSH) and luteinizing hormone by the anterior pituitary. The follicular phase FSH and midcycle surge of gonadotropins are inhibited. In addition, oral contraceptives produce alterations in the genital tract, including changes in the cervical mucus, rendering it unfavorable for sperm penetration even if ovulation occurs. Changes in the endometrium may also occur, producing an unfavorable environment for nidation. Oral contraceptive drugs may alter the tubal transport of the ova through the fallopian tubes. Progestational agents may also alter sperm fertility.

**Use** Prevention of pregnancy; treatment of hypermenorrhea, endometriosis, female hypogonadism

**USUAL DOSAGE** Adults: Female: Oral:
For 21-tablet cycle packs, with 21 active tablets (28-day packs have 21 active tablets and 7 inert tablets): Take 1 tablet daily starting on the fifth day of menstrual cycle, with day 1

being the first day of menstruation; begin taking a new cycle pack on the eighth day after taking the last tablet from the previous pack

With 28-tablet packages, dosage is 1 tablet daily without interruption; extra tablets are placebos or contain iron. If next menstrual period does not begin on schedule, rule out pregnancy before starting new dosing cycle. If menstrual period begins, start new dosing cycle 7 days after last tablet was taken. If all doses have been taken on schedule and one menstrual period is missed, continue dosing cycle. If two consecutive menstrual periods are missed, pregnancy test is required before new dosing cycle is started.

One dose missed: Take as soon as remembered or take 2 tablets next day

Two doses missed: Take 2 tablets as soon as remembered or 2 tablets next 2 days

Three doses missed: Begin new compact of tablets starting on day 1 of next cycle

Biphasic oral contraceptive (Jenest™-28, Ortho-Novum™ 10/11, Nelova™ 10/11): 1 color tablet/day for 10 days, then next color tablet for 11 days

Triphasic oral contraceptive (Ortho-Novum™ 7/7/7, Tri-Norinyl®, Triphasil®): 1 tablet/day in the sequence specified by the manufacturer

**Dosage Forms Tab:** Brevicon®, Genora® 0.5/35, Modicon™, Nelova® 0.5/35E: Ethinyl estradiol 0.035 mg and norethindrone 0.5 mg (21s, 28s)

Estrostep®: Triangular tab (white): Ethinyl estradiol 0.02 mg and norethindrone acetate 1 mg, Square tab (white): Ethinyl estradiol 0.03 mg and norethindrone acetate 1 mg, Round tab (white): Ethinyl estradiol 0.035 mg and norethindrone acetate 1 mg

Estrostep® Fe: Triangular tab (white): Ethinyl estradiol 0.02 mg and norethindrone acetate 1 mg, Square tab (white): Ethinyl estradiol 0.03 mg and norethindrone acetate 1 mg, Round tab (white): Ethinyl estradiol 0.035 mg and norethindrone acetate 1 mg, Brown tab: Ferrous fumarate 75 mg

Loestrin® 1.5/30: Ethinyl estradiol 0.03 mg and norethindrone acetate 1.5 mg (21s)

Loestrin® Fe 1.5/30: Ethinyl estradiol 0.03 mg and norethindrone acetate 1.5 mg with ferrous fumarate 75 mg in 7 inert tabs (28s)

Loestrin® 1/20: Ethinyl estradiol 0.02 mg and norethindrone acetate 1 mg (21s)

Loestrin® Fe 1/20: Ethinyl estradiol 0.02 mg and norethindrone acetate 1 mg with ferrous fumarate 75 mg in 7 inert tabs (28s)

Genora® 1/35, N.E.E.® 1/35, Nelova® 1/35E, Norethin™ 1/35E, Norinyl® 1+35, Ortho-Novum® 1/35: Ethinyl estradiol 0.035 mg and norethindrone 1 mg (21s, 28s)

Jenest-28™: Phase 1 (7 white tabs): Ethinyl estradiol 0.035 mg and norethindrone 0.5 mg; Phase 2 (14 peach tabs): Ethinyl estradiol 0.035 mg and norethindrone 1 mg and 7 green inert tabs (28s)

Ortho-Novum® 7/7/7: Phase 1 (7 white tabs): Ethinyl estradiol 0.035 mg and norethindrone 0.5 mg; Phase 2 (7 light peach tabs): Ethinyl estradiol 0.035 mg and norethindrone 0.75 mg; Phase 3 (7 peach tabs): Ethinyl estradiol 0.035 mg and norethindrone 1 mg (21s, 28s)

Ortho-Novum® 10/11: Phase 1 (10 white tabs): Ethinyl estradiol 0.035 mg and norethindrone 0.5 mg; Phase 2 (11 dark yellow tabs): Ethinyl estradiol 0.035 mg and norethindrone 1 mg (21s, 28s)

Ovcon® 35: Ethinyl estradiol 0.035 mg and norethindrone 0.4 mg (21s, 28s)

Ovcon® 50: Ethinyl estradiol 0.050 mg and norethindrone 1 mg (21s, 28s)

Tri-Norinyl®: Phase 1 (7 blue tabs): Ethinyl estradiol 0.035 mg and norethindrone 0.5 mg; Phase 2 (9 green tabs): Ethinyl estradiol 0.035 mg and norethindrone 1 mg; Phase 3 (5 blue tabs): Ethinyl estradiol 0.035 mg and norethindrone 0.5 mg (21s, 28s)

**Contraindications** Thrombophlebitis, cerebral vascular disease, coronary artery disease, known or suspected breast carcinoma, undiagnosed abnormal genital bleeding, hypersensitivity to any component; pregnancy

**Warnings/Precautions** Use of any progestin during the first 4 months of pregnancy is not recommended; in patients with a history of thromboembolism, stroke, myocardial infarction (especially >40 years of age who smoke), liver tumor, hypertension, cardiac, renal or hepatic insufficiency; risk of cardiovascular side effects increases in those women who smoke cigarettes and in women >35 years of age

**Pregnancy Risk Factor** X

**Adverse Reactions**

>10%:

Cardiovascular: Peripheral edema

Endocrine & metabolic: Enlargement of breasts, breast tenderness

Gastrointestinal: Nausea, anorexia, bloating

1% to 10%:

Central nervous system: Headache

Endocrine & metabolic: Increased libido

Gastrointestinal: Vomiting, diarrhea

<1%: Hypertension, thromboembolism, stroke, myocardial infarction, edema, depression, dizziness, anxiety, chloasma, melasma, rash, decreased glucose tolerance, breast tumors, amenorrhea, alterations in frequency and flow of menses, increased triglycerides and LDL, GI distress, cholestatic jaundice, intolerance to contact lenses, increased susceptibility to *Candida* infection

Minimize these effects by adjusting the estrogen/progestin balance or dosage. The table categorizes products by both their estrogenic and progestational potencies; because (Continued)

# Ethinyl Estradiol and Norethindrone *(Continued)*

overall activity is influenced by the interaction of components, it is difficult to precisely classify products; placement in the table is only approximate. Differences between products within a group are probably not clinically significant. See tables.

### Achieving Proper Hormonal Balance in an Oral Contraceptive

| Estrogen | | Progestin | |
|---|---|---|---|
| Excess | Deficiency | Excess | Deficiency |
| Nausea, bloating | Early or midcycle | Increased appetite | Late breakthrough |
| Cervical mucorrhea, | breakthrough | Weight gain | bleeding |
| polyposis | bleeding | Tiredness, fatigue | Amenorrhea |
| Melasma | Increased spotting | Hypomenorrhea | Hypermenorrhea |
| Migraine headache | Hypomenorrhea | Acne, oily scalp* | |
| Breast fullness or | | Hair loss, hirsutism* | |
| tenderness | | Depression | |
| Edema | | Monilial vaginitis | |
| Hypertension | | Breast regression | |

*Result of androgenic activity of progestins.

### Pharmacological Effects of Progestins Used in Oral Contraceptives

| | Progestin | Estrogen | Antiestrogen | Androgen |
|---|---|---|---|---|
| Norgestrel/levonorgestrel | +++ | 0 | ++ | +++ |
| Ethynodiol diacetate | ++ | +* | +* | + |
| Norethindrone acetate | + | + | +++ | + |
| Norethindrone | + | +* | +* | + |
| Norethynodrel | + | +++ | 0 | 0 |

*Has estrogenic effect at low doses; may have antiestrogenic effect at higher doses.

+++ = pronounced effect

++ = moderate effect

+ = slight effect

0 = no effect

**Drug Interactions** Ethinyl estradiol is a CYP3A3/4 and 3A5-7 enzyme substrate; CYP1A2 enzyme inhibitor

Decreased effect:

Potential contraceptive failure with barbiturates, hydantoins, and rifampin

Concomitant penicillins or tetracyclines may lead to contraceptive failure

Increased toxicity:

Increased toxicity of carbamazepine, tricyclic antidepressants, and corticosteroids

Increased thromboembolic potential with oral anticoagulants

**Special PA Issues**

**Patient Education:** Take exactly as directed; use additional method of birth control during first week of administration of first cycle; photosensitivity may occur. Women should inform their physicians if signs or symptoms of any of the following occur thromboembolic or thrombotic disorders including sudden severe headache or vomiting, disturbance of vision or speech, loss of vision, numbness or weakness in an extremity, sharp or crushing chest pain, calf pain, shortness of breath, severe abdominal pain or mass, mental depression, or unusual bleeding.

When any doses are missed, alternative contraceptive methods should be used for the next 2 days or until 2 days into the new cycle

Women should discontinue taking the medication if they suspect they are pregnant or become pregnant

# Ethinyl Estradiol and Norgestimate

(ETH in il es tra DYE ole & nor JES ti mate)

**Pharmacologic Class** Contraceptive, Oral

**Mechanism of Action** Combination oral contraceptives inhibit ovulation via a negative feedback mechanism on the hypothalamus, which alters the normal pattern of gonadotropin secretion of a follicle-stimulating hormone (FSH) and luteinizing hormone by the anterior pituitary. The follicular phase FSH and midcycle surge of gonadotropins are inhibited. In addition, oral contraceptives produce alterations in the genital tract, including changes in the cervical mucus, rendering it unfavorable for sperm penetration even if ovulation occurs. Changes in the endometrium may also occur, producing an unfavorable environment for nidation. Oral contraceptive drugs may alter the tubal transport of the ova through the fallopian tubes. Progestational agents may also alter sperm fertility.

**Use** Prevention of pregnancy

**USUAL DOSAGE**

Contraception: Oral: 1 tablet daily, beginning on day 5 of menstrual cycle (first day of menstrual flow is day 1). With 21-tablet packages, new dosing cycle begins 7 days after last tablet taken. With 28-tablet packages, dosage is 1 tablet daily without interruption; extra tablets are placebos or contain iron. If next menstrual period does not begin on schedule, rule out pregnancy before starting new dosing cycle. If menstrual period begins, start new dosing cycle 7 days after last tablet was taken. If all doses have been taken on schedule and one menstrual period is missed, continue dosing cycle. If two consecutive menstrual periods are missed, pregnancy test is required before new dosing cycle is started.

One dose missed: Take as soon as remembered or take 2 tablets next day

Two doses missed: Take 2 tablets as soon as remembered or 2 tablets next 2 days

Three doses missed: Begin new compact of tablets starting on day 1 of next cycle

Triphasic oral contraceptive: 1 tablet/day in the sequence specified by the manufacturer

**Dosage Forms Tab:** Ortho-Cyclen®: Ethinyl estradiol 0.035 mg and norgestimate 0.25 mg (21s, 28s)

Ortho Tri-Cyclen®: Phase 1 (7 white tablets): Ethinyl estradiol 0.035 mg and norgestimate 0.18 mg; Phase 2 (5 light blue tablets): Ethinyl estradiol 0.035 mg and norgestimate 0.215 mg; Phase 3 (10 blue tablets): Ethinyl estradiol 0.035 mg and norgestimate 0.25 mg (21s, 28s)

**Contraindications** Thrombophlebitis, undiagnosed vaginal bleeding, hypersensitivity to ethinyl estradiol or any component, known or suspected pregnancy, carcinoma of the breast, estrogen-dependent tumor

**Warnings/Precautions** Use of any progestin during the first 4 months of pregnancy is not recommended; use with caution in patients with asthma, seizure disorders, migraine, cardiac, renal or hepatic impairment, cerebrovascular disorders or history of breast cancer, past and present thromboembolic disease, smokers >35 years of age

**Pregnancy Risk Factor** X

**Drug Interactions** Ethinyl estradiol is a CYP3A3/4 and 3A5-7 enzyme substrate; CYP1A2 enzyme inhibitor

Anticonvulsants, rifampin, tetracyclines → ↓ efficacy of BCPs

**Special PA Issues**

**Patient Education:** Women should inform their physicians if signs or symptoms of any of the following occur: thromboembolic or thrombotic disorders including sudden severe headache or vomiting, disturbance of vision or speech, loss of vision, numbness or weakness in an extremity, sharp or crushing chest pain, calf pain, shortness of breath, severe abdominal pain or mass, mental depression or unusual bleeding. Women should be advised that when any doses are missed, alternative contraceptive methods should be used for the next 2 days or until 2 days into the new cycle; women should discontinue taking the medication if they suspect they are pregnant or become pregnant.

# Ethinyl Estradiol and Norgestrel (ETH in il es tra DYE ole & nor JES trel)

**Pharmacologic Class** Contraceptive, Oral (Intermediate Potency Estrogen, High Potency Progestin); Contraceptive, Oral (Low Potency Estrogen, Intermediate Potency Progestin); Contraceptive, Oral (Monophasic); Estrogen Derivative, Oral; Progestin

**U.S. Brand Names** Lo/Ovral®; Ovral®

**Mechanism of Action** Combination oral contraceptives inhibit ovulation via a negative feedback mechanism on the hypothalamus, which alters the normal pattern of gonadotropin secretion of a follicle-stimulating hormone (FSH) and luteinizing hormone by the anterior pituitary. The follicular phase FSH and midcycle surge of gonadotropins are inhibited. In addition, oral contraceptives produce alterations in the genital tract, including changes in the cervical mucus, rendering it unfavorable for sperm penetration even if ovulation occurs. Changes in the endometrium may also occur, producing an unfavorable environment for nidation. Oral contraceptive drugs may alter the tubal transport of the ova through the fallopian tubes. Progestational agents may also alter sperm fertility.

**Use** Prevention of pregnancy; oral: postcoital contraceptive or "morning after" pill; treatment of hypermenorrhea, endometriosis, female hypogonadism

**USUAL DOSAGE** Female: Oral: Contraceptive: 1 tablet daily, beginning on day 5 of menstrual cycle (first day of menstrual flow is day 1). With 20-tablet and 21-tablet packages, new dosing cycle begins 7 days after last tablet taken; with 28-tablet packages, dosage is 1 tablet daily without interruption; extra tablets are placebos or contain iron. If next menstrual period does not begin on schedule, rule out pregnancy before starting new dosing cycle; if menstrual period begins, start new dosing cycle 7 days after last tablet was taken; if all doses have been taken on schedule and one menstrual period is missed, continue dosing cycle; if two consecutive menstrual periods are missed, pregnancy test is required before new dosing cycle is started.

One dose missed: Take as soon as remembered or take 2 tablets next day

Two doses missed: Take 2 tablets as soon as remembered or 2 tablets next 2 days

Three doses missed: Begin new compact of tablets starting on day 1 of next cycle

Postcoital contraception or "morning after" pill: Oral (50 mcg ethinyl estradiol and 0.5 mg norgestrel): 2 tablets at initial visit and 2 tablets 12 hours later

(Continued)

## Ethinyl Estradiol and Norgestrel *(Continued)*

**Dosage Forms** Tab: Lo/Ovral®: Ethinyl estradiol 0.03 mg and norgestrel 0.3 mg (21s and 28s), Ovral®: Ethinyl estradiol 0.05 mg and norgestrel 0.5 mg (21s and 28s)

**Contraindications** Thromboembolic disorders, cerebrovascular or coronary artery disease; known or suspected breast cancer; undiagnosed abnormal vaginal bleeding; women smokers >35 years of age; all women >40 years of age, hypersensitivity to drug or components; pregnancy

**Warnings/Precautions** Use of any progestin during the first 4 months of pregnancy is not recommended; in patients with a history of thromboembolism, stroke, myocardial infarction (especially >40 years of age who smoke), liver tumor, hypertension, cardiac, renal or hepatic insufficiency; risk of cardiovascular side effects increases in those women who smoke cigarettes and in women >35 years of age

**Pregnancy Risk Factor** X

**Adverse Reactions** Effects can be minimized by adjusting the estrogen/progestin balance or dosage.

>10%:
Cardiovascular: Peripheral edema
Endocrine & metabolic: Enlargement of breasts, breast tenderness
Gastrointestinal: Nausea, anorexia, bloating
1% to 10%:
Central nervous system: Headache
Endocrine & metabolic: Increased libido
Gastrointestinal: Vomiting, diarrhea
<1%: Hypertension, thromboembolism, myocardial infarction, edema, depression, dizziness, anxiety, stroke, chloasma, melasma, rash, decreased glucose tolerance, breast tumors, amenorrhea, alterations in frequency and flow of menses, increased triglycerides and LDL, GI distress, cholestatic jaundice, intolerance to contact lenses, increased susceptibility to *Candida* infection

**Drug Interactions** Ethinyl estradiol is a CYP3A3/4 and 3A5-7 enzyme substrate; CYP1A2 enzyme inhibitor
Decreased effect:
Potential contraceptive failure with barbiturates, hydantoins, and rifampin
Concomitant penicillins or tetracyclines may lead to contraceptive failure
Increased toxicity:
Increased toxicity of carbamazepine, tricyclic antidepressants, and corticosteroids
Increased thromboembolic potential with oral anticoagulants

**Special PA Issues**

**Patient Education:** Take exactly as directed; use additional method of birth control during first week of administration of first cycle; photosensitivity may occur. Women should inform their physicians if signs or symptoms of any of the following occur: Thromboembolic or thrombotic disorders including sudden severe headache or vomiting, disturbance of vision or speech, loss of vision, numbness or weakness in an extremity, sharp or crushing chest pain, calf pain, shortness of breath, severe abdominal pain or mass, mental depression or unusual bleeding.

Women should be advised that when any doses are missed, alternative contraceptive methods should be used for the next 2 days or until 2 days into the new cycle

Women should discontinue taking the medication if they suspect they are pregnant or become pregnant

## Ethionamide (e thye on AM ide)

**Pharmacologic Class** Antitubercular Agent

**U.S. Brand Names** Trecator®-SC

**Mechanism of Action** Inhibits peptide synthesis

**Use** Treatment of tuberculosis and other mycobacterial diseases, in conjunction with other antituberculosis agents, when first-line agents have failed or resistance has been demonstrated

**USUAL DOSAGE** Oral:
Children: 15-20 mg/kg/day in 2 divided doses, not to exceed 1 g/day
Adults: 500-1000 mg/day in 1-3 divided doses
Dosing adjustment in renal impairment: $Cl_{cr}$ <50 mL/minute: Administer 50% of dose

**Dosage Forms** Tab, sugar coated: 250 mg

**Contraindications** Contraindicated in patients with severe hepatic impairment or in patients who are sensitive to the drug

**Warnings/Precautions** Use with caution in patients receiving cycloserine or isoniazid, in diabetics

**Pregnancy Risk Factor** C

**Adverse Reactions**
>10%: Gastrointestinal: Anorexia, nausea, vomiting
1% to 10%:
Cardiovascular: Postural hypotension

Central nervous system: Psychiatric disturbances, drowsiness
Gastrointestinal: Metallic taste, diarrhea
Hepatic: Hepatitis (5%), jaundice
Neuromuscular & skeletal: Weakness
<1%: Dizziness, seizures, headache, peripheral neuritis, rash, alopecia, hypothyroidism or goiter, hypoglycemia, gynecomastia, stomatitis, abdominal pain, thrombocytopenia, optic neuritis, blurred vision, olfactory disturbances

**Half-Life** 2-3 hours

**Special PA Issues**

**Patient Education:** Take this medication as prescribed; avoid missing doses and do not discontinue without contacting prescriber. You will need to schedule regular medical check-ups which will include blood tests. You may experience GI upset (small frequent meals may help), metallic taste and increased salivation (lozenges, frequent mouth care), dizziness, blurred vision (use caution when driving or engaging in dangerous tasks), postural hypotension (change position slowly), impotence and/or menstrual difficulties (these will go away when drug is discontinued). Report acute unresolved GI upset, changes in vision, numbness or pain in extremities, or unusual bleeding or bruising.

**Monitoring Parameters:** Initial and periodic serum ALT and AST

♦ **Ethmozine®** *see Moricizine on page 618*

## Ethosuximide (eth oh SUKS i mide)

**Pharmacologic Class** Anticonvulsant, Succinimide

**U.S. Brand Names** Zarontin®

**Use** Management of absence (petit mal) seizures, myoclonic seizures, and akinetic epilepsy; considered to be drug of choice for simple absence seizures

**USUAL DOSAGE** Oral:
Children 3-6 years: Initial: 250 mg/day (or 15 mg/kg/day) in 2 divided doses; increase every 4-7 days; usual maintenance dose: 15-40 mg/kg/day in 2 divided doses
Children >6 years and Adults: Initial: 250 mg twice daily; increase by 250 mg as needed every 4-7 days up to 1.5 g/day in 2 divided doses; usual maintenance dose: 20-40 mg/kg/day in 2 divided doses

**Dosage Forms Cap:** 250 mg; **Syr (raspberry flavor):** 250 mg/5 mL (473 mL)

**Contraindications** Known hypersensitivity to ethosuximide

**Pregnancy Risk Factor** C

**Drug Interactions** CYP3A3/4 enzyme substrate; CYP3A3/4 enzyme inducer

**Half-Life** 50-60 hours

**Special PA Issues**

**Patient Education:** Take exactly as directed (do not increase dose or frequency or discontinue without consulting prescriber). While using this medication, do not use alcohol and other prescription or OTC medications (especially pain medications, sedatives, antihistamines, or hypnotics) without consulting prescriber. Maintain adequate hydration (2-3 L/day of fluids unless instructed to restrict fluid intake). You may experience drowsiness, dizziness, or blurred vision (use caution when driving or engaging in hazardous tasks); nausea, vomiting, loss of appetite, or dry mouth (small frequent meals, good mouth care, chewing gum, or sucking on lozenges may help); constipation (increased exercise, fluids, or dietary fruit and fiber may help). Wear identification of epileptic status and medications. Report CNS changes, mentation changes, or changes in cognition; muscle cramping, weakness, tremors, or changes in gait; persistent GI symptoms (cramping, constipation, vomiting, anorexia); rash or skin irritations; unusual bruising or bleeding (mouth, urine, stool); worsening of seizure activity, or loss of seizure control.

♦ **Ethoxynaphthamido Penicillin Sodium** *see Nafcillin on page 630*

♦ **Ethyl Aminobenzoate** *see Benzocaine on page 105*

## Ethyl Chloride and Dichlorotetrafluoroethane
(ETH il KLOR ide & dye klor oh te tra floo or oh ETH ane)

**Pharmacologic Class** Local Anesthetic

**U.S. Brand Names** Fluro-Ethyl® Aerosol

**Dosage Forms Aero:** Ethyl chloride 25% and dichlorotetrafluoroethane 75% (225 g)

♦ **Ethylenediamine** *see Theophylline Salts on page 888*

♦ **Ethynodiol Diacetate and Ethinyl Estradiol** *see Ethinyl Estradiol and Ethynodiol Diacetate on page 345*

♦ **Etibi®** *see Ethambutol on page 342*

## Etidocaine (e TI doe kane)

**Pharmacologic Class** Local Anesthetic

**U.S. Brand Names** Duranest®

**Mechanism of Action** Blocks nervous conduction through the stabilization of neuronal membranes. By preventing the transient increase in membrane permeability to sodium, the
(Continued)

## Etidocaine *(Continued)*

ionic fluxes necessary for initiation and transmission of electrical impulses are inhibited and local anesthesia is induced.

**Use** Infiltration anesthesia; peripheral nerve blocks; central neural blocks

**USUAL DOSAGE** Varies with procedure; use 1% for peripheral nerve block, central nerve block, lumbar peridural caudal; use 1.5% for maxillary infiltration or inferior alveolar nerve block; use 1% or 1.5% for intra-abdominal or pelvic surgery, lower limb surgery, or caesarean section

**Dosage Forms Inj, as hydrochloride:** 1% [10 mg/mL] (30 mL); **Inj, as hydrochloride, with epinephrine 1:200,000** 1% [10 mg/mL] (30 mL), 1.5% [15 mg/mL] (20 mL)

**Contraindications** Heart block, severe hemorrhage, severe hypotension, known hypersensitivity to etidocaine or other amide local anesthetics

**Warnings/Precautions** Use with caution in patients with cardiac disease and hyperthyroidism; fetal bradycardia may occur up to 20% of the time; use with caution in areas of inflammation or sepsis, in debilitated or elderly patients, and those with severe cardiovascular disease or hepatic dysfunction; some products may contain sulfites

**Pregnancy Risk Factor** B

**Adverse Reactions** <1%: Myocardial depression, hypotension, bradycardia, cardiovascular collapse, anxiety, restlessness, disorientation, confusion, seizures, drowsiness, unconsciousness, chills, urticaria, nausea, vomiting, transient stinging or burning at injection site, tremor, blurred vision, tinnitus, respiratory arrest, anaphylactoid reactions, shivering

**Special PA Issues**

**Reference Range:** Toxic concentration: >0.1 μg/mL

♦ **Etidocaine Hydrochloride** *see* Etidocaine *on previous page*

## Etidronate Disodium (e ti DROE nate dye SOW dee um)

**Pharmacologic Class** Bisphosphonate Derivative

**U.S. Brand Names** Didronel®

**Mechanism of Action** Decreases bone resorption by inhibiting osteocystic osteolysis; decreases mineral release and matrix or collagen breakdown in bone

**Use** Symptomatic treatment of Paget's disease and heterotopic ossification due to spinal cord injury or after total hip replacement, hypercalcemia associated with malignancy

**USUAL DOSAGE** Adults Oral formulation should be taken on an empty stomach 2 hours before any meal.

Paget's disease: Oral

Initial: 5-10 mg/kg/day (not to exceed 6 months) or 11-20 mg/kg/day (not to exceed 3 months). Doses >10 mg/kg/day are **not** recommended.

Retreatment: Initiate only after etidronate-free period ≥90 days. Monitor patients every 3-6 months. Retreatment regimens are the same as for initial treatment.

Heterotopic ossification: Oral:

Caused by spinal cord injury: 20 mg/kg/day for 2 weeks, then 10 mg/kg/day for 10 weeks; total treatment period: 12 weeks

Complicating total hip replacement: 20 mg/kg/day for 1 month preoperatively then 20 mg/kg/day for 3 months postoperatively; total treatment period is 4 months

Hypercalcemia associated with malignancy:

I.V. (dilute dose in at least 250 mL NS): 7.5 mg/kg/day for 3 days; there should be at least 7 days between courses of treatment

Oral: Start 20 mg/kg/day on the last day of infusion and continue for 30-90 days

**Dosing adjustment in renal impairment:**

$S_{cr}$ 2.5-5 mg/dL: Use with caution

$S_{cr}$ >5 mg/dL: **Not recommended**

**Dosage Forms Inj:** 50 mg/mL (6 mL); **Tab:** 200 mg, 400 mg

**Contraindications** Patients with serum creatinine >5 mg/dL; hypersensitivity to biphosphonates

**Warnings/Precautions** Use with caution in patients with restricted calcium and vitamin D intake; dosage modification required in renal impairment; I.V. form may be nephrotoxic and should be used with caution, if at all, in patients with impaired renal function (serum creatinine: 2.5-4.9 mg/dL)

**Pregnancy Risk Factor** E (oral)/C (parenteral)

**Adverse Reactions**

1% to 10%:

Central nervous system: Fever, convulsions

Endocrine & metabolic: Hypophosphatemia, hypomagnesemia, fluid overload

Neuromuscular & skeletal: Bone pain

Respiratory: Dyspnea

<1%: Pain, angioedema, rash, abnormal taste, occult blood in stools, increased risk of fractures, nephrotoxicity, hypersensitivity reactions

**Onset** I.V.: 1-2 days; oral: 1-3 months

**Duration** Up to 12 months

**Special PA Issues**
   **Patient Education:** Maintain adequate intake of calcium and vitamin D; take medicine on an empty stomach 2 hours before meals
   **Monitoring Parameters:** Serum calcium and phosphorous; serum creatinine and BUN
   **Reference Range:** Calcium (total): Adults: 9.0-11.0 mg/dL

# Etodolac (ee toe DOE lak)

**Pharmacologic Class** Nonsteroidal Anti-Inflammatory Agent (NSAID)

**U.S. Brand Names** Lodine®; Lodine® XL

**Mechanism of Action** Inhibits prostaglandin synthesis by decreasing the activity of the enzyme, cyclo-oxygenase, which results in decreased formation of prostaglandin precursors

**Use** Acute and long-term use in the management of signs and symptoms of osteoarthritis and management of pain

   **Unapproved use:** Rheumatoid arthritis

**USUAL DOSAGE** Single dose of 76-100 mg is comparable to the analgesic effect of aspirin 650 mg; in patients ≥65 years, no substantial differences in the pharmacokinetics or side-effects profile were seen compared with the general population

   Adults: Oral:
      Acute pain: 200-400 mg every 6-8 hours, as needed, not to exceed total daily doses of 1200 mg; for patients weighing <60 kg, total daily dose should not exceed 20 mg/kg/day
      Osteoarthritis: Initial: 800-1200 mg/day given in divided doses: 400 mg 2 or 3 times/day; 300 mg 2, 3 or 4 times/day; 200 mg 3 or 4 times/day; total daily dose should not exceed 1200 mg; for patients weighing <60 kg, total daily dose should not exceed 20 mg/kg/day

**Dosage Forms Cap (Lodine®):** 200 mg, 300 mg; **Tab:** (Lodine®): 400 mg, 500 mg; **Tab, extended release (Lodine® XL):** 400 mg, 500 mg, 600 mg

**Contraindications** Hypersensitivity to etodolac, aspirin, or other NSAIDs

**Warnings/Precautions** Use with caution in patients with congestive heart failure, hypertension, decreased renal or hepatic function, history of GI disease, or those receiving anticoagulants

**Pregnancy Risk Factor** C

**Adverse Reactions**
   >10%:
      Central nervous system: Dizziness
      Dermatologic: Rash
      Gastrointestinal: Abdominal cramps, heartburn, indigestion, nausea
   1% to 10%:
      Central nervous system: Headache, nervousness
      Dermatologic: Itching
      Endocrine & metabolic: Fluid retention
      Gastrointestinal: Vomiting
      Otic: Tinnitus
   <1%: Congestive heart failure, hypertension, arrhythmia, tachycardia, confusion, hallucinations, aseptic meningitis, mental depression, drowsiness, insomnia, urticaria, erythema multiforme, toxic epidermal necrolysis, Stevens-Johnson syndrome, angioedema, polydipsia, hot flashes, gastritis, GI ulceration, cystitis, polyuria, agranulocytosis, anemia, hemolytic anemia, bone marrow suppression, leukopenia, thrombocytopenia, hepatitis, peripheral neuropathy, toxic amblyopia, blurred vision, conjunctivitis, dry eyes, decreased hearing, acute renal failure, allergic rhinitis, shortness of breath, epistaxis

**Drug Interactions**
   Decreased effect with aspirin
   Increased effect/toxicity with aspirin (GI irritation), probenecid; increased effect/toxicity of lithium, methotrexate, digoxin, cyclosporin (nephrotoxicity), warfarin (bleeding)

**Onset** Analgesia: 2-4 hours; Anti-inflammatory: A few days

**Half-Life** 7 hours

**Special PA Issues**
   **Patient Education:** Take this medication exactly as directed; do not increase dose without consulting prescriber. Do not crush tablets or break capsules. Take with food or milk to reduce GI distress. Maintain adequate fluid intake (2-3 L/day). Do not use alcohol, aspirin, or aspirin-containing medication, and all other anti-inflammatory medications without consulting prescriber. You may experience anorexia, nausea, vomiting, or heartburn (frequent small meals, frequent oral care, sucking on lozenges, or chewing gum may help); drowsiness, dizziness, nervousness, or headache (use caution when driving or performing hazardous tasks); fluid retention (weigh yourself weekly and report unusual (3-5 lb/week) weight gain). GI bleeding, ulceration, or perforation can occur with or without pain; discontinue medication and contact prescriber if persistent abdominal pain or cramping, or blood in stool occurs. Report breathlessness, difficulty breathing, or unusual cough; chest pain, rapid heartbeat, palpitations; unusual bruising/bleeding; blood
(Continued)

## Etodolac *(Continued)*

in urine, stool, mouth, or vomitus; swollen extremities; skin rash or itching; acute fatigue; or changes in hearing or ringing in ears.

**Monitoring Parameters:** Monitor CBC, liver enzymes; in patients receiving diuretics, monitor urine output and BUN/serum creatinine

**Related Information**

Nonsteroidal Anti-Inflammatory Agents *on page 1026*

♦ **Etodolic Acid** *see* Etodolac *on previous page*

♦ **Etrafon®** *see* Amitriptyline and Perphenazine *on page 59*

## Etretinate (e TRET i nate)

**Pharmacologic Class** Antipsoriatic Agent

**U.S. Brand Names** Tegison®

**Mechanism of Action** Unknown; related to retinoic acid and retinol (vitamin A)

**Use** Treatment of severe recalcitrant psoriasis in patients intolerant of or unresponsive to standard therapies

**USUAL DOSAGE** Adults: Oral: Individualized; Initial: 0.75-1 mg/kg/day in divided doses, increase by 0.25 mg/kg/day at weekly intervals up to 1.5 mg/kg/day; maintenance dose established after 8-10 weeks of therapy 0.5-0.75 mg/kg/day

**Dosage Forms Cap:** 10 mg, 25 mg

**Contraindications** Pregnancy, known hypersensitivity to etretinate; because of the high likelihood of long lasting teratogenic effects, do not prescribe etretinate for women who are or who are likely to become pregnant while or after using the drug

**Warnings/Precautions** Not to be used in severe obesity or women of childbearing potential unless woman is capable of complying with effective contraceptive measures; therapy is normally begun on the second or third day of next normal menstrual period; effective contraception must be used for at least 1 month before beginning therapy, during therapy, and for 1 month after discontinuation of therapy; pregnancy test must be performed prior to starting therapy

**Pregnancy Risk Factor** X

**Adverse Reactions**

>10%:

Central nervous system: Fatigue, headache, fever

Dermatologic: Chapped lips, alopecia

Endocrine & metabolic: Hypercholesterolemia, hypertriglyceridemia

Gastrointestinal: Nausea, appetite change, xerostomia, sore tongue

Neuromuscular & skeletal: Hyperostosis, bone pain, arthralgia

Ocular: Eye irritation

Respiratory: Epistaxis

1% to 10%:

Cardiovascular: Edema

Central nervous system: Dizziness, lethargy

Hepatic: Hepatitis

Neuromuscular & skeletal: Myalgia

Ocular: Blurred vision

Otic: Otitis externa

Respiratory: Dyspnea

<1%: Syncope, amnesia, confusion, pseudotumor cerebri, depression, urticaria, mouth ulcers, diarrhea, constipation, flatulence, weight loss, gingival bleeding, gout, dysuria, polyuria, phlebitis, hyperkinesia, hypertonia, photophobia, ear infection, kidney stones, rhinorrhea

**Drug Interactions**

Increased effect: Milk increases absorption of etretinate

Increased toxicity: Additive toxicity with vitamin A

**Half-Life** 4-8 days (with multiple doses)

**Special PA Issues**

**Patient Education:** Take with food. Do not take additional vitamin A supplements. You may experience dizziness, blurred vision, or fatigue; use caution when driving or engaging in tasks that require alertness until response to drug is known. Report persistent severe nausea, abdominal pain, visual disturbances, yellowing of skin or eyes, unusual bruising or bleeding, muscle pain or cramping, or unusual nosebleeds.

♦ **Euglucon®** *see* Glyburide *on page 419*

♦ **Eulexin®** *see* Flutamide *on page 393*

♦ **Eurax® Topical** *see* Crotamiton *on page 241*

♦ **Evac-Q-Mag® [OTC]** *see* Magnesium Citrate *on page 552*

♦ **Evalose®** *see* Lactulose *on page 512*

♦ **Everone® Injection** *see* Testosterone *on page 881*

♦ **Evista®** *see* Raloxifene *on page 792*

♦ **E-Vitamin® [OTC]** *see* Vitamin E *on page 963*

- **Excedrin™ IB [OTC]** *see* Ibuprofen *on page 466*
- **Exelderm®** *see* Sulconazole *on page 857*
- **Exidine® Scrub [OTC]** *see* Chlorhexidine Gluconate *on page 190*
- **Exna®** *see* Benzthiazide *on page 107*
- **Exosurf® Neonatal** *see* Colfosceril Palmitate *on page 235*
- **Exsel®** *see* Selenium Sulfide *on page 827*
- **Extendryl® SR** *see* Chlorpheniramine, Phenylephrine, and Methscopolamine *on page 196*
- **Extra Action Cough Syrup [OTC]** *see* Guaifenesin and Dextromethorphan *on page 428*
- **Extra Strength Adprin-B® [OTC]** *see* Aspirin *on page 80*
- **Extra Strength Bayer® Enteric 500 Aspirin [OTC]** *see* Aspirin *on page 80*
- **Extra Strength Bayer® Plus [OTC]** *see* Aspirin *on page 80*
- **Eye Balm** *see* Golden Seal *on page 421*
- **Eye Root** *see* Golden Seal *on page 421*
- **Eye-Sed® [OTC]** *see* Zinc Supplements *on page 975*
- **Ezide®** *see* Hydrochlorothiazide *on page 447*
- **F₃T** *see* Trifluridine *on page 935*
- **Factors Affecting Plasma Levels Obtained for Common Drugs** *see* Chart *on page 1128*
- **Factrel®** *see* Gonadorelin *on page 423*

## Famciclovir (fam SYE kloe veer)

**Pharmacologic Class** Antiviral Agent

**U.S. Brand Names** Famvir™

**Mechanism of Action** After undergoing rapid biotransformation to the active compound, penciclovir, famciclovir is phosphorylated by viral thymidine kinase in HSV-1, HSV-2, and VZV-infected cells to a monophosphate form; this is then converted to penciclovir triphosphate and competes with deoxyguanosine triphosphate to inhibit HSV-2 polymerase (ie, herpes viral DNA synthesis/replication is selectively inhibited)

**Use** Management of acute herpes zoster (shingles) and recurrent episodes of genital herpes; treatment of recurrent herpes simplex in immunocompetent patients

**USUAL DOSAGE** Adults: Oral:

Acute herpes zoster: 500 mg every 8 hours for 7 days

Recurrent herpes simplex in immunocompetent patients: 125 mg twice daily for 5 days

Genital herpes:

Recurrent episodes: 125 mg twice daily for 5 days

Prophylaxis: 250 mg twice daily

**Dosing interval in renal impairment:**

$Cl_{cr}$ 40-59 mL/minute: Administer 500 mg every 12 hours

$Cl_{cr}$ 20-39 mL/minute: Administer 500 mg every 24 hours

$Cl_{cr}$ <20 mL/minute: Unknown

**Dosage Forms** Tab: 125 mg, 250 mg, 500 mg

**Contraindications** Hypersensitivity to famciclovir

**Warnings/Precautions** Has not been studied in immunocompromised patients or patients with ophthalmic or disseminated zoster; dosage adjustment is required in patients with renal insufficiency ($Cl_{cr}$ <60 mL/minute) and in patients with noncompensated hepatic disease; safety and efficacy have not been established in children <18 years of age; animal studies indicated increases in incidence of carcinomas, mutagenic changes, and decreases in fertility with extremely large doses

**Pregnancy Risk Factor** B

**Pregnancy Implications**

Clinical effects on the fetus: Use only if the benefit to the patient clearly exceeds the potential risk to the fetus

Breast-feeding/lactation: Due to potential for excretion of famciclovir in breast milk and for its associated tumorigenicity, discontinue nursing or discontinue the drug during lactation

**Adverse Reactions**

1% to 10%:

Central nervous system: Fatigue (4% to 6%), fever (1% to 3%), dizziness (3% to 5%), somnolence (1% to 2%), headache

Dermatologic: Pruritus (1% to 4%)

Gastrointestinal: Diarrhea (4% to 8%), vomiting (1% to 5%), constipation (1% to 5%), anorexia (1% to 3%), abdominal pain (1% to 4%), nausea

Neuromuscular & skeletal: Paresthesia (1% to 3%)

Respiratory: Sinusitis/pharyngitis (2%)

<1%: Rigors, arthralgia, upper respiratory infection

**Drug Interactions** Increased effect/toxicity:

Cimetidine: Penciclovir AUC may increase due to impaired metabolism

Digoxin: $C_{max}$ of digoxin increases by ~19%

Probenecid: Penciclovir serum levels significantly increase

Theophylline: Penciclovir AUC/$C_{max}$ may increase and renal clearance decrease, although not clinically significant

(Continued)

## Famciclovir (Continued)

**Half-Life** Penciclovir: 2-3 hours (10, 20, and 7 hours in HSV-1, HSV-2, and VZV-infected cells); linearly decreased with reductions in renal failure

**Special PA Issues**

**Patient Education:** Take for prescribed length of time, even if condition improves. Do not discontinue without consulting prescriber. This is not a cure for genital herpes. You may experience mild GI disturbances (eg, nausea, vomiting, constipation, or diarrhea), fatigue, headaches, or muscle aches and pains. If these are severe, contact prescriber.

## Famotidine (fa MOE ti deen)

**Pharmacologic Class** Histamine $H_2$ Antagonist

**U.S. Brand Names** Pepcid®; Pepcid® AC Acid Controller [OTC]; Pepcid® RPD

**Mechanism of Action** Competitive inhibition of histamine at $H_2$ receptors of the gastric parietal cells, which inhibits gastric acid secretion

**Use**

Pepcid®: Therapy and treatment of duodenal ulcer, gastric ulcer, control gastric pH in critically ill patients, symptomatic relief in gastritis, gastroesophageal reflux, active benign ulcer, and pathological hypersecretory conditions

Pepcid® AC Acid Controller: Relieves heartburn, acid indigestion and sour stomach

**USUAL DOSAGE**

Children: Oral, I.V.: Doses of 1-2 mg/kg/day have been used; maximum dose: 40 mg

Adults:

Oral:

Duodenal ulcer, gastric ulcer: 40 mg/day at bedtime for 4-8 weeks

Hypersecretory conditions: Initial: 20 mg every 6 hours, may increase up to 160 mg every 6 hours

GERD: 20 mg twice daily for 6 weeks

I.V.: 20 mg every 12 hours

**Dosing adjustment in renal impairment:**

$Cl_{cr}$ <10 mL/minute: Administer every 24 hours or 50% of dose

**Dosage Forms Inf, premixed in NS:** 20 mg (50 mL); **Inj:** 10 mg/mL (2 mL, 4 mL); **Powder for oral susp (cherry-banana-mint flavor):** 40 mg/5 mL (50 mL); **Tab, film coated:** 20 mg, 40 mg, Pepcid® AC Acid Controller: 10 mg; **Tab, disintegrating:** 20 mg, 40 mg

**Contraindications** Hypersensitivity to famotidine or other $H_2$-antagonists

**Warnings/Precautions** Modify dose in patients with renal impairment

**Pregnancy Risk Factor** B

**Pregnancy Implications**

Clinical effects on the fetus: Crosses the placenta. No data on effects on the fetus (insufficient data).

Breast-feeding/lactation: Crosses into breast milk. American Academy of Pediatrics has NO RECOMMENDATIONS.

**Adverse Reactions**

1% to 10%:

Central nervous system: Dizziness, headache

Gastrointestinal: Constipation, diarrhea

<1%: Bradycardia, tachycardia, palpitations, hypertension, fever, fatigue, seizures, insomnia, drowsiness, acne, pruritus, urticaria, dry skin, abdominal discomfort, flatulence, belching, anorexia, agranulocytosis, neutropenia, thrombocytopenia, increased AST/ALT, paresthesia, weakness, increased BUN/creatinine, proteinuria, bronchospasm, allergic reaction

**Drug Interactions** Decreased effect of ketoconazole, itraconazole

**Onset** Onset of GI effect: Oral: Within 1 hour

**Duration** 10-12 hours

**Half-Life** 2.5-3.5 hours; increases with renal impairment, oliguric patient: 20 hours

**Special PA Issues**

**Patient Education:** Take as directed, for full dose as prescribed, even if feeling better. Take antacids 1 hour before or 2 hours after famotidine. Avoid alcohol and smoking (smoking decreases effectiveness of medication). You may experience some drowsiness or dizziness; use caution when driving or engaging in tasks that require alertness until response to drug is known. Increased exercise, increased dietary fluids, fruits, or fiber may reduce constipation; yogurt or buttermilk may help relieve diarrhea. Report acute headache, unresolved constipation or diarrhea, palpitations, black tarry stools, abdominal pain, rash, worsening of condition being treated, or recurrence of symptoms after therapy is completed.

♦ **Famvir™** see Famciclovir on previous page

♦ **Fareston®** see Toremifene on page 917

♦ **Fastin®** see Phentermine on page 716

## Fat Emulsion (fat e MUL shun)

**Pharmacologic Class** Caloric Agent

**U.S. Brand Names** Intralipid®; Liposyn®; Nutrilipid®; Soyacal®

**Mechanism of Action** Essential for normal structure and function of cell membranes

**Use** Source of calories and essential fatty acids for patients requiring parenteral nutrition of extended duration

**USUAL DOSAGE** Fat emulsion should not exceed 60% of the total daily calories

Premature Infants: Initial dose: 0.25-0.5 g/kg/day, increase by 0.25-0.5 g/kg/day to a maximum of 3 g/kg/day depending on needs/nutritional goals; limit to 1 g/kg/day if on phototherapy; maximum rate of infusion: 0.15 g/kg/hour (0.75 mL/kg/hour of 20% solution)

Infants and Children: Initial dose: 0.5-1 g/kg/day, increase by 0.5 g/kg/day to a maximum of 3 g/kg/day depending on needs/nutritional goals; maximum rate of infusion: 0.25 g/kg/hour (1.25 mL/kg/hour of 20% solution)

Adolescents and Adults: Initial dose: 1 g/kg/day, increase by 0.5-1 g/kg/day to a maximum of 2.5 g/kg/day of 10% and 3 g/kg/day of 20% depending on needs/nutritional goals; maximum rate of infusion: 0.25 g/kg/hour (1.25 mL/kg/hour of 20% solution); do not exceed 50 mL/hour (20%) or 100 mL/hour (10%)

Prevention of essential fatty acid deficiency (8% to 10% of total caloric intake): 0.5-1 g/kg/24 hours

Children: 5-10 mL/kg/day at 0.1 mL/minute then up to 100 mL/hour

Adults: 500 mL (10%) twice weekly at rate of 1 mL/minute for 30 minutes, then increase to 42 mL/hour (500 mL over 12 hours)

Note: At the onset of therapy, the patient should be observed for any immediate allergic reactions such as dyspnea, cyanosis, and fever; slower initial rates of infusion may be used for the first 10-15 minutes of the infusion (eg, 0.1 mL/minute of 10% or 0.05 mL/minute of 20% solution)

**Dosage Forms** Inj: 10% [100 mg/mL] (100 mL, 250 mL, 500 mL), 20% [200 mg/mL] (100 mL, 250 mL, 500 mL)

**Contraindications** Pathologic hyperlipidemia, lipoid nephrosis, known hypersensitivity to fat emulsion and severe egg or legume (soybean) allergies, pancreatitis with hyperlipemia

**Warnings/Precautions** Use caution in patients with severe liver damage, pulmonary disease, anemia, or blood coagulation disorder; use with caution in jaundiced, premature, and low birth weight children

**Pregnancy Risk Factor** B/C

**Adverse Reactions**

>10%: Local: Thrombophlebitis

1% to 10%: Endocrine & metabolic: Hyperlipemia

<1%: Cyanosis, flushing, chest pain, nausea, vomiting, diarrhea, hepatomegaly, dyspnea, sepsis

**Half-Life** 0.5-1 hour

**Special PA Issues**

**Patient Education:** Report pain at infusion site, difficulty breathing, chest pain, calf pain, or excessive sweating.

**Monitoring Parameters:** Serum triglycerides; before initiation of therapy and at least weekly during therapy

♦ **5-FC** see Flucytosine on page 376

♦ **Featherfew** see Feverfew on page 368

♦ **Featherfoil** see Feverfew on page 368

♦ **Feldene®** see Piroxicam on page 733

## Felodipine (fe LOE di peen)

**Pharmacologic Class** Calcium Channel Blocker

**U.S. Brand Names** Plendil®

**Mechanism of Action** Inhibits calcium ions from entering the "slow channels" or select voltage-sensitive areas of vascular smooth muscle and myocardium during depolarization, producing a relaxation of coronary vascular smooth muscle and coronary vasodilation; increases myocardial oxygen delivery in patients with vasospastic angina

**Use** Treatment of hypertension, congestive heart failure

**USUAL DOSAGE**

Adults: Oral: 2.5-10 mg once daily; usual initial dose: 5 mg; increase by 5 mg at 2-week intervals, as needed; maximum: 10 mg

Elderly: Begin with 2.5 mg/day

**Dosing adjustment/comments in hepatic impairment:** Begin with 2.5 mg/day; do not use doses >10 mg/day

**Dosage Forms** Tab, extended release: 2.5 mg, 5 mg, 10 mg

**Contraindications** Hypersensitivity to felodipine or any component or other calcium channel blocker; severe hypotension or second and third degree heart block

**Warnings/Precautions** Use with caution and titrate dosages for patients with impaired renal or hepatic function; use caution when treating patients with congestive heart failure, (Continued)

## Felodipine *(Continued)*

sick-sinus syndrome, severe left ventricular dysfunction, hypertrophic cardiomyopathy (especially obstructive), concomitant therapy with beta-blockers or digoxin, edema, or increased intracranial pressure with cranial tumors; do not abruptly withdraw (may cause chest pain); elderly may experience hypotension and constipation more readily.

**Pregnancy Risk Factor** C

**Adverse Reactions**

>10%:

Cardiovascular: Peripheral edema (22%)

Central nervous system: Headache (18%)

1% to 10%:

Cardiovascular: Chest pain, palpitations (2%), flushing (6%)

Central nervous system: Dizziness/lightheadedness (6%)

Dermatologic: Rash (1% to 2%)

Gastrointestinal: Constipation/diarrhea (1% to 2%), nausea (2%), abdominal pain (1% to 2%)

Neuromuscular & skeletal: Weakness (5%), paresthesia (2.5%)

Respiratory: Cough (3%), upper respiratory infection (5.5%)

<1%: Hypotension, arrhythmia, tachycardia, syncope, A-V block, myocardial infarction, angina, mental depression, nervousness, somnolence, insomnia, pruritus, sexual disorder, gingival hyperplasia, xerostomia, vomiting, flatulence, micturition disorder, anemia, marked elevations in LFTs, blurred vision, shortness of breath, rhinitis, epistaxis

**Drug Interactions** CYP3A3/4 enzyme substrate

Decreased effect:

Felodipine and carbamazepine may decrease felodipine effect

Felodipine and theophylline may decrease pharmacologic actions of theophylline

Increased toxicity/effect/levels:

Felodipine and metoprolol may increase cardiac depressant effects on A-V conduction

Felodipine and erythromycin inhibits felodipine (and other dihydropyridine calcium antagonist) metabolism resulting in a twofold increase in levels and consequent toxicity

**Onset** 2-5 hours

**Duration** 16-24 hours

**Half-Life** 11-16 hours

**Special PA Issues**

**Patient Education:** Take without food. Take as prescribed; do not stop abruptly without consulting prescriber immediately. Swallow whole; do not crush or chew. You may experience headache (if unrelieved, consult prescriber), nausea or vomiting (frequent small meals may help), constipation (increased dietary bulk and fluids may help), depression (should resolve when drug is discontinued). May cause dizziness or drowsiness; use caution when driving or engaging in hazardous activities. Report any chest pain or swelling of hands or feet, respiratory distress, sudden weight gain, or unresolved constipation.

**Dietary Considerations:** Should be taken without food; the bioavailability of felodipine is influenced by the presence of food and has been shown to increase more than twofold when taken with concentrated grapefruit juice

**Related Information**

Calcium Channel Blocking Agents *on page 1004*

♦ **Femara™** *see Letrozole on page 519*

♦ **Femcet®** *see Butalbital Compound on page 131*

♦ **Femguard®** *see Sulfabenzamide, Sulfacetamide, and Sulfathiazole on page 857*

♦ **Femiron® [OTC]** *see Ferrous Fumarate on page 366*

♦ **Femizole-7® [OTC]** *see Clotrimazole on page 228*

♦ **Femizol-M®** [OTC] *see Miconazole on page 604*

♦ **Femogen®** *see Estrone on page 338*

♦ **FemPatch® Transdermal** *see Estradiol on page 332*

♦ **Femstat®** *see Butoconazole on page 132*

♦ **Fenesin™** *see Guaifenesin on page 427*

♦ **Fenesin™ DM** *see Guaifenesin and Dextromethorphan on page 428*

## Fenofibrate *(fen oh FYE brate)*

**Pharmacologic Class** Antilipemic Agent (Fibric Acid)

**U.S. Brand Names** TriCor™

**Mechanism of Action** Fenofibric acid is believed to increase VLDL catabolism by enhancing the synthesis of lipoprotein lipase; as a result of a decrease in VLDL levels, total plasma triglycerides are reduced by 30% to 60%; modest increase in HDL occurs in some hypertriglyceridemic patients

**Use** Adjunct to dietary therapy for the treatment of adults with very high elevations of serum triglyceride levels (types IV and V hyperlipidemia) who are at risk of pancreatitis and who do not respond adequately to a determined dietary effort; its efficacy can be enhanced by combination with other hypolipidemic agents that have a different mechanism of action; safety and efficacy may be greater than that of clofibrate

**USUAL DOSAGE** Adults: Oral: Initial: 67 mg/day, up to 3 capsules (201 mg); requires 6-8 weeks of therapy to determine efficacy

**Dosing adjustment/comments in renal impairment:** Decrease dose or increase dosing interval for patients with renal failure

**Dosage Forms Cap:** 67 mg

**Warnings/Precautions** The hypoprothrombinemic effect of anticoagulants is significantly increased with concomitant fenofibrate administration; use with caution in patients with severe renal dysfunction

**Pregnancy Risk Factor** C

**Pregnancy Implications** Although teratogenicity and mutagenicity tests in animals have been negative, significant risk has been identified with clofibrate, an agent similar in action to fenofibrate. Use should be avoided, if possible, in pregnant women since the neonatal glucuronide conjugation pathways are immature.

**Adverse Reactions**
>10%: Gastrointestinal: Nausea, gastric discomfort
1% to 10%:
Dermatologic: Skin reactions
Gastrointestinal: Constipation, diarrhea
<1%: Dizziness, headache, fatigue, insomnia, transient increases in LFTs, arthralgia, myalgia

**Drug Interactions** Increased effect/toxicity: Increased hypolipidemic effect when used with cholestyramine or colestipol; increased hypoprothrombinemic effect when used with warfarin

**Half-Life** Fenofibrate: 21 hours (30 hours in the elderly, 44-54 hours in hepatic impairment)

**Special PA Issues**
**Patient Education:** Take with food. Do not change dosage without consulting prescriber. Maintain diet and exercise program as prescribed. You may experience mild GI disturbances (eg, gas, diarrhea, constipation, nausea); inform prescriber if these are severe. Report skin rash or irritation, insomnia, unusual muscle pain or tremors, or persistent dizziness.

**Monitoring Parameters:** Total serum cholesterol and triglyceride concentration and CLDL, LDL, and HDL levels should be measured periodically; if only marginal changes are noted in 6-8 weeks, the drug should be discontinued; serum transaminases should be measured every 3 months; if ALT values increase >100 units/L, therapy should be discontinued. Monitor LFTs prior to initiation, at 6 and 12 weeks after initiation of first dose, then periodically thereafter.

# Fenoprofen (fen oh PROE fen)

**Pharmacologic Class** Nonsteroidal Anti-Inflammatory Agent (NSAID)

**U.S. Brand Names** Nalfon®

**Mechanism of Action** Inhibits prostaglandin synthesis by decreasing the activity of the enzyme, cyclo-oxygenase, which results in decreased formation of prostaglandin precursors

**Use** Symptomatic treatment of acute and chronic rheumatoid arthritis and osteoarthritis; relief of mild to moderate pain

**USUAL DOSAGE** Adults: Oral:
Rheumatoid arthritis: 300-600 mg 3-4 times/day up to 3.2 g/day
Mild to moderate pain: 200 mg every 4-6 hours as needed

**Dosage Forms Cap:** 200 mg, 300 mg; **Tab:** 600 mg

**Contraindications** Known hypersensitivity to fenoprofen or other NSAIDs

**Warnings/Precautions** Use with caution in patients with congestive heart failure, hypertension, decreased renal or hepatic function, history of GI disease, or those receiving anticoagulants

**Pregnancy Risk Factor** B (D if used in the 3rd trimester or near delivery)

**Adverse Reactions**
>10%:
Central nervous system: Dizziness
Dermatologic: Rash
Gastrointestinal: Abdominal cramps, heartburn, indigestion, nausea
1% to 10%:
Central nervous system: Headache, nervousness
Dermatologic: Itching
Endocrine & metabolic: Fluid retention
Gastrointestinal: Vomiting
Otic: Tinnitus
<1%: Congestive heart failure, hypertension, arrhythmias, tachycardia, confusion, hallucinations, aseptic meningitis, mental depression, drowsiness, insomnia, urticaria, erythema multiforme, toxic epidermal necrolysis, Stevens-Johnson syndrome, angioedema, polydipsia, hot flashes, gastritis, GI ulceration, cystitis, polyuria, agranulocytosis, anemia, (Continued)

## Fenoprofen *(Continued)*

hemolytic anemia, bone marrow suppression, leukopenia, thrombocytopenia, hepatitis, peripheral neuropathy, toxic amblyopia, blurred vision, conjunctivitis, dry eyes, decreased hearing, acute renal failure, allergic rhinitis, shortness of breath, epistaxis

**Drug Interactions**

Decreased effect with phenobarbital

Increased effect/toxicity of phenytoin, sulfonamides, sulfonylureas

Increased toxicity with salicylates, oral anticoagulants

**Onset** Begins in a few days

**Half-Life** 2.5-3 hours

**Special PA Issues**

**Patient Education:** Take this medication exactly as directed; do not increase dose without consulting prescriber. Do not crush tablets or break capsules. Take with food or milk to reduce GI distress. Maintain adequate fluid intake (2-3 L/day). Do not use alcohol, aspirin, or aspirin-containing medication, and all other anti-inflammatory medications without consulting prescriber. You may experience drowsiness, dizziness, nervousness, or headache (use caution when driving or performing hazardous tasks); anorexia, nausea, vomiting, or heartburn (frequent small meals, frequent oral care, sucking on lozenges, or chewing gum may help); fluid retention (weigh yourself weekly and report unusual (3-5 lb/week) weight gain). GI bleeding, ulceration, or perforation can occur with or without pain; discontinue medication and contact prescriber if persistent abdominal pain or cramping, or blood in stool occurs. Report breathlessness, difficulty breathing, or unusual cough; chest pain, rapid heartbeat, palpitations; unusual bruising/bleeding; blood in urine, stool, mouth, or vomitus; swollen extremities; skin rash or itching; acute fatigue; or changes in hearing or ringing in ears.

**Monitoring Parameters:** Monitor CBC, liver enzymes; monitor urine output and BUN/serum creatinine in patients receiving diuretics

**Reference Range:** Therapeutic: 20-65 µg/mL (SI: 82-268 µmol/L)

**Related Information**

Nonsteroidal Anti-Inflammatory Agents *on page 1026*

♦ **Fenoprofen Calcium** *see* Fenoprofen *on previous page*

## Fentanyl *(FEN ta nil)*

**Pharmacologic Class** Analgesic, Narcotic; General Anesthetic

**U.S. Brand Names** Actiq®; Duragesic® Transdermal; Fentanyl Oralet®; Sublimaze® Injection

**Mechanism of Action** Binds with stereospecific receptors at many sites within the CNS, increases pain threshold, alters pain reception, inhibits ascending pain pathways

**Use** Sedation, relief of pain, preoperative medication, adjunct to general or regional anesthesia, management of chronic pain (transdermal product)

**USUAL DOSAGE** Doses should be titrated to appropriate effects; wide range of doses, dependent upon desired degree of analgesia/anesthesia

Children 1-12 years:

Sedation for minor procedures/analgesia:

I.M., I.V.: 1-2 mcg/kg/dose; may repeat at 30- to 60-minute intervals. **Note:** Children 18-36 months of age may require 2-3 mcg/kg/dose

Transmucosal (dosage strength is based on patient weight): 5 mcg/kg if child is not fearful; fearful children and some younger children may require doses of 5-15 mcg/kg (which also carries an increased risk of hypoventilation); drug effect begins within 10 minutes, with sedation beginning shortly thereafter

Continuous sedation/analgesia: Initial I.V. bolus: 1-2 mcg/kg then 1 mcg/kg/hour; titrate upward; usual: 1-3 mcg/kg/hour

Pain control: Transdermal: Not recommended

### Dosage Recommendations for Transmucosal Fentanyl (Oralet®)

| Patient Age/Weight | 5-10 mcg/kg/dose | 10-15 mcg/kg/dose |
|---|---|---|
| Children <2 years of age OR <15 kg | NOT RECOMMENDED | NOT RECOMMENDED |
| <15 kg | NOT AVAILABLE | 200 mcg |
| 20 kg | 200 mcg | 200-300 mcg |
| 25 kg | 200 mcg | 300 mcg |
| 30 kg | 300 mcg | 300-400 mcg |
| 35 kg | 300 mcg | 400 mcg |
| >40 kg | 400 mcg | 400 mcg |
| Adults | 400 mcg | 400 mcg |

Children >12 years and Adults:

Sedation for minor procedures/analgesia:

I.M., I.V.: 0.5-1 mcg/kg/dose; higher doses are used for major procedures

Transmucosal: 5 mcg/kg, suck on lozenge vigorously approximately 20-40 minutes before the start of procedure, drug effect begins within 10 minutes, with sedation beginning shortly thereafter; see table.

Preoperative sedation, adjunct to regional anesthesia, postoperative pain: I.M., I.V.: 50-100 mcg/dose

Adjunct to general anesthesia: I.M., I.V.: 2-50 mcg/kg

General anesthesia without additional anesthetic agents: I.V. 50-100 mcg/kg with $O_2$ and skeletal muscle relaxant

Pain control: Transdermal: Initial: 25 mcg/hour system; if currently receiving opiates, convert to fentanyl equivalent and administer equianalgesic dosage titrated to minimize the adverse effects and provide analgesia. To convert patients from oral or parenteral opioids to Duragesic®, the previous 24-hour analgesic requirement should be calculated. This analgesic requirement should be converted to the equianalgesic oral morphine dose. See tables.

**Equianalgesic Doses of Opioid Agonists**

| Drug | Equianalgesic Dose (mg) | |
|---|---|---|
| | I.M. | P.O. |
| Codeine | 130 | 200 |
| Hydromorphone | 1.5 | 7.5 |
| Levorphanol | 2 | 4 |
| Meperidine | 75 | — |
| Methadone | 10 | 20 |
| Morphine | 10 | 60 |
| Oxycodone | 15 | 30 |
| Oxymorphone | 1 | 10 (PR) |

From N Engl J Med, 1985, 313:84-95.

**Corresponding Doses of Oral/Intramuscular Morphine and Duragesic™**

| P.O. 24-Hour Morphine (mg/d) | I.M. 24-Hour Morphine (mg/d) | Duragesic™ Dose (mcg/h) |
|---|---|---|
| 45-134 | 8-22 | 25 |
| 135-224 | 28-37 | 50 |
| 225-314 | 38-52 | 75 |
| 315-404 | 53-67 | 100 |
| 405-494 | 68-82 | 125 |
| 495-584 | 83-97 | 150 |
| 585-674 | 98-112 | 175 |
| 675-764 | 113-127 | 200 |
| 765-854 | 128-142 | 225 |
| 855-944 | 143-157 | 250 |
| 945-1034 | 158-172 | 275 |
| 1035-1124 | 173-187 | 300 |

Product information, Duragesic™ — Janssen Pharmaceutica, January, 1991.

The dosage should not be titrated more frequently than every 3 days after the initial dose or every 6 days thereafter. The majority of patients are controlled on every 72-hour administration, however, a small number of patients require every 48-hour administration.

Elderly >65 years: Transmucosal: Dose should be reduced to 2.5-5 mcg/kg; elderly have been found to be twice as sensitive as younger patients to the effects of fentanyl

**Dosing adjustment in renal impairment:**

$Cl_{cr}$ 10-50 mL/minute: Administer at 75% of normal dose

$Cl_{cr}$ <10 mL/minute: Administer at 50% of normal dose

**Dosage Forms Inj, as citrate:** 0.05 mg/mL (2 mL, 5 mL, 10 mL, 20 mL, 50 mL); **Loz, oral transmucosal (raspberry flavored):** 200 mcg, 300 mcg, 400 mcg, 600 mcg, 800 mcg, 1200 mcg, 1600 mcg; **Transdermal system:** 25 mcg/hour [10 cm²], 50 mcg/hour [20 cm²], 75 mcg/hour [30 cm²], 100 mcg/hour [40 cm²] (all available in 5s)

(Continued)

## Fentanyl *(Continued)*

**Contraindications** Hypersensitivity to fentanyl or any component; increased intracranial pressure; severe respiratory depression; severe liver or renal insufficiency

Transmucosal is contraindicated in unmonitored settings where a risk of unrecognized hypoventilation exists or in treating acute or chronic pain

**Warnings/Precautions** Fentanyl shares the toxic potentials of opiate agonists, and precautions of opiate agonist therapy should be observed; use with caution in patients with bradycardia; rapid I.V. infusion may result in skeletal muscle and chest wall rigidity → impaired ventilation → respiratory distress → apnea, bronchoconstriction, laryngospasm; inject slowly over 3-5 minutes; nondepolarizing skeletal muscle relaxant may be required. Tolerance of drug dependence may result from extended use.

Transmucosal fentanyl: Fentanyl Oralet® is not indicated for use in unmonitored settings where there is a risk of unrecognized hypoventilation or in treating acute or chronic pain. Patients should be monitored by direct visual observation and by some means of measuring respiratory function such as pulse oximetry until they are recovered. Facilities for the administration of fluids, opioid antagonists, oxygen and resuscitation equipment (including facilities for endotracheal intubation) should be readily available.

Topical patches: Serum fentanyl concentrations may increase approximately one-third for patients with a body temperature of 40°C secondary to a temperature-dependent increase in fentanyl release from the system and increased skin permeability. Patients who experience adverse reactions should be monitored for at least 12 hours after removal of the patch.

The elderly may be particularly susceptible to the CNS depressant and constipating effects of narcotics

**Pregnancy Risk Factor** B (D if used for prolonged periods or in high doses at term)

**Adverse Reactions**

>10%:

Cardiovascular: Hypotension, bradycardia

Central nervous system: CNS depression, drowsiness, sedation

Gastrointestinal: Nausea, vomiting, constipation

Respiratory: Respiratory depression

1% to 10%:

Cardiovascular: Cardiac arrhythmias, orthostatic hypotension

Central nervous system: Confusion

Gastrointestinal: Biliary tract spasm

Ocular: Miosis

<1%: Circulatory depression, convulsions, dysesthesia, paradoxical CNS excitation or delirium; cold, clammy skin; dizziness, erythema, pruritus, rash, urticaria, itching, ADH release, urinary tract spasm, bronchospasm, laryngospasm, physical and psychological dependence with prolonged use

**Drug Interactions** CYP3A3/4 enzyme substrate

Increased toxicity: CNS depressants, phenothiazines, tricyclic antidepressants may potentiate fentanyl's adverse effects

**Onset** Respiratory depressant effect may last longer than analgesic effect

I.M.: 7-15 minutes

I.V.: Almost immediate

Transmucosal: 5-15 minutes with a maximum reduction in activity/apprehension; Peak analgesia: Within 20-30 minutes

**Duration** Respiratory depressant effect may last longer than analgesic effect.

I.M.: 1-2 hours; I.V.: 0.5-1 hour; Transmucosal: Related to blood level of the drug

**Half-Life** 2-4 hours; Transmucosal: 6.6 hours (range: 5-15 hours)

**Special PA Issues**

**Patient Education:** While using this medication, do not use alcohol and other prescription or OTC medications (especially sedatives, tranquilizers, antihistamines, or pain medications) without consulting prescriber. Maintain adequate hydration (2-3 L/day of fluids unless instructed to restrict fluid intake). May cause hypotension, dizziness, drowsiness, impaired coordination, or blurred vision (use caution when driving, climbing stairs, or changing position - rising from sitting or lying to standing, or when engaging in hazardous activities until response to medication is known); nausea or vomiting (frequent mouth care, small frequent meals, or sucking on lozenges may help); constipation (increased exercise, fluids, or dietary fruit and fiber may help - if constipation remains an unresolved problem, consult prescriber about use of stool softeners). Report acute dizziness, chest pain, slow or rapid heartbeat, acute headache; confusion or changes in mentation; changes in voiding frequency or amount, swelling of extremities, or unusual weight gain; shortness of breath or difficulty breathing; or changes in vision.

**Administration:** Transdermal: Apply to clean, dry skin, immediately after removing from package. Firmly press in place and hold for 20 seconds.

**Dietary Considerations:**

Alcohol: Additive CNS effects, avoid or limit alcohol; watch for sedation

Food: Glucose may cause hyperglycemia; monitor blood glucose concentrations

**Monitoring Parameters:** Respiratory and cardiovascular status, blood pressure, heart rate

**Related Information**
Narcotic Agonists *on page 1023*

## Ferric Gluconate (food THIK eh ner IN stant)

**Pharmacologic Class** Iron Salt

**U.S. Brand Names** Ferrlecit®

**Mechanism of Action** Supplies a source to elemental iron necessary to the function of hemoglobin, myoglobin and specific enzyme systems; allows transport of oxygen via hemoglobin

**Use** Repletion of total body iron content in patients with iron deficiency anemia who are undergoing hemodialysis in conjunction with erythropoietin therapy

**USUAL DOSAGE** Adults:

Test dose (recommended): 2 mL diluted in 50 mL 0.9% sodium chloride over 60 minutes
Repletion of iron in hemodialysis patients: I.V.: 125 mg (10 mL) in 100 mL 0.9% sodium chloride over 1 hour during hemodialysis. Most patients will require a cumulative dose of 1 g elemental iron over approximately 8 sequential dialysis treatments to achieve a favorable response.

**Dosage Forms Inj:** 12.5 mg/mL (5 mL ampuls)

**Contraindications** Hypersensitivity to ferric gluconate, benzyl alcohol, or any component of the formulation; use in any anemia not caused by iron deficiency, heart failure (of any severity)

**Warnings/Precautions** Potentially serious hypersensitivity reactions may occur. Fatal immediate hypersensitivity reactions have occurred with other iron carbohydrate complexes. Avoid rapid administration - flushing and hypotension may occur. Administration rate should not exceed 2.1 mg/minute. Do not administer to patients with iron overload. Use with caution in elderly patients.

**Pregnancy Risk Factor** B

**Pregnancy Implications** There are no well-controlled studies available. Should be used in pregnancy only when the potential benefit to the mother clearly outweighs the potential risk to the fetus. It is not known if ferrous gluconate is excreted in human milk. Use caution if the drug is administered to women who are breast-feeding.

**Adverse Reactions** Major adverse reactions which are likely to be related ferrous gluconate include hypotension and hypersensitivity reactions. Hypersensitivity reactions have included pruritus, chest pain, hypotension, nausea, abdominal pain, flank pain, fatigue and rash. Fatal hypersensitivity reactions have occurred with other iron polysaccharide complexes. A test dose is recommended.

1% to 10%:
Cardiovascular: Hypotension (serious hypotension in 1.3%), chest pain, hypertension, syncope, tachycardia, angina, myocardial infarction, pulmonary edema, hypovolemia, peripheral edema
Central nervous system: Headache, fatigue, fever, malaise, dizziness, paresthesia, insomnia, agitation, somnolence
Dermatologic: Pruritus, rash
Endocrine & metabolic: Hyperkalemia, hypoglycemia, hypokalemia
Gastrointestinal: Abdominal pain, nausea, vomiting, diarrhea, rectal disorder, dyspepsia, flatulence, melena
Genitourinary: Urinary tract infection
Hematologic: Anemia, abnormal erythrocytes, lymphadenopathy
Local: Injection site reactions, pain
Neuromuscular & skeletal: Weakness, back pain, leg cramps, myalgia, arthralgia, paresthesia
Ocular: Blurred vision, conjunctivitis
Respiratory: Dyspnea, cough, rhinitis, upper respiratory infection, pneumonia
Miscellaneous: Hypersensitivity reactions (3%), infection, rigors, chills, flu-like syndrome, sepsis, carcinoma, increased sweating, diaphoresis (increased)

<1% Epigastric pain, groin pain
(Continued)

## Ferric Gluconate *(Continued)*

### Special PA Issues
**Monitoring Parameters:** Hemoglobin and hematocrit, serum ferritin, iron saturation

♦ **Ferrlecit®** *see* Ferric Gluconate *on previous page*

♦ **Ferro-Sequels® [OTC]** *see* Ferrous Fumarate *on this page*

## Ferrous Fumarate *(FER us FYOO ma rate)*

**Pharmacologic Class** Iron Salt

**U.S. Brand Names** Femiron® [OTC]; Feostat® [OTC]; Ferro-Sequels® [OTC]; Fumasorb® [OTC]; Fumerin® [OTC]; Hemocyte® [OTC]; Ircon® [OTC]; Nephro-Fer™ [OTC]; Span-FF® [OTC]

**Mechanism of Action** Replaces iron found in hemoglobin, myoglobin, and enzymes; allows the transportation of oxygen via hemoglobin

**Use** Prevention and treatment of iron deficiency anemias

**USUAL DOSAGE Oral (dose expressed in terms of elemental iron):**
Children:
Severe iron deficiency anemia: 4-6 mg Fe/kg/day in 3 divided doses
Mild to moderate iron deficiency anemia: 3 mg Fe/kg/day in 1-2 divided doses
Prophylaxis: 1-2 mg Fe/kg/day
Adults:
Iron deficiency: 60-100 mg twice daily up to 60 mg 2 times/day
Prophylaxis: 60-100 mg/day
To avoid GI upset, start with a single daily dose and increase by 1 tablet/day each week or as tolerated until desired daily dose is achieved
Elderly: 200 mg 3-4 times/day

**Dosage Forms** Amount of elemental iron is listed in brackets **Cap, controlled release (Span-FF®):** 325 mg [106 mg]; **Drops (Feostat®):** 45 mg/0.6 mL [15 mg/0.6 mL] (60 mL); **Susp, oral (Feostat®):** 100 mg/5 mL [33 mg/5 mL] (240 mL); **Tab:** 325 mg [106 mg], Chewable (chocolate flavor) (Feostat®): 100 mg [33 mg], Femiron®: 63 mg [20 mg],
Fumerin®: 195 mg [64 mg] Fumasorb®, Ircon®: 200 mg [66 mg], Hemocyte®: 324 mg [106 mg], Nephro-Fer™: 350 mg [115 mg], Timed release (Ferro-Sequels®): Ferrous fumarate 150 mg [50 mg] and docusate sodium 100 mg

**Contraindications** Hemochromatosis, hemolytic anemia, known hypersensitivity to iron salts

**Warnings/Precautions** Avoid in patients with peptic ulcer, enteritis, or ulcerative colitis. Administration of iron for >6 months should be avoided except in patients with continuous bleeding or menorrhagia. Anemia in the elderly is often caused by "anemia of chronic disease" or associated with inflammation rather than blood loss. Iron stores are usually normal or increased, with a serum ferritin >50 ng/mL and a decreased total iron binding capacity. Hence, the "anemia of chronic disease" is not secondary to iron deficiency but the inability of the reticuloendothelial system to reclaim available iron stores.

**Pregnancy Risk Factor** A

**Adverse Reactions**
>10%: Gastrointestinal: Stomach cramping, constipation, nausea, vomiting, dark stools
1% to 10%:
Gastrointestinal: Heartburn, diarrhea, staining of teeth
Genitourinary: Discoloration of urine
<1%: Contact irritation

**Drug Interactions**
Decreased effect: Absorption of oral preparation of iron and tetracyclines are decreased when both of these drugs are given together; concurrent administration of antacids may decrease iron absorption; iron may decrease absorption of penicillamine when given at the same time; response to iron therapy may be delayed in patients receiving chloramphenicol
Milk may decrease absorption of iron
Increased effect: Current administration ≥200 mg vitamin C per 30 mg elemental iron increases absorption of oral iron

**Special PA Issues**
**Patient Education:** May color stool black, take between meals for maximum absorption; may take with food if GI upset occurs, do not take with milk or antacids; keep out of reach of children
**Reference Range:**
Serum iron:
Male: 75-175 µg/dL (SI: 13.4-31.3 µmol/L)
Female: 65-165 µg/dL (SI: 11.6-29.5 µmol/L)
Total iron binding capacity: 230-430 µg/dL
Transferrin: 204-360 mg/dL
Percent transferrin saturation: 20% to 50%
Iron levels >300 µg/dL can be considered toxic, should be treated as an overdose

## Ferrous Gluconate (FER us GLOO koe nate)

**Pharmacologic Class** Iron Salt

**U.S. Brand Names** Fergon® [OTC]; Ferralet® [OTC]; Simron® [OTC]

**Mechanism of Action** Replaces iron found in hemoglobin, myoglobin, and enzymes; allows the transportation of oxygen via hemoglobin

**Use** Prevention and treatment of iron deficiency anemias

**USUAL DOSAGE** Oral **(dose expressed in terms of elemental iron):**

Children:

Severe iron deficiency anemia: 4-6 mg Fe/kg/day in 3 divided doses

Mild to moderate iron deficiency anemia: 3 mg Fe/kg/day in 1-2 divided doses

Prophylaxis: 1-2 mg Fe/kg/day

Adults:

Iron deficiency: 60 mg twice daily up to 60 mg 4 times/day

Prophylaxis: 60 mg/day

**Dosage Forms** Amount of elemental iron is listed in brackets **Cap, soft gelatin (Simron®):** 86 mg [10 mg]; **Elix (Fergon®):** 300 mg/5 mL [34 mg/5 mL] with alcohol 7% (480 mL); **Tab:** 300 mg [34 mg]; 325 mg [38 mg], Fergon®, Ferralet®: 320 mg [37 mg], Sustained release (Ferralet® Slow Release): 320 mg [37 mg]

**Contraindications** Hemochromatosis, hemolytic anemia; known hypersensitivity to iron salts

**Warnings/Precautions** Administration of iron for >6 months should be avoided except in patients with continued bleeding, menorrhagia, or repeated pregnancies; avoid in patients with peptic ulcer, enteritis, or ulcerative colitis. Anemia in the elderly is often caused by "anemia of chronic disease" or associated with inflammation rather than blood loss. Iron stores are usually normal or increased, with a serum ferritin >50 ng/mL and a decreased total iron binding capacity. Hence, the "anemia of chronic disease" is not secondary to iron deficiency but the inability of the reticuloendothelial system to reclaim available iron stores.

**Pregnancy Risk Factor** A

**Adverse Reactions**

>10%: Gastrointestinal: Stomach cramping, constipation, nausea, vomiting, dark stools

1% to 10%:

Gastrointestinal: Heartburn, diarrhea, staining of teeth

Genitourinary: Discoloration of urine

<1%: Contact irritation

**Drug Interactions** Absorption of oral preparation of iron and tetracyclines is decreased when both of these drugs are given together; concurrent administration of antacids may decrease iron absorption; iron may decrease absorption of penicillamine when given at the same time. Response to iron therapy may be delayed in patients receiving chloramphenicol. Concurrent administration ≥200 mg vitamin C/30 mg elemental iron increases absorption of oral iron; milk may decrease absorption of iron.

**Special PA Issues**

**Patient Education:** May color stool black, take between meals for maximum absorption; may take with food if GI upset occurs, do not take with milk or antacids; keep out of reach of children

**Reference Range:** Therapeutic: Male: 75-175 µg/dL (SI: 13.4-31.3 µmol/L); Female: 65-165 µg/dL (SI: 11.6-29.5 µmol/L); serum iron level >300 µg/dL usually requires treatment of overdose due to severe toxicity

## Ferrous Sulfate (FER us SUL fate)

**Pharmacologic Class** Iron Salt

**U.S. Brand Names** Feosol® [OTC]; Feratab® [OTC]; Fer-Iron® [OTC]; Fero-Gradumet® [OTC]; Ferospace® [OTC]; Ferralyn® Lanacaps® [OTC]; Ferra-TD® [OTC]; Mol-Iron® [OTC]; Slow FE® [OTC]

**Mechanism of Action** Replaces iron, found in hemoglobin, myoglobin, and other enzymes; allows the transportation of oxygen via hemoglobin

**Use** Prevention and treatment of iron deficiency anemias

**USUAL DOSAGE** Oral:

Children **(dose expressed in terms of elemental iron):**

Severe iron deficiency anemia: 4-6 mg Fe/kg/day in 3 divided doses

Mild to moderate iron deficiency anemia: 3 mg Fe/kg/day in 1-2 divided doses

Prophylaxis: 1-2 mg Fe/kg/day up to a maximum of 15 mg/day

Adults **(dose expressed in terms of ferrous sulfate):**

Iron deficiency: 300 mg twice daily up to 300 mg 4 times/day or 250 mg (extended release) 1-2 times/day

Prophylaxis: 300 mg/day

**Dosage Forms** Amount of elemental iron is listed in brackets **Cap:** Exsiccated, timed release (Feosol®): 159 mg [50 mg], Exsiccated, timed release (Ferralyn® Lanacaps®, Ferra-TD®): 250 mg [50 mg], Ferospace®: 250 mg [50 mg]; **Drops, oral:** Fer-In-Sol®: 75 mg/0.6 mL [15 mg/0.6 mL] (50 mL), Fer-Iron®: 125 mg/mL [25 mg/mL] (50 mL); **Elix (Feosol®):** 220 mg/5 mL [44 mg/5 mL] with alcohol 5% (473 mL, 4000 mL); **Syr (Fer-In-Sol®):** 90 mg/5 mL [18 mg/5 mL] with alcohol 5% (480 mL); **Tab:** 324 mg [65 mg], Exsiccated (Feosol®) 200 mg (Continued)

## Ferrous Sulfate *(Continued)*

[65 mg], Exsiccated, timed release (Slow FE®): 160 mg [50 mg], Feratab®: 300 mg [60 mg], Mol-Iron®: 195 mg [39 mg], Timed release (Fero-Gradumet®): 525 mg [105 mg]

**Contraindications** Hemochromatosis, hemolytic anemia; known hypersensitivity to iron salts

**Warnings/Precautions** Administration of iron for >6 months should be avoided except in patients with continued bleeding, menorrhagia, or repeated pregnancies; avoid in patients with peptic ulcer, enteritis, or ulcerative colitis. Anemia in the elderly is often caused by "anemia of chronic disease" or associated with inflammation rather than blood loss. Iron stores are usually normal or increased, with a serum ferritin >50 ng/mL and a decreased total iron binding capacity. Hence, the "anemia of chronic disease" is not secondary to iron deficiency but the inability of the reticuloendothelial system to reclaim available iron stores.

**Pregnancy Risk Factor** A

**Adverse Reactions**

>10%: Gastrointestinal: GI irritation, epigastric pain, nausea, dark stool, vomiting, stomach cramping, constipation

1% to 10%:

Gastrointestinal: Heartburn, diarrhea

Genitourinary: Discoloration of urine

Miscellaneous: Liquid preparations may temporarily stain the teeth

<1%: Contact irritation

**Drug Interactions**

Decreased effect: Absorption of oral preparation of iron and tetracyclines are decreased when both of these drugs are given together; concurrent administration of antacids may decrease iron absorption; iron may decrease absorption of penicillamine when given at the same time; response to iron therapy may be delayed in patients receiving chloramphenicol; milk may decrease absorption of iron

Increased effect: Concurrent administration ≥200 mg vitamin C per 30 mg elemental Fe increases absorption of oral iron

**Special PA Issues**

**Patient Education:** May color stool black, take between meals for maximum absorption; may take with food if GI upset occurs, do not take with milk or antacids; keep out of reach of children

**Reference Range:**

Serum iron:

Male: 75-175 µg/dL (SI: 13.4-31.3 µmol/L)

Female: 65-165 µg/dL (SI: 11.6-29.5 µmol/L)

Total iron binding capacity: 230-430 µg/dL

Transferrin: 204-360 mg/dL

Percent transferrin saturation: 20% to 50%

## Ferrous Sulfate, Ascorbic Acid, Vitamin B-Complex, and Folic Acid

(FER us SUL fate, a SKOR bik AS id, VYE ta min bee KOM pleks, & FOE lik AS id)

**Pharmacologic Class** Vitamin

**U.S. Brand Names** Iberet-Folic-500®

**Dosage Forms Tab, controlled release:** Ferrous sulfate: 105 mg, Ascorbic acid: 500 mg, $B_1$: 6 mg, $B_2$: 6 mg, $B_3$: 30 mg, $B_5$: 10 mg, $B_6$: 5 mg, $B_{12}$: 25 mcg, Folic acid: 800 mcg

♦ **Fertinex™** *see Follitropins on page 397*

♦ **FeSO$_4$** *see Ferrous Sulfate on previous page*

♦ **Feverall™ [OTC]** *see Acetaminophen on page 21*

♦ **Feverall™ Sprinkle Caps [OTC]** *see Acetaminophen on page 21*

♦ **Fever Due to Drugs** *see Chart on page 1129*

## Feverfew

**Mechanism of Action** Active ingredient is parthenolide (~0.2% concentration), a sesquiterpene which is a serotonin antagonist; also, the plant may be an inhibitor of prostaglandin synthesis and platelet aggregation; has spasmolytic effect on cerebral blood vessels; other anti-inflammatory effects, antimicrobial, antifungal

**Use** Prophylaxis and treatment of migraine headaches; used to treat menstrual complaints and fever

**USUAL DOSAGE** 125 mg of a preparation standardized to 0.2% parthenolide (250 mcg) once or twice daily

**Contraindications** Pregnancy, breast-feeding; children <2 years of age; allergies to feverfew and other members of the Asteraceae, daisy, ragweed, chamomile

**Warnings/Precautions** Use with caution in patients taking medications with serotonergic properties

**Adverse Reactions**

>10%: Gastrointestinal: Mouth ulcerations

<10%:

Dermatologic: Contact dermatitis

Gastrointestinal: Swelling of tongue, lips, abdominal pain, nausea, vomiting, loss of taste

Post-feverfew syndrome: Nervousness, insomnia, stiff joints, headache

**Drug Interactions** Use with caution in patients taking aspirin or anticoagulants due to increased potential for bleeding

# Fexofenadine (feks oh FEN a deen)

**Pharmacologic Class** Antihistamine

**U.S. Brand Names** Allegra®

**Mechanism of Action** Fexofenadine is an active metabolite of terfenadine and like terfenadine it competes with histamine for $H_1$-receptor sites on effector cells in the gastrointestinal tract, blood vessels and respiratory tract; it appears that fexofenadine does not cross the blood brain barrier to any appreciable degree, resulting in a reduced potential for sedation

**Use** Nonsedating antihistamine indicated for the relief of seasonal allergic rhinitis

**USUAL DOSAGE** Oral:

Children <12 years: Not recommended

Children ≥12 years and Adults: 1 capsule (60 mg) twice daily

**Dosing adjustment in renal impairment:** Recommended initial doses of 60 mg once daily

**Dosage Forms Cap, as hydrochloride:** 60 mg

**Contraindications** Individuals demonstrating hypersensitivity to fexofenadine or any components of its formulation

**Warnings/Precautions** Safety and effectiveness in pediatric patients <12 years of age has not been established. Fexofenadine is classified in FDA pregnancy category C and no data is yet available evaluating its use in breast-feeding women.

**Pregnancy Risk Factor** C

**Adverse Reactions** 1% to 10%:

Central nervous system: Drowsiness (1.3%), fatigue (1.3%)

Endocrine & metabolic: Dysmenorrhea (1.5%)

Gastrointestinal: Nausea (1.5%), dyspepsia (1.3%)

Miscellaneous: Viral infection (2.5%)

**Drug Interactions** CYP3A3/4 enzyme substrate

Fexofenadine levels have increased with erythromycin (82% higher) and with ketoconazole (135% higher); this has not been associated with any increased incidence of side effects

In two separate studies, fexofenadine 120 mg twice daily (high doses) was coadministered with standard doses of erythromycin or ketoconazole to healthy volunteers and although fexofenadine peak plasma concentrations increased, no differences in adverse events or $QT_c$ intervals were observed. **It remains unknown if a similar interaction occurs with other azole antifungal agents (eg, itraconazole) or other macrolide antibiotics (eg, clarithromycin).**

**Onset** 1 hour

**Duration** Antihistaminic effect: At least 12 hours

**Half-Life** 14.4 hours

**Special PA Issues**

**Patient Education:** Take as directed; do not exceed recommended dose. Store at room temperature in a dry place. Avoid use of other depressants, alcohol, or sleep-inducing medications unless approved by prescriber. You may experience mild drowsiness or dizziness (use caution when driving or engaging in hazardous activity until response to medication is known); or nausea (frequent small meals, frequent mouth care, chewing gum, or sucking hard candy may help). Report persistent sedation or drowsiness, menstrual irregularities, or lack of improvement or worsening or condition.

**Monitoring Parameters:** Relief of symptoms

# Fexofenadine and Pseudoephedrine

(feks oh FEN a deen & soo doe e FED rin)

**Pharmacologic Class** Antihistamine/Decongestant Combination

**U.S. Brand Names** Allegra-D™

**Dosage Forms Tab, extended release:** Fexofenadine hydrochloride 60 mg and pseudoephedrine hydrochloride 120 mg

♦ **Fexofenadine Hydrochloride** see Fexofenadine on this page

♦ **Fiberall® Powder [OTC]** see Psyllium on page 781

♦ **Fiberall® Wafer [OTC]** see Psyllium on page 781

♦ **Fibrepur®** see Psyllium on page 781

# Fibrinolysin and Desoxyribonuclease

(fye brin oh LYE sin & des oks i rye boe NOO klee ase)

**Pharmacologic Class** Enzyme

**U.S. Brand Names** Elase-Chloromycetin® Topical; Elase® Topical

**Dosage Forms Oint, top:** Elase®: Fibrinolysin 1 unit and desoxyribonuclease 666.6 units per g (10 g, 30 g), Elase-Chloromycetin®: Fibrinolysin 1 unit and desoxyribonuclease 666.6 (Continued)

## Fibrinolysin and Desoxyribonuclease *(Continued)*

units per g with chloramphenicol 10 mg per g (10 g, 30 g); **Powder, dry:** Fibrinolysin 25 units and desoxyribonuclease 15,000 units per 30 g

## Filgrastim *(fil GRA stim)*

**Pharmacologic Class** Colony Stimulating Factor

**U.S. Brand Names** Neupogen® Injection

**Mechanism of Action** Simulates the production, maturation, and activation of neutrophils, G-CSF activates neutrophils to increase both their migration and cytotoxicity

**Use**

Patients with nonmyeloic malignancies receiving myelosuppressive anticancer drugs associated with a significant incidence of neutropenia (FDA-approved indication)

Cancer patients receiving bone marrow transplant (BMT) (FDA-approved indication)

Patients undergoing peripheral blood progenitor cell (PBPC) collection

Patients with severe chronic neutropenia (SCN) (FDA-approved indication)

Chronic administration in symptomatic patients with congenital neutropenia, cyclic neutropenia, or idiopathic neutropenic; filgrastim should not be started until the diagnosis of SCN is confirmed, as it may interfere with diagnostic efforts

Safety and efficacy of G-CSF given simultaneously with cytotoxic chemotherapy have not been established; concurrent treatment may increase myelosuppression; G-CSF should be avoided in patients receiving concomitant chemotherapy and radiation therapy

**USUAL DOSAGE** Children and Adults:

**Dosage should be based on actual body weight** (even in morbidly obese patients)

Existing clinical data suggest that starting G-CSF between 24 and 72 hours subsequent to chemotherapy may provide optimal neutrophil recovery; continue therapy until the occurrence of an absolute neutrophil count of 10,000 µL after the neutrophil nadir

**The available data suggest that rounding the dose to the nearest vial size may enhance patient convenience and reduce costs without clinical detriment**

Neonates: 5-10 mcg/kg/day once daily for 3-5 days has been administered to neutropenic neonates with sepsis; there was a rapid and significant increase in peripheral neutrophil counts and the neutrophil storage pool

Children and Adults:

**Myelosuppressive chemotherapy** S.C. or I.V. infusion: 5 mcg/kg/day

Doses may be increased in increments of 5 mcg/kg for each chemotherapy cycle, according to the duration and severity of the absolute neutrophil count (ANC) nadir

Bone marrow transplant patients: 5-10 mcg/kg/day as an I.V. infusion of 4 or 24 hours or as continuous 24-hour S.C. infusion; administer first dose at least 24 hours after cytotoxic chemotherapy and at least 24 hours after bone marrow infusion; if ANC decreases <1000/mm³ during the 5 mcg/kg/day dose, increase filgrastim to 10 mcg/kg/day and follow the steps in the table

### Filgrastim Dose Based on Neutrophil Response

| Absolute Neutrophil Count | Filgrastim Dose Adjustment |
|---|---|
| When ANC >1000/mm³ for 3 consecutive days | Reduce to 5 mcg/kg/day |
| If ANC remains >1000/mm³ for 3 more consecutive days | Discontinue filgrastim |
| If ANC decreases to <1000/mm³ | Resume at 5 mcg/kg/day |

If ANC decreases <1000/mm³ during the 5 mcg/kg/day dose, increase filgrastim to 10 mcg/kg/day and follow the above steps in the table.

**Peripheral blood progenitor cell (PBPC) collection:** 10 mcg/kg/day either S.C. or a bolus or continuous I.V. infusion. It is recommended that G-CSF be given for at least 4 days before the first leukapheresis procedure and continued until the last leukapheresis; although the optimal duration of administration and leukapheresis schedule have not been established, administration of G-CSF for 6-7 days with leukaphereses on days 5,6 and 7 was found to be safe and effective; neutrophil counts should be monitored after 4 days of G-CSF, and G-CSF dose-modification should be considered for those patients who develop a white blood cell count >100,000/mm³

**Severe chronic neutropenia:** S.C.:

Congenital neutropenia: 6 mcg/kg/dose twice daily

Idiopathic/cyclic neutropenia: 5 mcg/kg single dose daily

Chronic daily administration is required to maintain clinical benefit; adjust dose based on the patients' clinical course as well as ANC; in phase III studies, the target ANC was 1500-10,000/mm³. Reduce the dose if the ANC is persistently >10,000/mm³

Premature discontinuation of G-CSF therapy prior to the time of recovery from the expected neutrophil is generally not recommended; a transient increase in neutrophil counts is typically seen 1-2 days after initiation of therapy

Hemodialysis: Supplemental dose is not necessary

Peritoneal dialysis: Supplemental dose is not necessary

**Dosage Forms Inj, preservative free:** 300 mcg/mL (1 mL, 1.6 mL)

**Contraindications** Patients with known hypersensitivity to *E. coli*-derived proteins or G-CSF

**Warnings/Precautions** Complete blood count and platelet count should be obtained prior to chemotherapy. Do not use G-CSF in the period 12-24 hours before to 24 hours after administration of cytotoxic chemotherapy because of the potential sensitivity of rapidly dividing myeloid cells to cytotoxic chemotherapy. Precaution should be exercised in the usage of G-CSF in any malignancy with myeloid characteristics. G-CSF can potentially act as a growth factor for any tumor type, particularly myeloid malignancies. Tumors of nonhematopoietic origin may have surface receptors for G-CSF.

Allergic-type reactions have occurred in patients receiving G-CSF with first or later doses. Reactions tended to occur more frequently with intravenous administration and within 30 minutes of infusion. Most cases resolved rapidly with antihistamines, steroids, bronchodilators, and/or epinephrine. Symptoms recurred in >50% of patients on rechallenge.

**Pregnancy Risk Factor** C

**Adverse Reactions** Effects are generally mild and dose related
>10%:
  Central nervous system: Neutropenic fever, fever
  Dermatologic: Alopecia
  Gastrointestinal: Nausea, vomiting, diarrhea, mucositis,
    Splenomegaly: This occurs more commonly in patients with cyclic neutropenia/congenital agranulocytosis who received S.C. injections for a prolonged (>14 days) period of time; ~33% of these patients experience subclinical splenomegaly (detected by MRI or CT scan); ~3% of these patients experience clinical splenomegaly
  Neuromuscular & skeletal: Medullary bone pain (24% incidence): This occurs most commonly in lower back pain, posterior iliac crest, and sternum and is controlled with non-narcotic analgesics
1% to 10%:
  Cardiovascular: Chest pain, fluid retention
  Central nervous system: Headache
  Dermatologic: Skin rash
  Gastrointestinal: Anorexia, stomatitis, constipation
  Hematologic: Leukocytosis
  Local: Pain at injection site
  Neuromuscular & skeletal: Weakness
  Respiratory: Dyspnea, cough, sore throat
<1%: Transient supraventricular arrhythmia, pericarditis, thrombophlebitis, anaphylactic reaction

**Drug Interactions** Drugs which may potentiate the release of neutrophils (eg, lithium) should be used with caution

**Onset** Rapid elevation in neutrophil counts within the first 24 hours, reaching a plateau in 3-5 days

**Duration** ANC decreases by 50% within 2 days after discontinuing G-CSF; white counts return to the normal range in 4-7 days

**Half-Life** 1.8-3.5 hours

**Special PA Issues**
  **Patient Education:** Follow directions for proper storage and administration of S.C. medication. Never reuse syringes or needles. You may experience bone pain (request analgesic); nausea or vomiting (small frequent meals may help); hair loss (reversible); or sore mouth (frequent mouth care with soft toothbrush or cotton swab may help). Report unusual fever or chills; unhealed sores; severe bone pain; pain, redness, or swelling at injection site; unusual swelling of extremities or difficulty breathing; or chest pain and palpitations.
  **Monitoring Parameters:** Complete blood cell count and platelet count should be obtained twice weekly after chemotherapy or three times weekly after transplant. Leukocytosis (white blood cell counts of ≥100,000/mm³) has been observed in ~2% of patients receiving G-CSF at doses above 5 mcg/kg/day. Monitor platelets and hematocrit regularly. Monitor patients with pre-existing cardiac conditions closely as cardiac events (myocardial infarctions, arrhythmias) have been reported in premarketing clinical studies.
  **Reference Range:** No clinical benefit seen with ANC >10,000/mm³

♦ Filibon® [OTC] *see* Vitamins, Multiple *on page 964*

# Finasteride (fi NAS teer ide)
**Pharmacologic Class** Antiandrogen
**U.S. Brand Names** Propecia®; Proscar®
**Mechanism of Action** Finasteride is a 4-azo analog of testosterone and is a competitive inhibitor of both tissue and hepatic 5-alpha reductase. This results in inhibition of the conversion of testosterone to dihydrotestosterone and markedly suppresses serum dihydrotestosterone levels; depending on dose and duration, serum testosterone concentrations may or may not increase. Testosterone-dependent processes such as fertility, muscle strength, potency, and libido are not affected by finasteride.
**Use** Early data indicate that finasteride is useful in the treatment of symptomatic benign prostatic hyperplasia (BPH); male pattern baldness
(Continued)

## Finasteride *(Continued)*

**Unlabeled use:** Adjuvant monotherapy after radical prostatectomy in the treatment of prostatic cancer

**USUAL DOSAGE** Adults: Male:

Benign prostatic hyperplasia: Oral: 5 mg/day as a single dose; clinical responses occur within 12 weeks to 6 months of initiation of therapy; long-term administration is recommended for maximal response

Male pattern baldness: 1 mg daily

**Dosing adjustment in renal impairment:** No dosage adjustment is necessary

**Dosing adjustment in hepatic impairment:** Use with caution in patients with liver function abnormalities because finasteride is metabolized extensively in the liver

**Dosage Forms** Tab, film coated: Propecia®: 1 mg, Proscar®: 5 mg

**Contraindications** History of hypersensitivity to drug, pregnancy, lactation, children

**Warnings/Precautions** A minimum of 6 months of treatment may be necessary to determine whether an individual will respond to finasteride. Use with caution in those patients with liver function abnormalities. Carefully monitor patients with a large residual urinary volume or severely diminished urinary flow for obstructive uropathy. These patients may not be candidates for finasteride therapy.

**Pregnancy Risk Factor** X

**Adverse Reactions** 1% to 10%:

Endocrine & metabolic: Decreased libido

Genitourinary: <4% incidence of impotence, decreased volume of ejaculate

**Drug Interactions** CYP3A3/4 enzyme substrate

**Onset** Onset of clinical effect: Within 12 weeks to 6 months of ongoing therapy

**Duration**

After a single oral dose as small as 0.5 mg: 65% depression of plasma dihydrotestosterone levels persists 5-7 days.

After 6 months of treatment with 5 mg/day: Circulating dihydrotestosterone levels are reduced to castrate levels without significant effects on circulating testosterone. Levels return to normal within 14 days of discontinuation of treatment.

**Half-Life**

Half-life, serum: Parent drug: ~5-17 hours (mean: 1.9 fasting, 4.2 with breakfast)

Half-life: Adults: 6 hours (3-16); Elderly: 8 hours

**Special PA Issues**

**Patient Education:** Take on an empty stomach with fluids. Your may experience decreased libido or impotence during therapy. If no increase in urinary volume and decreased urgency and micturition occurs, notify prescriber.

**Dietary Considerations:** Food: Administration with food may delay the rate and reduce the extent of oral absorption

**Monitoring Parameters:** Objective and subjective signs of relief of benign prostatic hyperplasia, including improvement in urinary flow, reduction in symptoms of urgency, and relief of difficulty in micturition

- ♦ **Fiorgen PF®** *see* Butalbital Compound *on page 131*
- ♦ **Fioricet®** *see* Butalbital Compound *on page 131*
- ♦ **Fiorinal®** *see* Butalbital Compound *on page 131*
- ♦ **Fisalamine** *see* Mesalamine *on page 571*
- ♦ **FK506** *see* Tacrolimus *on page 869*
- ♦ **Flagyl ER® Oral** *see* Metronidazole *on page 601*
- ♦ **Flagyl® Oral** *see* Metronidazole *on page 601*
- ♦ **Flamazine®** *see* Silver Sulfadiazine *on page 835*
- ♦ **Flarex®** *see* Fluorometholone *on page 384*
- ♦ **Flavorcee® [OTC]** *see* Ascorbic Acid *on page 79*

## Flavoxate *(fla VOKS ate)*

**Pharmacologic Class** Antispasmodic Agent, Urinary

**U.S. Brand Names** Urispas®

**Mechanism of Action** Synthetic antispasmotic with similar actions to that of propantheline; it exerts a direct relaxant effect on smooth muscles via phosphodiesterase inhibition, providing relief to a variety of smooth muscle spasms; it is especially useful for the treatment of bladder spasticity, whereby it produces an increase in urinary capacity

**Use** Antispasmodic to provide symptomatic relief of dysuria, nocturia, suprapubic pain, urgency, and incontinence due to detrusor instability and hyper-reflexia in elderly with cystitis, urethritis, urethrocystitis, urethrotrigonitis, and prostatitis

**USUAL DOSAGE** Children >12 years and Adults: Oral: 100-200 mg 3-4 times/day; reduce the dose when symptoms improve

**Dosage Forms** Tab, film coated, as hydrochloride: 100 mg

**Contraindications** Pyloric or duodenal obstruction, GI hemorrhage, GI obstruction; ileus; achalasia; obstructive uropathies of lower urinary tract (BPH)

**Warnings/Precautions** May cause drowsiness, vertigo, and ocular disturbances; administer cautiously in patients with suspected glaucoma

**Pregnancy Risk Factor** B

**Adverse Reactions**

>10%:

Central nervous system: Drowsiness

Gastrointestinal: Xerostomia, dry throat

1% to 10%:

Cardiovascular: Tachycardia, palpitations,

Central nervous system: Nervousness, fatigue, vertigo, headache, hyperpyrexia

Gastrointestinal: Constipation, nausea, vomiting

<1%: Confusion (especially in the elderly), rash, leukopenia, increased intraocular pressure

**Onset** 55-60 minutes

**Special PA Issues**

**Patient Education:** Take exactly as directed, with water, preferably on an empty stomach (1 hour before or 2 hours after meals). Do not use alcohol or OTC medications without consulting prescriber. You may experience mild drowsiness, nervousness, or dizziness (use caution when driving or engaging in tasks that require alertness until response to medication is known); nausea, vomiting, dry mouth (small frequent meals, frequent oral care, chewing gum, or sucking hard candy may help); decreased ability to perspire (avoid extremes of heat); constipation (increased exercise or dietary fluid and fiber may help). Report vision changes (blurred vision); rapid heartbeat; or unresolved nausea, vomiting, or constipation.

**Monitoring Parameters:** Monitor I & O closely

♦ **Flavoxate Hydrochloride** *see* Flavoxate *on previous page*

# Flecainide (fle KAY nide)

**Pharmacologic Class** Antiarrhythmic Agent, Class I-C

**U.S. Brand Names** Tambocor™

**Mechanism of Action** Class Ic antiarrhythmic; slows conduction in cardiac tissue by altering transport of ions across cell membranes; causes slight prolongation of refractory periods; decreases the rate of rise of the action potential without affecting its duration; increases electrical stimulation threshold of ventricle, HIS-Purkinje system; possesses local anesthetic and moderate negative inotropic effects

**Use** Prevention and suppression of documented life-threatening ventricular arrhythmias (ie, sustained ventricular tachycardia); controlling symptomatic, disabling supravent.∪ular tachycardias in patients without structural heart disease in whom other agents fail

**USUAL DOSAGE** Oral:

Children:

Initial: 3 mg/kg/day or 50-100 mg/m²/day in 3 divided doses

Usual: 3-6 mg/kg/day or 100-150 mg/m²/day in 3 divided doses; up to 11 mg/kg/day or 200 mg/m²/day for uncontrolled patients with subtherapeutic levels

Adults:

Life-threatening ventricular arrhythmias:

Initial: 100 mg every 12 hours

Increase by 50-100 mg/day (given in 2 doses/day) every 4 days; maximum: 400 mg/day

Use of higher initial doses and more rapid dosage adjustments have resulted in an increased incidence of proarrhythmic events and congestive heart failure, particularly during the first few days. Do not use a loading dose. Use very cautiously in patients with history of congestive heart failure or myocardial infarction.

Prevention of paroxysmal supraventricular arrhythmias in patients with disabling symptoms but no structural heart disease:

Initial: 50 mg every 12 hours

Increase by 50 mg twice daily at 4-day intervals; maximum: 300 mg/day

**Dosing adjustment in severe renal impairment:** Cl_cr <35 mL/minute: Decrease initial dose to 50 mg every 12 hours; increase doses at intervals >4 days monitoring plasma levels closely

Dialysis: Not dialyzable (0% to 5%) via hemo- or peritoneal dialysis; no supplemental dose necessary

**Dosing adjustment/comments in hepatic impairment:** Monitoring of plasma levels is recommended because of significantly increased half-life

When transferring from another antiarrhythmic agent, allow for 2-4 half-lives of the agent to pass before initiating flecainide therapy

**Dosage Forms Tab, as acetate:** 50 mg, 100 mg, 150 mg

**Contraindications** Pre-existing second or third degree A-V block; right bundle-branch block associated with left hemiblock (bifascicular block) or trifascicular block; cardiogenic shock, myocardial depression; known hypersensitivity to the drug; concurrent use of ritonavir

**Warnings/Precautions** Pre-existing sinus node dysfunction, sick-sinus syndrome, history of congestive heart failure or myocardial dysfunction; increases in P-R interval ≥300 MS, QRS ≥180 MS, QT_c interval increases, and/or new bundle-branch block; patients with pacemakers, renal impairment, and/or hepatic impairment.

(Continued)

## Flecainide *(Continued)*

The manufacturer and FDA recommend that this drug be reserved for life-threatening ventricular arrhythmias unresponsive to conventional therapy. Its use for symptomatic nonsustained ventricular tachycardia, frequent premature ventricular complexes (PVCs), uniform and multiform PVCs and/or coupled PVCs is no longer recommended. Flecainide can worsen or cause arrhythmias with an associated risk of death. Proarrhythmic effects range from an increased number of PVCs to more severe ventricular tachycardias (eg, tachycardias that are more sustained or more resistant to conversion to sinus rhythm).

**Pregnancy Risk Factor** C

**Adverse Reactions**

>10%:

Central nervous system: Dizziness (19%)

Ocular: Visual disturbances (16%)

Respiratory: Dyspnea (~10%)

1% to 10%:

Cardiovascular: Palpitations (6%), chest pain (5%), edema (3.5%), tachycardia (1% to 3%)

Central nervous system: Headache (4%), fatigue (8%), fever (1% to 3%), malaise (1% to 3%)

Dermatologic: Rash (1% to 3%)

Gastrointestinal: Nausea (9%), constipation, abdominal pain (3%), anorexia (1% to 3%)

Neuromuscular & skeletal: Tremor (5%), weakness (5%)

Ocular: Diplopia (1% to 3%)

<1%: Bradycardia, heart block, increased P-R, QRS duration, worsening ventricular arrhythmias, congestive heart failure, flushing, A-V block, angina, hyper/hypotension, nervousness, hypoesthesia, ataxia, vertigo, somnolence, alopecia, flatulence, xerostomia, blood dyscrasias, possible hepatic dysfunction, paresthesia, eye pain, photophobia, tinnitus

**Drug Interactions** CYP2D6 enzyme substrate

Increased toxicity:

Flecainide increases the bioavailability/toxicity of propranolol

Digoxin, amiodarone increase plasma concentrations of flecainide and may increase toxicity

Beta-adrenergic blockers, disopyramide, verapamil (possible additive negative inotropic effects)

Alkalinizing agents (high dose antacids, cimetidine, carbonic anhydrase inhibitors or sodium bicarbonate) may decrease flecainide clearance

Avoid use with ritonavir due to increased risk of flecainide toxicity, especially cardiotoxicity

Decreased toxicity: Smoking and acid urine (increases flecainide clearance)

**Half-Life** 7-22 hours, increased with congestive heart failure or renal dysfunction; End-stage renal disease: 19-26 hours

**Special PA Issues**

**Patient Education:** Take exactly as directed, around-the-clock. Do not discontinue without consulting prescriber. You will require frequent monitoring while taking this medication. You may experience lightheadedness, nervousness, dizziness, visual disturbances (use caution when driving or performing hazardous tasks); or nausea, vomiting, or loss of appetite (small frequent meals may help). Report palpitations, chest pain, excessively slow or rapid heartbeat; acute nervousness, headache, or fatigue; unusual weight gain; unusual cough; difficulty breathing; swelling of hands or ankles; or muscle tremor, numbness, or weakness.

**Monitoring Parameters:** EKG, blood pressure, pulse, periodic serum concentrations, especially in patients with renal or hepatic impairment

**Reference Range:** Therapeutic: 0.2-1 µg/mL; pediatric patients may respond at the lower end of the recommended therapeutic range

♦ **Flubenisolone** *see* Betamethasone *on page 111*

# Fluconazole (floo KOE na zole)

**Pharmacologic Class** Antifungal Agent, Oral; Antifungal Agent, Parenteral

**U.S. Brand Names** Diflucan®

**Mechanism of Action** Interferes with cytochrome P-450 activity, decreasing ergosterol synthesis (principal sterol in fungal cell membrane) and inhibiting cell membrane formation

**Use** Oral fluconazole should be used in persons able to tolerate oral medications; parenteral fluconazole should be reserved for patients who are both unable to take oral medications and are unable to tolerate amphotericin B (eg, due to hypersensitivity or renal insufficiency)

**Indications for use in adult patients:**
Oral or vaginal candidiasis unresponsive to nystatin or clotrimazole
Nonlife-threatening *Candida* infections (eg, cystitis, esophagitis)
Treatment of hepatosplenic candidiasis
Treatment of other *Candida* infections in persons unable to tolerate amphotericin B
Treatment of cryptococcal infections
Secondary prophylaxis for cryptococcal meningitis in persons with AIDS
Antifungal prophylaxis in allogeneic bone marrow transplant recipients

**USUAL DOSAGE** The daily dose of fluconazole is the same for oral and I.V. administration

Neonates: First 2 weeks of life, especially premature neonates: Same dose as older children every 72 hours
Children: See table for once daily dosing

### Fluconazole — Once-Daily Dosing (Children)

| Indication | Day 1 | Daily Therapy | Minimum Duration of Therapy |
|---|---|---|---|
| Oropharyngeal candidiasis | 6 mg/kg | 3 mg/kg | 14 d |
| Esophageal candidiasis | 6 mg/kg | 3-12 mg/kg | 21 d and for at least 2 wks following resolution of symptoms |
| Systemic candidiasis | — | 6-12 mg/kg | 28 d |
| Cryptococcal meningitis<br>relapse | 12 mg/kg<br>6 mg/kg | 6-12 mg/kg<br>6 mg/kg | 10-12 wk after CSF culture becomes negative |

Adults: Oral, I.V.: See table for once daily dosing.

### Fluconazole — Once-Daily Dosing (Adults)

| Indication | Day 1 | Daily Therapy | Minimum Duration of Therapy |
|---|---|---|---|
| Oropharyngeal candidiasis | 200 mg | 100 mg | 14 d |
| Esophageal candidiasis | 200 mg | 100 mg | 21 d and for at least 14 d following resolution of symptoms |
| Prevention of candidiasis in bone marrow transplant | 400 mg | 400 mg | 3 d before neutropenia, 7 d after neutrophils >1000 cells/mm³ |
| Candidiasis UTIs, peritonitis | Twice daily dose | 50-200 mg | |
| Systemic candidiasis | 400 mg | 200 mg | 28 d |
| Cryptococcal meningitis<br>acute<br>relapse | 400 mg<br>200 mg | 200 mg<br>200 mg | 10-12 wk after CSF culture becomes negative |
| Vaginal candidiasis | 150 mg | Single dose | |

**Dosing adjustment/interval in renal impairment:**
No adjustment for vaginal candidiasis single-dose therapy
For multiple dosing, administer usual load then adjust daily doses
$Cl_{cr}$ 11-50 mL/minute: Administer 50% of recommended dose or administer every 48 hours
Hemodialysis: One dose after each dialysis
Continuous arteriovenous or venovenous hemodiafiltration (CAVH) effects: Dose as for $Cl_{cr}$ 11-50 mL/minute

**Dosage Forms Inj:** 2 mg/mL (100 mL, 200 mL); **Powder for oral susp:** 10 mg/mL (35 mL), 40 mg/mL (35 mL); **Tab:** 50 mg, 100 mg, 150 mg, 200 mg

**Contraindications** Known hypersensitivity to fluconazole or other azoles; concomitant administration with terfenadine

**Warnings/Precautions** Should be used with caution in patients with renal and hepatic dysfunction or previous hepatotoxicity from other azole derivatives. Patients who develop
(Continued)

## Fluconazole *(Continued)*

abnormal liver function tests during fluconazole therapy should be monitored closely and discontinued if symptoms consistent with liver disease develop. **Should be used with caution in patients receiving cisapride or astemizole.**

**Pregnancy Risk Factor** C

**Adverse Reactions**

1% to 10%:

Central nervous system: Headache

Dermatologic: Rash

Gastrointestinal: Nausea, vomiting, abdominal pain, diarrhea

<1%: Pallor, dizziness, hypokalemia, increased AST/ALT, or alkaline phosphatase

**Drug Interactions** CYP2C9 enzyme inducer; CYP2C9, 2C18, and 2C19 enzyme inhibitor and CYP3A3/4 enzyme inhibitor (weak)

Decreased effect: Rifampin and cimetidine decrease concentrations of fluconazole; fluconazole may decrease the effect of oral contraceptives

Increased toxicity:

Coadministration with terfenadine is contraindicated; use with caution with cisapride and astemizole due to increased risk of significant cardiotoxicity

Hydrochlorothiazide may decrease fluconazole clearance

Fluconazole may also inhibit warfarin, phenytoin, cyclosporine, and theophylline, zidovudine, sulfonylureas, and warfarin clearance

**Half-Life** 25-30 hours with normal renal function

**Special PA Issues**

**Patient Education:** Take as directed. Take full course of medication as ordered. Do not discontinue without consulting prescriber. Practice good hygiene measures to prevent reinfection. Frequent blood tests may be required. You may experience nausea and vomiting (small, frequent meals may help), or headache. Report unresolved headache, rash, respiratory difficulty, increased salivation, or yellowing of skin or eyes, and changes in color of stool or urine.

**Monitoring Parameters:** Periodic liver function tests (AST, ALT, alkaline phosphatase) and renal function tests, potassium

## Flucytosine *(floo SYE toe seen)*

**Pharmacologic Class** Antifungal Agent, Oral

**U.S. Brand Names** Ancobon®

**Mechanism of Action** Penetrates fungal cells and is converted to fluorouracil which competes with uracil interfering with fungal RNA and protein synthesis

**Use** Adjunctive treatment of susceptible fungal infections (usually *Candida* or *Cryptococcus*); synergy with amphotericin B for certain fungal infections (*Cryptococcus* spp., *Candida* spp.

**USUAL DOSAGE** Children and Adults: Oral: 50-150 mg/kg/day in divided doses every 6 hours

**Dosing interval in renal impairment:** Use lower initial dose:

$Cl_{cr}$ >50 mL/minute: Administer every 12 hours

$Cl_{cr}$ 10-50 mL/minute: Administer every 16 hours

$Cl_{cr}$ <10 mL/minute: Administer every 24 hours

Hemodialysis: Dialyzable (50% to 100%); administer dose posthemodialysis

Peritoneal dialysis: Adults: Administer 0.5-1 g every 24 hours

Continuous arteriovenous or venovenous hemodiafiltration (CAVH) effects: Dose as for $Cl_{cr}$ 10-50 mL/minute

**Dosage Forms Cap:** 250 mg, 500 mg

**Contraindications** Hypersensitivity to flucytosine or any component

**Warnings/Precautions** Use with extreme caution in patients with renal impairment, bone marrow suppression, or in patients with AIDS; dosage modification required in patients with impaired renal function

**Pregnancy Risk Factor** C

**Adverse Reactions**

1% to 10%:

Dermatologic: Rash

Gastrointestinal: Abdominal pain, diarrhea, loss of appetite, nausea, vomiting

Hematologic: Anemia, leukopenia, thrombocytopenia

Hepatic: Hepatitis, jaundice

<1%: Cardiac arrest, confusion, hallucinations, dizziness, drowsiness, headache, parkinsonism, psychosis, ataxia, photosensitivity, temporary growth failure, hypoglycemia, hypokalemia, bone marrow suppression, elevated liver enzymes, paresthesia, hearing loss, respiratory arrest, anaphylaxis

**Drug Interactions** Increased effect/toxicity with concurrent amphotericin administration; cytosine may inactivate flucytosine activity

**Half-Life** 3-8 hours; Anuria: May be as long as 200 hours; End-stage renal disease: 75-200 hours

**Special PA Issues**

**Patient Education:** Take capsules one at a time over a few minutes with food to reduce GI upset. Take full course of medication as ordered. Do not discontinue without consulting prescriber. Practice good hygiene measures to prevent reinfection. Frequent blood tests may be required. You may experience nausea and vomiting (small, frequent meals may help). Report rash, respiratory difficulty, CNS changes (eg, confusion, hallucinations, ataxia, acute headache), yellowing of skin or eyes, and changes in color of stool or urine, unresolved diarrhea or anorexia, or unusual bleeding or fatigue and weakness.

**Monitoring Parameters:** Serum creatinine, BUN, alkaline phosphatase, AST, ALT, CBC; serum flucytosine concentrations

**Reference Range:**

Therapeutic: 25-100 µg/mL (SI: 195-775 µmol/L); levels should not exceed 100-120 µg/mL to avoid toxic bone marrow depressive effects

Trough: Draw just prior to dose administration

Peak: Draw 2 hours after an oral dose administration

# Fludrocortisone Acetate (floo droe KOR ti sone AS e tate)

**Pharmacologic Class** Corticosteroid, Oral

**U.S. Brand Names** Florinef® Acetate

**Mechanism of Action** Promotes increased reabsorption of sodium and loss of potassium from renal distal tubules

**Use** Partial replacement therapy for primary and secondary adrenocortical insufficiency in Addison's disease; treatment of salt-losing adrenogenital syndrome

**USUAL DOSAGE** Oral:

Infants and Children: 0.05-0.1 mg/day

Adults: 0.1-0.2 mg/day with ranges of 0.1 mg 3 times/week to 0.2 mg/day

Addison's disease: Initial: 0.1 mg/day; if transient hypertension develops, reduce the dose to 0.05 mg/day. Preferred administration with cortisone (10-37.5 mg/day) or hydrocortisone (10-30 mg/day).

Salt-losing adrenogenital syndrome: 0.1-0.2 mg/day

**Dosage Forms** Tab, as acetate: 0.1 mg

**Contraindications** Known hypersensitivity to fludrocortisone; systemic fungal infections

**Warnings/Precautions** Taper dose gradually when therapy is discontinued; use with caution with Addison's disease, sodium retention and potassium loss

**Pregnancy Risk Factor** C

**Adverse Reactions** 1% to 10%:

Cardiovascular: Hypertension, edema, congestive heart failure

Central nervous system: Convulsions, headache, dizziness

Dermatologic: Acne, rash, bruising

Endocrine & metabolic: Hypokalemic alkalosis, suppression of growth, hyperglycemia, HPA suppression

Gastrointestinal: Peptic ulcer

Neuromuscular & skeletal: Muscle weakness

Ocular: Cataracts

Miscellaneous: Diaphoresis

**Drug Interactions Decreased effect:**

Anticholinesterases effects are antagonized

Decreased corticosteroid effects by rifampin, barbiturates, and hydantoins

Decreased salicylate levels

**Half-Life** Plasma: 30-35 minutes; Biological: 18-36 hours

**Special PA Issues**

**Patient Education:** Take exactly as directed. Do not take more than prescribed dose and do not discontinue abruptly; consult prescriber. Take with or after meals. Take once-a-day dose with food in the morning. Limit intake of caffeine or stimulants. Maintain adequate nutrition; consult prescriber for possibility of special dietary recommendations. If diabetic, monitor serum glucose closely and notify prescriber of changes; this medication can alter hypoglycemic requirements. Notify prescriber if you are experiencing higher than normal levels of stress; medication may need adjustment. Periodic ophthalmic examinations will be necessary with long-term use. You will be susceptible to infection; avoid crowds or infected persons or persons with contagious diseases. You may experience insomnia or nervousness; use caution when driving or engaging in tasks requiring alertness until response to medication is known. Report weakness, change in menstrual pattern, vision changes, signs of hyperglycemia, signs of infection (eg, fever, chills, mouth sores, perianal itching, vaginal discharge), other persistent side effects, or worsening of condition.

**Monitoring Parameters:** Monitor blood pressure and signs of edema when patient is on chronic therapy; very potent mineralocorticoid with high glucocorticoid activity; monitor serum electrolytes, serum renin activity, and blood pressure; monitor for evidence of infection

**Related Information**

Corticosteroids *on page 1007*

♦ **Flumadine®** *see* Rimantadine *on page 807*

# Flumazenil (FLO may ze nil)

**Pharmacologic Class** Antidote

**U.S. Brand Names** Romazicon™ Injection

**Mechanism of Action** Antagonizes the effect of benzodiazepines on the GABA/benzodiazepine receptor complex. Flumazenil is benzodiazepine specific and does not antagonize other nonbenzodiazepine GABA agonists (including ethanol, barbiturates, general anesthetics); flumazenil does not reverse the effects of opiates

**Use** Benzodiazepine antagonist - reverses sedative effects of benzodiazepines used in general anesthesia; for management of benzodiazepine overdose; flumazenil does **not** antagonize the CNS effects of other GABA agonists (such as ethanol, barbiturates, or general anesthetics), **does not** reverse narcotics

**USUAL DOSAGE** See table.

### Flumazenil

| Pediatric Dosage | |
|---|---|
| Further studies are needed | |
| Pediatric dosage for **reversal of conscious sedation**: Intravenously through a freely running intravenous infusion into a large vein to minimize pain at the injection site | |
| Initial dose | 0.01 mg/kg over 15 seconds (maximum dose of 0.2 mg) |
| Repeat doses | 0.005-0.01 mg/kg (maximum dose of 0.2 mg) repeated at 1-minute intervals |
| Maximum total cumulative dose | 1 mg |
| Pediatric dosage for **management of benzodiazepine overdose**: Intravenously through a freely running intravenous infusion into a large vein to minimize pain at the injection site | |
| Initial dose | 0.01 mg/kg (maximum dose: 0.2 mg) |
| Repeat doses | 0.01 mg/kg (maximum dose of 0.2 mg) repeated at 1-minute intervals |
| Maximum total cumulative dose | 1 mg |
| In place of repeat bolus doses, follow-up continuous infusions of 0.005-0.01 mg/kg/hour have been used; further studies are needed. | |

| Adult Dosage | |
|---|---|
| Adult dosage for **reversal of conscious sedation**: Intravenously through a freely running intravenous infusion into a large vein to minimize pain at the injection site | |
| Initial dose | 0.2 mg intravenously over 15 seconds |
| Repeat doses | If desired level of consciousness is not obtained, 0.2 mg may be repeated at 1-minute intervals. |
| Maximum total cumulative dose | 1 mg (usual dose 0.6-1 mg) **In the event of resedation**: Repeat doses may be given at 20-minute intervals with maximum of 1 mg/dose and 3 mg/hour |
| Adult dosage for **suspected benzodiazepine overdose**: Intravenously through a freely running intravenous infusion into a large vein to minimize pain at the injection site | |
| Initial dose | 0.2 mg intravenously over 30 seconds |
| Repeat doses | 0.5 mg over 30 seconds repeated at 1-minute intervals |
| Maximum total cumulative dose | 3 mg (usual dose 1-3 mg) Patients with a partial response at 3 mg may require additional titration up to a total dose of 5 mg. If a patient has not responded 5 minutes after cumulative dose of 5 mg, the major cause of sedation is not likely due to benzodiazepines. **In the event of resedation:** May repeat doses at 20-minute intervals with maximum of 1 mg/dose and 3 mg/hour |

Resedation: Repeated doses may be given at 20-minute intervals as needed; repeat treatment doses of 1 mg (at a rate of 0.5 mg/minute) should be given at any time and no more than 3 mg should be given in any hour. After intoxication with high doses of benzodiazepines, the duration of a single dose of flumazenil is not expected to exceed 1 hour; if desired, the period of wakefulness may be prolonged with repeated low intravenous doses of flumazenil, or by an infusion of 0.1-0.4 mg/hour. Most patients with benzodiazepine overdose will respond to a cumulative dose of 1-3 mg and doses >3 mg do not reliably produce additional effects. Rarely, patients with a partial response at 3 mg may require additional titration up to a total dose of 5 mg. **If a patient has not responded 5 minutes after receiving a cumulative dose of 5 mg, the major cause of sedation is not likely to be due to benzodiazepines.**

**Dosing in renal impairment:** Not significantly affected by renal failure ($Cl_{cr}$ <10 mL/minute) or hemodialysis beginning 1 hour after drug administration

**Dosing in hepatic impairment:** Initial dose of flumazenil used for initial reversal of benzo-diazepine effects is not changed; however, subsequent doses in liver disease patients should be reduced in size or frequency

**Dosage Forms** Inj: 0.1 mg/mL (5 mL, 10 mL)

**Contraindications** Known hypersensitivity to flumazenil or benzodiazepines; patients given benzodiazepines for control of potentially life-threatening conditions (eg, control of intracra-nial pressure or status epilepticus); patients who are showing signs of serious cyclic-antidepressant overdosage

**Warnings/Precautions**

Risk of seizures = high-risk patients:

Patients on benzodiazepines for long-term sedation

Tricyclic antidepressant overdose patients

Concurrent major sedative-hypnotic drug withdrawal

Recent therapy with repeated doses of parenteral benzodiazepines

Myoclonic jerking or seizure activity prior to flumazenil administration

Hypoventilation: Does not reverse respiratory depression/hypoventilation or cardiac depres-sion

Resedation: Occurs more frequently in patients where a large single dose or cumulative dose of a benzodiazepine is administered along with a neuromuscular blocking agent and multiple anesthetic agents

**Flumazenil should be used with caution in the intensive care unit because of increased risk of unrecognized benzodiazepine dependence in such settings.**

**Pregnancy Risk Factor** C

**Adverse Reactions**

>10%:

Central nervous system: Dizziness

Gastrointestinal: Vomiting, nausea

1% to 10%:

Central nervous system: Headache, asthenia, malaise, anxiety, nervousness, insomnia, abnormal crying, euphoria, depression

Endocrine & metabolic: Hot flashes

Gastrointestinal: Xerostomia

Local: Pain at injection site

Neuromuscular & skeletal: Tremor

Ocular: Abnormal vision

Respiratory: Dyspnea, hyperventilation

Miscellaneous: Increased sweating disorders

<1%: Bradycardia, tachycardia, chest pain, hypertension, ventricular extrasystoles, altered blood pressure (increases and decreases), anxiety and sensation of coldness, general-ized convulsions, somnolence, thick tongue, abnormal hearing, hiccups

**Drug Interactions** Increased toxicity: Use with caution in overdosage involving mixed drug overdose; toxic effects may emerge (especially with cyclic antidepressants) with the reversal of the benzodiazepine effect by flumazenil

**Onset** 1-3 minutes; 80% response within 3 minutes; Peak effect: 6-10 minutes

**Duration** Resedation occurs usually within 1 hour. Duration is related to dose given and benzodiazepine plasma concentrations. Reversal effects of flumazenil may wear off before effects of benzodiazepine.

**Half-Life** Alpha: 7-15 minutes; Terminal: 41-79 minutes

**Special PA Issues**

**Patient Education:** Avoid driving or activities requiring alertness for 18-24 hours after drug use. Memory and judgment may be impaired for 24-48 hours. Avoid alcohol or other CNS depressants for 2-3 days after treatment.

**Monitoring Parameters:** Monitor patients for return of sedation or respiratory depression

# Flunisolide (floo NIS oh lide)

**Pharmacologic Class** Corticosteroid, Oral Inhaler; Corticosteroid, Nasal

**U.S. Brand Names** AeroBid®-M Oral Aerosol Inhaler; AeroBid® Oral Aerosol Inhaler; Nasalide® Nasal Aerosol; Nasarel™

**Mechanism of Action** Decreases inflammation by suppression of migration of polymorpho-nuclear leukocytes and reversal of increased capillary permeability; does not depress hypothalamus

**Use** Steroid-dependent asthma; nasal solution is used for seasonal or perennial rhinitis

**USUAL DOSAGE**

Children >6 years:

Oral inhalation: 2 inhalations twice daily (morning and evening) up to 4 inhalations/day

Nasal: 1 spray each nostril twice daily (morning and evening), not to exceed 4 sprays/day each nostril

Adults:

Oral inhalation: 2 inhalations twice daily (morning and evening) up to 8 inhalations/day maximum

(Continued)

## Flunisolide (Continued)

Nasal: 2 sprays each nostril twice daily (morning and evening); maximum dose: 8 sprays/day in each nostril

**Dosage Forms** Inh: Nasal (Nasalide®): 25 mcg/actuation [200 sprays] (25 mL), Nasal (Nasarel™): 25 mcg/actuation [200 sprays] (25 mL); Oral: AeroBid®: 250 mcg/actuation [100 metered doses] (7 g), AeroBid-M® (menthol flavor): 250 mcg/actuation [100 metered doses] (7 g); **Soln, spray:** 0.025% [200 actuations] (25 mL)

**Contraindications** Known hypersensitivity to flunisolide, acute status asthmaticus; viral, tuberculosis, fungal or bacterial respiratory infections, or infections of nasal mucosa

**Warnings/Precautions** Use with caution in patients with hypothyroidism, cirrhosis, hypertension, congestive heart failure, ulcerative colitis, thromboembolic disorders; do not stop medication abruptly if on prolonged therapy; fatalities have occurred due to adrenal insufficiency in asthmatic patients during and after transfer from systemic corticosteroids to aerosol steroids; several months may be required for recovery of this syndrome; during this period, aerosol steroids do **not** provide the systemic steroid needed to treat patients having trauma, surgery or infections. When consumed in excessive quantities, systemic hypercorticism and adrenal suppression may occur; withdrawal and discontinuation of the corticosteroid should be done carefully. Controlled clinical studies have shown that inhaled and intranasal corticosteroids may cause a reduction in growth velocity in pediatric patients. Growth velocity provides a means of comparing the rate of growth among children of the same age.

In studies involving inhaled corticosteroids, the average reduction in growth velocity was approximately 1 cm (about $1/3$ of an inch) per year. It appears that the reduction is related to dose and how long the child takes the drug.

FDA's Pulmonary and Allergy Drugs and Metabolic and Endocrine Drugs advisory committees discussed this issue at a July 1998 meeting. They recommended that the agency develop class-wide labeling to inform healthcare providers so they would understand this potential side effect and monitor growth routinely in pediatric patients who are treated with inhaled corticosteroids, intranasal corticosteroids or both.

Long-term effects of this reduction in growth velocity on final adult height are unknown. Likewise, it also has not yet been determined whether patients' growth will "catch up" if treatment in discontinued. Drug manufacturers will continue to monitor these drugs to learn more about long-term effects. Children are prescribed inhaled corticosteroids to treat asthma. Intranasal corticosteroids are generally used to prevent and treat allergy-related nasal symptoms.

Patients are advised not to stop using their inhaled or intranasal corticosteroids without first speaking to their healthcare providers about the benefits of these drugs compared to their risks.

**Pregnancy Risk Factor** C

**Pregnancy Implications**

Clinical effects on the fetus  No data on crossing the placenta or effects on the fetus
Breast-feeding/lactation: No data on crossing into breast milk or effects on the infant

**Adverse Reactions**

>10%:

Cardiovascular: Pounding heartbeat
Central nervous system: Dizziness, headache, nervousness
Dermatologic: Itching, rash
Endocrine & metabolic: Adrenal suppression, menstrual problems
Gastrointestinal: GI irritation, anorexia, sore throat, bitter taste
Local: Nasal burning, Candida infections of the nose or pharynx, atrophic rhinitis
Respiratory: Sneezing, coughing, upper respiratory tract infection, bronchitis, nasal congestion, nasal dryness
Miscellaneous: Increased susceptibility to infections

1% to 10%:

Central nervous system: Insomnia, psychic changes
Dermatologic: Acne, urticaria
Gastrointestinal: Increase in appetite, xerostomia, dry throat, loss of taste perception
Ocular: Cataracts
Respiratory: Epistaxis
Miscellaneous: Diaphoresis, loss of smell

<1%: Abdominal fullness, bronchospasm, shortness of breath

**Drug Interactions** Expected interactions similar to other corticosteroids

**Half-Life** 1.8 hours

**Special PA Issues**

**Patient Education:** Use as directed; do not use nasal preparations for oral inhalation. Do not increase dosage or discontinue abruptly without consulting prescriber. Review use of inhaler or spray with prescriber or follow package insert for directions. Keep oral inhaler clean and unobstructed. Always rinse mouth and throat after use of inhaler to prevent opportunistic infection. If you are also using an inhaled bronchodilator, wait 10 minutes before using this steroid aerosol. You may experience dizziness, anxiety, or blurred vision (rise slowly from sitting or lying position and use caution when driving or engaging in hazardous tasks until response to drug is known); or taste disturbance or aftertaste (frequent mouth care and mouth rinses may help). Report pounding heartbeat or chest pain; acute nervousness or inability to sleep; severe sneezing or nosebleed; difficulty breathing, sore throat, hoarseness, or bronchitis; respiratory difficulty or bronchospasms; disturbed menstrual pattern; vision changes; loss of taste or smell perception; or worsening of condition or lack of improvement.

**Administration:** Inhaler: Sit when using. Take deep breaths for 3-5 minutes, and clear nasal passages before administration (use decongestant as needed). Hold breath for 5-10 seconds after use, and wait 1-3 minutes between inhalations. Follow package insert instructions for use. Do not exceed maximum dosage. If also using inhaled bronchodilator, use before flunisolide. Rinse mouth and throat after use to reduce aftertaste and prevent candidiasis.

**Related Information**
Asthma Therapy Guidelines *on page 1049*

# Fluocinolone (floo oh SIN oh lone)

**Pharmacologic Class** Corticosteroid, Shampoo; Corticosteroid, Topical

**U.S. Brand Names** Derma-Smoothe/FS®; Fluonid®; Flurosyn®; FS Shampoo®; Synalar®; Synalar-HP®; Synemol®

**Mechanism of Action** A synthetic corticosteroid which differs structurally from triamcinolone acetonide in the presence of an additional fluorine atom in the 6-alpha position on the steroid nucleus. The mechanism of action for all topical corticosteroids is not well defined, however, is believed to be a combination of three important properties: anti-inflammatory activity, immunosuppressive properties, and antiproliferative actions.

**Use** Relief of susceptible inflammatory dermatosis [low, medium, high potency topical corticosteroid]

**USUAL DOSAGE** Children and Adults: Topical: Apply a thin layer to affected area 2-4 times/day

**Dosage Forms Crm, top:** 0.01% (15 g, 60 g); 0.025% (15 g, 60 g), Flurosyn®, Synalar®: 0.01% (15 g, 30 g, 60 g, 425 g), Flurosyn®, Synalar®, Synemol®: 0.025% (15 g, 60 g, 425 g), Synalar-HP®: 0.2% (12 g); **Oint, top:** 0.025% (15 g, 60 g), Flurosyn®, Synalar®: 0.025% (15 g, 30 g, 60 g, 425 g); **Oil (Derma-Smoothe/FS®):** 0.01% (120 mL); **Shamp (FS Shampoo®):** 0.01% (180 mL); **Soln, top:** 0.01% (20 mL, 60 mL), Fluonid®, Synalar®: 0.01% (20 mL, 60 mL)

**Contraindications** Fungal infection, hypersensitivity to fluocinolone or any component, TB of skin, herpes (including varicella)

**Warnings/Precautions** Adverse systemic effects may occur when used on large areas of the body, denuded areas, for prolonged periods of time, with an occlusive dressing, and/or in infants or small children. Infants and small children may be more susceptible to adrenal axis suppression from topical corticosteroid therapy.

**Pregnancy Risk Factor** C

**Adverse Reactions** <1%: Acne, hypopigmentation, allergic dermatitis, maceration of the skin, skin atrophy, folliculitis, hypertrichosis, dry skin, itching, HPA suppression, Cushing's syndrome, growth retardation, burning, irritation, secondary infection

**Special PA Issues**
**Patient Education:** For external use only. Use exactly as directed; do not overuse. Do not apply to open wounds or weeping areas. Before using, wash and dry area gently. Apply a thin film to affected area and rub in gently. If dressing is necessary, use a porous dressing. Avoid contact with eyes. Avoid exposing treated area to direct sunlight; sunburn can occur. Report increased swelling, redness, rash, itching, signs of infection, worsening of condition, or lack of healing.

♦ **Fluocinolone Acetonide** *see* Fluocinolone *on this page*

# Fluocinonide (floo oh SIN oh nide)

**Pharmacologic Class** Corticosteroid, Topical

**U.S. Brand Names** Fluonex®; Lidex®; Lidex-E®

**Mechanism of Action** Fluorinated topical corticosteroid considered to be of high potency. The mechanism of action for all topical corticosteroids is not well defined, however, is felt to be a combination of three important properties: anti-inflammatory activity, immunosuppressive properties, and antiproliferative actions.

**Use** Anti-inflammatory, antipruritic, relief of inflammatory and pruritic manifestations [high potency topical corticosteroid]

**USUAL DOSAGE** Children and Adults: Topical: Apply thin layer to affected area 2-4 times/day depending on the severity of the condition

**Dosage Forms Crm:** 0.05% (15 g, 30 g, 60 g, 120 g), Anhydrous, emollient (Lidex®): 0.05% (15 g, 30 g, 60 g, 120 g), Aqueous, emollient (Lidex-E®): 0.05% (15 g, 30 g, 60 g, 120 g); **Gel, top:** 0.05% (15 g, 60 g), Lidex®: 0.05% (15 g, 30 g, 60 g, 120 g); **Oint, top:** 0.05% (15 g, 30 g, 60 g), Lidex®: 0.05% (15 g, 30 g, 60 g, 120 g); **Soln, top:** 0.05% (20 mL, 60 mL), Lidex®: 0.05% (20 mL, 60 mL)

(Continued)

# Fluocinonide *(Continued)*

**Contraindications** Viral, fungal, or tubercular skin lesions, herpes simplex, known hypersensitivity to fluocinonide

**Warnings/Precautions** Adverse systemic effects may occur when used on large areas of the body, denuded areas, for prolonged periods of time, with an occlusive dressing, and/or in infants or small children

**Pregnancy Risk Factor** C

**Adverse Reactions** < %: Intracranial hypertension, acne, hypopigmentation, allergic dermatitis, maceration of the skin, skin atrophy, dry skin, itching, folliculitis, hypertrichosis, HPA suppression, Cushing's syndrome, growth retardation, burning, irritation, secondary infection

**Special PA Issues**

**Patient Education:** For external use only. Use exactly as directed; do not overuse. Do not apply to open wounds or weeping areas. Before using, wash and dry area gently. Apply a thin film to affected area and rub in gently. If dressing is necessary, use a porous dressing. Avoid contact with eyes. Avoid exposing treated area to direct sunlight; sunburn can occur. Report increased swelling, redness, rash, itching, signs of infection, worsening of condition, or lack of healing.

+ **Fluohydrisone Acetate** *see* Fludrocortisone Acetate *on page 377*
+ **Fluohydrocortisone Acetate** *see* Fludrocortisone Acetate *on page 377*
+ **Fluonex®** *see* Fluocinonide *on previous page*
+ **Fluonid®** *see* Fluocinolone *on previous page*
+ **Fluoracaine® Ophthalmic** *see* Proparacaine and Fluorescein *on page 771*

# Fluorescein Sodium *(FLURE e seen SOW dee um)*

**Pharmacologic Class** Diagnostic Agent, Ophthalmic Dye

**U.S. Brand Names** AK-Fluor; Fluorescite®; Fluorets®; Fluor-I-Strip®; Fluor-I-Strip-AT®; Fluress®; Ful-Glo®; Funduscein®; Ophthifluor®

**Mechanism of Action** Yellow, water soluble, dibasic acid xanthine dye which penetrates any break in epithelial barrier to permit rapid penetration

**Use** Demonstrates defects of corneal epithelium; diagnostic aid in ophthalmic angiography

**USUAL DOSAGE**

Ophthalmic:

Solution: Instill 1-2 drops of 2% solution and allow a few seconds for staining; wash out excess with sterile water or irrigating solution

Strips: Moisten strip with sterile water. Place moistened strip at the fornix into the lower cul-de-sac close to the punctum. For best results, patient should close lid tightly over strip until desired amount of staining is obtained. Patient should blink several times after application.

Removal of foreign bodies, sutures or tonometry (Fluress®): Instill 1 or 2 drops (single instillations) into each eye before operating

Deep ophthalmic anesthesia (Fluress®): Instill 2 drops into each eye every 90 seconds up to 3 doses

Injection: Prior to use, perform intradermal skin test; have epinephrine 1:1000, an antihistamine, and oxygen available

Children: 3.5 mg/lb (7.5 mg/kg) injected rapidly into antecubital vein

Adults: 500-750 mg injected rapidly into antecubital vein

**Dosage Forms Inj (AK-Fluor, Fluorescite®, Funduscein®, Ophthifluor®):** 10% [100 mg/mL] (5 mL); 25% [250 mg/mL] (2 mL, 3 mL); **Ophth: Soln:** 2% [20 mg/mL] (1 mL, 2 mL, 15 mL), Fluress®: 0.25% [2.5 mg/mL] with benoxinate 0.4% (5 mL); **Strip:** (Ful-Glo®): 0.6 mg, Fluorets®, Fluor-I-Strip-AT®: mg, Fluor-I-Strip®: 9 mg

**Contraindications** Hypersensitivity to fluorescein or any other component of the product; do not use with soft contact lenses, as this will cause them to discolor; pregnancy with parenteral product

**Warnings/Precautions** Use with caution in patients with history of hypersensitivity, allergies, or asthma; avoid extravasation; should not be used in patients with soft contact lenses, will cause them to discolor

**Pregnancy Risk Factor** C (topical); X (parenteral)

**Adverse Reactions**

1% to 10%:

Dermatologic: Burning sensation

Local: Temporary stinging

<1%: Syncope, hypotension, cardiac arrest, basilar artery ischemia, severe shock, headache, nausea, GI distress, vomiting, thrombophlebitis

**Special PA Issues**

**Patient Education:** Do not replace soft contact lenses for at least 1 hour, flush eye before replacing; skin discoloration may last 6-12 hours, urine 24-36 hours if given systemically

+ **Fluorescite®** *see* Fluorescein Sodium *on this page*
+ **Fluorets®** *see* Fluorescein Sodium *on this page*

## Fluoride (FLOR ide)

**Pharmacologic Class** Mineral, Oral; Mineral, Oral Topical

**U.S. Brand Names** ACT® [OTC]; Fluorigard® [OTC]; Fluorinse®; Fluoritab®; Flura®; Flura-Drops®; Flura-Loz®; Gel Kam®; Gel-Tin® [OTC]; Karidium®; Karigel®; Karigel®-N; Listermint® with Fluoride [OTC]; Luride®; Luride Lozi-Tab®; Luride®-SF Lozi-Tab®; Minute-Gel®; Pediaflor®; Pharmaflur®; Phos-Flur®; Point-Two®; PreviDent®; Stop® [OTC]; Thera-Flur®; Thera-Flur-N®

**Mechanism of Action** Promotes remineralization of decalcified enamel; inhibits the cariogenic microbial process in dental plaque; increases tooth resistance to acid dissolution

**Use** Prevention of dental caries

**USUAL DOSAGE** Oral:

Recommended daily fluoride supplement (2.2 mg of sodium fluoride is equivalent to 1 mg of fluoride ion): See table.

**Fluoride Ion**

| Fluoride Content of Drinking Water | Daily Dose, Oral (mg) |
|---|---|
| **<0.3 ppm** | |
| Birth - 6 mo | 0 |
| 6 mo - 3 y | 0.25 |
| 3-6 y | 0.5 |
| 6-16 y | 1 |
| **0.3-0.6 ppm** | |
| Birth - 3 y | 0 |
| 3-6 y | 0.25 |
| 6-16 y | 0.5 |
| **>0.6 ppm** | |
| All ages | 0 |

Adapted from *AAP News*, 1995, 11(2):18.

Dental rinse or gel:

Children 6-12 years: 5-10 mL rinse or apply to teeth and spit daily after brushing

Adults: 10 mL rinse or apply to teeth and spit daily after brushing

**Dosage Forms** Fluoride ion content listed in brackets

Acidulated phosphate fluoride: **Rinse, top:** Minute-Gel®: 1.23% (480 mL)

Sodium fluoride; **Drops, oral:** Fluoritab®, Flura-Drops®: 0.55 mg/drop [0.25 mg/drop] (22.8 mL, 24 mL), Karidium®, Luride®: 0.275 mg/drop [0.125 mg/drop] (30 mL, 60 mL), Pediaflor®: 1.1 mg/mL [0.5 mg/mL] (50 mL); **Gel, top:** Karigel®, Karigel®-N, PreviDent®: 1.1% [0.5%] (24 g, 30 g, 60 g, 120 g, 130 g, 250 g); **Rinse, top:** ACT®, Fluorigard®: 0.05% [0.02%] (90 mL, 180 mL, 300 mL, 360 mL, 480 mL), Fluorinse®, Point-Two®: 0.2% [0.09%] (240 mL, 480 mL, 3780 mL), Listermint® with Fluoride: 0.02% [0.01%] (180 mL, 300 mL, 360 mL, 480 mL, 540 mL, 720 mL, 960 mL, 1740 mL); **Soln, oral, as sodium (Phos-Flur®):** 0.44 mg/mL [0.2 mg/mL] (250 mL, 500 mL, 3780 mL); **Tab: Chewable:** Fluoritab®, Luride® Lozi-Tab®, Pharmaflur®: 1.1 mg [0.5 mg]

Fluoritab®, Karidium®, Luride® Lozi-Tab®, Luride®-SF Lozi-Tab®, Pharmaflur®: 2.2 mg [1 mg]; **Oral:** Flura®, Karidium®: 2.2 mg [1 mg];

Stannous fluoride: **Rinse, top:** Gel-Kam®, Gel-Tin®, Stop®: 0.4% [0.1%] (60 g, 15 g, 105 g, 120 g)

**Contraindications** Hypersensitivity to fluoride, tartrazine, or any component; when fluoride content of drinking water exceeds 0.7 ppm; low sodium or sodium-free diets; do not use 1 mg tablets in children <3 years of age or when drinking water fluoride content is ≥0.3 ppm; do not use 1 mg/5 mL rinse (as supplement) in children <6 years of age

**Warnings/Precautions** Prolonged ingestion with excessive doses may result in dental fluorosis and osseous changes; do **not** exceed recommended dosage; some products contain tartrazine

**Pregnancy Risk Factor** C

**Adverse Reactions** <1%: Rash, nausea, vomiting, products containing stannous fluoride may stain the teeth

**Drug Interactions** Decreased effect/absorption with magnesium-, aluminum-, and calcium-containing products

**Special PA Issues**

**Patient Education:** Take with food (but not milk) to eliminate GI upset; with dental rinse or dental gel do **not** swallow, do **not** eat or drink for 30 minutes after use

♦ **Fluorigard® [OTC]** *see* Fluoride *on this page*

♦ **Fluori-Methane® Topical Spray** *see* Dichlorodifluoromethane and Trichloromonofluoromethane *on page 271*

♦ **Fluorinse®** *see* Fluoride *on this page*

- **Fluor-I-Strip®** *see* Fluorescein Sodium *on page 382*
- **Fluor-I-Strip-AT®** *see* Fluorescein Sodium *on page 382*
- **Fluoritab®** *see* Fluoride *on previous page*
- **9α-Fluorohydrocortisone Acetate** *see* Fludrocortisone Acetate *on page 377*

# Fluorometholone (flure oh METH oh lone)

**Pharmacologic Class** Corticosteroid, Ophthalmic; Corticosteroid, Topical

**U.S. Brand Names** Flarex®; Fluor-Op®; FML®; FML® Forte

**Mechanism of Action** Decreases inflammation by suppression of migration of polymorphonuclear leukocytes and reversal of increased capillary permeability

**Use** Inflammatory conditions of the eye, including keratitis, iritis, cyclitis, and conjunctivitis

**USUAL DOSAGE** Children >2 years and Adults: Ophthalmic:

Ointment: May be applied every 4 hours in severe cases; 1-3 times/day in mild to moderate cases

Solution: Instill 1-2 drops into conjunctival sac every hour during day, every 2 hours at night until favorable response is obtained, then use 1 drop every 4 hours; for mild to moderate inflammation, instill 1-2 drops into conjunctival sac 2-4 times/day

**Dosage Forms** Ophth: **Oint (FML®)**: 0.1% (3.5 g); **Susp:** Flarex®, Fluor-Op®, FML®: 0.1% (2.5 mL, 5 mL, 10 mL) FML® Forte: 0.25% (2 mL, 5 mL, 10 mL, 15 mL)

**Contraindications** Herpes simplex, keratitis, fungal diseases of ocular structures, most viral diseases, hypersensitivity to any component

**Warnings/Precautions** Not recommended in children <2 years of age, prolonged use may result in glaucoma, elevated intraocular pressure, or other ocular damage; some products contain sulfites

**Pregnancy Risk Factor** C

**Adverse Reactions**

1% to 10%: Ocular: Blurred vision

<1%: Stinging, burning eyes, increased intraocular pressure, open-angle glaucoma, defect in visual acuity and field of vision, cataracts

**Special PA Issues**

Patient Education: For ophthalmic use only. Store solution in refrigerator. Apply prescribed amount as often as directed. Wash hands before using and do not let tip of applicator touch eye or contaminate tip of applicator. Tilt head back and look upward. Gently pull down lower lid and put drop(s) in inner corner of eye. Close eye and roll eyeball in all directions. Do not blink for $1/2$ minute. Apply gentle pressure to inner corner of eye for 30 seconds. Wipe away excess from skin around eye. Do not use any other eye preparation for at least 10 minutes. Do not touch tip of applicator to eye or contaminate tip of applicator. Do not share medication with anyone else. May cause sensitivity to bright light (dark glasses may help); temporary stinging or blurred vision may occur. Inform prescriber if you experience eye pain, redness, burning, watering, dryness, double vision, puffiness around eye, vision disturbances, or other adverse eye response; worsening of condition or lack of improvement within 3-4 days.

- **Fluor-Op®** *see* Fluorometholone *on this page*
- **Fluoroplex® Topical** *see* Fluorouracil *on this page*

# Fluorouracil (flure oh YOOR a sil)

**Pharmacologic Class** Antineoplastic Agent, Antimetabolite

**U.S. Brand Names** Adrucil® Injection; Efudex® Topical; Fluoroplex® Topical

**Mechanism of Action** A pyrimidine antimetabolite that interferes with DNA synthesis by blocking the methylation of deoxyuridylic acid; 5-FU rapidly enters the cell and is activated to the nucleotide level; there it inhibits thymidylate synthetase (TS), or is incorporated into RNA (most evident during the GI phase of the cell cycle). The reduced folate cofactor is required for tight binding to occur between the 5-FdUMP and TS.

**Use** Treatment of carcinoma of stomach, colon, rectum, breast, and pancreas; also used topically for management of multiple actinic keratoses and superficial basal cell carcinomas

**USUAL DOSAGE** Refer to individual protocols

All dosages are based on the patient's actual weight. However, the estimated lean body mass (dry weight) is used if the patient is obese or if there has been a spurious weight gain due to edema, ascites or other forms of abnormal fluid retention.

Children and Adults:

I.V.: Initial: 400-500 mg/m²/day (12 mg/kg/day; maximum: 800 mg/day) for 4-5 days either as a single daily I.V. push or 4-day CIV

I.V.: Maintenance dose regimens:

200-250 mg/m² (6 mg/kg) every other day for 4 days repeated in 4 weeks

500-600 mg/m² (15 mg/kg) weekly as a CIV or I.V. push

I.V.: Concomitant with leucovorin:

370 mg/m²/day x 5 days

500-1000 mg/m² every 2 weeks

600 mg/m² weekly for 6 weeks

Although the manufacturer recommends no daily dose >800 mg, higher doses of up to 2 g/day are routinely administered by CIV; higher daily doses have been successfully used

Hemodialysis: Administer dose posthemodialysis

**Dosing adjustment/comments in hepatic impairment:** Bilirubin >5 mg/dL: Omit use

Topical:

Actinic or solar keratosis: Apply twice daily for 2-6 weeks

Superficial basal cell carcinomas: Apply 5% twice daily for at least 3-6 weeks and up to 10-12 weeks

**Dosage Forms Crm, top:** Efudex®: 5% (25 g), Fluoroplex®: 1% (30 g); **Inj (Adrucil®):** 50 mg/mL (10 mL, 20 mL, 50 mL, 100 mL); **Soln, top:** Efudex®: 2% (10 mL), 5% (10 mL), Fluoroplex®: 1% (30 mL)

**Contraindications** Hypersensitivity to fluorouracil or any component, poor nutritional status, bone marrow depression, or potentially serious infections; pregnancy with topical product

**Warnings/Precautions** The U.S. Food and Drug Administration (FDA) currently recommends that procedures for proper handling and disposal of antineoplastic agents be considered. Use with caution in patients with impaired kidney or liver function. The drug should be discontinued if intractable vomiting or diarrhea, precipitous falls in leukocyte or platelet counts, stomatitis, hemorrhage, or myocardial ischemia occurs. Use with caution in patients who have had high-dose pelvic radiation or previous use of alkylating agents. Patient should be hospitalized during initial course of therapy.

**Pregnancy Risk Factor** D (injection); X (topical)

**Adverse Reactions** Toxicity depends on route and duration of infusion

>10%:

Dermatologic: Dermatitis, pruritic maculopapular rash, alopecia

**Irritant chemotherapy**

Gastrointestinal (route and schedule dependent): Heartburn, nausea, vomiting, anorexia, stomatitis, esophagitis, anorexia, stomatitis, and diarrhea; bolus dosing produces milder GI problems, while continuous infusion tends to produce severe mucositis and diarrhea; vomiting is moderate, occurring in 30% to 60% of patients, and responds well to phenothiazines and dexamethasone

Emetic potential:

<1000 mg: Moderately low (10% to 30%)

≥1000 mg: Moderate (30% to 60%)

Hematologic: Myelosuppressive: Granulocytopenia occurs around 9-14 days after 5-FU and thrombocytopenia around 7-17 days. The marrow recovers after 22 days. Myelosuppression tends to be more pronounced in patients receiving bolus dosing of 5-FU.

WBC: Moderate

Platelets: Mild to moderate

Onset (days): 7-10

Nadir (days): 14

Recovery (days): 21

1% to 10%:

Dermatologic: Dry skin

Gastrointestinal: GI ulceration

<1%: Hypotension, chest pain, EKG changes similar to ischemic changes, and possibly cardiac enzyme abnormalities. Usually occurs within the first two days of therapy, and may resolve with nitroglycerin and calcium channel blockers. May be due to coronary vessel vasospasm induced by 5-FU.

Cerebellar ataxia, headache, somnolence, ataxia are seen primarily in intracarotid arterial infusions for head and neck tumors. This is believed to be caused by fluorocitrate, a neurotoxic metabolite of the parent compound.

Pruritic maculopapular rash, alopecia, hyperpigmentation of nailbeds, face, hands, and veins used in infusion; photosensitization with UV light; palmar-plantar syndrome (hand-foot syndrome); coagulopathy, hepatotoxicity, conjunctivitis, tear duct stenosis, excessive lacrimation, visual disturbances, shortness of breath

**Drug Interactions**

Methotrexate: This interaction is schedule dependent; **5-FU should be given following MTX, not prior to**

If MTX is given first: The cells exposed to MTX before 5-FU have a depleted reduced folate pool which inhibits the binding of the 5dUMP to TS. However, it does not interfere with FUTP incorporation into RNA. Polyglutamines, which accumulate in the presence of MTX may be substituted for the folates and allow binding of FdUMP to TS. MTX given prior to 5-FU may actually activate 5-FU due to MTX inhibition of purine synthesis.

If 5-FU is given first: 5-FU inhibits the TS binding and thus the reduced folate pool is not depleted, thereby negating the effect of MTX

Increased effect: Leucovorin: ↑ the folate pool and in certain tumors, may promote TS inhibition and ↑ 5-FU activity. Must be given before or with the 5-FU to prime the cells; it is not used as a rescue agent in this case.

(Continued)

## Fluorouracil *(Continued)*

Increased toxicity:

Allopurinol: Inhibits thymidine phosphorylase (an enzyme that activates 5-FU). The anti-tumor effect of 5-FU appears to be unaltered, but decreases toxicity

Cimetidine: Results in increased plasma levels of 5-FU due to drug metabolism inhibition and reduction of liver blood flow induced by cimetidine

**Duration** ~3 weeks

**Half-Life** Biphasic: Initial: 6-20 minutes; doses of 400-600 mg/m$^2$ produce drug concentrations above the threshold for cytotoxicity for normal tissue and remain there for 6 hours; two metabolites, FdUMP and FUTP, have prolonged half-lives depending on the type of tissue; the clinical effect of these metabolites has not been determined

**Special PA Issues**

**Patient Education:** Avoid alcohol and all OTC drugs unless approved by your oncologist. Maintain adequate hydration (2-3 L/day of fluids unless instructed to restrict fluid intake) and nutrition (small frequent meals may help). You may experience sensitivity to sunlight (use sunblock, wear protective clothing, or avoid direct sunlight); susceptibility to infection (avoid crowds or infected persons or persons with contagious diseases); nausea, vomiting, diarrhea, or loss of appetite (frequent small meals may help - request medication); weakness, lethargy, dizziness, decreased vision (use caution when driving or engaging in tasks that require alertness); headache (request medication). Report signs and symptoms of infection (eg, fever, chills, sore throat, burning urination, vaginal itching or discharge, fatigue, mouth sores); bleeding (eg, tarry stools, easy bruising, unusual bleeding); vision changes; unremitting nausea, vomiting, or abdominal pain; CNS changes; respiratory difficulty; chest pain or palpitations; severe skin reactions to topical application; or any other adverse reactions.

Topical: Use as directed; do not overuse. Wash hands thoroughly before and after applying medication. Avoid contact with eyes and mouth. Avoid occlusive dressings; use a porous dressing. May cause local reaction (pain, burning, or swelling); if severe contact prescriber.

**Monitoring Parameters:** CBC with differential and platelet count, renal function tests, liver function tests

♦ **5-Fluorouracil** *see Fluorouracil on page 384*

♦ **Fluostigmin** *see Isoflurophate on page 494*

## Fluoxetine *(floo OKS e teen)*

**Pharmacologic Class** Antidepressant, Selective Serotonin Reuptake Inhibitor

**U.S. Brand Names** Prozac®

**Mechanism of Action** Inhibits CNS neuron serotonin uptake; minimal or no effect on reuptake of norepinephrine or dopamine; does not significantly bind to alpha-adrenergic, histamine or cholinergic receptors; may therefore be useful in patients at risk from sedation, hypotension, and anticholinergic effects of tricyclic antidepressants

**Use** Treatment of major depression; treatment of binge-eating and vomiting in patients with moderate-to-severe bulimia nervosa; obsessive-compulsive disorder

**USUAL DOSAGE** Oral:

Children <18 years: Dose and safety not established; preliminary experience in children 6-14 years using initial doses of 20 mg/day have been reported

Adults: 20 mg/day in the morning; may increase after several weeks by 20 mg/day increments; maximum: 80 mg/day; doses >20 mg should be divided into morning and noon doses

Usual dosage range:

20-80 mg/day for depression and OCD

20-60 mg/day for obesity

60-80 mg/day for bulimia nervosa

**Note:** Lower doses of 5 mg/day have been used for initial treatment

Elderly: Some patients may require an initial dose of 10 mg/day with dosage increases of 10 and 20 mg every several weeks as tolerated; should not be taken at night unless patient experiences sedation

**Dosing adjustment in renal impairment:**

Single dose studies: Pharmacokinetics of fluoxetine and norfluoxetine were similar among subjects with all levels of impaired renal function, including anephric patients on chronic hemodialysis

Chronic administration: Additional accumulation of fluoxetine or norfluoxetine may occur in patients with severely impaired renal function

Hemodialysis: Not removed by hemodialysis

**Dosing adjustment in hepatic impairment:** Elimination half-life of fluoxetine is prolonged in patients with hepatic impairment; a lower or less frequent dose of fluoxetine should be used in these patients

Cirrhosis patients: Administer a lower dose or less frequent dosing interval

Compensated cirrhosis without ascites: Administer 50% of normal dose

**Dosage Forms** Fluoxetine hydrochloride: **Cap:** 10 mg, 20 mg; **Liq** (mint flavor): 20 mg/5 mL (120 mL)

**Contraindications** Hypersensitivity to fluoxetine; patients receiving MAO inhibitors currently or in past 2 weeks

**Warnings/Precautions** Use with caution in patients with hepatic impairment, history of seizures; MAO inhibitors should be discontinued at least 14 days before initiating fluoxetine therapy; add or initiate other antidepressants with caution for up to 5 weeks after stopping fluoxetine

**Pregnancy Risk Factor** B

**Adverse Reactions** Predominant adverse effects are CNS and GI

>10%:

Central nervous system: Headache, nervousness, insomnia, drowsiness

Gastrointestinal: Nausea, diarrhea, xerostomia

1% to 10%:

Central nervous system: Anxiety, dizziness, fatigue, sedation

Dermatologic: Rash, pruritus

Endocrine & metabolic: SIADH, hypoglycemia, hyponatremia (elderly or volume-depleted patients)

Gastrointestinal: Anorexia, dyspepsia, constipation

Neuromuscular & skeletal: Tremor

Miscellaneous: Diaphoresis (excessive)

<1%: Extrapyramidal reactions (rare), visual disturbances, anaphylactoid reactions, allergies, suicidal ideation

**Drug Interactions** CYP2D6 enzyme substrate (minor), CYP2C enzyme substrate (minor), CYP3A3/4 enzyme substrate; CYP2C9 enzyme inducer; CYP1A2, 2C9, 2C18, 2C19, 2D6, and 3A3/4 enzyme inhibitor

Increased effect with tricyclics (2 times increased plasma level)

Increased/decreased effect of lithium (both increased and decreased level has been reported)

Increased toxicity of diazepam, trazodone via decreased clearance; increased toxicity with MAO inhibitors (hyperpyrexia, tremors, seizures, delirium, coma)

May displace highly protein bound drugs (warfarin)

**Onset** >2-4 weeks for therapeutic effects

**Half-Life** 2-3 days; due to long half-life, resolution of adverse reactions after discontinuation may be slow

**Special PA Issues**

**Patient Education:** Take exactly as directed (do not increase dose or frequency); may take 2-3 weeks to achieve desired results; may cause physical and/or psychological dependence. Take once-a-day dose in the morning to reduce incidence of insomnia. Avoid excessive alcohol, caffeine, and other prescription or OTC medications not approved by prescriber. Maintain adequate hydration (2-3 L/day of fluids unless instructed to restrict fluid intake). You may experience drowsiness, lightheadedness, impaired coordination, dizziness, or blurred vision (use caution when driving or engaging in hazardous tasks until response to medication is known); constipation (increased exercise, fluids, or dietary fruit and fiber may help); anorexia (maintain regular dietary intake to avoid excessive weight loss); or postural hypotension (use caution when climbing stairs or changing position from lying or sitting to standing). If diabetic, monitor serum glucose closely (may cause hypoglycemia). Report persistent CNS effects (nervousness, restlessness, insomnia, anxiety, excitation, headache, sedation); rash or skin irritation; muscle cramping, tremors, or change in gait; respiratory depression or difficulty breathing; or worsening of condition.

**Dietary Considerations:** Alcohol: Avoid use

**Reference Range:** Therapeutic levels have not been well established

Therapeutic: Fluoxetine: 100-800 ng/mL (SI: 289-2314 nmol/L); Norfluoxetine: 100-600 ng/mL (SI: 289-1735 nmol/L)

Toxic: Fluoxetine plus norfluoxetine: >2000 ng/mL

**Related Information**

Antidepressant Agents *on page 998*

♦ **Fluoxetine Hydrochloride** *see* Fluoxetine *on previous page*

# Fluoxymesterone (floo oks i MES te rone)

**Pharmacologic Class** Androgen

**U.S. Brand Names** Halotestin®

**Mechanism of Action** Synthetic androgenic anabolic hormone responsible for the normal growth and development of male sex hormones and development of male sex organs and maintenance of secondary sex characteristics; synthetic testosterone derivative with significant androgen activity; stimulates RNA polymerase activity resulting in an increase in protein production; increases bone development

**Use** Replacement of endogenous testicular hormone; in females, used as palliative treatment of breast cancer; stimulation of erythropoiesis, angioneurotic edema, postpartum breast engorgement

**USUAL DOSAGE** Adults: Oral:

(Continued)

## Fluoxymesterone *(Continued)*

Male:
Hypogonadism: 5-20 mg/day
Delayed puberty: 2.5-20 mg/day for 4-6 months
Female:
Inoperable breast carcinoma: 10-40 mg/day in divided doses for 1-3 months
Breast engorgement: 2.5 mg after delivery, 5-10 mg/day in divided doses for 4-5 days

**Dosage Forms** Tab: 2 mg, 5 mg, 10 mg

**Contraindications** Serious cardiac disease, liver or kidney disease, hypersensitivity to fluoxymesterone or any component; pregnancy

**Warnings/Precautions** May accelerate bone maturation without producing compensatory gain in linear growth in children; in prepubertal children perform radiographic examination of the hand and wrist every 6 months to determine the rate of bone maturation and to assess the effect of treatment on the epiphyseal centers

**Pregnancy Risk Factor** X

**Adverse Reactions**
>10%:
Males: Priapism
Females: Menstrual problems (amenorrhea), virilism, breast soreness
Cardiovascular: Edema
Dermatologic: Acne
1% to 10%:
Males: Prostatic carcinoma, hirsutism (increase in pubic hair growth), impotence, testicular atrophy
Cardiovascular: Edema
Gastrointestinal: GI irritation, nausea, vomiting
Genitourinary: Prostatic hypertrophy
Hepatic: Hepatic dysfunction
<1%:
Males: Gynecomastia
Females: Amenorrhea
Hypercalcemia, leukopenia, polycythemia, hepatic necrosis, cholestatic hepatitis, hypersensitivity reactions

**Drug Interactions**
Decreased effect:
Fluphenazine effectiveness with anticholinergics
Barbiturate levels and decreased fluphenazine effectiveness when given together
Increased toxicity:
Anticoagulants: Fluoxymesterone may suppress clotting factors II, V, VII, and X; therefore, bleeding may occur in patients on anticoagulant therapy
Cyclosporine: May elevate cyclosporine serum levels
Insulin: May enhance hypoglycemic effect of insulin therapy
May decrease blood glucose concentrations and insulin requirements in patients with diabetes
With ethanol, effects of both drugs may increase
EPSEs and other CNS effects may increase when coadministered with lithium
May potentiate the effects of narcotics including respiratory depression

**Half-Life** 10-100 minutes

**Special PA Issues**
**Patient Education:** Take as directed, with meals. Do not discontinue abruptly without consulting prescriber. Diabetics should monitor serum glucose closely and report abnormal glucose tests so adjustments can be made in diabetic regimen. You may experience acne, growth of body hair or baldness, deepening of voice, loss of libido, impotence (most are reversible). You may experience drowsiness, dizziness, or blurred vision; use caution when driving or engaging in hazardous tasks. Small frequent meals and good mouth care may reduce any nausea or vomiting. Report persistent GI distress or diarrhea, change in color of urine or stool, yellowing of eyes or skin, unusual bruising or bleeding, fluid retention (swelling of ankles, feet, or hands, difficulty breathing), menstrual irregularity, persistent penile erection, or excessive growth of body hair.
**Monitoring Parameters:** In prepubertal children, perform radiographic examination of the head and wrist every 6 months

## Fluphenazine *(floo FEN a zeen)*

**Pharmacologic Class** Antipsychotic Agent, Phenothiazine, Piperazine

**U.S. Brand Names** Permitil® Oral; Prolixin Decanoate® Injection; Prolixin Enanthate® Injection; Prolixin® Injection; Prolixin® Oral

**Mechanism of Action** Blocks postsynaptic mesolimbic dopaminergic $D_1$ and $D_2$ receptors in the brain; exhibits a strong alpha-adrenergic blocking and anticholinergic effect, depresses the release of hypothalamic and hypophyseal hormones; believed to depress the reticular activating system thus affecting basal metabolism, body temperature, wakefulness, vasomotor tone, and emesis

**Use** Management of manifestations of psychotic disorders

**USUAL DOSAGE** Adults:

Oral: 0.5-10 mg/day in divided doses at 6- to 8-hour intervals; some patients may require up to 40 mg/day

I.M.: 2.5-10 mg/day in divided doses at 6- to 8-hour intervals (parenteral dose is $^1/_3$ to $^1/_2$ the oral dose for the hydrochloride salts)

I.M., S.C. (decanoate): 12.5 mg every 3 weeks

Conversion from hydrochloride to decanoate I.M. 0.5 mL (12.5 mg) decanoate every 3 weeks is approximately equivalent to 10 mg hydrochloride/day

I.M., S.C. (enanthate): 12.5-25 mg every 3 weeks

Hemodialysis: Not dialyzable (0% to 5%)

**Dosage Forms**

Fluphenazine decanoate: **Inj:** Prolixin Decanoate®: 25 mg/mL (1 mL, 5 mL)

Fluphenazine enanthate: **Inj:** Prolixin Enanthate®: 25 mg/mL (5 mL)

Fluphenazine hydrochloride: **Conc, oral:** Permitil®: 5 mg/mL with alcohol 1% (118 mL), Prolixin®: 5 mg/mL with alcohol 14% (120 mL); **Elix (Prolixin®):** 2.5 mg/5 mL with alcohol 14% (60 mL, 473 mL); **Inj:** Prolixin®: 2.5 mg/mL (10 mL); **Tab:** Permitil®: 2.5 mg, 5 mg, 10 mg, Prolixin®: 1 mg, 2.5 mg, 5 mg, 10 mg

**Contraindications** Hypersensitivity to fluphenazine or any component, cross-sensitivity with other phenothiazines may exist; avoid use in patients with narrow-angle glaucoma

**Warnings/Precautions** Safety in children <6 months of age has not been established; use with caution in patients with cardiovascular disease or seizures; benefits of therapy must be weighed against risks of therapy; adverse effects may be of longer duration with Depot® form; watch for hypotension when administering I.M. or I.V.; use with caution in patients with severe liver or renal disease

**Pregnancy Risk Factor** C

**Adverse Reactions**

>10%:

Cardiovascular: Orthostatic hypotension, hypotension, tachycardia, arrhythmias

Central nervous system: Parkinsonian symptoms, akathisia, dystonias, tardive dyskinesia (persistent), dizziness

Gastrointestinal: Constipation

Ocular: Pigmentary retinopathy

Respiratory: Nasal congestion

Miscellaneous: Diaphoresis (decreased)

1% to 10%:

Dermatologic: Increased sensitivity to sun, rash

Endocrine & metabolic: Changes in menstrual cycle, breast pain, amenorrhea, galactorrhea, gynecomastia, changes in libido

Gastrointestinal: Weight gain, nausea, vomiting, stomach pain

Genitourinary: Dysuria, ejaculatory disturbances

Neuromuscular & skeletal: Trembling of fingers

<1%: Sedation, drowsiness, restlessness, anxiety, extrapyramidal reactions, pseudoparkinsonian signs and symptoms, seizures, altered central temperature regulation, photosensitivity, hyperpigmentation, pruritus, rash, discoloration of skin (blue-gray), galactorrhea, xerostomia, priapism, urinary retention, agranulocytosis (more often in women between 4th and 10th weeks of therapy), leukopenia (usually in patients with large doses for prolonged periods), cholestatic jaundice, hepatotoxicity, cornea and lens changes, blurred vision

**Drug Interactions** CYP2D6 enzyme substrate; CYP2D6 enzyme inhibitor

Decreased effect: Barbiturate levels and decreased fluphenazine effectiveness when given together

Increased toxicity: With ethanol, effects of both drugs may be increased; EPSEs and other CNS effects may be increased when coadministered with lithium; may potentiate the effects of narcotics including respiratory depression

**Onset**

Following I.M. or S.C. administration (derivative dependent):

Decanoate (lasts the longest and requires 24-72 hours for onset of action): Onset of action: 24-72 hours; Peak neuroleptic effect: Within 48-96 hours

Hydrochloride salt (acts quickly and persists briefly): Onset of activity: Within 1 hour

**Duration** Hydrochloride salt: 6-8 hours

**Half-Life** Derivative dependent: Enanthate: 84-96 hours; Hydrochloride: 33 hours; Decanoate: 163-232 hours

**Special PA Issues**

**Patient Education:** Use exactly as directed (do not increase dose or frequency); may cause physical and/or psychological dependence. Do not discontinue without consulting prescriber. Dilute with water, milk, orange or grapefruit juice; do not dilute with beverages containing caffeine, tannin, or pactinate (eg, coffee, colas, tea, or apple juice). Do not take within 2 hours of any antacid. Avoid excess alcohol or caffeine and other prescription or OTC medications not approved by prescriber. Avoid skin contact with medication; may cause contact dermatitis (wash immediately with warm, soapy water). Maintain adequate

(Continued)

## Fluphenazine *(Continued)*

hydration (2-3 L/day of fluids unless instructed to restrict fluid intake). You may experience excess drowsiness, lightheadedness, dizziness, or blurred vision (use caution driving or when engaging in hazardous tasks until response to medication is known); dry mouth, upset stomach, nausea, vomiting (small frequent meals, frequent mouth care, or sucking lozenges may help); constipation (increased exercise, fluids, or dietary fruit and fiber may help); postural hypotension (use caution climbing stairs or when changing position from lying or sitting to standing); urinary retention (void before taking medication); ejaculatory dysfunction (reversible); decreased perspiration (avoid strenuous exercise in hot environments); or photosensitivity (use sunscreen, protective clothing, and avoid prolonged exposure to direct sunlight). Report persistent CNS effects (eg, trembling fingers, altered gait or balance, excessive sedation, seizures, unusual movements, anxiety, abnormal thoughts, confusion, personality changes); chest pain, palpitations, rapid heartbeat, severe dizziness; unresolved urinary retention or changes in urinary pattern; altered menstrual pattern, change in libido, swelling or pain in breasts (male or female); vision changes; skin rash or irritation or yellowing of skin; or worsening of condition.

**Dietary Considerations:** Alcohol: Additive CNS effect, avoid use

**Reference Range:** Therapeutic: 5-20 ng/mL; correlation of serum concentrations and efficacy is controversial; most often dosed to best response

**Related Information**

Antipsychotic Agents *on page 1001*

♦ **Fluphenazine Decanoate** *see* Fluphenazine *on page 388*

♦ **Fluphenazine Enanthate** *see* Fluphenazine *on page 388*

♦ **Fluphenazine Hydrochloride** *see* Fluphenazine *on page 388*

♦ **Flura®** *see* Fluoride *on page 383*

♦ **Flura-Drops®** *see* Fluoride *on page 383*

♦ **Flura-Loz®** *see* Fluoride *on page 383*

## Flurandrenolide *(flure an DREN oh lide)*

**Pharmacologic Class** Corticosteroid, Topical

**U.S. Brand Names** Cordran®; Cordran® SP

**Mechanism of Action** Decreases inflammation by suppression of migration of polymorphonuclear leukocytes and reversal of increased capillary permeability

**Use** Inflammation of corticosteroid-responsive dermatoses [medium potency topical corticosteroid]

**USUAL DOSAGE** Topical:

Children:

Ointment, cream: Apply sparingly 1-2 times/day

Tape: Apply once daily

Adults: Cream, lotion, ointment: Apply sparingly 2-3 times/day

**Dosage Forms Crm, emulsified base (Cordran® SP):** 0.025% (30 g, 60 g), 0.05% (15 g, 30 g, 60 g); **Lot (Cordran®):** 0.05% (15 mL, 60 mL); **Oint, top (Cordran®):** 0.025% (30 g, 60 g), 0.05% (15 g, 30 g, 60 g); **Tape, top (Cordran®):** 4 mcg/cm² (7.5 cm x 60 cm, 7.5 cm x 200 cm rolls)

**Contraindications** Viral, fungal, or tubercular skin lesions, known hypersensitivity to flurandrenolide

**Warnings/Precautions** Adverse systemic effects may occur when used on large areas of the body, denuded areas, for prolonged periods of time, with an occlusive dressing, and/or in infants or small children

**Pregnancy Risk Factor** C

**Adverse Reactions** <1%: Itching, dry skin, folliculitis, hypertrichosis, acneiform eruptions, hypopigmentation, perioral dermatitis, allergic contact dermatitis, skin atrophy, striae, miliaria, intracranial hypertension, acne, maceration of the skin; HPA suppression, Cushing's syndrome, growth retardation, burning, irritation, secondary infection

**Special PA Issues**

**Patient Education:** For external use only. Use exactly as directed; do not overuse. Do not apply to open wounds or weeping areas. Before using, wash and dry area gently. Apply a thin film to affected area and rub in gently. If dressing is necessary, use a porous dressing. Avoid contact with eyes. Avoid exposing treated area to direct sunlight; sunburn can occur. Report increased swelling, redness, rash, itching, signs of infection, worsening of condition, or lack of healing.

♦ **Flurandrenolone** *see* Flurandrenolide *on this page*

## Flurazepam *(flure AZ e pam)*

**Pharmacologic Class** Benzodiazepine

**U.S. Brand Names** Dalmane®

**Mechanism of Action** Depresses all levels of the CNS, including the limbic and reticular formation, probably through the increased action of gamma-aminobutyric acid (GABA), which is a major inhibitory neurotransmitter in the brain

**Use** Short-term treatment of insomnia

**USUAL DOSAGE** Oral:

Children:

&lt;15 years: Dose not established

&gt;15 years: 15 mg at bedtime

Adults: 15-30 mg at bedtime

**Dosage Forms Cap, as hydrochloride:** 15 mg, 30 mg

**Contraindications** Hypersensitivity to flurazepam or any component (there may be cross-sensitivity with other benzodiazepines); pregnancy, pre-existing CNS depression, respiratory depression, narrow-angle glaucoma

**Warnings/Precautions** Use with caution in patients receiving other CNS depressants, patients with low albumin, hepatic dysfunction, and in the elderly; do not use in pregnant women; may cause drug dependency; safety and efficacy have not been established in children &lt;15 years of age

**Pregnancy Risk Factor** X

**Adverse Reactions**

&gt;10%:

Cardiovascular: Tachycardia, chest pain

Central nervous system: Drowsiness, fatigue, ataxia, lightheadedness, memory impairment, insomnia, anxiety, depression, headache

Dermatologic: Rash

Endocrine & metabolic: Decreased libido

Gastrointestinal: Xerostomia, constipation, decreased salivation, nausea, vomiting, diarrhea, increased or decreased appetite

Neuromuscular & skeletal: Dysarthria

Ocular: Blurred vision

Miscellaneous: Diaphoresis

1% to 10%:

Cardiovascular: Syncope, hypotension

Central nervous system: Confusion, nervousness, dizziness, akathisia

Dermatologic: Dermatitis

Gastrointestinal: Weight gain or loss, increased salivation

Neuromuscular & skeletal: Rigidity, tremor, muscle cramps

Otic: Tinnitus

Respiratory: Hyperventilation, nasal congestion

&lt;1%: Menstrual irregularities, blood dyscrasias, reflex slowing, drug dependence

**Drug Interactions**

Decreased effect with enzyme inducers

Increased toxicity with other CNS depressants and cimetidine

**Onset** Onset of hypnotic effect: 15-20 minutes; Peak: 3-6 hours

**Duration** 7-8 hours

**Half-Life** 40-114 hours

**Special PA Issues**

**Patient Education:** Use exactly as directed (do not increase dose or frequency or discontinue without consulting prescriber); may cause physical and/or psychological dependence. May take with food to decrease GI upset. While using this medication, do not use alcohol or other prescription or OTC medications (especially, pain medications, sedatives, antihistamines, or hypnotics) without consulting prescriber. Maintain adequate hydration (2-3 L/day of fluids unless instructed to restrict fluid intake). You may experience drowsiness, dizziness, lightheadedness, or blurred vision (use caution when driving or engaging in hazardous tasks); dry mouth, nausea or vomiting (small frequent meals, good mouth care, chewing gum, or sucking lozenges may help); difficulty urinating (void before taking medication); or altered libido (resolves when medication is discontinued). Report CNS changes (confusion, depression, increased sedation, excitation, headache, abnormal thinking, insomnia, or nightmares, memory impairment, impaired coordination); muscle pain or weakness; difficulty breathing; persistent dizziness, chest pain, or palpitations; alterations in normal gait; vision changes; ringing in ears; or ineffectiveness of medication.

**Dietary Considerations:** Alcohol: Additive CNS effect, avoid use

**Monitoring Parameters:** Respiratory and cardiovascular status

**Reference Range:** Therapeutic: 0-4 ng/mL (SI: 0-9 nmol/L); Metabolite N-desalkyl-flurazepam: 20-110 ng/mL (SI: 43-240 nmol/L); Toxic: >0.12 µg/mL

♦ **Flurazepam Hydrochloride** *see* Flurazepam *on previous page*

# Flurbiprofen (flure BI proe fen)

**Pharmacologic Class** Nonsteroidal Anti-Inflammatory Agent (NSAID)

**U.S. Brand Names** Ansaid® Oral; Ocufen® Ophthalmic

(Continued)

## Flurbiprofen *(Continued)*

**Mechanism of Action** Inhibits prostaglandin synthesis by decreasing the activity of the enzyme, cyclo-oxygenase, which results in decreased formation of prostaglandin precursors

**Use** Inhibition of intraoperative miosis; acute or long-term treatment of signs and symptoms of rheumatoid arthritis and osteoarthritis; prevention and management of postoperative ocular inflammation and postoperative cystoid macular edema remains to be determined

### USUAL DOSAGE

Oral: Rheumatoid arthritis and osteoarthritis: 200-300 mg/day in 2, 3, or 4 divided doses

Ophthalmic: Instill 1 drop every 30 minutes, 2 hours prior to surgery (total of 4 drops to each affected eye)

**Dosage Forms** Soln, ophth (Ocufen®): 0.03% (2.5 mL, 5 mL, 10 mL); **Tab (Ansaid®):** 50 mg, 100 mg

**Contraindications** Dendritic keratitis, hypersensitivity to flurbiprofen or any component

**Warnings/Precautions** Should be used with caution in patients with a history of herpes simplex, keratitis, and patients who might be affected by inhibition of platelet aggregation; slowing of corneal wound healing patients in whom asthma, rhinitis, or urticaria is precipitated by aspirin or other NSAIDs.

**Pregnancy Risk Factor** C

### Adverse Reactions

Ophthalmic:

>10%: Ocular: Slowing of corneal wound healing, mild ocular stinging, itching and burning eyes, ocular irritation

1% to 10%: Ocular: Eye redness

Oral:

>10%:

Central nervous system: Dizziness

Dermatologic: Rash

Gastrointestinal: Abdominal cramps, heartburn, indigestion, nausea

1% to 10%:

Central nervous system: Headache, nervousness

Dermatologic: Itching

Endocrine & metabolic: Fluid retention

Gastrointestinal: Vomiting

Otic: Tinnitus

<1%: Congestive heart failure, hypertension, arrhythmias, tachycardia, confusion, hallucinations, aseptic meningitis, mental depression, drowsiness, insomnia, urticaria, erythema multiforme, toxic epidermal necrolysis, Stevens-Johnson syndrome, angioedema, polydipsia, hot flashes, gastritis, GI ulceration, cystitis, polyuria, agranulocytosis, anemia, hemolytic anemia, bone marrow suppression, leukopenia, thrombocytopenia, hepatitis, peripheral neuropathy, toxic amblyopia, blurred vision, conjunctivitis, dry eyes, decreased hearing, acute renal failure, shortness of breath, allergic rhinitis, epistaxis

**Drug Interactions** CYP2C9 enzyme substrate; CYP2C9 enzyme inhibitor

Decreased effect: When used concurrently with flurbiprofen, reports acetylcholine chloride and carbachol being ineffective

**Half-Life** 5.7 hours

**Special PA Issues**

**Patient Education:**

Oral: Take this medication exactly as directed; do not increase dose without consulting prescriber. Do not crush tablets or break capsules. Take with food or milk to reduce GI distress. Maintain adequate fluid intake (2-3 L/day). Do not use alcohol, aspirin, or aspirin-containing medication, and all other anti-inflammatory medications without consulting prescriber. You may experience drowsiness, dizziness, nervousness, or headache (use caution when driving or performing hazardous tasks); anorexia, nausea, vomiting, or heartburn (frequent small meals, frequent oral care, sucking on lozenges, or chewing gum may help); fluid retention (weigh yourself weekly and report unusual (3-5 lb/week) weight gain). GI bleeding, ulceration, or perforation can occur with or without pain; discontinue medication and contact prescriber if persistent abdominal pain or cramping, or blood in stool occurs. Report breathlessness, difficulty breathing, or unusual cough; chest pain, rapid heartbeat, palpitations; unusual bruising/bleeding; blood in urine, stool, mouth, or vomitus; swollen extremities; skin rash or itching; acute fatigue; changes in hearing or ringing in ears.

Ophthalmic: Wash hands before instilling. Sit or lie down to instill. Open eye, look at ceiling, and instill prescribed amount of medication. Close eye and roll eye in all directions, and apply gentle pressure to inner corner of eye. Do not let tip of applicator touch eye or contaminate tip of applicator. Use protective dark eyewear until healed; avoid direct sunlight. Temporary stinging or burning may occur. Report persistent pain, burning, redness, vision disturbances, swelling, itching, or worsening of condition.

**Related Information**

Nonsteroidal Anti-Inflammatory Agents *on page 1026*

- **Flurbiprofen Sodium** *see Flurbiprofen on page 391*
- **Fluress®** *see Fluorescein Sodium on page 382*
- **5-Flurocytosine** *see Flucytosine on page 376*
- **Fluro-Ethyl® Aerosol** *see Ethyl Chloride and Dichlorotetrafluoroethane on page 353*
- **Flurosyn®** *see Fluocinolone on page 381*

## Flutamide (FLOO ta mide)

**Pharmacologic Class** Antiandrogen

**U.S. Brand Names** Eulexin®

**Mechanism of Action** Nonsteroidal antiandrogen that inhibits androgen uptake or inhibits binding of androgen in target tissues

**Use** In combination therapy with LHRH agonist analogues in treatment of metastatic prostatic carcinoma. A study has shown that the addition of flutamide to leuprolide therapy in patients with advanced prostatic cancer increased median actuarial survival time to 34.9 months versus 27.9 months with leuprolide alone. To achieve benefit to combination therapy, both drugs need to be started simultaneously.

**USUAL DOSAGE** Adults: Oral: 2 capsules every 8 hours for a total daily dose of 750 mg

**Dosage Forms Cap:** 125 mg

**Contraindications** Known hypersensitivity to flutamide

**Warnings/Precautions** The U.S. Food and Drug Administration (FDA) currently recommends that procedures for proper handling and disposal of antineoplastic agents be considered. Animal data (based on using doses higher than recommended for humans) produced testicular interstitial cell adenoma. Do not discontinue therapy without physician's advice.

**Pregnancy Risk Factor** D

**Adverse Reactions**
>10%:
Gastrointestinal: Nausea, vomiting, diarrhea
Genitourinary: Impotence
Endocrine & metabolic: Loss of libido, hot flashes
1% to 10%:
Endocrine & metabolic: Gynecomastia
Gastrointestinal: Anorexia
Neuromuscular & skeletal: Numbness in extremities
<1%: Hypertension, edema, drowsiness, nervousness, confusion, hepatitis

**Drug Interactions** CYP3A3/4 enzyme substrate

**Half-Life** 5-6 hours

**Special PA Issues**
Patient Education: Flutamide and the LHRH analog used for medical castration should be administered concomitantly. Frequent blood tests may be needed to monitor therapy. Take as directed. Do not discontinue before consulting prescriber. You may experience decrease libido or impotence, swelling of breasts, decreased appetite; frequent, small meals may help. Report chest pain, acute abdominal pain, yellowing of skin or eyes, changes (darkening) in color of urine or stool, respiratory changes, or difficulty in urination.
Monitoring Parameters: LFTs, tumor reduction, testosterone/estrogen, and phosphatase serum levels

- **Flutex®** *see Triamcinolone on page 928*

## Fluticasone (floo TIK a sone)

**Pharmacologic Class** Corticosteroid, Oral Inhaler; Corticosteroid, Nasal

**U.S. Brand Names** Cutivate™; Flonase®; Flovent®

**Mechanism of Action** Fluticasone belongs to a new group of corticosteroids which utilizes a fluorocarbothioate ester linkage at the 17 carbon position; extremely potent vasoconstrictive and anti-inflammatory activity; has a weak hypothalamic -pituitary- adrenocortical axis (HPA) inhibitory potency when applied topically, which gives the drug a high therapeutic index. The mechanism of action for all topical corticosteroids is believed to be a combination of three important properties: anti-inflammatory activity, immunosuppressive properties, and antiproliferative actions.

**Use**
Inhalation: Maintenance treatment of asthma as prophylactic therapy. It is also indicated for patients requiring oral corticosteroid therapy for asthma to assist in total discontinuation or reduction of total oral dose. NOT indicated for the relief of acute bronchospasm.
Intranasal: Management of seasonal and perennial allergic rhinitis in patients ≥12 years of age
Topical: Relief of inflammation and pruritus associated with corticosteroid-responsive dermatoses [medium potency topical corticosteroid]

**USUAL DOSAGE** Flovent® Rotadisk can now be used in children ≥4 years; Flovent® is still indicated for use ≥12 years of age
Adolescents:
Topical: Apply sparingly in a thin film twice daily
(Continued)

# Fluticasone *(Continued)*

Intranasal: Initially 1 spray (50 mcg/spray) per nostril once daily. Patients not adequately responding or patients with more severe symptoms may use 2 sprays (200 mcg) per nostril. Depending on response, dosage may be reduced to 100 mcg daily. Total daily dosage should not exceed 4 sprays (200 mcg)/day.

Adults:

Topical: Apply sparingly in a thin film twice daily

Inhalation, Oral:

### Recommended Oral Inhalation Doses

| Previous Therapy | Recommended Starting Dose | Recommended Highest Dose |
|---|---|---|
| Bronchodilator alone | 88 mcg twice daily | 440 mcg twice daily |
| Inhaled corticosteroids | 88–220 mcg twice daily | 440 mcg twice daily |
| Oral corticosteroids | 880 mcg twice daily | 880 mcg twice daily |

Intranasal: Initial: 2 sprays (50 mcg/spray) per nostril once daily; after the first few days, dosage may be reduced to 1 spray per nostril once daily for maintenance therapy; maximum total daily dose should not exceed 4 sprays (200 mcg)/day

**Dosage Forms Spray, aerc, oral inh (Flovent®):** 44 mcg/actuation (17.9 g = 60 actuations or 13 g = 120 actuations), 110 mcg/actuation (13 g = 120 actuations); 220 mcg/actuation (13 g = 120 actuations); **Spray, intranasal (Flonase®):** 50 mcg/actuation (9 g = 60 actuations, 16 g = 120 actuations); **Top (Cutivate™):** Crm: 0.05% (15 g, 30 g, 60 g), **Oint:** 0.005% (15 g, 60 g)

**Contraindications** Hypersensitivity to any component, bacterial infections, ophthalmic use

**Warnings/Precautions** Adverse systemic effects may occur when used on large areas of the body, denuded areas, for prolonged periods of time, with an occlusive dressing, and/or in infants or small children Controlled clinical studies have shown that inhaled and intranasal corticosteroids may cause a reduction in growth velocity in pediatric patients. Growth velocity provides a means of comparing the rate of growth among children of the same age.

In studies involving inhaled corticosteroids, the average reduction in growth velocity was approximately 1 cm (about $1/2$ of an inch) per year. It appears that the reduction is related to dose and how long the child takes the drug.

FDA's Pulmonary and Allergy Drugs and Metabolic and Endocrine Drugs advisory committees discussed this issue at a July 1998 meeting. They recommended that the agency develop class-wide labeling to inform healthcare providers so they would understand this potential side effect and monitor growth routinely in pediatric patients who are treated with inhaled corticosteroids, intranasal corticosteroids or both.

Long-term effects of this reduction in growth velocity on final adult height are unknown. Likewise, it also has not yet been determined whether patients' growth will "catch up" if treatment is discontinued. Drug manufacturers will continue to monitor these drugs to learn more about long-term effects. Children are prescribed inhaled corticosteroids to treat asthma. Intranasal corticosteroids are generally used to prevent and treat allergy-related nasal symptoms.

Patients are advised not to stop using their inhaled or intranasal corticosteroids without first speaking to their healthcare providers about the benefits of these drugs compared to their risks.

**Pregnancy Risk Factor** C

**Adverse Reactions**

\>10%: Oral inhalation:

Central nervous system: Headache

Respiratory: Respiratory infection, pharyngitis, nasal congestion

1% to 10%: Oral Inhalation:

Central nervous system: Dysphonia

Gastrointestinal: Oral candidiasis

Respiratory: Sinusitis

<1%: Acne, hypopigmentation, allergic dermatitis, maceration of the skin, skin atrophy, folliculitis, hypertrichosis, itching, dry skin, HPA suppression, Cushing's syndrome, growth retardation, burning, irritation, secondary infection

**Special PA Issues**

**Patient Education:** Use as directed; do not overuse and use only for length of time prescribed.

Topical: For external use only. Apply thin film of cream to affected area only; rub in lightly. Do not apply occlusive covering unless advised by prescriber. Wash hand thoroughly after use; avoid contact with eyes. Notify prescriber if skin condition persists or worsens.

Nasal spray: Shake gently before use. Use at regular intervals, no more frequently than directed. Report unusual cough or spasm; persistent nasal bleeding, burning, or irritation; or worsening of condition.

**Related Information**
Asthma Therapy Guidelines *on page 1049*

♦ **Fluticasone Propionate** *see* Fluticasone *on page 393*

# Fluvastatin (FLOO va sta tin)

**Pharmacologic Class** Antilipemic Agent (HMG-CoA Reductase Inhibitor)
**U.S. Brand Names** Lescol®
**Mechanism of Action** Acts by competitively inhibiting 3-hydroxyl-3-methylglutaryl-coenzyme A (HMG-CoA) reductase, the enzyme that catalyzes the reduction of HMG-CoA to mevalonate; this is an early rate-limiting step in cholesterol biosynthesis. HDL is increased while total, LDL and VLDL cholesterols, apolipoprotein B, and plasma triglycerides are decreased.
**Use** Adjunct to dietary therapy to decrease elevated serum total and LDL cholesterol concentrations in primary hypercholesterolemia
**USUAL DOSAGE** Adults: Oral:
Initial dose: 20-40 mg at bedtime
Usual dose: 20-80 mg at bedtime
**Note:** Splitting the 80 mg dose into a twice daily regimen may provide a modest improvement in LDL response; maximum response occurs within 4-6 weeks; decrease dose and monitor effects carefully in patients with hepatic insufficiency
**Dosage Forms Cap:** 20 mg, 40 mg
**Contraindications** Pregnancy; myopathy or marked elevations of CPK
**Warnings/Precautions** Avoid combination of clofibrate and fluvastatin due to possible myopathy; consider temporarily withholding therapy in patients with risk of developing renal failure; avoid prolonged exposure to the sun or other ultraviolet light
**Pregnancy Risk Factor** X
**Pregnancy Implications**
Clinical effects on the fetus: Skeletal malformations have occurred in animals following agents with similar structure; avoid use in women of childbearing age; discontinue if pregnancy occurs
Breast-feeding/lactation: Avoid use in nursing mothers
**Adverse Reactions**
>10%: Respiratory: Upper respiratory infection (16%)
1% to 10%:
Central nervous system: Headache (9%), dizziness (2%), insomnia (2% to 3%), fatigue (2% to 3%)
Dermatologic: Rash (2% to 3%)
Gastrointestinal: Dyspepsia (8%), diarrhea (5%), nausea/vomiting (3%), constipation (2% to 3%), flatulence (2% to 3%), abdominal pain (5%)
Neuromuscular & skeletal: Back pain/myalgia (5% to 6%), arthropathy (2% to 4%)
Miscellaneous: Cold/flu symptoms (2% to 5%)
**Drug Interactions** CYP2C9 enzyme substrate; CYP2C9, 2C18, and 2C19 enzyme inhibitor
Anticoagulant effect of warfarin, digoxin may be increased
Concurrent use of erythromycin, cyclosporine, niacin, gemfibrozil, and HMG-CoA reductase inhibitors may result in rhabdomyolysis
Increased effect/toxicity of fluvastatin with alcohol, itraconazole
Decreased effect of fluvastatin or other HMG-CoA reductase inhibitors with bile acid sequestrants, nicotinic acid, propranolol, rifampin, and digoxin
**Half-Life** 1.2 hours
**Special PA Issues**
**Patient Education:** Take at bedtime since highest rate of cholesterol synthesis occurs between midnight and 5 AM. Follow diet and exercise regimen as prescribed. Have periodic ophthalmic exam to check for cataract development. Avoid prolonged exposure to the sun and other ultraviolet light. Report unexplained muscle pain or weakness, especially if accompanied by fever or malaise.
**Related Information**
Lipid-Lowering Agents *on page 1022*

# Fluvoxamine (floo VOKS ah meen)

**Pharmacologic Class** Antidepressant, Selective Serotonin Reuptake Inhibitor
**U.S. Brand Names** Luvox®
**Mechanism of Action** Inhibits CNS neuron serotonin uptake; minimal or no effect on reuptake of norepinephrine or dopamine; does not significantly bind to alpha-adrenergic, histamine or cholinergic receptors
**Use** Treatment of obsessive-compulsive disorder (OCD); effective in the treatment of major depression; may be useful for the treatment of panic disorder
**USUAL DOSAGE**
Adults: Initial: 50 mg at bedtime; adjust in 50 mg increments at 4- to 7-day intervals; usual dose range: 100-300 mg/day; divide total daily dose into 2 doses; administer larger portion at bedtime
Elderly or hepatic impairment: Reduce dose, titrate slowly
(Continued)

## Fluvoxamine *(Continued)*

**Dosage Forms** Tab: 50 mg, 100 mg

**Contraindications** Concomitant terfenadine or astemizole; during or within 14 days of MAO inhibitors; hypersensitivity to fluvoxamine or any congeners (eg, fluoxetine)

**Warnings/Precautions** Use with caution in patients with liver dysfunction, suicidal tendencies, history of seizures, mania, or drug abuse, ECT, cardiovascular disease, and the elderly

**Pregnancy Risk Factor** C

### Adverse Reactions
>10%: Gastrointestinal: Nausea

1% to 10%:

Cardiovascular: Palpitations

Central nervous system: Somnolence, headache, insomnia, dizziness, nervousness, mania, hypomania, vertigo, abnormal thinking, agitation, anxiety, malaise, amnesia

Endocrine & metabolic: Decreased libido

Gastrointestinal: Xerostomia, abdominal pain, vomiting, dyspepsia, constipation, diarrhea, abnormal taste, anorexia

Neuromuscular & skeletal: Tremors, weakness

Miscellaneous: Diaphoresis

<1%: Seizures, toxic epidermal necrolysis, thrombocytopenia, hepatic dysfunction, increases in serum creatinine, extrapyramidal reactions

**Drug Interactions** CYP1A2 enzyme substrate; CYP1A2, 2C9, 2C19, 2D6, and 3A3/4 enzyme inhibitor

Increased toxicity: Terfenadine, astemizole, and cisapride are metabolized by the CYP3A4 isozyme, increased levels of these drugs have been associated with prolongation of the Q-T interval and potentially fatal, torsade de pointes ventricular arrhythmias. Since fluvoxamine inhibits the enzyme responsible for their clearance, the concomitant use of these agents is contraindicated.

Potentiates triazolam and alprazolam (dose should be reduced by at least 50%), hypertensive crisis with MAO inhibitors, theophylline (doses should be reduced by 1/3 and plasma levels monitored), warfarin (reduce its dose and monitor PT/INR), carbamazepine (monitor levels), tricyclic antidepressants (monitor effects and reduce doses accordingly), methadone, beta-blockers (reduce dose of propranolol or metoprolol), diltiazem. Caution with other benzodiazepines, phenytoin, lithium, clozapine, alcohol, other CNS drugs, quinidine, ketoconazole.

**Onset** >2 weeks for therapeutic effect

**Half-Life** ~15 hours

### Special PA Issues
**Patient Education:** Take exactly as directed (do not increase dose or frequency); may take 2-3 weeks to achieve desired results; may cause physical and/or psychological dependence. Take once-a-day dose at bedtime. Avoid excessive alcohol, caffeine, and other prescription or OTC medications not approved by prescriber. Maintain adequate hydration (2-3 L/day of fluids unless instructed to restrict fluid intake). You may experience drowsiness, lightheadedness, impaired coordination, dizziness, or blurred vision (use caution when driving or engaging in hazardous tasks until response to medication is known); nausea, vomiting, or anorexia (small frequent meals, frequent mouth care, or sucking lozenges may help); constipation (increased exercise, fluids, or dietary fruit and fiber may help); diarrhea (buttermilk, yogurt, or boiled milk may help); postural hypotension (use caution when climbing stairs or changing position from lying or sitting to standing); or decreased sexual function or libido (reversible). Report persistent CNS effects (nervousness, restlessness, insomnia, anxiety, excitation, headache, sedation, seizures, mania, abnormal thinking); rash or skin irritation; muscle cramping, tremors, or change in gait; chest pain or palpitations; change in urinary pattern; or worsening of condition.

**Dietary Considerations:** Alcohol: Additive CNS effect, avoid use

**Monitoring Parameters:** Signs and symptoms of depression, anxiety, weight gain or loss, nutritional intake, sleep

### Related Information
Antidepressant Agents *on page 998*

## Folic Acid (FOE lik AS id)

**Pharmacologic Class** Vitamin, Water Soluble

**U.S. Brand Names** Folvite®

**Mechanism of Action** Folic acid is necessary for formation of a number of coenzymes in many metabolic systems, particularly for purine and pyrimidine synthesis; required for nucleoprotein synthesis and maintenance in erythropoiesis; stimulates WBC and platelet production in folate deficiency anemia

**Use** Treatment of megaloblastic and macrocytic anemias due to folate deficiency; dietary supplement to prevent neural tube defects

**USUAL DOSAGE**

Infants: 0.1 mg/day

Children <4 years: Up to 0.3 mg/day

Children >4 years and Adults: 0.4 mg/day

Pregnant and lactating women: 0.8 mg/day

RDA:

Adult male: 0.15-0.2 mg/day

Adult female: 0.15-0.18 mg/day

**Dosage Forms** Inj, as sodium folate: 5 mg/mL (10 mL); 10 mg/mL (10 mL), Folvite®: 5 mg/mL (10 mL); **Tab:** 0.1 mg, 0.4 mg, 0.8 mg, 1 mg, Folvite®: 1 mg

**Contraindications** Pernicious, aplastic, or normocytic anemias

**Warnings/Precautions** Doses >0.1 mg/day may obscure pernicious anemia with continuing irreversible nerve damage progression. Resistance to treatment may occur with depressed hematopoiesis, alcoholism, deficiencies of other vitamins. Injection contains benzyl alcohol (1.5%) as preservative (use care in administration to neonates).

**Pregnancy Risk Factor** A (C if dose exceeds RDA recommendation)

**Adverse Reactions** <1%: Slight flushing, general malaise, pruritus, rash, bronchospasm, allergic reaction

**Drug Interactions** Decreased effect: In folate-deficient patients, folic acid therapy may increase phenytoin metabolism. Phenytoin, primidone, para-aminosalicylic acid, and sulfasalazine may decrease serum folate concentrations and cause deficiency. Oral contraceptives may also impair folate metabolism producing depletion, but the effect is unlikely to cause anemia or megaloblastic changes. Concurrent administration of chloramphenicol and folic acid may result in antagonism of the hematopoietic response to folic acid; dihydrofolate reductase inhibitors (eg, methotrexate, trimethoprim) may interfere with folic acid utilization.

**Onset** Peak effect: Oral: Within 0.5-1 hour

**Special PA Issues**

**Patient Education:** Take as prescribed. Toxicity can occur from elevated doses. Do not self medicate. Increase intake of foods high in folic acid (eg, dried beans, nuts, bran, vegetables, fruits) as recommended by prescriber. Excessive use of alcohol increases requirement for folic acid. May turn urine more intensely yellow. Report skin rash.

**Reference Range:** Therapeutic: 0.005-0.015 μg/mL

♦ **Folinic Acid** *see* Leucovorin *on page 520*

♦ **Follistim™** *see* Follitropins *on this page*

♦ **Follitropin Alpha** *see* Follitropins *on this page*

♦ **Follitropin Beta** *see* Follitropins *on this page*

## Follitropins (foe li TRO pins)

**Pharmacologic Class** Ovulation Stimulator

**U.S. Brand Names** Fertinex™; Follistim™; Gonal-F®

**Mechanism of Action** Urofollitropin is a preparation of highly purified follicle-stimulating hormone (FSH) extracted from the urine of postmenopausal women. Follitropin alpha and follitropin beta are human FSH preparations of recombinant DNA origin. Follitropins stimulate ovarian follicular growth in women who do not have primary ovarian failure. FSH is required for normal follicular growth, maturation, and gonadal steroid production.

**Use**

**Urofollitropin (Fertinex™):**

Polycystic ovary syndrome: Give sequentially with hCG for the stimulation of follicular recruitment and development and the induction of ovulation in patients with polycystic ovary syndrome and infertility, who have failed to respond or conceive following adequate clomiphene citrate therapy

Follicle stimulation: Stimulate the development of multiple follicles in ovulatory patients undergoing Assisted Reproductive Technologies such as *in vitro* fertilization

**Follitropin alpha (Gonal-F™)/follitropin beta (Follistim™):**

Ovulation induction: For the induction of ovulation and pregnancy in anovulatory infertile patients in whom the cause of infertility is functional and not caused by primary ovarian failure

Follicle stimulation: To stimulate the development of multiple follicles in ovulatory patients undergoing Assisted Reproductive Technologies such as *in vitro* fertilization

(Continued)

## Follitropins (Continued)

### USUAL DOSAGE

**Urofollitropin (Fertinex™):** Adults: S.C.:

Polycystic ovary syndrome: Initial recommended dose of the first cycle: 75 IU/day; consider dose adjustment after 5-7 days; additional dose adjustments may be considered based on individual patient response. The dose should not be increased more than twice in any cycle or by more than 75 IU per adjustment. To complete follicular development and affect ovulation in the absence of an endogenous LH surge, give 5000 to 10,000 units hCG, 1 day after the last dose of urofollitropin. Withhold hCG if serum estradiol is >2000 pg/mL.

Individualize the initial dose administered in subsequent cycles for each patient based on her response in the preceding cycle. Doses of >300 IU of FSH/day are not routinely recommended. As in the initial cycle, 5000 to 10,000 units of hCG must be given 1 day after the last dose of urofollitropin to complete follicular development and induce ovulation.

Give the lowest dose consistent with the expectation of good results. Over the course of treatment, doses may range between 75 to 300 IU/day depending on individual patient response. Administer urofollitropin until adequate follicular development as indicated by serum estradiol and vaginal ultrasonography. A response is generally evident after 5-7 days.

Encourage the couple to have intercourse daily, beginning on the day prior to the administration of hCG until ovulation becomes apparent from the indices employed for determination of progestational activity. Take care to ensure insemination.

Follicle stimulation: For Assisted Reproductive Technologies, initiate therapy with urofollitropin in the early follicular phase (cycle day 2 or 3) at a dose of 150 IU/day, until sufficient follicular development is attained. In most cases, therapy should not exceed 10 days.

**Follitropin alpha (Gonal-F®):** Adults: S.C.:

Ovulation induction: Initial recommended dose of the first cycle: 75 IU/day. Consider dose adjustment after 5-7 days; additional dose adjustments of up to 37.5 IU may be considered after 14 days. Further dose increases of the same magnitude can be made, if necessary, every 7 days. To complete follicular development and affect ovulation in the absence of an endogenous LH surge, give 5000 to 10,000 units hCG, 1 day after the last dose of follitropin alpha. Withhold hCG if serum estradiol is >2000 pg/mL.

Individualize the initial dose administered in subsequent cycles for each patient based on her response in the preceding cycle. Doses of >300 IU of FSH/day are not routinely recommended. As in the initial cycle, 5000 to 10,000 units of hCG must be given 1 day after the last dose of urofollitropin to complete follicular development and induce ovulation.

Give the lowest dose consistent with the expectation of good results. Over the course of treatment, doses may range between 75 to 300 IU/day depending on individual patient response. Administer urofollitropin until adequate follicular development as indicated by serum estradiol and vaginal ultrasonography. A response is generally evident after 5-7 days.

Encourage the couple to have intercourse daily, beginning on the day prior to the administration of hCG until ovulation becomes apparent from the indices employed for determination of progestational activity. Take care to ensure insemination.

Follicle stimulation: Initiate therapy with follitropin alpha in the early follicular phase (cycle day 2 or 3) at a dose of 150 IU/day, until sufficient follicular development is attained. In most cases, therapy should not exceed 10 days.

In patients undergoing Assisted Reproductive Technologies, whose endogenous gonadotropin levels are suppressed, initiate follitropin alpha at a dose of 225 IU/day. Continue treatment until adequate follicular development is indicated as determined by ultrasound in combination with measurement of serum estradiol levels. Consider adjustments to dose after 5 days based on the patient's response; adjust subsequent dosage every 3-5 days by ≤75-150 IU additionally at each adjustment. Doses >450 IU/day are not recommended. Once adequate follicular development is evident, administer hCG (5000-10,000 units) to induce final follicular maturation in preparation for oocyte.

**Follitropin beta (Follistim™):** Adults: S.C. or I.M.:

Ovulation induction: Stepwise approach: Initiate therapy with 75 IU/day for up to 14 days. Increase by 37.5 IU at weekly intervals until follicular growth or serum estradiol levels indicate an adequate response. The maximum, individualized, daily dose that has been safely used for ovulation induction in patients during clinical trials is 300 IU. Treat the patient until ultrasonic visualizations or serum estradiol determinations indicate preovulatory conditions greater than or equal to normal values followed by 5000 to 10,000 units hCG.

During treatment and during a 2-week post-treatment period, examine patients at least every other day for signs of excessive ovarian stimulation. Discontinue follitropin beta administration if the ovaries become abnormally enlarged or abdominal pain occurs.

Encourage the couple to have intercourse daily, beginning on the day prior to the administration of hCG until ovulation becomes apparent from the indices employed for determination of progestational activity. Take care to ensure insemination.

Follicle stimulation: A starting dose of 150-225 IU of follitropin beta is recommended for at least the first 4 days of treatment. The dose may be adjusted for the individual patient based upon their ovarian response. Daily maintenance doses ranging from 75-300 IU for 6-12 days are usually sufficient, although longer treatment may be necessary. However, maintenance doses of up to 375-600 IU may be necessary according to individual response. The maximum daily dose used in clinical studies is 600 IU. When a sufficient number of follicles of adequate size are present, the final maturation of the follicles is induced by administering hCG at a dose of 5000-10,000 IU. Oocyte retrieval is performed 34-36 hours later. Withhold hCG in cases where the ovaries are abnormally enlarged on the last day of follitropin beta therapy.

**Dosage Forms Powder for inj**: Urofollitropin (Fertinex®): 75 international units (1, 10, 100 mL ampuls with diluent), 150 international units (1 mL ampuls with diluent); Follitropin alpha (Gonal-F®): 75 international units (1, 10, 100 mL ampuls with diluent), 150 international units (1 mL ampuls with diluent); Follitropin beta (Follistim®): 75 international units (1, 5 mL vials with diluent)

**Contraindications** High levels of FSH indicating primary ovarian failure; uncontrolled thyroid or adrenal dysfunction; the presence of any cause of infertility other than anovulation; tumor of the ovary, breast, uterus, hypothalamus, or pituitary gland; abnormal vaginal bleeding of undetermined origin; ovarian cysts or enlargement not due to polycystic ovary syndrome; hypersensitivity to the product or any of its components; pregnancy

**Warnings/Precautions** These medications should only be used by physicians who are thoroughly familiar with infertility problems and their management. To minimize risks, use only at the lowest effective dose. Monitor ovarian response with serum estradiol and vaginal ultrasound on a regular basis.

Ovarian enlargement which may be accompanied by abdominal distention or abdominal pain, occurs in ~20% of those treated with urofollitropin and hCG, and generally regresses without treatment within 2-3 weeks. Ovarian hyperstimulation syndrome, characterized by severe ovarian enlargement, abdominal pain/distention, nausea, vomiting, diarrhea, dyspnea, and oliguria, and may be accompanied by ascites, pleural effusion, hypovolemia, electrolyte imbalance, hemoperitoneum, and thromboembolic events is reported in about 6% of patients. If hyperstimulation occurs, stop treatment and hospitalize patient. This syndrome develops rapidly within 24 hours to several days and generally occurs during the 7-10 days immediately following treatment. Hemoconcentration associated with fluid loss into the abdominal cavity has occurred and should be assessed by fluid intake & output, weight, hematocrit, serum & urinary electrolytes, urine specific gravity, BUN and creatinine, and abdominal girth. Determinations should be performed daily or more often if the need arises. Treatment is primarily symptomatic and consists of bed rest, fluid and electrolyte replacement and analgesics. The ascitic, pleural and pericardial fluids should never be removed because of the potential danger of injury.

Serious pulmonary conditions (atelectasis, acute respiratory distress syndrome and exacerbation of asthma) have been reported. Thromboembolic events, both in association with and separate from ovarian hyperstimulation syndrome, have been reported.

Multiple pregnancies have been associated with these medications, including triplet and quintuplet gestations. Advise patient of the potential risk of multiple births before starting the treatment.

**Pregnancy Risk Factor** X

**Adverse Reactions** 1% to 10%:

Dermatologic: Dry skin, body rash, hair loss, hives

Endocrine & metabolic: Ovarian hyperstimulation syndrome, adnexal torsion, mild to moderate ovarian enlargement, abdominal pain, ovarian cysts, breast tenderness

Gastrointestinal: Nausea, vomiting, diarrhea, abdominal cramps, bloating

Local: Pain, rash, swelling, or irritation at the site of injection

Respiratory: Atelectasis, acute respiratory distress syndrome, exacerbation of asthma

Miscellaneous: Febrile reactions accompanied by chills, musculoskeletal, joint pains, malaise, headache, and fatigue

**Special PA Issues**

**Patient Education:** Discontinue immediately if possibility of pregnancy. Prior to therapy, inform patients of the following: Duration of treatment and monitoring required; possible adverse reactions; risk of multiple births.

**Monitoring Parameters:** Monitor sufficient follicular maturation. This may be directly estimated by sonographic visualization of the ovaries and endometrial lining or measuring serum estradiol levels. The combination of both ultrasonography and measurement of estradiol levels is useful for monitoring for the growth and development of follicles and timing hCG administration.

The clinical evaluation of estrogenic activity (changes in vaginal cytology and changes in appearance and volume of cervical mucus) provides an indirect estimate of the estrogenic effect upon the target organs and, therefore, it should only be used adjunctively

(Continued)

## Follitropins *(Continued)*

with more direct estimates of follicular development (ultrasonography and serum estradiol determinations).

The clinical confirmation of ovulation is obtained by direct and indirect indices of progesterone production. The indices most generally used are: rise in basal body temperature, increase in serum progesterone, and menstruation following the shift in basal body temperature.

♦ **Follutein®** *see* Chorionic Gonadotropin *on page 205*

♦ **Folvite®** *see* Folic Acid *on page 397*

# Fomivirsen *(foe MI vir sen)*

**Pharmacologic Class** Antiviral Agent, Ophthalmic

**U.S. Brand Names** Vitravene™

**Mechanism of Action** Inhibits synthesis of viral protein by binding to mRNA which blocks replication of cytomegalovirus through an antisense mechanism

**Use** Local treatment of cytomegalovirus (CMV) retinitis in patients with acquired immunodeficiency syndrome who are intolerant or insufficiently responsive to other treatments for CMV retinitis or when other treatments for CMV retinitis are contraindicated

**USUAL DOSAGE** Adults: Intravitreal injection: Induction: 330 mcg (0.05 mL) every other week for 2 doses, followed by maintenance dose of 330 mcg (0.05 mL) every 4 weeks

If progression occurs during maintenance, a repeat of the induction regimen may be attempted to establish resumed control. Unacceptable inflammation during therapy may be managed by temporary interruption, provided response has been established. Topical corticosteroids have been used to reduce inflammation.

**Dosage Forms Soln, for ocular inj:** 6.6 mg/mL (0.25 mL)

**Contraindications** Hypersensitivity to fomivirsen or any component

**Warnings/Precautions** For ophthalmic use via intravitreal injection only. Uveitis occurs frequently, particularly during induction dosing. Do not use in patients who have received intravenous or intravitreal cidofovir within 2-4 weeks (risk of exaggerated inflammation is increased). Patients should be monitored for CMV disease in the contralateral eye and/or extraocular disease. Commonly increases intraocular pressure - monitoring is recommended.

**Pregnancy Risk Factor** C

**Pregnancy Implications** Studies have not been conducted in pregnant women. Should be used in pregnancy only when potential benefit to the mother outweighs the potential risk to the fetus. Excretion in human milk is unknown. Use during breast-feeding is contraindicated - a decision to discontinue nursing or discontinue the drug is should be made.

**Adverse Reactions**

5% to 10%:

Central nervous system: Fever, headache

Gastrointestinal: Abdominal pain, diarrhea, nausea, vomiting

Hematologic: Anemia

Neuromuscular & skeletal: Asthenia

Ocular: Uveitis, abnormal vision, anterior chamber inflammation, blurred vision, cataract, conjunctival hemorrhage, decreased visual acuity, loss of color vision, eye pain, increased intraocular pressure, photophobia, retinal detachment, retinal edema, retinal hemorrhage, retinal pigment changes, vitreitis

Respiratory: Pneumonia, sinusitis

Miscellaneous: Systemic CMV, sepsis, infection

2% to 5%:

Cardiovascular: Chest pain

Central nervous system: Confusion, depression, dizziness, neuropathy, pain

Endocrine and metabolic: Dehydration

Gastrointestinal: Abnormal LFTs, pancreatitis, anorexia, weight loss

Hematologic: Thrombocytopenia, lymphoma

Neuromuscular & skeletal: Back pain, cachexia

Ocular: Application site reaction, conjunctival hyperemia, conjunctivitis, corneal edema, decreased peripheral vision, eye irritation, keratic precipitates, optic neuritis, photopsia, retinal vascular disease, visual field defect, vitreous hemorrhage, vitreous opacity

Renal: Kidney failure

Respiratory: Bronchitis, dyspnea, cough

Miscellaneous: Allergic reaction, flu-like syndrome, diaphoresis (increased)

**Drug Interactions** Drug interactions between fomivirsen and other medications have not been conducted.

**Special PA Issues**

**Monitoring Parameters:** Immediately after injection, light perception and optic nerve head perfusion should be monitored. Anterior chamber paracentesis may be necessary if perfusion is not complete within 7-10 minutes after injection. Subsequent patient evaluation should include monitoring for contralateral CMV infection or extraocular CMV disease, and intraocular pressure prior to each injection.

- **Fomivirsen Sodium** *see Fomivirsen on previous page*
- **Food-Drug Interactions, Key Summary** *see Chart on page 1130*
- **Formula Q®** *see Quinine on page 790*
- **Formulex®** *see Dicyclomine on page 273*
- **5-Formyl Tetrahydrofolate** *see Leucovorin on page 520*
- **Fortaz®** *see Ceftazidime on page 172*
- **Fortovase®** *see Saquinavir on page 821*
- **Fosamax®** *see Alendronate on page 38*

# Foscarnet (fos KAR net)

**Pharmacologic Class** Antiviral Agent

**U.S. Brand Names** Foscavir® Injection

**Mechanism of Action** Pyrophosphate analogue which acts as a noncompetitive inhibitor of many viral RNA and DNA polymerases as well as HIV reverse transcriptase. Similar to ganciclovir, foscarnet is a virostatic agent. Foscarnet does not require activation by thymidine kinase.

**Use**

Herpesvirus infections suspected to be caused by acyclovir - (HSV, VZV) or ganciclovir - (CMV) resistant strains (this occurs almost exclusively in immunocompromised persons, eg, with advanced AIDS), who have received prolonged treatment for a herpesvirus infection

CMV retinitis in persons with AIDS

Other CMV infections in persons unable to tolerate ganciclovir; may be given in combination with ganciclovir in patients who relapse after monotherapy with either drug

**USUAL DOSAGE** Adolescents and Adults: I.V.:

CMV retinitis:

Induction treatment: 60 mg/kg/dose every 8 hours **or** 100 mg/kg every 12 hours for 14-21 days

Maintenance therapy: 90-120 mg/kg/day as a single infusion

Acyclovir-resistant HSV induction treatment: 40 mg/kg/dose every 8-12 hours for 14-21 days

**Dosage adjustment in renal impairment:** Refer to tables

### Induction Dosing of Foscarnet in Patients with Abnormal Renal Function

| $Cl_{cr}$ (mL/min/kg) | HSV<br>Equivalent to 40 mg/kg q12h | HSV<br>Equivalent to 40 mg/kg q8h | CMV<br>Equivalent to 60 mg/kg q8h |
|---|---|---|---|
| <0.4 | not recommended | not recommended | not recommended |
| ≥0.4-0.5 | 20 mg/kg every 24 hours | 35 mg/kg every 24 hours | 50 mg/kg every 24 hours |
| ≥0.5-0.6 | 25 mg/kg every 24 hours | 40 mg/kg every 24 hours | 60 mg/kg every 24 hours |
| ≥0.6-0.8 | 35 mg/kg every 24 hours | 25 mg/kg every 12 hours | 40 mg/kg every 12 hours |
| ≥0.8-1.0 | 20 mg/kg every 12 hours | 35 mg/kg every 12 hours | 50 mg/kg every 12 hours |
| ≥1.0-1.4 | 30 mg/kg every 12 hours | 30 mg/kg every 8 hours | 45 mg/kg every 8 hours |
| 1.4 | 40 mg/kg every 12 hours | 40 mg/kg every 8 hours | 60 mg/kg every 8 hours |

### Maintenance Dosing of Foscarnet in Patients with Abnormal Renal Function

| $Cl_{cr}$ (mL/min/kg) | CMV<br>Equivalent to 90 mg/kg q24h | CMV<br>Equivalent to 120 mg/kg q24h |
|---|---|---|
| <0.4 | not recommended | not recommended |
| ≥0.4-0.5 | 50 mg/kg every 48 hours | 65 mg/kg every 48 hours |
| ≥0.5-0.6 | 60 mg/kg every 48 hours | 80 mg/kg every 48 hours |
| ≥0.6-0.8 | 80 mg/kg every 48 hours | 105 mg/kg every 48 hours |
| ≥0.8-1.0 | 50 mg/kg every 24 hours | 65 mg/kg every 24 hours |
| ≥1-1.4 | 70 mg/kg every 24 hours | 90 mg/kg every 24 hours |
| ≥1.4 | 90 mg/kg every 24 hours | 120 mg/kg every 24 hours |

**Hemodialysis:**

Foscarnet is highly removed by hemodialysis (30% in 4 hours HD)

(Continued)

## Foscarnet *(Continued)*

Doses of 50 mg/kg/dose posthemodialysis have been found to produce similar serum concentrations as doses of 90 mg/kg twice daily in patients with normal renal function

Doses of 60-90 mg/kg/dose loading dose (posthemodialysis) followed by 45 mg/kg/dose posthemodialysis (3 times/week) with the monitoring of weekly plasma concentrations to maintain peak plasma concentrations in the range of 400-800 µMolar has been recommended by some clinicians

Continuous arteriovenous or venovenous hemodiafiltration (CAVH) effects: Dose as for $Cl_{cr}$ 10-50 mL/minute

**Dosage Forms** Inj: 24 mg/mL (250 mL, 500 mL)

**Contraindications** Hypersensitivity to foscarnet, $Cl_{cr}$ <0.4 mL/minute/kg during therapy

**Warnings/Precautions** Renal impairment occurs to some degree in the majority of patients treated with foscarnet; renal impairment may occur at any time and is usually reversible within 1 week following dose adjustment or discontinuation of therapy, however, several patients have died with renal failure within 4 weeks of stopping foscarnet; therefore, renal function should be closely monitored. Foscarnet is deposited in teeth and bone of young, growing animals; it has adversely affected tooth enamel development in rats; safety and effectiveness in children have not been studied. Imbalance of serum electrolytes or minerals occurs in 6% to 18% of patients (hypocalcemia, low ionized calcium, hypo- or hyperphosphatemia, hypomagnesemia or hypokalemia).

Patients with a low ionized calcium may experience perioral tingling, numbness, paresthesias, tetany, and seizures. Seizures have been experienced by up to 10% of AIDS patients. Risk factors for seizures include a low baseline absolute neutrophil count (ANC), impaired baseline renal function and low total serum calcium. Some patients who have experienced seizures have died, while others have been able to continue or resume foscarnet treatment after their mineral or electrolyte abnormality has been corrected, their underlying disease state treated, or their dose decreased. Foscarnet has been shown to be mutagenic *in vitro* and in mice at very high doses. Information on the use of foscarnet is lacking in the elderly; dose adjustments and proper monitoring must be performed because of the decreased renal function common in older patients.

**Pregnancy Risk Factor** C

**Adverse Reactions**

>10%:

Central nervous system: Fever (65%), headache (26%), seizures (10%)

Gastrointestinal: Nausea (47%), diarrhea (30%), vomiting

Hematologic: Anemia (33%)

Renal: Abnormal renal function/decreased creatinine clearance (27%)

1% to 10%:

Central nervous system: Fatigue, malaise, dizziness, hypoesthesia, depression/confusion/anxiety (≥5%)

Dermatologic: Rash

Endocrine & metabolic: Electrolyte imbalance (especially potassium, calcium, magnesium, and phosphorus)

Gastrointestinal: Anorexia

Hematologic: Granulocytopenia, leukopenia (≥5%), thrombocytopenia, thrombosis

Local: Injection site pain

Neuromuscular & skeletal: Paresthesia, involuntary muscle contractions, rigors, neuropathy (peripheral), weakness

Ocular: Vision abnormalities

Respiratory: Coughing, dyspnea (≥5%)

Miscellaneous: Sepsis, diaphoresis (increased)

<1%: Cardiac failure, bradycardia, arrhythmias, cerebral edema, leg edema, peripheral edema, syncope, substernal chest pain, hypothermia, abnormal crying, malignant hyperpyrexia, vertigo, coma, speech disorders, gynecomastia, decreased gonadotropins, cholecystitis, cholelithiasis, hepatitis, hepatosplenomegaly, ascites, abnormal gait, dyskinesia, hypertonia, nystagmus, vocal cord paralysis

**Drug Interactions** Increased toxicity: Pentamidine increases hypocalcemia; concurrent use with ciprofloxacin increases seizure potential; acute renal failure (reversible) has been reported with cyclosporin due most likely to toxic synergistic effect; other nephrotoxic drugs (amphotericin B, I.V. pentamidine, aminoglycosides, etc) should be avoided, if possible, to minimize additive renal risk with foscarnet

**Half-Life** ~3 hours

**Special PA Issues**

**Patient Education:** Foscarnet is not a cure for the disease; progression may occur during or following therapy. Regular ophthalmic examinations will be necessary. While on the therapy it is important to maintain adequate nutrition and hydration (2-3 L/day of fluids unless instructed to restrict fluid intake) ; small frequent meals may help. Do not use alcohol or OTC medications without consulting prescriber. You may experience dizziness or confusion; use caution when driving or performing tasks that require alertness. Report unresolved diarrhea or vomiting, unusual fever, chills, sore throat, unhealed sores, swollen lymph glands or extreme, or malaise. Barrier contraceptives are recommended to reduce transmission of disease.

♦ **Foscavir® Injection** *see Foscarnet on page 401*

# Fosinopril (foe SIN oh pril)

**Pharmacologic Class** Angiotensin-Converting Enzyme (ACE) Inhibitors

**U.S. Brand Names** Monopril®

**Mechanism of Action** Competitive inhibitor of angiotensin-converting enzyme (ACE); prevents conversion of angiotensin I to angiotensin II, a potent vasoconstrictor; results in lower levels of angiotensin II which causes an increase in plasma renin activity and a reduction in aldosterone secretion; a CNS mechanism may also be involved in hypotensive effect as angiotensin II increases adrenergic outflow from CNS; vasoactive kallikreins may be decreased in conversion to active hormones by ACE inhibitors, thus reducing blood pressure

**Use** Treatment of hypertension, either alone or in combination with other antihypertensive agents; congestive heart failure; believed to prolong survival in heart failure

**USUAL DOSAGE** Adults: Oral:

Hypertension: Initial: 10 mg/day; most patients are maintained on 20-40 mg/day; may need to divide the dose into two if trough effect is inadequate; discontinue the diuretic, if possible 2-3 days before initiation of therapy; resume diuretic therapy carefully, if needed.

Heart failure: Initial: 10 mg/day (5 mg if renal dysfunction present) and increase, as needed, to a maximum of 40 mg once daily over several weeks; usual dose: 20-40 mg/day; if hypotension, orthostasis, or azotemia occur during titration, consider decreasing concomitant diuretic dose, if any

**Dosing adjustment/comments in renal impairment:** None needed since hepatobiliary elimination compensates adequately diminished renal elimination

Hemodialysis: Moderately dialyzable (20% to 50%)

**Dosage Forms Tab:** 10 mg, 20 mg

**Contraindications** Renal impairment, collagen vascular disease, hypersensitivity to fosinopril, any component, or other angiotensin-converting enzyme inhibitors

**Warnings/Precautions** Use with caution and modify dosage in patients with renal impairment (decrease dosage) (especially renal artery stenosis), severe congestive heart failure or with coadministered diuretic therapy; experience in children is limited. Severe hypotension may occur in patients who are sodium and/or volume depleted; initiate lower doses and monitor closely when starting therapy in these patients.

**Pregnancy Risk Factor** C (1st trimester); D (2nd and 3rd trimester)

**Adverse Reactions**

1% to 10%:

Cardiovascular: Orthostatic hypotension (especially after initial dose)

Central nervous system: Headache (3%), dizziness (1% to 2%), fatigue (1% to 2%)

Gastrointestinal: Diarrhea/nausea/vomiting (1% to 2%)

Respiratory: Cough (2%)

<1%: Syncope, hypotension, hypertensive crisis, claudication, edema, vertigo, insomnia, memory disturbance, drowsiness, angioedema, rash, hypoglycemia, hyperkalemia, abnormal taste, dysphagia, abdominal distention, dyspepsia, impotence, neutropenia, agranulocytosis, anemia, muscle cramps, tremor, deterioration in renal function, cold/flu symptoms

**Drug Interactions** Increased toxicity: See Drug-Drug Interactions With ACEIs *on page 997*

**Onset** 1 hour

**Duration** 24 hours

**Half-Life** Serum (fosinoprilat): 12 hours

**Special PA Issues**

**Patient Education:** Take as directed; do not change dosage or stop taking without consulting prescriber. Do not change amount of dietary salt without advice or consult of prescriber. You may experience dizziness, fainting, or fatigue (use caution when driving or performing hazardous tasks and use caution when changing position - rising from sitting or lying position) until response to therapy is established. You may experience sexual dysfunction (this will resolve when drug is discontinued), dry cough (not dangerous), or gastric upset and diarrhea (usually temporary). Report swelling of hands, feet, mouth, or face (or difficulty swallowing); persistent sore throat; fever; rash; respiratory difficulty; chest pains or irregular heartbeat; persistent cough; unresolved diarrhea or vomiting; excessive perspiration; or dehydration.

**Monitoring Parameters:** Blood pressure (supervise for at least 2 hours after the initial dose or any increase for significant orthostasis); serum potassium, calcium, creatinine, BUN, WBC

**Related Information**

ACE Inhibitors *on page 995*

Heart Failure: Management of Patients with Left Ventricular Systolic Dysfunction *on page 1064*

Drug-Drug Interactions With ACEIs *on page 997*

- **Fragmin®** *see* Dalteparin *on page 251*
- **Froben®** *see* Flurbiprofen *on page 391*
- **Froben-SR®** *see* Flurbiprofen *on page 391*
- **Frusemide** *see* Furosemide *on next page*
- **FS Shampoo®** *see* Fluocinolone *on page 381*
- **5-FU** *see* Fluorouracil *on page 384*
- **Ful-Glo®** *see* Fluorescein Sodium *on page 382*
- **Fulvicin® P/G** *see* Griseofulvin *on page 426*
- **Fulvicin-U/F®** *see* Griseofulvin *on page 426*
- **Fumasorb® [OTC]** *see* Ferrous Fumarate *on page 366*
- **Fumerin® [OTC]** *see* Ferrous Fumarate *on page 366*
- **Funduscein®** *see* Fluorescein Sodium *on page 382*
- **Fungoid® Creme** *see* Miconazole *on page 604*
- **Fungoid® Solution** *see* Clotrimazole *on page 228*
- **Fungoid® Tincture** *see* Miconazole *on page 604*
- **Furacin® Topical** *see* Nitrofurazone *on page 660*
- **Furadantin®** *see* Nitrofurantoin *on page 659*
- **Furalan®** *see* Nitrofurantoin *on page 659*
- **Furamide®** *see* Diloxanide Furoate *on page 286*
- **Furan®** *see* Nitrofurantoin *on page 659*
- **Furanite®** *see* Nitrofurantoin *on page 659*

## Furazolidone (fyoor a ZOE li done)

**Pharmacologic Class** Antiprotozoal

**U.S. Brand Names** Furoxone®

**Mechanism of Action** Inhibits several vital enzymatic reactions causing antibacterial and antiprotozoal action

**Use** Treatment of bacterial or protozoal diarrhea and enteritis caused by susceptible organisms *Giardia lamblia* and *Vibrio cholerae*

**USUAL DOSAGE** Oral:

Children >1 month: 5-8 mg/kg/day in 4 divided doses for 7 days, not to exceed 400 mg/day or 8.8 mg/kg/day

Adults: 100 mg 4 times/day for 7 days

**Dosage Forms Liq:** 50 mg/15 mL (60 mL, 473 mL); **Tab:** 100 mg

**Contraindications** Known hypersensitivity to furazolidone; concurrent use of alcohol; patients <1 month of age because of the possibility of producing hemolytic anemia

**Warnings/Precautions** Use caution in patients with G-6-PD deficiency when administering large doses for prolonged periods; furazolidone inhibits monoamine oxidase

**Pregnancy Risk Factor** C

**Adverse Reactions**

>10%: Genitourinary: Discoloration of urine (dark yellow to brown)

1% to 10%:

Central nervous system: Headache

Gastrointestinal: Abdominal pain, diarrhea, nausea, vomiting

<1%: Orthostatic hypotension, fever, dizziness, drowsiness, malaise, rash, hypoglycemia, disulfiram-like reaction after alcohol ingestion, leukopenia, agranulocytosis, hemolysis in patients with G-6-PD deficiency, arthralgia

**Drug Interactions**

Increases toxicity of sympathomimetic amines, tricyclic antidepressants, MAO inhibitors, meperidine, anorexiants, dextromethorphan, fluoxetine, paroxetine, sertraline, trazodone

Increased effect/toxicity of levodopa

Disulfiram-like reaction with alcohol

**Special PA Issues**

**Patient Education:** Take as directed. Avoid alcohol and tyramine-containing foods during and for 4 days following therapy. Do not take any other prescription or OTC medications without consulting prescriber. Your urine may turn dark brown or yellow (normal). If diabetic, use something other than Clinitest® for urine glucose testing. Report acute GI pain, unresolved diarrhea, unresolved nausea or vomiting, fever, dizziness, or unusual joint pain. Consult prescriber if condition is not resolved at the end of therapy.

**Dietary Considerations:**

Alcohol: Avoid use

Food: Marked elevation of blood pressure, hypertensive crisis, or hemorrhagic stroke may occur with foods high in amine content

**Monitoring Parameters:** CBC

**Related Information**

Tyramine-Containing Foods *on page 1148*

- **Furazosin** *see* Prazosin *on page 750*

## Furosemide (fyoor OH se mide)

**Pharmacologic Class** Diuretic, Loop

**U.S. Brand Names** Lasix®

**Mechanism of Action** Inhibits reabsorption of sodium and chloride in the ascending loop of Henle and distal renal tubule, interfering with the chloride-binding cotransport system, thus causing increased excretion of water, sodium, chloride, magnesium, and calcium

**Use** Management of edema associated with congestive heart failure and hepatic or renal disease; used alone or in combination with antihypertensives in treatment of hypertension

**USUAL DOSAGE**

Infants and Children:

    Oral: 1-2 mg/kg/dose increased in increments of 1 mg/kg/dose with each succeeding dose until a satisfactory effect is achieved to a maximum of 6 mg/kg/dose no more frequently than 6 hours

    I.M., I.V.: 1 mg/kg/dose, increasing by each succeeding dose at 1 mg/kg/dose at intervals of 6-12 hours until a satisfactory response up to 6 mg/kg/dose

Adults:

    Oral: 20-80 mg/dose initially increased in increments of 20-40 mg/dose at intervals of 6-8 hours; usual maintenance dose interval is twice daily or every day; may be titrated up to 600 mg/day with severe edematous states

    I.M., I.V.: 20-40 mg/dose, may be repeated in 1-2 hours as needed and increased by 20 mg/dose until the desired effect has been obtained; usual dosing interval: 6-12 hours; for acute pulmonary edema, the usual dose is 40 mg I.V. over 1-2 minutes; if not adequate, may increase dose to 80 mg

    Continuous I.V. infusion: Initial I.V. bolus dose of 0.1 mg/kg followed by continuous I.V. infusion doses of 0.1 mg/kg/hour doubled every 2 hours to a maximum of 0.4 mg/kg/hour if urine output is <1 mL/kg/hour have been found to be effective and result in a lower daily requirement of furosemide than with intermittent dosing. Other studies have used a rate of ≤4 mg/minute as a continuous I.V. infusion.

Elderly: Oral, I.M., I.V.: Initial: 20 mg/day; increase slowly to desired response

Refractory heart failure: Oral, I.V.: Doses up to 8 g/day have been used

**Dosing adjustment/comments in renal impairment:** Acute renal failure: High doses (up to 1-3 g/day - oral/I.V.) have been used to initiate desired response; avoid use in oliguric states

Dialysis: Not removed by hemo- or peritoneal dialysis; supplemental dose is not necessary

**Dosing adjustment/comments in hepatic disease:** Diminished natriuretic effect with increased sensitivity to hypokalemia and volume depletion in cirrhosis; monitor effects, particularly with high doses

**Dosage Forms Inj:** 10 mg/mL (2 mL, 4 mL, 5 mL, 6 mL, 8 mL, 10 mL, 12 mL); **Soln, oral:** 10 mg/mL (60 mL, 120 mL); 40 mg/5 mL (5 mL, 10 mL, 500 mL); **Tab:** 20 mg, 40 mg, 80 mg

**Contraindications** Hypersensitivity to furosemide, any component, or other sulfonamides; use with sparfloxacin; anuric patients

**Warnings/Precautions** Loop diuretics are potent diuretics; close medical supervision and dose evaluation is required to prevent fluid and electrolyte imbalance; use caution with other nephrotoxic or ototoxic drugs

**Pregnancy Risk Factor** C

**Pregnancy Implications**

Clinical effects on the fetus: Crosses the placenta. Increased fetal urine production, electrolyte disturbances reported. Generally, use of diuretics during pregnancy is avoided due to risk of decreased placental perfusion.

Breast-feeding/lactation: Crosses into breast milk; may suppress lactation. American Academy of Pediatrics has NO RECOMMENDATION.

**Adverse Reactions**

>10%:

    Cardiovascular: Orthostatic hypotension

    Central nervous system: Dizziness

1% to 10%:

    Central nervous system: Headache

    Dermatologic: Photosensitivity

    Endocrine & metabolic: Electrolyte imbalance (hypokalemia, hyponatremia, hypochloremia, hypercalciuria, hyperuricemia), alkalosis, dehydration

    Gastrointestinal: Diarrhea, loss of appetite, stomach cramps or pain

    Ocular: Blurred vision

<1%: Rash, pancreatitis, nausea, hepatic dysfunction, agranulocytosis, leukopenia, anemia, thrombocytopenia, redness at injection site, gout, xanthopsia, ototoxicity, nephrocalcinosis, interstitial nephritis, prerenal azotemia

**Drug Interactions**

Decreased effect:

    Furosemide interferes with hypoglycemic effect of antidiabetic agents; decreased furosemide concentrations with metformin have been observed

    Furosemide may antagonize the skeletal muscle relaxing effect of tubocurarine and decrease the responsiveness of norepinephrine (although not to a major extent)

    Indomethacin may reduce natriuretic and hypotensive effects of furosemide

(Continued)

## Furosemide *(Continued)*

Furosemide effects may be significantly decreased when given within 2 hours of sucralfate

Increased effect: Effects of antihypertensive agents may be enhanced

Increased toxicity:

High-dose salicylates with furosemide may predispose patients to salicylate toxicity due to competitive renal excretory sites

Lithium → renal clearance decreased; furosemide may increase toxicity of metformin (eg, ethacrynic acid)

Concomitant use of furosemide with aminoglycoside antibiotics or other ototoxic drugs should be avoided, especially with renal dysfunction

Avoid use with sparfloxacin due to increased risk of cardiotoxicity

Succinylcholine's action may be potentiated by furosemide as is ganglionic or peripheral adrenergic-blocking drugs

Aspirin and furosemide in combination may reduce temporarily $Cl_{cr}$ in patients with chronic renal insufficiency; other NSAIDs may result in increased BUN, creatinine, potassium, and weight gain when used in conjunction with furosemide

**Onset**

Onset of diuresis: Oral: Within 30-60 minutes; I.M.: 30 minutes; I.V.: Within 5 minutes

Peak effect: Oral: Within 1-2 hours

**Duration** Oral: 6-8 hours; I.V.: 2 hours

**Half-Life** Normal renal function: 0.5-1.1 hours; End-stage renal disease: 9 hours

**Special PA Issues**

**Patient Education:** Take as directed, with food or milk early in the day (daily), or if twice daily, take last dose in late afternoon in order to avoid sleep disturbance and achieve maximum therapeutic effect. Keep medication in original container, away from light; do not use discolored medication. Include bananas or orange juice (or other potassium-rich foods) in daily diet; do not take potassium supplements without advice of prescriber. Weigh yourself each day, at same time, in the same clothes when beginning therapy, and weekly on long-term therapy; report unusual or unanticipated weight gain or loss. You may experience dizziness, blurred vision, or drowsiness; use caution when driving or engaging in hazardous tasks until response is established. Use caution when rising or changing position. You may experience sensitivity to sunlight; use sunblock or wear protective clothing and sunglasses. Report signs of edema (eg, weight gains, swollen ankles, feet or hands), trembling, numbness or fatigue, any cramping or muscle weakness, palpitations, or unresolved nausea or vomiting.

**Monitoring Parameters:** Monitor weight and I & O daily; blood pressure, serum electrolytes, renal function; in high doses, monitor hearing

**Related Information**

Heart Failure: Management of Patients with Left Ventricular Systolic Dysfunction *on page 1064*

♦ **Furoside®** *see Furosemide on previous page*

♦ **Furoxone®** *see Furazolidone on page 404*

♦ **G-1®** *see Butalbital Compound on page 131*

## Gabapentin *(GA ba pen tin)*

**Pharmacologic Class** Anticonvulsant, Miscellaneous

**U.S. Brand Names** Neurontin®

**Mechanism of Action** Exact mechanism of action is not known, but does have properties in common with other anticonvulsants; although structurally related to GABA, it does not interact with GABA receptors

**Use** Adjunct for treatment of drug-refractory partial and secondarily generalized seizures in adults with epilepsy; not effective for absence seizures

**USUAL DOSAGE** If gabapentin is discontinued or if another anticonvulsant is added to therapy, it should be done slowly over a minimum of 1 week

Children >12 years and Adults: Oral:

Initial: 300 mg on day 1 (at bedtime to minimize sedation), then 300 mg twice daily on day 2, and then 300 mg 3 times/day on day 3

Total daily dosage range: 900-1800 mg/day administered in 3 divided doses at 8-hour intervals

Pain: 300-1800 mg/day given in 3 divided doses has been the most common dosage range

**Dosing adjustment in renal impairment:**

$Cl_{cr}$ >60 mL/minute: Administer 1200 mg/day

$Cl_{cr}$ 30-60 mL/minute: Administer 600 mg/day

$Cl_{cr}$ 15-30 mL/minute: Administer 300 mg/day

$Cl_{cr}$ <15 mL/minute: Administer 150 mg/day

Hemodialysis: 200-300 mg after each 4-hour dialysis following a loading dose of 300-400 mg

**Dosage Forms Cap:** 100 mg, 300 mg, 400 mg, 600 mg, 800 mg

**Contraindications** Hypersensitivity to the drug or its ingredients

**Warnings/Precautions** Avoid abrupt withdrawal, may precipitate seizures; may be associated with a slight incidence (0.6%) of status epilepticus and sudden deaths (0.0038 deaths/patient year); use cautiously in patients with severe renal dysfunction; rat studies demonstrated an association with pancreatic adenocarcinoma in male rats; clinical implication unknown

**Pregnancy Risk Factor** C

**Pregnancy Implications**

Clinical effects on the fetus: No data on crossing the placenta; 4 reports of normal pregnancy outcomes; 1 report of infant with respiratory distress, pyloric stenosis, inguinal hernia following 1st trimester exposure to gabapentin plus carbamazepine; epilepsy itself, number of medications, genetic factors, or a combination of these probably influence the teratogenicity of anticonvulsant therapy

Breast-feeding/lactation: No data available

**Adverse Reactions**

>10%: Central nervous system: Somnolence, dizziness, ataxia, fatigue

1% to 10%:

Cardiovascular: Peripheral edema

Central nervous system: Nervousness, amnesia, depression, anxiety, abnormal coordination

Dermatologic: Pruritus

Gastrointestinal: Dyspepsia, dry throat, xerostomia, nausea, constipation, appetite stimulation (weight gain)

Genitourinary: Impotence

Hematologic: Leukopenia

Neuromuscular & skeletal: Back pain, myalgia, dysarthria, tremor

Ocular: Diplopia, blurred vision, nystagmus

Respiratory: Rhinitis, bronchospasm

Miscellaneous: Hiccups

**Drug Interactions**

Gabapentin does not modify plasma concentrations of standard anticonvulsant medications (ie, valproic acid, carbamazepine, phenytoin, or phenobarbital)

Decreased effect: Antacids reduce the bioavailability of gabapentin by 20%

Increased toxicity: Cimetidine may decrease clearance of gabapentin; gabapentin may increase levels of norethindrone by 13%

**Half-Life** 5-6 hours

**Special PA Issues**

**Patient Education:** Take exactly as directed (do not increase dose or frequency or discontinue without consulting prescriber). While using this medication, do not use alcohol and other prescription or OTC medications (especially pain medications, sedatives, antihistamines, or hypnotics) without consulting prescriber. Maintain adequate hydration (2-3 L/day of fluids unless instructed to restrict fluid intake). You may experience drowsiness, dizziness, or blurred vision (use caution when driving or engaging in hazardous tasks); nausea, vomiting, loss of appetite, or dry mouth (small frequent meals, good mouth care, chewing gum, or sucking on lozenges may help). Wear identification of epileptic status. Report CNS changes, mentation changes, or changes in cognition; muscle cramping, weakness, tremors, changes in gait; persistent GI symptoms (cramping, constipation, vomiting, anorexia); difficulty breathing; impotence or changes in urinary pattern; worsening of seizure activity, or loss of seizure control.

**Dietary Considerations:**

Food: Does not change rate or extent of absorption; take without regard to meals

Serum lipids: May see increases in total cholesterol, HDL cholesterol and triglycerides. Hyperlipidemia and hypercholesterolemia have been reported with gabapentin.

**Monitoring Parameters:** Monitor serum levels of concomitant anticonvulsant therapy; routine monitoring of gabapentin levels is not mandatory

**Reference Range:** Minimum effective serum concentration may be 2 µg/mL; **routine monitoring of drug levels is not required**

♦ **Gabitril®** see Tiagabine on page 900

# Gallium Nitrate (GAL ee um NYE trate)

**Pharmacologic Class** Antidote

**U.S. Brand Names** Ganite™

**Mechanism of Action** Primarily via inhibition of bone resorption with associated reduction in urinary calcium excretion. Gallium has increased the calcium content of newly mineralized bone following short-term treatment in vitro, and this effect combined with its ability to inhibit bone resorption has suggested the use of gallium for other disorders associated with increased bone loss.

**Use** Treatment of clearly symptomatic cancer-related hypercalcemia that has not responded to adequate hydration

**USUAL DOSAGE** Adults:

I.V. infusion (over 24 hours): 200 mg/m² for 5 consecutive days in 1 L of NS or $D_5W$

Mild hypercalcemia/few symptoms: 100 mg/m²/day for 5 days in 1 L of NS or $D_5W$

**Dosing adjustment/comments in renal impairment:** $Cl_{cr}$ <30 mL/minute: Avoid use

(Continued)

## Gallium Nitrate *(Continued)*

**Dosage Forms Inj:** 25 mg/mL (20 mL)

**Contraindications** Should not be used in patients with a serum creatinine >2.5 mg/dL, hypersensitivity to any component

**Warnings/Precautions** Safety and efficacy in children have not been established. Concurrent use of gallium nitrate with other potentially nephrotoxic drugs may increase the risk for developing severe renal insufficiency in patients with cancer-related hypercalcemia; use with caution in patients with impaired renal function or dehydration

**Pregnancy Risk Factor** C

**Adverse Reactions**
>10%:
  Endocrine & metabolic: Hypophosphatemia
  Gastrointestinal: Nausea, vomiting, diarrhea, metallic taste
  Renal: Renal toxicity
1% to 10%: Endocrine & metabolic: Hypocalcemia
<1%: Anemia, optic neuritis, hearing impairment

**Drug Interactions** Increased toxicity: Nephrotoxic drugs (eg, aminoglycosides, amphotericin B)

**Special PA Issues**
  **Monitoring Parameters:** Serum creatinine, BUN, and calcium
  **Reference Range:** Steady-state gallium serum levels: Generally obtained within 2 days following initiation of continuous I.V. infusions of gallium nitrate

♦ **Gamimune® N** *see* Immune Globulin, Intravenous *on page 472*

♦ **Gamma Benzene Hexachloride** *see* Lindane *on page 534*

♦ **Gammagard® S/D** *see* Immune Globulin, Intravenous *on page 472*

♦ **Gamma Globulin** *see* Immune Globulin, Intramuscular *on page 472*

♦ **Gammar®-P I.V.** *see* Immune Globulin, Intravenous *on page 472*

♦ **Gamulin® Rh** *see* Rh$_o$(D) Immune Globulin (Intramuscular) *on page 800*

## Ganciclovir *(gan SYE kloe veer)*

**Pharmacologic Class** Antiviral Agent

**U.S. Brand Names** Cytovene®; Vitrasert®

**Mechanism of Action** Ganciclovir is phosphorylated to a substrate which competitively inhibits the binding of deoxyguanosine triphosphate to DNA polymerase resulting in inhibition of viral DNA synthesis

**Use**
Parenteral: Treatment of CMV retinitis in immunocompromised individuals, including patients with acquired immunodeficiency syndrome; prophylaxis of CMV infection in transplant patients; may be given in combination with foscarnet in patients who relapse after monotherapy with either drug
Oral: Alternative to the I.V. formulation for maintenance treatment of CMV retinitis in immunocompromised patients, including patients with AIDS, in whom retinitis is stable following appropriate induction therapy and for whom the risk of more rapid progression is balanced by the benefit associated with avoiding daily I.V. infusions.
Implant: Treatment of CMV retinitis

**USUAL DOSAGE**
CMV retinitis: Slow I.V. infusion (dosing is based on total body weight):
  Children >3 months and Adults:
    Induction therapy: 5 mg/kg/dose every 12 hours for 14-21 days followed by maintenance therapy
    Maintenance therapy: 5 mg/kg/day as a single daily dose for 7 days/week or 6 mg/kg/day for 5 days/week
CMV retinitis: Oral: 1000 mg 3 times/day with food **or** 500 mg 6 times/day with food
Prevention of CMV disease in patients with advanced HIV infection and normal renal function: Oral: 1000 mg 3 times/day with food
Prevention of CMV disease in transplant patients: Same initial and maintenance dose as CMV retinitis except duration of initial course is 7-14 days, duration of maintenance therapy is dependent on clinical condition and degree of immunosuppression
Intravitreal implant: One implant for 5- to 8-month period; following depletion of ganciclovir, as evidenced by progression of retinitis, implant may be removed and replaced

**Dosing adjustment in renal impairment:**
  I.V. (Induction):
    Cl$_{cr}$ 50-69 mL/minute: Administer 2.5 mg/kg/dose every 12 hours
    Cl$_{cr}$ 25-49 mL/minute: Administer 2.5 mg/kg/dose every 24 hours
    Cl$_{cr}$ 10-24 mL/minute: Administer 1.25 mg/kg/dose every 24 hours
    Cl$_{cr}$ <10 mL/minute: Administer 1.25 mg/kg/dose 3 times/week following hemodialysis
  I.V. (Maintenance):
    Cl$_{cr}$ 50-69 mL/minute: Administer 2.5 mg/kg/dose every 24 hours
    Cl$_{cr}$ 25-49 mL/minute: Administer 1.25 mg/kg/dose every 24 hours
    Cl$_{cr}$ 10-24 mL/minute: Administer 0.625 mg/kg/dose every 24 hours

Cl$_{cr}$ <10 mL/minute: Administer 0.625 mg/kg/dose 3 times/week following hemodialysis

Oral:

Cl$_{cr}$ 50-69 mL/minute: Administer 1500 mg/day or 500 mg 3 times/day

Cl$_{cr}$ 25-49 mL/minute: Administer 1000 mg/day or 500 mg twice daily

Cl$_{cr}$ 10-24 mL/minute: Administer 500 mg/day

Cl$_{cr}$ <10 mL/minute: Administer 500 mg 3 times/week following hemodialysis

Hemodialysis effects: Dialyzable (50%) following hemodialysis; administer dose postdialysis. During peritoneal dialysis, dose as for Cl$_{cr}$ <10 mL/minute. During continuous arteriovenous or venovenous hemofiltration (CAVH/CAVHD), administer 2.5 mg/kg/dose every 24 hours.

**Dosage Forms Cap:** 250 mg; **Implant, intravitreal:** 4.5 mg released gradually over 5-8 months; **Powder for inj, lyophilized:** 500 mg (10 mL)

**Contraindications** Absolute neutrophil count <500/mm$^3$; platelet count <25,000/mm$^3$; known hypersensitivity to ganciclovir or acyclovir

**Warnings/Precautions** Dosage adjustment or interruption of ganciclovir therapy may be necessary in patients with neutropenia and/or thrombocytopenia and patients with impaired renal function. Use with extreme caution in children since long-term safety has not been determined and due to ganciclovir's potential for long-term carcinogenic and adverse reproductive effects; ganciclovir may adversely affect spermatogenesis and fertility; due to its mutagenic potential, contraceptive precautions for female and male patients need to be followed during and for at least 90 days after therapy with the drug; take care to administer only into veins with good blood flow.

**Pregnancy Risk Factor** C

**Adverse Reactions**

>10%:

Central nervous system: Fever (38% to 48%)

Dermatologic: Rash (15% - oral, 10% - I.V.)

Gastrointestinal: Abdominal pain (17% to 19%), diarrhea (40%), nausea (25%), anorexia (15%), vomiting (13%)

Hematologic: Anemia (20% to 25%), leukopenia (30% to 40%)

1% to 10%:

Central nervous system: Confusion, neuropathy (8% to 9%), headache (4%)

Dermatologic: Pruritus (5%)

Hematologic: Thrombocytopenia (6%), neutropenia with ANC <500/mm$^3$ (5% - oral, 14% - I.V.)

Neuromuscular & skeletal: Paresthesia (6% to 10%), weakness (6%)

Miscellaneous: Sepsis (4% - oral, 15% - I.V.)

<1%: Arrhythmia, hypertension, hypotension, edema, ataxia, dizziness, nervousness, psychosis, malaise, coma, seizures, alopecia, urticaria, eosinophilia, hemorrhage, increased LFTs, increased serum creatinine, azotemia, inflammation or pain at injection site, tremor, retinal detachment, visual loss, hyphema, uveitis (intravitreal implant), creatinine increased 2.5%, dyspnea

**Drug Interactions**

Decreased effect: Didanosine: A decrease in steady-state ganciclovir AUC may occur

Increased toxicity:

Immunosuppressive agents may increase cytotoxicity of ganciclovir

Imipenem/cilastatin may increase seizure potential

Zidovudine: Oral ganciclovir increased the AUC of zidovudine, although zidovudine decreases steady state levels of ganciclovir. Since both drugs have the potential to cause neutropenia and anemia, some patients may not tolerate concomitant therapy with these drugs at full dosage.

Probenecid: The renal clearance of ganciclovir is decreased in the presence of probenecid

Didanosine levels are increased with concurrent ganciclovir

Other nephrotoxic drugs (eg, amphotericin and cyclosporine) may have additive nephrotoxicity with ganciclovir

**Half-Life** 1.7-5.8 hours; increases with impaired renal function; End-stage renal disease: 3.6 hours

**Special PA Issues**

**Patient Education:** Ganciclovir is not a cure for CMV retinitis. For oral administration, take as directed and maintain adequate hydration (2-3 L/day of fluids unless instructed to restrict fluid intake). You will need frequent blood tests and regular ophthalmic exams while taking this drug. You may experience increased susceptibility to infection; avoid crowds or exposure to infectious persons. You may experience photosensitivity; use sunblock and wear protective clothing. Report fever, chills, unusual bleeding or bruising, infection, or unhealed sores or white plaques in mouth.

**Monitoring Parameters:** CBC with differential and platelet count, serum creatinine, ophthalmologic exams

♦ **Ganite™** *see* Gallium Nitrate *on page 407*

♦ **Gantanol®** *see* Sulfamethoxazole *on page 861*

♦ **Garamycin®** *see* Gentamicin *on page 411*

## Garlic

**Mechanism of Action** Garlic bulbs contain alliin, a parent to the substance allicin (after the bulb is ground), which is odoriferous and may have some antioxidant activity; ajoene (a byproduct of allicin) has potent platelet inhibition effects; garlic can also decrease LDL cholesterol levels and increase fibrinolytic activity

**Use** Herbal medicine used for lowering LDL cholesterol and triglycerides, and raising HDL cholesterol; protection against atherosclerosis, hypertension, antiseptic agent; may lower blood glucose and decrease thrombosis; potential anti-inflammatory and antitumor effects

**USUAL DOSAGE** Adult dose: 4-12 mg allicin/day

Average daily dose for cardiovascular benefits: 0.25-1 g/kg or 1-4 cloves daily in an 80 kg individual in divided doses

Toxic dose: >5 cloves or >25 mL of extract can cause gastrointestinal symptoms

**Warnings/Precautions** Cholesterol lowering and hypotensive effects may require months. Use with caution in patients receiving treatment for hyperglycemia or hypertension.

**Pregnancy Implications** Avoid use

**Adverse Reactions**

Dermatologic: Skin blistering, eczema, systemic contact dermatitis, immunologic contact urticaria

Gastrointestinal: G.I. upset and changes in intestinal flora (in rare cases) per Commission E

Ocular: Lacrimation

Respiratory: Asthma (upon inhalation of garlic dust)

Miscellaneous: Allergic reactions (in rare cases); change in odor of skin and breath per Commission E

**Drug Interactions** Iodine uptake may be reduced with garlic ingestion; can exacerbate bleeding in patients taking aspirin or anticoagulant agents; may increase risk of hypoglycemia, may increase response to antihypertensives

**Additional Information** 1% as active as penicillin as an antibiotic; number one over-the-counter medication in Germany; enteric-coated products may demonstrate best results

♦ **Gastrocrom® Oral** see Cromolyn Sodium on page 240

♦ **Gastrosed™** see Hyoscyamine on page 463

♦ **G-CSF** see Filgrastim on page 370

♦ **GCV Sodium** see Ganciclovir on page 408

♦ **Gee Gee® [OTC]** see Guaifenesin on page 427

♦ **Gel Kam®** see Fluoride on page 383

♦ **Gel-Tin® [OTC]** see Fluoride on page 383

♦ **Gelucast®** see Zinc Gelatin on page 975

♦ **Gemcor®** see Gemfibrozil on this page

## Gemfibrozil (jem FI broe zil)

**Pharmacologic Class** Antilipemic Agent (Fibric Acid)

**U.S. Brand Names** Gemcor®; Lopid®

**Mechanism of Action** The exact mechanism of action of gemfibrozil is unknown, however, several theories exist regarding the VLDL effect; it can inhibit lipolysis and decrease subsequent hepatic fatty acid uptake as well as inhibit hepatic secretion of VLDL; together these actions decrease serum VLDL levels; increases HDL cholesterol; the mechanism behind HDL elevation is currently unknown

**Use** Treatment of hypertriglyceridemia in types IV and V hyperlipidemia for patients who are at greater risk for pancreatitis and who have not responded to dietary intervention; reduction of coronary heart disease in type IIB patients who have low HDL cholesterol, increased LDL cholesterol, and increased triglycerides

**USUAL DOSAGE** Adults: Oral: 1200 mg/day in 2 divided doses, 30 minutes before breakfast and dinner

Hemodialysis: Not removed by hemodialysis; supplemental dose is not necessary

**Dosage Forms Cap:** 300 mg; **Tab, film coated:** 600 mg

**Contraindications** Renal or hepatic dysfunction, gallbladder disease, hypersensitivity to gemfibrozil or any component

**Warnings/Precautions** Abnormal elevation of AST, ALT, LDH, bilirubin, and alkaline phosphatase has occurred; if no appreciable triglyceride or cholesterol lowering effect occurs after 3 months, the drug should be discontinued; not useful for type I hyperlipidemia; myositis may be more common in patients with poor renal function

**Pregnancy Risk Factor** B

**Adverse Reactions**

>10%:

Gastrointestinal: Dyspepsia (20%), abdominal pain (10%)

Hepatic: Cholelithiasis

1% to 10%:

Central nervous system: Fatigue (4%), vertigo (1.5%), headache (1.2%)

Dermatologic: Eczema/rash (1% to 2%)

Gastrointestinal: Diarrhea (7%), nausea/vomiting (2.5%), constipation (1.4%), acute appendicitis (1.2%)

<1%: Atrial fibrillation, hyperesthesia, dizziness, drowsiness, somnolence, mental depression, flatulence, paresthesia, blurred vision

**Drug Interactions** Increased toxicity:
May potentiate the effects of warfarin
Manufacturer warns against the use of gemfibrozil with concomitant lovastatin therapy

**Onset** May require several days

**Half-Life** 1.4 hours

**Special PA Issues**
**Patient Education:** You must return to provider for assessment of drug effectiveness. Should be taken 30 minutes before meals. Take with milk or meals if GI upset occurs. You may experience loss of appetite and flatulence (frequent small meals may help), muscle aches (mild, temporary pain relievers may be required), dizziness, faintness, or blurred vision (use caution when driving or engaging in hazardous tasks). Report severe stomach pain, nausea, vomiting, chills, sore throat, headache, and any vision changes.
**Monitoring Parameters:** Serum cholesterol, LFTs

**Related Information**
Lipid-Lowering Agents on page 1022

♦ **Genabid®** see Papaverine on page 696

♦ **Genagesic®** see Propoxyphene and Acetaminophen on page 774

♦ **Genahist® Oral** see Diphenhydramine on page 289

♦ **Genapap® [OTC]** see Acetaminophen on page 21

♦ **Genapax®** see Gentian Violet on page 413

♦ **Genaspor® [OTC]** see Tolnaftate on page 915

♦ **Genatuss® [OTC]** see Guaifenesin on page 427

♦ **Genatuss DM® [OTC]** see Guaifenesin and Dextromethorphan on page 428

♦ **Gencalc® 600 [OTC]** see Calcium Carbonate on page 139

♦ **Gen-Clobetasol** see Clobetasol on page 219

♦ **Gen-Glybe** see Glyburide on page 419

♦ **Gen-K®** see Potassium Chloride on page 742

♦ **Gen-Nifedipine** see Nifedipine on page 654

♦ **Genoptic® Ophthalmic** see Gentamicin on this page

♦ **Genoptic® S.O.P. Ophthalmic** see Gentamicin on this page

♦ **Genora® 0.5/35** see Ethinyl Estradiol and Norethindrone on page 348

♦ **Genora® 1/35** see Ethinyl Estradiol and Norethindrone on page 348

♦ **Genora® 1/50** see Mestranol and Norethindrone on page 573

♦ **Genotropin® Injection** see Human Growth Hormone on page 444

♦ **Gen-Pindolol** see Pindolol on page 728

♦ **Genpril® [OTC]** see Ibuprofen on page 466

♦ **Gentacidin® Ophthalmic** see Gentamicin on this page

♦ **Gentafair®** see Gentamicin on this page

♦ **Gentak® Ophthalmic** see Gentamicin on this page

# Gentamicin (jen ta MYE sin)

**Pharmacologic Class** Antibiotic, Aminoglycoside; Antibiotic, Ophthalmic; Antibiotic, Topical

**U.S. Brand Names** Garamycin®; Genoptic® Ophthalmic; Genoptic® S.O.P. Ophthalmic; Gentacidin® Ophthalmic; Gentafair®; Gentak® Ophthalmic; Gentrasul®; G-myticin® Topical; I-Gent®; Jenamicin® Injection; Ocumycin®

**Mechanism of Action** Interferes with bacterial protein synthesis by binding to 30S and 50S ribosomal subunits resulting in a defective bacterial cell membrane

**Use** Treatment of susceptible bacterial infections, normally gram-negative organisms including *Pseudomonas, Proteus, Serratia*, and gram-positive *Staphylococcus*; treatment of bone infections, respiratory tract infections, skin and soft tissue infections, as well as abdominal and urinary tract infections, endocarditis, and septicemia; used topically to treat superficial infections of the skin or ophthalmic infections caused by susceptible bacteria; prevention of bacterial endocarditis prior to dental or surgical procedures

**USUAL DOSAGE** Individualization is critical because of the low therapeutic index
**Use of ideal body weight (IBW) for determining the mg/kg/dose appears to be more accurate than dosing on the basis of total body weight (TBW).**
In morbid obesity, dosage requirement may best be estimated using a dosing weight of IBW + 0.4 (TBW - IBW)
Initial and periodic peak and trough plasma drug levels should be determined, particularly in critically ill patients with serious infections or in disease states known to significantly alter aminoglycoside pharmacokinetics (eg, cystic fibrosis, burns, or major surgery)
Newborns: Intrathecal: 1 mg every day
Infants >3 months: Intrathecal: 1-2 mg/day
Infants and Children <5 years: I.M., I.V.: 2.5 mg/kg/dose every 8 hours*
Cystic fibrosis: 2.5 mg/kg/dose every 6 hours
(Continued)

## Gentamicin *(Continued)*

Children >5 years: I.M., I.V.: 1.5-2.5 mg/kg/dose every 8 hours*

    Prevention of bacterial endocarditis: Dental, oral, upper respiratory procedures, GI/GU procedures: 2 mg/kg with ampicillin (50 mg/kg) 30 minutes prior to procedure

*Some patients may require larger or more frequent doses (eg, every 6 hours) if serum levels document the need (ie, cystic fibrosis or febrile granulocytopenic patients)

Adults: I.M., I.V.:

    Severe life-threatening infections: 2-2.5 mg/kg/dose

    Urinary tract infections: 1.5 mg/kg/dose

    Synergy (for gram-positive infections): 1 mg/kg/dose

    Prevention of bacterial endocarditis:

        Dental, oral, or upper respiratory procedures: 1.5 mg/kg not to exceed 80 mg with ampicillin (1-2 g) 30 minutes prior to procedure

        GI/GU surgery: 1.5 mg/kg not to exceed 80 mg with ampicillin 2 g 30 minutes prior to procedure

Children and Adults:

    Intrathecal: 4-8 mg/day

    Ophthalmic:

        Ointment: Instill ½" (1.25 cm) 2-3 times/day to every 3-4 hours

        Solution: Instill 1-2 drops every 2-4 hours, up to 2 drops every hour for severe infections

    Topical: Apply 3-4 times/day to affected area

Some clinicians suggest a daily dose of 4-7 mg/kg for all patients with normal renal function. This dose is at least as efficacious with similar, if not less, toxicity than conventional dosing.

**Dosing interval in renal impairment:**

    $Cl_{cr}$ ≥60 mL/minute: Administer every 8 hours

    $Cl_{cr}$ 40-60 mL/minute: Administer every 12 hours

    $Cl_{cr}$ 20-40 mL/minute: Administer every 24 hours

    $Cl_{cr}$ <20 mL/minute: Loading dose, then monitor levels

Hemodialysis: Dialyzable; removal by hemodialysis: 30% removal of aminoglycosides occurs during 4 hours of HD; administer dose after dialysis and follow levels

Removal by continuous ambulatory peritoneal dialysis (CAPD):

    Administration via CAPD fluid:

    Gram-negative infection: 4-8 mg/L (4-8 mcg/mL) of CAPD fluid

    Gram-positive infection (ie, synergy): 3-4 mg/L (3-4 mcg/mL) of CAPD fluid

    Administration via I.V., I.M. route during CAPD: Dose as for $Cl_{cr}$ <10 mL/minute and follow levels

Removal via continuous arteriovenous or venovenous hemofiltration (CAVH/CAVHD): Dose as for $Cl_{cr}$ 10-40 mL/minute and follow levels

**Dosing adjustment/comments in hepatic disease:** Monitor plasma concentrations

**Dosage Forms Crm, top, (Garamycin®, G-myticin®):** 0.1% (15 g); **Inf, in $D_5W$:** 60 mg, 80 mg, 100 mg; **Inf, in NS:** 40 mg, 60 mg, 80 mg, 90 mg, 100 mg, 120 mg; **Inj:** 40 mg/mL (1 mL, 1.5 mL, 2 mL); Pediatric: 10 mg/mL (2 mL); **Intrathecal, preservative free (Garamycin®):** 2 mg/mL (2 mL); **Oint: Ophth:** 0.3% [3 mg/g] (3.5 g), Garamycin®, Genoptic® S.O.P., Gentacidin®, Gentak®: 0.3% [3 mg/g] (3.5 g); **Top (Garamycin®, G-myticin®):** 0.1% (15 g); **Soln, ophth:** 0.3% (5 mL, 15 mL), Garamycin®, Genoptic®, Gentacidin®, Gentak®: 0.3% (1 mL, 5 mL, 15 mL)

**Contraindications** Hypersensitivity to gentamicin or other aminoglycosides

**Warnings/Precautions** Not intended for long-term therapy due to toxic hazards associated with extended administration; pre-existing renal insufficiency, vestibular or cochlear impairment, myasthenia gravis, hypocalcemia, conditions which depress neuromuscular transmission

Parenteral aminoglycosides have been associated with significant nephrotoxicity or ototoxicity; the ototoxicity may be directly proportional to the amount of drug given and the duration of treatment; tinnitus or vertigo are indications of vestibular injury and impending hearing loss; renal damage is usually reversible

**Pregnancy Risk Factor** C

**Adverse Reactions**

>10%:

    Central nervous system: Neurotoxicity (vertigo, ataxia)

    Neuromuscular & skeletal: Gait instability

    Otic: Ototoxicity (auditory), ototoxicity (vestibular)

    Renal: Nephrotoxicity, decreased creatinine clearance

1% to 10%:

    Cardiovascular: Edema

    Dermatologic: Skin itching, reddening of skin, rash

<1%: Drowsiness, headache, pseudomotor cerebri, photosensitivity, erythema, anorexia, nausea, vomiting, weight loss, increased salivation, enterocolitis, granulocytopenia, agranulocytosis, thrombocytopenia, elevated LFTs, burning, stinging, tremors, muscle cramps, weakness, dyspnea

**Drug Interactions** Increased toxicity:

Penicillins, cephalosporins, amphotericin B, loop diuretics may increase nephrotoxic potential

Neuromuscular blocking agents may increase neuromuscular blockade

**Half-Life** 1.5-3 hours; end-stage renal disease: 36-70 hours

**Special PA Issues**

**Patient Education:** Take exactly as directed and when prescribed. Drink adequate amounts of water (2-3 L/day). You may experience headaches, ringing in ears, dizziness, blurred vision (use caution when driving or engaging in hazardous tasks); GI upset, loss of appetite (small frequent meals and frequent mouth care may help); photosensitivity (wear sunscreen and protective clothing). Report severe headache, changes in hearing acuity or ringing in ears, changes in urine pattern, difficulty breathing, rash, fever, unhealed sores, sores in mouth, vaginal drainage, muscle or bone pain, change in gait, or worsening of condition.

Ophthalmic: Wash hands before instilling. Sit or lie down to instill. Open eye, look at ceiling, and instill prescribed amount of solution (Ointment: Pull lower lid down gently, instill thin ribbon of ointment inside lid.) Close eye and roll eye in all directions, and apply gentle pressure to inner corner of eye. Do not let tip of applicator touch eye or contaminate tip of applicator. Temporary stinging or blurred vision may occur. Report persistent pain, burning, vision disturbances, swelling, itching, or worsening of condition.

Topical: Apply thin film of ointment to affected area as often as recommended. May apply porous dressing. Report persistent burning, swelling, itching, worsening of condition, or lack of response to therapy.

**Dietary Considerations:** Calcium, magnesium, potassium: Renal wasting may cause hypocalcemia, hypomagnesemia, and/or hypokalemia

**Monitoring Parameters:** Urinalysis, urine output, BUN, serum creatinine; hearing should be tested before, during, and after treatment; particularly in those at risk for ototoxicity or who will be receiving prolonged therapy (>2 weeks)

**Reference Range:**

Timing of serum samples: Draw peak 30 minutes after 30-minute infusion has been completed or 1 hour after I.M. injection; draw trough immediately before next dose

Sample size: 0.5-2 mL blood (red top tube) or 0.1-1 mL serum (separated)

Therapeutic levels:

Peak:

Serious infections: 6-8 µg/mL (12-17 µmol/L)

Life-threatening infections: 8-10 µg/mL (17-21 µmol/L)

Urinary tract infections: 4-6 µg/mL

Synergy against gram-positive organisms: 3-5 µg/mL

Trough:

Serious infections: 0.5-1 µg/mL

Life-threatening infections: 1-2 µg/mL

Obtain drug levels after the third dose unless renal dysfunction/toxicity suspected

♦ **Gentamicin Sulfate** see Gentamicin on page 411

# Gentian Violet (JEN shun VYE oh let)

**Pharmacologic Class** Antibacterial, Topical; Antifungal Agent, Topical

**U.S. Brand Names** Genapax®

**Mechanism of Action** Topical antiseptic/germicide effective against some vegetative gram-positive bacteria, particularly *Staphylococcus* sp, and some yeast; it is much less effective against gram-negative bacteria and is ineffective against acid-fast bacteria

**Use** Treatment of cutaneous or mucocutaneous infections caused by *Candida albicans* and other superficial skin infections

**USUAL DOSAGE**

Children and Adults: Topical: Apply 0.5% to 2% locally with cotton to lesion 2-3 times/day for 3 days, do not swallow and avoid contact with eyes

Adults: Intravaginal: Insert one tampon for 3-4 hours once or twice daily for 12 days

**Dosage Forms Soln, top:** 1% (30 mL), 2% (30 mL); **Tampons:** 5 mg (12s)

**Contraindications** Known hypersensitivity to gentian violet; ulcerated areas; patients with porphyria

**Warnings/Precautions** Infants should be turned face down after application to minimize amount of drug swallowed; may result in tattooing of the skin when applied to granulation tissue; solution is for external use only; avoid contact with eyes

**Pregnancy Risk Factor** C

**Adverse Reactions** 1% to 10%: Esophagitis, burning, irritation, vesicle formation, sensitivity reactions, ulceration of mucous membranes, laryngitis, tracheitis, laryngeal obstruction

**Special PA Issues**

**Patient Education:** Drug stains skin and clothing purple; do not apply to an ulcerative lesion; may result in "tattooing" of the skin; when used for the treatment of vaginal candidiasis, coitus should be avoided; insert vaginal product high into vagina. Use condoms or refrain from sexual intercourse to avoid reinfection.

# Ginger

**Mechanism of Action** Unknown; may increase GI motility and thus block nausea feedback from the GI tract; appears to decrease prostaglandin synthesis; may have cardiotonic activity; may inhibit platelet aggregation

**Use** In herbal medicine as a digestive aid; for treatment of nausea (antiemetic) and motion sickness; also used as a menstruation promoter in Chinese herbal medicine; headaches, colds and flu; ginger oil is used as a flavoring agent in beverages and mouthwashes; may be useful in some forms of arthritis

**USUAL DOSAGE**

For preventing motion sickness or digestive aid: 1-4 g/day (250 mg of ginger root powder 4 times/day)

Per Commission E: 2-4 g/day or equivalent preparations

**Contraindications** Gallstones per Commission E

**Warnings/Precautions** Use with caution in diabetics, patients on cardiac glycosides, and patients receiving anticoagulants

**Pregnancy Risk Factor** No administration for morning sickness during pregnancy per Commission E; however, two-peer reviewed revision of the literature does not justify this caution; Commission E made its cautions based on animal studies and *in vitro* mutagenicity studies (2) on 1 compound, gingerol. Indian and Chinese women use large amounts of ginger routinely in their diet during pregnancy with no ill effects on pregnancy or fetus. High doses may be abortifacient.

**Drug Interactions** May alter response to cardiotonic, hypoglycemia, anticoagulant, anti-platelet agents

# Ginkgo Biloba

**Mechanism of Action** Inhibits platelet aggregation; ginkgo biloba leaf extract contain terpenoids and flavonoids which can allegedly inactivate oxygen-free radicals causing vaso-dilatation and antagonize effects of platelet activating factor (PAF); fruit pulp contains ginkolic acids which are allergens (seeds are not sensitizing)

**Use** Dilates blood vessels; plant/leaf extract has been used in Europe for intermittent claudi-cation, arterial insufficiency, and cerebral vascular disease (dementia); tinnitus, visual disor-ders, traumatic brain injury, vertigo of vascular origin

Per Commission E: Demential syndromes including memory deficits, etc (tinnitus, head-ache); depressive emotional conditions, primary degenerative dementia, vascular dementia, or both

**Investigational**: Asthma, impotence (male)

**USUAL DOSAGE** Beneficial effects for cerebral ischemia in the elderly occur after one month of use

Usual dosage: ~40 mg 3 times/day with meals; 60-80 mg twice daily to 3 times/day depending on indication; maximum dose: 360 mg/day

Cerebral ischemia: 120 mg/day in 2-3 divided doses (24% flavonoid-glycoside extract, 6% terpene glycosides)

**Contraindications** Pregnancy, patients with clotting disorders; hypersensitivity to ginkgo biloba preparations per Commission E

**Warnings/Precautions** Use with caution following recent surgery or trauma; effects may require 1-2 months

**Adverse Reactions**

Cardiovascular: Palpitations, bilateral subdural hematomas

Central nervous system: Headache (very seldom per Commission E), dizziness, seizures (in children), restlessness

Dermatologic: Urticaria, cheilitis

Gastrointestinal: Nausea, ciarrhea, vomiting, stomatitis, proctitis; very seldom stomach or intestinal upsets (per Commission E)

Ocular: Hyphema

Miscellaneous: Allergic skin reactions (very seldom per Commission E)

**Drug Interactions** Due to effects on PAF, use with caution in patients receiving anticoagu-lants or platelet inhibitors

**Additional Information** Seeds and pulp are poisonous; beneficial effects for cerebral ischemia in the elderly occur after one month of use

**Special PA Issues**

**Reference Range:** Maximum plasma level of ginkogolide A and ginkogolide B after an 80 mg oral dose was 15 mg/mL and 4 mg/mL respectively; maximum plasma level of bilobalide after a 120 mg oral dose is ~18.8 mg/mL

# Ginseng

**Mechanism of Action** The active agent (ginsenosides) may have CNS stimulant and estrogen-like effect, anti-inflammatory, antiplatelet; used as an adaptogen; may lower cholesterol; not effective as an aphrodesiac

**Use** A popular ingredient in herbal teas; has been advocated for its antistress and adaptogenic effects although these effects have not been scientifically confirmed, there's much "suggestive" scientific literature

**USUAL DOSAGE** Avoid in long-term use

Herbal tea: Usually about 1.75 g; 0.5-2 g/day

Dried root: 0.6-3 g/day of dried root or equivalent preparations

Ethanolic extract: 0.5-6 mL 1-3 times/day

Root: 1-2 g/day

Extract: (7% ginsenosides) 100-300 mg 3 times/day

**Contraindications** Estrogen-receptor positive breast cancer

**Warnings/Precautions** Nervousness may occur during first few days; use with caution in hypertensives, diabetes; avoid long-term use

**Pregnancy Implications** Not recommended in pregnancy or breast-feeding

**Adverse Reactions**

Cardiovascular: Tachycardia, hypertension, sinus tachycardia

Central nervous system: Nervousness, agitation, mania, headache, sciatic nerve inflammation

Dermatologic: Stevens Johnson syndrome

Endocrine & metabolic: Hypoglycemia, vaginal bleeding, breast nodules

**Drug Interactions** May decrease effects of loop diuretics (furosemide); theoretically may increase effect of antiplatelet agents, anticoagulants, hypoglycemics, and hypotensive agents

**Additional Information** There are three forms of ginseng (American, Asian, and Siberian); each has slightly different properties

# Glatiramer Acetate (gla TIR a mer AS e tate)

**Pharmacologic Class** Biological, Miscellaneous

**U.S. Brand Names** Copaxone®

**Mechanism of Action** Glatiramer is a mixture of random polymers of four amino acids; L-alanine, L-glutamic acid, L-lysine and L-tyrosine, the resulting mixture is antigenically similar to myelin basic protein, which is an important component of the myelin sheath of nerves; glatiramer is thought to suppress T-lymphocytes specific for a myelin antigen, it is also proposed that glatiramer interferes with the antigen-presenting function of certain immune cells opposing pathogenic T-cell function

**Use** Relapsing-remitting type multiple sclerosis; studies indicate that it reduces the frequency of attacks and the severity of disability; appears to be most effective for patients with minimal disability

**USUAL DOSAGE** Adults: S.C.: 20 mg daily

**Dosage Forms Inj:** 20 mg (2 mL)

**Contraindications** Previous hypersensitivity to any component of the copolymer formulation

**Pregnancy Risk Factor** B

**Adverse Reactions**

>10%:

Cardiovascular: Chest pain (26%)

Local: Pain

1% to 10%:

Cardiovascular: Chest tightness, flushing, tachycardia, vasodilitation

Central nervous system: Anxiety, depression, dizziness

Dermatologic: Erythema (4%), urticaria

Hematologic: Transient eosinophilia

Local: Injection site reactions (6.5%)

Neuromuscular & skeletal: Tremor

Respiratory: Dyspnea

Miscellaneous: Diaphoresis, unintended pregnancy

**Special PA Issues**

**Patient Education:** It is essential to provide the patient with proper handling and reconstitution instruction, since they will most likely have to self-administer the drug for an extended period

♦ **GlaucTabs®** see Methazolamide on page 581

♦ **Glibenclamide** see Glyburide on page 419

# Glimepiride (GLYE me pye ride)

**Pharmacologic Class** Antidiabetic Agent (Sulfonylurea)

**U.S. Brand Names** Amaryl®

**Mechanism of Action** Stimulates insulin release from the pancreatic beta cells; reduces glucose output from the liver; insulin sensitivity is increased at peripheral target sites

**Use**

Management of noninsulin-dependent diabetes mellitus (type II) as an adjunct to diet and exercise to lower blood glucose

Use in combination with insulin to lower blood glucose in patients whose hyperglycemia cannot be controlled by diet and exercise in conjunction with an oral hypoglycemic agent

**USUAL DOSAGE** Oral (allow several days between dose titrations):

Adults: Initial: 1-2 mg once daily, administered with breakfast or the first main meal; usual maintenance dose: 1-4 mg once daily; after a dose of 2 mg once daily, increase in increments of 2 mg at 1- to 2-week intervals based upon the patient's blood glucose response to a maximum of 8 mg once daily

Elderly: Initial: 1 mg/day

Combination with insulin therapy (fasting glucose level for instituting combination therapy is in the range of >150 mg/dL in plasma or serum depending on the patient): 8 mg once daily with the first main meal

After starting with low-dose insulin, upward adjustments of insulin can be done approximately weekly as guided by frequent measurements of fasting blood glucose. Once stable, combination-therapy patients should monitor their capillary blood glucose on an ongoing basis, preferably daily.

**Dosing adjustment/comments in renal impairment:** $Cl_{cr}$ <22 mL/minute: Initial starting dose should be 1 mg and dosage increments should be based on fasting blood glucose levels

**Dosing adjustment in hepatic impairment:** No data available

**Dosage Forms Tab:** 1 mg, 2 mg, 4 mg

**Contraindications** Hypersensitivity to glimepiride or any component, other sulfonamides; diabetic ketoacidosis (with or without coma)

**Warnings/Precautions**

The administration of oral hypoglycemic drugs (ie, tolbutamide) has been reported to be associated with increased cardiovascular mortality as compared to treatment with diet alone or diet plus insulin

All sulfonylurea drugs are capable of producing severe hypoglycemia. Hypoglycemia is more likely to occur when caloric intake is deficient, after severe or prolonged exercise, when alcohol is ingested, or when more than one glucose-lowering drug is used.

**Pregnancy Risk Factor** C

**Adverse Reactions**

1% to 10%: Central nervous system: Headache

<1%: Edema, rash, urticaria, photosensitivity, hypoglycemia, hyponatremia, anorexia, nausea, vomiting, diarrhea, epigastric fullness, constipation, heartburn, blood dyscrasias, aplastic anemia, hemolytic anemia, bone marrow suppression, thrombocytopenia, agranulocytosis, cholestatic jaundice, diuretic effect

**Drug Interactions** CYP2C9 enzyme substrate

Decreased effects: Cholestyramine, hydantoins, rifampin, thiazide diuretics, urinary alkalines, charcoal

Increased effects: $H_2$-antagonists, anticoagulants, androgens, beta-blockers, fluconazole, salicylates, gemfibrozil, sulfonamides, tricyclic antidepressants, probenecid, MAO inhibitors, methyldopa, NSAIDs, salicylates, sulfonamides, chloramphenicol, coumarins, probenecid, MAO inhibitors, digitalis glycosides, urinary acidifiers

Increased toxicity: Cimetidine may increase hypoglycemic effects; certain drugs tend to produce hyperglycemia and may lead to loss of control. These drugs include the thiazides and other diuretics, corticosteroids, phenothiazines, thyroid products, estrogens, oral contraceptives, phenytoin, nicotinic acid, sympathomimetics, and isoniazid.

**Onset** Peak blood glucose reductions: Within 2-3 hours

**Duration** 24 hours

**Half-Life** 5-9 hours

**Special PA Issues**

**Patient Education:** This medication is used to control diabetes; it is not a cure. Other components of treatment plan are important; follow prescribed diet, medication, and exercise regimen. You may be referred to a diabetic educator for diabetic counseling. May be taken with a meal or food. Do not alter dosage or discontinue current medications or introduce new medications without consulting prescriber. Eat regularly; do not skip meals. Carry quick sugar source; monitor serum glucose daily. Avoid alcohol intake (may cause disulfiram reactions) and OTC medications without consulting prescriber. Report acute headache or acute hyper- or hypoglycemic reactions.

**Monitoring Parameters:** Urine for glucose and ketones; monitor for signs and symptoms of hypoglycemia (fatigue, excessive hunger, profuse sweating, numbness of extremities), fasting blood glucose, hemoglobin $A_{1c}$, fructosamine

**Reference Range:** Target range: Adults: Fasting blood glucose: <120 mg/dL; Glycosylated hemoglobin: <7%

**Related Information**

Hypoglycemic Drugs *on page 1020*

# Glipizide (GLIP i zide)

**Pharmacologic Class** Antidiabetic Agent (Sulfonylurea)

**U.S. Brand Names** Glucotrol®; Glucotrol® XL

**Mechanism of Action** Stimulates insulin release from the pancreatic beta cells; reduces glucose output from the liver; insulin sensitivity is increased at peripheral target sites

**Use** Management of noninsulin-dependent diabetes mellitus (type II)

**USUAL DOSAGE** Oral (allow several days between dose titrations): Give ~30 minutes before a meal to obtain the greatest reduction in postprandial hyperglycemia

Adults: Initial: 5 mg/day; adjust dosage at 2.5-5 mg daily increments as determined by blood glucose response at intervals of several days. Maximum recommended once-daily dose: 15 mg; maximum recommended total daily dose: 40 mg.

Elderly: Initial: 2.5 mg/day; increase by 2.5-5 mg/day at 1- to 2-week intervals

**Dosing adjustment/comments in renal impairment:** $Cl_{cr}$ <10 mL/minute: Some investigators recommend not using

**Dosing adjustment in hepatic impairment:** Initial dosage should be 2.5 mg/day

**Dosage Forms Tab:** 5 mg, 10 mg; **Tab, extended release:** 5 mg, 10 mg

**Contraindications** Hypersensitivity to glipizide or any component, other sulfonamides, type I diabetes mellitus

**Warnings/Precautions** Use with caution in patients with severe hepatic disease; a useful agent since few drug to drug interactions and not dependent upon renal elimination of active drug

**Pregnancy Risk Factor** C

**Pregnancy Implications**

Clinical effects on the fetus: Crosses the placenta. Insulin is the drug of choice for the control of diabetes mellitus during pregnancy.

Breast-feeding/lactation: No data available

**Adverse Reactions**

>10%:

Central nervous system: Headache

Gastrointestinal: Anorexia, nausea, vomiting, diarrhea, epigastric fullness, constipation, heartburn

1% to 10%: Dermatologic: Rash, urticaria, photosensitivity

<1%: Edema, hypoglycemia, hyponatremia, blood dyscrasias, aplastic anemia, hemolytic anemia, bone marrow suppression, thrombocytopenia, agranulocytosis, cholestatic jaundice, diuretic effect

**Drug Interactions**

Decreased effects: Beta-blockers, cholestyramine, hydantoins, rifampin, thiazide diuretics, urinary alkalines, charcoal

Increased effects: $H_2$-antagonists, anticoagulants, androgens, fluconazole, salicylates, gemfibrozil, sulfonamides, tricyclic antidepressants, probenecid, MAO inhibitors, methyldopa, digitalis glycosides, urinary acidifiers

Increased toxicity: Cimetidine may increase hypoglycemic effects

**Onset** Peak blood glucose reductions: Within 1.5-2 hours

**Duration** 12-24 hours

**Half-Life** 2-4 hours

**Special PA Issues**

**Patient Education:** This medication is used to control diabetes; it is not a cure. Other components of treatment plan are important; follow prescribed diet, medication, and exercise regimen. You may be referred to a diabetic educator for diabetic counseling. Take once daily dose 30 minutes before breakfast, multiple doses 30 minutes before meals. Do not chew or crush extended release product. Do not alter dosage or discontinue current medications or introduce new medications without consulting prescriber. Eat regularly; do not skip meals. Carry quick sugar source; monitor serum glucose daily. Avoid alcohol intake (may cause disulfiram reaction) and OTC medications without consulting prescriber. You may be more sensitive to sunlight; avoid excessive exposure, wear sunblock or protective clothing. Report acute headache, unresolved diarrhea or constipation, unusual weight gain, excessive urination, or acute hyper- or hypoglycemic reactions.

**Dietary Considerations:**

Alcohol: A disulfiram-like reaction characterized by flushing, headache, nausea, vomiting, sweating, or tachycardia; avoid use

Food: Food delays absorption by 40%; take glipizide before meals

Glucose: Decreases blood glucose concentration. Hypoglycemia may occur. Educate patients how to detect and treat hypoglycemia. Monitor for signs and symptoms of hypoglycemia. Administer glucose if necessary. Evaluate patient's diet and exercise regimen. May need to decrease or discontinue dose of sulfonylurea.

(Continued)

## Glipizide *(Continued)*

Sodium: Reports of hyponatremia and SIADH. Those at increased risk include patients on medications or who have medical conditions that predispose them to hyponatremia. Monitor sodium serum concentration and fluid status. May need to restrict water intake.

**Monitoring Parameters:** Urine for glucose and ketones; monitor for signs and symptoms of hypoglycemia (fatigue, excessive hunger, profuse sweating, numbness of extremities), fasting blood glucose, hemoglobin A$_{1c}$, fructosamine

**Reference Range:** Target range: Adults: Fasting blood glucose: <120 mg/dL; Glycosylated hemoglobin: <7%

**Related Information**

Hypoglycemic Drugs *on page 1020*

## Glucagon *(GLOO ka gon)*

**Pharmacologic Class** Antidote; Diagnostic Agent, Gastrointestinal

**Mechanism of Action** Stimulates adenylate cyclase to produce increased cyclic AMP, which promotes hepatic glycogenolysis and gluconeogenesis, causing a raise in blood glucose levels

**Use** Management of hypoglycemia; diagnostic aid in the radiologic examination of GI tract when a hypnotic state is needed; used with some success as a cardiac stimulant in management of severe cases of beta-adrenergic blocking agent overdosage

**USUAL DOSAGE**

Hypoglycemia or insulin shock therapy: I.M., I.V., S.C.:

Children: 0.025-0.1 mg/kg/dose, not to exceed 1 mg/dose, repeated in 20 minutes as needed

Adults: 0.5-1 mg, may repeat in 20 minutes as needed

**If patient fails to respond to glucagon, I.V. dextrose must be given**

Diagnostic aid: Adults: I.M., I.V.: 0.25-2 mg 10 minutes prior to procedure

**Dosage Forms Powder for inj, lyophilized:** 1 mg [1 unit]; 10 mg [10 units]

**Contraindications** Hypersensitivity to glucagon or any component

**Warnings/Precautions** Use with caution in patients with a history of insulinoma and/or pheochromocytoma

**Pregnancy Risk Factor** B

**Adverse Reactions** 1% to 10%:

Cardiovascular: Hypotension

Dermatologic: Urticaria

Gastrointestinal: Nausea, vomiting

Respiratory: Respiratory distress

**Drug Interactions** Increased toxicity: Oral anticoagulant - hypoprothrombinemic effects may be increased possibly with bleeding

**Onset** Peak effect on blood glucose levels: Parenteral: Within 5-20 minutes

**Duration** 60-90 minutes

**Half-Life** Plasma: 3-10 minutes

**Special PA Issues**

**Patient Education:** Identify appropriate support person to administer glucagon if necessary. Follow prescribers instructions for administering glucagon. Review diet, insulin administration, and testing procedures with prescriber or diabetic educator.

**Monitoring Parameters:** Blood pressure, blood glucose

♦ **Glucocerebrosidase** *see* Alglucerase *on page 41*

♦ **Glucophage®** *see* Metformin *on page 577*

## Glucosamine

**Mechanism of Action** Glucosamine is an amino sugar which is a key component in the synthesis of proteoglycans, a group of proteins found in cartilage. These proteoglycans are negatively charged, and attract water so they can produce synovial fluid in the joints. The theory is that supplying the body with these precursors will replenish important synovial fluid, and lead to production of new cartilage. Glucosamine also appears to inhibit cartilage-destroying enzymes such as collagenase and phospholipase A2, thus stopping the degenerative processes of osteoarthritis. A third mechanism may be glucosamine's ability to prevent production of damaging superoxide radicals, which may lead to cartilage destruction.

**Use** Osteoarthritis, rheumatoid arthritis, tendonitis, gout, bursitis

**USUAL DOSAGE** 500 mg of the sulfate form 3 times/day

**Adverse Reactions** Gastrointestinal: Very few effects (eg, flatulence, nausea)

**Drug Interactions** None known

**Additional Information** Both a sulfate and a hydrochloride salt are available. Glucosamine appears more highly absorbed when administered in the sulfate form, and sulfate is also an important mineral in cartilage.

♦ **Glucotrol®** *see* Glipizide *on previous page*

- **Glucotrol®** XL *see* Glipizide *on page 417*
- **Glukor®** *see* Chorionic Gonadotropin *on page 205*
- **Glyate® [OTC]** *see* Guaifenesin *on page 427*
- **Glybenclamide** *see* Glyburide *on this page*
- **Glybenzcyclamide** *see* Glyburide *on this page*

## Glyburide (GLYE byoor ide)

**Pharmacologic Class** Antidiabetic Agent (Sulfonylurea)

**U.S. Brand Names** Diaβeta®; Glynase™ PresTab™; Micronase®

**Mechanism of Action** Stimulates insulin release from the pancreatic beta cells; reduces glucose output from the liver; insulin sensitivity is increased at peripheral target sites

**Use** Management of noninsulin-dependent diabetes mellitus (type II)

**USUAL DOSAGE** Oral:

Adults:

Initial: 2.5-5 mg/day, administered with breakfast or the first main meal of the day. In patients who are more sensitive to hypoglycemic drugs, start at 1.25 mg/day.

Increase in increments of no more than 2.5 mg/day at weekly intervals based on the patient's blood glucose response

Maintenance: 1.25-20 mg/day given as single or divided doses; maximum: 20 mg/day

Elderly: Initial: 1.25-2.5 mg/day, increase by 1.25-2.5 mg/day every 1-3 weeks

Micronized tablets (Glynase PresTab™): Adults:

Initial: 1.5-3 mg/day, administered with breakfast or the first main meal of the day in patients who are more sensitive to hypoglycemic drugs, start at 0.75 mg/day. Increase in increments of no more than 1.5 mg/day in weekly intervals based on the patient's blood glucose response.

Maintenance: 0.75-12 mg/day given as a single dose or in divided doses. Some patients (especially those receiving >6 mg/day) may have a more satisfactory response with twice-daily dosing.

**Dosing adjustment/comments in renal impairment:** Cl$_{cr}$ <50 mL/minute: **Not recommended**

**Dosing adjustment in hepatic impairment:** Use conservative initial and maintenance doses and avoid use in severe disease

**Dosage Forms Tab (Diaβeta®, Micronase®):** 1.25 mg, 2.5 mg, 5 mg; **Tab, micronized (Glynase™ PresTab™):** 1.5 mg, 3 mg, 4.5 mg, 6 mg

**Contraindications** Hypersensitivity to glyburide or any component, or other sulfonamides; type I diabetes mellitus, diabetic ketoacidosis with or without coma

**Warnings/Precautions** Use with caution in patients with hepatic impairment. Elderly: Rapid and prolonged hypoglycemia (>12 hours) despite hypertonic glucose injections have been reported; age and hepatic and renal impairment are independent risk factors for hypoglycemia; dosage titration should be made at weekly intervals. Use with caution in patients with renal and hepatic impairment, malnourished or debilitated conditions, or adrenal or pituitary insufficiency. The administration of oral hypoglycemic drugs (ie, tolbutamide) has been reported to be associated with increased cardiovascular mortality as compared to treatment with diet alone or diet plus insulin.

**Pregnancy Risk Factor** C

**Pregnancy Implications**

Clinical effects on the fetus: Crosses the placenta. Hypoglycemia; ear defects reported; other malformations reported but may have been secondary to poor maternal glucose control/diabetes. Insulin is the drug of choice for the control of diabetes mellitus during pregnancy.

Breast-feeding/lactation: No data available

**Adverse Reactions**

>10%:

Central nervous system: Headache, dizziness

Gastrointestinal: Nausea, epigastric fullness, heartburn, constipation, diarrhea, anorexia

Ocular: Blurred vision

1% to 10%: Dermatologic: Pruritus, rash, urticaria, photosensitivity reaction

<1%: Hypoglycemia, nocturia, leukopenia, thrombocytopenia, hemolytic anemia, aplastic anemia, bone marrow suppression, agranulocytosis, cholestatic jaundice, arthralgia, paresthesia, diuretic effect

**Drug Interactions** CYP3A3/4 enzyme substrate

Decreased effect: Thiazides may decrease effectiveness of glyburide

Increased effect: Possible interaction between glyburide and fluoroquinolone antibiotics has been reported resulting in a potentiation of hypoglycemic action of glyburide

Increased toxicity:

Since this agent is highly protein bound, the toxic potential is increased when given concomitantly with other highly protein bound drugs (ie, phenylbutazone, oral anticoagulants, hydantoins, salicylates, NSAIDs, beta-blockers, sulfonamides) - increase hypoglycemic effect

Alcohol increases disulfiram reactions

Phenylbutazone can increase hypoglycemic effects

(Continued)

## Glyburide (Continued)

Certain drugs tend to produce hyperglycemia and may lead to loss of control (ie, thiazides and other diuretics, corticosteroids, phenothiazines, thyroid products, estrogens, oral contraceptives, phenytoin, nicotinic acid, sympathomimetics, calcium channel blocking drugs, and isoniazid)

Possible interactions between glyburide and coumarin derivatives have been reported that may either potentiate or weaken the effects of coumarin derivatives

**Onset** Oral: Insulin levels in the serum begin to increase within 15-60 minutes after a single dose

**Duration** Up to 24 hours

**Half-Life** 5-16 hours; may be prolonged with renal insufficiency or hepatic insufficiency

**Special PA Issues**

**Patient Education:** This medication is used to control diabetes; it is not a cure. Other components of treatment plan are important; follow prescribed diet, medication, and exercise regimen. You may be referred to a diabetic educator for diabetic counseling. Take this medication with breakfast or first main meal of the day. Do not alter dosage or discontinue current medications or introduce new medications without consulting prescriber. Eat regularly; do not skip meals. Carry quick sugar source; monitor serum glucose daily. Avoid alcohol intake (possible disulfiram reaction) and OTC medications without consulting prescriber. You may be more sensitive to sunlight; avoid excessive exposure, wear sunblock or protective clothing. Report acute headache, unresolved diarrhea or constipation, unusual weight gain, excessive urination, rash, or acute hyper- or hypoglycemic reactions.

**Dietary Considerations:**

Alcohol: A disulfiram-like reaction characterized by flushing, headache, nausea, vomiting, sweating, or tachycardia; avoid use

Food: Food does not affect absorption; glyburide may be taken with food

Glucose: Decreases blood glucose concentration. Hypoglycemia may occur. Educate patients how to detect and treat hypoglycemia. Monitor for signs and symptoms of hypoglycemia. Administer glucose if necessary. Evaluate patient's diet and exercise regimen. May need to decrease or discontinue dose of sulfonylurea.

Sodium: Reports of hyponatremia and SIADH. Those at increased risk include patients on medications or who have medical conditions that predispose them to hyponatremia. Monitor sodium serum concentration and fluid status. May need to restrict water intake.

**Monitoring Parameters:** Signs and symptoms of hypoglycemia, fasting blood glucose, hemoglobin A$_{1c}$, fructosamine

**Reference Range:** Target range: Adults: Fasting blood glucose: <120 mg/dL; Glycosylated hemoglobin: <7%

**Related Information**

Hypoglycemic Drugs on page 1020

♦ **Glycerol Guaiacolate** see Guaifenesin on page 427

♦ **Glycerol-T®** see Theophylline and Guaifenesin on page 888

♦ **Glyceryl Trinitrate** see Nitroglycerin on page 660

## Glycopyrrolate (glye koe PYE roe late)

**Pharmacologic Class** Anticholinergic Agent

**U.S. Brand Names** Robinul®; Robinul® Forte

**Mechanism of Action** Blocks the action of acetylcholine at parasympathetic sites in smooth muscle, secretory glands, and the CNS

**Use** Adjunct in treatment of peptic ulcer disease; inhibit salivation and excessive secretions of the respiratory tract preoperatively; reversal of neuromuscular blockade; control of upper airway secretions

**USUAL DOSAGE**

Children:

Control of secretions:

Oral: 40-100 mcg/kg/dose 3-4 times/day

I.M., I.V.: 4-10 mcg/kg/dose every 3-4 hours; maximum: 0.2 mg/dose or 0.8 mg/24 hours

Intraoperative: I.V.: 4 mcg/kg not to exceed 0.1 mg; repeat at 2- to 3-minute intervals as needed

Preoperative: I.M.:

<2 years: 4.4-8.8 mcg/kg 30-60 minutes before procedure

>2 years: 4.4 mcg/kg 30-60 minutes before procedure

Children and Adults: Reverse neuromuscular blockade: I.V.: 0.2 mg for each 1 mg of neostigmine or 5 mg of pyridostigmine administered

Adults:

Intraoperative: I.V.: 0.1 mg repeated as needed at 2- to 3-minute intervals

Preoperative: I.M.: 4.4 mcg/kg 30-60 minutes before procedure

Peptic ulcer:

Oral: 1-2 mg 2-3 times/day

I.M., I.V.: 0.1-0.2 mg 3-4 times/day

**Dosage Forms Inj:** 0.2 mg/mL (1 mL, 2 mL, 5 mL, 20 mL), Robinul®: 0.2 mg/mL (1 mL, 2 mL, 5 mL, 20 mL); **Tab:** Robinul®: 1 mg, Robinul® Forte: 2 mg

**Contraindications** Narrow-angle glaucoma, acute hemorrhage, tachycardia, hypersensitivity to glycopyrrolate or any component; ulcerative colitis, obstructive uropathy, paralytic ileus, obstructive disease of GI tract

**Warnings/Precautions** Not recommended in children <12 years of age for the management of peptic ulcer; infants, patients with Down syndrome, and children with spastic paralysis or brain damage may be hypersensitive to antimuscarine effects. Use caution in elderly, patients with autonomic neuropathy, hepatic or renal disease, ulcerative colitis may predispose megacolon, hyperthyroidism, CAD, CHF, arrhythmias, tachycardia, BPH, hiatal hernia, with reflux.

**Pregnancy Risk Factor** B

**Adverse Reactions**
>10%:
Dermatologic: Dry skin
Gastrointestinal: Constipation, dry throat, xerostomia
Local: Irritation at injection site
Respiratory: Dry nose
Miscellaneous: Diaphoresis (decreased)
1% to 10%:
Dermatologic: Increased sensitivity to light
Endocrine & metabolic: Decreased flow of breast milk
Gastrointestinal: Dysphagia
<1%: Orthostatic hypotension, ventricular fibrillation, tachycardia, palpitations, confusion, drowsiness, headache, loss of memory, fatigue, ataxia, rash, bloated feeling, nausea, vomiting, dysuria, weakness, increased intraocular pain, blurred vision

**Drug Interactions**
Decreased effect of levodopa
Increased toxicity with amantadine, cyclopropane

**Onset**
Oral: Onset of action: Within 50 minutes; Peak effect: Within 1 hour
I.M.: 20-40 minutes
I.V.: 1 minute

**Duration**
Vagal effects: 2-3 hours
Inhibition of salivation: Up to 7 hours
Anticholinergic effects (after oral administration): 8-12 hours

**Half-Life** <10 minutes

**Special PA Issues**
**Patient Education:** Take as directed. Empty bladder before taking medication. Frequent mouth care and sips of water, chewing gum, or sucking on lozenges may reduce dry mouth. You may experience drowsiness, dizziness, or blurred vision; use caution when driving or engaging in hazardous tasks. You may be sensitive to light (wear sunglasses in bright sunlight), impotence (temporary), decreased sweating and increased sensitivity to heat (avoid excessively hot environments). Report rash, eye pain or acute sensitivity to light, unresolved constipation (increased fluids and dietary fiber may help), palpitations, respiratory problems, difficulty swallowing, loss of sensation, or CNS changes.

♦ **Glycopyrronium Bromide** see Glycopyrrolate on previous page
♦ **Glycotuss® [OTC]** see Guaifenesin on page 427
♦ **Glycotuss-DM® [OTC]** see Guaifenesin and Dextromethorphan on page 428
♦ **Glydiazinamide** see Glipizide on page 417
♦ **Glynase™ PresTab™** see Glyburide on page 419
♦ **Gly-Oxide® Oral [OTC]** see Carbamide Peroxide on page 150
♦ **Glytuss® [OTC]** see Guaifenesin on page 427
♦ **GM-CSF** see Sargramostim on page 822
♦ **G-myticin® Topical** see Gentamicin on page 411
♦ **GnRH** see Gonadorelin on page 423
♦ **Goatweed** see St Johns Wort on page 852

# Golden Seal

**Mechanism of Action** Contains the alkaloids hydrastine (4%) and berberine (6%), which at higher doses can cause vasoconstriction, hypertension, and mucosal irritation; berberine can produce hypotension

**Use** Gastrointestinal and peripheral vascular activity; also used in sterile eye washes, as a mouthwash, laxative, hemorrhoids, and to stop postpartum hemorrhage. Efficacy not established in clinical studies; has been used to treat mucosal inflammation/gastritis

**USUAL DOSAGE**
Root: 0.5-1 g 3 times/day
Solid form: Usual dosage: 5-10 grains
(Continued)

## Golden Seal *(Continued)*

**Contraindications** Pregnancy, breast-feeding

**Warnings/Precautions** Should not be used in patients with hypertension, glaucoma, diabetes, history of stroke, or heart disease

**Adverse Reactions** Generally high doses:
Central nervous system: Stimulation/agitation
Gastrointestinal: Nausea, vomiting, diarrhea, mouth and throat irritation
Neuromuscular & skeletal: Extremity numbness
Respiratory: Respiratory failure

**Drug Interactions** May interfere with vitamin B absorption

## Gold Sodium Thiomalate *(gold SOW dee um thye oh MAL ate)*

**Pharmacologic Class** Gold Compound

**U.S. Brand Names** Aurolate®

**Mechanism of Action** Unknown, may decrease prostaglandin synthesis or may alter cellular mechanisms by inhibiting sulfhydryl systems

**Use** Treatment of progressive rheumatoid arthritis

**USUAL DOSAGE** I.M.:
Children: Initial: Test dose of 10 mg is recommended, followed by 1 mg/kg/week for 20 weeks; maintenance: 1 mg/kg/dose at 2- to 4-week intervals thereafter for as long as therapy is clinically beneficial and toxicity does not develop. Administration for 2-4 months is usually required before clinical improvement is observed.
Adults: 10 mg first week; 25 mg second week; then 25-50 mg/week until 1 g cumulative dose has been given; if improvement occurs without adverse reactions, administer 25-50 mg every 2-3 weeks for 2-20 weeks, then every 3-4 weeks indefinitely

**Dosing adjustment in renal impairment:**
Cl$_{cr}$ 50-80 mL/minute: Administer 50% of normal dose
Cl$_{cr}$ <50 mL/minute: Avoid use

**Dosage Forms** Inj: 25 mg/mL (1 mL), 50 mg/mL (1 mL, 2 mL, 10 mL)

**Contraindications** Hypersensitivity to gold compounds or any component; systemic lupus erythematosus; history of blood dyscrasias; congestive heart failure, exfoliative dermatitis, colitis

**Warnings/Precautions** Frequent monitoring of patients for signs and symptoms of toxicity will prevent serious adverse reactions; nonsteroidal anti-inflammatory drugs (NSAIDs) and corticosteroids may be discontinued after initiating gold therapy; must not be injected I.V.

Explain the possibility of adverse reactions before initiating therapy; signs of gold toxicity include decrease in hemoglobin, leukopenia, granulocytes and platelets; proteinuria, hematuria, pigmentation, pruritus, stomatitis or persistent diarrhea, rash, metallic taste; advise patient to report any symptoms of toxicity; use with caution in patients with liver or renal disease

**Pregnancy Risk Factor** C

**Adverse Reactions**
>10%:
Dermatologic: Itching, rash
Gastrointestinal: Stomatitis, gingivitis, glossitis
Ocular: Conjunctivitis
1% to 10%:
Dermatologic: Urticaria, alopecia
Hematologic: Eosinophilia, leukopenia, thrombocytopenia
Renal: Proteinuria, hematuria
<1%: Angioedema, ulcerative enterocolitis, GI hemorrhage, dysphagia, metallic taste, agranulocytosis, anemia aplastic anemia, hepatotoxicity, peripheral neuropathy, interstitial pneumonitis

**Drug Interactions** Decreased effect with penicillamine, acetylcysteine

**Onset** Delayed; may require up to 3 months

**Half-Life** Single dose: 3-27 days; usual is approximately 5 days; After third dose: 14-40 days; After eleventh dose: Up to 168 days

**Special PA Issues**
**Patient Education:** This medication can only be administered I.M. Drug effects may not be seen for as long as 3 weeks to 3 months. Metallic taste or mouth sores may occur (frequent mouth care and lozenges may help); gray-blue color or irritation and reddening of skin may occur (avoid excessive exposure to sunlight, use sunscreen, sunglasses, and protective clothing). Report acute headache, fever; chest pain, palpitations, or irregular heartbeat; unusual bruising, blood in mouth, urine, stool, vomitus; persistent fatigue; persistent metallic taste; abdominal cramping, vomiting, diarrhea; sores in mouth; unresolved skin rash or itching.

**Monitoring Parameters** Signs and symptoms of gold toxicity, CBC with differential and platelet count, urinalysis

**Reference Range:** Gold: Normal: 0-0.1 µg/mL (SI: 0-0.0064 µmol/L); Therapeutic: 1-3 µg/mL (SI: 0.06-0.18 µmol/L); Urine: <0.1 µg/24 hour

♦ **GoLYTELY®** *see* Polyethylene Glycol-Electrolyte Solution *on page 736*

## Gonadorelin (goe nad oh REL in)

**Pharmacologic Class** Diagnostic Agent, Gonadotrophic Hormone; Gonadotropin
**U.S. Brand Names** Factrel®; Lutrepulse®
**Mechanism of Action** Stimulates the release of luteinizing hormone (LH) from the anterior pituitary gland
**Use** Evaluation of the functional capacity and response of gonadotrophic hormones; evaluate abnormal gonadotropin regulation as in precocious puberty and delayed puberty. Lutrepulse®: Induction of ovulation in females with hypothalamic amenorrhea.
**USUAL DOSAGE**
Diagnostic test: Children >12 years and Adults (female): I.V., S.C. hydrochloride salt: 100 mcg administered in women during early phase of menstrual cycle (day 1-7)
Primary hypothalamic amenorrhea: Female adults: Acetate: I.V.: 5 mcg every 90 minutes via Lutrepulse® pump kit at treatment intervals of 21 days (pump will pulsate every 90 minutes for 7 days)
**Dosage Forms Inj, as acetate (Lutrepulse®):** 0.8 mg, 3.2 mg; **Inj, as hydrochloride (Factrel®):** 100 mcg, 500 mcg
**Contraindications** Known hypersensitivity to gonadorelin, women with any condition that could be exacerbated by pregnancy; patients who have ovarian cysts or causes of anovulation other than those of hypothalamic origin; any condition that may worsened by reproductive hormones
**Warnings/Precautions** Hypersensitivity and anaphylactic reactions have occurred following multiple-dose administration; multiple pregnancy is a possibility; use with caution in women in whom pregnancy could worsen pre-existing conditions (eg, pituitary prolactinemia). Multiple pregnancy is a possibility with Lutrepulse®.
**Pregnancy Risk Factor** B
**Adverse Reactions**
1% to 10%: Local: Pain at injection site
<1%: Flushing, lightheadedness, headache, rash, nausea, abdominal discomfort
**Drug Interactions**
Decreased levels/effect: Oral contraceptives, digoxin, phenothiazines, dopamine antagonists
Increased levels/effect: Androgens, estrogens, progestins, glucocorticoids, spironolactone, levodopa
**Duration** 3-5 hours
**Half-Life** 4 minutes
**Special PA Issues**
**Patient Education:** If receiving this drug via pulsating pump, check all procedures with prescriber. Report any rash, pain, or inflammation at injection site, and any change in respiratory status.
**Monitoring Parameters:** LH, FSH

♦ **Gonadorelin Acetate** *see* Gonadorelin *on this page*
♦ **Gonadorelin Hydrochloride** *see* Gonadorelin *on this page*
♦ **Gonadotropin Releasing Hormone** *see* Gonadorelin *on this page*
♦ **Gonal-F®** *see* Follitropins *on page 397*
♦ **Gonic®** *see* Chorionic Gonadotropin *on page 205*
♦ **Gormel® Creme [OTC]** *see* Urea *on page 947*

## Goserelin (GOE se rel in)

**Pharmacologic Class** Antineoplastic Agent, Miscellaneous; Gonadotropin Releasing Hormone Analog; Luteinizing Hormone-Releasing Hormone Analog
**U.S. Brand Names** Zoladex® Implant
**Mechanism of Action** LHRH synthetic analog of luteinizing hormone-releasing hormone also known as gonadotropin-releasing hormone (GnRH) incorporated into a biodegradable depot material which allows for continuous slow release over 28 days; mechanism of action is similar to leuprolide
**Use**
Prostate carcinoma: Palliative treatment of advanced carcinoma of the prostate. An alternative treatment of prostatic cancer when orchiectomy or estrogen administration are either not indicated or unacceptable to the patient. Combination with flutamide for the management of locally confined stage T2b-T4 (stage B2-C) carcinoma of the prostate.
3.6 mg implant **only:**
Endometriosis: Management of endometriosis, including pain relief and reduction of endometriotic lesions for the duration of therapy
Advanced breast cancer: Palliative treatment of advanced breast cancer in pre- and perimenopausal women. Estrogen and progesterone receptor values may help to predict whether goserelin therapy is likely to be beneficial.
**Note:** The 10.8 mg implant is not indicated in women as the data are insufficient to support reliable suppression of serum estradiol
(Continued)

## Goserelin *(Continued)*

### USUAL DOSAGE
Adults: S.C.:

Monthly implant: 3.6 mg injected into upper abdomen every 28 days; do not try to aspirate with the goserelin syringe; if the needle is in a large vessel, blood will immediately appear in syringe chamber. While a delay of a few days is permissible, attempt to adhere to the 28-day schedule.

3-month implant: 10.8 mg injected into the upper abdominal wall every 12 weeks; do not try to aspirate with the goserelin syringe; if the needle is in a large vessel, blood will immediately appear in syringe chamber. While a delay of a few days is permissible, attempt to adhere to the 12-week schedule.

Prostate carcinoma: Intended for long-term administration

Endometriosis: Recommended duration: 6 months; retreatment is not recommended since safety data is not available. If symptoms recur after a course of therapy, and further treatment is contemplated, consider monitoring bone mineral density. Currently, there are no clinical data on the effect of treatment of benign gynecological conditions with goserelin for periods >6 months.

**Dosing adjustment in renal/hepatic impairment:** No adjustment is necessary

**Dosage Forms** Inj, implant, as acetate: 3.6 mg, 10.8 mg

**Contraindications** In women who are or may become pregnant, patients who are hypersensitive to the drug

**Warnings/Precautions** Initially, goserelin, transiently increases serum levels of testosterone. Transient worsening of signs and symptoms, usually manifested by an increase in cancer-related pain which was managed symptomatically, may develop during the first few weeks of treatment. Isolated cases of ureteral obstruction and spinal cord compression have been reported; patient's symptoms may initially worsen temporarily during first few weeks of therapy, cancer-related pain can usually be controlled by analgesics

**Pregnancy Risk Factor** X

### Adverse Reactions
General: Worsening of signs and symptoms may occur during the first few weeks of therapy and are usually manifested by an increase in bone pain, increased difficulty in urinating, hot flashes, injection site irritation, and weakness; this will subside, but patients should be aware

>10%:

Endocrine & metabolic: Gynecomastia, postmenopausal symptoms, sexual dysfunction, loss of libido, hot flashes

Genitourinary: Impotence, decreased erection

1% to 10%:

Cardiovascular: Edema

Central nervous system: Headache, spinal cord compression (possible result of tumor flare), lethargy, dizziness, insomnia

Dermatologic: Rash

Gastrointestinal: Nausea and vomiting, anorexia, diarrhea, weight gain

Genitourinary: Vaginal spotting and breakthrough bleeding, breast tenderness/enlargement

Local: Pain on injection

Neuromuscular & skeletal: Bone loss, increased bone pain

Miscellaneous: Diaphoresis

**Half-Life** Following a bolus S.C. dose: ~5 hours; prolonged in impaired renal function ~12 hours

### Special PA Issues
**Patient Education:** This drug must be implanted into your stomach every 28 days; it is important to maintain appointment schedule. You may experience systemic hot flashes (cool clothes and temperatures may help), headache (analgesic may help), constipation (increased bulk and water in diet or stool softener may help), sexual dysfunction (decreased libido, decreased erection). Symptoms may worsen temporarily during first weeks of therapy. Report unusual nausea or vomiting, any chest pain, respiratory difficulty, unresolved dizziness, or constipation.

♦ **Goserelin Acetate** *see* Goserelin *on previous page*

♦ **GR1222311X** *see* Ranitidine Bismuth Citrate *on page 794*

## Granisetron *(gra NI se tron)*

**Pharmacologic Class** Selective 5-HT$_3$ Receptor Antagonist

**U.S. Brand Names** Kytril™

**Mechanism of Action** Selective 5-HT$_3$-receptor antagonist, blocking serotonin, both peripherally on vagal nerve terminals and centrally in the chemoreceptor trigger zone

**Use** Prophylaxis and treatment of chemotherapy-related emesis; may be prescribed for patients who are refractory to or have severe adverse reactions to standard antiemetic therapy. Granisetron may be prescribed for young patients (ie, <45 years of age who are more likely to develop extrapyramidal reactions to high-dose metoclopramide) who are to receive highly emetogenic chemotherapeutic agents as listed:

Agents with high emetogenic potential (>90%) (dose/m²):
Amifostine
Azacitidine
Carmustine ≥200 mg/m²
Cisplatin ≥50 mg/m²
Cyclophosphamide ≥1 g/m²
Cytarabine ≥1500 mg/m²
Dacarbazine ≥500 mg/m²
Dactinomycin
Doxorubicin ≥60 mg/m²
Lomustine ≥60 mg/m²
Mechlorethamine
Melphalan ≥100 mg/m²
Streptozocin
Thiotepa ≥100 mg/m²

**or** two agents classified as having high or moderately high emetogenic potential as listed:

Agents with moderately high emetogenic potential (60% to 90%) (dose/m²):
Carboplatin 200-400 mg/m²
Carmustine <200 mg/m²
Cisplatin <50 mg/m²
Cyclophosphamide 600-999 mg/m²
Dacarbazine <500 mg/m²
Doxorubicin 21-59 mg/m²
Hexamethyl melamine
Ifosfamide ≥5000 mg/m²
Lomustine <60 mg/m²
Methotrexate ≥250 mg/m²
Pentostatin
Procarbazine

Granisetron should not be prescribed for chemotherapeutic agents with a low emetogenic potential (eg, bleomycin, busulfan, cyclophosphamide <1000 mg, etoposide, 5-fluorouracil, vinblastine, vincristine)

## USUAL DOSAGE
I.V.: Children and Adults: 10 mcg/kg for 1-3 doses. Doses should be administered as a single IVPB over 5 minutes to 1 hour or by undiluted IV push over 30 seconds, given just prior to chemotherapy (15-60 minutes before); as intervention therapy for breakthrough nausea and vomiting, during the first 24 hours following chemotherapy, 2 or 3 repeat infusions (same dose) have been administered, separated by at least 10 minutes

Oral: Adults: 1 mg twice daily; the first 1 mg dose should be given up to 1 hour before chemotherapy, and the second tablet, 12 hours after the first; alternatively may give a single dose of 2 mg, up to 1 hour before chemotherapy

**Note: Granisetron should only be given on the day(s) of chemotherapy**

**Dosing interval in renal impairment:** Creatinine clearance values have no relationship to granisetron clearance

**Dosing interval in hepatic impairment:** Kinetic studies in patients with hepatic impairment showed that total clearance was approximately halved, however, standard doses were very well tolerated

**Dosage Forms Inj:** 1 mg/mL; **Tab:** 1 mg (2s), (20s)

**Contraindications** Previous hypersensitivity to granisetron

**Warnings/Precautions** Use with caution in patients with liver disease or in pregnant patients

## Adverse Reactions
>10%: Central nervous system: Headache
1% to 10%:
Cardiovascular: Hyper/hypotension
Central nervous system: Dizziness, insomnia, anxiety
Gastrointestinal: Constipation, abdominal pain, diarrhea
Neuromuscular & skeletal: Weakness
<1%: Arrhythmias, somnolence, agitation, hot flashes, liver enzyme elevations

**Drug Interactions** CYP3A3/4 enzyme substrate

**Onset** Commonly controls emesis within 1-3 minutes of administration

**Duration** Effects generally last no more than a maximum of 24 hours

**Half-Life** Cancer patient: 10-12 hours; Healthy volunteer: 3-4 hours

## Special PA Issues
**Patient Education:** This drug will be administered on days when you receive chemotherapy to reduce nausea and vomiting. If outpatient chemotherapy, you may be given oral medication to take after return home; take as directed. You may experience drowsiness; use caution when driving. For persistent acute headache request analgesic from prescriber. Frequent mouth care, chewing gum, or sucking on lozenges may relieve persistent nausea. Report unrelieved headache, fever, diarrhea, or constipation.

♦ **Granulex** *see* Trypsin, Balsam Peru, and Castor Oil *on page 945*

♦ **Granulocyte Colony Stimulating Factor** *see* Filgrastim *on page 370*

♦ **Granulocyte-Macrophage Colony Stimulating Factor** *see* Sargramostim *on page 822*

# Grepafloxacin (grep a FLOX a sin)

**Pharmacologic Class** Antibiotic, Quinolone

**U.S. Brand Names** Raxar®

**Mechanism of Action** Inhibits DNA-gyrase in susceptible organisms; inhibits relaxation of supercoiled DNA and promotes breakage of double-stranded DNA

**Use** Treatment of acute bacterial exacerbations of chronic bronchitis caused by *Haemophilus influenzae*, *Streptococcus pneumoniae*, or *Moraxella catarrhalis*; community-acquired pneumonia caused by *Mycoplasma pneumoniae* or the organisms previously mentioned; uncomplicated gonorrhea caused by *Neisseria gonorrhoeae*, and nongonococcal cervicitis and urethritis caused by *Chlamydia trachomatis*

*In vitro* studies suggest similar or lesser activity against *Enterobacteriaceae* and *P. aeruginosa* but greater activity against gram-positive cocci, especially *S. pneumoniae*, and some anaerobes and *Chlamydia* spp.

**USUAL DOSAGE** Oral:

Bronchitis: 400-600 mg/day for 10 days

Community-acquired pneumonia: 600 mg/day for 10 days

Nongonococcal urethritis or cervicitis: 400 mg/day for 7 days

Uncomplicated gonorrhea: 400 mg as a single dose

**Dosage Forms Tab, as hydrochloride:** 200 mg

**Contraindications** Previous hypersensitivity to grepafloxacin and other quinolone derivatives; in patients with hepatic failure; given concomitantly with class I and III antiarrhythmics or bepridil due to the potential risk of cardiac arrhythmias (including torsade de pointes); patients with $QT_c$ prolongation and use with drugs which prolong $QT_c$ interval

**Warnings/Precautions** Use caution in patients with cerebral arteriosclerosis or epilepsy, and in patients with GI disorders or hepatic or renal dysfunction; there is no data to support safety and efficacy in children <18 years of age

**Pregnancy Risk Factor** C

**Adverse Reactions** Percentage unknown: Syncope, headache, dizziness, fatigue, nausea, emesis due to medicinal taste, hepatotoxicity (ie, elevated serum transaminases), abdominal pain, diarrhea, hypersensitivity

**Drug Interactions** CYP1A2 enzyme substrate

Antacids decrease grepafloxacin levels by 60%; grepafloxacin decreases theophylline clearance by 50%; may inhibit the metabolism of other drugs metabolized by cytochrome P-450 enzymes; may have additive effect of $Q-T_c$ prolongation when administered with other agent that may prolong $Q-T_c$ interval

**Half-Life** 15.7 hours (average)

**Special PA Issues**

**Patient Education:** Take per recommended schedule, preferably on an empty stomach (1 hour before or 2 hours after meals). Maintain adequate hydration (2-3 L/day of fluids unless instructed to restrict fluid intake). Take complete prescription; do not skip doses. If dose is missed, take as soon as possible; do not double dose. Do not take with antacids, or multivitamins with zinc or iron salts. Diabetics: If taking oral hypoglycemic agent, monitor blood sugars closely; may alter effect of oral hypoglycemic agent. You may experience dizziness, lightheadedness, anxiety, insomnia, or confusion (use caution when driving or engaging in tasks that require alertness). Small frequent meals and frequent mouth care may reduce nausea, vomiting, or taste disturbances. You may experience photosensitivity; use sunscreen, appropriate clothing, or avoid direct sun. Report immediately any CNS disturbances such as hallucinations, tremor, confusion, seizures, palpitations, or chest pain. Report persistent diarrhea or GI disturbances or abdominal pain; muscle tremor or pain; pain, inflammation, or rupture of tendon; yellowing of eyes or skin; easy bruising or bleeding; unusual fatigue; fever, chills, or signs of infection; or worsening of condition.

**Monitoring Parameters:** CBC, signs/symptoms of infection, liver/renal function tests

♦ **Grifulvin® V** *see* Griseofulvin *on this page*

♦ **Grisactin-500®** *see* Griseofulvin *on this page*

♦ **Grisactin® Ultra** *see* Griseofulvin *on this page*

# Griseofulvin (gri see oh FUL vin)

**Pharmacologic Class** Antifungal Agent, Oral

**U.S. Brand Names** Fulvicin® P/G; Fulvicin-U/F®; Grifulvin® V; Grisactin-500®; Grisactin® Ultra; Gris-PEG®

**Mechanism of Action** Inhibits fungal cell mitosis at metaphase; binds to human keratin making it resistant to fungal invasion

**Use** Treatment of susceptible tinea infections of the skin, hair, and nails

**USUAL DOSAGE** Oral:

Children >2 years:

Microsize: 10-15 mg/kg/day in single or divided doses

Ultramicrosize: 5.5-7.3 mg/kg/day in single or divided doses
Adults:
Microsize: 500 mg/day in single or divided doses for tinea corporis, cruris, capitis
Ultramicrosize: 330-375 mg/day in single or divided doses
Doses of 750-1000 mg (microsize) and 660-750 mg (ultramicrosize) have been used for infections more difficult to eradicate such as tinea unguium and tinea pedis
Duration of therapy depends on the site of infection:
Tinea corporis: 2-4 weeks
Tinea capitis: 4-6 weeks or longer
Tinea pedis: 4-8 weeks
Tinea unguium: 4-6 months

**Dosage Forms** Microsize: **Cap (Grisactin®):** 125 mg, 250 mg; **Susp, oral (Grifulvin® V):** 125 mg/5 mL with alcohol 0.2% (120 mL); **Tab:** Fulvicin-U/F®, Grifulvin® V: 250 mg, Fulvicin-U/F®, Grifulvin® V, Grisactin-500®: 500 mg

Ultramicrosize: **Tab:** Fulvicin® P/G: 165 mg, 330 mg, Fulvicin® P/G, Grisactin® Ultra, Gris-PEG®: 125 mg, 250 mg, Grisactin® Ultra: 330 mg

**Contraindications** Hypersensitivity to griseofulvin or any component; severe liver disease, porphyria (interferes with porphyrin metabolism)

**Warnings/Precautions** Safe use in children <2 years of age has not been established; during long-term therapy, periodic assessment of hepatic, renal, and hematopoietic functions should be performed; may cause fetal harm when administered to pregnant women; avoid exposure to intense sunlight to prevent photosensitivity reactions; hypersensitivity cross reaction between penicillins and griseofulvin is possible

**Pregnancy Risk Factor** C

**Adverse Reactions**
>10%: Dermatologic: Rash, urticaria
1% to 10%:
Central nervous system: Headache, fatigue, dizziness, insomnia, mental confusion
Dermatologic: Photosensitivity
Gastrointestinal: Nausea, vomiting, epigastric distress, diarrhea
Miscellaneous: Oral thrush
<1%: Angioneurotic edema, menstrual toxicity, GI bleeding, leukopenia, hepatotoxicity, proteinuria, nephrosis

**Drug Interactions**
Decreased effect:
Barbiturates may decrease levels of griseofulvin
Decreased warfarin, cyclosporine, and salicylate activity with griseofulvin
Griseofulvin decreases oral contraceptive effectiveness
Increased toxicity: With alcohol → tachycardia and flushing

**Half-Life** 9-22 hours

**Special PA Issues**
**Patient Education:** Take full course of medication as directed. High fat meals will enhance absorption. Do not discontinue without notifying prescriber. Practice good hygiene measures to prevent reinfection. Frequent blood tests may be required with prolonged therapy. You may experience nausea and vomiting (small, frequent meals may help). Avoid alcohol while taking this drug. Alcohol will cause "disulfiram"-type reaction consisting of flushing, headache, nausea, and in some patients, vomiting and chest pain, and/or abdominal pain. You may be sensitive to sun; avoid excessive exposure and use appropriate sunblock and clothing. Report rash, respiratory difficulty, CNS changes (eg, confusion, dizziness, acute headache), yellowing of skin or eyes, changes in color of stool or urine, or white plaques in mouth. Inform prescriber if you are or intend to be pregnant. Oral contraceptives may have decreased effectiveness with this medication.
**Monitoring Parameters:** Periodic renal, hepatic, and hematopoietic function tests

+ **Griseofulvin Microsize** see Griseofulvin on previous page
+ **Griseofulvin Ultramicrosize** see Griseofulvin on previous page
+ **Grisovin®-FP** see Griseofulvin on previous page
+ **Gris-PEG®** see Griseofulvin on previous page
+ **Growth Hormone** see Human Growth Hormone on page 444

# Guaifenesin (gwye FEN e sin)

**Pharmacologic Class** Expectorant

**U.S. Brand Names** Anti-Tuss® Expectorant [OTC]; Breonesin® [OTC]; Diabetic Tussin EX® [OTC]; Durafuss-G®; Fenesin™; Gee Gee® [OTC]; Genatuss® [OTC]; GG-Cen® [OTC]; Glyate® [OTC]; Glycotuss® [OTC]; Glytuss® [OTC]; Guaifenex LA®; GuiaCough® Expectorant [OTC]; Guiatuss® [OTC]; Halotussin® [OTC]; Humibid® L.A.; Humibid® Sprinkle; Hytuss® [OTC]; Hytuss-2X® [OTC]; Liquibid®; Malotuss® [OTC]; Medi-Tuss® [OTC]; Monafed®; Muco-Fen-LA®; Mytussin® [OTC]; Naldecon® Senior EX [OTC]; Organidin® NR; Pneumomist®; Respa-GF®; Robitussin® [OTC]; Scot-Tussin® [OTC]; Siltussin® [OTC]; Sinumist®-SR Capsulets®; Touro Ex®; Tusibron® [OTC]; Uni-Tussin® [OTC]
(Continued)

# Guaifenesin (Continued)

**Mechanism of Action** Thought to act as an expectorant by irritating the gastric mucosa and stimulating respiratory tract secretions, thereby increasing respiratory fluid volumes and decreasing phlegm viscosity

**Use** Temporary control of cough due to minor throat and bronchial irritation

**USUAL DOSAGE** Oral:

Children:

<2 years: 12 mg/kg/day in 6 divided doses

2-5 years: 50-100 mg every 4 hours, not to exceed 600 mg/day

6-11 years: 100-200 mg every 4 hours, not to exceed 1.2 g/day

Children >12 years and Adults: 200-400 mg every 4 hours to a maximum of 2.4 g/day

**Dosage Forms Caplet, sustained release (Touro Ex®):** 600 mg; **Cap (Breonesin®, GG-Cen®, Hytuss-2X®):** 200 mg, Sustained release (Humibid® Sprinkle): 300 mg; **Liq:** Diabetic Tussin® EX, Organidin® NR, Tusibron®: 100 mg/5 mL (118 mL), Naldecon® Senior EX: 200 mg/5 mL (118 mL, 480 mL); **Syr (Anti-Tuss® Expectorant, Genatuss®, Glyate®, GuiaCough® Expectorant, Guiatuss®, Halotussin®, Malotuss®, Medi-Tuss®, Mytussin®, Robitussin®, Scot-Tussin®, Siltussin®, Tusibron®, Uni-Tussin®):** 100 mg/5 mL with alcohol 3.5% (30 mL, 120 mL, 240 mL, 473 mL, 946 mL); **Tab:** Duratuss-G®: 1200 mg, Gee Gee®, Glytuss®, Organidin® NR: 200 mg, Glycotuss®, Hytuss®: 100 mg, Sustained release: Fenesin™, Guaifenex® LA, Humibid® L.A., Liquibid®, Monafed®, Muco-Fen-LA®, Pneumomist®, Respa-GF®, Sinumist®-SR; **Capsulets®:** 600 mg

**Contraindications** Hypersensitivity to guaifenesin or any component

**Warnings/Precautions** Not for persistent cough such as occurs with smoking, asthma, or emphysema or cough accompanied by excessive secretions

**Pregnancy Risk Factor** C

**Adverse Reactions** 1% to 10%:

Central nervous system: Drowsiness, headache

Dermatologic: Rash

Gastrointestinal: Nausea vomiting, stomach pain

**Special PA Issues**

**Patient Education:** Take only as prescribed; do not exceed prescribed dose or frequency. Do not chew or crush timed release capsule. Maintain adequate hydration (2-3 L/day of fluids unless instructed to restrict fluid intake). You may experience some drowsiness (use caution when driving or engaging in hazardous tasks until response to therapy is known). Report excessive drowsiness, difficulty breathing, or lack of improvement or worsening of condition.

# Guaifenesin and Codeine (gwye FEN e sin & KOE deen)

**Pharmacologic Class** Antitussive; Cough Preparation; Expectorant

**U.S. Brand Names** Brontex® Liquid; Brontex® Tablet; Cheracol®; Guaituss AC®; Guiatussin® With Codeine; Mytussin® AC; Robafen® AC; Robitussin® A-C; Tussi-Organidin® NR

**Dosage Forms Liq [C-V] (Brontex®):** Guaifenesin 75 mg and codeine phosphate 2.5 mg per 5 mL; **Syr [C-V] (Cheracol®, Guaituss AC®, Guiatussin® with Codeine, Mytussin® AC, Robafen® AC, Robitussin® A-C, Tussi-Organidin® NR):** Guaifenesin 100 mg and codeine phosphate 10 mg per 5 mL (60 mL, 120 mL, 480 mL); **Tab [C-III] (Brontex®):** Guaifenesin 300 mg and codeine phosphate 10 mg

# Guaifenesin and Dextromethorphan

(gwye FEN e sin & deks troe meth OR fan)

**Pharmacologic Class** Antitussive; Cough Preparation; Expectorant

**U.S. Brand Names** Benylin® Expectorant [OTC]; Cheracol® D [OTC]; Clear Tussin® 30; Contac® Cough Formula Liquid [OTC]; Diabetic Tussin DM® [OTC]; Extra Action Cough Syrup [OTC]; Fenesin™ DM; Genatuss DM® [OTC]; Glycotuss-DM® [OTC]; Guaifenex DM®; GuiaCough® [OTC]; Guiatuss-DM® [OTC]; Halotussin®-DM [OTC]; Humibid® DM [OTC]; Iobid DM®; Kolephrin® GG/DM [OTC]; Monafed® DM; Muco-Fen-DM®; Mytussin® DM [OTC]; Naldecon® Senior DX [OTC]; Phanatuss® Cough Syrup [OTC]; Phenadex® Senior [OTC]; Queltuss®; Respa-DM®; Rhinosyn-DMX® [OTC]; Robafen DM® [OTC]; Robitussin®-DM [OTC]; Safe Tussin® 30 [OTC]; Scot-Tussin® Senior Clear [OTC]; Siltussin DM® [OTC]; Synacol® CF [OTC]; Syracol-CF® [OTC]; Tolu-Sed® DM [OTC]; Tusibron-DM® [OTC]; Tuss-DM® [OTC]; Tussi-Organidin® DM NR [OTC]; Uni-tussin® DM [OTC]; Vicks® 44E [OTC]; Vicks® Pediatric Formula 44E [OTC]

**Use** Temporary control of cough due to minor throat and bronchial irritation

**USUAL DOSAGE** Oral:

Children: Dextromethorphan: 1-2 mg/kg/24 hours divided 3-4 times/day

Children >12 years and Adults: 5 mL every 4 hours or 10 mL every 6-8 hours not to exceed 40 mL/24 hours

**Dosage Forms Syr:** Benylin® Expectorant: Guaifenesin 100 mg and dextromethorphan hydrobromide 5 mg per 5 mL (118 mL, 236 mL), Cheracol® D, Clear Tussin® 30, Genatuss DM®, Mytussin® DM, Robitussin®-DM, Siltussin DM®, Tolu-Sed® DM, Tussi-Organidin® DM NR: Guaifenesin 100 mg and dextromethorphan hydrobromide 10 mg per 5 mL (5 mL, 10 mL, 120 mL, 240 mL, 360 mL, 480 mL, 3780 mL), Contac® Cough Formula Liquid: Guaifenesin 67 mg and dextromethorphan hydrobromide 10 mg per 5 mL (120 mL), Extra Action Cough Syrup, GuiaCough®, Guiatuss DM®, Halotussin® DM, Rhinosyn-DMX®, Tusibron-DM®, Uni-tussin® DM: Guaifenesin 100 mg and dextromethorphan hydrobromide 15 mg per 5 mL (120 mL, 240 mL, 480 mL), Kolephrin® GG/DM: Guaifenesin 150 mg and dextromethorphan hydrobromide 10 mg per 5 mL (120 mL), Naldecon® Senior DX: Guaifenesin 200 mg and dextromethorphan hydrobromide 15 mg per 5 mL (118 mL, 480 mL), Phanatuss®: Guaifenesin 85 mg and dextromethorphan hydrobromide 10 mg per 5 mL, Vicks® 44E: Guaifenesin 66.7 mg and dextromethorphan hydrobromide 6.7 mg per 5 mL; **Tab:** Extended release Guaifenex DM®, Iobid DM®, Fenesin™ DM, Humibid® DM, Monafed® DM, Respa-DM®: Guaifenesin 600 mg and dextromethorphan hydrobromide 30 mg, Glycotuss-dM®: Guaifenesin 100 mg and dextromethorphan hydrobromide 10 mg, Queltuss®: Guaifenesin 100 mg and dextromethorphan hydrobromide 15 mg, Syracol-CF®: Guaifenesin 200 mg and dextromethorphan hydrobromide 15 m, Tuss-DM®: Guaifenesin 200 mg and dextromethorphan hydrobromide 10 mg

**Contraindications** Hypersensitivity to guaifenesin, dextromethorphan or any component

**Warnings/Precautions** Should not be used for persistent or chronic cough such as that occurring with smoking, asthma, chronic bronchitis, or emphysema or for cough associated with excessive phlegm

**Pregnancy Risk Factor** C

**Adverse Reactions** 1% to 10%:
Central nervous system: Drowsiness, headache
Dermatologic: Rash
Gastrointestinal: Nausea, vomiting

## Guaifenesin and Phenylephrine (gwye FEN e sin & fen il EF rin)

**Pharmacologic Class** Cold Preparation

**U.S. Brand Names** Deconsal® Sprinkle®; Endal®; Sinupan®

**Dosage Forms Cap, sustained release:** Deconsal® Sprinkle®: Guaifenesin 300 mg and phenylephrine hydrochloride 10 mg, Sinupan®: Guaifenesin 200 mg and phenylephrine hydrochloride 40 mg; **Tab, timed release (Endal®):** Guaifenesin 300 mg and phenylephrine hydrochloride 20 mg

## Guaifenesin, Pseudoephedrine, and Codeine

(gwye FEN e sin, soo doe e FED rin, & KOE deen)

**Pharmacologic Class** Antitussive/Decongestant/Expectorant

**U.S. Brand Names** Codafed® Expectorant; Cycofed® Pediatric; Decohistine® Expectorant; Deproist® Expectorant With Codeine; Dihistine® Expectorant; Guiatuss DAC®; Guiatussin® DAC; Halotussin® DAC; Isoclor® Expectorant; Mytussin® DAC; Nucofed®; Nucofed® Pediatric Expectorant; Nucotuss®; Phenhist® Expectorant; Robitussin®-DAC; Ryna-CX®; Tussar® SF Syrup

**Dosage Forms Liq:** C-III: Nucofed®, Nucotuss®: Guaifenesin 200 mg, pseudoephedrine hydrochloride 60 mg, and codeine phosphate 20 mg per 5 mL (480 mL), C-V: Codafed® Expectorant, Decohistine® Expectorant, Deproist® Expectorant with Codeine, Dihistine® Expectorant, Guiatuss DAC®, Guiatussin® DAC, Halotussin® DAC, Isoclor® Expectorant, Mytussin® DAC, Nucofed® Pediatric Expectorant, Phenhist® Expectorant, Robitussin®-DAC, Ryna-CX®, Tussar® SF: Guaifenesin 100 mg, pseudoephedrine hydrochloride 30 mg, and codeine phosphate 10 mg per 5 mL (120 mL, 480 mL, 4000 mL)

◆ **Guaifenex DM**® *see* Guaifenesin and Dextromethorphan *on previous page*

◆ **Guaifenex LA**® *see* Guaifenesin *on page 427*

◆ **Guaituss AC**® *see* Guaifenesin and Codeine *on previous page*

## Guanabenz (GWAHN a benz)

**Pharmacologic Class** Alpha₂ Agonist

**U.S. Brand Names** Wytensin®

**Use** Management of hypertension

**USUAL DOSAGE** Adults: Oral: Initial: 4 mg twice daily, increase in increments of 4-8 mg/day every 1-2 weeks to a maximum of 32 mg twice daily

**Dosing adjustment in hepatic impairment:** Probably necessary

**Dosage Forms Tab, as acetate:** 4 mg, 8 mg

**Contraindications** Hypersensitivity to guanabenz or any component

**Pregnancy Risk Factor** C

**Onset** Onset of antihypertensive effect: Within 1 hour

**Half-Life** 7-10 hours

**Special PA Issues**

**Patient Education:** Take as directed. Do not skip dose or discontinue without consulting prescriber. Store medication container away from light. Follow recommended diet and exercise program. Do not use OTC medications which may affect blood pressure (eg, cough or cold remedies, diet pills, stay-awake medications) without consulting prescriber. This medication may cause drowsiness, dizziness, or impaired judgment (use caution when driving or engaging in tasks that require alertness until response is known); (Continued)

## Guanabenz *(Continued)*

decreased libido or sexual function (will resolve when drug is discontinued); postural hypotension (use caution when rising from sitting or lying position or when climbing stairs); or dry mouth or nausea (frequent mouth care or sucking lozenges may help). Report difficulty, pain, or burning on urination; increased nervousness or depression; sudden weight gain (weigh yourself in the same clothes at same time of day once a week); unusual or persistent swelling of ankles, feet, or extremities; wet cough or respiratory difficulty; chest pain or palpitations; muscle weakness, fatigue, or pain; or other persistent side effects.

♦ **Guanabenz Acetate** *see* Guanabenz *on previous page*

## Guanadrel (GWAHN a drel)

**Pharmacologic Class** False Neurotransmitter

**U.S. Brand Names** Hylorel®

**Use** Considered a second line agent in the treatment of hypertension, usually with a diuretic

**USUAL DOSAGE** Oral:

Adults: Initial: 10 mg/day (5 mg twice daily); adjust dosage weekly or monthly until blood pressure is controlled, usual dosage: 20-75 mg/day, given twice daily; for larger dosage, 3-4 times/day dosing may be needed

Elderly: Initial: 5 mg once daily

**Dosing interval in renal impairment:**

$Cl_{cr}$ 10-50 mL/minute: Administer every 12-24 hours

$Cl_{cr}$ <10 mL/minute: Administer every 24-48 hours

**Dosage Forms Tab, as sulfate:** 10 mg, 25 mg

**Contraindications** Known hypersensitivity to guanadrel, pheochromocytoma, patients taking MAO inhibitors

**Pregnancy Risk Factor** B

**Onset** Peak effect: Within 4-6 hours

**Duration** 4-14 hours

**Half-Life** Biphasic: Initial: 1-4 hours; Terminal: 5-45 hours

**Special PA Issues**

**Patient Education:** Take as directed. Do not skip dose or discontinue without consulting prescriber. Store medication container away from light. Follow recommended diet and exercise program. Do not use OTC medications which may affect blood pressure (eg, cough or cold remedies, diet pills, stay-awake medications) without consulting prescriber. This medication may cause drowsiness, dizziness, or impaired judgment (use caution when driving or engaging in tasks that require alertness until response is known); decreased libido or sexual function (will resolve when drug is discontinued); postural hypotension (use caution when rising from sitting or lying position or when climbing stairs); or dry mouth or nausea (frequent mouth care or sucking lozenges may help). Report difficulty, pain, or burning on urination; increased nervousness or depression; sudden weight gain (weigh yourself in the same clothes at same time of day once a week); unusual or persistent swelling of ankles, feet, or extremities; wet cough or respiratory difficulty; chest pain or palpitations; muscle weakness, fatigue, or pain; or other persistent side effects.

♦ **Guanadrel Sulfate** *see* Guanadrel *on this page*

## Guanethidine (gwahn ETH i deen)

**Pharmacologic Class** False Neurotransmitter

**U.S. Brand Names** Ismelin®

**Use** Treatment of moderate to severe hypertension

**USUAL DOSAGE** Oral:

Children: Initial: 0.2 mg/kg/day, increase by 0.2 mg/kg/day at 7- to 10-day intervals to a maximum of 3 mg/kg/day

Adults:

Ambulatory patients: Initial: 10 mg/day, increase at 5- to 7-day intervals to an average of 25-50 mg/day

Hospitalized patients: Initial: 25-50 mg/day, increase by 25-50 mg/day or every other day to desired therapeutic response

Elderly: Initial: 5 mg once daily

**Dosing interval in renal impairment:** $Cl_{cr}$ <10 mL/minute: Administer every 24-36 hours

**Dosage Forms Tab, as monosulfate:** 10 mg, 25 mg

**Contraindications** Pheochromocytoma, patients taking MAO inhibitors, hypersensitivity to guanethidine or any component

**Pregnancy Risk Factor** C

**Onset** Within 0.5-2 hours; Peak antihypertensive effect: Within 6-8 hours

**Duration** 24-48 hours

**Half-Life** 5-10 days

**Special PA Issues**
  **Patient Education:** Take as directed. Do not skip dose or discontinue without consulting prescriber. Store medication container away from light. Follow recommended diet and exercise program. Do not use OTC medications which may affect blood pressure (eg, cough or cold remedies, diet pills, stay-awake medications) without consulting prescriber. This medication may cause drowsiness, dizziness, or impaired judgment (use caution when driving or engaging in tasks that require alertness until response is known); decreased libido or sexual function (will resolve when drug is discontinued); postural hypotension (use caution when rising from sitting or lying position or when climbing stairs); or dry mouth or nausea (frequent mouth care or sucking lozenges may help). Report difficulty, pain, or burning on urination; increased nervousness or depression; sudden weight gain (weigh yourself in the same clothes at same time of day once a week); unusual or persistent swelling of ankles, feet, or extremities; wet cough or respiratory difficulty; chest pain or palpitations; muscle weakness, fatigue, or pain; or other persistent side effects.

♦ **Guanethidine Monosulfate** *see* Guanethidine *on previous page*

## Guanfacine (GWAHN fa seen)
  **Pharmacologic Class** Alpha₂ Agonist
  **U.S. Brand Names** Tenex®
  **Use** Management of hypertension
  **USUAL DOSAGE** Adults: Oral: 1 mg usually at bedtime, may increase if needed at 3- to 4-week intervals; 1 mg/day is most common dose
  **Dosage Forms Tab, as hydrochloride:** 1 mg
  **Contraindications** Hypersensitivity to guanfacine or any component
  **Pregnancy Risk Factor** B
  **Onset** Peak effect: Within 8-11 hours
  **Duration** 24 hours following a single dose
  **Half-Life** 17 hours
  **Special PA Issues**
  **Patient Education:** Take as directed, at bedtime. Do not skip dose or discontinue without consulting prescriber. Store medication container away from light. Follow recommended diet and exercise program. Do not use OTC medications which may affect blood pressure (eg, cough or cold remedies, diet pills, stay-awake medications) without consulting prescriber. This medication may cause drowsiness, dizziness, or impaired judgment (use caution when driving or engaging in tasks that require alertness until response is known); postural hypotension (use caution when rising from sitting or lying position or when climbing stairs); or dry mouth or nausea (frequent mouth care or sucking lozenges may help). Report increased nervousness or depression; sudden weight gain (weigh yourself in the same clothes at same time of day once a week); unusual or persistent swelling of ankles, feet, or extremities; wet cough or respiratory difficulty; chest pain or palpitations; muscle weakness, fatigue, or pain; or other persistent side effects.

♦ **GuiaCough® [OTC]** *see* Guaifenesin and Dextromethorphan *on page 428*
♦ **GuiaCough® Expectorant [OTC]** *see* Guaifenesin *on page 427*
♦ **Guiatuss® [OTC]** *see* Guaifenesin *on page 427*
♦ **Guiatuss DAC®** *see* Guaifenesin, Pseudoephedrine, and Codeine *on page 429*
♦ **Guiatuss-DM® [OTC]** *see* Guaifenesin and Dextromethorphan *on page 428*
♦ **Guiatussin® DAC** *see* Guaifenesin, Pseudoephedrine, and Codeine *on page 429*
♦ **Guiatussin® With Codeine** *see* Guaifenesin and Codeine *on page 428*
♦ **G-well®** *see* Lindane *on page 534*
♦ **Gynecort® [OTC]** *see* Hydrocortisone *on page 453*
♦ **Gyne-Lotrimin® [OTC]** *see* Clotrimazole *on page 228*
♦ **Gynergen®** *see* Ergotamine *on page 328*
♦ **Gyne-Sulf®** *see* Sulfabenzamide, Sulfacetamide, and Sulfathiazole *on page 857*
♦ **Gynix® Vaginal Tablets** *see* Clotrimazole *on page 228*
♦ **Gynogen L.A.® Injection** *see* Estradiol *on page 332*
♦ **Habitrol™ Patch** *see* Nicotine *on page 653*

## *Haemophilus* b Conjugate and Hepatitis b Vaccine
  (he MOF i lus bee KON joo gate & hep a TYE tis bee vak SEEN)
  **Pharmacologic Class** Vaccine
  **U.S. Brand Names** Comvax™
  **Mechanism of Action** Hib conjugate vaccines use covalent binding of capsular polysaccharide of *Haemophilus influenzae* type b to OMPC carrier to produce an antigen which is postulated to convert a T-independent antigen into a T-dependent antigen to result in enhanced antibody response and on immunologic memory. Recombinant hepatitis B vaccine is a noninfectious subunit viral vaccine. The vaccine is derived from hepatitis B surface antigen (HBₛAg) produced through recombinant DNA techniques from yeast cells. (Continued)

## *Haemophilus* b Conjugate and Hepatitis b Vaccine *(Continued)*

The portion of the hepatitis B gene which codes for HB$_s$Ag is cloned into yeast which is then cultured to produce hepatitis B vaccine.

**Use**

Immunization against invasive disease caused by *H. influenzae* type b and against infection caused by all known subtypes of hepatitis B virus in infants 8 weeks to 15 months of age born of HB$_s$Ag-negative mothers

Infants born of HB$_s$Ag-positive mothers or mothers of unknown HB$_s$Ag status should receive hepatitis B immune globulin and hepatitis B vaccine (Recombinant) at birth and should complete the hepatitis B vaccination series given according to a particular schedule

**USUAL DOSAGE** Infants (>8 weeks of age): I.M.: 0.5 mL at 2, 4, and 12-15 months of age (total of 3 doses)

If the recommended schedule cannot be followed, the interval between the first two doses should be at least 2 months and the interval between the second and third dose should be as close as possible to 8-11 months.

*Modified Schedule:* Children who receive one dose of hepatitis B vaccine at or shortly after birth may receive Comvax™ on a schedule of 2,4, and 12-15 months of age

**Dosage Forms Inj:** 7.5 mcg *Haemophilus* b PRP and 5 mcg HB$_s$Ag/0.5 mL

**Contraindications** Hypersensitivity to any component of the vaccine

**Warnings/Precautions** If used in persons with malignancies or those receiving immunosuppressive therapy or who are otherwise immunocompromised, the expected immune response may not be obtained.

Patients who develop symptoms suggestive of hypersensitivity after an injection should not receive further injections of the vaccine.

The decision to administer or delay vaccination because of current or recent febrile illness depends on the severity of symptoms and the etiology of the disease. Immunization should be delayed during the course of an acute febrile illness.

**Pregnancy Risk Factor** C

**Adverse Reactions** When administered during the same visit that DTP, OPV, IPV, Varicella Virus Vaccine, and M-M-R II vaccines are given, the rates of systemic reactions do not differ from those observed only when any of the vaccines are administered **All serious adverse reactions must be reported to the U.S. Department of Health and Human Services (DHHS) Vaccine Adverse Event Reporting System (VAERS) 1-800-822-7967.**

>10%: Central nervous system: Acute febrile reactions

1% to 10%:
Central nervous system: Fever (up to 102.2°F), irritability, lethargy
Gastrointestinal: Anorexia, diarrhea
Local: Irritation at injection site

<1%: Convulsions, fever (>102.2°F), vomiting, allergic or anaphylactic reactions (difficulty in breathing, hives, itching, swelling of eyes, face, unusual tiredness or weakness)

**Special PA Issues**

**Patient Education:** May use acetaminophen for postdose fever

## *Haemophilus* b Conjugate Vaccine

(hem OF fi lus bee KON joo gate vak SEEN)

**Pharmacologic Class** Vaccine

**U.S. Brand Names** ActHIB®; HibTITER®; OmniHIB™; PedvaxHIB™; ProHIBiT®; TriHIBiT®

**Mechanism of Action** Stimulates production of anticapsular antibodies and provides active immunity to *Haemophilus influenzae*

### Vaccination Schedule for *Haemophilus* b Conjugate Vaccines

| Age at 1st Dose (mo) | HibTITER® | | PedvaxHIB® | | ProHIBiT® | |
|---|---|---|---|---|---|---|
| | Primary Series | Booster | Primary Series | Booster | Primary Series | Booster |
| 2-6* | 3 doses, 2 months apart | 15 mo† | 2 doses, 2 months apart | 12 mo† | | |
| 7-11 | 2 doses, 2 months apart | 15 mo† | 2 doses, 2 months apart | 15 mo† | | |
| 12-14 | 1 dose | 15 mo† | 1 dose | 15 mo† | | |
| 15-60 | 1 dose | — | 1 dose | — | 1 dose | — |

*It is not currently recommended that the various *Haemophilus* b conjugate vaccines be interchanged (ie, the same brand should be used throughout the entire vaccination series). If the health care provider does not know which vaccine was previously used, it is prudent that an infant, 2-6 months of age, be given a primary series of three doses.

†At least 2 months after previous dose.

**Use** Routine immunization of children 2 months to 5 years of age against invasive disease caused by *H. influenzae*

Unimmunized children ≥5 years of age with a chronic illness known to be associated with increased risk of *Haemophilus influenzae* type b disease, specifically, persons with anatomic or functional asplenia or sickle cell anemia or those who have undergone splenectomy, should receive Hib vaccine.

*Haemophilus* b conjugate vaccines are not indicated for prevention of bronchitis or other infections due to *H. influenzae* in adults; adults with specific dysfunction or certain complement deficiencies who are at especially high risk of *H. influenzae* type b infection (HIV-infected adults); patients with Hodgkin's disease (vaccinated at least 2 weeks before the initiation of chemotherapy or 3 months after the end of chemotherapy)

**USUAL DOSAGE** Children: I.M.: 0.5 mL as a single dose should be administered according to one of the following "brand-specific" schedules; do not inject I.V.

**Dosage Forms Inj: (ActHIB®, HibTITER®, OmniHIB™):** Capsular oligosaccharide 10 mcg and diphtheria CRM$_{197}$ protein ~25 mcg per 0.5 mL (0.5 mL, 2.5 mL, 5 mL); **(PedvaxHIB™):** Purified capsular polysaccharide 15 mcg and *Neisseria meningitidis* OMPC 250 mcg per dose (0.5 mL); **ProHIBiT®:** Purified capsular polysaccharide 25 mcg and conjugated diphtheria toxoid protein 18 mcg per dose (0.5 mL, 2.5 mL, 5 mL); **TriHIBit® vaccine [Tripedia® vaccine used to reconstitute ActHIB®]:** 0.5 mL

**Contraindications** Children with any febrile illness or active infection, known hypersensitivity to *Haemophilus* b polysaccharide vaccine (thimerosal), children who are immunosuppressed or receiving immunosuppressive therapy

**Warnings/Precautions** Have epinephrine 1:1000 available; children in whom DTP or DT vaccination is deferred: The carrier proteins used in HbOC (but not PRP-OMP) are chemically and immunologically related to toxoids contained in DTP vaccine. Earlier or simultaneous vaccination with diphtheria or tetanus toxoids may be required to elicit an optimal anti-PRP antibody response to HbOC. In contrast, the immunogenicity of PRP-OMP is not affected by vaccination with DTP. In infants in whom DTP or DT vaccination is deferred, PRP-OMP may be advantageous for *Haemophilus influenzae* type b vaccination.

Children with immunologic impairment: Children with chronic illness associated with increased risk of *Haemophilus influenzae* type b disease may have impaired anti-PRP antibody responses to conjugate vaccination. Examples include those with HIV infection, immunoglobulin deficiency, anatomic or functional asplenia, and sickle cell disease, as well as recipients of bone marrow transplants and recipients of chemotherapy for malignancy. Some children with immunologic impairment may benefit from more doses of conjugate vaccine than normally indicated.

**Pregnancy Risk Factor** C

**Adverse Reactions** When administered during the same visit that DTP vaccine is given, the rates of systemic reactions do not differ from those observed only when DTP vaccine is administered. **All serious adverse reactions must be reported to the U.S. Department of Health and Human Services (DHHS) Vaccine Adverse Event Reporting System (VAERS) 1-800-822-7967.**

25%:
   Cardiovascular: Edema
   Dermatologic: Local erythema
   Local: Increased risk of *Haemophilus* b infections in the week after vaccination
   Miscellaneous: Warmth
>10%: Acute febrile reactions
1% to 10%:
   Central nervous system: Fever (up to 102.2°F), irritability, lethargy
   Gastrointestinal: Anorexia, diarrhea
   Local: Irritation at injection site
<1%: Edema of the eyes/face, convulsions, fever (>102.2°F), unusual fatigue, urticaria, itching, vomiting, weakness, dyspnea

**Drug Interactions** Decreased effect with immunosuppressive agents, immunoglobulins within 1 month may decrease antibody production

**Special PA Issues**
   **Patient Education:** May use acetaminophen for postdose fever

♦ *Haemophilus* b (meningococcal protein conjugate) Conjugate Vaccine *see Haemophilus* b Conjugate and Hepatitis b Vaccine *on page 431*

♦ *Haemophilus* b Oligosaccharide Conjugate Vaccine *see Haemophilus* b Conjugate Vaccine *on previous page*

♦ *Haemophilus* b Polysaccharide Vaccine *see Haemophilus* b Conjugate Vaccine *on previous page*

# Halazepam (hal AZ e pam)

**Pharmacologic Class** Benzodiazepine

**U.S. Brand Names** Paxipam®

**Use** Management of anxiety disorders; short-term relief of the symptoms of anxiety
*(Continued)*

## Halazepam *(Continued)*

**USUAL DOSAGE** Oral:

Adults: 20-40 mg 3-4 times/day; optimal dosage usually ranges from 80-160 mg/day. If side effects occur with the starting dose, lower the dose.

Elderly ≥70 years or debilitated patients: 20 mg 1-2 times/day and adjust dose accordingly

**Dosage Forms** Tab: 20 mg, 40 mg

**Contraindications** Hypersensitivity to halazepam or any component, cross-sensitivity with other benzodiazepines may exist; avoid using in patients with pre-existing CNS depression, severe uncontrolled pain, or angle-closure glaucoma

**Pregnancy Risk Factor** D

**Onset** Peak levels in 1-3 hours

**Half-Life** Parent: 14 hours; metabolite (desmethyldiazepam): 50-100 hours

## Halcinonide (hal SIN oh nide)

**Pharmacologic Class** Corticosteroid, Topical

**U.S. Brand Names** Halog®; Halog®-E

**Mechanism of Action** Decreases inflammation by suppression of migration of polymorphonuclear leukocytes and reversal of increased capillary permeability

**Use** Inflammation of corticosteroid-responsive dermatoses [high potency topical corticosteroid]

**USUAL DOSAGE** Children and Adults: Topical: Apply sparingly 1-3 times/day, occlusive dressing may be used for severe or resistant dermatoses; a thin film of cream or ointment is effective; do not overuse

**Dosage Forms Crm (Halog®):** 0.025% (15 g, 60 g, 240 g); 0.1% (15 g, 30 g, 60 g, 240 g); **Crm, emollient base (Halog®-E):** 0.1% (15 g, 30 g, 60 g); **Oint, top (Halog®):** 0.1% (15 g, 30 g, 60 g, 240 g); **Soln (Halog®):** 0.1% (20 mL, 60 mL)

**Contraindications** Viral, fungal, or tubercular skin lesions, known hypersensitivity to halcinonide or any component

**Warnings/Precautions** Adverse systemic effects may occur when used on large areas of the body, denuded areas, for prolonged periods of time, with an occlusive dressing, and/or in infants or small children

**Pregnancy Risk Factor** C

**Adverse Reactions** <1%: Itching, dry skin, folliculitis, hypertrichosis, acneiform eruptions, hypopigmentation, perioral dermatitis, allergic contact dermatitis, skin maceration, skin atrophy, striae; local burning, irritation, miliaria; secondary infection

**Special PA Issues**

**Patient Education:** For external use only. Use exactly as directed; do not overuse. Do not apply to open wounds or weeping areas. Before using, wash and dry area gently. Apply a thin film to affected area and rub in gently. If dressing is necessary, use a porous dressing. Avoid contact with eyes. Avoid exposing treated area to direct sunlight; sunburn can occur. Report increased swelling, redness, rash, itching, signs of infection, worsening of condition, or lack of healing.

♦ **Halcion®** *see Triazolam on page 931*

♦ **Haldol®** *see Haloperidol on next page*

♦ **Haldol® Decanoate** *see Haloperidol on next page*

♦ **Halenol® Childrens [OTC]** *see Acetaminophen on page 21*

♦ **Halfan®** *see Halofantrine on next page*

♦ **Halfprin® 81® [OTC]** *see Aspirin on page 80*

♦ **Hallucinogenic Drugs** *see Chart on page 1019*

## Halobetasol (hal oh BAY ta sol)

**Pharmacologic Class** Corticosteroid, Topical

**U.S. Brand Names** Ultravate™ Topical

**Mechanism of Action** Corticosteroids inhibit the initial manifestations of the inflammatory process (ie, capillary dilation and edema, fibrin deposition, and migration and diapedesis of leukocytes into the inflamed site) as well as later sequelae (angiogenesis, fibroblast proliferation)

**Use** Relief of inflammatory and pruritic manifestations of corticosteroid-response dermatoses [very high potency topical corticosteroid]

**USUAL DOSAGE** Children and Adults: Topical: Apply sparingly to skin twice daily, rub in gently and completely; treatment should not exceed 2 consecutive weeks and total dosage should not exceed 50 g/week

**Dosage Forms Crm:** 0.05% (15 g, 45 g); **Oint, top:** 0.05% (15 g, 45 g)

**Contraindications** Hypersensitivity to halobetasol or any component; viral, fungal, or tubercular skin lesions

**Warnings/Precautions** Not for ophthalmic use; may cause adrenal suppression or insufficiency; application to abraded or inflamed areas or too large of areas of the body may increase the risk of systemic absorption and the risk of adrenal suppression, as may prolonged use or the use of >50 g/week. Topical halobetasol should not be used for the treatment of rosacea or perioral dermatitis.

**Pregnancy Risk Factor** C

**Adverse Reactions** <1%: Itching, dry skin, folliculitis, hypertrichosis, acneiform eruptions, hypopigmentation, perioral dermatitis, allergic contact dermatitis, skin maceration, skin atrophy, striae; local burning, irritation, miliaria; secondary infection

**Special PA Issues**

**Patient Education:** For external use only. Use exactly as directed; do not overuse. Do not apply to open wounds or weeping areas. Before using, wash and dry area gently. Apply a thin film to affected area and rub in gently. If dressing is necessary, use a porous dressing. Avoid contact with eyes. Avoid exposing treated area to direct sunlight; sunburn can occur. Report increased swelling, redness, rash, itching, signs of infection, worsening of condition, or lack of healing.

♦ **Halobetasol Propionate** *see* Halobetasol *on previous page*

# Halofantrine (ha loe FAN trin)

**Pharmacologic Class** Antimalarial Agent

**U.S. Brand Names** Halfan®

**Mechanism of Action** Similar to mefloquine; destruction of asexual blood forms, possible inhibition of proton pump

**Use** Treatment of mild to moderate acute malaria caused by susceptible strains of *Plasmodium falciparum* and *Plasmodium vivax*

**USUAL DOSAGE** Oral:

Children <40 kg: 8 mg/kg every 6 hours for 3 doses; repeat in 1 week

Adults: 500 mg every 6 hours for 3 doses; repeat in 1 week

**Dosage Forms Susp:** 100 mg/5 mL; **Tab:** 250 mg

**Contraindications** Family history of congenital Q-T$_c$ prolongation; hypersensitivity to halofantrine

**Warnings/Precautions** Monitor closely for decreased hematocrit and hemoglobin, patients with chronic liver disease

**Pregnancy Risk Factor** C

**Adverse Reactions**

>10%: Dermatologic: Pruritus

1% to 10%:

Cardiovascular: Edema

Central nervous system: Malaise, headache

Gastrointestinal: Nausea, vomiting

Hematologic: Leukocytosis

Hepatic: Elevated LFTs

Local: Tenderness

Neuromuscular & skeletal: Myalgia

Respiratory: Cough

Miscellaneous: Lymphadenopathy

<1%: Tachycardia, hypotension, urticaria, hypoglycemia, sterile abscesses, asthma, anaphylactic shock

**Drug Interactions** CYP2D6 and 3A3/4 enzyme substrate

Increased toxicity (Q-T$_c$ interval prolongation) with other agents that cause Q-T$_c$ interval prolongation, especially mefloquine

**Special PA Issues**

**Patient Education:** Take on an empty stomach; avoid high fat meals; notify physician of persistent nausea, vomiting, abdominal pain, light stools, dark urine

**Monitoring Parameters:** CBC, LFTs, parasite counts

♦ **Halofantrine Hydrochloride** *see* Halofantrine *on this page*

♦ **Halog®** *see* Halcinonide *on previous page*

♦ **Halog®-E** *see* Halcinonide *on previous page*

# Haloperidol (ha loe PER i dole)

**Pharmacologic Class** Antipsychotic Agent, Butyrophenone

**U.S. Brand Names** Haldol®; Haldol® Decanoate

**Mechanism of Action** Blocks postsynaptic mesolimbic dopaminergic D$_1$ and D$_2$ receptors in the brain; exhibits a strong alpha-adrenergic blocking and anticholinergic effect, depresses the release of hypothalamic and hypophyseal hormones; believed to depress the reticular activating system thus affecting basal metabolism, body temperature, wakefulness, vasomotor tone, and emesis

**Use** Treatment of psychoses, Tourette's disorder, and severe behavioral problems in children; may be used for the emergency sedation of severely agitated or delirious patients; may be effective for infantile autism and has been commonly used to reduce disabling choreiform movements associated with Huntington's disease

(Continued)

435

# Haloperidol *(Continued)*

## USUAL DOSAGE

Children: 3-12 years (15-40 kg): Oral:

Initial: 0.05 mg/kg/day or 0.25-0.5 mg/day given in 2-3 divided doses; increase by 0.25-0.5 mg every 5-7 days; maximum: 0.15 mg/kg/day

Usual maintenance:

Agitation or hyperkinesia: 0.01-0.03 mg/kg/day once daily

Nonpsychotic disorders: 0.05-0.075 mg/kg/day in 2-3 divided doses

Psychotic disorders: 0.05-0.15 mg/kg/day in 2-3 divided doses

Children 6-12 years: I.M. (as lactate): 1-3 mg/dose every 4-8 hours to a maximum of 0.15 mg/kg/day; change over to oral therapy as soon as able

Adults:

Oral: 0.5-5 mg 2-3 times/day; usual maximum: 30 mg/day; some patients may require up to 100 mg/day

I.M. (as lactate): 2-5 mg every 4-8 hours as needed

I.M. (as decanoate): Initial: 10-15 times the daily oral dose administered at 3- to 4-week intervals

Sedation in the Intensive Care Unit:

I.M./IVP/IVPB: May repeat bolus doses after 30 minutes until calm achieved then administer 50% of the maximum dose every 6 hours

Mild agitation: 0.5-2 mg

Moderate agitation: 2-5 mg

Severe agitation: 10-20 mg

Continuous intravenous infusion (100 mg/100 mL $D_5W$) Rates of 1-40 mg/hour have been used

Elderly (nonpsychotic patients, dementia behavior):

Initial: Oral: 0.25-0.5 mg 1-2 times/day; increase dose at 4- to 7-day intervals by 0.25-0.5 mg/day; increase dosing intervals (twice daily, 3 times/day, etc) as necessary to control response or side effects

Maximum daily dose: 50 mg; gradual increases (titration) may prevent side effects or decrease their severity

Hemodialysis/peritoneal dialysis: Supplemental dose is not necessary

## Dosage Forms

Haloperidol lactate: **Conc, oral:** 2 mg/mL (5 mL, 10 mL, 15 mL, 120 mL, 240 mL); **Inj:** 5 mg/mL (1 mL, 2 mL, 2.5 mL, 10 mL)

Haloperidol decanoate: **Inj:** 50 mg/mL (1 mL, 5 mL); 100 mg/mL (1 mL, 5 mL); **Tab:** 0.5 mg, 1 mg, 2 mg, 5 mg, 10 mg, 20 mg

**Contraindications** Hypersensitivity to haloperidol or any component; narrow-angle glaucoma, bone marrow suppression, CNS depression, severe liver or cardiac disease, subcortical brain damage; circulatory collapse; severe hypotension or hypertension

**Warnings/Precautions** Safety and efficacy have not been established in children <3 years of age; watch for hypotension when administering I.M. or I.V.; use with caution in patients with cardiovascular disease or seizures; benefits of therapy must be weighed against risks of therapy; decanoate form should never be given I.V.; some tablets contain tartrazine which may cause allergic reactions; use caution with CNS depression and severe liver or cardiac disease

## Pregnancy Risk Factor C

**Adverse Reactions** EKG changes, retinal pigmentation are more common than with chlorpromazine

>10%:

Central nervous system: Restlessness, anxiety, extrapyramidal reactions, dystonic reactions, pseudoparkinsonian signs and symptoms, tardive dyskinesia, neuroleptic malignant syndrome (NMS), seizures, altered central temperature regulation, akathisia

Endocrine & metabolic: Edema of the breasts

Gastrointestinal: Weight gain, constipation

1% to 10%:

Cardiovascular: Hypotension (especially orthostatic), tachycardia, arrhythmias, abnormal T waves with prolonged ventricular repolarization

Central nervous system: Hallucinations, sedation, drowsiness, persistent tardive dyskinesia

Gastrointestinal: Nausea, vomiting

Genitourinary: Dysuria

<1%: Tardive dystonia, hyperpigmentation, pruritus, rash, contact dermatitis, alopecia, photosensitivity (rare), amenorrhea, galactorrhea, gynecomastia, sexual dysfunction, adynamic ileus, nausea, vomiting, xerostomia (problem for denture user), urinary retention, overflow incontinence, priapism, agranulocytosis, leukopenia (usually inpatients with large doses for prolonged periods), cholestatic jaundice, obstructive jaundice, blurred vision, retinal pigmentation, decreased visual acuity (may be irreversible), laryngospasm, respiratory depression, heat stroke

**Drug Interactions** CYP1A2 enzyme substrate, CYP2D6 enzyme substrate (minor); CYP2D6 enzyme inhibitor

Decreased effect: Carbamazepine and phenobarbital may increase metabolism and decreased effectiveness of haloperidol

Increased toxicity: CNS depressants may increase adverse effects; epinephrine may cause hypotension; haloperidol and anticholinergic agents may increase intraocular pressure; concurrent use with lithium has occasionally caused acute encephalopathy-like syndrome

**Onset** Onset of sedation: I.V.: Within 1 hour

**Duration** ~3 weeks for decanoate form

**Half-Life** 20 hours

**Special PA Issues**

**Patient Education:** Use exactly as directed (do not increase dose or frequency); may cause physical and/or psychological dependence. It may take 2-3 weeks to achieve desired results; do not discontinue without consulting prescriber. Dilute oral concentration with water or juice. Do not take within 2 hours of any antacid. Store away from light. Avoid excess alcohol or caffeine and other prescription or OTC medications not approved by prescriber. Maintain adequate hydration (2-3 L/day of fluids unless instructed to restrict fluid intake). Avoid skin contact with medication; may cause contact dermatitis (wash immediately with warm, soapy water). You may experience excess drowsiness, restlessness, dizziness, or blurred vision (use caution driving or when engaging in hazardous tasks until response to medication is known); nausea, vomiting (small frequent meals, frequent mouth care, or sucking lozenges may help); constipation (increased exercise, fluids, or dietary fruit and fiber may help); postural hypotension (use caution climbing stairs or when changing position from lying or sitting to standing); urinary retention (void before taking medication); decreased perspiration (avoid strenuous exercise in hot environments). Report persistent CNS effects (eg, trembling fingers, altered gait or balance, excessive sedation, seizures, unusual movements, anxiety, abnormal thoughts, confusion, personality changes); chest pain, palpitations, rapid heartbeat, severe dizziness; unresolved urinary retention or changes in urinary pattern; vision changes; skin rash or yellowing of skin; difficulty breathing; or worsening of condition.

**Dietary Considerations:** Alcohol: Additive CNS effect, avoid use

**Monitoring Parameters:** Monitor orthostatic blood pressures 3-5 days after initiation of therapy or a dose increase; observe for tremor and abnormal movement or posturing (extrapyramidal symptoms)

**Reference Range:** Therapeutic: 5-15 ng/mL (SI: 10-30 nmol/L) (psychotic disorders - less for Tourette's and mania); Toxic: >42 ng/mL (SI: >84 nmol/L)

**Related Information**

Antipsychotic Agents on page 1001

♦ **Haloperidol Decanoate** see Haloperidol on page 435
♦ **Haloperidol Lactate** see Haloperidol on page 435

# Haloprogin (ha loe PROE jin)

**Pharmacologic Class** Antifungal Agent, Topical

**U.S. Brand Names** Halotex®

**Mechanism of Action** Interferes with fungal DNA replication to inhibit yeast cell respiration and disrupt its cell membrane

**Use** Topical treatment of tinea pedis (athlete's foot), tinea cruris (jock itch), tinea corporis (ringworm), tinea manuum caused by *Trichophyton rubrum, Trichophyton tonsurans, Trichophyton mentagrophytes, Microsporum canis,* or *Epidermophyton floccosum;* topical treatment of *Malassezia furfur*

**USUAL DOSAGE** Topical: Children and Adults: Apply liberally twice daily for 2-3 weeks; intertriginous areas may require up to 4 weeks of treatment

**Dosage Forms Crm:** 1% (15 g, 30 g); **Soln, top:** 1% with alcohol 75% (10 mL, 30 mL)

**Contraindications** Hypersensitivity to haloprogin or any component

**Warnings/Precautions** Safety and efficacy have not been established in children

**Pregnancy Risk Factor** B

**Adverse Reactions** <1%: Pruritus, folliculitis, vesicle formation, erythema, irritation, burning sensation

**Special PA Issues**

**Patient Education:** Avoid contact with eyes; for external use only; improvement should occur within 4 weeks; discontinue use if sensitization or irritation occur

**Related Information**

Antifungal Agents, Topical on page 1000

♦ **Halotestin®** see Fluoxymesterone on page 387
♦ **Halotex®** see Haloprogin on this page
♦ **Halotussin®** [OTC] see Guaifenesin on page 427
♦ **Halotussin® DAC** see Guaifenesin, Pseudoephedrine, and Codeine on page 429
♦ **Halotussin®-DM** [OTC] see Guaifenesin and Dextromethorphan on page 428
♦ **Haltran®** [OTC] see Ibuprofen on page 466
♦ **Haw** see Hawthorn on next page

## Hawthorn

**Mechanism of Action** Contains flavonoids, catechin, and epicatechin which may be cardioprotective and have vasodilatory properties; shown to dilate coronary vessels

**Use** In herbal medicine to treat cardiovascular abnormalities (arrhythmia, angina), increased cardiac output, increased contractility of heart muscle; also used as a sedative

**USUAL DOSAGE** Daily dose of total flavonoids: 10 mg

Per Commission E: 160-900 mg native water-ethanol extract (ethanol 45% v/v or methanol 70% v/v, drug-extract ratio: 4-7:1, with defined flavonoid or procyanidin content), corresponding to 30-168.7 mg procyanidins, calculated as epicatechin, or 3.5-19.8 mg flavonoids, calculated as hyperoside in accordance with DAB 10 [German pharmacopoeia #10] in 2 or 3 individual doses; duration of administration: 6 weeks minimum

**Contraindications** Pregnancy and breast-feeding

**Pregnancy Implications** Do not use

**Adverse Reactions**

Cardiovascular: Hypotension, bradycardia, hypertension

Central nervous system: Depression, fatigue

Dermatologic: Rash

Gastrointestinal: Nausea

**Drug Interactions** Antihypertensives (effect enhanced), digoxin; effects with Viagra® unknown

- ◆ **HbCV** *see Haemophilus* b Conjugate Vaccine *on page 432*
- ◆ **HBIG** *see* Hepatitis B Immune Globulin *on page 440*
- ◆ **H-BIG**® *see* Hepatitis B Immune Globulin *on page 440*
- ◆ **25-HCC** *see* Calcifediol *on page 135*
- ◆ **HCFA Guidelines for Unnecessary Drugs in Long-Term Care Facilities** *see* Chart *on page 1132*
- ◆ **hCG** *see* Chorionic Gonadotropin *on page 205*
- ◆ **HCTZ** *see* Hydrochlorothiazide *on page 447*
- ◆ **Head & Shoulders**® **Intensive Treatment [OTC]** *see* Selenium Sulfide *on page 827*
- ◆ **Healon**® *see* Sodium Hyaluronate *on page 841*
- ◆ **Healon**® **GV** *see* Sodium Hyaluronate *on page 841*
- ◆ **Heart Failure: Management of Patients with Left Ventricular Systolic Dysfunction** *see* Chart *on page 1064*
- ◆ **Helicobacter pylori Treatment** *see* Chart *on page 1065*
- ◆ **Helidac**™ *see* Bismuth Subsalicylate, Metronidazole, and Tetracycline *on page 117*
- ◆ **Helistat**® *see* Microfibrillar Collagen Hemostat *on page 605*
- ◆ **Hemabate**™ *see* Carboprost Tromethamine *on page 153*
- ◆ **Hemocyte**® **[OTC]** *see* Ferrous Fumarate *on page 366*
- ◆ **Hemotene**® *see* Microfibrillar Collagen Hemostat *on page 605*
- ◆ **Hemril-HC**® **Uniserts**® *see* Hydrocortisone *on page 453*

## Heparin (HEP a rin)

**Pharmacologic Class** Anticoagulant

**U.S. Brand Names** Hep-Lock®; Liquaemin®

**Mechanism of Action** Potentiates the action of antithrombin III and thereby inactivates thrombin (as well as activated coagulation factors IX, X, XI, XII, and plasmin) and prevents the conversion of fibrinogen to fibrin; heparin also stimulates release of lipoprotein lipase (lipoprotein lipase hydrolyzes triglycerides to glycerol and free fatty acids)

**Use** Prophylaxis and treatment of thromboembolic disorders

**USUAL DOSAGE**

Line flushing: When using daily flushes of heparin to maintain patency of single and double lumen central catheters, 10 units/mL is commonly used for younger infants (eg, <10 kg) while 100 units/mL is used for older infants, children, and adults. Capped PVC catheters and peripheral heparin locks require flushing more frequently (eg, every 6-8 hours). Volume of heparin flush is usually similar to volume of catheter (or slightly greater). Additional flushes should be given when stagnant blood is observed in catheter, after catheter is used for drug or blood administration, and after blood withdrawal from catheter.

Addition of heparin (0.5-1 unit/mL) to peripheral and central TPN has been shown to increase duration of line patency. The final concentration of heparin used for TPN solutions may need to be decreased to 0.5 units/mL in small infants receiving larger amounts of volume in order to avoid approaching therapeutic amounts. Arterial lines are heparinized with a final concentration of 1 unit/mL.

Children:

Intermittent I.V.: Initial: 50-100 units/kg, then 50-100 units/kg every 4 hours

I.V. infusion: Initial: 50 units/kg, then 15-25 units/kg/hour; increase dose by 2-4 units/kg/hour every 6-8 hours as required

Adults:

Prophylaxis (low-dose heparin): S.C.: 5000 units every 8-12 hours

Intermittent I.V.: Initial: 10,000 units, then 50-70 units/kg (5000-10,000 units) every 4-6 hours

I.V. infusion: 50 units/kg to start, then 15-25 units/kg/hour as continuous infusion; increase dose by 5 units/kg/hour every 4 hours as required according to PTT results, usual range: 10-30 units/hour

Weight-based protocol: 80 units/kg I.V. push followed by continuous infusion of 18 units/kg/hour; see table.

### Standard Heparin Solution
### (25,000 units/500 mL D₅W)

| To Administer a Dose of | Set Infusion Rate at |
|---|---|
| 400 units/h | 8 mL/h |
| 500 units/h | 10 mL/h |
| 600 units/h | 12 mL/h |
| 700 units/h | 14 mL/h |
| 800 units/h | 16 mL/h |
| 900 units/h | 18 mL/h |
| 1000 units/h | 20 mL/h |
| 1100 units/h | 22 mL/h |
| 1200 units/h | 24 mL/h |
| 1300 units/h | 26 mL/h |
| 1400 units/h | 28 mL/h |
| 1500 units/h | 30 mL/h |
| 1600 units/h | 32 mL/h |
| 1700 units/h | 34 mL/h |
| 1800 units/h | 36 mL/h |
| 1900 units/h | 38 mL/h |
| 2000 units/h | 40 mL/h |

**Dosage Forms** Heparin sodium: **Lock flush inj:** Beef lung source: 10 units/mL (1 mL, 2 mL, 2.5 mL, 3 mL, 5 mL, 10 mL, 30 mL), 100 units/mL (1 mL, 2 mL, 2.5 mL, 3 mL, 5 mL, 10 mL, 30 mL), Porcine intestinal mucosa source: 10 units/mL (1 mL, 2 mL, 10 mL, 30 mL), 100 units/mL (1 mL, 2 mL, 10 mL, 30 mL), Porcine intestinal mucosa source, preservative free: 10 units/mL (1 mL), 100 units/mL (1 mL); **Multiple-dose vial inj:** Beef lung source, with preservative: 1000 units/mL (5 mL, 10 mL, 30 mL), 5000 units/mL (10 mL), 10,000 units/mL (4 mL, 5 mL, 10 mL), 20,000 units/mL (2 mL, 5 mL, 10 mL), 40,000 units/mL (5 mL), Porcine intestinal mucosa source, with preservative: 1000 units/mL (10 mL, 30 mL), 5000 units/mL (10 mL), 10,000 units/mL (4 mL), 20,000 units/mL (2 mL, 5 mL); **Single-dose vial inj:** Beef lung source: 1000 units/mL (1 mL), 5000 units/mL (1 mL), 10,000 units/mL (1 mL), 20,000 units/mL (1 mL), 40,000 units/mL (1 mL), Porcine intestinal mucosa: 1000 units/mL (1 mL), 5000 units/mL (1 mL), 10,000 units/mL (1 mL), 20,000 units/mL (1 mL), 40,000 units/mL (1 mL); **Unit dose inj:** Porcine intestinal mucosa source, with preservative: 1000 units/dose (1 mL, 2 mL), 2500 units/dose (1 mL), 5000 units/dose (0.5 mL, 1 mL), 7500 units/dose (1 mL), 10,000 units/dose (1 mL), 15,000 units/dose (1 mL), 20,000 units/dose (1 mL); **Heparin sodium inf, porcine intestinal mucosa source:** D₅W: 40 units/mL (500 mL), 50 units/mL (250 mL, 500 mL), 100 units/mL (100 mL, 250 mL), NaCl 0.45%: 2 units/mL (500 mL, 1000 mL), 50 units/mL (250 mL), 100 units/mL (250 mL), NaCl 0.9%: 2 units/mL (500 mL, 1000 mL), 5 units/mL (1000 mL), 50 units/mL (250 mL, 500 mL, 1000 mL); **Heparin calcium: Unit dose injection, porcine intestinal mucosa, preservative free:** 5000 units/dose (0.2 mL), 12,500 units/dose (0.5 mL), 20,000 units/dose (0.8 mL)

**Contraindications** Hypersensitivity to heparin or any component; severe thrombocytopenia, subacute bacterial endocarditis, suspected intracranial hemorrhage, uncontrollable bleeding (unless secondary to disseminated intravascular coagulation)

**Warnings/Precautions**

Use with caution as hemorrhaging may occur; risk factors for hemorrhage include I.M. injections, peptic ulcer disease, increased capillary permeability, menstruation; severe renal, hepatic or biliary disease; use with caution in patients with shock, severe hypotension

Some preparations contain benzyl alcohol as a preservative. In neonates, large amounts of benzyl alcohol (>100 mg/kg/day) have been associated with fatal toxicity (gasping syndrome). The use of preservative-free heparin is, therefore, recommended in neonates. Some preparations contain sulfite which may cause allergic reactions.

Heparin does not possess fibrinolytic activity and, therefore, cannot lyse established thrombi; discontinue heparin if hemorrhage occurs; severe hemorrhage or overdosage may require protamine

Use caution with white clot syndrome (new thrombus associated with thrombocytopenia) and heparin resistance

(Continued)

439

## Heparin *(Continued)*

### Pregnancy Risk Factor C

### Adverse Reactions

>10%:

Dermatologic: Unexplained bruising

Gastrointestinal: Constipation, vomiting of blood

Hematologic: Hemorrhage, blood in urine, bleeding from gums

1% to 10%:

Cardiovascular: Chest pain

Genitourinary: Frequent or persistent erection

Neuromuscular & skeletal: Peripheral neuropathy

Miscellaneous: Allergic reactions

<1%: Fever, headache, chills, urticaria, nausea, vomiting; thrombocytopenia (heparin-associated thrombocytopenia occurs in <1% of patients, immune thrombocytopenia occurs with progressive fall in platelet counts and, in some cases, thromboembolic complications; daily platelet counts for 5-7 days at initiation of therapy may help detect the onset of this complication); elevated liver enzymes, irritation, ulceration, cutaneous necrosis have been rarely reported with deep S.C. injections, osteoporosis (chronic therapy effect)

### Drug Interactions

Decreased effect with digoxin, tetracycline, nicotine, antihistamine, I.V. NTG

Increased toxicity with NSAIDs, ASA, dipyridamole, dextran, hydroxychloroquine

**Onset** Onset of anticoagulation: I.V.: Immediate with use; S.C.: Within 20-30 minutes

### Half-Life

Mean: 1.5 hours

Range: 1-2 hours; affected by obesity, renal function, hepatic function, malignancy, presence of pulmonary embolism, and infections

### Special PA Issues

**Patient Education:** Use caution to avoid activities that could cause injury or bruising. Avoid bleeding; use safety razor, soft toothbrush, thimble, etc. Report unresolved nausea or vomiting, constipation, blood in urine, bleeding gums, black or tarry stools, back pain, or unusual headaches.

**Monitoring Parameters:** Platelet counts, PTT, hemoglobin, hematocrit, signs of bleeding

For intermittent I.V. injections, PTT is measured 3.5-4 hours after I.V. injection

**Note:** Continuous I.V. infusion is preferred vs I.V. intermittent injections. For full-dose heparin (ie, nonlow-dose), the dose should be titrated according to PTT results. For anticoagulation, an APTT 1.5-2.5 times normal is usually desired. APTT is usually measured prior to heparin therapy, 6-8 hours after initiation of a continuous infusion (following a loading dose), and 6-8 hours after changes in the infusion rate; increase or decrease infusion by 2-4 units/kg/hour dependent on PTT. See table.

#### Heparin Infusion Dose Adjustment

| APTT | Adjustment |
|------|------------|
| >3x control | ↓ Infusion rate 50% |
| 2-3x control | ↓ Infusion rate 25% |
| 1.5-2x control | No change |
| <1.5x control | ↑ Rate of infusion 25%; max 2500 units/h |

**Reference Range:** Heparin: 0.3-0.5 unit/mL; APTT: 1.5-2.5 times **the patient's baseline**

♦ **Heparin Calcium** *see Heparin on page 438*

♦ **Heparin Lock Flush** *see Heparin on page 438*

♦ **Heparin Sodium** *see Heparin on page 438*

## Hepatitis B Immune Globulin *(hep a TYE tis bee i MYUN GLOB yoo lin)*

**Pharmacologic Class** Immune Globulin

**U.S. Brand Names** H-BIG®; Hep-B Gammagee®; HyperHep®

**Mechanism of Action** Hepatitis B immune globulin (HBIG) is a nonpyrogenic sterile solution containing 10% to 18% protein of which at least 80% is monomeric immunoglobulin G (IgG). HBIG differs from immune globulin in the amount of anti-HB$_s$. Immune globulin is prepared from plasma that is not preselected for anti-HB$_s$ content. HBIG is prepared from plasma preselected for high titer anti-HB$_s$. In the U.S., HBIG has an anti-HB$_s$ high titer >1:100,000 by IRA. There is no evidence that the causative agent of AIDS (HTLV-III/LAV) is transmitted by HBIG.

**Use** Provide prophylactic passive immunity to hepatitis B infection to those individuals exposed; newborns of mothers known to be hepatitis B surface antigen positive; hepatitis B immune globulin is not indicated for treatment of active hepatitis B infections and is ineffective in the treatment of chronic active hepatitis B infection

**USUAL DOSAGE** I.M.:

Newborns: Hepatitis B: 0.5 mL as soon after birth as possible (within 12 hours); may repeat at 3 months in order for a higher rate of prevention of the carrier state to be achieved; at this time an active vaccination program with the vaccine may begin

Adults: Postexposure prophylaxis: 0.06 mL/kg as soon as possible after exposure (ie, within 24 hours of needlestick, ocular, or mucosal exposure or within 14 days of sexual exposure); usual dose: 3-5 mL; repeat at 28-30 days after exposure

**Note:** HBIG may be administered at the same time (but at a different site) or up to 1 month preceding hepatitis B vaccination without impairing the active immune response

**Dosage Forms Inj:** H-BIG®: 4 mL, 5 mL, HyperHep®: 0.5 mL, 1 mL, 5 mL

**Contraindications** Hypersensitivity to hepatitis B immune globulin or any component; allergies to gamma globulin or anti-immunoglobulin antibodies; allergies to thimerosal; IgA deficiency; I.M. injections in patients with thrombocytopenia or coagulation disorders

**Pregnancy Risk Factor** C

**Adverse Reactions**

1% to 10%:

Central nervous system: Dizziness, malaise

Dermatologic: Urticaria, angioedema, rash, erythema

Local: Pain and tenderness at injection site

Neuromuscular & skeletal: Arthralgia

<1%: Anaphylaxis

**Drug Interactions** Interferes with immune response of live virus vaccines

♦ **Hep-B Gammagee®** *see* Hepatitis B Immune Globulin *on previous page*

♦ **Hep-Lock®** *see* Heparin *on page 438*

♦ **Heptalac®** *see* Lactulose *on page 512*

♦ **Herbals That May Alter Metabolism and GI Absorption of Drugs** *see* Chart *on page 1133*

♦ **Herceptin®** *see* Trastuzumab *on page 923*

♦ **HES** *see* Hetastarch *on this page*

♦ **Hespan®** *see* Hetastarch *on this page*

# Hetastarch (HET a starch)

**Pharmacologic Class** Plasma Volume Expander, Colloid

**U.S. Brand Names** Hespan®

**Mechanism of Action** Produces plasma volume expansion by virtue of its highly colloidal starch structure, similar to albumin

**Use** Blood volume expander used in treatment of shock or impending shock when blood or blood products are not available; does not have oxygen-carrying capacity and is not a substitute for blood or plasma

**USUAL DOSAGE** I.V. infusion (requires an infusion pump):

Children: Safety and efficacy have not been established

Adults: 500-1000 mL (up to 1500 mL/day) or 20 mL/kg/day (up to 1500 mL/day); larger volumes (15,000 mL/24 hours) have been used safely in small numbers of patients

**Dosing adjustment in renal impairment:** Cl$_{cr}$ <10 mL/minute: Initial dose is the same but subsequent doses should be reduced by 20% to 50% of normal

**Dosage Forms Inf, in sodium chloride 0.9%:** 6% (500 mL)

**Contraindications** Severe bleeding disorders, renal failure with oliguria or anuria, or severe congestive heart failure

**Warnings/Precautions** Anaphylactoid reactions have occurred; use with caution in patients with thrombocytopenia (may interfere with platelet function); large volume may cause drops in hemoglobin concentrations; use with caution in patients at risk from overexpansion of blood volume, including the very young or aged patients, those with congestive heart failure or pulmonary edema; large volumes may interfere with platelet function and prolong PT and PTT times

**Pregnancy Risk Factor** C

**Adverse Reactions** <1%: Peripheral edema, heart failure, circulatory overload, fever, chills, headaches, itching, pruritus, vomiting, bleeding, prolongation of PT, PTT, clotting time, and bleeding time, myalgia, hypersensitivity

**Onset** Onset of volume expansion: I.V.: Within 30 minutes

**Duration** 24-36 hours

**Special PA Issues**

Patient Education: This drug can only be given I.V. Report immediately any respiratory difficulty, acute headache, muscle pain, or abdominal cramping.

♦ **Hexachlorocyclohexane** *see* Lindane *on page 534*

# Hexachlorophene (heks a KLOR oh feen)

**Pharmacologic Class** Antibacterial, Topical; Soap

**U.S. Brand Names** pHisoHex®; Septisol®

**Mechanism of Action** Bacteriostatic polychlorinated biphenyl which inhibits membrane-bound enzymes and disrupts the cell membrane

(Continued)

## Hexachlorophene *(Continued)*

**Use** Surgical scrub and as a bacteriostatic skin cleanser; control an outbreak of gram-positive infection when other procedures have been unsuccessful

**USUAL DOSAGE** Children and Adults: Topical: Apply 5 mL cleanser and water to area to be cleansed; lather and rinse thoroughly under running water

**Dosage Forms Foam (Septisol®):** 0.23% with alcohol 56% (180 mL, 600 mL); **Liq, top (pHisoHex®):** 3% (8 mL, 150 mL, 500 mL, 3840 mL)

**Contraindications** Known hypersensitivity to halogenated phenol derivatives or hexachlorophene; use in premature infants; use on burned or denuded skin; occlusive dressing; application to mucous membranes

**Warnings/Precautions** Discontinue use if signs of cerebral irritability occur; exposure of preterm infants or patients with extensive burns has been associated with apnea, convulsions, agitation and coma; do not use for bathing infants, premature infants are particularly susceptible to hexachlorophene topical absorption

**Pregnancy Risk Factor** C

**Adverse Reactions** <1%: CNS injury, seizures, irritability, photosensitivity, dermatitis, redness, dry skin

**Special PA Issues**

**Patient Education:** Do not leave on skin for prolonged contact; for external use only; discontinue product if condition persists or worsens and call physician; if suds enter eye, rinse out thoroughly with water

## Histrelin *(his TREL in)*

**Pharmacologic Class** Gonadotropin Releasing Hormone Analog; Luteinizing Hormone-Releasing Hormone Analog

**U.S. Brand Names** Supprelin™ Injection

**Mechanism of Action** Histrelin is a synthetic long-acting gonadotropin-releasing hormone analog; with daily administration, it desensitizes the pituitary to endogenous gonadotropin-releasing hormone (ie, suppresses gonadotropin release by causing down regulation of the pituitary); this results in a decrease in gonadal sex steroid production which stops the secondary sexual development

**Use** Treatment of central idiopathic precocious puberty; treatment of estrogen-associated gynecological disorders such as acute intermittent porphyria, endometriosis, leiomyomata uteri, and premenstrual syndrome

**USUAL DOSAGE**

Central idiopathic precocious puberty: S.C.: Usual dose is 10 mcg/kg/day given as a single daily dose at the same time each day

Acute intermittent porphyria in women: S.C.: 5 mcg/day

Endometriosis: S.C.: 100 mcg/day

Leiomyomata uteri: S.C.: 20-50 mcg/day or 4 mcg/kg/day

**Dosage Forms Inj:** 7-day kits of single use: 120 mcg/0.6 mL; 300 mcg/0.6 mL; 600 mcg/0.6 mL

**Contraindications** Hypersensitivity to histrelin, pregnancy, breast-feeding

**Warnings/Precautions** The site of injection should be varied daily; the dose should be administered at the same time each day. In precocious puberty, changing the dosage schedule or noncompliance may result in inadequate control of the pubertal process.

**Pregnancy Risk Factor** X

**Adverse Reactions**
>10%:
Cardiovascular: Vasodilation
Central nervous system: Headache
Gastrointestinal: Abdominal pain
Genitourinary: Vaginal bleeding, vaginal dryness
Local: Skin reaction at injection site

1% to 10%:
Central nervous system: Mood swings, headache, pain
Dermatologic: Rashes, urticaria
Endocrine & metabolic: Breast tenderness, hot flashes
Gastrointestinal: Nausea, vomiting
Genitourinary: Increased urinary calcium excretion
Neuromuscular & skeletal: Joint stiffness

**Onset**
Precocious puberty: Onset of hormonal responses: Within 3 months of initiation of therapy
Acute intermittent porphyria associated with menses: Amelioration of symptoms: After 1-2 months of therapy
Treatment of endometriosis or leiomyomata uteri: Onset of responses: After 3-6 months of treatment

**Special PA Issues**
Patient Education: Use as directed - daily at the same time. Maintain regular follow-up schedule. You may experience headache and GI distress (analgesics may help), vaginal bleeding, pain, irritation (during first weeks of therapy), nausea or anorexia (small frequent meals may help), flushing or redness (cold clothes and cool environment may help). Report irregular or rapid heartbeat, unresolved nausea or vomiting, difficulty breathing, or infection at injection sites.

Monitoring Parameters: Precocious puberty: Prior to initiating therapy: Height and weight, hand and wrist x-rays, total sex steroid levels, beta-hCG level, adrenal steroid level, gonadotropin-releasing hormone stimulation test, pelvic/adrenal/testicular ultrasound/head CT; during therapy monitor 3 months after initiation and then every 6-12 months; serial levels of sex steroids and gonadotropin-releasing hormone testing; physical exam; secondary sexual development; histrelin may be discontinued when the patient reaches the appropriate age for puberty

♦ **Histussin D® Liquid** *see* Hydrocodone and Pseudoephedrine *on page 453*

♦ **Hivid®** *see* Zalcitabine *on page 971*

♦ **HMS Liquifilm®** *see* Medrysone *on page 562*

# Homatropine (hoe MA troe peen)

**Pharmacologic Class** Anticholinergic Agent, Ophthalmic; Ophthalmic Agent, Mydriatic

**U.S. Brand Names** AK-Homatropine® Ophthalmic; Isopto® Homatropine Ophthalmic

**Mechanism of Action** Blocks response of iris sphincter muscle and the accommodative muscle of the ciliary body to cholinergic stimulation resulting in dilation and loss of accommodation

**Use** Producing cycloplegia and mydriasis for refraction; treatment of acute inflammatory conditions of the uveal tract

**USUAL DOSAGE**
Children:
Mydriasis and cycloplegia for refraction: Instill 1 drop of 2% solution immediately before the procedure; repeat at 10-minute intervals as needed
Uveitis: Instill 1 drop of 2% solution 2-3 times/day

Adults:
Mydriasis and cycloplegia for refraction: Instill 1-2 drops of 2% solution or 1 drop of 5% solution before the procedure; repeat at 5- to 10-minute intervals as needed; maximum of 3 doses for refraction
Uveitis: Instill 1-2 drops of 2% or 5% 2-3 times/day up to every 3-4 hours as needed

**Dosage Forms Soln, ophth, as hydrobromide:** 2% (1 mL, 5 mL); 5% (1 mL, 2 mL, 5 mL), AK-Homatropine®: 5% (15 mL), Isopto® Homatropine 2% (5 mL, 15 mL); 5% (5 mL, 15 mL)

**Contraindications** Narrow-angle glaucoma, acute hemorrhage or hypersensitivity to the drug or any component in the formulation

**Warnings/Precautions** Use with caution in patients with hypertension, cardiac disease, or increased intraocular pressure; safety and efficacy not established in infants and young children, therefore, use with extreme caution due to susceptibility of systemic effects; use with caution in obstructive uropathy, paralytic ileus, ulcerative colitis, unstable cardiovascular status in acute hemorrhage

**Pregnancy Risk Factor** C
(Continued)

## Homatropine *(Continued)*

### Adverse Reactions

>10%: Ocular: Blurred vision, photophobia

1% to 10%:

Local: Stinging, local irritation

Ocular: Increased intraocular pressure

Respiratory: Congestion

<1%: Vascular congestion, edema, drowsiness, exudate, eczematoid dermatitis, follicular conjunctivitis

**Onset** Onset of accommodation and pupil effect: Maximum mydriatic effect: Within 10-30 minutes; Maximum cycloplegic effect: Within 30-90 minutes

**Duration** Mydriasis: 6 hours to 4 days; Cycloplegia: 10-48 hours

### Special PA Issues

**Patient Education:** Instill only as often as recommended; do not overuse. Wash hands before using. Sit or lie down, open eye, look at ceiling, and instill prescribed amount of solution. Do not blink for 30 seconds. Close eye and roll eye in all directions and apply gentle pressure to inner corner of eye for 1-2 minutes. Do not let tip of applicator touch eye or contaminate tip of applicator. Temporary stinging or blurred vision may occur. Report persistent pain, redness, burning, double vision, severe sensitivity to light, or respiratory congestion.

♦ **Homatropine and Hydrocodone** *see* Hydrocodone and Homatropine *on page 451*

♦ **Homatropine Hydrobromide** *see* Homatropine *on previous page*

♦ **Honvol**® *see* Diethylstilbestrol *on page 277*

♦ **Horse Anti-human Thymocyte Gamma Globulin** *see* Lymphocyte Immune Globulin *on page 550*

♦ **Humalog**® *see* Insulin Preparations *on page 479*

## Human Growth Hormone (HYU man grothe HOR mone)

**Pharmacologic Class** Growth Hormone

**U.S. Brand Names** Genotropin® Injection; Humatrope® Injection; Norditropin® Injection; Nutropin® AQ Injection; Nutropin® Injection; Protropin® Injection; Saizen® Injection; Serostim® Injection

**Mechanism of Action** Somatropin and somatrem are purified polypeptide hormones of recombinant DNA origin; somatropin contains the identical sequence of amino acids found in human growth hormone while somatrem's amino acid sequence is identical plus an additional amino acid, methionine; human growth hormone stimulates growth of linear bone, skeletal muscle, and organs; stimulates erythropoietin which increases red blood cell mass; exerts both insulin-like and diabetogenic effects

### Use

Long-term treatment of growth failure from lack of adequate endogenous growth hormone secretion

Nutropin®: Treatment of children who have growth failure associated with chronic renal insufficiency up until the time of renal transplantation

**USUAL DOSAGE** Children (individualize dose):

Somatrem (Protropin®): I.M., S.C.: Up to 0.1 mg (0.26 units)/kg/dose 3 times/week

Somatropin (Genotropin®): S.C.: Weekly dosage of 0.16-0.24 mg/kg divided into 6-7 doses

Somatropin (Humatrope®): I.M., S.C.: Up to 0.06 mg (0.16 units)/kg/dose 3 times/week

Somatropin (Nutropin®): S.C.:

Growth hormone inadequacy: Weekly dosage of 0.3 mg/kg (0.78 units/kg) administered daily

Chronic renal insufficiency: Weekly dosage of 0.35 mg/kg (0.91 units/kg) administered daily

Therapy should be discontinued when patient has reached satisfactory adult height, when epiphyses have fused, or when the patient ceases to respond

Growth of 5 cm/year or more is expected, if growth rate does not exceed 2.5 cm in a 6-month period, double the dose for the next 6 months, if there is still no satisfactory response, discontinue therapy

**Dosage Forms Powder for inj (lyophilized):** Somatropin: Genotropin®: 1.5 mg ~4.5 units (5 mL), 5.8 mg ~17.4 units (5 mL), Humatrope®: 5 mg ~15 units, Norditropin®: 4 mg ~12 units, 8 mg ~24 units, Nutropin®: 5 mg ~15 units (10 mL), 10 mg ~30 units (10 mL), Nutropin® AQ: 10 mg ~30 units (2 mL), Saizen® (rDNA origin): 5 mg ~15 units, Serostim®: 5 mg ~15 units (5 mL), 6 mg ~18 units (5 mL); Somatrem, Protropin®: 5 mg ~15 units (10 mL), 10 mg ~26 units (10 mL)

**Contraindications** Closed epiphyses, known hypersensitivity to drug, benzyl alcohol (somatrem), or m-Cresol or glycerin (somatropin); progression of any underlying intracranial lesion or actively growing intracranial tumor

**Warnings/Precautions** Use with caution in patients with diabetes; when administering to newborns, reconstitute with sterile water for injection

**Pregnancy Risk Factor** C

**Adverse Reactions** S.C. administration can cause local lipoatrophy or lipodystrophy and may enhance the development of neutralizing antibodies

1% to 10%: Endocrine & metabolic: Hypothyroidism

<1%: Rash, itching, hypoglycemia, pain at injection site, small risk for developing leukemia, pain in hip/knee

**Drug Interactions** Decreased effect: Glucocorticoid therapy may inhibit growth-promoting effects.

**Special PA Issues**

**Monitoring Parameters:** Growth curve, periodic thyroid function tests, bone age (annually), periodical urine testing for glucose, somatomedin C levels

- ◆ **Human Thyroid Stimulating Hormone** *see* Thyrotropin Alpha *on page 899*
- ◆ **Humatin®** *see* Paromomycin *on page 698*
- ◆ **Humatrope® Injection** *see* Human Growth Hormone *on previous page*
- ◆ **Humegon™** *see* Menotropins *on page 567*
- ◆ **Humibid® DM [OTC]** *see* Guaifenesin and Dextromethorphan *on page 428*
- ◆ **Humibid® L.A.** *see* Guaifenesin *on page 427*
- ◆ **Humibid® Sprinkle** *see* Guaifenesin *on page 427*
- ◆ **HuMist® Nasal Mist [OTC]** *see* Sodium Chloride *on page 839*
- ◆ **Humorsol® Ophthalmic** *see* Demecarium *on page 258*
- ◆ **Humulin® 50/50** *see* Insulin Preparations *on page 479*
- ◆ **Humulin® 70/30** *see* Insulin Preparations *on page 479*
- ◆ **Humulin® L** *see* Insulin Preparations *on page 479*
- ◆ **Humulin® N** *see* Insulin Preparations *on page 479*
- ◆ **Humulin® R** *see* Insulin Preparations *on page 479*
- ◆ **Humulin® U** *see* Insulin Preparations *on page 479*
- ◆ **Hurricaine®** *see* Benzocaine *on page 105*
- ◆ **Hyaluronic Acid** *see* Sodium Hyaluronate *on page 841*

# Hyaluronidase (hye al yoor ON i dase)

**Pharmacologic Class** Antidote

**U.S. Brand Names** Wydase® Injection

**Mechanism of Action** Modifies the permeability of connective tissue through hydrolysis of hyaluronic acid, one of the chief ingredients of tissue cement which offers resistance to diffusion of liquids through tissues

**Use** Increases the dispersion and absorption of other drugs; increases rate of absorption of parenteral fluids given by hypodermoclysis; enhances diffusion of locally irritating or toxic drugs in the management of I.V. extravasation

**USUAL DOSAGE**

Infants and Children:

Management of I.V. extravasation: Reconstitute the 150 unit vial of lyophilized powder with 1 mL normal saline; take 0.1 mL of this solution and dilute with 0.9 mL normal saline to yield 15 units/mL; using a 25- or 26-gauge needle, five 0.2 mL injections are made subcutaneously or intradermally into the extravasation site at the leading edge, changing the needle after each injection

Hypodermoclysis:

S.C.: 1 mL (150 units) is added to 1000 mL of infusion fluid and 0.5 mL (75 units) in injected into each clysis site at the initiation of the infusion

I.V.: 15 units is added to each 100 mL of I.V. fluid to be administered

Children <3 years: Limit volume of single clysis to 200 mL

Premature Infants: Do not exceed 25 mL/kg/day and not >2 mL/minute

Adults: Absorption and dispersion of drugs: 150 units are added to the vehicle containing the drug

**Dosage Forms Inj, stabilized soln:** 150 units/mL (1 mL, 10 mL); **Powder for inj, lyophilized:** 150 units, 1500 units

**Contraindications** Hypersensitivity to hyaluronidase or any component; do not inject in or around infected, inflamed, or cancerous areas

**Warnings/Precautions** Drug infiltrates in which hyaluronidase is contraindicated: Dopamine, alpha-adrenergic agonists; an intradermal skin test for sensitivity should be performed before actual administration using 0.02 mL of a 150 units/mL of hyaluronidase solution

**Pregnancy Risk Factor** C

**Adverse Reactions** <1%: Tachycardia, hypotension, dizziness, chills, urticaria, erythema, nausea, vomiting

**Drug Interactions** Decreased effect: Salicylates, cortisone, ACTH, estrogens, antihistamines

**Onset** Immediate by the subcutaneous or intradermal routes for the treatment of extravasation

**Duration** 24-48 hours

(Continued)

## Hyaluronidase *(Continued)*

### Special PA Issues
**Patient Education:** Report itching, pain, changes in respiration, or excessive dizziness.

◆ **Hybalamin®** *see* Hydroxocobalamin *on page 458*

◆ **Hybolin™ Decanoate Injection** *see* Nandrolone *on page 634*

◆ **Hybolin™ Improved Injection** *see* Nandrolone *on page 634*

◆ **HycoClear Tuss®** *see* Hydrocodone and Guaifenesin *on page 451*

◆ **Hycodan®** *see* Hydrocodone and Homatropine *on page 451*

◆ **Hycomine®** *see* Hydrocodone and Phenylpropanolamine *on page 453*

◆ **Hycomine® Compound** *see* Hydrocodone, Chlorpheniramine, Phenylephrine, Acetaminophen and Caffeine *on page 453*

◆ **Hycomine® Pediatric** *see* Hydrocodone and Phenylpropanolamine *on page 453*

◆ **Hycort®** *see* Hydrocortisone *on page 453*

◆ **Hycotuss® Expectorant Liquid** *see* Hydrocodone and Guaifenesin *on page 451*

◆ **Hydergine®** *see* Ergoloid Mesylates *on page 327*

◆ **Hydergine® LC** *see* Ergoloid Mesylates *on page 327*

## Hydralazine *(hye DRAL a zeen)*

**Pharmacologic Class** Vasodilator

**U.S. Brand Names** Apresoline®

**Mechanism of Action** Direct vasodilation of arterioles (with little effect on veins) with decreased systemic resistance

**Use** Management of moderate to severe hypertension, congestive heart failure, hypertension secondary to pre-eclampsia/eclampsia; also used to treat primary pulmonary hypertension

### USUAL DOSAGE
Children:

Oral: Initial: 0.75-1 mg/kg/day in 2-4 divided doses; increase over 3-4 weeks to maximum of 7.5 mg/kg/day in 2-4 divided doses; maximum daily dose: 200 mg/day

I.M., I.V.: 0.1-0.2 mg/kg/dose (not to exceed 20 mg) every 4-6 hours as needed, up to 1.7-3.5 mg/kg/day in 4-6 divided doses

Adults:

Oral: Hypertension:

Initial dose: 10 mg 4 times/day for first 2-4 days; increase to 25 mg 4 times/day for the balance of the first week

Increase by 10-25 mg/dose gradually to 50 mg 4 times/day; 300 mg/day may be required for some patients

Oral: Congestive heart failure:

Initial dose: 10-25 mg 3 times/day

Target dose: 75 mg 3 times/day

Maximum dose: 100 mg 3 times/day

I.M., I.V.:

Hypertension: Initial: 10-20 mg/dose every 4-6 hours as needed, may increase to 40 mg/dose; change to oral therapy as soon as possible

Pre-eclampsia/eclampsia: 5 mg/dose then 5-10 mg every 20-30 minutes as needed

Elderly: Oral: Initial: 10 mg 2-3 times/day; increase by 10-25 mg/day every 2-5 days

**Dosing interval in renal impairment:**

$Cl_{cr}$ 10-50 mL/minute: Administer every 8 hours

$Cl_{cr}$ <10 mL/minute: Administer every 8-16 hours in fast acetylators and every 12-24 hours in slow acetylators

Hemodialysis: Supplemental dose is not necessary

Peritoneal dialysis: Supplemental dose is not necessary

**Dosage Forms** Hydralazine hydrochloride: **Inj:** 20 mg/mL (1 mL); **Tab:** 10 mg, 25 mg, 50 mg, 100 mg

**Contraindications** Hypersensitivity to hydralazine or any component, dissecting aortic aneurysm, mitral valve rheumatic heart disease

**Warnings/Precautions** Discontinue hydralazine in patients who develop SLE-like syndrome or positive ANA. Use with caution in patients with severe renal disease or cerebral vascular accidents or with known or suspected coronary artery disease; monitor blood pressure closely with I.V. use; some formulations may contain tartrazines or sulfites. Slow acetylators, patients with decreased renal function, and patients receiving >200 mg/day (chronically) are at higher risk for SLE. Titrate dosage to patient's response. Usually administered with diuretic and a beta-blocker to counteract side effects of sodium and water retention and reflex tachycardia.

**Pregnancy Risk Factor** C

**Pregnancy Implications**

Clinical effects on the fetus: Crosses the placenta. One report of fetal arrhythmia; transient neonatal thrombocytopenia and fetal distress reported following late 3rd trimester use. A large amount of clinical experience with the use of these drugs for management of hypertension during pregnancy is available. Available evidence suggests safe use during pregnancy and breast-feeding.

Breast-feeding/lactation: Crosses into breast milk in extremely small amounts. American Academy of Pediatrics considers **compatible** with breast-feeding.

**Adverse Reactions**
>10%:
Cardiovascular: Palpitations, flushing, tachycardia, angina pectoris
Central nervous system: Headache
Gastrointestinal: Nausea, vomiting, diarrhea, anorexia
1% to 10%:
Cardiovascular: Hypotension, redness or flushing of face
Gastrointestinal: Constipation
Ocular: Lacrimation
Respiratory: Dyspnea, nasal congestion
<1%: Malaise, fever, dizziness, rash, edema, arthralgias, weakness, peripheral neuritis, positive ANA, positive LE cells
**Note:** Because of blunted beta-receptor response, the elderly are less likely to experience reflex tachycardia; this puts them at greater risk for orthostatic hypotension

**Drug Interactions** Increased toxicity: MAO inhibitors → significant decrease in blood pressure indomethacin may decrease hypotensive effects; hydralazine serum levels may be increased by beta-blockers (metoprolol, propranolol) while hydralazine increases serum levels/toxic risk of beta-blockers

**Onset** Oral: 20-30 minutes; I.V.: 5-20 minutes

**Duration** Oral: 2-4 hours; I.V.: 2-6 hours

**Half-Life** Normal renal function: 2-8 hours; End-stage renal disease: 7-16 hours

**Special PA Issues**
**Patient Education:** Take as directed, with meals. Do not use alcohol or OTC medication without consulting prescriber. Weigh daily at same time, in the same clothes. Report weight gain >5 lb/week, swelling of feet or ankles. May cause dizziness or weakness; change position slowly when rising from sitting or lying position and avoid driving or activities requiring alertness until response to drug is known. You may experience nausea (small frequent meals may help), impotence (reversible), or constipation (fluids, exercise, dietary fiber may help). This medication does not replace other antihypertensive interventions; follow instructions for diet and lifestyle changes. Report flu-like symptoms, difficulty breathing, skin rash, or numbness and tingling of extremities.

**Dietary Considerations:** Food enhances bioavailability of hydralazine

**Monitoring Parameters:** Blood pressure (monitor closely with I.V. use), standing and sitting/supine, heart rate, ANA titer

**Related Information**
Heart Failure: Management of Patients with Left Ventricular Systolic Dysfunction *on page 1064*

# Hydralazine and Hydrochlorothiazide
(hye DRAL a zeen & hye droe klor oh THYE a zide)
**Pharmacologic Class** Antihypertensive Agent, Combination
**U.S. Brand Names** Apresazide®
**Dosage Forms Cap:** 25/25: Hydralazine hydrochloride 25 mg and hydrochlorothiazide 25 mg, 50/50: Hydralazine hydrochloride 50 mg and hydrochlorothiazide 50 mg, 100/50: Hydralazine hydrochloride 100 mg and hydrochlorothiazide 50 mg

♦ **Hydralazine Hydrochloride** *see* Hydralazine *on previous page*

# Hydralazine, Hydrochlorothiazide, and Reserpine
(hye DRAL a zeen, hye droe klor oh THYE a zide, & re SER peen)
**Pharmacologic Class** Antihypertensive Agent, Combination
**U.S. Brand Names** Hydrap-ES®; Marpres®; Ser-Ap-Es®
**Dosage Forms Tab:** Hydralazine 25 mg, hydrochlorothiazide 15 mg, and reserpine 0.1 mg

♦ **Hydramyn® Syrup [OTC]** *see* Diphenhydramine *on page 289*
♦ **Hydrap-ES®** *see* Hydralazine, Hydrochlorothiazide, and Reserpine *on this page*
♦ *Hydrastis canadensis see* Golden Seal *on page 421*
♦ **Hydrated Chloral** *see* Chloral Hydrate *on page 186*
♦ **Hydrea®** *see* Hydroxyurea *on page 460*
♦ **Hydrex®** *see* Benzthiazide *on page 107*
♦ **Hydrocet®** *see* Hydrocodone and Acetaminophen *on page 449*

# Hydrochlorothiazide (hye droe klor oh THYE a zide)
**Pharmacologic Class** Diuretic, Thiazide
**U.S. Brand Names** Esidrix®; Ezide®; HydroDIURIL®; Hydro-Par®; Microzide™; Oretic®
**Mechanism of Action** Inhibits sodium reabsorption in the distal tubules causing increased excretion of sodium and water as well as potassium and hydrogen ions
**Use** Management of mild to moderate hypertension; treatment of edema in congestive heart failure and nephrotic syndrome
(Continued)

## Hydrochlorothiazide *(Continued)*

**USUAL DOSAGE** Oral (effect of drug may be decreased when used every day):
Children (In pediatric patients, chlorothiazide may be preferred over hydrochlorothiazide as there are more dosage formulations (eg, suspension) available):
<6 months: 2-3 mg/kg/day in 2 divided doses
>6 months: 2 mg/kg/day in 2 divided doses
Adults: 25-100 mg/day in 1-2 doses
Maximum: 200 mg/day
Elderly: 12.5-25 mg once daily
Minimal increase in response and more electrolyte disturbances are seen with doses >50 mg/day

**Dosing adjustment/comments in renal impairment:** $Cl_{cr}$ 25-50 mL/minute: Not effective

**Dosage Forms Cap:** 12.5 mg; **Soln, oral (mint flavor):** 50 mg/5 mL (50 mL); **Tab:** 25 mg, 50 mg, 100 mg

**Contraindications** Anuria, renal decompensation, hypersensitivity to hydrochlorothiazide or any component, cross-sensitivity with other thiazides and sulfonamide derivatives

**Warnings/Precautions** Use with caution in renal disease, hepatic disease, gout, lupus erythematosus, diabetes mellitus; some products may contain tartrazine. Hydrochlorothiazide is not effective in patients with a $Cl_{cr}$ 25-50 mL/minute, therefore, it may not be a useful agent in many elderly patients.

**Pregnancy Risk Factor** B

**Adverse Reactions**
1% to 10%: Endocrine & metabolic: Hypokalemia
<1%: Hypotension, photosensitivity, fluid and electrolyte imbalances, hyperglycemia, rarely blood dyscrasias, prerenal azotemia

**Drug Interactions**
Decreased effect:
Thiazides may decrease the effect of anticoagulants, antigout agents, sulfonylureas
Bile acid sequestrants, methenamine, and NSAIDs may decrease the effect of the thiazides
Increased effect: Thiazides may increase the toxicity of allopurinol, anesthetics, antineoplastics, calcium salts, diazoxide, digitalis, lithium, loop diuretics, methyldopa, nondepolarizing muscle relaxants, vitamin D; amphotericin B and anticholinergics may increase the toxicity of thiazides

**Onset** Diuretic effect within 2 hours; Peak effect: 4-6 hours

**Duration** 6-12 hours

**Half-Life** 5.6-14.8

**Special PA Issues**
**Patient Education:** This medication does not replace other antihypertensive recommendations (diet and lifestyle changes). Take as directed, with meals, early in the day to avoid nocturia. Avoid alcohol or OTC medication unless approved by prescriber. Include bananas and/or orange juice in daily diet; do not take potassium supplements unless recommended by prescriber. May cause dizziness or postural hypotension (use caution when rising from sitting or lying position, when driving, climbing stairs, or engaging in hazardous tasks); nausea or vomiting (small frequent meals, frequent mouth care, or sucking on lozenges may help); impotence (reversible); constipation (increased exercise or dietary fruit, fiber, or fluids will help); photosensitivity (use sunblock, wear protective clothing and eyewear, or avoid protracted exposure to bright sunlight). If diabetic, monitor serum glucose closely; this medication may increase serum glucose levels. Report persistent flu-like symptoms, chest pain, palpitations, muscle cramping, difficulty breathing, skin rash or itching, unusual bruising or easy bleeding, or excessive fatigue.
**Monitoring Parameters:** Assess weight, I & O reports daily to determine fluid loss; blood pressure, serum electrolytes, BUN, creatinine

**Related Information**
Heart Failure: Management of Patients with Left Ventricular Systolic Dysfunction *on page 1064*

♦ **Hydrochlorothiazide and Irbesartan** see Irbesartan and Hydrochlorothiazide *on page 492*

# Hydrochlorothiazide and Reserpine
(hye droe klor oh THYE a zide & re SER peen)
**Pharmacologic Class** Antihypertensive Agent, Combination
**U.S. Brand Names** Hydropres®; Hydro-Serp®; Hydroserpine®
**Dosage Forms Tab:** 25: Hydrochlorothiazide 25 mg and reserpine 0.125 mg, 50: Hydrochlorothiazide 50 mg and reserpine 0.125 mg

# Hydrochlorothiazide and Spironolactone
(hye droe klor oh THYE a zide & speer on oh LAK tone)
**Pharmacologic Class** Antihypertensive Agent, Combination
**U.S. Brand Names** Aldactazide®

**Dosage Forms Tab:** 25/25: Hydrochlorothiazide 25 mg and spironolactone 25 mg, 50/50: Hydrochlorothiazide 50 mg and spironolactone 50 mg

## Hydrochlorothiazide and Triamterene
(hye droe klor oh THYE a zide & trye AM ter een)

**Pharmacologic Class** Antihypertensive Agent, Combination; Diuretic, Potassium Sparing; Diuretic, Thiazide

**U.S. Brand Names** Dyazide®; Maxzide®

**Dosage Forms Cap (Dyazide®):** Hydrochlorothiazide 25 mg and triamterene 37.5 mg; **Tab:** Maxzide®-25: Hydrochlorothiazide 25 mg and triamterene 37.5 mg, Maxzide®: Hydrochlorothiazide 50 mg and triamterene 75 mg

♦ **Hydrocil® [OTC]** see Psyllium on page 781

♦ **Hydro-Cobex®** see Hydroxocobalamin on page 458

## Hydrocodone and Acetaminophen
(hye droe KOE done & a seet a MIN oh fen)

**Pharmacologic Class** Analgesic, Narcotic

**U.S. Brand Names** Anexsia®; Anodynos-DHC®; Bancap HC®; Co-Gesic®; Dolacet®; DuoCet™; Duradyne DHC®; Hydrocet®; Hydrogesic®; Hy-Phen®; Lorcet®-HD; Lorcet® Plus; Lortab®; Margesic® H; Medipain 5®; Norcet®; Stagesic®; T-Gesic®; Vicodin®; Vicodin® ES; Vicodin® HP; Zydone®

**Mechanism of Action** See individual agents

**Use** Relief of moderate to severe pain; antitussive (hydrocodone)

**USUAL DOSAGE** Oral (doses should be titrated to appropriate analgesic effect):
Children:
Antitussive (hydrocodone): 0.6 mg/kg/day in 3-4 divided doses
A single dose should not exceed 10 mg in children >12 years, 5 mg in children 2-12 years, and 1.25 mg in children <2 years of age
Analgesic (acetaminophen): Refer to Acetaminophen monograph
Adults: Analgesic: 1-2 tablets or capsules every 4-6 hours or 5-10 mL solution every 4-6 hours as needed for pain

**Dosage Forms Cap:** Bancap HC®, Dolacet®, Hydrocet®, Hydrogesic®, Lorcet®-HD, Margesic® H, Medipain 5®, Norcet®, Stagesic®, T-Gesic®, Zydone®: Hydrocodone bitartrate 5 mg and acetaminophen 500 mg; **Elix (tropical fruit punch flavor) (Lortab®):** Hydrocodone bitartrate 2.5 mg and acetaminophen 167 mg per 5 mL with alcohol 7% (480 mL); **Soln, oral (tropical fruit punch flavor) (Lortab®):** Hydrocodone bitartrate 2.5 mg and acetaminophen 167 mg per 5 mL with alcohol 7% (480 mL); **Tab:** Lortab® 2.5/500: Hydrocodone bitartrate 2.5 mg and acetaminophen 500 mg, Anexsia® 5/500, Anodynos-DHC®, Co-Gesic®, DuoCet™, DHC®, Hy-Phen®, Lortab®® 5/500, Vicodin®: Hydrocodone bitartrate 5 mg and acetaminophen 500 mg, Lortab® 7.5/500: Hydrocodone bitartrate 7.5 mg and acetaminophen 500 mg, Anexsia® 7.5/650, Lorcet® Plus: Hydrocodone bitartrate 7.5 mg and acetaminophen 650 mg, Vicodin® ES: Hydrocodone bitartrate 7.5 mg and acetaminophen 750 mg, Norco®: Hydrocodone bitartrate 10 mg and acetaminophen 325 mg, Lortab® 10/500: Hydrocodone bitartrate 10 mg and acetaminophen 500 mg, Lorcet® 10/650: Hydrocodone bitartrate 10 mg and acetaminophen 650 mg, Vicodin® HP: Hydrocodone bitartrate 10 mg and acetaminophen 660 mg

**Contraindications** CNS depression, hypersensitivity to hydrocodone, acetaminophen or any component; severe respiratory depression

**Warnings/Precautions** Use with caution in patients with hypersensitivity reactions to other phenanthrene derivative opioid agonists (morphine, hydrocodone, hydromorphone, levorphanol, oxycodone, oxymorphone); tablets contain metabisulfite which may cause allergic reactions; tolerance or drug dependence may result from extended use

**Pregnancy Risk Factor** C

**Adverse Reactions**
>10%:
Cardiovascular: Hypotension
Central nervous system: Lightheadedness, dizziness, sedation, drowsiness, fatigue
Neuromuscular & skeletal: Weakness
1% to 10%:
Cardiovascular: Bradycardia
Central nervous system: Confusion
Gastrointestinal: Nausea, vomiting
Genitourinary: Decreased urination
Respiratory: Shortness of breath, dyspnea
<1%: Hypertension, hallucinations, xerostomia, anorexia, biliary tract spasm, urinary tract spasm, diplopia, miosis, histamine release, physical and psychological dependence with prolonged use

**Drug Interactions**
Decreased effect with phenothiazines
Increased effect with dextroamphetamine
Increased toxicity with CNS depressants, TCAs; effect of warfarin may be enhanced
(Continued)

## Hydrocodone and Acetaminophen *(Continued)*

**Onset** Onset of narcotic analgesia: Within 10-20 minutes

**Duration** 3-6 hours

**Half-Life** Hydrocodone: 3.8 hours

**Special PA Issues**

**Patient Education:** If self-administered, use exactly as directed (do not increase dose or frequency); may cause physical and/or psychological dependence. Take with food or milk. While using this medication, do not use alcohol and other prescription or OTC medications (especially sedatives, tranquilizers, antihistamines, or pain medications) without consulting prescriber. Maintain adequate hydration (2-3 L/day of fluids unless instructed to restrict fluid intake). May cause dizziness, lightheadedness, confusion, or drowsiness (use caution when driving, climbing stairs, or changing position - rising from sitting or lying to standing, or when engaging in hazardous activities until response to medication is known); nausea or vomiting (frequent mouth care, frequent sips of fluids, chewing gum, or sucking on lozenges may help). Report chest pain or palpitations; persistent dizziness, shortness of breath, or difficulty breathing; unusual bleeding or bruising; or unusual fatigue and weakness.

**Monitoring Parameters:** Pain relief, respiratory and mental status, blood pressure

## Hydrocodone and Aspirin *(hye droe KOE done & AS pir in)*

**Pharmacologic Class** Analgesic, Narcotic

**U.S. Brand Names** Alor® 5/500; Azdone®; Damason-P®; Lortab® ASA; Panasal® 5/500

**Mechanism of Action** Refer to individual agents

**Use** Relief of moderate to moderately severe pain

**USUAL DOSAGE** Adults: Oral: 1-2 tablets every 4-6 hours as needed for pain

**Dosage Forms Tab:** Hydrocodone bitartrate 5 mg and aspirin 500 mg

**Warnings/Precautions** Use with caution in patients with impaired renal function, erosive gastritis, or peptic ulcer disease; children and teenagers should not use for chickenpox or flu symptoms before a physician is consulted about Reye's syndrome; tolerance or drug dependence may result from extended use

**Pregnancy Risk Factor** D

**Adverse Reactions**

>10%:

Cardiovascular: Hypotension

Central nervous system: Lightheadedness, dizziness, sedation, drowsiness, fatigue

Gastrointestinal: Nausea, heartburn, stomach pains, dyspepsia, epigastric discomfort

Neuromuscular & skeletal: Weakness

1% to 10%:

Cardiovascular: Bradycardia

Central nervous system: Confusion

Dermatologic: Rash

Gastrointestinal: Vomiting, gastrointestinal ulceration

Genitourinary: Decreased urination

Hematologic: Hemolytic anemia

Respiratory: Shortness of breath, dyspnea

Miscellaneous: Anaphylactic shock

<1%: Hypertension, hallucinations, insomnia, nervousness, jitters, xerostomia, anorexia, biliary tract spasm, urinary tract spasm, occult bleeding, prolonged bleeding time, leukopenia, thrombocytopenia, iron deficiency anemia, hepatotoxicity, diplopia, miosis, impaired renal function, bronchospasm, histamine release, physical and psychological dependence with prolonged use

**Drug Interactions** Increased toxicity with CNS depressants, warfarin (bleeding)

**Special PA Issues**

**Patient Education:** If self-administered, use exactly as directed (do not increase dose or frequency); may cause physical and/or psychological dependence. Take with food or milk. While using this medication, do not use alcohol, excessive amounts of vitamin C, or salicylate-containing foods (curry powder, prunes, raisins, tea, or licorice), other aspirin- or salicylate-containing medications, and other prescription or OTC medications (especially sedatives, tranquilizers, antihistamines, or pain medications) without consulting prescriber. Maintain adequate hydration (2-3 L/day of fluids unless instructed to restrict fluid intake). May cause hypotension, dizziness, drowsiness, impaired coordination, or blurred vision (use caution when driving, climbing stairs, or changing position - rising from sitting or lying to standing, or when engaging in hazardous activities until response to medication is known); nausea, vomiting, or dry mouth (frequent mouth care, small frequent meals, or sucking on lozenges may help); constipation (increased exercise, fluids, or dietary fruit and fiber may help - if constipation remains an unresolved problem, consult prescriber about use of stool softeners). Report ringing in ears; persistent pain in stomach; unresolved nausea or vomiting; difficulty breathing or shortness of breath; yellowing of skin or eyes; changes in color of stool or urine; or unusual bruising or bleeding.

**Dietary Considerations:** Alcohol: Additive CNS effect, avoid use
**Monitoring Parameters:** Observe patient for excessive sedation, respiratory depression

# Hydrocodone and Chlorpheniramine
(hye droe KOE done & klor fen IR a meen)
**Pharmacologic Class** Antihistamine/Antitussive
**U.S. Brand Names** Tussionex®
**Dosage Forms Syr, alcohol free:** Hydrocodone polistirex 10 mg and chlorpheniramine polistirex 8 mg per 5 mL (480 mL, 900 mL)
**Duration** Hydrocodone: 4-6 hours
**Half-Life** Hydrocodone: 3.8 hours

# Hydrocodone and Guaifenesin (hye droe KOE done & gwye FEN e sin)
**Pharmacologic Class** Antitussive/Expectorant
**U.S. Brand Names** Codiclear® DH; HycoClear Tuss®; Hycotuss® Expectorant Liquid; Kwelcof®
**Dosage Forms Liq:** Hydrocodone bitartrate 5 mg and guaifenesin 100 mg per 5 mL (120 mL, 480 mL)
**Duration** Hydrocodone: 4-6 hours
**Half-Life** Hydrocodone: 3.8 hours

# Hydrocodone and Homatropine (hye droe KOE done & hoe MA troe peen)
**Pharmacologic Class** Antitussive; Cough Preparation
**U.S. Brand Names** Hycodan®; Hydromet®; Hydropane®; Hydrotropine®; Oncet®; Tussigon®
**Use** Symptomatic relief of cough
**USUAL DOSAGE** Oral (based on hydrocodone component):
  Children: 0.6 mg/kg/day in 3-4 divided doses; do not administer more frequently than every 4 hours
    A single dose should not exceed 1.25 mg in children <2 years of age, 5 mg in children 2-12 years, and 10 mg in children >12 years
  Adults: 5-10 mg every 4-6 hours, a single dose should not exceed 15 mg; do not administer more frequently than every 4 hours
**Dosage Forms Syr (Hycodan®, Hydromet®, Hydropane®, Hydrotropine®):** Hydrocodone bitartrate 5 mg and homatropine methylbromide 1.5 mg per 5 mL (120 mL, 480 mL, 4000 mL); **Tab (Hycodan®, Tussigon®):** Hydrocodone bitartrate 5 mg and homatropine methylbromide 1.5 mg
**Contraindications** Increased intracranial pressure, narrow-angle glaucoma, depressed ventilation, hypersensitivity to hydrocodone, homatropine, or any component
**Warnings/Precautions** Use with caution in patients with hypersensitivity to other phenanthrene derivatives; use with caution in patients with respiratory diseases, or severe liver or renal failure; use with caution in children with spastic paralysis, in the elderly, and in patients with prostatic hypertrophy
**Pregnancy Risk Factor** C
**Adverse Reactions**
  >10%:
    Cardiovascular: Hypotension
    Central nervous system: Lightheadedness, dizziness, sedation, drowsiness, fatigue
    Neuromuscular & skeletal: Weakness
  1% to 10%:
    Cardiovascular: Bradycardia, tachycardia
    Central nervous system: Confusion
    Gastrointestinal: Nausea, vomiting
    Genitourinary: Decreased urination
    Respiratory: Shortness of breath, dyspnea
  <1%: Hallucinations, hypertension, dry hot skin, xerostomia, anorexia, impaired GI motility, biliary tract spasm, urinary tract spasm, diplopia, miosis, mydriasis, blurred vision, histamine release, physical and psychological dependence with prolonged use
**Duration** Hydrocodone: 4-6 hours
**Half-Life** Hydrocodone: 3.8 hours
**Special PA Issues**
  **Patient Education:** Take only as prescribed; do not exceed prescribed dose or frequency. May be habit-forming. Maintain adequate hydration (2-3 L/day of fluids unless instructed to restrict fluid intake). Avoid use of other depressants, alcohol, or sleep-inducing medications, or tranquilizers or pain medications unless approved by prescriber. You may experience orthostatic hypotension (change position slowly when rising from sitting or lying or when climbing stairs); drowsiness, impaired coordination, or blurred vision (use caution when driving or engaging in hazardous tasks until response to therapy is known); nausea or vomiting (frequent small meals, frequent mouth care, chewing gum, or sucking hard candy may help); or constipation (increased exercise, fluids, or dietary fruit and fiber may help). Report persistent CNS changes (dizziness, sedation, tremor, or
(Continued)

## Hydrocodone and Homatropine *(Continued)*

agitation), difficulty breathing, persistent abdominal cramping, visual changes, or lack of improvement or worsening or condition.

**Dietary Considerations:** Alcohol: Additive CNS effect, avoid use

## Hydrocodone and Ibuprofen *(hye droe KOE done & eye byoo PROE fen)*

**Pharmacologic Class** Analgesic, Narcotic

**U.S. Brand Names** Vicoprofen®

**Mechanism of Action** Refer to individual agents

**Use** Short-term (generally <10 days) management of moderate to severe acute pain; is not indicated for treatment of such conditions as osteoarthritis or rheumatoid arthritis

**USUAL DOSAGE** Adults: Oral: 1-2 tablets every 4-6 hours as needed for pain; maximum: 5 tablets/day

**Dosage Forms Tab:** Hydrocodone bitartrate 7.5 mg and ibuprofen 200 mg

**Contraindications** Hypersensitivity to any of the ingredients, aspirin allergy, and 3rd trimester pregnancy

**Warnings/Precautions** As with any opioid analgesic agent, this agent should be used with caution in elderly or debilitated patients, and those with severe impairment of hepatic or renal function, hypothyroidism, Addison's disease, prostatic hypertrophy, or urethral stricture. The usual precautions should be observed and the possibility of respiratory depression should be kept in mind. Patients with head injury, increased intracranial pressure, acute abdomen, active peptic ulcer disease, history of upper GI disease, impaired thyroid function, asthma, hypertension, edema, heart failure, and any bleeding disorder should use this agent cautiously. Hydrocodone suppresses the cough reflex; as with opioids, caution should be exercised when this agent is used postoperatively and in patients with pulmonary disease.

**Pregnancy Risk Factor** C

**Pregnancy Implications** Clinical effects on the fetus: As with other NSAID-containing products, this agent should be avoided in late pregnancy because it may cause premature closure of the ductus arteriosus

**Adverse Reactions**

>10%:

Cardiovascular: Hypotension

Central nervous system: Lightheadedness, dizziness, sedation, drowsiness, fatigue

Dermatologic: Rash, urticaria

Gastrointestinal: Abdominal cramps, heartburn, indigestion, nausea

Neuromuscular & skeletal: Weakness

1% to 10%:

Cardiovascular: Bradycardia

Central nervous system: Headache, nervousness, confusion

Dermatologic: Itching

Endocrine & metabolic: Fluid retention

Gastrointestinal: Dyspepsia, vomiting, abdominal pain, GI ulceration

Genitourinary: Decreased urination

Otic: Tinnitus

Respiratory: Shortness of breath, dyspnea

<1%: Edema, congestive heart failure, arrhythmias, tachycardia, hypertension, confusion, hallucinations, mental depression, insomnia, aseptic meningitis, urticaria, erythema multiforme, toxic epidermal necrolysis, Stevens-Johnson syndrome, polydipsia, hot flashes, gastritis, xerostomia, anorexia, biliary tract spasm, cystitis, urinary tract spasm, neutropenia, anemia, agranulocytosis, inhibition of platelet aggregation, hemolytic anemia, bone marrow suppression, leukopenia, thrombocytopenia, hepatitis, peripheral neuropathy, vision changes, blurred vision, conjunctivitis, dry eyes, toxic amblyopia, diplopia, miosis, decreased hearing, acute renal failure, polyuria, allergic rhinitis, shortness of breath, epistaxis, histamine release, physical and psychological dependence with prolonged use

**Drug Interactions**

Decreased effect: May decrease efficacy of ACE inhibitors and diuretics

Increased toxicity potential: Aspirin, other CNS depressants, alcohol, MAO inhibitors, ACE inhibitors, tricyclic antidepressants, lithium, anticoagulants, anticholinergics, methotrexate

**Half-Life** Ibuprofen: 2.2 hours; Hydrocodone: 4.5 hours

**Special PA Issues**

**Patient Education:** If self-administered, use exactly as directed (do not increase dose or frequency); may cause physical and/or psychological dependence. Take with food or milk. While using this medication, do not use alcohol and other prescription or OTC medications (especially sedatives, tranquilizers, antihistamines, or pain medications) without consulting prescriber. Maintain adequate hydration (2-3 L/day of fluids unless instructed to restrict fluid intake). May cause dizziness, drowsiness, confusion, nervousness, or anxiety (use caution when driving, climbing stairs, or changing position - rising from sitting or lying to standing, or when engaging in hazardous activities until response to medication is known); nausea, dry mouth, decreased appetite, or gastric distress (frequent mouth care, frequent sips of fluids, chewing gum, or sucking on lozenges may help); constipation (increased exercise, fluids, or dietary fruit and fiber may help - if constipation remains an unresolved problem, consult prescriber about use of stool softeners). Report chest pain or palpitations; persistent dizziness, shortness of breath, or difficulty breathing; unusual bleeding (stool, mouth, urine) or bruising; unusual fatigue and weakness; change in elimination patterns; or change in color of urine or stool.

# Hydrocodone and Phenylpropanolamine
(hye droe KOE done & fen il proe pa NOLE a meen)

**Pharmacologic Class** Antitussive/Decongestant

**U.S. Brand Names** Codamine®; Codamine® Pediatric; Hycomine®; Hycomine® Pediatric; Hydrocodone PA® Syrup

**Dosage Forms Syr:** Codamine®, Hycomine®: Hydrocodone bitartrate 5 mg and phenylpropanolamine hydrochloride 25 mg per 5 mL (480 mL), Codamine® Pediatric, Hycomine® Pediatric: Hydrocodone bitartrate 2.5 mg and phenylpropanolamine hydrochloride 12.5 mg per 5 mL (480 mL)

**Duration** Hydrocodone: 4-6 hours

**Half-Life** Hydrocodone: 3.8 hours

# Hydrocodone and Pseudoephedrine
(hye droe KOE done & soo doe e FED rin)

**Pharmacologic Class** Cough and Cold Combination

**U.S. Brand Names** Detussin® Liquid; Entuss-D® Liquid; Histussin D® Liquid; Tyrodone® Liquid

**Dosage Forms Liq:** Hydrocodone bitartrate 5 mg and pseudoephedrine hydrochloride 30 mg per 5 mL; hydrocodone bitartrate 5 mg and pseudoephedrine hydrochloride 60 mg per 5 mL

# Hydrocodone, Chlorpheniramine, Phenylephrine, Acetaminophen and Caffeine
(hye droe KOE done, klor fen IR a meen, fen il EF rin, a seet a MIN oh fen, & KAF een)

**Pharmacologic Class** Antitussive

**U.S. Brand Names** Hycomine® Compound

**Dosage Forms Tab:** Hydrocodone bitartrate 5 mg, chlorpheniramine maleate 2 mg, phenylephrine hydrochloride 10 mg, acetaminophen 250 mg, and caffeine 30 mg

**Duration** Hydrocodone: 4-6 hours

**Half-Life** Hydrocodone: 3.8 hours

♦ **Hydrocodone PA® Syrup** see Hydrocodone and Phenylpropanolamine on this page

# Hydrocodone, Phenylephrine, Pyrilamine, Phenindamine, Chlorpheniramine, and Ammonium Chloride
(hye droe KOE done, fen il EF rin, peer IL a meen, fen IN da meen, klor fen IR a meen, & a MOE nee um KLOR ide)

**Pharmacologic Class** Antihistamine/Decongestant/Antitussive

**U.S. Brand Names** P-V-Tussin®

**Dosage Forms Syr:** Hydrocodone bitartrate 2.5 mg, phenylephrine hydrochloride 5 mg, pyrilamine maleate 6 mg, phenindamine tartrate 5 mg, chlorpheniramine maleate 2 mg, and ammonium chloride 50 mg per 5 mL with alcohol 5% (480 mL, 3780 mL)

# Hydrocodone, Pseudoephedrine, and Guaifenesin
(hye droe KOE done, soo doe e FED rin & gwye FEN e sin)

**Pharmacologic Class** Antitussive/Decongestant/Expectorant

**U.S. Brand Names** Cophene XP®; Detussin® Expectorant; SRC® Expectorant; Tussafin® Expectorant

**Dosage Forms Liq:** Hydrocodone bitartrate 5 mg, pseudoephedrine hydrochloride 60 mg, and guaifenesin 200 mg per 5 mL with alcohol 12.5% (480 mL)

**Duration** Hydrocodone: 4-6 hours

**Half-Life** Hydrocodone: 3.8 hours

♦ **Hydrocort®** see Hydrocortisone on this page

# Hydrocortisone (hye droe KOR ti sone)

**Pharmacologic Class** Corticosteroid, Oral; Corticosteroid, Parenteral; Corticosteroid, Rectal

**U.S. Brand Names** Acticort 100®; Aeroseb-HC®; A-hydroCort®; Ala-Cort®; Ala-Scalp®; Anucort-HC® Suppository; Anuprep HC® Suppository; Anusol® HC-1 [OTC]; Anusol® HC-2.5% [OTC]; Anusol-HC® Suppository; CaldeCORT®; CaldeCORT® Anti-Itch Spray; Cetacort®; Clocort® Maximum Strength; CortaGel® [OTC]; Cortaid® Maximum Strength [OTC]; Cortaid® With Aloe [OTC]; Cort-Dome®; Cortef®; Cortef® Feminine Itch; Cortenema®; Cortifoam®; Cortizone®-5 [OTC]; Cortizone®-10 [OTC]; Delcort®; Dermacort®; Dermarest Dricort®; DermiCort®; Dermolate® [OTC]; Dermtex® HC With Aloe; Eldecort®; Gynecort® (Continued)

## Hydrocortisone *(Continued)*

[OTC]; Hemril-HC® Uniserts®; Hi-Cor-1.0®; Hi-Cor-2.5®; Hycort®; Hydrocort®; Hydrocortone® Acetate; Hydrocortone® Phosphate; HydroSKIN®; Hydro-Tex® [OTC]; Hytone®; Lacti-Care-HC®; Lanacort® [OTC]; Locoid®; Nutracort®; Orabase® HCA; Pandel®; Penecort®; Procort® [OTC]; Proctocort™; Scalpicin®; Solu-Cortef®; S-T Cort®; Synacort®; Tegrin®-HC [OTC]; U-Cort™; Westcort®

**Mechanism of Action** Decreases inflammation by suppression of migration of polymorpho-nuclear leukocytes and reversal of increased capillary permeability

**Use** Management of adrenocortical insufficiency; relief of inflammation of corticosteroid-responsive dermatoses (low and medium potency topical corticosteroid); adjunctive treatment of ulcerative colitis

**USUAL DOSAGE** Dose should be based on severity of disease and patient response
Acute adrenal insufficiency: I.M., I.V.:
  Infants and young Children: Succinate: 1-2 mg/kg/dose bolus, then 25-150 mg/day in divided doses every 6-8 hours
  Older Children: Succinate: 1-2 mg/kg bolus then 150-250 mg/day in divided doses every 6-8 hours
  Adults: Succinate: 100 mg I.V. bolus, then 300 mg/day in divided doses every 8 hours or as a continuous infusion for 48 hours; once patient is stable change to oral, 50 mg every 8 hours for 6 doses, then taper to 30-50 mg/day in divided doses
Chronic adrenal corticoid insufficiency: Adults: Oral: 20-30 mg/day
Anti-inflammatory or immunosuppressive:
  Infants and Children:
    Oral: 2.5-10 mg/kg/day **or** 75-300 mg/m²/day every 6-8 hours
    I.M., I.V.: Succinate: 1-5 mg/kg/day **or** 30-150 mg/m²/day divided every 12-24 hours
  Adolescents and Adults: Oral, I.M., I.V.: Succinate: 15-240 mg every 12 hours
Congenital adrenal hyperplasia: Oral: Initial: 30-36 mg/m²/day with ⅓ of dose every morning and ⅔ every evening or ¼ every morning and mid-day and ½ every evening; maintenance: 20-25 mg/m²/day in divided doses
Physiologic replacement: Children:
  Oral: 0.5-0.75 mg/kg/day **or** 20-25 mg/m²/day every 8 hours
  I.M.: Succinate: 0.25-0.35 mg/kg/day **or** 12-15 mg/m²/day once daily
Shock: I.M., I.V.: Succinate:
  Children: Initial: 50 mg/kg, then repeated in 4 hours and/or every 24 hours as needed
  Adolescents and Adults: Succinate: 500 mg to 2 g every 2-6 hours
Status asthmaticus: Children and Adults: I.V.: Succinate: 1-2 mg/kg/dose every 6 hours for 24 hours, then maintenance of 0.5-1 mg/kg every 6 hours
Rheumatic diseases:
  Adults: Intralesional, intra-articular, soft tissue injection: Acetate:
    Large joints: 25 mg (up to 37.5 mg)
    Small joints: 10-25 mg
    Tendon sheaths: 5-12.5 mg
    Soft tissue infiltration: 25-50 mg (up to 75 mg)
    Bursae: 25-37.5 mg
    Ganglia: 12.5-25 mg
Dermatosis: Children >2 years and Adults: Topical: Apply to affected area 3-4 times/day (Buteprate: Apply once or twice daily)
Ulcerative colitis: Adults: Rectal: 10-100 mg 1-2 times/day for 2-3 weeks

**Dosage Forms** Acetate: **Aero, rectal (Cortifoam®):** 10% [90 mg/applicatorful] 20 g; **Crm:** CaldeCORT®, Gynecort®, Cortaid® with Aloe, Cortef® Feminine Itch, Lanacort®: 0.5% (15 g, 22.5 g, 30 g), Anusol-HC-1®, CaldeCORT®, Clocort® Maximum Strength, Cortaid® Maximum Strength, Dermarest Dricort®, U-Cort™: 1% (15 g, 21 g, 30 g, 120 g); **Oint, top:** Cortaid® with Aloe, Lanacort® 5: 0.5% (15 g, 30 g), Gynecort® 10, Lanacort® 10: 1% (15 g, 30 g); **Inj, susp (Hydrocortone® Acetate):** 25 mg/mL (5 mL, 10 mL), 50 mg/mL (5 mL, 10 mL); **Paste (Orabase® HCA):** 0.5% (5 g); **Soln, top (Scalpicin®):** 1%; **Supp, rectal (Anucort-HC®, Anuprep HC®, Anusol-HC®, Hemril-HC® Uniserts®):** 25 mg; Base: **Aero, top:** Aeroseb-HC®, CaldeCORT® Anti-Itch Spray, Cortaid®: 0.5% (45 g, 58 g), Cortaid® Maximum Strength: 1% (45 mL); **Crm:** Cort-Dome®, Cortizone®-5, DermiCort®, Dermolate®, Dermtex® HC with Aloe, HydroSKIN®, Hydro-Tex®: 0.5% (15 g, 30 g, 120 g, 454 g), Ala-Cort®, Cort-Dome®, Delcort®, Dermacort®, DermiCort®, Eldecort®, Hi-Cor 1.0®, Hycort®, Hytone®, Nutracort®, Penecort®, Synacort®: 1% (15 g, 20 g, 30 g, 60 g, 120 g, 240 g, 454 g), Anusol-HC-2.5%®, Eldecort®, Hi-Cor-2.5®, Hydrocort®, Hytone®: 2.5% (15 g, 20 g, 30 g, 60 g, 120 g, 240 g, 454 g); Rectal (Proctocort™): 1% (30 g); **Gel:** CortaGel® 0.5% (15 g, 30 g), CortaGel® Extra Strength: 1% (15 g, 30 g); **Lot:** Cetacort®, DermiCort®, HydroSKIN®, S-T Cort®: 0.5% (60 mL, 120 mL), Acticort 100®, Cetacort®, Cortizone-10®, Dermacort®, HydroSKIN® Maximum Strength, Hytone®, LactiCare-HC®, Nutracort®: 1% (60 mL, 120 mL), Ala-Scalp: 2% (30 mL), Hytone®, LactiCare-HC®, Nutracort®: 2.5% (60 mL, 120 mL); **Oint, top:** Cortizone®-5, HydroSKIN®: 0.5% (30 g), Cortizone®-10, Hycort®, HydroSKIN®, Hydro-Tex®, Hytone®, Tegrin®-HC: 1% (15 g, 20 g, 30 g, 60 g, 120 g, 240 g, 454 g), Hytone®: 2.5% (20 g, 30 g); **Susp, rectal (Cortenema®):** 100 mg/60 mL (7s); **Tab:** Cortef®: 5 mg, 10 mg, 20 mg, Hydrocortone®: 10 mg, 20 mg,

Butyrate (Locoid®): **Crm:** 0.1% (15 g, 45 g); **Oint, top:** 0.1% (15 g, 45 g); **Soln, top:** 0.1% (20 mL, 60 mL)

Cypionate: **Susp, oral (Cortef®):** 10 mg/5 mL (120 mL)

Sodium phosphate: **Inj (Hydrocortone® Phosphate):** 50 mg/mL (2 mL, 10 mL)

Sodium succinate: **Inj (A-hydroCort®, Solu-Cortef®):** 100 mg, 250 mg, 500 mg, 1000 mg

Valerate (Westcort®): **Crm:** 0.2% (15 g, 45 g, 60 g); **Oint, top:** 0.2% (15 g, 45 g, 60 g, 120 g)

**Contraindications** Serious infections, except septic shock or tuberculous meningitis; known hypersensitivity to hydrocortisone; viral, fungal, or tubercular skin lesions

**Warnings/Precautions**

Use with caution in patients with hyperthyroidism, cirrhosis, nonspecific ulcerative colitis, hypertension, osteoporosis, thromboembolic tendencies, CHF, convulsive disorders, myasthenia gravis, thrombophlebitis, peptic ulcer, diabetes

Acute adrenal insufficiency may occur with abrupt withdrawal after long-term therapy or with stress; young pediatric patients may be more susceptible to adrenal axis suppression from topical therapy

Because of the risk of adverse effects, systemic corticosteroids should be used cautiously in the elderly, in the smallest possible dose, and for the shortest possible time

**Pregnancy Risk Factor** C

**Adverse Reactions**

>10%:

Central nervous system: Insomnia, nervousness

Gastrointestinal: Increased appetite, indigestion

1% to 10%:

Dermatologic: Hirsutism

Endocrine & metabolic: Diabetes mellitus

Neuromuscular & skeletal: Arthralgia

Ocular: Cataracts

Respiratory: Epistaxis

<1%: Hypertension, edema, euphoria, headache, delirium, hallucinations, seizures, mood swings, acne, dermatitis, skin atrophy, bruising, hyperpigmentation, hypokalemia, hyperglycemia, Cushing's syndrome, sodium and water retention, bone growth suppression, amenorrhea, peptic ulcer, abdominal distention, ulcerative esophagitis, pancreatitis, muscle wasting, hypersensitivity reactions, immunosuppression

**Drug Interactions** CYP2D6 and 3A3/4 enzyme substrate

Decreased effect:

Insulin decreases hypoglycemic effect

Phenytoin, phenobarbital, ephedrine, and rifampin increase metabolism of hydrocortisone and decrease steroid blood level

Increased toxicity:

Oral anticoagulants change prothrombin time; potassium-depleting diuretics increase risk of hypokalemia

Cardiac glucosides increase risk of arrhythmias or digitalis toxicity secondary to hypokalemia

**Onset**

Hydrocortisone acetate: Slow onset but long duration of action when compared with more soluble preparations.

Hydrocortisone sodium phosphate: A water soluble salt with a rapid onset but short duration of action.

Hydrocortisone sodium succinate: A water soluble salt which is rapidly active.

**Half-Life** Biologic: 8-12 hours

**Special PA Issues**

**Patient Education:**

Systemic: Take as directed; do not increase doses and do not stop abruptly without consulting prescribed. Dosage of systemic hydrocortisone is usually tapered off gradually. Take oral dose with food to reduce GI upset. Hydrocortisone may cause immunosuppression and mask symptoms of infection; avoid exposure to contagion and notify prescriber of any signs of infection (eg, fever, chills, sore throat, injury) and notify dentist or surgeon (if necessary) that you are taking this medication. You may experience increased appetite, indigestion, or increased nervousness. Report any sudden weight gain (>5 lb/week), swelling of extremities or difficulty breathing, abdominal pain, severe vomiting, tarry stools, fatigue, anorexia, weakness, or unusual mood swings.

Topical: Before applying, wash area gently and thoroughly. Apply gel, cream, or ointment in thin film to cleansed area and rub in gently until medication vanishes. Avoid exposing affected area to sunlight; you will be more sensitive and severe sunburn may occur. Consult prescriber if breast-feeding.

Rectal: Insert suppository gently as high as possible with gloved finger while lying down. Avoid injury with long or sharp fingernails. Remain in resting position for 10 minutes after insertion.

**Monitoring Parameters:** Blood pressure, weight, serum glucose, and electrolytes

**Reference Range:** Therapeutic: AM: 5-25 µg/dL (SI: 138-690 nmol/L), PM: 2-9 µg/dL (SI: 55-248 nmol/L) depending on test, assay

(Continued)

## Hydrocortisone *(Continued)*
**Related Information**
Corticosteroids *on page 1007*

♦ **Hydrocortisone Acetate** *see Hydrocortisone on page 453*
♦ **Hydrocortisone Buteprate** *see Hydrocortisone on page 453*
♦ **Hydrocortisone Butyrate** *see Hydrocortisone on page 453*
♦ **Hydrocortisone Cypionate** *see Hydrocortisone on page 453*
♦ **Hydrocortisone Sodium Phosphate** *see Hydrocortisone on page 453*
♦ **Hydrocortisone Sodium Succinate** *see Hydrocortisone on page 453*
♦ **Hydrocortisone Valerate** *see Hydrocortisone on page 453*
♦ **Hydrocortone® Acetate** *see Hydrocortisone on page 453*
♦ **Hydrocortone® Phosphate** *see Hydrocortisone on page 453*
♦ **Hydro-Crysti-12®** *see Hydroxocobalamin on page 458*
♦ **HydroDIURIL®** *see Hydrochlorothiazide on page 447*
♦ **Hydrogesic®** *see Hydrocodone and Acetaminophen on page 449*
♦ **Hydromet®** *see Hydrocodone and Homatropine on page 451*
♦ **Hydromorph Contin®** *see Hydromorphone on this page*

## Hydromorphone *(hye droe MOR fone)*
**Pharmacologic Class** Analgesic, Narcotic
**U.S. Brand Names** Dilaudid®; Dilaudid-5®; Dilaudid-HP®; HydroStat IR®
**Mechanism of Action** Binds to opiate receptors in the CNS, causing inhibition of ascending pain pathways, altering the perception of and response to pain; causes cough supression by direct central action in the medulla; produces generalized CNS depression
**Use** Management of moderate to severe pain; antitussive at lower doses
**USUAL DOSAGE**
Doses should be titrated to appropriate analgesic effects; when changing routes of adminis-tration, note that oral doses are less than half as effective as parenteral doses (may be only one-fifth as effective)
Pain: Older Children and Adults:
Oral, I.M., I.V., S.C.: 1-4 mg/dose every 4-6 hours as needed; usual adult dose: 2 mg/dose
Rectal: 3 mg every 6-8 hours
Antitussive: Oral:
Children 6-12 years: 0.5 mg every 3-4 hours as needed
Children >12 years and Adults: 1 mg every 3-4 hours as needed
**Dosing adjustment in hepatic impairment:** Should be considered
**Dosage Forms Inj:** Dilaudid®: 1 mg/mL (1 mL), 2 mg/mL (1 mL, 20 mL), 3 mg/mL (1 mL), 4 mg/mL (1 mL), Dilaudid-HP®: 10 mg/mL (1 mL, 2 mL, 5 mL); **Liq:** 5 mg/5 mL (480 mL); **Powder for inj:** (Dilaudid-HP®): 250 mg; **Supp, rectal:** 3 mg (6s); **Tab:** 1 mg, 2 mg, 3 mg, 4 mg, 8 mg
**Contraindications** Hypersensitivity to hydromorphone or any component or other phenan-threne derivative
**Warnings/Precautions** Tablet and cough syrup contain tartrazine which may cause allergic reactions; hydromorphone shares toxic potential of opiate agonists, and precaution of opiate agonist therapy should be observed; extreme caution should be taken to avoid confusing the highly concentrated injection with the less concentrated injectable product, injection contains benzyl alcohol; use with caution in patients with hypersensitivity to other phenanthrene opiates, in patients with respiratory disease, or severe liver or renal failure; tolerance or drug dependence may result from extended use
**Pregnancy Risk Factor** B (D if used for prolonged periods or in high doses at term)
**Adverse Reactions**
Percentage unknown: Antidiuretic hormone release, biliary tract spasm, urinary tract spasm, miosis, histamine release, physical and psychological dependence, increased AST, ALT
>10%:
Cardiovascular: Palpitations, hypotension, peripheral vasodilation
Central nervous system: Dizziness, lightheadedness, drowsiness
Gastrointestinal: Anorexia
1% to 10%:
Cardiovascular: Tachycardia, bradycardia, flushing of face
Central nervous system: CNS depression, increased intracranial pressure, fatigue, head-ache, nervousness, restlessness
Gastrointestinal: Nausea, vomiting, constipation, stomach cramps, xerostomia
Genitourinary: Decreased urination, ureteral spasm
Hepatic: Increased LFTs
Neuromuscular & skeletal: Trembling, weakness
Respiratory: Respiratory depression, dyspnea, shortness of breath
<1%: Hallucinations, mental depression, pruritus, rash, urticaria, paralytic ileus

**Drug Interactions** Increased toxicity: CNS depressants, phenothiazines, tricyclic antidepressants may potentiate the adverse effects of hydromorphone

**Onset** Analgesic effect: Within 15-30 minutes; Peak effect: Within 0.5-1.5 hours

**Duration** 4-5 hours

**Half-Life** 1-3 hours

**Special PA Issues**

**Patient Education:** If self-administered, use exactly as directed (do not increase dose or frequency); may cause physical and/or psychological dependence. While using this medication, do not use alcohol and other prescription or OTC medications (especially sedatives, tranquilizers, antihistamines, or pain medications) without consulting prescriber. Maintain adequate hydration (2-3 L/day of fluids unless instructed to restrict fluid intake). May cause dizziness, drowsiness, impaired coordination, or blurred vision (use caution when driving, climbing stairs, or changing position - rising from sitting or lying to standing, or when engaging in hazardous activities until response to medication is known); loss of appetite, nausea, or vomiting (frequent mouth care, small frequent meals, or sucking on lozenges may help); constipation (increased exercise, fluids, or dietary fruit and fiber may help - if constipation remains an unresolved problem, consult prescriber about use of stool softeners). Report chest pain, slow or rapid heartbeat, acute dizziness, or persistent headache; swelling of extremities or unusual weight gain; changes in urinary elimination; acute headache; back or flank pain or spasms; or other adverse reactions.

**Dietary Considerations:**

Alcohol: Additive CNS effects, avoid or limit alcohol; watch for sedation

Food: Glucose may cause hyperglycemia; monitor blood glucose concentrations

**Monitoring Parameters:** Pain relief, respiratory and mental status, blood pressure

**Related Information**

Narcotic Agonists *on page 1023*

♦ **Hydromorphone Hydrochloride** *see* Hydromorphone *on previous page*

♦ **Hydropane®** *see* Hydrocodone and Homatropine *on page 451*

♦ **Hydro-Par®** *see* Hydrochlorothiazide *on page 447*

♦ **Hydrophed®** *see* Theophylline, Ephedrine, and Hydroxyzine *on page 888*

♦ **Hydropres®** *see* Hydrochlorothiazide and Reserpine *on page 448*

♦ **Hydroquinol** *see* Hydroquinone *on this page*

# Hydroquinone (HYE droe kwin one)

**Pharmacologic Class** Depigmenting Agent

**U.S. Brand Names** Ambi® Skin Tone [OTC]; Eldopaque® [OTC]; Eldopaque Forte®; Eldoquin® [OTC]; Eldoquin® Forte®; Esoterica® Facial [OTC]; Esoterica® Regular, Porcelana®: 2% [OTC] (14.2 g, 28.4 g, 60 g, 85 g, 120 g), Eldopaque Forte®, Eldoquin® Forte®, Melquin HP®: 4% (14.2 g, 28.4 g); **Crm, top, with sunblock:** Esoterica® Sunscreen, Porcelana®, Solaquin®: 2% [OTC] (28.4 g, 120 g), Melpaque HP®, Nuquin HP®, Solaquin Forte®: 4% (14.2 g, 28.4 g); **Gel, top, with sunscreen (Solaquin Forte®):** 4% (14.2 g, 28.4 g); **Sol, top (Melanex®):** 3% (30 mL)

**Mechanism of Action** Produces reversible depigmentation of the skin by suppression of melanocyte metabolic processes, in particular the inhibition of the enzymatic oxidation of tyrosine to DOPA (3,4-dihydroxyphenylalanine); sun exposure reverses this effect and will cause repigmentation.

**Use** Gradual bleaching of hyperpigmented skin conditions

**USUAL DOSAGE** Children >12 years and Adults: Topical: Apply thin layer and rub in twice daily

**Dosage Forms Crm, top:** Esoterica® Sensitive Skin Formula: 1.5% [OTC] (85 g), Eldopaque®, Eldoquin®, Esoterica® Facial, Esoterica® Regular, Porcelana®: 2% [OTC] (14.2 g, 28.4 g, 60 g, 85 g, 120 g), Eldopaque Forte®, Eldoquin® Forte®, Melquin HP®: 4% (14.2 g, 28.4 g); **Crm, top, with sunblock:** Esoterica® Sunscreen, Porcelana®, Solaquin®: 2% [OTC] (28.4 g, 120 g), Melpaque HP®, Nuquin HP®, Solaquin Forte®: 4% (14.2 g, 28.4 g); **Gel, top, with sunscreen (Solaquin Forte®):** 4% (14.2 g, 28.4 g); **Sol, top (Melanex®):** 3% (30 mL)

**Contraindications** Sunburn, depilatory usage, known hypersensitivity to hydroquinone

**Warnings/Precautions** Limit application to area no larger than face and neck or hands and arms

**Pregnancy Risk Factor** C

**Adverse Reactions** 1% to 10%:

Dermatologic: Dermatitis, dryness, erythema, stinging, inflammatory reaction, sensitization

Local: Irritation

**Onset** Onset of depigmentation produced by hydroquinone varies among individuals.

**Duration** Duration of depigmentation produced by hydroquinone varies among individuals

**Special PA Issues**

**Patient Education:** Use exactly as directed; do not overuse. Therapeutic effect may take several weeks. Test response by applying to small area of unbroken skin and check in 24 hours; if irritation or blistering occurs do not use. Avoid contact with eyes. Do not apply to open wounds or weeping areas. Before using, wash and dry area gently. Apply a thin film to affected area and rub in gently. Avoid direct sunlight or use sunblock or protective

(Continued)

## Hydroquinone *(Continued)*

clothing to prevent repigmentation. Report swelling, redness, rash, itching, signs of infection, worsening of condition, or lack of healing.

- ◆ **Hydro-Serp®** *see Hydrochlorothiazide and Reserpine on page 448*
- ◆ **Hydroserpine®** *see Hydrochlorothiazide and Reserpine on page 448*
- ◆ **HydroSKIN®** *see Hydrocortisone on page 453*
- ◆ **HydroStat IR®** *see Hydromorphone on page 456*
- ◆ **Hydro-Tex® [OTC]** *see Hydrocortisone on page 453*
- ◆ **Hydrotropine®** *see Hydrocodone and Homatropine on page 451*

## Hydroxocobalamin (hye droks oh koe BAL a min)

**Pharmacologic Class** Vitamin, Water Soluble

**U.S. Brand Names** Alphamin®; Codroxomin®; Hybalamin®; Hydro-Cobex®; Hydro-Crysti-12®; LA-12®

**Mechanism of Action** Coenzyme for various metabolic functions, including fat and carbohydrate metabolism and protein synthesis, used in cell replication and hematopoiesis

**Use** Treatment of pernicious anemia, vitamin $B_{12}$ deficiency, increased $B_{12}$ requirements due to pregnancy, thyrotoxicosis, hemorrhage, malignancy, liver or kidney disease

**USUAL DOSAGE** Vitamin $B_{12}$ deficiency: I.M.:

Children: 1-5 mg given in single doses of 100 mcg over 2 or more weeks, followed by 30-50 mcg/month

Adults: 30 mcg/day for 5-10 days, followed by 100-200 mcg/month

**Dosage Forms Inj:** 1000 mcg/mL (10 mL, 30 mL)

**Contraindications** Hypersensitivity to cyanocobalamin or any component, cobalt; patients with hereditary optic nerve atrophy

**Warnings/Precautions** Some products contain benzoyl alcohol; avoid use in premature infants; an intradermal test dose should be performed for hypersensitivity; use only if oral supplementation not possible or when treating pernicious anemia

**Pregnancy Risk Factor** C

**Adverse Reactions**

1% to 10%:

Dermatologic: Itching

Gastrointestinal: Diarrhea

<1%: Peripheral vascular thrombosis, urticaria, anaphylaxis

**Special PA Issues**

**Patient Education:** Use exactly as directed. Pernicious anemia may require monthly injections for life. Report skin rash; swelling, pain, or redness in extremities; or acute persistent diarrhea.

## Hydroxyamphetamine and Tropicamide

(hye droks ee am FET a meen & troe PIK a mide)

**Pharmacologic Class** Adrenergic Agonist Agent

**U.S. Brand Names** Paremyd® Ophthalmic

**Dosage Forms Soln, ophth:** Hydroxyamphetamine hydrobromide 1% and tropicamide 0.25% (5 mL, 15 mL)

- ◆ **Hydroxycarbamide** *see Hydroxyurea on page 460*

## Hydroxychloroquine (hye droks ee KLOR oh kwin)

**Pharmacologic Class** Aminoquinoline (Antimalarial)

**U.S. Brand Names** Plaquenil®

**Mechanism of Action** Interferes with digestive vacuole function within sensitive malarial parasites by increasing the pH and interfering with lysosomal degradation of hemoglobin; inhibits locomotion of neutrophils and chemotaxis of eosinophils; impairs complement-dependent antigen-antibody reactions

**Use** Suppresses and treats acute attacks of malaria; treatment of systemic lupus erythematosus and rheumatoid arthritis

**USUAL DOSAGE** Note: Hydroxychloroquine sulfate 200 mg is equivalent to 155 mg hydroxychloroquine base and 250 mg chloroquine phosphate. Oral:

Children:

Chemoprophylaxis of malaria: 5 mg/kg (base) once weekly; should not exceed the recommended adult dose; begin 2 weeks before exposure; continue for 4-6 weeks after leaving endemic area; if suppressive therapy is not begun prior to the exposure, double the initial dose and give in 2 doses, 6 hours apart

Acute attack: 10 mg/kg (base) initial dose; followed by 5 mg/kg at 6, 24, and 48 hours

JRA or SLE: 3-5 mg/kg/day divided 1-2 times/day; avoid exceeding 7 mg/kg/day

Adults:

Chemoprophylaxis of malaria: 310 mg base weekly on same day each week; begin 2 weeks before exposure; continue for 4-6 weeks after leaving endemic area; if suppressive therapy is not begun prior to the exposure, double the initial dose and give in 2 doses, 6 hours apart

Acute attack: 620 mg first dose day 1; 310 mg in 6 hours day 1; 310 mg in 1 dose day 2; and 310 mg in 1 dose on day 3

Rheumatoid arthritis: 310-465 mg/day to start taken with food or milk; increase dose until optimum response level is reached; usually after 4-12 weeks dose should be reduced by $1/2$ and a maintenance dose of 155-310 mg/day given

Lupus erythematosus: 310 mg every day or twice daily for several weeks depending on response; 155-310 mg/day for prolonged maintenance therapy

**Dosage Forms** Tab, as sulfate: 200 mg [base 155 mg]

**Contraindications** Retinal or visual field changes attributable to 4-aminoquinolines; hypersensitivity to hydroxychloroquine, 4-aminoquinoline derivatives, or any component

**Warnings/Precautions** Use with caution in patients with hepatic disease, G-6-PD deficiency, psoriasis, and porphyria; long-term use in children is not recommended; perform baseline and periodic (6 months) ophthalmologic examinations; test periodically for muscle weakness

**Pregnancy Risk Factor** C

**Adverse Reactions**

>10%:

Central nervous system: Headache

Dermatologic: Itching

Gastrointestinal: Diarrhea, loss of appetite, nausea, stomach cramps, vomiting

Ocular: Ciliary muscle dysfunction

1% to 10%:

Central nervous system: Dizziness, lightheadedness, nervousness, restlessness

Dermatologic: Bleaching of hair, rash, discoloration of skin (black-blue)

Ocular: Ocular toxicity, keratopathy, retinopathy

<1%: Emotional changes, seizures, agranulocytosis, aplastic anemia, neutropenia, thrombocytopenia, neuromyopathy, ototoxicity

**Drug Interactions**

Chloroquine and other 4-aminoquinolones may be decreased due to GI binding with kaolin or magnesium trisilicate

Increased effect: Cimetidine increases levels of chloroquine and probably other 4-aminoquinolones

**Onset** In rheumatic disease, may require 4-6 weeks to respond (maximum after several months)

**Half-Life** 32-50 days

**Special PA Issues**

**Patient Education:** It is important to complete full course of therapy which may take up to 6 months for full effect. May be taken with meals to decrease GI upset and bitter aftertaste. Avoid alcohol. You should have regular ophthalmic exams (every 4-6 months) if using this medication over extended periods. You may experience skin discoloration (blue/black), hair bleaching, or skin rash. If you have psoriasis, you may experience exacerbation. You may experience dizziness, headache, nervousness, or lightheadedness (use caution when driving or engaging in tasks requiring alertness until response is known); nausea, vomiting, or loss of appetite (small frequent meals, frequent mouth care, or sucking lozenges may help); or increased sensitivity to sunlight (wear dark glasses and protective clothing, use sunblock, and avoid direct exposure to sunlight). Report vision changes, rash or itching, persistent diarrhea or GI disturbances, change in hearing acuity or ringing in the ears, chest pain or palpitation, CNS changes, unusual fatigue, easy bruising or bleeding, or any other persistent adverse reactions.

**Monitoring Parameters:** Ophthalmologic exam, CBC

♦ **Hydroxychloroquine Sulfate** *see* Hydroxychloroquine *on previous page*

♦ **25-Hydroxycholecalciferol** *see* Calcifediol *on page 135*

♦ **Hydroxyethyl Starch** *see* Hetastarch *on page 441*

# Hydroxyprogesterone Caproate

(hye droks ee proe JES te rone KAP roe ate)

**Pharmacologic Class** Progestin

**U.S. Brand Names** Hylutin® Injection; Hyprogest® 250 Injection

**Mechanism of Action** Natural steroid hormone that induces secretory changes in the endometrium, promotes mammary gland development, relaxes uterine smooth muscle, blocks follicular maturation and ovulation and maintains pregnancy

**Use** Treatment of amenorrhea, abnormal uterine bleeding, endometriosis, uterine carcinoma

**USUAL DOSAGE** Adults: Female: I.M.: *Long-acting progestin*

Amenorrhea: 375 mg; if no bleeding, begin cyclic treatment with estradiol valerate

(Continued)

## Hydroxyprogesterone Caproate *(Continued)*

Production of secretory endometrium and desquamation: (Medical D and C): 125-250 mg administered on day 10 of cycle; repeat every 7 days until suppression is no longer desired.

Uterine carcinoma: 1 g one or more times/day (1-7 g/week) for up to 12 weeks

**Dosage Forms** Inj: 125 mg/mL (10 mL), Hylutin®, Hyprogest®: 250 mg/mL (5 mL)

**Contraindications** Thrombophlebitis, thromboembolic disorders, cerebral hemorrhage, liver impairment, carcinoma of the breast, hypersensitivity to hydroxyprogesterone or any component, undiagnosed vaginal bleeding

**Warnings/Precautions** Use with caution in patients with asthma, seizure disorders, migraine, cardiac or renal impairment, history of mental depression; use of any progestin during the first 4 months of pregnancy is not recommended; observe patients closely for signs and symptoms of thrombotic disorders

**Pregnancy Risk Factor** D

**Adverse Reactions**

>10%:

Cardiovascular: Edema

Endocrine & metabolic: Breakthrough bleeding, spotting, changes in menstrual flow, amenorrhea

Gastrointestinal: Anorexia

Local: Pain at injection site

Neuromuscular & skeletal: Weakness

1% to 10%:

Central nervous system: Mental depression, insomnia, fever

Dermatologic: Melasma or chloasma, allergic rash with or without pruritus

Gastrointestinal: Weight gain or loss

Genitourinary: Changes in cervical erosion and secretions, increased breast tenderness

Hepatic: Cholestatic jaundice

**Drug Interactions** Decreased effect: Rifampin may increase clearance of hydroxyprogesterone

**Special PA Issues**

**Patient Education:** Maintain a regular schedule of injections as prescribed. This drug can only be given deep I.M. injection. If diabetic, monitor serum glucose closely. You may experience some sensitivity to sunlight; wear protective clothing, use sunblock, or avoid sunlight. You may experience dizziness; use caution when driving or engaging in hazardous tasks. Report rash, alopecia, radically increased weight gain or swelling, anorexia, muscular weakness, fever, or unresolved nausea or vomiting. Report immediately any swelling or warmth in calves, chest pain or respiratory difficulty, severe headache or acute dizziness, numbness and/or tingling in extremities.

## Hydroxyurea *(hye droks ee yoor EE a)*

**Pharmacologic Class** Antineoplastic Agent, Antimetabolite

**U.S. Brand Names** Droxia™; Hydrea®

**Mechanism of Action** Thought to interfere (unsubstantiated hypothesis) with synthesis of DNA, during the S phase of cell division, without interfering with RNA synthesis; inhibits ribonucleoside diphosphate reductase, preventing conversion of ribonucleotides to deoxyribonucleotides; cell-cycle specific for the S phase and may hold other cells in the $G_1$ phase of the cell cycle.

**Use** CML in chronic phase; radiosensitizing agent in the treatment of primary brain tumors, head and neck tumors, uterine cervix and nonsmall cell lung cancer, psoriasis, sickle cell anemia and other hemoglobinopathies; treatment of hematologic conditions such as essential thrombocythemia, polycythemia vera, hypereosinophilia, and hyperleukocytosis due to acute leukemia. Has shown activity against renal cell cancer, melanoma, ovarian cancer, head and neck cancer, and prostate cancer. Management of sickle cell anemia - to reduce the frequency of painful crises and to reduce the need for blood transfusions in adult patients with sickle cell anemia with recurrent moderate to severe painful crises (generally at least 3 during the preceding 12 months). Has been used in combination with didanosine and other antiretrovirals in the treatment of HIV.

**USUAL DOSAGE** Oral (refer to individual protocols): All dosage should be based on ideal or actual body weight, whichever is less:

Children:

No FDA-approved dosage regimens have been established; dosages of 1500-3000 mg/$m^2$ as a single dose in combination with other agents every 4-6 weeks have been used in the treatment of pediatric astrocytoma, medulloblastoma, and primitive neuroectodermal tumors

CML: Initial: 10-20 mg/kg/day once daily; adjust dose according to hematologic response

Adults: Dose should always be titrated to patient response and WBC counts; usual oral doses range from 10-30 mg/kg/day or 500-3000 mg/day; if WBC count falls to <2500 cells/mm³, or the platelet count to <100,000/mm³, therapy should be stopped for at least 3 days and resumed when values rise toward normal

Solid tumors:
Intermittent therapy: 80 mg/kg as a single dose every third day
Continuous therapy: 20-30 mg/kg/day given as a single dose/day
Concomitant therapy with irradiation: 80 mg/kg as a single dose every third day starting at least 7 days before initiation of irradiation
Resistant chronic myelocytic leukemia: 20-30 mg/kg/day divided daily
HIV: 1000-1500 mg daily in a single dose or divided doses
Sickle cell anemia (moderate/severe disease): Initial: 15 mg/kg/day, increased by 5 mg/kg every 12 weeks if blood counts are in an acceptable range until the maximum tolerated dose of 35 mg/kg/day is achieved or the dose that does not produce toxic effects

*Acceptable range:*
Neutrophils ≥2500 cells/mm$^3$
Platelets ≥95,000/mm$^3$
Hemoglobin >5.3 g/dL, and
Reticulocytes ≥95,000/mm$^3$ if the hemoglobin concentration is <9 g/dL

*Toxic range:*
Neutrophils <2000 cells/mm$^3$
Platelets <80,000/mm$^3$
Hemoglobin <4.5 g/dL
Reticulocytes <80,000/mm$^3$ if the hemoglobin concentration is <9 g/dL
Monitor for toxicity every 2 weeks; if toxicity occurs, stop treatment until the bone marrow recovers; restart at 2.5 mg/kg/day less than the dose at which toxicity occurs; if no toxicity occurs over the next 12 weeks, then the subsequent dose should be increased by 2.5 mg/kg/day; reduced dosage of hydroxyurea alternating with erythropoietin may decrease myelotoxicity and increase levels of fetal hemoglobin in patients who have not been helped by hydroxyurea alone

**Dosing adjustment in renal impairment:**
Cl$_{cr}$ 10-50 mL/minute: Administer 50% of normal dose
Cl$_{cr}$ <10 mL/minute: Administer 20% of normal dose
Hemodialysis: Supplemental dose is not necessary. Hydroxyurea is a low molecular weight compound with high aqueous solubility that may be freely dialyzable, however, clinical studies confirming this hypothesis have not been performed; peak serum concentrations are reached within 2 hours after oral administration and by 24 hours, the concentration in the serum is zero
CAPD effects: Unknown
CAVH effects: Unknown

**Dosage Forms Cap:** 500 mg; **Cap (Droxia™):** 200 mg, 300 mg, 400 mg

**Contraindications** Severe anemia, severe bone marrow suppression; WBC <2500/mm$^3$ or platelet count <100,000/mm$^3$; hypersensitivity to hydroxyurea

**Warnings/Precautions** The U.S. Food and Drug Administration (FDA) currently recommends that procedures for proper handling and disposal of antineoplastic agents be considered. Use with caution in patients with renal impairment, in patients who have received prior irradiation therapy, and in the elderly.

**Pregnancy Risk Factor** D

**Adverse Reactions**
>10%:
Central nervous system: Drowsiness
Gastrointestinal: Mild to moderate nausea and vomiting may occur, as well as diarrhea, constipation, mucositis, ulceration of the GI tract, anorexia, and stomatitis
Hematologic: Myelosuppression: Dose-limiting toxicity, causes a rapid drop in leukocyte count (seen in 4-5 days in nonhematologic malignancy and more rapidly in leukemia); thrombocytopenia and anemia occur less often; reversal of WBC count occurs rapidly, but the platelet count may take 7-10 days to recover
WBC: Moderate
Platelets: Moderate
Onset (days): 7
Nadir (days): 10
Recovery (days): 21
1% to 10%:
Dermatologic: Dermatologic changes (hyperpigmentation, erythema of the hands and face, maculopapular rash, or dry skin), alopecia
Hepatic: Abnormal LFTs and hepatitis
Renal: Increased creatinine and BUN due to impairment of renal tubular function
Miscellaneous: Carcinogenic potential
<1%: Neurotoxicity, dizziness, disorientation, hallucination, seizures, headache, fever, facial erythema, hyperuricemia, dysuria, elevated hepatic enzymes, rarely, acute diffuse pulmonary infiltrates; dyspnea

**Drug Interactions**
Increased effect: Zidovudine, zalcitabine, didanosine: Synergy
Increased toxicity:
Fluorouracil: The potential for neurotoxicity may increase with concomitant administration
(Continued)

## Hydroxyurea *(Continued)*

Cytarabine: Modulation of its metabolism and cytotoxicity → reduction of cytarabine dose is recommended

**Half-Life** 3-4 hours

**Special PA Issues**

**Patient Education:** Take capsules exactly on schedule directed by prescriber (dosage and timing will be specific to purpose of therapy). Contents of capsule may be emptied into a glass of water and taken immediately. You will require frequent monitoring and blood tests while taking this medication to assess effectiveness and monitor adverse reactions. You will be susceptible to infection; avoid crowds, infected persons, and persons with contagious diseases. You may experience nausea, vomiting, or loss of appetite (small frequent meals, sucking lozenges may help); constipation (increased exercise, fluid, or dietary fiber may help); diarrhea (buttermilk, boiled milk, or yogurt may help); mouth sores (frequent mouth care will help). Report persistent vomiting, diarrhea, constipation, stomach pain, or mouth sores; skin rash, redness, irritation, or sores; painful or difficult urination; increased confusion, depression, hallucinations, lethargy, or seizures; persistent fever or chills, unusual fatigue, white plaques in mouth, vaginal discharge, or unhealed sores; unusual lassitude, weakness, or muscle tremors; easy bruising/bleeding; or blood in vomitus, stool, or urine. People not taking hydroxyurea should not be exposed to it; if powder from capsule is spilled, wipe up with damp, disposable towel immediately, and discard the towel in a closed container, such as a plastic bag. Wash hands thoroughly.

**Monitoring Parameters:** CBC with differential, platelets, hemoglobin, renal function and liver function tests, serum uric acid

♦ **25-Hydroxyvitamin D₃** *see Calcifediol on page 135*

## Hydroxyzine *(hye DROKS i zeen)*

**Pharmacologic Class** Antiemetic; Antihistamine

**U.S. Brand Names** Anxanil®; Atarax®; Atozine®; Durrax®; Hy-Pam®; Hyzine-50®; Neucalm®; Quiess®; QYS®; Rezine®; Vamate®; Vistacon-50®; Vistaject-25®; Vistaject-50®; Vistaquel®; Vistaril®; Vistazine®

**Mechanism of Action** Competes with histamine for H₁-receptor sites on effector cells in the gastrointestinal tract, blood vessels, and respiratory tract

**Use** Treatment of anxiety, as a preoperative sedative, an antipruritic, an antiemetic, and in alcohol withdrawal symptoms

**USUAL DOSAGE**

Children:

Oral: 0.6 mg/kg/dose every 6 hours

I.M.: 0.5-1 mg/kg/dose every 4-6 hours as needed

Adults:

Antiemetic: I.M.: 25-100 mg/dose every 4-6 hours as needed

Anxiety: Oral: 25-100 mg 4 times/day; maximum dose: 600 mg/day

Preoperative sedation:

Oral: 50-100 mg

I.M.: 25-100 mg

Management of pruritus: Oral: 25 mg 3-4 times/day

**Dosing interval in hepatic impairment:** Change dosing interval to every 24 hours in patients with primary biliary cirrhosis

**Dosage Forms** Hydroxyzine hydrochloride: **Inj:** Vistaril®: 25 mg/mL (1 mL, 2 mL, 10 mL); Hyzine-50®, Neucalm®, Quiess®, Vistacon-50®, Vistaquel®, Vistaril®, Vistazine®: 50 mg/mL (1 mL, 2 mL, 10 mL); **Syr (Atarax®):** 10 mg/5 mL (120 mL, 480 mL, 4000 mL); **Tab:** Anxanil®: 25 mg, Atarax®: 10 mg, 25 mg, 50 mg, 100 mg, Atozine®: 10 mg, 25 mg, 50 mg, Durrax®: 10 mg, 25 mg

Hydroxyzine pamoate: **Cap:** Hy-Pam®: 25 mg, 50 mg, Vamate®: 25 mg, 50 mg, 100 mg, Vistaril®: 25 mg, 50 mg, 100 mg (Vistaril®): 25 mg, 50 mg, 100 mg; **Susp, oral (Vistaril®):** 25 mg/5 mL (120 mL, 480 mL)

**Contraindications** Hypersensitivity to hydroxyzine or any component

**Warnings/Precautions** S.C., intra-arterial and I.V. administration **not** recommended since thrombosis and digital gangrene can occur; extravasation can result in sterile abscess and marked tissue induration; should be used with caution in patients with narrow-angle glaucoma, prostatic hypertrophy, and bladder neck obstruction; should also be used with caution in patients with asthma or COPD

Anticholinergic effects are not well tolerated in the elderly. Hydroxyzine may be useful as a short-term antipruritic, but it is not recommended for use as a sedative or anxiolytic in the elderly.

**Pregnancy Risk Factor** C

**Adverse Reactions**

>10%:

Central nervous system: Slight to moderate drowsiness

Respiratory: Thickening of bronchial secretions

1% to 10%:
Central nervous system: Headache, fatigue, nervousness, dizziness
Gastrointestinal: Appetite increase, weight gain, nausea, diarrhea, abdominal pain, xerostomia
Neuromuscular & skeletal: Arthralgia
Respiratory: Pharyngitis
<1%: Palpitations, hypotension, edema, depression, sedation, paradoxical excitement, insomnia, angioedema, photosensitivity, rash, urinary retention, hepatitis, myalgia, tremor, paresthesia, blurred vision, bronchospasm, epistaxis

**Drug Interactions**
Decreased effect: Epinephrine decreased vasopressor effect
Increased toxicity: CNS depressants, anticholinergics

**Onset** Within 15-30 minutes

**Duration** 4-6 hours

**Half-Life** 3-7 hours

**Special PA Issues**
**Patient Education:** Take this drug as prescribed; do not increase dosage or discontinue without consulting prescriber. Store medication away from light. Maintain adequate hydration (2-3 L/day of fluids unless instructed to restrict fluid intake). Void before taking medication. Do not use excessive alcohol or other CNS depressants or sleeping aids without consulting prescriber. May cause dizziness, drowsiness, or blurred vision (use caution when driving or engaging in hazardous activities until effect of medication is known); or nausea, dry mouth, appetite disturbances (small frequent meals, frequent mouth care, or sucking hard candy may help). Report unusual weight gain, unresolved nausea or diarrhea, chest pain or palpitations, muscle or joint pain, excess sedation, sore throat, or difficulty breathing.
**Dietary Considerations:** Alcohol: Additive CNS effect, avoid use
**Monitoring Parameters:** Relief of symptoms, mental status, blood pressure

♦ **Hydroxyzine Hydrochloride** *see* Hydroxyzine *on previous page*
♦ **Hydroxyzine Pamoate** *see* Hydroxyzine *on previous page*
♦ **Hygroton®** *see* Chlorthalidone *on page 200*
♦ **Hylorel®** *see* Guanadrel *on page 430*
♦ **Hylutin® Injection** *see* Hydroxyprogesterone Caproate *on page 459*
♦ **Hyoscine** *see* Scopolamine *on page 824*

# Hyoscyamine (hye oh SYE a meen)

**Pharmacologic Class** Anticholinergic Agent

**U.S. Brand Names** Anaspaz®; A-Spas® S/L; Cystospaz®; Cystospaz-M®; Donnamar®; ED-SPAZ®; Gastrosed™; Levbid®; Levsin®; Levsinex®; Levsin/SL®

**Mechanism of Action** Blocks the action of acetylcholine at parasympathetic sites in smooth muscle, secretory glands and the CNS; increases cardiac output, dries secretions, antagonizes histamine and serotonin

**Use** Treatment of GI tract disorders caused by spasm, adjunctive therapy for peptic ulcers

**USUAL DOSAGE**
Children: Oral, S.L.: Dose as per table repeated every 4 hours as needed

### Hyoscyamine

| Weight (kg) | Dose (mcg) | Maximum 24-Hour Dose (mcg) |
|---|---|---|
| **Children <2 y** | | |
| 2.3 | 12.5 | 75 |
| 3.4 | 16.7 | 100 |
| 5 | 20.8 | 125 |
| 7 | 25 | 150 |
| 10 | 31.3-33.3 | 200 |
| 15 | 45.8 | 275 |
| **Children 2-10 y** | | |
| 10 | 31.3-33.3 | |
| 20 | 62.5 | Do not exceed |
| 40 | 93.8 | 0.75 mg |
| 50 | 125 | |

Adults:
Oral or S.L.: 0.125-0.25 mg 3-4 times/day before meals or food and at bedtime
Oral: 0.375-0.75 mg (timed release) every 12 hours
I.M., I.V., S.C.: 0.25-0.5 mg every 6 hours
(Continued)

## Hyoscyamine *(Continued)*

**Dosage Forms** Cap, as sulfate, timed release (Cystospaz-M®, Levsinex®): 0.375 mg; **Elix, as sulfate (Levsin®):** 0.125 mg/5 mL with alcohol 20% (480 mL); **Inj, as sulfate (Levsin®):** 0.5 mg/mL (1 mL, 10 mL); **Soln, oral (Gastrosed™, Levsin®):** 0.125 mg/mL (15 mL); **Tab, as sulfate:** Anaspaz®, Gastrosed™, Levsin®: 0.125 mg, Cystospaz®: 0.15 mg

**Contraindications** Narrow-angle glaucoma, obstructive uropathy, obstructive GI tract disease, myasthenia gravis, known hypersensitivity to belladonna alkaloids

**Warnings/Precautions** Use with caution in children with spastic paralysis; use with caution in elderly patients. Low doses cause a paradoxical decrease in heart rates. Some commercial products contain sodium metabisulfite, which can cause allergic-type reactions. May accumulate with multiple inhalational administration, particularly in the elderly. Heat prostration may occur in hot weather. Use with caution in patients with autonomic neuropathy, prostatic hypertrophy, hyperthyroidism, congestive heart failure, cardiac arrhythmias, chronic lung disease, biliary tract disease.

**Pregnancy Risk Factor** C

**Adverse Reactions**
> 10%:
  Dermatologic: Dry skin
  Gastrointestinal: Dry throat, xerostomia
  Local: Irritation at injection site
  Respiratory: Dry nose
  Miscellaneous: Diaphoresis (decreased)
1% to 10%:
  Dermatologic: Photosensitivity
  Gastrointestinal: Constipation, dysphagia
  Ocular: Blurred vision, mydriasis
<1%: Palpitations, orthostatic hypotension, headache, lightheadedness, memory loss, fatigue, delirium, restlessness, ataxia, rash, dysuria, tremor, increased intraocular pressure

**Drug Interactions**
Decreased effect with antacids
Increased toxicity with amantadine, antimuscarinics, haloperidol, phenothiazines, TCAs, MAO inhibitors

**Onset** 2-3 minutes

**Duration** 4-6 hours

**Half-Life** 13% to 38%

**Special PA Issues**
**Patient Education:** Take as directed. You may experience drowsiness, blurred vision, or dizziness (avoid driving or engaging in hazardous activities until response is evaluated). Avoid excessive heat (heat stroke), maintain adequate fluid intake. Maintain good oral hygiene, lack of saliva (dry mouth) may increase chance of dental carries. Report rash, flushing, eye pain, difficulty urinating (void before taking medication), unresolved constipation, or persistent sensitivity to light or blurred vision.

## Hyoscyamine, Atropine, Scopolamine, and Phenobarbital

(hye oh SYE a meen, A troe peen, skoe POL a meen & fee noe BAR bi tal)

**Pharmacologic Class** Anticholinergic Agent; Antispasmodic Agent, Gastrointestinal

**U.S. Brand Names** Barbidonna®; Barophen®; Donnapine®; Donna-Sed®; Donnatal®; Hyosophen®; Kinesed®; Malatal®; Relaxadon®; Spaslin®; Spasmolin®; Spasmophen®; Spasquid®; Susano®

**Mechanism of Action** Refer to individual agents

**Use** Adjunct in treatment of peptic ulcer disease, irritable bowel, spastic colitis, spastic bladder, and renal colic

**USUAL DOSAGE** Oral:
Children 2-12 years: Kinesed® dose: ½ to 1 tablet 3-4 times/day
Children: Donnatal® elixir: 0.1 mL/kg/dose every 4 hours; maximum dose: 5 mL or see table for alternative.

#### Hyoscyamine, Atropine, Scopolamine, and Phenobarbital

| Weight (kg) | Dose (mL) | |
|---|---|---|
| | q4h | q6h |
| 4.5 | 0.5 | 0.75 |
| 10 | 1 | 1.5 |
| 14 | 1.5 | 2 |
| 23 | 2.5 | 3.8 |
| 34 | 3.8 | 5 |
| ≥45 | 5 | 7.5 |

Adults: 1-2 capsules or tablets 3-4 times/day; or 1 Donnatal® Extentab® in sustained release form every 12 hours; or 5-10 mL elixir 3-4 times/day or every 8 hours

**Dosage Forms** Cap (Donnatal®, Spasmolin®): Hyoscyamine sulfate 0.1037 mg, atropine sulfate 0.0194 mg, scopolamine hydrobromide 0.0065 mg, and phenobarbital 16.2 mg; **Elix (Donnatal®, Hyosophen®, Spasmophen®):** Hyoscyamine sulfate 0.1037 mg, atropine sulfate 0.0194 mg, scopolamine hydrobromide 0.0065 mg, and phenobarbital 16.2 mg per 5 mL (120 mL, 480 mL, 4000 mL); **Tab:** Barbidonna®: Hyoscyamine hydrobromide 0.1286 mg, atropine sulfate 0.025 mg, scopolamine hydrobromide 0.0074 mg, and phenobarbital 16 mg, Barbidonna® No. 2: Hyoscyamine hydrobromide 0.1286 mg, atropine sulfate 0.025 mg, scopolamine hydrobromide 0.0074 mg, and phenobarbital 32 mg, Donnatal®, Hyosophen®: Hyoscyamine sulfate 0.1037 mg, atropine sulfate 0.0194 mg, scopolamine hydrobromide 0.0065 mg, and phenobarbital 16.2 mg, Long-acting (Donnatal®): Hyoscyamine sulfate 0.3111 mg, atropine sulfate 0.0582 mg, scopolamine hydrobromide 0.0195 mg, and phenobarbital 48.6 mg, Spasmophen®: Hyoscyamine sulfate 0.1037 mg, atropine sulfate 0.0194 mg, scopolamine hydrobromide 0.0065 mg, and phenobarbital 15 mg

**Contraindications** Hypersensitivity to hyoscyamine, atropine, scopolamine, phenobarbital, or any component; narrow-angle glaucoma, tachycardia, GI and GU obstruction, myasthenia gravis

**Warnings/Precautions** Use with caution in patients with hepatic or renal disease, hyperthyroidism, cardiovascular disease, hypertension, prostatic hypertrophy, autonomic neuropathy in the elderly; abrupt withdrawal may precipitate status epilepticus. Because of the anticholinergic effects of this product, it is not recommended for use in the elderly.

**Pregnancy Risk Factor** C

**Adverse Reactions**
>10%:
  Dermatologic: Dry skin
  Gastrointestinal: Constipation, dry throat, xerostomia
  Local: Irritation at injection site
  Respiratory: Dry nose
  Miscellaneous: Diaphoresis (decreased)
1% to 10%:
  Dermatologic: Increased sensitivity to light
  Endocrine & metabolic: Decreased flow of breast milk
  Gastrointestinal: Dysphagia
<1%: Orthostatic hypotension, ventricular fibrillation, tachycardia, palpitations, confusion, drowsiness, headache, loss of memory, fatigue, ataxia, rash, bloated feeling, nausea, vomiting, dysuria, increased intraocular pain, blurred vision

**Drug Interactions** Increased toxicity: CNS depressants, coumarin anticoagulants, amantadine, antihistamine, phenothiazides, antidiarrheal suspensions, corticosteroids, digitalis, griseofulvin, tetracyclines, anticonvulsants, MAO inhibitors, tricyclic antidepressants

# Hyoscyamine, Atropine, Scopolamine, Kaolin, Pectin, and Opium

(hye oh SYE a meen, A troe peen, skoe POL a meen, KAY oh lin, PEK tin, & OH pee um)

**Pharmacologic Class** Anticholinergic Agent

**U.S. Brand Names** Donnapectolin-PG®; Kapectolin PG®

**Dosage Forms** Susp, oral: Hyoscyamine sulfate 0.1037 mg, atropine sulfate 0.0194 mg, scopolamine hydrobromide 0.0065 mg, kaolin 6 g, pectin 142.8 mg, and powdered opium 24 mg per 30 mL with alcohol 5%

+ **Hytuss-2X®** [OTC] *see* Guaifenesin *on page 427*
+ **Hyzaar®** *see* Losartan and Hydrochlorothiazide *on page 545*
+ **Hyzine-50®** *see* Hydroxyzine *on page 462*
+ **Ibenzmethyzin** *see* Procarbazine *on page 761*
+ **Iberet-Folic-500®** *see* Vitamins, Multiple *on page 964*
· + **Iberet-Folic-500®** *see* Ferrous Sulfate, Ascorbic Acid, Vitamin B-Complex, and Folic Acid *on page 368*
+ **Ibidomide Hydrochloride** *see* Labetalol *on page 510*
+ **Ibuprin®** [OTC] *see* Ibuprofen *on this page*

## Ibuprofen (eye byoo PROE fen)

**Pharmacologic Class** Nonsteroidal Anti-Inflammatory Agent (NSAID)

**U.S. Brand Names** Aches-N-Pain® [OTC]; Advil® [OTC]; Children's Advil® Oral Suspension [OTC]; Children's Motrin® Oral Suspension [OTC]; Excedrin® IB [OTC]; Genpril® [OTC]; Haltran® [OTC]; Ibuprin® [OTC]; Ibuprohm® [OTC]; Ibu-Tab®; Junior Strength Motrin® [OTC]; Medipren® [OTC]; Menadol® [OTC]; Midol® 200 [OTC]; Motrin®; Motrin® IB [OTC]; Nuprin® [OTC]; Pamprin IB® [OTC]; PediaProfen™; Saleto-200® [OTC]; Saleto-400®; Trendar® [OTC]; Uni-Pro® [OTC]

**Mechanism of Action** Inhibits prostaglandin synthesis by decreasing the activity of the enzyme, cyclo-oxygenase, which results in decreased formation of prostaglandin precursors

**Use** Inflammatory diseases and rheumatoid disorders including juvenile rheumatoid arthritis, mild to moderate pain, fever, dysmenorrhea, gout, ankylosing spondylitis, acute migraine headache

**USUAL DOSAGE** Oral:

Children:

Antipyretic: 6 months to 12 years: Temperature <102.5°F (39°C): 5 mg/kg/dose; temperature >102.5°F: 10 mg/kg/dose given every 6-8 hours; maximum daily dose: 40 mg/kg/day

Juvenile rheumatoid arthritis: 30-70 mg/kg/24 hours divided every 6-8 hours

<20 kg: Maximum: 400 mg/day

20-30 kg: Maximum: 600 mg/day

30-40 kg: Maximum: 800 mg/day

>40 kg: Adult dosage

Start at lower end of dosing range and titrate upward; maximum: 2.4 g/day

Analgesic: 4-10 mg/kg/dose every 6-8 hours

Adults:

Inflammatory disease: 400-800 mg/dose 3-4 times/day; maximum dose: 3.2 g/day

Analgesia/pain/fever/dysmenorrhea: 200-400 mg/dose every 4-6 hours; maximum daily dose: 1.2 g (unless directed by physician)

**Dosage adjustment/comments in severe hepatic impairment:** Avoid use

**Dosage Forms Caplet:** 100 mg; **Drops, oral (berry flavor):** 40 mg/mL (15 mL); **Supp, rectal:** 80 mg; **Susp, oral:** 100 mg/5 mL [OTC] (60 mL, 120 mL, 480 mL); **Drops:** 40 mg/mL [OTC], **Tab:** 100 mg [OTC], 200 mg [OTC], 300 mg, 400 mg, 600 mg, 800 mg; Chewable: 50 mg, 100 mg

**Contraindications** Hypersensitivity to ibuprofen, any component, aspirin, or other nonsteroidal anti-inflammatory drugs (NSAIDs)

**Warnings/Precautions** Do not exceed 3200 mg/day; use with caution in patients with congestive heart failure, hypertension, decreased renal or hepatic function, history of GI disease (bleeding or ulcers), or those receiving anticoagulants; safety and efficacy in children <6 months of age have not yet been established; elderly are a high-risk population for adverse effects from nonsteroidal anti-inflammatory agents. As much as 60% of elderly can develop peptic ulceration and/or hemorrhage asymptomatically.

Use lowest effective dose for shortest period possible. Use of NSAIDs can compromise existing renal function especially when $Cl_{cr}$ is <30 mL/minute. CNS adverse effects such as confusion, agitation, and hallucination are generally seen in overdose or high dose situations; but elderly may demonstrate these adverse effects at lower doses than younger adults.

**Pregnancy Risk Factor** B (D if used in the 3rd trimester)

**Adverse Reactions**

>10%:

Central nervous system: Dizziness, fatigue

Dermatologic: Rash, urticaria

Gastrointestinal: Abdominal cramps, heartburn, indigestion, nausea

1% to 10%:

Central nervous system: Headache, nervousness

Dermatologic: Itching

Endocrine & metabolic: Fluid retention

Gastrointestinal: Dyspepsia, vomiting, abdominal pain, peptic ulcer, GI bleed, GI perforation

Otic: Tinnitus

<1%: Edema, congestive heart failure, arrhythmias, tachycardia, hypertension, confusion, hallucinations, mental depression, drowsiness, insomnia, aseptic meningitis, erythema multiforme, toxic epidermal necrolysis, Stevens-Johnson syndrome, polydipsia, hot flashes, gastritis, GI ulceration, cystitis, polyuria, neutropenia, anemia, agranulocytosis, inhibition of platelet aggregation, hemolytic anemia, bone marrow suppression, leukopenia, thrombocytopenia, hepatitis, peripheral neuropathy, vision changes, blurred vision, conjunctivitis, dry eyes, toxic amblyopia, decreased hearing, acute renal failure, allergic rhinitis, shortness of breath, epistaxis

**Drug Interactions** CYP2C8 and 2C9 enzyme substrate

Decreased effect: Aspirin may decrease ibuprofen serum concentrations

Increased toxicity: May increase digoxin, methotrexate, and lithium serum concentrations; other nonsteroidal anti-inflammatories may increase adverse gastrointestinal effects

**Onset** Onset of analgesia: 30-60 minutes; Onset of anti-inflammatory effect: Up to 7 days; Peak action: 1-2 weeks

**Duration** 4-6 hours

**Half-Life** 2-4 hours; End-stage renal disease: Unchanged

**Special PA Issues**

**Patient Education:** If self-administered, use exactly as directed (do not increase dose or frequency); adverse reactions can occur with overuse. Do not take longer than 3 days for fever, or 10 days for pain without consulting medical advisor. Take with food or milk. While using this medication, do not use alcohol, excessive amounts of vitamin C, or salicylate containing foods (curry powder, prunes, raisins, tea, or licorice), other prescription or OTC medications containing aspirin or salicylate, or other NSAIDs without consulting prescriber. Maintain adequate hydration (2-3 L/day of fluids unless instructed to restrict fluid intake). You may experience nausea, vomiting, gastric discomfort (frequent mouth care, small frequent meals, or sucking on lozenges may help). GI bleeding, ulceration, or perforation can occur with or without pain. Stop taking medication and report ringing in ears; persistent cramping or pain in stomach; unresolved nausea or vomiting; difficulty breathing or shortness of breath; unusual bruising or bleeding (mouth, urine, stool); skin rash; unusual swelling of extremities; chest pain; or palpitations.

**Dietary Considerations:** Food: May decrease the rate but not the extent of oral absorption; drug may cause GI upset, bleeding, ulceration, perforation; take with food or milk to minimize GI upset

**Monitoring Parameters:** CBC; occult blood loss and periodic liver function tests; monitor response (pain, range of motion, grip strength, mobility, ADL function), inflammation; observe for weight gain, edema; monitor renal function (urine output, serum BUN and creatinine); observe for bleeding, bruising; evaluate gastrointestinal effects (abdominal pain, bleeding, dyspepsia); mental confusion, disorientation; with long-term therapy, periodic ophthalmic exams

**Reference Range:** Plasma concentrations >200 µg/mL may be associated with severe toxicity

**Related Information**

Nonsteroidal Anti-Inflammatory Agents *on page 1026*

♦ **Ibuprohm® [OTC]** *see* Ibuprofen *on previous page*

♦ **Ibu-Tab®** *see* Ibuprofen *on previous page*

# Ibutilide (i BYOO ti lide)

**Pharmacologic Class** Antiarrhythmic Agent, Class III

**U.S. Brand Names** Corvert®

**Mechanism of Action** Exact mechanism of action is unknown; prolongs the action potential in cardiac tissue

**Use** Acute termination of atrial fibrillation or flutter of recent onset; the effectiveness of ibutilide has not been determined in patients with arrhythmias of >90 days in duration

**USUAL DOSAGE** I.V.: Initial:

<60 kg: 0.01 mg/kg over 10 minutes

≥60 kg: 1 mg over 10 minutes

If the arrhythmia does not terminate within 10 minutes after the end of the initial infusion, a second infusion of equal strength may be infused over a 10-minute period

**Dosage Forms Inj, as fumarate:** 0.1 mg/mL (10 mL)

**Contraindications** Hypersensitivity to the drug or any component

**Warnings/Precautions** Potentially fatal arrhythmias (eg, polymorphic ventricular tachycardia) can occur with ibutilide, **usually** in association with torsade de pointes (Q-T prolongation). Studies indicate a 1.7% incidence of arrhythmias in treated patients. The drug should be given in a setting of continuous EKG monitoring and by personnel trained in treating arrhythmias particularly polymorphic ventricular tachycardia. Patients with chronic atrial fibrillation may not be the best candidates for ibutilide since they often revert after conversion and the risks of treatment may not be justified when compared to alternative management. Dosing adjustments in patients with renal or hepatic dysfunction since a maximum of only two 10-minute infusions are indicated and drug distribution is one of the primary mechanisms responsible for termination of the pharmacologic effect; safety and efficacy in children have not been established.

(Continued)

## Ibutilide *(Continued)*

**Pregnancy Risk Factor** C

**Pregnancy Implications**

Clinical effects on the fetus: Teratogenic and embryocidal in rats; avoid use in pregnancy
Breast-feeding/lactation: Avoid breast-feeding during therapy

**Adverse Reactions**

1% to 10%:

Cardiovascular: Sustained polymorphic ventricular tachycardia (ie, torsade de pointes) (1.7%), often requiring cardioversion, nonsustained polymorphic ventricular tachycardia (2.7%), nonsustained monomorphic ventricular extrasystoles (5.1%), nonsustained monomorphic VT (4.9%), tachycardia/supraventricular tachycardia, hypotension (2%), bundle branch block (1.9%), A-V block (1.5%), bradycardia, Q-T segment prolongation, hypertension (1.2%), palpitations (1%)

Central nervous system: Headache (3.6%)

Gastrointestinal: Nausea (>1%)

<1%: Supraventricular extrasystoles (0.9%), nodal arrhythmia (0.7%), congestive heart failure (0.5%), syncope, idioventricular rhythm, sustained monomorphic VT (0.2%), renal failure (0.3%)

**Drug Interactions** Increased toxicity: Class Ia antiarrhythmic drugs (disopyramide, quinidine, and procainamide) and other class III drugs such as amiodarone and sotalol, should not be given concomitantly with ibutilide due to their potential to prolong refractoriness; the potential for prolongation of the Q-T interval may occur if ibutilide is given concurrently with phenothiazines, tricyclic and tetracyclic antidepressants, and the nonsedating antihistamines (terfenadine and astemizole); signs of digoxin toxicity may be masked when coadministered with ibutilide

**Onset** Within 90 minutes after start of infusion ($\frac{1}{2}$ of conversions to sinus rhythm occur during infusion)

**Half-Life** 2-12 hours (average: 6 hours)

**Special PA Issues**

**Patient Education:** This drug is only given I.V. and you will be on continuous cardiac monitoring during and for several hours following administration. You may experience headache or irregular heartbeat during infusion. Report chest pain or respiratory difficulty immediately.

**Monitoring Parameters:** Observe patient with continuous EKG monitoring for at least 4 hours following infusion or until $QT_c$ has returned to baseline; skilled personnel and proper equipment should be available during administration of ibutilide and subsequent monitoring of the patient

♦ **Ibutilide Fumarate** *see* Ibutilide *on previous page*

♦ **Ideal Body Weight Calculation** *see* Chart *on page 987*

♦ **IFLrA** *see* Interferon Alfa-2a *on page 481*

♦ **IFN** *see* Interferon Alfa-2a *on page 481*

♦ **IG** *see* Immune Globulin, Intramuscular *on page 472*

♦ **I-Gent®** *see* Gentamicin *on page 411*

♦ **IGIM** *see* Immune Globulin, Intramuscular *on page 472*

♦ **IL-2** *see* Aldesleukin *on page 36*

♦ **IL-11** *see* Oprelvekin *on page 678*

♦ **Ilopan®** *see* Dexpanthenol *on page 267*

♦ **Ilopan-Choline®** *see* Dexpanthenol *on page 267*

♦ **Ilosone®** *see* Erythromycin *on page 329*

♦ **Ilozyme®** *see* Pancrelipase *on page 694*

♦ **Imdur™** *see* Isosorbide Mononitrate *on page 499*

♦ **I-Methasone®** *see* Dexamethasone *on page 264*

♦ **Imipemide** *see* Imipenem and Cilastatin *on this page*

## Imipenem and Cilastatin (i mi PEN em & sye la STAT in)

**Pharmacologic Class** Antibiotic, Carbapenem

**U.S. Brand Names** Primaxin®

**Mechanism of Action** Inhibits bacterial cell wall synthesis by binding to one or more of the penicillin binding proteins (PBPs); which in turn inhibits the final transpeptidation step of peptidoglycan synthesis in bacterial cell walls, thus inhibiting cell wall biosynthesis. Bacteria eventually lyse due to ongoing activity of cell wall autolytic enzymes (autolysins and murein hydrolases) while cell wall assembly is arrested. Cilastatin prevents renal metabolism of imipenem by competitive inhibition of dehydropeptidase along the brush border of the renal tubules.

**Use** Treatment of respiratory tract, urinary tract, intra-abdominal, gynecologic, bone and joint, skin structure, and polymicrobic infections as well as bacterial septicemia and endocarditis. Antibacterial activity includes resistant gram-negative bacilli (*Pseudomonas aeruginosa* and *Enterobacter* sp), gram-positive bacteria (methicillin-sensitive *Staphylococcus aureus* and *Streptococcus* sp) and anaerobes.

**USUAL DOSAGE** Dosing based on imipenem component:
Children: I.V.:
  3 months to 3 years: 25 mg/kg every 6 hours; maximum: 2 g/day
  ≥3 years: 15 mg/kg/every 6 hours
Adults: I.V.:
  Mild to moderate infection: 250-500 mg every 6-8 hours
  Severe infections with only **moderately susceptible** organisms: 1 g every 6-8 hours
  Mild to moderate infection **only**: I.M.: 500-750 mg every 12 hours (**Note:** 750 mg is recommended for intra-abdominal and more severe respiratory, dermatologic, or gynecologic infections; total daily I.M. dosages >1500 mg are not recommended; deep I.M. injection should be carefully made into a large muscle mass only)
**Dosing adjustment in renal impairment:** See table.

### Imipenem/Cilastatin

| Creatinine Clearance (mL/min/1.73 m²) | Frequency | Dose (mg) |
|---|---|---|
| 30-70 | q8h | 500 |
| 20-30 | q12h | 500 |
| 5-20 | q12h | 250 |

Hemodialysis: Imipenem (**not cilastatin**) is moderately dialyzable (20% to 50%); administer dose postdialysis

Peritoneal dialysis: Dose as for $Cl_{cr}$ <10 mL/minute

Continuous arteriovenous or venovenous hemofiltration (CAVH/CAVHD): Dose as for $Cl_{cr}$ 20-30 mL/minute; monitor for seizure activity; imipenem is well removed by CAVH but cilastatin is not; removes 20 mg of imipenem per liter of filtrate per day

**Dosage Forms Powder for inj: I.M.:** Imipenem 500 mg and cilastatin 500 mg, Imipenem 750 mg and cilastatin 750 mg; **I.V.:** Imipenem 250 mg and cilastatin 250 mg, Imipenem 500 mg and cilastatin 500 mg

**Contraindications** Hypersensitivity to imipenem/cilastatin or any component

**Warnings/Precautions** Dosage adjustment required in patients with impaired renal function; safety and efficacy in children <12 years of age have not yet been established; prolonged use may result in superinfection; use with caution in patients with a history of seizures or hypersensitivity to beta-lactams; elderly patients often require lower doses

**Pregnancy Risk Factor** C

**Adverse Reactions**
1% to 10%:
  Gastrointestinal: Nausea/diarrhea/vomiting (1% to 2%)
  Local: Phlebitis (3%)
  <1%: Hypotension, palpitations, seizures, rash, pseudomembranous colitis, neutropenia (including agranulocytosis), eosinophilia, anemia, (+) Coombs' test, thrombocytopenia, increased PT, increased LFTs, pain at injection site, increased BUN/creatine, abnormal urinalysis, emergence of resistant strains of *P. aeruginosa*

**Drug Interactions** Increased toxicity: Beta-lactam antibiotics, probenecid may increase toxic potential

**Half-Life** Imipenem: 1 hour, extended with renal insufficiency; Cilastatin: 1 hour, extended with renal insufficiency

**Special PA Issues**
  **Patient Education:** Report warmth, swelling, irritation at infusion or injection site. Maintain adequate hydration (2-3 L/day of fluids unless instructed to restrict fluid intake) and nutrition. Report unresolved nausea or vomiting (small, frequent meals may help). Diabetics must use serum glucose testing rather than Clinitest®. Report feelings of excessive dizziness, palpitations, visual disturbances, and CNS changes. Report chills, or unusual discharge, or foul-smelling urine.
  **Monitoring Parameters:** Periodic renal, hepatic, and hematologic function tests; monitor for signs of anaphylaxis during first dose

## Imipramine (im IP ra meen)

**Pharmacologic Class** Antidepressant, Tricyclic (Tertiary Amine)

**U.S. Brand Names** Janimine®; Tofranil®; Tofranil-PM®

**Mechanism of Action** Traditionally believed to increase the synaptic concentration of serotonin and/or norepinephrine in the central nervous system by inhibition of their reuptake by the presynaptic neuronal membrane. However, additional receptor effects have been found including desensitization of adenyl cyclase, down regulation of beta-adrenergic receptors, and down regulation of serotonin receptors.

**Use** Treatment of various forms of depression, often in conjunction with psychotherapy; enuresis in children; certain types of chronic and neuropathic pain

**USUAL DOSAGE** Maximum antidepressant effect may not be seen for 2 or more weeks after initiation of therapy.
(Continued)

# Imipramine *(Continued)*

Children: Oral:

Depression: 1.5 mg/kg/day with dosage increments of 1 mg/kg every 3-4 days to a maximum dose of 5 mg/kg/day in 1-4 divided doses; monitor carefully especially with doses ≥3.5 mg/kg/day

Enuresis: ≥6 years: Initial: 10-25 mg at bedtime; if inadequate response still seen after 1 week of therapy, increase by 25 mg/day; dose should not exceed 2.5 mg/kg/day or 50 mg at bedtime if 6-12 years of age or 75 mg at bedtime if ≥12 years of age

Adjunct in the treatment of cancer pain: Initial: 0.2-0.4 mg/kg at bedtime; dose may be increased by 50% every 2-3 days up to 1-3 mg/kg/dose at bedtime

Adolescents: Oral: Initial: 25-50 mg/day; increase gradually; maximum: 100 mg/day in single or divided doses

Adults:

Oral: Initial: 25 mg 3-4 times/day, increase dose gradually, total dose may be given at bedtime; maximum: 300 mg/day

I.M.: Initial: Up to 100 mg/day in divided doses; change to oral as soon as possible

Elderly: Initial: 10-25 mg at bedtime; increase by 10-25 mg every 3 days for inpatients and weekly for outpatients if tolerated; average daily dose to achieve a therapeutic concentration: 100 mg/day; range: 50-150 mg/day

**Dosage Forms** Imipramine hydrochloride: **Inj (Tofranil®):** 12.5 mg/mL (2 mL); **Tab (Janimine®, Tofranil®):** 10 mg, 25 mg, 50 mg

Imipramine pamoate: **Cap (Tofranil-PM®):** 75 mg, 100 mg, 125 mg, 150 mg

**Contraindications** Hypersensitivity to imipramine (cross-sensitivity with other tricyclics may occur); patients receiving MAO inhibitors or fluoxetine within past 14 days; narrow-angle glaucoma

**Warnings/Precautions** Use with caution in patients with cardiovascular disease, conduction disturbances, seizure disorders, urinary retention, hyperthyroidism or those receiving thyroid replacement; do not discontinue abruptly in patients receiving long-term, high-dose therapy; some oral preparations contain tartrazine and injection contains sulfites, both of which can cause allergic reactions

Orthostatic hypotension is a concern with this agent, especially in patients taking other medications that may affect blood pressure; may precipitate arrhythmias in predisposed patients; may aggravate seizures; a less anticholinergic antidepressant may be a better choice

**Pregnancy Risk Factor** D

**Adverse Reactions** Less sedation and anticholinergic effects than amitriptyline

>10%:

Central nervous system: Dizziness, drowsiness, headache

Gastrointestinal: Increased appetite, nausea, unpleasant taste, weight gain, xerostomia, constipation

Genitourinary: Urinary retention

Neuromuscular & skeletal: Weakness

1% to 10%:

Cardiovascular: Postural hypotension, arrhythmias, tachycardia

Central nervous system: Confusion, delirium, hallucinations, nervousness, restlessness, parkinsonian syndrome, insomnia

Endocrine & metabolic: Sexual dysfunction

Gastrointestinal: Diarrhea, heartburn

Genitourinary: Dysuria

Neuromuscular & skeletal: Fine muscle tremors

Ocular: Blurred vision, eye pain

Miscellaneous: Diaphoresis (excessive)

<1%: Anxiety, seizures, alopecia, photosensitivity, breast enlargement, galactorrhea, SIADH, trouble with gums, decreased lower esophageal sphincter tone may cause GE reflux, testicular edema, leukopenia, eosinophilia, rarely agranulocytosis, increased liver enzymes, cholestatic jaundice, increased intraocular pressure, tinnitus, allergic reactions, has been associated with falls, sudden death

**Drug Interactions** CYP1A2, 2C9, 2C18, 2C19, 2D6, and 3A3/4 enzyme substrate

Decreased effect: Imipramine inhibits the antihypertensive effects of clonidine

Increased toxicity: MAO inhibitors: Hyperpyrexia, hypertension, tachycardia, confusion, seizures, and death; may increase the prothrombin time in patients stabilized on warfarin; may potentiate the action of other CNS depressants; potentiates the pressor and cardiac effects of sympathomimetic agents such as isoproterenol, epinephrine, etc; additive anticholinergic effects seen with other anticholinergic agents; cimetidine reduces the hepatic metabolism of imipramine; tricyclic antidepressants like imipramine may enhance the hypertensive response associated with abrupt clonidine withdrawal

**Onset** Peak antidepressant effect: Usually after ≥2 weeks

**Half-Life** 6-18 hours

**Special PA Issues**

**Patient Education:** Oral: Take exactly as directed (do not increase dose or frequency); may take 2-3 weeks to achieve desired results; may cause physical and/or psychological dependence. Take in the evening. Avoid excessive alcohol, caffeine, and other prescription or OTC medications not approved by prescriber. Maintain adequate hydration (2-3 L/day of fluids unless instructed to restrict fluid intake). You may experience drowsiness, lightheadedness, impaired coordination, dizziness, or blurred vision (use caution when driving or engaging in hazardous tasks until response to medication is known); nausea, vomiting, altered taste, dry mouth (small frequent meals, frequent mouth care, or sucking lozenges may help); constipation (increased exercise, fluids, or dietary fruit and fiber may help); diarrhea (buttermilk, yogurt, or boiled milk may help); postural hypotension (use caution when climbing stairs or changing position from lying or sitting to standing); or urinary retention (void before taking medication). Report persistent insomnia; muscle cramping or tremors; chest pain, palpitations, rapid heartbeat, swelling of extremities, or severe dizziness; unresolved urinary retention; rash or skin irritation; yellowing of eyes or skin; pale stools/dark urine; or worsening of condition.

**Dietary Considerations:** Alcohol: Additive CNS effect, avoid use

**Monitoring Parameters:** Monitor blood pressure and pulse rate prior to and during initial therapy; EKG, CBC; evaluate mental status

**Reference Range:** Therapeutic: Imipramine and desipramine: 150-250 ng/mL (SI: 530-890 nmol/L); desipramine: 150-300 ng/mL (SI: 560-1125 nmol/L); Toxic: >500 ng/mL (SI: 446-893 nmol/L); utility of serum level monitoring controversial

**Related Information**

Antidepressant Agents *on page 998*

♦ **Imipramine Hydrochloride** *see* Imipramine *on page 469*

♦ **Imipramine Pamoate** *see* Imipramine *on page 469*

# Imiquimod (i mi KWI mod)

**Pharmacologic Class** Skin and Mucous Membrane Agent; Topical Skin Product

**U.S. Brand Names** Aldara™

**Mechanism of Action** Mechanism of action is unknown; however, induces cytokines, including interferon-alpha and others

**Use** Treatment of external genital and perianal warts/condyloma acuminata in adults

**USUAL DOSAGE**

Adults: Topical: Apply 3 times/week prior to normal sleeping hours and leave on the skin for 6-10 hours. Following treatment period, remove cream by washing the treated area with mild soap and water. Examples of 3 times/week application schedules are: Monday, Wednesday, Friday; or Tuesday, Thursday, Saturday. Continue imiquimod treatment until there is total clearance of the genital/perianal warts for ≤16 weeks. A rest period of several days may be taken if required by the patient's discomfort or severity of the local skin reaction. Treatment may resume once the reaction subsides.

Nonocclusive dressings such as cotton gauze or cotton underwear may be used in the management of skin reactions. Handwashing before and after cream application is recommended. Imiquimod is packaged in single-use packets that contain sufficient cream to cover a wart area of up to 20 cm²; avoid use of excessive amounts of cream. Instruct patients to apply imiquimod to external or perianal warts. Apply a thin layer to the wart area and rub in until the cream is no longer visible. Do not occlude the application site.

**Dosage Forms Crm:** 5% (250 mg single dose packets)

**Contraindications** Hypersensitivity to imiquimod

**Warnings/Precautions** Imiquimod has not been evaluated for the treatment of urethral, intravaginal, cervical, rectal, or intra-anal human papilloma viral disease and is not recommended for these conditions. Topical imiquimod is not intended for ophthalmic use. Topical imiquimod administration is not recommended until genital/perianal tissue is healed from any previous drug or surgical treatment. Imiquimod has the potential to exacerbate inflammatory conditions of the skin.

**Pregnancy Risk Factor** B

**Adverse Reactions**

>10%: Local, mild/moderate: Erythema, itching, erosion, burning, excoriation/flaking, edema

1% to 10%:

Local, severe: Erythema, erosion, edema

Local, mild/moderate: Pain, induration, ulceration, scabbing, vesicles, soreness

**Special PA Issues**

**Patient Education:** Imiquimod may weaken condoms and vaginal diaphragms; therefore, concurrent use is not recommended. This medication is for external use only; avoid contact with eyes. Do not occlude the treatment area with bandages or other covers or wraps. Avoid sexual (genital, anal, oral) contact while the cream is on the skin. Wash the treatment area with mild soap and water 6-10 hours following application of imiquimod.

Patients commonly experience local skin reactions such as erythema, erosion, excoriation/flaking, and edema at the site of application or surrounding areas. Most skin reactions are mild to moderate. Severe skin reactions can occur; promptly report severe reactions to physician. Uncircumcised males treating warts under the foreskin should retract the foreskin and clean the area daily.

(Continued)

## Imiquimod *(Continued)*

Imiquimod is not a cure; new warts may develop during therapy.

**Monitoring Parameters:** Reduction in wart size is indicative of a therapeutic response; patients should be monitored for signs and symptoms of hypersensitivity to imiquimod

♦ **Imitrex**® *see* Sumatriptan Succinate *on page 866*

## Immune Globulin, Intramuscular

(i MYUN GLOB yoo lin, IN tra MUS kyoo ler)

**Pharmacologic Class** Immune Globulin

**Mechanism of Action** Provides passive immunity by increasing the antibody titer and antigen-antibody reaction potential

**Use** Household and sexual contacts of persons with hepatitis A, measles, varicella, and possibly rubella; travelers to high-risk areas outside tourist routes; staff, attendees, and parents of diapered attendees in day-care center outbreaks

For travelers, IG is no an alternative to careful selection of foods and water; immune globulin can interfere with the antibody response to parenterally administered live virus vaccines. Frequent travelers should be tested for hepatitis A antibody, immune hemolytic anemia, and neutropenia (with ITP, I.V. route is usually used).

**USUAL DOSAGE** I.M.:

Hepatitis A:

Pre-exposure prophylaxis upon travel into endemic areas (hepatitis A vaccine preferred):

0.02 mL/kg for anticipated risk 1-3 months

0.06 mL/kg for anticipated risk >3 months

Repeat approximate dose every 4-6 months if exposure continues

Postexposure prophylaxis: 0.02 mL/kg given within 2 weeks of exposure

Measles:

Prophylaxis: 0.25 mL/kg/dose (maximum dose: 15 mL) given within 6 days of exposure followed by live attenuated measles vaccine in 3 months or at 15 months of age (whichever is later)

For patients with leukemia, lymphoma, immunodeficiency disorders, generalized malignancy, or receiving immunosuppressive therapy: 0.5 mL/kg (maximum dose: 15 mL)

Poliomyelitis: Prophylaxis 0.3 mL/kg/dose as a single dose

Rubella: Prophylaxis: 0.55 mL/kg/dose within 72 hours of exposure

Varicella:: Prophylaxis: 0.6-1.2 mL/kg (varicella zoster immune globulin preferred) within 72 hours of exposure

IgG deficiency: 1.3 mL/kg, then 0.66 mL/kg in 3-4 weeks

Hepatitis B: Prophylaxis: 0.06 mL/kg/dose (HBIG preferred)

**Dosage Forms Inj:** I.M.: 165±15 mg (of protein)/mL (2 mL, 10 mL)

**Contraindications** Thrombocytopenia, hypersensitivity to immune globulin, thimerosal, IgA deficiency

**Warnings/Precautions** Skin testing should not be performed as local irritation can occur and be misinterpreted as a positive reaction; do not administer I.V.; IG should **not** be used to control outbreaks of measles; epidemiologic and laboratory data indicate current IMIG products do not have a discernible risk of transmitting HIV

**Pregnancy Risk Factor** C

**Adverse Reactions**

>10%: Local: Pain, tenderness, muscle stiffness at I.M. site

1% to 10%:

Cardiovascular: Flushing

Central nervous system: Chills

Gastrointestinal: Nausea

<1%: Lethargy, fever, urticaria, angioedema, erythema, vomiting, myalgia, hypersensitivity reactions

**Drug Interactions** Increased toxicity: Live virus, vaccines (measles, mumps, rubella); do not administer within 3 months after administration of these vaccines

## Immune Globulin, Intravenous (i MYUN GLOB yoo lin, IN tra VEE nus)

**Pharmacologic Class** Immune Globulin

**U.S. Brand Names** Gamimune® N; Gammagard® S/D; Gammar®-P I.V.; Polygam®; Polygam® S/D; Sandoglobulin®; Venoglobulin®-I; Venoglobulin®-S

**Mechanism of Action** Replacement therapy for primary and secondary immunodeficiencies; interference with $F_c$ receptors on the cells of the reticuloendothelial system for autoimmune cytopenias and ITP; possible role of contained antiviral-type antibodies

**Use** Treatment of immunodeficiency sufficiency (hypogammaglobulinemia, agammaglobulinemia, IgG subclass deficiencies, severe combined immunodeficiency syndromes (SCIDS), Wiskott-Aldrich syndrome), idiopathic thrombocytopenic purpura; used in conjunction with appropriate anti-infective therapy *to prevent or modify acute bacterial or viral infections* in patients with iatrogenically-induced or disease-associated immunodepression; *chronic lymphocytic leukemia (CLL) - chronic prophylaxis autoimmune neutropenia, bone marrow* *transplantation patients, autoimmune hemolytic anemia or neutropenia, refractory dermato-myositis/polymyositis, autoimmune diseases (myasthenia gravis, SLE, bullous pemphigoid, severe rheumatoid arthritis), Guillain-Barré syndrome; pediatric HIV infection to decrease frequency of serious bacterial infections*

**USUAL DOSAGE** Children and Adults: I.V.:

**Dosages should be based on ideal body weight** and not actual body weight in morbidly obese patients; approved doses and regimens may vary between brands; check manufacturer guidelines

Primary immunodeficiency disorders: 200-400 mg/kg every 4 weeks or as per monitored serum IgG concentrations

Chronic lymphocytic leukemia (CLL): 400 mg/kg/dose every 3 weeks

Idiopathic thrombocytopenic purpura (ITP): Maintenance dose:
400 mg/kg/day for 2-5 consecutive days; or 1000 mg/kg every other day for 3 doses, if needed or
1000 mg/kg/day for 2 consecutive days; or up to 2000 mg/kg/day over 2-7 consecutive days

Chronic ITP: 400-2000 mg/kg/dose as needed to maintain appropriate platelet counts

Kawasaki disease:
400 mg/kg/day for 4 days within 10 days of onset of fever
800 mg/kg/day for 1-2 days within 10 days of onset of fever
2 g/kg for one dose only

Acquired immunodeficiency syndrome (patients must be symptomatic):
200-250 mg/kg/dose every 2 weeks
400-500 mg/kg/dose every month or every 4 weeks

Pediatric HIV: 400 mg/kg every 28 days

Autoimmune hemolytic anemia and neutropenia: 1000 mg/kg/dose for 2-3 days

Autoimmune diseases: 400 mg/kg/day for 4 days

Bone marrow transplant: 500 mg/kg beginning on days 7 and 2 pretransplant, then 500 mg/kg/week for 90 days post-transplant

Adjuvant to severe cytomegalovirus infections: 500 mg/kg/dose every other day for 7 doses

Severe systemic viral and bacterial infections: Children: 500-1000 mg/kg/week

Prevention of gastroenteritis: Infants and Children: Oral: 50 mg/kg/day divided every 6 hours

Guillain-Barré syndrome:
400 mg/kg/day for 4 days
1000 mg/kg/day for 2 days
2000 mg/kg/day for one day

Refractory dermatomyositis: 2 g/kg/dose every month x 3-4 doses

Refractory polymyositis: 1 g/kg/day x 2 days every month x 4 doses

Chronic inflammatory demyelinating polyneuropathy:
400 mg/kg/day for 5 doses once each month
800 mg/kg/day for 3 doses once each month
1000 mg/kg/day for 2 days once each month

**Dosing adjustment/comments in renal impairment:** $Cl_{cr}$ <10 mL/minute: Avoid use

**Dosage Forms** Inj: Gamimune® N: 5% [50 mg/mL] (10 mL, 50 mL, 100 mL); 10% [100 mg/mL] (50 mL, 100 mL, 200 mL); **Powder for inj, lyophilized:** Gammar-P®-IV: 1 g, 2.5 g, 5 g, Sandoglobulin®: 1 g, 3 g, 6 g, Venoglobulin®-I: 2.5 g, 5 g; **Detergent treated:** Gammagard® S/D: 2.5 g, 5 g, 10 g, Polygam® S/D: 2.5 g, 5 g, 10 g, Venoglobulin®-S: 2.5 g, 5 g, 10 g

**Contraindications** Hypersensitivity to immune globulin or any component, IgA deficiency (except with the use of Gammagard®, Polygam®)

**Warnings/Precautions** Anaphylactic hypersensitivity reactions can occur, especially in IgA-deficient patients; studies indicate that the currently available products have no discernible risk of transmitting HIV or hepatitis B; aseptic meningitis may occur with high doses (≥2 g/kg)

**Pregnancy Risk Factor** C

**Adverse Reactions**
1% to 10%:
Cardiovascular: Flushing of the face, tachycardia
Central nervous system: Chills
Gastrointestinal: Nausea
Respiratory: Dyspnea
<1%: Hypotension, tightness in the chest, dizziness, fever, headache, diaphoresis, hypersensitivity reactions

**Drug Interactions** Increased toxicity: Live virus, vaccines (measles, mumps, rubella); do not administer within 3 months after administration of these vaccines

**Onset** I.V. provides immediate antibody levels.

**Half-Life** 21-24 days

**Special PA Issues**

**Patient Education:** This medication can only be administered by infusion. You will be monitored closely during the infusion. If you experience nausea ask for assistance, do not get up alone. Do not have any vaccinations for the next 3 months without consulting
(Continued)

## Immune Globulin, Intravenous *(Continued)*

prescriber. Immediately report chills; chest pain, tightness, or rapid heartbeat; acute back pain; or difficulty breathing.

### Intravenous Immune Globulin Product Comparison

| | Gamimune® N | Gammagard® SD | Gammar®-IV | Polygam® | Sandoglobulin® | Venoglobulin®-I |
|---|---|---|---|---|---|---|
| FDA indication | Primary immunodeficiency, ITP | Primary immunodeficiency, ITP, CLL prophylaxis | Primary immunodeficiency | Primary immunodeficiency, ITP, CLL | Primary immunodeficiency, ITP | Primary immunodeficiency, ITP |
| Contraindication | IgA deficiency | None (caution with IgA deficiency) | IgA deficiency | None (caution with IgA deficiency) | IgA deficiency | IgA deficiency |
| IgA content | 270 mcg/mL | 0.92-1.6 mcg/mL | <20 mcg/mL | 0.74±0.33 mcg/mL | 720 mcg/mL | 20-24 mcg/mL |
| Adverse reactions (%) | 5.2 | 6 | 15 | 6 | 2.5-6.6 | 6 |
| Plasma source | >2000 paid donors | 4000-5000 paid donors | >8000 paid donors | 50,000 voluntary donors | 8000-15,000 voluntary donors | 6000-9000 paid donors |
| Half-life | 21 d | 24 d | 21-24 d | 21-25 d | 21-23 d | 29 d |
| IgG subclass (%) | | | | | | |
| $IgG_1$ (60-70) | 60 | 67 (66.8)[1] | 69 | 67 | 60.5 (55.3)[1] | 62.3[2] |
| $IgG_2$ (19-31) | 29.4 | 25 (25.4) | 23 | 25 | 30.2 (35.7) | 32.8 |
| $IgG_3$ (5-8.4) | 6.5 | 5 (7.4) | 6 | 5 | 6.6 (6.3) | 2.9 |
| $IgG_4$ (0.7-4) | 4.1 | 3 (0.3) | 2 | 3 | 2.6 (2.6) | 2 |
| Monomers (%) | >95 | >95 | >98 | >95 | >92 | >98 |
| Gammaglobulin (%) | >98 | >90 | >98 | >90 | >96 | >98 |
| Storage | Refrigerate | Room temp | Room temp | Room temp | Room temp | Room temp |
| Recommendations for initial infusion rate | 0.01-0.02 mL/kg/min | 0.5 mL/kg/h | 0.01-0.02 mL/kg/min | 0.5 mL/kg/h | 0.01-0.03 mL/kg/min | 0.01-0.02 mL/kg/min |
| Maximum infusion rate | 0.08 mL/kg/min | 4 mL/kg/h | 0.06 mL/kg/min | 4 mL/kg/h | 2.5 mL/kg/min | 0.04 mL/kg/min |
| Maximum concentration for infusion (%) | 10 | 5 | 5 | 10 | 12 | 10 |

[1]Skvaril F and Gardi A, "Differences Among Available Immunoglobulin Preparations for Intravenous Use," *Pediatr Infect Dis J*, 1988, 7:543-48.
[2]Roemer J, Morgenthaler JJ, Scherz R, et al, "Characterization of Various Immunoglobulin Preparations for Intravenous Application," *Vox Sang*, 1982, 42:62-73.

◆ **Immune Serum Globulin** *see* Immune Globulin, Intramuscular *on page 472*

◆ **Immunization Recommendations** *see* Chart *on page 1081*

◆ **Imodium®** *see* Loperamide *on page 540*

◆ **Imodium® A-D [OTC]** *see* Loperamide *on page 540*

◆ **Imogam®** *see* Rabies Immune Globulin (Human) *on page 791*

- **Imuran®** *see* Azathioprine *on page 90*
- **I-Naphline®** *see* Naphazoline *on page 635*
- **Inapsine®** *see* Droperidol *on page 308*
- **Indanyl Sodium** *see* Carbenicillin *on page 151*

## Indapamide (in DAP a mide)
**Pharmacologic Class** Diuretic, Thiazide
**U.S. Brand Names** Lozol®
**Mechanism of Action** Diuretic effect is localized at the proximal segment of the distal tubule of the nephron; it does not appear to have significant effect on glomerular filtration rate nor renal blood flow; like other diuretics, it enhances sodium, chloride, and water excretion by interfering with the transport of sodium ions across the renal tubular epithelium
**Use** Management of mild to moderate hypertension; treatment of edema in congestive heart failure and nephrotic syndrome
**USUAL DOSAGE** Adults: Oral:
  Edema: 2.5-5 mg/day. **Note:** There is little therapeutic benefit to increasing the dose >5 mg/day; there is, however, an increased risk of electrolyte disturbances
  Hypertension: 1.25 mg in the morning, may increase to 5 mg/day by increments of 1.25-2.5 mg; consider adding another antihypertensive and decreasing the dose if response is not adequate
**Dosage Forms Tab:** 1.25 mg, 2.5 mg
**Contraindications** Anuria, hypersensitivity to indapamide or any component, cross-sensitivity with other thiazides and sulfonamide derivatives
**Warnings/Precautions** Use with caution in patients with renal or hepatic disease, gout, lupus erythematosus, or diabetes mellitus
**Pregnancy Risk Factor** D
**Adverse Reactions**
  1% to 10%: Endocrine & metabolic: Hypokalemia
  <1%: Arrhythmia, weak pulse, hypotension, mood changes, photosensitivity, fluid and electrolyte imbalances (hypocalcemia, hypomagnesemia, hyponatremia), hyperglycemia, xerostomia, rarely blood dyscrasias, numbness or paresthesia in hands, feet or lips, muscle cramps or pain, unusual weakness, prerenal azotemia, shortness of breath, increased thirst
**Drug Interactions**
  Decreased effect:
    Thiazides may decrease the effect of anticoagulants, antigout agents, sulfonylureas
    Bile acid sequestrants, methenamine, and NSAIDs may decrease the effect of the thiazides
  Increased effect: Thiazides may increase the toxicity of allopurinol, anesthetics, antineoplastics, calcium salts, diazoxide, digitalis, lithium, loop diuretics, methyldopa, nondepolarizing muscle relaxants, vitamin D; amphotericin B and anticholinergics may increase the toxicity of thiazides
**Onset** 1-2 hours
**Duration** Up to 36 hours
**Half-Life** 14-18 hours
**Special PA Issues**
  **Patient Education:** Take as directed, early in the day (last dose late afternoon). Do not exceed recommended dosage. Noninsulin-dependent diabetics should monitor serum glucose closely (medication may decrease effect of oral hypoglycemics). Monitor weight on a regular basis. Report sudden or excessive weight gain, swelling of ankles or hands, or difficulty breathing. You may experience dizziness, weakness, or drowsiness; use caution when changing position (rising from sitting or lying position) and when driving or engaging in hazardous activities. Use may experience sensitivity to sunlight (use sunblock, wear protective clothing or sunglasses), impotence (reversible), dry mouth or thirst (frequent mouth care, chewing gum or sucking on lozenges may help). Report unusual bleeding, palpitations, numbness or tingling or cramping.
  **Monitoring Parameters:** Blood pressure (both standing and sitting/supine), serum electrolytes, renal function, assess weight, I & O reports daily to determine fluid loss

- **Inderal®** *see* Propranolol *on page 775*
- **Inderal® LA** *see* Propranolol *on page 775*
- **Inderide®** *see* Propranolol and Hydrochlorothiazide *on page 777*
- **Indian Eye: Orange Root** *see* Golden Seal *on page 421*
- **Indian Head** *see* Echinacea *on page 310*

## Indinavir (in DIN a veer)
**Pharmacologic Class** Antiretroviral Agent, Protease Inhibitor
**U.S. Brand Names** Crixivan®
**Mechanism of Action** Indinavir is a human immunodeficiency virus protease inhibitor, binding to the protease activity site and inhibiting the activity of this enzyme. HIV protease is an enzyme required for the cleavage of viral polyprotein precursors into individual functional
(Continued)

## Indinavir *(Continued)*

proteins found in infectious HIV. Inhibition prevents cleavage of these polyproteins resulting in the formation of immature noninfectious viral particles.

**Use** Treatment of HIV infection; should always be used as part of a multidrug regimen (at least three antiretroviral agents)

**USUAL DOSAGE** Adults: Oral: 800 mg every 8 hours

**Dosage adjustment in hepatic impairment:** 600 mg every 8 hours with mild/medium impairment due to cirrhosis or with ketoconazole coadministration

**Dosage Forms Cap:** 200 mg, 400 mg

**Contraindications** Hypersensitivity to the drug or its components

**Warnings/Precautions** Because indinavir may cause nephrolithiasis the drug should be discontinued if signs and symptoms occur. Indinavir should not be administered concurrently with terfenadine, astemizole, cisapride, triazolam, and midazolam because of competition for metabolism of these drugs through the CYP3A4 system, and potential serious or life-threatening events. Patients with hepatic insufficiency due to cirrhosis should have dose reduction.

**Pregnancy Risk Factor** C

**Pregnancy Implications**

Clinical effects on the fetus: Administer during pregnancy only if benefits to mother outweigh risks to the fetus; hyperbilirubinemia may be exacerbated in neonates

Breast-feeding/lactation: HIV-infected mothers are discouraged from breast-feeding to decrease potential transmission of HIV

**Adverse Reactions** Protease inhibitors cause dyslipidemia which includes elevated cholesterol and triglycerides and a redistribution of body fat centrally to cause "protease paunch", buffalo hump, facial atrophy, and breast enlargement. These agents also cause hyperglycemia.

1% to 10%:

Central nervous system: Headache (5.6%), insomnia (3.1%)

Gastrointestinal: Mild elevation of indirect bilirubin (10%), abdominal pain (8.7%), nausea (11.7%), diarrhea/vomiting (4% to 5%), taste perversion (2.6%)

Neuromuscular & skeletal: Weakness (3.6%), flank pain (2.6%)

Renal: Kidney stones (2% to 3%)

<1%: Malaise, dizziness, somnolence, anorexia, xerostomia, decreased hemoglobin

**Drug Interactions** CYP3A3/4 enzyme substrate; CYP3A3/4 enzyme inhibitor

Decreased effect: Concurrent use of rifampin and rifabutin may decrease the effectiveness of indinavir (dosage increase of indinavir is recommended), dosage decreases of rifampin/rifabutin is recommended; the efficacy of protease inhibitors may be decreased when given with nevirapine

Increased toxicity: Gastric pH is lowered and absorption may be decreased when didanosine and indinavir are taken <1 hour apart; a reduction of dose is often required when coadministered with ketoconazole; terfenadine, astemizole, cisapride should be avoided with indinavir due to life-threatening cardiotoxicity; benzodiazepines with indinavir may result in prolonged sedation and respiratory depression

**Half-Life** 1.8 ±0.4 hour

**Special PA Issues**

**Patient Education:** Take as directed, around-the-clock, with a large glass of water, preferably 1 hour before or 2 hours after meals. Maintain adequate hydration (2-3 L/day of fluids unless instructed to restrict fluid intake). If indinavir and didanosine are prescribed together, take at least 1 hour apart on an empty stomach.

**Dietary Considerations:** Meals high in calories, fat, and protein result in a significant decrease in drug levels; grapefruit juice may decrease indinavir's AUC

**Monitoring Parameters:** Monitor viral load, CD4 count, triglycerides, cholesterol, glucose

- ♦ **Indochron E-R®** *see* Indomethacin *on this page*
- ♦ **Indocid®** *see* Indomethacin *on this page*
- ♦ **Indocid® SR** *see* Indomethacin *on this page*
- ♦ **Indocin®** *see* Indomethacin *on this page*
- ♦ **Indocin® I.V.** *see* Indomethacin *on this page*
- ♦ **Indocin® SR** *see* Indomethacin *on this page*
- ♦ **Indometacin** *see* Indomethacin *on this page*

## Indomethacin *(in doe METH a sin)*

**Pharmacologic Class** Nonsteroidal Anti-Inflammatory Agent (NSAID)

**U.S. Brand Names** Indochron E-R®; Indocin®; Indocin® I.V.; Indocin® SR

**Mechanism of Action** Inhibits prostaglandin synthesis by decreasing the activity of the enzyme, cyclo-oxygenase, which results in decreased formation of prostaglandin precursors

**Use** Management of inflammatory diseases and rheumatoid disorders; moderate pain; acute gouty arthritis; I.V. form used as alternative to surgery for closure of patent ductus arteriosus in neonates

## USUAL DOSAGE

Patent ductus arteriosus: Neonates: I.V.: Initial: 0.2 mg/kg; followed with: 2 doses of 0.1 mg/kg at 12- to 24-hour intervals if age <48 hours at time of first dose; 0.2 mg/kg 2 times if 2-7 days old at time of first dose; or 0.25 mg/kg 2 times if over 7 days at time of first dose; discontinue if significant adverse effects occur. Dose should be withheld if patient has anuria or oliguria.

Analgesia:

Children: Oral: Initial: 1-2 mg/kg/day in 2-4 divided doses; maximum: 4 mg/kg/day; not to exceed 150-200 mg/day

Adults: Oral, rectal: 25-50 mg/dose 2-3 times/day; maximum dose: 200 mg/day; extended release capsule should be given on a 1-2 times/day schedule

**Dosage Forms** Cap: 25 mg, 50 mg, Indocin®: 25 mg, 50 mg; **Cap, sustained release (Indocin® SR):** 75 mg; **Powder for inj, as sodium trihydrate (Indocin® I.V.):** 1 mg; **Supp, rectal (Indocin®):** 50 mg; **Susp, oral (Indocin®):** 25 mg/5 mL (5 mL, 10 mL, 237 mL, 500 mL)

**Contraindications** Hypersensitivity to indomethacin, any component, aspirin, or other nonsteroidal anti-inflammatory drugs (NSAIDs); active GI bleeding, ulcer disease; premature neonates with necrotizing enterocolitis, impaired renal function, active bleeding, thrombocytopenia

**Warnings/Precautions** Use with caution in patients with cardiac dysfunction, hypertension, renal or hepatic impairment, epilepsy, history of GI bleeding, patients receiving anticoagulants, and for treatment of JRA in children (fatal hepatitis has been reported); may have adverse effects on fetus; may affect platelet and renal function in neonates; elderly are a high-risk population for adverse effects from nonsteroidal anti-inflammatory agents. As much as 60% of elderly can develop peptic ulceration and/or hemorrhage asymptomatically.

Use lowest effective dose for shortest period possible. Use of NSAIDs can compromise existing renal function especially when $Cl_{cr}$ is <30 mL/minute.

CNS adverse effects such as confusion, agitation, and hallucination are generally seen in overdose or high-dose situations; but elderly may demonstrate these adverse effects at lower doses than younger adults.

**Pregnancy Risk Factor** B (D if used longer than 48 hours or after 34-week gestation)

**Adverse Reactions**

>10%:

Central nervous system: Dizziness

Dermatologic: Rash

Gastrointestinal: Nausea, epigastric pain, abdominal pain, anorexia, GI bleeding, ulcers, perforation, abdominal cramps, heartburn, indigestion

1% to 10%:

Central nervous system: Headache, nervousness

Dermatologic: Itching

Endocrine & metabolic: Fluid retention

Gastrointestinal: Vomiting

Otic: Tinnitus

<1%: Hypertension, congestive heart failure, arrhythmias, tachycardia, somnolence, fatigue, depression, confusion, drowsiness, hallucinations, aseptic meningitis, urticaria, erythema multiforme, toxic epidermal necrolysis, Stevens-Johnson syndrome, angioedema, hyperkalemia, dilutional hyponatremia (I.V.), hypoglycemia (I.V.), polydipsia, hot flashes, gastritis, GI ulceration, cystitis, polyuria, hemolytic anemia, bone marrow suppression, agranulocytosis, thrombocytopenia, inhibition of platelet aggregation, anemia, leukopenia, hepatitis, peripheral neuropathy, corneal opacities, blurred vision, conjunctivitis, dry eyes, toxic amblyopia, decreased hearing, oliguria, renal failure, shortness of breath, allergic rhinitis, epistaxis, hypersensitivity reactions

**Drug Interactions** CYP2C9 enzyme substrate

Decreased effect: May decrease antihypertensive effects of beta-blockers, hydralazine and captopril; indomethacin may decrease antihypertensive and diuretic effects of furosemide and thiazides

Increased toxicity: May increase serum potassium with potassium-sparing diuretics; probenecid may increase indomethacin serum concentrations; other NSAIDs may increase GI adverse effects; may increase nephrotoxicity of cyclosporin

Indomethacin may increase serum concentrations of digoxin, methotrexate, lithium, and aminoglycosides (reported with I.V. use in neonates)

**Onset** Within 30 minutes

**Duration** 4-6 hours

**Half-Life** 4.5 hours, longer in neonates

(Continued)

## Indomethacin *(Continued)*

### Special PA Issues

**Patient Education:**

Oral: Take this medication exactly as directed; do not increase dose without consulting prescriber. Do not crush, break, or chew capsules. Take with food or milk to reduce GI distress. Maintain adequate fluid intake (2-3 L/day).

Rectal: Suppositories do not need to be refrigerated. Wash hands before inserting unwrapped suppository high up in rectum. Wearing glove is recommended. (Use caution to avoid damage with long fingernails.)

Do not use alcohol, aspirin, or aspirin-containing medication, and all other anti-inflammatory medications without consulting prescriber. You may experience drowsiness, dizziness, nervousness, or headache (use caution when driving or performing hazardous tasks); anorexia, nausea, vomiting, or heartburn (frequent small meals, frequent oral care, sucking on lozenges, or chewing gum may help); fluid retention (weigh yourself weekly and report unusual (3-5 lb/week) weight gain). GI bleeding, ulceration, or perforation can occur with or without pain; discontinue medication and contact prescriber if persistent abdominal pain or cramping, or blood in stool occurs. Report breathlessness, difficulty breathing, or unusual cough; chest pain, rapid heartbeat, palpitations; unusual bruising/bleeding; blood in urine, stool, gums, or vomitus; swollen extremities; skin rash, irritation, or itching; acute fatigue; or changes in hearing or ringing in ears.

**Dietary Considerations:**

Food: May decrease the rate but not the extent of oral absorption. Drug may cause GI upset, bleeding, ulceration, perforation; take with food or milk to minimize GI upset.

Potassium: Hyperkalemia has been reported. The elderly and those with renal insufficiency are at greatest risk. Monitor potassium serum concentration in those at greatest risk. Avoid salt substitutes.

Sodium: Hyponatremia from sodium retention. Suspect secondary to suppression of renal prostaglandin. Monitor serum concentration and fluid status. May need to restrict fluid.

**Monitoring Parameters:** Monitor response (pain, range of motion, grip strength, mobility, ADL function), inflammation; observe for weight gain, edema; monitor renal function (serum creatinine, BUN); observe for bleeding, bruising; evaluate gastrointestinal effects (abdominal pain, bleeding, dyspepsia); mental confusion, disorientation, CBC, liver function tests

### Related Information

Nonsteroidal Anti-Inflammatory Agents *on page 1026*

- ♦ **Indomethacin Sodium Trihydrate** *see* Indomethacin *on page 476*
- ♦ **INF** *see* Interferon Alfa-2b *on page 483*
- ♦ **INF-alpha 2** *see* Interferon Alfa-2b *on page 483*
- ♦ **Infants Feverall™ [OTC]** *see* Acetaminophen *on page 21*
- ♦ **Infants' Silapap® [OTC]** *see* Acetaminophen *on page 21*
- ♦ **InFed™ Injection** *see* Iron Dextran Complex *on page 492*
- ♦ **Inflamase® Forte Ophthalmic** *see* Prednisolone *on page 752*
- ♦ **Inflamase® Mild Ophthalmic** *see* Prednisolone *on page 752*

## Infliximab *(in FLIKS e mab)*

**Pharmacologic Class** Gastrointestinal Agent, Miscellaneous; Monoclonal Antibody

**U.S. Brand Names** Remicade™

**Use** Treatment of moderately to severely active Crohn's disease for the reduction of the signs and symptoms in patients who have an inadequate response to conventional therapy or for the treatment of patients with fistulizing Crohn's disease for the reduction in the number of draining enterocutaneous fistula(s)

**USUAL DOSAGE**

Moderately to severely active Crohn's disease: Adults: I.V.: 5 mg/kg as a single infusion over a minimum of 2 hours

Fistulizing Crohn's disease: 5 mg/kg as an infusion over a minimum of 2 hours, dose repeated at 2 and 6 weeks after the initial infusion

**Dosing adjustment in renal impairment:** No specific adjustment recommended

**Dosing adjustment in hepatic impairment:** No specific adjustment recommended

**Dosage Forms Powder for inj:** 100 mg

**Contraindications** Known hypersensitivity to murine proteins or any component

**Warnings/Precautions** Hypersensitivity reactions, including urticaria, dyspnea, and hypotension have occurred; discontinue the drug if a reaction occurs. Medications for the treatment of hypersensitivity reactions should be available for immediate use. Autoimmune antibodies and a lupus-like syndrome have been reported; if antibodies to double-stranded DNA are confirmed in a patient with lupus-like symptoms, treatment should be discontinued. May affect normal immune responses; effects on development of lymphoma and infection in Crohn's patients are unknown. Treatment may result in the development of human antichimeric antibodies (HACA); presence of these antibodies may predispose patients to infusion reactions.

**Pregnancy Risk Factor** C

**Pregnancy Implications** It is not known whether infliximab is secreted in human milk. Because many immunoglobulins are secreted in milk, and the potential for serious adverse reactions exists, a decision should be made whether to discontinue nursing or discontinue the drug, taking into account the importance of the drug to the mother.

**Adverse Reactions**

>10%:

Central nervous system: Headache (22.6%), fatigue (10.6%), fever (10.1%)

Gastrointestinal: Nausea (16.6%), abdominal pain (12.1%)

Local: Infusion reactions (16%)

Respiratory: Upper respiratory tract infection (16.1%)

Miscellaneous: Infections (21%)

1% to 10%:

Cardiovascular: Chest pain (5.5%)

Central nervous system: Pain (8.5%), dizziness (8%)

Dermatologic: Rash (6%), pruritus (5%)

Gastrointestinal: Vomiting (8.5%)

Neuromuscular & skeletal: Myalgia (5%), back pain (5%)

Respiratory: Pharyngitis (8.5%), bronchitis (7%), rhinitis (6%), cough (5%), sinusitis (5%)

Miscellaneous: Development of antibodies to double-stranded DNA (9%), candidiasis (5%), serious infection (3%)

<1%: Lupus-like syndrome (2 patients); a proportion of patients (12%) with fistulizing disease developed new abscess 8-16 weeks after the last infusion of infliximab

**Drug Interactions** Specific drug interaction studies have not been conducted

**Onset** Within 2 weeks

**Half-Life** 9.5 days

**Special PA Issues**

**Patient Education:** This drug can only be administered by infusion. Report adverse symptoms: headache or unusual fatigue; increased nausea or abdominal pain; cough, runny nose, difficulty breathing; chest pain or persistent dizziness; fatigue, muscle pain or weakness, back pain; fever or chills, mouth sores, vaginal itching or discharge, sore throat, unhealed sores, or frequent infections.

♦ **Infufer®** see Iron Dextran Complex on page 492

♦ **Infumorph™ Injection** see Morphine Sulfate on page 619

♦ **INH** see Isoniazid on page 494

♦ **Innovar®** see Droperidol and Fentanyl on page 309

♦ **Inocor®** see Amrinone on page 68

♦ **Insta-Char® [OTC]** see Charcoal on page 184

# Insulin Preparations (IN su lin prep a RAY shuns)

**Pharmacologic Class** Antidiabetic Agent (Insulin); Antidote

**U.S. Brand Names** Humalog®; Humulin® 50/50; Humulin® 70/30; Humulin® L; Humulin® N; Humulin® R; Humulin® U; Lente® Iletin® I; Lente® Iletin® II; Lente® Insulin; Lente® L; Novolin® 70/30; Novolin® L; Novolin® N; Novolin® R; NPH Iletin® I; NPH Insulin; NPH-N; Pork NPH Iletin® II; Pork Regular Iletin® II; Regular (Concentrated) Iletin® II U-500; Regular Iletin® I; Regular Insulin; Regular Purified Pork Insulin; Velosulin® Human

**Mechanism of Action** The principal hormone required for proper glucose utilization in normal metabolic processes; it is obtained from beef or pork pancreas or a biosynthetic process converting pork insulin to human insulin; insulins are categorized into 3 groups related to promptness, duration, and intensity of action

**Use** Treatment of insulin-dependent diabetes mellitus, also noninsulin-dependent diabetes mellitus unresponsive to treatment with diet and/or oral hypoglycemics; to assure proper utilization of glucose and reduce glucosuria in nondiabetic patients receiving parenteral nutrition whose glucosuria cannot be adequately controlled with infusion rate adjustments or those who require assistance in achieving optimal caloric intakes; hyperkalemia (use with glucose to shift potassium into cells to lower serum potassium levels)

**USUAL DOSAGE** Dose requires continuous medical supervision; may administer I.V. (regular), I.M., S.C.

Diabetes mellitus: The number and size of daily doses, time of administration, and diet and exercise require continuous medical supervision. Lispro should be given within 15 minutes of a meal and human regular insulin should be given within 30-60 minutes before a meal. Maintenance doses should be administered subcutaneously and sites should be rotated to prevent lipodystrophy.

Children and Adults: 0.5-1 unit/kg/day in divided doses

Adolescents (growth spurts): 0.8-1.2 units/kg/day in divided doses

Adjust dose to maintain premeal and bedtime blood glucose of 80-140 mg/dL (children <5 years: 100-200 mg/dL)

Hyperkalemia: Administer calcium gluconate and NaHCO$_3$ first then 50% dextrose at 0.5-1 mL/kg and insulin 1 unit for every 4-5 g dextrose given

Diabetic ketoacidosis: Children and Adults: Regular Insulin: I.V. loading dose: 0.1 unit/kg, then maintenance continuous infusion: 0.1 unit/kg/hour (range: 0.05-0.2 units/kg/hour (Continued)

## Insulin Preparations *(Continued)*

depending upon the rate of decrease of serum glucose - too rapid decrease of serum glucose may lead to cerebral edema).

Optimum rate of decrease (serum glucose): 80-100 mg/dL/hour

**Note:** Newly diagnosed patients with IDDM presenting in DKA and patients with blood sugars <800 mg/dL may be relatively "sensitive" to insulin and should receive loading and initial maintenance doses approximately $1/2$ of those indicated above.

**Dosing adjustment in renal impairment (regular):** Insulin requirements are reduced due to changes in insulin clearance or metabolism

$Cl_{cr}$ 10-50 mL/minute: Administer at 75% of normal dose

$Cl_{cr}$ <10 mL/minute: Administer at 25% to 50% of normal dose and monitor glucose closely

Hemodialysis: Because of a large molecular weight (6000 daltons), insulin is not significantly removed by either peritoneal or hemodialysis

Supplemental dose is not necessary

Peritoneal dialysis: Supplemental dose is not necessary

Continuous arteriovenous or venovenous hemofiltration effects: Supplemental dose is not necessary

**Dosage Forms** All insulins are 100 units/mL (10 mL) except where indicated:

RAPID ACTING: **Insulin lispro rDNA origin:** Humalog® [*Lilly*] (1.5 mL, 10 mL); **Insulin Inj** (Regular Insulin), Beef and pork: Regular Iletin® I [*Lilly*]; Human: rDNA: Humulin® R [*Lilly*], Novolin® R [*Novo Nordisk*], Semisynthetic: Velosulin® Human [*Novo Nordisk*], Pork: Regular Insulin [*Novo Nordisk*], Purified pork: Pork Regular Iletin® II [*Lilly*], Regular Purified Pork Insulin [*Novo Nordisk*], Regular (Concentrated) Iletin® II U-500 (*Lilly*): 500 units/mL

INTERMEDIATE-ACTING: **Insulin Zinc Susp** (Lente), Beef and pork: Lente® Iletin® I [*Lilly*], Human, rDNA: Humulin® L [*Lilly*], Novolin® L [*Novo Nordisk*], Purified pork: Lente® Iletin® II [*Lilly*], Lente® L [*Novo Nordisk*], **Isophane Insulin Susp** (NPH), Beef and pork: NPH Iletin® I [*Lilly*], Human, rDNA: Humulin® N [*Lilly*], Novolin® N [*Novo Nordisk*], Purified pork: Pork NPH Iletin® II [*Lilly*], NPH-N [*Novo Nordisk*]

LONG-ACTING: **Insulin zinc susp, extended** (Ultralente®), Human, rDNA: Humulin® U [*Lilly*]

COMBINATIONS: **Isophane Insulin Susp and Insulin Inj**, Isophane insulin susp (50%) and insulin inj (50%) human (rDNA): Humulin® 50/50 [*Lilly*], Isophane insulin susp (70%) and insulin inj (30%) human (rDNA): Humulin® 70/30 [*Lilly*], Novolin® 70/30 [*Novo Nordisk*]

**Warnings/Precautions** Any change of insulin should be made cautiously; changing manufacturers, type and/or method of manufacture, may result in the need for a change of dosage; human insulin differs from animal-source insulin; regular insulin is the only insulin to be used I.V.; hypoglycemia may result from increased work or exercise without eating

**Pregnancy Risk Factor** B

**Pregnancy Implications**

Clinical effects on the fetus: Does not cross the placenta. Insulin is the drug of choice for the control of diabetes mellitus during pregnancy.

Breast-feeding/lactation: The gastrointestinal tract destroys insulin when administered orally and therefore would not be expected to be absorbed intact by the breast-feeding infant.

### Drug Interactions With Insulin Injection

| Decrease Hypoglycemic Effect of Insulin | Increase Hypoglycemic Effect of Insulin |
|---|---|
| Contraceptives, oral | Alcohol |
| Corticosteroids | Alpha-blockers |
| Dextrothyroxine | Anabolic steroids |
| Diltiazem | Beta-blockers* |
| Dobutamine | Clofibrate |
| Epinephrine | Fenfluramine |
| Niacin | Guanethidine |
| Smoking | MAO inhibitors |
| Thiazide diuretics | Pentamidine |
| Thyroid hormone | Phenylbutazone |
| | Salicylates |
| | Sulfinpyrazone |
| | Tetracyclines |

*Nonselective beta-blockers may delay recovery from hypoglycemic episodes and mask signs/symptoms of hypoglycemia. Cardioselective agents may be alternatives.

**Adverse Reactions** 1% to 10%:

Cardiovascular: Palpitation, tachycardia, pallor

Central nervous system: Fatigue, mental confusion, loss of consciousness, headache, hypothermia

Dermatologic: Urticaria, redness

Endocrine & metabolic: Hypoglycemia

Gastrointestinal: Hunger, nausea, numbness of mouth

Local: Itching, edema, stinging, or warmth at injection site, atrophy or hypertrophy of S.C. fat tissue

Neuromuscular & skeletal: Muscle weakness, paresthesia, tremors

Ocular: Transient presbyopia or blurred vision, blurred vision

Miscellaneous: Diaphoresis, anaphylaxis

**Drug Interactions** See table.

**Onset**

Onset and duration of hypoglycemic effects depend upon preparation administered. See table.

**Pharmacokinetics/Pharmacodynamics: Onset and Duration of Hypoglycemic Effects Depend Upon Preparation Administered**

| | Onset (h) | Peak (h) | Duration (h) |
|---|---|---|---|
| Insulin, regular (Novolin® R) | 0.5–1 | 2-3 | 5–7 |
| Isophane insulin suspension (NPH) (Novolin® N) | 1–1.5 | 4–12 | 18–24 |
| Insulin zinc suspension (Lente®) | 1–2.5 | 8–12 | 18–24 |
| Isophane insulin suspension and regular insulin injection (Novolin® 70/30) | 0.5 (0.5) | 4-8 (2-12) | 24 (24) |
| Prompt zinc insulin suspension (PZI) | 4-8 | 14-24 | 36 |
| Extended insulin zinc suspension (Ultralente®) | 4-8 | 16–18 | >36 |

Onset and duration: Insulin lispro may begin to act in 15-30 minutes. Biosynthetic NPH human insulin shows a more rapid onset and shorter duration of action than corresponding porcine insulins; human insulin and purified porcine regular insulin are similarly efficacious following S.C. administration. The duration of action of highly purified porcine insulins is shorter than that of conventional insulin equivalents. Duration depends on type of preparation and route of administration as well as patient related variables. In general, the larger the dose of insulin, the longer the duration of activity.

**Special PA Issues**

**Patient Education:** Follow instructions of prescriber exactly. Appropriate diet should be followed. Smoking and alcohol intake will effect insulin activity. You will most likely be referred to a diabetic educator. Do not change insulins or brands without consulting prescriber. Roll bottle gently in hand; do not shake. Store in a cool place. When mixing insulin, draw up regular insulin first. Monitor urine or serum glucose as recommended; more frequently with unusual exercise, stress, or illness. Report fever, rash, or hypoglycemic or hyperglycemic reactions.

**Dietary Considerations:**

Alcohol: Increase in hypoglycemic effect of insulin; monitor blood glucose concentration; avoid or limit use

Food:

Potassium: Shifts potassium from extracellular to intracellular space. Decreases potassium serum concentration; monitor potassium serum concentration.

Sodium: SIADH; water retention and dilutional hyponatremia may occur. Patients at greatest risk are those with CHF or hepatic cirrhosis. Monitor sodium serum concentration and fluid status.

**Monitoring Parameters:** Urine sugar and acetone, serum glucose, electrolytes

**Reference Range:**

Therapeutic, serum insulin (fasting): 5-20 μIU/mL (SI: 35-145 pmol/L)

Glucose, fasting: Newborns: 60-110 mg/dL; Adults: 60-110 mg/dL; Elderly: 100-180 mg/dL

♦ **Intal® Nebulizer Solution** *see* Cromolyn Sodium *on page 240*

♦ **Intal® Oral Inhaler** *see* Cromolyn Sodium *on page 240*

♦ **α-2-interferon** *see* Interferon Alfa-2b *on page 483*

# Interferon Alfa-2a (in ter FEER on AL fa too aye)

**Pharmacologic Class** Biological Response Modulator

**U.S. Brand Names** Roferon-A®

**Mechanism of Action** Alpha interferons are a family of proteins, produced by nucleated cells, that have antiviral, antiproliferative, and immune-regulating activity. There are 16 known subtypes of alpha interferons. Interferons interact with cells through high affinity cell surface receptors. Following activation, multiple effects can be detected including induction of gene transcription. Inhibits cellular growth, alters the state of cellular differentiation, (Continued)

## Interferon Alfa-2a (Continued)

interferes with oncogene expression, alters cell surface antigen expression, increases phagocytic activity of macrophages, and augments cytotoxicity of lymphocytes for target cells

**Use** Patients >18 years of age: Hairy cell leukemia, AIDS-related Kaposi's sarcoma, chronic myelogenous leukemia (CML), chronic hepatitis C, adjuvant treatment to surgery for primary or recurrent malignant melanoma; multiple unlabeled uses; indications and dosage regimens are specific for a particular brand of interferon

**USUAL DOSAGE** Refer to individual protocols

Infants and Children: Hemangiomas of infancy, pulmonary hemangiomatosis: S.C.: 1-3 million units/m²/day once daily

Adults >18 years: I.M., S.C.:

Hairy cell leukemia:

Induction: 3 million units/day for 16-24 weeks.

Maintenance: 3 million units 3 times/week (may be treated for up to 20 consecutive weeks)

AIDS-related Kaposi's sarcoma:

Induction: 36 million units/day for 10-12 weeks

Maintenance: 36 million units 3 times/week (may begin with dose escalation from 3-9-18 million units each day over 3 consecutive days followed by 36 million units/day for the remainder of the 10-12 weeks of induction)

If severe adverse reactions occur, modify dosage (50% reduction) or temporarily discontinue therapy until adverse reactions abate

**Dosage Forms Inj:** 3 million units/mL (1 mL), 6 million units/mL (3 mL), 9 million units/mL (0.9 mL, 3 mL), 36 million units/mL (1 mL); **Powder for inj:** 6 million units/mL when reconstituted

**Contraindications** Hypersensitivity to alfa-2a interferon or any component of the product

**Warnings/Precautions** Use with caution in patients with seizure disorders, brain metastases, compromised CNS, multiple sclerosis, and patients with pre-existing cardiac disease, severe renal or hepatic impairment, or myelosuppression; safety and efficacy in children <18 years of age have not been established. Higher doses in the elderly or in malignancies other than hairy cell leukemia may result in severe obtundation.

**Pregnancy Risk Factor** C

**Adverse Reactions**

>10%:

Central nervous system: Dizziness, fatigue, malaise, fever (usually within 4-6 hours), chills

Dermatologic: Rash

Gastrointestinal: Xerostomia, nausea, vomiting, diarrhea, abdominal cramps, weight loss, metallic taste

Hematologic: Mildly myelosuppressive and well tolerated if used without adjunct antineoplastic agents; thrombocytosis has been reported, leukopenia (mainly neutropenia), anemia, thrombocytopenia, decreased hemoglobin, hematocrit, platelets

Myelosuppressive:

WBC: Mild

Platelets: Mild

Onset (days): 7-10

Nadir (days): 14

Recovery (days): 21

Neuromuscular & skeletal: Rigors, arthralgia

Miscellaneous: Flu-like syndrome, diaphoresis

1% to 10%:

Central nervous system: Headache, delirium, somnolence, neurotoxicity

Dermatologic: Alopecia, dry skin

Gastrointestinal: Anorexia, stomatitis

Hepatic: Hepatotoxicity

Neuromuscular & skeletal: Peripheral neuropathy, leg cramps

Ocular: Blurred vision

Miscellaneous: Diaphoresis

<1%: Tachycardia, arrhythmias, chest pain, hypotension, SVT, edema, confusion, sensory neuropathy, psychiatric effects, EEG abnormalities, depression, hypothyroidism, increased uric acid level, change in taste, increased hepatic transaminase, myalgia, visual disturbances, proteinuria, increased BUN/creatinine, coughing, dyspnea, nasal congestion, neutralizing antibodies, local sensitivity to injection; usually patient can build up a tolerance to side effects

**Drug Interactions**

Increased effect:

Cimetidine: May augment the antitumor effects of interferon in melanoma

Theophylline: Clearance has been reported to be decreased in hepatitis patients receiving interferon

Increased toxicity: Vinblastine: Enhances interferon toxicity in several patients; increased incidence of paresthesia has also been noted

**Half-Life** I.M., I.V.: 2 hours after administration; S.C.: 3 hours

**Special PA Issues**

**Patient Education:** Use as directed; do not change dosage or schedule of administration without consulting prescriber. Maintain adequate hydration (2-3 L/day of fluids unless instructed to restrict fluid intake). You may experience flu-like syndrome (acetaminophen may help); nausea, vomiting, dry mouth, or metallic taste (frequent small meals, frequent oral care, sucking on lozenges or chewing gum may help); drowsiness, dizziness, agitation, abnormal thinking (use caution when driving or performing hazardous tasks). Report unusual bruising or bleeding; persistent abdominal disturbances; unusual fatigue; muscle pain or tremors; chest pain or palpitation; swelling of extremities or unusual weight gain; difficulty breathing; pain, swelling, or redness at injection site; or other unusual symptoms.

**Monitoring Parameters:** Baseline chest x-ray, EKG, CBC with differential, liver function tests, electrolytes, platelets, weight; patients with pre-existing cardiac abnormalities, or in advanced stages of cancer should have EKGs taken before and during treatment

# Interferon Alfa-2b (in ter FEER on AL fa too bee)

**Pharmacologic Class** Biological Response Modulator

**U.S. Brand Names** Intron® A

**Mechanism of Action** Alpha interferons are a family of proteins, produced by nucleated cells, that have antiviral, antiproliferative, and immune-regulating activity. There are 16 known subtypes of alpha interferons. Interferons interact with cells through high affinity cell surface receptors. Following activation, multiple effects can be detected including induction of gene transcription. Inhibits cellular growth, alters the state of cellular differentiation, interferes with oncogene expression, alters cell surface antigen expression, increases phagocytic activity of macrophages, and augments cytotoxicity of lymphocytes for target cells

**Use** Hairy-cell leukemia in patients >18 years, condylomata acuminata, AIDS-related Kaposi's sarcoma in patients >18 years, chronic non-A/non-B/C hepatitis in patients >18 years, chronic hepatitis B in patients >18 years (indications and dosage are specific for a particular brand of interferon)

**USUAL DOSAGE** Adults (refer to individual protocols):

Hairy cell leukemia: I.M., S.C.: 2 million units/m$^2$ 3 times/week for 2 to ≥6 months of therapy

AIDS-related Kaposi's sarcoma: I.M., S.C. (use 50 million IU vial): 30 million units/m$^2$ 3 times/week

*Condylomata acuminata*: Intralesionally (use 10 million IU vial): 1 million units/lesion 3 times/week for 4-8 weeks; not to exceed 5 million units per treatment (maximum: 5 lesions at one time)

Chronic hepatitis C (non-A/non-B): I.M., S.C.: 3 million units 3 times/week for approximately a 6-month course

Chronic hepatitis B: I.M., S.C.: 5 million IU/day or 10 million IU 3 times/week for 16 weeks; if severe adverse reactions occur, reduce dosage 50% or temporarily discontinue therapy until adverse reactions abate; when platelet/granulocyte count returns to normal, reinstitute therapy

Hemodialysis: Supplemental dose is not necessary

Peritoneal dialysis: Supplemental dose is not necessary

**Dosage Forms Inj, albumin free:** 3 million units (0.5 mL), 5 million units (0.5 mL), 10 million units (1 mL), 25 million units; **Powder for inj, lyophilized:** 18 million units, 50 million units

**Contraindications** Known hypersensitivity to interferon alfa-2b or any components, patients with pre-existing thyroid disease uncontrolled by medication, coagulation disorders, diabetics prone to DKA, pulmonary disease

**Warnings/Precautions** Use with caution in patients with seizure disorders, brain metastases, compromised CNS, multiple sclerosis, and patients with pre-existing cardiac disease, severe renal or hepatic impairment, or myelosuppression; safety and efficacy in children <18 years has not been established. Higher doses in the elderly or in malignancies other than hairy cell leukemia may result in severe obtundation. A baseline ocular exam is recommended in patients with diabetes or hypertension.

**Pregnancy Risk Factor** C

**Adverse Reactions**

>10%:

Central nervous system: Dizziness, fatigue, malaise, fever (usually within 4-6 hours), chills

Dermatologic: Skin rash

Gastrointestinal: Xerostomia, nausea, vomiting, diarrhea, dizziness, abdominal cramps, weight loss, metallic taste, anorexia

Hematologic: Mildly myelosuppressive and well tolerated if used without adjunct antineoplastic agents; thrombocytosis has been reported, leukopenia (mainly neutropenia), anemia, thrombocytopenia, decreased hemoglobin, hematocrit, platelets

Myelosuppressive:

WBC: Mild

Platelets: Mild

Onset (days): 7-10

Nadir (days): 14

(Continued)

## Interferon Alfa-2b (Continued)

Recovery (days): 21
Neuromuscular & skeletal: Rigors, arthralgia
Miscellaneous: Flu-like syndrome, diaphoresis
1% to 10%:
Central nervous system: Neurotoxicity
Dermatologic: Dry skin, alopecia
Gastrointestinal: Stomatitis
Hepatic: Hepatotoxicity
Neuromuscular & skeletal: Peripheral neuropathy, leg cramps
Ocular: Blurred vision
Miscellaneous: Diaphoresis
<1%: Cardiotoxicity, tachycardia, arrhythmias, hypotension, SVT, arrhythmias, chest pain, edema, EEG abnormalities, confusion, sensory neuropathy, headache, psychiatric effects, delirium, somnolence, partial alopecia, rash, increased uric acid level, hypothyroidism, change in taste, increased hepatic transaminase, increased ALT/AST, sensitivity to injection, myalgia, rigors, visual disturbances, proteinuria, increased creatinine, increased BUN, coughing, dyspnea, nasal congestion, neutralizing antibodies; usually patient can build up a tolerance to side effects

**Drug Interactions**
Increased effect: Cimetidine: May augment the antitumor effects of interferon in melanoma
Increased toxicity:
Theophylline: Clearance has been reported to be decreased in hepatitis patients receiving interferon
Vinblastine: Enhances interferon toxicity in several patients; increased incidence of paresthesia has also been noted
Zidovudine: Increased myelosuppression

**Half-Life** I.M., I.V.: 2 hours; S.C.: 3 hours

**Special PA Issues**
**Patient Education:** Use as directed; do not change dosage or schedule of administration without consulting prescriber. Maintain adequate hydration (2-3 L/day of fluids unless instructed to restrict fluid intake). You may experience flu-like syndrome (acetaminophen may help); nausea, vomiting, dry mouth, or metallic taste (frequent small meals, frequent oral care, sucking on lozenges or chewing gum may help); drowsiness, dizziness, agitation, abnormal thinking (use caution when driving or performing hazardous tasks). Report unusual bruising or bleeding; persistent abdominal disturbances; unusual fatigue; muscle pain or tremors; chest pain or palpitation; swelling of extremities or unusual weight gain; difficulty breathing; pain, swelling, or redness at injection site; or other unusual symptoms.
**Monitoring Parameters:** Baseline chest x-ray, EKG, CBC with differential, liver function tests, electrolytes, thyroid function tests, platelets, weight; patients with pre-existing cardiac abnormalities, or in advanced stages of cancer should have EKGs taken before and during treatment

## Interferon Alfa-2b and Ribavirin Combination Pack

(in ter FEER on AL fa too bee)
**Pharmacologic Class** Antiviral Agent; Biological Response Modulator
**U.S. Brand Names** Rebetron™
**Dosage Forms** Combination package:
For patients ≤75 kg:
Each Rebetron™ combination package consists of:
A box containing 6 vials of Intron® A (3 million int. units in 0.5 mL per vial) and 6 syringes and alcohol swabs; two boxes containing 35 Rebetrol® capsules each for a total of 70 capsules (5 capsules per blister card)
One 18 million int. units multidose vial of Intron® A injection (22.8 million int. units/3.8 mL; 3 million int. units/0.5 mL) and 6 syringes and alcohol swabs; two boxes containing 35 Rebetrol® capsules each for a total of 70 capsules (5 capsules per blister card)
One 18 million int. units Intron A injection multidose pen (22.5 million int. units per 1.5 mL; 3 million int. units/0.2 mL) and 6 disposable needles and alcohol swabs; two boxes containing 35 Rebetrol® capsules each for a total of 70 capsules (5 capsules per blister card)
For patients >75 kg:
A box containing 6 vials of Intron® A injection (3 million int. units in 0.5 mL per vial) and 6 syringes and alcohol swabs; two boxes containing 42 Rebetrol® capsules each for a total of 84 capsules (6 capsules per blister card)
One 18 million int. units multidose vial of Intron® A injection (22.5 million int. units per 3.8 mL; 3 million int. units/0.5 mL) and 6 syringes and alcohol swabs; two boxes containing 42 Rebetrol® capsules each for a total of 84 capsules (6 capsules per blister card)
One 18 million int. units Intron® A injection multidose pen (22.5 million int. units per 1.5 mL; 3 million int. units/0.2 mL) and 6 disposable needles and alcohol swabs; two boxes containing 42 Rebetrol® capsules each for a total of 84 capsules (6 capsules per blister card)

For Rebetrol® dose reduction:

A box containing 6 vials of Intron® A injection (3 million int. units in 0.5 mL per vial) and 6 syringes and alcohol swabs; one box containing 42 Rebetrol® capsules (6 capsules per blister card)

One 18 million int. units multidose vial of Intron® A injection (22.8 million int. units per 3.8 mL; 3 million int. units/0.5 mL) and 6 syringes and alcohol swabs; one box containing 42 Rebetrol® capsules (6 capsules per blister card)

One 18 million int. units Introl® A injection multidose pen (22.5 million int. units per 1.5 mL; 3 million int. units/0.2 mL) and 6 disposable needles and alcohol swabs; one box containing 42 Rebetrol® capsules (6 capsules per blister card)

# Interferon Alfa-n3 (in ter FEER on AL fa en three)

**Pharmacologic Class** Biological Response Modulator

**U.S. Brand Names** Alferon® N

**Mechanism of Action** Interferons interact with cells through high affinity cell surface receptors. Following activation, multiple effects can be detected including induction of gene transcription. Inhibits cellular growth, alters the state of cellular differentiation, interferes with oncogene expression, alters cell surface antigen expression, increases phagocytic activity of macrophages, and augments cytotoxicity of lymphocytes for target cells

**Use** Patients ≥18 years of age: Condylomata acuminata, intralesional treatment of refractory or recurring genital or venereal warts; useful in patients who do not respond or are not candidates for usual treatments; indications and dosage regimens are specific for a particular brand of interferon

**USUAL DOSAGE** Adults: Inject 250,000 units (0.05 mL) in each wart twice weekly for a maximum of 8 weeks; therapy should not be repeated for at least 3 months after the initial 8-week course of therapy

**Dosage Forms Inj:** 5 million units (1 mL)

**Contraindications** Patients with known hypersensitivity to alpha interferon, mouse immunoglobulin, or any component of the product

**Warnings/Precautions** Use with caution in patients with seizure disorders, brain metastases, compromised CNS function, cardiac disease, severe renal or hepatic impairment, multiple sclerosis; safety and efficacy in children <18 years have not been established.

**Pregnancy Risk Factor** C

**Adverse Reactions**

>10%:

Central nervous system: Fatigue, malaise, fever (usually within 4-6 hours), chills, dizziness

Dermatologic: Rash

Gastrointestinal: Xerostomia, nausea, vomiting, diarrhea, abdominal cramps, weight loss, metallic taste, anorexia

Hematologic: Mildly myelosuppressive and well tolerated if used without adjunct antineoplastic agents; thrombocytosis has been reported, leukopenia (mainly neutropenia), anemia, thrombocytopenia, decreased hemoglobin, hematocrit, platelets

Myelosuppressive:

WBC: Mild

Platelets: Mild

Onset (days): 7-10

Nadir (days): 14

Recovery (days): 21

Neuromuscular & skeletal: Arthralgia, rigors

Miscellaneous: Flu-like syndrome, diaphoresis

1% to 10%:

Central nervous system: Headache, delirium, somnolence, neurotoxicity

Dermatologic: Alopecia, dry skin

Gastrointestinal: Stomatitis

Hepatic: Hepatotoxicity

Neuromuscular & skeletal: Peripheral neuropathy, leg cramps

Ocular: Blurred vision

Miscellaneous: Diaphoresis

<1%: Tachycardia, arrhythmias, chest pain, hypotension, SVT, edema, EEG abnormalities, confusion, sensory neuropathy, confusion, psychiatric effects, depression, hypothyroidism, increased uric acid level, change in taste, increased hepatic transaminase, increased ALT/AST, sensitivity to injection, myalgia, visual disturbances, proteinuria, increased BUN/creatinine, coughing, dyspnea, cough, nasal congestion, neutralizing antibodies, usually patient can build up a tolerance to side effects

**Drug Interactions**

Increased effect: Cimetidine: May augment the antitumor effects of interferon in melanoma
Increased toxicity:

Vinblastine: Enhances interferon toxicity in several patients; increased incidence of paresthesia has also been noted

Theophylline: Clearance has been reported to be decreased in hepatitis patients receiving interferon

(Continued)

## Interferon Alfa-n3 (Continued)

### Special PA Issues

**Patient Education:** Warts are highly contagious until they completely disappear, abstain from sexual activity or use barrier protection; inform nurse or physician if allergy exists to eggs, neomycin, mouse immunoglobulin, or to human interferon alpha; acetaminophen can be used to treat flu-like symptoms

## Interferon Beta-1a (in ter FEER on BAY ta won aye)

**Pharmacologic Class** Biological Response Modulator

**U.S. Brand Names** Avonex™

**Mechanism of Action** Interferon beta differs from naturally occurring human protein by a single amino acid substitution and the lack of carbohydrate side chains; alters the expression and response to surface antigens and can enhance immune cell activities. Properties of interferon beta that modify biologic responses are mediated by cell surface receptor interactions; mechanism in the treatment of MS is unknown.

**Use** Treatment of relapsing forms of multiple sclerosis (MS); to slow the accumulation of physical disability and decrease the frequency of clinical exacerbations

**USUAL DOSAGE** Adults >18 years: I.M.: 30 mcg once weekly

**Dosage Forms Powder for inj, lyophilized:** 33 mcg [6.6 million units]

**Contraindications** History of hypersensitivity to natural or recombinant interferon beta, human albumin, or any other component of the formulation

**Warnings/Precautions** Interferon beta-1a should be used with caution in patients with a history of depression, seizures, or cardiac disease; because its use has not been evaluated during lactation, its use in breast-feeding mothers may not be safe and should be warned against

**Pregnancy Risk Factor** C

**Adverse Reactions** 1% to 10%:

Cardiovascular: CHF (rare) tachycardia, syncope

Central nervous system: Headache, lethargy, depression, emotional lability, anxiety, suicidal ideations, somnolence, agitation, confusion

Dermatologic: Alopecia (rare)

Endocrine & metabolic: Hypocalcemia

Gastrointestinal: Nausea, anorexia, vomiting, diarrhea, chronic weight loss

Hematologic: Leukopenia, thrombocytopenia, anemia (frequent, dose-related, but not usually severe)

Hepatic: Elevated liver enzymes (mild, transient)

Local: Pain/redness at injection site (80%)

Neuromuscular & skeletal: Weakness

Ocular: Retinal toxicity/visual changes

Renal: Elevated BUN and $S_{cr}$

Miscellaneous: Flu-like syndrome (fever, nausea, malaise, myalgia) occurs in most patients, but is usually controlled by acetaminophen or NSAIDs; dose related abortifacient activity was reported in Rhesus monkeys

**Drug Interactions** Decreases clearance of zidovudine thus increasing zidovudine toxicity

**Half-Life** I.M.: 10 hours; S.C.: 8.6 hours

### Special PA Issues

**Patient Education:** This is not a cure for MS; you will continue to receive regular treatment and follow-up for MS. Use as directed; do not change dosage or schedule of administration without consulting prescriber. Maintain adequate hydration (2-3 L/day of fluids unless instructed to restrict fluid intake). You may experience flu-like syndrome (acetaminophen may help); nausea, vomiting, or loss of appetite (frequent small meals, frequent oral care, sucking on lozenges, or chewing gum may help); drowsiness, dizziness, agitation, or abnormal thinking (use caution when driving or performing hazardous tasks). Report unusual bruising or bleeding; persistent abdominal disturbances; unusual fatigue; muscle pain or tremors; chest pain or palpitations; swelling of extremities; visual disturbances; pain, swelling, or redness at injection site; or other unusual symptoms.

**Monitoring Parameters:** Hemoglobin, liver function, and blood chemistries

## Interferon Beta-1b (in ter FEER on BAY ta won bee)

**Pharmacologic Class** Biological Response Modulator

**U.S. Brand Names** Betaseron®

**Mechanism of Action** Interferon beta-1b differs from naturally occurring human protein by a single amino acid substitution and the lack of carbohydrate side chains; alters the expression and response to surface antigens and can enhance immune cell activities. Properties of interferon beta-1b that modify biologic responses are mediated by cell surface receptor interactions; mechanism in the treatment of MS is unknown.

**Use** Reduces the frequency of clinical exacerbations in ambulatory patients with relapsing-remitting multiple sclerosis (MS)

**USUAL DOSAGE** S.C.:

Children <18 years: Not recommended

Adults >18 years: 0.25 mg (8 million units) every other day

**Dosage Forms** Powder for inj, lyophilized: 0.3 mg [9.6 million units]

**Contraindications** Hypersensitivity to *E. coli* derived products, natural or recombinant interferon beta, albumin human or any other component of the formulation

**Warnings/Precautions** The safety and efficacy of interferon beta-1b in chronic progressive MS have not been evaluated; use with caution in women who are breast-feeding; flu-like symptoms complex (ie, myalgia, fever, chills, malaise, sweating) is reported in 53% of patients who receive interferon beta-1b

**Pregnancy Risk Factor** C

**Adverse Reactions** Due to the pivotal position of interferon in the immune system, toxicities can affect nearly every organ system: Injection site reactions, injection site necrosis, flu-like symptoms, menstrual disorders, depression (with suicidal ideations), somnolence, palpitations, peripheral vascular disorders, hypertension, blood dyscrasias, dyspnea, laryngitis, cystitis, gastrointestinal complaints, seizures, headache, and liver enzyme elevations

**Special PA Issues**

**Patient Education:** This is not a cure for MS; you will continue to receive regular treatment and follow-up for MS. Use as directed; do not change dosage or schedule of administration without consulting prescriber. Maintain adequate hydration (2-3 L/day of fluids unless instructed to restrict fluid intake). You may experience flu-like syndrome (acetaminophen may help); nausea, vomiting, or loss of appetite (frequent small meals, frequent oral care, sucking on lozenges, or chewing gum may help); drowsiness, dizziness, agitation, or abnormal thinking (use caution when driving or performing hazardous tasks). Report unusual bruising or bleeding; persistent abdominal disturbances; unusual fatigue; muscle pain or tremors; chest pain or palpitations; swelling of extremities; visual disturbances; pain, swelling, or redness at injection site; or other unusual symptoms.

**Monitoring Parameters:** Hemoglobin, liver function, and blood chemistries

- ◆ **Interleukin-2** *see* Aldesleukin *on page 36*
- ◆ **Interleukin-11** *see* Oprelvekin *on page 678*
- ◆ **Intralipid®** *see* Fat Emulsion *on page 359*
- ◆ **Intravenous Fat Emulsion** *see* Fat Emulsion *on page 359*
- ◆ **Intron® A** *see* Interferon Alfa-2b *on page 483*
- ◆ **Intropin® Injection** *see* Dopamine *on page 301*
- ◆ **Invirase®** *see* Saquinavir *on page 821*
- ◆ **Iobid DM®** *see* Guaifenesin and Dextromethorphan *on page 428*
- ◆ **Iodex® [OTC]** *see* Povidone-Iodine *on page 747*
- ◆ **Iodex-p® [OTC]** *see* Povidone-Iodine *on page 747*

## Iodinated Glycerol (EYE oh di nay ted GLI ser ole)

**Pharmacologic Class** Expectorant

**U.S. Brand Names** Iophen®; Organidin®; Par Glycerol®; R-Gen®

**Mechanism of Action** Increases respiratory tract secretions by decreasing surface tension and thereby decreases the viscosity of mucus, which aids in removal of the mucus

**Use** Mucolytic expectorant in adjunctive treatment of bronchitis, bronchial asthma, pulmonary emphysema, cystic fibrosis, or chronic sinusitis

**USUAL DOSAGE** Oral:

Children: Up to 30 mg 4 times/day

Adults: 60 mg 4 times/day

**Dosage Forms** Organically bound iodine in brackets. Elix: 60 mg/5 mL [30 mg/5 mL] (120 mL, 480 mL); Soln: 50 mg/mL [25 mg/mL] (30 mL); Tab: 30 mg [15 mg]

**Contraindications** Hypersensitivity to inorganic iodides, iodinated glycerol, or any component; pregnancy, newborns

**Warnings/Precautions** Use with caution in patients with thyroid disease or renal impairment

**Pregnancy Risk Factor** X

**Adverse Reactions**

1% to 10%: Gastrointestinal: Diarrhea, nausea, vomiting

<1%: Headache, acne, dermatitis, acute parotitis, thyroid gland enlargement, GI irritation, eyelid edema, pulmonary edema, hypersensitivity

**Drug Interactions** Increased toxicity: Disulfiram, metronidazole, procarbazine, MAO inhibitors, CNS depressants, lithium

**Special PA Issues**

**Patient Education:** Take with a full glass of water; not for use in coughs lasting longer than 1 week or associated with a fever

- ◆ **Iodochlorhydroxyquin** *see* Clioquinol *on page 219*

## Iodoquinol (eye oh doe KWIN ole)

**Pharmacologic Class** Amebicide

**U.S. Brand Names** Yodoxin®

**Mechanism of Action** Contact amebicide that works in the lumen of the intestine by an unknown mechanism

(Continued)

## Iodoquinol *(Continued)*

**Use** Treatment of acute and chronic intestinal amebiasis; asymptomatic cyst passers; *Blastocystis hominis* infections; ineffective for amebic hepatitis or hepatic abscess

**USUAL DOSAGE** Oral:

Children: 30-40 mg/kg/day (maximum: 650 mg/dose) in 3 divided doses for 20 days; not to exceed 1.95 g/day

Adults: 650 mg 3 times/day after meals for 20 days; not to exceed 1.95 g/day

**Dosage Forms Powder:** 25 g; **Tab:** 210 mg, 650 mg

**Contraindications** Known hypersensitivity to iodine or iodoquinol; hepatic damage; preexisting optic neuropathy

**Warnings/Precautions** Optic neuritis, optic atrophy, and peripheral neuropathy have occurred following prolonged use; avoid long-term therapy

**Pregnancy Risk Factor** C

**Adverse Reactions**

>10%: Gastrointestinal: Diarrhea, nausea, vomiting, stomach pain

1% to 10%:

Central nervous system: Fever, chills, agitation, retrograde amnesia, headache

Dermatologic: Rash, urticaria

Endocrine & metabolic: Thyroid gland enlargement

Neuromuscular & skeletal: Peripheral neuropathy, weakness

Ocular: Optic neuritis, optic atrophy, visual impairment

Miscellaneous: Itching of rectal area

**Special PA Issues**

**Patient Education:** Take as directed; complete full course of therapy. Maintain adequate hydration (2-3 L/day of fluids unless instructed to restrict fluid intake) and nutrition. If GI upset occurs, small frequent meals, frequent mouth care, and sucking on lozenges may help. Report unresolved or severe nausea or vomiting, skin rash, fever, or fatigue.

**Monitoring Parameters** Ophthalmologic exam

## Iodoquinol and Hydrocortisone

(eye oh doe KWIN ole & hye droe KOR ti sone)

**Pharmacologic Class** Antifungal Agent, Topical; Corticosteroid, Topical

**U.S. Brand Names** Vytone® Topical

**Dosage Forms Crm:** Iodoquinol 1% and hydrocortisone 1% (30 g)

♦ **Iofran ODT®** *see* Ondansetron *on page 675*

♦ **Ionamin®** *see* Phentermine *or page 716*

♦ **Iophen®** *see* Iodinated Glycerol *on previous page*

♦ **Iopidine®** *see* Apraclonidine *on page 76*

## Ioxilan (eye OKS ee lan)

**Pharmacologic Class** Radiopaque Agents

**U.S. Brand Names** Oxilan®

**Mechanism of Action** Ioxilan is a nonionic, water soluble, tri-iodinated x-ray contrast agent for intravascular injection. Intravascular injection of a radiopaque diagnostic agent opacifies those vessels in the path of flow of the contrast medium, permitting radiographic visualization of the internal structures of the human body until significant hemodilution occurs.

**Use**

Intra-arterial: Ioxilan 300 mg/mL is indicated for cerebral arteriography. Ioxilan 350 mg/mL is indicated for coronary arteriography and left ventriculography, visceral angiography, aortography, and peripheral arteriography

Intravenous: Both products are indicated for excretory urography and contrast enhanced computed tomographic (CECT) imaging of the head and body

**USUAL DOSAGE**

Intra-arterial: Coronary arteriography and left ventriculography: For visualization of coronary arteries and left ventricle, ioxilan injection with a concentration of 350 mg iodine/mL is recommended

Usual injection volumes:

Left and right coronary: 2-10 mL (0.7-3.5 g iodine)

Left ventricle: 25-50 mL (8.75-17.5 g iodine)

Total doses should not exceed 250 mL; the injection rate of ioxilan should approximate the flow rate in the vessel injected

Cerebral arteriography: For evaluation of arterial lesions of the brain, a concentration of 300 mg iodine/mL is indicated

Recommended doses: 8-12 mL (2.4-3.6 g iodine)

Total dose should not exceed 150 mL

**Dosage Forms Soln, for inj:** 300 mg/mL, 350 mg/mL

**Contraindications** Ioxilan injection is not indicated for intrathecal use

**Warnings/Precautions** Clotting has been reported when blood remains in contact with syringes containing ioxilan; use of plastic syringes in place of glass syringes has been reported to decrease, but not eliminate, the likelihood of *in vitro* clotting. Serious, rarely fatal, thromboembolic events causing myocardial infarction and stroke have been reported during angiographic procedures with both ionic and nonionic contrast media. Therefore, meticulous intravascular administration technique is necessary; caution must be exercised in patients with severely impaired renal function, combined renal and hepatic disease, combined renal and cardiac disease, severe thyrotoxicosis, myelomatosis, or anuria, particularly when large doses are administered.

Intravascularly administered ioxilan is potentially hazardous in patients with multiple myeloma or other paraproteinacious diseases, who are prone to disease-induced renal insufficiency and/or failure. Partial dehydration in the preparation of these patients prior to injection is not recommended since this may predispose the patient to precipitation of the myeloma protein. Reports of thyroid storm following the intravascular use of iodinated radiopaque agents in patients with hyperthyroidism, or with an autonomously functioning thyroid nodule, suggest that this additional risk be evaluated in such patients before use of any contrast agent. Administration of radiopaque materials to patients with known or suspected pheochromocytoma should be performed with extreme caution. Contrast agents may promote sickling in individuals who are homozygous for sickle cell disease when administered intravascularly.

**Pregnancy Risk Factor** B

**Adverse Reactions**
1% to 10%:
Cardiovascular: Angina (1.3%), hypertension (1.1%)
Central nervous system: Headache (3.6%), fever (1.7%)
Gastrointestinal: Nausea (1.5%)
<1%: Bradycardia (0.8%), hypotension (0.9%), dizziness (0.8%), chills (0.6%), urticaria (0.8%), rash (0.6%), vomiting (0.9%), diarrhea (0.9%), injection site hematomas (0.8%)

**Drug Interactions** Increased toxicity: Renal toxicity has been reported in a few patients with liver dysfunction who were given an oral cholecystographic agent followed by intravascular contrast agents such as ioxilan

**Special PA Issues**
**Patient Education:** Patients receiving iodinated intravascular contrast agents should be instructed to:
Inform physician if pregnant
Inform physician if diabetic or have multiple myeloma, pheochromocytoma, homozygous sickle cell disease, or known thyroid disorder
Inform physician if allergic to any drugs or food, or have immune, autoimmune, or immune deficiency disorders; also inform physician if previous reactions to injections of dyes used for x-ray procedures
Inform physician about all medications currently being taken, including nonprescription (over-the-counter) drugs, before having this procedure
**Monitoring Parameters:** Prior to and 24-48 hours after intravascular administration: Thyroid function tests, renal function tests, blood counts, serum electrolytes, and urinalysis should be monitored for and blood pressure, heart rate, electrocardiogram, and temperature should be monitored throughout the procedure

♦ **I-Paracaine®** see Proparacaine on page 771

# Ipecac Syrup (IP e kak SIR up)

**Pharmacologic Class** Antidote

**Mechanism of Action** Irritates the gastric mucosa and stimulates the medullary chemoreceptor trigger zone to induce vomiting

**Use** Treatment of acute oral drug overdosage and in certain poisonings

**USUAL DOSAGE** Oral:
Children:
6-12 months: 5-10 mL followed by 10-20 mL/kg of water; repeat dose one time if vomiting does not occur within 20 minutes
1-12 years: 15 mL followed by 10-20 mL/kg of water; repeat dose one time if vomiting does not occur within 20 minutes
If emesis does not occur within 30 minutes after second dose, ipecac must be removed from stomach by gastric lavage
Adults: 15-30 mL followed by 200-300 mL of water; repeat dose one time if vomiting does not occur within 20 minutes

**Dosage Forms Syr:** 70 mg/mL (15 mL, 30 mL, 473 mL, 4000 mL)

**Contraindications** Do not use in unconscious patients when time elapsed since exposure is >1 hour, patients with no gag reflex; following ingestion of strong bases or acids, volatile oils; when seizures are likely

**Warnings/Precautions** Do not confuse ipecac syrup with ipecac fluid extract, which is 14 times more potent; use with caution in patients with cardiovascular disease and bulimics; may not be effective in antiemetic overdose

**Pregnancy Risk Factor** C

**Adverse Reactions** 1% to 10%:
Cardiovascular: Cardiotoxicity
Central nervous system: Lethargy
(Continued)

## Ipecac Syrup *(Continued)*

Gastrointestinal: Protracted vomiting, diarrhea
Neuromuscular & skeletal: Myopathy

**Drug Interactions**
Decreased effect: Activated charcoal, milk, carbonated beverages
Increased toxicity: Phenothiazines (chlorpromazine has been associated with serious dystonic reactions)

**Onset** Within 15-30 minutes

**Duration** 20-25 minutes; can last longer, 60 minutes in some cases

**Special PA Issues**
**Patient Education:** The Poison Control Center should be contacted before administration. Take only as directed; do not take more than recommended or more often than recommended. Follow with 8 oz of water. If vomiting does not occur within 30 minutes, contact the Poison Control Center or emergency services again. Do not administer if vomiting. If vomiting occurs after taking, do not eat or drink until vomiting subsides.

♦ **I-Pentolate®** *see* Cyclopentolate *on page 244*

♦ **I-Phrine® Ophthalmic Solution** *see* Phenylephrine *on page 718*

## Ipratropium *(i pra TROE pee um)*

**Pharmacologic Class** Anticholinergic Agent

**U.S. Brand Names** Atrovent®

**Mechanism of Action** Blocks the action of acetylcholine at parasympathetic sites in bronchial smooth muscle causing bronchodilation

**Use** Anticholinergic bronchodilator in bronchospasm associated with COPD, bronchitis, and emphysema

**USUAL DOSAGE**
Children:
<2 years: Nebulization 250 mcg 3 times/day
3-14 years: Metered dose inhaler: 1-2 inhalations 3 times/day, up to 6 inhalations/24 hours
Children >12 years and Adults: Nebulization: 500 mcg (1 unit-dose vial) administered 3-4 times/day by oral nebulization, with doses 6-8 hours apart
Children >14 years and Adults: Metered dose inhaler: 2 inhalations 4 times/day every 4-6 hours up to 12 inhalations in 24 hours

**Dosage Forms Soln, as bromide:** Inhalation: 18 mcg/actuation (14 g), Nasal spray: 0.03% (30 mL); 0.06% (15 mL), Nebulizing: 0.02% (2.5 mL)

**Contraindications** Hypersensitivity to atropine or its derivatives

**Warnings/Precautions** Not indicated for the initial treatment of acute episodes of bronchospasm; use with caution in patients with narrow-angle glaucoma, prostatic hypertrophy, or bladder neck obstruction; ipratropium has not been specifically studied in the elderly, but it is poorly absorbed from the airways and appears to be safe in this population.

**Pregnancy Risk Factor** 3

**Adverse Reactions Note** Ipratropium is poorly absorbed from the lung, so systemic effects are rare
>10%:
Central nervous system: Nervousness, dizziness, fatigue, headache
Gastrointestinal: Nausea, xerostomia, stomach upset
Respiratory: Cough
1% to 10%:
Cardiovascular: Palpitations, hypotension
Central nervous system: Insomnia
Genitourinary: Urinary retention
Neuromuscular & skeletal: Trembling
Ocular: Blurred vision
Respiratory: Nasal congestion
<1%: Rash, urticaria, stomatitis

**Drug Interactions**
Increased effect with albuterol
Increased toxicity with anticholinergics or drugs with anticholinergic properties, dronabinol

**Onset** Onset of bronchodilation: 1-3 minutes after administration; Peak effect: Within 1.5-2 hours

**Duration** Up to 4-6 hours

**Special PA Issues**
**Patient Education:** Use exactly as directed (see below). Do not use more often than recommended. Store solution away from light. Maintain adequate hydration (2-3 L/day of fluids unless instructed to restrict fluid intake). You may experience sensitivity to heat (avoid extremes in temperature); nervousness, dizziness, or fatigue (use caution when driving or engaging in hazardous activities until response to treatment is known); dry mouth, unpleasant taste, stomach upset (frequent small meals, frequent mouth care, chewing gum, or sucking hard candy may help); or difficulty urinating (always void before

treatment). Report unresolved GI upset, dizziness or fatigue, vision changes, palpitations, persistent inability to void, nervousness, or insomnia.

**Administration:**
Inhaler: Follow instructions for use accompanying the product. Close eyes when administering ipratropium; blurred vision may result if sprayed into eyes. Effects are enhanced by holding breath 10 seconds after inhalation; wait at least 1 full minute between inhalations.

Nebulizer: Wash hands before and after treatment. Wash and dry nebulizer after each treatment. Twist open the top of one unit dose vial and squeeze the contents into the nebulizer reservoir. Connect the nebulizer reservoir to the mouthpiece or face mask. Connect the nebulizer reservoir to the mouthpiece or face mask. Connect nebulizer to compressor. Sit in a comfortable, upright position. Place mouthpiece in your mouth or put on the face mask and turn on the compressor. If a face mask is used, avoid leakage around the mask (temporary blurring of vision, worsening of narrow-angle glaucoma, or eye pain may occur if mist gets into eyes). Breathe calmly and deeply until no more mist is formed in the nebulizer (about 5 minutes). At this point, treatment is finished.

# Ipratropium and Albuterol (i pra TROE pee um & al BYOO ter ole)
**Pharmacologic Class** Bronchodilator
**U.S. Brand Names** Combivent®
**Dosage Forms Aero:** Ipratropium bromide 18 mcg and albuterol sulfate 103 mcg per actuation [200 doses] (14.7 g)

♦ **Ipratropium Bromide** see Ipratropium on previous page

♦ **Iproveratril Hydrochloride** see Verapamil on page 959

# Irbesartan (ir be SAR tan)
**Pharmacologic Class** Angiotensin II Antagonists
**U.S. Brand Names** Avapro®
**Mechanism of Action** Irbesartan is an angiotensin receptor antagonist. Angiotensin II acts as a vasoconstrictor. In addition to causing direct vasoconstriction, angiotensin II also stimulates the release of aldosterone. Once aldosterone is released, sodium as well as water are reabsorbed. The end result is an elevation in blood pressure. Irbesartan binds to the AT1 angiotensin II receptor. This binding prevents angiotensin II from binding to the receptor thereby blocking the vasoconstriction and the aldosterone secreting effects of angiotensin II.

**Use** Treatment of hypertension alone or in combination with other antihypertensives
**USUAL DOSAGE** Adults: Oral: 150 mg once daily with or without food; patients may be titrated to 300 mg once daily
**Dosage Forms Tab:** 75 mg, 150 mg, 300 mg
**Contraindications** Hypersensitivity to any component
**Warnings/Precautions** Avoid use or use a much smaller dose in patients who are intravascularly volume-depleted; use caution in patients with unilateral or bilateral renal artery stenosis to avoid a decrease in renal function; AUCs of irbesartan (not the active metabolite) are about 50% greater in patients with $Cl_{cr}$ <30 mL/minute and are doubled in hemodialysis patients
**Pregnancy Risk Factor** C (1st trimester); D (2nd and 3rd trimesters)
**Adverse Reactions** 1% to 10%:
Cardiovascular: Edema, chest pain, tachycardia
Central nervous system: Dizziness, headache, fatigue, anxiety, nervousness
Dermatologic: Rash
Gastrointestinal: Diarrhea, dyspepsia/heartburn, nausea, vomiting, abdominal pain
Genitourinary: Urinary tract infection
Neuromuscular & skeletal: Pain, trauma
Respiratory: Upper respiratory infection, cough, sinus disorder, pharyngitis, rhinitis, influenza
**Drug Interactions** CYP2C9 enzyme substrate
**Onset** Peak levels in 1-2 hours
**Duration** >24 hours
**Half-Life** 11-15 hours
**Special PA Issues**
**Patient Education:** Take exactly as directed with or without food. Do not change dosage or stop taking without consulting prescriber. Do not change amount of dietary salt or increase potassium intake without advice or consult of prescriber. You may experience dizziness, fainting, or lightheadedness; use caution when driving or performing hazardous tasks and use caution when changing position (rising from sitting or lying position) until response to therapy is established. Report sore throat, fever, rash; chest pain, unusual heartbeat, palpitations or swelling of hands, feet, or legs; respiratory difficulty or unusual cough; persistent vomiting, diarrhea, sweating, or perspiration; or any changes in urinary pattern.

## Irbesartan and Hydrochlorothiazide
(ir be SAR tan & hye droe klor oh THYE a zide)

**Pharmacologic Class** Antihypertensive Agent, Combination

**U.S. Brand Names** Avapro® HCT

**Dosage Forms Tab:** Irbesartan 150 mg and hydrochlorothiazide 12.5 mg; irbesartan 300 mg and hydrochlorothiazide 12.5 mg

• **Ircon®** [OTC] see Ferrous Fumarate on page 366

## Iron Dextran Complex (EYE ern DEKS tran KOM pleks)

**Pharmacologic Class** Iron Salt

**U.S. Brand Names** Dexferrum®; InFed™ Injection

**Mechanism of Action** The released iron, from the plasma, eventually replenishes the depleted iron stores in the bone marrow where it is incorporated into hemoglobin

**Use** Treatment of microcytic hypochromic anemia resulting from iron deficiency in whom oral administration is infeasible or ineffective

**USUAL DOSAGE** I.M. (Z-track method should be used for I.M. injection), I.V.:

A 0.5 mL test dose (0.25 mL in infants) should be given prior to starting iron dextran therapy; total dose should be divided into a daily schedule for I.M., total dose may be given as a single continuous infusion

Iron deficiency anemia: Dose (mL) = 0.0476 x wt (kg) x (normal hemoglobin - observed hemoglobin) + (1 mL/5 kg) to maximum of 14 mL for iron stores

Iron replacement therapy for blood loss: Replacement iron (mg) = blood loss (mL) x hematocrit

Maximum daily dose (can administer total dose at one time I.V.):

Infants <5 kg: 25 mg iron (0.5 mL)

Children:

5-10 kg: 50 mg iron (1 mL)

10-50 kg: 100 mg iron (2 mL)

Adults >50 kg: 100 mg iron (2 mL)

**Dosage Forms Inj:** 50 mg/mL (2 mL, 10 mL)

**Contraindications** Hypersensitivity to iron dextran, all anemias that are not involved with iron deficiency, hemochromatosis, hemolytic anemia

**Warnings/Precautions** Use with caution in patients with history of asthma, hepatic impairment, rheumatoid arthritis; not recommended in children <4 months of age; deaths associated with parenteral administration following anaphylactic-type reactions have been reported; use only in patients where the iron deficient state is not amenable to oral iron therapy. A test dose of 0.5 mL I.V. or I.M. should be given to observe for adverse reactions. Anemia in the elderly is often caused by "anemia of chronic disease" or associated with inflammation rather than blood loss. Iron stores are usually normal or increased, with a serum ferritin >50 ng/mL and a decreased total iron binding capacity. I.V. administration of iron dextran is often preferred over I.M. in the elderly secondary to a decreased muscle mass and the need for daily injections.

**Pregnancy Risk Factor** C

**Adverse Reactions**

Cardiovascular: Cardiovascular collapse, hypotension

Dermatologic: Urticaria

Hematologic: Leukocytosis

>10%:

Cardiovascular: Flushing

Central nervous system: Dizziness, fever, headache, pain

Gastrointestinal: Nausea, vomiting, metallic taste

Local: Staining of skin at the site of I.M. injection, phlebitis,

Miscellaneous: Diaphoresis

1% to 10%:

Gastrointestinal: Diarrhea

Genitourinary: Discoloration of urine

<1%: Chills, phlebitis, arthralgia, respiratory difficulty, lymphadenopathy

**Note:** Diaphoresis, urticaria, arthralgia, fever, chills, dizziness, headache, and nausea may be delayed 24-48 hours after I.V. administration or 3-4 days after I.M. administration

Anaphylactoid reactions: Respiratory difficulties and cardiovascular collapse have been reported and occur most frequently within the first several minutes of administration

**Drug Interactions** Decreased effect with chloramphenicol

**Special PA Issues**

**Patient Education:** You will need frequent blood tests while on this therapy. If you have rheumatoid arthritis you may experience increased swelling or joint pain; consult prescriber for medication adjustment. If you experience dizziness or severe headache, use caution when driving or engaging in hazardous activities. Small frequent meals, frequent mouth care, or sucking on lozenges may relieve nausea and metallic taste. You may experience increased sweating. Report acute GI problems, fever, difficulty breathing, rapid heartbeat, yellowing of skin or eyes, or swelling of hands and feet.

**Monitoring Parameters:** Hemoglobin, hematocrit, reticulocyte count, serum ferritin
**Reference Range:**
Hemoglobin 14.8 mg % (for weight >15 kg), hemoglobin 12.0 mg % (for weight <15 kg)
Serum iron: 40-160 µg/dL
Total iron binding capacity: 230-430 µg/dL
Transferrin: 204-360 mg/dL
Percent transferrin saturation: 20% to 50%

## Isoetharine (eye soe ETH a reen)

**Pharmacologic Class** Adrenergic Agonist Agent; Bronchodilator; Sympathomimetic
**U.S. Brand Names** Arm-a-Med® Isoetharine; Beta-2®; Bronkometer®; Bronkosol®; Dey-Lute® Isoetharine
**Mechanism of Action** Relaxes bronchial smooth muscle by action on beta$_2$-receptors with very little effect on heart rate
**Use** Bronchodilator in bronchial asthma and for reversible bronchospasm occurring with bronchitis and emphysema
**USUAL DOSAGE** Treatments are not usually repeated more than every 4 hours, except in severe cases

Nebulizer: Children: 0.01 mL/kg; minimum dose 0.1 mL; maximum dose: 0.5 mL diluted in 2-3 mL normal saline

Inhalation: Oral: Adults: 1-2 inhalations every 4 hours as needed
**Dosage Forms** Isoetharine hydrochloride: **Soln, inh:** 0.062% (4 mL), 0.08% (3.5 mL), 0.1% (2.5 mL, 5 mL), 0.125% (4 mL), 0.167% (3 mL), 0.17% (3 mL), 0.2% (2.5 mL), 0.25% (2 mL, 3.5 mL), 0.5% (0.5 mL), 1% (0.5 mL, 0.25 mL, 10 mL, 14 mL, 30 mL);
Isoetharine mesylate: **Aero, oral:** 340 mcg/metered spray
**Contraindications** Known hypersensitivity to isoetharine
**Warnings/Precautions** Excessive or prolonged use may result in decreased effectiveness
**Pregnancy Risk Factor** C
**Adverse Reactions**
1% to 10%:
Cardiovascular: Tachycardia, hypertension, pounding heartbeat
Central nervous system: Dizziness, lightheadedness, headache, nervousness, insomnia
Gastrointestinal: Xerostomia, nausea, vomiting
Neuromuscular & skeletal: Trembling, weakness
<1%: Paradoxical bronchospasm
**Drug Interactions**
Decreased effect with beta-blockers
Increased toxicity with other sympathomimetics (eg, epinephrine)
**Onset** Peak effect: Inhaler: Within 5-15 minutes
**Duration** 1-4 hours
**Special PA Issues**
**Patient Education:** Use as directed (see below). Do not use more often than recommended. Store solution away from light. You may experience nervousness, dizziness, or fatigue; use caution when driving or engaging in hazardous activities until response to treatment is known. Frequent small meals may reduce incidence of nausea or vomiting. Report unresolved/persistent GI upset, rapid heartbeat or palpitations, dizziness or fatigue, trembling, or difficulty breathing.

**Administration:** Shake canister well before use. Administer pressurized inhalation during the second half of inspiration. If more than one inhalation per dose is necessary, wait at least 1 full minute between inhalations; second inhalation is best delivered after 10 minutes.

**Monitoring Parameters:** Heart rate, blood pressure, respiratory rate

## Isoflurophate (eye soe FLURE oh fate)

**Pharmacologic Class** Acetylcholinesterase Inhibitor (Central); Ophthalmic Agent, Antiglaucoma; Ophthalmic Agent, Miotic

**U.S. Brand Names** Floropryl® Ophthalmic

**Mechanism of Action** Cholinesterase inhibitor that causes contraction of the iris and ciliary muscles producing miosis, reduced intraocular pressure, and increased aqueous humor outflow

**Use** Treat primary open-angle glaucoma and conditions that obstruct aqueous outflow and to treat accommodative convergent strabismus

**USUAL DOSAGE** Adults: Ophthalmic:

Glaucoma: Instill 0.25" strip in eye every 8-72 hours

Strabismus: Instill 0.25" strip to each eye every night for 2 weeks then reduce to 0.25" every other night to once weekly for 2 months

**Dosage Forms** Oint, ophth: 0.025% in polyethylene mineral oil gel (3.5 g)

**Contraindications** Active uveal inflammation, angle-closure (narrow-angle) glaucoma, known hypersensitivity to isoflurophate, pregnancy

**Warnings/Precautions** May retard corneal healing; because of the tendency to produce more severe adverse effects, use the lowest dose possible; keep frequency of use to a minimum to avoid cyst formation; some products may contain sulfites

**Pregnancy Risk Factor** X

**Adverse Reactions**

1% to 10%: Ocular: Stinging, burning eyes, myopia, visual blurring

<1%: Bradycardia, hypotension, flushing, nausea, vomiting, diarrhea, muscle weakness, retinal detachment, browache, miosis, twitching eyelids, watering eyes, dyspnea, diaphoresis

**Drug Interactions** Increased toxicity: Succinylcholine, systemic anticholinesterases, carbamate or organic phosphate insecticides, may decrease cholinesterase levels

**Onset** Peak IOP reduction: 24 hours; Onset of miosis: Within 5-10 minutes

**Duration** IOP reduction: 1 week; Miosis: Up to 4 weeks

**Special PA Issues**

**Patient Education:** For ophthalmic use only. Apply prescribed amount as often as directed. Wash hands before using and do not touch tip of applicator to eye or contaminate tip of applicator. Tilt head back and look upward. Gently pull down lower lid and put drop(s) inside lower eyelid at inner corner. Close eye and roll eyeball in all directions. Do not blink for 1/2 minute. Apply gentle pressure to inner corner of eye for 30 seconds. Wipe away excess from skin around eye. Do not use any other eye preparation for at least 10 minutes. Do not share medication with anyone else. Temporary stinging or blurred vision may occur. Immediately report any adverse cardiac or CNS effects (usually signifies overdose). Report persistent eye pain, redness, burning, watering, dryness, double vision, puffiness around eye, vision disturbances, other adverse eye response, worsening of condition or lack of improvement.

♦ **Isollyl® Improved** *see* Butalbital Compound *on page 131*

## Isoniazid (eye soe NYE a zid)

**Pharmacologic Class** Antitubercular Agent

**U.S. Brand Names** Laniazid®; Nydrazid®

**Mechanism of Action** Unknown, but may include the inhibition of myocolic acid synthesis resulting in disruption of the bacterial cell wall

**Use** Treatment of susceptible tuberculosis infections and prophylactically to those individuals exposed to tuberculosis

**USUAL DOSAGE** Recommendations often change due to resistant strains and newly developed information; consult *MMWR* for current CDC recommendations: **Oral** (intramuscular is available in patients who are unable to either take or absorb oral therapy):

**Note:** A four-drug regimen (isoniazid, rifampin, pyrazinamide, and either streptomycin or ethambutol) is preferred for the initial, empiric treatment of TB. When the drug susceptibility results are available, the regimen should be altered as appropriate.

Infants and Children:

Prophylaxis: 10 mg/kg/day in 1-2 divided doses (maximum: 300 mg/day) 6 months in patients who do not have HIV infection and 12 months in patients who have HIV infection

Treatment:

Daily therapy: 10-20 mg/kg/day in 1-2 divided doses (maximum: 300 mg/day)

Directly observed therapy (DOT): Twice weekly therapy: 20-40 mg/kg (maximum: 900 mg/day); 3 times/week therapy: 20-40 mg/kg (maximum: 900 mg)

Adults:

Prophylaxis: 300 mg/day for 6 months in patients who do not have HIV infection and 12 months in patients who have HIV infection

Treatment:

Daily therapy: 5 mg/kg/day given daily (usual dose: 300 mg/day); 10 mg/kg/day in 1-2 divided doses in patients with disseminated disease

Directly observed therapy (DOT): Twice weekly therapy: 15 mg/kg (maximum: 900 mg); 3 times/week therapy: 15 mg/kg (maximum: 900 mg)

**Note:** Concomitant administration of 6-50 mg/day pyridoxine is recommended in malnourished patients or those prone to neuropathy (eg, alcoholics, diabetics)

**Hemodialysis:** Dialyzable (50% to 100%)

Administer dose postdialysis

**Peritoneal dialysis effects:** Dose for $Cl_{cr}$ <10 mL/minute

**Continuous arteriovenous or venovenous hemofiltration (CAVH/CAVHD):** Dose for $Cl_{cr}$ <10 mL/minute

**Dosing adjustment in hepatic impairment:** Dose should be reduced in severe hepatic disease

**Dosage Forms Inj:** 100 mg/mL (10 mL); **Syr** (orange flavor): 50 mg/5 mL (473 mL); **Tab:** 50 mg, 100 mg, 300 mg

**Contraindications** Acute liver disease; hypersensitivity to isoniazid or any component; previous history of hepatic damage during isoniazid therapy

**Warnings/Precautions** Use with caution in patients with renal impairment and chronic liver disease. Severe and sometimes fatal hepatitis may occur or develop even after many months of treatment; patients must report any prodromal symptoms of hepatitis, such as fatigue, weakness, malaise, anorexia, nausea, or vomiting. Children with low milk and low meat intake should receive concomitant pyridoxine therapy. Periodic ophthalmic examinations are recommended even when usual symptoms do not occur; pyridoxine (10-50 mg/day) is recommended in individuals likely to develop peripheral neuropathies.

**Pregnancy Risk Factor** C

**Adverse Reactions**

>10%:

Gastrointestinal: Loss of appetite, nausea, vomiting, stomach pain

Hepatic: Mild increased LFTs (10% to 20%)

Neuromuscular & skeletal: Weakness, peripheral neuropathy (dose-related incidence, 10% to 20% incidence with 10 mg/kg/day)

1% to 10%:

Central nervous system: Dizziness, slurred speech, lethargy

Hepatic: Progressive liver damage (increases with age; 2.3% in patients >50 years of age)

Neuromuscular & skeletal: Hyper-reflexia

<1%: Fever, seizures, mental depression, psychosis, rash, blood dyscrasias, arthralgia, blurred vision, loss of vision

**Drug Interactions** CYP2E1 enzyme substrate; CYP2E1 enzyme inducer; and CYP1A2, 2C, 2C9, 2C18, 2C19, and 3A3/4 enzyme inhibitor

Decreased effect of ketoconazole with isoniazid

Decreased effect/levels of isoniazid with aluminum salts

Increased toxicity/levels of oral anticoagulants, carbamazepine, cycloserine, meperidine, hydantoins, hepatically metabolized benzodiazepines with isoniazid; reaction with disulfiram occurs; enflurane with isoniazid may result in renal failure especially in rapid acetylators

Increased hepatic toxicity with alcohol or with rifampin and isoniazid

**Half-Life**

Fast acetylators: 30-100 minutes

Slow acetylators: 2-5 hours; half-life may be prolonged in patients with impaired hepatic function or severe renal impairment

**Special PA Issues**

**Patient Education:** Best if taken on an empty stomach (1 hour before or 2 hours after meals). Avoid missing any dose and do not discontinue without notifying prescriber. Avoid alcohol and tyramine-containing foods (eg, fish, preserved meats or sausages, tuna, sauerkraut, aged cheeses, broad beans, liver pate, wine, protein supplements, etc). Increase dietary intake of folate, niacin, magnesium. If diabetic, use serum testing (isoniazid may affect Clinitest® results). You may experience GI distress (taking dose with meals may help). Use caution to prevent injury. You will need to have frequent ophthalmic exams and periodic medical check-ups to evaluate drug effects. Report tingling or numbness in hands or feet, loss of sensation, unusual weakness, fatigue, nausea or vomiting, dark colored urine, change in urinary pattern, yellowing skin or eyes, or change in color of stool.

**Monitoring Parameters:** Periodic liver function tests; monitoring for prodromal signs of hepatitis

**Reference Range:** Therapeutic: 1-7 µg/mL (SI: 7-51 µmol/L); Toxic: 20-710 µg/mL (SI: 146-5176 µmol/L)

**Related Information**

Tyramine-Containing Foods *on page 1148*

- ◆ **Isonicotinic Acid Hydrazide** *see* Isoniazid *on previous page*
- ◆ **Isonipecaine Hydrochloride** *see* Meperidine *on page 567*
- ◆ **Isopap®** *see* Acetaminophen, Isometheptene, and Dichloralphenazone *on page 23*
- ◆ **Isoprenaline Hydrochloride** *see* Isoproterenol *on next page*

♦ **Isopro®** see Isoproterenol *on this page*

# Isoproterenol (eye soe proe TER e nole)

**Pharmacologic Class** Beta₁, Beta₂ Agonist

**U.S. Brand Names** Aerolone®; Arm-a-Med® Isoproterenol; Dey-Dose® Isoproterenol; Dispos-a-Med® Isoproterenol; Isopro®; Isuprel®; Medihaler-Iso®; Norisodrine®; Vapo-Iso®

**Mechanism of Action** Stimulates beta₁- and beta₂-receptors resulting in relaxation of bronchial, GI, and uterine smooth muscle, increased heart rate and contractility, vasodilation of peripheral vasculature

**Use** Treatment of reversible airway obstruction as in asthma or COPD; used parenterally in ventricular arrhythmias due to A-V nodal block; hemodynamically compromised bradyarrhythmias or atropine-resistant bradyarrhythmias; temporary use in third degree A-V block until pacemaker insertion; low cardiac output; vasoconstrictive shock states

## USUAL DOSAGE

Children:

Bronchodilation: Inhalation: Metered dose inhaler: 1-2 metered doses up to 5 times/day

Bronchodilation (using 1:200 inhalation solution) 0.01 mL/kg/dose every 4 hours as needed (maximum: 0.05 mL/dose) diluted with NS to 2 mL

Sublingual: 5-10 mg every 3-4 hours, not to exceed 30 mg/day

Cardiac arrhythmias: I.V.: Start 0.1 mcg/kg/minute (usual effective dose 0.2-2 mcg/kg/minute)

Adults:

Bronchodilation: Inhalation: Metered dose inhaler: 1-2 metered doses 4-6 times/day

Bronchodilation: 1-2 inhalations of a 0.25% solution, no more than 2 inhalations at any one time (1-5 minutes between inhalations); no more than 6 inhalations in any hour during a 24-hour period: maintenance therapy: 1-2 inhalations 4-6 times/day. Alternatively: 0.5% solution via hand bulb nebulizer is 5-15 deep inhalations repeated once in 5-10 minutes if necessary; treatments may be repeated up to 5 times/day.

Sublingual: 10-20 mg every 3-4 hours; not to exceed 60 mg/day

Cardiac arrhythmias: I.V.: 5 mcg/minute initially, titrate to patient response (2-20 mcg/minute)

Shock: I.V.: 0.5-5 mcg/minute; adjust according to response

**Dosage Forms** Isoprenaline hydrochloride: **Inh: Aero:** 0.2% (1:500) (15 mL, 22.5 mL), 0.25% (1:400) (15 mL); **Soln for nebulization:** 0.031% (4 mL), 0.062% (4 mL), 0.25% (0.5 mL, 30 mL), 0.5% (0.5 mL, 10 mL, 60 mL), 1% (10 mL); **Inj:** 0.2 mg/mL (1:5000) (1 mL, 5 mL, 10 mL); **Tab, sublingual:** 10 mg, 15 mg

**Contraindications** Angina, pre-existing cardiac arrhythmias (ventricular); tachycardia or A-V block caused by cardiac glycoside intoxication; allergy to sulfites or isoproterenol or other sympathomimetic amines

**Warnings/Precautions** Elderly patients, diabetics, renal or cardiovascular disease, hyperthyroidism; excessive or prolonged use may result in decreased effectiveness

**Pregnancy Risk Factor** C

**Adverse Reactions**

>10%:

Central nervous system: Insomnia, restlessness

Gastrointestinal: Dry throat, xerostomia, discoloration of saliva (pinkish-red)

1% to 10%:

Cardiovascular: Flushing of the face or skin, ventricular arrhythmias, tachycardias, profound hypotension, hypertension

Central nervous system: Nervousness, anxiety, dizziness, headache, lightheadedness

Gastrointestinal: Vomiting, nausea

Neuromuscular & skeletal: Trembling, tremor, weakness

Miscellaneous: Diaphoresis

<1%: Arrhythmias, chest pain, paradoxical bronchospasm

**Drug Interactions** Increased toxicity: Sympathomimetic agents may cause headaches and elevate blood pressure; general anesthetics may cause arrhythmias

**Onset** Onset of bronchodilation: Oral inhalation: Immediately

**Duration** Oral inhalation: 1 hour; S.C.: Up to 2 hours

**Half-Life** 2.5-5 minutes

**Special PA Issues**

**Patient Education:**

Sublingual: Do not chew or swallow tables, let them dissolve under the tongue.

Inhalant: Shake canister before use. Administer pressurized inhalation during the second half of inspiration. If more than one dose is necessary, wait at least 1 full minute between inhalations; second inhalation is best delivered after 5-10 minutes. Do not use more often than recommended. Store solution away from light or excess heat or cold.

You may experience nervousness, dizziness, or fatigue. Use caution when driving or engaging in hazardous activities until response to treatment is known. Frequent small meals may reduce the incidence of nausea or vomiting. Report chest pain, rapid heartbeat or palpitations, unresolved/persistent GI upset, dizziness, fatigue, trembling, increased anxiety, sleeplessness, or difficulty breathing.

**Monitoring Parameters:** EKG, heart rate, respiratory rate, arterial blood gas, arterial blood pressure, CVP

# Isoproterenol and Phenylephrine (eye soe proe TER e nole & fen il EF rin)

**Pharmacologic Class** Adrenergic Agonist Agent

**U.S. Brand Names** Duo-Medihaler® Aerosol

**Dosage Forms Aero:** Each actuation releases isoproterenol hydrochloride 0.16 mg and phenylephrine bitartrate 0.24 mg (15 mL, 22.5 mL)

♦ **Isoproterenol Hydrochloride** *see* Isoproterenol *on previous page*

♦ **Isoproterenol Sulfate** *see* Isoproterenol *on previous page*

♦ **Isoptin®** *see* Verapamil *on page 959*

♦ **Isoptin® SR** *see* Verapamil *on page 959*

♦ **Isopto® Atropine Ophthalmic** *see* Atropine *on page 87*

♦ **Isopto® Carbachol Ophthalmic** *see* Carbachol *on page 148*

♦ **Isopto® Carpine Ophthalmic** *see* Pilocarpine *on page 726*

♦ **Isopto® Cetamide Ophthalmic** *see* Sulfacetamide Sodium *on page 858*

♦ **Isopto® Cetapred® Ophthalmic** *see* Sulfacetamide Sodium and Prednisolone *on page 859*

♦ **Isopto® Eserine** *see* Physostigmine *on page 724*

♦ **Isopto® Frin Ophthalmic Solution** *see* Phenylephrine *on page 718*

♦ **Isopto® Homatropine Ophthalmic** *see* Homatropine *on page 443*

♦ **Isopto® Hyoscine Ophthalmic** *see* Scopolamine *on page 824*

♦ **Isordil®** *see* Isosorbide Dinitrate *on next page*

# Isosorbide (eye soe SOR bide)

**Pharmacologic Class** Diuretic, Osmotic; Ophthalmic Agent, Antiglaucoma; Ophthalmic Agent, Osmotic

**U.S. Brand Names** Ismotic®

**Mechanism of Action** Elevates osmolarity of glomerular filtrate to hinder the tubular resorption of water and increase excretion of sodium and chloride to result in diuresis; creates an osmotic gradient between plasma and ocular fluids

**Use** Short-term emergency treatment of acute angle-closure glaucoma and short-term reduction of intraocular pressure prior to and following intraocular surgery; may be used to interrupt an acute glaucoma attack; preferred agent when need to avoid nausea and vomiting

**USUAL DOSAGE** Adults: Oral: Initial: 1.5 g/kg with a usual range of 1-3 g/kg 2-4 times/day as needed

**Dosage Forms Soln:** 45% [450 mg/mL] (220 mL)

**Contraindications** Severe renal disease, anuria, severe dehydration, acute pulmonary edema, severe cardiac decompensation, known hypersensitivity to isosorbide

**Warnings/Precautions** Use with caution in patients with impending pulmonary edema and in the elderly due to the elderly's predisposition to dehydration and the fact that they frequently have concomitant diseases which may be aggravated by the use of isosorbide; hypernatremia and dehydration may begin to occur after 72 hours of continuous administration. Maintain fluid/electrolyte balance with multiple doses; monitor urinary output; if urinary output declines, need to review clinical status.

**Pregnancy Risk Factor** B

**Adverse Reactions**

1% to 10%:

Central nervous system: Headache, confusion, disorientation

Gastrointestinal: Vomiting

<1%: Syncope, lethargy, vertigo, dizziness, lightheadedness, irritability, rash, hypernatremia, hyperosmolarity, nausea, abdominal/gastric discomfort (infrequently), anorexia, hiccups, thirst

**Onset** Onset of action: Within 10-30 minutes; Peak action: 1-1.5 hours

**Duration** 5-6 hours

**Half-Life** 5-9.5 hours

**Special PA Issues**

**Patient Education:** This is for short-term treatment, it is not for long-term use. Pour over cracked ice and sip. Take all of medication. You may experience frequent urination (maintain adequate hydration - 2-3 L/day of fluids unless instructed to restrict fluid intake); gastric upset (small frequent meals may help); dizziness, drowsiness, or confusion (use caution when driving); or dry mouth (chewing gum, frequent oral care, sucking on lozenges may help). Report difficulty breathing, unrelieved headache, changes in CNS (eg, confusion or disorientation).

**Monitoring Parameters:** Monitor for signs of dehydration, blood pressure, renal output, intraocular pressure reduction

# Isosorbide Dinitrate (eye soe SOR bide dye NYE trate)

**Pharmacologic Class** Vasodilator

**U.S. Brand Names** Dilatrate®-SR; Isordil®; Sorbitrate®

**Mechanism of Action** Stimulation of intracellular cyclic-GMP results in vascular smooth muscle relaxation of both arterial and venous vasculature. Increased venous pooling decreases left ventricular pressure (preload) and arterial dilatation decreases arterial resistance (afterload). Therefore, this reduces cardiac oxygen demand by decreasing left ventricular pressure and systemic vascular resistance by dilating arteries. Additionally, coronary artery dilation improves collateral flow to ischemic regions; esophageal smooth muscle is relaxed via the same mechanism.

**Use** Prevention and treatment of angina pectoris; for congestive heart failure; to relieve pain, dysphagia, and spasm in esophageal spasm with GE reflux

**USUAL DOSAGE** Adults (elderly should be given lowest recommended daily doses initially and titrate upward): Oral:

Angina: 5-40 mg 4 times/day or 40 mg every 8-12 hours in sustained-release dosage form

Congestive heart failure:

Initial dose: 10 mg 3 times/day

Target dose: 40 mg 3 times/day

Maximum dose: 80 mg 3 times/day

Sublingual: 2.5-10 mg every 4-6 hours

Chew: 5-10 mg every 2-3 hours

**Tolerance to nitrate effects develops with chronic exposure**

Dose escalation does not overcome this effect. Tolerance can only be overcome by short periods of nitrate absence from the body. Short periods (14 hours) or nitrate withdrawal help minimize tolerance

Hemodialysis: During hemodialysis, administer dose postdialysis or administer supplemental 10-20 mg dose

Peritoneal dialysis: Supplemental dose is not necessary

**Dosage Forms Cap, sustained release:** 40 mg; **Tab: Chewable:** 5 mg, 10 mg; **Oral:** 5 mg, 10 mg, 20 mg, 30 mg; **Subl:** 2.5 mg, 5 mg, 10 mg; **Sustained release:** 40 mg

**Contraindications** Severe anemia, closed-angle glaucoma, postural hypotension, cerebral hemorrhage, head trauma, hypersensitivity to isosorbide dinitrate or any component

**Warnings/Precautions** Use with caution in patients with increased intracranial pressure, hypotension, hypovolemia, glaucoma; sustained release products may be absorbed erratically in patients with GI hypermotility or malabsorption syndrome; do not crush or chew sublingual dosage form; abrupt withdrawal may result in angina; tolerance may develop (adjust dose or change agent)

**Pregnancy Risk Factor** C

**Adverse Reactions**

>10%:

Cardiovascular: Flushing, postural hypotension

Central nervous system: Headache, lightheadedness, dizziness

Neuromuscular & skeletal: Weakness

1% to 10%: Dermatologic: Drug rash, exfoliative dermatitis

<1%: Nausea, vomiting methemoglobinemia (overdose)

**Onset**

Sublingual tablet: 2-10 minutes

Chewable tablet: 3 minutes

Oral tablet: 45-60 minutes

Sustained release tablet: 30 minutes

**Duration** Sublingual tablet: 1-2 hours; Chewable tablet: 0.5-2 hours; Oral tablet: 4-6 hours; Sustained release tablet: 6-12 hours

**Half-Life** Parent drug: 1-4 hours; Metabolite (5-mononitrate): 4 hours

**Special PA Issues**

**Patient Education:** Take as directed, at same time each day. Do not chew or swallow sublingual tablets; allow them to dissolve under your tongue. Do not change brands without consulting prescriber. Do not discontinue abruptly. Keep medication in original container, tightly closed. Avoid alcohol; combination may cause severe hypotension. Take medication while sitting down and use caution when changing position (rise from sitting or lying position slowly). May cause dizziness; use caution when driving or engaging in hazardous activities until response to drug is known. If chest pain is unresolved in 15 minutes, seek emergency medical help at once. Report acute headache, rapid heartbeat, unusual restlessness or dizziness, muscular weakness, or blurring vision.

**Monitoring Parameters:** Monitor for orthostasis

**Related Information**

Heart Failure: Management of Patients with Left Ventricular Systolic Dysfunction *on page 1064*

## Isosorbide Mononitrate (eye soe SOR bide mon oh NYE trate)

**Pharmacologic Class** Vasodilator

**U.S. Brand Names** Imdur™; Ismo®; Monoket®

**Mechanism of Action** Prevailing mechanism of action for nitroglycerin (and other nitrates) is systemic venodilation, decreasing preload as measured by pulmonary capillary wedge pressure and left ventricular end diastolic volume and pressure; the average reduction in left ventricular end diastolic volume is 25% at rest, with a corresponding increase in ejection fractions of 50% to 60%. This effect improves congestive symptoms in heart failure and improves the myocardial perfusion gradient in patients with coronary artery disease.

**Use** Long-acting metabolite of the vasodilator isosorbide dinitrate used for the prophylactic treatment of angina pectoris

**USUAL DOSAGE** Adults: Oral:

Regular tablet: 20 mg twice daily separated by 7 hours; may initiate with 5-10 mg

Extended release tablet (Imdur™): Initial: 30-60 mg once daily; after several days the dosage may be increased to 120 mg/day (given as two 60 mg tablets); daily dose should be taken in the morning upon arising; rarely, 240 mg may be needed

Asymmetrical dosing regimen of 7 AM and 3 PM or 9 AM and 5 PM to allow for a nitrate-free dosing interval to minimize nitrate tolerance

**Dosing adjustment in renal impairment:** Not necessary for elderly or patients with altered renal or hepatic function

**Dosage Forms Tab (Ismo®, Monoket®):** 10 mg, 20 mg; **Tab, extended release (Imdur™):** 30 mg, 60 mg, 120 mg

**Contraindications** Contraindicated due to potential increases in intracranial pressure in patients with head trauma or cerebral hemorrhage; hypersensitivity or idiosyncrasy to nitrates

**Warnings/Precautions** Postural hypotension, transient episodes of weakness, dizziness, or syncope may occur even with small doses; alcohol accentuates these effects; tolerance and cross-tolerance to nitrate antianginal and hemodynamic effects may occur during prolonged isosorbide mononitrate therapy; (minimized by using the smallest effective dose, by alternating coronary vasodilators or offering drug-free intervals of as little as 12 hours). Excessive doses may result in severe headache, blurred vision, or dry mouth; increased anginal symptoms may be a result of dosage increases.

**Adverse Reactions**

>10%: Central nervous system: Headache

1% to 10%: Gastrointestinal: Dizziness, nausea, vomiting

<1%: Angina pectoris, arrhythmias, atrial fibrillation, hypotension, palpitations, postural hypotension, premature ventricular contractions, supraventricular tachycardia, syncope, edema, malaise, agitation, anxiety, confusion, hypoesthesia, insomnia, nervousness, nightmares, pruritus, rash, abdominal pain, diarrhea, dyspepsia, tenesmus, increased appetite, tooth disorder, impotence, polyuria, dysuria, methemoglobinemia (rarely with very high doses), neck stiffness, rigors, arthralgia, dyscoordination, weakness, blurred vision, diplopia, bronchitis, pneumonia, upper respiratory tract infection, cold sweat

**Onset** Oral: 30-60 minutes

**Half-Life** Mononitrate: ~4 hours (8 times that of dinitrate)

**Special PA Issues**

**Patient Education:** Take as directed, at same time each day. Do not chew or crush extended release capsules; swallow with 8 oz of water. Do not change brands without consulting prescriber. Do not discontinue abruptly. Keep medication in original container, tightly closed. Avoid alcohol; combination may cause severe hypotension. Take medication while sitting down and use caution when changing position (rise from sitting or lying position slowly). May cause dizziness; use caution when driving or engaging in hazardous activities until response to drug is known. If chest pain is unresolved in 15 minutes, seek emergency medical help at once. Report acute headache, rapid heartbeat, unusual restlessness or dizziness, muscular weakness, or blurring vision.

**Dietary Considerations:** Alcohol: Has been found to exhibit additive effects of this variety

**Monitoring Parameters:** Monitor for orthostasis

## Isotretinoin (eye soe TRET i noyn)

**Pharmacologic Class** Retinoic Acid Derivative

**U.S. Brand Names** Accutane®

**Mechanism of Action** Reduces sebaceous gland size and reduces sebum production; regulates cell proliferation and differentiation

**Use** Treatment of severe recalcitrant cystic and/or conglobate acne unresponsive to conventional therapy

**Investigational:** Treatment of children with metastatic neuroblastoma or leukemia that does not respond to conventional therapy

**USUAL DOSAGE** Oral:

Children: Maintenance therapy for neuroblastoma: 100-250 mg/m$^2$/day in 2 divided doses has been used investigationally

(Continued)

## Isotretinoin *(Continued)*

Children and Adults: 0.5-2 mg/kg/day in 2 divided doses (dosages as low as 0.05 mg/kg/day have been reported to be beneficial) for 15-20 weeks or until the total cyst count decreases by 70%, whichever is sooner

**Dosing adjustment in hepatic impairment:** Dose reductions empirically are recommended in hepatitis disease

**Dosage Forms** Cap: 10 mg, 20 mg, 40 mg

**Contraindications** Sensitivity to parabens, vitamin A, or other retinoids; patients who are pregnant or intend to become pregnant during treatment

**Warnings/Precautions** Use with caution in patients with diabetes mellitus, hypertriglyceridemia; **not to be used in women of childbearing potential** unless woman is capable of complying with effective contraceptive measures; therapy is normally begun on the second or third day of next normal menstrual period; effective contraception must be used for at least 1 month before beginning therapy, during therapy, and for 1 month after discontinuation of therapy. Because of the high likelihood of teratogenic effects (~20%), do not prescribe isotretinoin for women who are or who are likely to become pregnant while using the drug. Isolated reports of depression, psychosis and rarely suicidal thoughts and actions have been reported during isotretinoin usage.

**Pregnancy Risk Factor** X

**Adverse Reactions**

>10%:

Dermatologic: Redness, cheilitis, inflammation of lips, dry skin, pruritus, photosensitivity

Endocrine & metabolic: Increased serum concentration of triglycerides

Gastrointestinal: Xerostomia

Local: Burning

Neuromuscular & skeletal: Bone pain, arthralgia, myalgia

Ocular: Itching eyes

Respiratory: Epistaxis, cry nose

1% to 10%:

Cardiovascular: Facial edema, pallor

Central nervous system: Fatigue, headache, mental depression, hypothermia

Dermatologic: Skin peeling on hands or soles of feet, rash, cellulitis

Endocrine & metabolic: Fluid imbalance, acidosis

Gastrointestinal: Stomach upset

Hepatic: Ascites

Neuromuscular & skeletal: Flank pain

Ocular: Dry eyes, photophobia

Miscellaneous: Lymph disorders

<1%: Mood change, pseudomotor cerebri, alopecia, pruritus, hyperuricemia, xerostomia, anorexia, nausea, vomiting, inflammatory bowel syndrome, bleeding of gums, increase in erythrocyte sedimentation rate, decrease in hemoglobin and hematocrit, hepatitis, conjunctivitis, corneal opacities, optic neuritis, cataracts

**Drug Interactions**

Decreased effect: Increased clearance of carbamazepine

Increased toxicity: Avoid other vitamin A products; may interfere with medications used to treat hypertriglyceridemia

**Half-Life** Parent drug: 10-20 hours; Metabolite: 11-50 hours

**Special PA Issues**

**Patient Education:** Use exactly as directed; do not take more than recommended. Capsule can be chewed and swallowed, swallowed, or opened with a large needle and contents sprinkled on applesauce or ice cream. Do not take any other vitamin A products, limit vitamin A intake, and increase exercise during therapy. Exacerbations of acne may occur during first weeks of therapy. You may experience headache, loss of night vision, lethargy, or visual disturbances (use caution when driving or engaging in hazardous tasks until response to therapy is known); photosensitivity (avoid sunlamps and use sunscreen, sunglasses, and protective clothing); dry mouth or nausea (small frequent meals, sucking hard candy, or chewing gum may may help); dryness, redness, or itching of skin, eye irritation, or increased sensitivity to contact lenses (wear regular glasses). Discontinue therapy and report acute vision changes, rectal bleeding, abdominal cramping, or unresolved diarrhea.

**Monitoring Parameters:** CBC with differential and platelet count, baseline sedimentation rate, serum triglycerides, liver enzymes

♦ **Isotrex®** *see* Isotretinoin *on previous page*

## Isradipine *(iz RA di peen)*

**Pharmacologic Class** Calcium Channel Blocker

**U.S. Brand Names** DynaCirc®

**Mechanism of Action** Inhibits calcium ion from entering the "slow channels" or select voltage-sensitive areas of vascular smooth muscle and myocardium during depolarization, producing a relaxation of coronary vascular smooth muscle and coronary vasodilation; increases myocardial oxygen delivery in patients with vasospastic angina

**Use** Treatment of hypertension, congestive heart failure, migraine prophylaxis

**USUAL DOSAGE** Adults: 2.5 mg twice daily; antihypertensive response occurs in 2-3 hours; maximal response in 2-4 weeks; increase dose at 2- to 4-week intervals at 2.5-5 mg increments; usual dose range: 5-20 mg/day. **Note:** Most patients show no improvement with doses >10 mg/day except adverse reaction rate increases

**Dosage Forms** Cap: 2.5 mg, 5 mg

**Contraindications** Sinus bradycardia; advanced heart block; ventricular tachycardia; cardiogenic shock, hypotension, congestive heart failure; hypersensitivity to isradipine or any component, hypersensitivity to calcium channel blockers and adenosine; atrial fibrillation or flutter associated with accessory conduction pathways; not to be given within a few hours of I.V. beta-blocking agents

**Warnings/Precautions** Avoid use in hypotension, congestive heart failure, cardiac conduction defects, PVCs, idiopathic hypertrophic subaortic stenosis; may cause platelet inhibition; do not abruptly withdraw (chest pain); may cause hepatic dysfunction or increased angina; increased intracranial pressure with cranial tumors; elderly may have greater hypotensive effect

**Pregnancy Risk Factor** C

**Pregnancy Implications**
Clinical effects on the fetus: No data on crossing the placenta
Breast-feeding/lactation: No data on crossing into breast milk. Not recommended due to potential harm to infant.

**Adverse Reactions**
>10%: Central nervous system: Headache (14%)
1% to 10%:
Cardiovascular: Edema (7%), palpitations (4%), flushing (2.6%), angina (2.4%), tachycardia (1.5%), hypotension
Central nervous system: Dizziness (7%), fatigue (4%)
Dermatologic: Rash (1.5%)
Gastrointestinal: Nausea (1.8%), abdominal discomfort (1.7%), vomiting/diarrhea (1%)
Neuromuscular & skeletal: Weakness (1% to 2%)
Respiratory: Dyspnea (1.8%)
<1%: Heart failure, atrial and ventricular fibrillation, TIAs, A-V block, myocardial infarction, abnormal EKG, disturbed sleep, pruritus, urticaria, rash, xerostomia, nocturia, leukopenia, foot cramps, paresthesia, numbness, visual disturbance, cough

**Drug Interactions** CYP3A3/4 enzyme substrate
Decreased effect:
Isradipine and NSAIDs (diclofenac) may decrease antihypertensive response
Isradipine and lovastatin causes decrease lovastatin effect
Increased toxicity/effect/levels:
Isradipine and beta-blockers may increase cardiovascular adverse effects; with fentanyl, isradipine therapy may cause severe hypotension
Isradipine and cyclosporine may minimally increase cyclosporine levels

**Onset** Peak serum concentration in 1-2 hours

**Duration** 8-16 hours

**Half-Life** 8 hours

**Special PA Issues**
**Patient Education:** Take as prescribed; do not stop abruptly without consulting prescriber immediately. You may experience headache (if unrelieved, consult prescriber), nausea or vomiting (frequent small meals may help), constipation (increased dietary bulk and fluids may help), or depression (should resolve when drug is discontinued). May cause dizziness or drowsiness; use caution when driving or engaging in hazardous activities. Report unrelieved headache, vomiting, constipation, palpitations, swelling of hands or feet, or sudden weight gain.

**Related Information**
Calcium Channel Blocking Agents *on page 1004*

♦ **Isuprel®** *see* Isoproterenol *on page 496*

# Itraconazole (i tra KOE na zole)

**Pharmacologic Class** Antifungal Agent, Oral

**U.S. Brand Names** Sporanox®

**Mechanism of Action** Interferes with cytochrome P-450 activity, decreasing ergosterol synthesis (principal sterol in fungal cell membrane) and inhibiting cell membrane formation

**Use** Treatment of susceptible fungal infections in immunocompromised and immunocompetent patients including blastomycosis and histoplasmosis; indicated for aspergillosis, and onychomycosis of the toenail; treatment of onychomycosis of the fingernail without concomitant toenail infection via a pulse-type dosing regimen; has activity against *Aspergillus*, *Candida*, *Coccidioides*, *Cryptococcus*, *Sporothrix*, tinea unguium

Oral solution (not capsules) is marketed for oral and esophageal candidiasis

Useful in superficial mycoses including dermatophytoses (eg, tinea capitis), pityriasis versicolor, sebopsoriasis, vaginal and chronic mucocutaneous candidiases; systemic mycoses
(Continued)

## Itraconazole *(Continued)*

including candidiasis, meningeal and disseminated cryptococcal infections, paracoccidioidomycosis, coccidioidomycoses; miscellaneous mycoses such as sporotrichosis, chromomycosis, leishmaniasis, fungal keratitis, alternariosis, zygomycosis

Intravenous solution is indicated in the treatment of blastomycosis, histoplasmosis (nonmeningeal), and aspergillosis (in patients intolerant or refractory to amphotericin B therapy)

**USUAL DOSAGE** Oral: Capsule: Absorption is best if taken with food, therefore, it is best to administer itraconazole after meals; Solution: Should be taken on an empty stomach. Absorption of both products is significantly increased when taken with a cola beverage.

Children: Efficacy and safety have not been established; a small number of patients 3-16 years of age have been treated with 100 mg/day for systemic fungal infections with no serious adverse effects reported

Adults:

Oral:

Blastomycosis/histoplasmosis: 200 mg once daily, if no obvious improvement or there is evidence of progressive fungal disease, increase the dose in 100 mg increments to a maximum of 400 mg/day; doses >200 mg/day are given in 2 divided doses; length of therapy varies from 1 day to >6 months depending on the condition and mycological response

Aspergillosis: 200-400 mg/day

Onychomycosis: 200 mg once daily for 12 consecutive weeks

Life-threatening infections: Loading dose: 200 mg 3 times/day (600 mg/day) should be given for the first 3 days of therapy

Oropharyngeal and esophageal candidiasis: Oral solution: 100-200 mg once daily

I.V.: 200 mg twice daily for 4 doses, followed by 200 mg daily

**Dosing adjustment in renal impairment:** Not necessary; intraconazole injection is not recommended in patients with $Cl_{cr}$ <30 mL/minute

Hemodialysis: Not dialyzable

**Dosing adjustment in hepatic impairment:** May be necessary, but specific guidelines are not available

**Dosage Forms** Cap: 100 mg; Inj kit: 10 mg/mL - 25 mL ampul, one 50 mL (100 mL capacity) bag 0.9% sodium chloride, one filtered infusion set; **Soln, oral:** 100 mg/10 mL (150 mL)

**Contraindications** Known hypersensitivity to other azoles; concurrent administration with astemizole, cisapride, lovastatin, midazolam, simvastatin, or triazolam

**Warnings/Precautions** Rare cases of serious cardiovascular adverse event, including death, ventricular tachycardia and torsade de pointes have been observed due to increased terfenadine and cisapride concentrations induced by itraconazole; patients who develop abnormal liver function tests during itraconazole therapy should be monitored and therapy discontinued if symptoms of liver disease develop

**Pregnancy Risk Factor** C

**Adverse Reactions** Listed incidences are for higher doses appropriate for systemic fungal infections

>10%: Gastrointestinal: Nausea (10.6%)

1% to 10%:

Cardiovascular: Edema (3.5%), hypertension (3.2%)

Central nervous system: Headache (4%), fatigue (2% to 3%), malaise (1.2%), fever (2.5%)

Dermatologic: Rash (8.6%)

Endocrine & metabolic: Decreased libido (1.2%), hypertriglyceridemia

Gastrointestinal: Abdominal pain (1.5%), vomiting (5%), diarrhea (3%)

Hepatic: Abnormal LFTs (2.7%), hepatitis

<1%: Fatigue, dizziness, somnolence, pruritus, hypokalemia, anorexia, impotence, adrenal suppression, gynecomastia, albuminuria

**Drug Interactions** CYP3A3/4 enzyme substrate; CYP3A3/4 enzyme inhibitor

Decreased effect:

Decreased serum levels with carbamazepine, didanosine, isoniazid, phenobarbital, phenytoin, rifabutin, and rifampin; may cause a decreased effect of oral contraceptives; alternative birth control is recommended

Decreased/undetectable serum levels with rifampin - **should not be administered concomitantly with rifampin**

Absorption requires gastric acidity; therefore, antacids, $H_2$-antagonists (cimetidine and ranitidine), omeprazole, and sucralfate significantly reduce bioavailability resulting in treatment failures and should not be administered concomitantly; amphotericin B or fluconazole should be used instead

Increased toxicity:

May increase cyclosporine or tacrolimus levels (by 50%) when high doses are used

Itraconazole increases serum levels of lovastatin (possibly 20-fold) and other HMG-CoA inhibitors due to inhibition of CYP3A4

May increase phenytoin serum concentration

May inhibit warfarins metabolism

May increase digoxin serum levels

May increase astemizole, busulfan, cisapride, terfenadine, and vinca alkaloid levels - **concomitant administration is not recommended** due to increased risk of cardiotoxicity

Itraconazole may increase astemizole levels resulting in prolonged Q-T intervals - concomitant administration is contraindicated

Itraconazole may increase levels of cisapride - concomitant administration is contraindicated due to increased risk of cardiotoxicity

May increase amlodipine, benzodiazepine, buspirone, corticosteroids, and oral hypoglycemic levels; use with caution in patients prescribed medications eliminated by CYP3A4 metabolism

**Half-Life** After single 200 mg dose: 21 ±5 hours; 64 hours at steady-state; I.V. steady-state: 35 hours

**Special PA Issues**

**Patient Education:** Take as directed, around-the-clock, with food or after meals. Take full course of medication; some infections may require long periods of therapy. Frequent blood tests may be required with long-term therapy. Practice good hygiene measures to reduce incidence of reinfection. If diabetic, test serum glucose regularly; can cause hypoglycemia when given with sulfonylureas. You may experience nausea and vomiting (small, frequent meals, frequent mouth care, or sucking on lozenges may help); or headache (mild analgesic may be necessary). Report unresolved headache, rash or itching, yellowing of eyes or skin, changes in color of urine or stool, or chest pain or palpitations.

Topical: Wash and dry area before applying medication thinly. Do not cover with occlusive dressing.

**Dietary Considerations:** Food increases absorption of capsule and decreases absorption of the solution

♦ **I-Tropine® Ophthalmic** see Atropine on page 87

# Ivermectin (eye ver MEK tin)

**Pharmacologic Class** Antibiotic, Miscellaneous

**U.S. Brand Names** Mectizan®; Stromectol®

**Mechanism of Action** Ivermectin is a semisynthetic antihelminthic agent; it binds selectively and with strong affinity to glutamate-gated chloride ion channels which occur in invertebrate nerve and muscle cells. This leads to increased permeability of cell membranes to chloride ions then hyperpolarization of the nerve or muscle cell, and death of the parasite.

**Use** Treatment of the following infections: Strongyloidiasis of the intestinal tract due the nematode parasite *Strongyloides stercoralis*. Onchocerciasis due to the nematode parasite *Onchocerca volvulus*. Ivermectin is only active against the immature form of *Onchocerca volvulus*, and the intestinal forms of *Strongyloides stercoralis*. Ivermectin has been used for other parasitic infections including *Ascaris lumbricoides*, bancroftian filariasis, *Brugia malayi*, scabies, *Enterobius vermicularis*, *Mansonella ozzardi*, *Trichuris trichiura*.

**USUAL DOSAGE** Oral:

Children ≥5 years: 150 mcg/kg as a single dose; treatment for onchocerciasis may need to be repeated every 3-12 months until the adult worms die

Adults:

Strongyloidiasis: 200 mcg/kg as a single dose; follow-up stool examinations

Onchocerciasis: 150 mcg/kg as a single dose; retreatment may be required every 3-12 months until the adult worms die

**Dosage Forms Tab:** 6 mg

**Contraindications** Hypersensitivity to ivermectin or any component

**Warnings/Precautions** Data have shown that antihelmintic drugs like ivermectin may cause cutaneous and/or systemic reactions (Mazzoti reaction) of varying severity including ophthalmological reactions in patients with onchocerciasis. These reactions are probably due to allergic and inflammatory responses to the death of microfilariae. Patients with hyper-reactive onchodermatitis may be more likely than others to experience severe adverse reactions, especially edema and aggravation of the onchodermatitis. Repeated treatment may be required in immunocompromised patients (eg, HIV); control of extraintestinal strongyloidiasis may necessitate suppressive (once monthly) therapy

**Pregnancy Risk Factor** C

**Adverse Reactions**

Percentage unknown: Transient tachycardia, peripheral and facial edema, hypotension, mild EKG changes, dizziness, headache, somnolence, vertigo, insomnia, hyperthermia, pruritus, rash, urticaria, diarrhea, nausea, abdominal pain, vomiting, leukopenia, eosinophilia, increased ALT/AST, weakness, myalgia, tremor, limbitis, punctate opacity, mild conjunctivitis, blurred vision

Mazzotti reaction (with onchocerciasis): Pruritus, edema, rash, fever, lymphadenopathy, ocular damage

(Continued)

## Ivermectin *(Continued)*

### Special PA Issues

**Patient Education:** If infected with strongyloidiasis, repeated stool examinations are required to document clearance of the organisms; repeated follow-up and retreatment is usually required in the treatment of onchocerciasis

**Monitoring Parameters:** Skin and eye microfilarial counts, periodic ophthalmologic exams

♦ **IVIG** *see* Immune Globulin, Intravenous *on page 472*

♦ **IvyBlock®** *see* Bentoquatam *on page 104*

♦ **Jaa Amp® Trihydrate** *see* Ampicillin *on page 64*

♦ **Jaa-Prednisone®** *see* Prednisone *on page 754*

♦ **Janimine®** *see* Imipramine *on page 469*

♦ **Jaundice Root** *see* Golden Seal *on page 421*

♦ **Jenamicin® Injection** *see* Gentamicin *on page 411*

♦ **Jenest-28™** *see* Ethinyl Estradiol and Norethindrone *on page 348*

♦ **Junior Strength Motrin® [OTC]** *see* Ibuprofen *on page 466*

♦ **Junior Strength Panadol® [OTC]** *see* Acetaminophen *on page 21*

♦ **K+ 10®** *see* Potassium Chloride *on page 742*

♦ **Kabikinase®** *see* Streptokinase *on page 853*

♦ **Kadian™** *see* Morphine Sulfate *on page 619*

♦ **Kalcinate®** *see* Calcium Gluconate *on page 143*

## Kanamycin *(kan a MYE sin)*

**Pharmacologic Class** Antibiotic, Aminoglycoside

**U.S. Brand Names** Kantrex®

**Mechanism of Action** Interferes with protein synthesis in bacterial cell by binding to ribosomal subunit

### Use

Oral: Preoperative bowel preparation in the prophylaxis of infections and adjunctive treatment of hepatic coma (oral kanamycin is not indicated in the treatment of systemic infections); treatment of susceptible bacterial infection including gram-negative aerobes, gram-positive *Bacillus* as well as some mycobacteria

Parenteral: Rarely used in antibiotic irrigations during surgery

### USUAL DOSAGE

Children: Infections: I.M., I.V.: 15 mg/kg/day in divided doses every 8-12 hours

Adults:

Infections: I.M., I.V.: 5-7.5 mg/kg/dose in divided doses every 8-12 hours (<15 mg/kg/day)

Preoperative intestinal antisepsis: Oral: 1 g every 4-6 hours for 36-72 hours

Hepatic coma: Oral: 8-12 g/day in divided doses

Intraperitoneal: After contamination in surgery: 500 mg diluted in 20 mL distilled water; other irrigations: 0.25% solutions

Aerosol: 250 mg 2-4 times/day (250 mg diluted with 3 mL of NS and nebulized)

**Dosing adjustment/interval in renal impairment:**

$Cl_{cr}$ 50-80 mL/minute: Administer 60% to 90% of dose or administer every 8-12 hours

$Cl_{cr}$ 10-50 mL/minute: Administer 30% to 70% of dose or administer every 12 hours

$Cl_{cr}$ <10 mL/minute: Administer 20% to 30% of dose or administer every 24-48 hours

Hemodialysis: Dialyzable (50% to 100%)

**Dosage Forms Cap:** 500 mg; **Inj:** Pediatrics: 75 mg (2 mL), Adults: 500 mg (2 mL); 1 g (3 mL)

**Contraindications** Hypersensitivity to kanamycin or any component or other aminoglycosides

**Warnings/Precautions** Use with caution in patients with pre-existing renal insufficiency, vestibular or cochlear impairment, myasthenia gravis, conditions which depress neuromuscular transmission

Parenteral aminoglycosides are associated with nephrotoxicity or ototoxicity; the ototoxicity may be proportional to the amount of drug given and the duration of treatment; tinnitus or vertigo are indications of vestibular injury and impending hearing loss; renal damage is usually reversible

**Pregnancy Risk Factor** D

**Adverse Reactions** Percentage unknown: Edema, neurotoxicity, drowsiness, headache, pseudomotor cerebri, skin itching, redness, rash, photosensitivity, erythema, nausea, vomiting, diarrhea (most common with oral form), malabsorption syndrome with prolonged and high-dose therapy of hepatic coma; anorexia, weight loss, increased salivation, enterocolitis, granulocytopenia, agranulocytosis, thrombocytopenia, burning, stinging, weakness, tremors, muscle cramps, ototoxicity (auditory), ototoxicity (vestibular), nephrotoxicity, dyspnea

**Drug Interactions**
Increased toxicity:
Penicillins, cephalosporins, amphotericin B, diuretics may increase nephrotoxicity; poly-peptide antibiotics may increase risk of respiratory paralysis and renal dysfunction
Neuromuscular blocking agents with oral kanamycin may increase neuromuscular blockade; a small increase in warfarin's effect may occur due to decreased absorption of vitamin K
Decreased toxicity: Methotrexate with kanamycin (oral) may be less well absorbed as may digoxin (minor) and vitamin A

**Half-Life** 2-4 hours, increases in anuria to 80 hours; End-stage renal disease: 40-96 hours

**Special PA Issues**
**Patient Education:** It is important to maintain adequate hydration (2-3 L/day) unless informed by prescriber to restrict fluid intake. Report change in hearing acuity, ringing or roaring in ears, alteration in balance, vertigo, feeling of fullness in head; pain, tingling, or numbness of any body part; change in urinary pattern or decrease in urine; signs of opportunistic infection (eg, white plaques in mouth, vaginal discharge, unhealed sores, sore throat, unusual fever, chills); pain, redness, or swelling at injection site; skin rash; or other adverse reactions.
**Monitoring Parameters:** Serum creatinine and BUN every 2-3 days; peak and trough concentrations; hearing
**Reference Range:** Therapeutic: Peak: 25-35 µg/mL; Trough: 4-8 µg/mL; Toxic: Peak: >35 µg/mL; Trough: >10 µg/mL

- **Kanamycin Sulfate** see Kanamycin on previous page
- **Kantrex®** see Kanamycin on previous page
- **Kaochlor®** see Potassium Chloride on page 742
- **Kaochlor-Eff®** see Potassium Bicarbonate, Potassium Chloride, and Potassium Citrate on page 742
- **Kaochlor® SF** see Potassium Chloride on page 742

## Kaolin and Pectin With Opium (KAY oh lin & PEK tin with OH pee um)
**Pharmacologic Class** Antidiarrheal
**U.S. Brand Names** Parepectolin®
**Dosage Forms Susp, oral:** Kaolin 5.5 g, pectin 162 mg, and opium 15 mg per 30 mL [3.7 mL paregoric] (240 mL)

- **Kaon®** see Potassium Gluconate on page 744
- **Kaon-Cl®** see Potassium Chloride on page 742
- **Kaon Cl-10®** see Potassium Chloride on page 742
- **Kaopectate® II [OTC]** see Loperamide on page 540
- **Kapectolin PG®** see Hyoscyamine, Atropine, Scopolamine, Kaolin, Pectin, and Opium on page 465
- **Karidium®** see Fluoride on page 383
- **Karigel®** see Fluoride on page 383
- **Karigel®-N** see Fluoride on page 383
- **Kasof® [OTC]** see Docusate on page 298

## Kava
**Mechanism of Action** Contains alpha-pyrones in root extracts; may possess central dopaminergic antagonistic properties
**Use** Conditions of nervous anxiety, stress, and restlessness per Commission E; used for sleep inducement and to reduce anxiety
**USUAL DOSAGE** Per Commission E: Herb and preparations equivalent to 60-120 mg kavalactones
**Contraindications** Per Commission E: Pregnancy, breast-feeding, endogenous depression. "Extended continuous intake can cause a temporary yellow discoloration of skin, hair and nails. In this case, further application must be discontinued. In rare cases, allergic skin reactions occur. Also, accommodative disturbances (eg, enlargement of the pupils and disturbances of the oculomotor equilibrium) have been described."
**Pregnancy Implications** Do not use
**Adverse Reactions**
Central nervous system: Euphoria, depression, somnolence
Dermatologic: Skin discoloration (prolonged use)
Neuromuscular & skeletal: Muscle weakness
Ocular: Eye disturbances
**Drug Interactions** Coma can occur from concomitant administration of kava and alprazolam; may potentiate alcohol or CNS depressants, barbiturates, psychopharmacological agents

- **Kaybovite-1000®** see Cyanocobalamin on page 242
- **Kay Ciel®** see Potassium Chloride on page 742
- **Kayexalate®** see Sodium Polystyrene Sulfonate on page 843

## Ketoconazole (kee toe KOE na zole)

**Pharmacologic Class** Antifungal Agent, Oral; Antifungal Agent, Topical

**U.S. Brand Names** Nizoral®

**Mechanism of Action** Alters the permeability of the cell wall by blocking fungal cytochrome P-450; inhibits biosynthesis of triglycerides and phospholipids by fungi; inhibits several fungal enzymes that results in a build-up of toxic concentrations of hydrogen peroxide

**Use** Treatment of susceptible fungal infections, including candidiasis, oral thrush, blastomycosis, histoplasmosis, paracoccidioidomycosis, coccidioidomycosis, chromomycosis, candiduria, chronic mucocutaneous candidiasis, as well as, certain recalcitrant cutaneous dermatophytoses; used topically for treatment of tinea corporis, tinea cruris, tinea versicolor, and cutaneous candidiasis, seborrheic dermatitis

**USUAL DOSAGE**

Oral:

Children ≥2 years: 3.3-6.5 mg/kg/day as a single dose for 1-2 weeks for candidiasis, for at least 4 weeks in recalcitrant dermatophyte infections, and for up to 6 months for other systemic mycoses

Adults: 200-400 mg/day as a single daily dose for durations as stated above

Shampoo: Apply twice weekly for 4 weeks with at least 3 days between each shampoo

Topical: Rub gently into the affected area once daily to twice daily

**Dosing adjustment in hepatic impairment:** Dose reductions should be considered in patients with severe liver disease

Hemodialysis: Not dialyzable (0% to 5%)

**Dosage Forms Crm:** 2% (15 g, 30 g, 60 g); **Shamp:** 2% (120 mL); **Tab:** 200 mg

**Contraindications** Hypersensitivity to ketoconazole or any component; CNS fungal infections (due to poor CNS penetration); coadministration with terfenadine, astemizole, or cisapride is contraindicated due to risk of potentially fatal cardiac arrhythmias

**Warnings/Precautions** Rare cases of serious cardiovascular adverse event, including death, ventricular tachycardia and torsade de pointes have been observed due to increased terfenadine concentrations induced by ketoconazole. Use with caution in patients with impaired hepatic function; has been associated with hepatotoxicity, including some fatalities; perform periodic liver function tests; high doses of ketoconazole may depress adrenocortical function.

**Pregnancy Risk Factor** C

**Adverse Reactions**

Oral:

1% to 10%:

Dermatologic: Pruritus (1.5%)

Gastrointestinal: Nausea/vomiting (3% to 10%), abdominal pain (1.2%)

<1%: Headache, dizziness, somnolence, fever, chills, bulging fontanelles, depression, gynecomastia, diarrhea, impotence, thrombocytopenia, leukopenia, hemolytic anemia, hepatotoxicity, photophobia

Cream: Severe irritation, pruritus, stinging (~5%)

Shampoo: Increases in normal hair loss, irritation (<1%), abnormal hair texture, scalp pustules, mild dryness of skin, itching, oiliness/dryness of hair

**Drug Interactions** CYP3A3/4 enzyme substrate; CYP1A2, 2C, 2C9, 2C18, 2C19, 3A3/4, and 3A5-7 enzyme inhibitor

Decreased effect:

Decreased ketoconazole serum levels with isoniazid and phenytoin; decreased/undetectable serum levels with rifampin - **should not be administered concomitantly with rifampin**; theophylline and oral hypoglycemic serum levels may be decreased

Absorption requires gastric acidity; therefore, antacids, $H_2$-antagonists (cimetidine and ranitidine), omeprazole, and sucralfate significantly reduce bioavailability resulting in treatment failures; should not be administered concomitantly

Increased toxicity:

May increase cyclosporine levels (by 50%) when high doses are used

Inhibits warfarin metabolism resulting in increased anticoagulant effect

Increases corticosteroid bioavailability and decreases steroid clearance

Increases phenytoin, digoxin, terfenadine, astemizole, and cisapride concentrations; **concomitant administration with astemizole or cisapride is contraindicated**; may significantly increase levels and toxicity of lovastatin and simvastatin due to CYP3A4 inhibition; a disulfiram-type reaction may occur with concomitant ethanol

**Half-Life** Biphasic: Initial: 2 hours; Terminal: 8 hours

**Special PA Issues**

**Patient Education:**

Oral: May take with food; at least 2 hours before any antacids. Take full course of medication as directed; some infections may require long periods of therapy. Frequent blood tests may be required with long-term therapy. Practice good hygiene measures to reduce incidence of reinfection. If diabetic, test serum glucose regularly. You may experience nausea and vomiting (small, frequent meals, frequent mouth care, or sucking on lozenges may help); headache (mild analgesic may be necessary); or dizziness (use caution when driving). Report unresolved headache, rash or itching, yellowing of eyes or skin, changes in color of urine or stool, chest pain or palpitations, or sense of fullness or ringing in ears.

Topical: Wash and dry area before applying medication thinly. Do not cover with occlusive dressing. Report severe skin irritation or if condition does not improve.

Shampoo: Allow 3 days between shampoos. You may experience some hair loss, scalp irritation, itching, change in hair texture, or scalp pustules. Report severe side effects or if infestation persists.

**Monitoring Parameters:** Liver function tests

# Ketoprofen (kee toe PROE fen)

**Pharmacologic Class** Nonsteroidal Anti-Inflammatory Agent (NSAID)

**U.S. Brand Names** Actron® [OTC]; Orudis®; Orudis® KT [OTC]; Oruvail®

**Mechanism of Action** Inhibits prostaglandin synthesis by decreasing the activity of the enzyme, cyclo-oxygenase, which results in decreased formation of prostaglandin precursors

**Use** Acute or long-term treatment of rheumatoid arthritis and osteoarthritis; primary dysmenorrhea; mild to moderate pain

**USUAL DOSAGE** Oral:

Children 3 months to 14 years: Fever: 0.5-1 mg/kg every 6-8 hours

Children >12 years and Adults:

Rheumatoid arthritis or osteoarthritis: 50-75 mg 3-4 times/day up to a maximum of 300 mg/day

Mild to moderate pain: 25-50 mg every 6-8 hours up to a maximum of 300 mg/day

**Dosage Forms** Cap: 25 mg, 50 mg, 75 mg; Orudis®: 25 mg, 50 mg, 75 mg, Actron®, Orudis® KT [OTC]: 12.5 mg; **Cap, extended release (Oruvail®):** 100 mg, 200 mg

**Contraindications** Known hypersensitivity to ketoprofen or other NSAIDs/aspirin

**Warnings/Precautions** Use with caution in patients with congestive heart failure, hypertension, decreased renal or hepatic function, history of GI disease (bleeding or ulcers), or those receiving anticoagulants; safety and efficacy in children <6 months of age have not yet been established

**Pregnancy Risk Factor** B

**Adverse Reactions**

>10%:

Central nervous system: Dizziness

Dermatologic: Rash

Gastrointestinal: Abdominal cramps, heartburn, indigestion, nausea

1% to 10%:

Central nervous system: Headache, nervousness

Dermatologic: Itching

Endocrine & metabolic: Fluid retention

Gastrointestinal: Vomiting

Otic: Tinnitus

<1%: Congestive heart failure, hypertension, arrhythmias, tachycardia, confusion, hallucinations, mental depression, drowsiness, insomnia, aseptic meningitis, urticaria, erythema multiforme, toxic epidermal necrolysis, Stevens-Johnson syndrome, angioedema, polydipsia, hot flashes, gastritis, GI ulceration, cystitis, polyuria, agranulocytosis, anemia, hemolytic anemia, bone marrow suppression, leukopenia, thrombocytopenia, hepatitis, (Continued)

## Ketoprofen *(Continued)*

peripheral neuropathy, toxic amblyopia, blurred vision, conjunctivitis, dry eyes, decreased hearing, acute renal failure, allergic rhinitis, shortness of breath, epistaxis

**Drug Interactions** CYP2C and 2C9 enzyme inhibitor

Decreased effect of diuretics

Increased effect/toxicity with probenecid, lithium, anticoagulants

Increased toxicity of methotrexate

**Onset** Peak levels in 1-2 hours

**Half-Life** 1-4 hours

**Special PA Issues**

**Patient Education:** Take this medication exactly as directed; do not increase dose without consulting prescriber. Do not crush tablets or break capsules. Take with food or milk to reduce GI distress. Maintain adequate fluid intake (2-3 L/day). Do not use alcohol, aspirin, or aspirin-containing medication, and all other anti-inflammatory medications without consulting prescriber. You may experience drowsiness, dizziness, nervousness, or headache (use caution when driving or performing hazardous tasks); anorexia, nausea, vomiting, or heartburn (frequent small meals, frequent oral care, sucking on lozenges, or chewing gum may help); fluid retention (weigh yourself weekly and report unusual (3-5 lb/week) weight gain). GI bleeding, ulceration, or perforation can occur with or without pain; discontinue medication and contact prescriber if persistent abdominal pain or cramping, or blood in stool occurs. Report breathlessness, difficulty breathing, or unusual cough; chest pain, rapid heartbeat, palpitations; unusual bruising/bleeding; blood in urine, stool, mouth, or vomitus; swollen extremities; skin rash or itching; acute fatigue; or changes in hearing or ringing in ears.

**Related Information**

Nonsteroidal Anti-Inflammatory Agents *on page 1026*

## Ketorolac Tromethamine (KEE toe role ak troe METH a meen)

**Pharmacologic Class** Nonsteroidal Anti-Inflammatory Agent (NSAID)

**U.S. Brand Names** Acular® Ophthalmic; Toradol® Injection; Toradol® Oral

**Mechanism of Action** Inhibits prostaglandin synthesis by decreasing the activity of the enzyme, cyclo-oxygenase which results in decreased formation of prostaglandin precursors

**Use** Short-term (<5 days) management of pain; first parenteral NSAID for analgesia; 30 mg provides the analgesia comparable to 12 mg of morphine or 100 mg of meperidine

**USUAL DOSAGE Note:** The use of ketorolac in children <16 years of age is outside of product labeling

Children 2-16 years: Dosing guidelines are not established; **do not exceed adult doses**
Single-dose treatment:

I.M., I.V.: 0.4-1 mg/kg as a single dose; **Note:** Limited information exists. Single I.V. doses of 0.5 mg/kg, 0.75 mg/kg, 0.9 mg/kg and 1 mg/kg have been studied in children 2-16 years of age for postoperative analgesia. One study (Maunuksela, 1992) used a titrating dose starting with 0.2 mg/kg up to a total of 0.5 mg/kg (median dose required: 0.4 mg/kg).

Oral: One study used 1 mg/kg as a single dose for analgesia in 30 children (mean ±SD age: 3 ±2.5 years) undergoing bilateral myringotomy

Multiple-dose treatment: I.M., I.V., Oral: No pediatric studies exist; one report (Buck, 1994) of the clinical experience with ketorolac in 112 children, 6 months to 19 years of age (mean: 9 years), described usual I.V. maintenance doses of 0.5 mg/kg every 6 hours (mean dose: 0.52 mg/kg; range: 0.17-1 mg/kg)

Adults (pain relief usually begins within 10 minutes with parenteral forms):

Oral: 10 mg every 4-6 hours as needed for a maximum of 40 mg/day; on day of transition from I.M. to oral: maximum oral dose: 40 mg (or 120 mg combined oral and I.M.); maximum 5 days administration

I.M.: Initial: 30-60 mg, then 15-30 mg every 6 hours as needed for up to 5 days maximum; maximum dose in the first 24 hours: 150 mg with 120 mg/24 hours for up to 5 days total

I.V.: Initial: 30 mg, then 15-30 mg every 6 hours as needed for up to 5 days **maximum**; maximum daily dose: 120 mg for up to 5 days total

Ophthalmic: Instill 1 drop in eye(s) 4 times/day for up to 7 days

Elderly >65 years: Renal insufficiency or weight <50 kg:

I.M.: 30 mg, then 15 mg every 6 hours

I.V.: 15 mg every 6 hours as needed for up to 5 days total; maximum daily dose: 60 mg

**Dosage Forms Inj:** 15 mg/mL (1 mL); 30 mg/mL (1 mL, 2 mL); **Soln, ophth:** 0.5% (5 mL); **Tab:** 10 mg

**Contraindications** In patients who have developed nasal polyps, angioedema, or bronchospastic reactions to other NSAIDs, active peptic ulcer disease, recent GI bleeding or perforation, patients with advanced renal disease or risk of renal failure, labor and delivery, nursing mothers, patients with hypersensitivity to ketorolac, aspirin, or other NSAIDs, **prophylaxis before major surgery**, suspected or confirmed cerebrovascular bleeding, hemorrhagic diathesis, concurrent ASA or other NSAIDs, epidural or intrathecal administration, concomitant probenecid

**Warnings/Precautions** Use extra caution and reduce dosages in the elderly because it is cleared renally somewhat slower, and the elderly are also more sensitive to the renal effects of NSAIDs; use with caution in patients with congestive heart failure, hypertension, decreased renal or hepatic function, history of GI disease (bleeding or ulcers), or those receiving anticoagulants

**Pregnancy Risk Factor** B (D if used in the 3rd trimester)

**Adverse Reactions**

Percentage unknown: Renal impairment, wound bleeding (with I.M.), postoperative hematomas

1% to 10%:

Cardiovascular: Edema

Central nervous system: Drowsiness, dizziness, headache, pain

Gastrointestinal: Nausea, dyspepsia, diarrhea, gastric ulcers, indigestion

Local: Pain at injection site

Miscellaneous: Diaphoresis (increased)

<1%: Mental depression, purpura, aphthous stomatitis, rectal bleeding, peptic ulceration, change in vision, oliguria, dyspnea

**Drug Interactions**

Decreased effect of diuretics

Increased toxicity: Lithium, methotrexate increased drug level; increased effect/toxicity with salicylates, probenecid, anticoagulants

**Onset** Analgesic effect: Onset of action: I.M.: Within 10 minutes; Peak effect: Within 75-150 minutes

**Duration** Analgesic effect: 6-8 hours

**Half-Life** 2-8 hours; increased 30% to 50% in the elderly

**Special PA Issues**

**Patient Education:** If self-administered, use exactly as directed (do not increase dose or frequency); adverse reactions can occur with overuse. Do not take longer than 5 days without consulting medical advisor. Take with food or milk. While using this medication, do not use alcohol, other prescription or OTC medications including aspirin, aspirin-containing medications, or other NSAIDs without consulting prescriber. Maintain adequate hydration (2-3 L/day of fluids unless instructed to restrict fluid intake). You may experience nausea, vomiting, gastric discomfort (frequent mouth care, small frequent meals, or sucking on lozenges may help). GI bleeding, ulceration, or perforation can occur with or without pain. Stop taking medication and report ringing in ears; persistent cramping or pain in stomach; unresolved nausea or vomiting; difficulty breathing or shortness of breath; unusual bruising or bleeding (mouth, urine, stool); skin rash; unusual swelling of extremities; chest pain; or palpitations.

Ophthalmic: Instill drops as often as recommended. Wash hands before instilling. Sit or lie down to instill. Open eye, look at ceiling, and instill prescribed amount of solution. Close eye and roll eye in all directions, and apply gentle pressure to inner corner of eye for 1-2 minutes after instillation. Do not let tip of applicator touch eye or contaminate tip of applicator. Temporary stinging or blurred vision may occur. Report persistent pain, burning, double vision, swelling, itching, worsening of condition. Inform prescriber if you are or intend to be pregnant. Do not breast-feed.

**Dietary Considerations:**

Potassium: Hyperkalemia has been reported. The elderly and those with renal insufficiency are at greatest risk. Monitor potassium serum concentration in those at greatest risk. Avoid salt substitutes.

Sodium: Hyponatremia from sodium retention. Suspect secondary to suppression of renal prostaglandin. Monitor serum concentration and fluid status. May need to restrict fluid.

**Monitoring Parameters:** Monitor response (pain, range of motion, grip strength, mobility, ADL function), inflammation; observe for weight gain, edema; monitor renal function (serum creatinine, BUN, urine output); observe for bleeding, bruising; evaluate gastrointestinal effects (abdominal pain, bleeding, dyspepsia); mental confusion, disorientation, CBC, liver function tests

**Reference Range:** Serum concentration: Therapeutic: 0.3-5 µg/mL; Toxic: >5 µg/mL

**Related Information**

Nonsteroidal Anti-Inflammatory Agents on page 1026

- ◆ **Kew** see Kava on page 505
- ◆ **Kew Tree** see Ginkgo Biloba on page 414
- ◆ **Key-Pred® Injection** see Prednisolone on page 752
- ◆ **Key-Pred-SP® Injection** see Prednisolone on page 752
- ◆ **K-G®** see Potassium Gluconate on page 744
- ◆ **KI** see Potassium Iodide on page 744
- ◆ **K-Ide®** see Potassium Bicarbonate and Potassium Citrate, Effervescent on page 741
- ◆ **Kinesed®** see Hyoscyamine, Atropine, Scopolamine, and Phenobarbital on page 464
- ◆ **Klamath Weed** see St Johns Wort on page 852
- ◆ **Klaron® Lotion** see Sulfacetamide Sodium on page 858

- **Klean-Prep®** *see* Polyethylene Glycol-Electrolyte Solution *on page 736*
- **K-Lease®** *see* Potassium Chloride *on page 742*
- **Klonopin™** *see* Clonazepam *on page 224*
- **K-Lor™** *see* Potassium Chloride *on page 742*
- **Klor-Con®** *see* Potassium Chloride *on page 742*
- **Klor-Con® 8** *see* Potassium Chloride *on page 742*
- **Klor-Con® 10** *see* Potassium Chloride *on page 742*
- **Klor-Con/25®** *see* Potassium Chloride *on page 742*
- **Klor-Con®/EF** *see* Potassium Bicarbonate and Potassium Citrate, Effervescent *on page 741*
- **Klorvess®** *see* Potassium Chloride *on page 742*
- **Klorvess® Effervescent** *see* Potassium Bicarbonate and Potassium Chloride, Effervescent *on page 742*
- **Klotrix®** *see* Potassium Chloride *on page 742*
- **K-Lyte®** *see* Potassium Bicarbonate and Potassium Citrate, Effervescent *on page 741*
- **K-Lyte/Cl®** *see* Potassium Chloride *on page 742*
- **K/Lyte/CL®** *see* Potassium Bicarbonate and Potassium Chloride, Effervescent *on page 741*
- **K-Norm®** *see* Potassium Chloride *on page 742*
- **Kolephrin® GG/DM [OTC]** *see* Guaifenesin and Dextromethorphan *on page 428*
- **Kolyum®** *see* Potassium Chloride and Potassium Gluconate *on page 743*
- **Konakion® Injection** *see* Phytonadione *on page 725*
- **Kondon's Nasal® [OTC]** *see* Ephedrine *on page 321*
- **Konsyl® [OTC]** *see* Psyllium *on page 781*
- **Konsyl-D® [OTC]** *see* Psyllium *on page 781*
- **K-Phos® Neutral** *see* Potassium Phosphate and Sodium Phosphate *on page 747*
- **K-Phos® Original** *see* Potassium Acid Phosphate *on page 740*
- **K-Tab®** *see* Potassium Chloride *on page 742*
- **Ku-Zyme® HP** *see* Pancrelipase *on page 694*
- **K-Vescent®** *see* Potassium Bicarbonate and Potassium Citrate, Effervescent *on page 741*
- **Kwelcof®** *see* Hydrocodone and Guaifenesin *on page 451*
- **Kwell®** *see* Lindane *on page 534*
- **Kwellada™** *see* Lindane *on page 534*
- **Kytril™** *see* Granisetron *on page 424*
- **L-3-Hydroxytyrosine** *see* Levodopa *on page 524*
- **LA-12®** *see* Hydroxocobalamin *on page 458*

## Labetalol (la BET a lole)

**Pharmacologic Class** Alpha-/Beta- Blocker

**U.S. Brand Names** Normodyne®; Trandate®

**Mechanism of Action** Blocks alpha-, beta₁-, and beta₂-adrenergic receptor sites; elevated renins are reduced

**Use** Treatment of mild to severe hypertension with or without other agents; I.V. for hypertensive emergencies

**Unlabeled use** Pheochromocytoma, clonidine withdrawal hypertension

**USUAL DOSAGE** Due to limited documentation of its use, labetalol should be initiated cautiously in pediatric patients with careful dosage adjustment and blood pressure monitoring

Children:

Oral: Limited information regarding labetalol use in pediatric patients is currently available in literature. Some centers recommend initial oral doses of 4 mg/kg/day in 2 divided doses. Reported oral doses have started at 3 mg/kg/day and 20 mg/kg/day and have increased up to 40 mg/kg/day.

I.V., intermittent bolus doses of 0.3-1 mg/kg/dose have been reported

For treatment of pediatric hypertensive emergencies, initial continuous infusions of 0.4-1 mg/kg/hour with a maximum of 3 mg/kg/hour have been used; administration requires the use of an infusion pump

Adults:

Oral: Initial: 100 mg twice daily, may increase as needed every 2-3 days by 100 mg until desired response is obtained; usual dose: 200-400 mg twice daily; may require up to 2.4 g/day

I.V.: 20 mg (0.25 mg/kg or an 80 kg patient) IVP over 2 minutes, may administer 40-80 mg at 10-minute intervals, up to 300 mg total dose

I.V. infusion: Initial: 2 mg/minute; titrate to response up to 300 mg total dose, if needed; administration requires the use of an infusion pump

I.V. infusion (500 mg/250 mL D₅W) rates:

1 mg/minute: 30 mL/hour

2 mg/minute: 60 mL/hour

3 mg/minute: 90 mL/hour

    4 mg/minute: 120 mL/hour
    5 mg/minute: 150 mL/hour
    6 mg/minute: 180 mL/hour
    Dialysis: Not removed by hemo- or peritoneal dialysis; supplemental dose is not necessary
    **Dosage adjustment in hepatic impairment:** Dosage reduction may be necessary

**Dosage Forms** Labetalol hydrochloride: **Inj:** 5 mg/mL (20 mL, 40 mL, 60 mL); **Tab:** 100 mg, 200 mg, 300 mg

**Contraindications** Cardiogenic shock, uncompensated congestive heart failure, bradycardia, pulmonary edema, or heart block

**Warnings/Precautions** Paradoxical increase in blood pressure has been reported with treatment of pheochromocytoma or clonidine withdrawal syndrome; use with caution in patients with hyper-reactive airway disease, congestive heart failure, diabetes mellitus, hepatic dysfunction; orthostatic hypotension may occur with I.V. administration; patient should remain supine during and for up to 3 hours after I.V. administration; use with caution in impaired hepatic function (discontinue if signs of liver dysfunction occur); may mask the signs and symptoms of hypoglycemia; a lower hemodynamic response rate and higher incidence of toxicity may be observed with administration to elderly patients.

**Pregnancy Risk Factor** C

**Pregnancy Implications**

    Clinical effects on the fetus: Crosses the placenta. Bradycardia, hypotension, hypoglycemia, intrauterine growth rate (IUGR). IUGR probably related to maternal hypertension. Available evidence suggests safe use during pregnancy and breast-feeding. Monitor breast-fed infant for symptoms of beta-blockade.

    Breast-feeding/lactation: Crosses into breast milk. American Academy of Pediatrics considers **compatible** with breast-feeding.

**Adverse Reactions**

    1% to 10%:
        Cardiovascular: Orthostatic hypotension (dose-related, usual 1% to 5%), edema (1%)
        Central nervous system: Dizziness (11%), fatigue (2% to 5%), vertigo (2%), headache (2%)
        Endocrine & metabolic: Decreased sexual ability (1% to 2%)
        Gastrointestinal: Nausea (1% to 4%), stomach discomfort (3%), abnormal taste (1%)
        Neuromuscular & skeletal: Paresthesia (1% to 2%)
        Respiratory: Dyspnea (2%), nasal congestion (1% to 3%)
    <1%: Drowsiness, rash (1%), diarrhea, vomiting, vision abnormality

**Drug Interactions** CYP2D6 enzyme substrate; CYP2D6 enzyme inhibitor

    Decreased effect of beta-blockers with aluminum salts, barbiturates, calcium salts, cholestyramine, colestipol, NSAIDs, penicillins (ampicillin), rifampin, salicylates and sulfinpyrazone due to decreased bioavailability and plasma levels

    Beta-blockers may decrease the effect of sulfonylureas and bronchodilators

    Increased effect/toxicity of beta-blockers with calcium blockers (diltiazem, felodipine, nicardipine), contraceptives, flecainide, $H_2$-antagonists (cimetidine), quinidine (in extensive metabolizers), ciprofloxacin, nitroglycerin, and halothane

    Beta-blockers may increase the effect/toxicity of flecainide, haloperidol (hypotensive effects), hydralazine, phenothiazines, acetaminophen, benzodiazepines (not atenolol), clonidine (hypertensive crisis after or during withdrawal of either agent), epinephrine (initial hypertensive episode followed by bradycardia), nifedipine and verapamil, lidocaine, ergots, prazosin

    Beta-blockers may affect the action or levels of ethanol, disopyramide, nondepolarizing muscle relaxants and theophylline although the effects are difficult to predict

**Onset**

    Oral: 20 minutes to 2 hours
    I.V.: 2-5 minutes
    Peak effect: Oral: 1-4 hours; I.V.: 5-15 minutes

**Duration** Oral: 8-24 hours (dose-dependent); I.V.: 2-4 hours

**Half-Life** Normal renal function: 6-8 hours

**Special PA Issues**

    **Patient Education:** For I.V. use in emergency situations - patient information is included in general instruction. Oral: Take as directed, with meals. Do not skip dose or discontinue without consulting prescriber. Follow recommended diet and exercise program. Do not use alcohol or OTC medications which may affect blood pressure (eg, cough or cold remedies, diet pills, stay-awake medications) without consulting prescriber. If diabetic, monitor serum glucose closely and notify prescriber of changes; this medication can alter hypoglycemic requirements. You may experience drowsiness, dizziness, or impaired judgment (use caution when driving or engaging in tasks that require alertness until response is known); postural hypotension (use caution when rising from sitting or lying position or when climbing stairs); dry mouth, nausea, or loss of appetite (frequent mouth care or sucking lozenges may help); or sexual dysfunction (reversible, may resolve with continued use). Report altered CNS status (eg, fatigue, depression, numbness or tingling of fingers, toes, or skin); palpitations or slowed heartbeat; difficulty breathing; edema or cold extremities; or other persistent side effects.

    (Continued)

## Labetalol *(Continued)*

**Monitoring Parameters:** Blood pressure, standing and sitting/supine, pulse, cardiac monitor and blood pressure monitor required for I.V. administration

**Related Information**
Beta-Blockers *on page 1002*

◆ **Labetalol Hydrochloride** *see* Labetalol *on page 510*

◆ **LaBID®** *see* Theophylline Salts *on page 888*

◆ **LactiCare-HC®** *see* Hydrocortisone *on page 453*

◆ **Lactinex® [OTC]** *see* Lactobacillus acidophilus and Lactobacillus bulgaricus *on this page*

## *Lactobacillus acidophilus* and *Lactobacillus bulgaricus*

(lak toe ba SIL us as i DOF fil us & lak toe ba SIL us bul GAR i cus)

**Pharmacologic Class** Antidiarrheal

**U.S. Brand Names** Bacid® [OTC]; Lactinex® [OTC]; More-Dophilus® [OTC]

**Mechanism of Action** Creates an environment unfavorable to potentially pathogenic fungi or bacteria through the production of lactic acid, and favors establishment of an aciduric flora, thereby suppressing the growth of pathogenic microorganisms; helps re-establish normal intestinal flora

**Use** Treatment of uncomplicated diarrhea particularly that caused by antibiotic therapy; re-establish normal physiologic and bacterial flora of the intestinal tract

**USUAL DOSAGE** Children >3 years and Adults: Oral:

Capsules: 2 capsules 2-4 times/day

Granules: 1 packet added to or taken with cereal, food, milk, fruit juice, or water, 3-4 times/day

Powder: 1 teaspoonful daily with liquid

Tablet, chewable: 4 tablets 3-4 times/day; may follow each dose with a small amount of milk, fruit juice, or water

**Dosage Forms Cap:** Bacid®: *Lactobacillus acidophilus* cultured strain ≥500 million viable (50s, 100s), Pro-Bionate®: *Lactobacillus acidophilus* strain NAS 2 billion units/g; **Granules (Lactinex®):** *Lactobacillus acidophilus* and *Lactobacillus bulgaricus* mixed culture (1 g/packet-12s); **Powder:** MoreDophilus®: Acidophilus-carrot derivative 4 billion units/g; Pro-Bionate®: *Lactobacillus acidophilus* strain NAS 2 billion units/g; **Tab, chewable (Lactinex®):** *Lactobacillus acidophilus* and *Lactobacillus bulgaricus* mixed culture (50s)

**Contraindications** Allergy to milk or lactose

**Warnings/Precautions** Discontinue if high fever present; do not use in children <3 years of age

**Adverse Reactions** 1% to 10%: Gastrointestinal: Intestinal flatus

**Special PA Issues**

**Patient Education:** Refrigerate; granules may be added to or taken with cereal, food, milk, fruit juice, or water

◆ **Lactoflavin** *see* Riboflavin *on page 802*

## Lactulose (LAK tyoo lose)

**Pharmacologic Class** Ammonium Detoxicant; Laxative, Miscellaneous

**U.S. Brand Names** Cephulac®; Cholac®; Chronulac®; Constilac®; Constulose®; Duphalac®; Enulose®; Evalose®; Heptalac®; Lactulose PSE®

**Mechanism of Action** The bacterial degradation of lactulose resulting in an acidic pH inhibits the diffusion of $NH_3$ into the blood by causing the conversion of $NH_3$ to $NH_4+$; also enhances the diffusion of $NH_3$ from the blood into the gut where conversion to $NH_4+$ occurs; produces an osmotic effect in the colon with resultant distention promoting peristalsis

**Use** Adjunct in the prevention and treatment of portal-systemic encephalopathy (PSE); treatment of chronic constipation

**USUAL DOSAGE** Diarrhea may indicate overdosage and responds to dose reduction
Prevention of portal systemic encephalopathy (PSE): Oral:

Infants: 2.5-10 mL/day divided 3-4 times/day; adjust dosage to produce 2-3 stools/day

Older Children: Daily dose of 40-90 mL divided 3-4 times/day; if initial dose causes diarrhea, then reduce it immediately; adjust dosage to produce 2-3 stools/day

Constipation:

Children: 5 g/day (7.5 mL) after breakfast

Adults:

Acute PSE:

Oral: 20-30 g (30-45 mL) every 1-2 hours to induce rapid laxation; adjust dosage daily to produce 2-3 soft stools; doses of 30-45 mL may be given hourly to cause rapid laxation, then reduce to recommended dose; usual daily dose: 60-100 g (90-150 mL) daily

Rectal administration: 200 g (300 mL) diluted with 700 mL of $H_2O$ or NS; administer rectally via rectal balloon catheter and retain 30-60 minutes every 4-6 hours

Constipation: Oral: 15-30 mL/day increased to 60 mL/day if necessary

**Dosage Forms** Syr: 10 g/15 mL (15 mL, 30 mL, 237 mL, 473 mL, 946 mL, 1890 mL)

**Contraindications** Patients with galactosemia and require a low galactose diet, hypersensitivity to any component

**Warnings/Precautions** Use with caution in patients with diabetes mellitus; monitor periodically for electrolyte imbalance when lactulose is used >6 months or in patients predisposed to electrolyte abnormalities (eg, elderly); patients receiving lactulose and an oral anti-infective agent should be monitored for possible inadequate response to lactulose

**Pregnancy Risk Factor** B

**Adverse Reactions**

>10%: Gastrointestinal: Flatulence, diarrhea (excessive dose)

1% to 10%: Gastrointestinal: Abdominal discomfort, nausea, vomiting

**Drug Interactions** Decreased effect: Oral neomycin, laxatives, antacids

**Special PA Issues**

**Patient Education:** Not for long-term use. Take as directed, alone, or diluted with water, juice or milk, or take with food. Laxative results may not occur for 24-48 hours; do not take more often than recommended or for a longer time than recommended. Do not use any other laxatives while taking lactulose. Increased fiber, fluids, and exercise may help reduce constipation. Do not use if experiencing abdominal pain, nausea, or vomiting. Diarrhea may indicate overdose. May cause flatulence, belching, or abdominal cramping. Report persistent or severe diarrhea or abdominal cramping.

**Monitoring Parameters:** Blood pressure, standing/supine; serum potassium, bowel movement patterns, fluid status, serum ammonia

♦ **Lactulose PSE®** see Lactulose on previous page

♦ **Lamictal®** see Lamotrigine on next page

♦ **Lamisil®** see Terbinafine on page 878

# Lamivudine (la MI vyoo deen)

**Pharmacologic Class** Antiretroviral Agent, Reverse Transcriptase Inhibitor (Non-Nucleoside)

**U.S. Brand Names** Epivir®; Epivir® HBV

**Mechanism of Action** After lamivudine is triphosphorylated, the principle mode of action is inhibition of HIV reverse transcription via viral DNA chain termination; inhibits RNA- and DNA-dependent DNA polymerase activities of reverse transcriptase. The monophosphate form of lamivudine is incorporated into the viral DNA by hepatitis B virus polymerase, resulting in DNA chain termination.

**Use** Treatment of HIV infection when antiretroviral therapy is warranted; should always be used as part of a multidrug regimen (at least three antiretroviral agents); indicated for the treatment of chronic hepatitis B associated with evidence of hepatitis B viral replication and active liver inflammation

**USUAL DOSAGE** Oral: Use with at least two other antiretroviral agents when treating HIV

Children 3 months to 12 years: 4 mg/kg twice daily (maximum: 150 mg twice daily)

Adolescents 12-16 years and Adults: 150 mg twice daily

Prevention of HIV following needlesticks: 150 mg twice daily (with zidovudine and a protease inhibitor)

Adults <50 kg: 2 mg/kg twice daily

Treatment of hepatitis B: 100 mg/day

**Dosing interval in renal impairment in patients >16 years for HIV:**

$Cl_{cr}$ 30-49 mL/minute: Administer 150 mg once daily

$Cl_{cr}$ 15-29 mL/minute: Administer 150 mg first dose, then 100 mg once daily

$Cl_{cr}$ 5-14 mL/minute: Administer 150 mg first dose, then 50 mg once daily

$Cl_{cr}$ <5 mL/minute: Administer 50 mg first dose, then 25 mg once daily

**Dosing interval in renal impairment in patients with hepatitis B:**

$Cl_{cr}$ 30-49: Administer 100 mg first dose then 50 mg once daily

$Cl_{cr}$ 15-29: Administer 100 mg first dose then 25 mg once daily

$Cl_{cr}$ 5-14: Administer 35 mg first dose then 15 mg once daily

$Cl_{cr}$ <5: Administer 35 mg first dose then 10 mg once daily

Dialysis: No data available

**Dosage Forms** Soln, oral: 10 mg/mL (240 mL); **Tab:** 150 mg

**Contraindications** Hypersensitivity to lamivudine or any component

**Warnings/Precautions** A decreased dosage is recommended in patients with renal dysfunction since AUC, $C_{max}$, and half-life increased with diminishing renal function; use with extreme caution in children with history of pancreatitis or risk factors for development of pancreatitis. Do not use as monotherapy in treatment of HIV.

**Pregnancy Risk Factor** C

**Pregnancy Implications**

Clinical effects on the fetus: Use only if the potential benefits outweigh the risks. Combination therapy with zidovudine and lamivudine is currently being investigated to decrease the maternal/fetal transmission of HIV.

Breast-feeding/lactation: HIV-infected mothers are discouraged from breast-feeding to decrease postnatal transmission of HIV

(Continued)

## Lamivudine *(Continued)*

### Adverse Reactions

>10%:

Central nervous system: Headache, insomnia, malaise, fatigue, pain
Gastrointestinal: Nausea, diarrhea, vomiting
Neuromuscular & skeletal: Peripheral neuropathy, paresthesia
Respiratory: Nasal signs and symptoms, cough

1% to 10%:

Central nervous system: Dizziness, depression, fever, chills
Dermatologic: Rashes
Gastrointestinal: Anorexia, abdominal pain, dyspepsia, increased amylase
Hematologic: Neutropenia, anemia
Hepatic: Elevated AST/ALT
Neuromuscular & skeletal: Myalgia, arthralgia

<1%: Pancreatitis, thrombocytopenia, hyperbilirubinemia

**Drug Interactions** Increased effect: Zidovudine concentrations increase (~39%) with coadministration with lamivudine; trimethoprim/sulfamethoxazole increases lamivudine's AUC and decreases its renal clearance by 44% and 29%, respectively; although the AUC was not significantly affected, absorption of lamivudine was slowed and $C_{max}$ was 40% lower when administered to patients in the fed versus the fasted state

**Half-Life** 5-7 hours

### Special PA Issues

**Patient Education:** This is not a cure for AIDS or AIDS complex, nor will it reduce the risk of transmission to others. Long-term effects are unknown. You will need frequent blood tests to adjust dosage for maximum therapeutic effect. Take as directed for full course of therapy; do not discontinue (even if feeling better). You may experience loss of appetite; change in taste (sucking on lozenges, chewing gum, or small frequent meals may help); dizziness or numbness (use caution when driving or engaging in hazardous activities); headache, fever, or muscle pain (an analgesic may be recommended). Report persistent lethargy, acute headache, severe nausea or vomiting, difficulty breathing, loss of sensation, or rash.

**Monitoring Parameters:** Amylase, bilirubin, liver enzymes, hematologic parameters, viral load, and CD4 count; signs and symptoms of pancreatitis

## Lamotrigine *(la MOE tri jeen)*

**Pharmacologic Class** Anticonvulsant, Miscellaneous

**U.S. Brand Names** Lamictal®

**Mechanism of Action** A triazine derivative which inhibits release of glutamate (an excitatory amino acid) and inhibits voltage-sensitive sodium channels, which stabilizes neuronal membranes

**Use** Partial/secondary generalized seizures in adults; childhood epilepsy, including Lennox-Gastaut disorder **(not approved for use in children <2 years of age)**

**USUAL DOSAGE** Oral:

Children 2-12 years:

With concomitant AEDs including valproic acid therapy: Initial: 0.15 mg/kg/day in 1-2 divided doses for 2 weeks; may increase by 0.3 mg/kg/day in 1-2 divided doses for 2 weeks; may increase by 0.3 mg/kg/day at 1- to 2-week intervals in 1-2 divided doses; see table

With concomitant AEDs without valproic acid therapy: Initial: 0.6 mg/kg/day in 2 divided doses for 2 weeks, then 1-2 mg/kg/day in 2 divided doses for 2 weeks; may increase by 1.2 mg/kg/day (round down to nearest 5 mg) at 1- to 2-week intervals; usual maintenance dose: 5-15 mg/kg/day; maximum: 400 mg/day in 2 divided doses

### Lamictal Added to an AED Regimen Containing VPA in Patients 2-12 Years of Age

| Weeks 1 and 2 | 0.15 mg/kg/day in 1 or 2 divided doses, rounded down to the nearest 5 mg; if the initial calculated daily dose is 2.5-5 mg, then 5 mg should be taken on alternate days for the first 2 weeks |
|---|---|
| Weeks 3 and 4 | 0.3 mg/kg/day in 1 or 2 divided doses, rounded down to the nearest 5 mg |

Usual maintenance dose: 1-5 mg/kg/day (maximum: 200 mg/day in 1-2 divided doses). To achieve usual maintenance dose, subsequent doses should be increased every 1-2 weeks as follows: Calculate 0.3 mg/kg/day, round this amount down to the nearest 5 mg, and add this amount to the previously administered daily dose.

Adults: Initial: 50-100 mg/day then titrate to daily maintenance dose of 100-400 mg/day in 1-2 divided daily doses

With concomitant valproic acid therapy: Start initial dose at 25 mg/day then titrate to maintenance dose of 50-200 mg/day in 1-2 divided daily doses

**Dosage Forms** Tab: 25 mg, 100 mg, 150 mg, 200 mg; **Tab, chew:** 5 mg, 25 mg
**Contraindications** History of hypersensitivity to lamotrigine or any component
**Warnings/Precautions** Lactation, impaired renal, hepatic, or cardiac function; avoid abrupt cessation, taper over at least 2 weeks if possible. Severe and potentially life-threatening skin rashes have been reported; this appears to occur most frequently in pediatric patients.
**Pregnancy Risk Factor** C
**Adverse Reactions** 1% to 10%:
Central nervous system: Dizziness, sedation, ataxia
Dermatologic: Hypersensitivity rash, Stevens-Johnson syndrome, angioedema
Ocular: Nystagmus, diplopia
Renal: Hematuria
**Drug Interactions**
Decreased effect: Acetaminophen (increased renal clearance); carbamazepine, phenobarbital, and phenytoin (increased metabolic clearance)
Increased effect: Valproic acid increases half-life of lamotrigine (decreased metabolic clearance)
**Half-Life** 24 hours; increases to 59 hours with concomitant valproic acid therapy; decreases with concomitant phenytoin or carbamazepine therapy to 15 hours
**Special PA Issues**
**Patient Education:** Take exactly as directed (do not increase dose or frequency or discontinue without consulting prescriber). While using this medication, do not use alcohol and other prescription or OTC medications (especially pain medications, sedatives, antihistamines, or hypnotics) without consulting prescriber. Maintain adequate hydration (2-3 L/day of fluids unless instructed to restrict fluid intake). You may experience drowsiness, dizziness, or blurred vision (use caution when driving or engaging in hazardous tasks); nausea, vomiting, loss of appetite, heartburn, or dry mouth (small frequent meals, good mouth care, chewing gum, or sucking on lozenges may help). Wear identification of epileptic status and medications. Report CNS changes, mentation changes, or changes in cognition; persistent GI symptoms (cramping, constipation, vomiting, anorexia); skin rash; swelling of face, lips, or tongue; easy bruising or bleeding (mouth, urine, stool); vision changes; worsening of seizure activity, or loss of seizure control.
**Dietary Considerations:** Food: Has no effect on absorption, take without regard to meals; drug may cause GI upset
**Monitoring Parameters:** Seizure (frequency and duration); serum levels of concurrent anticonvulsants; hypersensitivity reactions (especially rash)
**Reference Range:** Therapeutic range: 2-4 µg/mL

♦ **Lamprene®** see Clofazimine on page 220
♦ **Lanacane® [OTC]** see Benzocaine on page 105
♦ **Lanacort® [OTC]** see Hydrocortisone on page 453
♦ **Lanaphilic® Topical [OTC]** see Urea on page 947
♦ **Laniazid®** see Isoniazid on page 494
♦ **Lanorinal®** see Butalbital Compound on page 131
♦ **Lanoxicaps®** see Digoxin on page 281
♦ **Lanoxin®** see Digoxin on page 281

## Lansoprazole (lan SOE pra zole)
**Pharmacologic Class** Proton Pump Inhibitor
**U.S. Brand Names** Prevacid®
**Use** Short-term treatment (up to 4 weeks) for healing and symptom relief of active duodenal ulcers (should not be used for maintenance therapy of duodenal ulcers); as part of a multiple drug regimen for H. pylori eradication; short-term treatment of symptomatic GERD; up to 8 weeks of treatment for all grades of erosive esophagitis (8 additional weeks can be given for incompletely healed esophageal erosions or for recurrence); and long-term treatment of pathological hypersecretory conditions, including Zollinger-Ellison syndrome
**USUAL DOSAGE**
Duodenal ulcer: 15 mg once daily for 4 weeks; maintenance therapy: 15 mg once daily
Gastric ulcer: 30 mg once daily for up to 8 weeks
GERD: 15 mg once daily for up to 8 weeks
Erosive esophagitis: 30 mg once daily for up to 8 weeks, continued treatment for an additional 8 weeks may be considered for recurrence or for patients that do not heal after the first 8 weeks of therapy. Maintenance therapy: 15 mg once daily.
Hypersecretory conditions: Initial: 60 mg once daily; adjust dose based upon patient response and to reduce acid secretion to <10 mEq/hour (5 mEq/hour in patients with prior gastric surgery); doses of 90 mg twice daily have been used; administer doses >120 mg/day in divided doses.
Helicobacter pylori-associated antral gastritis: 30 mg/day for 2 weeks (in combination with 1 g amoxicillin and 500 mg clarithromycin given twice daily for 14 days). Alternatively, in patients allergic to or intolerant of clarithromycin or in whom resistance to clarithromycin is known or suspected, lansoprazole 30 mg every 8 hours and amoxicillin 1 g every 8 hours may be given for 2 weeks
(Continued)

## Lansoprazole *(Continued)*

**Dosing adjustment in hepatic impairment:** Dose reduction is necessary for severe hepatic impairment

**Dosage Forms Cap, delayed release:** 15 mg, 30 mg

**Contraindications** Should not be taken by anyone with a known hypersensitivity to lansoprazole or any of the formulation's components

**Warnings/Precautions** Liver disease may require dosage reductions

**Pregnancy Risk Factor** B

**Adverse Reactions**
1% to 10%:
  Central nervous system: Fatigue, dizziness, headache
  Gastrointestinal: Abdominal pain, diarrhea, nausea, increased appetite, hypergastrinoma
<1%: Rash, tinnitus, proteinuria

**Drug Interactions** CYP2C19 enzyme substrate, CYP3A3/4 enzyme substrate (minor)
Decreased effect: Ketoconazole, itraconazole, and other drugs dependent upon acid for absorption; theophylline clearance increased slightly; sucralfate delays and reduces lansoprazole absorption by 30%

**Duration** 1 day

**Half-Life** Healthy patient: 1.5 hours; Elderly: 2.9 hours; Cirrhosis: 7 hours

**Special PA Issues**
  **Patient Education:** Take as directed, before eating. Do not crush or chew capsules. Report unresolved fatigue, diarrhea, or constipation, and appetite changes.
  **Monitoring Parameters:** Patients with Zollinger-Ellison syndrome should be monitored for gastric acid output, which should be maintained at 10 mEq/hour or less during the last hour before the next lansoprazole dose; lab monitoring should include CBC, liver function, renal function, and serum gastrin levels

♦ **Largactil®** *see* Chlorpromazine *on page 197*

♦ **Lariam®** *see* Mefloquine *on page 563*

♦ **Larodopa®** *see* Levodopa *on page 524*

♦ **Lasix®** *see* Furosemide *on page 405*

## Latanoprost (la TAN oh prost)

**Pharmacologic Class** Ophthalmic Agent, Antiglaucoma; Prostaglandin, Ophthalmic

**U.S. Brand Names** Xalatan®

**Mechanism of Action** Latanoprost is a prostaglandin $F_2$-alpha analog believed to reduce intraocular pressure by increasing the outflow of the aqueous humor

**Use** Reduction of elevated intraocular pressure in patients with open-angle glaucoma and ocular hypertension who are intolerant of the other IOP lowering medications or insufficiently responsive (failed to achieve target IOP determined after multiple measurements over time) to another IOP lowering medication

**USUAL DOSAGE** Adults: Ophthalmic: 1 drop (1.5 mcg) in the affected eye(s) once daily in the evening; do not exceed the once daily dosage because it has been shown that more frequent administration may decrease the IOP lowering effect

**Dosage Forms Soln, ophth:** 0.005% (2.5 mL)

**Contraindications** Hypersensitivity to any component of product

**Warnings/Precautions** Latanoprost may gradually change eye color, increasing the amount of brown pigment in the iris by increasing the number of melanosome in melanocytes. The long-term effects on the melanocytes and the consequences of potential injury to the melanocytes or deposition of pigment granules to other areas of the eye is currently unknown. Patients should be examined regularly, and depending on the clinical situation, treatment may be stopped if increased pigmentation ensues.

There have been reports of bacterial keratitis associated with the use of multiple-dose containers of topical ophthalmic products. Do not administer while wearing contact lenses.

**Pregnancy Risk Factor** C

**Adverse Reactions**
>10%: Ocular: Blurred vision, burning and stinging, conjunctival hyperemia, foreign body sensation, itching, increased pigmentation of the iris, and punctate epithelial keratopathy
1% to 10%:
  Cardiovascular: Chest pain, angina pectoris
  Dermatologic: Rash, allergic skin reaction
  Neuromuscular & skeletal: Myalgia, arthralgia, back pain
  Ocular: Dry eye, excessive tearing, eye pain, lid crusting, lid edema, lid erythema, lid discomfort/pain, photophobia
  Respiratory: Upper respiratory tract infection, cold, flu
<1%: Conjunctivitis, diplopia, discharge from the eye, retinal artery embolus, retinal detachment, vitreous hemorrhage from diabetic retinopathy

**Drug Interactions** Decreased effect: *In vitro* studies have shown that precipitation occurs when eye drops containing thimerosal are mixed with latanoprost. If such drugs are used, administer with an interval of at least 5 minutes between applications

**Onset** 3-4 hours; Maximum effect: 8-12 hours

**Half-Life** 17 minutes

**Special PA Issues**

**Patient Education:** For ophthalmic use only. Store in cool place. If you wear soft contact lenses, remove before using medication and wait at least 15 minutes before replacing. Apply prescribed amount as often as directed. Wash hands before using and do not touch tip of applicator to eye or contaminate tip of applicator. Tilt head back and look upward. Gently pull down lower lid and put drop(s) inside lower eyelid at inner corner. Close eye and roll eyeball in all directions. Do not blink for $1/2$ minute. Apply gentle pressure to inner corner of eye for 30 seconds. Wipe away excess from skin around eye. Do not use any other eye preparation for at least 10 minutes. Do not share medication with anyone else. Stinging or blurred vision may occur (this is temporary). Your iris may change color with use of medication (this may be more noticeable if you have green, brown, blue, gray, or combination-colored iris - notify prescriber if iris changes color). You may experience sensitivity to sunlight (wearing dark glasses may help). Report systemic effects (chest, muscle, or back pain, or symptoms of upper respiratory infection); persistent eye pain, redness, burning, watering, dryness, double vision, puffiness around eye, vision disturbances, other adverse eye response, worsening of condition or lack of improvement.

- **Laxatives: Classification and Properties** *see* Chart *on page 1021*
- **LazerSporin-C® Otic** *see* Neomycin, Polymyxin B, and Hydrocortisone *on page 645*
- **l-Bunolol Hydrochloride** *see* Levobunolol *on page 523*
- **L-Deprenyl** *see* Selegiline *on page 826*
- **L-Dopa** *see* Levodopa *on page 524*

# Leflunomide (le FLU no mide)

**Pharmacologic Class** Antimetabolite

**U.S. Brand Names** Arava™

**Mechanism of Action** Inhibits pyrimidine synthesis, resulting in antiproliferative and anti-inflammatory effects

**Use** Treatment of active rheumatoid arthritis to reduce signs and symptoms and to retard structural damage as evidenced by x-ray erosions and joint space narrowing

**USUAL DOSAGE**

**Adults:** Oral: Initial: 100 mg/day for 3 days, followed by 20 mg/day; dosage may be decreased to 10 mg/day in patients who have difficulty tolerating the 20 mg dose. Due to the long half-life of the active metabolite, plasma levels may require a prolonged period to decline after dosage reduction.

**Dosing adjustment in renal impairment:** No specific dosage adjustment is recommended. There is no clinical experience in the use of leflunomide in patients with renal impairment. The free fraction of MI is doubled in dialysis patients. Patients should be monitored closely for adverse effects requiring dosage adjustment.

**Dosing adjustment in hepatic impairment:** No specific dosage adjustment is recommended. Since the liver is involved in metabolic activation and subsequent metabolism/elimination of leflunomide, patients with hepatic impairment should be monitored closely for adverse effects requiring dosage adjustment.

Guidelines for dosage adjustment or discontinuation based on the severity and persistence of ALT elevation secondary to leflunomide have been developed. For ALT elevations >2 times the upper limit of normal, dosage reduction to 10 mg/day may allow continued administration. Cholestyramine 8 g 3 times/day for 1-3 days may be administered to decrease plasma levels. If elevations >2 times but ≤3 times the upper limit of normal persist, liver biopsy is recommended. If elevations >3 times the upper limit of normal persist despite cholestyramine administration and dosage reduction, leflunomide should be discontinued and drug elimination should be enhanced with additional cholestyramine as indicated.

**Elderly:** Although hepatic function may decline with age, no specific dosage adjustment is recommended. Patients should be monitored closely for adverse effects which may require dosage adjustment.

**Dosage Forms Tab:** 10 mg, 20 mg, 100 mg

**Contraindications** Pregnancy/breast-feeding; known hypersensitivity to leflunomide or any component

**Warnings/Precautions** Hepatic disease (including seropositive hepatitis B or C patients) may increase risk of hepatotoxicity; immunosuppression may increase the risk of lymphoproliferative disorders or other malignancies; women of childbearing potential should not receive leflunomide until pregnancy has been excluded, patients have been counseled concerning fetal risk and reliable contraceptive measures have been confirmed. Caution in renal impairment, immune deficiency, bone marrow dysplasia or severe, uncontrolled infection. Use of live vaccines is not recommended; will increase uric acid excretion.

**Pregnancy Risk Factor** X

**Pregnancy Implications** Has been associated with teratogenic and embryolethal effects in animal models at low doses. Leflunomide is contraindicated in pregnant women or women of childbearing potential who are not using reliable contraception. Pregnancy must be (Continued)

# Leflunomide *(Continued)*

excluded prior to initiating treatment. Following treatment, pregnancy should be avoided until the drug elimination procedure is completed.

Breast-feeding is contraindicated. It is not known whether leflunomide is secreted in human milk; however, there is a potential for serious adverse reactions in nursing infants. A decision should be made whether to discontinue nursing or discontinue the drug, taking into account the importance of the drug to the mother.

## Adverse Reactions

>10%:

Gastrointestinal: Diarrhea (17%)

Respiratory: Respiratory tract infection (15%)

1% to 10%:

Cardiovascular: Hypertension (10%), chest pain (2%), palpitation, tachycardia, vasculitis, vasodilation, varicose vein, edema (peripheral)

Central nervous system: Headache (7%), dizziness (4%), pain (2%), fever, malaise, migraine, anxiety, depression, insomnia, sleep disorder

Dermatologic: Alopecia (10%), rash (10%), pruritus (4%), dry skin (2%), eczema (2%), acne, dermatitis, hair discoloration, hematoma, herpes infection, nail disorder, subcutaneous nodule, skin disorder/discoloration, skin ulcer, bruising

Endocrine & metabolic: Hypokalemia (1%), diabetes mellitus, hyperglycemia, hyperlipidemia, hyperthyroidism, menstrual disorder

Gastrointestinal: Nausea (9%), abdominal pain (5%), dyspepsia (5%), weight loss (4%), anorexia (3%), gastroenteritis (3%), stomatitis (3%), vomiting (3%), cholelithiasis, colitis, constipation, esophagitis, flatulence, gastritis, gingivitis, melena, candidiasis (oral), enlarged salivary gland, tooth disorder, xerostomia, taste disturbance

Genitourinary: Urinary tract infection (5%), albuminuria, cystitis, dysuria, hematuria, vaginal candidiasis, prostate disorder, urinary frequency

Hematologic: Anemia

Hepatic: Abnormal LFTs (5%)

Neuromuscular & skeletal: Back pain (5%), joint disorder (4%), weakness (3%), tenosynovitis (3%), synovitis (2%), arthralgia (1%), paresthesia (2%), muscle cramps (2%), neck pain, pelvic pain, increased CPK, arthrosis, bursitis, myalgia, bone necrosis, bone pain, tendon rupture, neuralgia, neuritis

Ocular: Blurred vision, cataract, conjunctivitis, eye disorder

Respiratory: Bronchitis (7%), cough (3%), pharyngitis (3%), pneumonia (2%), rhinitis (2%), sinusitis (2%), asthma, dyspnea, epistaxis, lung disorder

Miscellaneous: Infection (4%), accidental injury (5%), allergic reactions (2%), diaphoresis

<1%: Anaphylaxis, urticaria, eosinophilia, thrombocytopenia, leukopenia

**Drug Interactions** Cytochrome P-450 2C9 enzyme inhibitor

Increased effect: Theoretically, the concomitant use of drugs metabolized by this enzyme, which includes many NSAIDs, may result in increased serum concentrations. Coadministration with methotrexate increases the risk of hepatotoxicity. Leflunomide may also enhance the hepatotoxicity of other drugs. Tolbutamide free fraction may be increased. Rifampin may increase the serum concentrations of the active metabolite of leflunomide. Leflunomide has uricosuric activity and may enhance activity of other uricosuric agents.

Decreased effect: Administration of cholestyramine and activated charcoal enhance the elimination of leflunomide's active metabolite

**Half-Life** Mean 14-15 days; enterohepatic recycling appears to contribute to the long half-life of this agent, since activated charcoal and cholestyramine substantially reduce plasma half-life

## Special PA Issues

**Patient Education:** Take as directed; do not increase dose without consulting prescriber. Maintain adequate hydration (2-3 L/day of fluids unless instructed to restrict fluid intake). Store medication away from light. You may experience diarrhea (buttermilk, boiled milk, or yogurt may help); nausea, vomiting, loss of appetite, and flatulence (small frequent meals, frequent mouth care, or sucking lozenges may help); dizziness (use caution when driving or engaging in hazardous tasks until response is known). If diabetic, monitor blood sugars closely; this medication may alter glucose levels. Report chest pain, palpitations, rapid heartbeat, or swelling of extremities; persistent gastrointestinal problems; skin rash, redness, irritation, acne, ulcers, or easy bruising; frequency, painful or difficult urination, or genital itching or irritation; depression, acute headache, anxiety, or difficulty sleeping; weakness, muscle tremors, cramping or weakness, back pain, or altered gait; cough, cold symptoms, wheezing, or difficulty breathing; easy bruising/bleeding; blood in vomitus, stool, urine; or other unusual effects related to this medication.

**Dietary Considerations:** No interactions with food have been noted

**Monitoring Parameters:** Serum transaminase determinations at baseline and monthly during the initial phase of treatment; if stable, monitoring frequency may be decreased to intervals determined by the individual clinical situation

♦ **Lenoltec No 1, 2, 3, 4** *see* Acetaminophen and Codeine *on page 22*

♦ **Lente® Iletin® I** *see* Insulin Preparations *on page 479*

♦ **Lente® Iletin® II** *see* Insulin Preparations *on page 479*

♦ **Lente® Insulin** *see* Insulin Preparations *on page 479*
♦ **Lente® L** *see* Insulin Preparations *on page 479*
♦ **Lescol®** *see* Fluvastatin *on page 395*

# Letrozole (LET roe zole)

**Pharmacologic Class** Antineoplastic Agent, Miscellaneous; Aromatase Inhibitor
**U.S. Brand Names** Femara™
**Mechanism of Action** Nonsteroidal, competitive inhibitor of the aromatase enzyme system which binds to the heme group of aromatase, a cytochrome P-450 enzyme which catalyzes conversion of androgens to estrogens (specifically, androstenedione to estrone and testosterone to estradiol). This leads to inhibition of the enzyme and a significant reduction in plasma estrogen levels. Approximately 30% of breast cancers are sensitive to this estrogen deprivation.
**Use** Treatment of advanced breast cancer in postmenopausal women with disease progression following antiestrogen therapy
**USUAL DOSAGE** Oral (refer to individual protocols):
**Adults:** 2.5 mg once daily without regard to meals; continue treatment until tumor progression is evident. Patients treated with letrozole do not require glucocorticoid or mineralocorticoid replacement therapy.
**Dosage adjustment in renal impairment:** No dosage adjustment is required in patients with renal impairment if $Cl_{cr}$ ≥10 mL/minute
**Dosage adjustment in hepatic impairment:** No dosage adjustment is recommended for patients with mild-to-moderate hepatic impairment. Patients with severe impairment of liver function have not been studied; dose patients with severe impairment of liver function with caution.
**Dosage Forms Tab:** 2.5 mg
**Contraindications** Hypersensitivity to letrozole or any of its excipients
**Warnings/Precautions** Letrozole was not mutagenic in *in vitro* tests but was observed to be a potential clastogen in *in vitro* assays. Repeated dosing caused sexual inactivity in females and atrophy in the reproductive tract in males and females at doses of 0.6 mg/kg, 0.1 mg/kg, and 0.03 mg/kg in mice, rats, and dogs, respectively (~1 mg/kg, 0.4 mg/kg, and 0.4 mg/kg the maximum recommended human doses, respectively).

Moderate decreases in lymphocyte counts, of uncertain clinical significance, were observed in some patients receiving letrozole 2.5 mg. This depression was transient in ~50% of those affected. Two patients on letrozole developed thrombocytopenia; relationship to the drug was unclear.

Increases in AST, ALT, and GGT ≥5 times the upper limit of normal (ULN) and of bilirubin ≥1.5 times the ULN were most often associated with metastatic disease in the liver.
**Pregnancy Risk Factor** D
**Pregnancy Implications**
Clinical effects on the fetus: Letrozole may cause fetal harm when administered to pregnant women. Letrozole is embryotoxic and fetotoxic when administered to rats. There are no studies in pregnant women and letrozole is indicated for postmenopausal women.
Breast-feeding/lactation: It is not known if letrozole is excreted in breast milk; exercise caution when letrozole is administered to nursing women
**Adverse Reactions**
>10%: Gastrointestinal: Nausea
1% to 10%:
Central nervous system: Headache, somnolence, dizziness
Dermatologic: Hot flashes, rash, pruritus
Gastrointestinal: Vomiting, constipation, diarrhea, abdominal pain, anorexia, dyspepsia
Neuromuscular: Arthralgia
Respiratory: Dyspnea, coughing
<1%: Thromboembolic events, vaginal bleeding
**Drug Interactions** CYP3A3/4 and 2A6 enzyme substrate; CYP2A6 and 2C19 enzyme inhibitor
**Half-Life** 2 days
**Special PA Issues**
**Patient Education:** Take as directed, without regard to food. You may experience nausea, vomiting, or loss of appetite (frequent mouth care, frequent small meals, chewing gum, or sucking on lozenges may help); musculoskeletal pain or headache (mild analgesics may offer relief); sleepiness, fatigue, or dizziness (use caution when driving, climbing stairs, or engaging in tasks that require alertness); constipation (increased exercise, or dietary fruit or fluids may help); diarrhea (boiled milk or yogurt may help); loss of hair (will grow back). Report chest pain, palpitations, or swollen extremities; vaginal bleeding or hot flashes; unusual coughing or difficulty breathing; severe nausea; muscle pain; or skin rash.
**Monitoring Parameters:** Clinical/radiologic evidence of tumor regression in advanced breast cancer patients. Until the toxicity has been defined in larger patient populations, monitor the following laboratory tests periodically during therapy: complete blood counts, thyroid function tests, serum electrolytes, serum transaminases, and serum creatinine.

# Leucovorin (loo koe VOR in)

**Pharmacologic Class** Antidote; Vitamin, Water Soluble

**U.S. Brand Names** Wellcovorin®

**Mechanism of Action** A reduced form of folic acid, but does not require a reduction reaction by an enzyme for activation, allows for purine and thymidine synthesis, a necessity for normal erythropoiesis; leucovorin supplies the necessary cofactor blocked by MTX, enters the cells via the same active transport system as MTX

**Use** Antidote for folic acid antagonists (methotrexate [>100 mg/m²], trimethoprim, pyrimethamine); treatment of megaloblastic anemias when folate is deficient as in infancy, sprue, pregnancy, and nutritional deficiency when oral folate therapy is not possible; in combination with fluorouracil in the treatment of malignancy

**USUAL DOSAGE** Children and Adults:

Treatment of folic acid antagonist overdosage (eg, pyrimethamine or trimethoprim): Oral: 2-15 mg/day for 3 days or until blood counts are normal or 5 mg every 3 days; doses of 6 mg/day are needed for patients with platelet counts <100,000/mm³

Folate-deficient megaloblastic anemia: I.M.: 1 mg/day

Megaloblastic anemia secondary to congenital deficiency of dihydrofolate reductase: I.M.: 3-6 mg/day

Rescue dose (rescue therapy should start within 24 hours of MTX therapy): I.V.: 10 mg/m² to start, then 10 mg/m² every 6 hours orally for 72 hours until serum MTX concentration is <10⁻⁸ molar; if serum creatinine 24 hours after methotrexate is elevated 50% or more above the pre-MTX serum creatinine or the serum MTX concentration is >5 x 10⁻⁶ molar (see graph), increase dose to 100 mg/m²/dose (preservative-free) every 3 hours until serum methotrexate level is <1 x 10⁻⁸ molar

Investigational: Post I.T. methotrexate: Oral: 12 mg/m² as a single dose; post high-dose methotrexate: 100-1000 mg/m²/dose until the serum methotrexate level is less than 1 x 10⁻⁷ molar

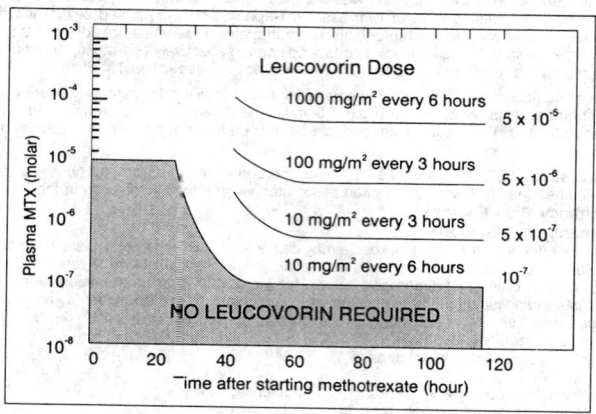

The drug should be given parenterally instead of orally in patients with GI toxicity, nausea, vomiting, and when individual doses are >25 mg

**Dosage Forms** Inj: 3 mg/mL (1 mL); **Powder for inj:** 25 mg, 50 mg, 100 mg, 350 mg; **Powder for oral soln:** 1 mg/mL (60 mL); **Tab:** 5 mg, 10 mg, 15 mg, 25 mg

**Contraindications** Pernicious anemia or vitamin $B_{12}$ deficient megaloblastic anemias; should **NOT** be administered Intrathecally/Intraventricularly

**Warnings/Precautions** Use with caution in patients with a history of hypersensitivity

**Pregnancy Risk Factor** C

**Adverse Reactions** <1%: Rash, pruritus, erythema, urticaria, thrombocytosis, wheezing, anaphylactoid reactions

**Onset** Onset of activity: Oral: Within 30 minutes; I.V.: Within 5 minutes

**Half-Life** Leucovorin: 15 minutes; Metabolite 5MTHF: 33-35 minutes

**Special PA Issues**

**Patient Education:** Take as directed, at evenly spaced intervals around-the-clock. Maintain hydration (2-3 L of water/day while taking for rescue therapy). For folic acid deficiency, eat foods high in folic acid (eg, meat proteins, bran, dried beans, asparagus, green leafy vegetables). Report respiratory difficulty, lethargy, or rash or itching.

**Monitoring Parameters:** Plasma MTX concentration as a therapeutic guide to high-dose MTX therapy with leucovorin factor rescue

Leucovorin is continued until the plasma MTX level is <1 x $10^{-7}$ molar

Each dose of leucovorin is increased if the plasma MTX concentration is excessively high (see graph)

With 4- to 6-hour high-dose MTX infusions, plasma drug values in excess of 5 x $10^{-5}$ and $10^{-6}$ molar at 24 and 48 hours after starting the infusion, respectively, are often predictive of delayed MTX clearance; see graph.

♦ **Leucovorin Calcium** *see Leucovorin on previous page*

♦ **Leukeran®** *see Chlorambucil on page 187*

♦ **Leukine™** *see Sargramostim on page 822*

## Leuprolide Acetate (loo PROE lide AS e tate)

**Pharmacologic Class** Antineoplastic Agent, Miscellaneous; Luteinizing Hormone-Releasing Hormone Analog

**U.S. Brand Names** Lupron®; Lupron Depot®; Lupron Depot®-3 Month; Lupron Depot®-4 Month; Lupron Depot-Ped®

**Mechanism of Action** Continuous daily administration results in suppression of ovarian and testicular steroidogenesis due to decreased levels of LH and FSH with subsequent decrease in testosterone (male) and estrogen (female) levels

**Use** Palliative treatment of advanced prostate carcinoma (alternative when orchiectomy or estrogen administration are not indicated or are unacceptable to the patient); combination therapy with flutamide for treating metastatic prostatic carcinoma; endometriosis (3.75 mg depot only); central precocious puberty (may be used an agent to treat precocious puberty because of its effect in lowering levels of LH and FSH, testosterone, and estrogen).

**Unlabeled use:** Treatment of breast, ovarian, and endometrial cancer; leiomyoma uteri; infertility; prostatic hypertrophy

**USUAL DOSAGE** Requires parenteral administration

Children: Precocious puberty:

S.C.: 20-45 mcg/kg/day

I.M. (Depot®) formulation: 0.3 mg/kg/dose given every 28 days

≤25 kg: 7.5 mg

>25-37.5 kg: 11.25 mg

>37.5 kg: 15 mg

Adults:

Male: Advanced prostatic carcinoma:

S.C.: 1 mg/day **or**

I.M., Depot® (suspension): 7.5 mg/dose given monthly (every 28-33 days)

Female: Endometriosis: I.M., Depot® (suspension): 3.75 mg monthly for up to 6 months

**Dosage Forms Inj:** 5 mg/mL (2.8 mL); **Powder for inj (depot):** Depot®: 3.75 mg, 7.5 mg, Depot-3® Month: 11.25 mg, 22.5 mg, Depot-Ped™: 7.5 mg, 11.25 mg, 15 mg

**Contraindications** Hypersensitivity to leuprolide; spinal cord compression (orchiectomy suggested); undiagnosed abnormal vaginal bleeding; women who are or may be pregnant should not receive Lupron® Depot®

**Warnings/Precautions** Use with caution in patients hypersensitive to benzyl alcohol; after 6 months use of Depot® leuprolide, vertebral bone density decreased (average 13.5%); long-term safety of leuprolide in children has not been established; urinary tract obstruction may occur upon initiation of therapy. Closely observe patients for weakness, paresthesias, and urinary tract obstruction in first few weeks of therapy. Tumor flare and bone pain may occur at initiation of therapy; transient weakness and paresthesia of lower limbs, hematuria, and urinary tract obstruction in first week of therapy; animal studies have shown dose-related benign pituitary hyperplasia and benign pituitary adenomas after 2 years of use.

**Pregnancy Risk Factor** X

**Adverse Reactions**

>10%:

Central nervous system: Depression, pain

Endocrine & metabolic: Hot flashes

Gastrointestinal: Weight gain, nausea, vomiting

1% to 10%:

Cardiovascular: Cardiac arrhythmias, edema

Central nervous system: Dizziness, lethargy, insomnia, headache

Dermatologic: Rash

Endocrine: Estrogenic effects (gynecomastia, breast tenderness)

Gastrointestinal: Nausea, vomiting, diarrhea, GI bleed

Hematologic: Decreased hemoglobin and hematocrit

Neuromuscular & skeletal: Paresthesia, myalgia

Ocular: Blurred vision

<1%: Myocardial infarction, thrombophlebitis, pulmonary embolism

**Onset** Serum testosterone levels first increase within 3 days of therapy.

**Duration** Levels decrease after 2-4 weeks with continued therapy.

**Half-Life** 3-4.25 hours

(Continued)

## Leuprolide Acetate (Continued)

### Special PA Issues

**Patient Education:** Use as directed. Do not discontinue abruptly; consult prescriber. You may experience disease flare (increased bone pain) and urinary retention during early treatment (usually resolves), dizziness, headache, lethargy, or faintness (use caution when driving or engaging in hazardous tasks), nausea or vomiting (small frequent meals or analgesics may help), hot flashes - flushing or redness (cold clothes and cool environment may help). Report irregular or rapid heartbeat, unresolved nausea or vomiting, numbness of extremities, breast swelling or pain, difficulty breathing, or infection at injection sites.

**Monitoring Parameters:** Precocious puberty: GnRH testing (blood LH and FSH levels), testosterone in males and estradiol in females; closely monitor patients with prostatic carcinoma for weakness, paresthesias, and urinary tract obstruction in first few weeks of therapy

♦ **Leuprorelin Acetate** see Leuprolide Acetate on previous page

♦ **Leustatin™** see Cladribine on page 214

## Levamisole (lee VAM i soe)

**Pharmacologic Class** Immune Modulator

**U.S. Brand Names** Ergamisol®

**Mechanism of Action** Clinically, combined therapy with levamisole and 5-fluorouracil has been effective in treating colon cancer patients, whereas demonstrable activity has been demonstrated. Due to the broad range of pharmacologic activities of levamisole, it has been suggested that the drug may act as a biochemical modulator (of fluorouracil, for example, in colon cancer), an effect entirely independent of immune modulation. Further studies are needed to evaluate the mechanisms of action of the drug in cancer patients.

**Use** Adjuvant treatment with fluorouracil in Dukes stage C colon cancer

**USUAL DOSAGE** Adults: Oral: Initial: 50 mg every 8 hours for 3 days, then 50 mg every 8 hours for 3 days every 2 weeks (fluorouracil is always given concomitantly)

**Dosing adjustment in hepatic impairment:** May be necessary in patients with liver disease, but no specific guidelines are available

**Dosage Forms** Tab, as base: 50 mg

**Contraindications** Previous hypersensitivity to the drug

**Warnings/Precautions** Agranulocytosis can occur asymptomatically and flu-like symptoms can occur without hematologic adverse effects; frequent hematologic monitoring is necessary

**Pregnancy Risk Factor** C

**Adverse Reactions**

>10%: Gastrointestinal: Nausea, diarrhea

1% to 10%:

Cardiovascular: Edema

Central nervous system: Fatigue, fever, dizziness, headache, somnolence, depression, nervousness, insomnia

Dermatologic: Dermatitis, alopecia

Gastrointestinal: Stomatitis, vomiting, anorexia, abdominal pain, constipation, taste perversion

Hematologic: Leukopenia

Neuromuscular & skeletal: Rigors, arthralgia, myalgia, paresthesia

Miscellaneous: Infection

<1%: Chest pain, anxiety, pruritus, urticaria, flatulence, dyspepsia, thrombocytopenia, anemia, granulocytopenia, abnormal tearing, blurred vision, conjunctivitis, epistaxis, altered sense of smell

**Drug Interactions**

Increased toxicity/serum levels of phenytoin

Disulfiram-like reaction with alcohol

**Half-Life** 2-6 hours

### Special PA Issues

**Patient Education:** Take as directed, at regular intervals around-the-clock. Avoid alcohol (may cause disulfiram-like effect). Avoid all aspirin-containing medications. You may experience GI upset (small frequent meals may help); diarrhea (request medication); sensitivity to sun (use sunblock, wear protective clothing, and avoid direct sun); or dizziness, drowsiness, or impaired judgment (use caution when driving, performing hazardous tasks, climbing stairs). You will be more susceptible to infection; avoid crowds or infected persons. Report chills or fever, confusion, persistent or violent vomiting, persistent diarrhea, or respiratory difficulty.

**Monitoring Parameters:** CBC with platelet count prior to therapy and weekly prior to treatment; LFTs every 3 months

♦ **Levamisole Hydrochloride** see Levamisole on this page

♦ **Levaquin™** see Levofloxacin on page 526

- **Levate®** *see* Amitriptyline *on page 57*
- **Levbid®** *see* Hyoscyamine *on page 463*
- **Levlen®** *see* Ethinyl Estradiol and Levonorgestrel *on page 347*
- **Levlite®** *see* Ethinyl Estradiol and Levonorgestrel *on page 347*

## Levobunolol (lee voe BYOO noe lole)

**Pharmacologic Class** Beta Blocker, Nonselective; Ophthalmic Agent, Antiglaucoma

**U.S. Brand Names** AKBeta®; Betagan® Liquifilm®

**Mechanism of Action** A nonselective beta-adrenergic blocking agent that lowers intraocular pressure by reducing aqueous humor production and possibly increases the outflow of aqueous humor

**Use** To lower intraocular pressure in chronic open-angle glaucoma or ocular hypertension

**USUAL DOSAGE** Adults: Instill 1 drop in the affected eye(s) 1-2 times/day

**Dosage Forms** Soln, ophth, as hydrochloride: 0.25% (5 mL, 10 mL, 15 mL), 0.5% (2 mL, 5 mL, 10 mL, 15 mL)

**Contraindications** Known hypersensitivity to levobunolol; bronchial asthma, severe COPD, sinus bradycardia, second or third degree A-V block, cardiac failure, cardiogenic shock

**Warnings/Precautions** Use with caution in patients with congestive heart failure, diabetes mellitus, hyperthyroidism; contains metabisulfite. Because systemic absorption does occur with ophthalmic administration, the elderly with other disease states or syndromes that may be affected by a beta-blocker (CHF, COPD, etc) should be monitored closely.

**Pregnancy Risk Factor** C

**Adverse Reactions**

>10%: Ocular: Stinging/burning eyes

1% to 10%:

Cardiovascular: Bradycardia, arrhythmia, hypotension

Central nervous system: Dizziness, headache

Dermatologic: Alopecia, erythema

Local: Stinging, burning

Ocular: Blepharoconjunctivitis, conjunctivitis

Respiratory: Bronchospasm

<1%: Rash, itching, visual disturbances, keratitis, decreased visual acuity

**Drug Interactions** Increased toxicity:

Systemic beta-adrenergic blocking agents

Ophthalmic epinephrine (increased blood pressure/loss of IOP effect)

Quinidine (sinus bradycardia)

Verapamil (bradycardia and asystole have been reported)

**Onset** Decrease in intraocular pressure (IOP) can be noted within 1 hour; Peak effect: 2-6 hours

**Duration** 1-7 days

**Special PA Issues**

**Patient Education:** For ophthalmic use only. Apply prescribed amount as often as directed. Wash hands before using and do not touch tip of applicator to eye or contaminate tip of applicator. Tilt head back and look upward. Gently pull down lower lid and put drop(s) inside lower eyelid at inner corner. Close eye and roll eyeball in all directions. Do not blink for ½ minute. Apply gentle pressure to inner corner of eye for 30 seconds. Wipe away excess from skin around eye. Do not use any other eye preparation for at least 10 minutes. Do not share medication with anyone else. Temporary stinging or blurred vision may occur. Immediately report any adverse cardiac or CNS effects (usually signifies overdose). Report persistent eye pain, redness, burning, watering, dryness, double vision, puffiness around eye, vision disturbances, other adverse eye response, or worsening of condition or lack of improvement.

**Monitoring Parameters:** Intraocular pressure, heart rate, funduscopic exam, visual field testing

- **Levobunolol Hydrochloride** *see* Levobunolol *on this page*

## Levocabastine (LEE voe kab as teen)

**Pharmacologic Class** Antihistamine; Antihistamine, H₁ Blocker, Ophthalmic

**U.S. Brand Names** Livostin®

**Mechanism of Action** Potent, selective histamine $H_1$-receptor antagonist for topical ophthalmic use

**Use** Treatment of allergic conjunctivitis

**USUAL DOSAGE** Children >12 years and Adults: Instill 1 drop in affected eye(s) 4 times/day for up to 2 weeks

**Dosage Forms** Susp, ophth, as hydrochloride: 0.05% (2.5 mL, 5 mL, 10 mL)

**Contraindications** Hypersensitivity to any component of product; while soft contact lenses are being worn

**Warnings/Precautions** Safety and efficacy in children <12 years of age have not been established; not for injection; not for use in patients wearing soft contact lenses during treatment

(Continued)

## Levocabastine *(Continued)*

**Pregnancy Risk Factor** B
**Adverse Reactions**
>10%: Local: Transient burning, stinging, discomfort
1% to 10%:
Central nervous system: Headache, somnolence, fatigue
Dermatologic: Rash
Gastrointestinal: Xerostomia
Ocular: Blurred vision, eye pain, somnolence, red eyes, eyelid edema
Respiratory: Dyspnea

♦ **Levocabastine Hydrochloride** *see Levocabastine on previous page*

## Levodopa *(lee voe DOE pa)*

**Pharmacologic Class** Ant-Parkinson's Agent (Dopamine Agonist)
**U.S. Brand Names** Dopar®; Larodopa®
**Mechanism of Action** Increases dopamine levels in the brain, then stimulates dopaminergic receptors in the basal ganglia to improve the balance between cholinergic and dopaminergic activity
**Use** Treatment of Parkinson's disease; used as a diagnostic agent for growth hormone deficiency
**USUAL DOSAGE** Oral:
Children (administer as a single dose to evaluate growth hormone deficiency):
0.5 g/m² **or**
<30 lbs: 125 mg
30-70 lbs: 250 mg
>70 lbs: 500 mg
Adults: 500-1000 mg/day in divided doses every 6-12 hours; increase by 100-750 mg/day every 3-7 days until response or total dose of 8,000 mg is reached
A significant therapeutic response may not be obtained for 6 months
**Dosage Forms Cap:** 100 mg, 250 mg, 500 mg; **Tab:** 100 mg, 250 mg, 500 mg
**Contraindications** Hypersensitivity to levodopa or any component; narrow-angle glaucoma, MAO inhibitor therapy, melanomas or any undiagnosed skin lesions
**Warnings/Precautions** Use with caution in patients with history of myocardial infarction, arrhythmias, asthma, wide-angle glaucoma, peptic ulcer disease; sudden discontinuation of levodopa may cause a worsening of Parkinson's disease; some products may contain tartrazine. Elderly may be more sensitive to CNS effects of levodopa.
**Pregnancy Risk Factor** C
**Adverse Reactions**
>10%:
Cardiovascular: Orthostatic hypotension, arrhythmias
Central nervous system: Dizziness, anxiety, confusion, nightmares
Gastrointestinal: Anorexia, nausea, vomiting, constipation
Genitourinary: Dysuria
Neuromuscular & skeletal: Choreiform and involuntary movements
Ocular: Blepharospasm
1% to 10%:
Central nervous system: Headache
Gastrointestinal: Anorexia, diarrhea, xerostomia
Genitourinary: Discoloration of urine
Neuromuscular & skeletal: Muscle twitching
Ocular: Eyelid spasms
Miscellaneous: Discoloration of sweat
<1%: Hypertension, duodenal ulcer, GI bleeding, hemolytic anemia, blurred vision
**Drug Interactions**
Decreased effect:
Hydantoins may decrease effectiveness
Phenothiazines and hypotensive agents may decrease effect of levodopa
Pyridoxine may increase peripheral conversion, may decrease levodopa effectiveness
Increased toxicity with antacids
Monoamine oxidase inhibitors → hypertensive reactions
**Onset** Peak serum concentrations in 1-2 hours
**Duration** Variable, usually 6-12 hours
**Half-Life** 1.2-2.3 hours
**Special PA Issues**
Patient Education: Take exactly as directed; do not change dosage or discontinue without consulting prescriber. Therapeutic effects may take several weeks or months to achieve and you may need frequent monitoring during first weeks of therapy. Take with meals if GI upset occurs, before meals if dry mouth occurs, after eating if drooling or if nausea occurs. Take at same time each day. Maintain adequate hydration (2-3 L/day of fluids unless instructed to restrict fluid intake); void before taking medication. Do not use alcohol and prescription or OTC sedatives or CNS depressants without consulting

prescriber. Urine or perspiration may appear darker. You may experience drowsiness, dizziness, confusion, or vision changes (use caution when driving, climbing stairs, or engaging in hazardous tasks); orthostatic hypotension (use caution when changing position - rising to standing from sitting or lying); increased susceptibility to heat stroke, decreased perspiration (use caution in hot weather - maintain adequate fluids and reduce exercise activity); constipation (increased exercise, fluids, or dietary fruit and fiber may help); dry skin or nasal passages (consult prescriber for appropriate relief); nausea, vomiting, loss of appetite, or stomach discomfort (small frequent meals, chewing gum, or sucking on lozenges may help). Report unresolved constipation or vomiting; chest pain or irregular heartbeat; difficulty breathing; acute headache or dizziness; CNS changes (hallucination, loss of memory, nervousness, etc); painful or difficult urination; abdominal pain or blood in stool; increased muscle spasticity or rigidity; skin rash; or significant worsening of condition.

**Monitoring Parameters:** Serum growth hormone concentration

# Levodopa and Carbidopa (lee voe DOE pa & kar bi DOE pa)

**Pharmacologic Class** Anti-Parkinson's Agent (Dopamine Agonist)

**U.S. Brand Names** Atamet®; Sinemet®; Sinemet® CR

**Mechanism of Action** Parkinson's symptoms are due to a lack of striatal dopamine; levodopa circulates in the plasma to the blood-brain-barrier (BBB), where it crosses, to be converted by striatal enzymes to dopamine; carbidopa inhibits the peripheral plasma breakdown of levodopa by inhibiting its decarboxylation, and thereby increases available levodopa at the BBB

**Use** Treatment of parkinsonian syndrome; 50-100 mg/day of carbidopa is needed to block the peripheral conversion of levodopa to dopamine. "On-off" can be managed by giving smaller, more frequent doses of Sinemet® or adding a dopamine agonist or selegiline; when adding a new agent, doses of Sinemet® should usually be decreased.

**USUAL DOSAGE** Oral:

Adults: Initial: 25/100 2-4 times/day, increase as necessary to a maximum of 200/2000 mg/day

Elderly: Initial: 25/100 twice daily, increase as necessary

**Conversion from Sinemet® to Sinemet® CR (50/200):** (Sinemet® [total daily dose of levodopa] / Sinemet® CR)

300-400 mg / 1 tablet twice daily

500-600 mg / 1½ tablets twice daily or one 3 times/day

700-800 mg / 4 tablets in 3 or more divided doses

900-1000 mg / 5 tablets in 3 or more divided doses

Intervals between doses of Sinemet® CR should be 4-8 hours while awake

**Dosage Forms Tab:** 10/100: Carbidopa 10 mg and levodopa 100 mg, 25/100: Carbidopa 25 mg and levodopa 100 mg, 25/250: Carbidopa 25 mg and levodopa 250 mg, **Sustained release:** Carbidopa 25 mg and levodopa 100 mg; carbidopa 50 mg and levodopa 200 mg

**Contraindications** Narrow-angle glaucoma, MAO inhibitors, hypersensitivity to levodopa, carbidopa, or any component; do not use in patients with malignant melanoma or undiagnosed skin lesions

**Warnings/Precautions** Use with caution in patients with history of myocardial infarction, arrhythmias, asthma, wide angle glaucoma, peptic ulcer disease; sudden discontinuation of levodopa may cause a worsening of Parkinson's disease; some tablets may contain tartrazine. The elderly may be more sensitive to the CNS effects of levodopa. Protein in the diet should be distributed throughout the day to avoid fluctuations in levodopa absorption.

**Pregnancy Risk Factor** C

**Adverse Reactions**

>10%:

Cardiovascular: Orthostatic hypotension, palpitations, cardiac arrhythmias

Central nervous system: Confusion, nightmares, dizziness, anxiety

Gastrointestinal: Nausea, vomiting, anorexia, constipation

Neuromuscular & skeletal: Dystonic movements, "on-off", choreiform and involuntary movements

Ocular: Blepharospasm

Renal: Dysuria

1% to 10%:

Central nervous system: Headache

Gastrointestinal: Diarrhea, xerostomia

Genitourinary: Discoloration of urine

Neuromuscular & skeletal: Muscle twitching

Ocular: Eyelid spasms

Miscellaneous: Discoloration of sweat

<1%: Hypertension, memory loss, nervousness, insomnia, fatigue, hallucinations, ataxia, duodenal ulcer, GI bleeding, hemolytic anemia, blurred vision

**Drug Interactions**

Decreased effect:

Hydantoins, pyridoxine

Phenothiazines and hypotensive agents may decrease effects of levodopa

(Continued)

## Levodopa and Carbidopa *(Continued)*

Increased toxicity with antacids

Monoamine oxidase inhibitors → hypertensive reactions

**Duration** Variable, 6-12 hours; longer with CR dosage forms

**Half-Life** Carbidopa: 1-2 hours; Levodopa: 1.2-2.3 hours

**Special PA Issues**

**Patient Education:** Take exactly as directed; do not change dosage or discontinue without consulting prescriber. Therapeutic effects may take several weeks or months to achieve and you may need frequent monitoring during first weeks of therapy. Take with meals if GI upset occurs, before meals if dry mouth occurs, after eating if drooling or if nausea occurs. Take at same time each day. Maintain adequate hydration (2-3 L/day of fluids unless instructed to restrict fluid intake); void before taking medication. Do not use alcohol and prescription or OTC sedatives or CNS depressants without consulting prescriber. Urine or perspiration may appear darker. You may experience drowsiness, dizziness, confusion, or vision changes (use caution when driving, climbing stairs, or engaging in hazardous tasks); orthostatic hypotension (use caution when changing position - rising to standing from sitting or lying); increased susceptibility to heat stroke, decreased perspiration (use caution in hot weather - maintain adequate fluids and reduce exercise activity); constipation (increased exercise, fluids, or dietary fruit and fiber may help); dry skin or nasal passages (consult prescriber for appropriate relief); nausea, vomiting, loss of appetite, or stomach discomfort (small frequent meals, chewing gum, or sucking on lozenges may help). Report unresolved constipation or vomiting; chest pain or irregular heartbeat; difficulty breathing; acute headache or dizziness; CNS changes (hallucination, loss of memory, nervousness, etc); painful or difficult urination; abdominal pain or blood in stool; increased muscle spasticity or rigidity; skin rash; or significant worsening of condition.

**Monitoring Parameters:** Blood pressure, standing and sitting/supine; symptoms of parkinsonism, dyskinesias, mental status

♦ **Levo-Dromoran®** *see* Levorphanol *on page 528*

## Levofloxacin *(lee voe FLOKS a sin)*

**Pharmacologic Class** Antibiotic, Quinolone

**U.S. Brand Names** Levaquin™

**Mechanism of Action** As the S (-) enantiomer of the fluoroquinolone, ofloxacin, levofloxacin, inhibits DNA-gyrase in susceptible organisms thereby inhibits relaxation of supercoiled DNA and promotes breakage of DNA strands. DNA gyrase (topoisomerase II), is an essential bacterial enzyme that maintains the superhelical structure of DNA and is required for DNA replication and transcription, DNA repair, recombination, and transposition.

**Use** Acute maxillary sinusitis due to *S. pneumoniae, H. influenzae,* or *M. catarrhalis;* uncomplicated urinary tract infection due to *E. coli, K. pneumoniae,* or *S. saprophyticus;* also for acute bacterial exacerbation of chronic bronchitis and community-acquired pneumonia due to *S. aureus, S. pneumoniae, H. influenzae, H. parainfluenza,* or *M. catarrhalis, C. pneumoniae, L. pneumophila,* or *M. pneumoniae;* may be used for uncomplicated skin and skin structure infection (due to *S. aureus* or *S. pyogenes*) and complicated urinary tract infection due to gram-negative *Enterobacter* sp, including acute pyelonephritis (caused by *E. coli*)

**USUAL DOSAGE** Adults: Oral, I.V. solution over 60 minutes):

Acute bacterial exacerbation of chronic bronchitis: 500 mg every 24 hours for at least 7 days

Community acquired pneumonia: 500 mg every 24 hours for 7-14 days

Acute maxillary sinusitis: 500 mg every 24 hours for 10-14 days

Uncomplicated skin infections: 500 mg every 24 hours for 7-10 days

Uncomplicated urinary tract infections: 250 mg once daily for 3 days

Complicated urinary tract infections include acute pyelonephritis: 250 mg every 24 hours for 10 days

**Dosing adjustment in renal impairment:**

$Cl_{cr}$ 20-49 mL/minute: Administer 250 mg every 24 hours (initial: 500 mg)

$Cl_{cr}$ 10-19 mL/minute: Administer 250 mg every 48 hours (initial: 500 mg for most infections; 250 mg for renal infections)

Hemodialysis/CAPD: 250 mg every 48 hours (initial: 500 mg)

**Dosage Forms** Inf, in $D_5W$: 5 mg/mL (50 mL, 100 mL); **Inj:** 25 mg/mL (20 mL); **Tab:** 250 mg, 500 mg

**Contraindications** Hypersensitivity to levofloxacin, any component, or other quinolones; pregnancy, lactation

**Warnings/Precautions** Not recommended in children <18 years of age; other quinolones have caused transient arthropathy in children; CNS stimulation may occur (tremor, restlessness, confusion, and very rarely hallucinations or seizures); use with caution in patients with known or suspected CNS disorders or renal dysfunction; prolonged use may result in superinfection; if an allergic reaction (itching, urticaria, dyspnea, pharyngeal or facial edema, loss of consciousness, tingling, cardiovascular collapse) occurs, discontinue the drug immediately; use caution to avoid possible photosensitivity reactions during and for several days following fluoroquinolone therapy; pseudomembranous colitis may occur and should be considered in patients who present with diarrhea

**Pregnancy Risk Factor** C

**Pregnancy Implications**

Clinical effects on the fetus: Avoid use in pregnant women unless the benefit justifies the potential risk to the fetus

Breast-feeding/lactation: Quinolones are known to distribute well into breast milk; consequently, use during lactation should be avoided, if possible

**Adverse Reactions** >1%:

Central nervous system: Dizziness, headache, insomnia

Dermatologic: Rash

Gastrointestinal: Nausea, vomiting, increased transaminases

Hematologic: Leukopenia, thrombocytopenia

Neuromuscular & skeletal: Tremor, arthralgia

**Drug Interactions** CYP1A2 enzyme inhibitor (minor)

Decreased effect: Decreased absorption with antacids containing aluminum, magnesium, and/or calcium (by up to 98% if given at the same time); phenytoin serum levels may be reduced by quinolones; antineoplastic agents may also decrease serum levels of fluoroquinolones

Increased toxicity/serum levels: Quinolones may cause increased levels of digoxin, caffeine, warfarin, cyclosporine. Cimetidine and probenecid increase quinolone levels; an increased incidence of seizures may occur with foscarnet.

**Half-Life** 6 hours; prolonged in renal impairment

**Special PA Issues**

**Patient Education:** Oral: Take per recommended schedule, preferably on an empty stomach (1 hour before or 2 hours after meals). Maintain adequate hydration (2-3 L/day of fluids unless instructed to restrict fluid intake). Take complete prescription; do not skip doses. Do not take with antacids. You may experience dizziness, lightheadedness, or confusion; use caution when driving or engaging in tasks that require alertness. Small frequent meals and frequent mouth care may reduce nausea or vomiting. You may experience photosensitivity; use sunblock, wear appropriate clothing, or avoid direct sun. Report palpitations or chest pain, persistent diarrhea, GI disturbances or abdominal pain, muscle tremor or pain, yellowing of eyes or skin, easy bruising or bleeding, unusual fatigue, fever, chills, signs of infection, or worsening of condition. Report immediately any rash; itching; unusual CNS changes; pain, inflammation, or rupture of tendon; or any facial swelling.

**Monitoring Parameters:** Evaluation of organ system functions (renal, hepatic, ophthalmologic, and hematopoietic) is recommended periodically during therapy; the possibility of crystalluria should be assessed; WBC and signs of infection

# Levomethadyl Acetate Hydrochloride

(lee voe METH a dil AS e tate hye droe KLOR ide)

**Pharmacologic Class** Analgesic, Narcotic

**U.S. Brand Names** ORLAAM®

**Use** Management of opiate dependence

**USUAL DOSAGE** Adults: Oral: 20-40 mg 3 times/week, with ranges of 10 mg to as high as 140 mg 3 times/week; always dilute before administration and mix with diluent prior to dispensing

**Dosage Forms Soln, oral:** 10 mg/mL (474 mL)

**Warnings/Precautions** Not recommended for use outside of the treatment of opiate addiction; shall be dispensed only by treatment programs approved by FDA, DEA, and the designated state authority. Approved treatment programs shall dispense and use levomethadyl in oral form only and according to the treatment requirements stipulated in federal regulations. Failure to abide by these requirements may result in injunction precluding operation of the program, seizure of the drug supply, revocation of the program approval, and possible criminal prosecution.

**Adverse Reactions**

>10%:

Cardiovascular: Bradycardia, hypotension

Central nervous system: Drowsiness

Gastrointestinal: Nausea, vomiting

Respiratory: Respiratory depression

1% to 10%:

Cardiovascular: Peripheral vasodilation, orthostatic hypotension, increased intracranial pressure

Central nervous system: Dizziness/vertigo, CNS depression, confusion, sedation

Endocrine & metabolic: Antidiuretic hormone release

Gastrointestinal: Constipation, biliary tract spasm

Genitourinary: Urinary tract spasm

Ocular: Miosis, blurred vision

**Drug Interactions** Decreased effect/levels with phenobarbital

**Special PA Issues**

**Monitoring Parameters:** Patient adherence with regimen and avoidance of illicit substances; random drug testing is recommended

## Levonorgestrel (LEE voe nor jes trel)

**Pharmacologic Class** Contraceptive

**U.S. Brand Names** Norplant® Implant

**Mechanism of Action** First, ovulation is inhibited in about 50% to 60% of implant users from a negative feedback mechanism on the hypothalamus, leading to reduced secretion of follicle stimulating hormone (FSH) and luteinizing hormone (LH). An insufficient luteal phase has also been demonstrated with levonorgestrel administration and may result from defective gonadotropin stimulation of the ovary or from a direct effect of the drug on progesterone synthesis by the corpora utea.

**Use** Prevention of pregnancy. The net cumulative 5-year pregnancy rate for levonorgestrel implant use has been reported to be from 1.5-3.9 pregnancies/100 users. Norplant® is a very efficient, yet reversible, method of contraception. The long duration of action may be particularly advantageous in women who desire an extended period of contraceptive protection without sacrificing the possibility of future fertility.

**USUAL DOSAGE** Total administration doses (implanted): 216 mg in 6 capsules which should be implanted during the first 7 days of onset of menses subdermally in the upper arm; each Norplant® silastic capsule releases 80 mcg of drug/day for 6-18 months, following which a rate of release of 25-30 mcg/day is maintained for ≤5 years; capsules should be removed by end of 5th year

**Dosage Forms** Cap, subdermal implantation: 36 mg (6s)

**Contraindications** Women with undiagnosed abnormal uterine bleeding, hemorrhagic diathesis, known or suspected pregnancy, active hepatic disease, active thrombophlebitis, thromboembolic disorders, or known or suspected carcinoma of the breast

**Warnings/Precautions** Patients presenting with lower abdominal pain should be evaluated for follicular atresia and ectopic pregnancy

**Pregnancy Risk Factor** X

**Adverse Reactions**

>10%: Hormonal: Prolonged menstrual flow, spotting

1% to 10%:

Central nervous system: Headache, nervousness, dizziness

Dermatologic: Dermatitis, acne

Endocrine & metabolic: Amenorrhea, irregular menstrual cycles, scanty bleeding, breast discharge

Gastrointestinal: Nausea, change in appetite, weight gain

Genitourinary: Vaginitis, leukorrhea

Local: Pain or itching at implant site

Neuromuscular & skeletal: Myalgia

<1%: Infection at implant site

**Drug Interactions** Decreased effect: Carbamazepine/phenytoin

**Half-Life** 11-45 hours

**Special PA Issues**

**Patient Education:** Do not attempt to remove implants - see prescriber. You may experience photosensitivity (avoid excessive sunlight, wear protective clothing, use sunblock), dizziness or sleeplessness (use caution when driving or engaging in hazardous tasks until response is evaluated), skin rash, change in skin color, loss of hair, or unusual menses (breakthrough bleeding, irregularity, excessive bleeding - these should resolve after the first month). Report swelling, pain, or excessive feelings of warmth in calves, sudden acute headache, or visual disturbance, unusual nausea or vomiting, and any loss of feeling in arms or legs, unusual menses (if they persist past first month), and irritation at insertion site.

♦ **Levonorgestrel and Ethinyl Estradiol** see Ethinyl Estradiol and Levonorgestrel on page 347

♦ **Levora®** see Ethinyl Estradiol and Levonorgestrel on page 347

## Levorphanol (lee VOR fa nole)

**Pharmacologic Class** Analgesic, Narcotic

**U.S. Brand Names** Levo-Dromoran®

**Mechanism of Action** Levorphanol tartrate is a synthetic opioid agonist that is classified as a morphinan derivative. Opioids interact with stereospecific opioid receptors in various parts of the central nervous system and other tissues. Analgesic potency parallels the affinity for these binding sites. These drugs do not alter the threshold or responsiveness to pain, but the perception of pain.

**Use** Relief of moderate to severe pain; also used parenterally for preoperative sedation and an adjunct to nitrous oxide/oxygen anesthesia; 2 mg levorphanol produces analgesia comparable to that produced by 10 mg of morphine

**USUAL DOSAGE** Adults:

Oral: 2 mg every 6-24 hours as needed

S.C.: 2 mg, up to 3 mg if necessary, every 6-8 hours

**Dosing adjustment in hepatic disease:** Reduction is necessary in patients with liver disease

**Dosage Forms** Inj: 2 mg/mL (1 mL, 10 mL); **Tab:** 2 mg

**Contraindications** Hypersensitivity to levorphanol or any component

**Warnings/Precautions** Use with caution in patients with hypersensitivity reactions to other phenanthrene derivative opioid agonists (morphine, hydrocodone, hydromorphone, levorphanol, oxycodone, oxymorphone); respiratory diseases including asthma, emphysema, COPD or severe liver or renal insufficiency; some preparations contain sulfites which may cause allergic reactions; tolerance or dependence may result from extended use; dextromethorphan has equivalent antitussive activity but has much lower toxicity in accidental overdose. Elderly may be particularly susceptible to the CNS depressant and constipating effects of narcotics.

**Pregnancy Risk Factor** B (D if used for prolonged periods or in high doses at term)

**Adverse Reactions**

>10%:
  Cardiovascular: Palpitations, hypotension, bradycardia, peripheral vasodilation
  Central nervous system: CNS depression, fatigue, drowsiness, dizziness
  Dermatologic: Pruritus
  Gastrointestinal: Nausea, vomiting
  Neuromuscular & skeletal: Weakness

1% to 10%:
  Central nervous system: Nervousness, headache, restlessness, anorexia, malaise, confusion
  Gastrointestinal: Stomach cramps, xerostomia, constipation
  Endocrine & metabolic: Antidiuretic hormone release
  Gastrointestinal: Biliary tract spasm
  Genitourinary: Decreased urination, urinary tract spasm
  Local: Pain at injection site
  Ocular: Miosis
  Respiratory: Respiratory depression

<1%: Paralytic ileus, mental depression, hallucinations, paradoxical CNS stimulation, increased intracranial pressure, rash, urticaria, histamine release, physical and psychological dependence, histamine release

**Drug Interactions** Increased toxicity: CNS depressants increase CNS depression

**Onset** Oral: 10-60 minutes

**Duration** 4-8 hours

**Half-Life** 12-16 hours

**Special PA Issues**

**Patient Education:** If self-administered, use exactly as directed (do not increase dose or frequency); may cause physical and/or psychological dependence. While using this medication, do not use alcohol and other prescription or OTC medications (especially sedatives, tranquilizers, antihistamines, or pain medications) without consulting prescriber. Maintain adequate hydration (2-3 L/day of fluids unless instructed to restrict fluid intake). May cause hypotension, dizziness, drowsiness, impaired coordination, or blurred vision (use caution when driving, climbing stairs, or changing position - rising from sitting or lying to standing, or when engaging in hazardous activities until response to medication is known); loss of appetite, nausea, or vomiting (frequent mouth care, small frequent meals, or sucking on lozenges may help); constipation (increased exercise, fluids, or dietary fruit and fiber may help - if constipation remains an unresolved problem, consult prescriber about use of stool softeners). Report chest pain, slow or rapid heartbeat, acute dizziness, or persistent headache; swelling of extremities or unusual weight gain; changes in urinary elimination; acute headache; back or flank pain or spasms; blurred vision; skin rash; or shortness of breath.

**Dietary Considerations:**
  Alcohol: Additive CNS effects, avoid or limit alcohol; watch for sedation
  Food: Glucose may cause hyperglycemia; monitor blood glucose concentrations

**Monitoring Parameters:** Pain relief, respiratory and mental status, blood pressure

**Related Information**
  Narcotic Agonists *on page 1023*

♦ **Levorphanol Tartrate** *see* Levorphanol *on previous page*

♦ **Levorphan Tartrate** *see* Levorphanol *on previous page*

♦ **Levo-T™** *see* Levothyroxine *on this page*

♦ **Levothroid®** *see* Levothyroxine *on this page*

# Levothyroxine (lee voe thye ROKS een)

**Pharmacologic Class** Thyroid Product

**U.S. Brand Names** Eltroxin®; Levo-T™; Levothroid®; Levoxyl®; Synthroid®

**Mechanism of Action** Exact mechanism of action is unknown; however, it is believed the thyroid hormone exerts its many metabolic effects through control of DNA transcription and protein synthesis; involved in normal metabolism, growth, and development; promotes gluconeogenesis, increases utilization and mobilization of glycogen stores, and stimulates protein synthesis, increases basal metabolic rate

(Continued)

## Levothyroxine *(Continued)*

**Use** Replacement or supplemental therapy in hypothyroidism; some clinicians suggest levothyroxine is the drug of choice for replacement therapy

**USUAL DOSAGE**

Children: Congenital hypothyroidism:

Oral:

0-6 months: 8-10 mcg/kg/day **or** 25-50 mcg/day

6-12 months: 6-8 mcg/kg/day **or** 50-75 mcg/day

1-5 years: 5-6 mcg/kg/day **or** 75-100 mcg/day

6-12 years: 4-5 mcg/kg/day **or** 100-150 mcg/day

>12 years: 2-3 mcg/kg/day **or** ≥150 mcg/day

I.M., I.V.: 50% to 75% of the oral dose

Adults:

Oral: Initial: 0.05 mg/day, then increase by increments of 25 mcg/day at intervals of 2-3 weeks; average adult dose: 100-200 mcg/day; maximum dose: 200 mcg/day

I.M., I.V.: 50% of the oral dose

Myxedema coma or stupor: I.V.: 200-500 mcg one time, then 100-300 mcg the next day if necessary

Thyroid suppression therapy: Oral: 2-6 mcg/kg/day for 7-10 days

**Dosage Forms** Powder for inj, lyophilized: 200 mcg/vial (6 mL, 10 mL), 500 mcg/vial (6 mL, 10 mL); Tab: 25 mcg, 50 mcg, 75 mcg, 88 mcg, 100 mcg, 112 mcg, 125 mcg, 150 mcg, 175 mcg, 200 mcg, 300 mcg

**Contraindications** Recent myocardial infarction or thyrotoxicosis, uncorrected adrenal insufficiency, hypersensitivity to levothyroxine sodium or any component

**Warnings/Precautions** Ineffective for weight reduction; high doses may produce serious or even life-threatening toxic effects particularly when used with some anorectic drugs. Use with caution and reduce dosage in patients with angina pectoris or other cardiovascular disease; levothyroxine tablets contain tartrazine dye which may cause allergic reactions in susceptible individuals; use cautiously in elderly since they may be more likely to have compromised cardiovascular functions. Patients with adrenal insufficiency, myxedema, diabetes mellitus and insidious may have symptoms exaggerated or aggravated; thyroid replacement requires periodic assessment of thyroid status. Chronic hypothyroidism predisposes patients to coronary artery disease.

**Pregnancy Risk Factor** A

**Adverse Reactions** <1%: Palpitations, cardiac arrhythmias, tachycardia, chest pain, nervousness, headache, insomnia, fever, ataxia, alopecia, changes in menstrual cycle, weight loss, increased appetite, diarrhea, abdominal cramps, constipation, myalgia, hand tremors, tremor, shortness of breath, diaphoresis

**Drug Interactions**

Decreased effect:

Phenytoin may decrease levothyroxine levels

Cholestyramine may decrease absorption of levothyroxine

Increased oral hypoglycemic requirements

Increased effect: Increased effects of oral anticoagulants

Increased toxicity: Tricyclic antidepressants may increase toxic potential of both drugs

**Onset**

Onset of therapeutic effect: Oral: 3-5 days; I.V. Within 6-8 hours

Peak effect: I.V.: Within 24 hours

**Half-Life** 6-7 days

**Special PA Issues**

**Patient Education:** Thyroid replacement therapy is generally for life. Take as directed, in the morning before breakfast. Do not change brands and do not discontinue without consulting prescriber. Consult prescriber if drastically increasing or decreasing intake of goitrogenic food (eg, asparagus, cabbage, peas, turnip greens, broccoli, spinach, Brussels sprouts, lettuce, soybeans). Report chest pain, rapid heart rate, palpitations, heat intolerance, excessive sweating, increased nervousness, agitation, or lethargy.

**Monitoring Parameters:** Thyroid function test (serum thyroxine, thyrotropin concentrations), resin triiodothyronine uptake ($RT_3U$), free thyroxine index (FTI), $T_4$, TSH, heart rate, blood pressure, clinical signs of hypo- and hyperthyroidism; TSH is the most reliable guide for evaluating adequacy of thyroid replacement dosage. TSH may be elevated during the first few months of thyroid replacement despite patients being clinically euthyroid. In cases where $T_4$ remains low and TSH is within normal limits, an evaluation of "free" (unbound) $T_4$ is needed to evaluate further increase in dosage

**Reference Range:** Pediatrics: Cord $T_4$ and values in the first few weeks are much higher, falling over the first months and years. ≥10 years: ~5.8-11 µg/dL (SI: 75-142 nmol/L). Borderline low: ≤4.5-5.7 µg/dL (SI: 58-73 nmol/L); low: ≤4.4 µg/dL (SI: 57 nmol/L); results <2.5 µg/dL (SI: <32 nmol/L) are strong evidence for hypothyroidism.

Approximate adult normal range: 4-12 µg/dL (SI: 51-154 nmol/L). Borderline high: 11.1-13 µg/dL (SI: 143-167 nmol/L); high: ≥13.1 µg/dL (SI: 169 nmol/L). Normal range is increased in women on birth control pills (5.5-12 µg/dL); normal range in pregnancy: ~5.5-16 µg/dL (SI: ~71-206 nmol/L). TSH: 0.4-10 (for those ≥80 years) mIU/L; $T_4$: 4-12 µg/dL (SI: 51-154 nmol/L); $T_3$ (RIA) (total $T_3$): 80-230 ng/dL (SI: 1.2-3.5 nmol/L); $T_4$ free (free $T_4$): 0.7-1.8 ng/dL (SI: 9-23 pmol/L).

## Lidocaine (LYE doe kane)

**Pharmacologic Class** Analgesic, Topical; Antiarrhythmic Agent, Class I-B; Local Anesthetic

**U.S. Brand Names** Anestacon®; Dermaflex® Gel; Dilocaine®; Dr Scholl's® Cracked Heel Relief Cream [OTC]; Duo-Trach®; LidoPen® Auto-Injector; Nervocaine®; Octocaine®; Solarcaine® Aloe Extra Burn Relief [OTC]; Xylocaine®; Zilactin-L® [OTC]

**Mechanism of Action** Class IB antiarrhythmic; suppresses automaticity of conduction tissue, by increasing electrical stimulation threshold of ventricle, HIS-Purkinje system, and spontaneous depolarization of the ventricles during diastole by a direct action on the tissues; blocks both the initiation and conduction of nerve impulses by decreasing the neuronal membrane's permeability to sodium ions, which results in inhibition of depolarization with resultant blockade of conduction

**Use** Local anesthetic and acute treatment of ventricular arrhythmias from myocardial infarction, cardiac manipulation, digitalis intoxication; topical local anesthetic; drug of choice for ventricular ectopy, ventricular tachycardia, ventricular fibrillation; for pulseless VT or VF preferably administer **after** defibrillation and epinephrine; control of premature ventricular contractions, wide-complex PSVT

### USUAL DOSAGE

Topical: Apply to affected area as needed; maximum: 3 mg/kg/dose; do not repeat within 2 hours

Injectable local anesthetic: Varies with procedure, degree of anesthesia needed, vascularity of tissue, duration of anesthesia required, and physical condition of patient; maximum: 4.5 mg/kg/dose; do not repeat within 2 hours

I.M.: Adults: 300 mg (best in deltoid muscle; only 10% solution)

Children: Endotracheal, I.O., I.V.: Loading dose: 1 mg/kg; may repeat in 10-15 minutes x 2 doses; after loading dose, start I.V. continuous infusion 20-50 mcg/kg/minute (300 mcg/kg/minute per American Heart Association)

   Use 20 mcg/kg/minute in patients with shock, hepatic disease, mild congestive heart failure (CHF)

   Moderate to severe CHF may require ½ loading dose and lower infusion rates to avoid toxicity

Adults: Antiarrhythmic:

   I.V.: 1-1.5 mg/kg bolus over 2-3 minutes; may repeat doses of 0.5-0.75 mg/kg in 5-10 minutes up to a total of 3 mg/kg; continuous infusion: 1-4 mg/minute

   I.V. (2 g/250 mL $D_5W$) infusion rates (infusion pump should be used for I.V. infusion administration):

      1 mg/minute: 7 mL/hour
      2 mg/minute: 15 mL/hour
      3 mg/minute: 21 mL/hour
      4 mg/minute: 30 mL/hour

   Ventricular fibrillation (after defibrillation and epinephrine): Initial dose: 1.5 mg/kg, may repeat boluses as above; follow with continuous infusion after return of perfusion

   Prevention of ventricular fibrillation: I.V.: Initial bolus: 0.5 mg/kg; repeat every 5-10 minutes to a total dose of 2 mg/kg

      Refractory ventricular fibrillation: Repeat 1.5 mg/kg bolus may be given 3-5 minutes after initial dose

   **Endotracheal: 2-2.5 times the I.V. dose**

**Decrease dose in patients with CHF, shock, or hepatic disease**

**Dosing adjustment/comments in hepatic disease:** Reduce dose in acute hepatitis and decompensated cirrhosis by 50%

(Continued)

## Lidocaine *(Continued)*

Dialysis: Not dialyzable (0% to 5%) by hemo- or peritoneal dialysis; supplemental dose not necessary; supplemental dose is not necessary

**Dosage Forms Crm:** 2% (56 g); **Inj:** 0.5% [5 mg/mL] (50 mL), 1% [10 mg/mL] (2 mL, 5 mL, 10 mL, 20 mL, 30 mL, 50 mL), 1.5% [15 mg/mL] (20 mL), 2% [20 mg/mL] (2 mL, 5 mL, 10 mL, 20 mL, 30 mL, 50 mL), 4% [40 mg/mL] (5 mL), 10% [100 mg/mL] (10 mL), 20% [200 mg/mL] (10 mL, 20 mL); **Inj** I.M. use: 10% [100 mg/mL] (3 mL, 5 mL), Direct I.V.: 1% [10 mg/mL] (5 mL, 10 mL); 20 mg/mL (5 mL), I.V. admixture, preservative free: 4% [40 mg/mL] (25 mL, 30 mL); 10% [100 mg/mL] (10 mL); 20% [200 mg/mL] (5 mL, 10 mL), I.V. infusion, in D₅W: 0.2% [2 mg/mL] (500 mL), 0.4% [4 mg/mL] (250 mL, 500 mL, 1000 mL), 0.8% [8 mg/mL] (250 mL, 500 mL); **Gel, top:** 2% (30 mL), 2.5% (15 mL); **Liq, top:** 2.5% (7.5 mL); **Liq, viscous:** 2% (20 mL, 100 mL); **Oint, top:** 2.5% [OTC], 5% (35 g); **Soln, top:** 2% (15 mL, 240 mL), 4% (50 mL)

**Contraindications** Known hypersensitivity to amide-type local anesthetics; patients with Adams-Stokes syndrome or with severe degree of S-A, A-V, or intraventricular heart block (without a pacemaker)

**Warnings/Precautions** Avoid use of preparations containing preservatives for spinal or epidural (including caudal anesthesia). Use extreme caution in patients with hepatic disease, heart failure, marked hypoxia, severe respiratory depression, hypovolemia or shock, incomplete heart block or bradycardia, and atrial fibrillation.

Due to decreases in phase I metabolism and possibly decrease in splanchnic perfusion with age, there may be a decreased clearance or increased half-life in elderly and increased risk for CNS side effects and cardiac effects

**Pregnancy Risk Factor** B

**Adverse Reactions**

1% to 10%:

Cardiovascular: Hypotension

Central nervous system: Positional headache

Miscellaneous: Shivering

<1%: Heart block, arrhythmias, cardiovascular collapse, lethargy, coma, agitation, slurred speech, seizures, anxiety, euphoria, hallucinations, itching, rash, edema of the skin, nausea, vomiting, paresthesias, blurred vision, diplopia, dyspnea, respiratory depression or arrest

**Drug Interactions** CYP3A3/4 enzyme substrate

Increased toxicity:

Concomitant cimetidine or beta-blockers may result in increased serum concentrations of lidocaine with resultant toxicity; procainamide and tocainide may result in additive cardiodepressant action

Effect of succinylcholine may be enhanced

**Onset** Single bolus dose: 45-90 seconds

**Duration** 10-20 minutes

**Half-Life** Biphasic: Increased with CHF, liver disease, shock, severe renal disease; Initial: 7-30 minutes; Terminal: 1.5-2 hours

**Special PA Issues**

**Patient Education:** I.V. You will be monitored during infusion. Do not get up without assistance. Report dizziness, numbness, double vision, nausea, pain or burning at infusion site, nightmares, hearing strange noises, seeing unusual visions, or difficulty breathing.

Dermatologic: You will experience decreased sensation to pain, heat, or cold in the area and/or decreased muscle strength (depending on area of application) until effects wear off; use necessary caution to reduce incidence of possible injury until full sensation returns. Report irritation, pain, burning at injection site, persistent numbness, tingling, swelling; restlessness, dizziness, acute weakness; blurred vision; ringing in ears; or difficulty breathing.

Oral: Lidocaine can cause numbness of tongue, cheeks, and throat. Do not eat or drink for 1 hour after use. Take small sips of water at first to ensure that you can swallow without difficulty. Your tongue and mouth may be numb; use caution avoid biting yourself. Immediately report swelling of face, lips, or tongue.

**Reference Range:**

Therapeutic: 1.5-5.0 μg/mL (SI: 6-21 μmol/L)

Potentially toxic: >6 μg/mL (SI: >26 μmol/L)

Toxic: >9 μg/mL (SI: >38 μmol/L)

## Lidocaine and Epinephrine *(LYE doe kane & ep i NEF rin)*

**Pharmacologic Class** Local Anesthetic

**U.S. Brand Names** Octocaine® With Epinephrine; Xylocaine® With Epinephrine

**Mechanism of Action** Lidocaine blocks both the initiation and conduction of nerve impulses via decreased permeability of sodium ions; epinephrine increases the duration of action of lidocaine by causing vasoconstriction (via alpha effects) which slows the vascular absorption of lidocaine

**Use** Local infiltration anesthesia; AVS for nerve block

## USUAL DOSAGE

Children: Use lidocaine concentrations of 0.5% to 1% (or even more diluted) to decrease possibility of toxicity; lidocaine dose should not exceed 7 mg/kg/dose; do not repeat within 2 hours

Adults: Dosage varies with the anesthetic procedure, degree of anesthesia needed, vascularity of tissue, duration of anesthesia required, and physical condition of patient

**Dosage Forms Inj, with epinephrine: 1:200,000:** Lidocaine hydrochloride 0.5% [5 mg/mL] (50 mL), 1% [10 mg/mL] (30 mL), 1.5% [15 mg/mL] (5 mL, 10 mL, 30 mL), 2% [20 mg/mL] (20 mL); **1:100,000:** Lidocaine hydrochloride 1% [10 mg/mL] (20 mL, 50 mL), 2% [20 mg/mL] (1.8 mL, 20 mL, 50 mL); **1:50,000:**Lidocaine hydrochloride 2% [20 mg/mL] (1.8 mL)

**Contraindications** Hypersensitivity to local anesthetics of the amide type, myasthenia gravis, shock, or cardiac conduction disease

**Warnings/Precautions** Do not use solutions in distal portions of the body (digits, nose, ears, penis); use with caution in endocrine, heart, hepatic, or thyroid disease

**Pregnancy Risk Factor** B

**Adverse Reactions** Refer to Lidocaine monograph

# Lidocaine and Hydrocortisone (LYE doe kane & hye droe KOR ti sone)

**Pharmacologic Class** Anesthetic/Corticosteroid

**U.S. Brand Names** Lida-Mantle HC® Topical

**Dosage Forms Crm:** Lidocaine 3% and hydrocortisone 0.5% (15 g, 30 g)

# Lidocaine and Prilocaine (LYE doe kane & PRIL oh kane)

**Pharmacologic Class** Analgesic, Topical; Anesthetic, Topical; Local Anesthetic

**U.S. Brand Names** EMLA®

**Mechanism of Action** Local anesthetic action occurs by stabilization of neuronal membranes and inhibiting the ionic fluxes required for the initiation and conduction of impulses

**Use** Topical anesthetic for use on normal intact skin to provide local analgesia for minor procedures such as I.V. cannulation or venipuncture; has also been used for painful procedures such as lumbar puncture and skin graft harvesting

**USUAL DOSAGE** Children and Adults:

**EMLA® cream should not be used in infants under the age of 1 month or in infants, under the age of 12 months, who are receiving treatment with methemogloblin-inducing agents**

Choose 2 application sites available for intravenous access

Apply a thick layer (2.5 g/site ~½ of a 5 g tube) of cream to each designated site of intact skin

Cover each site with the occlusive dressing (Tegaderm®)

Mark the time on the dressing

**Allow at least 1 hour for optimum therapeutic effect.** Remove the dressing and wipe off excess EMLA® cream (gloves should be worn).

**EMLA® Cream Maximum Recommended Application Area* for Infants and Children Based on Application to Intact Skin**

| Body Weight (kg) | Maximum Application Area (cm²)† |
|---|---|
| <10 | 100 |
| 10-20 | 600 |
| >20 | 2000 |

*These are broad guidelines for avoiding systemic toxicity in applying EMLA® to patients with normal intact skin and with normal renal and hepatic function.

†For more individualized calculation of how much lidocaine and prilocaine may be absorbed, use the following estimates of lidocaine and prilocaine absorption for children and adults:

Estimated mean (±SD) absorption of lidocaine: 0.045 (±0.016) mg/cm²/h.

Estimated mean (±SD) absorption of prilocaine: 0.077 (±0.036) mg/cm²/h.

**Debilitated patients, small children or patients with impaired elimination (ie, hepatic or renal dysfunction):** Smaller areas of treatment are recommended

**Dosage Forms Crm:** Lidocaine 2.5% and prilocaine 2.5% [2 Tegaderm® dressings] (5 g, 30 g)

## Contraindications

Children <1 month of age

Administration on mucous membranes

Administration on broken or inflamed skin

Children with congenital or idiopathic methemoglobinemia, or in children who are receiving medications associated with drug-induced methemoglobinemia [ie, acetaminophen (overdosage), benzocaine, chloroquine, dapsone, nitrofurantoin, nitroglycerin, nitroprusside, phenazopyridine, phenelzine, phenobarbital, phenytoin, quinine, sulfonamides]

(Continued)

## Lidocaine and Prilocaine *(Continued)*

Patients with a documented hypersensitivity to amide type anesthetic agents [ie, lidocaine, prilocaine, dibucaine, mepivacaine, bupivacaine, etidocaine]

Patients with a documented hypersensitivity to any components of EMLA® cream or Tegaderm®

**Pregnancy Risk Factor** B

**Adverse Reactions**
1% to 10%:
Dermatologic: Angioedema, contact dermatitis
Local: Burning, stinging
<1%: Bradycardia, hypotension, shock, edema, nervousness, euphoria, confusion, dizziness, drowsiness, convulsions, CNS excitation, erythema, itching, rash, urticaria, methemoglobinemia in infants, blanching, alteration in temperature sensation, tenderness, tremors, blurred vision, innitus, respiratory depression, bronchospasm

**Drug Interactions** Increased toxicity:
Class I antiarrhythmic drugs (tocainide, mexiletine): Effects are additive and potentially synergistic
Drugs known to induce methemoglobinemia

**Onset** 1 hour for sufficient dermal analgesia; Peak effect: 2-3 hours

**Duration** 1-2 hours after removal of the cream

**Half-Life**
Lidocaine: 65-150 minutes, prolonged with cardiac or hepatic dysfunction
Prilocaine: 10-150 minutes, prolonged in hepatic or renal dysfunction

**Special PA Issues**
**Patient Education:** This drug will block sensation to the applied area. Report irritation, pain, burning at application site.

+ **Lidocaine Hydrochloride** *see* Lidocaine *on page 531*
+ **LidoPen® Auto-Injector** *see* Lidocaine *on page 531*
+ **Lignocaine Hydrochloride** *see* Lidocaine *on page 531*
+ **Limbitrol® DS 10-25** *see* Amitriptyline and Chlordiazepoxide *on page 59*
+ **Linctus Codeine Blac** *see* Codeine *on page 232*
+ **Linctus With Codeine Phosphate** *see* Codeine *on page 232*

## Lindane *(LIN dane)*

**Pharmacologic Class** Antiparasitic Agent, Topical; Pediculocide; Scabicidal Agent

**U.S. Brand Names** G-well®; Kwell®; Scabene®

**Mechanism of Action** Directly absorbed by parasites and ova through the exoskeleton; stimulates the nervous system resulting in seizures and death of parasitic arthropods

**Use** Treatment of scabies (*Sarcoptes scabiei*), *Pediculus capitis* (head lice), and *Pediculus pubis* (crab lice); FDA recommends reserving lindane as a second-line agent or with inadequate response to other therapies

**USUAL DOSAGE** Children and Adults: Topical:
Scabies: Apply a thin layer of lotion or cream and massage it on skin from the neck to the toes (head to toe in infants). For adults, bathe and remove the drug after 8-12 hours; for children, wash off 6-8 hours after application (for infants, wash off 6 hours after application); repeat treatment in 7 days if lice or nits are still present
Pediculosis, capitis and pubis: 15-30 mL of shampoo is applied and lathered for 4-5 minutes; rinse hair thoroughly and comb with a fine tooth comb to remove nits; repeat treatment in 7 days if lice or nits are still present

**Dosage Forms** Crm: 1% (60 g, 454 g); **Lot:** 1% (60 mL, 473 mL, 4000 mL); **Shamp:** 1% (60 mL, 473 mL, 4000 mL)

**Contraindications** Hypersensitivity to lindane or any component; premature neonates; acutely inflamed skin or raw, weeping surfaces

**Warnings/Precautions** Not considered a drug of first choice; use with caution in infants and small children, and patients with a history of seizures; avoid contact with face, eyes, mucous membranes, and urethral meatus. Because of the potential for systemic absorption and CNS side effects, lindane should be used with caution; consider permethrin or crotamiton agent first.

**Pregnancy Risk Factor** B

**Pregnancy Implications** Clinical effects on the fetus: There are no well controlled studies in pregnant women; treat no more than twice during a pregnancy

**Adverse Reactions** <1%: Cardiac arrhythmia, dizziness, restlessness, seizures, headache, ataxia, eczematous eruptions, contact dermatitis, skin and adipose tissue may act as repositories, nausea, vomiting, aplastic anemia, hepatitis, burning and stinging, hematuria, pulmonary edema

**Drug Interactions** Increased toxicity: Oil-based hair dressing may increase toxic potential

**Special PA Issues**
**Patient Education:** For external use only. Do not apply to face and avoid getting in eyes. Do not apply immediately after hot soapy bath. Apply from neck to toes. Bathe to remove drug after 8-12 hours. Repeat in 7 days if lice or nits are still present. Clothing and

bedding must be washed in hot water or dry cleaned to kill nits. Wash combs and brushes with lindane shampoo and thoroughly rinse. May need to treat all members of household and all sexual contacts concurrently. Report if condition persists or infection occurs.

- ♦ **Lioresal®** *see* Baclofen *on page 97*
- ♦ **Lipancreatin** *see* Pancrelipase *on page 694*
- ♦ **Lipid-Lowering Agents** *see* Chart *on page 1022*
- ♦ **Lipitor®** *see* Atorvastatin *on page 85*
- ♦ **Liposyn®** *see* Fat Emulsion *on page 359*
- ♦ **Liquaemin®** *see* Heparin *on page 438*
- ♦ **Liquibid®** *see* Guaifenesin *on page 427*
- ♦ **Liqui-Char® [OTC]** *see* Charcoal *on page 184*
- ♦ **Liquid Antidote** *see* Charcoal *on page 184*
- ♦ **Liquid Pred®** *see* Prednisone *on page 754*
- ♦ **Liquiprin® [OTC]** *see* Acetaminophen *on page 21*

# Lisinopril (lyse IN oh pril)

**Pharmacologic Class** Angiotensin-Converting Enzyme (ACE) Inhibitors

**U.S. Brand Names** Prinivil®; Zestril®

**Mechanism of Action** Competitive inhibitor of angiotensin-converting enzyme (ACE); prevents conversion of angiotensin I to angiotensin II, a potent vasoconstrictor; results in lower levels of angiotensin II which causes an increase in plasma renin activity and a reduction in aldosterone secretion; a CNS mechanism may also be involved in hypotensive effect as angiotensin II increases adrenergic outflow from CNS; vasoactive kallikreins may be decreased in conversion to active hormones by ACE inhibitors, thus reducing blood pressure

**Use** Treatment of hypertension, either alone or in combination with other antihypertensive agents; adjunctive therapy in treatment of CHF (afterload reduction); treatment of hemodynamically stable patients within 24 hours of acute myocardial infarction, to improve survival

## USUAL DOSAGE

Hypertension:

Adults: Initial: 10 mg/day; increase doses 5-10 mg/day at 1- to 2-week intervals; maximum daily dose: 40 mg

Elderly: Initial: 2.5-5 mg/day; increase doses 2.5-5 mg/day at 1- to 2-week intervals; maximum daily dose: 40 mg

Patients taking diuretics should have them discontinued 2-3 days prior to initiating lisinopril if possible; restart diuretic after blood pressure is stable if needed; if diuretic cannot be discontinued prior to therapy, begin with 5 mg with close supervision until stable blood pressure; in patients with hyponatremia (<130 mEq/L), start dose at 2.5 mg/day

Congestive heart failure: Adults: 5 mg initially with diuretics and digitalis; usual maintenance: 5-20 mg/day as a single dose

Acute myocardial infarction (within 24 hours in hemodynamically stable patients): Oral: 5 mg immediately, then 5 mg at 24 hours, 10 mg at 48 hours, and 10 mg every day thereafter for 6 weeks; patients should continue to receive standard treatments such as thrombolytics, aspirin, and beta-blockers

**Dosing adjustment in renal impairment:**

$Cl_{cr}$ 10-50 mL/minute: Administer 50% to 75% of normal dose

$Cl_{cr}$ <10 mL/minute: Administer 25% to 50% of normal dose

Hemodialysis: Dialyzable (50%)

**Dosage Forms Tab:** 2.5 mg, 5 mg, 10 mg, 20 mg, 40 mg

**Contraindications** Hypersensitivity to lisinopril or any component or other ACE inhibitors

**Warnings/Precautions** Use with caution and modify dosage in patients with renal impairment (decrease dosage) (especially renal artery stenosis), severe congestive heart failure, or with coadministered diuretic therapy; experience in children is limited. Severe hypotension may occur in patients who are sodium and/or volume depleted, initiate lower doses and monitor closely when starting therapy in these patients.

**Pregnancy Risk Factor** C (1st trimester); D (2nd and 3rd trimester)

**Pregnancy Implications**

Clinical effects on the fetus: No data available on crossing the placenta. Cranial defects, hypocalvaria/acalvaria, oligohydramnios, persistent anuria following delivery, hypotension, renal defects, renal dysgenesis/dysplasia, renal failure, pulmonary hypoplasia, limb contractures secondary to oligohydramnios and stillbirth reported. ACE inhibitors should be avoided during pregnancy.

Breast-feeding/lactation: Crosses into breast milk. American Academy of Pediatrics considers **compatible** with breast-feeding.

## Adverse Reactions

1% to 10%:

Cardiovascular: Hypotension (1% to 5%)

Central nervous system: Dizziness (6%), headache (5%), fatigue (3%)

Dermatologic: Rash (1.5%)

(Continued)

## Lisinopril *(Continued)*

Gastrointestinal: Diarrhea/vomiting/nausea (1% to 3%)
Renal: Increased BUN/serum creatinine (transient)
Respiratory: Upper respiratory symptoms, cough (3% to 5%)
<1%: Chest discomfort (~1%), flushing, myocardial infarction, angina pectoris, orthostatic hypotension, rhythm disturbances, tachycardia, peripheral edema, vasculitis, palpitations, syncope, fever, malaise, depression, somnolence, insomnia, urticaria, pruritus, angioedema, gout, pancreatitis, abdominal pain, anorexia, constipation, flatulence, xerostomia, neutropenia, bone marrow suppression, hepatitis, arthralgia, shoulder pain, blurred vision, bronchitis, sinusitis, pharyngeal pain, diaphoresis

**Drug Interactions** Increased toxicity:
Probenecid increases blood levels of captopril
Captopril and diuretics have additive hypotensive effects
Increased toxicity: See Drug-Drug Interactions With ACEIs *on page 997*

**Onset** 1 hour; Peak hypotensive effect: Oral: Within 6 hours

**Duration** 24 hours

**Half-Life** 11-12 hours

**Special PA Issues**

**Patient Education:** Take as directed; do not change dosage or stop taking without consulting prescriber. Do not change amount of dietary salt without advice or consult of prescriber. You may experience headache, dizziness, fainting, or fatigue (use caution when driving or performing hazardous tasks and use caution when rising from sitting or lying position) until response to therapy is established. You may experience dry cough or gastric upset and diarrhea (usually temporary). Report swelling of hands, feet, mouth, or face (or difficulty swallowing); persistent sore throat; fever; rash; respiratory difficulty; chest pains or irregular heartbeat; persistent cough; unresolved diarrhea or vomiting; excessive sweating, perspiration, or dehydration.

**Monitoring Parameters:** Serum calcium levels, BUN, serum creatinine, renal function, WBC, and potassium

**Related Information**
ACE Inhibitors *on page 995*
Heart Failure: Management of Patients with Left Ventricular Systolic Dysfunction *on page 1064*
Drug-Drug Interactions With ACEIs *on page 997*

## Lisinopril and Hydrochlorothiazide

(lyse IN oh pril & hye droe klor oh THYE a zide)

**Pharmacologic Class** Antihypertensive Agent, Combination

**U.S. Brand Names** Prinzide®; Zestoretic®

**Dosage Forms Tab:** Lisinopril 10 mg and hydrochlorothiazide 12.5 mg, [12.5]-Lisinopril 20 mg and hydrochlorothiazide 12.5 mg, [25]-Lisinopril 20 mg and hydrochlorothiazide 25 mg

♦ **Listermint® with Fluoride [OTC]** *see Fluoride on page 383*

♦ **Lithane®** *see Lithium on this page*

## Lithium (LITH ee um)

**Pharmacologic Class** Lithium

**U.S. Brand Names** Eskalith®; Eskalith CR®; Lithane®; Lithobid®; Lithonate®; Lithotabs®

**Mechanism of Action** Alters cation transport across cell membrane in nerve and muscle cells and influences reuptake of serotonin and/or norepinephrine

**Use** Management of acute manic episodes, bipolar disorders, and depression

**USUAL DOSAGE** Oral: Monitor serum concentrations and clinical response (efficacy and toxicity) to determine proper dose

Children 6-12 years: 15-60 mg/kg/day in 3-4 divided doses; dose not to exceed usual adult dosage

Adults: 300-600 mg 3-4 times/day; usual maximum maintenance dose: 2.4 g/day or 450-900 mg of sustained release twice daily

Elderly: Initial dose: 300 mg twice daily; increase weekly in increments of 300 mg/day, monitoring levels; rarely need >900-1200 mg/day

**Dosing adjustment in renal impairment:**
$Cl_{cr}$ 10-50 mL/minute: Administer 50% to 75% of normal dose
$Cl_{cr}$ <10 mL/minute: Administer 25% to 50% of normal dose
Hemodialysis: Dialyzable (50% to 100%)

**Dosage Forms** Lithium carbonate: **Cap:** 150 mg, 300 mg, 600 mg; **Tab:** 300 mg; **Tab, controlled release:** 450 mg (Eskalith CR®); **Tab, slow release:** 300 mg (Lithobid®)
Lithium citrate: **Syr:** 300 mg/5 mL (5 mL, 10 mL, 480 mL)

**Contraindications** Hypersensitivity to lithium or any component; severe cardiovascular or renal disease

**Warnings/Precautions** Lithium toxicity is closely related to serum levels and can occur at therapeutic doses; serum lithium determinations are required to monitor therapy. Use with caution in patients with cardiovascular or thyroid disease, severe debilitation, dehydration or sodium depletion, or in patients receiving diuretics. Some elderly patients may be extremely sensitive to the effects of lithium.

**Pregnancy Risk Factor** D

**Adverse Reactions**

>10%:

Endocrine & metabolic: Polydipsia, stress

Gastrointestinal: Nausea, diarrhea, abnormal taste

Neuromuscular & skeletal: Trembling

1% to 10%:

Central nervous system: Fatigue

Dermatologic: Rash

Gastrointestinal: Bloated feeling, weight gain

Neuromuscular & skeletal: Muscle twitching, weakness

<1%: Lethargy, dizziness, vertigo, pseudotumor cerebri, eruptions, hypothyroidism, goiter, acneiform, diabetes insipidus, anorexia, xerostomia, nonspecific nephron atrophy, renal tubular acidosis, leukocytosis, cogwheel rigidity, chronic movements of the limbs, tremor, vision problems, discoloration of fingers and toes

**Drug Interactions**

Decreased effect with xanthines (eg, theophylline, caffeine)

Increased effect/toxicity of CNS depressants, alfentanil, iodide salts increased hypothyroid effect

Increased toxicity with thiazide diuretics (dose may need to be reduced by 30%), NSAIDs, haloperidol, phenothiazines (neurotoxicity), neuromuscular blockers, carbamazepine, fluoxetine, ACE inhibitors

**Onset** Peak serum concentration: 30 minutes to 2 hours

**Half-Life** 18-24 hours; can increase to more than 36 hours in the elderly or in patients with renal impairment

**Special PA Issues**

**Patient Education:** Take exactly as directed; do not change dosage without consulting prescriber. Do not crush or chew tablets or capsules. Maintain adequate fluid intake (2-3 L/day) especially in summer. Frequent blood test and monitoring will be necessary. You may experience decreased appetite or altered taste sensation (small frequent meals may help maintain nutrition); or drowsiness or dizziness, especially during early therapy (use caution when driving or engaging in hazardous activities). Immediately report unresolved diarrhea, abrupt changes in weight, muscular tremors or lack of coordination, fever, or changes in urinary volume.

Dietary: Avoid changes in sodium content (eg, low sodium diets); reduction of sodium can increase lithium toxicity. Limit caffeine intake (diuresis can increase lithium toxicity).

**Monitoring Parameters:** Serum lithium every 3-4 days during initial therapy; draw lithium serum concentrations 8-12 hours postdose; renal, hepatic, thyroid, and cardiovascular function; fluid status; serum electrolytes; CBC with differential, urinalysis; monitor for signs of toxicity

**Reference Range:** Levels should be obtained twice weekly until both patient's clinical status and levels are stable then levels may be obtained every 1-2 months

Timing of serum samples: Draw trough just before next dose

Therapeutic levels:

Acute mania: 0.6-1.2 mEq/L (SI: 0.6-1.2 mmol/L)

Protection against future episodes in most patients with bipolar disorder: 0.8-1 mEq/L (SI: 0.8-1.0 mmol/L); a higher rate of relapse is described in subjects who are maintained at <0.4 mEq/L (SI: 0.4 mmol/L)

Elderly patients can usually be maintained at lower end of therapeutic range (0.6-0.8 mEq/L)

Toxic concentration: >2 mEq/L (SI: >2 mmol/L)

Adverse effect levels:

GI complaints/tremor: 1.5-2 mEq/L

Confusion/somnolence: 2-2.5 mEq/L

Seizures/death: >2.5 mEq/L

## Lodoxamide Tromethamine (loe DOKS a mide troe METH a meen)

**Pharmacologic Class** Mast Cell Stabilizer

**U.S. Brand Names** Alomide® Ophthalmic

**Mechanism of Action** Mast cell stabilizer that inhibits the *in vivo* type I immediate hypersensitivity reaction to increase cutaneous vascular permeability associated with IgE and antigen-mediated reactions

**Use** Treatment of vernal keratoconjunctivitis, vernal conjunctivitis, and vernal keratitis

**USUAL DOSAGE** Children >2 years and Adults: Instill 1-2 drops in eye(s) 4 times/day for up to 3 months

**Dosage Forms Soln, ophth:** 0.1% (10 mL)

**Contraindications** Hypersensitivity to any component of product

**Warnings/Precautions** Safety and efficacy in children <2 years of age have not been established; not for injection; not for use in patients wearing soft contact lenses during treatment

**Pregnancy Risk Factor** B

**Adverse Reactions**

>10%: Local: Transient burning, stinging, discomfort

1% to 10%:

Central nervous system: Headache

Ocular: Blurred vision, corneal erosion/ulcer, eye pain, corneal abrasion, blepharitis

<1%: Dizziness, somnolence, rash, nausea, stomach discomfort, sneezing, dry nose

**Special PA Issues**

**Patient Education:** For ophthalmic use only. Apply prescribed amount as often as directed. Wash hands before using and do not touch tip of applicator to eye or contaminate tip of applicator. Tilt head back and look upward. Gently pull down lower lid and put drop(s) inside lower eyelid at inner corner. Close eye and roll eyeball in all directions. Do not blink for 1/2 minute. Apply gentle pressure to inner corner of eye for 30 seconds. Wipe away excess from skin around eye. Do not use any other eye preparation for at least 10 minutes. Do not share medication with anyone else. Temporary stinging or blurred vision may occur. Immediately report any adverse cardiac or CNS effects (usually signifies overdose). Report persistent eye pain, redness, burning, watering, dryness, double vision, puffiness around eye, vision disturbances, other adverse eye response, worsening of condition or lack of improvement.

- **Loestrin®** *see* Ethinyl Estradiol and Norethindrone *on page 348*
- **Lofene®** *see* Diphenoxylate and Atropine *on page 290*
- **Logen®** *see* Diphenoxylate and Atropine *on page 290*
- **Lomanate®** *see* Diphenoxylate and Atropine *on page 290*

## Lomefloxacin (loe me FLOKS a sin)

**Pharmacologic Class** Antibiotic, Quinolone

**U.S. Brand Names** Maxaquin®

**Mechanism of Action** Inhibits DNA-gyrase in susceptible organisms thereby inhibits relaxation of supercoiled DNA and promotes breakage of DNA strands. DNA gyrase (topoisomerase II), is an essential bacterial enzyme that maintains the superhelical structure of DNA and is required for DNA replication and transcription, DNA repair, recombination, and transposition.

**Use** Lower respiratory infections, acute bacterial exacerbation of chronic bronchitis, skin infections, sexually transmitted diseases, and urinary tract infections caused by *E. coli, K. pneumoniae, P. mirabilis, P. aeruginosa*; also has gram-positive activity including *S. pneumoniae* and some staphylococci

**USUAL DOSAGE**

Lower respiratory and urinary tract infections (UTI): Adults: Oral: 400 mg once daily for 10-14 days

Urinary tract infection (UTI) due to susceptible organisms:

Uncomplicated cystitis caused by *Escherichia coli*: Adult female: Oral: 400 mg once daily for 3 successive days

Uncomplicated cystitis caused by *Klebsiella pneumoniae, Proteus mirabilis*, or *Staphylococcus saprophyticus*: Adult female: 400 mg once daily for 10 successive days

Complicated UTI caused by *Escherichia coli, Klebsiella penumoniae, Proteus mirabilis*, or *Pseudomonas aeruginosa*: Adults: Oral: 400 mg once daily for 14 successive days

Surgical prophylaxis: 400 mg 2-6 hours before surgery

Uncomplicated gonorrhea: 400 mg as a single dose

No dosage adjustment is needed for elderly patients with normal renal function

**Dosing adjustment in renal impairment:**

Cl$_{cr}$ 11-39 mL/minute: Loading dose: 400 mg; then 200 mg every day

Hemodialysis: Same as above

**Dosage Forms Tab, as hydrochloride:** 400 mg

**Contraindications** Hypersensitivity to lomefloxacin or other members of the quinolone group such as nalidixic acid, oxolinic acid, cinoxacin, norfloxacin, and ciprofloxacin; avoid use in children <18 years of age due to association of other quinolones with transient arthropathies

**Warnings/Precautions** Use with caution in patients with epilepsy or other CNS diseases which could predispose them to seizures

**Pregnancy Risk Factor** C

**Adverse Reactions**

1% to 10%:

Central nervous system: Headache, dizziness

Dermatologic: Photosensitivity

Gastrointestinal: Nausea

<1%: Flushing, chest pain, hypotension, hypertension, edema, syncope, tachycardia, bradycardia, arrhythmia, extrasystoles, cyanosis, cardiac failure, angina pectoris, myocardial infarction, facial edema, fatigue, malaise, chills, convulsions, vertigo, coma, purpura, rash, gout, hypoglycemia, abdominal pain, vomiting, flatulence, constipation, xerostomia, discoloration of tongue, abnormal taste, urinary disorders, dysuria, thrombocytopenia, increased fibrinolysis, back pain, hyperkinesia, tremor, paresthesias, leg cramps, myalgia, weakness, earache, hematuria, anuria, dyspnea, cough, epistaxis, diaphoresis (increased), allergic reaction, flu-like symptoms, decreased heat tolerance, thirst

**Drug Interactions**

Decreased effect: Decreased absorption with antacids containing aluminum, magnesium, and/or calcium (by up to 98% if given at the same time)

Increased toxicity/serum levels: Quinolones cause increased levels of caffeine, warfarin, cyclosporine, and theophylline; cimetidine, probenecid increase quinolone levels

**Half-Life** 5-7.5 hours

**Special PA Issues**

Patient Education: Take as directed, preferably on an empty stomach 1 hour before or 2 hours after meals. Complete entire prescription even if feeling better. Maintain adequate hydration (2-3 L/day of fluids unless instructed to restrict fluid intake). You may experience dizziness or drowsiness; use caution when driving or engaging in tasks that require alertness. You may experience photosensitivity (use sunblock, wear protective clothing and dark glasses, or avoid direct sunlight). Report any signs of opportunistic infection (eg, fever, chills, vaginal itching or foul-smelling vaginal discharge, oral thrush, easy bruising). Report immediately any signs of allergic reaction (eg, rash, itching or tingling of skin); join pain; difficulty breathing; CNS changes (excitability, seizures); pain, inflammation, or rupture of tendon; or abdominal cramping or pain.

Dietary Considerations: May be taken without regard to meals

♦ **Lomefloxacin Hydrochloride** see Lomefloxacin on previous page

♦ **Lomodix®** see Diphenoxylate and Atropine on page 290

♦ **Lomotil®** see Diphenoxylate and Atropine on page 290

# Lomustine (loe MUS teen)

**Pharmacologic Class** Antineoplastic Agent, Alkylating Agent

**U.S. Brand Names** CeeNU®

**Mechanism of Action** Inhibits DNA and RNA synthesis via carbamylation of DNA polymerase, alkylation of DNA, and alteration of RNA, proteins, and enzymes

**Use** Treatment of brain tumors and Hodgkin's disease, non-Hodgkin's lymphoma, melanoma, renal carcinoma, lung cancer, colon cancer

**USUAL DOSAGE** Oral (refer to individual protocols):

Children: 75-150 mg/m² as a single dose every 6 weeks; subsequent doses are readjusted after initial treatment according to platelet and leukocyte counts

Adults: 100-130 mg/m² as a single dose every 6 weeks; readjust after initial treatment according to platelet and leukocyte counts

With compromised marrow function: Initial dose: 100 mg/m² as a single dose every 6 weeks

Repeat courses should only be administered after adequate recovery: WBC >4000 and platelet counts >100,000

**Subsequent dosing adjustment based on nadir**:

Leukocytes 2000-2900/mm³, platelets 25,000-74,999/mm³: Administer 70% of prior dose

Leukocytes <2000/mm³, platelets <25,000/mm³: Administer 50% of prior dose

**Dosage adjustment in renal impairment**:

Cl_cr 10-50 mL/minute: Administer 75% of normal dose

Cl_cr <10 mL/minute: Administer 50% of normal dose

Hemodialysis: Supplemental dose is not necessary

Peritoneal dialysis: Significant drug removal is unlikely based on physiochemical characteristics

**Dosage Forms Cap:** 10 mg, 40 mg, 100 mg; **Dose Pack:** 10 mg (2s), 100 mg (2s), 40 mg (2s)

**Contraindications** Hypersensitivity to lomustine or any component

**Warnings/Precautions** The U.S. Food and Drug Administration (FDA) currently recommends that procedures for proper handling and disposal for antineoplastic agents be considered. Bone marrow suppression, notably thrombocytopenia and leukopenia, may (Continued)

## Lomustine *(Continued)*

lead to bleeding and overwhelming infections in an already compromised patient; will last for at least 6 weeks after a dose, do not administer courses more frequently than every 6 weeks because the toxicity is cumulative. Use with caution in patients with depressed platelet, leukocyte or erythrocyte counts, liver function abnormalities.

**Pregnancy Risk Factor** D

**Adverse Reactions**

>10%:

Gastrointestinal: Nausea and vomiting occur 3-6 hours after oral administration; this is due to a centrally mediated mechanism, not a direct effect on the GI lining; if vomiting occurs, it is not necessary to replace the dose unless it occurs immediately after drug administration

Emetic potential:

<60 mg: Moderately high (60% to 90%)

≥60 mg: High (>90%)

Time course of nausea/vomiting: Onset: 2-6 hours; Duration: 4-6 hours

Hematologic: Myelosuppression: Anemia; effects occur 4-6 weeks after a dose and may persist for 1-2 weeks

WBC: Moderate

Platelets: Severe

Onset (days): 14

Nadir (weeks): 4-5

Recovery (weeks): 6

1% to 10%:

Central nervous system: Neurotoxicity

Dermatologic: Skin rash

Gastrointestinal: Stomatitis, diarrhea

Hematologic: Anemia

<1%: Disorientation, lethargy, ataxia, alopecia, hepatotoxicity, dysarthria, pulmonary fibrosis with cumulative doses >600 mg, renal failure

**Drug Interactions** CYP2D6 enzyme inhibitor

Decreased effect with phenobarbital, resulting in decreased efficacy of both drugs

Increased toxicity with cimetidine, reported to cause bone marrow suppression or to potentiate the myelosuppressive effects of lomustine

**Duration** Marrow recovery may require 6 weeks

**Half-Life** Parent drug: 16-72 hours; Active metabolite: 1.3-2 days

**Special PA Issues**

**Patient Education:** Take with fluids on an empty stomach; do not eat or drink for 2 hours following administration Do not use alcohol, aspirin, or aspirin-containing medications and OTC medications without consulting prescriber. Maintain adequate fluid balance (2-3 L/day). May cause hair loss (reversible); easy bleeding or bruising (use soft toothbrush or cotton swabs and frequent mouth care, use electric razor, avoid sharp knives or scissors); increased susceptibility to infection (avoid crowds or exposure to infection - do not have any vaccinations unless approved by prescriber). Report unusual bleeding or bruising or persistent fever or sore throat; blood in urine, stool, or vomitus; delayed healing of any wounds; skin rash; yellowing of skin or eyes; changes in color of urine of stool.

**Monitoring Parameters:** CBC with differential and platelet count, hepatic and renal function tests, pulmonary function tests

♦ **Loniten®** *see* Minoxidil *on page 610*

♦ **Lonox®** *see* Diphenoxylate and Atropine *on page 290*

♦ **Lo/Ovral®** *see* Ethinyl Estradiol and Norgestrel *on page 351*

## Loperamide *(loe PER a mide)*

**Pharmacologic Class** Antidiarrheal

**U.S. Brand Names** Diar-aid® [OTC]; Imodium®; Imodium® A-D [OTC]; Kaopectate® II [OTC]; Pepto® Diarrhea Control [OTC]

**Mechanism of Action** Acts directly on intestinal muscles to inhibit peristalsis and prolongs transit time enhancing fluid and electrolyte movement through intestinal mucosa; reduces fecal volume, increases viscosity, and diminishes fluid and electrolyte loss; demonstrates antisecretory activity; exhibits peripheral action

**Use** Treatment of acute diarrhea and chronic diarrhea associated with inflammatory bowel disease; chronic functional diarrhea (idiopathic), chronic diarrhea caused by bowel resection or organic lesions; to decrease the volume of ileostomy discharge

**Unlabeled use:** Treatment of traveler's diarrhea in combination with trimethoprim-sulfamethoxazole (co-trimoxazole) (3 days therapy)

**USUAL DOSAGE** Oral:

Children:

Acute diarrhea: Initial doses (in first 24 hours):

2-6 years: 1 mg 3 times/day

6-8 years: 2 mg twice daily

8-12 years: 2 mg 3 times/day

Maintenance: After initial dosing, 0.1 mg/kg doses after each loose stool, but not exceeding initial dosage

Chronic diarrhea: 0.08-0.24 mg/kg/day divided 2-3 times/day, maximum: 2 mg/dose

Adults: Initial: 4 mg (2 capsules), followed by 2 mg after each loose stool, up to 16 mg/day (8 capsules)

**Dosage Forms** Loperamide hydrochloride: **Caplet:** 2 mg; **Cap:** 2 mg; **Liq, oral:** 1 mg/5 mL (60 mL, 90 mL, 120 mL); **Tab:** 2 mg

**Contraindications** Patients who must avoid constipation, diarrhea resulting from some infections, or in patients with pseudomembranous colitis, hypersensitivity to specific drug or component, bloody diarrhea

**Warnings/Precautions** Large first-pass metabolism, use with caution in hepatic dysfunction; should not be used if diarrhea accompanied by high fever, blood in stool

**Pregnancy Risk Factor** B

**Adverse Reactions**

Central nervous system: Sedation, fatigue, dizziness, drowsiness

Dermatologic: Rash

Gastrointestinal: Nausea, vomiting, constipation, abdominal cramping, xerostomia, abdominal distention

**Drug Interactions** Increased toxicity: CNS depressants, phenothiazines, tricyclic antidepressants may potentiate the adverse effects

**Onset** Oral: Within 0.5-1 hour

**Half-Life** 7-14 hours

**Special PA Issues**

**Patient Education:** Do not take more than 8 capsules or 80 mL in 24 hours. May cause drowsiness. If acute diarrhea lasts longer than 48 hours, consult prescriber. Do not take if diarrhea is bloody.

♦ **Loperamide Hydrochloride** see Loperamide on previous page

♦ **Lopid®** see Gemfibrozil on page 410

♦ **Lopressor®** see Metoprolol on page 599

♦ **Loprox®** see Ciclopirox on page 205

♦ **Lorabid™** see Loracarbef on this page

# Loracarbef (lor a KAR bef)

**Pharmacologic Class** Antibiotic, Carbacephem

**U.S. Brand Names** Lorabid™

**Mechanism of Action** Inhibits bacterial cell wall synthesis by binding to one or more of the penicillin binding proteins (PBPs); inhibits the final transpeptidation step of peptidoglycan synthesis in bacterial cell walls, thus inhibiting cell wall biosynthesis. It is thought that beta-lactam antibiotics inactivate transpeptidase via acylation of the enzyme with cleavage of the CO-N bond of the beta-lactam ring. Upon exposure to beta-lactam antibiotics, bacteria eventually lyse due to ongoing activity of cell wall autolytic enzymes (autolysins and murein hydrolases) while cell wall assembly is arrested.

**Use** Infections caused by susceptible organisms involving the respiratory tract, acute otitis media, sinusitis, skin and skin structure, bone and joint, and urinary tract and gynecologic

**USUAL DOSAGE** Oral:

Children:

Acute otitis media: 15 mg/kg twice daily for 10 days

Pharyngitis and impetigo: 7.5-15 mg/kg twice daily for 10 days

Adults:

Uncomplicated urinary tract infections: 200 mg once daily for 7 days

Skin and soft tissue: 200-400 mg every 12-24 hours

Uncomplicated pyelonephritis: 400 mg every 12 hours for 14 days

Upper/lower respiratory tract infection: 200-400 mg every 12-24 hours for 7-14 days

**Dosing comments in renal impairment:**

$Cl_{cr}$ 10-49 mL/minute: 50% of usual dose at usual interval or usual dose given half as often

$Cl_{cr}$ <10 mL/minute: Administer usual dose every 3-5 days

Hemodialysis: Doses should be administered after dialysis sessions

**Dosage Forms Cap:** 200 mg, 400 mg; **Susp, oral:** 100 mg/5 mL (50 mL, 100 mL), 200 mg/5 mL (50 mL, 100 mL)

**Contraindications** Patients with a history of hypersensitivity to loracarbef or cephalosporins

**Warnings/Precautions** Modify dosage in patients with severe renal impairment; prolonged use may result in superinfection; use with caution in patients with a previous history of hypersensitivity to other beta-lactam antibiotics (eg, penicillins, cephalosporins)

**Pregnancy Risk Factor** B

**Adverse Reactions**

>1%: Gastrointestinal: Diarrhea

<1%: Seizures (with high doses and renal dysfunction), headache, nervousness, rash, urticaria, pruritus, Stevens-Johnson syndrome, nausea, vomiting, pseudomembranous (Continued)

## Loracarbef *(Continued)*

colitis, eosinophilia, hemolytic anemia, neutropenia, positive Coombs' test, thrombocytopenia, cholestatic jaundice, slightly increased AST/ALT, arthralgia, nephrotoxicity with transient elevations of BUN/creatinine, interstitial nephritis, serum sickness, candidiasis

**Drug Interactions**

Increased effect: Probenecid may decrease cephalosporin elimination

Increased toxicity: Furosemide, aminoglycosides may be a possible additive to nephrotoxicity

**Half-Life** ~1 hour; prolonged in renal impairment

**Special PA Issues**

**Patient Education:** Take as directed, preferably on an empty stomach 1 hour before or 2 hours after meals. Complete entire prescription even if feeling better. Maintain adequate hydration (2-3 L/day of fluids unless instructed to restrict fluid intake). You may experience nausea, vomiting, or loss of appetite; frequent small meals, frequent mouth care, or sucking on lozenges may help. Buttermilk or yogurt may relieve diarrhea. Report fever, chills, vaginal itching or foul-smelling vaginal discharge, oral thrush, yellowing of skin or eyes, easy bruising, or unusual bleeding. Report immediately any signs of allergic reaction such as rash, itching or tingling of skin, join pain, or difficulty breathing.

## Loratadine (lor AT a deen)

**Pharmacologic Class** Antihistamine

**U.S. Brand Names** Claritin®

**Mechanism of Action** Long-acting tricyclic antihistamine with selective peripheral histamine $H_1$-receptor antagonistic properties

**Use** Relief of nasal and non-nasal symptoms of seasonal allergic rhinitis

**USUAL DOSAGE** Children ≥6 years and Adults: Oral: 10 mg/day on an empty stomach

**Dosing interval in hepatic impairment:** 10 mg every other day to start

**Dosage Forms** Soln, ora: 1 mg/mL; **Tab:** 10 mg; **Rapid-disintegrating tab:** 10 mg (RediTabs®)

**Contraindications** Patients hypersensitive to loratadine or any of its components

**Warnings/Precautions** Patients with liver impairment should start with a lower dose (10 mg every other day), since their ability to clear the drug will be reduced; use with caution in lactation, safety in children <12 years of age has not been established

**Pregnancy Risk Factor** B

**Adverse Reactions**

>10%:

Central nervous system: Headache, somnolence, fatigue

Gastrointestinal: Xerostomia

1% to 10%:

Cardiovascular: Hypotension, hypertension, palpitations, tachycardia

Central nervous system: Anxiety, depression

Endocrine & metabolic: Breast pain

Neuromuscular & skeletal: Hyperkinesia, arthralgias

Respiratory: Nasal dryness, pharyngitis, dyspnea

Miscellaneous: Diaphoresis

**Drug Interactions** CYP2D6 and 3A3/4 enzyme substrate

Increased plasma concentrations of loratadine and its active metabolite with ketoconazole; erythromycin increases the AUC of loratadine and its active metabolite; no change in $QT_c$ interval was seen

Increased toxicity: Procarbazine, other antihistamines, alcohol

**Onset** Within 1-3 hours; Peak effect: 8-12 hours

**Duration** >24 hours

**Half-Life** 12-15 hours

**Special PA Issues**

**Patient Education:** Take as directed; do not exceed recommended dose. Avoid use of other depressants, alcohol, or sleep-inducing medications unless approved by prescriber. You may experience drowsiness or dizziness (use caution when driving or engaging in hazardous activity until response to medication is known); or dry mouth or nausea (frequent small meals, frequent mouth care, chewing gum, or sucking hard candy may help). Report persistent dizziness, sedation, or seizures; chest pain, rapid heartbeat, or palpitations; swelling of face, mouth, lips, or tongue; difficulty breathing; changes in urinary pattern; yellowing of skin or eyes, dark urine, or pale stool; or lack of improvement or worsening or condition.

## Loratadine and Pseudoephedrine (lor AT a deen & soo doe e FED rin)

**Pharmacologic Class** Antihistamine/Decongestant Combination

**U.S. Brand Names** Claritin-D®; Claritin-D® 24-Hour

**Dosage Forms Tab:** Loratadine 5 mg and pseudoephedrine sulfate 120 mg; **Tab, extended release:** Loratadine 10 mg and pseudoephedrine sulfate 240 mg

# Lorazepam (lor A ze pam)

**Pharmacologic Class** Benzodiazepine

**U.S. Brand Names** Ativan®

**Mechanism of Action** Depresses all levels of the CNS, including the limbic and reticular formation, probably through the increased action of gamma-aminobutyric acid (GABA), which is a major inhibitory neurotransmitter in the brain

**Use** Management of anxiety, status epilepticus, preoperative sedation, for desired amnesia, and as an antiemetic adjunct

**Unapproved uses:** Alcohol detoxification, insomnia, psychogenic catatonia, partial complex seizures

## USUAL DOSAGE

Antiemetic:

Children 2-15 years: I.V.: 0.05 mg/kg (up to 2 mg/dose) prior to chemotherapy

Adults: Oral, I.V.: 0.5-2 mg every 4-6 hours as needed

Anxiety and sedation:

Infants and Children: Oral, I.V.: Usual: 0.05 mg/kg/dose (range: 0.02-0.09 mg/kg) every 4-8 hours

Adults: Oral: 1-10 mg/day in 2-3 divided doses; usual dose: 2-6 mg/day in divided doses

Insomnia: Adults: Oral: 2-4 mg at bedtime

Preoperative: Adults:

I.M.: 0.05 mg/kg administered 2 hours before surgery; maximum: 4 mg/dose

I.V.: 0.044 mg/kg 15-20 minutes before surgery; usual maximum: 2 mg/dose

Operative amnesia: Adults: I.V.: Up to 0.05 mg/kg; maximum: 4 mg/dose

Status epilepticus: I.V.:

Infants and Children: 0.1 mg/kg slow I.V. over 2-5 minutes, do not exceed 4 mg/single dose; may repeat second dose of 0.05 mg/kg slow I.V. in 10-15 minutes if needed

Adolescents: 0.07 mg/kg slow I.V. over 2-5 minutes; maximum: 4 mg/dose; may repeat in 10-15 minutes

Adults: 4 mg/dose given slowly over 2-5 minutes; may repeat in 10-15 minutes; usual maximum dose: 8 mg

**Dosage Forms Inj:** 2 mg/mL (1 mL, 10 mL), 4 mg/mL (1 mL, 10 mL); **Soln, oral concentrated, alcohol and dye free:** 2 mg/mL (30 mL); **Tab:** 0.5 mg, 1 mg, 2 mg

**Contraindications** Hypersensitivity to lorazepam or any component; there may be a cross-sensitivity with other benzodiazepines; do not use in a comatose patient, those with pre-existing CNS depression, narrow-angle glaucoma, severe uncontrolled pain, severe hypotension

**Warnings/Precautions** Use caution in patients with renal or hepatic impairment, organic brain syndrome, myasthenia gravis, or Parkinson's disease. Dilute injection prior to I.V. use with equal volume of compatible diluent (D $_5$W, 0.9% sodium chloride, sterile water for injection); do **not** inject intra-arterially, arteriospasm and gangrene may occur; injection contains benzyl alcohol 2%, polyethylene glycol and propylene glycol, which may be toxic to newborns in high doses, may reduce effectiveness of ECT; oral doses >0.09 mg/kg produced increased ataxia without increased sedative benefit versus lower doses

**Pregnancy Risk Factor** D

**Pregnancy Implications**

Clinical effects on the fetus: Crosses the placenta. Respiratory depression or hypotonia if administered near time of delivery.

Breast-feeding/lactation: Crosses into breast milk and no data on clinical effects on the infant. American Academy of Pediatrics states MAY BE OF CONCERN.

## Adverse Reactions

Respiratory: Decrease in respiratory rate, apnea, laryngospasm

>10%:

Cardiovascular: Tachycardia, chest pain

Central nervous system: Drowsiness, confusion, ataxia, amnesia, slurred speech, paradoxical excitement, rage, headache, depression, anxiety, fatigue, lightheadedness, insomnia

Dermatologic: Rash

Endocrine & metabolic: Decreased libido

Gastrointestinal: Xerostomia, constipation, diarrhea, nausea, vomiting, increased or decreased appetite, decreased salivation

Local: Phlebitis, pain with injection

Neuromuscular & skeletal: Dysarthria

Ocular: Blurred vision, diplopia

Miscellaneous: Diaphoresis

1% to 10%:

Cardiovascular: Cardiac arrest, hypotension, bradycardia, cardiovascular collapse, syncope

Central nervous system: Confusion, nervousness, dizziness, akathisia

Neuromuscular & skeletal: Rigidity, tremor, muscle cramps

Dermatologic: Dermatitis

Gastrointestinal: Weight gain or loss

Otic: Tinnitus

(Continued)

## Lorazepam (Continued)

Respiratory: Nasal congestion, hyperventilation

<1%: Menstrual irregularities, increased salivation, blood dyscrasias, reflex slowing, physical and psychological dependence with prolonged use

**Drug Interactions**

Decreased effect with oral contraceptives (combination products), cigarette smoking; decreased effect of levodopa

Increased effect with morphine

Increased toxicity with alcohol, CNS depressants, MAO inhibitors, loxapine, TCAs

**Onset**

Onset of hypnosis: I.M.: 20-30 minutes

Sedation, anticonvulsant: I.V.: 5 minutes; oral: 30 minutes to 1 hour

**Duration** 6-8 hours

**Half-Life** Adults: 12.9 hours; Elderly: 15.9 hours; End-stage renal disease: 32-70 hours

**Special PA Issues**

**Patient Education:**

Oral: Take exactly as directed (do not increase dose or frequency); may cause physical and/or psychological dependence. Do not use excessive alcohol or other prescription or OTC medications -especially pain medications, sedatives, antihistamines, or hypnotics) without consulting prescriber. Maintain adequate hydration (2-3 L/day of fluids unless instructed to restrict fluid intake). You may experience drowsiness, lightheadedness, impaired coordination, dizziness, or blurred vision (use caution when driving or engaging in hazardous tasks until response to medication is known); nausea, vomiting, or dry mouth (small frequent meals, good mouth care, chewing gum, or sucking lozenges may help); constipation (increased exercise, fluids, or dietary fruit and fiber may help); altered sexual drive or ability (reversible); or photosensitivity (use sunscreen, protective clothing, and avoid extended exposure to direct sunlight). Report persistent CNS effects (eg, confusion, depression, increased sedation, excitation, headache, agitation, insomnia or nightmares, dizziness, fatigue, impaired coordination, changes in personality, or changes in cognition); changes in urinary pattern; chest pain, palpitations, or rapid heartbeat; muscle cramping, weakness, tremors, or rigidity; ringing in ears or visual disturbances; excessive perspiration, or excessive GI symptoms (cramping, constipation, vomiting, anorexia); or worsening of condition.

**Dietary Considerations** Alcohol: Additive CNS depression has been reported with benzodiazepines; avoid or limit alcohol

**Monitoring Parameters** Respiratory and cardiovascular status, blood pressure, heart rate, symptoms of anxiety

**Reference Range:** Therapeutic: 50-240 ng/mL (SI: 156-746 nmol/L)

♦ **Lorcet®-HD** see Hydrocodone and Acetaminophen on page 449

♦ **Lorcet® Plus** see Hydrocodone and Acetaminophen on page 449

♦ **Lortab®** see Hydrocodone and Acetaminophen on page 449

♦ **Lortab® ASA** see Hydrocodone and Aspirin on page 450

## Losartan (loe SAR tan)

**Pharmacologic Class** Angiotensin II Antagonists

**U.S. Brand Names** Cozaar®

**Mechanism of Action** As a selective and competitive, nonpeptide angiotensin II receptor antagonist, losartan blocks the vasoconstrictor and aldosterone-secreting effects of angiotensin II; losartan interacts reversibly at the AT1 and AT2 receptors of many tissues and has slow dissociation kinetics; its affinity for the AT1 receptor is 1000 times greater than the AT2 receptor. Angiotensin II receptor antagonists may induce a more complete inhibition of the renin-angiotensin system than ACE inhibitors, they do not affect the response to bradykinin, and are less likely to be associated with nonrenin-angiotensin effects (eg, cough and angioedema). Losartan increases urinary flow rate and in addition to being natriuretic and kaliuretic, increases excretion of chloride, magnesium, uric acid, calcium, and phosphate.

**Use** Treatment of hypertension with or without concurrent use of thiazide diuretics; may prolong survival in heart failure; recommended for patients unable to tolerated ACE inhibitors

**USUAL DOSAGE**

Oral: The usual starting dose is 50 mg once daily; can be administered once or twice daily with total daily doses ranging from 25 mg to 100 mg

Usual initial doses in patients receiving diuretics or those with intravascular volume depletion: 25 mg

Patients not receiving diuretics: 50 mg

**Dosing adjustment in renal impairment:** None necessary

**Dosing adjustment in hepatic impairment or geriatric patients:** Reduce the initial dose to 25 mg; divide dosage intervals into two

Not removed via hemodialysis

**Dosage Forms Tab, film coated, as potassium:** 25 mg, 50 mg

**Contraindications** Hypersensitivity to losartan or any components; pregnancy

**Warnings/Precautions** Avoid use or use a much smaller dose in patients who are intravascularly volume-depleted; use caution in patients with unilateral or bilateral renal artery stenosis to avoid a decrease in renal function; AUCs of losartan (not the active metabolite) are about 50% greater in patients with $Cl_{cr}$ <30 mL/minute and are doubled in hemodialysis patients

**Pregnancy Risk Factor** C (1st trimester); D (2nd and 3rd trimester)

**Pregnancy Implications** Breast-feeding/lactation: Avoid use in the nursing mother, if possible, since it is postulated that losartan is excreted in breast milk

**Adverse Reactions**

1% to 10%:

Cardiovascular: Hypotension without reflex tachycardia

Central nervous system: Dizziness, insomnia

Endocrine & metabolic: Hyperkalemia

Gastrointestinal: Diarrhea, dyspepsia

Hematologic: Slight decreases in hemoglobin and hematocrit

Neuromuscular & skeletal: Back/leg pain, myalgia

Renal: Hypouricemia (with large doses)

Respiratory: Cough (less than ACE inhibitors), nasal congestion, sinus disorders, sinusitis

<1%: Orthostatic effects, angina, second degree A-V block, CVA, palpitations, sinus bradycardia, tachycardia, flushing, facial edema, anxiety, ataxia, confusion, depression, dream abnormality, migraine headache, sleep disorders, vertigo, fever, alopecia, dermatitis, dry skin, bruising, erythema, photosensitivity, pruritus, rash, urticaria, gout, anorexia, constipation, flatulence, vomiting, abnormal taste, gastritis, impotence, decreased libido, polyuria, nocturia, slightly elevated LFTs and bilirubin, paresthesia, tremor; arm, hip, shoulder, and knee pain, joint edema, fibromyalgia, muscle weakness, blurred vision, burning and stinging eyes, conjunctivitis, decreased visual acuity, tinnitus, urinary tract infection, nocturia, mild increases in BUN/creatinine, dyspnea, bronchitis, pharyngeal discomfort, epistaxis, rhinitis, respiratory congestion, diaphoresis

**Drug Interactions** CYP2C9 and 3A3/4 enzyme substrate

Decreased effect: Phenobarbital, troleandomycin, sulfaphenazole

Increased effect: Cimetidine

**Onset** 6 hours

**Half-Life** Losartan: 1.5-2 hours; Metabolite (E-3174): 6-9 hours

**Special PA Issues**

**Patient Education:** Take as directed; do not change dosage or stop taking without consulting prescriber. Do not change amount of dietary salt without advice or consult of prescriber. You may experience dizziness, fainting, or lightheadedness (use caution when driving or performing hazardous tasks and use caution rising from sitting or lying position) until response to therapy is established. Report immediately any swelling of face, lips, throat, or tongue, or difficulty breathing. Report sore throat; fever; rash; swelling of hands, feet, or legs; respiratory difficulty; chest pains or irregular heartbeat; unusual cough; persistent vomiting, diarrhea, or perspiration; or flu-like symptoms.

**Monitoring Parameters:** Supine blood pressure, electrolytes, serum creatinine, BUN, urinalysis, symptomatic hypotension and tachycardia, CBC

# Losartan and Hydrochlorothiazide

(loe SAR tan & hye droe klor oh THYE a zide)

**Pharmacologic Class** Antihypertensive Agent, Combination

**U.S. Brand Names** Hyzaar®

**Dosage Forms Tab:** Losartan potassium 50 mg and hydrochlorothiazide 12.5 mg

♦ **Losartan Potassium** see Losartan on previous page

♦ **Losec®** see Omeprazole on page 674

♦ **Lotemax®** see Loteprednol on this page

♦ **Lotensin®** see Benazepril on page 103

♦ **Lotensin® HCT** see Benazepril and Hydrochlorothiazide on page 104

# Loteprednol (loe te PRED nol)

**Pharmacologic Class** Corticosteroid, Ophthalmic

**U.S. Brand Names** Alrex™; Lotemax®

**Mechanism of Action** Corticosteroids inhibit the inflammatory response including edema, capillary dilation, leukocyte migration, and scar formation. Loteprednol is highly lipid soluble and penetrates cells readily to induce the production of lipocortins. These proteins modulate the activity of prostaglandins and leukotrienes.

**Use**

0.2% suspension (Alrex™): Temporary relief of signs and symptoms of seasonal allergic conjunctivitis

0.5% suspension (Lotemax®): Inflammatory conditions (treatment of steroid-responsive inflammatory conditions of the palpebral and bulbar conjunctiva, cornea, and anterior segment of the globe such as allergic conjunctivitis, acne rosacea, superficial punctate keratitis, herpes zoster keratitis, iritis, cyclitis, selected infective conjunctivitis, when the (Continued)

## Loteprednol *(Continued)*

inherent hazard of steroid use is accepted to obtain an advisable diminution in edema and inflammation) and treatment of postoperative inflammation following ocular surgery

**USUAL DOSAGE** Adults: Ophthalmic:

0.2% suspension (Alrex™): Instill 1 drop into affected eye(s) 4 times/day

0.5% suspension (Lotemax®):

Inflammatory conditions: Apply 1-2 drops into the conjunctival sac of the affected eye(s) 4 times/day. During the initial treatment within the first week, the dosing may be increased up to 1 drop every hour. Advise patients not to discontinue therapy prematurely. If signs and symptoms fail to improve after 2 days, re-evaluate the patient.

Postoperative inflammation: Apply 1-2 drops into the conjunctival sac of the operated eye(s) 4 times/day beginning 24 hours after surgery and continuing throughout the first 2 weeks of the postoperative period

**Dosage Forms** Susp, ophth, as etabonate: 0.2% (5 mL, 10 mL), 0.5% (2.5 mL, 5 mL, 10 mL, 15 mL)

**Contraindications** Viral diseases of the cornea and conjunctiva; mycobacterial infection of the eye; fungal diseases of ocular structures; hypersensitivity to loteprednol and any ingredients; hypersensitivity to other corticosteroids

**Warnings/Precautions** For ophthalmic use only; patients should be re-evaluated if symptoms fail to improve after 2 days. Intraocular pressure should be monitored if this product is used >10 days. Prolonged use may result in glaucoma and injury to the optic nerve. Visual defects in acuity and field of vision may occur. Posterior subcapsular cataracts may form after long-term use. Use with caution in presence of glaucoma (steroids increase intraocular pressure). Perforation may occur with topical steroids in diseases which thin the cornea or sclera. Steroids may mask infection or enhance existing infection. Steroid use may delay healing after cataract surgery.

**Pregnancy Risk Factor** C

**Adverse Reactions**

Ocular: Increased intraocular pressure, changes in visual acuity and/or field defects, cataract formation, secondary ocular infection, globe perforation in disease which thins cornea or sclera

10% to 15%:

Central nervous system: Headache

Respiratory: Rhinitis, pharyngitis

5% to 10%: Ocular: Abnormal vision/blurring, burning on instillation, chemosis, dry eyes, itching, injection

<5%: Ocular: Conjunctivitis/irritation, corneal abnormalities, eyelid erythema, papillae uveitis

**Special PA Issues**

**Patient Education:** Solution: Store in a cool place. Tilt head back, place medication in conjunctival sac, and close eyes. Apply finger pressure at corner of eye for 1 minute following application. Do not allow tip of applicator to touch eye or any contaminated surface.

May cause temporary sensitivity to bright light, blurring or stinging, changes in visual acuity, headache, runny nose, or sore throat. Do not discontinue therapy prematurely. If improvement is not noted within 2 days, notify prescriber. Report persistent vision changes, signs of increased infection, swollen eyelids, extreme itching, or if inflammation does not improve.

**Monitoring Parameters:** Intraocular pressure (if >10 days)

- **Loteprednol Etabonate** *see* Loteprednol *on previous page*
- **Lotrel®** *see* Amlodipine and Benazepril *on page 60*
- **Lotrimin®** *see* Clotrimazole *on page 228*
- **Lotrimin® AF Cream [OTC]** *see* Clotrimazole *on page 228*
- **Lotrimin® AF Lotion [OTC]** *see* Clotrimazole *on page 228*
- **Lotrimin® AF Powder [OTC]** *see* Miconazole *on page 604*
- **Lotrimin® AF Solution [OTC]** *see* Clotrimazole *on page 228*
- **Lotrimin® AF Spray Liquid [OTC]** *see* Miconazole *on page 604*
- **Lotrimin® AF Spray Powder [OTC]** *see* Miconazole *on page 604*
- **Lotrisone®** *see* Betamethasone and Clotrimazole *on page 113*

## Lovastatin *(LOE va sta tin)*

**Pharmacologic Class** Antilipemic Agent (HMG-CoA Reductase Inhibitor)

**U.S. Brand Names** Mevacor®

**Mechanism of Action** Lovastatin acts by competitively inhibiting 3-hydroxyl-3-methylglutaryl-coenzyme A (HMG-CoA) reductase, the enzyme that catalyzes the rate-limiting step in cholesterol biosynthesis

**Use** Adjunct to dietary therapy to decrease elevated serum total and LDL cholesterol concentrations in primary hypercholesterolemia

**USUAL DOSAGE** Adults: Oral: Initial: 20 mg with evening meal, then adjust at 4-week intervals; maximum dose: 80 mg/day; before initiation of therapy, patients should be placed on a standard cholesterol-lowering diet for 3-6 months and the diet should be continued during drug therapy

**Dosage Forms** Tab: 10 mg, 20 mg, 40 mg

**Contraindications** Pregnancy; active liver disease, hypersensitivity to lovastatin or any component

**Warnings/Precautions** May elevate aminotransferases; LFTs should be performed before and every 4- 6 weeks during the first 15 months of therapy and periodically thereafter; can also cause myalgia and rhabdomyolysis; use with caution in patients who consume large quantities of alcohol or who have a history of liver disease

**Pregnancy Risk Factor** X

**Adverse Reactions**

1% to 10%:

Central nervous system: Headache, dizziness

Dermatologic: Rash, pruritus

Gastrointestinal: Flatulence, abdominal pain, cramps, diarrhea, pancreatitis, constipation, nausea, dyspepsia, heartburn

Neuromuscular & skeletal: Myalgia, increased CPK

<1%: Abnormal taste, gynecomastia, blurred vision, myositis, lenticular opacities

**Drug Interactions** CYP3A3/4 and 3A5-7 enzyme substrate

Increased toxicity: Gemfibrozil (musculoskeletal effects such as myopathy, myalgia, and/or muscle weakness accompanied by markedly elevated CK concentrations, rash, and/or pruritus); clofibrate, niacin (myopathy), erythromycin, cyclosporine, oral anticoagulants (elevated PT)

Increased effect/toxicity of lovastatin (20-fold increase in serum levels) with concurrent itraconazole or ketoconazole; interactions may also occur with simvastatin

Increased effect/toxicity of levothyroxine

Concurrent use of erythromycin and lovastatin may result in elevated lovastatin levels and rhabdomyolysis

**Onset** 3 days of therapy required for LDL cholesterol concentration reductions

**Half-Life** 1.1-1.7 hours

**Special PA Issues**

**Patient Education:** Take with evening meal (highest rate of cholesterol synthesis occurs from midnight to morning). If sleep disturbances occur, take earlier in the day. Do not change dosage without consulting prescriber. Maintain diet and exercise program as identified by prescriber. Have periodic ophthalmic exams while taking lovastatin (check for cataracts). You may experience mild GI disturbances (eg, gas, diarrhea, constipation); inform prescriber if these are severe or if you experience severe muscle pain or tenderness accompanied with malaise, blurred vision, or chest pain.

**Monitoring Parameters:** Plasma triglycerides, cholesterol, and liver function tests

**Related Information**

Lipid-Lowering Agents *on page 1022*

- **Lovenox® Injection** *see* Enoxaparin *on page 319*
- **Low-Quel®** *see* Diphenoxylate and Atropine *on page 290*
- **Loxapac®** *see* Loxapine *on this page*

# Loxapine (LOKS a peen)

**Pharmacologic Class** Antipsychotic Agent, Dibenzoxazepine

**U.S. Brand Names** Loxitane®; Loxitane® C; Loxitane® I.M.

**Mechanism of Action** Unclear, thought to be similar to chlorpromazine

**Use** Management of psychotic disorders

**USUAL DOSAGE** Adults:

Oral: 10 mg twice daily, increase dose until psychotic symptoms are controlled; usual dose range: 60-100 mg/day in divided doses 2-4 times/day; dosages >250 mg/day are not recommended

I.M.: 12.5-50 mg every 4-6 hours or longer as needed and change to oral therapy as soon as possible

**Dosage Forms** Loxapine hydrochloride: **Conc, oral:** 25 mg/mL (120 mL dropper bottle); **Inj:** 50 mg/mL (1 mL)

Loxapine succinate: **Cap:** 5 mg, 10 mg, 25 mg, 50 mg

**Contraindications** Hypersensitivity to chlorpromazine or any component, cross-sensitivity with other phenothiazines may exist; avoid use in patients with narrow-angle glaucoma, bone marrow suppression, severe liver or cardiac disease, severe CNS depression, coma

**Warnings/Precautions** Watch for hypotension when administering I.M.; safety in children <6 months of age has not been established; use with caution in patients with cardiovascular disease or seizures; benefits of therapy must be weighed against risks of therapy; should not be given I.V.

**Pregnancy Risk Factor** C

(Continued)

## Loxapine *(Continued)*

### Adverse Reactions

>10%:

Cardiovascular: Orthostatic hypotension

Central nervous system: Drowsiness, extrapyramidal effects (parkinsonian), confusion, persistent tardive dyskinesia

Gastrointestinal: Xerostomia

Ocular: Blurred vision

1% to 10%:

Dermatologic: Rash

Endocrine & metabolic: Enlargement of breasts

Gastrointestinal: Constipation, nausea, vomiting

<1%: Tachycardia, arrhythmias, abnormal T-waves with prolonged ventricular repolarization, neuroleptic malignant syndrome (NMS), sedation, restlessness, anxiety, seizures, altered central temperature regulation, hyperpigmentation, pruritus, photosensitivity, galactorrhea, amenorrhea, gynecomastia, weight gain, adynamic ileus, urinary retention, overflow incontinence, priapism, sexual dysfunction, agranulocytosis (more often in women between fourth and tenth week of therapy), leukopenia (usually in patients with large doses for prolonged periods), cholestatic jaundice, retinal pigmentation

### Drug Interactions

Decreased effect of guanethidine, phenytoin

Increased toxicity with CNS depressants, metrizamide (increased seizure potential), guanabenz, MAO inhibitors

**Onset** Onset of neuroleptic effect: Oral: Within 20-30 minutes; Peak effect: 1.5-3 hours

**Duration** ~12 hours

**Half-Life** Half-life, biphasic: Initial: 5 hours; Terminal: 12-19 hours

### Special PA Issues

**Patient Education:** Use exactly as directed (do not increase dose or frequency); may cause physical and/or psychological dependence. It may take 2-3 weeks to achieve desired results; do not discontinue without consulting prescriber. Dilute oral concentration with water or juice. Do not take within 2 hours of any antacid. Avoid excess alcohol or caffeine and other prescription and other OTC medications not approved by prescriber. Maintain adequate hydration (2-3 L/day of fluids unless instructed to restrict fluid intake). You may experience excess drowsiness, restlessness, dizziness, or blurred vision (use caution driving or when engaging in hazardous tasks until response to medication is known); nausea, vomiting (small frequent meals, frequent mouth care, or sucking lozenges may help); constipation (increased exercise, fluids, or dietary fruit and fiber may help); postural hypotension (use caution climbing stairs or when changing position from lying or sitting to standing); urinary retention (void before taking medication); or decreased perspiration (avoid strenuous exercise in hot environments). Report persistent CNS effects (eg, trembling fingers, altered gait or balance, excessive sedation, seizures, unusual movements, anxiety, abnormal thoughts, confusion, personality changes); chest pain, palpitations, rapid heartbeat, severe dizziness; unresolved urinary retention or changes in urinary pattern; vision changes; skin rash or yellowing of skin; difficulty breathing; or worsening of condition.

**Dietary Considerations:** Alcohol: Additive CNS effect, avoid use

### Related Information

Antipsychotic Agents *on page 1001*

# Lyme Disease Vaccine (LIME dee seas vak SEEN)

**Pharmacologic Class** Vaccine

**U.S. Brand Names** LYMErix®

**Mechanism of Action** Lyme disease vaccine is a recombinant, noninfectious lipoprotein (OspA) derived from the outer surface of *Borrelia burgdorfi*, the causative agent of Lyme disease. Vaccination stimulates production of antibodies directed against this organism, including antibodies against the LA-2 epitope, which have bactericidal activity. Since OspA expression is down-regulated after inoculation into the human host, at least part of the vaccine's efficacy may be related to neutralization of bacteria within the midgut of the tick vector, preventing transmission to the human host.

**Use** Active immunization against Lyme disease in individuals between 15-70 years of age. Individuals most at risk are those who live, work, or travel to *B. burgdorfi*-infected, tick-infested, grassy/wooded areas.

**USUAL DOSAGE** Adults: I.M.: Vaccination with 3 doses of 30 mcg (0.5 mL), administered at 0, 1, and 12 months, is recommended for optimal protection

**Dosage Forms Inj:** Vial: 30 mcg/0.5 mL; Prefilled syringe (Tip-Lok™): 30 mcg/0.5 mL

**Contraindications** Known hypersensitivity to any component of the vaccine. Vaccination should be postponed during acute moderate to severe febrile illness (minor illness is generally not a contraindication). Safety and efficacy in patients <15 years of age have not been established.

**Warnings/Precautions** Do not administer to patients with treatment-resistant Lyme arthritis. Will not prevent disease in patients with prior infection and offers no protection against other tick-borne diseases. Immunosuppressed patients or those receiving immuno-suppressive therapy (vaccine may not be effective) - defer vaccination until 3 months after therapy. Avoid in patients receiving anticoagulant therapy (due to intramuscular injection). The physician should take all known precautions for prevention of allergic or other reactions. Administer with caution to patients with known or suspected latex allergy (applies only to the LMErix Tip-Lok™ syringe, vaccine vial does not contain natural rubber). Duration of immunity has not been established.

**Pregnancy Risk Factor** C

**Pregnancy Implications** It is not known whether Lyme disease vaccine is excreted in human milk. Because many drugs are excreted in milk, caution should be exercised when the vaccine is given to nursing mothers. Healthcare professionals are encouraged to register pregnant women who receive the vaccine with the SKB vaccination pregnancy registry (1-800-8900, ext 5231).

**Adverse Reactions** (Limited to overall self-reported events occurring within 30 days following a dose)

>10%: Local: Injection site pain (21.9%)

1% to 10%:

Central nervous system: Headache (5.6%), fatigue (3.9%), fever (2.6%), chills (2%), dizziness (1%)

Dermatologic: Rash (1.4%)

Gastrointestinal: Nausea (1.1%)

Neuromuscular & skeletal: Arthralgia (6.8%), myalgia (4.8%), muscle aches (2.8%), back pain (1.9%), stiffness (1%)

Respiratory: Upper respiratory tract infection (4.4%), sinusitis (3.2%), pharyngitis (2.5%), rhinitis (2.4%), cough (1.5%), bronchitis (1.1%)

Miscellaneous: Viral infection (2.8%), flu-like syndrome (2.5%)

Solicited adverse event rates were higher than unsolicited event rates (above). These included local reactions of soreness (93.5%), redness (41.8%), and swelling (29.9%). In addition, general systemic symptoms included fatigue (40.8%), headache (38.6%), arthralgia (25.6%), rash (11.7%), and fever (3.5%)

Patients with a history of Lyme disease were noted to experience a higher frequency of early musculoskeletal reactions. Other differences in the observed rate of adverse reactions were not significantly different between vaccine and placebo recipients.

**Drug Interactions** No data available

**Special PA Issues**

**Patient Education:** You will require two more injections over the next 12 months; schedule appointments for those injections as directed by prescriber. You may experience headache, mild nausea, chills, fever, or dizziness following injection. These should

(Continued)

## Lyme Disease Vaccine *(Continued)*

subside, if not contact prescriber. Report persistent redness, swelling, or pain at injection site; skin rash; persistent flu-like symptoms; or muscle aches of stiffness.

♦ **Lyme Disease Vaccine (Recombinant OspA)** *see Lyme Disease Vaccine on previous page*

♦ **LYMErix®** *see Lyme Disease Vaccine on previous page*

## Lymphocyte Immune Globulin (LIM foe site i MYUN GLOB yoo lin)

**Pharmacologic Class** Immunosuppressant Agent

**U.S. Brand Names** Atgam®

**Mechanism of Action** May involve elimination of antigen-reactive T-lymphocytes (killer cells) in peripheral blood or alteration of T-cell function

**Use** Prevention and treatment of acute renal and other solid organ allograft rejection; treatment of moderate to severe aplastic anemia in patients not considered suitable candidates for bone marrow transplantation; prevention of graft-versus-host disease following bone marrow transplantation

**USUAL DOSAGE** An intradermal skin test is recommended prior to administration of the initial dose of ATG; use 0.1 mL of a 1:1000 dilution of ATG in normal saline. A positive skin reaction consists of a wheal ≥10 mm in diameter. If a positive skin test occurs, the first infusion should be administered in a controlled environment with intensive life support immediately available. A systemic reaction precludes further administration of the drug. The absence of a reaction does not preclude the possibility of an immediate sensitivity reaction.

First dose: Premedicate with diphenhydramine 50 mg orally 30 minutes prior to and hydrocortisone 100 mg I.V. 15 minutes prior to infusion and acetaminophen 650 mg 2 hours after start of infusion

Children: I.V.:

Aplastic anemia protocol: 10-20 mg/kg/day for 8-14 days; then administer every other day for 7 more doses; addition doses may be given every other day for 21 total doses in 28 days

Renal allograft: 5-25 mg/kg/day

Adults: I.V.:

Aplastic anemia protocol: 10-20 mg/kg/day for 8-14 days, then administer every other day for 7 more doses

Renal allograft:

Rejection prophylaxis: 15 mg/kg/day for 14 days followed by 14 days of alternative day therapy at the same dose; the first dose should be administered within 24 hours before or after transplantation

Rejection treatment: 10-15 mg/kg/day for 14 days, then administer every other day for 10-14 days up to 21 doses in 28 days

**Dosage Forms Inj:** 50 mg/mL (5 mL)

**Contraindications** Known hypersensitivity to ATG, thimerosal, or other equine gamma globulins; severe, unremitting leukopenia and/or thrombocytopenia

**Warnings/Precautions** Must be administered via central line due to chemical phlebitis; should only be used by physicians experienced in immunosuppressive therapy or management of solid organ or bone marrow transplant patients; adequate laboratory and supportive medical resources must be readily available in the facility for patient management; rash, dyspnea, hypotension, or anaphylaxis precludes further administration of the drug. Dose must be administered over at least 4 hours; patient may need to be pretreated with an antipyretic, antihistamine, and/or corticosteroid. Intradermal skin testing is recommended prior to first-dose administration.

**Pregnancy Risk Factor** C

**Adverse Reactions**

>10%:

Central nervous system: Fever, chills

Dermatologic: Rash

Hematologic: Leukopenia, thrombocytopenia

Miscellaneous: Systemic infection

1% to 10%:

Cardiovascular: Hypotension, hypertension, tachycardia, edema, chest pain

Central nervous system: Headache, malaise, pain

Gastrointestinal: Diarrhea, nausea, stomatitis, GI bleeding

Respiratory: Dyspnea

Local: Edema or redness at injection site, thrombophlebitis

Neuromuscular & skeletal: Myalgia, back pain, arthralgia

Renal: Abnormal renal function tests

Miscellaneous: Sensitivity reactions: Anaphylaxis may be indicated by hypotension, respiratory distress; serum sickness, viral infection

<1%: Seizures, pruritus, urticaria, hemolysis, anemia, arthralgia, weakness, acute renal failure, lymphadenopathy

**Half-Life** Plasma: 1.5-12 days

**Special PA Issues**

**Patient Education:** This medication can only be administered by infusion. You will be monitored closely during the infusion. Do not get up alone; ask for assistance if you must get up or change position. Do not have any vaccinations for the next 3 months without consulting prescriber. Immediately report chills; persistent dizziness or nausea; itching or stinging; acute back pain; chest pain or tightness or rapid heartbeat; or difficulty breathing.

**Monitoring Parameters:** Lymphocyte profile, CBC with differential and platelet count, vital signs during administration

♦ **Lyphocin®** *see* Vancomycin *on page 954*

# Lypressin (lye PRES in)

**Pharmacologic Class** Antidiuretic Hormone Analog

**U.S. Brand Names** Diapid® Nasal Spray

**Mechanism of Action** Increases cyclic adenosine monophosphate (cAMP) which increases water permeability at the renal tubule resulting in decreased urine volume and increased osmolality; causes peristalsis by directly stimulating the smooth muscle in the GI tract

**Use** Controls or prevents signs and complications of neurogenic diabetes insipidus

**USUAL DOSAGE** Children and Adults: Instill 1-2 sprays into one or both nostrils whenever frequency of urination increases or significant thirst develops; usual dosage is 1-2 sprays 4 times/day; range: 1 spray/day at bedtime to 10 sprays each nostril every 3-4 hours

**Dosage Forms Spr:** 0.185 mg/mL (equivalent to 50 USP posterior pituitary units/mL) (8 mL)

**Contraindications** Known hypersensitivity to lypressin

**Warnings/Precautions** Use with caution in patients with coronary artery disease

**Pregnancy Risk Factor** C

**Adverse Reactions**

1% to 10%:

Cardiovascular: Chest tightness

Central nervous system: Dizziness, headache

Endocrine & metabolic: Water intoxication

Gastrointestinal: Abdominal cramping, increased bowel movements

Local: Irritation or burning

Respiratory: Coughing, dyspnea, rhinorrhea, nasal congestion

<1%: Inadvertent inhalation

**Drug Interactions** Increased effect: Chlorpropamide, clofibrate, carbamazepine → prolongation of antidiuretic effects

**Onset** Onset of antidiuretic effect: Intranasal spray: Within 0.5-2 hours

**Duration** 3-8 hours

**Half-Life** 15-20 minutes

**Special PA Issues**

**Patient Education:** To control nocturia, an additional dose may be given at bedtime. Notify prescriber if drowsiness, fatigue, headache, shortness of breath, abdominal cramps, or severe nasal irritation occurs.

♦ **Lysatec-rt-PA®** *see* Alteplase *on page 46*

♦ **Macrobid®** *see* Nitrofurantoin *on page 659*

♦ **Macrodantin®** *see* Nitrofurantoin *on page 659*

# Mafenide (MA fe nide)

**Pharmacologic Class** Antibacterial, Topical; Antibiotic, Topical

**U.S. Brand Names** Sulfamylon® Topical

**Mechanism of Action** Interferes with bacterial folic acid synthesis through competitive inhibition of para-aminobenzoic acid

**Use** Adjunct in the treatment of second and third degree burns to prevent septicemia caused by susceptible organisms such as *Pseudomonas aeruginosa*; prevention of graft loss of meshed autografts on excised burn wounds

**USUAL DOSAGE** Children and Adults: Topical: Apply once or twice daily with a sterile gloved hand; apply to a thickness of approximately 16 mm; the burned area should be covered with cream at all times

**Dosage Forms Crm, top, as acetate:** 85 mg/g (56.7 g, 113.4 g, 411 g); **Powder for top soln:** 5% (50 g)

**Contraindications** Hypersensitivity to mafenide, sulfites, or any component

**Warnings/Precautions** Use with caution in patients with renal impairment and in patients with G-6-PD deficiency; prolonged use may result in superinfection

**Pregnancy Risk Factor** C

**Adverse Reactions**

>10%:

Central nervous system: Pain

Local: Burning sensation, excoriation

(Continued)

## Mafenide *(Continued)*

1% to 10%:
Cardiovascular: Facial edema
Dermatologic: Rash
Miscellaneous: Dyspnea
<1%: Erythema, hyperchloremia, metabolic acidosis, bone marrow suppression, hemolytic anemia, bleeding, porphyria, hyperventilation, tachypnea, hypersensitivity

### Special PA Issues

**Patient Education:** For external use only. Apply exactly as directed with sterile gloved hand so that burned areas are covered with cream at all times. Avoid getting in eyes. Report facial swelling, skin rash, unusual bleeding, difficulty breathing, or signs of infections.

**Monitoring Parameters:** Acid base balance

♦ **Mafenide Acetate** *see* Mafenide *on previous page*
♦ **Magnesia Magma** *see* Magnesium Hydroxide *on this page*
♦ **Magnesium Chloride** *see* Magnesium Salts (Other) *on page 554*

## Magnesium Citrate (mag NEE zhum SIT rate)

**Pharmacologic Class** Laxative, Saline
**U.S. Brand Names** Evac-Q-Mag® [OTC]
**Mechanism of Action** Promotes bowel evacuation by causing osmotic retention of fluid which distends the colon with increased peristaltic activity
**Use** Evacuation of bowel prior to certain surgical and diagnostic procedures or overdose situations
**USUAL DOSAGE** Cathartic Oral:

Children:
<6 years: 0.5 mL/kg up to a maximum of 200 mL repeated every 4-6 hours until stools are clear
6-12 years: 100-150 mL
Adults ≥12 years: ½ to 1 full bottle (120-300 mL)

**Dosage Forms Soln, oral:** 300 mL
**Contraindications** Renal failure, appendicitis, abdominal pain, intestinal impaction, obstruction or perforation, diabetes mellitus, complications in gastrointestinal tract, patients with colostomy, ileostomy, ulcerative colitis or diverticulitis
**Warnings/Precautions** Use with caution in patients with impaired renal function, especially if $Cl_{cr}$ <30 mL/minute (accumulation of magnesium which may lead to magnesium intoxication); use with caution in digitalized patients (may alter cardiac conduction leading to heart block); use with caution in patients with lithium administration; use with caution with neuromuscular blocking agents, CNS depressants

**Pregnancy Risk Factor** B
**Adverse Reactions** 1% to 10%:
Cardiovascular: Hypotension
Endocrine & metabolic: Hypermagnesemia
Gastrointestinal: Abdominal cramps, diarrhea, gas formation
Respiratory: Respiratory depression

### Special PA Issues

**Patient Education:** Take with a glass of water, fruit juice, or citrus flavored carbonated beverage to improve taste, chill before using; report severe abdominal pain to physician
**Reference Range:** Serum magnesium: Children: 1.5-1.9 mg/dL ~1.2-1.6 mEq/L; Adults: 2.2-2.8 mg/dL ~1.8-2.3 mEq/L

♦ **Magnesium Gluconate** *see* Magnesium Salts (Other) *on page 554*

## Magnesium Hydroxide (mag NEE zhum hye DROKS ide)

**Pharmacologic Class** Antacid; Laxative, Saline; Magnesium Salt
**U.S. Brand Names** Phillips'® Milk of Magnesia [OTC]
**Mechanism of Action** Promotes bowel evacuation by causing osmotic retention of fluid which distends the colon with increased peristaltic activity; reacts with hydrochloric acid in stomach to form magnesium chloride
**Use** Short-term treatment of occasional constipation and symptoms of hyperacidity, magnesium replacement therapy
**USUAL DOSAGE** Oral:

Average daily intakes of dietary magnesium have declined in recent years due to processing of food; the latest estimate of the average American dietary intake was 349 mg/day

Laxative:
<2 years: 0.5 mL/kg/dose
2-5 years: 5-15 mL/day or in divided doses
6-12 years: 15-30 mL/day or in divided doses
≥12 years: 30-60 mL/day or in divided doses

Antacid:

Children: 2.5-5 mL as needed up to 4 times/day

Adults: 5-15 mL up to 4 times/day as needed

**Dosing in renal impairment:** Patients in severe renal failure should not receive magnesium due to toxicity from accumulation. Patients with a $Cl_{cr}$ <25 mL/minute receiving magnesium should be monitored by serum magnesium levels.

**Dosage Forms Liq:** 390 mg/5 mL (10 mL, 15 mL, 20 mL, 30 mL, 100 mL, 120 mL, 180 mL, 360 mL, 720 mL); **Liq, conc:** 10 mL equivalent to 30 mL milk of magnesia USP (3 times as potent as regular strength product); **Susp, oral:** 2.5 g/30 mL (10 mL, 15 mL, 30 mL); **Tab:** 300 mg, 600 mg

**Contraindications** Patients with colostomy or an ileostomy, intestinal obstruction, fecal impaction, renal failure, appendicitis, hypersensitivity to any component

**Warnings/Precautions** Use with caution in patients with severe renal impairment, (especially when doses are >50 mEq magnesium/day); hypermagnesemia and toxicity may occur due to decreased renal clearance of absorbed magnesium. Decreased renal function ($Cl_{cr}$ <30 mL/minute) may result in toxicity; monitor for toxicity.

**Pregnancy Risk Factor** B

**Adverse Reactions**

>10%: Gastrointestinal: Diarrhea

1% to 10%:

Cardiovascular: Hypotension

Endocrine & metabolic: Hypermagnesemia

Gastrointestinal: Abdominal cramps

Neuromuscular & skeletal: Muscle weakness

Respiratory: Respiratory depression

**Drug Interactions** Decreased effect: Decreased absorption of tetracyclines, digoxin, indomethacin, or iron salts

**Onset** Onset of laxative action: 4-8 hours

**Special PA Issues**

**Patient Education:** Take as directed, with water or juice. Shake liquid well before using. Take 1 hour prior to or after other medications. You may experience excessive diarrhea, gastric cramping, dizziness (use fall precautions). Report rectal bleeding, tarry stools, unresolved abdominal cramps, or unrelieved constipation.

**Reference Range:** Serum magnesium: Children: 1.5-1.9 mg/dL (1.2-1.6 mEq/L); Adults: 1.5-2.5 mg/dL (1.2-2.0 mEq/L)

# Magnesium Oxide (mag NEE zhum OKS ide)

**Pharmacologic Class** Antacid; Electrolyte Supplement, Oral; Laxative, Saline; Magnesium Salt

**U.S. Brand Names** Maox®

**Mechanism of Action** Promotes bowel evacuation by causing osmotic retention of fluid which distends the colon with increased peristaltic activity

**Use** Short-term treatment of occasional constipation and symptoms of hyperacidity

**USUAL DOSAGE** Adults: Oral:

Dietary supplement: 20-40 mEq (1-2 tablets) 2-3 times

Antacid: 140 mg 3-4 times/day **or** 400-840 mg/day

Laxative: 2-4 g at bedtime with full glass of water

**Dosing in renal impairment:** Patients in severe renal failure should not receive magnesium due to toxicity from accumulation. Patients with a $Cl_{cr}$ <25 mL/minute should be monitored by serum magnesium levels.

**Note:** Oral magnesium is not generally adequate for repletion in patients with serum magnesium concentrations <1.5 mEq/L

**Dosage Forms Cap:** 140 mg; **Tab:** 400 mg, 425 mg

**Contraindications** Patients with colostomy or an ileostomy, appendicitis, ulcerative colitis, diverticulitis, heart block, myocardial damage, serious renal impairment, hepatitis, Addison's disease, hypersensitivity to any component

**Warnings/Precautions** Hypermagnesemia and toxicity may occur due to decreased renal clearance ($Cl_{cr}$ <30 mL/minute) of absorbed magnesium; monitor serum magnesium level, respiratory rate, deep tendon reflex, renal function when $MgSO_4$ is administered parenterally; use with caution in digitalized patients (may alter cardiac conduction leading heart block); use with caution in patients with lithium administration; elderly, due to disease or drug therapy, may be predisposed to diarrhea; diarrhea may result in electrolyte imbalance; monitor for toxicity

**Pregnancy Risk Factor** B

**Adverse Reactions**

>10%: Gastrointestinal: Diarrhea

1% to 10%:

Cardiovascular: Hypotension, EKG changes

Central nervous system: Mental depression, coma

Gastrointestinal: Nausea, vomiting

Respiratory: Respiratory depression

(Continued)

## Magnesium Oxide *(Continued)*

**Drug Interactions** Decreased effect: Tetracyclines, digoxin, indomethacin, iron salts, isoni-azid, quinolones

**Onset** Onset of laxative action: 4-8 hours

**Special PA Issues**

**Patient Education:** Use as a laxative should be short-term. Electrolyte imbalance can occur with long-term therapy. Chew tablets before swallowing. Take with full glass of water after meals. Notify prescriber if relief not obtained or if any signs of bleeding occur (eg, black tarry stools, "coffee ground" vomit).

**Reference Range:** Serum magnesium: Children: 1.5-1.9 mg/dL (1.2-1.6 mEq/L); Adults: 1.5-2.5 mg/dL (1.2-2.0 mEq/L)

## Magnesium Salts (Other) (mag NEE zhum GLOO koe nate)

**Pharmacologic Class** Magnesium Salt

**U.S. Brand Names** Almora® (Gluconate); Magonate® (Gluconate) [OTC]; Magtrate® (Gluconate); Slow-Mag® (Chloride)

**Mechanism of Action** Magnesium is important as a cofactor in many enzymatic reactions in the body involving protein synthesis and carbohydrate metabolism, (at least 300 enzymatic reactions require magnesium). Actions on lipoprotein lipase have been found to be important in reducing serum cholesterol and on sodium/potassium ATPase in promoting polarization (ie, neuromuscular functioning).

**Use** Dietary supplement for treatment of magnesium deficiencies

**USUAL DOSAGE** Oral:

Average daily intakes of dietary magnesium have declined in recent years due to processing of food; the latest estimate of the average American dietary intake was 349 mg/day

Adequate intakes:

Infants:

0-6 months: 30 mg

7-12 months: 75 mg

Recommended dietary allowance:

Children:

1-3 years: 80 mg/day

4-8 years: 130 mg/day

Male:

9-13 years: 240 mg/day

14-18 years: 130 mg/day

19-30 years: 400 mg/day

≥31 years: 420 mg/day

Female:

9-13 years: 240 mg/day

14-18 years: 360 mg/day

19-30 years: 310 mg/day

≥31 years: 320 mg/day

Female: Pregnancy:

≤18 years: 400 mg/day

19-30 years: 350 mg/day

31-50 years: 360 mg/day

Female: Lactation:

≤18 years: 360 mg/day

19-30 years: 310 mg/day

31-50 years: 320 mg/day

Hypomagnesemia: There are no specific dosage recommendations for this product in replacement of magnesium. Extrapolation from dosage recommendations of magnesium sulfate are as follows:

Children: 10-20 mg/kg/dose **elemental** magnesium 4 times/day

Adults: 300 mg **elemental** magnesium 4 times/day

The recommended dietary allowance (RDA) of magnesium is 4.5 mg/kg which is a total daily allowance of 350-400 mg for adult men and 280-300 mg for adult women. During pregnancy the RDA is 300 mg and during lactation the RDA is 355 mg.

Dietary supplement: Oral:

Children: 3-6 mg/kg/day in divided doses 3-4 times/day; maximum: 400 mg/day

Adults: 54-483 mg/day in divided doses; refer to product labeling

**Dosing in renal impairment:** Patients in severe renal failure should not receive magnesium due to toxicity from accumulation. Patients with a $Cl_{cr}$ <25 mL/minute receiving magnesium should be monitored by serum magnesium levels.

**Dosage Forms Tab:** 500 mg [elemental magnesium 27 mg]

**Contraindications** Patients with heart block, severe renal disease

**Warnings/Precautions** Use with caution in patients with impaired renal function; hypermagnesemia and toxicity may occur due to decreased renal clearance of absorbed magnesium

**Adverse Reactions**

1% to 10%: Gastrointestinal: Diarrhea (excessive dose)

<1%: Hypotension, hypermagnesemia, abdominal cramps, muscle weakness, respiratory depression

**Drug Interactions**

Increased effect of nondepolarizing neuromuscular blockers

Decreased absorption of aminoquinolones, digoxin, nitrofurantoin, penicillamine, and tetracyclines may occur with magnesium salts

**Special PA Issues**

**Reference Range:** Serum magnesium: Children: 1.5-1.9 mg/dL ~1.2-1.6 mEq/L; Adults: 2.2-2.8 mg/dL ~1.8-2.3 mEq/L

# Magnesium Sulfate (mag NEE zhum SUL fate)

**Pharmacologic Class** Antacid; Anticonvulsant, Miscellaneous; Electrolyte Supplement, Parenteral; Laxative, Saline; Magnesium Salt

**Mechanism of Action** Promotes bowel evacuation by causing osmotic retention of fluid which distends the colon with increased peristaltic activity when taken orally; parenterally, decreases acetylcholine in motor nerve terminals and acts on myocardium by slowing rate of S-A node impulse formation and prolonging conduction time

**Use** Treatment and prevention of hypomagnesemia and in seizure prevention in severe preeclampsia or eclampsia, pediatric acute nephritis; also used as short-term treatment of constipation, postmyocardial infarction, and torsade de pointes

**USUAL DOSAGE** The recommended dietary allowance (RDA) of magnesium is 4.5 mg/kg which is a total daily allowance of 350-400 mg for adult men and 280-300 mg for adult women. During pregnancy the RDA is 300 mg and during lactation the RDA is 355 mg. Average daily intakes of dietary magnesium have declined in recent years due to processing of food. The latest estimate of the average American dietary intake was 349 mg/day. Dose represented as $MgSO_4$ unless stated otherwise.

**Note:** Serum magnesium is poor reflection of repletional status as the majority of magnesium is intracellular; serum levels may be transiently normal for a few hours after a dose is given, therefore, aim for consistently high normal serum levels in patients with normal renal function for most efficient repletion

Hypomagnesemia:

Neonates: I.V.: 25-50 mg/kg/dose (0.2-0.4 mEq/kg/dose) every 8-12 hours for 2-3 doses

Children: I.M., I.V.: 25-50 mg/kg/dose (0.2-0.4 mEq/kg/dose) every 4-6 hours for 3-4 doses, maximum single dose: 2000 mg (16 mEq), may repeat if hypomagnesemia persists (higher dosage up to 100 mg/kg/dose $MgSO_4$ I.V. has been used); maintenance: I.V.: 30-60 mg/kg/day (0.25-0.5 mEq/kg/day)

Adults:

Oral: 3 g every 6 hours for 4 doses as needed

I.M., I.V.: 1 g every 6 hours for 4 doses; for severe hypomagnesemia: 8-12 g $MgSO_4$/day in divided doses has been used

Management of seizures and hypertension: Children: I.M., I.V.: 20-100 mg/kg/dose every 4-6 hours as needed; in severe cases doses as high as 200 mg/kg/dose have been used

Eclampsia, pre-eclampsia: Adults:

I.M.: 1-4 g every 4 hours

I.V.: Initial: 4 g, then switch to I.M. or 1-4 g/hour by continuous infusion

Maximum dose should not exceed 30-40 g/day; maximum rate of infusion: 1-2 g/hour

Maintenance electrolyte requirements:

Daily requirements: 0.2-0.5 mEq/kg/24 hours or 3-10 mEq/1000 kcal/24 hours

Maximum: 8-16 mEq/24 hours

Cathartic: Oral:

Children: 0.25 g/kg every 4-6 hours

Adults: 10-15 g in a glass of water

**Dosing adjustment/comments in renal impairment:** $Cl_{cr}$ <25 mL/minute: Do not administer or monitor serum magnesium levels carefully

**Dosage Forms Granules:** ~40 mEq magnesium/5 g (240 g); **Inj:** 100 mg/mL (20 mL), 125 mg/mL (8 mL), 250 mg/mL (150 mL), 500 mg/mL (2 mL, 5 mL, 10 mL, 30 mL, 50 mL); **Soln, oral:** 50% [500 mg/mL] (30 mL)

**Contraindications** Heart block, serious renal impairment, myocardial damage, hepatitis, Addison's disease

**Warnings/Precautions** Use with caution in patients with impaired renal function (accumulation of magnesium which may lead to magnesium intoxication); use with caution in digitalized patients (may alter cardiac conduction leading to heart block); monitor serum magnesium level, respiratory rate, deep tendon reflex, renal function when $MgSO_4$ is administered parenterally

**Pregnancy Risk Factor** B

(Continued)

## Magnesium Sulfate *(Continued)*

**Adverse Reactions** 1% to 10%:
Serum magnesium levels >3 mg/dL:
 Central nervous system: Depressed CNS
 Gastrointestinal: Diarrhea
 Neuromuscular & skeletal: Blocked peripheral neuromuscular transmission leading to anticonvulsant effects
Serum magnesium levels >5 mg/dL:
 Cardiovascular: Flushing
 Central nervous system: Somnolence
Serum magnesium levels >12.5 mg/dL:
 Cardiovascular: Complete heart block
 Respiratory: Respiratory paralysis

**Drug Interactions**
Decreased effect: Nifedipine decreased blood pressure and neuromuscular blockade
Increased toxicity: Aminoglycosides increased neuromuscular blockade; CNS depressants increased CNS depression; neuromuscular antagonists, betamethasone (pulmonary edema), ritodrine increased cardiotoxicity

**Onset** Oral: Onset of cathartic action: Within 1-2 hours; I.M.: 1 hour; I.V.: Immediate

**Duration** I.M.: 3-4 hours; I.V.: 30 minutes

**Special PA Issues**
**Patient Education:** Oral: Take as directed, with adequate fluids, for short-term only. Do not take if abdominal cramping, vomiting, or diarrhea is present. Report unusual sweating or flushed skin, muscle twitching, weakness or inability to move extremities.

**Monitoring Parameters** Monitor blood pressure when administering $MgSO_4$ I.V.; serum magnesium levels should be monitored to avoid overdose; monitor for diarrhea; monitor for arrhythmias, hypotension, respiratory and CNS depression during rapid I.V. administration

**Reference Range:** Serum magnesium: Children: 1.5-1.9 mg/dL (1.2-1.6 mEq/L); Adults: 1.5-2.5 mg/dL (1.2-2.0 mEq/L)

**Note:** Serum magnesium is poor reflection of repletional status as the majority of magnesium is intracellular; serum levels may be transiently normal for a few hours after a dose is given, therefore, aim for consistently high normal serum levels in patients with normal renal function for most efficient repletion

- **Magonate® (Gluconate) [OTC]** *see* Magnesium Salts (Other) *on page 554*
- **Magtrate® (Gluconate)** *see* Magnesium Salts (Other) *on page 554*
- **Maindenhair Tree** *see* Ginkgo Biloba *on page 414*
- **Malatal®** *see* Hyoscyamine, Atropine, Scopolamine, and Phenobarbital *on page 464*

## Malathion *(mal a THYE on)*

**Pharmacologic Class** Pediculocide

**U.S. Brand Names** Ovide™

**Use** Treatment of head lice and their ova

**USUAL DOSAGE** Sprinkle Ovide™ lotion on dry hair and rub gently until the scalp is thoroughly moistened; pay special attention to the back of the head and neck. Allow to dry naturally - use no heat and leave uncovered. After 8-12 hours, the hair should be washed with a nonmedicated shampoo; rinse and use a fine-toothed comb to remove dead lice and eggs. If required, repeat with second application in 7-9 days. Further treatment is generally not necessary. Other family members should be evaluated to determine if infested and if so, receive treatment.

**Dosage Forms** Lot: 0.5% (59 mL)

**Contraindications** Known hypersensitivity to malathion

**Pregnancy Risk Factor** B

**Special PA Issues**
**Patient Education:** Topical use only

- **Mallamint® [OTC]** *see* Calcium Carbonate *on page 139*
- **Mallisol® [OTC]** *see* Povidone-Iodine *on page 747*
- **Malotuss® [OTC]** *see* Guaifenesin *on page 427*
- **Mandelamine®** *see* Methenamine *on page 582*
- **Mandol®** *see* Cefamandole *on page 160*
- **Mandrake** *see* Podophyllum Resin *on page 735*

## Manganese *(MAN ga nees)*

**Pharmacologic Class** Trace Element; Trace Element, Parenteral

**U.S. Brand Names** Chelated Manganese® [OTC]

**Mechanism of Action** Cofactor in many enzyme systems, stimulates synthesis of cholesterol and fatty acids in liver, and influences mucopolysaccharide synthesis

**Use** Trace element added to TPN (total parenteral nutrition) solution to prevent manganese deficiency; orally as a dietary supplement

**USUAL DOSAGE**

Infants: I.V.: 2-10 mcg/kg/day usually administered in TPN solutions

Adults:

Oral: 20-50 mg/day

RDA: 2-5 mg/day

I.V.: 150-800 mcg/day usually administered in TPN solutions

**Dosage Forms Inj, as chloride:** 0.1 mg/mL (10 mL); **Inj, as sulfate:** 0.1 mg/mL (10 mL, 30 mL); **Tab:** 20 mg, 50 mg

**Contraindications** High manganese levels; patients with severe liver dysfunction or cholestasis (conjugated bilirubin >2 mg/dL) due to reduced biliary excretion

**Pregnancy Risk Factor** C

**Special PA Issues**

**Monitoring Parameters:** Periodic manganese plasma level

**Reference Range:** 4-14 µg/L

- **Manganese Chloride** *see* Manganese *on previous page*
- **Manganese Sulfate** *see* Manganese *on previous page*

# Mannitol (MAN i tole)

**Pharmacologic Class** Diuretic, Osmotic

**U.S. Brand Names** Osmitrol® Injection; Resectisol® Irrigation Solution

**Mechanism of Action** Increases the osmotic pressure of glomerular filtrate, which inhibits tubular reabsorption of water and electrolytes and increases urinary output

**Use** Reduction of increased intracranial pressure associated with cerebral edema; promotion of diuresis in the prevention and/or treatment of oliguria or anuria due to acute renal failure; reduction of increased intraocular pressure; promoting urinary excretion of toxic substances; genitourinary irrigant in transurethral prostatic resection or other transurethral surgical procedures

**USUAL DOSAGE** I.V.:

Children:

Test dose (to assess adequate renal function): 200 mg/kg over 3-5 minutes to produce a urine flow of at least 1 mL/kg for 1-3 hours

Initial: 0.5-1 g/kg

Maintenance: 0.25-0.5 g/kg given every 4-6 hours

Adults:

Test dose (to assess adequate renal function): 12.5 g (200 mg/kg) over 3-5 minutes to produce a urine flow of at least 30-50 mL of urine per hour over the next 2-3 hours

Initial: 0.5-1 g/kg

Maintenance: 0.25-0.5 g/kg every 4-6 hours; usual adult dose: 20-200 g/24 hours

Intracranial pressure: Cerebral edema: 1.5-2 g/kg/dose I.V. as a 15% to 20% solution over ≥30 minutes; maintain serum osmolality 310-320 mOsm/kg

Preoperative for neurosurgery: 1.5-2 g/kg administered 1-1.5 hours prior to surgery

Transurethral irrigation: Use urogenital solution as required for irrigation

**Dosage Forms Inj:** 5% [50 mg/mL] (1000 mL), 10% [100 mg/mL] (500 mL, 1000 mL), 15% [150 mg/mL] (150 mL, 500 mL), 20% [200 mg/mL] (150 mL, 250 mL, 500 mL); 25% [250 mg/mL] (50 mL); **Soln, urogenital:** 0.54% [5.4 mg/mL] (2000 mL)

**Contraindications** Severe renal disease (anuria), dehydration, or active intracranial bleeding, severe pulmonary edema or congestion, hypersensitivity to any component

**Warnings/Precautions** Should not be administered until adequacy of renal function and urine flow is established; cardiovascular status should also be evaluated; do not administer electrolyte-free mannitol solutions with blood

**Pregnancy Risk Factor** C

**Adverse Reactions**

>10%:

Central nervous system: Headache

Gastrointestinal: Nausea, vomiting

Genitourinary: Polyuria

1% to 10%:

Central nervous system: Dizziness

Dermatologic: Rash

Ocular: Blurred vision

<1%: Circulatory overload, congestive heart failure, convulsions, headache, chills, fluid and electrolyte imbalance, water intoxication, dehydration and hypovolemia secondary to rapid diuresis, xerostomia, dysuria, tissue necrosis, pulmonary edema, allergic reactions

**Onset** Onset of diuresis: Injection: Within 1-3 hours; Onset of reduction in intracerebral pressure: Within 15 minutes

**Duration** Duration of reduction in intracerebral pressure: 3-6 hours

**Half-Life** 1.1-1.6 hours

(Continued)

## Mannitol *(Continued)*

### Special PA Issues

**Patient Education:** This medication can only be given by infusion. Report immediately any muscle weakness, numbness, tingling, acute headache, nausea, dizziness, blurred vision, eye pain, difficulty breathing, chest pain, or pain at infusion site.

**Monitoring Parameters:** Renal function, daily fluid I & O, serum electrolytes, serum and urine osmolality; for treatment of elevated intracranial pressure, maintain serum osmolality 310-320 mOsm/kg

- **Mantoux** *see* Tuberculin Tests *on page 945*
- **Maox**® *see* Magnesium Oxide *on page 553*
- **Mapap**® **[OTC]** *see* Acetaminophen *on page 21*
- **Maranox**® **[OTC]** *see* Acetaminophen *on page 21*
- **Marax**® *see* Theophylline, Ephedrine, and Hydroxyzine *on page 888*
- **Marazide**® *see* Benzthiazide *on page 107*
- **Marbaxin**® *see* Methocarbamol *on page 585*
- **Marcaine**® *see* Bupivacaine *on page 126*
- **Marcillin**® *see* Ampicillin *on page 64*
- **Margesic**® **H** *see* Hydrocodone and Acetaminophen *on page 449*
- **Marinol**® *see* Dronabinol *on page 307*
- **Marnal**® *see* Butalbital Compound *on page 131*
- **Marpres**® *see* Hydralazine, Hydrochlorothiazide, and Reserpine *on page 447*
- **Marthritic**® *see* Salsalate *on page 820*

## Masoprocol *(ma SOE pro kole)*

**Pharmacologic Class** Topical Skin Product, Acne

**U.S. Brand Names** Actinex® Topical

**Mechanism of Action** Antiproliferative activity against keratinocytes

**Use** Treatment of actinic keratosis

**USUAL DOSAGE** Adults: Topical: Wash and dry area; gently massage into affected area every morning and evening for 28 days

**Dosage Forms Crm:** 10% (30 g)

**Contraindications** Hypersensitivity to masoprocol or any component

**Warnings/Precautions** Occlusive dressings should not be used; for external use only

**Pregnancy Risk Factor** E

### Adverse Reactions

>10%:

Dermatologic: Erythema, flaking, dryness, itching

Local: Burning

1% to 10%:

Dermatologic: Soreness, rash

Neuromuscular & skeletal: Paresthesia

Ocular: Eye irritation

<1%: Blistering, excoriation, skin roughness, wrinkling

### Special PA Issues

**Patient Education:** For external use only. Apply with gloves in thin film to thoroughly clean/dry skin; avoid area around eyes or mouth. Do not cover with occlusive dressing. Results make take some time to appear. May stain clothing or fabrics. You may experience transient stinging or burning after application. Report worsening of condition; eye irritation; or skin redness, dryness, peeling, or burning that persists between applications.

- **Massengill**® **Medicated Douche w/Cepticin [OTC]** *see* Povidone-Iodine *on page 747*
- **Matricaria chamomilla** *see* Chamomile *on page 184*
- **Matricarta recutita** *see* Chamomile *on page 184*
- **Matulane**® *see* Procarbazine *on page 761*
- **Mavik**® *see* Trandolapril *on page 920*
- **Maxair**™ **Autohaler**™ *see* Pirbuterol *on page 732*
- **Maxair**™ **Inhalation Aerosol** *see* Pirbuterol *on page 732*
- **Maxalt**® *see* Rizatriptan *on page 814*
- **Maxalt-MLT**™ *see* Rizatriptan *on page 814*
- **Maxaquin**® *see* Lomefloxacin *on page 538*
- **Maxeran**® *see* Metoclopramide *on page 597*
- **Maxidex**® *see* Dexamethasone *on page 264*
- **Maxiflor**® *see* Diflorasone *on page 278*
- **Maximum Strength Anbesol**® **[OTC]** *see* Benzocaine *on page 105*
- **Maximum Strength Desenex**® **Antifungal Cream [OTC]** *see* Miconazole *on page 604*
- **Maximum Strength Dex-A-Diet**® **[OTC]** *see* Phenylpropanolamine *on page 720*
- **Maximum Strength Dexatrim**® **[OTC]** *see* Phenylpropanolamine *on page 720*

- **Maximum Strength Nytol®** [OTC] *see* Diphenhydramine *on page 289*
- **Maximum Strength Orajel®** [OTC] *see* Benzocaine *on page 105*
- **Maxipime®** *see* Cefepime *on page 162*
- **Maxitrol®** *see* Neomycin, Polymyxin B, and Dexamethasone *on page 644*
- **Maxivate®** *see* Betamethasone *on page 111*
- **Maxolon®** *see* Metoclopramide *on page 597*
- **Maxzide®** *see* Hydrochlorothiazide and Triamterene *on page 449*
- **May Apple** *see* Podophyllum Resin *on page 735*
- **Maybush** *see* Hawthorn *on page 438*
- **Mazepine®** *see* Carbamazepine *on page 148*
- **MCH** *see* Microfibrillar Collagen Hemostat *on page 605*
- **Mebaral®** *see* Mephobarbital *on page 569*

## Mebendazole (me BEN da zole)

**Pharmacologic Class** Anthelmintic

**U.S. Brand Names** Vermox®

**Mechanism of Action** Selectively and irreversibly blocks glucose uptake and other nutrients in susceptible adult intestine-dwelling helminths

**Use** Treatment of pinworms (*Enterobius vermicularis*), whipworms (*Trichuris trichiura*), roundworms (*Ascaris lumbricoides*), and hookworms (*Ancylostoma duodenale*)

**USUAL DOSAGE** Children and Adults: Oral:

Pinworms: 100 mg as a single dose; may need to repeat after 2 weeks; treatment should include family members in close contact with patient

Whipworms, roundworms, hookworms: One tablet twice daily, morning and evening on 3 consecutive days; if patient is not cured within 3-4 weeks, a second course of treatment may be administered

Capillariasis: 200 mg twice daily for 20 days

**Dosing adjustment in hepatic impairment:** Dosage reduction may be necessary in patients with liver dysfunction

Hemodialysis: Not dialyzable (0% to 5%)

**Dosage Forms Tab, chewable:** 100 mg

**Contraindications** Hypersensitivity to mebendazole or any component

**Warnings/Precautions** Pregnancy and children <2 years of age are relative contraindications since safety has not been established; not effective for hydatid disease

**Pregnancy Risk Factor** C

**Adverse Reactions**

1% to 10%: Gastrointestinal: Abdominal pain, diarrhea, nausea, vomiting

<1%: Fever, dizziness, headache, rash, angioedema, seizures, itching, alopecia (with high doses), neutropenia (sore throat, unusual fatigue), unusual weakness

**Drug Interactions** Decreased effect: Anticonvulsants such as carbamazepine and phenytoin may increase metabolism of mebendazole

**Half-Life** 2.8-9 hours

**Special PA Issues**

**Patient Education:** Take exactly as directed for full course of medication. Tablets may be chewed, swallowed whole, or crushed and mixed with food. May need to be repeated in 2-3 weeks. All family members and friends should also be treated. To reduce possibility of reinfection, wash hands and scrub nails carefully with soap and hot water before handling food, before eating, and before and after toileting. Keep hands out of mouth. Do not go barefoot in house or outside and do not sit directly on ground or grass. Disinfect toilet daily and launder bed linens, undergarments, and nightclothes daily with hot water and soap. Report acute nausea, vomiting, or diarrhea; skin rash; signs of infection; or flu-like symptoms.

**Monitoring Parameters:** Check for helminth ova in feces within 3-4 weeks following the initial therapy

- **Meclan® Topical** *see* Meclocycline *on next page*

## Meclizine (MEK li zeen)

**Pharmacologic Class** Antihistamine

**U.S. Brand Names** Antivert®; Antrizine®; Bonine® [OTC]; Dizmiss® [OTC]; Dramamine® II [OTC]; Meni-D®; Nico-Vert® [OTC]; Ru-Vert-M®; Vergon® [OTC]

**Mechanism of Action** Has central anticholinergic action by blocking chemoreceptor trigger zone; decreases excitability of the middle ear labyrinth and blocks conduction in the middle ear vestibular-cerebellar pathways

**Use** Prevention and treatment of symptoms of motion sickness; management of vertigo with diseases affecting the vestibular system

**USUAL DOSAGE** Children >12 years and Adults: Oral:

Motion sickness: 12.5-25 mg 1 hour before travel, repeat dose every 12-24 hours if needed; doses up to 50 mg may be needed

Vertigo: 25-100 mg/day in divided doses

(Continued)

## Meclizine *(Continued)*

**Dosage Forms** Meclizine hydrochloride: **Cap:** 15 mg, 25 mg, 30 mg; **Tab:** 12.5 mg, 25 mg, 50 mg; **Tab:** Chewable: 25 mg, Film coated: 25 mg

**Contraindications** Hypersensitivity to meclizine or any component; pregnancy

**Warnings/Precautions** Use with caution in patients with angle-closure glaucoma, prostatic hypertrophy, pyloric or duodenal obstruction, or bladder neck obstruction; use with caution in hot weather, and during exercise; elderly may be at risk for anticholinergic side effects such as glaucoma, prostatic hypertrophy, constipation, gastrointestinal obstructive disease; if vertigo does not respond in 1-2 weeks, it is advised to discontinue use

### Pregnancy Risk Factor B
### Pregnancy Implications

Clinical effects on the fetus: No data available on crossing the placenta. Probably no effect on the fetus (insufficient data). Available evidence suggests safe use during pregnancy.
Breast-feeding/lactation: No data available

### Adverse Reactions

>10%:
　Central nervous system: Slight to moderate drowsiness
　Respiratory: Thickening of bronchial secretions
1% to 10%:
　Central nervous system: Headache, fatigue, nervousness, dizziness
　Gastrointestinal: Appetite increase, weight gain, nausea, diarrhea, abdominal pain, xerostomia
　Neuromuscular & skeletal: Arthralgia
　Respiratory: Pharyngitis
<1%: Palpitations, hypotension, depression, sedation, photosensitivity, rash, angioedema, urinary retention, hepatitis, myalgia, tremor, paresthesia, blurred vision, bronchospasm, epistaxis

**Drug Interactions** Increased toxicity: CNS depressants, neuroleptics, anticholinergics
**Onset** Oral: Within 1 hour
**Duration** 8-24 hours
**Half-Life** 6 hours

### Special PA Issues

**Patient Education:** Take this drug as prescribed; do not increase dosage. Do not use alcohol, other CNS depressant, or sleeping aids without consulting prescriber. May cause dizziness, drowsiness, or blurred vision; use caution when driving or engaging in hazardous activities until effect of medication is known. Frequent mouth care and sucking on lozenges may reduce dry mouth. Adequate dietary fiber and fluids may reduce constipation. You may develop heat intolerance; avoid excessive heat and maintain adequate fluid intake. Report unusual weight gain, unresolved nausea or diarrhea, palpitations, muscle pain, or changes in urinary pattern.

**Dietary Considerations:** Alcohol: Additive CNS effect, avoid use

♦ **Meclizine Hydrochloride** *see* Meclizine *on previous page*

## Meclocycline *(me kloe SYE kleen)*

**Pharmacologic Class** Antibiotic, Topical; Topical Skin Product, Acne
**U.S. Brand Names** Meclan® Topical

**Mechanism of Action** Inhibits bacterial protein synthesis by binding with the 30S and possibly the 50S ribosomal subunit(s) of susceptible bacteria; may also cause alterations in the cytoplasmic membrane

**Use** Topical treatment of inflammatory acne vulgaris

**USUAL DOSAGE** Children >11 years and Adults: Topical: Apply generously to affected areas twice daily

**Dosage Forms** Crm, top, as sulfosalicylate: 1% (20 g, 45 g)

**Contraindications** Known hypersensitivity to tetracyclines or any component

**Warnings/Precautions** Use with caution in patients allergic to formaldehyde; for external use only

### Pregnancy Risk Factor B
### Adverse Reactions

>10%: Topical: Follicular staining, yellowing of the skin, burning/stinging feeling
1% to 10%: Topical: Pain, redness, skin irritation, dermatitis

### Special PA Issues

**Patient Education:** For external use only. Apply with gloves to thoroughly clean/dry skin until skin is wet; avoid area around eyes or mouth. Do not cover with occlusive dressing. Results make take some time to appear. May stain clothing or fabrics. You may experience transient stinging or burning after application. If skin turns yellow, washing with soap and water will remove color. Report worsening of condition; eye irritation; or skin redness, dryness, peeling, or burning that persists between applications.

♦ **Meclocycline Sulfosalicylate** *see* Meclocycline *on this page*

## Meclofenamate (me kloe fen AM ate)

**Pharmacologic Class** Nonsteroidal Anti-Inflammatory Agent (NSAID)

**U.S. Brand Names** Meclomen®

**Mechanism of Action** Inhibits prostaglandin synthesis by decreasing the activity of the enzyme, cyclo-oxygenase, which results in decreased formation of prostaglandin precursors

**Use** Treatment of inflammatory disorders

**USUAL DOSAGE** Children >14 years and Adults: Oral:
Mild to moderate pain: 50 mg every 4-6 hours, not to exceed 400 mg/day
Rheumatoid arthritis/osteoarthritis: 200-400 mg/day in 3-4 equal doses

**Dosage Forms Cap, as sodium:** 50 mg, 100 mg

**Contraindications** Active GI bleeding, ulcer disease, hypersensitivity to aspirin, meclofenamate, or other NSAIDs

**Warnings/Precautions** May have adverse effects on fetus

**Pregnancy Risk Factor** B (D if used in the 3rd trimester)

**Adverse Reactions**
>10%:
Central nervous system: Dizziness
Dermatologic: Rash
Gastrointestinal: Abdominal cramps, heartburn, indigestion, nausea
1% to 10%:
Central nervous system: Headache, nervousness
Dermatologic: Itching
Endocrine & metabolic: Fluid retention
Gastrointestinal: Vomiting
Otic: Tinnitus
<1%: Congestive heart failure, hypertension, arrhythmia, tachycardia, confusion, hallucinations, aseptic meningitis, mental depression, drowsiness, insomnia, urticaria, erythema multiforme, toxic epidermal necrolysis, Stevens-Johnson syndrome, angioedema, polydipsia, hot flashes, gastritis, GI ulceration, cystitis, polyuria, agranulocytosis, anemia, hemolytic anemia, bone marrow suppression, leukopenia, thrombocytopenia, hepatitis, peripheral neuropathy, toxic amblyopia, blurred vision, conjunctivitis, dry eyes, decreased hearing, acute renal failure, allergic rhinitis, shortness of breath, epistaxis

**Drug Interactions**
Decreased effect with aspirin; decreased effect of diuretics, antihypertensives
Increased effect/toxicity of warfarin, methotrexate

**Onset** Peak concentration: 1-2 hours

**Duration** 2-4 hours

**Special PA Issues**
Patient Education: Take with food, milk, or with antacids

**Related Information**
Nonsteroidal Anti-Inflammatory Agents on page 1026

♦ **Meclofenamate Sodium** see Meclofenamate on this page

♦ **Meclomen®** see Meclofenamate on this page

♦ **Meclozine Hydrochloride** see Meclizine on page 559

♦ **Mectizan®** see Ivermectin on page 503

♦ **Medicinal Carbon** see Charcoal on page 184

♦ **Medicinal Charcoal** see Charcoal on page 184

♦ **Medigesic®** see Butalbital Compound on page 131

♦ **Medihaler-Iso®** see Isoproterenol on page 496

♦ **Medilium®** see Chlordiazepoxide on page 189

♦ **Medimet®** see Methyldopa on page 590

♦ **Medipain 5®** see Hydrocodone and Acetaminophen on page 449

♦ **Medipren® [OTC]** see Ibuprofen on page 466

♦ **Medi-Quick® Topical Ointment [OTC]** see Bacitracin, Neomycin, and Polymyxin B on page 97

♦ **Meditran®** see Meprobamate on page 570

♦ **Medi-Tuss® [OTC]** see Guaifenesin on page 427

♦ **Medralone® Injection** see Methylprednisolone on page 593

♦ **Medrol® Oral** see Methylprednisolone on page 593

## Medroxyprogesterone Acetate (me DROKS ee proe JES te rone AS e tate)

**Pharmacologic Class** Contraceptive; Progestin

**U.S. Brand Names** Amen®; Curretab®; Cycrin®; Depo-Provera® Injection; Provera®

**Mechanism of Action** Inhibits secretion of pituitary gonadotropins, which prevents follicular maturation and ovulation, stimulates growth of mammary tissue

**Use** Endometrial carcinoma or renal carcinoma as well as secondary amenorrhea or abnormal uterine bleeding due to hormonal imbalance; prevention of pregnancy
(Continued)

## Medroxyprogesterone Acetate (Continued)

### USUAL DOSAGE
Adolescents and Adults: Oral:
Amenorrhea: 5-10 mg/day for 5-10 days or 2.5 mg/day
Abnormal uterine bleeding: 5-10 mg for 5-10 days starting on day 16 or 21 of cycle
Accompanying cyclic estrogen therapy, postmenopausal: 2.5-10 mg the last 10-13 days of estrogen dosing each month
Adults: I.M.:
Endometrial or renal carcinoma: 400-1000 mg/week
Contraception: 150 mg every 3 months
**Dosing adjustment in hepatic impairment:** Dose needs to be lowered in patients with alcoholic cirrhosis

**Dosage Forms** Inj, susp: 100 mg/mL (5 mL), 150 mg/mL (1 mL), 400 mg/mL (1 mL, 2.5 mL, 10 mL); **Tab:** 2.5 mg, 5 mg, 10 mg

**Contraindications** Pregnancy, thrombophlebitis; hypersensitivity to medroxyprogesterone or any component; cerebral apoplexy, undiagnosed vaginal bleeding, liver dysfunction

**Warnings/Precautions** Use with caution in patients with depression, diabetes, epilepsy, asthma, migraines, renal or cardiac dysfunction; pretreatment exams should include PAP smear, physical exam of breasts and pelvic areas. May increase serum cholesterol, LDL, decrease HDL and triglycerides; use of any progestin during the first 4 months of pregnancy is not recommended; monitor patient closely for loss of vision, sudden onset of proptosis, diplopia, migraine, and signs and symptoms of thromboembolic disorders.

### Pregnancy Risk Factor X

### Adverse Reactions
>10%:
Cardiovascular: Edema
Endocrine & metabolic: Breakthrough bleeding, spotting, changes in menstrual flow, amenorrhea
Gastrointestinal: Anorexia
Local: Pain at injection site
Neuromuscular & skeletal: Weakness
1% to 10%:
Cardiovascular: Embolism, central thrombosis
Central nervous system: Mental depression, fever, insomnia
Dermatologic: Melasma or chloasma, allergic rash with or without pruritus
Endocrine & metabolic: Changes in cervical erosion and secretions, increased breast tenderness
Gastrointestinal: Weight gain or loss
Hepatic: Cholestatic jaundice
Local: Thrombophlebitis

**Drug Interactions** Decreased effect: Aminoglutethimide may decrease effects by increasing hepatic metabolism

### Special PA Issues
**Patient Education:** Follow dosage schedule and do not take more than prescribed. You may experience sensitivity to sunlight (use sunblock, wear protective clothing and eyewear, and avoid extensive exposure to direct sunlight); dizziness, anxiety, depression (use caution when driving or engaging in hazardous tasks); changes in appetite (maintain adequate hydration and diet - 2-3 L/day of fluids unless instructed to restrict fluid intake); decreased libido or increased body hair (reversible when drug is discontinued); hot flashes (cool clothes and environment may help). Report swelling of face, lips, or mouth; absence or altered menses; abdominal pain; vaginal itching, irritation, or discharge; heat, warmth, redness, or swelling of extremities; or sudden onset change in vision.

**Monitoring Parameters:** Monitor patient closely for loss of vision, sudden onset of proptosis, diplopia, migraine, and signs and symptoms of thromboembolic disorders

## Medrysone (ME dri sone)

**Pharmacologic Class** Corticosteroid, Ophthalmic

**U.S. Brand Names** HMS Liquifilm®

**Mechanism of Action** Decreases inflammation by suppression of migration of polymorphonuclear leukocytes and reversal of increased capillary permeability

**Use** Treatment of allergic conjunctivitis, vernal conjunctivitis, episcleritis, ophthalmic epinephrine sensitivity reaction

**USUAL DOSAGE** Children and Adults: Ophthalmic: Instill 1 drop in conjunctival sac 2-4 times/day up to every 4 hours; may use every 1-2 hours during first 1-2 days

**Dosage Forms Soln, ophth:** 1% (5 mL, 10 mL)

**Contraindications** Fungal, viral, or untreated pus-forming bacterial ocular infections; not for use in iritis and uveitis

**Warnings/Precautions** Prolonged use has been associated with the development of corneal or scleral perforation and posterior subcapsular cataracts; may mask or enhance the establishment of acute purulent untreated infections of the eye; effectiveness and safety have not been established in children. Medrysone is a synthetic corticosteroid; structurally related to progesterone; if no improvement after several days of treatment, discontinue medrysone and institute other therapy; duration of therapy: 3-4 days to several weeks dependent on type and severity of disease; taper dose to avoid disease exacerbation.

**Pregnancy Risk Factor** C

**Adverse Reactions**

1% to 10%: Ocular: Temporary mild blurred vision

<1%: Stinging, burning eyes, corneal thinning, increased intraocular pressure, glaucoma, damage to the optic nerve, defects in visual activity, cataracts, secondary ocular infection

**Special PA Issues**

**Patient Education:** For ophthalmic use only. Shake before using. Apply prescribed amount as often as directed. Wash hands before using and do not let tip of applicator touch eye or contaminate tip of applicator. Tilt head back and look upward. Gently pull down lower lid and put drop(s) in inner corner of eye. Close eye and roll eyeball in all directions. Do not blink for 1/2 minute. Apply gentle pressure to inner corner of eye for 30 seconds. Wipe away excess from skin around eye. Do not use any other eye preparation for at least 10 minutes. Do not touch tip of applicator to eye or contaminate tip of applicator. Do not share medication with anyone else. May cause sensitivity to bright light (dark glasses may help); temporary stinging or blurred vision may occur. Inform prescriber if you experience eye pain, redness, burning, watering, dryness, double vision, puffiness around eye, vision disturbances, or other adverse eye response; worsening of condition or lack of improvement within 3-4 days.

**Monitoring Parameters:** Intraocular pressure and periodic examination of lens (with prolonged use)

# Mefloquine (ME floe kwin)

**Pharmacologic Class** Antimalarial Agent

**U.S. Brand Names** Lariam®

**Mechanism of Action** Mefloquine is a quinoline-methanol compound structurally similar to quinine; mefloquine's effectiveness in the treatment and prophylaxis of malaria is due to the destruction of the asexual blood forms of the malarial pathogens that affect humans, *Plasmodium falciparum, P. vivax, P. malariae, P. ovale*

**Use** Treatment of acute malarial infections and prevention of malaria

**USUAL DOSAGE** Oral:

Children: Malaria prophylaxis:

15-19 kg: 1/4 tablet

20-30 kg: 1/2 tablet

31-45 kg: 3/4 tablet

>45 kg: 1 tablet

Administer weekly starting 1 week before travel, continuing weekly during travel and for 4 weeks after leaving endemic area

Adults:

Treatment of mild to moderate malaria infection: 5 tablets (1250 mg) as a single dose with at least 8 oz of water

Malaria prophylaxis: 1 tablet (250 mg) weekly starting 1 week before travel, continuing weekly during travel and for 4 weeks after leaving endemic area

**Dosage Forms Tab, as hydrochloride:** 250 mg

**Contraindications** Hypersensitivity to any component

**Warnings/Precautions** Caution is warranted with lactation; discontinue if unexplained neuropsychiatric disturbances occur, caution in epilepsy patients or in patients with significant cardiac disease. If mefloquine is to be used for a prolonged period, periodic evaluations including liver function tests and ophthalmic examinations should be performed. (Retinal abnormalities have not been observed with mefloquine in humans; however, it has with long-term administration to rats.) In cases of life-threatening, serious, or overwhelming malaria infections due to *Plasmodium falciparum*, patients should be treated with intravenous antimalarial drug. Mefloquine may be given orally to complete the course. Caution should be exercised with regard to driving, piloting airplanes, and operating machines since dizziness, disturbed sense of balance; neuropsychiatric reactions have been reported with mefloquine.

**Pregnancy Risk Factor** C

**Adverse Reactions**

1% to 10%:

Central nervous system: Difficulty concentrating, headache, insomnia, lightheadedness, vertigo

Gastrointestinal: Vomiting (3%), diarrhea, stomach pain, nausea

Ocular: Visual disturbances

Otic: Tinnitus

<1%: Bradycardia, extrasystoles, syncope, anxiety, dizziness, confusion, seizures, hallucinations, mental depression, psychosis

**Drug Interactions**

Decreased effect of valproic acid

Increased toxicity of beta-blockers; chloroquine, quinine, and quinidine (hold treatment until at least 12 hours after these later drugs)

(Continued)

## Mefloquine *(Continued)*

**Half-Life** 21-22 days

**Special PA Issues**

**Patient Education:** Take on schedule as directed, with a full 8 oz of water. Ophthalmic exams will be necessary when used long-term. When taking for prophylaxis, begin 1 week before traveling to endemic areas, continue during travel period, and for 4 weeks following return. You may experience GI distress (frequent, small meals may help). You may experience dizziness, changes in mentation, insomnia, headache, visual disturbances (use caution when driving or operating dangerous machinery).

**Monitoring Parameters:** LFTS; ocular examination

- ♦ **Mefloquine Hydrochloride** *see Mefloquine on previous page*
- ♦ **Mefoxin®** *see Cefoxitin on page 169*
- ♦ **Mega-B® [OTC]** *see Vitamins, Multiple on page 964*
- ♦ **Megace®** *see Megestrol Acetate on this page*
- ♦ **Megacillin® Susp** *see Penicillin G Benzathine, Parenteral on page 704*

## Megestrol Acetate *(me JES trole AS e tate)*

**Pharmacologic Class** Antineoplastic Agent, Miscellaneous; Progestin

**U.S. Brand Names** Megace®

**Mechanism of Action** A synthetic progestin with antiestrogenic properties which disrupt the estrogen receptor cycle. Megace® interferes with the normal estrogen cycle and results in a lower LH titer. May also have a direct effect on the endometrium. Megestrol is an antineoplastic progestin thought to act through an antileutenizing effect mediated via the pituitary.

**Use** Palliative treatment of breast and endometrial carcinomas, appetite stimulation, and promotion of weight gain in cachexia

**USUAL DOSAGE** Adults: Oral (refer to individual protocols):

Female:

Breast carcinoma: 40 mg 4 times/day

Endometrial: 40-320 mg/day in divided doses; use for 2 months to determine efficacy; maximum doses used have been up to 800 mg/day

Uterine bleeding: 40 mg 2-4 times/day

Male/Female: HIV-related cachexia: Initial dose: 800 mg/day; daily doses of 400 and 800 mg/day were found to be clinically effective

**Dosing adjustment in renal impairment:** No data available; however, the urinary excretion of megestrol acetate administered in doses of 4-90 mg ranged from 56% to 78% within 10 days

Hemodialysis: Megestrol acetate has not been tested for dialyzability; however, due to its low solubility, it is postulated that dialysis would not be an effective means of treating an overdose

**Dosage Forms Susp, oral** 40 mg/mL with alcohol 0.06% (240 mL); **Tab:** 20 mg, 40 mg

**Contraindications** Hypersensitivity to megestrol or any component; pregnancy

**Warnings/Precautions** The U.S. Food and Drug Administration (FDA) currently recommends that procedures for proper handling and disposal of antineoplastic agents be considered. Use during the first few months of pregnancy is not recommended. Use with caution in patients with a history of thrombophlebitis. Elderly females may have vaginal bleeding or discharge and need to be forewarned of this side effect and inconvenience.

**Pregnancy Risk Factor** X

**Adverse Reactions**

>10%:

Cardiovascular: Edema

Endocrine & metabolic: Breakthrough bleeding and amenorrhea, spotting, changes in menstrual flow

Neuromuscular & skeletal: Weakness

1% to 10%:

Central nervous system: Insomnia, depression, fever, headache

Dermatologic: Allergic rash with or without pruritus, melasma or chloasma, rash, and rarely alopecia

Endocrine & metabolic: Changes in cervical erosion and secretions, increased breast tenderness, amenorrhea, changes in vaginal bleeding pattern, edema, fluid retention, hyperglycemia

Gastrointestinal: Weight gain (not attributed to edema or fluid retention), nausea, vomiting, stomach cramps

Hepatic: Cholestatic jaundice, hepatotoxicity

Hematologic: Myelosuppressive:

WBC: None

Platelets: None

Local: Thrombophlebitis

Neuromuscular & skeletal: Carpal tunnel syndrome

Respiratory: Hyperpnea

**Onset** At least 2 months of continuous therapy is necessary.

**Half-Life** 15-20 hours
**Special PA Issues**

**Patient Education:** Follow dosage schedule and do not take more than prescribed. You may experience sensitivity to sunlight (use sunblock, wear protective clothing, and avoid extended exposure to direct sunlight); dizziness, anxiety, depression (use caution when driving or engaging in hazardous tasks); change in appetite (maintain adequate hydration and diet - 2-3 L/day of fluids unless instructed to restrict fluid intake); decreased libido or increased body hair (reversible when drug is discontinued); hot flashes (cool clothes and environment may help). Report swelling of face, lips, or mouth; absence or altered menses; abdominal pain; vaginal itching, irritation, or discharge; heat, warmth, redness, or swelling of extremities; or sudden onset change in vision.

**Monitoring Parameters:** Monitor for tumor response; observe for signs of thromboembolic phenomena; monitor for thromboembolism

## Melaleuca Oil

**Mechanism of Action** Consists of plant terpenes, pinenes, and cineole, derived from the *Melaleuca alternifolia* tree, the colorless or pale yellow oil can cause CNS depression; may be bacteriostatic

**Use** Marketed as having fungicidal, bactericidal properties; also used as a topical dermal agent for burns

**USUAL DOSAGE** Minimal toxic dose: Infant: <10 mL applied topically

**Adverse Reactions** Dermatologic: Rarely causes allergic reactions or dermatitis

♦ **Melanex®** *see* Hydroquinone *on page 457*

## Melatonin (mel ah TOE nin)

**Mechanism of Action** Melatonin is a hormone responsible for regulating the body's circadian rhythm and sleep patterns. Its release is prompted by darkness and inhibited by light. Secretion appears to peak during childhood, and declines gradually through adolescence and adulthood. Melatonin receptors have been found in blood cells, the brain, gut, and ovaries. This substance may also have a role in regulating cardiovascular and reproductive function through its antioxidant properties.

**Use** Sleep disorders (eg, jet lag, insomnia, neurologic problems, shift work); aging; cancer; immune system support

**USUAL DOSAGE** Sleep disturbances: 0.3-5 mg/day

**Contraindications** Patients with immune disorders

**Pregnancy Implications** Do not use if thinking about becoming pregnant, during pregnancy, or lactation

**Adverse Reactions** Central nervous system: Reduced alertness, headache, irritability, increased fatigue, drowsiness, sedation

**Drug Interactions** Medications commonly used as sedatives or hyphotics, or those that induce sedation, drowsiness (eg, benzodiazepines, narcotics); CNS depressants (prescription, supplements such as 5-HTP); other herbs known to cause sedation include kava kava, valerian

♦ **Mellaril®** *see* Thioridazine *on page 895*

♦ **Mellaril-S®** *see* Thioridazine *on page 895*

♦ **Melpaque HP®** *see* Hydroquinone *on page 457*

## Melphalan (MEL fa lan)

**Pharmacologic Class** Antineoplastic Agent, Alkylating Agent

**U.S. Brand Names** Alkeran®

**Mechanism of Action** Alkylating agent which is a derivative of mechlorethamine that inhibits DNA and RNA synthesis via formation of carbonium ions; cross-links strands of DNA

**Use** Palliative treatment of multiple myeloma and nonresectable epithelial ovarian carcinoma; neuroblastoma, rhabdomyosarcoma, breast cancer

**USUAL DOSAGE**
Oral (refer to individual protocols); dose should always be adjusted to patient response and weekly blood counts:
Children: 4-20 mg/m$^2$/day for 1-21 days
Adults:
Multiple myeloma: 6 mg/day initially adjusted as indicated **or** 0.15 mg/kg/day for 7 days **or** 0.25 mg/kg/day for 4 days; repeat at 4- to 6-week intervals
Ovarian carcinoma: 0.2 mg/kg/day for 5 days, repeat every 4-5 weeks
Intravenous (refer to individual protocols):
Children:
Pediatric rhabdomyosarcoma: 10-35 mg/m$^2$/dose every 21-28 days
High-dose melphalan with bone marrow transplantation for neuroblastoma: 70-100 mg/m$^2$/day on day 7 and 6 before BMT **or** 140-220 mg/m$^2$ single dose before BMT **or** 50 mg/m$^2$/day for 4 days **or** 70 mg/m$^2$/day for 3 days

(Continued)

## Melphalan *(Continued)*

Adults:

Multiple myeloma: 16 mg/m² administered at 2-week intervals for 4 doses, then repeat monthly as per protocol for multiple myeloma

**Dosing adjustment in renal impairment:**

Cl$_{cr}$ 10-50 mL/minute: Administer at 75% of normal dose

Cl$_{cr}$ <10 mL/minute: Administer at 50% of normal dose

**or**

BUN >30 mg/dL: Reduce dose by 50%

Serum creatinine >1.5 mg/dL: Reduce dose by 50%

Hemodialysis: Unknown

CAPD effects: Unknown

CAVH effects: Unknown

**Dosage Forms** Powder for inj: 50 mg; **Tab:** 2 mg

**Contraindications** Hypersensitivity to melphalan or any component; severe bone marrow suppression; patients whose disease was resistant to prior therapy

**Warnings/Precautions** The U.S. Food and Drug Administration (FDA) currently recommends that procedures for proper handling and disposal for antineoplastic agents be considered. Is potentially mutagenic, carcinogenic, and teratogenic; produces amenorrhea. Reduce dosage or discontinue therapy if leukocyte count <3000/mm³ or platelet count <100,000/mm³; use with caution in patients with bone marrow suppression, impaired renal function, or who have received prior chemotherapy or irradiation; will cause amenorrhea. Toxicity to immunosuppressives is increased in elderly. Start with lowest recommended adult doses. Signs of infection, such as fever and WBC rise, may not occur. Lethargy and confusion may be more prominent signs of infection.

**Pregnancy Risk Factor** D

**Adverse Reactions**

>10%:

Hematologic: Myelosuppressive: Leukopenia and thrombocytopenia are the most common effects of melphalan. Irreversible bone marrow failure has been reported.

WBC: Moderate

Platelets: Moderate

Onset (days): 7

Nadir (days): 8-10 and 27-32

Recovery (days): 42-50

Second malignancies: Reported are melphalan more frequently

1% to 10%:

Cardiovascular: Vasculitis

Dermatologic: Vesiculation of skin, alopecia, pruritus, rash

Endocrine & metabolic: SIADH, sterility and amenorrhea

Gastrointestinal: Nausea and vomiting are mild; stomatitis and diarrhea are infrequent

Genitourinary: Bladder irritation, hemorrhagic cystitis

Hematologic: Anemia, agranulocytosis, hemolytic anemia

Respiratory: Pulmonary fibrosis, interstitial pneumonitis

Miscellaneous: Hypersensitivity

**Drug Interactions**

Decreased effect: Cimetidine and other H$_2$-antagonists: The reduction in gastric pH has been reported to decrease bioavailability of melphalan by 30%

Increased toxicity: Cyclosporine: Increased incidence of nephrotoxicity

**Half-Life** 1.5 hours

**Special PA Issues**

**Patient Education:** Infusion: Report promptly any pain, irritation, or redness at infusion site. Oral: Preferable to take on an empty stomach, 1 hour prior to or 2 hours after meals. Do not take alcohol, aspirin or aspirin-containing medications, and OTC medications without consulting prescriber. Inform prescriber of all prescription medication you are taking. Maintain adequate fluid balance (2-3 L/day). May cause hair loss (reversible); easy bleeding or bruising (use soft toothbrush or cotton swabs and frequent mouth care, use electric razor, avoid sharp knives or scissors); increased susceptibility to infection (avoid crowds or exposure to infection - do not have any vaccinations unless approved by prescriber). Report unusual bleeding or bruising or persistent fever or sore throat; blood in urine, stool, or vomitus; delayed healing of any wounds; skin rash; yellowing of skin or eyes; changes in color of urine of stool; pain or burning on urination; respiratory difficulty; or other severe adverse reactions.

**Monitoring Parameters:** CBC with differential and platelet count, serum electrolytes, serum uric acid

♦ **Melquin HP®** *see* Hydroquinone *on page 457*

♦ **Menadol® [OTC]** *see* Ibuprofen *on page 466*

♦ **Menest®** *see* Estrogens, Esterified *on page 337*

♦ **Meni-D®** *see* Meclizine *on page 559*

## Menotropins (men oh TROE pins)

**Pharmacologic Class** Gonadotropin; Ovulation Stimulator

**U.S. Brand Names** Humegon™; Pergonal®; Repronex™

**Mechanism of Action** Actions occur as a result of both follicle stimulating hormone (FSH) effects and luteinizing hormone (LH) effects; menotropins stimulate the development and maturation of the ovarian follicle (FSH), cause ovulation (LH), and stimulate the development of the corpus luteum (LH); in males it stimulates spermatogenesis (LH)

**Use** Sequentially with hCG to induce ovulation and pregnancy in the infertile woman with functional anovulation; used with hCG in men to stimulate spermatogenesis in those with primary hypogonadotropic hypogonadism

**USUAL DOSAGE** Adults: I.M.:

Male: Following pretreatment with hCG, 1 ampul 3 times/week and hCG 2000 units twice weekly until sperm is detected in the ejaculate (4-6 months) then may be increased to 2 ampuls of menotropins (150 units FSH/150 units LH) 3 times/week

Female: 1 ampul/day (75 units of FSH and LH) for 9-12 days followed by 10,000 units hCG 1 day after the last dose; repeated at least twice at same level before increasing dosage to 2 ampuls (150 units FSH/150 units LH)

**Dosage Forms Inj:** Follicle stimulating hormone activity 75 units and luteinizing hormone activity 75 units per 2 mL ampul, Follicle stimulating hormone activity 150 units and luteinizing hormone activity 150 units per 2 mL ampul

**Contraindications** Primary ovarian failure, overt thyroid and adrenal dysfunction, abnormal bleeding, pregnancy, men with normal urinary gonadotropin concentrations, elevated gonadotropin levels indicating primary testicular failure

**Warnings/Precautions** Advise patient of frequency and potential hazards of multiple pregnancy; to minimize the hazard of abnormal ovarian enlargement, use the lowest possible dose

**Pregnancy Risk Factor** X

**Adverse Reactions**

Male:

>10%: Endocrine & metabolic: Gynecomastia

1% to 10%: Erythrocytosis (shortness of breath, dizziness, anorexia, syncope, epistaxis)

Female:

>10%:

Endocrine & metabolic: Ovarian enlargement

Gastrointestinal: Abdominal distention

Local: Pain/rash at injection site

1% to 10%: Ovarian hyperstimulation syndrome

<1%: Thromboembolism, pain, febrile reactions

**Special PA Issues**

**Patient Education:** Self injection: Follow prescriber's recommended schedule for injections. Multiple ovulations resulting in multiple pregnancies have been reported. Male infertility and/or breast enlargement may occur. Report pain at injection site; enlarged breasts (male); difficulty breathing; nosebleeds; acute abdominal discomfort; or fever, pain, redness, or swelling of calves.

♦ **Mentax®** *see* Butenafine *on page 132*

♦ **Mepergan®** *see* Meperidine and Promethazine *on page 569*

## Meperidine (me PER i deen)

**Pharmacologic Class** Analgesic, Narcotic

**U.S. Brand Names** Demerol®

**Mechanism of Action** Binds to opiate receptors in the CNS, causing inhibition of ascending pain pathways, altering the perception of and response to pain; produces generalized CNS depression

**Use** Management of moderate to severe pain; adjunct to anesthesia and preoperative sedation

**USUAL DOSAGE** Doses should be titrated to appropriate analgesic effect; when changing route of administration, note that oral doses are about half as effective as parenteral dose

Children: Oral, I.M., I.V., S.C.: 1-1.5 mg/kg/dose every 3-4 hours as needed; 1-2 mg/kg as a single dose preoperative medication may be used; maximum 100 mg/dose

Adults: Oral, I.M., I.V.: S.C.: 50-150 mg/dose every 3-4 hours as needed

Elderly:

Oral: 50 mg every 4 hours

I.M.: 25 mg every 4 hours

**Dosing adjustment in renal impairment:**

$Cl_{cr}$ 10-50 mL/minute: Administer at 75% of normal dose

$Cl_{cr}$ <10 mL/minute: Administer at 50% of normal dose

**Dosing adjustment/comments in hepatic disease:** Increased narcotic effect in cirrhosis; reduction in dose more important for oral than I.V. route

**Dosage Forms Inj:** Multiple dose vials: 50 mg/mL (30 mL), 100 mg/mL (20 mL), Single dose: 10 mg/mL (5 mL, 10 mL, 30 mL), 25 mg/dose (0.5 mL, 1 mL), 50 mg/dose (1 mL), 75 (Continued)

## Meperidine *(Continued)*

mg/dose (1 mL, 1.5 mL), 100 mg/dose (1 mL); **Syr:** 50 mg/5 mL (500 mL); **Tab:** 50 mg, 100 mg

**Contraindications** Hypersensitivity to meperidine or any component; patients receiving MAO inhibitors presently or in the past 14 days

**Warnings/Precautions** Use with caution in patients with pulmonary, hepatic, renal disorders, or increased intracranial pressure; use with caution in patients with renal failure or seizure disorders or those receiving high-dose meperidine; normeperidine (an active metabolite and CNS stimulant) may accumulate and precipitate twitches, tremors, or seizures; some preparations contain sulfites which may cause allergic reaction; not recommended as a drug of first choice for the treatment of chronic pain in the elderly due to the accumulation of normeperidine; for acute pain, its use should be limited to 1-2 doses; tolerance or drug dependence may result from extended use

**Pregnancy Risk Factor** B D if used for prolonged periods or in high doses at term)

**Adverse Reactions**

> 10%:

  Cardiovascular: Hypotension

  Central nervous system: Fatigue, drowsiness, dizziness

  Gastrointestinal: Nausea, vomiting, constipation

  Neuromuscular & skeletal: Weakness

  Miscellaneous: Histamine release

1% to 10%:

  Central nervous system: Nervousness, headache, restlessness, malaise, confusion

  Gastrointestinal: Anorexia, stomach cramps, xerostomia, biliary spasm

  Genitourinary: Ureteral spasms, decreased urination

  Local: Pain at injection site

  Respiratory: Dyspnea, shortness of breath

<1%: Mental depression, hallucinations, paradoxical CNS stimulation, increased intracranial pressure, rash, urticaria, paralytic ileus, physical and psychological dependence

**Drug Interactions** CYP2D6 enzyme substrate

Decreased effect: Phenytoin may decrease the analgesic effects

Increased toxicity: May aggravate the adverse effects of isoniazid; MAO inhibitors, fluoxetine, and other serotonin uptake inhibitors greatly potentiate the effects of meperidine; acute opioid overdosage symptoms can be seen, including severe toxic reactions; CNS depressants, tricyclic antidepressants, phenothiazines may potentiate the effects of meperidine

**Onset**

Oral, S.C., I.M.: Onset of analgesic effect: Within 10-15 minutes; Peak effect: Within 1 hour

I.V.: Onset of effects: Within 5 minutes

**Duration** 2-4 hours

**Half-Life**

Parent drug: Terminal phase: Adults: 2.5-4 hours; Adults with liver disease: 7-11 hours

Normeperidine (active metabolite): 15-30 hours; is dependent on renal function and can accumulate with high doses or in patients with decreased renal function

**Special PA Issues**

**Patient Education:** If self-administered, use exactly as directed (do not increase dose or frequency); may cause physical and/or psychological dependence. While using this medication, do not use alcohol and other prescription or OTC medications (especially sedatives, tranquilizers, antihistamines, or pain medications) without consulting prescriber. Maintain adequate hydration (2-3 L/day of fluids unless instructed to restrict fluid intake). May cause hypotension dizziness, drowsiness, impaired coordination, or blurred vision (use caution when driving, climbing stairs, or changing position - rising from sitting or lying to standing, or when engaging in hazardous activities until response to medication is known); loss of appetite, nausea, or vomiting (frequent mouth care, small frequent meals, or sucking on lozenges may help); constipation (increased exercise, fluids, or dietary fruit and fiber may help - if constipation remains an unresolved problem, consult prescriber about use of stool softeners). Report chest pain, slow or rapid heartbeat, acute dizziness or persistent headache changes in mental status; swelling of extremities or unusual weight gain; changes in urinary elimination; acute headache; back or flank pain or muscle spasms; blurred vision; skin rash; or shortness of breath.

**Dietary Considerations:**

Alcohol: Additive CNS effects, avoid or limit alcohol; watch for sedation

Food: Glucose may cause hyperglycemia; monitor blood glucose concentrations

**Monitoring Parameters:** Pain relief, respiratory and mental status, blood pressure; observe patient for excessive sedation, CNS depression, seizures, respiratory depression

**Reference Range:** Therapeutic: 70-500 ng/mL (SI: 283-2020 nmol/L); Toxic: >1000 ng/mL (SI: >4043 nmol/L)

**Related Information**

Narcotic Agonists *on page 1023*

## Meperidine and Promethazine (me PER i deen & proe METH a zeen)
**Pharmacologic Class** Analgesic, Narcotic
**U.S. Brand Names** Mepergan®
**Dosage Forms Cap:** Meperidine hydrochloride 50 mg and promethazine hydrochloride 25 mg; **Inj:** Meperidine hydrochloride 25 mg and promethazine hydrochloride 25 per mL (2 mL, 10 mL)

♦ **Meperidine Hydrochloride** *see* Meperidine *on page 567*

## Mephobarbital (me foe BAR bi tal)
**Pharmacologic Class** Barbiturate
**U.S. Brand Names** Mebaral®
**Use** Sedative; treatment of grand mal and petit mal epilepsy
**USUAL DOSAGE** Oral:
Epilepsy:
Children: 6-12 mg/kg/day in 2-4 divided doses
Adults: 200-600 mg/day in 2-4 divided doses
Sedation:
Children:
<5 years: 16-32 mg 3-4 times/day
>5 years: 32-64 mg 3-4 times/day
Adults: 32-100 mg 3-4 times/day
**Dosing adjustment in renal or hepatic impairment:** Use with caution and reduce dosages
**Dosage Forms Tab:** 32 mg, 50 mg, 100 mg
**Contraindications** Hypersensitivity to mephobarbital, other barbiturates, or any component; pre-existing CNS depression; respiratory depression; severe uncontrolled pain; history of porphyria
**Pregnancy Risk Factor** D
**Drug Interactions** CYP2C, 2C8, and 2C19 enzyme substrate

♦ **Mephyton® Oral** *see* Phytonadione *on page 725*

## Mepivacaine (me PIV a kane)
**Pharmacologic Class** Local Anesthetic
**U.S. Brand Names** Carbocaine®; Isocaine® HCl; Polocaine®
**Mechanism of Action** Mepivacaine is an amino amide local anesthetic similar to lidocaine; like all local anesthetics, mepivacaine acts by preventing the generation and conduction of nerve impulses
**Use** Local anesthesia by nerve block; infiltration in dental procedures; **not** for use in spinal anesthesia
**USUAL DOSAGE** Children and Adults: Injectable local anesthetic: Varies with procedure, degree of anesthesia needed, vascularity of tissue, duration of anesthesia required, and physical condition of patient
**Dosage Forms Inj, as hydrochloride:** 1% [10 mg/mL] (30 mL, 50 mL); 1.5% [15 mg/mL] (30 mL); 2% [20 mg/mL] (20 mL, 50 mL); 3% [30 mg/mL] (1.8 mL)
**Contraindications** Hypersensitivity to mepivacaine or any component or other amide anesthetics, allergy to sodium bisulfate
**Warnings/Precautions** Use with caution in patients with cardiac disease, renal disease, and hyperthyroidism; convulsions due to systemic toxicity leading to cardiac arrest have been reported presumably due to intravascular injection
**Pregnancy Risk Factor** C
**Adverse Reactions** <1%: Bradycardia, myocardial depression, hypotension, cardiovascular collapse, edema, anxiety, restlessness, disorientation, confusion, seizures, drowsiness, unconsciousness, chills, urticaria, nausea, vomiting, transient stinging or burning at injection site, tremors, blurred vision, tinnitus, respiratory arrest, anaphylactoid reactions, shivering
**Onset** Epidural: Within 7-15 minutes
**Duration** 2-2.5 hours; similar onset and duration is seen following infiltration
**Half-Life** 1.9 hours
**Special PA Issues**
**Patient Education:** You will experience decreased sensation to pain, heat, or cold in the area and/or decreased muscle strength (depending on area of application) until effects wear off; use necessary caution to reduce incidence of possible injury until full sensation returns. Report irritation, pain, burning at injection site; chest pain or palpitations; or difficulty breathing.

Oral: This will cause numbness of your mouth. Do not eat or drink for 1 hour after use. Take small sips of water at first to ensure that you can swallow without difficulty. Your tongue and/or mouth may be numb - use caution to avoid biting yourself. Report irritation, pain, burning at injection site; chest pain or palpitations; or difficulty breathing.

♦ **Mepivacaine Hydrochloride** *see* Mepivacaine *on this page*

## Meprobamate (me proe BA mate)

**Pharmacologic Class** Antianxiety Agent, Miscellaneous

**U.S. Brand Names** Equanil®; Miltown®; Neuramate®

**Mechanism of Action** Precise mechanism is not yet clear, but many effects have been ascribed to its central depressant actions

**Use** Management of anxiety disorders; insomnia; preprocedure sedation and relaxation

**Unlabeled use:** Demonstrated value for muscle contraction, headache, premenstrual tension, external sphincter spasticity, muscle rigidity, opisthotonos-associated with tetanus

**USUAL DOSAGE** Oral:

Children 6-12 years: 100-200 mg 2-3 times/day

Sustained release: 200 mg twice daily

Adults: 400 mg 3-4 times/day, up to 2400 mg/day

Sustained release: 400-800 mg twice daily

**Dosing interval in renal impairment:**

$Cl_{cr}$ 10-50 mL/minute: Administer every 9-12 hours

$Cl_{cr}$ <10 mL/minute: Administer every 12-18 hours

Hemodialysis: Moderately dialyzable (20% to 50%)

**Dosing adjustment in hepatic impairment:** Probably necessary in patients with liver disease

**Dosage Forms Cap, sustained release:** 200 mg, 400 mg; **Tab:** 200 mg, 400 mg, 600 mg

**Contraindications** Acute intermittent porphyria; hypersensitivity to meprobamate or any component; do not use in patients with pre-existing CNS depression, narrow-angle glaucoma, or severe uncontrolled pain

**Warnings/Precautions** Physical and psychological dependence and abuse may occur; not recommended in children <6 years of age; allergic reaction may occur in patients with history of dermatological condition (usually by fourth dose); use with caution in patients with renal or hepatic impairment, or with a history of seizures

**Pregnancy Risk Factor** D

**Adverse Reactions**

>10%: Central nervous system: Drowsiness, ataxia

1% to 10%:

Central nervous system: Dizziness

Dermatologic: Rashes

Gastrointestinal: Diarrhea, vomiting

Ocular: Blurred vision

Respiratory: Wheezing

<1%: Syncope, peripheral edema, paradoxical excitement, confusion, slurred speech, headache, euphoria, chills, purpura, dermatitis, Stevens-Johnson syndrome, stomatitis, thrombocytopenia, leukopenia, renal failure, dyspnea, bronchospasm

**Drug Interactions** Increased toxicity: CNS depressants may increase CNS depression

**Onset** Onset of sedation: Oral: Within 1 hour

**Half-Life** 10 hours

**Special PA Issues**

**Patient Education:** Take exactly as directed (do not increase dose or frequency); may cause physical and/or psychological dependence. Do not chew or crush extended release capsule. Do not use excessive alcohol or other prescription or OTC medications (especially pain medications, sedatives, antihistamines, or hypnotics) without consulting prescriber. Maintain adequate hydration (2-3 L/day of fluids unless instructed to restrict fluid intake). You may experience drowsiness, lightheadedness, impaired coordination, dizziness, or blurred vision (use caution when driving or engaging in hazardous tasks until response to medication is known); nausea, vomiting, or dry mouth (small frequent meals, good mouth care, chewing gum, or sucking lozenges may help); or diarrhea (boiled milk, yogurt, or buttermilk may help). Report persistent CNS effects, skin rash or irritation, changes in urinary pattern, wheezing or respiratory difficulty, or worsening of condition.

**Dietary Considerations:** Alcohol: Additive CNS effect, avoid use

**Monitoring Parameters:** Mental status

**Reference Range:** Therapeutic: 6-12 µg/mL (SI: 28-55 µmol/L); Toxic: >60 µg/mL (SI: >275 µmol/L)

♦ **Mepron™** see Atovaquone on page 86

♦ **Mercapturic Acid** see Acetylcysteine on page 26

♦ **Meridia®** see Sibutramine on page 832

♦ **Meronem®** see Meropenem on this page

## Meropenem (mer oh PEN em)

**Pharmacologic Class** Antibiotic, Carbapenem

**U.S. Brand Names** Meronem®; Merrem® I.V.

**Mechanism of Action** Inhibits bacterial cell wall synthesis by binding to several of the penicillin-binding proteins, which in turn inhibit the final transpeptidation step of peptidoglycan synthesis in bacterial cell walls, thus inhibiting cell wall biosynthesis; bacteria eventually lyse due to ongoing activity of cell wall autolytic enzymes (autolysins and murein hydrolases) while cell wall assembly is arrested

**Use** Intra-abdominal infections (complicated appendicitis and peritonitis) caused by viridans group streptococci, *E. coli, K. pneumoniae, P. aeruginosa, B. fragilis, B. thetaiotaomicron,* and *Peptostreptococcus* sp; also indicated for bacterial meningitis in pediatric patients >3 months of age caused by *S. pneumoniae, H. influenzae,* and *N. meningitidis;* meropenem has also been used to treat soft tissue infections, febrile neutropenia, and urinary tract infections

## USUAL DOSAGE I.V.:

Neonates:

Preterm: 20 mg/kg/dose every 12 hours (may be increased to 40 mg/kg/dose if treating a highly resistant organism such as *Pseudomonas aeruginosa*)

Full-term (<3 months of age): 20 mg/kg/dose every 8 hours (may be increased to 40 mg/kg/dose if treating a highly resistant organism such as *Pseudomonas aeruginosa*)

Children >3 months (<50 kg):

Intra-abdominal infections: 20 mg/kg every 8 hours (maximum dose: 1 g every 8 hours)

Meningitis: 40 mg/kg every 8 hours (maximum dose: 2 g every 8 hours)

Children >50 kg:

Intra-abdominal infections: 1 g every 8 hours

Meningitis: 2 g every 8 hours

Adults: 1 g every 8 hours

**Dosing adjustment in renal impairment:** Adults:

$Cl_{cr}$ 26-50 mL/minute: Administer 1 g every 12 hours

$Cl_{cr}$ 10-25 mL/minute: Administer 500 mg every 12 hours

$Cl_{cr}$ <10 mL/minute: Administer 500 mg every 24 hours

Dialysis: Meropenem and its metabolites are readily dialyzable

Continuous arteriovenous or venovenous hemodiafiltration (CAVH) effects: Dose as $Cl_{cr}$ 10-50 mL/minute

**Dosage Forms Inf:** 500 mg (100 mL); 1 g (100 mL); **Inf, ADD-vantage®:** 500 mg (15 mL), 1 g (15 mL); **Inj:** 25 mg/mL (20 mL), 33.3 mg/mL (30 mL)

**Contraindications** Patients with known hypersensitivity to meropenem, any component, or other carbapenems (eg, imipenem); patients who have experienced anaphylactic reactions to other beta-lactams

**Warnings/Precautions** Pseudomembranous colitis and hypersensitivity reactions have occurred and often require immediate drug discontinuation; thrombocytopenia has been reported in patients with significant renal dysfunction; seizures have occurred in patients with underlying neurologic disorders (less frequent than with Primaxin®); safety and efficacy have not been established for children <3 months of age; superinfection possible with long courses of therapy

**Pregnancy Risk Factor** B

**Pregnancy Implications** Although no teratogenic or infant harm has been found in studies, excretion in breast milk is not known and this drug should be used during pregnancy and lactation only if clearly indicated

## Adverse Reactions

1% to 10%:

Central nervous system: Headache (2.8%)

Dermatologic: Rash, pruritus (1% to 2%)

Gastrointestinal: Diarrhea (5%), nausea/vomiting (4%), constipation (1.2%)

Local: Pain at injection site (3%), phlebitis, thrombophlebitis (1%)

Respiratory: Apnea (1.2%)

<1%: Hypotension, heart failure (MI and arrhythmias), tachycardia, hypertension, edema, seizures, insomnia, agitation, confusion, hallucinations, depression, seizures, fever, urticaria, anorexia, flatulence, ileus, oral moniliasis, glossitis, dysuria, RBCs in urine, cholestatic jaundice, hepatic failure, increase LFTs, anemia, hypo- and hypercytosis, bleeding events (epistaxis, melena, etc), paresthesia, whole body pain, renal failure, increased creatinine/BUN

**Drug Interactions** Increased effect: Probenecid competes with meropenem for active tubular secretion and inhibits the renal excretion of meropenem (half-life increased by 38%)

**Half-Life** ~1 hour

**Special PA Issues**

**Patient Education:** Report pain at infusion/injection site, rash, or respiratory difficulty. You may experience gastric distress, diarrhea, mouth sores, respiratory difficulty, or headache (consult prescriber for appropriate medication).

**Monitoring Parameters:** Monitor for signs of anaphylaxis during first dose

♦ **Merrem® I.V.** *see* Meropenem *on previous page*

# Mesalamine (me SAL a meen)

**Pharmacologic Class** 5-Aminosalicylic Acid Derivative

**U.S. Brand Names** Asacol® Oral; Pentasa® Oral; Rowasa® Rectal

(Continued)

## Mesalamine *(Continued)*

**Mechanism of Action** Mesalamine (5-aminosalicylic acid) is the active component of sulfasalazine; the specific mechanism of action of mesalamine is unknown; however, it is thought that it modulates local chemical mediators of the inflammatory response, especially leukotrienes; action appears topical rather than systemic

**Use**

Oral: Remission and treatment of mildly to moderately active ulcerative colitis

Rectal: Treatment of active mild to moderate distal ulcerative colitis, proctosigmoiditis, or proctitis

**USUAL DOSAGE** Adults (usual course of therapy is 3-6 weeks):

Oral:

Capsule: 1 g 4 times/day

Tablet: 800 mg 3 times/day

Retention enema: 60 mL (4 g) at bedtime, retained overnight, approximately 8 hours

Rectal suppository: Insert 1 suppository in rectum twice daily

Some patients may require rectal and oral therapy concurrently

**Dosage Forms** Cap, controlled release (Pentasa®): 250 mg; Supp, rectal (Rowasa®): 500 mg; Susp, rectal (Rowasa®): 4 g/60 mL (7s); Tab, enteric coated (Asacol®): 400 mg

**Contraindications** Known hypersensitivity to mesalamine, sulfasalazine, sulfites, or salicylates

**Warnings/Precautions** Pericarditis should be considered in patients with chest pain; pancreatitis should be considered in any patient with new abdominal complaints. Elderly may have difficulty administering and retaining rectal suppositories. Given renal function decline with aging, monitor serum creatinine often during therapy. Use caution in patients with impaired hepatic function.

**Pregnancy Risk Factor** B

**Adverse Reactions**

>10%:

Central nervous system: Headache, malaise

Gastrointestinal: Abdominal pain, cramps, flatulence, gas

1% to 10%: Dermatologic: Alopecia, rash

<1%: Anal irritation, acute intolerance syndrome (bloody diarrhea, severe abdominal cramps, severe headache)

**Drug Interactions** Decreased effect: Decreased digoxin bioavailability

**Half-Life** 5-ASA: 0.5-1.5 hours; Acetyl 5-ASA: 5-10 hours

**Special PA Issues**

**Patient Education:** Take as directed. Oral: Do not chew or break tablets. Enemas: Shake well before using, retain for 8 hours or as long as possible. Suppository: After removing foil wrapper, insert high in rectum without excessive handling (warmth will melt suppository). You may experience flatulence, headache, or hair loss (reversible). Report abdominal pain, unresolved diarrhea, severe headache, or chest pain.

♦ **Mesalazine** *see* Mesalamine *on previous page*

♦ **M-Eslon®** *see* Morphine Sulfate *on page 619*

## Mesoridazine (mez o RID a zeen)

**Pharmacologic Class** Antipsychotic Agent, Phenothiazine, Piperidine

**U.S. Brand Names** Serentil®

**Mechanism of Action** Blockade of postsynaptic CNS dopamine receptors

**Use** Symptomatic management of psychotic disorders, including schizophrenia, behavioral problems, alcoholism as well as reducing anxiety and tension occurring in neurosis

**USUAL DOSAGE** Concentrate may be diluted just prior to administration with distilled water, acidified tap water, orange or grape juice; do not prepare and store bulk dilutions

Adults:

Oral: 25-50 mg 3 times/day; maximum: 100-400 mg/day

I.M.: Initial: 25 mg, repeat in 30-60 minutes as needed; optimal dosage range: 25-200 mg/day

Hemodialysis: Not dialyzable (0% to 5%)

**Dosage Forms** Mesoridazine besylate: Inj: 25 mg/mL (1 mL); Liq, oral: 25 mg/mL (118 mL); Tab: 10 mg, 25 mg, 50 mg, 100 mg

**Contraindications** Hypersensitivity to mesoridazine or any component, cross-sensitivity with other phenothiazines may exist

**Warnings/Precautions** Safety in children <6 months of age has not been established; use with caution in patients with cardiovascular disease or seizures; benefits of therapy must be weighed against risks of therapy; doses >1 g/day frequently cause pigmentary retinopathy; some products contain sulfites and/or tartrazine; use with caution in patients with narrow-angle glaucoma, bone marrow suppression, severe liver disease

**Pregnancy Risk Factor** C

**Adverse Reactions**

>10%:

Cardiovascular: Hypotension, orthostatic hypotension

    Central nervous system: Pseudoparkinsonism, akathisia, dystonias, tardive dyskinesia (persistent), dizziness
    Gastrointestinal: Constipation
    Ocular: Pigmentary retinopathy
    Respiratory: Nasal congestion
    Miscellaneous: Diaphoresis (decreased)

1% to 10%:
    Dermatologic: Increased sensitivity to sun, rash
    Endocrine & metabolic: Changes in menstrual cycle, changes in libido, breast pain
    Gastrointestinal: Weight gain, nausea, vomiting, stomach pain
    Genitourinary: Dysuria, ejaculatory disturbances
    Neuromuscular & skeletal: Trembling of fingers

<1%: Neuroleptic malignant syndrome (NMS), impairment of temperature regulation, lowering of seizures threshold, discoloration of skin (blue-gray), galactorrhea, priapism, agranulocytosis, leukopenia, cholestatic jaundice, hepatotoxicity, cornea and lens changes

**Drug Interactions**
    Decreased effect with anticonvulsants, anticholinergics
    Increased toxicity with CNS depressants, metrizamide (increases seizures), propranolol

**Duration** 4-6 hours

**Half-Life** Time to steady-state serum: 4-7 days

**Special PA Issues**
    **Patient Education:** Use exactly as directed (do not increase dose or frequency); may cause physical and/or psychological dependence. It may take 2-3 weeks to achieve desired results; do not discontinue without consulting prescriber. Dilute oral concentration with water, orange or grape juice. Do not take within 2 hours of any antacid. Avoid excess alcohol or caffeine and other prescription or OTC medications not approved by prescriber. Maintain adequate hydration (2-3 L/day of fluids unless instructed to restrict fluid intake). Avoid skin contact with medication; may cause contact dermatitis (wash immediately with warm, soapy water). You may experience excess drowsiness, restlessness, dizziness, or blurred vision (use caution driving or when engaging in hazardous tasks until response to medication is known); dry mouth, nausea, vomiting (small frequent meals, frequent mouth care, or sucking lozenges may help); constipation (increased exercise, fluids, or dietary fruit and fiber may help); postural hypotension (use caution climbing stairs or when changing position from lying or sitting to standing); urinary retention (void before taking medication); photosensitivity (use sunscreen, protective clothing, and avoid prolonged exposure to direct sunlight); decreased perspiration (avoid strenuous exercise in hot environments); or changes in menstrual cycle, libido, ejaculation (will resolve when medication is discontinued). Report persistent CNS effects (eg, trembling fingers, altered gait or balance, excessive sedation, seizures, unusual movements, anxiety, abnormal thoughts, confusion, personality changes); chest pain, palpitations, rapid heartbeat, severe dizziness; unresolved urinary retention or changes in urinary pattern; menstrual pattern, change in libido, swelling or pain in breasts (male or female); vision changes; skin rash or yellowing of skin; difficulty breathing; or worsening of condition.

    **Dietary Considerations:** Alcohol: Additive CNS effect, avoid use

**Related Information**
    Antipsychotic Agents *on page 1001*

♦ **Mesoridazine Besylate** *see* Mesoridazine *on previous page*

♦ **Mestatin®** *see* Nystatin *on page 669*

♦ **Mestinon®** *see* Pyridostigmine *on page 783*

♦ **Mestinon Time-Span®** *see* Pyridostigmine *on page 783*

# Mestranol and Norethindrone (MES tra nole & nor eth IN drone)

**Pharmacologic Class** Contraceptive

**U.S. Brand Names** Genora® 1/50; Nelova™ 1/50M; Norethin™ 1/50M; Norinyl® 1+50; Ortho-Novum™ 1/50

**Mechanism of Action** Combination oral contraceptives inhibit ovulation via a negative feedback mechanism on the hypothalamus, which alters the normal pattern of gonadotropin secretion of a follicle-stimulating hormone (FSH) and luteinizing hormone by the anterior pituitary. The follicular phase FSH and midcycle surge of gonadotropins are inhibited. In addition, oral contraceptives produce alterations in the genital tract, including changes in the cervical mucus, rendering it unfavorable for sperm penetration even if ovulation occurs. Changes in the endometrium may also occur, producing an unfavorable environment for nidation. Oral contraceptive drugs may alter the tubal transport of the ova through the fallopian tubes. Progestational agents may also alter sperm fertility.

**Use** Prevention of pregnancy; treatment of hypermenorrhea, endometriosis, female hypogonadism [monophasic oral contraceptive]

**USUAL DOSAGE** Adults: Female: Oral:
    Contraception: 1 tablet daily, beginning on day 5 of menstrual cycle (first day of menstrual flow is day 1). With 20-tablet and 21-tablet packages, new dosing cycle begins 7 days
    (Continued)

## Mestranol and Norethindrone *(Continued)*

after last tablet taken. Wi h 28-tablet packages, dosage is 1 tablet daily without interruption; extra tablets are placebos or contain iron. If next menstrual period does not begin on schedule, rule out pregnancy before starting new dosing cycle. If menstrual period begins, start new dosing cycle 7 days after last tablet was taken. If all doses have been taken on schedule and one menstrual period is missed, continue dosing cycle. If two consecutive menstrual periods are missed, pregnancy test is required before new dosing cycle is started.

One dose missed: Take as soon as remembered or take 2 tablets next day

Two doses missed: Take 2 tablets as soon as remembered or 2 tablets next 2 days

Three doses missed: Begin new compact of tablets starting on day 1 of next cycle

**Dosage Forms Tab:** Mestranol 0.05 mg and norethindrone 1 mg (21s and 28s)

**Contraindications** Known or suspected breast cancer, undiagnosed abnormal vaginal bleeding, carcinoma of the breast, estrogen-dependent tumor, pregnancy

**Warnings/Precautions** Use with caution in patients with a history of thromboembolism, stroke, myocardial infarction, liver tumor, hypertension, cardiac, renal or hepatic insufficiency; use of any progestin during the first 4 months of pregnancy is not recommended; risk of cardiovascular side effects increases in those women who smoke cigarettes and in women >35 years of age

**Pregnancy Risk Factor** X

**Adverse Reactions**

>10%:

Cardiovascular: Peripheral edema

Central nervous system: Headache

Endocrine: Enlargement of breasts, breast tenderness, increased libido

Gastrointestinal: Nausea, anorexia, bloating

1% to 10%: Gastrointestinal: Vomiting, diarrhea

<1%: Hypertension, thromboembolism, edema, stroke, myocardial infarction, depression, dizziness, anxiety, chloasma, melasma, rash, decreased glucose tolerance, amenorrhea, alterations in frequency and flow of menses, increased triglycerides and LDL, GI distress, cholestatic jaundice, intolerance to contact lenses, increased susceptibility to *Candida* infection, breast tumors

See tables.

### Achieving Proper Hormonal Balance in an Oral Contraceptive

| Estrogen | | Progestin | |
|---|---|---|---|
| Excess | Deficiency | Excess | Deficiency |
| Nausea, bloating | Early or midcycle | Increased appetite | Late breakthrough |
| Cervical mucorrhea, | breakthrough | Weight gain | bleeding |
| polyposis | bleeding | Tiredness, fatigue | Amenorrhea |
| Melasma | Increased spotting | Hypomenorrhea | Hypermenorrhea |
| Migraine headache | Hypomenorrhea | Acne, oily scalp* | |
| Breast fullness or | | Hair loss, hirsutism* | |
| tenderness | | Depression | |
| Edema | | Monilial vaginitis | |
| Hypertension | | Breast regression | |

*Result of androgenic activity of progestins.

### Pharmacological Effects of Progestins Used in Oral Contraceptives

| | Progestin | Estrogen | Antiestrogen | Androgen |
|---|---|---|---|---|
| Norgestrel/levonorgestrel | +++ | 0 | ++ | +++ |
| Ethynodiol diacetate | ++ | +* | +* | + |
| Norethindrone acetate | + | + | +++ | + |
| Norethindrone | + | +* | +* | + |
| Norethynodrel | + | +++ | 0 | 0 |

*Has estrogenic effect at low doses; may have antiestrogenic effect at higher doses.

+++ = pronounced effect

++ = moderate effect

+ = slight effect

0 = no effect

### Drug Interactions

Decreased effect:

Tetracyclines, penicillins, griseofulvin, rifampin, acetaminophen, barbiturates, hydantoins may increase contraceptive failures

Decreases acetaminophen, estrogen levels, and anticoagulants

Increased toxicity: Increases benzodiazepines, caffeine, metoprolol, theophyllines, and tricyclic antidepressants

**Special PA Issues**

**Patient Education:** Take exactly as directed; use additional method of birth control during first week of administration of first cycle; photosensitivity may occur

Women should inform their physicians if signs or symptoms of any of the following occur thromboembolic or thrombotic disorders including sudden severe headache or vomiting, disturbance of vision or speech, loss of vision, numbness or weakness in an extremity, sharp or crushing chest pain, calf pain, shortness of breath, severe abdominal pain or mass, mental depression or unusual bleeding

Women should be advised that if they miss one daily dose, they should take the tablet as soon as remembered. If 2 daily doses are missed, 2 tablets should be taken daily for 2 days and the regular schedule resumed. If 3 or more daily doses are missed, therapy should be discontinued. Therapy with a new cycle can be resumed in 7 or 8 days. When any doses are missed, alternative contraceptive methods should be used for the next 2 days or until 2 days into the new cycle.

Women should discontinue taking the medication if they suspect they are pregnant or become pregnant

♦ **Metacortandralone** see Prednisolone on page 752
♦ **Metahydrin®** see Trichlormethiazide on page 932
♦ **Metamucil® [OTC]** see Psyllium on page 781
♦ **Metamucil® Instant Mix [OTC]** see Psyllium on page 781
♦ **Metandren®** see Methyltestosterone on page 595
♦ **Metaprel® Syrup** see Metaproterenol on this page

# Metaproterenol (met a proe TER e nol)

**Pharmacologic Class** Beta$_2$ Agonist

**U.S. Brand Names** Alupent®; Arm-a-Med® Metaproterenol; Dey-Dose® Metaproterenol; Metaprel® Syrup; Prometa®

**Mechanism of Action** Relaxes bronchial smooth muscle by action on beta$_2$-receptors with very little effect on heart rate

**Use** Bronchodilator in reversible airway obstruction due to asthma or COPD; because of its delayed onset of action (1 hour) and prolonged effect (4 or more hours), this may not be the drug of choice for assessing response to a bronchodilator

**USUAL DOSAGE**

Oral:

Children:

<2 years: 0.4 mg/kg/dose given 3-4 times/day; in infants, the dose can be given every 8-12 hours

2-6 years: 1-2.6 mg/kg/day divided every 6 hours

6-9 years: 10 mg/dose 3-4 times/day

Children >9 years and Adults: 20 mg 3-4 times/day

Elderly: Initial: 10 mg 3-4 times/day, increasing as necessary up to 20 mg 3-4 times/day

Inhalation: Children >12 years and Adults: 2-3 inhalations every 3-4 hours, up to 12 inhalations in 24 hours

Nebulizer:

Infants and Children: 0.01-0.02 mL/kg of 5% solution; minimum dose: 0.1 mL; maximum dose: 0.3 mL diluted in 2-3 mL normal saline every 4-6 hours (may be given more frequently according to need)

Adolescents and Adults: 5-20 breaths of full strength 5% metaproterenol **or** 0.2 to 0.3 mL 5% metaproterenol in 2.5-3 mL normal saline until nebulized every 4-6 hours (can be given more frequently according to need)

**Dosage Forms** Aero, oral: 0.65 mg/dose (5 mL, 10 mL); **Soln for inh, preservative free:** 0.4% [4 mg/mL] (2.5 mL), 0.6 [6 mg/mL] (2.5 mL), 5% [50 mg/mL] (10 mL, 30 mL); **Syr:** 10 mg/5 mL (480 mL); **Tab:** 10 mg, 20 mg

**Contraindications** Hypersensitivity to metaproterenol or any components, pre-existing cardiac arrhythmias associated with tachycardia

**Warnings/Precautions** Use with caution in patients with hypertension, CHF, hyperthyroidism, CAD, diabetes, or sensitivity to sympathomimetics; excessive prolonged use may result in decreased efficacy or increased toxicity and death; use caution in patients with pre-existing cardiac arrhythmias associated with tachycardia. Metaproterenol has more beta$_1$ activity than other sympathomimetics such as albuterol and, therefore, may no longer be the beta agonist of first choice. All patients should utilize a spacer device when using a metered dose inhaler. Oral use should be avoided due to the increased incidence of adverse effects.

**Pregnancy Risk Factor** C

**Pregnancy Implications**

Clinical effects on the fetus: No data on crossing the placenta. Reported association with polydactyly in 1 study; may be secondary to severe maternal disease or chance.

Breast-feeding/lactation: No data on crossing into breast milk or clinical effects on the infant

(Continued)

## Metaproterenol *(Continued)*

### Adverse Reactions
>10%:

Central nervous system: Nervousness

Neuromuscular & skeletal: Tremor

1% to 10%:

Cardiovascular: Tachycardia, palpitations, hypertension

Central nervous system: Headache, dizziness

Gastrointestinal: Nausea, vomiting, bad taste

Neuromuscular & skeletal: Trembling, muscle cramps, weakness

Respiratory: Coughing

Miscellaneous: Diaphoresis (increased)

<1%: Paradoxical bronchospasm

### Drug Interactions
Decreased effect: Beta-blockers

Increased toxicity: Sympathomimetics, TCAs, MAO inhibitors

### Onset
Oral: Onset of bronchodilation: Within 15 minutes; Peak effect: Within 1 hour

Inhalation: Onset of bronchodilation: Within 60 seconds

**Duration** Oral or inhalation: ~1-5 hours, regardless of route administered

### Special PA Issues

**Patient Education:** Use exactly as directed (see Administration below). Do not use more often than recommended. Maintain adequate hydration (2-3 L/day of fluids unless instructed to restrict fluid intake). You may experience nervousness, dizziness, or fatigue (use caution when driving or engaging in hazardous activities until response to treatment is known); dry mouth, unpleasant aftertaste, stomach upset (frequent small meals, frequent mouth care, chewing gum, or sucking hard candy may help); or increased perspiration. Report unresolved GI upset; dizziness or fatigue; vision changes; chest pain, rapid heartbeat, or palpitations; nervousness or insomnia; muscle cramping or tremor; or unusual cough.

**Administration:**

Self-administered inhalation: Store canister upside down; do not freeze. Shake canister before using. Sit when using medication. Close eyes when administering metaproterenol to avoid spray getting into eyes. Exhale slowly and completely through nose; inhale deeply through mouth while administering aerosol. Hold breath for 1-3 seconds after inhalation. Wait at least 1 full minute between inhalations. Wash mouthpiece between use. If more than one inhalation medication is used, use bronchodilator first and wait 5 minutes between medications.

Self-administered nebulizer: Wash hands before and after treatment. Wash and dry nebulizer after each treatment. Twist open the top of one unit dose vial and squeeze contents into nebulizer reservoir. Connect nebulizer reservoir to the mouthpiece or face-mask. Connect nebulizer to compressor. Sit in comfortable, upright position. Place mouthpiece in your mouth or put on face-mask and turn on compressor. If face-mask is used, avoid leakage around the mask to avoid mist getting into eyes which may cause vision problems. Breath calmly and deeply until no more mist is formed in nebulizer (about 5 minutes). At this point treatment is finished.

**Monitoring Parameters:** Assess lung sounds, pulse, and blood pressure before administration and during peak of medication; observe patient for wheezing after administration, if this occurs, call physician; monitor heart rate, respiratory rate, blood pressure, and arterial or capillary blood gases if applicable

♦ **Metaproterenol Sulfate** *see* Metaproterenol *on previous page*

♦ **Metastron®** *see* Strontium-89 *on page 855*

## Metaxalone *(me TAKS a lone)*

**Pharmacologic Class** Skeletal Muscle Relaxant

**U.S. Brand Names** Skelaxin®

**Mechanism of Action** Does not have a direct effect on skeletal muscle; most of its therapeutic effect comes from actions on the central nervous system

**Use** Relief of discomfort associated with acute, painful musculoskeletal conditions

**USUAL DOSAGE** Children >12 years and Adults: Oral: 800 mg 3-4 times/day

**Dosage Forms Tab:** 400 mg

**Contraindications** Impaired hepatic or renal function, known hypersensitivity to metaxalone, history of drug-induced hemolytic anemias or other anemias

**Warnings/Precautions** Use with caution in patients with impaired hepatic function

**Pregnancy Risk Factor** C

### Adverse Reactions
>10%:

Gastrointestinal: Nausea, vomiting, stomach cramps

Central nervous system: Paradoxical stimulation, headache, drowsiness, dizziness

<1%:
    Dermatologic: Allergic dermatitis
    Hematologic: Leukopenia, hemolytic anemia
    Hepatic: Hepatotoxicity
    Miscellaneous: Anaphylaxis
**Drug Interactions** Increased effect of alcohol, CNS depressants
**Special PA Issues**
    **Patient Education:** Avoid alcohol and other CNS depressants; may cause drowsiness, impairment of judgment, or coordination; notify physician of dark urine, pale stools, yellowing of eyes, severe nausea, vomiting, or abdominal pain

# Metformin (met FOR min)

**Pharmacologic Class** Antidiabetic Agent (Biguanide)
**U.S. Brand Names** Glucophage®
**Mechanism of Action** Decreases hepatic glucose production, decreasing intestinal absorption of glucose and improves insulin sensitivity (increases peripheral glucose uptake and utilization)
**Use** Management of noninsulin-dependent diabetes mellitus (type II) as monotherapy when hyperglycemia cannot be managed on diet alone. May be used concomitantly with a sulfonylurea when diet and metformin or sulfonylurea alone do not result in adequate glycemic control.
    **Investigational:** Data suggests that some patients with NIDDM with secondary failure to sulfonylurea therapy may obtain significant improvement in metabolic control when metformin in combination with insulin and a sulfonylurea is used in lieu of insulin alone
**USUAL DOSAGE** Oral (allow 1-2 weeks between dose titrations): Generally, clinically significant responses are not seen at doses <1500 mg daily; however, a lower recommended starting dose and gradual increased dosage is recommended to minimize gastrointestinal symptoms
    Adults:
        500 mg tablets: Initial: 500 mg twice daily (give with the morning and evening meals). Dosage increases should be made in increments of 1 tablet every week, given in divided doses, up to a maximum of 2500 mg/day. Doses of up to 2000 mg/day may be given twice daily. If a dose of 2500 mg/day is required, it may be better tolerated 3 times/day (with meals).
        850 mg tablets: Initial: 850 mg once daily (give with the morning meal). Dosage increases should be made in increments of 1 tablet every **other** week, given in divided doses, up to a maximum of 2550 mg/day. Usual maintenance dose: 850 mg twice daily (with the morning and evening meals). Some patients may be given 850 mg 3 times/day (with meals).
    Elderly: The initial and maintenance dosing should be conservative, due to the potential for decreased renal function. Generally, elderly patients should not be titrated to the maximum dose of metformin.
    **Transfer from other antidiabetic agents:** No transition period is generally necessary except when transferring from chlorpropamide. When transferring from chlorpropamide, care should be exercised during the first 2 weeks because of the prolonged retention of chlorpropamide in the body, leading to overlapping drug effects and possible hypoglycemia.
    **Concomitant metformin and oral sulfonylurea therapy:** If patients have not responded to 4 weeks of the maximum dose of metformin monotherapy, consideration to a gradual addition of an oral sulfonylurea while continuing metformin at the maximum dose, even if prior primary or secondary failure to a sulfonylurea has occurred.
    **Dosing adjustment/comments in renal impairment:** The plasma and blood half-life of metformin is prolonged and the renal clearance is decreased in proportion to the decrease in creatinine clearance. Metformin is contraindicated in the presence of renal dysfunction defined as a serum creatinine >1.5 mg/dL in males or >1.4 mg/dL in females or an abnormal creatinine clearance.
    **Dosing adjustment in hepatic impairment:** No studies have been conducted, however, metformin should be avoided because the presence of liver disease is a risk factor for the development of lactic acidosis during metformin therapy.
**Dosage Forms Tab, as hydrochloride:** 500 mg, 625 mg, 750 mg, 850 mg, 1000 mg
**Contraindications** Hypersensitivity to metformin or any component; renal disease or renal dysfunction (serum creatinine ≥1.5 mg/dL in males or ≥1.4 mg/dL in females or creatinine clearance <60 mL/minute) which may also result from conditions such as cardiovascular collapse, acute myocardial infarction, and septicemia; acute or chronic metabolic acidosis with or without coma (including diabetic ketoacidosis); should be temporarily withheld (at the time or prior to the procedure and withheld for 48 hours subsequent to the procedure and reinstituted only after renal function has been re-evaluated and found to be normal) in patients undergoing radiologic studies involving the parenteral administration of iodinated contrast materials (potential for acute alteration in renal function)
**Warnings/Precautions** Administration of oral antidiabetic drugs has been reported to be associated with increased cardiovascular mortality as compared to treatment with diet alone
(Continued)

## Metformin (Continued)

or diet plus insulin. Metformin is substantially excreted by the kidney - the risk of accumulation and lactic acidosis increases with the degree of impairment of renal function. Patients with renal function below the limit of normal for their age should not receive metformin. In elderly patients, renal function should be monitored regularly. Use of concomitant medications that may affect renal function (ie, affect tubular secretion) may affect metformin disposition. Therapy should be suspended for any surgical procedures. Avoid use in patients with impaired liver function. Metformin should be discontinued at the time of or prior to the procedure in patients undergoing radiologic studies in which intravascular iodinated contrast materials are utilized, and withheld for 48 hours subsequent to the procedure, and reinstituted only after renal function has been re-evaluated and found to be normal.

**Pregnancy Risk Factor** B

**Adverse Reactions**

>10%: Gastrointestinal: Anorexia, nausea, vomiting, diarrhea, epigastric fullness, constipation, heartburn

1% to 10%:

Dermatologic: Rash, urticaria, photosensitivity

Miscellaneous: Decreased vitamin $B_{12}$ levels

<1%: Blood dyscrasias, aplastic anemia, hemolytic anemia, bone marrow suppression, thrombocytopenia, agranulocytosis

**Drug Interactions**

Decreased effect: Drugs which tend to produce hyperglycemia (eg, diuretics, corticosteroids, phenothiazines, thyroid products, estrogens, oral contraceptives, phenytoin, nicotinic acid, sympathomimetics, calcium channel blocking drugs, isoniazid) may lead to a loss of glycemic control

Increased effect: Furosemide increased the metformin plasma and blood $C_{max}$ without altering metformin renal clearance in a single dose study

Increased toxicity:

Cationic drugs (eg, amilcride, digoxin, morphine, procainamide, quinidine, quinine, ranitidine, triamterene, trimethoprim, and vancomycin) which are eliminated by renal tubular secretion could have the potential for interaction with metformin by competing for common renal tubular transport systems

Cimetidine increases (by 60%) peak metformin plasma and whole blood concentrations

**Onset** Within days, maximum effects up to 2 weeks

**Half-Life** 6.2 hours; prolonged in renal impairment

**Special PA Issues**

Patient Education: Ideally, you will probably be referred to a diabetic educator for diabetic counseling. Eat regularly; do not skip meals. Carry a quick sugar source. Monitor serum glucose as directed. Do not alter dosage or discontinue current medications or introduce new medications without consulting prescriber. Avoid alcohol while taking this drug (disulfiram reactions). You may be sensitive to sun; avoid excessive exposure and use appropriate sunblock and clothing. Report unresolved nausea or vomiting, constipation or diarrhea, headache, anorexia, or skin rash.

**Dietary Considerations:**

Alcohol: Incidence of lactic acidosis may be increased; avoid or limit use

Food: Food decreases the extent and slightly delays the absorption. Drug may cause GI upset; take with food to decrease GI upset.

Glucose: Decreases blood glucose concentration. Hypoglycemia does not usually occur unless a patient is predisposed. Monitor blood glucose concentration. Exercise caution with administration in patients predisposed to hypoglycemia (eg, cases of reduced caloric intake, strenuous exercise without repletion of calories, alcohol ingestion or when metformin is combined with another oral antidiabetic agent).

Vitamin $B_{12}$: Decreases absorption of Vitamin $B_{12}$; monitor for signs and symptoms of vitamin $B_{12}$ deficiency

Folic acid: Decreases absorption of folic acid; monitor for signs and symptoms of folic acid deficiency

Monitoring Parameters: Urine for glucose and ketones, fasting blood glucose, hemoglobin $A_{1c}$, and fructosamine. Initial and periodic monitoring of hematologic parameters (eg, hemoglobin/hematocrit and red blood cell indices) and renal function should be performed, at least annually. While megaloblastic anemia has been rarely seen with metformin, if suspected, vitamin $B_{12}$ deficiency should be excluded.

Reference Range: Target range: Adults: Fasting blood glucose: <120 mg/dL; Glycosylated hemoglobin: <7%

**Related Information**

Hypoglycemic Drugs on page 1020

♦ **Metformin Hydrochloride** see Metformin on previous page

## Methacholine (meth a KOLE leen)

Pharmacologic Class Cholinergic Agonist; Diagnostic Agent, Bronchial Airway Hyperactivity

U.S. Brand Names Provocholine®

**Mechanism of Action** Methacholine chloride is a cholinergic (parasympathomimetic) synthetic analogue of acetylcholine. The drug stimulates muscarinic, postganglionic parasympathetic receptors, which results in smooth muscle contraction of the airways and increased tracheobronchial secretions.

**Use** Diagnosis of bronchial airway hyperactivity in subjects who do not have clinically apparent asthma

**USUAL DOSAGE** Before inhalation challenge, perform baseline pulmonary function tests; the patient must have an $FEV_1$ of at least 70% of the predicted value. The following is a suggested schedule for administration of methacholine challenge. Calculate cumulative units by multiplying number of breaths by concentration given. Total cumulative units is the sum of cumulative units for each concentration given. See table.

**Methacholine**

| Vial | Serial Concentration (mg/mL) | No. of Breaths | Cumulative Units per Concentration | Total Cumulative Units |
|------|------|------|------|------|
| E | 0.025 | 5 | 0.125 | 0.125 |
| D | 0.25 | 5 | 1.25 | 1.375 |
| C | 2.5 | 5 | 12.5 | 13.88 |
| B | 10 | 5 | 50 | 63.88 |
| A | 25 | 5 | 125 | 188.88 |

Determine $FEV_1$ within 5 minutes of challenge, a positive challenge is a 20% reduction in $FEV_1$

**Dosage Forms Powder for reconstitution, inhalation, as chloride:** 100 mg/5 mL

**Contraindications** Concomitant use of beta-blockers; hypersensitivity to the drug; because of the potential for severe bronchoconstriction, methacholine challenge should not be performed on any patient with clinically apparent asthma, wheezing, or very low baseline pulmonary function tests (forced expiratory volume in one second less than 70% of predicted value).

**Warnings/Precautions** Methacholine is a bronchoconstrictor for diagnostic purposes only. Perform inhalation challenge under the supervision of a physician trained in and thoroughly familiar with all aspects of the technique, all contraindications, warnings, and precautions of methacholine challenge and the management of respiratory distress. Have emergency equipment and medication immediately available to treat acute respiratory distress. Administer only by inhalation; severe bronchoconstriction and reduction in respiratory function can result. Patients with severe hyper-reactivity of the airways can experience bronchoconstriction at a dosage as low as 0.025 mg/mL (0.125 cumulative units). If severe bronchoconstriction occurs, reverse immediately by administration of a rapid-acting inhaled bronchodilator (beta-agonist).

**Pregnancy Risk Factor** C

**Adverse Reactions** <1%: Hypotension, complete heart block, substernal pain, tightness of the chest, syncope, headache, lightheadedness, throat irritation, itching, cough, dyspnea, wheezing

♦ **Methacholine Chloride** see Methacholine on previous page

# Methadone (METH a done)

**Pharmacologic Class** Analgesic, Narcotic

**U.S. Brand Names** Dolophine®

**Mechanism of Action** Binds to opiate receptors in the CNS, causing inhibition of ascending pain pathways, altering the perception of and response to pain; produces generalized CNS depression

**Use** Management of severe pain, used in narcotic detoxification maintenance programs

**USUAL DOSAGE** Doses should be titrated to appropriate effects

Children: Analgesia:

Oral, I.M., S.C.: 0.7 mg/kg/24 hours divided every 4-6 hours as needed or 0.1-0.2 mg/kg every 4-12 hours as needed; maximum: 10 mg/dose

I.V.: 0.1 mg/kg every 4 hours initially for 2-3 doses, then every 6-12 hours as needed; maximum: 10 mg/dose

Adults:

Analgesia: Oral, I.M., S.C.: 2.5-10 mg every 3-8 hours as needed, up to 5-20 mg every 6-8 hours

Detoxification: Oral: 15-40 mg/day; should not exceed 21 days and may not be repeated earlier than 4 weeks after completion of preceding course

Maintenance of opiate dependence: Oral: 20-120 mg/day

**Dosing adjustment in renal impairment:** $Cl_{cr}$ <10 mL/minute: Administer at 50% to 75% of normal dose

**Dosing adjustment/comments in hepatic disease:** Avoid in severe liver disease

(Continued)

## Methadone *(Continued)*

**Important note:** Methadone accumulates with repeated doses and dosage may need to be adjusted downward after 3-5 days to prevent toxic effects. Some patients may benefit from every 8- to 12-hour dosing interval (pain control).

**Dosage Forms Inj:** 10 mg/mL (1 mL, 10 mL, 20 mL); **Soln:** Oral: 5 mg/5 mL (5 mL, 500 mL); 10 mg/5 mL (500 mL), Oral, concentrate: 10 mg/mL (30 mL); **Tab:** 5 mg, 10 mg; **Tab, dispersible:** 40 mg

**Contraindications** Hypersensitivity to methadone or any component

**Warnings/Precautions** Tablets are to be used only for oral administration and **must not** be used for injection; use with caution in patients with respiratory diseases including asthma, emphysema, or COPD and in patients with severe liver disease; because methadone's effects on respiration last much longer than its analgesic effects, the dose must be titrated slowly; because of its long half-life and risk of accumulation, it is not considered a drug of first choice in the elderly, who may be particularly susceptible to its CNS depressant and constipating effects; tolerance or drug dependence may result from extended use

**Pregnancy Risk Factor** B (D if used for prolonged periods or in high doses at term)

**Adverse Reactions**

Percentage unknown: CNS depression, antidiuretic hormone release, miosis, respiratory depression

>10%:

Cardiovascular: Palpitations, hypotension, bradycardia, peripheral vasodilation

Central nervous system: Fatigue, drowsiness, dizziness

Gastrointestinal: Nausea, vomiting, constipation

Neuromuscular & skeletal: Weakness

Miscellaneous: Histamine release

1% to 10%:

Central nervous system: Nervousness, headache, restlessness, anorexia, malaise, confusion, increased intracranial pressure

Gastrointestinal: Stomach cramps, xerostomia, biliary tract spasm

Genitourinary: Decreased urination, urinary tract spasm

Local: Pain at injection site

Respiratory: Dyspnea, shortness of breath

<1%: Mental depression, hallucinations, paradoxical CNS stimulation, pruritus, rash, urticaria, paralytic ileus, physical and psychological dependence, increased LFTs

**Drug Interactions** CYP1A2, 2D6, and 3A3/4 enzyme substrate; CYP2D6 inhibitor

Decreased effect: Phenytoin, pentazocine and rifampin may increase the metabolism of methadone and may precipitate withdrawal

Increased toxicity: CNS depressants, phenothiazines, tricyclic antidepressants, MAO inhibitors may potentiate the adverse effects of methadone

**Onset**

Oral: Onset of analgesia: Within 0.5-1 hour

Parenteral: Onset of analgesia: Within 10-20 minutes; Peak effect: Within 1-2 hours

**Duration** Oral: 6-8 hours, increases to 22-48 hours with repeated doses

**Half-Life** 15-29 hours, may be prolonged with alkaline pH

**Special PA Issues**

**Patient Education:** If self-administered, use exactly as directed (do not increase dose or frequency); may cause physical and/or psychological dependence. While using this medication, do not use alcohol and other prescription or OTC medications (especially sedatives, tranquilizers, antihistamines, or pain medications) without consulting prescriber. Maintain adequate hydration (2-3 L/day of fluids unless instructed to restrict fluid intake). May cause hypotension, dizziness, drowsiness, impaired coordination, or blurred vision (use caution when driving, climbing stairs, or changing position - rising from sitting or lying to standing, or when engaging in hazardous activities until response to medication is known); loss of appetite, nausea, or vomiting (frequent mouth care, small frequent meals, or sucking on lozenges may help); constipation (increased exercise, fluids, or dietary fruit and fiber may help - if constipation remains an unresolved problem, consult prescriber about use of stool softeners). Report chest pain, slow or rapid heartbeat, acute dizziness or persistent headache; changes in mental status; swelling of extremities or unusual weight gain; changes in urinary elimination; acute headache; back or flank pain or muscle spasms; blurred vision, skin rash; or shortness of breath.

**Dietary Considerations:**

Alcohol: Additive CNS effects, avoid or limit alcohol; watch for sedation

Food: Glucose may cause hyperglycemia; monitor blood glucose concentrations

**Monitoring Parameters:** Pain relief, respiratory and mental status, blood pressure

**Reference Range:** Therapeutic: 100-400 ng/mL (SI: 0.32-1.29 µmol/L); Toxic: >2 µg/mL (SI: >6.46 µmol/L)

**Related Information**

Narcotic Agonists *on page 1023*

♦ **Methadone Hydrochloride** *see* Methadone *on previous page*

♦ **Methadose®** *see* Methadone *on previous page*

◆ **Methaminodiazepoxide Hydrochloride** *see* Chlordiazepoxide *on page 189*

# Methamphetamine *(meth am FET a meen)*
**Pharmacologic Class** Stimulant
**U.S. Brand Names** Desoxyn®; Desoxyn Gradumet®
**Use** Treatment of narcolepsy, exogenous obesity, abnormal behavioral syndrome in children (minimal brain dysfunction)
**USUAL DOSAGE**
   Attention deficit disorder: Children >6 years: 2.5-5 mg 1-2 times/day, may increase by 5 mg increments weekly until optimum response is achieved, usually 20-25 mg/day
   Exogenous obesity: Children >12 years and Adults: 5 mg, 30 minutes before each meal; long-acting formulation: 10-15 mg in morning; treatment duration should not exceed a few weeks
**Dosage Forms** Methamphetamine hydrochloride: **Tab:** 5 mg; **Tab, extended release (Gradumet®):** 5 mg, 10 mg, 15 mg
**Contraindications** Known hypersensitivity to methamphetamine
**Warnings/Precautions** Cardiovascular disease, nephritis, angina pectoris, hypertension, glaucoma, patients with a history of drug abuse, known hypersensitivity to amphetamine
**Pregnancy Risk Factor** C
**Adverse Reactions**
   >10%:
      Cardiovascular: Arrhythmia
      Central nervous system: False feeling of well being, nervousness, restlessness, insomnia
   1% to 10%:
      Cardiovascular: Hypertension
      Central nervous system: Mood or mental changes, dizziness, lightheadedness, headache
      Endocrine & metabolic: Changes in libido
      Gastrointestinal: Diarrhea, nausea, vomiting, stomach cramps, constipation, anorexia, weight loss, xerostomia
      Ocular: Blurred vision
      Miscellaneous: Diaphoresis (increased)
   <1%: Chest pain, CNS stimulation (severe), Tourette's syndrome, hyperthermia, seizures, paranoia, rash, urticaria, tolerance and withdrawal with prolonged use
**Drug Interactions** CYP2D6 enzyme substrate
   Increased toxicity with MAO inhibitors (hypertensive crisis)
**Duration** 12-24 hours
**Half-Life** 4-5 hours
**Special PA Issues**
   **Patient Education:** Take exactly as directed (do not increase dose or frequency without consulting prescriber); may cause physical and/or psychological dependence. Do not crush extended release tablets. Take early in day to avoid sleep disturbance, 30 minutes before meals. Avoid alcohol, caffeine, or OTC medications that act as stimulants. You may experience restlessness, false sense of euphoria, or impaired judgment (use caution when driving or engaging in hazardous activities); dry mouth (frequent mouth care, sucking on lozenges, or chewing gum may help); nausea or vomiting (small frequent meals, frequent mouth care may help); constipation (increased exercise, dietary fiber, fruit, or fluid may help); diarrhea (buttermilk, boiled milk, or yogurt may help); or altered libido (reversible). Diabetics need to monitor serum glucose closely (may alter antidiabetic medication requirements). Report chest pain, palpitations, or irregular heartbeat; extreme fatigue or depression; CNS changes (aggressiveness, restlessness, euphoria, sleep disturbances); severe unremitting abdominal distress or cramping; changes in sexual activity; or blurred vision.
   **Monitoring Parameters:** Heart rate, respiratory rate, blood pressure, and CNS activity

◆ **Methamphetamine Hydrochloride** *see* Methamphetamine *on this page*

# Methazolamide *(meth a ZOE la mide)*
**Pharmacologic Class** Carbonic Anhydrase Inhibitor; Diuretic, Carbonic Anhydrase Inhibitor; Ophthalmic Agent, Antiglaucoma
**U.S. Brand Names** GlaucTabs®; Neptazane®
**Mechanism of Action** Noncompetitive inhibition of the enzyme carbonic anhydrase; thought that carbonic anhydrase is located at the luminal border of cells of the proximal tubule. When the enzyme is inhibited, there is an increase in urine volume and a change to an alkaline pH with a subsequent decrease in the excretion of titratable acid and ammonia.
**Use** Adjunctive treatment of open-angle or secondary glaucoma; short-term therapy of narrow-angle glaucoma when delay of surgery is desired
**USUAL DOSAGE** Adults: Oral: 50-100 mg 2-3 times/day
**Dosage Forms** Tab: 25 mg, 50 mg
**Contraindications** Marked kidney or liver dysfunction, severe pulmonary obstruction, hypersensitivity to methazolamide or any component
**Warnings/Precautions** Sulfonamide-type reactions, melena, anorexia, nausea, vomiting, constipation, hematuria, glycosuria, urinary frequency, renal colic, renal calculi, crystalluria, *(Continued)*

## Methazolamide *(Continued)*

polyuria, hepatic insufficiency, various CNS effects, transient myopia, bone marrow suppression, thrombocytopenia/purpura, hemolytic anemia, leukopenia, pancytopenia, agranulocytosis, urticaria, pruritus, rash, Stevens-Johnson syndrome, weight loss, fever, acidosis; use with caution in patients with respiratory acidosis and diabetes mellitus; impairment of mental alertness and/or physical coordination. Malaise and complaints of tiredness and myalgia are signs of excessive dosing and acidosis in the elderly.

**Pregnancy Risk Factor** C

**Adverse Reactions**
>10%:
    Central nervous system: Malaise
    Gastrointestinal: Metallic taste, anorexia
    Genitourinary: Polyuria
    Neuromuscular & skeletal: Weakness
1% to 10%:
    Central nervous system: Mental depression, drowsiness, dizziness
    Genitourinary: Crystalluria
<1%: Fever, headache, seizures, fatigue, rash, sulfonamide rash, Stevens-Johnson syndrome, hyperchloremic metabolic acidosis, hypokalemia, hyperglycemia, GI irritation, constipation, xerostomia, black tarry stools, bone marrow suppression, dysuria, paresthesia, trembling, unsteadiness, myopia, tinnitus, loss of smell, hypersensitivity

**Drug Interactions**
Increased toxicity:
    May induce hypokalemia which would sensitize a patient to digitalis toxicity
    May increase the potential for salicylate toxicity
    Hypokalemia may be compounded with concurrent diuretic use or steroids
    Primidone absorption may be delayed
Decreased effect: Increased lithium excretion and altered excretion of other drugs by alkalinization of the urine, such as amphetamines, quinidine, procainamide, methenamine, phenobarbital, salicylates

**Onset** Slow in comparison with acetazolamide (2-4 hours); Peak effect: 6-8 hours

**Duration** 10-18 hours

**Half-Life** ~14 hours

**Special PA Issues**
**Patient Education:** Take with food; swallow whole, do not chew or crush. You may experience gastrointestinal upset and loss of appetite; frequent small meals are advised to reduce these effects and the metallic taste that sometimes occurs with this medication. You may experience lightheadedness, depression, dizziness, or weakness for a few days; use caution when driving or engaging in hazardous tasks until this disappears. Report excessive tiredness; loss of appetite; cramping, pain, or weakness in muscles; acute GI symptoms; changes in CNS (depression, drowsiness); difficulty or pain on urination; visual changes; or skin rash.

## Methenamine *(meth EN a meen)*

**Pharmacologic Class** Antibiotic, Miscellaneous

**U.S. Brand Names** Hiprex®; Mandelamine®; Urex®

**Mechanism of Action** Methenamine is hydrolyzed to formaldehyde and ammonia in acidic urine; formaldehyde has nonspecific bactericidal action

**Use** Prophylaxis or suppression of recurrent urinary tract infections; urinary tract discomfort secondary to hypermotility

**USUAL DOSAGE** Oral:
Children:
    <6 years: 0.25 g/30 lb 4 times/day
    6-12 years:
        Hippurate: 25-50 mg/kg/day divided every 12 hours or 0.5-1 g twice daily
        Mandelate: 50-75 mg/kg/day divided every 6 hours or 0.5 g 4 times/day
Children >12 years and Adults:
    Hippurate: 1 g twice daily
    Mandelate: 1 g 4 times/day after meals and at bedtime
**Dosing adjustment/comments in renal impairment:** Cl$_{cr}$ <50 mL/minute: Avoid use

**Dosage Forms** Methenamine hippurate: **Tab, (Hiprex®, Urex®):** 1 g (Hiprex® contains tartrazine dye)
Methenamine mandelate: **Tab, enteric coated:** 250 mg, 500 mg, 1 g

**Contraindications** Severe dehydration, renal insufficiency, hepatic insufficiency in patients receiving hippurate salt, hypersensitivity to methenamine or any component; patients receiving sulfonamides

**Warnings/Precautions** Use with caution in patients with hepatic disease, gout, and the elderly; doses of 8 g/day for 3-4 weeks may cause bladder irritation, some products may contain tartrazine; methenamine should not be used to treat infections outside of the lower urinary tract. Use care to maintain an acid pH of the urine, especially when treating infections due to urea splitting organisms (eg, *Proteus* and strains of *Pseudomonas*);

reversible increases in LFTs have occurred during therapy especially in patients with hepatic dysfunction.

**Pregnancy Risk Factor** C

**Adverse Reactions**
1% to 10%:
Dermatologic: Rash (3.5%)
Gastrointestinal: Nausea, dyspepsia (3.5%)
Genitourinary: Dysuria (3.5%)
<1%: Bladder irritation, crystalluria (especially with large doses), increased AST/ALT (reversible, rare)

**Drug Interactions**
Decreased effect: Sodium bicarbonate and acetazolamide will decrease effect secondary to alkalinization of urine
Increased toxicity: Sulfonamides (may precipitate)

**Half-Life** 3-6 hours

**Special PA Issues**
**Patient Education:** Take with food or cranberry juice at intervals around-the-clock. Maintain adequate hydration (2-3 L/day of fluids unless instructed to restrict fluid intake). Avoid excessive alkalizing food or medications (eg, citrus fruits, milk products, sodium bicarbonate). Small frequent meals may help reduce nausea or vomiting. Report painful urination, rash, unresolved GI distress, or blood in urine.
**Monitoring Parameters:** Urinalysis, periodic liver function tests in patients

♦ **Methenamine Hippurate** *see* Methenamine *on previous page*

♦ **Methenamine Mandelate** *see* Methenamine *on previous page*

♦ **Methergine®** *see* Methylergonovine *on page 592*

# Methicillin (meth i SIL in)

**Pharmacologic Class** Antibiotic, Penicillin

**U.S. Brand Names** Staphcillin®

**Mechanism of Action** Inhibits bacterial cell wall synthesis by binding to one or more of the penicillin binding proteins (PBPs); which in turn inhibits the final transpeptidation step of peptidoglycan synthesis in bacterial cell walls, thus inhibiting cell wall biosynthesis. Bacteria eventually lyse due to ongoing activity of cell wall autolytic enzymes (autolysins and murein hydrolases) while cell wall assembly is arrested.

**Use** Treatment of susceptible bacterial infections such as osteomyelitis, septicemia, endocarditis, and CNS infections due to penicillinase-producing strains of *Staphylococcus*; other antistaphylococcal penicillins are usually preferred

**USUAL DOSAGE** I.M., I.V.:
Infants:
>7 days and >2000 g: 100 mg/kg/day in divided doses every 6 hours (for meningitis: 200 mg/kg/day)
>7 days and <2000 g: 75 mg/kg/day in divided doses every 8 hours (for meningitis: 150 mg/kg/day)
<7 days and >2000 g: Same as above
<7 days and <2000 g: 50 mg/kg/day in divided doses every 12 hours (for meningitis: 100 mg/kg/day)
Children: 100-300 mg/kg/day in divided doses every 4-6 hours
Adults: 4-12 g/day in divided doses every 4-6 hours
**Dosing interval in renal impairment:**
Cl$_{cr}$ 10-50 mL/minute: Administer every 6-8 hours
Cl$_{cr}$ <10 mL/minute: Administer every 8-12 hours
Hemodialysis: Not dialyzable (0% to 5%)

**Dosage Forms Powder for inj, as sodium:** 1 g, 4 g, 6 g, 10 g

**Contraindications** Known hypersensitivity to methicillin or any penicillin

**Warnings/Precautions** Elimination rate will be slow in neonates; modify dosage in patients with renal impairment and in the elderly; use with caution in patients with cephalosporin hypersensitivity

**Pregnancy Risk Factor** B

**Adverse Reactions**
1% to 10%:
Dermatologic: Rash
Renal: Acute interstitial nephritis
<1%: Fever, rash, hemorrhagic cystitis, eosinophilia, anemia, leukopenia, neutropenia, thrombocytopenia, phlebitis, serum sickness-like reactions

**Drug Interactions**
Decreased effect: Efficacy of oral contraceptives may be reduced
Increased effect: Disulfiram, probenecid may increase penicillin levels, increased effect of anticoagulants

**Half-Life** Normal renal function: 0.4-0.5 hour
(Continued)

## Methicillin *(Continued)*

### Special PA Issues

**Patient Education:** This medication can only be administered by injection. Maintain adequate hydration (2-3 L/day of fluids unless instructed to restrict fluid intake). Small frequent meals, frequent mouth care, and adequate fluids may reduce the incidence of nausea or vomiting. If diabetic, drug may cause false tests with Clinitest® urine glucose monitoring; use of glucose oxidase methods (Clinistix®) or serum glucose monitoring is preferable. This drug may interfere with oral contraceptives; an alternate form of birth control should be used. Report difficulty breathing, acute diarrhea, systemic rash, fever, white plaques in mouth or mouth sores.

**Monitoring Parameters:** Observe for signs and symptoms of anaphylaxis during first dose

♦ **Methicillin Sodium** *see Methicillin on previous page*

## Methimazole *(meth IM a zole)*

**Pharmacologic Class** Antithyroid Agent

**U.S. Brand Names** Tapazole®

**Mechanism of Action** Inhibits the synthesis of thyroid hormones by blocking the oxidation of iodine in the thyroid gland, blocking iodine's ability to combine with tyrosine to form thyroxine and triiodothyronine ($T_3$), does not inactivate circulating $T_4$ and $T_3$

**Use** Palliative treatment of hyperthyroidism, return the hyperthyroid patient to a normal metabolic state prior to thyroidectomy, and to control thyrotoxic crisis that may accompany thyroidectomy. The use of antithyroid thioamides is as effective in elderly as they are in younger adults; however, the expense, potential adverse effects, and inconvenience (compliance, monitoring) make them undesirable. The use of radioiodine due to ease of administration and less concern for long-term side effects and reproduction problems (some older males) makes it a more appropriate therapy.

**USUAL DOSAGE** Oral: Administer in 3 equally divided doses at approximately 8-hour intervals

Children: Initial: 0.4 mg/kg/day in 3 divided doses; maintenance: 0.2 mg/kg/day in 3 divided doses up to 30 mg/24 hours maximum

Alternatively: Initial: 0.5-0.7 mg/kg/day or 15-20 mg/m²/day in 3 divided doses

Maintenance: $1/3$ to $2/3$ of the initial dose beginning when the patient is euthyroid

Maximum: 30 mg/24 hours

Adults: Initial: 15 mg/day for mild hyperthyroidism; 30-40 mg/day in moderately severe hyperthyroidism; 60 mg/day in severe hyperthyroidism; maintenance: 5-15 mg/day

Adjust dosage as required to achieve and maintain serum $T_3$, $T_4$, and TSH levels in the normal range. An elevated $T_3$ may be the sole indicator of inadequate treatment. An elevated TSH indicates excessive antithyroid treatment.

**Dosing adjustment in renal impairment:** Adjustment is not necessary

**Dosage Forms** Tab: 5 mg, 10 mg

**Contraindications** Hypersensitivity to methimazole or any component, nursing mothers

**Warnings/Precautions** Use with extreme caution in patients receiving other drugs known to cause myelosuppression particularly agranulocytosis, patients >40 years of age; avoid doses >40 mg/day (↑ myelosuppression); may cause acneiform eruptions or worsen the condition of the thyroid

**Pregnancy Risk Factor** D

**Adverse Reactions**

>10%:

Central nervous system: Fever

Dermatologic: Rash

Hematologic: Leukopenia

1% to 10%:

Central nervous system: Dizziness

Gastrointestinal: Nausea, vomiting, stomach pain, abnormal taste

Hematologic: Agranulocytosis

Miscellaneous: SLE-like syndrome

<1%: Edema, drowsiness, vertigo, headache, rash, urticaria, pruritus, alopecia, goiter, constipation, weight gain, nephrotic syndrome, thrombocytopenia, aplastic anemia, cholestatic jaundice, arthralgia, paresthesia, swollen salivary glands

**Drug Interactions** Increased toxicity: Iodinated glycerol, lithium, potassium iodide; anticoagulant activity increased

**Onset** Onset of antithyroid effect: Oral: Within 30-40 minutes

**Duration** 2-4 hours

**Half-Life** 4-13 hours

### Special PA Issues

**Patient Education:** Take as directed, at same time each day around-the-clock; do not miss doses or make up missed doses. This drug will need to be taken for an extended period of time to achieve appropriate results. You may experience nausea or vomiting (small frequent meals may help), dizziness or drowsiness (use caution when driving or engaging in hazardous activities). Report rash, fever, unusual bleeding or bruising, unresolved headache, yellowing of eyes or skin, or changes in color of urine or feces, unresolved malaise.

**Monitoring Parameters:** Monitor for signs of hypothyroidism, hyperthyroidism, $T_4$, $T_3$; CBC with differential, liver function (baseline and as needed), serum thyroxine, free thyroxine index

## Methocarbamol (meth oh KAR ba mole)

**Pharmacologic Class** Skeletal Muscle Relaxant

**U.S. Brand Names** Delaxin®; Marbaxin®; Robaxin®; Robomol®

**Mechanism of Action** Causes skeletal muscle relaxation by reducing the transmission of impulses from the spinal cord to skeletal muscle

**Use** Treatment of muscle spasm associated with acute painful musculoskeletal conditions, supportive therapy in tetanus

**USUAL DOSAGE**

Children: Recommended **only** for use in tetanus I.V.: 15 mg/kg/dose or 500 mg/m²/dose, may repeat every 6 hours if needed; maximum dose: 1.8 g/m²/day for 3 days only

Adults: Muscle spasm:

Oral: 1.5 g 4 times/day for 2-3 days, then decrease to 4-4.5 g/day in 3-6 divided doses

I.M., I.V.: 1 g every 8 hours if oral not possible

**Dosing adjustment/comments in renal impairment:** Do not administer parenteral formulation to patients with renal dysfunction

**Dosage Forms Inj:** 100 mg/mL in polyethylene glycol 50% (10 mL); **Tab:** 500 mg, 750 mg

**Contraindications** Renal impairment, hypersensitivity to methocarbamol or any component

**Warnings/Precautions** Rate of injection should not exceed 3 mL/minute; solution is hypertonic; avoid extravasation; use with caution in patients with a history of seizures

**Pregnancy Risk Factor** C

**Adverse Reactions**

>10%: Central nervous system: Drowsiness, dizziness, lightheadedness

1% to 10%:

Cardiovascular: Flushing of face, bradycardia

Dermatologic: Allergic dermatitis

Gastrointestinal: Nausea, vomiting

Ocular: Nystagmus

Respiratory: Nasal congestion

<1%: Syncope, convulsion, leukopenia, pain at injection site, thrombophlebitis, blurred vision, renal impairment, allergic manifestations

**Drug Interactions** Increased effect/toxicity with CNS depressants

**Onset** Onset of muscle relaxation: Oral: Within 30 minutes

**Half-Life** 1-2 hours

**Special PA Issues**

**Patient Education:** Take exactly as directed. Do not increase dose or discontinue without consulting prescriber. Do not use alcohol, prescriptive or OTC antidepressants, sedatives, or pain medications without consulting prescriber. You may experience drowsiness, dizziness, lightheadedness (avoid driving or engaging in tasks that require alertness until response to therapy is known); or nausea or vomiting (small, frequent meals, frequent mouth care, or sucking hard candy may help). Report excessive drowsiness or mental agitation, chest pain, skin rash, swelling of mouth/face, difficulty speaking, or vision disturbances.

**Dietary Considerations:** Alcohol: Additive CNS effect, avoid use

## Methocarbamol and Aspirin (meth oh KAR ba mole & AS pir in)

**Pharmacologic Class** Skeletal Muscle Relaxant

**U.S. Brand Names** Robaxisal®

**Dosage Forms Tab:** Methocarbamol 400 mg and aspirin 325 mg

## Methotrexate (meth oh TREKS ate)

**Pharmacologic Class** Antineoplastic Agent, Antimetabolite

**U.S. Brand Names** Folex® PFS; Rheumatrex®

**Mechanism of Action** An antimetabolite that inhibits DNA synthesis and cell reproduction in malignant cells

Folates must be in the reduced form ($FH_4$) to be active

Folates are activated by dihydrofolate reductase (DHFR)

DHFR is inhibited by MTX (by binding irreversibly), causing an increase in the intracellular dihydrofolate pool (the inactive cofactor) and inhibition of both purine and thymidylate synthesis (TS)

MTX enters the cell through an energy-dependent and temperature-dependent process which is mediated by an intramembrane protein; this carrier mechanism is also used by naturally occurring reduced folates, including folinic acid (leucovorin), making this a competitive process

(Continued)

## Methotrexate *(Continued)*

At high drug concentrations (>20 µM), MTX enters the cell by a second mechanism which is not shared by reduced olates; the process may be passive diffusion or a specific, saturable process, and provides a rationale for high-dose MTX

A small fraction of MTX is converted intracellularly to polyglutamates, which leads to a prolonged inhibition of DHFR

The MOA in the treatment of rheumatoid arthritis is unknown, but may affect immune function

In psoriasis, methotrexate is thought to target rapidly proliferating epithelial cells in the skin

**Use** Treatment of trophoblastic neoplasms; leukemias; psoriasis; rheumatoid arthritis; breast, head and neck, and lung carcinomas; osteosarcoma; sarcomas; carcinoma of gastric, esophagus, testes; lymphomas

**USUAL DOSAGE** Refer to individual protocols. May be administered orally, I.M., intra-arterially, intrathecally, or I.V.

Leucovorin may be administered concomitantly or within 24 hours of methotrexate - refer to Leucovorin *on page 520* for details

Children:

Dermatomyositis: Oral: 15-20 mg/m²/week as a single dose once weekly or 0.3-1 mg/kg/dose once weekly

Juvenile rheumatoid arthritis: Oral, I.M.: 5-15 mg/m²/week as a single dose **or** as 3 divided doses given 12 hours apart

Antineoplastic dosage range:

Oral, I.M.: 7.5-30 mg/m²/week **or** every 2 weeks

I.V.: 10-18,000 mg/m² bolus dosing **or** continuous infusion over 6-42 hours

### Methotrexate Dosing Schedules

| Dose | Route | Frequency |
|---|---|---|
| Conventional | | |
| 15-20 mg/m² | P.O. | Twice weekly |
| 30-50 mg/m² | P.O., I.V. | Weekly |
| 15 mg/day for 5 days | P.O., I.M. | Every 2-3 weeks |
| Intermediate | | |
| 50-150 mg/m² | I.V. push | Every 2-3 weeks |
| 240 mg/m²* | I.V. infusion | Every 4-7 days |
| 0.5-1 g/m²* | I.V. infusion | Every 2-3 weeks |
| High | | |
| 1-12 g/m²* | I.V. infusion | Every 1-3 weeks |

*Followed with leucovorin rescue - refer to Leucovorin monograph for details.

Pediatric solid tumors (high-dose): I.V.:

<12 years: 12 g/m² (dosage range: 12-18 g)

≥12 years: 8 g/m² (maximum: 18 g)

Acute lymphocytic leukemia (intermediate-dose): I.V.: Loading: 100 mg/m² over 1 hour, followed by a 35-hour infusion of 900 mg/m²/day

Meningeal leukemia: I.T.: 10-15 mg/m² (maximum dose: 15 mg) **or**

≤3 months: 3 mg/dose

4-11 months: 6 mg/dose

1 year: 8 mg/dose

2 years: 10 mg/dose

≥3 years: 12 mg/dose

I.T. doses are prepared with preservative-free MTX only. Hydrocortisone may be added to the I.T. preparation; total volume should range from 3-6 mL. Doses should be repeated at 2- to 5-day intervals until CSF counts return to normal followed by a dose once weekly for 2 weeks then monthly thereafter.

Adults: I.V.: Range is wide from 30-40 mg/m²/week to 100-12,000 mg/m² with leucovorin rescue

Doses **not** requiring leucovorin rescue range from 30-40 mg/m² I.V. or I.M. repeated weekly, or oral regimens of 10 mg/m² twice weekly

**High-dose MTX is considered to be >100 mg/m²** and can be as high as 1500-7500 mg/m². These doses **require** leucovorin rescue. Patients receiving doses ≥1000 mg/m² should have their urine alkalinized with bicarbonate or Bicitra® prior to and following MTX therapy.

Trophoblastic neoplasms: Oral, I.M.: 15-30 mg/day for 5 days; repeat in 7 days for 3-5 courses

Head and neck cancer: Oral, I.M., I.V.: 25-50 mg/m² once weekly

Rheumatoid arthritis: Oral: 7.5 mg once weekly **OR** 2.5 mg every 12 hours for 3 doses/week; not to exceed 20 mg/week

Psoriasis: Oral: 2.5-5 mg/dose every 12 hours for 3 doses given weekly **or** Oral, I.M.: 10-25 mg/dose given once weekly

Ectopic pregnancy: I.M./I.V.: 50 mg/m² single-dose without leucovorin rescue

Elderly: Rheumatoid arthritis/psoriasis: Oral: Initial: 5 mg once weekly; if nausea occurs, split dose to 2.5 mg every 12 hours for the day of administration; dose may be increased to 7.5 mg/week based on response, not to exceed 20 mg/week

**Dosing adjustment in renal impairment:**

Cl$_{cr}$ 61-80 mL/minute: Reduce dose to 75% of usual dose

Cl$_{cr}$ 51-60 mL/minute: Reduce dose to 70% of usual dose

Cl$_{cr}$ 10-50 mL/minute: Reduce dose to 30% to 50% of usual dose

Cl$_{cr}$ <10 mL/minute: Avoid use

Hemodialysis: Not dialyzable (0% to 5%); supplemental dose is not necessary

Peritoneal dialysis: Supplemental dose is not necessary

**Dosage adjustment in hepatic impairment:**

Bilirubin 3.1-5 mg/dL OR AST >180 units: Administer 75% of usual dose

Bilirubin >5 mg/dL: Do not use

**Dosage Forms Inj:** 2.5 mg/mL (2 mL), 25 mg/mL (2 mL, 4 mL, 8 mL, 10 mL); **Inj, preservative free:** 25 mg (2 mL, 4 mL, 8 mL, 10 mL); **Powder, for inj:** 20 mg, 25 mg, 50 mg, 100 mg, 250 mg, 1 g; **Tab:** 2.5 mg; **Tab, dose pack:** 2.5 mg (4 cards with 2, 3, 4, 5, or 6 tabs each)

**Contraindications** Hypersensitivity to methotrexate or any component; severe renal or hepatic impairment; pre-existing profound bone marrow suppression in patients with psoriasis or rheumatoid arthritis, alcoholic liver disease, AIDS, pre-existing blood dyscrasias

**Warnings/Precautions** The U.S. Food and Drug Administration (FDA) currently recommends that procedures for proper handling and disposal of antineoplastic agents be considered

May cause photosensitivity type reaction. Reduce dosage in patients with renal or hepatic impairment; drain ascites and pleural effusions prior to treatment; use with caution in patients with peptic ulcer disease, ulcerative colitis, pre-existing bone marrow suppression. Monitor closely for pulmonary disease; use with caution in the elderly.

Because of the possibility of severe toxic reactions, fully inform patient of the risks involved. Do not use in women of childbearing age unless benefit outweighs risks; may cause hepatotoxicity, fibrosis, and cirrhosis, along with marked bone marrow depression. Death from intestinal perforation may occur.

Patients should receive 1-2 L of I.V. fluid prior to initiation of high-dose methotrexate. Patients should receive sodium bicarbonate to alkalinize their urine during and after high-dose methotrexate (urine SG <1.010 and pH >7 should be maintained for at least 24 hours after infusion).

Toxicity to methotrexate or any immunosuppressive is increased in elderly; must monitor carefully. For rheumatoid arthritis and psoriasis, immunosuppressive therapy should only be used when disease is active and less toxic, traditional therapy is ineffective. Recommended doses should be reduced when initiating therapy in elderly due to possible decreased metabolism, reduced renal function, and presence of interacting diseases and drugs.

Methotrexate penetrates slowly into 3rd space fluids, such as pleural effusions or ascites, and exits slowly from these compartments (slower than from plasma).

**Pregnancy Risk Factor** D

**Adverse Reactions**

>10%:

Cardiovascular: Vasculitis

Central nervous system (with I.T. administration only):

Arachnoiditis: Acute reaction manifested as severe headache, nuchal rigidity, vomiting, and fever; may be alleviated by reducing the dose

Subacute toxicity: 10% of patients treated with 12-15 mg/m² I.T. MTX may develop this in the second or third week of therapy; consists of motor paralysis of extremities, cranial nerve palsy, seizures, or coma. This has also been seen in pediatric cases receiving very high-dose I.V. MTX (when enough MTX can get across into the CSF).

Demyelinating encephalopathy: Seen months or years after receiving MTX; usually in association with cranial irradiation or other systemic chemotherapy

Dermatologic: Reddening of skin

Endocrine & metabolic: Hyperuricemia, defective oogenesis or spermatogenesis

Gastrointestinal: Ulcerative stomatitis, glossitis, gingivitis, nausea, vomiting, diarrhea, anorexia, intestinal perforation, mucositis (dose-dependent; appears in 3-7 days after therapy, resolving within 2 weeks)

Emetic potential:

<100 mg: Moderately low (10% to 30%)

≥100 mg or <250 mg: Moderate (30% to 60%)

≥250 mg: Moderately high (60% to 90%)

Hematologic: Leukopenia, thrombocytopenia

Renal: Renal failure, azotemia, nephropathy

Respiratory: Pharyngitis

(Continued)

# Methotrexate (Continued)

1% to 10%:

Cardiovascular: Vasculitis

Central nervous system: Dizziness, malaise, encephalopathy, seizures, fever, chills

Dermatitis: Alopecia, rash, photosensitivity, depigmentation or hyperpigmentation of skin

Endocrine & metabolic: Diabetes

Genitourinary: Cystitis

Hematologic: Hemorrhage

Myelosuppressive: This is the primary dose-limiting factor (along with mucositis) of MTX; occurs about 5-7 days after MTX therapy, and should resolve within 2 weeks

WBC: Mild

Platelets: Moderate

Onset (days): 7

Nadir (days): 10

Recovery (days): 21

Hepatic: Cirrhosis and portal fibrosis have been associated with chronic MTX therapy; acute elevation of liver enzymes are common after high-dose MTX, and usually resolve within 10 days

Neuromuscular & skeletal: Arthralgia

Ocular: Blurred vision

Renal: Renal dysfunction: Manifested by an abrupt rise in serum creatinine and BUN and a fall in urine output; more common with high-dose MTX, and may be due to precipitation of the drug. The best treatment is prevention: Aggressively hydrate with 3 L/m²/day starting 12 hours before therapy and continue for 24-36 hours; alkalinize the urine by adding 50 mEq of bicarbonate to each liter of fluid; keep urine flow >100 mL/hour and urine pH >7.

Respiratory: Pneumonitis: Associated with fever, cough, and interstitial pulmonary infiltrates; treatment is to withhold MTX during the acute reaction

Miscellaneous: Anaphylaxis, decreased resistance to infection

## Drug Interactions

Decreased effect:

Corticosteroids: Reported to decrease uptake of MTX into leukemia cells. Administration of these drugs should be separated by 12 hours. Dexamethasone has been reported to not affect methotrexate influx into cells.

Decreases phenytoin, 5-FU

Increased toxicity:

Live virus vaccines → vaccinia infections

Vincristine: Inhibits MTX efflux from the cell, leading to increased and prolonged MTX levels in the cell; the dose of VCR needed to produce this effect is not achieved clinically

Organic acids: Salicylates, sulfonamides, probenecid, and high doses of penicillins compete with MTX for transport and reduce renal tubular secretion. Salicylates and sulfonamides may also displace MTX from plasma proteins, ↑ MTX levels.

Ara-C: Increases formation of the Ara-C nucleotide can occur when MTX precedes Ara-C, thus promoting the action of Ara-C

Cyclosporine: CSA and MTX interfere with each others renal elimination, which may result in increased toxicity

Nonsteroidal anti-inflammatory drugs (NSAIDs): Should not be used during moderate or high-dose methotrexate due to increased and prolonged methotrexate levels may increase toxicity

**Onset** Antirheumatic effects may require several weeks

**Half-Life** 8-12 hours with high doses and 3-10 hours with low doses

## Special PA Issues

**Patient Education:** Avoid alcohol to prevent serious side effects. Avoid intake of extra dietary folic acid, maintain adequate hydration (2-3 L/day of fluids unless instructed to restrict fluid intake) and adequate nutrition (frequent small meals may help). You may experience nausea and vomiting (small frequent meals may help or request antiemetic from prescriber); drowsiness, tingling, numbness, or blurred vision (avoid driving or tasks that require focused concentration); mouth sores (frequent oral care is necessary); loss of hair; permanent sterility; skin rash; photosensitivity (avoid direct sun, use sunblock, and wear protective clothing). Report tarry stools, fever, chills, unusual bleeding or bruising, shortness of breath or difficulty breathing, yellowing of skin or eyes, dark or bloody urine, or acute joint pain or other side effects you may experience.

**Dietary Considerations:** Alcohol: Avoid use

**Monitoring Parameters:** For prolonged use (especially rheumatoid arthritis, psoriasis) a baseline liver biopsy, repeated at each 1-1.5 g cumulative dose interval, should be performed; WBC and platelet counts every 4 weeks; CBC and creatinine, LFTs every 3-4 months; chest x-ray

**Reference Range:** Refer to chart in Leucovorin Calcium monograph. Therapeutic levels: Variable; Toxic concentration: Variable; therapeutic range is dependent upon therapeutic approach.

High-dose regimens produce drug levels between 10⁻⁶Molar and 10⁻⁷Molar 24-72 hours after drug infusion

**10⁻⁶ Molar unit = 1 microMolar unit**

Toxic: Low-dose therapy: >9.1 ng/mL; high-dose therapy: >454 ng/mL

◆ **Methotrexate Sodium** *see* Methotrexate *on page 585*

# Methoxamine (meth OKS a meen)

**Pharmacologic Class** Alpha₁ Agonist

**U.S. Brand Names** Vasoxyl®

**Mechanism of Action** Direct-acting sympathomimetic amine with similar actions as phenylephrine; causes vasoconstriction primarily via alpha-adrenergic stimulation

**Use** Treatment of hypotension occurring during general anesthesia; to terminate episodes of supraventricular tachycardia; treatment of shock

**USUAL DOSAGE** Adults:

Emergencies: I.V.: 3-5 mg

Supraventricular tachycardia: I.V.: 10 mg

During spinal anesthesia: I.M.: 10-20 mg

**Dosage Forms Inj, as hydrochloride:** 20 mg/mL (1 mL)

**Contraindications** Hypersensitivity to methoxamine or any component

**Pregnancy Risk Factor** C

**Adverse Reactions**

1% to 10%:

Cardiovascular: Hypertension (severe)

Gastrointestinal: Vomiting

<1%: Ventricular ectopic beats, fetal bradycardia, headache, urinary urgency, diaphoresis

◆ **Methoxamine Hydrochloride** *see* Methoxamine *on this page*

# Methoxsalen (meth OKS a len)

**Pharmacologic Class** Psoralen

**U.S. Brand Names** 8-MOP®; Oxsoralen® Topical; Oxsoralen-Ultra® Oral; Uvadex®

**Mechanism of Action** Bonds covalently to pyrimidine bases in DNA, inhibits the synthesis of DNA, and suppresses cell division. The augmented sunburn reaction involves excitation of the methoxsalen molecule by radiation in the long-wave ultraviolet light (UVA), resulting in transference of energy to the methoxsalen molecule producing an excited state ("triplet electronic state"). The molecule, in this "triplet state", then reacts with cutaneous DNA.

**Use**

Oral: Symptomatic control of severe, recalcitrant disabling psoriasis, not responsive to other therapy when to diagnosis has been supported by biopsy. Administer only in conjunction with a schedule of controlled doses of long wave ultraviolet (UV) radiation; also used with long wave ultraviolet (UV) radiation for repigmentation of idiopathic vitiligo.

Topical: Repigmenting agent in vitiligo, used in conjunction with controlled doses of UVA or sunlight

**USUAL DOSAGE**

Psoriasis: Adults: Oral: 10-70 mg 1½-2 hours before exposure to ultraviolet light, 2-3 times at least 48 hours apart; dosage is based upon patient's body weight and skin type

Vitiligo: Children >12 years and Adults:

Oral: 20 mg 2-4 hours before exposure to UVA light or sunlight; limit exposure to 15-40 minutes based on skin basic color and exposure

Topical: Apply lotion 1-2 hours before exposure to UVA light, no more than once weekly

**Dosage Forms Cap:** 10 mg; **Lot:** 1% (30 mL); **Soln:** 20 mcg/mL

**Contraindications** Diseases associated with photosensitivity, cataract, invasive squamous cell cancer, known hypersensitivity to methoxsalen (psoralens), and children <12 years of age

**Warnings/Precautions** Family history of sunlight allergy or chronic infections; lotion should only be applied under direct supervision of a physician and should not be dispensed to the patient; for use only if inadequate response to other forms of therapy, serious burns may occur from UVA or sunlight even through glass if dose and or exposure schedule is not maintained; some products may contain tartrazine; use caution in patients with hepatic or cardiac disease

**Pregnancy Risk Factor** C

**Adverse Reactions**

>10%:

Dermatologic: Itching

Gastrointestinal: Nausea

1% to 10%:

Cardiovascular: Severe edema, hypotension

Central nervous system: Nervousness, vertigo, depression

Dermatologic: Painful blistering, burning, and peeling of skin; pruritus, freckling, hypopigmentation, rash, cheilitis, erythema

Neuromuscular & skeletal: Loss of muscle coordination

(Continued)

## Methoxsalen *(Continued)*

**Drug Interactions** Increased toxicity: Concomitant therapy with other photosensitizing agents such as anthralin, coal tar, griseofulvin, phenothiazines, nalidixic acid, sulfanilamides, tetracyclines, thiazides

**Special PA Issues**

**Patient Education:** This medication is used in conjunction with specific ultraviolet treatment. Follow prescriber's directions exactly for oral medication which can be taken with food or milk to reduce nausea. Consult prescriber for specific dietary instructions. Avoid use of any other skin treatments unless approved by prescriber. Control exposure to direct sunlight as per prescriber's instructions. If sunlight cannot be avoided, use sunblock (consult prescriber for specific SPF level), wear protective clothing and wraparound protective eyewear. Consult prescriber immediately if burning, blistering, or skin irritation occur.

♦ **Methoxypsoralen** *see Methoxsalen on previous page*

♦ **8-Methoxypsoralen** *see Methoxsalen on previous page*

♦ **Methylacetoxyprogesterone** *see Medroxyprogesterone Acetate on page 561*

## Methyldopa *(meth il DOE pa)*

**Pharmacologic Class** False Neurotransmitter

**U.S. Brand Names** Aldomet®

**Mechanism of Action** Stimulation of central alpha-adrenergic receptors by a false transmitter that results in a decreased sympathetic outflow to the heart, kidneys, and peripheral vasculature

**Use** Management of moderate to severe hypertension

**USUAL DOSAGE**

Children:

Oral: Initial: 10 mg/kg/day in 2-4 divided doses; increase every 2 days as needed to maximum dose of 65 mg/kg/day; do not exceed 3 g/day

I.V.: 5-10 mg/kg/dose every 6-8 hours up to a total dose of 65 mg/kg/24 hours or 3 g/24 hours

Adults:

Oral: Initial: 250 mg 2-3 times/day; increase every 2 days as needed; usual dose 1-1.5 g/day in 2-4 divided doses; maximum dose: 3 g/day

I.V.: 250-500 mg every 6-8 hours; maximum dose: 1 g every 6 hours

**Dosing interval in renal impairment:**

$Cl_{cr}$ >50 mL/minute: Administer every 8 hours

$Cl_{cr}$ 10-50 mL/minute: Administer every 8-12 hours

$Cl_{cr}$ <10 mL/minute: Administer every 12-24 hours

Hemodialysis: Slightly dialyzable (5% to 20%)

**Dosage Forms** Susp, oral: 250 mg/5 mL (5 mL, 473 mL); **Tab:** 125 mg, 250 mg, 500 mg; Methyldopate hydrochloride: **Inj:** 50 mg/mL (5 mL, 10 mL)

**Contraindications** Hypersensitivity to methyldopa or any component; (oral suspension contains benzoic acid and sodium bisulfite; injection contains sodium bisulfite); liver disease, pheochromocytoma, coadministration with MAO inhibitors

**Warnings/Precautions** May rarely produce hemolytic anemia and liver disorders; positive Coombs' test occurs in 10% to 20% of patients (perform periodic CBCs); sedation usually transient may occur during initial therapy or whenever the dose is increased. Use with caution in patients with previous liver disease or dysfunction, the active metabolites of methyldopa accumulate in uremia. Patients with impaired renal function may respond to smaller doses. Elderly patients may experience syncope (avoid by giving smaller doses). Tolerance may occur usually between the second and third month of therapy. Adding a diuretic or increasing the dosage of methyldopa frequently restores blood pressure control. Because of its CNS effects, methyldopa is not considered a drug of first choice in the elderly.

**Pregnancy Risk Factor** B (oral); C (I.V.)

**Pregnancy Implications**

Clinical effects on the fetus: Crosses the placenta. Hypotension reported. A large amount of clinical experience with the use of these drugs for the management of hypertension during pregnancy is available. Available evidence suggests safe use during pregnancy and breast-feeding.

Breast-feeding/lactation: Crosses into breast milk at extremely low levels. American Academy of Pediatrics considers **compatible** with breast-feeding.

**Adverse Reactions**

Cardiovascular: Peripheral edema, orthostatic hypotension, bradycardia (sinus)

Central nervous system: Drug fever, mental depression, anxiety, nightmares, drowsiness, headache, fever, chills, sedation, vertigo, depression, memory lapse

Dermatologic: Rash

Endocrine & metabolic: Sodium retention, sexual dysfunction, gynecomastia, hyperprolactinemia

Gastrointestinal: Xerostomia, colitis, pancreatitis, diarrhea, nausea, vomiting, "black" tongue

Genitourinary: Decreased libido

Hematologic: Thrombocytopenia, hemolytic anemia, positive Coombs' test, leukopenia, transient leukopenia or granulocytopenia

Hepatic: Cholestasis or hepatitis and heptocellular injury, increased liver enzymes, jaundice, cirrhosis

Neuromuscular & skeletal: Paresthesias, weakness

Respiratory: Dyspnea

Miscellaneous: SLE-like syndrome

**Drug Interactions**

Decreased effect: Iron supplements can interact and cause a significant **increase** in blood pressure; reduced effects of methyldopa may occur with barbiturates and tricyclic antidepressants; hypertension, sometimes severe, may occur with beta-blockers, MAO inhibitors, phenothiazines, and sympathomimetics

Increased toxicity: Methyldopa may increase lithium toxicity; tolbutamide, haloperidol, anesthetic, and levodopa effects/toxicity increased with methyldopa

**Onset** Peak hypotensive effect: Oral, parenteral: Within 3-6 hours

**Duration** 12-24 hours

**Half-Life** 75-80 minutes; End-stage renal disease: 6-16 hours

**Special PA Issues**

**Patient Education:** Take as directed. Do not skip dose or discontinue without consulting prescriber. Follow recommended diet and exercise program. Do not use OTC medications which may affect blood pressure (eg, cough or cold remedies, diet pills, stay-awake medications) without consulting prescriber. This medication may cause altered color of urine (normal); drowsiness, dizziness, or impaired judgment (use caution when driving or engaging in tasks that require alertness until response is known); postural hypotension (use caution when rising from sitting or lying position or when climbing stairs); or dry mouth or nausea (frequent mouth care or sucking lozenges may help). Report altered CNS status (eg, nightmares, depression, anxiety, increased nervousness); sudden weight gain (weigh yourself in the same clothes at same time of day once a week); unusual or persistent swelling of ankles, feet, or extremities; palpitations or rapid heartbeat; persistent weakness, fatigue, or unusual bleeding; or other persistent side effects.

**Monitoring Parameters:** Blood pressure, standing and sitting/lying down, CBC, liver enzymes, Coombs' test (direct); blood pressure monitor required during I.V. administration

# Methyldopa and Hydrochlorothiazide

(meth il DOE pa & hye droe klor oh THYE a zide)

**Pharmacologic Class** Antihypertensive Agent, Combination

**U.S. Brand Names** Aldoril®

**Dosage Forms Tab:** 15: Methyldopa 250 mg and hydrochlorothiazide 15 mg, 25: Methyldopa 250 mg and hydrochlorothiazide 25 mg, D30: Methyldopa 500 mg and hydrochlorothiazide 30 mg, D50: Methyldopa 500 mg and hydrochlorothiazide 50 mg

♦ **Methyldopate Hydrochloride** see Methyldopa on previous page

# Methylene Blue (METH i leen bloo)

**Pharmacologic Class** Antidote

**U.S. Brand Names** Urolene Blue®

**Mechanism of Action** Weak germicide in low concentrations, hastens the conversion of methemoglobin to hemoglobin; has opposite effect at high concentrations by converting ferrous ion of reduced hemoglobin to ferric ion to form methemoglobin; in cyanide toxicity, it combines with cyanide to form cyanmethemoglobin preventing the interference of cyanide with the cytochrome system

**Use** Antidote for cyanide poisoning and drug-induced methemoglobinemia, indicator dye, chronic urolithiasis.

**Unlabeled use:** Has been used topically (0.1% solutions) in conjunction with polychromatic light to photoinactivate viruses such as herpes simplex; has been used alone or in combination with vitamin C for the management of chronic urolithiasis

**USUAL DOSAGE**

Children: NADPH-methemoglobin reductase deficiency: Oral: 1-1.5 mg/kg/day (maximum: 300 mg/day) given with 5-8 mg/kg/day of ascorbic acid

Children and Adults: Methemoglobinemia: I.V.: 1-2 mg/kg or 25-50 mg/m² over several minutes; may be repeated in 1 hour if necessary

Adults: Genitourinary antiseptic: Oral: 65-130 mg 3 times/day with a full glass of water (maximum: 390 mg/day)

**Dosage Forms Inj:** 10 mg/mL (1 mL, 10 mL); **Tab:** 65 mg

**Contraindications** Renal insufficiency, hypersensitivity to methylene blue or any component, intraspinal injection

**Warnings/Precautions** Do not inject S.C. or intrathecally; use with caution in young patients and in patients with G-6-PD deficiency; continued use can cause profound anemia

**Pregnancy Risk Factor** C (D if injected intra-amniotically)

(Continued)

## Methylene Blue *(Continued)*

### Adverse Reactions
>10%:
Gastrointestinal: Fecal discoloration (blue-green)
Genitourinary: Discoloration of urine (blue-green)
1% to 10%: Hematologic: Anemia
<1%: Hypertension, precordial pain, dizziness, mental confusion, headache, fever, stains skin, nausea, vomiting, abdominal pain, bladder irritation, diaphoresis

### Special PA Issues
**Patient Education:** May discolor urine and feces blue-green; take oral formulation after meals with a glass of water; skin stains may be removed using a hypochlorite solution

♦ **Methylergometrine Maleate** *see* Methylergonovine *on this page*

## Methylergonovine (meth il er goe NOE veen)

**Pharmacologic Class** Ergot Derivative

**U.S. Brand Names** Methergine®

**Mechanism of Action** Similar smooth muscle actions as seen with ergotamine; however, it affects primarily uterine smooth muscles producing sustained contractions and thereby shortens the third stage of labor

**Use** Prevention and treatment of postpartum and postabortion hemorrhage caused by uterine atony or subinvolution

**USUAL DOSAGE** Adults:
Oral: 0.2 mg 3-4 times/day for 2-7 days
I.M.: 0.2 mg after delivery of anterior shoulder, after delivery of placenta, or during puerperium; may be repeated as required at intervals of 2-4 hours
I.V.: Same dose as I.M., but should not be routinely administered I.V. because of possibility of inducing sudden hypertension and cerebrovascular accident

**Dosage Forms Inj:** 0.2 mg/mL (1 mL); **Tab:** 0.2 mg

**Contraindications** Induction of labor, threatened spontaneous abortion, hypertension, toxemia, hypersensitivity to methylergonovine or any component, pregnancy

**Warnings/Precautions** Use caution in patients with sepsis, obliterative vascular disease, hepatic, or renal involvement, hypertension; administer with extreme caution if using I.V.

**Pregnancy Risk Factor** C

### Adverse Reactions
>10%: Cardiovascular: Hypertension
1% to 10%: Gastrointestinal: Nausea, vomiting
<1%: Temporary chest pain, palpitations, hallucinations, dizziness, seizures, headache, water intoxication, diarrhea, thrombophlebitis, leg cramps, tinnitus, hematuria, dyspnea, nasal congestion, diaphoresis, foul taste

**Drug Interactions** Augmented effects may occur with concurrent use of methylergonovine and vasoconstrictors or ergot alkaloids

**Onset** Onset of oxytocic effect: Oral: 5-10 minutes; I.M.: 2-5 minutes; I.V.: Immediately

**Duration** Oral: ~3 hours  I.M.: ~3 hours; I.V.: 45 minutes

**Half-Life** Biphasic: Initial: 1-5 minutes; Terminal: 30 minutes to 2 hours

### Special PA Issues
**Patient Education:** This drug will generally not be needed for more than a week. You may experience nausea and vomiting (small frequent meals may help), dizziness, headache, or ringing in the ears (will reverse when drug is discontinued). Report any respiratory difficulty, acute headache, or numb cold extremities, or severe abdominal cramping.

♦ **Methylergonovine Maleate** *see* Methylergonovine *on this page*

♦ **Methylmorphine** *see* Codeine *on page 232*

♦ **Methylone®** *see* Methylprednisolone *on next page*

## Methylphenidate (meth il FEN i date)

**Pharmacologic Class** Stimulant

**U.S. Brand Names** Ritalin®; Ritalin-SR®

**Mechanism of Action** Blocks the reuptake mechanism of dopaminergic neurons; appears to stimulate the cerebral cortex and subcortical structures similar to amphetamines

**Use** Treatment of attention deficit disorder and symptomatic management of narcolepsy; many unlabeled uses

**USUAL DOSAGE** Oral: (Discontinue periodically to re-evaluate or if no improvement occurs within 1 month)

Children ≥6 years: Attention deficit disorder: Initial: 0.3 mg/kg/dose or 2.5-5 mg/dose given before breakfast and lunch; increase by 0.1 mg/kg/dose or by 5-10 mg/day at weekly intervals; usual dose: 0.5-1 mg/kg/day; maximum dose: 2 mg/kg/day or 60 mg/day
Adults:
Narcolepsy: 10 mg 2-3 times/day, up to 60 mg/day

Depression: Initial: 2.5 mg every morning before 9 AM; dosage may be increased by 2.5-5 mg every 2-3 days as tolerated to a maximum of 20 mg/day; may be divided (ie, 7 AM and 12 noon), but should not be given after noon; do not use sustained release product

**Dosage Forms** Methylphenidate hydrochloride: **Tab:** 5 mg, 10 mg, 20 mg; **Tab, sustained release:** 20 mg

**Contraindications** Hypersensitivity to methylphenidate or any components; glaucoma, motor tics, Tourette's syndrome, patients with marked agitation, tension, and anxiety

**Warnings/Precautions** Use with caution in patients with hypertension, dementia (may worsen agitation or confusion) seizures; has high potential for abuse. Treatment should include "drug holidays" or periodic discontinuation in order to assess the patient's requirements and to decrease tolerance and limit suppression of linear growth and weight; it is often useful in treating elderly patients who are discouraged, withdrawn, apathetic, or disinterested in their activities. In particular, it is useful in patients who are starting a rehabilitation program but have resigned themselves to fail; these patients may not have a major depressive disorder; will not improve memory or cognitive function.

**Pregnancy Risk Factor** C

**Adverse Reactions**

>10%:
Cardiovascular: Tachycardia
Central nervous system: Nervousness, insomnia
Gastrointestinal: Anorexia

1% to 10%:
Central nervous system: Dizziness, drowsiness
Gastrointestinal: Stomach pain
Miscellaneous: Hypersensitivity reactions

<1%: Hypertension, hypotension, palpitations, cardiac arrhythmias, movement disorders, precipitation of Tourette's syndrome, and toxic psychosis (rare), fever, headache, convulsions, rash, nausea, weight loss, vomiting, growth retardation, thrombocytopenia, anemia, leukopenia, blurred vision

**Drug Interactions**

Decreased effect: Effects of guanethidine, bretylium may be antagonized by methylphenidate

Increased toxicity: May increase serum concentrations of tricyclic antidepressants, warfarin, phenytoin, phenobarbital, and primidone; MAO inhibitors may potentiate effects of methylphenidate

**Onset** Immediate release tablet: Peak cerebral stimulation effect: Within 2 hours; Sustained release tablet: Peak effect: Within 4-7 hours

**Duration** Immediate release tablet: 3-6 hours; Sustained release tablet: 8 hours

**Half-Life** 2-4 hours

**Special PA Issues**

**Patient Education:** Take exactly as directed; do not change dosage or discontinue without consulting prescriber. Response may take some time. Do not crush or chew sustained release tables. Avoid alcohol, caffeine, or other stimulants. Maintain adequate fluid intake (2-3 L/day). You may experience decreased appetite or weight loss (small frequent meals may help maintain adequate nutrition); restlessness, impaired judgment, or dizziness, especially during early therapy (use caution when driving or engaging in hazardous activities). Report unresolved rapid heartbeat; excessive agitation, nervousness, insomnia, tremors, or dizziness; skin rash or irritation; or altered gait or movement.

♦ **Methylphenidate Hydrochloride** see Methylphenidate on previous page

♦ **Methylphenobarbital** see Mephobarbital on page 569

♦ **Methylphenyl Isoxazolyl Penicillin** see Oxacillin on page 682

♦ **Methylphytyl Napthoquinone** see Phytonadione on page 725

# Methylprednisolone (meth il pred NIS oh lone)

**Pharmacologic Class** Corticosteroid, Parenteral

**U.S. Brand Names** Adlone® Injection; A-methaPred® Injection; depMedalone® Injection; Depoject® Injection; Depo-Medrol® Injection; Depopred® Injection; D-Med® Injection; Duralone® Injection; Medralone® Injection; Medrol® Oral; Methylone®; M-Prednisol® Injection; Solu-Medrol® Injection

**Mechanism of Action** In a tissue-specific manner, corticosteroids regulate gene expression subsequent to binding specific intracellular receptors and translocation into the nucleus. Corticosteroids exert a wide array of physiologic effects including modulation of carbohydrate, protein, and lipid metabolism and maintenance of fluid and electrolyte homeostasis. Moreover cardiovascular, immunologic, musculoskeletal, endocrine, and neurologic physiology are influenced by corticosteroids. Decreases inflammation by suppression of migration of polymorphonuclear leukocytes and reversal of increased capillary permeability.

**Use** Primarily as an anti-inflammatory or immunosuppressant agent in the treatment of a variety of diseases including those of hematologic, allergic, inflammatory, neoplastic, and autoimmune origin. Prevention and treatment of graft-versus-host disease following allogeneic bone marrow transplantation.

(Continued)

## Methylprednisolone *(Continued)*

**USUAL DOSAGE** Dosing should be based on the lesser of ideal body weight or actual body weight

**Only sodium succinate may be given I.V.;** methylprednisolone sodium succinate is highly soluble and has a rapid effect by I.M. and I.V. routes. Methylprednisolone acetate has a low solubility and has a sustained I.M. effect.

Children:

Anti-inflammatory or immunosuppressive: Oral, I.M., I.V. (sodium succinate): 0.5-1.7 mg/kg/day **or** 5-25 mg/m²/day in divided doses every 6-12 hours; "Pulse" therapy: 15-30 mg/kg/dose over ≥30 minutes given once daily for 3 days

Status asthmaticus: I.V. (sodium succinate): Loading dose: 2 mg/kg/dose, then 0.5-1 mg/kg/dose every 6 hours for up to 5 days

Acute spinal cord injury: I.V. (sodium succinate): 30 mg/kg over 15 minutes, followed in 45 minutes by a continuous infusion of 5.4 mg/kg/hour for 23 hours

Lupus nephritis: I.V. (sodium succinate): 30 mg/kg over ≥30 minutes every other day for 6 doses

High-dose therapy for acute spinal cord injury: I.V. bolus: 30 mg/kg over 15 minutes, followed 45 minutes later by an infusion of 5.4 mg/kg/hour for 23 hours

Adults:

Anti-inflammatory or immunosuppressive: Oral: 2-60 mg/day in 1-4 divided doses to start, followed by gradual reduction in dosage to the lowest possible level consistent with maintaining an adequate clinical response

I.M. (sodium succinate): 10-80 mg/day once daily

I.M. (acetate): 10-80 mg every 1-2 weeks

I.V. (sodium succinate): 10-40 mg over a period of several minutes and repeated I.V. or I.M. at intervals depending on clinical response; when high dosages are needed, administer 30 mg/kg over a period of ≥30 minutes and may be repeated every 4-6 hours for 48 hours

Status asthmaticus: I.V. (sodium succinate): Loading dose: 2 mg/kg/dose, then 0.5-1 mg/kg/dose every 6 hours for up to 5 days

High-dose therapy for acute spinal cord injury: I.V. bolus: 30 mg/kg over 15 minutes, followed 45 minutes later by an infusion of 5.4 mg/kg/hour for 23 hours

Lupus nephritis: High-dose "pulse" therapy: I.V. (sodium succinate): 1 g/day for 3 days

Aplastic anemia: I.V. (sodium succinate): 1 mg/kg/day or 40 mg/day (whichever dose is higher), for 4 days. After 4 days, change to oral and continue until day 10 or until symptoms of serum sickness resolve, then rapidly reduce over approximately 2 weeks.

Hemodialysis: Slightly dialyzable (5% to 20%); administer dose posthemodialysis

Intra-articular (acetate): Administer every 1-5 weeks

Large joints: 20-80 mg

Small joints: 4-10 mg

Intralesional (acetate): 20-60 mg every 1-5 weeks

**Dosage Forms Inj:** As acetate: 20 mg/mL (5 mL, 10 mL), 40 mg/mL (1 mL, 5 mL, 10 mL), 80 mg/mL (1 mL, 5 mL); As sodium succinate: 40 mg (1 mL, 3 mL), 125 mg (2 mL, 5 mL), 500 mg (1 mL, 4 mL, 8 mL, 20 mL), 1000 mg (1 mL, 8 mL, 50 mL), 2000 mg (30.6 mL); **Tab:** 2 mg, 4 mg, 8 mg, 16 mg, 24 mg, 32 mg, Dose pack: 4 mg (21s)

**Contraindications** Serious infections, except septic shock or tuberculous meningitis; known hypersensitivity to methylprednisolone; viral, fungal, or tubercular skin lesions; administration of live virus vaccines. Methylprednisolone formulations containing benzyl alcohol preservative are contraindicated in infants.

**Warnings/Precautions** Use with caution in patients with hyperthyroidism, cirrhosis, nonspecific ulcerative colitis, hypertension, osteoporosis, thromboembolic tendencies, CHF, convulsive disorders, myasthenia gravis, thrombophlebitis, peptic ulcer, diabetes; because of the risk of adverse effects, systemic corticosteroids should be used cautiously in the elderly, in the smallest possible dose, and for the shortest possible time

Acute adrenal insufficiency may occur with abrupt withdrawal after long-term therapy or with stress; young pediatric patients may be more susceptible to adrenal axis suppression from topical therapy

**Pregnancy Risk Factor** C

**Adverse Reactions**

>10%:

Central nervous system: Insomnia, nervousness

Gastrointestinal: Increased appetite, indigestion

1% to 10%:

Dermatologic: Hirsutism

Endocrine & metabolic: Diabetes mellitus, adrenal suppression, hyperlipidemia

Hematologic: Transient leukocytosis

Neuromuscular & skeletal: Arthralgia

Ocular: Cataracts, glaucoma

Miscellaneous: Infections

<1%: Edema, hypertension, vertigo, seizures, psychoses, pseudotumor cerebri, headache, mood swings, delirium, hallucinations, euphoria, acne, skin atrophy, bruising, hyperpigmentation, Cushing's syndrome, pituitary-adrenal axis suppression, growth suppression,

glucose intolerance, hypokalemia, alkalosis, amenorrhea, sodium and water retention, hyperglycemia, peptic ulcer, nausea, vomiting, abdominal distention, ulcerative esophagitis, pancreatitis, muscle weakness, osteoporosis, fractures, hypersensitivity reactions , arrhythmias, avascular necrosis, secondary malignancy, intractable hiccups

**Drug Interactions** CYP3A enzyme inducer

Decreased effect:

Phenytoin, phenobarbital, rifampin increase clearance of methylprednisolone

Potassium depleting diuretics enhance potassium depletion

Increased toxicity:

Skin test antigens, immunizations decrease response and increase potential infections

Methylprednisolone may increase circulating glucose levels and may need adjustments of insulin or oral hypoglycemics

**Onset** Methylprednisolone sodium succinate is highly soluble and has a rapid effect by I.M. and I.V. routes. Methylprednisolone acetate has a low solubility and has a sustained I.M. effect.

**Duration**

Peak effect: Oral: 1-2 hours; I.M.: 4-8 days; Intra-articular: 1 week

Duration: Oral: 30-36 hours; I.M.: 1-4 weeks; Intra-articular: 1-5 weeks

**Half-Life** 3-3.5 hours

**Special PA Issues**

**Patient Education:** Maintain adequate nutritional intake; consult prescriber for possibility of special dietary instructions. If diabetic, monitor serum glucose closely and notify prescriber of any changes; this medication can alter hypoglycemic requirements. Inform prescriber if you are experiencing unusual stress; dosage may need to be adjusted. You will be susceptible to infection; avoid crowds or infected persons or persons with contagious diseases. You may experience insomnia or nervousness; use caution when driving or engaging in tasks requiring alertness until response to medication is known. Report increased pain, swelling, or redness in area being treated; excessive or sudden weight gain; swelling of extremities; difficulty breathing; muscle pain or weakness; change in menstrual pattern; vision changes; signs of hyperglycemia; signs of infection (eg, fever, chills, mouth sores, perianal itching, vaginal discharge); other persistent side effects; or worsening of condition.

Oral: Take as directed, with food or milk. Take once-a-day dose in the morning. Do not take more than prescribed or discontinue without consulting prescriber.

Intra-articular: Refrain from excessive use of joint following therapy, even if pain is gone.

**Monitoring Parameters:** Blood pressure, blood glucose, electrolytes

**Related Information**

Corticosteroids on page 1007

♦ **6-α-Methylprednisolone** see Methylprednisolone on page 593

♦ **Methylprednisolone Acetate** see Methylprednisolone on page 593

♦ **Methylprednisolone Sodium Succinate** see Methylprednisolone on page 593

♦ **Methylrosaniline Chloride** see Gentian Violet on page 413

# Methyltestosterone (meth il tes TOS te rone)

**Pharmacologic Class** Androgen

**U.S. Brand Names** Android®; Metandren®; Oreton® Methyl; Testred®; Virilon®

**Mechanism of Action** Stimulates receptors in organs and tissues to promote growth and development of male sex organs and maintains secondary sex characteristics in androgen-deficient males

**Use**

Male: Hypogonadism; delayed puberty; impotence and climacteric symptoms

Female: Palliative treatment of metastatic breast cancer; postpartum breast pain and/or engorgement

**USUAL DOSAGE** Adults (buccal absorption produces twice the androgenic activity of oral tablets):

Male:

Hypogonadism, male climacteric and impotence: Oral: 10-40 mg/day

Androgen deficiency:

Oral: 10-50 mg/day

Buccal: 5-25 mg/day

Postpubertal cryptorchidism: Oral: 30 mg/day

Female:

Breast pain/engorgement:

Oral: 80 mg/day for 3-5 days

Buccal: 40 mg/day for 3-5 days

Breast cancer:

Oral: 50-200 mg/day

Buccal: 25-100 mg/day

(Continued)

## Methyltestosterone (Continued)

**Dosage Forms Cap:** 10 mg; **Tab:** 10 mg, 25 mg; **Buccal:** 5 mg, 10 mg

**Contraindications** Hypersensitivity to methyltestosterone or any component, known or suspected carcinoma of the breast or the prostate, pregnancy

**Warnings/Precautions** Use with extreme caution in patients with liver or kidney disease or serious heart disease; may accelerate bone maturation without producing compensatory gain in linear growth

**Pregnancy Risk Factor** X

**Adverse Reactions**

>10%:
  Cardiovascular: Edema
  Males: Virilism, priapism
  Females: Virilism, menstrual problems (amenorrhea), breast soreness
  Dermatologic: Acne

1% to 10%:
  Males: Prostatic hypertrophy, prostatic carcinoma, impotence, testicular
  Females: Hirsutism (increase in pubic hair growth) atrophy
  Gastrointestinal: GI irritation, nausea, vomiting
  Hepatic: Hepatic dysfunction

<1%: Gynecomastia, amenorrhea, hypercalcemia, leukopenia, polycythemia, hepatic necrosis, cholestatic hepatitis, hypersensitivity reactions

**Drug Interactions** Decreased effect: Oral anticoagulant effect or decrease insulin requirements

**Special PA Issues**

**Patient Education:** Take as directed; do not exceed recommended dosage. Diabetics must monitor serum glucose closely and report abnormal glucose tests so adjustments can be made in diabetic regimen. You may experience acne, growth of body hair or baldness, deepening of voice, loss of libido, menstrual irregularity, impotence (most are reversible). You may experience drowsiness, dizziness, or blurred vision; use caution when driving or engaging in hazardous tasks. Small frequent meals and good mouth care may reduce any nausea or vomiting. Report persistent GI distress or diarrhea; change in color of urine or stool; yellowing of eyes or skin; swelling of ankles, feet, or hands; unusual bruising or bleeding; severe menstrual irregularity (amenorrhea) or persistent penile erection; and excessive growth of body hair.

## Methysergide (meth i SER jide)

**Pharmacologic Class** Ergot Derivative

**U.S. Brand Names** Sansert®

**Use** Prophylaxis of vascular headache

**USUAL DOSAGE** Adults: Oral: 4-8 mg/day with meals; if no improvement is noted after 3 weeks, drug is unlikely to be beneficial; must not be given continuously for longer than 6 months, and a drug-free interval of 3-4 weeks must follow each 6-month course

**Dosage Forms Tab, as maleate:** 2 mg

**Contraindications** Peripheral vascular disease, severe arteriosclerosis, pulmonary disease, severe hypertension, phlebitis, serious infections, pregnancy

**Pregnancy Risk Factor** X

**Half-Life** ~10 hours

**Special PA Issues**

**Patient Education:** This drug is meant to prevent migraine headaches, not treat acute attacks. Take as directed; do not take more than recommended and do not discontinue without consulting prescriber (must be discontinued slowly). You may experience weight gain (monitor dietary intake and exercise) or dizziness or vertigo (use caution when driving or engaging in tasks that require alertness). Small frequent meals may reduce nausea or vomiting. Diarrhea will lessen with use. Report cold, numb, tingling, or painful extremities or leg cramps, chest pain, difficulty breathing or shortness of breath, or pain on urination.

♦ **Meticorten®** see Prednisone on page 754

♦ **Metimyd® Ophthalmic** see Sulfacetamide Sodium and Prednisolone on page 859

## Metipranolol (met i PRAN oh lol)

**Pharmacologic Class** Beta Blocker, Nonselective; Ophthalmic Agent, Antiglaucoma

**U.S. Brand Names** OptiPranolol® Ophthalmic

**Mechanism of Action** Beta-adrenoceptor-blocking agent; lacks intrinsic sympathomimetic activity and membrane-stabilizing effects and possesses only slight local anesthetic activity; mechanism of action of metipranolol in reducing intraocular pressure appears to be via reduced production of aqueous humor. This effect may be related to a reduction in blood flow to the iris root-ciliary body. It remains unclear if the reduction in intraocular pressure observed with beta-blockers is actually secondary to beta-adrenoceptor blockade.

**Use** Agent for lowering intraocular pressure in patients with chronic open-angle glaucoma

**USUAL DOSAGE** Ophthalmic: Adults: Instill 1 drop in the affected eye(s) twice daily

**Dosage Forms** Soln, ophth, as hydrochloride: 0.3% (5 mL, 10 mL)

**Contraindications** Bronchial asthma, sinus bradycardia, second and third degree A-V block, cardiac failure, cardiogenic shock, hypersensitivity to betaxolol or any component, pregnancy

**Warnings/Precautions** Use with caution in patients with cardiac failure or diabetes mellitus, asthma, bradycardia, or A-V block

**Pregnancy Risk Factor** C

**Adverse Reactions**

>10%: Ocular: Mild ocular stinging and discomfort, eye irritation

1% to 10%: Ocular: Blurred vision, browache

<1%: Bradycardia, A-V block, congestive heart failure, erythema, weakness, conjunctivitis, blepharitis, tearing, itching eyes, keratitis, photophobia, decreased corneal sensitivity, bronchospasm

**Onset** ≤30 minutes; Maximum effects: ~2 hours

**Duration** Intraocular pressure reduction has persisted for 24 hours following ocular instillation.

**Half-Life** ~3 hours

**Special PA Issues**

**Patient Education:** For ophthalmic use only. Apply prescribed amount as often as directed. Wash hands before using and do not touch tip of applicator to eye or contaminate tip of applicator. Tilt head back and look upward. Gently pull down lower lid and put drop(s) inside lower eyelid at inner corner. Close eye and roll eyeball in all directions. Do not blink for ½ minute. Apply gentle pressure to inner corner of eye for 30 seconds. Wipe away excess from skin around eye. Do not use any other eye preparation for at least 10 minutes. Do not share medication with anyone else. Temporary stinging or blurred vision may occur. Immediately report any adverse cardiac or CNS effects (usually signifies overdose). Report persistent eye pain, redness, burning, watering, dryness, double vision, puffiness around eye, vision disturbances, other adverse eye response, worsening of condition or lack of improvement.

♦ **Metipranolol Hydrochloride** see Metipranolol *on previous page*

# Metoclopramide (met oh kloe PRA mide)

**Pharmacologic Class** Gastrointestinal Agent, Prokinetic

**U.S. Brand Names** Clopra®; Maxolon®; Octamide®; Reglan®

**Mechanism of Action** Blocks dopamine receptors in chemoreceptor trigger zone of the CNS; enhances the response to acetylcholine of tissue in upper GI tract causing enhanced motility and accelerated gastric emptying without stimulating gastric, biliary, or pancreatic secretions

**Use** Symptomatic treatment of diabetic gastric stasis, gastroesophageal reflux; prevention of nausea associated with chemotherapy or postsurgery and facilitates intubation of the small intestine

**USUAL DOSAGE**

Children:

Gastroesophageal reflux: Oral: 0.1-0.2 mg/kg/dose up to 4 times/day; efficacy of continuing metoclopramide beyond 12 weeks in reflux has not been determined; total daily dose should not exceed 0.5 mg/kg/day

Gastrointestinal hypomotility (gastroparesis): Oral, I.M., I.V.: 0.1 mg/kg/dose up to 4 times/day, not to exceed 0.5 mg/kg/day

Antiemetic (chemotherapy-induced emesis): I.V.: 1-2 mg/kg 30 minutes before chemotherapy and every 2-4 hours

Facilitate intubation: I.V.:

<6 years: 0.1 mg/kg

6-14 years: 2.5-5 mg

Adults:

Gastroesophageal reflux: Oral: 10-15 mg/dose up to 4 times/day 30 minutes before meals or food and at bedtime; single doses of 20 mg are occasionally needed for provoking situations; efficacy of continuing metoclopramide beyond 12 weeks in reflux has not been determined

Gastrointestinal hypomotility (gastroparesis):

Oral: 10 mg 30 minutes before each meal and at bedtime for 2-8 weeks

I.V. (for severe symptoms): 10 mg over 1-2 minutes; 10 days of I.V. therapy may be necessary for best response

Antiemetic (chemotherapy-induced emesis): I.V.: 1-2 mg/kg 30 minutes before chemotherapy and every 2-4 hours to every 4-6 hours (and usually given with diphenhydramine 25-50 mg I.V./oral)

Postoperative nausea and vomiting: I.M.: 10 mg near end of surgery; 20 mg doses may be used

Facilitate intubation: I.V.: 10 mg

Elderly:

Gastroesophageal reflux: Oral: 5 mg 4 times/day (30 minutes before meals and at bedtime); increase dose to 10 mg 4 times/day if no response at lower dose

(Continued)

## Metoclopramide *(Continued)*

Gastrointestinal hypomotility:

Oral: Initial: 5 mg 30 minutes before meals and at bedtime for 2-8 weeks; increase if necessary to 10 mg doses

I.V.: Initiate at 5 mg over 1-2 minutes; increase to 10 mg if necessary

Postoperative nausea and vomiting: I.M.: 5 mg near end of surgery; may repeat dose if necessary

**Dosing adjustment in renal impairment:**

$Cl_{cr}$ 10-40 mL/minute: Administer at 50% of normal dose

$Cl_{cr}$ <10 mL/minute: Administer at 25% of normal dose

Hemodialysis: Not dialyzable (0% to 5%); supplemental dose is not necessary

**Dosage Forms Inj:** 5 mg/mL (2 mL, 10 mL, 30 mL, 50 mL, 100 mL); **Soln, oral, concentrated:** 10 mg/mL (10 mL, 30 mL); **Syr, sugar free:** 5 mg/5 mL (10 mL, 480 mL); **Tab:** 5 mg, 10 mg

**Contraindications** Hypersensitivity to metoclopramide or any component; GI obstruction, perforation or hemorrhage, pheochromocytoma, history of seizure disorder

**Warnings/Precautions** Use with caution in patients with Parkinson's disease and in patients with a history of mental illness; dosage and/or frequency of administration should be modified in response to degree of renal impairment; extrapyramidal reactions, depression; may exacerbate seizures in seizure patients; to prevent extrapyramidal reactions, patients may be pretreated with diphenhydramine; elderly are more likely to develop dystonic reactions than younger adults; use lowest recommended doses initially

**Pregnancy Risk Factor** B

**Pregnancy Implications**

Clinical effects on the fetus: Crosses the placenta. Available evidence suggests safe use during pregnancy and breast-feeding.

Breast-feeding/lactation: Crosses into breast milk

Clinical effects on the infant: Increased milk production; 2 reports of mild intestinal discomfort; American Academy of Pediatrics states MAY BE OF CONCERN

**Adverse Reactions**

>10%:

Central nervous system: Restlessness, drowsiness

Gastrointestinal: Diarrhea

Neuromuscular & skeletal: Weakness

1% to 10%:

Central nervous system: Insomnia, depression

Dermatologic: Rash

Endocrine & metabolic: Breast tenderness, prolactin stimulation

Gastrointestinal: Nausea, xerostomia

<1%: Tachycardia, hypertension or hypotension, extrapyramidal reactions*, tardive dyskinesia, fatigue, anxiety, agitation, constipation, methemoglobinemia

*Note: A recent study suggests the incidence of extrapyramidal reactions due to metoclopramide may be as high as 34% and the incidence appears more often in the elderly

**Drug Interactions** CYP1A2 and CYP2D6 enzyme substrate

Decreased effect: Anticholinergic agents antagonize metoclopramide's actions

Increased toxicity: Opiate analgesics may increase CNS depression

**Onset** Oral: Within 0.5-1 hour; I.V.: Within 1-3 minutes

**Duration** Duration of therapeutic effect: 1-2 hours, regardless of route administered

**Half-Life** Normal renal function: 4-7 hours (may be dose-dependent)

**Special PA Issues**

**Patient Education:** Take this drug as prescribed, 30 minutes prior to eating. Do not increase dosage. Do not use alcohol or other CNS depressant or sleeping aids without consulting prescriber. May cause dizziness, drowsiness, or blurred vision; use caution when driving or engaging in hazardous activities until effect of medication is known. May cause restlessness, anxiety, depression, or insomnia (will reverse when medication is discontinued). Report any CNS changes, involuntary movements, unresolved diarrhea. If diabetic, monitor serum glucose regularly.

**Dietary Considerations:** Alcohol: Additive CNS effect, avoid use

**Monitoring Parameters:** Periodic renal function test; monitor for dystonic reactions; monitor for signs of hypoglycemia in patients using insulin and those being treated for gastroparesis; monitor for agitation and irritable confusion

## Metolazone *(me TOLE a zone)*

**Pharmacologic Class** Diuretic, Thiazide

**U.S. Brand Names** Mykrox®; Zaroxolyn®

**Mechanism of Action** Inhibits sodium reabsorption in the distal tubules causing increased excretion of sodium and water, as well as, potassium and hydrogen ions

**Use** Management of mild to moderate hypertension; treatment of edema in congestive heart failure and nephrotic syndrome, impaired renal function

**USUAL DOSAGE** Adults: Oral:

Edema: 5-20 mg/dose every 24 hours

Hypertension: 2.5-5 mg/dose every 24 hours

Hypertension (Mykrox®): 0.5 mg/day; if response is not adequate, increase dose to maximum of 1 mg/day

Dialysis: Not dialyzable (0% to 5%) via hemo- or peritoneal dialysis; supplemental dose is not necessary

**Dosage Forms** Tab: Zaroxolyn® (slow acting): 2.5 mg, 5 mg, 10 mg, Mykrox® (rapidly acting): 0.5 mg

**Contraindications** Hypersensitivity to metolazone or any component, other thiazides, and sulfonamide derivatives; patients with hepatic coma, anuria

**Warnings/Precautions** Use with caution in renal disease, hepatic disease, gout, lupus erythematosus, diabetes mellitus; some products may contain tartrazine. **Mykrox® is not bioequivalent to Zaroxolyn® and should not be interchanged for one another.**

**Pregnancy Risk Factor** D

**Adverse Reactions**

1% to 10%:

Cardiovascular: Chest pain (3% with fast-acting product)

Central nervous system: Dizziness (10%), headache (9%)

Endocrine & metabolic: Hypokalemia

Neuromuscular & skeletal: Muscle cramps/spasms (6%)

<1%: Hypotension, drowsiness, photosensitivity, rash, fluid and electrolyte imbalances (hypocalcemia, hypomagnesemia, hyponatremia), hyperglycemia, nausea, vomiting, anorexia, polyuria, rarely blood dyscrasias, aplastic anemia, hemolytic anemia, leukopenia, agranulocytosis, thrombocytopenia, hepatitis, paresthesia, prerenal azotemia, uremia

**Drug Interactions**

Decreased effect:

Thiazides may decrease the effect of anticoagulants, antigout agents, sulfonylureas

Bile acid sequestrants, methenamine, and NSAIDs may decrease the effect of the thiazides

Increased effect: Thiazides may increase the toxicity of allopurinol, anesthetics, antineoplastics, calcium salts, diazoxide, digitalis, lithium, loop diuretics, methyldopa, nondepolarizing muscle relaxants, vitamin D; amphotericin B and anticholinergics may increase the toxicity of thiazides

**Onset** Onset of diuresis: Within 60 minutes

**Duration** 12-24 hours

**Half-Life** 6-20 hours, renal function dependent

**Special PA Issues**

**Patient Education:** Take exactly as directed - with meals. May take early in day to avoid nocturia. Include bananas or orange juice in daily diet but do not take dietary supplements without advice or consultation of prescriber. Do not use alcohol or OTC medication without consulting prescriber. Weigh weekly at same time, in the same clothes. Report weight gain >5 lb/week. May cause dizziness or weakness (change position slowly when rising from sitting or lying, avoid driving or activities requiring alertness until response to drug is known). You may experience nausea or loss of appetite (small frequent meals may help), impotence (reversible), constipation (fluids, exercise, dietary fiber may help), photosensitivity (use sunblock and wear protective clothing). This medication does not replace other antihypertensive interventions; follow instructions for diet and lifestyle changes. Report flu-like symptoms, headache, joint soreness or weakness, difficulty breathing, skin rash, excessive fatigue, swelling of extremities, or difficulty breathing.

**Monitoring Parameters:** Serum electrolytes (potassium, sodium, chloride, bicarbonate), renal function, blood pressure (standing, sitting/supine)

**Related Information**

Heart Failure: Management of Patients with Left Ventricular Systolic Dysfunction *on page 1064*

# Metoprolol (me toe PROE lole)

**Pharmacologic Class** Beta Blocker, Beta₁ Selective

**U.S. Brand Names** Lopressor®; Toprol XL®

**Mechanism of Action** Selective inhibitor of beta₁-adrenergic receptors; competitively blocks beta₁-receptors, with little or no effect on beta₂-receptors at doses <100 mg; does not exhibit any membrane stabilizing or intrinsic sympathomimetic activity

**Use** Treatment of hypertension and angina pectoris; prevention of myocardial infarction, atrial fibrillation, flutter, symptomatic treatment of hypertrophic subaortic stenosis

**Unlabeled use:** Treatment of ventricular arrhythmias, atrial ectopy, migraine prophylaxis, essential tremor, aggressive behavior

**USUAL DOSAGE**

Children: Oral: 1-5 mg/kg/24 hours divided twice daily; allow 3 days between dose adjustments

Adults:

Oral: 100-450 mg/day in 2-3 divided doses, begin with 50 mg twice daily and increase doses at weekly intervals to desired effect

Extended release: Same daily dose administered as a single dose

(Continued)

## Metoprolol *(Continued)*

> I.V.: 5 mg every 2 minutes for 3 doses in early treatment of myocardial infarction; thereafter administer 50 mg orally every 6 hours 15 minutes after last I.V. dose and continue for 48 hours; then administer a maintenance dose of 100 mg twice daily
>
> Elderly: Oral: Initial: 25 mg/day; usual range: 25-300 mg/day
>
> Hemodialysis: Administer dose posthemodialysis or administer 50 mg supplemental dose; supplemental dose is not necessary following peritoneal dialysis
>
> **Dosing adjustment/comments in hepatic disease:** Reduced dose probably necessary

**Dosage Forms** Metoprolol succinate: **Tab, sustained release:** 50 mg, 100 mg, 200 mg

> Metoprolol tartrate: **Inj:** 1 mg/mL (5 mL), **Tab:** 50 mg, 100 mg

**Contraindications** Hypersensitivity to beta-blocking agents, uncompensated congestive heart failure; cardiogenic shock; bradycardia (heart rate <45 bpm) or heart block; sinus node dysfunction; A-V conduction abnormalities, systolic blood pressure <100 mm Hg; diabetes mellitus. Although metoprolol primarily blocks beta$_1$-receptors, high doses can result in beta$_2$-receptor blockage; therefore, use with caution in elderly with bronchospastic lung disease.

**Warnings/Precautions** Use with caution in patients with inadequate myocardial function; those undergoing anesthesia, patients with CHF, myasthenia gravis, impaired hepatic or renal function, severe peripheral vascular disease, bronchospastic disease, diabetes mellitus or hyperthyroidism. Abrupt withdrawal of the drug should be avoided (may result in an exaggerated cardiac beta-adrenergic response, tachycardia, hypertension, ischemia, angina, myocardial infarction, and sudden death), drug should be discontinued over 1-2 weeks; do not use in pregnant or nursing women; may potentiate hypoglycemia in a diabetic patient and mask signs and symptoms; sweating will continue.

**Pregnancy Risk Factor** C

**Pregnancy Implications**

> Clinical effects on the fetus: Crosses the placenta. None; mild IUGR probably secondary to maternal hypertension. Available evidence suggests safe use during pregnancy and breast-feeding. Monitor breast-fed infant for symptoms of beta-blockade.
>
> Breast-feeding/lactation: Crosses into breast milk. American Academy of Pediatrics considers **compatible** with breast-feeding.

**Adverse Reactions**

> \>10%:
>
> Central nervous system: Fatigue/dizziness (10%)
>
> Neuromuscular & skeletal: Weakness
>
> 1% to 10%:
>
> Cardiovascular: Bradycardia (3%), arrhythmia, hypotension/reduced peripheral circulation (1%)
>
> Central nervous system: Mental depression (5%)
>
> Dermatologic: Pruritus/ash (5%)
>
> Gastrointestinal: Heartburn (1%), diarrhea (5%), nausea, xerostomia, abdominal pain (1%)
>
> Respiratory: Wheezing (1%), dyspnea (3%)
>
> <1%: Chest pain, heart failure, Raynaud's phenomenon, insomnia, nightmares, confusion, headache, memory loss, decreased sexual activity, constipation, nausea, vomiting, stomach discomfort, impotence, cold extremities

**Drug Interactions** CYP2D6 enzyme substrate

> Decreased effect of beta-blockers with aluminum salts, barbiturates, calcium salts, cholestyramine, colestipol, NSAIDs, penicillins (ampicillin), rifampin, salicylates and sulfinpyrazone due to decreased bioavailability and plasma levels; thyroid hormones, when hypothyroid patient is converted to euthyroid state
>
> Beta-blockers may decrease the effect of sulfonylureas
>
> Increased effect/toxicity of beta-blockers with calcium blockers (diltiazem, felodipine, nicardipine), oral contraceptives, flecainide, H$_2$-antagonists (cimetidine, possibly ranitidine), hydralazine, MAO inhibitors, phenothiazines, propafenone, quinidine (in extensive metabolizers), ciprofloxacin
>
> Beta-blockers may increase the effect/toxicity of flecainide, hydralazine, benzodiazepines (not atenolol), clonidine (hypertensive crisis after or during withdrawal of either agent), epinephrine (initial hypertensive episode followed by bradycardia), nifedipine, verapamil, lidocaine, ergots (peripheral ischemia), prazosin (postural hypotension)
>
> Beta-blockers may affect the action or levels of ethanol, disopyramide, nondepolarizing muscle relaxants and theophylline although the effects are difficult to predict

**Onset** Peak antihypertensive effect: Oral: Within 1.5-4 hours

**Duration** 10-20 hours

**Half-Life** 3-4 hours; End-stage renal disease: 2.5-4.5 hours

**Special PA Issues**

> **Patient Education:** I.V. use in emergency situations - patient information is included in general instructions.
>
> Oral: Take exactly as directed. Do not increase, decrease, or adjust dosage without consulting prescriber. Take pulse daily, prior to medication and follow prescriber's instruction about holding medication. Do not take with antacids. Do not use alcohol or OTC medications (eg, cold remedies) without consulting prescriber. If diabetic, monitor

serum sugars closely (may alter glucose tolerance or mask signs of hypoglycemia). May cause fatigue, dizziness, or postural hypotension; use caution when changing position from lying or sitting to standing, when driving, or when climbing stairs until response to medication is known. May cause alteration in sexual performance (reversible). Report unresolved swelling of extremities, difficulty breathing or new cough, unresolved fatigue, unusual weight gain, unresolved constipation, or unusual muscle weakness.

**Monitoring Parameters:** Blood pressure, apical and radial pulses, fluid I & O, daily weight, respirations, mental status, and circulation in extremities before and during therapy

**Related Information**
Beta-Blockers *on page 1002*

♦ **Metoprolol Succinate** *see* Metoprolol *on page 599*

♦ **Metoprolol Tartrate** *see* Metoprolol *on page 599*

♦ **Metreton® Ophthalmic** *see* Prednisolone *on page 752*

♦ **MetroGel® Topical** *see* Metronidazole *on this page*

♦ **MetroGel®-Vaginal** *see* Metronidazole *on this page*

♦ **Metro I.V.® Injection** *see* Metronidazole *on this page*

# Metronidazole (me troe NI da zole)

**Pharmacologic Class** Amebicide; Antibiotic, Topical; Antibiotic, Miscellaneous; Antiprotozoal

**U.S. Brand Names** Flagyl ER® Oral; Flagyl® Oral; MetroGel® Topical; MetroGel®-Vaginal; Metro I.V.® Injection; Noritate® Cream; Protostat® Oral

**Mechanism of Action** Reduced to a product which interacts with DNA to cause a loss of helical DNA structure and strand breakage resulting in inhibition of protein synthesis and cell death in susceptible organisms

**Use** Treatment of susceptible anaerobic bacterial and protozoal infections in the following conditions: amebiasis, symptomatic and asymptomatic trichomoniasis; skin and skin structure infections; CNS infections; intra-abdominal infections; systemic anaerobic infections; topically for the treatment of acne rosacea; treatment of antibiotic-associated pseudomembranous colitis (AAPC), bacterial vaginosis; used in combination with other agents (eg, tetracycline, bismuth subsalicylate, and an $H_2$-antagonist) to treat duodenal ulcer disease due to *Helicobacter pylori*; also used in Crohn's disease and hepatic encephalopathy

## USUAL DOSAGE

Neonates: Anaerobic infections: Oral, I.V.:

0-4 weeks: <1200 g: 7.5 mg/kg/dose every 48 hours

Postnatal age <7 days:

1200-2000 g: 7.5 mg/kg/day every 24 hours

>2000 g: 15 mg/kg/day in divided doses every 12 hours

Postnatal age >7 days:

1200-2000 g: 15 mg/kg/day in divided doses every 12 hours

>2000 g: 30 mg/kg/day in divided doses every 12 hours

Infants and Children:

Amebiasis: Oral: 35-50 mg/kg/day in divided doses every 8 hours for 10 days

Trichomoniasis: Oral: 15-30 mg/kg/day in divided doses every 8 hours for 7 days

Anaerobic infections:

Oral: 15-35 mg/kg/day in divided doses every 8 hours

I.V.: 30 mg/kg/day in divided doses every 6 hours

*Clostridium difficile* (antibiotic-associated colitis): Oral: 20 mg/kg/day divided every 6 hours

Maximum dose: 2 g/day

Adults:

Amebiasis: Oral: 500-750 mg every 8 hours for 5-10 days

Trichomoniasis: Oral: 250 mg every 8 hours for 7 days or 2 g as a single dose

Anaerobic infections: Oral, I.V.: 500 mg every 6-8 hours, not to exceed 4 g/day

Antibiotic-associated pseudomembranous colitis: Oral: 250-500 mg 3-4 times/day for 10-14 days

*H. pylori*: 1 capsule with meals and at bedtime for 14 days in combination with other agents (eg, tetracycline, bismuth subsalicylate, and $H_2$-antagonist)

Vaginosis: 1 applicatorful (~37.5 mg metronidazole) intravaginally once or twice daily for 5 days; apply once in morning and evening if using twice daily, if daily, use at bedtime

Elderly: Use lower end of dosing recommendations for adults, do not administer as a single dose

Topical (acne rosacea therapy): Apply and rub a thin film twice daily, morning and evening, to entire affected areas after washing. Significant therapeutic results should be noticed within 3 weeks. Clinical studies have demonstrated continuing improvement through 9 weeks of therapy.

**Dosing adjustment in renal impairment:** $Cl_{cr}$ <10 mL/minute: Administer every 12 hours

Hemodialysis: Extensively removed by hemodialysis and peritoneal dialysis (50% to 100%); administer dose posthemodialysis

(Continued)

## Metronidazole *(Continued)*

Peritoneal dialysis: Dose as or Cl<sub>cr</sub> <10 mL/minute

Continuous arteriovenous or venovenous hemofiltration (CAVH/CAVHD): Administer usual dose

**Dosing adjustment/comments in hepatic disease:** Unchanged in mild liver disease; reduce dosage in severe liver disease

**Dosage Forms Cap:** 375 mg **Gel, top:** 0.75% [7.5 mg/mL] (30 g); **Gel, vaginal:** 0.75% (5 g applicator delivering 37.5 mg in 70 g tube); **Inj, ready to use:** 5 mg/mL (100 mL); **Tab:** 250 mg, 500 mg;

Metronidazole hydrochloride **Powder for inj:** 500 mg

**Contraindications** Hypersensitivity to metronidazole or any component, 1st trimester of pregnancy since found to be carcinogenic in rats

**Warnings/Precautions** Use with caution in patients with liver impairment due to potential accumulation, blood dyscrasias; history of seizures, congestive heart failure, or other sodium retaining states; reduce dosage in patients with severe liver impairment, CNS disease, and severe renal failure (Cl<sub>cr</sub> <10 mL/minute); if *H. pylori* is not eradicated in patients being treated with metronidazole in a regimen, it should be assumed that metronidazole-resistance has occurred and it should not again be used; seizures and neuropathies have been reported especially with increased doses and chronic treatment; if this occurs, discontinue therapy

**Pregnancy Risk Factor** B

**Adverse Reactions**

>10%:

Central nervous system: Dizziness, headache

Gastrointestinal (12%): Nausea, diarrhea, loss of appetite, vomiting

<1%: Ataxia, seizures, disulfiram-type reaction with alcohol, pancreatitis, xerostomia, metallic taste, furry tongue, vaginal candidiasis, leukopenia, thrombophlebitis, neuropathy, hypersensitivity, change in taste sensation, dark urine

**Drug Interactions** CYP2C9 enzyme substrate; CYP2C9, 3A3/4, and 3A5-7 enzyme inhibitor

Decreased effect: Phenytoin, phenobarbital may decrease metronidazole half-life

Increased toxicity: Alcohol or disulfiram results in disulfiram-like reactions; metronidazole increases P-T prolongation with warfarin and increases lithium levels/toxicity; cimetidine may increase metronidazole levels

**Half-Life** 6-8 hours, increases with hepatic impairment; End-stage renal disease: 21 hours

**Special PA Issues**

**Patient Education:** Take exactly as directed, with meals. Avoid alcohol during and for 24 hours after last dose. With alcohol your may experience severe flushing, headache, nausea, vomiting, or chest and abdominal pain. Urine may be reddish or dark brown in color (normal). You may experience "metallic" taste disturbance or nausea or vomiting (small frequent meals, chewing gum, or sucking on lozenges may help). Refrain from intercourse or use a barrier contraceptive if being treated for trichomoniasis. Report unresolved or severe fatigue; weakness; fever or chills; mouth or vaginal sores; numbness, tingling, or swelling of extremities; difficulty breathing; or lack of improvement or worsening of condition.

Topical: Wash hands and area before applying and medication thinly. Wash hands after applying. Avoid contact with eyes. Do not cover with occlusive dressing. Report severe skin irritation or if condition does not improve.

**Dietary Considerations:**

Alcohol: A disulfiram-like reaction characterized by flushing, headache, nausea, vomiting, sweating or tachycardia; patients should be warned to avoid alcohol during and 72 hours after therapy

Food: Peak antibiotic serum concentration lowered and delayed, but total drug absorbed not affected. Take on an empty stomach. Drug may cause GI upset; if GI upset occurs, take with food.

♦ **Metronidazole Hydrochloride** *see* Metronidazole *on previous page*

♦ **Mevacor®** *see* Lovastatin *on page 546*

♦ **Meval®** *see* Diazepam *on page 269*

♦ **Mevinolin** *see* Lovastatin *or page 546*

## Mexiletine *(MEKS i le teen)*

**Pharmacologic Class** Antiarrhythmic Agent, Class I-B

**U.S. Brand Names** Mexitil®

**Mechanism of Action** Class IB antiarrhythmic, structurally related to lidocaine, which inhibits inward sodium current, decreases rate of rise of phase 0, increases effective refractory period/action potential duration ratio

**Use** Management of serious ventricular arrhythmias; use with lesser arrhythmias is generally not recommended

**Unlabeled use:** Diabetic neuropathy, reduction of ventricular tachycardia and other arrhythmias in the acute phase of myocardial infarction (mortality may not be reduced)

**USUAL DOSAGE** Adults: Oral: Initial: 200 mg every 8 hours (may load with 400 mg if necessary); adjust dose every 2-3 days; usual dose: 200-300 mg every 8 hours; maximum dose: 1.2 g/day (some patients respond to every 12-hour dosing); patients with hepatic impairment or CHF may require dose reduction; when switching from another antiarrhythmic, initiate a 200 mg dose 6-12 hours after stopping former agents, 3-6 hours after stopping procainamide

**Dosage Forms** Cap: 150 mg, 200 mg, 250 mg

**Contraindications** Cardiogenic shock, second or third degree heart block, hypersensitivity to mexiletine or any component

**Warnings/Precautions** Exercise extreme caution in patients with pre-existing sinus node dysfunction; mexiletine can worsen CHF, bradycardias, and other arrhythmias; mexiletine, like other antiarrhythmic agents, is proarrhythmic; CAST study indicates a trend toward increased mortality with antiarrhythmics in the face of cardiac disease (myocardial infarction); elevation of AST/ALT; hepatic necrosis reported; leukopenia, agranulocytopenia, and thrombocytopenia; seizures; alterations in urinary pH may change urinary excretion; electrolyte disturbances (hypokalemia, hyperkalemia, etc) after drug response

**Pregnancy Risk Factor** C

**Adverse Reactions**
>10%:
Central nervous system: Lightheadedness (10.5%), dizziness (20% to 25%), nervousness (5% to 10%), incoordination (10.2%)
Gastrointestinal: GI distress (41%), nausea/vomiting (40%)
Neuromuscular & skeletal: Trembling, unsteady gait, tremor (12.6%)
1% to 10%:
Cardiovascular: Chest pain (2.5% to 7.5%), premature ventricular contractions (1% to 2%), palpitations (4% to 8%)
Central nervous system: Confusion, headache, insomnia (5% to 7%)
Dermatologic: Rash (3.8% to 4.2%)
Gastrointestinal: Constipation or diarrhea (4% to 5%), xerostomia (2.8%), abdominal pain (1.2%)
Neuromuscular & skeletal: Weakness, numbness of fingers or toes (2% to 4%)
Ocular: Blurred vision (5% to 7%)
Otic: Tinnitus (2% to 2.5%)
Respiratory: Shortness of breath
<1%: Leukopenia, agranulocytosis, thrombocytopenia, positive antinuclear antibody, increased LFTs, diplopia

**Drug Interactions** CYP2D6 enzyme substrate; CYP1A2 enzyme inhibitor
Decreased plasma levels: Phenobarbital, phenytoin, rifampin, and other hepatic enzyme inducers, cimetidine and drugs which make the urine acidic
Increased effect: Allopurinol
Increased toxicity/levels of caffeine and theophylline

**Half-Life** 10-14 hours (average: 14.4 hours elderly, 12 hours in younger adults); increase in half-life with hepatic or heart failure

**Special PA Issues**
Patient Education: Take exactly as directed, with food or antacids, around-the-clock. Do not take additional doses or discontinue without consulting prescriber. Do not change diet without consulting prescriber. You will need regular cardiac check-ups and blood tests while taking this medication. You may experience drowsiness or dizziness, numbness, or visual changes (use caution when driving or performing tasks that require alertness until response to drug is determined); nausea, vomiting, or heartburn (small frequent meals, frequent mouth care, or sucking lozenges may help); or headaches or sleep disturbances (usually temporary, if persistent consult prescriber). Report chest pain, palpitation, or erratic heartbeat; increased weight or swelling of hands or feet; chills, fever, or persistent sore throat; numbness, weakness, trembling, or unsteady gait; blurred vision or ringing in ears; or difficulty breathing.

Reference Range: Therapeutic range: 0.5-2 µg/mL; potentially toxic: >2 µg/mL

♦ **Mexitil®** see Mexiletine on previous page

♦ **Mezlin®** see Mezlocillin on this page

## Mezlocillin (mez loe SIL in)

**Pharmacologic Class** Antibiotic, Penicillin

**U.S. Brand Names** Mezlin®

**Mechanism of Action** Inhibits bacterial cell wall synthesis by binding to one or more of the penicillin binding proteins (PBPs); which in turn inhibits the final transpeptidation step of peptidoglycan synthesis in bacterial cell walls, thus inhibiting cell wall biosynthesis. Bacteria eventually lyse due to ongoing activity of cell wall autolytic enzymes (autolysins and murein hydrolases) while cell wall assembly is arrested.

**Use** Treatment of infections caused by susceptible gram-negative aerobic bacilli (*Klebsiella, Proteus, Escherichia coli, Enterobacter, Pseudomonas aeruginosa, Serratia*) involving the skin and skin structure, bone and joint, respiratory tract, urinary tract, gastrointestinal tract, as well as, septicemia
(Continued)

## Mezlocillin *(Continued)*

**USUAL DOSAGE** I.M., I.V.:

Infants:

≤7 days, ≤2000 g: 75 mg/kg every 12 hours

≤7 days, >2000 g: Same as above

>7 days, ≤2000 g: 75 mg/kg every 8 hours

>7 days, >2000 g: 75 mg/kg every 6 hours

Children: 300 mg/kg/day divided every 4-6 hours; maximum: 24 g/day

Adults: Usual: 3-4 g every 4-6 hours

Uncomplicated urinary tract infection: 1.5-2 g every 6 hours

Serious infections: 200-300 mg/kg/day in 4-6 divided doses

**Dosing interval in renal impairment:**

Cl$_{cr}$ 10-30 mL/minute: Administer every 6-8 hours

Cl$_{cr}$ <10 mL/minute: Administer every 8 hours

Hemodialysis: Moderately dialyzable (20% to 50%)

**Dosing adjustment in hepatic impairment:** Reduce dose by 50%

**Dosage Forms** Powder for inj, as sodium: 1 g, 2 g, 3 g, 4 g, 20 g

**Contraindications** Hypersensitivity to mezlocillin, any component, or penicillins

**Warnings/Precautions** If bleeding occurs during therapy, mezlocillin should be discontinued; dosage modification required in patients with impaired renal function; use with caution in patients with renal impairment or biliary obstruction, or history of allergy to cephalosporins

**Pregnancy Risk Factor** B

**Adverse Reactions**

1% to 10%: Gastrointestinal: Nausea, diarrhea

<1%: Fever, seizures, dizziness, headache, rash, exfoliative dermatitis, hypokalemia, hypernatremia, vomiting eosinophilia, leukopenia, neutropenia, thrombocytopenia, agranulocytosis, hemolytic anemia, prolonged bleeding time, positive Coombs' [direct], hepatotoxicity, elevated liver enzymes, hematuria, elevated BUN/serum creatinine, interstitial nephritis, serum sickness-like reactions

**Drug Interactions** Aminoglycosides (synergy), probenecid (decreased clearance), vecuronium (increased duration of neuromuscular blockade), heparin (increased risk of bleeding); possible decrease in effectiveness of oral contraceptives; bacteriostatic action of tetracycline may impair bactericidal effects of the penicillins

**Half-Life** Dose dependent: 50-70 minutes, increased in renal impairment

**Special PA Issues**

**Patient Education:** This medication can only be administered by infusion or injection. Maintain adequate hydration (2-3 L/day of fluids unless instructed to restrict fluid intake). Small frequent meals, frequent mouth care, and adequate fluids may reduce incidence of nausea or vomiting. If diabetic, drug may cause false tests with Clinitest® urine glucose monitoring; use of glucose oxidase methods (Clinistix®) or serum glucose monitoring is preferable. This drug may interfere with oral contraceptives; an alternate form of birth control should be used. Report difficulty breathing, acute diarrhea, systemic rash, fever, white plaques in mouth, or mouth sores.

**Monitoring Parameters:** Observe for signs and symptoms of anaphylaxis during first dose

♦ **Mezlocillin Sodium** *see Mezlocillin on previous page*

♦ **Miacalcin® Injection** *see Calcitonin on page 136*

♦ **Miacalcin® Nasal Spray** *see Calcitonin on page 136*

♦ **Micanol® Cream** *see Anthralin on page 72*

♦ **Micardis®** *see Telmisartan on page 875*

♦ **Micatin® Topical [OTC]** *see Miconazole on this page*

## Miconazole (mi KON a zole)

**Pharmacologic Class** Antifungal Agent, Parenteral; Antifungal Agent, Topical; Antifungal Agent, Vaginal

**U.S. Brand Names** Absorbine® Antifungal Foot Powder [OTC]; Breezee® Mist Antifungal [OTC]; Femizol-M® [OTC]; Fungoid® Creme; Fungoid® Tincture; Lotrimin® AF Powder [OTC]; Lotrimin® AF Spray Liquid [OTC]; Lotrimin® AF Spray Powder [OTC]; Maximum Strength Desenex® Antifungal Cream [OTC]; Micatin® Topical [OTC]; Monistat-Derm™ Topical; Monistat i.v.™ Injection; Monistat™ Vaginal; M-Zole® 7 Dual Pack [OTC]; Ony-Clear® Spray; Prescription Strength Desenex® [OTC]; Zeasorb-AF® Powder [OTC]

**Mechanism of Action** Inhibits biosynthesis of ergosterol, damaging the fungal cell wall membrane, which increases permeability causing leaking of nutrients

**Use**

I.V.: Treatment of severe systemic fungal infections and fungal meningitis that are refractory to standard treatment

Topical: Treatment of vulvovaginal candidiasis and a variety of skin and mucous membrane fungal infections

**USUAL DOSAGE**

Children:

<1 year: 15-30 mg/kg/day

1-12 years:

I.V.: 20-40 mg/kg/day divided every 8 hours (do not exceed 15 mg/kg/dose)

Topical: Apply twice daily for up to 1 month

Adults:

Topical: Apply twice daily for up to 1 month

I.T.: 20 mg every 1-2 days

I.V.: Initial: 200 mg, then 0.6-3.6 g/day divided every 8 hours for up to 20 weeks

Bladder candidal infections: 200 mg diluted solution instilled in the bladder

Vaginal: Insert contents of 1 applicator of vaginal cream (100 mg) or 100 mg suppository at bedtime for 7 days, or 200 mg suppository at bedtime for 3 days

Hemodialysis: Not dialyzable (0% to 5%)

**Dosage Forms Inj:** 1% [10 mg/mL] (20 mL); **Tinct:** 2% with alcohol (7.39 mL, 29.57 mL)

Miconazole nitrate: **Crm: Topical:** 2% (15 g, 30 g, 56.7 g, 85 g); **Vag:** 2% (45 g is equivalent to 7 doses); **Lot:** 2% (30 mL, 60 mL); **Powder, top:** 2% (45 g, 90 g, 113 g); **Spray, top:** 2% (105 mL); **Supp, vag:** 100 mg (7s); 200 mg (3s)

**Contraindications** Hypersensitivity to miconazole, fluconazole, ketoconazole, polyoxyl 35 castor oil, or any component; concomitant administration with cisapride

**Warnings/Precautions** Administer I.V. with caution to patients with hepatic insufficiency; the safety of miconazole in patients <1 year of age has not been established; cardiorespiratory and anaphylaxis have occurred with excessively rapid administration

**Pregnancy Risk Factor** C

**Adverse Reactions**

>10%:

Central nervous system: Fever, chills (10%)

Dermatologic: Rash, itching, pruritus (21%)

Gastrointestinal: Anorexia, diarrhea, nausea (18%), vomiting (7%)

Local: Pain at injection site

1% to 10%: Dermatologic: Rash (9%)

<1%: Flushing of face or skin, drowsiness, anemia, thrombocytopenia

**Drug Interactions** CYP3A3/4 enzyme substrate; CYP2C enzyme inhibitor, CYP3A3/4 enzyme inhibitor (moderate), and CYP3A5-7 enzyme inhibitor

Warfarin (increased anticoagulant effect), oral sulfonylureas, amphotericin B (decreased antifungal effect of both agents), phenytoin (levels may be increased)

Increased risk of significant cardiotoxicity with concurrent administration of cisapride - concomitant administration is contraindicated

**Half-Life** I.V.: Multiphasic: Initial: 40 minutes; Secondary: 126 minutes; Terminal phase: 24 hours

**Special PA Issues**

**Patient Education:** Take full course of therapy as directed; do not discontinue without consulting prescriber. Some infections may require long periods of therapy. Practice good hygiene measures to prevent reinfection.

Topical: Wash and dry area before applying medication; apply thinly. Do not get in or near eyes.

Vaginal: Insert high in vagina. Refrain from intercourse during treatment.

If you are diabetic you should test serum glucose regularly at same time of day. You may experience nausea and vomiting (small, frequent meals may help) or headache, dizziness (use caution when driving). Report unresolved headache, rash, burning, itching, anorexia, unusual fatigue, diarrhea, nausea, or vomiting.

◆ **Miconazole Nitrate** *see* Miconazole *on previous page*

◆ **MICRhoGAM™** *see* Rh₀(D) Immune Globulin (Intramuscular) *on page 800*

# Microfibrillar Collagen Hemostat

(mye kro FI bri lar KOL la jen HEE moe stat)

**Pharmacologic Class** Hemostatic Agent

**U.S. Brand Names** Avitene®; Helistat®; Hemotene®

**Mechanism of Action** Microfibrillar collagen hemostat is an absorbable topical hemostatic agent prepared from purified bovine corium collagen and shredded into fibrils. Physically, microfibrillar collagen hemostat yields a large surface area. Chemically, it is collagen with hydrochloric acid noncovalently bound to some of the available amino groups in the collagen molecules. When in contact with a bleeding surface, microfibrillar collagen hemostat attracts platelets which adhere to its fibrils and undergo the release phenomenon. This triggers aggregation of the platelets into thrombi in the interstices of the fibrous mass, initiating the formation of a physiologic platelet plug.

**Use** Adjunct to hemostasis when control of bleeding by ligature is ineffective or impractical

**USUAL DOSAGE** Apply dry directly to source of bleeding

**Dosage Forms Fibrous:** 1 g, 5 g; **Nonwoven web:** 70 mm x 70 mm x 1 mm; 70 mm x 35 mm x 1 mm; **Sponge:** 1" x 2" (10s); 3" x 4" (10s); 9" x 10" (5s)

(Continued)

## Microfibrillar Collagen Hemostat *(Continued)*

**Contraindications** Closure of skin incisions, contaminated wounds

**Warnings/Precautions** Fragments of MCH may pass through filters of blood scavenging systems, avoid reintroduction of blood from operative sites treated with MCH; after several minutes remove excess material

**Pregnancy Risk Factor** C

**Adverse Reactions** 1% to 10%: Miscellaneous: Potentiation of infection, allergic reaction, adhesion formation

♦ **Micro-K® 10** *see* Potassium Chloride *on page 742*

♦ **Micro-K® Extencaps®** *see* Potassium Chloride *on page 742*

♦ **Micro-K® LS®** *see* Potassium Chloride *on page 742*

♦ **Micronase®** *see* Glyburide *on page 419*

♦ **Microsulfon®** *see* Sulfadiazine *on page 859*

♦ **Microzide™** *see* Hydrochlorothiazide *on page 447*

♦ **Midamor®** *see* Amiloride *on page 51*

## Midazolam (MID aye zoe am)

**Pharmacologic Class** Benzodiazepine

**U.S. Brand Names** Versed®

**Mechanism of Action** Depresses all levels of the CNS, including the limbic and reticular formation, probably through the increased action of gamma-aminobutyric acid (GABA), which is a major inhibitory neurotransmitter in the brain

**Use** Preoperative sedation and provides conscious sedation prior to diagnostic or radiographic procedures

**Unlabeled use:** Anxiety, status epilepticus

**USUAL DOSAGE** The dose of midazolam needs to be individualized based on the patient's age, underlying diseases, and concurrent medications. Decrease dose (by ~30%) if narcotics or other CNS depressants are administered concomitantly. **Personnel and equipment needed for standard respiratory resuscitation should be immediately available during midazolam administration.**

Neonates: Conscious sedation during mechanical ventilation: I.V. continuous infusion: 0.15-1 mcg/kg/minute. Use smallest dose possible; use lower doses (up to 0.5 mcg/kg/minute) for preterm neonates

Infants <2 months and Children: Status epilepticus refractory to standard therapy: I.V.: Loading dose: 0.15 mg/kg followed by a continuous infusion of 1 mcg/kg/minute; titrate dose upward very 5 minutes until clinical seizure activity is controlled; mean infusion rate required in 24 children was 2.3 mcg/kg/minute with a range of 1-18 mcg/kg/minute

Children:

Preoperative sedation:

Oral: Single dose preprocedure: 0.25-0.5 mg/kg, up to a maximum of 20 mg, depending on the status of the patient and desired effect; patients between 6 months and younger than 6 years, or less cooperative patients may require as much as 0.1 mg/kg as a single dose

I.M.: 0.07-0.08 mg/kg 30-60 minutes presurgery

I.V.: 0.035 mg/kg/dose, repeat over several minutes as required to achieve the desired sedative effect up to a total dose of 0.1-0.2 mg/kg

Conscious sedation during mechanical ventilation: I.V.: Loading dose: 0.05-0.2 mg/kg then follow with initial continuous infusion: 1-2 mcg/kg/minute; titrate to the desired effect; usual range: 0.4-6 mcg/kg/minute

Conscious sedation for procedures:

Oral, Intranasal: 0.2-0.4 mg/kg (maximum: 15 mg) 30-45 minutes before the procedure

I.V.: 0.05 mg/kg 3 minutes before procedure

Adolescents >12 years: I.V.: 0.5 mg every 3-4 minutes until effect achieved

Adults:

Preoperative sedation: I.M.: 0.07-0.08 mg/kg 30-60 minutes presurgery; usual dose: 5 mg

Conscious sedation: I.V.: Initial: 0.5-2 mg slow I.V. over at least 2 minutes; slowly titrate to effect by repeating doses every 2-3 minutes if needed; usual total dose: 2.5-5 mg; use decreased doses in elderly

Healthy Adults <60 years: Some patients respond to doses as low as 1 mg; no more than 2.5 mg should be administered over a period of 2 minutes. Additional doses of midazolam may be administered after a 2-minute waiting period and evaluation of sedation after each dose increment. A total dose >5 mg is generally not needed. If narcotics or other CNS depressants are administered concomitantly, the midazolam dose should be reduced by 30%.

Elderly: I.V.: Conscious sedation: Initial: 0.5 mg slow I.V.; give no more than 1.5 mg in a 2-minute period; if additional titration is needed, give no more than 1 mg over 2 minutes, waiting another 2 or more minutes to evaluate sedative effect; a total dose of >3.5 mg is rarely necessary

Sedation in mechanically intubated patients: I.V. continuous infusion: 100 mg in 250 mL D$_5$W or NS, (if patient is fluid-restricted, may concentrate up to a maximum of 0.5 mg/mL);

initial dose: 0.01-0.05 mg/kg (~0.5-4 mg for a typical adult) initially and either repeated at 10-15 minute intervals until adequate sedation is achieved or continuous infusion rates of 0.02-0.1 mg/kg/hour (1-7 mg/hour) and titrate to reach desired level of sedation

Hemodialysis: Supplemental dose is not necessary

Peritoneal dialysis: Significant drug removal is unlikely based on physiochemical characteristics

**Dosage Forms Inj, as hydrochloride:** 1 mg/mL (2 mL, 5 mL, 10 mL), 5 mg/mL (1 mL, 2 mL, 5 mL, 10 mL); **Syr:** 2 mg/mL (118 mL)

**Contraindications** Hypersensitivity to midazolam or any component (cross-sensitivity with other benzodiazepines may occur); uncontrolled pain; existing CNS depression; shock; narrow-angle glaucoma

**Warnings/Precautions** Use with caution in patients with congestive heart failure, renal impairment, pulmonary disease, hepatic dysfunction, the elderly, and those receiving concomitant narcotics; midazolam may cause respiratory depression/arrest; deaths and hypoxic encephalopathy have resulted when these were not promptly recognized and treated appropriately. Serious respiratory reactions have occurred after midazolam syrup, most often when used in combination with other CNS depressants. It should only be used in hospital or ambulatory care settings that are equipped with the capabilities to monitor cardiac and respiratory function.

**Pregnancy Risk Factor** D

**Adverse Reactions**

>10%:

Local: Pain and local reactions at injection site (severity less than diazepam)

Miscellaneous: Hiccups

1% to 10%:

Cardiovascular: Cardiac arrest, hypotension, bradycardia

Central nervous system: Drowsiness, ataxia, amnesia, dizziness, paradoxical excitement, sedation, headache

Gastrointestinal: Nausea, vomiting

Ocular: Blurred vision, diplopia

Respiratory: Respiratory depression, apnea, laryngospasm, bronchospasm

Miscellaneous: Physical and psychological dependence with prolonged use

<1%: Tachycardia, delirium, rash, wheezing

**Drug Interactions** CYP3A3/4 enzyme substrate

Decreased effect: Theophylline may antagonize the sedative effects of midazolam

Increased toxicity: CNS depressants, may increase sedation and respiratory depression; doses of anesthetic agents should be reduced when used in conjunction with midazolam; cimetidine may increase midazolam serum concentrations

**If narcotics or other CNS depressants are administered concomitantly, the midazolam dose should be reduced by 30%, if <65 years of age or by at least 50%, if >65 years of age.**

**Onset**

I.M.: Within 15 minutes; Peak effect: 0.5-1 hour

I.V.: Within 1-5 minutes

**Duration** I.M.: 2 hours mean, up to 6 hours

**Half-Life** 1-4 hours, increased with cirrhosis, CHF, obesity, elderly

## Causes of Orthostatic Hypotensin

| **Primary Autonomic Causes** |
| --- |
| Pure autonomic failure (Bradbury-Eggleston syndrome, idiopathic orthostatic hypotension) |
| Autonomic failure with multiple system atrophy (Shy-Drager syndrome) |
| Familial dysautonomia (Riley-Day syndrome) |
| Dopamine beta-hydroxylase deficiency |
| **Secondary Autonomic Causes** |
| Chronic alcoholism |
| Parkinson's disease |
| Diabetes mellitus |
| Porphyria |
| Amyloidosis |
| Various carcinomas |
| Vitamin $B_1$ or $B_{12}$ deficiency |
| **Nonautonomic Causes** |
| Hypovolemia (such as associated with hemorrhage, burns, or hemodialysis) and dehydration |
| Diminished homeostatic regulation (such as associated with aging, pregnancy, fever, or prolonged best rest) |
| Medications (eg, antihypertensives, insulin, tricyclic antidepressants) |

(Continued)

## Midazolam *(Continued)*

### Special PA Issues

**Patient Education:** Avoid use of alcohol or prescription or OTC sedatives or hypnotics for a minimum of 24 hours after administration. Avoid driving or engaging in any tasks that require alertness for 24 hours following administration. You may experience some loss of memory following administration.

**Monitoring Parameters:** Respiratory and cardiovascular status, blood pressure, blood pressure monitor required during I.V. administration

♦ **Midazolam Hydrochloride** *see Midazolam on page 606*

♦ **Midchlor®** *see Acetaminophen, Isometheptene, and Dichloralphenazone on page 23*

## Midodrine *(MI doe dreen)*

**Pharmacologic Class** Alpha₁ Agonist

**U.S. Brand Names** ProAmatine®

**Mechanism of Action** Midodrine forms an active metabolite, desglymidodrine, that is an alpha₁-agonist. This agent increases arteriolar and venous tone resulting in a rise in standing, sitting, and supine systolic and diastolic blood pressure in patients with orthostatic hypotension.

**Use** Treatment of symptomatic orthostatic hypotension

**Investigational:** Management of urinary incontinence

**USUAL DOSAGE** Adults: Oral: 10 mg 3 times/day during daytime hours (every 3-4 hours) when patient is upright (maximum: 40 mg/day)

**Dosing adjustment in renal impairment:** 2.5 mg 3 times/day, gradually increasing as tolerated

**Dosage Forms Tab, as hydrochloride:** 2.5 mg, 5 mg

**Contraindications** Severe organic heart disease, urinary retention, pheochromocytoma, thyrotoxicosis, persistent and significant supine hypertension; hypersensitivity to midodrine or any component; concurrent use of fludrocortisone

**Warnings/Precautions** Only indicated for patients for whom orthostatic hypotension significantly impairs their daily life. Use is not recommended with supine hypertension and caution should be exercised in patients with diabetes, visual problems, urinary retention (reduce initial dose) or hepatic dysfunction; monitor renal and hepatic function prior to and periodically during therapy; safety and efficacy has not been established in children; discontinue and re-evaluate therapy if signs of bradycardia occur.

**Pregnancy Risk Factor C**

**Pregnancy Implications** Clinical effects on the fetus: No studies are available; use during pregnancy and lactation should be avoided unless the potential benefit outweighs the risk to the fetus

**Adverse Reactions**

>10%:

Dermatologic: Piloerection (13%), pruritus (12%)

Genitourinary: Urinary urgency, retention, or polyuria, dysuria (up to 13%)

Neuromuscular & skeletal: Paresthesia (18.3%)

1% to 10%:

Cardiovascular: Supine hypertension, (7%) facial flushing

Central nervous system: Confusion, anxiety, dizziness, chills (5%)

Dermatologic: Rash, dry skin (2%)

Gastrointestinal: Xerostomia, nausea, abdominal pain

Neuromuscular & skeletal: Pain (5%)

<1%: Flushing, headache, insomnia, flatulence, leg cramps, visual changes

**Drug Interactions** Increased effect: Concomitant fludrocortisone results in hypernatremia or an increase in intraocular pressure and glaucoma; bradycardia may be accentuated with concomitant administration of cardiac glycosides, psychotherapeutics, and beta-blockers; alpha-agonists may increase the pressure effects and alpha-antagonists may negate the effects of midodrine

**Onset** Within 1 hour

**Duration** May last for 2-3 hours

**Half-Life** ~3-4 hours (active drug); 25 minutes (prodrug)

**Special PA Issues**

**Patient Education:** This drug may relieve positional hypotension; effects must be evaluated regularly. Take prescribed amount 3 times daily (shortly before rising in the morning, at midday, and in late afternoon); do not take after 6 PM or within 4 hours of bedtime or when lying down for any length of time. Follow recommended diet and exercise program. Do not use OTC medications which may affect blood pressure (eg, cough or cold remedies, diet pills, stay-awake medications) without consulting prescriber. You may experience urinary urgency or retention (void before taking or consult prescriber if difficulty persists); or dizziness, drowsiness, or headache (use caution when driving or engaging in tasks that require alertness until response to drug is known). Report skin rash, severe gastric upset or pain, muscle weakness or pain, or other persistent side effects.

**Monitoring Parameters:** Blood pressure, renal and hepatic parameters

♦ **Midodrine Hydrochloride** *see* Midodrine *on previous page*

♦ **Midol® 200 [OTC]** *see* Ibuprofen *on page 466*

♦ **Midrin®** *see* Acetaminophen, Isometheptene, and Dichloralphenazone *on page 23*

♦ **Migranal® Nasal Spray** *see* Dihydroergotamine *on page 285*

♦ **Migratine®** *see* Acetaminophen, Isometheptene, and Dichloralphenazone *on page 23*

♦ **Miles Nervine® Caplets [OTC]** *see* Diphenhydramine *on page 289*

♦ **Milk of Magnesia** *see* Magnesium Hydroxide *on page 552*

♦ **Milliequivalent and Millimole Calculations & Conversions** *see* Chart *on page 981*

♦ **Milophene®** *see* Clomiphene *on page 222*

## Milrinone (MIL ri none)

**Pharmacologic Class** Phosphodiesterase Enzyme Inhibitor

**U.S. Brand Names** Primacor®

**Mechanism of Action** Phosphodiesterase inhibitor resulting in vasodilation

**Use** Short-term I.V. therapy of congestive heart failure; used for calcium antagonist intoxication

**USUAL DOSAGE** Adults: I.V.: Loading dose: 50 mcg/kg administered over 10 minutes followed by a maintenance dose titrated according to the hemodynamic and clinical response, see table.

| Maintenance Dosage | Dose Rate (mcg/kg/min) | Total Dose (mg/kg/24 h) |
|---|---|---|
| Minimum | 0.375 | 0.59 |
| Standard | 0.500 | 0.77 |
| Maximum | 0.750 | 1.13 |

**Dosing adjustment in renal impairment:**

$Cl_{cr}$ 50 mL/minute/1.73 m$^2$: Administer 0.43 mcg/kg/minute

$Cl_{cr}$ 40 mL/minute/1.73 m$^2$: Administer 0.38 mcg/kg/minute

$Cl_{cr}$ 30 mL/minute/1.73 m$^2$: Administer 0.33 mcg/kg/minute

$Cl_{cr}$ 20 mL/minute/1.73 m$^2$: Administer 0.28 mcg/kg/minute

$Cl_{cr}$ 10 mL/minute/1.73 m$^2$: Administer 0.23 mcg/kg/minute

$Cl_{cr}$ 5 mL/minute/1.73 m$^2$: Administer 0.2 mcg/kg/minute

**Dosage Forms Inj, as lactate:** 1 mg/mL (5 mL, 10 mL, 20 mL)

**Contraindications** Hypersensitivity to drug or amrinone

**Warnings/Precautions** Severe obstructive aortic or pulmonic valvular disease, history of ventricular arrhythmias; atrial fibrillation, flutter; renal dysfunction. Life-threatening arrhythmias were infrequent and have been associated with pre-existing arrhythmias, metabolic abnormalities, abnormal digoxin levels, and catheter insertion

**Pregnancy Risk Factor** C

**Adverse Reactions**

>10%: Cardiovascular: Ventricular arrhythmias (12.1%)

1% to 10%:

Cardiovascular: Supraventricular arrhythmias, hypotension (2.9%), angina/chest pain (1.2), ventricular tachycardia (1% to 3%)

Central nervous system: Headache (3%)

<1%: Ventricular fibrillation, hypokalemia, thrombocytopenia, tremor

**Half-Life** I.V.: 136 minutes in patients with CHF; patients with severe CHF have a more prolonged half-life, with values ranging from 1.7-2.7 hours. Patients with CHF have a reduction in the systemic clearance of milrinone, resulting in a prolonged elimination half-life. Alternatively, one study reported that 1 month of therapy with milrinone did not change the pharmacokinetic parameters for patients with CHF despite improvement in cardiac function.

**Special PA Issues**

**Patient Education:** This drug can only be given intravenously. If you experience increased voiding call for assistance. Report pain at infusion site, numbness or tingling of extremities, or difficulty breathing.

**Monitoring Parameters:** Cardiac monitor and blood pressure monitor required; serum potassium

Therapeutic: Patients should be monitored for improvement in the clinical signs and symptoms of congestive heart failure

Toxic: Patients should be monitored for ventricular arrhythmias and exacerbation of anginal symptoms; during I.V. therapy with milrinone, blood pressure and heart rate should be monitored

♦ **Milrinone Lactate** *see* Milrinone *on this page*

♦ **Miltown®** *see* Meprobamate *on page 570*

- **Minidyne® [OTC]** *see* Povidone-Iodine *on page 747*
- **Mini-Gamulin® Rh** *see* Rh₀(D) Immune Globulin (Intramuscular) *on page 800*
- **Minims® Pilocarpine** *see* Pilocarpine *on page 726*
- **Minipress®** *see* Prazosin *on page 750*
- **Minitran® Patch** *see* Nitroglycerin *on page 660*
- **Minizide®** *see* Prazosin and Polythiazide *on page 751*
- **Minocin® IV Injection** *see* Minocycline *on this page*
- **Minocin® Oral** *see* Minocycline *on this page*

# Minocycline (mi noe SYE kleen)

**Pharmacologic Class** Antibiotic, Tetracycline Derivative

**U.S. Brand Names** Dynacin® Oral; Minocin® IV Injection; Minocin® Oral

**Mechanism of Action** Inhibits bacterial protein synthesis by binding with the 30S and possibly the 50S ribosomal subunit(s) of susceptible bacteria; cell wall synthesis is not affected

**Use** Treatment of susceptible bacterial infections of both gram-negative and gram-positive organisms; acne, meningococcal carrier state

## USUAL DOSAGE

Children >8 years: Oral, I.V.: Initial: 4 mg/kg followed by 2 mg/kg/dose every 12 hours

Adults:

Infection: Oral, I.V.: 200 mg stat, 100 mg every 12 hours not to exceed 400 mg/24 hours

Acne: Oral: 50 mg 1-3 times/day

Hemodialysis: Not dialyzable (0% to 5%)

**Dosage Forms Cap:** 50 mg, 100 mg; **Cap (Dynacin®):** 50 mg, 100 mg; **Cap, pellet-filled (Minocin®):** 50 mg, 100 mg; **Inj (Minocin® IV):** 100 mg; **Susp, oral (Minocin®):** 50 mg/5 mL (60 mL)

**Contraindications** Hypersensitivity to minocycline, other tetracyclines, or any component; children <8 years of age

**Warnings/Precautions** Should be avoided in renal insufficiency, children ≤8 years of age, pregnant and nursing women; photosensitivity reactions can occur with minocycline

**Pregnancy Risk Factor D**

## Adverse Reactions

>10%: Miscellaneous: Discoloration of teeth in children

1% to 10%:

Dermatologic: Photosensitivity

Gastrointestinal: Nausea, diarrhea

<1%: Pericarditis, increased intracranial pressure, bulging fontanels in infants, dermatologic effects, pruritus, exfoliative dermatitis, rash, pigmentation of nails, diabetes insipidus syndrome, vomiting, esophagitis, anorexia, abdominal cramps, paresthesia, acute renal failure, azotemia, superinfections, anaphylaxis

## Drug Interactions

Decreased effect with antacids (aluminum, calcium, zinc, or magnesium), bismuth salts, sodium bicarbonate, barbiturates, carbamazepine, hydantoins; decreased effect of oral contraceptives

Increased effect of warfarin

**Half-Life** 15 hours

## Special PA Issues

**Patient Education:** Take as directed, at regular intervals around-the-clock. May be taken with food or milk. Complete full course of therapy; do not discontinue even if condition is resolved. You may experience sensitivity to sun; avoid sun, use sunblock, or wear protective clothing. Frequent small meals may help reduce nausea, vomiting or diarrhea. If diabetic, drug may cause false tests with Clinitest® urine glucose monitoring; use of glucose oxidase methods (Clinistix®) or serum glucose monitoring is preferable. Report rash or itching, respiratory difficulty, yellowing of skin or eyes, change in color of urine or stool, fever or chills, unusual bruising or bleeding, or unresolved diarrhea.

- **Minocycline Hydrochloride** *see* Minocycline *on this page*

# Minoxidil (mi NOKS i dil)

**Pharmacologic Class** Topical Skin Product; Vasodilator

**U.S. Brand Names** Loniten®; Rogaine® Extra Strength for Men [OTC]; Rogaine® for Men [OTC]; Rogaine® for Women [OTC]

**Mechanism of Action** Produces vasodilation by directly relaxing arteriolar smooth muscle, with little effect on veins; effects may be mediated by cyclic AMP; stimulation of hair growth is secondary to vasodilation, increased cutaneous blood flow and stimulation of resting hair follicles

**Use** Management of severe hypertension (usually in combination with a diuretic and beta-blocker); treatment of male pattern baldness (alopecia androgenetica)

## USUAL DOSAGE

Children <12 years: Hypertension: Oral: Initial: 0.1-0.2 mg/kg once daily; maximum: 5 mg/day; increase gradually every 3 days; usual dosage: 0.25-1 mg/kg/day in 1-2 divided doses; maximum: 50 mg/day

Children >12 years and Adults:

Hypertension: Oral: Initial: 5 mg once daily, increase gradually every 3 days; usual dose: 10-40 mg/day in 1-2 divided doses; maximum: 100 mg/day

Alopecia: Topical: Apply twice daily; 4 months of therapy may be necessary for hair growth

Elderly: Initial: 2.5 mg once daily; increase gradually

**Note:** Dosage adjustment is needed when added to concomitant therapy

Dialysis: Supplemental dose is not necessary via hemo- or peritoneal dialysis

**Dosage Forms Soln, top:** 2% = 20 mg/metered dose (60 mL), 5% = 50 mg/metered dose (60 mL); **Tab:** 2.5 mg, 10 mg

**Contraindications** Pheochromocytoma, hypersensitivity to minoxidil or any component

**Warnings/Precautions Note:** Minoxidil can cause pericardial effusion, occasionally progressing to tamponade and it can exacerbate angina pectoris; use with caution in patients with pulmonary hypertension, significant renal failure, or congestive heart failure; use with caution in patients with coronary artery disease or recent myocardial infarction; renal failure or dialysis patients may require smaller doses; usually used with a beta-blocker (to treat minoxidil-induced tachycardia) and a diuretic (for treatment of water retention/edema); may take 1-6 months for hypertrichosis to totally reverse after minoxidil therapy is discontinued.

## Pregnancy Risk Factor C

## Adverse Reactions

>10%:

Cardiovascular: EKG changes (60%), tachycardia, congestive heart failure

Dermatologic: Hypertrichosis (commonly occurs within 1-2 months of therapy)

Hematologic: Transient H/H decrease

1% to 10%:

Cardiovascular: Edema (7%)

Endocrine & metabolic: Fluid and electrolyte imbalance

<1%: Angina, pericardial effusion tamponade, dizziness, breast tenderness, rashes, headache, coarsening facial features, dermatologic reactions, Stevens-Johnson syndrome, sunburn, weight gain, thrombocytopenia, leukopenia

**Drug Interactions** Increased toxicity:

Concurrent administration with guanethidine may cause profound orthostatic hypotensive effects

Additive hypotensive effects with other hypotensive agents or diuretics

**Onset** Oral: Within 30 minutes

**Duration** Up to 2-5 days

**Half-Life** 3.5-4.2 hours

## Special PA Issues

**Patient Education:** Topical product must be used every day. Hair growth usually takes 4 months. Notify physician if any of the following occur: Heart rate ≥20 beats per minute over normal; rapid weight gain >5 lb (2 kg); unusual swelling of extremities, face, or abdomen; breathing difficulty, especially when lying down; rise slowly from prolonged lying or sitting; new or aggravated angina symptoms (chest, arm, or shoulder pain); severe indigestion; dizziness, lightheadedness, or fainting; nausea or vomiting may occur. Do not make up for missed doses.

**Monitoring Parameters:** Blood pressure, standing and sitting/supine; fluid and electrolyte balance and body weight should be monitored

- **Mintezol®** see Thiabendazole on page 893
- **Minute-Gel®** see Fluoride on page 383
- **Miochol-E®** see Acetylcholine on page 26
- **Miostat® Intraocular** see Carbachol on page 148
- **Mirapex®** see Pramipexole on page 748
- **Mireze®** see Nedocromil Sodium on page 639

# Mirtazapine (mir TAZ a peen)

**Pharmacologic Class** Antidepressant, Alpha-2 Antagonist

**U.S. Brand Names** Remeron®

**Mechanism of Action** Mirtazapine is a tetracyclic antidepressant that works by its central presynaptic alpha$_2$-adrenergic antagonist effects, which results in increased release of norepinephrine and serotonin. It is also a potent antagonist of 5-HT$_2$ and 5-HT$_3$ serotonin receptors and H$_1$ histamine receptors and a moderate peripheral alpha$_1$-adrenergic and muscarinic antagonist; it does not inhibit the reuptake of norepinephrine or serotonin.

**Use** Treatment of depression

**USUAL DOSAGE** Adults: Oral: Initial: 15 mg nightly, titrate up to 15-45 mg/day with dose increases made no more frequently than every 1-2 weeks

(Continued)

## Mirtazapine *(Continued)*

**Dosage Forms** Tab: 15 mg, 30 mg

**Contraindications** Patients with a known hypersensitivity to mirtazapine, use during or within 14 days of monoamine oxidase inhibitor therapy

**Warnings/Precautions** Hepatic or renal dysfunction, predisposition to conditions that could be exacerbated by hypotension, history of mania or hypomania, seizure disorders, immunocompromized patients, the elderly, or during pregnancy or nursing

**Pregnancy Risk Factor** C

**Adverse Reactions**

>10%:

Central nervous system: Somnolence

Endocrine & metabolic: Increased cholesterol

Gastrointestinal: Constipation, xerostomia, increased appetite, weight gain

1% to 10%:

Cardiovascular: Hypertension, vasodilatation, peripheral edema, edema

Central nervous system: Dizziness, abnormal dreams, abnormal thoughts, confusion, malaise

Endocrine & metabolic: Increased triglycerides

Gastrointestinal: Vomiting, anorexia, eructation, glossitis, cholecystitis

Genitourinary: Polyuria

Neuromuscular & skeletal: Myalgia, back pain, arthralgia, tremor, weakness

Respiratory: Dyspnea

Miscellaneous: Flu-like symptoms, thirst

<1%: Orthostatic hypotension, seizures (1 case reported), dehydration, weight loss, agranulocytosis, neutropenia, lymphadenopathy, increased LFTs

**Drug Interactions** CYP1A2, 2C9, 2D6, and 3A3/4 enzyme substrate

Increased toxicity: Impairment of cognitive and motor skills are additive with those produced by alcohol, benzodiazepines, and other CNS depressants; possibly serious or fatal reactions can occur when given with or when given within 14 days of a monoamine oxidase inhibitor.

**Onset** Therapeutic effects general >2 weeks

**Half-Life** 20-40 hours

**Special PA Issues**

**Patient Education:** Take exactly as directed (do not increase dose or frequency); may take 2-3 weeks to achieve desired results; may cause physical and/or psychological dependence. Take once-a-day dose at bedtime. Avoid excessive alcohol, caffeine, and other prescription or OTC medications not approved by prescriber. Maintain adequate hydration (2-3 L/day of fluids unless instructed to restrict fluid intake). You may experience drowsiness, dizziness, or lightheadedness (use caution when driving or engaging in hazardous tasks until response to medication is known); nausea, vomiting, anorexia, or dry mouth (small frequent meals, frequent mouth care, or sucking lozenges may help); or orthostatic hypotension (use caution when climbing stairs or changing position from lying or sitting to standing). Report persistent insomnia, agitation, or confusion; muscle cramping, tremors, weakness, or change in gait; breathlessness or difficulty breathing; chest pain, palpitations, or rapid heartbeat; change in urinary pattern; vision changes or eye pain; yellowing of eyes or skin; pale stools/dark urine; or worsening of condition.

**Dietary Considerations:** Alcohol: Additive CNS effect, avoid use

**Monitoring Parameters:** Patients should be monitored for signs of agranulocytosis or severe neutropenia such as sore throat, stomatitis or other signs of infection or a low WBC; monitor for improvement in clinical signs and symptoms of depression, improvement may be observed within 1-4 weeks after initiating therapy

**Related Information**

Antidepressant Agents *on page 998*

## Misoprostol *(mye soe PROST ole)*

**Pharmacologic Class** Prostaglandin

**U.S. Brand Names** Cytotec®

**Mechanism of Action** Misoprostol is a synthetic prostaglandin $E_1$ analog that replaces the protective prostaglandins consumed with prostaglandin-inhibiting therapies eg, nonsteroidal anti-inflammatory drugs

**Use** Prevention of NSAID-induced gastric ulcers

**USUAL DOSAGE** Adults: Oral: 200 mcg 4 times/day with food; if not tolerated, may decrease dose to 100 mcg 4 times/day with food or 200 mcg twice daily with food

**Dosage Forms** Tab: 100 mcg, 200 mcg

**Contraindications** Pregnancy; hypersensitivity to misoprostol or any component

**Warnings/Precautions** Safety and efficacy have not been established in children <18 years of age; use with caution in patients with renal impairment and the elderly; not to be used in pregnant women or women of childbearing potential unless woman is capable of complying with effective contraceptive measures; therapy is normally begun on the second or third day of next normal menstrual period

**Pregnancy Risk Factor** X

**Adverse Reactions**

>10%: Gastrointestinal: Diarrhea, abdominal pain

1% to 10%:

Central nervous system: Headache

Gastrointestinal: Constipation, flatulence

<1%: Nausea, vomiting, uterine stimulation, vaginal bleeding

**Half-Life** Parent and metabolite combined: 1.5 hours

**Special PA Issues**

**Patient Education:** Take as directed; continue taking your NSAIDs while taking this medication. Take with meals or after meals to prevent nausea, diarrhea, and flatulence. Avoid using antacids. You may experience increased menstrual pain, or cramping; request analgesics. Report abnormal menstrual periods, spotting (may occur even in postmenstrual women), or severe menstrual bleeding.

♦ **Mitran® Oral** *see* Chlordiazepoxide *on page 189*

♦ **Mivacron®** *see* Mivacurium *on this page*

# Mivacurium (mye va KYOO ree um)

**Pharmacologic Class** Neuromuscular Blocker Agent, Nondepolarizing; Skeletal Muscle Relaxant

**U.S. Brand Names** Mivacron®

**Mechanism of Action** Mivacurium is a short-acting, nondepolarizing, neuromuscular-blocking agent. Like other nondepolarizing drugs, mivacurium antagonizes acetylcholine by competitively binding to cholinergic sites on motor endplates in skeletal muscle. This inhibits contractile activity in skeletal muscle leading to muscle paralysis. This effect is reversible with cholinesterase inhibitors such as edrophonium, neostigmine, and physostigmine.

**Use** Short-acting nondepolarizing neuromuscular blocking agent; an adjunct to general anesthesia; facilitates endotracheal intubation; provides skeletal muscle relaxation during surgery or mechanical ventilation

**USUAL DOSAGE** Continuous infusion requires an infusion pump; dose should be based on ideal body weight

Children 2-12 years (duration of action is shorter and dosage requirements are higher): 200 mcg/kg I.V. bolus; 5-31 mcg/kg/minute I.V. infusion

Adults: Initial: I.V.: 0.15 mg/kg bolus; for prolonged neuromuscular block, infusions of 1-15 mcg/kg/minute are used

**Dosing adjustment in renal impairment:** 150 mcg/kg I.V. bolus; duration of action of blockade: 1.5 times longer in ESRD, may decrease infusion rates by as much as 50%, dependent on degree of renal impairment

**Dosing adjustment in hepatic impairment:** 150 mcg/kg I.V. bolus; duration of blockade: 3 times longer in ESLD, may decrease rate of infusion by as much as 50% in ESLD, dependent on the degree of impairment

**Dosage Forms Inf, in D₅W:** 0.5 mg/mL (50 mL); **Inj:** 2 mg/mL (5 mL, 10 mL)

**Contraindications** Hypersensitivity to mivacurium chloride or other benzylisoquinolinium agents; pre-existing tachycardia

**Pregnancy Risk Factor** C

**Adverse Reactions**

>10%: Cardiovascular: Flushing of face

1% to 10%: Cardiovascular: Hypotension

<1%: Bradycardia, tachycardia, dizziness, cutaneous erythema, rash, injection site reaction, muscle spasms, bronchospasm, wheezing, hypoxemia, endogenous histamine release

**Drug Interactions** Prolonged neuromuscular blockade: Inhaled anesthetics; local anesthetics; calcium channel blockers; antiarrhythmics (eg, quinidine or procainamide); antibiotics (eg, aminoglycosides, tetracyclines, vancomycin, clindamycin); immunosuppressants (eg, cyclosporine)

♦ **Mivacurium Chloride** *see* Mivacurium *on this page*

♦ **MK 462** *see* Rizatriptan *on page 814*

♦ **MK594** *see* Losartan *on page 544*

♦ **Moban®** *see* Molindone *on page 616*

♦ **Mobenol®** *see* Tolbutamide *on page 911*

# Modafinil (moe DAF i nil)

**Pharmacologic Class** Central Nervous System Stimulant, Nonamphetamine

**U.S. Brand Names** Provigil®

**Mechanism of Action** The exact mechanism of action is unclear, it does not appear to alter the release of dopamine or norepinephrine, it may exert its stimulant effects by decreasing GABA-mediated neurotransmission, although this theory has not yet been fully evaluated; several studies also suggest that an intact central alpha-adrenergic system is required for modafinil's activity; the drug increases high-frequency alpha waves while decreasing both delta and theta wave activity, and these effects are consistent with generalized increases in mental alertness

(Continued)

## Modafinil *(Continued)*

**Use** Improve wakefulness in patients with excessive daytime sleepiness associated with narcolepsy

**USUAL DOSAGE**

Narcolepsy: Initial: 200 mg as a single daily dose in the morning

Doses of 400 mg/day, given as a single dose, have been well tolerated, but there is no consistent evidence that this dose confers additional benefit

**Dosing adjustment in elderly:** Elimination of modafinil and its metabolites may be reduced as a consequence of aging and as a result, lower doses should be considered.

**Dosing adjustment in renal impairment:** Inadequate data to determine safety and efficacy in severe renal impairment

**Dosing adjustment in hepatic impairment:** Dose should be reduced to one-half of that recommended for patients with normal liver function

**Dosage Forms Tab:** 100 mg, 200 mg

**Contraindications** Hypersensitivity to modafinil or any component

**Warnings/Precautions** History of angina, ischemic EKG changes, left ventricular hypertrophy, or clinically significant mitral valve prolapse in association with CNS stimulant use; caution should be exercised when modafinil is given to patients with a history of psychosis, recent history of myocardial nfarction, and because it has not yet been adequately studied in patients with hypertension, periodic monitoring of hypertensive patients receiving modafinil may be appropriate; caution is warranted when operating machinery or driving, although functional impairment has not been demonstrated with modafinil, all CNS-active agents may alter judgment, thinking and/or motor skills. Efficacy of oral contraceptives may be reduced, therefore, use of alternative contraception should be considered.

**Pregnancy Risk Factor** C

**Pregnancy Implications** Currently, there are no studies in humans evaluating its teratogenicity. Embryotoxicity of modafinil has been observed in animal models at dosages above those employed therapeutically. As a result, it should be used cautiously during pregnancy and should be used only when the potential risk of drug therapy is outweighed by the drug's benefits. It remains unknown if modafinil is secreted into human milk and, therefore, should be used cautiously in nursing women.

**Adverse Reactions** Limited to reports that were equal to or greater than placebo-related events:

<10%:

Cardiovascular: Chest pain (2%), hypertension (2%), hypotension (2%), vasodilation (1%), arrhythmia (1%), syncope (1%)

Central nervous system: Headache (50%, compared to 40% with placebo), nervousness (8%), dizziness (5%), depression (4%), anxiety (4%), cataplexy (3%), insomnia (3%), paresthesias (3%), dyskinesia (2%), chills (2%), fever (1%), confusion (1%), amnesia (1%), emotional lability (1%), ataxia (1%)

Dermatologic: Dry skin (1%)

Endocrine & metabolic: Hyperglycemia (1%), albuminuria (1%)

Gastrointestinal: Diarrhea (8%), Nausea (13%, compared to 4% with placebo), dry mouth (5%), anorexia (5%), vomiting (1%), mouth ulceration (1%), gingivitis (1%)

Genitourinary: Abnormal urine (1%), urinary retention (1%), ejaculatory disturbance (1%)

Hematologic: Eosinophilia (1%)

Hepatic: Abnormal LFTs (3%)

Neuromuscular & skeletal: Neck pain (2%), hypertonia (2%), neck rigidity (1%), joint disorder (1%), tremor (1%)

Ocular: Amblyopia (2%), abnormal vision (2%)

Respiratory: Pharyngitis (6%), rhinitis (11%, compared to 8% with placebo), lung disorder (4%), dyspnea (2%), asthma (1%), epistaxis (1%)

**Drug Interactions** Modafinil may interact with drugs that inhibit, induce, or are metabolized by cytochrome P-450 isoenzymes; specifically modafinil is a 3A4 isoenzyme substrate and induces CYP1A2, CYP2B6, and CYP3A4 isoenzymes, as a result modafinil may decrease serum concentrations of 3A4 metabolized drugs such as oral contraceptives, cyclosporine, and to a lesser degree, theophylline; agents that induce CYP3A4, including phenobarbital, carbamazepine, and rifampin may result in decreased modafinil levels; there is evidence to suggest that modafinil may induce its own metabolism.

**Increased effects:** As a result of its inhibition of CYP2C19 isoenzymes, serum concentrations of drugs metabolized by this enzyme can be increased, these agents include diazepam, mephenytoin, phenytoin, and propranolol and due to modafinil's potential inhibition of the CYP2C9 isoenzyme, warfarin and phenytoin levels may be increased; in populations deficient in the CYP2D6 isoenzyme, where CYP2C19 acts as a secondary metabolic pathway, concentrations of tricyclic antidepressants and selective serotonin reuptake inhibitors may be increased during coadministration

**Half-Life** 15 hours

**Special PA Issues**

**Patient Education:** Take exactly as prescribed; do not exceed recommended dosage without consulting prescriber. Maintain healthy sleep hygiene. Do not share medication with anyone else. Void before taking medication. You may experience headache, nervousness, confusion, or dizziness (use caution when driving or engaging in hazardous tasks until response to medication is known); diarrhea (yogurt or buttermilk may help); or dry mouth or sore mouth, loss of appetite, or vomiting (small frequent meals, frequent mouth care, chewing gum, or sucking lozenges may help). Diabetics should monitor glucose levels closely. Report chest pain or palpitations; difficulty breathing; excessive insomnia; CNS agitation, depression, or memory disturbances; vision changes; changes in urinary pattern or ejaculation disturbances; or persistent joint pain or stiffness.

♦ **Modane® Bulk [OTC]** *see* Psyllium *on page 781*

♦ **Modane® Soft [OTC]** *see* Docusate *on page 298*

♦ **Modecate®** *see* Fluphenazine *on page 388*

♦ **Modecate® Enanthate** *see* Fluphenazine *on page 388*

♦ **Modicon™** *see* Ethinyl Estradiol and Norethindrone *on page 348*

♦ **Modified Dakin's Solution** *see* Sodium Hypochlorite Solution *on page 842*

♦ **Modified Shohl's Solution** *see* Sodium Citrate and Citric Acid *on page 840*

♦ **Moditen® Hydrochloride** *see* Fluphenazine *on page 388*

♦ **Moduretic®** *see* Amiloride and Hydrochlorothiazide *on page 52*

## Moexipril (mo EKS i pril)

**Pharmacologic Class** Angiotensin-Converting Enzyme (ACE) Inhibitors

**U.S. Brand Names** Univasc®

**Mechanism of Action** Competitive inhibitor of angiotensin-converting enzyme (ACE); prevents conversion of angiotensin I to angiotensin II, a potent vasoconstrictor; results in lower levels of angiotensin II which causes an increase in plasma renin activity and a reduction in aldosterone secretion

**Use** Treatment of hypertension, alone or in combination with thiazide diuretics in a once daily dosing regimen

**USUAL DOSAGE** Adults: Oral: Initial: 7.5 mg once daily (in patients **not** receiving diuretics), one hour prior to a meal **or** 3.75 mg once daily (when combined with thiazide diuretics); maintenance dose: 7.5-30 mg/day in 1 or 2 divided doses one hour before meals

**Dosage adjustment in renal impairment:** $Cl_{cr}$ ≤40 mL/minute: Patients may be cautiously placed on 3.75 mg once daily, then upwardly titrated to a maximum of 15 mg/day

**Dosage Forms Tab, as hydrochloride:** 7.5 mg, 15 mg

**Contraindications** Hypersensitivity to moexipril, moexiprilat, or component; hypersensitivity or allergic reactions or angioedema related to an ACE inhibitor

**Warnings/Precautions** Do not administer in pregnancy; use with caution and modify dosage in patients with renal impairment especially renal artery stenosis, severe congestive heart failure, or with coadministered diuretic therapy; experience in children is limited. Severe hypotension may occur in patients who are sodium and/or volume depleted; initiate lower doses and monitor closely when starting therapy in these patients; ACE inhibitors may be preferred agents in elderly patients with congestive heart failure and diabetes mellitus (diabetic proteinuria is reduced, minimal CNS effects, and enhanced insulin sensitivity), however due to decreased renal function, tolerance must be carefully monitored; if possible, discontinue the diuretic 2-3 days prior to initiating moexipril in patients receiving them to reduce the risk of symptomatic hypotension.

**Pregnancy Risk Factor** C (1st trimester); D (2nd and 3rd trimester)

**Adverse Reactions**

1% to 10%:

Central nervous system: Headache, dizziness, fatigue

Dermatologic: Rash, pruritus, alopecia, flushing, rash

Endocrine & metabolic: Hyperkalemia

Gastrointestinal: Diarrhea

Genitourinary: Polyuria

Renal: Oliguria, reversible increases in creatinine or BUN

Respiratory: Nonproductive cough (6%), pharyngitis, upper respiratory infections, rhinitis

Miscellaneous: Flu-like symptoms

<1%: Symptomatic hypotension, chest pain, angina, peripheral edema, myocardial infarction, palpitations, arrhythmias, sleep disturbances, anxiety, mood changes, angioedema, photosensitivity, pemphigus, hypercholesterolemia, abdominal pain, taste disturbance, constipation, vomiting, xerostomia, changes in appetite, pancreatitis, abnormal taste, neutropenia, elevated LFTs, myalgia, arthralgia, proteinuria, bronchospasm, dyspnea

**Drug Interactions** Increased toxicity: See Drug-Drug Interactions With ACEIs *on page 997*

**Onset** Peak concentrations in 1-2 hours

**Duration** >24 hours

**Half-Life** Moexipril: 1 hour; Moexiprilat: 2-10 hours

**Special PA Issues**

**Patient Education:** This medication does not replace recommended dietary and lifestyle changes to reduce hypertension. Take as directed, 1 hour before or 2 hours after meals. Do not change dosage or stop taking without consulting prescriber. You may experience dizziness, fainting, or lightheadedness (use caution when driving or performing hazardous tasks and use caution when changing position - rising from sitting or lying (Continued)

## Moexipril *(Continued)*

position) until response to therapy is established. Report sore throat; fever; rash; swelling of hands, feet, or legs; respiratory difficulty; chest pains or irregular heartbeat; unusual cough; persistent vomiting, diarrhea, sweating, or perspiration; or flu-like symptoms.

**Monitoring Parameters:** Blood pressure, heart rate, electrolytes, CBC, symptoms of hypotension

**Related Information**
ACE Inhibitors *on page 995*
Drug-Drug Interactions With ACEIs *on page 997*

## Moexipril and Hydrochlorothiazide

(mo EKS i pril & hye droe klor oh THYE a zide)

**Pharmacologic Class** Angiotensin-Converting Enzyme (ACE) Inhibitors; Diuretic, Thiazide

**U.S. Brand Names** Uniretic™

**Dosage Forms Tab:** Moexipril hydrochloride 7.5 mg and hydrochlorothiazide 12.5 mg, moexipril hydrochloride 15 mg and hydrochlorothiazide 25 mg

♦ **Moexipril Hydrochloride** *see* Moexipril *on previous page*

## Molindone (moe LIN done)

**Pharmacologic Class** Antipsychotic Agent, Dihydroindoline

**U.S. Brand Names** Moban®

**Mechanism of Action** Mechanism of action mimics that of chlorpromazine; however, it produces more extrapyramidal effects and less sedation than chlorpromazine

**Use** Management of psychotic disorder

**USUAL DOSAGE** Oral:

Children:

3-5 years: 1-2.5 mg/day divided into 4 doses

5-12 years: 0.5-1 mg/kg/day in 4 divided doses

Adults: 50-75 mg/day increase at 3- to 4-day intervals up to 225 mg/day

**Dosage Forms** Molindone hydrochloride: **Conc, oral:** 20 mg/mL (120 mL); **Tab:** 5 mg, 10 mg, 25 mg, 50 mg, 100 mg

**Contraindications** Narrow-angle glaucoma, hypersensitivity to molindone or any component

**Warnings/Precautions** Use with caution in patients with cardiovascular disease or seizures, CNS depression, or hepatic impairment

**Pregnancy Risk Factor** C

**Adverse Reactions**

>10%:

Cardiovascular: Orthostatic hypotension

Central nervous system: Akathisia, extrapyramidal effects, persistent tardive dyskinesia

Gastrointestinal: Constipation, xerostomia

Ocular: Blurred vision

Miscellaneous: Diaphoresis (decreased)

1% to 10%:

Central nervous system: Mental depression, altered central temperature regulation

Endocrine & metabolic: Change in menstrual periods, edema of the breasts

<1%: Tachycardia, arrhythmias, sedation, drowsiness, restlessness, anxiety, seizures, neuroleptic malignant syndrome (NMS), hyperpigmentation, pruritus, rash, photosensitivity, galactorrhea, gynecomastia, weight gain, urinary retention, agranulocytosis (more often in women between fourth and tenth weeks of therapy), leukopenia (usually in patients with large doses for prolonged periods), retinal pigmentation

**Drug Interactions** CYP2D6 enzyme substrate

Increased toxicity: CNS depressants, antihypertensives, anticonvulsants

**Half-Life** 1.5 hours

**Special PA Issues**

**Patient Education:** Use exactly as directed (do not increase dose or frequency); may cause physical and/or psychological dependence. It may take 2-3 weeks to achieve desired results; do not discontinue without consulting prescriber. Avoid excess alcohol or caffeine and other prescription or OTC medications not approved by prescriber. Maintain adequate hydration (2-3 L/day of fluids unless instructed to restrict fluid intake). You may experience excess drowsiness, restlessness, dizziness, or blurred vision (use caution driving or when engaging in hazardous tasks until response to medication is known); constipation (increased exercise, fluids, or dietary fruit and fiber may help); postural hypotension (use caution climbing stairs or when changing position from lying or sitting to standing); or decreased perspiration (avoid strenuous exercise in hot environments). Report persistent CNS effects (eg, trembling fingers, altered gait or balance, excessive sedation, seizures, unusual movements, anxiety, abnormal thoughts, confusion, personality changes); chest pain, palpitations, rapid heartbeat, severe dizziness; unresolved urinary retention or changes in urinary pattern; changes in menstrual pattern or breast tenderness; vision changes; skin rash or yellowing of skin; difficulty breathing; or worsening of condition.

**Dietary Considerations:** Alcohol: Avoid use

**Monitoring Parameters:** Monitor blood pressure and pulse rate prior to and during initial therapy evaluate mental status; monitor weight

**Related Information**

Antipsychotic Agents *on page 1001*

◆ **Molindone Hydrochloride** *see Molindone on previous page*

◆ **Mol-Iron® [OTC]** *see Ferrous Sulfate on page 367*

◆ **Mollifene® Ear Wax Removing Formula [OTC]** *see Carbamide Peroxide on page 150*

◆ **MOM** *see Magnesium Hydroxide on page 552*

## Mometasone Furoate (moe MET a sone FYOOR oh ate)

**Pharmacologic Class** Corticosteroid, Topical

**U.S. Brand Names** Elocon® Topical

**Mechanism of Action** May depress the formation, release, and activity of endogenous chemical mediators of inflammation (kinins, histamine, liposomal enzymes, prostaglandins). Leukocytes and macrophages may have to be present for the initiation of responses mediated by the above substances. Inhibits the margination and subsequent cell migration to the area of injury, and also reverses the dilatation and increased vessel permeability in the area resulting in decreased access of cells to the sites of injury.

**Use** Relief of the inflammatory and pruritic manifestations of corticosteroid-responsive dermatoses (medium potency topical corticosteroid)

**USUAL DOSAGE** Adults: Topical: Apply sparingly to area once daily, do not use occlusive dressings

**Dosage Forms Crm:** 0.1% (15 g, 45 g); **Lot:** 0.1% (30 mL, 60 mL); **Oint, top:** 0.1% (15 g, 45 g)

**Contraindications** Hypersensitivity to mometasone or any component; fungal, viral, or tubercular skin lesions, herpes simplex or zoster

**Warnings/Precautions** Adverse systemic effects may occur when used on large areas of the body, denuded areas, for prolonged periods of time, with an occlusive dressing, and/or in infants or small children

**Pregnancy Risk Factor** C

**Adverse Reactions** <1%: Acne, hypopigmentation, allergic dermatitis, maceration of the skin, skin atrophy, striae, miliaria, itching, folliculitis, hypertrichosis, HPA suppression, Cushing's syndrome, growth retardation, burning, irritation, dryness, secondary infection

**Special PA Issues**

**Patient Education:** For external use only. Use exactly as directed; do not overuse. Do not apply to open wounds or weeping areas. Before using, wash and dry area gently. Apply a thin film to affected area and rub in gently. If dressing is necessary, use a porous dressing. Avoid contact with eyes. Avoid exposing treated area to direct sunlight; sunburn can occur. Report increased swelling, redness, rash, itching, signs of infection, worsening of condition, or lack of healing.

◆ **Monacolin K** *see Lovastatin on page 546*

◆ **Monafed®** *see Guaifenesin on page 427*

◆ **Monafed® DM** *see Guaifenesin and Dextromethorphan on page 428*

◆ **Monazole-7®** *see Miconazole on page 604*

◆ **Monistat-Derm™ Topical** *see Miconazole on page 604*

◆ **Monistat i.v.™ Injection** *see Miconazole on page 604*

◆ **Monistat™ Vaginal** *see Miconazole on page 604*

◆ **Monitan®** *see Acebutolol on page 20*

◆ **Monocid®** *see Cefonicid on page 165*

◆ **Monoclonal Antibody** *see Muromonab-CD3 on page 622*

◆ **Mono-Gesic®** *see Salsalate on page 820*

◆ **Monoket®** *see Isosorbide Mononitrate on page 499*

◆ **Monopril®** *see Fosinopril on page 403*

## Montelukast (mon te LOO kast)

**Pharmacologic Class** Leukotriene Receptor Antagonist

**U.S. Brand Names** Singulair®

**Mechanism of Action** Selective leukotriene receptor antagonist that inhibits the cysteinyl leukotriene receptor. Cysteinyl leukotrienes and leukotriene receptor occupation have been correlated with the pathophysiology of asthma, including airway edema, smooth muscle contraction, and altered cellular activity associated with the inflammatory process, which contribute to the signs and symptoms of asthma.

**Use** Prophylaxis and chronic treatment of asthma in adults and children ≥6 years

**USUAL DOSAGE** Oral:

Children:

<6 years: Safety and efficacy have not been established

(Continued)

## Montelukast *(Continued)*

6 to 14 years: Chew one 5 mg chewable tablet/day, taken in the evening
Children ≥15 years and Adults: 10 mg/day, taken in the evening
**Dosing adjustment in hepatic impairment:** Mild moderate: No adjustment necessary
**Dosage Forms Tab:** 10 mg; **Tab, chewable:** 5 mg

**Contraindications** Hypersensitivity to any component

**Warnings/Precautions** Montelukast is not indicated for use in the reversal of broncho-spasm in acute asthma attacks, including status asthmaticus. Should not be used as monotherapy for the treatment and management of exercise-induced bronchospasm. Advise patients to have appropriate rescue medication available. Appropriate clinical monitoring and caution are recommended when systemic corticosteroid reduction is considered in patients receiving montelukast. Inform phenylketonuric patients that the chewable tablet contains phenylalanine 0.842 mg/5 mg chewable tablet.

In rare cases, patients on therapy with montelukast may present with systemic eosinophilia, sometimes presenting with clinical features of vasculitis consistent with Churg-Strauss syndrome, a condition which is often treated with systemic corticosteroid therapy. See Adverse Reactions.

**Pregnancy Risk Factor** B

**Adverse Reactions**
>10%: Central nervous system: Headache
1% to 10%:
Central nervous system: Dizziness, fatigue, fever
Dermatologic: Rash
Gastrointestinal: Dyspepsia, dental pain, gastroenteritis, diarrhea, nausea, abdominal pain
Neuromuscular & skeletal: Weakness
Respiratory: Cough, nasal congestion, laryngitis, pharyngitis
Miscellaneous: Flu-like symptoms, trauma

In rare cases, patients on therapy with montelukast may present with systemic eosinophilia, sometimes presenting with clinical features of vasculitis consistent with Churg-Strauss syndrome, a condition which is often treated with systemic corticosteroid therapy. Physicians should be alert to eosinophilia, vasculitic rash, worsening pulmonary symptoms, cardiac complications, and/or neuropathy presenting in their patients. A casual association between montelukast and these underlying conditions has not been established.

**Drug Interactions** CYP2A3, and 2C9, 3A3/4, enzyme substrate

Decreased effect: Phenobarbital, rifampin induce hepatic metabolism and decrease the AUC of montelukast

**Onset** Time to peak: 2-4 hours

**Duration** >24 hours

**Special PA Issues**
**Patient Education:** This medication is not for an acute asthmatic attack; in acute attack, follow instructions of prescriber. Do not stop other asthma medication unless advised by prescriber. Take every evening on a continuous basis; do not discontinue even if feeling better (this medication may help reduce incidence of acute attacks). You may experience mild headache (mild analgesic may help); fatigue or dizziness (use caution when driving). Report skin rash or itching, abdominal pain or persistent GI upset, unusual cough or congestion, or worsening of asthmatic condition.

- **Montelukast Sodium** *see Montelukast on previous page*
- **8-MOP** *see Methoxsalen on page 589*
- **8-MOP®** *see Methoxsalen on page 589*
- **More-Dophilus® [OTC]** *see Lactobacillus acidophilus and Lactobacillus bulgaricus on page 512*

## Moricizine *(mor I siz een)*

**Pharmacologic Class** Antiarrhythmic Agent, Class I
**U.S. Brand Names** Ethmozine®
**Mechanism of Action** Class I antiarrhythmic agent; reduces the fast inward current carried by sodium ions, shortens Phase I and Phase II repolarization, resulting in decreased action potential duration and effective refractory period

**Moricizine**

| Transferred From | Start Ethmozine® |
| --- | --- |
| Encainide, propafenone, tocainide, or mexiletine | 8-12 hours after last dose |
| Flecainide | 12-24 hours after last dose |
| Procainamide | 3-6 hours after last dose |
| Quinidine, disopyramide | 6-12 hours after last dose |

**Use** Treatment of ventricular tachycardia and life-threatening ventricular arrhythmias
**Unlabeled use:** PVCs, complete and nonsustained ventricular tachycardia

**USUAL DOSAGE** Adults: Oral: 200-300 mg every 8 hours, adjust dosage at 150 mg/day at 3-day intervals. See table for dosage recommendations of transferring from other antiarrhythmic agents to Ethmozine®.

**Dosing interval in renal or hepatic impairment:** Start at 600 mg/day or less

**Dosage Forms Tab, as hydrochloride:** 200 mg, 250 mg, 300 mg

**Contraindications** Pre-existing second or third degree A-V block and in patients with right bundle-branch block when associated with left hemiblock, unless pacemaker is present; cardiogenic shock; known hypersensitivity to the drug

**Warnings/Precautions** Considering the known proarrhythmic properties and lack of evidence of improved survival for any antiarrhythmic drug in patients without life-threatening arrhythmias, it is prudent to reserve the use for patients with life-threatening ventricular arrhythmias; CAST II trial demonstrated a trend towards decreased survival for patients treated with moricizine; proarrhythmic effects occur as with other antiarrhythmic agents; hypokalemia, hyperkalemia, hypomagnesemia may effect response to class I agents; use with caution in patients with sick-sinus syndrome, hepatic, and renal impairment

**Pregnancy Risk Factor** B

**Adverse Reactions**

>10%: Central nervous system: Dizziness (15%)

1% to 10%:
    Cardiovascular: Proarrhythmia, palpitations (5.8%), cardiac death (2% to 5%), EKG abnormalities (1.6%), congestive heart failure (1%)
    Central nervous system: Headache (8%), fatigue (6%), insomnia (2% to 5%)
    Gastrointestinal: Nausea (3% to 9%), diarrhea (2% to 5%)
    Ocular: Blurred vision (2% to 5%)
    Respiratory: Dyspnea (6%)

<1%: Ventricular tachycardia, cardiac chest pain, hypotension or hypertension, syncope, supraventricular arrhythmias, myocardial infarction, anxiety, drug fever, confusion, loss of memory, vertigo, anorexia, rash, dry skin, GI upset, vomiting, dyspepsia, flatulence, bitter taste, urinary retention, urinary incontinence, impotence, tremor, tinnitus, apnea, diaphoresis

**Drug Interactions**

Decreased levels of theophylline (50%) with moricizine due to increased clearance
Increased levels of moricizine with concomitant cimetidine (50%)
Diltiazem increases moricizine levels resulting in an increased incidence of side effects
Moricizine decreases diltiazem plasma levels and decreases its half-life
Digoxin and moricizine concurrent administration may result in additive prolongation of the PR interval (but not rate of second and third degree A-V block)

**Half-Life** Normal patient: 3-4 hours; Cardiac disease patient: 6-13 hours

**Special PA Issues**
**Patient Education:** Take exactly as directed; do not take additional doses or discontinue without consulting prescriber. You will need regular cardiac check-ups and blood tests while taking this medication. You may experience dizziness or visual changes (use caution when driving or performing tasks that require alertness until response to drug is determined); nausea or vomiting (small frequent meals, frequent mouth care, or sucking lozenges may help); or headaches, sleep disturbances, or decreased libido (usually temporary, if persistent consult prescriber). Report chest pain, palpitation, or erratic heartbeat; increased weight or swelling of hands or feet; blurred vision or facial swelling; acute diarrhea; changes in bowel or bladder patterns; or difficulty breathing.

♦ **Moricizine Hydrochloride** see Moricizine on previous page
♦ **Morning After Pill** see Ethinyl Estradiol and Norgestrel on page 351
♦ **Morphine-HP®** see Morphine Sulfate on this page

# Morphine Sulfate (MOR feen SUL fate)

**Pharmacologic Class** Analgesic, Narcotic

**U.S. Brand Names** Astramorph™ PF Injection; Duramorph® Injection; Infumorph™ Injection; Kadian™; MS Contin® Oral; MSIR® Oral; MS/L®; MS/S®; OMS® Oral; Oramorph SR™ Oral; RMS® Rectal; Roxanol™ Oral; Roxanol Rescudose®; Roxanol SR™ Oral

**Mechanism of Action** Binds to opiate receptors in the CNS, causing inhibition of ascending pain pathways, altering the perception of and response to pain; produces generalized CNS depression

**Use** Relief of moderate to severe acute and chronic pain; pain of myocardial infarction; relieves dyspnea of acute left ventricular failure and pulmonary edema; preanesthetic medication

**USUAL DOSAGE** Doses should be titrated to appropriate effect; when changing routes of administration in chronically treated patients, please note that oral doses are approximately one-half as effective as parenteral dose
(Continued)

## Morphine Sulfate *(Continued)*

Infants and Children:

Oral: Tablet and solution (prompt release): 0.2-0.5 mg/kg/dose every 4-6 hours as needed; tablet (controlled release): 0.3-0.6 mg/kg/dose every 12 hours

I.M., I.V., S.C.: 0.1-0.2 mg kg/dose every 2-4 hours as needed; usual maximum: 15 mg/dose; may initiate at 0.05 mg/kg/dose

I.V., S.C. continuous infusion: Sickle cell or cancer pain: 0.025-2 mg/kg/hour; postoperative pain: 0.01-0.04 mg/kg/hour

Sedation/analgesia for procedures: I.V.: 0.05-0.1 mg/kg 5 minutes before the procedure

Adolescents >12 years: Sedation/analgesia for procedures: I.V.: 3-4 mg and repeat in 5 minutes if necessary

Adults:

Oral: Prompt release: 10-30 mg every 4 hours as needed; controlled release: 15-30 mg every 8-12 hours

I.M., I.V., S.C.: 2.5-20 mg/dose every 2-6 hours as needed; usual: 10 mg/dose every 4 hours as needed

I.V., S.C. continuous infusion: 0.8-10 mg/hour; may increase depending on pain relief/adverse effects; usual range: up to 80 mg/hour

Epidural: Initial: 5 mg in lumbar region; if inadequate pain relief within 1 hour, administer 1-2 mg, maximum dose: 10 mg/24 hours

Intrathecal ($\frac{1}{10}$ of epidural dose): 0.2-1 mg/dose; repeat doses **not** recommended

Rectal: 10-20 mg every 4 hours

**Dosing adjustment in renal impairment:**

$Cl_{cr}$ 10-50 mL/minute: Administer at 75% of normal dose

$Cl_{cr}$ <10 mL/minute: Administer at 50% of normal dose

**Dosing adjustment/comments in hepatic disease:** Unchanged in mild liver disease; substantial extrahepatic metabolism may occur; excessive sedation may occur in cirrhosis

**Dosage Forms Cap (MSIR®):** 15 mg, 30 mg; **Cap, sustained release (Kadian™):** 20 mg, 50 mg, 100 mg; **Inj:** 0.5 mg/mL (10 mL), 1 mg/mL (10 mL, 30 mL, 60 mL), 2 mg/mL (1 mL, 2 mL, 60 mL), 3 mg/mL (50 mL), 4 mg/mL (1 mL, 2 mL), 5 mg/mL (1 mL, 30 mL), 8 mg/mL (1 mL, 2 mL), 10 mg/mL (1 mL, 2 mL, 10 mL), 15 mg/mL (1 mL, 2 mL, 20 mL), 25 mg/mL (4 mL, 10 mL, 20 mL, 40 mL), 50 mg/mL (10 mL, 20 mL, 40 mL); **Inj: Preservative free (Astramorph™ PF, Duramorph®):** 0.5 mg/mL (2 mL, 10 mL), 1 mg/mL (2 mL, 10 mL), 10 mg/mL (20 mL), 25 mg/mL 20 mL); **I.V. via PCA pump:** 1 mg/mL (10 mL, 30 mL, 60 mL), 5 mg/mL (30 mL); **I.V. infusion preparation:** 25 mg/mL (4 mL, 10 mL, 20 mL); **Soln, oral:** 10 mg/5 mL (5 mL, 10 mL, 100 mL, 120 mL, 500 mL), 20 mg/5 mL (5 mL, 100 mL, 120 mL, 500 mL), MSIR®: 10 mg/5 mL (5 mL, 120 mL, 500 mL), 20 mg/5 mL (5 mL 120 mL, 500 mL), 20 mg/mL (30 mL, 120 mL), MS/L®: 100 mg/5 mL (120 mL) 20 mg/5 mL, OMS®: 20 mg/mL (30 mL, 120 mL), Roxanol™: 10 mg/2.5 mL (2.5 mL), 20 mg/mL (1 mL, 1.5 mL, 30 mL, 120 mL, 240 mL); **Supp, rectal:** 5 mg, 10 mg, 20 mg, 30 mg, MS/S®, RMS®, Roxanol™: 5 mg, 10 mg, 20 mg, 30 mg; **Tab:** 15 mg, 30 mg, MSIR®: 15 mg, 30 mg, **Controlled release:** MS Contin®: 15 mg, 30 mg, 60 mg, 100 mg, 200 mg, Roxanol™ SR: 30 mg; **Soluble:** 10 mg, 15 mg, 30 mg; **Sustained release (Oramorph SR™):** 30 mg, 60 mg, 100 mg

**Contraindications** Known hypersensitivity to morphine sulfate; increased intracranial pressure; severe respiratory depression

**Warnings/Precautions** Some preparations contain sulfites which may cause allergic reactions; infants <3 months of age are more susceptible to respiratory depression, use with caution and generally in reduced doses in this age group; use with caution in patients with impaired respiratory function or severe hepatic dysfunction and in patients with hypersensitivity reactions to other phenanthrene derivative opioid agonists (codeine, hydrocodone, hydromorphone, levorphanol, oxycodone, oxymorphone). Morphine shares the toxic potential of opiate agonists and usual precautions of opiate agonist therapy should be observed; may cause hypotension in patients with acute myocardial infarction. Tolerance or drug dependence may result from extended use.

Elderly may be particularly susceptible to the CNS depressant and constipating effects of narcotics

**Pregnancy Risk Factor** B (D if used for prolonged periods or in high doses at term)

**Adverse Reactions**

Percentage unknown: Flushing, CNS depression, drowsiness, sedation, increased intracranial pressure, antidiuretic hormone release, physical and psychological dependence, diaphoresis

>10%:

Cardiovascular: Palpitations, hypotension, bradycardia

Central nervous system: Dizziness

Gastrointestinal: Nausea, vomiting, constipation, xerostomia

Local: Pain at injection site

Neuromuscular & skeletal: Weakness

Miscellaneous: Histamine release

1% to 10%:

Central nervous system: Restlessness, headache, false feeling of well being, confusion

Gastrointestinal: Anorexia, GI irritation, paralytic ileus
Genitourinary: Decreased urination
Neuromuscular & skeletal: Trembling
Ocular: Vision problems
Respiratory: Respiratory depression, shortness of breath
<1%: Peripheral vasodilation, insomnia, mental depression, hallucinations, paradoxical CNS stimulation, increased intracranial pressure, pruritus, biliary tract spasm, urinary tract spasm, muscle rigidity, miosis, increased LFTs

**Drug Interactions** CYP2D6 enzyme substrate
Decreased effect: Phenothiazines may antagonize the analgesic effect of morphine and other opiate agonists
Increased toxicity: CNS depressants, tricyclic antidepressants may potentiate the effects of morphine and other opiate agonists; dextroamphetamine may enhance the analgesic effect of morphine and other opiate agonists

**Onset** Oral: 1 hour; I.V.: 5-10 minutes
**Duration** 3-5 hours (up to 12 hours for extended release)
**Half-Life** 2-4 hours
**Special PA Issues**
Patient Education: If self-administered, use exactly as directed (do not increase dose or frequency); may cause physical and/or psychological dependence. While using this medication, do not use alcohol and other prescription or OTC medications (especially sedatives, tranquilizers, antihistamines, or pain medications) without consulting prescriber. Maintain adequate hydration (2-3 L/day of fluids unless instructed to restrict fluid intake). May cause hypotension, dizziness, drowsiness, impaired coordination, or blurred vision (use caution when driving, climbing stairs, or changing position - rising from sitting or lying to standing, or when engaging in hazardous activities until response to medication is known); loss of appetite, nausea, or vomiting (frequent mouth care, small frequent meals, or sucking on lozenges may help); constipation (increased exercise, fluids, or dietary fruit and fiber may help - if constipation remains an unresolved problem, consult prescriber about use of stool softeners). Report chest pain, slow or rapid heartbeat, acute dizziness, or persistent headache; changes in mental status; swelling of extremities or unusual weight gain; changes in urinary elimination or pain on urination; acute headache; back or flank pain or muscle spasms; blurred vision; skin rash; or shortness of breath.

Dietary Considerations:
Alcohol: Additive CNS effects, avoid or limit alcohol; watch for sedation
Food:
Glucose may cause hyperglycemia; monitor blood glucose concentrations
Administration of oral morphine solution with food may increase bioavailability (ie, a report of 34% increase in morphine AUC when morphine oral solution followed a high-fat meal). Morphine may cause GI upset. Be consistent when taking morphine with or without meals. Take with food if GI upset.

Monitoring Parameters: Pain relief, respiratory and mental status, blood pressure
Reference Range: Therapeutic: Surgical anesthesia: 65-80 ng/mL (SI: 227-280 nmol/L); Toxic: 200-5000 ng/mL (SI: 700-17,500 nmol/L)

**Related Information**
Hallucinogenic Drugs *on page 1019*
Narcotic Agonists *on page 1023*

♦ **Multi Vit**® **Drops [OTC]** *see* Vitamins, Multiple *on page 964*

## Mupirocin (myoo PEER oh sin)

**Pharmacologic Class** Antibiotic, Topical

**U.S. Brand Names** Bactroban®; Bactroban® Nasal

**Mechanism of Action** Binds to bacterial isoleucyl transfer-RNA synthetase resulting in the inhibition of protein and RNA synthesis

**Use** Topical treatment of impetigo due to *Staphylococcus aureus*, beta-hemolytic *Streptococcus*, and *S. pyogenes*

**USUAL DOSAGE**

Topical: Children and Adults Apply small amount to affected area 2-5 times/day for 5-14 days

Nasal: In adults (12 years of age and older), approximately one-half of the ointment from the single-use tube should be applied into one nostril and the other half into the other nostril twice daily for 5 days

**Dosage Forms Oint:** Intranasal: 2% (1 g single use tube); **Top:** 2% (15 g, 30 g)

**Contraindications** Known hypersensitivity to mupirocin or polyethylene glycol

**Warnings/Precautions** Potentially toxic amounts of polyethylene glycol contained in the vehicle may be absorbed percutaneously in patients with extensive burns or open wounds; prolonged use may result in over growth of nonsusceptible organisms; for external use only; not for treatment of pressure sores

**Pregnancy Risk Factor** B

**Adverse Reactions** 1% to 10%:

Dermatologic: Pruritus, rash, erythema, dry skin

Local: Burning, stinging, tenderness, edema, pain

**Half-Life** 17-36 minutes

**Special PA Issues**

**Patient Education:** For external use only. Wash hands before and after application. Apply this film over affected areas exactly as directed. Avoid getting in eyes. Report rash; persistent burning, stinging, swelling, itching, or pain.

♦ **Mupirocin Calcium** *see* Mupirocin *on this page*

♦ **Murine**® **Ear Drops [OTC]** *see* Carbamide Peroxide *on page 150*

♦ **Muro 128**® **Ophthalmic [OTC]** *see* Sodium Chloride *on page 839*

♦ **Murocoll-2**® **Ophthalmic** *see* Phenylephrine and Scopolamine *on page 720*

## Muromonab-CD3 (myoo roe MOE nab see dee three)

**Pharmacologic Class** Immunosuppressant Agent

**U.S. Brand Names** Orthoclone® OKT3

**Mechanism of Action** Reverses graft rejection by binding to T cells and interfering with their function by binding T-cell receptor-associated CD3 glycoprotein

**Use** Treatment of acute allograft rejection in renal transplant patients; treatment of acute hepatic, kidney, and pancreas rejection episodes resistant to conventional treatment. Acute graft-versus-host disease following bone marrow transplantation resistant to conventional treatment.

**USUAL DOSAGE** I.V. (refer to individual protocols):

Children <30 kg: 2.5 mg/day once daily for 7-14 days

Children >30 kg: 5 mg/day once daily for 7-14 days

**OR**

Children <12 years: 0.1 mg/kg/day once daily for 10-14 days

Children ≥12 years and Adults: 5 mg/day once daily for 10-14 days

Hemodialysis: Molecular size of OKT3 is 150,000 daltons; not dialyzed by most standard dialyzers; however, may be dialyzed by high flux dialysis; OKT3 will be removed by plasmapheresis; administer following dialysis treatments

Peritoneal dialysis: Significant drug removal is unlikely based on physiochemical characteristics

**Dosage Forms Inj:** 5 mg/5 mL

**Contraindications** Hypersensitivity to OKT3 or any murine product; patients in fluid overload or those with >3% weight gain within 1 week prior to start of mouse antibody titers >1:1000

**Warnings/Precautions** It is imperative, especially prior to the first few doses, that there be no clinical evidence of volume overload, uncontrolled hypertension, or uncompensated heart failure, including a clear chest x-ray and weight restriction of ≤3% above the patient's minimum weight during the week prior to injection.

May result in an increased susceptibility to infection; dosage of concomitant immunosuppressants should be reduced during OKT3 therapy; cyclosporine should be decreased to 50% usual maintenance dose and maintenance therapy resumed about 4 days before stopping OKT3.

Severe pulmonary edema has occurred in patients with fluid overload.

**First dose effect** (flu-like symptoms, anaphylactic-type reaction): may occur within 30 minutes to 6 hours up to 24 hours after the first dose and may be minimized by using the recommended regimens. See table.

### Suggested Prevention/Treatment of Muromonab-CD3 First-Dose Effects

| Adverse Reaction | Effective Prevention or Palliation | Supportive Treatment |
|---|---|---|
| Severe pulmonary edema | Clear chest x-ray within 24 hours preinjection; weight restriction to ≤3% gain over 7 days preinjection | Prompt intubation and oxygenation 24 hours close observation |
| Fever, chills | 15 mg/kg methylprednisolone sodium succinate 1 hour preinjection; fever reduction to <37.8°C (100°F) 1 hour preinjection; acetaminophen (1 g orally) and diphenhydramine (50 mg orally) 1 hour preinjection | Cooling blanket Acetaminophen prn |
| Respiratory effects | 100 mg hydrocortisone sodium succinate 30 minutes postinjection | Additional 100 mg hydrocortisone sodium succinate prn for wheezing; if respiratory distress, give epinephrine 1:1000 (0.3 mL S.C.) |

Cardiopulmonary resuscitation may be needed. If the patient's temperature is >37.8°C, reduce before administering OKT3

**Pregnancy Risk Factor** C

**Adverse Reactions**

>10%:

**"First-dose" (cytokine release) effects:** Onset: 1-3 hours after the dose; duration: 12-16 hours. Severity is mild to life-threatening. Signs and symptoms include fever, chilling, dyspnea, wheezing, chest pain, chest tightness, nausea, vomiting, and diarrhea. Hypervolemic pulmonary edema, nephrotoxicity, meningitis, and encephalopathy are possible. Reactions tend to decrease with repeated doses.

Cardiovascular: Tachycardia (including ventricular)

Central nervous system: Dizziness, faintness

Gastrointestinal: Diarrhea, nausea, vomiting

Hematologic: Transient lymphopenia

Neuromuscular & skeletal: Trembling

Respiratory: Shortness of breath

1% to 10%:

Central nervous system: Headache

Neuromuscular & skeletal: Stiff neck

Ocular: Photophobia

Respiratory: Pulmonary edema

<1%: Hypertension, hypotension, chest pain, tightness, aseptic meningitis, seizures, fatigue, confusion, coma, hallucinations, pyrexia, pruritus, rash, arthralgia, tremor, increased BUN and creatinine, dyspnea, wheezing. Sensitivity reactions: Anaphylactic-type reactions, flu-like symptoms (ie, fever, chills); infection, pancytopenia, secondary lymphoproliferative disorder or lymphoma, thrombosis of major vessels in renal allograft.

**Drug Interactions** Decreased effect: Immunosuppressive drugs; it is recommended to decrease dose of azathioprine to 1 mg/kg and decrease dose of cyclosporine by 50% until 4 days prior to stopping OKT3

**Half-Life** Time to steady-state: Trough level: 3-14 days; pretreatment levels are restored within 7 days after treatment is terminated.

**Special PA Issues**

**Patient Education:** There may be a severe reaction to the first infusion of this medication. You may experience high fever, chills, difficulty breathing, or congestion. You will be closely monitored and comfort measures provided. Effects are substantially reduced with subsequent infusions. During the period of therapy and for some time after the regimen of infusions you will be susceptible to infection. People may wear masks and gloves while caring for you to protect you as much as possible from infection (avoid crowds and people with infections or contagious diseases). You may experience dizziness, faintness, or trembling (use caution until response to medication is known); nausea or vomiting (frequent small meals, frequent mouth care); sensitivity to direct sunlight (wear dark glasses, and protective clothing, use sunscreen, or avoid exposure to direct sunlight). Report chest pain or tightness; symptoms of respiratory infection, wheezing, or difficulty breathing; vision change; or muscular trembling.

**Monitoring Parameters:** Chest x-ray, weight gain, CBC with differential, temperature, vital signs (blood pressure, temperature, pulse, respiration); immunologic monitoring of T cells, serum levels of OKT3

(Continued)

## Muromonab-CD3 *(Continued)*

### Reference Range:

**OKT3 serum concentrations:**

Serum level monitoring should be performed in conjunction with lymphocyte subset determinations; Trough concentration sampling best correlates with clinical outcome. Serial monitoring may provide a better early indicator of inadequate dosing during induction or rejection.

Mean serum trough levels rise during the first 3 days, then average 0.9 mcg/mL on days 3-14

Circulating levels ≥0.8 mcg/mL block the function of cytotoxic T cells *in vitro* and *in vivo*

Several recent analysis have suggested appropriate dosage adjustments of OKT3 induction course are better determined with OKT3 serum levels versus lymphocyte subset determination; however, no prospective controlled trials have been performed to validate the equivalency of these tests in predicting clinical outcome.

**Lymphocyte subset monitoring: CD3+ cells:** Trough sample measurement is preferable and reagent utilized defines reference range.

OKT3-FITC: <10-50 cells/mm$^3$ or <3% to 5%

CD3 (IgG1)-FITC: similar to OKT3-FITC

Leu-4a: Higher number of CD3+ cells appears acceptable

Dosage adjustments should be made in conjunction with clinical response and based upon trends over several consecutive days

- ♦ **Muroptic-5® [OTC]** *see Sodium Chloride on page 839*
- ♦ **Muro's Opcon®** *see Naphazoline on page 635*
- ♦ **Muse® Pellet** *see Alprostadil on page 45*
- ♦ **M.V.I.®** *see Vitamins, Multiple on page 964*
- ♦ **M.V.I.®-12** *see Vitamins, Multiple on page 964*
- ♦ **M.V.I.® Concentrate** *see Vitamins, Multiple on page 964*
- ♦ **M.V.I.® Pediatric** *see Vitamins, Multiple on page 964*
- ♦ **Myambutol®** *see Ethambutol on page 342*
- ♦ **Mycelex®** *see Clotrimazole on page 228*
- ♦ **Mycelex®-7** *see Clotrimazole on page 228*
- ♦ **Mycelex®-G** *see Clotrimazole on page 228*
- ♦ **Mycifradin® Sulfate Oral** *see Neomycin on page 642*
- ♦ **Mycifradin® Sulfate Topical** *see Neomycin on page 642*
- ♦ **Mycinettes® [OTC]** *see Benzocaine on page 105*
- ♦ **Mycitracin® Topical [OTC]** *see Bacitracin, Neomycin, and Polymyxin B on page 97*
- ♦ **Mycobutin®** *see Rifabutin on page 803*
- ♦ **Mycogen II Topical** *see Nystatin and Triamcinolone on page 670*
- ♦ **Mycolog®-II Topical** *see Nystatin and Triamcinolone on page 670*
- ♦ **Myconel® Topical** *see Nystatin and Triamcinolone on page 670*

## Mycophenolate *(mye koe FEN oh late)*

**Pharmacologic Class** Immunosuppressant Agent

**U.S. Brand Names** CellCept®

**Mechanism of Action** Inhibition of purine synthesis of human lymphocytes and proliferation of human lymphocytes

**Use** Immunosuppressant used with corticosteroids and cyclosporine to prevent organ rejection in patients receiving allogenic renal and cardiac transplants; treatment of rejection in liver transplant patients unable to tolerate tacrolimus or cyclosporine due to neurotoxicity; mild rejection in heart transplant patients; treatment of moderate-severe psoriasis

Intravenous formulation is an alternative dosage form to oral capsules and tablets

### USUAL DOSAGE

**Oral:**

Children: 600 mg/m$^2$/dose twice daily; **Note:** Limited information regarding mycophenolate use in pediatric patients is currently available in the literature: 32 pediatric patients (14 underwent living donor and 18 receiving cadaveric donor renal transplants) received mycophenolate 8-30 mg/kg/dose orally twice daily with cyclosporine, prednisone, and Atgam® induction; however, pharmacokinetic studies suggest that doses of mycophenolate adjusted to body surface area resulted in AUCs which better approximated those of adults versus doses adjusted for body weight which resulted in lower AUCs in pediatric patients

Adults: 1 g twice daily within 72 hours of transplant (although 3 g daily has been given in some clinical trials, there was decreased tolerability and no efficacy advantage)

**Dosing adjustment in renal impairment:** Doses >2 g/day are not recommended in these patients because of the possibility for enhanced immunosuppression as well as toxicities

**Dosing adjustment in severe chronic renal impairment:** Cl$_{cr}$ <25 mL/minute/1.73 m$^2$: Doses of >1 g administered twice daily should be avoided; patients should also be carefully observed; no dose adjustments are needed in renal transplant patients experiencing delayed graft function postoperatively

Hemodialysis: Not removed; supplemental dose is not necessary

Peritoneal dialysis: Supplemental dose is not necessary

**Dosing adjustment for neutropenia:** ANC <1.3 x $10^3$/μL: Dosing should be interrupted or the dose reduced, appropriate diagnostic tests performed and patients managed appropriately

### Mycophenolate Adverse Reactions Reported in >10%

| Adverse Reaction | MM 2 g/day | MM 3 g/day |
|---|---|---|
| **Body as a Whole** | | |
| Pain | 33 | 31.2 |
| Abdominal pain | 12.1-24.7 | 11.9-27.6 |
| Fever | 20.4 | 23.3 |
| Headache | 20.1 | 16.1 |
| Infection | 12.7-18.2 | 15.6-20.9 |
| Sepsis | 17.6-20.8 | 17.5-19.7 |
| Asthenia | 13.7 | 16.1 |
| Chest pain | 13.4 | 13.3 |
| Back pain | 11.6 | 12.1 |
| Hypertension | 17.6-32.4 | 16.9-28.2 |
| **Central Nervous System** | | |
| Tremor | 11 | 11.8 |
| Insomnia | 8.9 | 11.8 |
| Dizziness | 5.7 | 11.2 |
| **Dermatologic** | | |
| Acne | 10.1 | 9.7 |
| Rash | 7.7 | 6.4 |
| **Gastrointestinal** | | |
| Diarrhea | 16.4-31 | 18.8-36.1 |
| Constipation | 21.9 | 18.5 |
| Nausea | 19.9 | 23.6 |
| Dyspepsia | 17.6 | 13.6 |
| Vomiting | 12.5 | 13.6 |
| Nausea & vomiting | 10.4 | 9.7 |
| Oral monoliasis | 10.1 | 12.1 |
| **Hemic/Lymphatic** | | |
| Anemia | 25.6 | 25.8 |
| Leukopenia | 11.5-23.2 | 16.3-34.5 |
| Thrombocytopenia | 10.1 | 8.2 |
| Hypochromic anemia | 7.4 | 11.5 |
| Leukocytosis | 7.1 | 10.9 |
| **Metabolic/Nutritional** | | |
| Peripheral edema | 28.6 | 27 |
| Hypercholesterolemia | 12.8 | 8.5 |
| Hypophosphatemia | 12.5 | 15.8 |
| Edema | 12.2 | 11.8 |
| Hypokalemia | 10.1 | 10 |
| Hyperkalemia | 8.9 | 10.3 |
| Hyperglycemia | 8.6 | 12.4 |
| **Respiratory** | | |
| Infection | 15.8-21 | 13.1-23.9 |
| Dyspnea | 15.5 | 17.3 |
| Cough increase | 15.5 | 13.3 |
| Pharyngitis | 9.5 | 11.2 |
| Bronchitis | 8.5 | 11.9 |
| Pneumonia | 3.6 | 10.6 |
| **Urogenital** | | |
| UTI | 37.2-45.5 | 37-44.4 |
| Hematuria | 14 | 12.1 |
| Kidney tubular necrosis | 6.3 | 10 |
| Urinary tract disorder | 6.7 | 10.6 |

(Continued)

## Mycophenolate (Continued)

### Dosage Forms Cap, as mofetil: 250 mg, 500 mg

**Contraindications** Hypersensitivity to mycophenolate mofetil, mycophenolic acid or any ingredient; intravenous is contraindicated in patients who are allergic to polysorbate 80

**Warnings/Precautions** Increased risk for infection and development of lymphoproliferative disorders. Patients should be monitored appropriately and given supportive treatment should these conditions occur. Increased toxicity in patients with renal impairment. Should be used with caution in patients with active peptic ulcer disease.

Because mycophenolate mofetil has demonstrated teratogenic effects in rats and rabbits, tablets should not be crushed and capsules should not be opened or crushed. Avoid inhalation or direct contact with skin or mucous membranes of the powder contained in the capsules. Caution should be exercised in the handling and preparation of solutions of intravenous mycophenolate. Avoid skin contact with the solution. If such contact occurs, wash thoroughly with soap and water, rinse eyes with plain water.

### Pregnancy Risk Factor C

**Adverse Reactions** 1% to 10%: Thrombophlebitis and thrombosis (4%) with intravenous administration

See table.

### Drug Interactions

Decreased effect: Antacids decrease $C_{max}$ and AUC, **do not administer together**; cholestyramine decreases AUC, **do not administer together**

Increased toxicity: Acyclovir and ganciclovir levels may increase due to competition for tubular secretion of these drugs; probenecid may increase mycophenolate levels due to inhibition of tubular secretion; salicylates: high doses may increase free fraction of mycophenolic acid

**Half-Life** 18 hours; Serum concentrations: Correlation of toxicity or efficacy is still being developed, however, one study indicated that 12-hour AUCs >40 mcg/mL/hour were correlated with efficacy and decreased episodes of rejection.

### Special PA Issues

**Patient Education:** Take as directed, preferably 1 hour before or 2 hours after meals. Do not take within 1 hour before or 2 hours after antacids or cholestyramine medications. Do not alter dose and do not discontinue without consulting prescriber. Maintain adequate hydration (2-3 L/day of fluids unless instructed to restrict fluid intake) during entire course of therapy. You will be susceptible to infection (avoid crowds and people with infections or contagious diseases). If you are diabetic, monitor glucose levels closely (may alter glucose levels). You may experience dizziness or trembling (use caution until response to medication is known); nausea or vomiting (frequent small meals, frequent mouth care may help); diarrhea (boiled milk, yogurt, or buttermilk may help); sores or white plaques in mouth (frequent rinsing or mouth and frequent mouth care may help); or muscle or back pain (mild analgesics may be recommended). Report chest pain; acute headache or dizziness; symptoms of respiratory infection, cough, or difficulty breathing; unresolved gastrointestinal effects; fatigue, chills, fever unhealed sores, white plaques in mouth; irritation in genital area or unusual discharge; unusual bruising or bleeding; or other unusual effects related to this medication.

- **Mycophenolate Mofetil** see Mycophenolate on page 624
- **Mycostatin®** see Nystatin on page 669
- **Myco-Triacet® II** see Nystatin and Triamcinolone on page 670
- **Mydfrin® Ophthalmic Solution** see Phenylephrine on page 718
- **Mydriacyl®** see Tropicamide on page 943
- **Mykrox®** see Metolazone on page 598
- **Mylanta® Gelcaps®** see Calcium Carbonate and Magnesium Carbonate on page 140
- **Myleran®** see Busulfan on page 129
- **Myotonachol™** see Bethanechol on page 114
- **Myphetane DC®** see Brompheniramine, Phenylpropanolamine, and Codeine on page 123
- **Mysoline®** see Primidone on page 756
- **Mytrex® F Topical** see Nystatin and Triamcinolone on page 670
- **Mytussin® [OTC]** see Guaifenesin on page 427
- **Mytussin® AC** see Guaifenesin and Codeine on page 428
- **Mytussin® DAC** see Guaifenesin, Pseudoephedrine, and Codeine on page 429
- **Mytussin® DM [OTC]** see Guaifenesin and Dextromethorphan on page 428
- **M-Zole® 7 Dual Pack [OTC]** see Miconazole on page 604

## Nabumetone (na BYOO me tone)

**Pharmacologic Class** Nonsteroidal Anti-Inflammatory Agent (NSAID)
**U.S. Brand Names** Relafen®

**Mechanism of Action** Nabumetone is a nonacidic, nonsteroidal anti-inflammatory drug that is rapidly metabolized after absorption to a major active metabolite, 6-methoxy-2-naphthylacetic acid. As found with previous nonsteroidal anti-inflammatory drugs, nabumetone's active metabolite inhibits the cyclo-oxygenase enzyme which is indirectly responsible for the production of inflammation and pain during arthritis by way of enhancing the production of endoperoxides and prostaglandins $E_2$ and $I_2$ (prostacyclin). The active metabolite of nabumetone is felt to be the compound primarily responsible for therapeutic effect. Comparatively, the parent drug is a poor inhibitor of prostaglandin synthesis.

**Use** Management of osteoarthritis and rheumatoid arthritis

    **Unlabeled use:** Sunburn, mild to moderate pain

**USUAL DOSAGE** Adults: Oral: 1000 mg/day; an additional 500-1000 mg may be needed in some patients to obtain more symptomatic relief; may be administered once or twice daily

    **Dosing adjustment in renal impairment:** None necessary; however, adverse effects due to accumulation of inactive metabolites of nabumetone that are renally excreted have not been studied and should be considered

**Dosage Forms Tab:** 500 mg, 750 mg

**Contraindications** Hypersensitivity to nabumetone; should not be administered to patients with active peptic ulceration and those with severe hepatic impairment or in patients in whom nabumetone, aspirin, or other NSAIDs have induced asthma, urticaria, or other allergic-type reactions; fatal asthmatic reactions have occurred following NSAID administration

**Warnings/Precautions** Elderly patients may sometimes require lower doses; patients with impaired renal function may need a dose reduction; use with caution in patients with severe hepatic impairment

**Pregnancy Risk Factor** C

**Adverse Reactions**

    >10%:

        Central nervous system: Dizziness

        Dermatologic: Rash

        Gastrointestinal: Abdominal cramps, heartburn, indigestion, nausea

    1% to 10%:

        Central nervous system: Headache, nervousness

        Dermatologic: Itching

        Endocrine & metabolic: Fluid retention

        Gastrointestinal: Vomiting

        Otic: Tinnitus

    <1%: Congestive heart failure, hypertension, arrhythmia, tachycardia, confusion, hallucinations, aseptic meningitis, mental depression, drowsiness, insomnia, angioedema, urticaria, erythema multiforme, toxic epidermal necrolysis, Stevens-Johnson syndrome, polydipsia, hot flashes, gastritis, GI ulceration, cystitis, polyuria, agranulocytosis, anemia, hemolytic anemia, bone marrow suppression, leukopenia, thrombocytopenia, hepatitis, peripheral neuropathy, toxic amblyopia, blurred vision, conjunctivitis, dry eyes, decreased hearing, acute renal failure, allergic rhinitis, shortness of breath, epistaxis

**Onset** May require several days to maximum effect

**Half-Life** Major metabolite: 24 hours

**Special PA Issues**

    **Patient Education:** Take this medication exactly as directed; do not increase dose without consulting prescriber. Do not crush tablets or break capsules. Take with food or milk to reduce GI distress. Maintain adequate fluid intake (2-3 L/day). Do not use alcohol, aspirin, or aspirin-containing medication, and all other anti-inflammatory medications without consulting prescriber. You may experience drowsiness, dizziness, nervousness, or headache (use caution when driving or performing hazardous tasks); anorexia, nausea, vomiting, or heartburn (frequent small meals, frequent oral care, sucking on lozenges, or chewing gum may help); fluid retention (weigh yourself weekly and report unusual (3-5 lb/week) weight gain). GI bleeding, ulceration, or perforation can occur with or without pain; discontinue medication and contact prescriber if persistent abdominal pain or cramping, or blood in stool occurs. Report breathlessness, difficulty breathing, or unusual cough; chest pain, rapid heartbeat, palpitations; unusual bruising/bleeding; blood in urine, stool, mouth, or vomitus; swollen extremities; skin rash or itching; acute fatigue; or changes in hearing or ringing in ears.

    **Dietary Considerations:**

        Alcohol: May add to irritant action in the stomach, avoid use if possible

        Food: Increases the rate but not the extent of oral absorption. Take without regard to meals OR take with food or milk to minimize GI upset.

**Related Information**

    Nonsteroidal Anti-Inflammatory Agents *on page 1026*

  &#9670; **NAC** *see* Acetylcysteine *on page 26*

  &#9670; ***N*-Acetylcysteine** *see* Acetylcysteine *on page 26*

  &#9670; ***N*-Acetyl-L-cysteine** *see* Acetylcysteine *on page 26*

  &#9670; **N-Acetyl-P-Aminophenol** *see* Acetaminophen *on page 21*

  &#9670; **NaCl** *see* Sodium Chloride *on page 839*

# Nadolol (nay DOE lole)

**Pharmacologic Class** Beta Blocker, Nonselective

**U.S. Brand Names** Corgard®

**Mechanism of Action** Competitively blocks response to beta$_1$- and beta$_2$-adrenergic stimulation; does not exhibit any membrane stabilizing or intrinsic sympathomimetic activity

**Use** Treatment of hypertension and angina pectoris; prevention of myocardial infarction; prophylaxis of migraine headaches

**USUAL DOSAGE** Oral:

Adults: Initial: 40 mg/day, increase dosage gradually by 40-80 mg increments at 3- to 7-day intervals until optimum clinical response is obtained with profound slowing of heart rate; doses up to 160-240 mg/day in angina and 240-320 mg/day in hypertension may be necessary

Elderly: Initial: 20 mg/day; increase doses by 20 mg increments at 3- to 7-day intervals; usual dosage range: 20-240 mg/day

**Dosing adjustment in renal impairment:**

Cl$_{cr}$ 31-40 mL/minute: Administer every 24-36 hours or administer 50% of normal dose

Cl$_{cr}$ 10-30 mL/minute: Administer every 24-48 hours or administer 50% of normal dose

Cl$_{cr}$ <10 mL/minute: Administer every 40-60 hours or administer 25% of normal dose

Hemodialysis: Moderately dialyzable (20% to 50%); administer dose postdialysis or administer 40 mg supplemental dose

Peritoneal dialysis: Supplemental dose is not necessary

**Dosing adjustment/comments in hepatic disease:** Reduced dose probably necessary

**Dosage Forms Tab:** 20 mg 40 mg, 80 mg, 120 mg, 160 mg

**Contraindications** Uncompensated congestive heart failure, cardiogenic shock, bradycardia or heart block, hypersensitivity to any component, bronchial asthma, bronchospasms, diabetes mellitus

**Warnings/Precautions** Increase dosing interval in patients with renal dysfunction; abrupt withdrawal of beta-blockers may result in an exaggerated cardiac beta-adrenergic responsiveness; symptomatology has included reports of tachycardia, hypertension, ischemia, angina, myocardial infarction, and sudden death; it is recommended that patients be tapered gradually off of beta-blockers over a period of 1-2 weeks rather than via abrupt discontinuation; use with caution in patients with bronchial asthma, bronchospasms, CHF, or diabetes mellitus

## Pregnancy Risk Factor C

## Pregnancy Implications

Clinical effects on the fetus: No data available on crossing the placenta. Bradycardia, hypotension, hypoglycemia, respiratory depression, hypothermia, IUGR reported. IUGR probably related to maternal hypertension. Alternative beta-blockers are preferred for use during pregnancy due to limited data. Monitor breast-fed infant for symptoms of beta-blockade.

Breast-feeding/lactation: Crosses into breast milk. American Academy of Pediatrics considers compatible with breast-feeding.

## Adverse Reactions

Cardiovascular: Bradycardia, reduced peripheral circulation, congestive heart failure, chest pain, orthostatic hypotension, Raynaud's syndrome, edema

Central nervous system: Mental depression, dizziness, drowsiness, nightmares, vivid dreams, paresthesia of toes and fingers, insomnia, lethargy, fatigue, confusion, headache

Dermatologic: Itching, rash

Endocrine & metabolic: Decreased sexual ability

Gastrointestinal: Constipation, vomiting, stomach discomfort, diarrhea, nausea

Genitourinary: Impotence

Hematologic: Thrombocytopenia

Neuromuscular & skeletal: Weakness

Ocular: Dry eyes

Respiratory: Dyspnea, wheezing, nasal congestion

Miscellaneous: Cold extremities

## Drug Interactions

Decreased effect of beta-blockers with aluminum salts, barbiturates, calcium salts, cholestyramine, colestipol, NSAIDs, penicillins (ampicillin), rifampin, salicylates and sulfinpyrazone due to decreased bioavailability and plasma levels

Beta-blockers may decrease the effect of sulfonylureas, beta agonists

Increased effect/toxicity of beta-blockers with calcium blockers (diltiazem, felodipine, nicardipine), contraceptives, flecainide, MAO inhibitors, quinidine (in extensive metabolizers), ciprofloxacin

Beta-blockers may increase the effect/toxicity of flecainide, phenothiazines, acetaminophen, clonidine (hypertensive crisis after or during withdrawal of either agent), epinephrine (initial hypertensive episode followed by bradycardia), nifedipine and verapamil, lidocaine, ergots (peripheral ischemia), prazosin (postural hypotension)

Beta-blockers may affect the action or levels of ethanol, disopyramide, nondepolarizing muscle relaxants and theophylline although the effects are difficult to predict

**Duration** 24 hours

**Half-Life** 10-24 hours; increased half-life with decreased renal function; End-stage renal disease: 45 hours

**Special PA Issues**

**Patient Education:** Check pulse daily prior to taking medication. If pulse is <50, hold medication and consult prescriber. Do not adjust dosage without consulting prescriber. May cause dizziness, fatigue, blurred vision; change position slowly (lying/sitting to standing) and use caution when driving or engaging in tasks that need alertness until response to medication is known. Exercise and increasing bulk or fiber in diet may help resolve constipation. If diabetic, monitor serum glucose closely (the drug may mask symptoms of hypoglycemia). Report swelling in feet or legs, difficulty breathing or persistent cough, unresolved fatigue, unusual weight gain >5 lb/week, or unresolved constipation.

**Related Information**
Beta-Blockers *on page 1002*

♦ **Nadopen-V®** *see* Penicillin V Potassium *on page 706*

♦ **Nadostine®** *see* Nystatin *on page 669*

# Nafarelin (NAF a re lin)

**Pharmacologic Class** Hormone, Posterior Pituitary; Luteinizing Hormone-Releasing Hormone Analog

**U.S. Brand Names** Synarel®

**Mechanism of Action** Potent synthetic decapeptide analogue of gonadotropin-releasing hormone (GnRH; LHRH) which is approximately 200 times more potent than GnRH in terms of pituitary release of luteinizing hormone (LH) and follicle-stimulating hormone (FSH). Effects on the pituitary gland and sex hormones are dependent upon its length of administration. After acute administration, an initial stimulation of the release of LH and FSH from the pituitary is observed; an increase in androgens and estrogens subsequently follows. Continued administration of nafarelin, however, suppresses gonadotrope responsiveness to endogenous GnRH resulting in reduced secretion of LH and FSH and, secondarily, decreased ovarian and testicular steroid production.

**Use** Treatment of endometriosis, including pain and reduction of lesions; treatment of central precocious puberty (gonadotropin-dependent precocious puberty) in children of both sexes

**USUAL DOSAGE**

Endometriosis: Adults: Female: 1 spray (200 mcg) in 1 nostril each morning and the other nostril each evening starting on days 2-4 of menstrual cycle for 6 months

Central precocious puberty: Children: Males/Females: 2 sprays (400 mcg) into each nostril in the morning 2 sprays (400 mcg) into each nostril in the evening. If inadequate suppression, may increase dose to 3 sprays (600 mcg) into alternating nostrils 3 times/day.

**Dosage Forms Soln, nasal, as acetate:** 2 mg/mL (10 mL)

**Contraindications** Hypersensitivity to GnRH, GnRH-agonist analogs or any components of this product; undiagnosed abnormal vaginal bleeding; pregnancy; lactation

**Warnings/Precautions** Use with caution in patients with risk factors for decreased bone mineral content, nafarelin therapy may pose an additional risk; hypersensitivity reactions occur in 0.2% of the patients; safety and efficacy in children have not been established

**Pregnancy Risk Factor** X

**Adverse Reactions**

>10%:
Central nervous system: Headache, emotional lability
Dermatologic: Acne
Endocrine & metabolic: Hot flashes, decreased libido, decreased breast size
Genitourinary: Vaginal dryness
Neuromuscular & skeletal: Myalgia
Respiratory: Nasal irritation

1% to 10%:
Cardiovascular: Edema, chest pain
Central nervous system: Insomnia
Dermatologic: Urticaria, rash, pruritus, seborrhea
Respiratory: Shortness of breath

<1%: Increased libido, weight loss

**Special PA Issues**

**Patient Education:** You will begin this treatment between days 2-4 of your regular menstrual cycle. Use as directed - daily at same time (arising and bedtime), and rotate nostrils. Maintain regular follow-up schedule. You may experience hot flashes, flushing or redness (cold clothes and cool environment may help), decreased or increased libido, emotional lability, weight gain, decreased breast size, or hirsutism. Report any breakthrough bleeding or continuing menstruation or musculoskeletal pain. Do not use a nasal decongestant within 30 minutes after nafarelin.

♦ **Nafarelin Acetate** *see* Nafarelin *on this page*

♦ **Nafazair®** *see* Naphazoline *on page 635*

♦ **Nafcil™ Injection** *see* Nafcillin *on next page*

# Nafcillin (naf SIL in)

**Pharmacologic Class** Antibiotic, Penicillin

**U.S. Brand Names** Nafcil™ Injection; Nallpen® Injection; Unipen® Injection; Unipen® Oral

**Mechanism of Action** Interferes with bacterial cell wall synthesis during active multiplication, causing cell wall death and resultant bactericidal activity against susceptible bacteria

**Use** Treatment of infections such as osteomyelitis, septicemia, endocarditis, and CNS infections caused by susceptible strains of staphylococcal species

## USUAL DOSAGE

Neonates:

&lt;2000 g, &lt;7 days: 50 mg/kg/day divided every 12 hours

&lt;2000 g, &gt;7 days: 75 mg/kg/day divided every 8 hours

&gt;2000 g, &lt;7 days: 50 mg/kg/day divided every 8 hours

&gt;2000 g, &gt;7 days: 75 mg/kg/day divided every 6 hours

Children:

Oral: 25-50 mg/kg/day in 4 divided doses

I.M.: 25 mg/kg twice daily

I.V.:

Mild to moderate infections: 50-100 mg/kg/day in divided doses every 6 hours

Severe infections: 100-200 mg/kg/day in divided doses every 4-6 hours

Maximum dose: 12 g/day

Adults:

Oral: 250-500 mg (up to g) every 4-6 hours

I.M.: 500 mg every 4-6 hours

I.V.: 500-2000 mg every 4-6 hours

**Dosing adjustment in renal impairment:** Not necessary

Dialysis: Not dialyzable (0% to 5%) via hemodialysis; supplemental dosage not necessary with hemo- or peritoneal dialysis or continuous arteriovenous or venovenous hemofiltration (CAVH/CAVHD)

**Dosage Forms Cap:** 250 mg; **Powder for inj:** 500 mg, 1 g, 2 g, 4 g, 10 g; **Soln:** 250 mg/5 mL (100 mL); **Tab:** 500 mg

**Contraindications** Hypersensitivity to nafcillin or any component or penicillins

**Warnings/Precautions** Extravasation of I.V. infusions should be avoided; modification of dosage is necessary in patients with both severe renal and hepatic impairment; elimination rate will be slow in neonates; use with caution in patients with cephalosporin hypersensitivity

## Pregnancy Risk Factor B

**Adverse Reactions** Percentage unknown: Fever, pain, rash, nausea, diarrhea, neutropenia, thrombophlebitis; oxacillin (less likely to cause phlebitis) is often preferred in pediatric patients, acute interstitial nephritis, hypersensitivity reactions

## Drug Interactions

Decreased effect: Efficacy of oral contraceptives may be reduced; warfarin/anticoagulants

Increased effect: Disulfiram, probenecid may increase penicillin levels

**Half-Life** 0.5-1.5 hours, with normal hepatic function; End-stage renal disease: 1.2 hours

## Special PA Issues

**Patient Education:** Oral: Take at regular intervals around-the-clock, preferably on and empty stomach with full glass of water. Take complete course of treatment as prescribed. You may experience nausea or vomiting; small frequent meals and good mouth care may help. If diabetic, drug may cause false tests with Clinitest® urine glucose monitoring; use of glucose oxidase methods (Clinistix®) or serum glucose monitoring is preferable. This drug may interfere with oral contraceptives; an alternate form of birth control should be used. Report persistent fever, sore throat, sores in mouth, diarrhea, unusual bleeding or bruising. Report difficulty breathing or skin rash. Notify prescriber if condition does not respond to treatment.

**Monitoring Parameters:** Periodic CBC, urinalysis, BUN, serum creatinine, AST and ALT; observe for signs and symptoms of anaphylaxis during first dose

♦ **Nafcillin Sodium** *see* Nafcillin *on this page*

# Naftifine (NAF ti feen)

**Pharmacologic Class** Antifungal Agent, Topical

**U.S. Brand Names** Naftin®

**Mechanism of Action** Synthetic, broad-spectrum antifungal agent in the allylamine class; appears to have both fungistatic and fungicidal activity. Exhibits antifungal activity by selectively inhibiting the enzyme squalene epoxidase in a dose-dependent manner which results in the primary sterol, ergosterol, within the fungal membrane not being synthesized.

**Use** Topical treatment of tinea cruris (jock itch), tinea corporis (ringworm), and tinea pedis (athlete's foot)

**USUAL DOSAGE** Adults: Topical: Apply cream once daily and gel twice daily (morning and evening) for up to 4 weeks

**Dosage Forms Crm:** 1% 15 g, 30 g, 60 g); **Gel, top:** 1% (20 g, 40 g, 60 g)

**Contraindications** Hypersensitivity to any component

**Warnings/Precautions** For external use only

**Pregnancy Risk Factor** B
**Adverse Reactions**
>10%: Local: Burning, stinging
1% to 10%:
Dermatologic: Erythema, itching
Local: Dryness, irritation
**Special PA Issues**
**Patient Education:** External use only; avoid eyes, mouth, and other mucous membranes; do not use occlusive dressings unless directed to do so; discontinue if irritation or sensitivity develops; wash hands after application
**Related Information**
Antifungal Agents, Topical *on page 1000*

♦ **Naftifine Hydrochloride** *see* Naftifine *on previous page*

♦ **Naftin®** *see* Naftifine *on previous page*

♦ **NaHCO₃** *see* Sodium Bicarbonate *on page 838*

# Nalbuphine (NAL byoo feen)

**Pharmacologic Class** Analgesic, Narcotic
**U.S. Brand Names** Nubain®
**Mechanism of Action** Binds to opiate receptors in the CNS, causing inhibition of ascending pain pathways, altering the perception of and response to pain; produces generalized CNS depression
**Use** Relief of moderate to severe pain; preoperative analgesia, postoperative and surgical anesthesia, and obstetrical analgesia during labor and delivery
**USUAL DOSAGE** I.M., I.V., S.C.:
Children 10 months to 14 years: Premedication: 0.2 mg/kg;  maximum: 20 mg/dose
Adults: 10 mg/70 kg every 3-6 hours; maximum single dose: 20 mg; maximum daily dose: 160 mg
**Dosing adjustment/comments in hepatic impairment:** Use with caution and reduce dose
**Dosage Forms Inj, as hydrochloride:** 10 mg/mL (1 mL, 10 mL), 20 mg/mL (1 mL, 10 mL)
**Contraindications** Hypersensitivity to nalbuphine or any component, including sulfites
**Warnings/Precautions** Use with caution in patients with recent myocardial infarction, biliary tract surgery, or sulfite sensitivity; may produce respiratory depression; use with caution in women delivering premature infants; use with caution in patients with a history of drug dependence, head trauma or increased intracranial pressure, decreased hepatic or renal function, or pregnancy; tolerance or drug dependence may result from extended use
**Pregnancy Risk Factor** B (D if used for prolonged periods or in high doses at term)
**Adverse Reactions**
>10%:
Central nervous system: Drowsiness, CNS depression, narcotic withdrawal
Miscellaneous: Histamine release
1% to 10%:
Cardiovascular: Hypotension, flushing
Central nervous system: Dizziness, headache
Dermatologic: Urticaria, rash
Gastrointestinal: Nausea, vomiting, anorexia, xerostomia
Local: Pain at injection site
Neuromuscular & skeletal: Weakness
Respiratory: Pulmonary edema
<1%: Hypertension, tachycardia, mental depression, hallucinations, confusion, paradoxical CNS stimulation, nervousness, restlessness, nightmares, insomnia GI irritation, biliary spasm, decreased urination, toxic megacolon, ureteral spasm, blurred vision, shortness of breath, respiratory depression
**Drug Interactions** Increased toxicity: Barbiturate anesthetics may increase CNS depression
**Onset** Peak effect: I.M.: 30 minutes; I.V.: 1-3 minutes
**Half-Life** 3.5-5 hours
**Special PA Issues**
**Patient Education:** If self-administered, use exactly as directed (do not increase dose or frequency); may cause physical and/or psychological dependence. While using this medication, do not use alcohol and other prescription or OTC medications (especially sedatives, tranquilizers, antihistamines, or pain medications) without consulting prescriber. Maintain adequate hydration (2-3 L/day of fluids unless instructed to restrict fluid intake). May cause hypotension, dizziness, drowsiness, impaired coordination, or blurred vision (use caution when driving, climbing stairs, or changing position - rising from sitting or lying to standing, or when engaging in hazardous activities until response to medication is known); loss of appetite, nausea, or vomiting (frequent mouth care, small frequent meals, or sucking on lozenges may help); constipation (increased exercise, fluids, or dietary fruit and fiber may help - if constipation remains an unresolved problem, consult prescriber about use of stool softeners). Report chest pain, slow or rapid heartbeat, acute dizziness or persistent headache; changes in mental status; swelling of extremities or unusual
(Continued)

## Nalbuphine *(Continued)*

weight gain; changes in urinary elimination or pain on urination; acute headache; back or flank pain or muscle spasms; blurred vision; skin rash; or shortness of breath.

**Dietary Considerations:** Alcohol: Additive CNS effects, avoid or limit alcohol; watch for sedation

**Monitoring Parameters:** Relief of pain, respiratory and mental status, blood pressure

**Related Information**

Narcotic Agonists *on page 1023*

♦ **Nalbuphine Hydrochloride** *see* Nalbuphine *on previous page*

♦ **Naldecon®** *see* Chlorpheniramine, Phenyltoloxamine, Phenylpropanolamine, and Phenylephrine *on page 196*

♦ **Naldecon® Senior DX [OTC]** *see* Guaifenesin and Dextromethorphan *on page 428*

♦ **Naldecon® Senior EX [OTC]** *see* Guaifenesin *on page 427*

♦ **Naldelate®** *see* Chlorpheniramine, Phenyltoloxamine, Phenylpropanolamine, and Phenylephrine *on page 196*

♦ **Nalfon®** *see* Fenoprofen *on page 361*

♦ **Nalgest®** *see* Chlorpheniramine, Phenyltoloxamine, Phenylpropanolamine, and Phenylephrine *on page 196*

♦ **Nallpen® Injection** *see* Nafcillin *on page 630*

♦ **N-allylnoroxymorphine Hydrochloride** *see* Naloxone *on next page*

## Nalmefene *(NAL me feen)*

**Pharmacologic Class** Antidote

**U.S. Brand Names** Revex®

**Mechanism of Action** As a 6-methylene analog of naltrexone, nalmefene acts as a competitive antagonist at opioid receptor sites, preventing or reversing the respiratory depression, sedation, and hypotension induced by opiates; no pharmacologic activity of its own (eg, opioid agonist activity) has been demonstrated

**Use** Complete or partial reversal of opioid drug effects, including respiratory depression induced by natural or synthetic opioids; reversal of postoperative opioid depression; management of known or suspected opioid overdose (if opioid dependence is suspected, nalmefene should only be used in opioid overdose if the likelihood of overdose is high based on history or the clinical presentation of respiratory depression with concurrent pupillary constriction is present)

**USUAL DOSAGE**

Reversal of postoperative opioid depression: Blue labeled product (100 mcg/mL): Titrate to reverse the undesired effects of opioids; initial dose for nonopioid dependent patients: 0.25 mcg/kg followed by 0.25 mcg/kg incremental doses at 2- to 5-minute intervals; after a total dose of >1 mcg/kg, further therapeutic response is unlikely

Management of known/suspected opioid overdose: Green labeled product (1000 mcg/mL): Initial dose: 0.5 mg/70 kg may repeat with 1 mg/70 kg in 2-5 minutes; further increase beyond a total dose of 1.5 mg/70 kg will not likely result in improved response and may result in cardiovascular stress and precipitated withdrawal syndrome. (If opioid dependency is suspected, administer a challenge dose of 0.1 mg/70 kg; if no withdrawal symptoms are observed in 2 minutes, the recommended doses can be administered.)

**Dosing adjustment in renal or hepatic impairment:** Not necessary with single uses, however, slow administration (over 60 seconds) of incremental doses is recommended to minimize hypertension and dizziness

**Dosage Forms Inj, as hydrochloride:** 100 mcg/mL [blue label] (1 mL), 1000 mcg/mL [green label] (2 mL)

**Contraindications** Hypersensitivity to nalmefene, naltrexone, or components

**Warnings/Precautions** May induce symptoms of acute withdrawal in opioid-dependent patients; recurrence of respiratory depression is possible if the opioid involved is long-acting; observe patients until there is no reasonable risk of recurrent respiratory depression; dosage may need to be decreased in renal and hepatic impairment; safety and efficacy have not been established in children; avoid abrupt reversal of opioid effects in patients of high cardiovascular risk or who have received potentially cardiotoxic drugs; animal studies indicate nalmefene may not completely reverse buprenorphine-induced respiratory depression

**Pregnancy Risk Factor** B

**Pregnancy Implications** Limited information available; do not use in pregnant or lactating women if possible

**Adverse Reactions**

>10%: Gastrointestinal: Nausea (18%)

1% to 10%:

Cardiovascular: Tachycardia/hypertension (5%)

Central nervous system: Fever/dizziness (3%)

Gastrointestinal: Vomiting (9%)

Miscellaneous: Postoperative pain (4%)

<1%: Hypotension, vasodilation, arrhythmia, bradycardia, headache, chills, nervousness, confusion, somnolence, depression, pruritus, diarrhea, xerostomia, urinary retention, increased AST, tremor, myoclonus, pharyngitis, withdrawal syndrome

**Drug Interactions** Increased effect: Potential increased risk of seizures exists with use of flumazenil and nalmefene coadministration

**Onset** I.M., S.C.: 5-15 minutes

**Half-Life** 10.8 hours

**Special PA Issues**

**Patient Education:** This drug can only be administered I.V. You may experience drowsiness, dizziness, or blurred vision for several days; use caution when driving or engaging in hazardous tasks. Small frequent meals and good mouth care may reduce any nausea or vomiting. Report yellowing of eyes or skin, unusual bleeding, dark or tarry stools, acute headache, or palpitations.

♦ **Nalmefene Hydrochloride** *see* Nalmefene *on previous page*

# Naloxone (nal OKS one)

**Pharmacologic Class** Antidote

**U.S. Brand Names** Narcan® Injection

**Mechanism of Action** Competes and displaces narcotics at narcotic receptor sites

**Use** Reverses CNS and respiratory depression in suspected narcotic overdose; neonatal opiate depression; coma of unknown etiology

**Investigational:** Shock, PCP and alcohol ingestion

**USUAL DOSAGE** I.M., I.V. (preferred), intratracheal, S.C.:

Postanesthesia narcotic reversal: Infants and Children: 0.01 mg/kg; may repeat every 2-3 minutes as needed based on response

Opiate intoxication:

Birth (including premature infants) to 5 years or <20 kg: 0.1 mg/kg; repeat every 2-3 minutes if needed; may need to repeat doses every 20-60 minutes

>5 years or ≥20 kg: 2 mg/dose; if no response, repeat every 2-3 minutes; may need to repeat doses every 20-60 minutes

Continuous infusion: I.V.: Children and Adults: If continuous infusion is required, calculate dosage/hour based on effective intermittent dose used and duration of adequate response seen, titrate dose 0.04-0.16 mg/kg/hour for 2-5 days in children, up to 0.8 mg/kg/hour in adults; alternatively, continuous infusion utilizes $2/3$ of the initial naloxone bolus on an hourly basis; add 10 times this dose to each liter of $D_5W$ and infuse at a rate of 100 mL/hour; $1/2$ of the initial bolus dose should be readministered 15 minutes after initiation of the continuous infusion to prevent a drop in naloxone levels; increase infusion rate as needed to assure adequate ventilation

Narcotic overdose: Adults: I.V.: 0.4-2 mg every 2-3 minutes as needed; may need to repeat doses every 20-60 minutes, if no response is observed after 10 mg, question the diagnosis. **Note:** Use 0.1-0.2 mg increments in patients who are opioid dependent and in postoperative patients to avoid large cardiovascular changes.

**Dosage Forms Inj, as hydrochloride:** 0.4 mg/mL (1 mL, 2 mL, 10 mL), 1 mg/mL (2 mL, 10 mL)

**Contraindications** Hypersensitivity to naloxone or any component

**Warnings/Precautions** Use with caution in patients with cardiovascular disease; excessive dosages should be avoided after use of opiates in surgery, because naloxone may cause an increase in blood pressure and reversal of anesthesia; may precipitate withdrawal symptoms in patients addicted to opiates, including pain, hypertension, sweating, agitation, irritability, shrill cry, failure to feed

**Pregnancy Risk Factor** B

**Adverse Reactions** 1% to 10%:

Cardiovascular: Hypertension, hypotension, tachycardia, ventricular arrhythmias

Central nervous system: Insomnia, irritability, anxiety, narcotic withdrawal

Dermatologic: Rash

Gastrointestinal: Nausea, vomiting

Ocular: Blurred vision

Miscellaneous: Diaphoresis

**Drug Interactions** Decreased effect of narcotic analgesics

**Onset** Endotracheal, I.M., S.C.: Within 2-5 minutes; I.V.: Within 2 minutes

**Duration** 20-60 minutes; since shorter than that of most opioids, repeated doses are usually needed

**Half-Life** 1-1.5 hours

**Special PA Issues**

**Patient Education:** If patient is responsive, instructions are individualized. This drug can only be administered I.V. Report difficulty breathing, palpitations, or tremors.

**Monitoring Parameters:** Respiratory rate, heart rate, blood pressure

**Related Information**

Narcotic Agonists *on page 1023*

♦ **Naloxone Hydrochloride** *see* Naloxone *on this page*

♦ **Nalspan®** *see* Chlorpheniramine, Phenyltoloxamine, Phenylpropanolamine, and Phenylephrine *on page 196*

# Naltrexone (nal TREKS one)

**Pharmacologic Class** Antidote

**U.S. Brand Names** ReVia®

**Mechanism of Action** Naltexone is a cyclopropyl derivative of oxymorphone similar in structure to naloxone and nalorphine (a morphine derivative); it acts as a competitive antagonist at opioid recepto sites

**Use** Adjunct to the maintenance of an opioid-free state in detoxified individual; alcoholism

**USUAL DOSAGE** Do not give until patient is opioid-free for 7-10 days as required by urine analysis; Adults: Oral:

25 mg; if no withdrawal signs within 1 hour give another 25 mg; maintenance regimen is flexible, variable and individualized (50 mg/day to 100-150 mg 3 times/week)

Adjunct in the management of alcoholism: A flexible approach to dosing is recommended by the manufacturer; the following are acceptable regimens:

50 mg once daily

50 mg once daily on weekdays and 100 mg on Saturdays

100 mg every other day

150 mg every third day

**Dosage Forms** Tab, as hydrochloride: 50 mg

**Contraindications** Acute hepatitis, liver failure, known hypersensitivity to naltrexone

**Warnings/Precautions** Dose-related hepatocellular injury is possible; the margin of separation between the apparent safe and hepatotoxic doses appear to be only fivefold or less

**Pregnancy Risk Factor** C

**Adverse Reactions**

>10%:

Central nervous system: Insomnia, nervousness, headache

Gastrointestinal: Abdominal cramping, nausea, vomiting

Neuromuscular & skeletal: Arthralgia

1% to 10%:

Central nervous system: Dizziness

Dermatologic: Rash

Endocrine & metabolic: Polydipsia

Gastrointestinal: Anorexia

Respiratory: Sneezing

<1%: Insomnia, irritability, anxiety, narcotic withdrawal, thrombocytopenia, agranulocytosis, hemolytic anemia, blurred vision

**Duration** 50 mg: 24 hours; 100 mg: 48 hours; 150 mg: 72 hours

**Half-Life** 4 hours; active metabolite, 6-β-naltrexol: 13 hours

**Special PA Issues**

**Patient Education:** This medication will help you achieve abstinence from opiates if taken as directed. Do not increase or change dose. Do not use opiates or any medications not approved by your prescriber during naltrexone therapy. You may experience drowsiness, dizziness, or blurred vision (use caution when driving or engaging in hazardous tasks); nausea or vomiting (small frequent meals, good mouth care, chewing gum, or sucking on lozenges may help); decreased sexual function (reversible when drug is discontinued). Report yellowing of skin or eyes, change in color of stool or urine, increased perspiration or chills, acute headache, palpitations, or unusual joint pain.

♦ **Naltrexone Hydrochloride** *see* Naltrexone *on this page*

# Nandrolone (NAN droe lone)

**Pharmacologic Class** Androgen

**U.S. Brand Names** Anabolin® Injection; Androlone®-D Injection; Androlone® Injection; Deca-Durabolin® Injection; Durabolin® Injection; Hybolin™ Decanoate Injection; Hybolin™ Improved Injection; Neo-Durabolic Injection

**Mechanism of Action** Promotes tissue-building processes, increases production of erythropoietin, causes protein anabolism; increases hemoglobin and red blood cell volume

**Use** Control of metastatic breast cancer; management of anemia of renal insufficiency

**USUAL DOSAGE** Deep I.M. (into gluteal muscle):

Children 2-13 years: (decanoate): 25-50 mg every 3-4 weeks

Adults:

Male:

Breast cancer (phenpropionate): 50-100 mg/week

Anemia of renal insufficiency (decanoate): 100-200 mg/week

Female: 50-100 mg/week

Breast cancer (phenpropionate): 50-100 mg/week

Anemia of renal insufficiency (decanoate): 50-100 mg/week

**Dosage Forms** Nandrolone phenpropionate: Inj in oil: 25 mg/mL (5 mL), 50 mg/mL (2 mL) Nandrolone decanoate: In. in oil: 50 mg/mL (1 mL, 2 mL), 100 mg/mL (1 mL, 2 mL), 200 mg/mL (1 mL); Inj, repository: 50 mg/mL (2 mL), 100 mg/mL (2 mL), 200 mg/mL (2 mL)

**Contraindications** Carcinoma of breast or prostate, nephrosis, pregnancy and infants, hypersensitivity to any component

**Warnings/Precautions** Monitor diabetic patients carefully; anabolic steroids may cause peliosis hepatis, liver cell tumors, and blood lipid changes with increased risk of arteriosclerosis; use with caution in elderly patients, they may be at greater risk for prostatic hypertrophy; use with caution in patients with cardiac, renal, or hepatic disease or epilepsy

**Pregnancy Risk Factor** X

**Adverse Reactions**

**Male:**

Postpubertal:

>10%:

Dermatologic: Acne

Endocrine & metabolic: Gynecomastia

Genitourinary: Bladder irritability, priapism

1% to 10%:

Central nervous system: Insomnia, chills

Endocrine & metabolic: Decreased libido, hepatic dysfunction

Gastrointestinal: Nausea, diarrhea

Genitourinary: Prostatic hypertrophy (elderly)

Hematologic: Iron deficiency anemia, suppression of clotting factors

<1%: Hepatic necrosis, hepatocellular carcinoma

Prepubertal:

>10%:

Dermatologic: Acne

Endocrine & metabolic: Virilism

1% to 10%:

Central nervous system: Chills, insomnia

Dermatologic: Hyperpigmentation

Gastrointestinal: Diarrhea, nausea

Hematologic: Iron deficiency anemia, suppression of clotting

<1%: Hepatocellular carcinoma, necrosis

**Female:**

>10%: Endocrine & metabolic: Virilism

1% to 10%:

Central nervous system: Chills, insomnia

Endocrine & metabolic: Hypercalcemia

Gastrointestinal: Nausea, diarrhea

Hematologic: Iron deficiency anemia, suppression of clotting factors

Hepatic: Hepatic dysfunction

<1%: Hepatic necrosis, hepatocellular carcinoma

**Drug Interactions** Increased toxicity: Oral anticoagulants, insulin, oral hypoglycemic agents, adrenal steroids, ACTH

**Special PA Issues**

**Patient Education:** This drug can only be given I.M. Diabetics must monitor serum glucose closely; glucose tolerance may change while on this drug. Report abnormal glucose tests so adjustments can be made in diabetic regimen. You may experience acne, growth of body hair or baldness, deepening of voice, loss of libido, impotence (most are reversible). Report menstrual irregularity or persistent penile erection. You may experience drowsiness, dizziness, or blurred vision; use caution when driving or engaging in hazardous tasks. Small frequent meals and good mouth care may reduce any nausea or vomiting. Report persistent GI distress or diarrhea; change in color of urine or stool; yellowing of eyes or skin; or swelling of ankles, feet, or hands.

♦ **Nandrolone Decanoate** *see* Nandrolone *on previous page*

♦ **Nandrolone Phenpropionate** *see* Nandrolone *on previous page*

## Naphazoline (naf AZ oh leen)

**Pharmacologic Class** Alpha₁ Agonist; Ophthalmic Agent; Vasoconstrictor

**U.S. Brand Names** AK-Con®; Albalon® Liquifilm®; Allerest® Eye Drops [OTC]; Clear Eyes® [OTC]; Comfort® [OTC]; Degest® 2 [OTC]; Estivin® II [OTC]; I-Naphline®; Muro's Opcon®; Nafazair®; Naphcon® [OTC]; Naphcon Forte®; Opcon®; Privine®; VasoClear® [OTC]; Vasocon Regular®

**Mechanism of Action** Stimulates alpha-adrenergic receptors in the arterioles of the conjunctiva and the nasal mucosa to produce vasoconstriction

**Use** Topical ocular vasoconstrictor; will temporarily relieve congestion, itching, and minor irritation, and to control hyperemia in patients with superficial corneal vascularity; treatment of nasal congestion; adjunct for sinusitis

**USUAL DOSAGE**

Nasal:

Children:

<6 years: Intranasal: Not recommended (especially infants) due to CNS depression

(Continued)

## Naphazoline *(Continued)*

6-12 years: 1 spray of 0.05% into each nostril every 6 hours if necessary; therapy should not exceed 3-5 days

Children >12 years and Adults: 0.05%, instill 1-2 drops or sprays every 6 hours if needed; therapy should not exceed 3-5 days

Ophthalmic:

Children <6 years: Not recommended for use due to CNS depression (especially in infants)

Children >6 years and Adults: Instill 1-2 drops into conjunctival sac of affected eye(s) every 3-4 hours; therapy generally should not exceed 3-4 days

**Dosage Forms Soln, as hydrochloride: Nasal:** Drops: 0.05% (20 mL), Spray: 0.05% (15 mL); **Ophth:** 0.012% (7.5 mL, 30 mL), 0.02% (15 mL), 0.03% (15 mL), 0.1% (15 mL)

**Contraindications** Hypersensitivity to naphazoline or any component, narrow-angle glaucoma, prior to peripheral iridectomy (in patients susceptible to angle block)

**Warnings/Precautions** Rebound congestion may occur with extended use; use with caution in the presence of hypertension, diabetes, hyperthyroidism, heart disease, coronary artery disease, cerebral arteriosclerosis, or long-standing bronchial asthma

**Pregnancy Risk Factor** C

**Adverse Reactions** 1% to 10%:

Cardiovascular: Systemic cardiovascular stimulation

Central nervous system: Dizziness, headache, nervousness

Gastrointestinal: Nausea

Local: Transient stinging, nasal mucosa irritation, dryness, rebound congestion

Ocular: Mydriasis, increased intraocular pressure, blurring of vision

Respiratory: Sneezing

**Drug Interactions** Increased toxicity: Anesthetics (discontinue mydriatic prior to use of anesthetics that sensitize the myocardium to sympathomimetics, ie, cyclopropane, halothane), MAO inhibitors, tricyclic antidepressants → hypertensive reactions

**Special PA Issues**

**Patient Education:** Do not use discolored solutions; discontinue eye drops if visual changes or ocular pain occur; notify physician of insomnia, tremor, or irregular heartbeat; stinging, burning, or drying of the nasal mucosa may occur; do not use beyond 72 hours

♦ **Naphazoline Hydrochloride** *see* Naphazoline *on previous page*

♦ **Naphcon® [OTC]** *see* Naphazoline *on previous page*

♦ **Naphcon Forte®** *see* Naphazoline *on previous page*

♦ **Naprelan®** *see* Naproxen *on this page*

♦ **Naprosyn®** *see* Naproxen *on this page*

## Naproxen *(na PROKS er)*

**Pharmacologic Class** Nonsteroidal Anti-Inflammatory Agent (NSAID)

**U.S. Brand Names** Aleve® [OTC]; Anaprox®; Naprelan®; Naprosyn®

**Mechanism of Action** Inhibits prostaglandin synthesis by decreasing the activity of the enzyme, cyclo-oxygenase which results in decreased formation of prostaglandin precursors

**Use** Management of inflammatory disease and rheumatoid disorders (including juvenile rheumatoid arthritis); acute gout; mild to moderate pain; dysmenorrhea; fever; migraine headache

**USUAL DOSAGE** Oral:

Children >2 years:

Fever: 2.5-10 mg/kg/dose; maximum: 10 mg/kg/day

Juvenile arthritis: 10 mg/kg/day in 2 divided doses

Adults:

Rheumatoid arthritis, osteoarthritis, and ankylosing spondylitis: 500-1000 mg/day in 2 divided doses; may increase to 1.5 g/day of naproxen base for limited time period

Mild to moderate pain or dysmenorrhea: Initial: 500 mg, then 250 mg every 6-8 hours; maximum: 1250 mg/day naproxen base

**Dosing adjustment in hepatic impairment:** Reduce dose to 50%

**Dosage Forms Susp, oral:** 125 mg/5 mL (15 mL, 30 mL, 480 mL); **Tab:** Aleve®: 200 mg, Naprosyn®: 250 mg, 375 mg, 500 mg; **Tab, controlled release (Naprelan®):** 375 mg, 500 mg

Naproxen sodium: **Tab, as sodium:** 220 mg (200 mg base), Anaprox®: 220 mg (200 mg base), 275 mg (250 mg base), 550 mg (500 mg base)

**Contraindications** Hypersensitivity to naproxen, aspirin, or other nonsteroidal anti-inflammatory drugs (NSAIDs)

**Warnings/Precautions** Use with caution in patients with GI disease (bleeding or ulcers), cardiovascular disease (CHF, hypertension), renal or hepatic impairment, and patients receiving anticoagulants; perform ophthalmologic evaluation for those who develop eye complaints during therapy (blurred vision, diminished vision, changes in color vision, retinal changes); NSAIDs may mask signs/symptoms of infections; photosensitivity reported; elderly are at especially high-risk for adverse effects

**Pregnancy Risk Factor** B (D if used in the 3rd trimester or near delivery)
**Adverse Reactions**
>10%:
Central nervous system: Dizziness
Dermatologic: Pruritus, rash
Gastrointestinal: Abdominal discomfort, nausea, heartburn, constipation, GI bleeding, ulcers, perforation, indigestion
1% to 10%:
Central nervous system: Headache, nervousness
Dermatologic: Itching
Endocrine & metabolic: Fluid retention
Gastrointestinal: Vomiting
Otic: Tinnitus
<1%: Edema, congestive heart failure, arrhythmias, tachycardia, hypertension, confusion, hallucinations, mental depression, fatigue, drowsiness, insomnia, aseptic meningitis, urticaria, erythema multiforme, toxic epidermal necrolysis, Stevens-Johnson syndrome, angioedema, polydipsia, hot flashes, gastritis, GI ulceration, cystitis, renal dysfunction, polyuria, anemia, hemolytic anemia, bone marrow suppression, leukopenia, thrombocytopenia, inhibits platelet aggregation, prolongs bleeding time, agranulocytosis, hepatitis, peripheral neuropathy, toxic amblyopia, blurred vision, conjunctivitis, dry eyes, decreased hearing, acute renal failure, shortness of breath, epistaxis, allergic rhinitis

**Drug Interactions** CYP2C8, 2C9, and 2C18 enzyme substrate
Decreased effect of furosemide
Increased toxicity:
Naproxen could displace other highly protein bound drugs, such as oral anticoagulants, hydantoins, salicylates, sulfonamides, and sulfonylureas
Naproxen and warfarin may cause a slight increase in free warfarin
Naproxen and probenecid may cause increased plasma half-life of naproxen
Naproxen and methotrexate may significantly increase and prolong blood methotrexate concentration, which may be severe or fatal

**Onset** Analgesia: 1 hour; Anti-inflammatory: Within 2 weeks

**Duration** Analgesia: Up to 7 hours; Anti-inflammatory: Peak: 2-4 weeks

**Half-Life** Normal renal function: 12-15 hours; End-stage renal disease: Unchanged

**Special PA Issues**
**Patient Education:** Take this medication exactly as directed; do not increase dose without consulting prescriber. Do not crush tablets or break capsules. Take with food or milk to reduce GI distress. Maintain adequate fluid intake (2-3 L/day). Do not use alcohol, aspirin, or aspirin-containing medication, and all other anti-inflammatory medications without consulting prescriber. You may experience drowsiness, dizziness, lightheadedness, or headache (use caution when driving or performing hazardous tasks); anorexia, nausea, vomiting, or heartburn (frequent small meals, frequent oral care, sucking on lozenges, or chewing gum may help); fluid retention (weigh yourself weekly and report unusual (3-5 lb/week) weight gain). GI bleeding, ulceration, or perforation can occur with or without pain; discontinue medication and contact prescriber if persistent abdominal pain or cramping, or blood in stool occurs. Report breathlessness, difficulty breathing, or unusual cough; chest pain, rapid heartbeat, palpitations; unusual bruising/bleeding; blood in urine, stool, mouth, or vomitus; swollen extremities; skin rash or itching; acute fatigue; or changes in eyesight (double vision, color changes, blurred vision), hearing, or ringing in ears.

**Dietary Considerations:**
Alcohol: Additive impairment of mental alertness and physical coordination, avoid or limit use
Food: Food may decrease the rate but not the extent of oral absorption. Drug may cause GI upset, bleeding, ulceration, perforation; take with food or milk to minimize GI upset.
**Monitoring Parameters:** Occult blood loss, periodic liver function test, CBC, BUN, serum creatinine

**Related Information**
Nonsteroidal Anti-Inflammatory Agents *on page 1026*

♦ **Naproxen Sodium** *see* Naproxen *on previous page*
♦ **Naqua®** *see* Trichlormethiazide *on page 932*

# Naratriptan (NAR a trip tan)

**Pharmacologic Class** Serotonin 5-HT$_{1D}$ Receptor Agonist
**U.S. Brand Names** Amerge®
**Mechanism of Action** The therapeutic effect for migraine is due to serotonin agonist activity
**Use** Treatment of acute migraine headache with or without aura
**USUAL DOSAGE**
Adults: Oral: 1-2.5 mg at the onset of headache; it is recommended to use the lowest possible dose to minimize adverse effects. If headache returns or does not fully resolve, the dose may be repeated after 4 hours; do not exceed 5 mg in 24 hours.
(Continued)

## Naratriptan *(Continued)*

Elderly: Not recommended for use in the elderly

**Dosing in renal impairment:**

$Cl_{cr}$: 18-39 mL/minute: Initial: 1 mg; do not exceed 2.5 mg in 24 hours

$Cl_{cr}$: <15 mL/minute: Do not use

**Dosing in hepatic impairment:** Contraindicated in patients with severe liver failure; maximum dose: 2.5 mg in 24 hours for patients with mild or moderate liver failure; recommended starting dose: 1 mg

**Dosage Forms Tab, as hydrochloride:** 1 mg, 2.5 mg

**Contraindications** Hypersensitivity to naratriptan or any component; cerebrovascular, peripheral vascular disease (ischemic bowel disease), ischemic heart disease (angina pectoris, history of myocardial infarction, or proven silent ischemia); or in patients with symptoms consistent with ischemic heart disease, coronary artery vasospasm, or Prinzmetal's variant angina; uncontrolled hypertension or patients who have received within 24 hours another 5-HT agonist (sumatriptan, zolmitriptan) or ergotamine-containing product; patients with known risk factors associated with coronary artery disease; patients with severe hepatic or renal disease ($Cl_{cr}$ <15 mL/minute); do not administer naratriptan to patients with hemiplegic or basilar migraine

**Warnings/Precautions** Use only if there is a clear diagnosis of migraine. Patients who are at risk of CAD but have had a satisfactory cardiovascular evaluation may receive naratriptan but with extreme caution (ie, in a physician's office where there are adequate precautions in place to protect the patient). Blood pressure may increase with the administration of naratriptan. Monitor closely, especially with the first administration of the drug. If the patient does not respond to the first dose, re-evaluate the diagnosis of migraine before trying a second dose.

**Pregnancy Risk Factor** C

**Adverse Reactions**

1% to 10%:

Central nervous system: Dizziness, drowsiness, malaise/fatigue, paresthesias

Gastrointestinal: Nausea, vomiting

Miscellaneous: Pain or pressure in throat or neck

<1% (limited to important or life-threatening symptoms): Coronary artery vasospasm, transient myocardial ischemia, myocardial infarction, ventricular tachycardia, ventricular fibrillation, palpitations, hypertension, EKG changes (PR prolongation, QTc prolongation, premature ventricular contractions, atrial flutter or atrial fibrillation) hypotension, heart murmurs, bradycardia, hyperlipidemia, hypercholesterolemia, hypothyroidism, hyperglycemia, glycosuria, ketonuria, eye hemorrhage, abnormal liver function tests, abnormal bilirubin tests, convulsions, allergic reaction, panic, hallucinations

**Drug Interactions**

Decreased effect: Smoking increases the clearance of naratriptan

Increased effect/toxicity: Ergot-containing drugs (dihydroergotamine or methysergide) may cause vasospastic reactions when taken with naratriptan. Avoid concomitant use with ergots; separate dose of naratriptan and ergots by at least 24 hours. Oral contraceptives taken with naratriptan reduced the clearance of naratriptan +30% which may contribute to adverse effects. Selective serotonin reuptake inhibitors (SSRIs) (eg, fluoxetine, fluvoxamine, paroxetine, sertraline) may cause lack of coordination, hyper-reflexia, or weakness and should be avoided when taking naratriptan.

**Onset** 30 minutes

**Special PA Issues**

**Patient Education:** This drug is to be used to reduce your migraine, not to prevent or reduce the number of attacks. If headache returns or is not fully resolved, the dose may be repeated after 4 hours. If you have no relief with first dose, do not take a second dose without consulting prescriber. **Do not exceed 5 mg in 24 hours. Do not take within 24 hours of any other migraine medication without first consulting prescriber.** You may experience some dizziness, fatigue, or drowsiness; use caution when driving or engaging in tasks that require alertness. Frequent mouth care and sucking on lozenges may relieve dry mouth. Report immediately any chest pain, heart throbbing, tightness in throat, skin rash or hives, hallucinations, anxiety, or panic.

♦ **Narcan® Injection** *see* Naloxone *on page 633*

♦ **Narcotic Agonists** *see Chart on page 1023*

♦ **Nardil®** *see* Phenelzine *on page 715*

♦ **Naropin™** *see* Ropivacaine *on page 816*

♦ **Nasacort®** *see* Triamcinolone *on page 928*

♦ **Nasacort® AQ** *see* Triamcinolone *on page 928*

♦ **NāSal™ [OTC]** *see* Sodium Chloride *on page 839*

♦ **Nasalcrom® Nasal Solution** *see* Cromolyn Sodium *on page 240*

♦ **Nasalide® Nasal Aerosol** *see* Flunisolide *on page 379*

♦ **Nasal Moist® [OTC]** *see* Sodium Chloride *on page 839*

♦ **Nasarel™** *see* Flunisolide *on page 379*

♦ **Nascobal®** *see* Cyanocobalamin *on page 242*

- **Natabec**® **[OTC]** *see* Vitamins, Multiple *on page 964*
- **Natabec**® **FA [OTC]** *see* Vitamins, Multiple *on page 964*
- **Natabec**® **Rx** *see* Vitamins, Multiple *on page 964*
- **Natacyn**® **Ophthalmic** *see* Natamycin *on this page*
- **Natalins**® **[OTC]** *see* Vitamins, Multiple *on page 964*
- **Natalins**® **Rx** *see* Vitamins, Multiple *on page 964*

## Natamycin (na ta MYE sin)

**Pharmacologic Class** Antifungal Agent, Ophthalmic

**U.S. Brand Names** Natacyn® Ophthalmic

**Mechanism of Action** Increases cell membrane permeability in susceptible fungi

**Use** Treatment of blepharitis, conjunctivitis, and keratitis caused by susceptible fungi (*Aspergillus, Candida*), *Cephalosporium, Curvularia, Fusarium, Penicillium, Microsporum, Epidermophyton, Blastomyces dermatitidis, Coccidioides immitis, Cryptococcus neoformans, Histoplasma capsulatum, Sporothrix schenckii,* and *Trichomonas vaginalis*

**USUAL DOSAGE** Adults: Ophthalmic: Instill 1 drop in conjunctival sac every 1-2 hours, after 3-4 days reduce to one drop 6-8 times/day; usual course of therapy is 2-3 weeks.

**Dosage Forms** Susp, ophth: 5% (15 mL)

**Contraindications** Known hypersensitivity to natamycin or any component

**Warnings/Precautions** Failure to improve (keratitis) after 7-10 days of administration suggests infection caused by a microorganism not susceptible to natamycin; inadequate as a single agent in fungal endophthalmitis

**Pregnancy Risk Factor** C

**Adverse Reactions** <1%: Blurred vision, photophobia, eye pain, eye irritation not present before therapy

**Drug Interactions** Increased toxicity: Topical corticosteroids (concomitant use contraindicated)

**Special PA Issues**

**Patient Education:** For ophthalmic use only. Store at room temperature. Shake before using. Apply prescribed amount as often as directed. Wash hands before using and do not let tip of applicator touch eye or contaminate tip of applicator. Tilt head back and look upward. Gently pull down lower lid and put drop(s) in inner corner of eye. Close eye and roll eyeball in all directions. Do not blink for ½ minute. Apply gentle pressure to inner corner of eye for 30 seconds. Wipe away excess from skin around eye. Do not use any other eye preparation for at least 10 minutes. Do not touch tip of applicator to eye or contaminate tip of applicator. Do not share medication with anyone else. May cause sensitivity to bright light (dark glasses may help); temporary stinging or blurred vision may occur. Inform prescriber if you experience eye pain, redness, burning, watering, dryness, double vision, puffiness around eye, vision disturbances, or other adverse eye response; worsening of condition or lack of improvement within 7-10 days.

- **Natural/Herbal Products and Dietary Supplements** *see* Chart *on page 1134*
- **Natural Lung Surfactant** *see* Beractant *on page 110*
- **Navane**® *see* Thiothixene *on page 896*
- **Naxen**® *see* Naproxen *on page 636*
- **Nebcin**® **Injection** *see* Tobramycin *on page 907*
- **NebuPent**™ **Inhalation** *see* Pentamidine *on page 707*
- **Nectar of the Gods** *see* Garlic *on page 410*

## Nedocromil Sodium (ne doe KROE mil SOW dee um)

**Pharmacologic Class** Antihistamine, Inhalation

**U.S. Brand Names** Tilade® Inhalation Aerosol

**Mechanism of Action** Inhibits the activation of and mediator release from a variety of inflammatory cell types associated with asthma including eosinophils, neutrophils, macrophages, mast cells, monocytes, and platelets; it inhibits the release of histamine, leukotrienes, and slow-reacting substance of anaphylaxis; it inhibits the development of early and late bronchoconstriction responses to inhaled antigen

**Use** Maintenance therapy in patients with mild to moderate bronchial asthma

**USUAL DOSAGE** Children >12 years and Adults: Inhalation: 2 inhalations 4 times/day; may reduce dosage to 2-3 times/day once desired clinical response to initial dose is observed

**Dosage Forms** Aero, as sodium: 1.75 mg/activation (16.2 g)

**Contraindications** Hypersensitivity to nedocromil or other ingredients in the preparation

**Warnings/Precautions** Safety and efficacy in children <12 years of age have not been established; if systemic or inhaled steroid therapy is at all reduced, monitor patients carefully; nedocromil is **not** a bronchodilator and, therefore, should not be used for reversal of acute bronchospasm

**Pregnancy Risk Factor** B

**Adverse Reactions** 1% to 10%:

Cardiovascular: Chest pain

Central nervous system: Dizziness, dysphonia, headache, fatigue

(Continued)

## Nedocromil Sodium *(Continued)*

Dermatologic: Rash

Gastrointestinal: Nausea, vomiting, dyspepsia, diarrhea, abdominal pain, xerostomia, unpleasant taste

Hepatic: Increased ALT

Neuromuscular & skeletal: Arthritis, tremor

Respiratory: Cough, pharyngitis, rhinitis, bronchitis, upper respiratory infection, broncho-spasm, increased sputum production

**Duration** 2 hours

**Half-Life** 1.5-2 hours

**Special PA Issues**

**Patient Education:** Do not use during acute bronchospasm. Use exactly as directed; do not use more often than instructed or discontinue without consulting prescriber. You may experience drowsiness, dizziness, fatigue, especially during early therapy (use caution when driving or engaging in hazardous tasks); dry mouth, nausea, or vomiting (small frequent meals, good mouth care, chewing gum, or sucking lozenges may help). Report persistent runny nose, cough, cold symptoms; unresolved gastrointestinal effects; skin rash; joint pain or tremor; or if breathing difficulty persists or worsens.

Use: Review use of inhalator with prescriber or follow package insert for directions. Prime with three activations prior to first use or if unused more than 7 days. Keep inhalator clean and unobstructed. Always rinse mouth and throat after use of inhaler to prevent advantageous infection. If you are also using a steroid bronchodilator, wait 10 minutes before using this aerosol.

♦ **N.E.E.**® **1/35** *see Ethinyl Estradiol and Norethindrone on page 348*

## Nefazodone *(nef AY zoe done)*

**Pharmacologic Class** Antidepressant, Serotonin Reuptake Inhibitor/Antagonist

**U.S. Brand Names** Serzone®

**Mechanism of Action** Inhibits serotonin (5-HT) reuptake and is a potent antagonist at type 2 serotonin (5-HT) receptors; minimal affinity for cholinergic, histaminic, or alpha$_1$-adrenergic receptors

**Use** Treatment of depression

**USUAL DOSAGE** Oral: Adults: 200 mg/day, administered in two divided doses initially, with a range of 300-600 mg/day in two divided doses thereafter

**Dosage Forms Tab, as hydrochloride:** 50 mg, 100 mg, 150 mg, 200 mg, 250 mg

**Contraindications** Hypersensitivity to nefazodone or any component; concomitant use of any MAO inhibitors, astemizole, or terfenadine

**Warnings/Precautions** Safety and efficacy in children <18 years of age have not been established; monitor closely and use with extreme caution in patients with cardiac disease, cerebrovascular disease or seizures; very sedating and can be dehydrating; therapeutic effects may take up to 4 weeks to occur; therapy is normally maintained for several months and optimum response is reached to prevent recurrence of depression, discontinue therapy and re-evaluate if priapism occurs

**Pregnancy Risk Factor** C

**Adverse Reactions**

>10%:

Central nervous system: Headache, drowsiness, insomnia, agitation, dizziness, confusion

Gastrointestinal: Xerostomia, nausea

Neuromuscular & skeletal: Tremor

1% to 10%:

Cardiovascular: Postural hypotension

Gastrointestinal: Constipation, vomiting

Neuromuscular & skeletal: Weakness

Ocular: Blurred vision, amblyopia

<1%: Diarrhea, prolonged priapism

**Drug Interactions** CYP3A3/4 enzyme substrate; CYP3A3/4 enzyme inhibitor

Decreased effect: Clonidine, methyldopa, diuretics, oral hypoglycemics, anticoagulants

Increased toxicity: Terfenadine, astemizole, and cisapride (increased concentrations have been associated with serious ventricular arrhythmias and death), fluoxetine, triazolam (reduce triazolam dose by 75%), alprazolam (reduce alprazolam dose by 50%), haloperidol, phenytoin, MAO inhibitors (allow 14 days after MAO inhibitors are stopped or 7 days after nefazodone is stopped); carbamazepine (40% increase); digoxin

**Onset** Therapeutic effects take at least 2 weeks to appear

**Half-Life** 2-4 hours (parent compound), active metabolites persist longer

**Special PA Issues**

**Patient Education:** Take exactly as directed (do not increase dose or frequency); may take 2-3 weeks to achieve desired results; may cause physical and/or psychological dependence. Avoid excessive alcohol, caffeine, and other prescription or OTC medications not approved by prescriber. Maintain adequate hydration (2-3 L/day of fluids unless instructed to restrict fluid intake). You may experience drowsiness, dizziness, or light-headedness (use caution when driving or engaging in hazardous tasks until response to medication is known); nausea or vomiting (small frequent meals, frequent mouth care, or sucking lozenges may help); or orthostatic hypotension (use caution when climbing stairs or changing position from lying or sitting to standing). Report persistent insomnia or excessive daytime sedation; muscle cramping, tremors, weakness, or change in gait; chest pain, palpitations, or rapid heartbeat; vision changes or eye pain; difficulty breathing or breathlessness; abdominal pain or blood in stool; or worsening of condition.

**Dietary Considerations:** Alcohol: Additive CNS effect, avoid use

**Reference Range:** Therapeutic plasma levels have not yet been defined

**Related Information**

Antidepressant Agents *on page 998*

♦ **Nefazodone Hydrochloride** *see* Nefazodone *on previous page*

# Nelfinavir (nel FIN a veer)

**Pharmacologic Class** Antiretroviral Agent, Protease Inhibitor

**U.S. Brand Names** Viracept®

**Mechanism of Action** Inhibits the HIV-1 protease; inhibition of the viral protease prevents cleavage of the gag-pol polyprotein resulting in the production of immature, noninfectious virus

**Use** In combination with other antiretroviral therapy in the treatment of HIV infection

**USUAL DOSAGE** Oral:

Children 2-13 years: 20-30 mg/kg 3 times/day with a meal or light snack; if tablets are unable to be taken, use oral powder in small amount of water, milk, formula, or dietary supplements; do not use acidic food/juice or store for >6 hours

Adults: 750 mg 3 times/day with meals

**Dosing adjustment in renal impairment:** No adjustment needed

**Dosing adjustment in hepatic impairment:** Use caution when administering to patients with hepatic impairment since eliminated predominantly by the liver

**Dosage Forms Powder, oral:** 50 mg/g [144 g] (contains 11.2 mg phenylalanine); **Tab:** 250 mg

**Contraindications** Hypersensitivity to nelfinavir or product components; phenylketonuria; concurrent therapy with terfenadine, astemizole, cisapride, triazolam, or midazolam

**Warnings/Precautions** Avoid use of powder in phenylketonurics since contains phenylala-nine; use extreme caution when administered to patients with hepatic insufficiency since nelfinavir is metabolized in the liver and excreted predominantly in the feces; avoid use, if possible, with terfenadine, astemizole, cisapride, triazolam, or midazolam. Concurrent use with some anticonvulsants may significantly limit nelfinavir's effectiveness.

**Pregnancy Risk Factor** B

**Pregnancy Implications** Breast-feeding/lactation: Animal studies suggest that nelfinavir may be excreted in human milk; the CDC advises against breast-feeding by HIV-infected mothers to avoid postnatal transmission of the virus to the infant

**Adverse Reactions** Protease inhibitors cause dyslipidemia which includes elevated choles-terol and triglycerides and a redistribution of body fat centrally to cause "protease paunch", buffalo hump, facial atrophy, and breast enlargement. These agents also cause hypergly-cemia.

>10%: Gastrointestinal: Diarrhea (19%)

1% to 10%:

Central nervous system: Decreased concentration

Dermatologic: Rash

Gastrointestinal: Nausea, flatulence, abdominal pain

Neuromuscular & skeletal: Weakness

<1%: Anxiety, depression, dizziness, emotional lability, hyperkinesia, insomnia, migraine, seizures, sleep disorder, somnolence, suicide ideation, fever, headache, malaise, derma-titis, pruritus, urticaria, increased LFTs, hyperlipemia, hyperuricemia, hypoglycemia, anorexia, dyspepsia, epigastric pain, mouth ulceration, GI bleeding, pancreatitis, vomiting, kidney calculus, sexual dysfunction, anemia, leukopenia, thrombocytopenia, hepatitis, arthralgia, arthritis, cramps, myalgia, myasthenia, myopathy, paresthesia, back pain, dyspnea, pharyngitis, rhinitis, sinusitis, diaphoresis, allergy

**Drug Interactions** CYP3A3/4 enzyme substrate; CYP3A3/4 enzyme inducer; CYP3A3/4 enzyme inhibitor

Increased effect:

Nelfinavir inhibits the metabolism of cisapride and astemizole and should, therefore, not be administered concurrently due to risk of life-threatening cardiac arrhythmias.

A 20% increase in rifabutin plasma AUC has been observed when coadministered with nelfinavir (decrease rifabutin's dose by 50%).

An increase in midazolam and triazolam serum levels may occur resulting in significant oversedation when administered with nelfinavir. These drugs should not be adminis-tered together.

Indinavir and ritonavir may increase nelfinavir plasma concentrations resulting in potential increases in side effects (the safety of these combinations have not been established).

(Continued)

## Nelfinavir *(Continued)*

Decreased effect:

Rifampin decreases nelfinavir's plasma AUC by ~82%; the two drugs should not be administered together.

Serum levels of the hormones in oral contraceptives may decrease significantly with administration of nelfinavir. Patients should use alternative methods of contraceptives during nelfinavir therapy

Phenobarbital, phenytoin, and carbamazepine may decrease serum levels and consequently effectiveness of nelfinavir.

Nelfinavir's effectiveness may be decreased with concomitant nevirapine

**Half-Life** 3.5-5 hours

**Special PA Issues**

**Patient Education:** This is not a cure for HIV and has not been shown to reduce the risk of transmitting HIV to others. The long-term effects of use are not known. Should be taken as scheduled with food (mix powder with nonacidic, noncitric fluids and do not store reconstituted powder mixture for longer than 6 hours). If you miss a dose, take as soon as possible and return to regular schedule (never take a double dose). Frequent blood tests may be required with prolonged therapy. You may experience nausea and vomiting (small, frequent meals, frequent mouth care, and sucking on lozenges may help). Report rash; respiratory difficulty; CNS changes (migraine, confusion, suicidal ideation); muscular or skeletal pain, weakness, or tremors; or other adverse reactions. Use appropriate barrier contraceptive measures (as alternative to oral contraceptives) to reduce risk of transmitting infection and potential pregnancy.

**Monitoring Parameters:** LFTs, viral load, CD4 count, triglycerides, cholesterol, glucose

- ◆ **Nelova™ 0.5/35E** *see* Ethinyl Estradiol and Norethindrone *on page 348*
- ◆ **Nelova™ 1/50M** *see* Mestranol and Norethindrone *on page 573*
- ◆ **Nelova™ 10/11** *see* Ethinyl Estradiol and Norethindrone *on page 348*
- ◆ **Neo-Calglucon® [OTC]** *see* Calcium Glubionate *on page 141*
- ◆ **Neo-Codema®** *see* Hydrochlorothiazide *on page 447*
- ◆ **Neo-Cortef®** *see* Neomycin and Hydrocortisone *on next page*
- ◆ **NeoDecadron® Ophthalmic** *see* Neomycin and Dexamethasone *on next page*
- ◆ **NeoDecadron® Topical** *see* Neomycin and Dexamethasone *on next page*
- ◆ **Neo-Dexameth® Ophthalmic** *see* Neomycin and Dexamethasone *on next page*
- ◆ **Neo-Durabolic Injection** *see* Nandrolone *on page 634*
- ◆ **Neo-Estrone®** *see* Estrone *on page 338*
- ◆ **Neo-Estrone®** *see* Estrogens, Esterified *on page 337*
- ◆ **Neofed® [OTC]** *see* Pseudoephedrine *on page 780*
- ◆ **Neo-fradin® Oral** *see* Neomycin *on this page*
- ◆ **Neomixin® Topical [OTC]** *see* Bacitracin, Neomycin, and Polymyxin B *on page 97*

## Neomycin *(nee oh MYE sin)*

**Pharmacologic Class** Ammonium Detoxicant; Antibiotic, Aminoglycoside; Antibiotic, Topical

**U.S. Brand Names** Mycifradin® Sulfate Oral; Mycifradin® Sulfate Topical; Neo-fradin® Oral; Neo-Tabs® Oral

**Mechanism of Action** Interferes with bacterial protein synthesis by binding to 30S ribosomal subunits

**Use** Orally to prepare GI tract for surgery; topically to treat minor skin infections; treat diarrhea caused by *E. coli*; adjunct in the treatment of hepatic encephalopathy

**USUAL DOSAGE**

Children: Oral:

Preoperative intestinal antisepsis: 90 mg/kg/day divided every 4 hours for 2 days; or 25 mg/kg at 1 PM, 2 PM, and 11 PM on the day preceding surgery as an adjunct to mechanical cleansing of the intestine and in combination with erythromycin base

Hepatic coma: 50-100 mg/kg/day in divided doses every 6-8 hours or 2.5-7 g/m²/day divided every 4-6 hours for 5-6 days not to exceed 12 g/day

Children and Adults: Topical: Apply ointment 1-4 times/day; topical solutions containing 0.1% to 1% neomycin have been used for irrigation

Adults: Oral:

Preoperative intestinal antisepsis: 1 g each hour for 4 doses then 1 g every 4 hours for 5 doses; or 1 g at 1 PM, 2 PM, and 11 PM on day preceding surgery as an adjunct to mechanical cleansing of the bowel and oral erythromycin; or 6 g/day divided every 4 hours for 2-3 days

Hepatic coma: 500-2000 mg every 6-8 hours or 4-12 g/day divided every 4-6 hours for 5-6 days

Chronic hepatic insufficiency: 4 g/day for an indefinite period

Hemodialysis: Dialyzable (50% to 100%)

**Dosage Forms Crm:** 0.5% (15 g); **Oint, top:** 0.5% (15 g, 30 g, 120 g); **Soln, oral:** 125 mg/5 mL (480 mL); **Tab:** 500 mg [base 300 mg]

**Contraindications** Hypersensitivity to neomycin or any component, or other aminoglycosides; patients with intestinal obstruction

**Warnings/Precautions** Use with caution in patients with renal impairment, pre-existing hearing impairment, neuromuscular disorders; neomycin is more toxic than other aminoglycosides when given parenterally; **do not administer parenterally**; topical neomycin is a contact sensitizer with sensitivity occurring in 5% to 15% of patients treated with the drug; symptoms include itching, reddening, edema, and failure to heal; **do not use as peritoneal lavage** due to significant systemic adsorption of the drug

**Pregnancy Risk Factor** C

**Adverse Reactions**
1% to 10%:
Dermatologic: Dermatitis, rash, urticaria, erythema
Local: Burning
Ocular: Contact conjunctivitis
<1%: Nausea, vomiting, diarrhea, neuromuscular blockade, ototoxicity, nephrotoxicity

**Drug Interactions**
Decreased effect: May decrease GI absorption of digoxin and methotrexate
Increased effect: Synergistic effects with penicillins
Increased toxicity:
Oral neomycin may potentiate the effects of oral anticoagulants
Increased adverse effects with other neurotoxic, ototoxic, or nephrotoxic drugs

**Half-Life** 3 hours (age and renal function dependent)

**Special PA Issues**
**Patient Education:**
Oral: Take as directed. Maintain adequate hydration (2-3 L/day of fluids unless instructed to restrict fluid intake). You may experience nausea or vomiting (small frequent meals or sucking on lozenges may help); constipation (exercise, increased fluid or fiber in diet may help, or consult prescriber); or diarrhea (buttermilk, boiled milk, or yogurt may help). Report immediately any change in hearing,; ringing or sense of fullness in ears; persistent diarrhea; changes in voiding patterns; or numbness, tingling, or pain in any extremity.
Topical: Apply a thin film of cream or ointment; do not overuse. Report rash, itching, redness, or failure of condition to improve.
**Monitoring Parameters:** Renal function tests, audiometry in symptomatic patients

# Neomycin and Dexamethasone (nee oh MYE sin & deks a METH a sone)

**Pharmacologic Class** Antibiotic/Corticosteroid, Ophthalmic; Antibiotic/Corticosteroid, Topical

**U.S. Brand Names** AK-Neo-Dex® Ophthalmic; NeoDecadron® Ophthalmic; NeoDecadron® Topical; Neo-Dexameth® Ophthalmic

**Dosage Forms Crm:** Neomycin sulfate 0.5% [5 mg/g] and dexamethasone 0.1% [1 mg/g] (15 g, 30 g); **Oint, ophth:** Neomycin sulfate 0.35% [3.5 mg/g] and dexamethasone 0.05% [0.5 mg/g] (3.5 g); **Soln, ophth:** Neomycin sulfate 0.35% [3.5 mg/mL] and dexamethasone 0.1% [1 mg/mL] (5 mL)

# Neomycin and Hydrocortisone (nee oh MYE sin & hye droe KOR ti sone)

**Pharmacologic Class** Antibiotic/Corticosteroid, Ophthalmic; Antibiotic/Corticosteroid, Topical

**U.S. Brand Names** Neo-Cortef®

**Dosage Forms Crm:** Neomycin sulfate 0.5% and hydrocortisone 1% (20 g); **Oint, top:** Neomycin sulfate 0.5% and hydrocortisone 0.5% (20 g), neomycin sulfate 0.5% and hydrocortisone 1% (20 g); **Soln, ophth:** Neomycin sulfate 0.5% and hydrocortisone 0.5% (5 mL)

# Neomycin and Polymyxin B (nee oh MYE sin & pol i MIKS in bee)

**Pharmacologic Class** Antibiotic, Topical

**U.S. Brand Names** Neosporin® Cream [OTC]; Neosporin® G.U. Irrigant

**Mechanism of Action** Refer to individual monographs for Neomycin and Polymyxin

**Use** Short-term as a continuous irrigant or rinse in the urinary bladder to prevent bacteriuria and gram-negative rod septicemia associated with the use of indwelling catheters; to help prevent infection in minor cuts, scrapes, and burns

**USUAL DOSAGE** Children and Adults:
Bladder irrigation: **Not for injection**; add 1 mL irrigant to 1 liter isotonic saline solution and connect container to the inflow of lumen of 3-way catheter. Continuous irrigant or rinse in the urinary bladder for up to a maximum of 10 days with administration rate adjusted to patient's urine output; usually no more than 1 L of irrigant is used per day.
Topical: Apply cream 1-4 times/day to affected area

**Dosage Forms Crm:** Neomycin sulfate 3.5 mg and polymyxin B sulfate 10,000 units per g (0.94 g, 15 g); **Soln, irrigant:** Neomycin sulfate 40 mg and polymyxin B sulfate 200,000 units per mL (1 mL, 20 mL)

**Contraindications** Known hypersensitivity to neomycin or polymyxin B or any component; ophthalmic use for topical cream
(Continued)

## Neomycin and Polymyxin B *(Continued)*

**Warnings/Precautions** Use with caution in patients with impaired renal function, infants with diaper rash involving large area of abraded skin, dehydrated patients, burn patients, and patients receiving a high-dose for prolonged periods; topical neomycin is a contact sensitizer; contains methylparaben

**Pregnancy Risk Factor** C (D G.U. irrigant)

**Adverse Reactions** 1% to 10%:
  Dermatologic: Contact dermatitis, erythema, rash, urticaria
  Genitourinary: Bladder irritation
  Local: Burning
  Neuromuscular & skeletal: Neuromuscular blockade
  Otic: Ototoxicity
  Renal: Nephrotoxicity

**Special PA Issues**
  **Monitoring Parameters:** Urinalysis

# Neomycin, Polymyxin B, and Dexamethasone

(nee oh MYE sin, pol i MIKS in bee, & deks a METH a sone)

**Pharmacologic Class** Antibiotic, Ophthalmic; Corticosteroid, Ophthalmic

**U.S. Brand Names** AK-Trol®; Dexacidin®; Dexasporin®; Maxitrol®

**Mechanism of Action** Refer to individual monographs for Neomycin Sulfate, Polymyxin B Sulfate, and Dexamethasone

**Use** Steroid-responsive inflammatory ocular conditions in which a corticosteroid is indicated and where bacterial infection or a risk of bacterial infection exists

**USUAL DOSAGE** Children and Adults: Ophthalmic:
  Ointment: Place a small amount (~½") in the affected eye 3-4 times/day or apply at bedtime as an adjunct with drops
  Solution: Instill 1-2 drops into affected eye(s) every 3-4 hours; in severe disease, drops may be used hourly and tapered to discontinuation

**Dosage Forms Oint, ophth:** Neomycin sulfate 3.5 mg, polymyxin B sulfate 10,000 units, and dexamethasone 0.1% per g (3.5 g); **Susp, ophth:** Neomycin sulfate 3.5 mg, polymyxin B sulfate 10,000 units, and dexamethasone 0.1% per mL (5 mL)

**Contraindications** Hypersensitivity to dexamethasone, polymyxin B, neomycin or any component; herpes simplex, vaccinia, and varicella

**Warnings/Precautions** Prolonged use may result in glaucoma, defects in visual acuity, posterior subcapsular cataract formation, and secondary ocular infections

**Pregnancy Risk Factor** C

**Adverse Reactions** 1% to 10%:
  Dermatologic: Contact dermatitis, delayed wound healing
  Ocular: Cutaneous sensitization, eye pain, development of glaucoma, cataract, increased intraocular pressure, optic nerve damage

**Special PA Issues**
  **Monitoring Parameters:** Intraocular pressure with use >10 days

# Neomycin, Polymyxin B, and Gramicidin

(nee oh MYE sin, pol i MIKS in bee, & gram i SYE din)

**Pharmacologic Class** Antibiotic, Ophthalmic

**U.S. Brand Names** AK-Spore® Ophthalmic Solution; Neosporin® Ophthalmic Solution; Ocutricin® Ophthalmic Solution

**Mechanism of Action** Interferes with bacterial protein synthesis by binding to 30S ribosomal subunits; binds to phospholipids, alters permeability, and damages the bacterial cytoplasmic membrane permitting leakage of intracellular constituents

**Use** Treatment of superficial ocular infection, infection prophylaxis in minor skin abrasions

**USUAL DOSAGE** Children and Adults: Ophthalmic: Instill 1-2 drops 4-6 times/day or more frequently as required for severe infections

**Dosage Forms Soln, ophth:** Neomycin sulfate 1.75 mg, polymyxin B sulfate 10,000 units, and gramicidin 0.025 mg per mL (2 mL, 10 mL)

**Contraindications** Hypersensitivity to neomycin, polymyxin B, gramicidin or any component

**Warnings/Precautions** Symptoms of neomycin sensitization include itching, reddening, edema, failure to heal; prolonged use may result in glaucoma, defects in visual acuity, posterior subcapsular cataract formation, and secondary ocular infections

**Pregnancy Risk Factor** C

**Adverse Reactions** 1% to 10%:
  Cardiovascular: Edema
  Dermatologic: Itching
  Local: Reddening, failure to heal
  Ocular: Low grade conjunctivitis

**Special PA Issues**
  **Patient Education:** For ophthalmic use only. Store at room temperature. Apply prescribed amount as often as directed. Wash hands before using and do not let tip of

applicator touch eye or contaminate tip of applicator. Tilt head back and look upward. Gently pull down lower lid and put drop(s) in inner corner of eye. Close eye and roll eyeball in all directions. Do not blink for $1/2$ minute. Apply gentle pressure to inner corner of eye for 30 seconds. Wipe away excess from skin around eye. Do not use any other eye preparation for at least 10 minutes. Do not touch tip of applicator to eye or contaminate tip of applicator. Do not share medication with anyone else. May cause sensitivity to bright light (dark glasses may help); temporary stinging or blurred vision may occur. Inform prescriber if you experience eye pain, redness, burning, watering, dryness, double vision, puffiness around eye, vision disturbances, or other adverse eye response; worsening of condition or lack of improvement within 7-10 days.

## Neomycin, Polymyxin B, and Hydrocortisone
(nee oh MYE sin, pol i MIKS in bee, & hye droe KOR ti sone)

**Pharmacologic Class** Antibiotic, Ophthalmic; Antibiotic, Otic; Antibiotic, Topical; Corticosteroid, Ophthalmic; Corticosteroid, Otic; Corticosteroid, Topical

**U.S. Brand Names** AK-Spore H.C.® Ophthalmic Suspension; AK-Spore H.C.® Otic; Antibi-Otic® Otic; Bacticort® Otic; Cortatrigen® Otic; Cortisporin® Ophthalmic Suspension; Cortisporin® Otic; Cortisporin® Topical Cream; Drotic® Otic; Ear-Eze® Otic; LazerSporin-C® Otic; Octicair® Otic; Otic-Care® Otic; OtiTricin® Otic; Otocort® Otic; Otomycin-HPN® Otic; Otosporin® Otic; PediOtic® Otic; UAD® Otic

**Mechanism of Action** Refer to individual monographs for Neomycin, Polymyxin B, and Hydrocortisone

**Use** Steroid-responsive inflammatory condition for which a corticosteroid is indicated and where bacterial infection or a risk of bacterial infection exists

**USUAL DOSAGE** Duration of use should be limited to 10 days unless otherwise directed by the physician

Otic solution is used **only** for swimmer's ear (infections of external auditory canal)

Otic:

Children: Instill 3 drops into affected ear 3-4 times/day

Adults: Instill 4 drops 3-4 times/day; otic suspension is the preferred otic preparation

Children and Adults:

Ophthalmic: Drops: Instill 1-2 drops 2-4 times/day, or more frequently as required for severe infections; in acute infections, instill 1-2 drops every 15-30 minutes gradually reducing the frequency of administration as the infection is controlled

Topical: Apply a thin layer 1-4 times/day

**Dosage Forms Crm, top:** Neomycin sulfate 5 mg, polymyxin B sulfate 10,000 units, and hydrocortisone 10 mg per mL (7.5 g); **Soln, otic:** Neomycin sulfate 5 mg, polymyxin B sulfate 10,000 units, and hydrocortisone 10 mg per mL (10 mL); **Susp: Ophth:** Neomycin sulfate 5 mg, polymyxin B sulfate 10,000 units, and hydrocortisone 10 mg per mL (7.5 mL), **Otic:** Neomycin sulfate 5 mg, polymyxin B sulfate 10,000 units, and hydrocortisone 10 mg per mL (10 mL)

**Contraindications** Known hypersensitivity to hydrocortisone, polymyxin B sulfate or neomycin sulfate; otic use when drum is perforated; herpes simplex, vaccinia, and varicella

**Warnings/Precautions** Prolonged use can lead to skin thinning, atrophy, sensitization, and development of resistant infections; neomycin may cause cutaneous and conjunctival sensitization; children are more susceptible to topical corticosteroid-induced hypothalamic - pituitary - adrenal axis suppression and Cushing's syndrome. Otic suspension is the preferred otic preparation; otic suspension can be used for the treatment of infections of mastoidectomy and fenestration cavities caused by susceptible organisms; otic solution is used **only** for superficial infections of the external auditory canal (ie, swimmer's ear).

**Pregnancy Risk Factor** C

**Adverse Reactions**

>10%: Hypersensitivity

1% to 10%:

Dermatologic: Contact dermatitis, erythema, rash, urticaria, itching

Genitourinary: Bladder irritation

Local: Burning, pain, edema, stinging

Neuromuscular & skeletal: Neuromuscular blockade

Ocular: Elevation of intraocular pressure, glaucoma, cataracts, conjunctival erythema

Otic: Ototoxicity

Renal: Nephrotoxicity

Miscellaneous: Sensitization to neomycin, secondary infections

## Neomycin, Polymyxin B, and Prednisolone
(nee oh MYE sin, pol i MIKS in bee, & pred NIS oh lone)

**Pharmacologic Class** Antibiotic, Ophthalmic; Corticosteroid, Ophthalmic

**U.S. Brand Names** Poly-Pred® Ophthalmic Suspension

**Mechanism of Action** Refer to individual monographs for Neomycin, Polymyxin B, and Prednisolone

**Use** Steroid-responsive inflammatory ocular condition in which bacterial infection or a risk of bacterial ocular infection exists

(Continued)

## Neomycin, Polymyxin B, and Prednisolone *(Continued)*

**USUAL DOSAGE** Children and Adults: Ophthalmic: Instill 1-2 drops every 3-4 hours; acute infections may require every 30-minute instillation initially with frequency of administration reduced as the infection is brought under control. To treat the lids: Instill 1-2 drops every 3-4 hours, close the eye and rub the excess on the lids and lid margins.

**Dosage Forms** Susp, ophth: Neomycin sulfate 0.35%, polymyxin B sulfate 10,000 units, and prednisolone acetate 0.5% per mL (5 mL, 10 mL)

**Contraindications** Known hypersensitivity to neomycin, polymyxin B, or prednisolone; dendritic keratitis, viral disease of the cornea and conjunctiva, mycobacterial infection of the eye, fungal disease of the ocular structure, or after uncomplicated removal of a corneal foreign body

**Warnings/Precautions** Prolonged use may result in overgrowth of nonsusceptible organisms, glaucoma, damage to the optic nerve, defects in visual acuity, and cataract formation; symptoms of neomycin sensitization include itching, reddening, edema, or failure to heal

**Pregnancy Risk Factor** C

**Adverse Reactions** 1% to 10%:
  Dermatologic: Cutaneous sensitization, rash, delayed wound healing
  Ocular: Increased intraocular pressure, glaucoma, optic nerve damage, cataracts, conjunctival sensitization

- ♦ **Neomycin Sulfate** *see* Neomycin *on page 642*
- ♦ **Neopap®** [OTC] *see* Acetaminophen *on page 21*
- ♦ **Neoral®** Oral *see* Cyclosporine *on page 245*
- ♦ **Neosporin® Cream** [OTC] *see* Neomycin and Polymyxin B *on page 643*
- ♦ **Neosporin® G.U. Irrigant** *see* Neomycin and Polymyxin B *on page 643*
- ♦ **Neosporin® Ophthalmic Ointment** *see* Bacitracin, Neomycin, and Polymyxin B *on page 97*
- ♦ **Neosporin® Ophthalmic Solution** *see* Neomycin, Polymyxin B, and Gramicidin *on page 644*
- ♦ **Neosporin® Topical Ointment** [OTC] *see* Bacitracin, Neomycin, and Polymyxin B *on page 97*

## Neostigmine *(nee oh STIG meen)*

**Pharmacologic Class** Acetylcholinesterase Inhibitor (Central)

**U.S. Brand Names** Prostigmin®

**Mechanism of Action** Inhibits destruction of acetylcholine by acetylcholinesterase which facilitates transmission of impulses across myoneural junction

**Use** Diagnosis and treatment of myasthenia gravis and prevent and treat postoperative bladder distention and urinary retention; reversal of the effects of nondepolarizing neuromuscular blocking agents after surgery

**USUAL DOSAGE**
Myasthenia gravis: Diagnosis: I.M.:
  Children: 0.04 mg/kg as a single dose
  Adults: 0.02 mg/kg as a single dose
Myasthenia gravis: Treatment:
  Children:
    Oral: 2 mg/kg/day divided every 3-4 hours
    I.M., I.V., S.C.: 0.01-0.04 mg/kg every 2-4 hours
  Adults:
    Oral: 15 mg/dose every 3-4 hours up to 375 mg/day maximum
    I.M., I.V., S.C.: 0.5-2.5 mg every 1-3 hours up to 10 mg/24 hours maximum
Reversal of nondepolarizing neuromuscular blockade after surgery in conjunction with atropine: I.V.:
  Infants: 0.025-0.1 mg/kg/dose
  Children: 0.025-0.08 mg/kg/dose
  Adults: 0.5-2.5 mg; total dose not to exceed 5 mg
Bladder atony: Adults: I.M., S.C.:
  Prevention: 0.25 mg every 4-6 hours for 2-3 days
  Treatment: 0.5-1 mg every 3 hours for 5 doses after bladder has emptied
**Dosing adjustment in renal impairment:**
  $Cl_{cr}$ 10-50 mL/minute: Administer 50% of normal dose
  $Cl_{cr}$ <10 mL/minute: Administer 25% of normal dose

**Dosage Forms** Inj, as methylsulfate: 0.25 mg/mL (1 mL), 0.5 mg/mL (1 mL, 10 mL), 1 mg/mL (10 mL); Tab, as bromide: 15 mg

**Contraindications** Hypersensitivity to neostigmine, bromides or any component; GI or GU obstruction

**Warnings/Precautions** Does not antagonize and may prolong the phase I block of depolarizing muscle relaxants (eg, succinylcholine); use with caution in patients with epilepsy, asthma, bradycardia, hyperthyroidism, cardiac arrhythmias, or peptic ulcer; adequate facilities should be available for cardiopulmonary resuscitation when testing and adjusting dose for myasthenia gravis; have atropine and epinephrine ready to treat hypersensitivity reactions; overdosage may result in cholinergic crisis, this must be distinguished from myasthenic crisis; anticholinesterase insensitivity can develop for brief or prolonged periods

**Pregnancy Risk Factor** C

**Adverse Reactions**
Respiratory: Bronchoconstriction
>10%:
Gastrointestinal: Hyperperistalsis, nausea, vomiting, salivation, diarrhea, stomach cramps
Miscellaneous: Diaphoresis (increased)
1% to 10%:
Genitourinary: Urge to urinate
Ocular: Small pupils, lacrimation
Respiratory: Increased bronchial secretions
<1%: A-V block, bradycardia, hypotension, bradyarrhythmias, asystole, dysphoria, restlessness, agitation, seizures, headache, drowsiness, thrombophlebitis, muscle spasms, tremor, weakness, fasciculations, diplopia, miosis, laryngospasm, respiratory paralysis, hypersensitivity, hyper-reactive cholinergic responses

**Drug Interactions**
Decreased effect: Antagonizes effects of nondepolarizing muscle relaxants (eg, pancuronium, tubocurarine); atropine antagonizes the muscarinic effects of neostigmine
Increased effect: Neuromuscular blocking agents effects are increased

**Onset** I.M.: Within 20-30 minutes; I.V.: Within 1-20 minutes

**Duration** I.M.: 2.5-4 hours; I.V.: 1-2 hours

**Half-Life** Normal renal function: 0.5-2.1 hours; End-stage renal disease: Prolonged

**Special PA Issues**
Patient Education: Take this drug exactly as prescribed. You may experience visual difficulty (eg, blurring and dark adaptation - use caution at night) or urinary frequency. Promptly report any muscle weakness, respiratory difficulty, severe or unresolved diarrhea, persistent abdominal cramping or vomiting, sweating, or tearing.

- **Neostigmine Bromide** see Neostigmine on previous page
- **Neostigmine Methylsulfate** see Neostigmine on previous page
- **Neostrata™ HQ** see Hydroquinone on page 457
- **Neo-Synephrine® Nasal Solution [OTC]** see Phenylephrine on page 718
- **Neo-Synephrine® Ophthalmic Solution** see Phenylephrine on page 718
- **Neo-Tabs® Oral** see Neomycin on page 642
- **Neotopic** see Bacitracin, Neomycin, and Polymyxin B on page 97
- **Neotricin HC® Ophthalmic Ointment** see Bacitracin, Neomycin, Polymyxin B, and Hydrocortisone on page 97
- **NeoVadrin® [OTC]** see Vitamins, Multiple on page 964
- **Nephro-Calci® [OTC]** see Calcium Carbonate on page 139
- **Nephrocaps®** see Vitamin B Complex With Vitamin C and Folic Acid on page 963
- **Nephro-Fer™ [OTC]** see Ferrous Fumarate on page 366
- **Nephronex®** see Nitrofurantoin on page 659
- **Nephrox Suspension [OTC]** see Aluminum Hydroxide on page 47
- **Neptazane®** see Methazolamide on page 581
- **Nervocaine®** see Lidocaine on page 531
- **Nesacaine®** see Chloroprocaine on page 191
- **Nesacaine®-MPF** see Chloroprocaine on page 191
- **Nestrex®** see Pyridoxine on page 784
- **1-N-Ethyl Sisomicin** see Netilmicin on this page

## Netilmicin (ne til MYE sin)

**Pharmacologic Class** Antibiotic, Aminoglycoside

**U.S. Brand Names** Netromycin®

**Mechanism of Action** Interferes with protein synthesis in bacterial cell by binding to 30S ribosomal subunits

**Use** Short-term treatment of serious or life-threatening infections including septicemia, peritonitis, intra-abdominal abscess, lower respiratory tract infections, urinary tract infections; skin, bone, and joint infections caused by susceptible organisms; active against Pseudomonas aeruginoasa, E. coli, Proteus, Klebsiella, Serratia, Enterobacter, Citrobacter, and other gram-negative bacilli

**USUAL DOSAGE** Individualization is critical because of the low therapeutic index. Use of ideal body weight (IBW) for determining the mg/kg/dose appears to be more accurate than dosing on the basis of total body weight (TBW). In morbid obesity, dosage requirement may best be estimated using a dosing weight of IBW + 0.4 (TBW - IBW). Peak and trough plasma drug levels should be determined, particularly in critically ill patients with serious infections or in disease states known to significantly alter aminoglycoside pharmacokinetics (eg, cystic fibrosis, burns, or major surgery).
(Continued)

## Netilmicin (Continued)

I.M., I.V.:

Neonates <6 weeks: 2-3.25 mg/kg/dose every 12 hours

Children 6 weeks to 12 years: 1-2.5 mg/kg/dose every 8 hours

Children >12 years and Adults: 1.5-2 mg/kg/dose every 8-12 hours

Some clinicians suggest a daily dose of 4-7 mg/kg for all patients with normal renal function. This dose is at least as efficacious with similar, if not less, toxicity than conventional dosing.

**Dosing adjustment in renal impairment:** Initial dose:

All patients should receive a loading dose of at least 2 mg/kg (subsequent dosing should be base on serum concentrations)

$Cl_{cr}$ ≥60 mL/minute: Administer every 8 hours

$Cl_{cr}$ 40-60 mL/minute: Administer every 12 hours

$Cl_{cr}$ 20-40 mL/minute: Administer every 24 hours

Continuous arteriovenous or venovenous hemodiafiltration (CAVH) effects: Dose as for $Cl_{cr}$ 20-40 mL/minute and follow levels

**Dosage Forms** Inj, as sulfate: 100 mg/mL (1.5 mL)

**Contraindications** Known hypersensitivity to netilmicin (aminoglycosides, bisulfites)

**Warnings/Precautions** Use with caution in patients with pre-existing renal insufficiency, vestibular or cochlear impairment, myasthenia gravis, hypocalcemia, conditions which depress neuromuscular transmission. Parenteral aminoglycosides are associated with nephrotoxicity or ototoxicity; the ototoxicity may be proportional to the amount of drug given and the duration of treatment; tinnitus or vertigo are indications of vestibular injury and impending hearing loss; renal damage is usually reversible.

**Pregnancy Risk Factor** D

**Adverse Reactions**

>10%:

Central nervous system: Neurotoxicity

Otic: Ototoxicity (auditory), ototoxicity (vestibular)

Renal: Nephrotoxicity, decreased creatinine clearance

1% to 10%: Dermatologic: Skin itching, redness, rash, swelling

<1%: Difficulty in breathing, drowsiness, weakness, headache, tremors, muscle cramps, pseudomotor cerebri, anorexia, nausea, vomiting, weight loss, increased salivation, enterocolitis, granulocytopenia, agranulocytosis, thrombocytopenia, photosensitivity, erythema, burning, stinging

**Drug Interactions**

Increased/prolonged effect of depolarizing and nondepolarizing neuromuscular blocking agents

Increased toxicity: Concurrent use of amphotericin, vancomycin, ethacrynic acid, furosemide and other nephrotoxic agents may increase nephrotoxicity

**Half-Life** 2-3 hours (age and renal function dependent)

**Special PA Issues**

**Patient Education:** This drug can only be administered I.V. or I.M. It is important to maintain adequate hydration (2-3 L/day) unless informed by prescriber to restrict fluid intake. Report change in hearing acuity, ringing or roaring in ears, alteration in balance, vertigo, or feeling of fullness in head; pain, tingling or numbness of any body part; change in urinary pattern or decrease in urine; signs of opportunistic infection (eg, white plaques in mouth, vaginal discharge, unhealed sores, sore throat, unusual fever, chills); pain, redness, or swelling at injection site; skin rash or itching; or other adverse reactions.

**Reference Range:** Therapeutic: Peak: 4-10 µg/mL (SI: 8-21 µmol/L); Trough: <2 µg/mL (SI: 4 µmol/L); Toxic: Peak: >10 µg/mL (SI: >21 µmol/L); Trough: >2 µg/mL (SI: >4.2 µmol/L)

◆ **Netromicina®** see Netilmicin on previous page

◆ **Netromycin®** see Netilmicin on previous page

◆ **Neucalm®** see Hydroxyzine on page 462

◆ **Neumega®** see Oprelvekin on page 678

◆ **Neupogen® Injection** see Filgrastim on page 370

◆ **Neuramate®** see Meprobamate on page 570

◆ **Neurontin®** see Gabapentin on page 406

◆ **Neut® Injection** see Sodium Bicarbonate on page 838

◆ **Neutra-Phos®** see Potassium Phosphate and Sodium Phosphate on page 747

◆ **Neutra-Phos®-K** see Potassium Phosphate on page 745

◆ **Neutrexin® Injection** see Trimetrexate Glucuronate on page 938

## Nevirapine (ne VYE ra peen)

**Pharmacologic Class** An iretroviral Agent, Reverse Transcriptase Inhibitor (Non-Nucleoside)

**U.S. Brand Names** Viramune®

**Mechanism of Action** As a non-nucleoside reverse transcriptase inhibitor, nevirapine has activity against HIV-1 by binding to reverse transcriptase. It consequently blocks the RNA-dependent and DNA-dependent DNA polymerase activities including HIV-1 replication. It does not require intracellular phosphorylation for antiviral activity.

**Use** In combination therapy with other antiretroviral agents for the treatment of HIV-1 in adults

**USUAL DOSAGE** Adults: Oral:

Initial: 200 mg once daily for 14 days

Maintenance: 200 mg twice daily (in combination with an additional antiretroviral agent)

**Dosage Forms Tab:** 200 mg

**Contraindications** Previous hypersensitivity to nevirapine or its components; concurrent use with oral contraceptives and protease inhibitors (indinavir, nelfinavir, ritonavir, saquinavir)

**Warnings/Precautions** Consider alteration of antiretroviral therapies if disease progression occurs while patients are receiving nevirapine. Resistant HIV virus emerges rapidly and uniformly when nevirapine is administered as monotherapy. Therefore, always administer in combination with at least 1 additional antiretroviral agent. Severe skin reactions (eg, Stevens-Johnson syndrome) have occurred, usually within 6 weeks. Therapy should be discontinued if any rash which develops does not resolve; mild to moderate alterations in LFTs are not uncommon, however, severe hepatotoxic reactions may occur rarely, and if abnormalities reoccur after temporarily discontinuing therapy, treatment should be permanently halted. Safety and efficacy have not been established in children.

**Pregnancy Risk Factor** C

**Pregnancy Implications**

Clinical effects on the fetus: Administer nevirapine during pregnancy only if benefits to the mother outweigh the risk to the fetus

Breast-feeding/lactation: Avoid use during lactation, if possible

**Adverse Reactions**

>10%:

Central nervous system: Headache (11%), fever (8% to 11%)

Dermatologic: Rash (15% to 20%)

Gastrointestinal: Diarrhea (15% to 20%)

Hematologic: Neutropenia (10% to 11%)

1% to 10%:

Gastrointestinal: Ulcerative stomatitis (4%), nausea, abdominal pain (2%)

Hematologic: Anemia

Hepatic: Hepatitis, increased LFTs (2% to 4%)

Neuromuscular & skeletal: Peripheral neuropathy, paresthesia (2%), myalgia

<1%: Thrombocytopenia, Stevens-Johnson syndrome, hepatotoxicity, hepatic necrosis

**Drug Interactions** CYP3A3/4 enzyme substrate; CYP3A3/4 enzyme inducer; CYP3A3/4 enzyme inhibitor

Decreased effect: Rifampin and rifabutin may decrease nevirapine trough concentrations due to induction of CYP3A; since nevirapine may decrease concentrations of protease inhibitors, they should not be administered concomitantly or doses should be increased; nevirapine may decrease the effectiveness of oral contraceptives - suggest alternate method of birth control; decreased effect of ketoconazole

Increased effect/toxicity with cimetidine, macrolides, ketoconazole

**Special PA Issues**

**Patient Education:** If rash develops, contact prescriber

**Monitoring Parameters:** Liver function tests periodically throughout therapy; observe for CNS side effects

◆ **New Decongestant®** *see* Chlorpheniramine, Phenyltoloxamine, Phenylpropanolamine, and Phenylephrine *on page 196*

◆ **N.G.T.® Topical** *see* Nystatin and Triamcinolone *on page 670*

# Niacin (NYE a sin)

**Pharmacologic Class** Antilipemic Agent (Miscellaneous); Vitamin, Water Soluble

**U.S. Brand Names** Nicobid® [OTC]; Nicolar® [OTC]; Nicotinex [OTC]; Slo-Niacin® [OTC]

**Mechanism of Action** Component of two coenzymes which is necessary for tissue respiration, lipid metabolism, and glycogenolysis; inhibits the synthesis of very low density lipoproteins

**Use** Adjunctive treatment of hyperlipidemias; peripheral vascular disease and circulatory disorders; treatment of pellagra; dietary supplement

**USUAL DOSAGE** Administer I.M., I.V., or S.C. only if oral route is unavailable and use only for vitamin deficiencies (not for hyperlipidemia)

Children: Oral:

Pellagra: 50-100 mg/dose 3 times/day

Recommended daily allowances:

0-0.5 years: 5 mg/day

0.5-1 year: 6 mg/day

1-3 years: 9 mg/day

4-6 years: 12 mg/day

7-10 years: 13 mg/day

(Continued)

## Niacin *(Continued)*

Children and Adolescents: Oral: Recommended daily allowances:

Male:

11-14 years: 17 mg/day

15-18 years: 20 mg/day

19-24 years: 19 mg/day

Female: 11-24 years: 15 mg/day

Adults: Oral:

Recommended daily allowances:

Male: 25-50 years: 19 mg/day; >51 years: 15 mg/day

Female: 25-50 years: 15 mg/day; >51 years: 13 mg/day

Hyperlipidemia: 1.5-6 g/day in 3 divided doses with or after meals

Pellagra: 50-100 mg 3-4 times/day, maximum: 500 mg/day

Niacin deficiency: 10-20 mg/day, maximum: 100 mg/day

**Dosage Forms** Cap, timed release: 125 mg, 250 mg, 300 mg, 400 mg, 500 mg; **Elix:** 50 mg/5 mL (473 mL, 4000 mL); **Inj:** 100 mg/mL (30 mL); **Tab:** 25 mg, 50 mg, 100 mg, 250 mg, 500 mg; Extended release: 500 mg, 750 mg, 1000 mg; Timed release: 150 mg, 250 mg, 500 mg, 750 mg

**Contraindications** Liver disease, peptic ulcer, severe hypotension, arterial hemorrhaging, hypersensitivity to niacin

**Warnings/Precautions** Monitor liver function tests, blood glucose; may elevate uric acid levels; use with caution in patients predisposed to gout; large doses should be administered with caution to patients with gallbladder disease, jaundice, liver disease, or diabetes; some products may contain tartrazine

**Pregnancy Risk Factor** A (C if used in doses greater than RDA suggested doses)

**Adverse Reactions**

1% to 10%:

Cardiovascular: Generalized flushing

Central nervous system: Headache

Gastrointestinal: Bloating, flatulence, nausea

Hepatic: Abnormalities of hepatic function tests, jaundice

Neuromuscular & skeletal: Paresthesia in extremities

Miscellaneous: Increased sebaceous gland activity, sensation of warmth

<1%: Tachycardia, syncope, vasovagal attacks, dizziness, rash, liver damage (dose-related incidence), blurred vision, wheezing

**Drug Interactions**

Decreased effect of oral hypoglycemics; may inhibit uricosuric effects of sulfinpyrazone and probenecid

Decreased toxicity (flush) with aspirin

Increased toxicity with lovastatin (myopathy) and possibly with other HMG-CoA reductase inhibitors; adrenergic blocking agents → additive vasodilating effect and postural hypotension

**Special PA Issues**

**Patient Education:** May experience transient cutaneous flushing and sensation of warmth, especially of face and upper body; itching or tingling, and headache may occur, these adverse effects may be decreased by increasing the dose slowly or by taking aspirin or a NSAID 30 minutes to 1 hour prior to taking niacin; may cause GI upset, take with food; if dizziness occurs, avoid sudden changes in posture; report any persistent nausea, vomiting, abdominal pain, dark urine, or pale stools to the physician; do not crush sustained release capsule

**Monitoring Parameters:** Blood glucose, liver function tests (with large doses or prolonged therapy), serum cholesterol

**Related Information**

Lipid-Lowering Agents *on page 1022*

## Niacinamide *(nye a SIN e mide)*

**Pharmacologic Class** Vitamin, Water Soluble

**Mechanism of Action** Used by the body as a source of niacin; is a component of two coenzymes which is necessary for tissue respiration, lipid metabolism, and glycogenolysis; inhibits the synthesis of very low density lipoproteins; does not have hypolipidemia or vasodilating effects

**Use** Prophylaxis and treatment of pellagra

**USUAL DOSAGE** Oral:

Children: Pellagra: 100-300 mg/day in divided doses

Adults: 50 mg 3-10 times/day

Pellagra: 300-500 mg/day

Recommended daily allowance: 13-19 mg/day

**Dosage Forms Tab:** 50 mg, 100 mg, 125 mg, 250 mg, 500 mg

**Contraindications** Liver disease, peptic ulcer, known hypersensitivity to niacin

**Warnings/Precautions** Large doses should be administered with caution to patients with gallbladder disease or diabetes; monitor blood glucose; may elevate uric acid levels; use with caution in patients predisposed to gout; some products may contain tartrazine

**Pregnancy Risk Factor** A (C if used in doses greater than RDA suggested doses)

**Adverse Reactions**

Cardiovascular: Tachycardia

Dermatologic: Rash

Gastrointestinal: Bloating, flatulence, nausea

Neuromuscular & skeletal: Paresthesia in extremities

Ocular: Blurred vision

Respiratory: Wheezing

Miscellaneous: Increased sebaceous gland activity

# Nicardipine (nye KAR de peen)

**Pharmacologic Class** Calcium Channel Blocker

**U.S. Brand Names** Cardene®; Cardene® SR; Cardene® I.V.

**Mechanism of Action** Inhibits calcium ion from entering the "slow channels" or select voltage-sensitive areas of vascular smooth muscle and myocardium during depolarization, producing a relaxation of coronary vascular smooth muscle and coronary vasodilation; increases myocardial oxygen delivery in patients with vasospastic angina

**Use** Chronic stable angina (immediate-release product only); management of essential hypertension (immediate and sustained release; parenteral only for short time that oral treatment is not feasible), migraine prophylaxis

**Unlabeled use:** Congestive heart failure

**USUAL DOSAGE** Adults:

Oral:

Immediate release: Initial: 20 mg 3 times/day; usual: 20-40 mg 3 times/day (allow 3 days between dose increases)

Sustained release: Initial: 30 mg twice daily, titrate up to 60 mg twice daily

I.V. (dilute to 0.1 mg/mL): Initial: 5 mg/hour increased by 2.5 mg/hour every 15 minutes to a maximum of 15 mg/hour

**Dosing adjustment in renal impairment:** Titrate dose beginning with 20 mg 3 times/day (immediate release) or 30 mg twice daily (sustained release)

**Dosing adjustment in hepatic impairment:** Starting dose: 20 mg twice daily (immediate release) with titration

### Equivalent Oral vs I.V. Infusion Doses

| Oral Dose | Equivalent I.V. Infusion |
|-----------|--------------------------|
| 20 mg q8h | 0.5 mg/h |
| 30 mg q8h | 1.2 mg/h |
| 40 mg q8h | 2.2 mg/h |

**Dosage Forms** Nicardipine hydrochloride: **Cap:** 20 mg, 30 mg; **Cap, sustained release:** 30 mg, 45 mg, 60 mg; **Inj:** 2.5 mg/mL (10 mL)

**Contraindications** Contraindicated in severe hypotension or second and third degree heart block, sinus bradycardia, advanced heart block, ventricular tachycardia, cardiogenic shock, atrial fibrillation or flutter associated with accessory conduction pathways, CHF; hypersensitivity to nicardipine or any component, calcium channel blockers, and adenosine; not to be given within a few hours of I.V. beta-blocking agents

**Warnings/Precautions** Use with caution in titrating dosages for impaired renal or hepatic function patients; may increase frequency, severity, and duration of angina during initiation of therapy; do not abruptly withdraw (chest pain); may have a greater hypotensive effect in the elderly

**Pregnancy Risk Factor** C

**Pregnancy Implications**

Clinical effects on the fetus: Crosses the placenta; may exhibit tocolytic effect

Breast-feeding/lactation: No data available

**Adverse Reactions**

1% to 10%:

Cardiovascular: Flushing (6% to 10%), palpitations, tachycardia (1% to 3.4%), peripheral edema (7% to 8%), syncope (3% to 4%)

Central nervous system: Headache (6.4% to 8%), dizziness (4% to 7%), somnolence (4.2% to 6%)

Gastrointestinal: Nausea (1.9% to 2.2%), abdominal pain (0.8% to 1.5%)

Neuromuscular & skeletal: Weakness (4.2% to 6%)

<1%: Abnormal EKG, insomnia, malaise, abnormal dreams, rash, vomiting, constipation, dyspepsia, xerostomia, nocturia, tremor

**Drug Interactions** CYP3A3/4 enzyme substrate

(Continued)

## Nicardipine *(Continued)*

Increased toxicity/effect/levels:

Nicardipine and $H_2$ blockers (cimetidine, ranitidine) may increase bioavailability of nicardipine

Nicardipine and propranolol or metoprolol (and possibly other beta-blockers) may increase cardiac depressant effects on A-V conduction

Nicardipine and cyclosporine may increase cyclosporine levels

**Onset** Oral: 1-2 hours; I.V.: 10 minutes

**Duration** 2-6 hours

**Half-Life** 2-4 hours

**Special PA Issues**

**Patient Education:** Take as directed; do not alter dosage regimen or increase, decrease, or discontinue without consulting prescriber. Do not crush or chew tablets or capsules. Take with nonfatty food. Avoid caffeine and alcohol. Consult prescriber before increasing exercise routine (decreased angina does not mean it is safe to increase exercise). Change position slowly to prevent orthostatic events. May cause dizziness or fatigue; use caution when driving or engaging in hazardous activities until effect of medication is known. Frequent, small meals or sucking on lozenges may reduce nausea. Report swelling, difficulty breathing or new cough, unresolved fatigue, unusual weight gain, or unresolved dizziness.

**Dietary Considerations:** Alcohol: Avoid use

**Related Information**

Calcium Channel Blocking Agents *on page 1004*

♦ **Nicardipine Hydrochloride** *see* Nicardipine *on previous page*
♦ **N'ice® Vitamin C Drops [OTC]** *see* Ascorbic Acid *on page 79*
♦ **Niclocide®** *see* Niclosamide *on this page*

## Niclosamide *(ni KLOE sa mide)*

**Pharmacologic Class** Anthelmintic

**U.S. Brand Names** Niclocide®

**Mechanism of Action** Inhibits the synthesis of ATP through inhibition of oxidative phosphorylation in the mitochondria of cestodes

**Use** Treatment of intestinal beef and fish tapeworm infections and dwarf tapeworm infections

**USUAL DOSAGE** Oral:

Beef and fish tapeworm:

Children:

11-34 kg: 1 g (2 tablets) as a single dose

>34 kg: 1.5 g (3 tablets) as a single dose

Adults: 2 g (4 tablets) in a single dose

May require a second course of treatment 7 days later

Dwarf tapeworm:

Children:

11-34 g: 1 g (2 tablets) chewed thoroughly in a single dose the first day, then 500 mg/day (1 tablet) for next 6 days

>34 g: 1.5 g (3 tablets) in a single dose the first day, then 1 g/day for 6 days

Adults: 2 g (4 tablets) in a single daily dose for 7 days

**Dosage Forms** Tab, chewable (vanilla flavor): 500 mg

**Contraindications** Known hypersensitivity to niclosamide

**Warnings/Precautions** Affects cestodes of the intestine only; it is without effect in cysticercosis

**Pregnancy Risk Factor** B

**Adverse Reactions**

1% to 10%:

Central nervous system: Drowsiness, dizziness, headache

Gastrointestinal: Nausea, vomiting, loss of appetite, diarrhea

<1%: Rash, pruritus ani, oral irritation, fever, rectal bleeding, weakness, bad taste in mouth, sweating, palpitations, constipation, alopecia, edema in the arm, backache

**Special PA Issues**

**Patient Education:** Chew tablets thoroughly; tablets can be pulverized and mixed with water to form a paste for administration to children; can be taken with food; a mild laxative can be used for constipation

**Monitoring Parameters:** Stool cultures

♦ **Nicobid® [OTC]** *see* Niacin *on page 649*
♦ **Nicoderm® Patch** *see* Nicotine *on next page*
♦ **Nicolar® [OTC]** *see* Niacin *on page 649*
♦ **Nicorette®** *see* Nicotine *on next page*
♦ **Nicorette® DS Gum** *see* Nicotine *on next page*
♦ **Nicorette® Gum** *see* Nicotine *on next page*
♦ **Nicorette® Plus** *see* Nicotine *on next page*

♦ **Nicotinamide** *see* Niacinamide *on page 650*

# Nicotine (nik oh TEEN)

**Pharmacologic Class** Smoking Cessation Aid

**U.S. Brand Names** Habitrol™ Patch; Nicoderm® Patch; Nicorette® DS Gum; Nicorette® Gum; Nicotrol® NS Nasal Spray; Nicotrol® Patch [OTC]; ProStep® Patch

**Mechanism of Action** Nicotine is one of two naturally-occurring alkaloids which exhibit their primary effects via autonomic ganglia stimulation. The other alkaloid is lobeline which has many actions similar to those of nicotine but is less potent. Nicotine is a potent ganglionic and central nervous system stimulant, the actions of which are mediated via nicotine-specific receptors. Biphasic actions are observed depending upon the dose administered. The main effect of nicotine in small doses is stimulation of all autonomic ganglia; with larger doses, initial stimulation is followed by blockade of transmission. Biphasic effects are also evident in the adrenal medulla; discharge of catecholamines occurs with small doses, whereas prevention of catecholamines release is seen with higher doses as a response to splanchnic nerve stimulation. Stimulation of the central nervous system (CNS) is characterized by tremors and respiratory excitation. However, convulsions may occur with higher doses, along with respiratory failure secondary to both central paralysis and peripheral blockade to respiratory muscles.

**Use** Treatment aid to smoking cessation while participating in a behavioral modification program under medical supervision

**USUAL DOSAGE** Patients should be advised to completely stop smoking upon initiation of therapy

Gum: Chew 1 piece of gum when urge to smoke, up to 30 pieces/day; most patients require 10-12 pieces of gum/day

Transdermal patch: Apply new patch every 24 hours to nonhairy, clean, dry skin on the upper body or upper outer arm; each patch should be applied to a different site

24-hour patches (some 24-hour duration patches may be worn for 16 hours/day and then removed at bedtime):

Initial starting dose: 21 mg/day for 4-8 weeks for most patients

First weaning dose: 14 mg/day for 2-4 weeks

Second weaning dose: 7 mg/day for 2-4 weeks

Initial starting dose for patients <100 pounds, smoke <10 cigarettes/day, have a history of cardiovascular disease: 14 mg/day for 4-8 weeks followed by 7 mg/day for 2-4 weeks

In patients who are receiving >600 mg/day of cimetidine: Decrease to the next lower patch size

16-hour patches:

One patch worn for 16 hours daily (remove at bedtime) for 6 weeks, then discontinue; these patches are not intended for lighter smokers

Benefits of use of nicotine transdermal patches beyond 3 months have not been demonstrated

Spray: 1-2 sprays/hour; do not exceed more than 5 doses (10 sprays) per hour; each dose (2 sprays) contains 1 mg of nicotine. **Warning:** A dose of 40 mg can cause fatalities.

Inhaler: Patients may self-titrate doses; most patients use between 6 and 16 cartridges daily during the first 3 months of therapy and then gradually reduce their daily dose over the ensuing 6-12 weeks; no tapering strategy has been shown to be superior to any other; the best clinical effects are seen with frequent continuous inhaler puffing (20 minutes). The recommended duration of treatment is 3 months and some patients may require up to 6 months of therapy.

**Dosage Forms Patch, transdermal:** Habitrol™: 21 mg/day, 14 mg/day, 7 mg/day (30 systems/box), Nicoderm®: 21 mg/day, 14 mg/day, 7 mg/day (14 systems/box), Nicotrol® [OTC]: 15 mg/day (gradually released over 16 hours), ProStep®: 22 mg/day, 11 mg/day (7 systems/box), **Pieces, chewing gum, as polacrilex:** 2 mg/square [OTC] (96 pieces/box), 4 mg/square (96 pieces/box); **Spray, nasal:** 0.5 mg/actuation [10 mg/mL - 200 actuations] (10 mL)

**Contraindications** Nonsmokers, patients with a history of hypersensitivity or allergy to nicotine or any components used in the transdermal system, pregnant or nursing women, patients who are smoking during the postmyocardial infarction period, patients with life-threatening arrhythmias, or severe or worsening angina pectoris, active temporomandibular joint disease (gum)

**Warnings/Precautions** Use with caution in oropharyngeal inflammation and in patients with history of esophagitis, peptic ulcer, coronary artery disease, vasospastic disease, angina, hypertension, hyperthyroidism, diabetes, and hepatic dysfunction; nicotine is known to be one of the most toxic of all poisons; while the gum is being used to help the patient overcome a health hazard, it also must be considered a hazardous drug vehicle. Nicotine nasal spray: Fatal dose: 40 mg

**Pregnancy Risk Factor** D (transdermal)/X (chewing gum)

**Adverse Reactions**

Chewing gum:

>10%:

Cardiovascular: Tachycardia

(Continued)

## Nicotine *(Continued)*

Central nervous system: Headache (mild)
Gastrointestinal: Nausea, vomiting, indigestion, excessive salivation, belching, increased appetite, mouth or throat soreness
Neuromuscular & skeletal: Jaw muscle ache
Miscellaneous: Hiccups
1% to 10%:
Central nervous system: Insomnia, dizziness, nervousness
Endocrine & metabolic: Dysmenorrhea
Gastrointestinal: GI distress, eructation
Neuromuscular & skeletal: Myalgia
Respiratory: Hoarseness
Miscellaneous: Hiccups
<1%: Atrial fibrillation, erythema, itching, hypersensitivity reactions

Transdermal systems:
>10%:
Cardiovascular: Tachycardia
Central nervous system: Headache (mild)
Dermatologic: Pruritus erythema
Gastrointestinal: Increased appetite
1% to 10%:
Central nervous system: Insomnia, nervousness
Endocrine & metabolic: Dysmenorrhea
Neuromuscular & skeletal: Myalgia
<1%: Atrial fibrillation, itching, hypersensitivity reactions

**Drug Interactions** CYP2A6, 2B6 enzyme substrate; CYP1A2 enzyme inducer
**Onset** Intranasal nicotine may more closely approximate the time course of plasma nicotine levels observed after cigarette smoking than other dosage forms.
**Duration** Transdermal: 24 hours
**Half-Life** 4 hours
**Special PA Issues**
**Patient Education:** Use exactly as directed; do not use more often than prescribed. Stop smoking completely during therapy.
Gum: Chew slowly for 30 minutes. Discard chewed gum away from access by children.
Transdermal patch: Follow directions in package for dosing schedule and use. Do not cut patches. Apply to clean, dry skin in different site each day. Do not touch eyes; wash hands after application. You may experience dizziness or lightheadedness; use caution driving or when engaging in tasks that require alertness. For nausea, vomiting or GI upset, small frequent meals, chewing gum, frequent oral care may help. Report persistent vomiting, diarrhea, chills, sweating, chest pain or palpitations, or burning or redness at application site.
Spray: Follow directions in package. Blow nose gently before use. Use 1-2 sprays/hour; do not exceed 5 doses (10 sprays) per hour. Excessive use can result in severe (even life-threatening) reactions. You may experience temporary stinging or burning after spray.

♦ **Nicotinex [OTC]** *see* Niacin *on page 649*
♦ **Nicotinic Acid** *see* Niacin *on page 649*
♦ **Nicotiramide** *see* Niacin *on page 649*
♦ **Nicotrol® NS Nasal Spray** *see* Nicotine *on previous page*
♦ **Nicotrol® Patch [OTC]** *see* Nicotine *on previous page*
♦ **Nico-Vert® [OTC]** *see* Meclizine *on page 559*

## Nifedipine *(nye FED i peen)*

**Pharmacologic Class** Calcium Channel Blocker
**U.S. Brand Names** Adalat®; Adalat® CC; Procardia®; Procardia XL®
**Mechanism of Action** Inhibits calcium ion from entering the "slow channels" or select voltage-sensitive areas of vascular smooth muscle and myocardium during depolarization, producing a relaxation of coronary vascular smooth muscle and coronary vasodilation; increases myocardial oxygen delivery in patients with vasospastic angina
**Use** Angina, hypertrophic cardiomyopathy, hypertension (sustained release only), pulmonary hypertension; Raynaud's disease, migraine headaches.
**USUAL DOSAGE** Oral or "bite and swallow" (eg, patient bites capsule to release liquid contents and then swallows): **Note:** Doses are usually titrated upward at 7- to 14-day intervals; may increase every 3 days if clinically necessary

Children: Hypertrophic cardiomyopathy: 0.6-0.9 mg/kg/24 hours in 3-4 divided doses
Adolescents and Adults: (note: when switching from immediate release to sustained release formulations, total daily dose will start the same)
Initial: 10 mg 3 times/day as capsules or 30 mg once daily as sustained release
Usual dose: 10-30 mg 3 times/day as capsules or 30-60 mg once daily as sustained release

Maximum dose: 120-180 mg/day
*Increase sustained release at 7- to 14-day intervals*
**Hemodialysis:** Supplemental dose is not necessary
**Peritoneal dialysis effects:** Supplemental dose is not necessary
**Dosing adjustment in hepatic impairment:** Reduce oral dose by 50% to 60% in patients with cirrhosis

**Dosage Forms Cap, liquid-filled (Adalat®, Procardia®):** 10 mg, 20 mg; **Tab, extended release (Adalat® CC):** 30 mg, 60 mg, 90 mg; **Tab, sustained release (Procardia XL®):** 30 mg, 60 mg, 90 mg

**Contraindications** Known hypersensitivity to nifedipine or any other calcium channel blocker and adenosine; sick-sinus syndrome, 2nd or 3rd degree A-V block, hypotension (<90 mm Hg systolic); advanced aortic stenosis; acute myocardial infarction

**Warnings/Precautions** The routine use of short-acting nifedipine capsules in hypertensive emergencies and pseudoemergencies is not recommended. **The FDA has concluded that the use of sublingual short-acting nifedipine in hypertensive emergencies is neither safe or effective and SHOULD BE ABANDONED!** Serious adverse events (cerebrovascular ischemia, syncope, heart block, stroke, sinus arrest, severe hypotension, acute myocardial infarction, ECG changes, and fetal distress) have been reported in relation to the administration of short-acting nifedipine in hypertensive emergencies.

Increased angina may be seen upon starting or increasing doses; may increase frequency, duration, and severity of angina during initiation of therapy; use with caution in patients with congestive heart failure or aortic stenosis (especially with concomitant beta-adrenergic blocker); severe left ventricular dysfunction, hepatic or renal impairment, hypertrophic cardiomyopathy (especially obstructive), concomitant therapy with beta-blockers or digoxin, edema

Mild and transient elevations in liver function enzymes may be apparent within 8 weeks of therapy initiation.

Therapeutic potential of sustained-release formulation (elementary osmotic pump, gastrointestinal therapeutic system [GITS]) may be decreased in patients with certain GI disorders that accelerate intestinal transit time (eg, short bowel syndrome, inflammatory bowel disease, severe diarrhea).

**Note:** Elderly patients may experience a greater hypotensive response and the use of the immediate release formulation in patients >71 years of age has been associated with a nearly fourfold increased risk for all-cause mortality when compared to β-blockers, ACE inhibitors, or other classes of calcium channel blockers

**Pregnancy Risk Factor** C
**Pregnancy Implications**
Clinical effects on the fetus: Use in pregnancy only when clearly needed and when the benefits outweigh the potential hazard to the fetus. No data on crossing the placenta. Hypotension, IUGR reported. IUGR probably related to maternal hypertension. May exhibit tocolytic effects. Available evidence suggests safe use during pregnancy and breast-feeding.
Breast-feeding/lactation: Crosses into breast milk. American Academy of Pediatrics considers **compatible** with breast-feeding.

**Adverse Reactions**
>10%:
Cardiovascular: Flushing (3% to 25%), peripheral edema (10% to 30%)
Central nervous system: Dizziness/lightheadedness (4% to 27%), giddiness, headache (10% to 23%)
Gastrointestinal: Nausea (3% to 11%), heartburn
Neuromuscular & skeletal: Weakness/jitteriness (≤12%)
Miscellaneous: Heat sensation
1% to 10%:
Cardiovascular: Congestive heart failure (2% to 7%), palpitations (≤7%), hypotension (<5%), myocardial infarction (4% to 7%)
Central nervous system: Nervousness (<7%), mood changes, somnolence(<3%)
Dermatologic: Rash/urticaria (≤3%)
Gastrointestinal: Sore throat, diarrhea (<3%), constipation (~3%), abdominal discomfort/flatulence (≤3%)
Neuromuscular & skeletal: Muscle cramps (<8%), arthritis (≤3%), paresthesia/weakness (<3%)
Respiratory: Dyspnea (≤8%), cough (6%), nasal congestion (≤6%), pulmonary edema (7%)
<1%: Tachycardia, syncope, fever, chills, dermatitis, urticaria, purpura, diarrhea, constipation, gingival hyperplasia, thrombocytopenia, leukopenia, anemia, joint stiffness, arthritis with increased ANA, blurred vision, transient blindness, diaphoresis
**Drug Interactions** CYP3A3/4 and 3A5-7 enzyme substrate
Decreased toxicity:
Nifedipine and phenobarbital may decrease nifedipine levels as observed with other calcium antagonists
Nifedipine and quinidine may decrease quinidine levels
(Continued)

## Nifedipine *(Continued)*

Nifedipine and rifampin may result in decreased nifedipine levels as with verapamil
Increased toxicity:

Nifedipine and beta-blockers may increase cardiovascular adverse effects

Nifedipine and digoxin may increase digoxin levels

Nifedipine and $H_2$-antagonists (cimetidine) increase bioavailability and may increase nifedipine serum concentration

Nifedipine and quinidine may increase nifedipine levels and toxicity

Nifedipine and theophylline may increase theophylline levels

Nifedipine and vincristine may increase vincristine levels

Nifedipine rarely increases PT time with concomitant warfarin administration

Neuromuscular blockade and hypotension may occur with coadministration of nifedipine and parenteral magnesium sulfate

Severe hypotension and fluid volume requirements may increase with concomitant fentanyl

**Onset** Oral: Within 20 minutes; S.L.: Within 1-5 minutes

**Half-Life** Adults, normal: 2-5 hours; Adults with cirrhosis: 7 hours

**Special PA Issues**

**Patient Education:** Take as directed; do not alter dosage regimen or increase, decrease, or discontinue without consulting prescriber. Do not crush or chew tablets or capsules. Consult prescriber before increasing exercise routine (decreased angina does not mean it is safe to increase exercise). Change position slowly to prevent orthostatic events. May cause dizziness or fatigue; use caution when driving or engaging in hazardous activities until effect of medication is known. Maintain good oral care and inspect gums for swelling or redness. May cause frequent urination at night. Report irregular heartbeat, swelling, difficulty breathing or new cough, unresolved fatigue, unusual weight gain, unresolved dizziness or constipation, and swollen or bleeding gums.

**Dietary Considerations:** Alcohol: Avoid use

**Monitoring Parameters:** Heart rate, blood pressure, signs and symptoms of CHF, peripheral edema

**Related Information**

Calcium Channel Blocking Agents *on page 1004*

♦ **Niferex®-PN** *see* Vitamins, Multiple *on page 964*

♦ **Nilandron™** *see* Nilutamide *on this page*

♦ **Nilstat®** *see* Nystatin *on page 669*

## Nilutamide *(ni LU ta mide)*

**Pharmacologic Class** Antineoplastic Agent, Miscellaneous

**U.S. Brand Names** Nilandron™

**Mechanism of Action** Nonsteroidal antiandrogen that inhibits androgen uptake or inhibits binding of androgen in target tissues

**Use** In combination with surgical castration in treatment of metastatic prostatic carcinoma (Stage $D_2$); for maximum benefit, nilutamide treatment must begin on the same day as or on the day after surgical castration

**USUAL DOSAGE** Adults: Oral: 6 tablets (50 mg each) once a day for a total daily dose of 300 mg for 30 days followed thereafter by 3 tablets (50 mg each) once a day for a total daily dose of 150 mg

**Dosage Forms** Tab: 50 mg

**Contraindications** Severe hepatic impairment; severe respiratory insufficiency; hypersensitivity to nilutamide or any component of this preparation

**Warnings/Precautions** The U.S. Food and Drug Administration (FDA) currently recommends that procedures for proper handling and disposal of antineoplastic agents be considered.

Interstitial pneumonitis has been reported in 2% of patients exposed to nilutamide. Patients typically experienced progressive exertional dyspnea, and possibly cough, chest pain and fever. X-rays showed interstitial or alveolo-interstitial changes. The suggestive signs of pneumonitis most often occurred within the first 3 months of nilutamide treatment.

Hepatitis or marked increases in liver enzymes leading to drug discontinuation occurred in 1% of nilutamide patients. There has been a report of elevated hepatic enzymes followed by death in a 65 year old patient treated with nilutamide.

Foreign postmarketing surveillance has revealed isolated cases of aplastic anemia in which a causal relationship with nilutamide could not be ascertained.

13% to 57% of patients receiving nilutamide reported a delay in adaptation to the dark, ranging from seconds to a few minutes. This effect sometimes does not abate as drug treatment is continued. Caution patients who experience this effect about driving at night or through tunnels. This effect can be alleviated by wearing tinted glasses.

**Pregnancy Risk Factor** C

**Adverse Reactions**

>10%:

Central nervous system: Pain, headache, insomnia

Gastrointestinal: Nausea, constipation, anorexia

Genitourinary: Impotence, testicular atrophy, gynecomastia

Endocrine & metabolic: Loss of libido, hot flashes

Neuromuscular & skeletal: Weakness

Ocular: Impaired adaption to dark

1% to 10%:

Cardiovascular: Hypertension

Central nervous system: Flu syndrome, fever, dizziness, depression, hypesthesia

Dermatologic: Alopecia, dry skin, rash

Gastrointestinal: Dyspepsia, vomiting, abdominal pain

Genitourinary: Urinary tract infection, hematuria, urinary tract disorder, nocturia

Respiratory: Dyspnea, upper respiratory infection, pneumonia

Ocular: Chromatopsia, impaired adaption to light, abnormal vision

Miscellaneous: Diaphoresis

**Half-Life** 38-59 hours

**Special PA Issues**

**Patient Education:** Take as prescribed; do not change dosing schedule or stop taking without consulting prescriber. Avoid alcohol while taking this medication; may cause severe reaction. Periodic laboratory tests are necessary while taking this medication. You may experience dizziness, confusion, or blurred vision (avoid driving or engaging in tasks that require alertness until response to drug is known); loss of light accommodation (avoid night driving and use caution in poorly lighted or changing light situations); impotence; or loss of libido (discuss with prescriber). Report any decreased respiratory function (eg, dyspnea, increased cough); yellowing of skin or eyes; change in color of urine or stool; unusual bruising or bleeding; chest pain; difficulty or painful voiding.

**Dietary Considerations:** Food: Can be taken without regard to food

**Monitoring Parameters:**

Perform routine chest x-rays before treatment, and tell patients to report immediately any dyspnea or aggravation of pre-existing dyspnea. At the onset of dyspnea or worsening of pre-existing dyspnea any time during therapy, interrupt nilutamide until it can be determined if respiratory symptoms are drug-related. Obtain a chest x-ray, and if there are findings suggestive of interstitial pneumonitis, discontinue treatment with nilutamide. The pneumonitis is almost always reversible when treatment is discontinued. If the chest x-ray appears normal, perform pulmonary function tests.

Measure serum hepatic enzyme levels at baseline and at regular intervals (3 months); if transaminases increase over 2-3 times the upper limit of normal, discontinue treatment. Perform appropriate laboratory testing at the first symptom/sign of liver injury (eg, jaundice, dark urine, fatigue, abdominal pain or unexplained GI symptoms ) and nilutamide treatment must be discontinued immediately if transaminases exceed 3 times the upper limit of normal.

# Nimodipine (nye MOE di peen)

**Pharmacologic Class** Calcium Channel Blocker

**U.S. Brand Names** Nimotop®

**Mechanism of Action** Nimodipine shares the pharmacology of other calcium channel blockers; animal studies indicate that nimodipine has a greater effect on cerebral arterials than other arterials; this increased specificity may be due to the drug's increased lipophilicity and cerebral distribution as compared to nifedipine; inhibits calcium ion from entering the "slow channels" or select voltage sensitive areas of vascular smooth muscle and myocardium during depolarization

**Use** Improvement of neurological deficits due to spasm following subarachnoid hemorrhage from ruptured congenital intracranial aneurysms in patients who are in good neurological condition postictus

**USUAL DOSAGE** Adults: Oral: 60 mg every 4 hours for 21 days, start therapy within 96 hours after subarachnoid hemorrhage

Dialysis: Not removed by hemo- or peritoneal dialysis; supplemental dose is not necessary

**Dosing adjustment in hepatic impairment:** Reduce dosage to 30 mg every 4 hours in patients with liver failure

**Dosage Forms Cap, liquid-filled:** 30 mg

**Contraindications** Hypersensitivity to nimodipine or any component

**Warnings/Precautions** Use with caution and titrate dosages for patients with impaired renal or hepatic function; use caution when treating patients with congestive heart failure, sick-sinus syndrome, PVCs, severe left ventricular dysfunction, hypertrophic cardiomyopathy (especially obstructive, IHSS), concomitant therapy with beta-blockers or digoxin, edema, or increased intracranial pressure with cranial tumors; do not abruptly withdraw (may cause chest pain); elderly may experience hypotension and constipation more readily

**Pregnancy Risk Factor** C

(Continued)

## Nimodipine *(Continued)*

### Pregnancy Implications

Clinical effects on the fetus: Use in pregnancy only when clearly needed and when the benefits outweigh the potential hazard to the fetus. Teratogenic and embryotoxic effects have been demonstrated in small animals. No well controlled studies have been conducted in pregnant women.

Breast milk/lactation: Appears in breast milk at levels higher than maternal plasma levels; no recommendations are currently available on breast-feeding

### Adverse Reactions

1% to 10%:

Cardiovascular: Reductions in systemic blood pressure (1.2% to 8.1%)

Central nervous system: Headache (1.4% to 4.1%)

Dermatologic: Rash (0.6% to 2.4%)

Gastrointestinal: Diarrhea (1.7% to 4.2%), abdominal discomfort (2%)

<1%: Edema (0.4% to 1.2%), EKG abnormalities (0.6% to 1.4%), tachycardia, bradycardia, depression, acne, nausea (0.6% to 1.4%), hemorrhage, hepatitis, muscle cramps (0.2% to 1.4%), dyspnea

### Drug Interactions CYP3A3/4 enzyme substrate

Increased toxicity/effect/levels:

Nimodipine and cimetidine may increase bioavailability of nimodipine as with other calcium blockers

Nimodipine and omeprazole may increase bioavailability of nimodipine

Nimodipine, propranolol, and other beta-blockers may have minimal increase of depressant effects on A-V conduction

### Half-Life 3 hours, increases with reduced renal function

### Special PA Issues

Patient Education: Take as prescribed, for the length of time prescribed; do not discontinue without consulting prescriber. You may experience headache (if unrelieved, consult prescriber), nausea or vomiting (frequent small meals may help), constipation (increased dietary bulk and fluids may help). Promptly report any chest pain or swelling of hands or feet, respiratory distress, sudden weight gain, or unresolved constipation.

♦ **Nimotop®** see Nimodipine *on previous page*

## Nisoldipine (NYE sole di peen)

**Pharmacologic Class** Calcium Channel Blocker

**U.S. Brand Names** Sular®

**Mechanism of Action** As a dihydropyridine calcium channel blocker, structurally similar to nifedipine, nisoldipine impedes the movement of calcium ions into vascular smooth muscle and cardiac muscle. Dihydropyridines are potent vasodilators and are not as likely to suppress cardiac contractility and slow cardiac conduction as other calcium antagonists such as verapamil and diltiazem; nisoldipine is 5-10 times as potent a vasodilator as nifedipine.

**Use** Management of hypertension, may be used alone or in combination with other antihypertensive agents

**USUAL DOSAGE** Adults: Oral: Initial: 20 mg once daily, then increase by 10 mg/week (or longer intervals) to attain adequate control of blood pressure; doses >60 mg once daily are not recommended. A starting dose not exceeding 10 mg/day is recommended for the elderly and those with hepatic impairment.

**Dosage Forms Tab, extended release:** 10 mg, 20 mg, 30 mg, 40 mg

**Contraindications** Hypersensitivity to nisoldipine or any component or other dihydropyridine calcium channel blocker

**Warnings/Precautions** Increased angina and/or myocardial infarction in patients with coronary artery disease

**Pregnancy Risk Factor** C

**Adverse Reactions**

Cardiovascular: Peripheral edema, tachycardia

Central nervous system: Dizziness, headache

**Drug Interactions** CYP3A3/4 enzyme substrate

Increased toxicity:

Nisoldipine and digoxin may increase digoxin effect

Nisoldipine, propranolol, and other beta-blockers may increase cardiovascular adverse effects

Nisoldipine and $H_2$-antagonists (cimetidine) increase bioavailability and may increase nisoldipine serum concentration

Nisoldipine and omeprazole increase bioavailability and may increase nisoldipine serum concentration

**Duration** >24 hours

**Half-Life** 7-12 hours

**Special PA Issues**

**Patient Education:** Take as prescribed - swallow whole (do not crush or break). May be taken with food but avoid grapefruit products and high fat foods. Do not stop abruptly without consulting prescriber. You may experience headache (if unrelieved, consult prescriber), nausea or vomiting (frequent small meals may help), constipation (increased dietary bulk and fluids may help), depression (should resolve when drug is discontinued). May cause dizziness or drowsiness; use caution when driving or engaging in hazardous activities. Promptly report any chest pain or swelling of hands or feet, respiratory distress, sudden weight gain, or unresolved constipation.

**Dietary Considerations:** Avoid grapefruit products before and after dosing

**Related Information**

Calcium Channel Blocking Agents *on page 1004*

- ◆ **Nitalapram** *see* Citalopram *on page 213*
- ◆ **Nitrek® Patch** *see* Nitroglycerin *on next page*
- ◆ **Nitro-Bid® I.V. Injection** *see* Nitroglycerin *on next page*
- ◆ **Nitro-Bid® Ointment** *see* Nitroglycerin *on next page*
- ◆ **Nitrodisc® Patch** *see* Nitroglycerin *on next page*
- ◆ **Nitro-Dur® Patch** *see* Nitroglycerin *on next page*
- ◆ **Nitrofural** *see* Nitrofurazone *on next page*

## Nitrofurantoin (nye troe fyoor AN toyn)

**Pharmacologic Class** Antibiotic, Miscellaneous

**U.S. Brand Names** Furadantin®; Furalan®; Furan®; Furanite®; Macrobid®; Macrodantin®

**Mechanism of Action** Inhibits several bacterial enzyme systems including acetyl coenzyme A interfering with metabolism and possibly cell wall synthesis

**Use** Prevention and treatment of urinary tract infections caused by susceptible gram-negative and some gram-positive organisms; *Pseudomonas*, *Serratia*, and most species of *Proteus* are generally resistant to nitrofurantoin

**USUAL DOSAGE** Oral:

Children >1 month: 5-7 mg/kg/day in divided doses every 6 hours; maximum: 400 mg/day
Chronic therapy: 1-2 mg/kg/day in divided doses every 12-24 hours; maximum dose: 100 mg/day

Adults: 50-100 mg/dose every 6 hours

Macrocrystal/monohydrate: 100 mg twice daily

Prophylaxis or chronic therapy: 50-100 mg/dose at bedtime

**Dosing adjustment in renal impairment:** Cl$_{cr}$ <50 mL/minute: Avoid use

Avoid use in hemo and peritoneal dialysis and continuous arteriovenous or venovenous hemofiltration (CAVH/CAVHD)

**Dosage Forms Cap:** 50 mg, 100 mg; **Capsule: Macrocrystal:** 25 mg, 50 mg, 100 mg; **Macrocrystal/monohydrate:** 100 mg; **Susp, oral:** 25 mg/5 mL (470 mL)

**Contraindications** Hypersensitivity to nitrofurantoin or any component; renal impairment; infants <1 month (due to the possibility of hemolytic anemia)

**Warnings/Precautions** Use with caution in patients with G-6-PD deficiency, patients with anemia, vitamin B deficiency, diabetes mellitus or electrolyte abnormalities; therapeutic concentrations of nitrofurantoin are not attained in urine of patients with Cl$_{cr}$ <40 mL/minute (elderly); use with caution if prolonged therapy is anticipated due to possible pulmonary toxicity; acute, subacute, or chronic (usually after 6 months of therapy) pulmonary reactions have been observed in patients treated with nitrofurantoin; if these occur, discontinue therapy; monitor closely for malaise, dyspnea, cough, fever, radiologic evidence of diffuse interstitial pneumonitis or fibrosis

**Pregnancy Risk Factor** B

**Adverse Reactions** Percentage unknown: Chest pains, chills, fever, fatigue, drowsiness, headache, dizziness, rash, itching, lupus-like syndrome, exfoliative dermatitis, stomach upset, diarrhea, loss of appetite/vomiting/nausea (most common), sore throat, hemolytic anemia, hepatitis, hypersensitivity, increased LFTs, weakness, paresthesia, numbness, arthralgia, cough, dyspnea, hypersensitivity

**Drug Interactions**

Decreased effect: Antacids, especially magnesium salts, decrease absorption of nitrofurantoin; nitrofurantoin may antagonize effects of norfloxacin

Increased toxicity: Probenecid (decreases renal excretion of nitrofurantoin); anticholinergic drugs increase absorption of nitrofurantoin

**Half-Life** 20-60 minutes; prolonged with renal impairment

**Special PA Issues**

**Patient Education:** Take as directed, at regular intervals, around-the-clock, with food or milk. Maintain adequate hydration (2-3 L/day of fluids unless instructed to restrict fluid intake). Avoid alcohol. Diabetics should not use Clinitest®; consult prescriber for alternative method of glucose testing. This may discolor urine dark yellow or brown (normal). Small frequent meals, sucking on lozenges, or chewing gum may relieve nausea or vomiting. If experiencing blurred vision or dizziness, avoid driving or other hazardous activities. Report rash, painful urination, fever or chills, cough or difficulty breathing, numbness or tingling in hands or feet.

(Continued)

## Nitrofurantoin *(Continued)*

**Dietary Considerations:** Alcohol: Avoid use

**Monitoring Parameters:** Signs of pulmonary reaction, signs of numbness or tingling of the extremities, periodic liver function tests

## Nitrofurazone *(nye troe FYOOR a zone)*

**Pharmacologic Class** Antibiotic, Topical

**U.S. Brand Names** Furacin® Topical

**Mechanism of Action** A broad antibacterial spectrum; it acts by inhibiting bacterial enzymes involved in carbohydrate metabolism; effective against a wide range of gram-negative and gram-positive organisms; bactericidal against most bacteria commonly causing surface infections including *Staphylococcus aureus*, *Streptococcus*, *Escherichia coli*, *Enterobacter cloacae*, *Clostridium perfringens*, *Aerobacter aerogenes*, and *Proteus* sp; not particularly active against most *Pseudomonas aeruginosa* strains and does not inhibit viruses or fungi. Topical preparations of nitrofurazone are readily soluble in blood, pus, and serum and are nonmacerating.

**Use** Antibacterial agent in second and third degree burns and skin grafting

**USUAL DOSAGE** Children and Adults: Topical: Apply once daily or every few days to lesion or place on gauze

**Dosage Forms Crm:** 0.2% (4 g, 28 g); **Oint, soluble dressing:** 0.2% (28 g, 56 g, 454 g, 480 g); **Soln, top:** 0.2% (480 mL, 3780 mL)

**Contraindications** Hypersensitivity to nitrofurazone or any component

**Warnings/Precautions** Use with caution in patients with renal impairment and patients with G-6-PD deficiency

**Pregnancy Risk Factor** C

**Adverse Reactions** Women should inform their physicians if signs or symptoms of any of the following occur thromboembolic or thrombotic disorders including sudden severe headache or vomiting, disturbance of vision or speech, loss of vision, numbness or weakness in an extremity, sharp or crushing chest pain, calf pain, shortness of breath, severe abdominal pain or mass, mental depression or unusual bleeding

Women should discontinue taking the medication if they suspect they are pregnant or become pregnant. Notify physician if area under dermal patch becomes irritated or a rash develops.

**Drug Interactions** Decreased effect: Sutilains decrease activity of nitrofurazone

**Special PA Issues**

**Patient Education:** Follow specific prescriber instructions for application. Protect skin around treated areas with Vaseline® or zinc ointment. Do not apply to skin around eyes. Report signs of sensitization reaction (eg, swelling, redness, itching, burning).

♦ **Nitrogard® Buccal** *see* Nitroglycerin *on this page*

## Nitroglycerin *(nye troe GLI ser in)*

**Pharmacologic Class** Vasodilator

**U.S. Brand Names** Deponit® Patch; Minitran® Patch; Nitrek® Patch; Nitro-Bid® I.V. Injection; Nitro-Bid® Ointment; Nitrodisc® Patch; Nitro-Dur® Patch; Nitrogard® Buccal; Nitroglyn® Oral; Nitrolingual® Translingual Spray; Nitrol® Ointment; Nitrong® Oral Tablet; Nitrostat® Sublingual; Nitro-Time® Capsules; Transderm-NTG® Patch; Transderm-Nitro® Patch; Tridil® Injection

**Mechanism of Action** Reduces cardiac oxygen demand by decreasing left ventricular pressure and systemic vascular resistance; dilates coronary arteries and improves collateral flow to ischemic regions

**Use** Treatment and prevention of angina pectoris; I.V. for congestive heart failure (especially when associated with acute myocardial infarction); pulmonary hypertension; hypertensive emergencies occurring perioperatively (especially during cardiovascular surgery)

**USUAL DOSAGE Note:** Hemodynamic and antianginal tolerance often develop within 24-48 hours of continuous nitrate administration

Children: Pulmonary hypertension: Continuous infusion: Start 0.25-0.5 mcg/kg/minute and titrate by 1 mcg/kg/minute at 20- to 60-minute intervals to desired effect; usual dose: 1-3 mcg/kg/minute; maximum: 5 mcg/kg/minute

Adults:

Buccal: Initial: 1 mg every 3-5 hours while awake (3 times/day); titrate dosage upward if angina occurs with tablet in place

Oral: 2.5-9 mg 2-4 times/day (up to 26 mg 4 times/day)

I.V.: 5 mcg/minute, increase by 5 mcg/minute every 3-5 minutes to 20 mcg/minute; if no response at 20 mcg/minute increase by 10 mcg/minute every 3-5 minutes, up to 200 mcg/minute

Ointment: ½" upon rising and ½" 6 hours later; the dose may be doubled and even doubled again as needed

Patch, transdermal: Initial: 0.2-0.4 mg/hour, titrate to doses of 0.4-0.8 mg/hour; tolerance is minimized by using a patch-on period of 12-14 hours and patch-off period of 10-12 hours

Sublingual: 0.2-0.6 mg every 5 minutes for maximum of 3 doses in 15 minutes; may also use prophylactically 5-10 minutes prior to activities which may provoke an attack

Translingual: 1-2 sprays into mouth under tongue every 3-5 minutes for maximum of 3 doses in 15 minutes, may also be used 5-10 minutes prior to activities which may provoke an attack prophylactically

Hemodialysis: Supplemental dose is not necessary

Peritoneal dialysis: Supplemental dose is not necessary

**May need to use nitrate-free interval (10-12 hours/day) to avoid tolerance development; gradually decrease dose in patients receiving NTG for prolonged period to avoid withdrawal reaction**

**Dosage Forms Cap, sustained release:** 2.5 mg, 6.5 mg, 9 mg; **Inj:** 0.5 mg/mL (10 mL), 0.8 mg/mL (10 mL), 5 mg/mL (1 mL, 5 mL, 10 mL, 20 mL), 10 mg/mL (5 mL, 10 mL); **Oint, top (Nitrol®):** 2% [20 mg/g] (30 g, 60 g); **Patch, transdermal, top:** Systems designed to deliver 2.5, 5, 7.5, 10, or 15 mg NTG over 24 hours; **Spray, translingual:** 0.4 mg/metered spray (13.8 g); **Tab: Buccal, controlled release:** 1 mg, 2 mg, 3 mg; **Sublingual (Nitrostat®):** 0.3 mg, 0.4 mg, 0.6 mg; **Sustained release:** 2.6 mg, 6.5 mg, 9 mg

**Contraindications** Hypersensitivity to nitroglycerin or any component; pericardial tamponade, restrictive cardiomyopathy, or constrictive pericarditis; allergy to adhesive (transdermal), uncorrected hypovolemia (I.V.); transdermal NTG is not effective for immediate relief of angina

**Warnings/Precautions** Do not use extended release preparations in patients with GI hypermotility or malabsorptive syndrome; use with caution in patients with hepatic impairment, CHF, or acute myocardial infarction; available preparations of I.V. nitroglycerin differ in concentration or volume; pay attention to dilution and dosage; I.V. preparations contain alcohol and/or propylene glycol; avoid loss of nitroglycerin in standard PVC tubing; dosing instructions must be followed with care when the appropriate infusion sets are used

Hypotension may occur, use with caution in patients who are volume-depleted, are hypotensive, have inadequate circulation; nitrate therapy may aggravate angina caused by hypertrophic cardiomyopathy

**Pregnancy Risk Factor** C

**Adverse Reactions**

Cardiovascular: Reflex tachycardia, hypotension, syncope, angina, rebound hypertension, bradycardia

Central nervous system: Headache (especially at higher doses, may be recurrent with each daily dose), lightheadedness

Dermatologic: Contact dermatitis, fixed drug eruptions (with ointments or patches)

Hematologic: Methemoglobinemia (very rare)

**Drug Interactions**

Decreased effect: I.V. nitroglycerin may antagonize the anticoagulant effect of heparin, monitor closely; may need to decrease heparin dosage when nitroglycerin is discontinued

Increased toxicity: Alcohol, other vasodilators (eg, calcium channel blockers) may enhance nitroglycerin's hypotensive effect

**Onset**

Sublingual tablet: 1-3 minutes

Translingual spray: 2 minutes

Buccal tablet: 2-5 minutes

Sustained release: 20-45 minutes

Topical: 15-60 minutes

Transdermal: 40-60 minutes

I.V. drip: Immediate

**Duration**

Sublingual tablet: 30-60 minutes

Translingual spray: 30-60 minutes

Buccal tablet: 2 hours

Sustained release: 4-8 hours

Topical: 2-12 hours

Transdermal: 18-24 hours

I.V. drip: 3-5 minutes

**Half-Life** 1-4 minutes

**Special PA Issues**

**Patient Education:**

Oral: Take as directed. Do not chew or swallow sublingual tablets; allow to dissolve under tongue. Do not chew or crush extended release capsules; swallow with 8 oz of water.

Spray. Spray directly on mucous members; do not inhale.

Topical: Spread prescribed amount thinly on applicator; rotate application sites.

Transdermal: Place on hair-free area of skin, rotate sites.

Do not change brands without consulting prescriber. Do not discontinue abruptly. Keep medication in original container, tightly closed. Take medication while sitting down and use caution when changing position (rise from sitting or lying position slowly). May cause dizziness; use caution when driving or engaging in hazardous activities until response to drug is known. If chest pain is unresolved in 15 minutes, seek emergency medical help at (Continued)

## Nitroglycerin *(Continued)*

once. Report acute headache, rapid heartbeat, unusual restlessness or dizziness, muscular weakness, or blurring vision.

**Monitoring Parameters:** Blood pressure, heart rate

- ◆ **Nitroglycerol** *see Nitroglycerin on page 660*
- ◆ **Nitroglyn® Oral** *see Nitroglycerin on page 660*
- ◆ **Nitrolingual® Translingual Spray** *see Nitroglycerin on page 660*
- ◆ **Nitrol® Ointment** *see Nitroglycerin on page 660*
- ◆ **Nitrong® Oral Tablet** *see Nitroglycerin on page 660*
- ◆ **Nitropress®** *see Nitroprusside on this page*

## Nitroprusside *(nye troe PRUS ide)*

**Pharmacologic Class** Vasodilator

**U.S. Brand Names** Nitropress®

**Mechanism of Action** Causes peripheral vasodilation by direct action on venous and arteriolar smooth muscle, thus reducing peripheral resistance; will increase cardiac output by decreasing afterload; reduces aortal and left ventricular impedance

**Use** Management of hypertensive crises; congestive heart failure; used for controlled hypotension to reduce bleeding during surgery

**USUAL DOSAGE** Administration requires the use of an infusion pump. Average dose: 5 mcg/kg/minute

Children: Pulmonary hypertension: I.V.: Initial: 1 mcg/kg/minute by continuous I.V. infusion; increase in increments of 1 mcg/kg/minute at intervals of 20-60 minutes; titrating to the desired response; usual dose: 3 mcg/kg/minute, rarely need >4 mcg/kg/minute; maximum: 5 mcg/kg/minute.

Adults: I.V. Initial: 0.3-0.5 mcg/kg/minute; increase in increments of 0.5 mcg/kg/minute, titrating to the desired hemodynamic effect or the appearance of headache or nausea; usual dose: 3 mcg/kg/minute; rarely need >4 mcg/kg/minute; maximum: 10 mcg/kg/minute. When >500 mcg/kg is administered by prolonged infusion of faster than 2 mcg/kg/minute, cyanide is generated faster than an unaided patient can handle.

**Dosage Forms Inj, as sodium:** 10 mg/mL (5 mL); 25 mg/mL (2 mL)

**Contraindications** Hypersensitivity to nitroprusside or components; decreased cerebral perfusion; arteriovenous shunt or coarctation of the aorta (ie, compensatory hypertension)

**Warnings/Precautions** Use with caution in patients with increased intracranial pressure (head trauma, cerebral hemorrhage); severe renal impairment, hepatic failure, hypothyroidism; use only as an infusion with 5% dextrose in water; continuously monitor patient's blood pressure; excessive amounts of nitroprusside can cause cyanide toxicity (usually in patients with decreased liver function) or thiocyanate toxicity (usually in patients with decreased renal function, or in patients with normal renal function but prolonged nitroprusside use)

**Pregnancy Risk Factor** C

**Adverse Reactions**

Cardiovascular: Excessive hypotensive response, palpitations, substernal distress

Central nervous system: Disorientation, psychosis, headache, restlessness

Endocrine & metabolic: Thyroid suppression

Gastrointestinal: Nausea, vomiting

Hematologic: Methemoglobinemia (in high-dose and prolonged infusions)

Neuromuscular & skeletal: Weakness, muscle spasm

Otic: Tinnitus

Respiratory: Hypoxia

Miscellaneous: Diaphoresis, thiocyanate toxicity

**Onset** Onset of hypotensive effect: <2 minutes

**Duration** Within 1-10 minutes following discontinuation of therapy, effects cease

**Half-Life** Parent drug: <10 minutes; Thiocyanate: 2.7-7 days

**Special PA Issues**

**Patient Education:** Patient condition should indicate extent of education and instruction needed. This drug can only be given I.V. You will be monitored at all times during infusion. Promptly report any chest pain or pain/burning at site of infusion.

**Monitoring Parameters:** Blood pressure, heart rate; monitor for cyanide and thiocyanate toxicity; monitor acid-base status as acidosis can be the earliest sign of cyanide toxicity; monitor thiocyanate levels if requiring prolonged infusion (>3 days) or dose ≥4 mcg/kg/minute or patient has renal dysfunction; monitor cyanide blood levels in patients with decreased hepatic function; cardiac monitor and blood pressure monitor required

**Reference Range:** Monitor thiocyanate levels if requiring prolonged infusion (>4 days) or ≥4 µg/kg/minute; not to exceed 100 µg/mL (or 10 mg/dL) plasma thiocyanate

Thiocyanate:
Therapeutic: 6-29 µg/mL
Toxic: 35-100 µg/mL
Fatal: >200 µg/mL

Cyanide: Normal <0.2 µg/mL; normal (smoker): <0.4 µg/mL
Toxic: >2 µg/mL
Potentially lethal: >3 µg/mL

♦ **Nitroprusside Sodium** *see* Nitroprusside *on previous page*
♦ **Nitrostat® Sublingual** *see* Nitroglycerin *on page 660*
♦ **Nitro-Time® Capsules** *see* Nitroglycerin *on page 660*
♦ **Nix™ Creme Rinse** *see* Permethrin *on page 712*

# Nizatidine (ni ZA ti deen)

**Pharmacologic Class** Histamine $H_2$ Antagonist

**U.S. Brand Names** Axid® AR [OTC]; Axid®

**Mechanism of Action** Nizatidine is an $H_2$-receptor antagonist. In healthy volunteers, nizatidine has been effective in suppressing gastric acid secretion induced by pentagastrin infusion or food. Nizatidine reduces gastric acid secretion by 29.4% to 78.4%. This compares with a 60.3% reduction by cimetidine. Nizatidine 100 mg is reported to provide equivalent acid suppression as cimetidine 300 mg.

**Use** Treatment and maintenance of duodenal ulcer; treatment of gastroesophageal reflux disease (GERD); OTC tablet used for the prevention of meal-induced heartburn, acid indigestion, and sour stomach

**USUAL DOSAGE** Adults: Oral:

Active duodenal ulcer:
Treatment: 300 mg at bedtime or 150 mg twice daily
Maintenance: 150 mg/day

Meal-induced heartburn, acid indigestion, and sour stomach:
75 mg tablet [OTC] twice daily, 30 to 60 minutes prior to consuming food or beverages

**Dosing adjustment in renal impairment:**
$Cl_{cr}$ 50-80 mL/minute: Administer 75% of normal dose
$Cl_{cr}$ 10-50 mL/minute: Administer 50% of normal dose or 150 mg/day for active treatment and 150 mg every other day for maintenance treatment
$Cl_{cr}$ <10 mL/minute: Administer 25% of normal dose or 150 mg every other day for treatment and 150 mg every 3 days for maintenance treatment

**Dosage Forms Cap:** 150 mg, 300 mg; **Tab:** 75 mg

**Contraindications** Hypersensitivity to nizatidine or any component of the preparation; hypersensitivity to other $H_2$-antagonists since a cross-sensitivity has been observed with this class of drugs

**Warnings/Precautions** Use with caution in children <12 years of age; use with caution in patients with liver and renal impairment; dosage modification required in patients with renal impairment

**Pregnancy Risk Factor** C

**Adverse Reactions**

1% to 10%:
Central nervous system: Dizziness, headache
Gastrointestinal: Constipation, diarrhea

<1%: Bradycardia, tachycardia, palpitations, hypertension, fever, fatigue, seizures, insomnia, drowsiness, acne, pruritus, urticaria, dry skin, abdominal discomfort, flatulence, belching, anorexia, agranulocytosis, neutropenia, thrombocytopenia, increased AST/ALT, paresthesia, weakness, increased BUN/creatinine, proteinuria, bronchospasm, allergic reaction

**Half-Life** Normal renal function: 1-2 hours; End-stage renal disease: 3.5-11 hours

**Special PA Issues**

**Patient Education:** Take as directed; do not increase dose. It may take several days before you notice relief. If antacids approved by prescriber, take 1 hour between antacid and nizatidine. Avoid OTC medications, especially cold or cough medication and aspirin or anything containing aspirin. Follow ulcer diet as prescriber recommends. May cause drowsiness; use caution when driving or engaging in hazardous activities. Report fever, sore throat, tarry stools, changes in CNS, or muscle or joint pain.

♦ **Nizoral®** *see* Ketoconazole *on page 506*
♦ **N-Methylhydrazine** *see* Procarbazine *on page 761*
♦ **Nobesine®** *see* Diethylpropion *on page 277*
♦ **Nolamine®** *see* Chlorpheniramine, Phenindamine, and Phenylpropanolamine *on page 196*
♦ **Nolvadex®** *see* Tamoxifen *on page 871*
♦ **Nonsteroidal Anti-Inflammatory Agents** *see* Chart *on page 1026*
♦ **Norcet®** *see* Hydrocodone and Acetaminophen *on page 449*
♦ **Nordeoxyguanosine** *see* Ganciclovir *on page 408*
♦ **Nordette®** *see* Ethinyl Estradiol and Levonorgestrel *on page 347*
♦ **Norditropin® Injection** *see* Human Growth Hormone *on page 444*
♦ **Nordryl® Injection** *see* Diphenhydramine *on page 289*
♦ **Nordryl® Oral** *see* Diphenhydramine *on page 289*
♦ **Norethin™ 1/35E** *see* Ethinyl Estradiol and Norethindrone *on page 348*

♦ **Norethin™ 1/50M** *see* Mestranol and Norethindrone *on page 573*

♦ **Norethindrone Acetate and Ethinyl Estradiol** *see* Ethinyl Estradiol and Norethindrone *on page 348*

♦ **Norethindrone and Mestranol** *see* Mestranol and Norethindrone *on page 573*

♦ **Norflex™** *see* Orphenadrine *on page 680*

## Norfloxacin (nor FLOKS a sin)

**Pharmacologic Class** Antibiotic, Quinolone

**U.S. Brand Names** Chibroxin™ Ophthalmic; Noroxin® Oral

**Mechanism of Action** Norfloxacin is a DNA gyrase inhibitor. DNA gyrase is an essential bacterial enzyme that maintains the superhelical structure of DNA. DNA gyrase is required for DNA replication and transcription, DNA repair, recombination, and transposition; bactericidal

**Use** Uncomplicated urinary tract infections and cystitis caused by susceptible gram-negative and gram-positive bacteria; sexually transmitted disease (eg, uncomplicated urethral and cervical gonorrhea) caused by *N. gonorrhoeae*; prostatitis due to *E. coli*; ophthalmic solution for conjunctivitis

**USUAL DOSAGE**

Ophthalmic: Children >1 year and Adults: Instill 1-2 drops in affected eye(s) 4 times/day for up to 7 days

Oral: Adults:

Urinary tract infections: 400 mg twice daily for 3-21 days depending on severity of infection or organism sensitivity; maximum: 800 mg/day

Uncomplicated gonorrhea: 800 mg as a single dose (CDC recommends as an alternative regimen to ciprofloxacin or ofloxacin)

Prostatitis: 400 mg every 12 hours for 4 weeks

**Dosing interval in renal impairment:**

$Cl_{cr}$ 10-30 mL/minute: Administer every 24 hours

$Cl_{cr}$ <10 mL/minute: Do not use

**Dosage Forms Soln, ophth:** 0.3% [3 mg/mL] (5 mL); **Tab:** 400 mg

**Contraindications** Known hypersensitivity to quinolones

**Warnings/Precautions** Not recommended in children <18 years of age; other quinolones have caused transient arthropathy in children; CNS stimulation may occur which may lead to tremor, restlessness, confusion, and very rarely to hallucinations or convulsive seizures; use with caution in patients with known or suspected CNS disorders; has rarely caused ruptured tendons (discontinue immediately with signs of inflammation or tendon pain)

**Pregnancy Risk Factor** C

**Adverse Reactions**

1% to 10%:

Central nervous system: Headache (2.7%), dizziness (1.8%), fatigue

Gastrointestinal: Nausea (2.8%)

<1%: Somnolence, depression, insomnia, fever, pruritus, hyperhidrosis, erythema, rash, abdominal pain, dyspepsia, constipation, flatulence, heartburn, xerostomia, diarrhea, vomiting, loose stools, anorexia, bitter taste, GI bleeding, increased liver enzymes, back pain, ruptured tendons, weakness, increased serum creatinine/BUN, acute renal failure

**Drug Interactions** CYP1A2 and 3A3/4 enzyme inhibitor

Decreased effect: Decreased absorption with antacids containing aluminum, magnesium, and/or calcium (by up to 98% if given at the same time); decreased serum levels of fluoroquinolones by antineoplastics; nitrofurantoin may antagonize effects of norfloxacin; phenytoin serum levels may be decreased by fluoroquinolones

Increased toxicity/serum levels: Quinolones cause increased levels or toxicity of digoxin, caffeine, warfarin, cyclosporine, and possibly theophylline. Cimetidine and probenecid increase quinolone levels.

**Half-Life** 4.8 hours (can be higher with reduced glomerular filtration rates)

**Special PA Issues**

**Patient Education:**

Oral: Take per recommended schedule, preferably on empty stomach (1 hour before or 2 hours after meals). Maintain adequate hydration (2-3 L/day of fluids unless instructed to restrict fluid intake). Take complete prescription; do not skip doses. Do not take with antacids. You may experience dizziness, lightheadedness; use caution when driving or engaging in tasks that require alertness. Small frequent meals and frequent mouth care may reduce nausea or vomiting. You may experience photosensitivity; use sunblock, wear protective clothing, or avoid direct sun. Report persistent diarrhea or GI disturbances; excessive sleepiness or agitation; tremors; rash; pain, inflammation, or rupture of tendon; or changes in vision.

Ophthalmic: Tilt head back and instill 1-2 drops in affected eye 4 times a day for length of time prescribed. Do not allow tip of applicator to touch eye or any contaminated surface.

♦ **Norgesic™** *see* Orphenadrine, Aspirin, and Caffeine *on page 681*

♦ **Norgesic™ Forte** *see* Orphenadrine, Aspirin, and Caffeine *on page 681*

♦ **Norgestimate and Ethinyl Estradiol** *see* Ethinyl Estradiol and Norgestimate *on page 350*

## Norgestrel (nor JES trel)

**Pharmacologic Class** Contraceptive

**U.S. Brand Names** Ovrette®

**Mechanism of Action** Inhibits secretion of pituitary gonadotropin (LH) which prevents follicular maturation and ovulation

**Use** Prevention of pregnancy; **progestin only products have higher risk of failure in contraceptive use**

**USUAL DOSAGE** Administer daily, starting the first day of menstruation, take 1 tablet at the same time each day, every day of the year. If one dose is missed, take as soon as remembered, then next tablet at regular time; if two doses are missed, take 1 tablet and discard the other, then take daily at usual time; if three doses are missed, use an additional form of birth control until menses or pregnancy is ruled out.

**Dosage Forms Tab:** 0.075 mg

**Contraindications** Known hypersensitivity to norgestrel; thromboembolic disorders, severe hepatic disease, breast cancer, undiagnosed vaginal bleeding, pregnancy

**Warnings/Precautions** Discontinue if sudden loss of vision or if diplopia or proptosis occur; use with caution in patients with a history of mental depression; use of any progestin during the first 4 months of pregnancy is not recommended

**Pregnancy Risk Factor** X

**Adverse Reactions**

>10%:

Cardiovascular: Edema

Endocrine & metabolic: Breakthrough bleeding, spotting, changes in menstrual flow, amenorrhea

Gastrointestinal: Anorexia

Neuromuscular & skeletal: Weakness

1% to 10%:

Cardiovascular: Embolism, central thrombosis

Central nervous system: Mental depression, fever, insomnia

Dermatologic: Melasma or chloasma, allergic rash with or without pruritus

Endocrine & metabolic: Changes in cervical erosion and secretions, increased breast tenderness

Gastrointestinal: Weight gain or loss

Hepatic: Cholestatic jaundice

Local: Thrombophlebitis

**Drug Interactions** Decreased effect: Aminoglutethimide may decrease effects by increasing hepatic metabolism

**Special PA Issues**

**Patient Education:** Take this medicine only as directed; do not take more of it and do not take it for a longer period of time; if you suspect you may have become pregnant, stop taking this medicine; report any loss of vision or vision changes immediately; avoid excessive exposure to sunlight

♦ **Norgestrel and Ethinyl Estradiol** see Ethinyl Estradiol and Norgestrel on page 351

♦ **Norinyl® 1+35** see Ethinyl Estradiol and Norethindrone on page 348

♦ **Norinyl® 1+50** see Mestranol and Norethindrone on page 573

♦ **Norisodrine®** see Isoproterenol on page 496

♦ **Noritate® Cream** see Metronidazole on page 601

♦ **Normal Human Serum Albumin** see Albumin on page 34

♦ **Normal Saline** see Sodium Chloride on page 839

♦ **Normal Serum Albumin (Human)** see Albumin on page 34

♦ **Normiflo®** see Ardeparin on page 77

♦ **Normodyne®** see Labetalol on page 510

♦ **Noroxin® Oral** see Norfloxacin on previous page

♦ **Norpace®** see Disopyramide on page 295

♦ **Norplant® Implant** see Levonorgestrel on page 528

♦ **Norpramin®** see Desipramine on page 260

♦ **Nor-tet® Oral** see Tetracycline on page 885

## Nortriptyline (nor TRIP ti leen)

**Pharmacologic Class** Antidepressant, Tricyclic (Secondary Amine)

**U.S. Brand Names** Aventyl® Hydrochloride; Pamelor®

**Mechanism of Action** Traditionally believed to increase the synaptic concentration of serotonin and/or norepinephrine in the central nervous system by inhibition of their reuptake by the presynaptic neuronal membrane. However, additional receptor effects have been found including desensitization of adenyl cyclase, down regulation of beta-adrenergic receptors, and down regulation of serotonin receptors.

**Use** Treatment of various forms of depression, often in conjunction with psychotherapy. Maximum antidepressant effect may not be seen for 2 or more weeks after initiation of therapy; has also demonstrated effectiveness for chronic pain.

(Continued)

## Nortriptyline *(Continued)*

**USUAL DOSAGE** Oral:

Nocturnal enuresis:

Children:

6-7 years (20-25 kg): 10 mg/day

8-11 years (25-35 kg): 10-20 mg/day

>11 years (35-54 kg): 25-35 mg/day

Depression:

Adolescents: 30-50 mg/day in divided doses

Adults: 25 mg 3-4 times/day up to 150 mg/day

Elderly:

Initial: 10-25 mg at bedtime

Dosage can be increased by 25 mg every 3 days for inpatients and weekly for outpatients if tolerated

Usual maintenance dose: 75 mg as a single bedtime dose, however, lower or higher doses may be required to stay within the therapeutic window

**Dosing adjustment in hepatic impairment:** Lower doses and slower titration dependent on individualization of dosage is recommended

**Dosage Forms Cap:** 10 mg, 25 mg, 50 mg, 75 mg; **Soln:** 10 mg/5 mL (473 mL)

**Contraindications** Narrow-angle glaucoma, avoid use during pregnancy and lactation, hypersensitivity to tricyclic antidepressants

**Warnings/Precautions** Use with caution in patients with cardiac conduction disturbances, history of hyperthyroid; should not be abruptly discontinued in patients receiving high doses for prolonged periods; use with caution with renal or hepatic impairment

**Pregnancy Risk Factor** D

**Adverse Reactions**

>10%:

Central nervous system: Dizziness, drowsiness, headache

Gastrointestinal: Xerostomia, constipation, increased appetite, nausea, unpleasant taste, weight gain

Neuromuscular & skeletal: Weakness

1% to 10%:

Cardiovascular: Postural hypotension, arrhythmias, tachycardia

Central nervous system: Confusion, delirium, hallucinations, nervousness, restlessness, parkinsonian syndrome, insomnia

Endocrine & metabolic: Sexual dysfunction

Gastrointestinal: Diarrhea, heartburn, constipation

Genitourinary: Dysuria, urinary retention

Ocular: Blurred vision, eye pain, increased intraocular pressure

Neuromuscular & skeletal: Fine muscle tremors

Miscellaneous: Diaphoresis (excessive)

<1%: Anxiety, seizures, alopecia, photosensitivity, breast enlargement, galactorrhea, SIADH, trouble with gums, decreased lower esophageal sphincter tone may cause GE reflux, testicular edema, leukopenia, rarely agranulocytosis, eosinophilia, increased liver enzymes, cholestatic jaundice, increased intraocular pressure, tinnitus, allergic reactions, sudden death

**Drug Interactions** CYP1A2 and 2D6 enzyme substrate

Blocks the uptake of guanethidine and thus prevents the hypotensive effect of guanethidine; may be additive with or may potentiate the action of other CNS depressants such as sedatives or hypnotics; potentiates the pressor and cardiac effects of sympathomimetic agents such as isoproterenol, epinephrine, etc

With MAO inhibitors, hyperpyrexia, hypertension, tachycardia, confusion, seizures, and death have been reported

Additive anticholinergic effect seen with other anticholinergic agents

Cimetidine reduces the metabolism of nortriptyline

May increase prothrombin time in patients stabilized on warfarin

**Onset** 1-3 weeks before therapeutic effects are seen

**Half-Life** 28-31 hours

**Special PA Issues**

**Patient Education:** Oral: Take exactly as directed (do not increase dose or frequency); may take 2-3 weeks to achieve desired results; may cause physical and/or psychological dependence. Take once-a-day dose at bedtime. Avoid excessive alcohol, caffeine, and other prescription or OTC medications not approved by prescriber. Maintain adequate hydration (2-3 L/day of fluids unless instructed to restrict fluid intake). You may experience drowsiness, lightheadedness, impaired coordination, dizziness, or blurred vision (use caution when driving or engaging in hazardous tasks until response to medication is known); nausea, vomiting, altered taste, dry mouth (small frequent meals, frequent mouth care, or sucking lozenges may help); constipation (increased exercise, fluids, or dietary fruit and fiber may help); diarrhea (buttermilk, yogurt, or boiled milk may help); increased appetite (monitor dietary intake to avoid excess weight gain); postural hypotension (use caution when climbing stairs or changing position from lying or sitting to standing); urinary retention (void before taking medication); or sexual dysfunction (reversible). Report persistent CNS effects (eg, insomnia, nervousness, restlessness, hallucinations, daytime sedation, impaired cognitive function); muscle cramping or tremors; chest pain, palpitations, rapid heartbeat, swelling of extremities, or severe dizziness; blurred vision or eye pain; yellowing of eyes or skin; pale stools/dark urine; or worsening of condition.

**Dietary Considerations:** Alcohol: Additive CNS effect, avoid use

**Monitoring Parameters:** Monitor blood pressure and pulse rate prior to and during initial therapy; evaluate mental status; monitor weight

**Reference Range:** Plasma levels do not always correlate with clinical effectiveness
Therapeutic: 50-150 ng/mL (SI: 190-570 nmol/L); Toxic: >500 ng/mL (SI: >1900 nmol/L)

**Related Information**
Antidepressant Agents *on page 998*

♦ **Nortriptyline Hydrochloride** *see* Nortriptyline *on page 665*

♦ **Norvasc®** *see* Amlodipine *on page 59*

♦ **Norvir®** *see* Ritonavir *on page 811*

♦ **Norzine®** *see* Thiethylperazine *on page 894*

♦ **Nosebleed** *see* Feverfew *on page 368*

♦ **Nostril® Nasal Solution [OTC]** *see* Phenylephrine *on page 718*

♦ **Novacet® Topical** *see* Sulfur and Sulfacetamide Sodium *on page 865*

♦ **Novahistine® Decongestant** *see* Phenylephrine *on page 718*

♦ **Novamoxin®** *see* Amoxicillin *on page 61*

♦ **Novasen** *see* Aspirin *on page 80*

♦ **Novo-Alprazol** *see* Alprazolam *on page 43*

♦ **Novo-Atenol** *see* Atenolol *on page 84*

♦ **Novo-AZT** *see* Zidovudine *on page 972*

♦ **Novo-Butamide** *see* Tolbutamide *on page 911*

♦ **Novocain® Injection** *see* Procaine *on page 760*

♦ **Novo-Captopril** *see* Captopril *on page 146*

♦ **Novo-Carbamaz** *see* Carbamazepine *on page 148*

♦ **Novo-Chlorhydrate** *see* Chloral Hydrate *on page 186*

♦ **Novo-Chlorpromazine** *see* Chlorpromazine *on page 197*

♦ **Novo-Cimetine** *see* Cimetidine *on page 208*

♦ **Novo-Clobetasol** *see* Clobetasol *on page 219*

♦ **Novo-Clonidine** *see* Clonidine *on page 225*

♦ **Novo-Clopate** *see* Clorazepate *on page 227*

♦ **Novo-Cloxin** *see* Cloxacillin *on page 229*

♦ **Novo-Cromolyn** *see* Cromolyn Sodium *on page 240*

♦ **Novo-Cycloprine** *see* Cyclobenzaprine *on page 243*

♦ **Novo-Difenac®** *see* Diclofenac *on page 271*

♦ **Novo-Difenac®-SR** *see* Diclofenac *on page 271*

♦ **Novo-Diflunisal** *see* Diflunisal *on page 279*

♦ **Novo-Digoxin** *see* Digoxin *on page 281*

♦ **Novo-Diltazem** *see* Diltiazem *on page 286*

♦ **Novo-Dipam** *see* Diazepam *on page 269*

♦ **Novo-Dipiradol** *see* Dipyridamole *on page 293*

♦ **Novo-Doxepin** *see* Doxepin *on page 304*

♦ **Novo-Doxylin** *see* Doxycycline *on page 306*

♦ **Novo-Famotidine** *see* Famotidine *on page 358*

♦ **Novo-Fibrate** *see* Clofibrate *on page 221*

♦ **Novo-Flupam** *see* Flurazepam *on page 390*

♦ **Novo-Flurprofen** *see* Flurbiprofen *on page 391*

♦ **Novo-Flutamide** *see* Flutamide *on page 393*

♦ **Novo-Folacid** *see* Folic Acid *on page 397*

♦ **Novo-Furan** *see* Nitrofurantoin *on page 659*

♦ **Novo-Gesic-C8** *see* Acetaminophen and Codeine *on page 22*

♦ **Novo-Gesic-C15** *see* Acetaminophen and Codeine *on page 22*

♦ **Novo-Gesic-C30** *see* Acetaminophen and Codeine *on page 22*

♦ **Novo-Glyburide** *see* Glyburide *on page 419*

♦ **Novo-Hexidyl** *see* Trihexyphenidyl *on page 935*

♦ **Novo-Hydrazide** *see* Hydrochlorothiazide *on page 447*

♦ **Novo-Hydroxyzin** *see* Hydroxyzine *on page 462*

♦ **Novo-Hylazin** *see* Hydralazine *on page 446*

♦ **Novo-Keto-EC** *see* Ketoprofen *on page 507*

♦ **Novo-Lexin** *see* Cephalexin *on page 179*

♦ **Novolin® 70/30** *see* Insulin Preparations *on page 479*

♦ **Novolin® L** *see* Insulin Preparations *on page 479*

- **Nu-Clonidine** *see* Clonidine *on page 225*
- **Nu-Cloxi** *see* Cloxacillin *on page 229*
- **Nucofed**® *see* Guaifenesin, Pseudoephedrine, and Codeine *on page 429*
- **Nucofed**® **Pediatric Expectorant** *see* Guaifenesin, Pseudoephedrine, and Codeine *on page 429*
- **Nu-Cotrimox** *see* Co-Trimoxazole *on page 238*
- **Nucotuss**® *see* Guaifenesin, Pseudoephedrine, and Codeine *on page 429*
- **Nu-Diclo** *see* Diclofenac *on page 271*
- **Nu-Diflunisal** *see* Diflunisal *on page 279*
- **Nu-Diltiaz** *see* Diltiazem *on page 286*
- **Nu-Doxycycline** *see* Doxycycline *on page 306*
- **Nu-Famotidine** *see* Famotidine *on page 358*
- **Nu-Flurprofen** *see* Flurbiprofen *on page 391*
- **Nu-Gemfibrozil** *see* Gemfibrozil *on page 410*
- **Nu-Glyburide** *see* Glyburide *on page 419*
- **Nu-Hydral** *see* Hydralazine *on page 446*
- **Nu-Ibuprofen** *see* Ibuprofen *on page 466*
- **Nu-Indo** *see* Indomethacin *on page 476*
- **Nu-Ketoprofen** *see* Ketoprofen *on page 507*
- **Nu-Ketoprofen-E** *see* Ketoprofen *on page 507*
- **Nu-Loraz** *see* Lorazepam *on page 543*
- **NuLytely**® *see* Polyethylene Glycol-Electrolyte Solution *on page 736*
- **Nu-Medopa** *see* Methyldopa *on page 590*
- **Nu-Metop** *see* Metoprolol *on page 599*
- **Numorphan**® *see* Oxymorphone *on page 689*
- **Numzitdent**® **[OTC]** *see* Benzocaine *on page 105*
- **Numzit Teething**® **[OTC]** *see* Benzocaine *on page 105*
- **Nu-Naprox** *see* Naproxen *on page 636*
- **Nu-Nifedin** *see* Nifedipine *on page 654*
- **Nu-Pen-VK** *see* Penicillin V Potassium *on page 706*
- **Nu-Pindol** *see* Pindolol *on page 728*
- **Nu-Pirox** *see* Piroxicam *on page 733*
- **Nu-Prazo** *see* Prazosin *on page 750*
- **Nuprin**® **[OTC]** *see* Ibuprofen *on page 466*
- **Nu-Prochlor** *see* Prochlorperazine *on page 763*
- **Nu-Propranolol** *see* Propranolol *on page 775*
- **Nuquin HP**® *see* Hydroquinone *on page 457*
- **Nu-Ranit** *see* Ranitidine Hydrochloride *on page 794*
- **Nu-Sulfinpyrazone** *see* Sulfinpyrazone *on page 863*
- **Nu-Tetra** *see* Tetracycline *on page 885*
- **Nu-Timolol** *see* Timolol *on page 905*
- **Nutracort**® *see* Hydrocortisone *on page 453*
- **Nutraplus**® **Topical [OTC]** *see* Urea *on page 947*
- **Nu-Triazide** *see* Hydrochlorothiazide and Triamterene *on page 449*
- **Nu-Triazo** *see* Triazolam *on page 931*
- **Nutrilipid**® *see* Fat Emulsion *on page 359*
- **Nu-Trimipramine** *see* Trimipramine *on page 938*
- **Nutropin**® **AQ Injection** *see* Human Growth Hormone *on page 444*
- **Nutropin**® **Injection** *see* Human Growth Hormone *on page 444*
- **Nu-Verap** *see* Verapamil *on page 959*
- **Nyaderm** *see* Nystatin *on this page*
- **Nydrazid**® *see* Isoniazid *on page 494*

## Nystatin (nye STAT in)

**Pharmacologic Class** Antifungal Agent, Oral Nonabsorbed; Antifungal Agent, Topical; Antifungal Agent, Vaginal

**U.S. Brand Names** Mycostatin®; Nilstat®; Nystat-Rx®; Nystex®; O-V Staticin®

**Mechanism of Action** Binds to sterols in fungal cell membrane, changing the cell wall permeability allowing for leakage of cellular contents

**Use** Treatment of susceptible cutaneous, mucocutaneous, and oral cavity fungal infections normally caused by the *Candida* species

**USUAL DOSAGE**

Oral candidiasis:

Suspension (swish and swallow orally):

Premature infants: 100,000 units 4 times/day

Infants: 200,000 units 4 times/day or 100,000 units to each side of mouth 4 times/day

(Continued)

## Nystatin *(Continued)*

Children and Adults: 400,000-600,000 units 4 times/day

Troche: Children and Adults: 200,000-400,000 units 4-5 times/day

Powder for compounding: Children and Adults: 1/8 teaspoon (500,000 units) to equal approximately 1/2 cup of water; give 4 times/day

Mucocutaneous infections: Children and Adults: Topical: Apply 2-3 times/day to affected areas; very moist topical lesions are treated best with powder

Intestinal infections: Adults: Oral tablets: 500,000-1,000,000 units every 8 hours

Vaginal infections: Adults: Vaginal tablets: Insert 1 tablet/day at bedtime for 2 weeks

**Dosage Forms Crm:** 100,000 units/g (15 g, 30 g); **Oint, top:** 100,000 units/g (15 g, 30 g); **Powder, for preparation of oral susp:** 50 million units, 1 billion units, 2 billion units, 5 billion units; **Powder, top:** 100,000 units/g (15 g); **Susp, oral:** 100,000 units/mL (5 mL, 60 mL, 480 mL); **Tab:** Oral: 500,000 units; **Vaginal:** 100,000 units (15 and 30/box with applicator); **Troche:** 200,000 units

**Contraindications** Hypersensitivity to nystatin or any component

**Pregnancy Risk Factor** B/C (oral)

**Adverse Reactions**

Percentage unknown: Contact dermatitis, Stevens-Johnson syndrome

1% to 10%: Gastrointestinal: Nausea, vomiting, diarrhea, stomach pain

<1%: Hypersensitivity reactions

**Onset** Onset of symptomatic relief from candidiasis: Within 24-72 hours

**Special PA Issues**

**Patient Education:** Take as directed. Maintain adequate hydration (2-3 L/day of fluids unless instructed to restrict fluid intake). Do not allow medication to come in contact with eyes. Report persistent nausea, vomiting, or diarrhea; or if condition being treated worsens or does not improve.

Oral tablets: Swallow whole; do not crush or chew.

Oral suspension: Shake well before using. Remove dentures, clean mouth (do not replace dentures until after using medications). Swish suspension in mouth for several minutes before swallowing.

Oral troches: Remove dentures, clean mouth (do not replace dentures until after using medication). Allow troche to dissolve in mouth; do not chew or swallow whole.

Topical: Wash and dry area before applying (do not reuse towels without washing, apply clean clothing after use). Report unresolved burning, redness, or swelling in treated areas.

Vaginal tablets: Wash hands before using. Lie down to insert high into vagina at bedtime.

## Nystatin and Triamcinolone *(nye STAT in & trye am SIN oh lone)*

**Pharmacologic Class** Antifungal Agent, Topical; Corticosteroid, Topical

**U.S. Brand Names** Mycogen II Topical; Mycolog®-II Topical; Myconel® Topical; Myco-Triacet® II; Mytrex® F Topical; N.G.T.® Topical; Tri-Statin® II Topical

**Mechanism of Action** Refer to individual monographs for Nystatin and Triamcinolone

**Use** Treatment of cutaneous candidiasis

**USUAL DOSAGE** Children and Adults: Topical: Apply sparingly 2-4 times/day

**Dosage Forms Crm:** Nystatin 100,000 units and triamcinolone acetonide 0.1% (15 g, 30 g, 45 g, 60 g, 240 g); **Oint, top:** Nystatin 100,000 units and triamcinolone acetonide 0.1% (15 g, 30 g, 60 g, 120 g)

**Contraindications** Known hypersensitivity to nystatin or triamcinolone

**Warnings/Precautions** Avoid use of occlusive dressings; limit therapy to least amount necessary for effective therapy, pediatric patients may be more susceptible to HPA axis suppression due to larger BSA to weight ratio

**Pregnancy Risk Factor** C

**Adverse Reactions** 1% to 10%:

Dermatologic: Dryness, folliculitis, hypertrichosis, acne, hypopigmentation, allergic dermatitis, maceration of the skin, skin atrophy, itching

Local: Burning, irritation

Miscellaneous: Increased incidence of secondary infection

- ◆ **Nystat-Rx®** *see* Nystatin *on previous page*
- ◆ **Nystex®** *see* Nystatin *on previous page*
- ◆ **Nytol® Extra Strength** *see* Diphenhydramine *on page 289*
- ◆ **Nytol® Oral [OTC]** *see* Diphenhydramine *on page 289*
- ◆ **Occlucort®** *see* Betamethasone *on page 111*
- ◆ **Ocean Nasal Mist [OTC]** *see* Sodium Chloride *on page 839*
- ◆ **OCL®** *see* Polyethylene Glycol-Electrolyte Solution *on page 736*
- ◆ **Octamide®** *see* Metoclopramide *on page 597*
- ◆ **Octicair® Otic** *see* Neomycin, Polymyxin B, and Hydrocortisone *on page 645*
- ◆ **Octocaine®** *see* Lidocaine *on page 531*

♦ **Octocaine® With Epinephrine** *see* Lidocaine and Epinephrine *on page 532*

♦ **Octostim®** *see* Desmopressin Acetate *on page 261*

# Octreotide Acetate (ok TREE oh tide AS e tate)

**Pharmacologic Class** Antidiarrheal; Antisecretory Agent; Somatostatin Analog

**U.S. Brand Names** Sandostatin®; Sandostatin LAR® Depot

**Mechanism of Action** Mimics natural somatostatin by inhibiting serotonin release, and the secretion of gastrin, VIP, insulin, glucagon, secretin, motilin, and pancreatic polypeptide

**Use** Control of symptoms in patients with metastatic carcinoid and vasoactive intestinal peptide-secreting tumors (VIPomas); pancreatic tumors, gastrinoma, secretory diarrhea, acromegaly

> **Unlabeled use:** AIDS-associated secretory diarrhea, control of bleeding of esophageal varices, breast cancer, cryptosporidiosis, Cushing's syndrome, insulinomas, small bowel fistulas, postgastrectomy dumping syndrome, chemotherapy-induced diarrhea, graft-versus-host disease (GVHD) induced diarrhea, Zollinger-Ellison syndrome

**USUAL DOSAGE** Adults: S.C.: Initial: 50 mcg 1-2 times/day and titrate dose based on patient tolerance and response

Carcinoid: 100-600 mcg/day in 2-4 divided doses

VIPomas: 200-300 mcg/day in 2-4 divided doses

Diarrhea: Initial: I.V.: 50-100 mcg every 8 hours; increase by 100 mcg/dose at 48-hour intervals; maximum dose: 500 mcg every 8 hours

Esophageal varices bleeding: I.V. bolus: 25-50 mcg followed by continuous I.V. infusion of 25-50 mcg/hour

Acromegaly, carcinoid tumors, and VIPomas (depot injection): Patients must be stabilized on subcutaneous octreotide for at least 2 weeks before switching to the long-acting depot: Upon switch: 20 mg I.M. intragluteally every 4 weeks for 2-3 months, then the dose may be modified based upon response

**Dosage adjustment for acromegaly:** After 3 months of depot injections the dosage may be continued or modified as follows:

GH ≤2.5 ng/mL, IGF-1 is normal, symptoms are controlled: Maintain octreotide LAR® at 20 mg I.M. every 4 weeks

GH >2.5 ng/mL, IGF-1 is elevated, or symptoms controlled: Increase octreotide LAR® to 10 mg I.M. every 4 weeks

GH ≤1 ng/mL, IGF-1 is normal, symptoms controlled: Reduce octreotide LAR® to 10 mg I.M. every 4 weeks

Dosages >40 mg are not recommended

**Dosage adjustment for carcinoid tumors and VIPomas:** After 2 months of depot injections the dosage may be continued or modified as follows:

Increase to 30 mg I.M. every 4 weeks if symptoms are inadequately controlled

Decrease to 10 mg I.M. every 4 weeks, for a trial period, if initially responsive to 20 mg dose

Dosage >30 mg is not recommended

**Dosage Forms** Inj, as acetate: 0.05 mg/mL (1 mL), 0.1 mg/mL (1 mL), 0.2 mg/mL (5 mL), 0.5 mg/mL (1 mL), 1 mg/mL (5 mL); **Inj, as depot:** 10 mg, 20 mg, 30 mg

**Contraindications** Known hypersensitivity to octreotide or any component

**Warnings/Precautions** Dosage adjustment may be required to maintain symptomatic control; insulin requirements may be reduced as well as sulfonylurea requirements; monitor patients for cholelithiasis, hyper- or hypoglycemia; use with caution in patients with renal impairment

**Pregnancy Risk Factor** B

**Adverse Reactions**

1% to 10%:

Cardiovascular: Flushing, edema

Central nervous system: Fatigue, headache, dizziness, vertigo, anorexia, depression

Endocrine & metabolic: Hypoglycemia or hyperglycemia (1%), hypothyroidism, galactorrhea

Gastrointestinal: Nausea, vomiting, diarrhea, constipation, abdominal pain, cramping, discomfort, fat malabsorption, loose stools, flatulence

Hepatic: Jaundice, hepatitis, increase LFTs, cholelithiasis has occurred, presumably by altering fat absorption and decreasing the motility of the gallbladder

Local: Pain at injection site (dose related)

Neuromuscular & skeletal: Weakness

<1%: Chest pain, hypertensive reaction, anxiety, fever, hyperesthesia, alopecia, wheal/erythema, rash, thrombophlebitis, leg cramps, Bell's palsy, muscle cramping, burning eyes, throat discomfort, rhinorrhea, shortness of breath

**Drug Interactions** CYP2D6 (high dose) and 3A enzyme inhibitor

Decreased effect: Cyclosporine (case report of a transplant rejection due to reduction of serum cyclosporine levels)

**Duration** 6-12 hours (S.C.)

**Half-Life** 60-110 minutes

(Continued)

## Octreotide Acetate *(Continued)*

### Special PA Issues

**Patient Education:** Schedule injections between meals to decrease GI effects. May affect dietary fat and vitamin B$_{12}$. Consult prescriber about appropriate diet. Diabetic patients should monitor serum glucose closely (this drug may increase the effects of insulin or sulfonylureas); report abnormal glucose levels so appropriate adjustment can be made. You may experience skin flushing; nausea or vomiting (small frequent meals, frequent mouth care, or sucking on lozenges may help); dizziness, fatigue, or drowsiness (use caution when driving or with tasks that require alertness). Report weight gain, swelling of extremities, or respiratory difficulty; acute or persistent GI distress (eg, diarrhea, vomiting, constipation, abdominal pain); muscle weakness or tremors or loss of motor function; chest pain or palpitations; blurred vision; pain, redness, or swelling at injection site; or emotional depression.

**Administration:** Slowly warm solution to room temperature. Inject slowly to reduce local reaction. Rotate injection sites, using hip, thigh, or abdomen. Dispose of syringes in closed container away from access of other persons.

**Reference Range:** Vasoactive intestinal peptide: <75 ng/L; levels vary considerably between laboratories

- ◆ **Ocu-Carpine® Ophthalmic** *see* Pilocarpine *on page 726*
- ◆ **Ocu-Dex®** *see* Dexamethasone *on page 264*
- ◆ **Ocufen® Ophthalmic** *see* Flurbiprofen *on page 391*
- ◆ **Ocuflox™ Ophthalmic** *see* Ofloxacin *on this page*
- ◆ **Ocumycin®** *see* Gentamicin *on page 411*
- ◆ **Ocupress® Ophthalmic** *see* Carteolol *on page 155*
- ◆ **Ocusert Pilo-20® Ophthalmic** *see* Pilocarpine *on page 726*
- ◆ **Ocusert Pilo-40® Ophthalmic** *see* Pilocarpine *on page 726*
- ◆ **Ocusulf-10® Ophthalmic** *see* Sulfacetamide Sodium *on page 858*
- ◆ **Ocutricin® Ophthalmic Solution** *see* Neomycin, Polymyxin B, and Gramicidin *on page 644*
- ◆ **Ocutricin® Topical Ointment** *see* Bacitracin, Neomycin, and Polymyxin B *on page 97*
- ◆ **Ocu-Tropine® Ophthalmic** *see* Atropine *on page 87*
- ◆ **Oestrilin®** *see* Estrone *on page 338*

## Ofloxacin *(oh FLOKS a sin)*

**Pharmacologic Class** Antibiotic, Quinolone

**U.S. Brand Names** Floxin®; Ocuflox™ Ophthalmic

**Mechanism of Action** Ofloxacin is a DNA gyrase inhibitor. DNA gyrase is an essential bacterial enzyme that maintains the superhelical structure of DNA. DNA gyrase is required for DNA replication and transcription, DNA repair, recombination, and transposition; bactericidal

### Use

Quinolone antibiotic for skin and skin structure, lower respiratory and urinary tract infections and sexually transmitted diseases. Active against many gram-positive and gram-negative aerobic bacteria.

Ophthalmic: Treatment of superficial ocular infections involving the conjunctiva or cornea due to strains of susceptible organisms

### USUAL DOSAGE

Children >1 year and Adults: Ophthalmic: Instill 1-2 drops in affected eye(s) every 2-4 hours for the first 2 days, then use 4 times/day for an additional 5 days

Adults:

Lower respiratory tract infection: 400 mg every 12 hours for 10 days

Gonorrhea: 400 mg as a single dose

Cervicitis due to *C. trachomatis* and/or *N. gonorrhoeae*: 300 mg every 12 hours for 7 days

Skin/skin structure: 400 mg every 12 hours for 10 days

Urinary tract infection: 200-400 mg every 12 hours for 3-10 days

Prostatitis: 300 mg every 12 hours for 6 weeks

**Dosing adjustment/interval in renal impairment:** Adults: I.V., Oral:

Cl$_{cr}$ 10-50 mL/minute: Administer 200-400 mg every 24 hours

Cl$_{cr}$ <10 mL/minute: Administer 100-200 mg every 24 hours

Continuous arteriovenous or venovenous hemodiafiltration (CAVH) effects: Administer 300 mg every 24 hours

**Dosage Forms Inj:** 200 mg (50 mL), 400 mg (10 mL, 20 mL, 100 mL); **Soln, ophth:** 0.3% (5 mL); **Tab:** 200 mg, 300 mg, 400 mg

**Contraindications** Hypersensitivity to ofloxacin or other members of the quinolone group such as nalidixic acid, oxolinic acid, cinoxacin, norfloxacin, and ciprofloxacin

**Warnings/Precautions** Use with caution in patients with epilepsy or other CNS diseases which could predispose seizures; use with caution in patients with renal impairment; failure to respond to an ophthalmic antibiotic after 2-3 days may indicate the presence of resistant organisms, or another causative agent; use caution with systemic preparation in children

<18 years of age due to association of other quinolones with transient arthropathy; has rarely caused ruptured tendons (discontinue immediately with signs of inflammation or tendon pain)

**Pregnancy Risk Factor** C

**Adverse Reactions**

1% to 10%:

Cardiovascular: Chest pain (1% to 3%)

Central nervous system: Headache (1% to 9%), insomnia (3% to 7%), dizziness (1% to 5%), fatigue (1% to 3%), somnolence (1% to 3%), sleep disorders, nervousness (1% to 3%), pyrexia (1% to 3%), pain

Dermatologic: Rash/pruritus (1% to 3%)

Gastrointestinal: Diarrhea (1% to 4%), vomiting (1% to 3%), GI distress, cramps, abdominal cramps (1% to 3%), flatulence (1% to 3%), abnormal taste (1% to 3%), xerostomia (1% to 3%), decreased appetite, nausea (3% to 10%)

Genitourinary: Vaginitis (1% to 3%), external genital pruritus in women

Local: Pain at injection site

Ocular: Superinfection (ophthalmic), photophobia, lacrimation, dry eyes, stinging, visual disturbances (1% to 3%)

Miscellaneous: Trunk pain

<1%: Syncope, vasculitis, edema, hypertension, palpitations, vasodilation, anxiety, cognitive change, depression, dream abnormality, euphoria, hallucinations, vertigo, chills, malaise, extremity pain, weight loss, paresthesia, ruptured tendons, Tourette's syndrome, weakness, photophobia, photosensitivity, hepatitis, decreased hearing acuity, tinnitus, cough, thirst

**Drug Interactions**

Decreased effect: Decreased absorption with antacids containing aluminum, magnesium, and/or calcium (by up to 98% if given at the same time); fluoroquinolones may be decreased by antineoplastic agents

Increased toxicity/serum levels: Quinolones cause increased caffeine, warfarin, cyclosporine, procainamide, and possibly theophylline levels. Cimetidine and probenecid increase quinolone levels.

**Half-Life** 5-7.5 hours; prolonged in renal impairment

**Special PA Issues**

Patient Education:

Oral: Take per recommended schedule, preferably on empty stomach (1 hour before or 2 hours after meals). Maintain adequate hydration (2-3 L/day of fluids unless instructed to restrict fluid intake). Take complete prescription; do not skip doses. Do not take with antacids. You may experience dizziness, lightheadedness; use caution when driving or engaging in tasks that require alertness. Small frequent meals and frequent mouth care may reduce nausea or vomiting. You may experience photosensitivity; use sunblock, wear protective clothing, or avoid direct sun. Report persistent diarrhea or GI disturbances; excessive sleepiness or agitation; tremors; rash; pain, inflammation, or rupture of tendon; or changes in vision.

Ophthalmic: Tilt head back and instill 1-2 drops in affected eye 4 times a day for length of time prescribed. Do not allow tip of applicator to touch eye or any contaminated surface. You may experience some stinging or burning or a bad taste in your mouth after instillation. Report persistent pain, burning, double vision, swelling, itching, feeling of something in your eye, or worsening of condition.

- ◆ **Ogen® Oral** *see* Estropipate *on page 339*
- ◆ **Ogen® Vaginal** *see* Estropipate *on page 339*
- ◆ **OKT3** *see* Muromonab-CD3 *on page 622*

# Olanzapine (oh LAN za peen)

**Pharmacologic Class** Antipsychotic Agent, Thienobenzodiaepine

**U.S. Brand Names** Zyprexa™

**Mechanism of Action** Olanzapine is a thienobenzodiazepine neuroleptic; thought to work by antagonizing dopamine and serotonin activities. It is a selective monoaminergic antagonist with high affinity binding to serotonin $5\text{-HT}_{2A}$ and $5\text{-HT}_{2C}$, dopamine $D_{1\text{-}4}$, muscarinic $M_{1\text{-}5}$, histamine $H_1$ and alpha$_1$-adrenergic receptor sites.

**Use** Treatment of the manifestations of psychotic disorders

**USUAL DOSAGE** Adults >18 years: Oral: Usual starting dose: 5-10 mg once daily; increase to 10 mg once daily within 5-7 days, thereafter adjust by 5 mg/day at 1-week intervals, up to a maximum of 20 mg/day

**Dosage Forms Tab:** 2.5 mg, 5 mg, 7.5 mg, 10 mg

**Warnings/Precautions** Use with caution in patients with cardiovascular disease, cerebrovascular disease, hypovolemia, dehydration, seizure disorders, Alzheimer's disease, hepatic impairment, prostatic hypertrophy, narrow-angle glaucoma, history of paralytic ileus or a history of breast cancer, the elderly, and in pregnancy or with nursing patients

**Adverse Reactions**

>10%: Central nervous system: Headache, somnolence, insomnia, agitation, nervousness, hostility, dizziness

(Continued)

## Olanzapine *(Continued)*

1% to 10%:

Central nervous system: Dystonic reactions, Parkinsonian events, akathisia, anxiety, personality changes, fever

Gastrointestinal: Xerostomia, constipation, abdominal pain, weight gain

Neuromuscular & skeletal: Arthralgia

Ocular: Amblyopia

Respiratory: Rhinitis, cough, pharyngitis

<1%: Peripheral edema, tardive dyskinesia, neuroleptic malignant syndrome

**Drug Interactions** CYP1A2 enzyme substrate, CYP2C19 enzyme substrate (minor), and CYP2D6 enzyme substrate (minor)

Decreased effect: Cigarette smoking, levodopa, pergolide, bromocriptine, charcoal, and reduction of effects may be seen with cytochrome P-450 enzyme inducers such as rifampin, omeprazole, carbamazepine

Increased effect: Effects may be potentiated with CYP1A2 inhibitors such as fluvoxamine

Increased toxicity: Increased sedation with alcohol or other CNS depressants, increased risk of hypotension with orthostatic hypotension with antihypertensives

**Half-Life** 21-54 hours (mean 30 hours)

**Special PA Issues**

**Patient Education:** Use exactly as directed (do not increase dose or frequency); may cause physical and/or psychological dependence. It may take 2-3 weeks to achieve desired results; do not discontinue without consulting prescriber. Avoid excess alcohol or caffeine and other prescription or OTC medications not approved by prescriber. Maintain adequate hydration (2-3 L/day of fluids unless instructed to restrict fluid intake). You may experience excess drowsiness, restlessness, dizziness, or blurred vision (use caution driving or when engaging in hazardous tasks until response to medication is known); or constipation (increased exercise, fluids, or dietary fruit and fiber may help). Report persistent CNS effects (eg, trembling fingers, altered gait or balance, excessive sedation, seizures, unusual movements, anxiety, abnormal thoughts, confusion, personality changes); unresolved constipation or gastrointestinal effects; vision changes; difficulty breathing; unusual cough or flu-like symptoms; or worsening of condition.

**Related Information**

Antipsychotic Agents *on page 1001*

♦ **Oleovitamin A** *see* Vitamin A *on page 962*

## Olsalazine *(ole SAL a zeen)*

**Pharmacologic Class** 5-Aminosalicylic Acid Derivative

**U.S. Brand Names** Dipentum®

**Mechanism of Action** The mechanism of action appears to be topical rather than systemic

**Use** Maintenance of remission of ulcerative colitis in patients intolerant to sulfasalazine

**USUAL DOSAGE** Adults: Oral: 1 g/day in 2 divided doses

**Dosage Forms Cap, as sodium:** 250 mg

**Contraindications** Hypersensitivity to salicylates

**Warnings/Precautions** Diarrhea is a common adverse effect of olsalazine; use with caution in patients with hypersensitivity to salicylates, sulfasalazine, or mesalamine

**Pregnancy Risk Factor** C

**Adverse Reactions**

>10%: Gastrointestinal: Diarrhea, cramps, abdominal pain

1% to 10%:

Central nervous system: Headache, fatigue, depression

Dermatologic: Rash, itching

Gastrointestinal: Nausea, dyspepsia, bloating, anorexia

Neuromuscular & skeletal: Arthralgia

<1%: Fever, bloody diarrhea, blood dyscrasias, hepatitis

**Special PA Issues**

**Patient Education:** Take as directed, with meals, in evenly divided doses. You may experience flu-like symptoms or muscle pain (a mild analgesic may help); diarrhea (boiled milk or yogurt may help); or nausea or loss of appetite (small frequent meals, frequent mouth care, or sucking lozenges may help). Report persistent diarrhea or abdominal cramping, skin rash or itching, or other adverse reactions.

♦ **Olsalazine Sodium** *see* Olsalazine *on this page*

## Omeprazole *(oh ME pray zol)*

**Pharmacologic Class** Proton Pump Inhibitor

**U.S. Brand Names** Prilosec™

**Mechanism of Action** Suppresses gastric acid secretion by inhibiting the parietal cell H+/ K+ ATP pump

**Use** Short-term (4-8 weeks) treatment of severe erosive esophagitis (grade 2 or above), diagnosed by endoscopy and short-term treatment of symptomatic gastroesophageal reflux disease (GERD) poorly responsive to customary medical treatment; pathological hypersecretory conditions; peptic ulcer disease; gastric ulcer therapy; approved for combination use in the eradication of *H. pylori* in patients with active duodenal ulcer.

**Unlabeled use:** Healing NSAID-induced ulcers

**USUAL DOSAGE** Adults: Oral:

Active duodenal ulcer: 20 mg/day for 4-8 weeks

GERD or severe erosive esophagitis: 20 mg/day for 4-8 weeks

Pathological hypersecretory conditions: 60 mg once daily to start; doses up to 120 mg 3 times/day have been administered; administer daily doses >80 mg in divided doses

*Helicobacter pylori:* Combination therapy with bismuth subsalicylate, tetracycline, clarithromycin, and $H_2$-antagonist; or with clarithromycin. Adult dose: Oral: 20 mg twice daily

Gastric ulcers: 40 mg/day for 4-8 weeks

**Dosage Forms Cap, delayed release:** 10 mg, 20 mg

**Contraindications** Known hypersensitivity to omeprazole

**Warnings/Precautions** In long-term (2-year) studies in rats, omeprazole produced a dose-related increase in gastric carcinoid tumors. While available endoscopic evaluations and histologic examinations of biopsy specimens from human stomachs have not detected a risk from short-term exposure to omeprazole, further human data on the effect of sustained hypochlorhydria and hypergastrinemia are needed to rule out the possibility of an increased risk for the development of tumors in humans receiving long-term therapy. Bioavailability may be increased in the elderly.

**Pregnancy Risk Factor** C

**Pregnancy Implications**

Clinical effects on the fetus: Crosses the placenta

Breast-feeding/lactation: No data available. American Academy of Pediatrics makes NO RECOMMENDATION.

**Adverse Reactions**

1% to 10%:

Cardiovascular: Angina, tachycardia, bradycardia, edema

Central nervous system: Headache (7%), dizziness

Dermatologic: Rash, urticaria, pruritus, dry skin, purpura, petechiae

Gastrointestinal: Diarrhea, nausea, abdominal pain, vomiting, constipation, anorexia, irritable colon, fecal discoloration, esophageal candidiasis, xerostomia, abnormal taste

Genitourinary: Testicular pain, urinary tract infection, polyuria

Neuromuscular & skeletal: Back pain, muscle cramps, myalgia, arthralgia, leg pain, weakness occurred in more frequently than 1% of patients

Renal: Pyuria, proteinuria, hematuria, glycosuria

Respiratory: Cough

<1%: Chest pain, fever, fatigue, malaise, apathy, somnolence, nervousness, anxiety, pain, abdominal swelling, rarely anaphylaxis

**Drug Interactions** CYP2C8, 2C9, 2C18, 2C19, and 3A3/4 enzyme substrate; CYP1A2 enzyme inducer; CYP2C19, 2C8, 2C9, and 2C19 enzyme inhibitor, CYP3A3/4 enzyme inhibitor (weak)

Decreased effect: Decreased ketoconazole; decreased itraconazole

Increased toxicity: Diazepam may increase half-life; increased digoxin, increased phenytoin, increased warfarin

**Onset** Onset of antisecretory action: Oral: Within 1 hour; Peak effect: 2 hours

**Duration** 72 hours

**Half-Life** 30-90 minutes

**Special PA Issues**

**Patient Education:** Take as directed, before eating. Do not crush or chew capsules. You may experience anorexia; small frequent meals may help to maintain adequate nutrition. Report changes in urination or pain on urination, unresolved severe diarrhea, testicular pain, or changes in respiratory status.

♦ **Omnicef®** *see* Cefdinir *on page 161*

♦ **OmniHIB™** *see* Haemophilus b Conjugate Vaccine *on page 432*

♦ **Omnipen®** *see* Ampicillin *on page 64*

♦ **Omnipen®-N** *see* Ampicillin *on page 64*

♦ **OMS® Oral** *see* Morphine Sulfate *on page 619*

♦ **Oncet®** *see* Hydrocodone and Homatropine *on page 451*

# Ondansetron (on DAN se tron)

**Pharmacologic Class** Selective 5-$HT_3$ Receptor Antagonist

**U.S. Brand Names** Iofran ODT®; Zofran®

**Mechanism of Action** Selective 5-$HT_3$-receptor antagonist, blocking serotonin, both peripherally on vagal nerve terminals and centrally in the chemoreceptor trigger zone

**Use** May be prescribed for patients who are refractory to or have severe adverse reactions to standard antiemetic therapy. Ondansetron may be prescribed for young patients (ie, <45 years of age who are more likely to develop extrapyramidal reactions to high-dose metoclopramide) who are to receive highly emetogenic chemotherapeutic agents as listed:
(Continued)

## Ondansetron *(Continued)*

Agents with high emetogenic potential (>90%) (dose/m$^2$):
    Amifostine
    Azacitidine
    Carmustine ≥200 mg/m$^2$
    Cisplatin ≥50 mg/m$^2$
    Cyclophosphamide ≥1 g/m$^2$
    Cytarabine ≥1500 mg/m$^2$
    Dacarbazine ≥500 mg/m$^2$
    Dactinomycin
    Doxorubicin ≥60 mg/m$^2$
    Lomustine ≥60 mg/m$^2$
    Mechlorethamine
    Melphalan ≥100 mg/m$^2$
    Streptozocin
    Thiotepa ≥100 mg/m$^2$

**or** two agents classified as having high or moderately high emetogenic potential as listed:

Agents with moderately high emetogenic potential (60% to 90%) (dose/m$^2$):
    Carboplatin 200-400 mg/m$^2$
    Carmustine <200 mg/m$^2$
    Cisplatin <50 mg/m$^2$
    Cyclophosphamide 600-999 mg/m$^2$
    Dacarbazine <500 mg/m$^2$
    Doxorubicin 21-59 mg/m$^2$
    Hexamethyl melamine
    Ifosfamide ≥5000 mg/m$^2$
    Lomustine <60 mg/m$^2$
    Methotrexate ≥250 mg/m$^2$
    Pentostatin
    Procarbazine

Ondansetron should not be prescribed for chemotherapeutic agents with a low emetogenic potential (eg, bleomycin, busulfan, cyclophosphamide <1000 mg, etoposide, 5-fluorouracil, vinblastine, vincristine)

### USUAL DOSAGE

Chemotherapy-induced emesis: Oral:
    Children 4-11 years: 4 mg 30 minutes before chemotherapy; repeat 4 and 8 hours after initial dose, then 4 mg every 8 hours for 1-2 days after chemotherapy completed
    Children >11 years and Adults: 8 mg every 8 hours for 2 doses beginning 30 minutes before chemotherapy, then 8 mg every 12 hours for 1-2 days after chemotherapy completed
    Total body irradiation: Adults: 8 mg 1-2 hours before each fraction of radiotherapy administered each day
    Single high-dose fraction radiotherapy to abdomen: 8 mg 1-2 hours before irradiation, then 8 mg every 8 hours after first dose for 1-2 days after completion of radiotherapy
    Daily fractionated radiotherapy to abdomen: 8 mg 1-2 hours before irradiation, then 8 mg every 8 hours after first dose for each day of radiotherapy
    Prophylaxis with moderate-emetogenic chemotherapy (not FDA-approved): 8 mg twice daily has been shown to be as effective as doses given 3 times/day
I.V.: Administer either three 0.15 mg/kg doses or a single 32 mg dose; with the 3-dose regimen, the initial dose is given 30 minutes prior to chemotherapy with subsequent doses administered 4 and 8 hours after the first dose. With the single-dose regimen 32 mg is infused over 15 minutes beginning 30 minutes before the start of emetogenic chemotherapy. Dosage should be calculated based on weight:
    Children: Pediatric dosing should follow the manufacturer's guidelines for 0.15 mg/kg/ dose administered 30 minutes prior to chemotherapy, 4 and 8 hours after the first dose. While not as yet FDA-approved, literature supports the day's total dose administered as a single dose 30 minutes prior to chemotherapy.
    Adults:
        >80 kg: 12 mg IVPB
        45-80 kg: 8 mg IVPB
        <45 kg: 0.15 mg/kg/dose IVPB
Postoperative emesis: I.V.:
    Children >2 years: 0.1 mg/kg I.V. slow push; if over 40 kg weight, administer 4 mg IVP over 2-5 minutes (no faster than 30 seconds); give I.V. as s single dose immediately before induction of anesthesia or shortly following procedure if vomiting occurs
    Adults (infuse in not less than 30 seconds, preferably over 2-5 minutes, as undiluted drug): 4 mg as a single dose immediately before induction of anesthesia; or shortly following procedure if vomiting occurs
**Dosing in hepatic impairment:** Maximum daily dose: 8 mg in cirrhotic patients with severe liver disease

**Dosage Forms** Ondansetron hydrochloride: **Inj:** 2 mg/mL (20 mL), 32 mg (single-dose vials); **Soln, oral:** 4 mg/5 mL; **Tab:** 4 mg, 8 mg; **Tab, disintegrating:** 4 mg, 8 mg

**Contraindications** Hypersensitivity to ondansetron or any component

**Warnings/Precautions Ondansetron should be used on a scheduled basis, not as an "as needed" (PRN) basis,** since data supports the use of this drug in the prevention of nausea and vomiting and not in the rescue of nausea and vomiting. Ondansetron should only be used in the first 24-48 hours of receiving chemotherapy. Data does not support any increased efficacy of ondansetron in delayed nausea and vomiting.

**Pregnancy Risk Factor** B

**Pregnancy Implications**

Clinical effects on the fetus: No data available on crossing the placenta; no effects on the fetus from 2 case reports

Breast-feeding/lactation: No data available. American Academy of Pediatrics has NO RECOMMENDATION.

**Adverse Reactions**

>10%:

Central nervous system: Headache, fever

Gastrointestinal: Constipation, diarrhea

1% to 10%:

Central nervous system: Dizziness

Gastrointestinal: Abdominal cramps, xerostomia

Hepatic: AST/ALT elevations (5%)

Neuromuscular & skeletal: Weakness

<1%: Tachycardia, lightheadedness, seizures, rash, hypokalemia, transient elevations in serum levels of aminotransferases and bilirubin, bronchospasm, shortness of breath, wheezing, angina

**Drug Interactions** CYP1A2, 2D6, 2E1, and 3A3/4 enzyme substrate

Decreased effect: Metabolized by the hepatic cytochrome P-450 enzymes; therefore, the drug's clearance and half-life may be changed with concomitant use of cytochrome P-450 inducers (eg, barbiturates, carbamazepine, rifampin, phenytoin, and phenylbutazone)

Increased toxicity: Inhibitors (eg, cimetidine, allopurinol, and disulfiram)

**Onset** Within 30 minutes

**Half-Life** 4 hours

**Special PA Issues**

**Patient Education:** This drug may cause drowsiness; use caution when driving or engaging in hazardous activities. You may experience constipation and headache (request appropriate treatment from prescriber). Do not change position rapidly (rise slowly). Good mouth care and sucking on lozenges may help relieve nausea. Report persistent headache, excessive drowsiness, fever, numbness or tingling, or severe changes in elimination patterns (constipation or diarrhea), chest pain, or palpitations.

**Dietary Considerations:**

Food: Increases the extent of absorption. The $C_{max}$ and $T_{max}$ does not change much; take without regard to meals

Potassium: Hypokalemia; monitor potassium serum concentration

♦ **Ondansetron Hydrochloride** *see* Ondansetron *on page 675*

♦ **Ony-Clear® Spray** *see* Miconazole *on page 604*

♦ **Onyvul®** *see* Urea *on page 947*

♦ **OPC13013** *see* Cilostazol *on page 207*

♦ **OPC-17116** *see* Grepafloxacin *on page 426*

♦ **Opcon®** *see* Naphazoline *on page 635*

♦ **Operand® [OTC]** *see* Povidone-Iodine *on page 747*

♦ **Ophthetic®** *see* Proparacaine *on page 771*

♦ **Ophthifluor®** *see* Fluorescein Sodium *on page 382*

♦ **Opium and Belladonna** *see* Belladonna and Opium *on page 102*

# Opium Tincture (OH pee um TING chur)

**Pharmacologic Class** Analgesic, Narcotic; Antidiarrheal

**Mechanism of Action** Contains many narcotic alkaloids including morphine; its mechanism for gastric motility inhibition is primarily due to this morphine content; it results in a decrease in digestive secretions, an increase in GI muscle tone, and therefore a reduction in GI propulsion

**Use** Treatment of diarrhea or relief of pain

**USUAL DOSAGE** Oral:

Children:

Diarrhea: 0.005-0.01 mL/kg/dose every 3-4 hours for a maximum of 6 doses/24 hours

Analgesia: 0.01-0.02 mL/kg/dose every 3-4 hours

Adults:

Diarrhea: 0.3-1 mL/dose every 2-6 hours to maximum of 6 mL/24 hours

Analgesia: 0.6-1.5 mL/dose every 3-4 hours

**Dosage Forms** Liq: 10% [0.6 mL equivalent to morphine 6 mg] with alcohol 19%

**Contraindications** Increased intracranial pressure, severe respiratory depression, severe liver or renal insufficiency, known hypersensitivity to morphine sulfate

(Continued)

## Opium Tincture *(Continued)*

**Warnings/Precautions** Opium shares the toxic potential of opiate agonists, and usual precautions of opiate agonist therapy should be observed; some preparations contain sulfites which may cause allergic reactions; infants <3 months of age are more susceptible to respiratory depression, use with caution and generally in reduced doses in this age group; this is **not** paregoric, dose accordingly

**Pregnancy Risk Factor** B (C if used for prolonged periods or in high doses at term)

**Adverse Reactions**

>10%:

Cardiovascular: Palpitations, hypotension, bradycardia

Central nervous system: Drowsiness, dizziness

Neuromuscular & skeletal: Weakness

1% to 10%:

Central nervous system: Restlessness, headache, malaise

Genitourinary: Decreased urination

Miscellaneous: Histamine release

<1%: Peripheral vasodilation, CNS depression, increased intracranial pressure, insomnia, mental depression, nausea, vomiting, constipation, anorexia, stomach cramps, biliary tract spasm, urinary tract spasm, miosis, respiratory depression, physical and psychological dependence

**Drug Interactions**

Decreased effect: Phenothiazines may antagonize the analgesic effect of opiate agonists

Increased toxicity: CNS depressants, MAO inhibitors, tricyclic antidepressants may potentiate the effects of opiate agonists; dextroamphetamine may enhance the analgesic effect of opiate agonists

**Duration** 4-5 hours

**Special PA Issues**

**Patient Education:** If self-administered, use exactly as directed (do not increase dose or frequency); may cause physical and/or psychological dependence. While using this medication, do not use alcohol and other prescription or OTC medications (especially sedatives, tranquilizers, antihistamines, or pain medications) without consulting prescriber. Maintain adequate hydration (2-3 L/day of fluids unless instructed to restrict fluid intake). May cause hypotension, dizziness, drowsiness, impaired coordination, or blurred vision (use caution when driving, climbing stairs, or changing position - rising from sitting or lying to standing, or when engaging in hazardous activities until response to medication is known); dry mouth (frequent mouth care, small frequent meals, or sucking on lozenges may help). Report slow or rapid heartbeat, acute dizziness, or persistent headache; changes in mental status; swelling of extremities or unusual weight gain; changes in urinary elimination or pain on urination; acute headache; trembling or muscle spasms; blurred vision; skin rash; or shortness of breath.

**Dietary Considerations:** Alcohol: Additive CNS effect, avoid use

**Monitoring Parameters:** Observe patient for excessive sedation, respiratory depression, implement safety measures, assist with ambulation

## Oprelvekin *(oh PREL ve kir )*

**Pharmacologic Class** Biological Response Modulator; Human Growth Factor

**U.S. Brand Names** Neumega®

**Mechanism of Action** Oprelvekin stimulates multiple stages of megakaryocytopoiesis and thrombopoiesis, resulting in proliferation of megakaryocyte progenitors and megakaryocyte maturation

**Use** Prevention of severe thrombocytopenia and the reduction of the need for platelet transfusions following myelosuppressive chemotherapy in patients with nonmyeloid malignancies who are at high risk of severe thrombocytopenia.

**USUAL DOSAGE** S.C.:

Children: 75-100 mcg/kg once daily for 10-21 days (until postnadir platelet count ≥50,000 cells/µL)

Adults: 50 mcg/kg once daily for 10-21 days (until postnadir platelet count ≥50,000 cells/µL)

**Dosage Forms** Powder for inj, lyophilized: 5 mg

**Contraindications** Hypersensitivity to oprelvekin, or any component

**Warnings/Precautions** Oprelvekin should be used cautiously in patients with conditions where expansion of plasma volume should be avoided (eg, left ventricular dysfunction, congestive heart failure, hypertension); cardiac arrhythmias or conduction defects, respiratory disease; history of thromboembolic problems; hepatic or renal dysfunction; not indicated following myeloablative chemotherapy

**Pregnancy Risk Factor** C

**Adverse Reactions**

>10%:

Cardiovascular: Tachycardia (19% to 30%), palpitations (14% to 24%), atrial arrhythmias (12%), peripheral edema (60% to 75%)

Central nervous system: Headache (41%), dizziness (38%), insomnia (33%), fatigue (30%), fever (36%)

Dermatologic: Rash (25%)
Endocrine & metabolic: Fluid retention
Gastrointestinal: Nausea (50% to 77%), vomiting, anorexia
Hematologic: Anemia (100%), probably a dilutional phenomena; appears within 3 days of initiation of therapy, resolves in about 2 weeks after cessation of oprelvekin
Neuromuscular & skeletal: Arthralgia, myalgias
Respiratory: Dyspnea (48%), pleural effusions (10%)

1% to 10%:
Cardiovascular: Syncope (6% to 13%)
Gastrointestinal: Weight gain (5%)

**Special PA Issues**
**Patient Education:** Report any swelling in the arms or legs (peripheral edema), shortness of breath (congestive failure, anemia), irregular heartbeat, headaches
**Monitoring Parameters:** Monitor fluid balance during therapy, appropriate medical management is advised. If a diuretic is used, carefully monitor fluid and electrolyte balance. Obtain a CBC prior to chemotherapy and at regular intervals during therapy. Monitor platelet counts during the time of the expected nadir and until adequate recovery has occurred (postnadir counts ≥50,000 cells/μL).

- **Opticrom®** see Cromolyn Sodium on page 240
- **Opticyl®** see Tropicamide on page 943
- **Optimine®** see Azatadine on page 90
- **OptiPranolol® Ophthalmic** see Metipranolol on page 596
- **Orabase®-B [OTC]** see Benzocaine on page 105
- **Orabase® HCA** see Hydrocortisone on page 453
- **Orabase®-O [OTC]** see Benzocaine on page 105
- **Oracit®** see Sodium Citrate and Citric Acid on page 840
- **Orafen** see Ketoprofen on page 507
- **Orajel® Brace-Aid Oral Anesthetic [OTC]** see Benzocaine on page 105
- **Orajel® Maximum Strength [OTC]** see Benzocaine on page 105
- **Orajel® Mouth-Aid [OTC]** see Benzocaine on page 105
- **Orajel® Perioseptic® [OTC]** see Carbamide Peroxide on page 150
- **Oramorph SR™ Oral** see Morphine Sulfate on page 619
- **Orap™** see Pimozide on page 727
- **Orasept® [OTC]** see Benzocaine on page 105
- **Orasol® [OTC]** see Benzocaine on page 105
- **Orasone®** see Prednisone on page 754
- **Oratect™ [OTC]** see Benzocaine on page 105
- **Orazinc® [OTC]** see Zinc Supplements on page 975
- **Orbenin®** see Cloxacillin on page 229
- **Orciprenaline Sulfate** see Metaproterenol on page 575
- **Ordrine AT® Extended Release Capsule** see Caramiphen and Phenylpropanolamine on page 148
- **Oretic®** see Hydrochlorothiazide on page 447
- **Oreton® Methyl** see Methyltestosterone on page 595
- **Organidin®** see Iodinated Glycerol on page 487
- **Organidin® NR** see Guaifenesin on page 427
- **Orgaran®** see Danaparoid on page 251
- **Orinase® Diagnostic Injection** see Tolbutamide on page 911
- **Orinase® Oral** see Tolbutamide on page 911
- **ORLAAM®** see Levomethadyl Acetate Hydrochloride on page 527

# Orlistat (OR li stat)
**Pharmacologic Class** Lipase Inhibitor
**U.S. Brand Names** Xenical®
**Use** Management of obesity, including weight loss and weight management when used in conjunction with a reduced-calorie diet; reduce the risk of weight regain after prior weight loss; indicated for obese patients with an initial body mass index (BMI) ≥30 kg/m² or ≥27 kg/m² in the presence of other risk factors; see table
**USUAL DOSAGE** 120 mg 3 times daily with each main meal containing fat (during or up to 1 hour after the meal); omit dose if meal is occasionally missed or contains no fat
**Dosage Forms Cap:** 120 mg
**Contraindications** Chronic malabsorption syndrome or cholestasis; hypersensitivity to orlistat or any component
**Warnings/Precautions** Patients should be advised to adhere to dietary guidelines; gastrointestinal adverse events may increase if taken with a diet high in fat (>30% total daily calories from fat). The daily intake of fat should be distributed over three main meals. If taken with any one meal very high in fat, the possibility of gastrointestinal effects increases.

Patients should be counselec to take a multivitamin supplement that contains fat-soluble vitamins to ensure adequate nutrition because orlistat has been shown to reduce the absorption of some fat-soluble vitamins and beta-carotene. The supplement should be taken once daily at least 2 hours before or after the administration of orlistat (ie, bedtime). Some patients may develop increased levels of urinary oxalate following treatment; caution should be exercised when prescribing it to patients with a history of hyperoxaluria or calcium oxalate nephrolithias-s. As with any weight-loss agent, the potential exists for misuse in appropriate patient populations (eg, patients with anorexia nervosa or bulimia).

### Body Mass Index (BMI), kg/m$^2$
### Height (feet, inches)

| Weight (pounds) | 5'0' | 5'3' | 5'6' | 5'9' | 6'0' | 6'3' |
|---|---|---|---|---|---|---|
| 140 | 27 | 25 | 23 | 21 | 19 | 18 |
| 150 | 29 | 27 | 24 | 22 | 20 | 19 |
| 160 | 31 | 28 | 26 | 24 | 22 | 20 |
| 170 | 33 | 30 | 28 | 25 | 23 | 21 |
| 180 | 35 | 32 | 29 | 27 | 25 | 23 |
| 190 | 37 | 34 | 31 | 28 | 26 | 24 |
| 200 | 39 | 36 | 32 | 30 | 27 | 25 |
| 210 | 41 | 37 | 34 | 31 | 29 | 26 |
| 220 | 43 | 39 | 36 | 33 | 30 | 28 |
| 230 | 45 | 41 | 37 | 34 | 31 | 29 |
| 240 | 47 | 43 | 39 | 36 | 33 | 30 |
| 250 | 49 | 44 | 40 | 37 | 34 | 31 |

**Pregnancy Risk Factor** B

**Pregnancy Implications** There are no adequate and well-controlled studies of orlistat in pregnant women. Because animal reproductive studies are not always predictive of human response, orlistat is not recommended for use during pregnancy. Teratogenicity studies were conducted in rats and rabbits at doses up to 800 mg/kg/day. Neither study showed embryotoxicity or teratogenicty. This dose is 23 and 47 times the daily human dose calculated on a body surface area basis for rats and rabbits, respectively. It is not know if orlistat is secreted in human milk. Therefore, it should not be taken by nursing women.

**Adverse Reactions** Percentage unknown:
Central nervous system: Headache, dizziness, sleep disorder, anxiety, depression
Dermatitis: Dry skin, rash
Gastrointestinal: Oily spotting, flatus with discharge, fecal urgency, fatty/oily stool, oily evacuation, increased defecation, fecal incontinence
Neuromuscular & skeletal: Back pain, pain of lower extremities, arthritis, myalgia, joint disorder, tendonitis
Otic: Otitis
Respiratory: Influenza; respiracory tract infection; ear, nose, and throat symptoms

**Drug Interactions** Decreased effect: Vitamin K absorption may be decreased when taken with orlistat

**Special PA Issues**
**Patient Education:** Patient should be on a nutritionally balanced, reduced-calorie diet that contains approximately 30% of calories from fat; daily intake of fat, carbohydrate, and protein should be distributed over the three main meals
**Monitoring Parameters:** Changes in coagulation parameters

♦ **Ormazine** *see* Chlorpromazine *on page 197*

♦ **Ornidyl®** *see* Eflornithine *on page 315*

## Orphenadrine (or FEN a dreen)

**Pharmacologic Class** Anti-Parkinson's Agent (Anticholinergic); Skeletal Muscle Relaxant
**U.S. Brand Names** Norflex™
**Mechanism of Action** Indirect skeletal muscle relaxant thought to work by central atropine-like effects; has some euphorigenic and analgesic properties
**Use** Treatment of muscle spasm associated with acute painful musculoskeletal conditions; supportive therapy in tetanus
**USUAL DOSAGE** Adults:
Oral: 100 mg twice daily
I.M., I.V.: 60 mg every 12 hours
**Dosage Forms Inj:** 30 mg/mL (2 mL, 10 mL); **Tab:** 100 mg; **Tab, sustained release:** 100 mg
**Contraindications** Glaucoma, GI obstruction, cardiospasm, myasthenia gravis, hypersensitivity to orphenadrine or any component
**Warnings/Precautions** Use with caution in patients with CHF or cardiac arrhythmias; some products contain sulfites

**Pregnancy Risk Factor** C
**Adverse Reactions**
>10%:
Central nervous system: Drowsiness, dizziness
Ocular: Blurred vision
1% to 10%:
Cardiovascular: Flushing of face, tachycardia, syncope
Dermatologic: Rash
Gastrointestinal: Nausea, vomiting, constipation
Genitourinary: Decreased urination
Neuromuscular & skeletal: Weakness
Ocular: Nystagmus, increased intraocular pressure
Respiratory: Nasal congestion
<1%: Hallucinations, aplastic anemia
**Drug Interactions** CYP2B6, 2D6, and 3A3/4 enzyme substrate; CYP2B6 enzyme inhibitor
**Onset** Peak effect: Oral: Within 2-4 hours
**Duration** 4-6 hours
**Half-Life** 14-16 hours
**Special PA Issues**
**Patient Education:** Take exactly as directed. Do not increase dose or discontinue without consulting prescriber. Do not chew or crush sustained release tablets. Do not use alcohol, prescriptive or OTC antidepressants, sedatives, or pain medications without consulting prescriber. You may experience drowsiness, dizziness, lightheadedness (avoid driving or engaging in tasks that require alertness until response to therapy is known); nausea or vomiting (small, frequent meals, frequent mouth care, or sucking hard candy may help); constipation (increased dietary fluids and fibers or increased exercise may help); or decreased urination (void before taking medication). Report excessive drowsiness or mental agitation, chest pain, skin rash, swelling of mouth/face, difficulty speaking, or vision disturbances.
**Dietary Considerations:** Alcohol: Additive CNS effect, avoid use

# Orphenadrine, Aspirin, and Caffeine
(or FEN a dreen, AS pir in, & KAF een)
**Pharmacologic Class** Skeletal Muscle Relaxant
**U.S. Brand Names** Norgesic™; Norgesic™ Forte
**Dosage Forms Tab:** Orphenadrine citrate 25 mg, aspirin 385 mg, and caffeine 30 mg; **Tab (Norgesic® Forte):** Orphenadrine citrate 50 mg, aspirin 770 mg, and caffeine 60 mg

♦ **Ovrette**® *see Norgestrel on page 665*

♦ **O-V Staticin**® *see Nystatin on page 669*

# Oxacillin (oks a SIL in)

**Pharmacologic Class** Antibiotic, Penicillin

**U.S. Brand Names** Bactocill®; Prostaphlin®

**Mechanism of Action** Inhibits bacterial cell wall synthesis by binding to one or more of the penicillin binding proteins (PBPs); which in turn inhibits the final transpeptidation step of peptidoglycan synthesis in bacterial cell walls, thus inhibiting cell wall biosynthesis. Bacteria eventually lyse due to ongoing activity of cell wall autolytic enzymes (autolysins and murein hydrolases) while cell wall assembly is arrested.

**Use** Treatment of infections such as osteomyelitis, septicemia, endocarditis, and CNS infections caused by susceptible strains of *Staphylococcus*

**USUAL DOSAGE**

Neonates: I.M., I.V.:

Postnatal age <7 days:

<2000 g: 25 mg/kg/dose every 12 hours

>2000 g: 25 mg/kg/dose every 8 hours

Postnatal age >7 days:

<1200 g: 25 mg/kg/dose every 12 hours

1200-2000 g: 30 mg/kg/dose every 8 hours

>2000 g: 37.5 mg/kg/dose every 6 hours

Infants and Children:

Oral: 50-100 mg/kg/day divided every 6 hours

I.M., I.V.: 150-200 mg/kg/day in divided doses every 6 hours; maximum dose: 12 g/day

Adults:

Oral: 500-1000 mg every 4-6 hours for at least 5 days

I.M., I.V.: 250 mg to 2 g/dose every 4-6 hours

**Dosing adjustment in renal impairment:** Cl$_{cr}$ <10 mL/minute: Use lower range of the usual dosage

Hemodialysis: Not dialyzable (0% to 5%)

**Dosage Forms Cap:** 250 mg, 500 mg; **Powder for inj:** 250 mg, 500 mg, 1 g, 2 g, 4 g, 10 g; **Powder for oral soln:** 250 mg/5 mL (100 mL)

**Contraindications** Hypersensitivity to oxacillin or other penicillins or any component

**Warnings/Precautions** Elimination rate will be slow in neonates; modify dosage in patients with renal impairment and in the elderly; use with caution in patients with cephalosporin hypersensitivity

**Pregnancy Risk Factor** B

**Adverse Reactions**

1% to 10%: Gastrointestinal: Nausea, diarrhea

<1%: Fever, rash, vomiting, eosinophilia, leukopenia, neutropenia, thrombocytopenia, agranulocytosis, hepatotoxicity, increased AST, hematuria, acute interstitial nephritis, serum sickness-like reactions

**Drug Interactions**

Decreased effect: Efficacy of oral contraceptives may be reduced; effects of penicillins may be impaired by tetracycline

Increased effect: Disulfiram, probenecid may increase penicillin levels, increased effect of anticoagulants are possible with large I.V. doses

**Half-Life** Absorption: Oral: 35% to 67%; Adults: 23-60 minutes (prolonged with reduced renal function and in neonates)

**Special PA Issues**

**Patient Education:** Take at regular intervals around-the-clock, preferably on empty stomach with a full glass of water. Take complete course of treatment as prescribed. You may experience nausea or vomiting; small frequent meals and good mouth care may help. If diabetic, drug may cause false tests with Clinitest® urine glucose monitoring; use of glucose oxidase methods (Clinistix®) or serum glucose monitoring is preferable. This drug may interfere with oral contraceptives; an alternate form of birth control should be used. Report persistent fever, sore throat, sores in mouth, diarrhea, unusual bleeding or bruising, difficulty breathing, or skin rash. Notify prescriber if condition does not respond to treatment.

**Monitoring Parameters:** Observe for signs and symptoms of anaphylaxis during first dose

♦ **Oxacillin Sodium** *see Oxacillin on this page*

# Oxamniquine (oks AM ni kwin)

**Pharmacologic Class** Anthelmintic

**U.S. Brand Names** Vansil™

**Mechanism of Action** Not fully elucidated; causes worms to dislodge from their usual site of residence (mesenteric veins to the liver) by paralysis and contraction of musculature and subsequently phagocytized

**Use** Treatment of all stages of *Schistosoma mansoni* infection

**USUAL DOSAGE** Oral:
  Children <30 kg: 20 mg/kg in 2 divided doses of 10 mg/kg at 2- to 8-hour intervals
  Adults: 12-15 mg/kg as a single dose

**Dosage Forms Cap:** 250 mg

**Warnings/Precautions** Rare epileptiform convulsions have been observed within the first few hours of administration, especially in patients with a history of CNS pathology

**Pregnancy Risk Factor** C

**Adverse Reactions**
  >10%: Central nervous system: Dizziness, drowsiness, headache
  <10%:
    Central nervous system: Insomnia, malaise, hallucinations, behavior changes
    Gastrointestinal: GI effects, orange/red discoloration of urine
    Hepatic: Elevated LFTs
    Dermatologic: Rash, urticaria, pruritus
    Renal: Proteinuria

**Drug Interactions** May be synergistic with praziquantel

**Special PA Issues**
  **Patient Education:** Take with food

♦ **Oxandrin®** *see* Oxandrolone *on this page*

# Oxandrolone (oks AN droe lone)

**Pharmacologic Class** Androgen

**U.S. Brand Names** Oxandrin®

**Mechanism of Action** Synthetic testosterone derivative with similar androgenic and anabolic actions

**Use** Adjunctive therapy to promote weight gain after weight loss following extensive surgery, chronic infections, or severe trauma, and in some patients who, without definite pathophysiologic reasons, fail to gain or to maintain normal weight

**USUAL DOSAGE**
  Children: Total daily dose: ≤0.1 mg/kg **or** ≤0.045 mg/lb
  Adults: 2.5 mg 2-4 times/day; however, since the response of individuals to anabolic steroids varies, a daily dose of as little as 2.5 mg or as much as 20 mg may be required to achieve the desired response. A course of therapy of 2-4 weeks is usually adequate. This may be repeated intermittently as needed.
  **Dosing adjustment in renal impairment:** Caution is recommended because of the propensity of oxandrolone to cause edema and water retention
  **Dosing adjustment in hepatic impairment:** Caution is advised but there are not specific guidelines for dosage reduction

**Dosage Forms Tab:** 2.5 mg

**Contraindications** Nephrosis, carcinoma of breast or prostate, pregnancy, hypersensitivity to oxandrolone or any component

**Warnings/Precautions** May stunt bone growth in children; anabolic steroids may cause peliosis hepatis, liver cell tumors, and blood lipid changes with increased risk of arteriosclerosis; monitor diabetic patients carefully; use with caution in elderly patients, they may be at greater risk for prostatic hypertrophy; use with caution in patients with cardiac, renal, or hepatic disease or epilepsy

**Pregnancy Risk Factor** X

**Adverse Reactions**
  **Male:**
  Postpubertal:
    >10%:
      Dermatologic: Acne
      Endocrine & metabolic: Gynecomastia
      Genitourinary: Bladder irritability, priapism
    1% to 10%:
      Central nervous system: Insomnia, chills
      Endocrine & metabolic: Decreased libido, hepatic dysfunction,
      Gastrointestinal: Nausea, diarrhea
      Genitourinary: Prostatic hypertrophy (elderly)
      Hematologic: Iron deficiency anemia, suppression of clotting factors
    <1%: Hepatic necrosis, hepatocellular carcinoma
  Prepubertal:
    >10%:
      Dermatologic: Acne
      Endocrine & metabolic: Virilism
    1% to 10%:
      Central nervous system: Chills, insomnia, factors
      Dermatologic: Hyperpigmentation
      Gastrointestinal: Diarrhea, nausea
      Hematologic: Iron deficiency anemia, suppression of clotting
    <1%: Hepatic necrosis, hepatocellular carcinoma

(Continued)

## Oxandrolone *(Continued)*

**Female:**
>10%: Endocrine & metabolic: Virilism
1% to 10%:
  Central nervous system: Chills, insomnia
  Endocrine & metabolic: Hypercalcemia
  Gastrointestinal: Nausea, diarrhea
  Hematologic: Iron deficiency anemia, suppression of clotting factors
  Hepatic: Hepatic dysfunction
<1%: Hepatic necrosis, hepatocellular carcinoma

**Drug Interactions** Increased toxicity: ACTH, adrenal steroids may increase risk of edema and acne; stanozolol enhances the hypoprothrombinemic effects of oral anticoagulants; enhances the hypoglycemic effects of insulin and sulfonylureas (oral hypoglycemics)

**Special PA Issues**
**Patient Education:** High protein, high caloric diet is suggested, restrict salt intake; glucose tolerance may be altered in diabetics

## Oxaprozin *(oks a PROE zin)*

**Pharmacologic Class** Nonsteroidal Anti-Inflammatory Agent (NSAID)
**U.S. Brand Names** Daypro™
**Mechanism of Action** Inhibits prostaglandin synthesis by decreasing the activity of the enzyme, cyclo-oxygenase, which results in decreased formation of prostaglandin precursors
**Use** Acute and long-term use in the management of signs and symptoms of osteoarthritis and rheumatoid arthritis
**USUAL DOSAGE** Adults: Oral (individualize dosage to lowest effective dose to minimize adverse effects):
Osteoarthritis: 600-1200 mg once daily
Rheumatoid arthritis: 1200 mg once daily
Maximum dose: 1800 mg/day or 26 mg/kg (whichever is lower) in divided doses
**Dosage Forms** Tab: 600 mg
**Contraindications** Aspirin allergy, 3rd trimester pregnancy or allergy to oxaprozin, history of GI disease, renal or hepatic dysfunction, bleeding disorders, cardiac failure, elderly, debilitated, nursing mothers
**Pregnancy Risk Factor** C
**Adverse Reactions**
1% to 10%:
  Central nervous system: CNS inhibition, disturbance of sleep
  Dermatologic: Rash
  Gastrointestinal: Nausea, dyspepsia, abdominal pain, anorexia, flatulence, vomiting
  Genitourinary: Dysuria or frequency
<1%: Anaphylaxis, serum sickness, edema, change in blood pressure, peptic ulcer and/or GI bleed, LFT abnormalities, stomatitis, rectal bleeding, pancreatitis, anemia, thrombocytopenia, leukopenia, ecchymosis, agranulocytosis, pancytopenia, weight gain, weight loss, weakness, malaise, symptoms of upper respiratory infection, pruritus, urticaria, photosensitivity, exfoliative dermatitis, erythema multiforme, Stevens-Johnson syndrome, blurred vision, conjunctivitis, acute interstitial nephritis, nephrotic syndrome, hematuria, renal insufficiency, acute renal failure, decreased menstrual flow

**Drug Interactions** Increased toxicity: Aspirin, oral anticoagulants, diuretics
**Onset** Steady-state 4-7 days
**Duration** Absorption: Almost completely; Protein binding: >99%; Half-life: 40-50 hours; Time to peak: 2-4 hours
**Half-Life** 40-50 hours
**Special PA Issues**
**Patient Education:** Take this medication exactly as directed; do not increase dose without consulting prescriber. Do not crush tablets or break capsules. Take with food or milk to reduce GI distress. Maintain adequate fluid intake (2-3 L/day). Do not use alcohol, aspirin, or aspirin-containing medication, and all other anti-inflammatory medications without consulting prescriber. You may experience drowsiness, dizziness, or nervousness (use caution when driving or performing hazardous tasks); anorexia, nausea, vomiting, or heartburn (frequent small meals, frequent oral care, sucking on lozenges, or chewing gum may help). GI bleeding, ulceration, or perforation can occur with or without pain; discontinue medication and contact prescriber if persistent abdominal pain or cramping, or blood in stool occurs. Report vaginal bleeding; breathlessness, difficulty breathing, or unusual cough; chest pain, rapid heartbeat, palpitations; unusual bruising/bleeding; blood in urine, stool, mouth, or vomitus; swollen extremities; skin rash or itching; acute fatigue; or swelling of face, lips, tongue, or throat.
**Monitoring Parameters:** Monitor blood, hepatic, renal, and ocular function
**Related Information**
Nonsteroidal Anti-Inflammatory Agents *on page 1026*

## Oxazepam (oks A ze pam)

**Pharmacologic Class** Benzodiazepine

**U.S. Brand Names** Serax®

**Mechanism of Action** Benzodiazepine anxiolytic sedative that produces CNS depression at the subcortical level, except at high doses, whereby it works at the cortical level

**Use** Treatment of anxiety and management of alcohol withdrawal; may also be used as an anticonvulsant in management of simple partial seizures

**USUAL DOSAGE** Oral:

Children: 1 mg/kg/day has been administered

Adults:

Anxiety: 10-30 mg 3-4 times/day

Alcohol withdrawal: 15-30 mg 3-4 times/day

Hypnotic: 15-30 mg

Hemodialysis: Not dialyzable (0% to 5%)

**Dosage Forms Cap:** 10 mg, 15 mg, 30 mg; **Tab:** 15 mg

**Contraindications** Hypersensitivity to oxazepam or any component, cross-sensitivity with other benzodiazepines may exist

**Warnings/Precautions** Avoid using in patients with pre-existing CNS depression, severe uncontrolled pain, or narrow-angle glaucoma; use with caution in patients using other CNS depressants and in the elderly

**Pregnancy Risk Factor** D

**Adverse Reactions**

>10%:

Cardiovascular: Tachycardia, chest pain

Central nervous system: Drowsiness, fatigue, ataxia, lightheadedness, memory impairment, insomnia, anxiety, depression, headache

Dermatologic: Rash

Endocrine & metabolic: Decreased libido

Gastrointestinal: Xerostomia, constipation, diarrhea, decreased salivation, nausea, vomiting, increased or decreased appetite

Neuromuscular & skeletal: Dysarthria

Ocular: Blurred vision

Miscellaneous: Diaphoresis

1% to 10%:

Cardiovascular: Syncope, hypotension

Central nervous system: Confusion, nervousness, dizziness, akathisia

Dermatologic: Dermatitis

Gastrointestinal: Increased salivation, weight gain or loss

Neuromuscular & skeletal: Rigidity, tremor, muscle cramps

Ocular: Blurred vision

Otic: Tinnitus

Respiratory: Nasal congestion, hyperventilation

<1%: Menstrual irregularities, blood dyscrasias, reflex slowing, drug dependence

**Drug Interactions** Increased toxicity with CNS depressants (eg, barbiturates, MAO inhibitors, TCAs, alcohol, narcotics, phenothiazines, and other sedative-hypnotics)

**Onset** Peak serum concentration: 1-2 hours

**Half-Life** 2.8-5.7 hours

**Special PA Issues**

**Patient Education:** Take exactly as directed (do not increase dose or frequency); may take 2-3 weeks to achieve desired results; may cause physical and/or psychological dependence. Do not use excessive alcohol or other prescription or OTC medications (especially pain medications, sedatives, antihistamines, or hypnotics) without consulting prescriber. Maintain adequate hydration (2-3 L/day of fluids unless instructed to restrict fluid intake). You may experience drowsiness, lightheadedness, impaired coordination, dizziness, or blurred vision (use caution when driving or engaging in hazardous tasks until response to medication is known); nausea, vomiting, or dry mouth (small frequent meals, good mouth care, chewing gum, or sucking lozenges may help); constipation (increased exercise, fluids, or dietary fruit and fiber may help); altered sexual drive or ability (reversible); or photosensitivity (use sunscreen, protective clothing, and avoid extended exposure to direct sunlight). Report persistent CNS effects (eg, confusion, depression, increased sedation, excitation, headache, agitation, insomnia or nightmares, dizziness, fatigue, impaired coordination, changes in personality, or changes in cognition); changes in urinary pattern; muscle cramping, weakness, tremors, or rigidity; ringing in ears or visual disturbances; chest pain, palpitations, or rapid heartbeat; excessive perspiration, excessive GI symptoms (cramping, constipation, vomiting, anorexia); or worsening of condition.

(Continued)

## Oxazepam *(Continued)*

**Dietary Considerations:** Alcohol: Additive CNS effect, avoid use
**Monitoring Parameters:** Respiratory and cardiovascular status
**Reference Range:** Therapeutic: 0.2-1.4 µg/mL (SI: 0.7-4.9 µmol/L)

## Oxiconazole (oks i KON a zole)

**Pharmacologic Class** Antifungal Agent, Topical
**U.S. Brand Names** Oxistat®

**Mechanism of Action** The cytoplasmic membrane integrity of fungi is destroyed by oxiconazole which exerts a fungicidal activity through inhibition of ergosterol synthesis. Effective for treatment of tinea pedis, tinea cruris, and tinea corporis. Active against *Trichophyton rubrum*, *Trichophyton mentagrophytes*, *Trichophyton violaceum*, *Microsporum canis*, *Microsporum audouini*, *Microsporum gypseum*, *Epidermophyton floccosum*, *Candida albicans*, and *Malassezia furfur*.

**Use** Treatment of tinea pedis (athlete's foot), tinea cruris (jock itch), and tinea corporis (ringworm)

**USUAL DOSAGE** Children and Adults: Topical: Apply once to twice daily to affected areas for 2 weeks (tinea corporis/tinea cruris) to 1 month (tinea pedis)

**Dosage Forms Crm:** 1% (15 g, 30 g, 60 g); **Lot:** 1% (30 mL)

**Contraindications** Hypersensitivity to this agent; not for ophthalmic use

**Warnings/Precautions** May cause irritation during therapy; if a sensitivity to oxiconazole occurs, therapy should be discontinued; avoid contact with eyes or vagina

**Pregnancy Risk Factor** B

**Adverse Reactions** 1% to 10%:
Dermatologic: Itching, erythema
Local: Transient burning, local irritation, stinging, dryness

**Drug Interactions** CYP3A3/4 enzyme inhibitor

**Special PA Issues**
**Patient Education:** External use only; discontinue if sensitivity or chemical irritation occurs, contact physician if condition fails to improve in 3-4 days

**Related Information**
Antifungal Agents, Topical *on page 1000*

♦ **Oxiconazole Nitrate** *see* Oxiconazole *on this page*
♦ **Oxilan®** *see* Ioxilan *on page 488*
♦ **Oxilapine Succinate** *see* Loxapine *on page 547*
♦ **Oxistat®** *see* Oxiconazole *on this page*
♦ **Oxpam®** *see* Oxazepam *on previous page*
♦ **Oxpentifylline** *see* Pentoxifylline *on page 709*
♦ **Oxsoralen® Topical** *see* Methoxsalen *on page 589*
♦ **Oxsoralen-Ultra® Oral** *see* Methoxsalen *on page 589*
♦ **Oxtriphylline** *see* Theophylline Salts *on page 888*

## Oxybutynin (oks i BYOO ti nin)

**Pharmacologic Class** Antispasmodic Agent, Urinary
**U.S. Brand Names** Ditropan®; Ditropan XL®

**Mechanism of Action** Direct antispasmodic effect on smooth muscle, also inhibits the action of acetylcholine on smooth muscle (exhibits $1/5$ the anticholinergic activity of atropine, but is 4-10 times the antispasmodic activity); does not block effects at skeletal muscle or at autonomic ganglia; increases bladder capacity, decreases uninhibited contractions, and delays desire to void; therefore, decreases urgency and frequency

**Use** Antispasmodic for neurogenic bladder (urgency, frequency, urge incontinence) and uninhibited bladder

**USUAL DOSAGE** Oral:
Children:
1-5 years: 0.2 mg/kg/dose 2-4 times/day
>5 years: 5 mg twice daily, up to 5 mg 4 times/day maximum
Adults: 5 mg 2-3 times/day up to 5 mg 4 times/day maximum
Extended release: Initial: 5 mg once daily, may increase in 5-10 mg increments; maximum: 30 mg daily
Elderly: 2.5-5 mg twice daily; increase by 2.5 mg increments every 1-2 days
**Note:** Should be discontinued periodically to determine whether the patient can manage without the drug and to minimize resistance to the drug

**Dosage Forms Syr:** 5 mg/5 mL (473 mL); **Tab:** 5 mg; **Tab, ext release:** 5 mg, 10 mg

**Contraindications** Glaucoma, myasthenia gravis, partial or complete GI obstruction, GU obstruction, ulcerative colitis, hypersensitivity to drug or specific component, intestinal atony, megacolon, toxic megacolon

**Warnings/Precautions** Use with caution in patients with urinary tract obstruction, angle-closure glaucoma, hyperthyroidism, reflux esophagitis, heart disease, hepatic or renal disease, prostatic hypertrophy autonomic neuropathy, ulcerative colitis (may cause ileus and toxic megacolon), hypertension, hiatal hernia. Caution should be used in elderly due to anticholinergic activity (eg, confusion, constipation, blurred vision, and tachycardia).

**Pregnancy Risk Factor** B

**Adverse Reactions**

>10%:

Central nervous system: Drowsiness

Gastrointestinal: Xerostomia, constipation

Miscellaneous: Diaphoresis (decreased)

1% to 10%:

Cardiovascular: Tachycardia, palpitations

Central nervous system: Dizziness, insomnia, fever, headache

Dermatologic: Rash

Endocrine & metabolic: Decreased flow of breast milk, decreased sexual ability, hot flashes

Gastrointestinal: Nausea, vomiting

Genitourinary: Urinary hesitancy or retention

Neuromuscular & skeletal: Weakness

Ocular: Blurred vision, mydriatic effect

<1%: Increased intraocular pressure, allergic reaction

**Drug Interactions** Increased toxicity:

Additive sedation with CNS depressants and alcohol

Additive anticholinergic effects with antihistamines and anticholinergic agents

**Onset** Oral: 30-60 minutes; Peak effect: 3-6 hours

**Duration** 6-10 hours

**Half-Life** 1-2.3 hours

**Special PA Issues**

**Patient Education:** Take prescribed dose preferably on an empty stomach (1 hour before or 2 hours after meals). You may experience dizziness, lightheadedness, or drowsiness (use caution when driving or with tasks that require alertness); dry mouth or changes in appetite (small frequent meals, frequent mouth care, sucking on lozenges, or chewing gum may help); constipation (frequent exercise or increased dietary fiber, fruit, and fluid or stool softener may help); decreased sexual ability (reversible with discontinuance of drug); decreased sweating (use caution in hot weather, avoid extreme exercise or activity). Report rapid heartbeat, palpitations, or chest pain; difficulty voiding; or vision changes.

**Monitoring Parameters:** Incontinence episodes, postvoid residual (PVR)

♦ **Oxybutynin Chloride** see Oxybutynin on previous page

♦ **Oxycocet** see Oxycodone and Acetaminophen on next page

♦ **Oxycodan** see Oxycodone and Aspirin on next page

# Oxycodone (oks i KOE done)

**Pharmacologic Class** Analgesic, Narcotic

**U.S. Brand Names** OxyContin®; OxyIR™; Percolone™; Roxicodone™

**Mechanism of Action** Binds to opiate receptors in the CNS, causing inhibition of ascending pain pathways, altering the perception of and response to pain; produces generalized CNS depression

**Use** Management of moderate to severe pain, normally used in combination with non-narcotic analgesics

**USUAL DOSAGE** Oral:

Immediate release:

Children:

6-12 years: 1.25 mg every 6 hours as needed

>12 years: 2.5 mg every 6 hours as needed

Adults: 5 mg every 6 hours as needed

Controlled release: Adults: 10 mg every 12 hours around-the-clock

**Dosing adjustment in hepatic impairment:** Reduce dosage in patients with severe liver disease

**Dosage Forms Cap, as hydrochloride, immediate release (OxyIR™):** 5 mg; **Liq, oral, as hydrochloride:** 5 mg/5 mL (500 mL); **Soln, oral concentrate, as hydrochloride:** 20 mg/mL (30 mL); **Tab, as hydrochloride:** 5 mg, Percolone™: 5 mg; **Tab, controlled release, as hydrochloride (OxyContin®):** 10 mg, 20 mg, 40 mg, 80 mg, (Roxicodone™): 10 mg, 30 mg

**Contraindications** Hypersensitivity to oxycodone or any component

**Warnings/Precautions** Use with caution in patients with hypersensitivity reactions to other phenanthrene derivative opioid agonists (morphine, hydrocodone, hydromorphone, levorphanol, oxycodone, oxymorphone); respiratory diseases including asthma, emphysema, COPD, or severe liver or renal insufficiency; some preparations contain sulfites which may cause allergic reactions; dextromethorphan has equivalent antitussive activity but has much lower toxicity in accidental overdose; tolerance or drug dependence may result from extended use

**Pregnancy Risk Factor** B (D if used for prolonged periods or in high doses at term)

(Continued)

## Oxycodone *(Continued)*

### Adverse Reactions

>10%:

Cardiovascular: Hypotension

Central nervous system: Fatigue, drowsiness, dizziness

Gastrointestinal: Nausea, vomiting

Neuromuscular & skeletal: Weakness

1% to 10%:

Central nervous system: Nervousness, headache, restlessness, malaise, confusion

Gastrointestinal: Anorexia, stomach cramps, xerostomia, constipation, biliary spasm

Genitourinary: Ureteral spasms, decreased urination

Local: Pain at injection site

Respiratory: Dyspnea, shortness of breath

<1%: Mental depression, hallucinations, paradoxical CNS stimulation, increased intracranial pressure, skin rash, urticaria, paralytic ileus, histamine release, physical and psychological dependence

### Drug Interactions CYP2D6 enzyme substrate

Decreased effect: Phenothiazines may antagonize the analgesic effect of opiate agonists

Increased toxicity: CNS depressants, monoamine oxidase inhibitors, general anesthetics, and tricyclic antidepressants may potentiate the effects of opiate agonists; dextroamphetamine may enhance the analgesic effect of opiate agonists

### Onset Oral: Within 10-15 minutes

### Duration 4-5 hours; up to 12 hours for controlled release

### Special PA Issues

**Patient Education:** If self-administered, use exactly as directed (do not increase dose or frequency); may cause physical and/or psychological dependence. While using this medication, do not use alcohol and other prescription or OTC medications (especially sedatives, tranquilizers, antihistamines, or pain medications) without consulting prescriber. Maintain adequate hydration (2-3 L/day of fluids unless instructed to restrict fluid intake). May cause hypotension, dizziness, drowsiness, impaired coordination, or blurred vision (use caution when driving, climbing stairs, or changing position - rising from sitting or lying to standing, or when engaging in hazardous activities until response to medication is known); nausea, vomiting or dry mouth (frequent mouth care, small frequent meals, or sucking on lozenges may help); constipation (increased exercise, fluids, or dietary fruit and fiber may help - if constipation remains an unresolved problem, consult prescriber about use of stool softeners) Report persistent dizziness or headache; excessive fatigue or sedation; changes in mental status; changes in urinary elimination or pain on urination; weakness or trembling; blurred vision; or shortness of breath.

**Dietary Considerations:** Alcohol: Additive CNS effect, avoid use

**Monitoring Parameters:** Pain relief, respiratory and mental status, blood pressure

**Reference Range:** Blood level of 5 mg/L associated with fatality

### Related Information

Narcotic Agonists *on page 1020*

## Oxycodone and Acetaminophen (oks i KOE done & a seet a MIN oh fen)

**Pharmacologic Class** Analgesic, Narcotic

**U.S. Brand Names** Percocet®; Roxicet® 5/500; Roxilox®; Tylox®

**Dosage Forms Caplet:** Oxycodone hydrochloride 5 mg and acetaminophen 500 mg; **Cap:** Oxycodone hydrochloride 5 mg and acetaminophen 500 mg; **Soln, oral:** Oxycodone hydrochloride 5 mg and acetaminophen 325 mg per 5 mL (5 mL, 500 mL); **Tab:** Oxycodone hydrochloride 5 mg and acetaminophen 325 mg

## Oxycodone and Aspirin (oks i KOE done & AS pir in)

**Pharmacologic Class** Analgesic, Narcotic

**U.S. Brand Names** Codoxy®; Fercodan®; Percodan®-Demi; Roxiprin®

**Dosage Forms Tab:** Percodan®: Oxycodone hydrochloride 4.5 mg, oxycodone terephthalate 0.38 mg, and aspirin 325 mg, Percodan®-Demi: Oxycodone hydrochloride 2.25 mg, oxycodone terephthalate 0.19 mg, and aspirin 325 mg

- ♦ **Oxycodone Hydrochloride** *see Oxycodone on previous page*
- ♦ **OxyContin®** *see Oxycodone on previous page*
- ♦ **Oxydess® II** *see Dextroamphetamine on page 268*
- ♦ **OxyIR™** *see Oxycodone on previous page*

## Oxymetholone (oks i METH oh lone)

**Pharmacologic Class** Anabolic Steroid

**U.S. Brand Names** Anadrol®

**Mechanism of Action** Stimulates receptors in organs and tissues to promote growth and development of male sex organs and maintains secondary sex characteristics in androgen-deficient males

**Use** Anemias caused by the administration of myelotoxic drugs

**USUAL DOSAGE** Adults: Erythropoietic effects: Oral: 1-5 mg/kg/day in one daily dose; usual effective dose: 1-2 mg/kg/day; give for a minimum trial of 3-6 months because response may be delayed

**Dosing adjustment in hepatic impairment:**
> Mild to moderate hepatic impairment: Oxymetholone should be used with caution in patients with liver dysfunction because of it's hepatotoxic potential
> Severe hepatic impairment: Oxymetholone should **not** be used

**Dosage Forms Tab:** 50 mg

**Contraindications** Carcinoma of breast or prostate, nephrosis, pregnancy, hypersensitivity to any component

**Warnings/Precautions** Anabolic steroids may cause peliosis hepatis, liver cell tumors, and blood lipid changes with increased risk of arteriosclerosis; monitor diabetic patients carefully; use with caution in elderly patients, they may be at greater risk for prostatic hypertrophy; use with caution in patients with cardiac, renal, or hepatic disease or epilepsy

**Pregnancy Risk Factor** X

**Adverse Reactions**
**Male:**
Postpubertal:
>10%:
Dermatologic: Acne
Endocrine & metabolic: Gynecomastia
Genitourinary: Bladder irritability, priapism
1% to 10%:
Central nervous system: Insomnia, chills
Endocrine & metabolic: Decreased libido
Gastrointestinal: Nausea, diarrhea
Genitourinary: Prostatic hypertrophy (elderly)
Hematologic: Iron deficiency anemia, suppression of clotting factors
Hepatic: Hepatic dysfunction
<1%: Hepatic necrosis, hepatocellular carcinoma
Prepubertal:
>10%:
Dermatologic: Acne
Endocrine & metabolic: Virilism
1% to 10%:
Central nervous system: Chills, insomnia
Dermatologic: Hyperpigmentation
Gastrointestinal: Diarrhea, nausea
Hematologic: Iron deficiency anemia, suppression of clotting factors
<1%: Hepatic necrosis, hepatocellular carcinoma

**Female:**
>10%: Endocrine & metabolic: Virilism
1% to 10%:
Central nervous system: Chills, insomnia
Endocrine & metabolic: Hypercalcemia
Gastrointestinal: Nausea, diarrhea
Hematologic: Iron deficiency anemia, suppression of clotting factors
Hepatic: Hepatic dysfunction
<1%: Hepatic necrosis, hepatocellular carcinoma

**Drug Interactions** Increased toxicity: Increased oral anticoagulants, insulin requirements may be decreased

**Half-Life** 9 hours

**Special PA Issues**
**Patient Education:** Take as directed; do not exceed recommended dosage. If diabetic, monitor serum glucose closely and notify prescriber of changes; this medication can alter hypoglycemic requirements. You may experience acne, growth of body hair or baldness, deepening of voice, loss of libido, impotence, swelling of breasts, menstrual irregularity, or priapism (most are reversible); drowsiness, dizziness, or blurred vision (use caution driving or when engaging in hazardous tasks); or nausea or vomiting (small frequent meals and good mouth care may help). Report persistent GI distress or diarrhea; change in color of urine or stool; yellowing of eyes or skin; swelling of ankles, feet, or hands; unusual bruising or bleeding; or other adverse reactions.

**Monitoring Parameters:** Liver function tests

# Oxymorphone (oks i MOR fone)

**Pharmacologic Class** Analgesic, Narcotic

**U.S. Brand Names** Numorphan®

**Mechanism of Action** Oxymorphone hydrochloride (Numorphan®) is a potent narcotic analgesic with uses similar to those of morphine. The drug is a semisynthetic derivative of morphine (phenanthrene derivative) and is closely related to hydromorphone chemically (Dilaudid®).
(Continued)

## Oxymorphone *(Continued)*

**Use** Management of moderate to severe pain and preoperatively as a sedative and a supplement to anesthesia

**USUAL DOSAGE** Adults:

I.M., S.C.: 0.5 mg initially, 1-1.5 mg every 4-6 hours as needed

I.V.: 0.5 mg initially

Rectal: 5 mg every 4-6 hours

**Dosage Forms Inj:** 1 mg (1 mL); 1.5 mg/mL (1 mL, 10 mL); **Supp, rectal:** 5 mg

**Contraindications** Hypersensitivity to oxymorphone or any component, increased intracranial pressure; severe respiratory depression

**Warnings/Precautions** Some preparations contain sulfites which may cause allergic reactions; infants <3 months of age are more susceptible to respiratory depression, use with caution and generally in reduced doses in this age group; use with caution in patients with impaired respiratory function or severe hepatic dysfunction and in patients with hypersensitivity reactions to other phenanthrene derivative opioid agonists (codeine, hydrocodone, hydromorphone, levorphanol, oxycodone, oxymorphone); tolerance or drug dependence may result from extended use

**Pregnancy Risk Factor** B (D if used for prolonged periods or in high doses at term)

**Adverse Reactions**

>10%:

Cardiovascular: Hypotension

Central nervous system: Fatigue, drowsiness, dizziness

Gastrointestinal: Nausea, vomiting, constipation

Neuromuscular & skeletal: Weakness

Miscellaneous: Histamine release

1% to 10%:

Central nervous system: Nervousness, headache, restlessness, malaise, confusion

Gastrointestinal: Anorexia, stomach cramps, xerostomia, biliary spasm

Genitourinary: Decreased urination, ureteral spasms

Local: Pain at injection site

Respiratory: Dyspnea, shortness of breath

<1%: Mental depression, hallucinations, paradoxical CNS stimulation, increased intracranial pressure, rash, urticaria, paralytic ileus, histamine release, physical and psychological dependence

**Drug Interactions**

Decreased effect with phenothiazines

Increased effect/toxicity with CNS depressants, TCAs, dextroamphetamine

**Onset** Onset of analgesia: I.V., .M., S.C.: Within 5-10 minutes; Rectal: Within 15-30 minutes

**Duration** Duration of analgesia: Parenteral, rectal: 3-4 hours

**Special PA Issues**

**Patient Education:** If self-administered, use exactly as directed (do not increase dose or frequency); may cause physical and/or psychological dependence. While using this medication, do not use alcohol and other prescription or OTC medications (especially sedatives, tranquilizers, antihistamines, or pain medications) without consulting prescriber. Maintain adequate hydration (2-3 L/day of fluids unless instructed to restrict fluid intake). May cause hypotension, dizziness, drowsiness, impaired coordination, or blurred vision (use caution when driving, climbing stairs, or changing position - rising from sitting or lying to standing, or when engaging in hazardous activities until response to medication is known); nausea, vomiting or dry mouth (frequent mouth care, small frequent meals, or sucking on lozenges may help); constipation (increased exercise, fluids, or dietary fruit and fiber may help - if constipation remains an unresolved problem, consult prescriber about use of stool softeners). Report persistent dizziness or headache; excessive fatigue or sedation; changes in mental status; changes in urinary elimination or pain on urination; weakness or trembling; blurred vision; or shortness of breath.

**Dietary Considerations:** Alcohol: Additive CNS effect, avoid use

**Monitoring Parameters:** Respiratory rate, heart rate, blood pressure, CNS activity

**Related Information**

Narcotic Agonists *on page 1023*

♦ **Oxymorphone Hydrochloride** *see* Oxymorphone *on previous page*

## Oxytetracycline *(oks i tet ra SYE kleen)*

**Pharmacologic Class** Antibiotic, Tetracycline Derivative

**U.S. Brand Names** Terramycin® I.M. Injection; Terramycin® Oral; Uri-Tet® Oral

**Mechanism of Action** Inhibits bacterial protein synthesis by binding with the 30S and possibly the 50S ribosomal subunit(s) of susceptible bacteria, cell wall synthesis is not affected

**Use** Treatment of susceptible bacterial infections; both gram-positive and gram-negative, as well as, *Rickettsia* and *Mycoplasma* organisms

**USUAL DOSAGE**

Oral:

Children >8 years: 40-50 mg/kg/day in divided doses every 6 hours (maximum: 2 g/24 hours)

Adults: 250-500 mg/dose every 6-12 hours depending on severity of the infection

I.M.:

Children >8 years: 15-25 mg/kg/day (maximum: 250 mg/dose) in divided doses every 8-12 hours

Adults: 250 mg every 24 hours or 300 mg/day divided every 8-12 hours

Syphilis: 30-40 g in divided doses over 10-15 days

Gonorrhea: 1.5 g, then 500 mg every 6 hours for total of 9 g

Uncomplicated chlamydial infections: 500 mg every 6 hours for 7 days

Severe acne: 1 g/day then decrease to 125-500 mg/day

**Dosing interval in renal impairment:**

$Cl_{cr}$ <10 mL/minute: Administer every 24 hours or avoid use if possible

**Dosing adjustment/comments in hepatic impairment:** Avoid use in patients with severe liver disease

**Dosage Forms Cap:** 250 mg; **Inj with lidocaine 2%:** 5% [50 mg/mL] (2 mL, 10 mL), 12.5% [125 mg/mL] (2 mL)

**Contraindications** Hypersensitivity to tetracycline or any component

**Warnings/Precautions** Avoid in children ≤8 years of age, pregnant and nursing women; photosensitivity can occur with oxytetracycline

**Pregnancy Risk Factor** D

**Adverse Reactions**

>10%: Miscellaneous: Discoloration of teeth and enamel hypoplasia (infants)

1% to 10%:

Dermatologic: Photosensitivity

Gastrointestinal: Nausea, diarrhea

<1%: Pericarditis, increased intracranial pressure, bulging fontanels in infants, pseudotumor cerebri, pruritus, exfoliative dermatitis, dermatologic effects, diabetes insipidus syndrome, vomiting, esophagitis, anorexia, abdominal cramps, antibiotic-associated pseudomembranous colitis, staphylococcal enterocolitis, hepatotoxicity, thrombophlebitis, paresthesia, renal damage, acute renal failure, azotemia, superinfections, anaphylaxis, pigmentation of nails, hypersensitivity reactions, candidal superinfection

**Drug Interactions**

Decreased effect with antacids containing aluminum, calcium or magnesium

Iron and bismuth subsalicylate may decrease doxycycline bioavailability

Barbiturates, phenytoin, and carbamazepine decrease doxycycline's half-life

Increased effect of warfarin

**Half-Life** 8.5-9.6 hours (increases with renal impairment)

**Special PA Issues**

**Patient Education:** Take as directed, around-the-clock. Finish all doses; do not skip doses. May take with food to reduce GI upset. Do not take with antacids, iron products, or dairy products. You may be sensitive to sunlight; use sunblock, wear protective clothing, or avoid direct sun. If diabetic, drug may cause false tests with Clinitest® urine glucose monitoring; use of glucose oxidase methods (Clinistix®) or serum glucose monitoring is preferable. Report rash, difficulty breathing, yellowing of skin or eyes, change in color of urine or stool, easy bruising or bleeding, fever, chills, perianal itching, purulent vaginal discharge, white plaques in mouth, or persistent diarrhea.

# Oxytetracycline and Hydrocortisone

(oks i tet ra SYE kleen & hye droe KOR ti sone)

**Pharmacologic Class** Antibiotic/Corticosteroid, Ophthalmic

**U.S. Brand Names** Terra-Cortril® Ophthalmic Suspension

**Dosage Forms Susp, ophth:** Oxytetracycline hydrochloride 0.5% and hydrocortisone 0.5% (5 mL)

# Oxytetracycline and Polymyxin B

(oks i tet ra SYE kleen & pol i MIKS in bee)

**Pharmacologic Class** Antibiotic, Ophthalmic

**U.S. Brand Names** Terak® Ophthalmic Ointment; Terramycin® Ophthalmic Ointment; Terramycin® w/Polymyxin B Ophthalmic Ointment

**Dosage Forms Oint, ophth/otic:** Oxytetracycline hydrochloride 5 mg and polymyxin B 10,000 units per g (3.5 g); **Tab, vag:** Oxytetracycline hydrochloride 100 mg and polymyxin B 100,000 units (10s)

♦ **Oxytetracycline Hydrochloride** *see* Oxytetracycline *on previous page*

# Oxytocin (oks i TOE sin)

**Pharmacologic Class** Oxytocic Agent

**U.S. Brand Names** Pitocin® Injection; Syntocinon® Injection; Syntocinon® Nasal Spray

(Continued)

## Oxytocin *(Continued)*

**Mechanism of Action** Produces the rhythmic uterine contractions characteristic to delivery and stimulates breast milk flow during nursing

**Use** Induces labor at term; controls postpartum bleeding; nasal preparation used to promote milk letdown in lactating females

**USUAL DOSAGE** I.V. administration requires the use of an infusion pump

Adults:

Induction of labor: I.V.: 0.001-0.002 units/minute; increase by 0.001-0.002 units every 15-30 minutes until contraction pattern has been established; maximum dose should not exceed 20 milliunits/minute

Postpartum bleeding:

I.M.: Total dose of 10 units after delivery

I.V.: 10-40 units by I.V. infusion in 1000 mL of intravenous fluid at a rate sufficient to control uterine atony

Promotion of milk letdown: Intranasal: 1 spray or 3 drops in one or both nostrils 2-3 minutes before breast-feeding

**Dosage Forms Inj:** 10 units/mL (1 mL, 10 mL); **Soln, nasal:** 40 units/mL (2 mL, 5 mL)

**Contraindications** Hypersensitivity to oxytocin or any component; significant cephalopelvic disproportion, unfavorable fetal positions, fetal distress, hypertonic or hyperactive uterus, contraindicated vaginal delivery, prolapse, total placenta previa, and vasa previa

**Warnings/Precautions** To be used for medical rather than elective induction of labor; may produce antidiuretic effect (ie, water intoxication and excess uterine contractions); high doses or hypersensitivity to oxytocin may cause uterine hypertonicity, spasm, tetanic contraction, or rupture of the uterus; severe water intoxication with convulsions, coma, and death is associated with a slow oxytocin infusion over 24 hours

**Pregnancy Risk Factor** X

**Adverse Reactions**

Fetal: <1%: Bradycardia, arrhythmias, intracranial hemorrhage, brain damage, neonatal jaundice, hypoxia, death

Maternal: <1%: Cardiac arrhythmias, premature ventricular contractions, hypotension, tachycardia, arrhythmias, seizures, coma, SIADH with hyponatremia, nausea, vomiting, pelvic hematoma, postpartum hemorrhage, increased uterine motility, fatal afibrinogenemia, increased blood loss, death, anaphylactic reactions

**Drug Interactions** Sympathomimetic pressor effects may be increased by oxytocin resulting in postpartum hypertension

**Onset** Onset of uterine contractions: I.V.: Within 1 minute

**Duration** <30 minutes

**Half-Life** 1-5 minutes

**Special PA Issues**

**Patient Education:**

I.V., I.M.: Generally used in emergency situations. Drug teaching should be incorporated in other situational teaching.

Intranasal spray: While sitting up, hold bottle upright and squeeze into nostril.

**Monitoring Parameters:** Fluid intake and output during administration; fetal monitoring

♦ **Oyst-Cal 500 [OTC]** *see* Calcium Carbonate *on page 139*

♦ **Oystercal® 500** *see* Calcium Carbonate *on page 139*

♦ **P-071** *see* Cetirizine *on page 183*

♦ **Pacerone®** *see* Amiodarone *on page 55*

## Palivizumab *(pah li VIZ u mab)*

**Pharmacologic Class** Monoclonal Antibody

**U.S. Brand Names** Synagis®

**Mechanism of Action** Exhibits neutralizing and fusion-inhibitory activity against RSV; these activities inhibit RSV replication in laboratory and clinical studies

**Use** Prevention of serious lower respiratory tract disease caused by respiratory syncytial virus (RSV) in pediatric patients at high risk of RSV disease; safety and efficacy were established in infants with bronchopulmonary dysplasia (BPD) and infants with a history of prematurity ≤35 weeks gestational age

**USUAL DOSAGE** Children: I.M.: 15 mg/kg of body weight, monthly throughout RSV season (First dose administered prior to commencement of RSV season)

**Dosage Forms Inj, lyophilized:** 100 mg

**Contraindications** Patients with a history of severe prior reaction to palivizumab or other components of the product

**Warnings/Precautions** Anaphylactoid reactions have not been observed following palivizumab administration; however, can occur after administration of proteins. Safety and efficacy of palivizumab have not been demonstrated in the treatment of established RSV disease.

**Pregnancy Risk Factor** C

**Pregnancy Implications** Animal reproduction studies have not been conducted; it is not known whether palivizumab can cause fetal harm when administered to a pregnant woman or could affect reprocuctive capacity

**Adverse Reactions** The incidence of adverse events was similar between the palivizumab and placebo groups

>1%:

Central nervous system: Nervousness

Dermatologic: Fungal dermatitis, eczema, seborrhea

Gastrointestinal: Diarrhea, vomiting, gastroenteritis

Hematologic: Anemia

Hepatic: ALT increase, abnormal LFTs

Local: Injection site reaction

Ocular: Conjunctivitis

Respiratory: Cough, wheezing, bronchiolitis, pneumonia, bronchitis, asthma, croup, dyspnea, sinusitis, apnea

Miscellaneous: Oral moniliasis, failure to thrive, viral infection, flu syndrome

**Drug Interactions** No formal drug interaction studies have been conducted

♦ **Palmetto Scrub** *see* Saw Palmetto *on page 824*

♦ **Palmitate-A® 5000 [OTC]** *see* Vitamin A *on page 962*

♦ **Pamelor®** *see* Nortriptyline *on page 665*

# Pamidronate (pa mi DROE nate)

**Pharmacologic Class** Antidote; Bisphosphonate Derivative

**U.S. Brand Names** Aredia™

**Mechanism of Action** A biphosphonate which inhibits bone resorption via actions on osteoclasts or on osteoclast precursors. Does not appear to produce any significant effects on renal tubular calcium handling and is poorly absorbed following oral administration (high oral doses have been reported effective); therefore, I.V. therapy is preferred.

**Use** Treatment of hypercalcemia associated with malignancy; treatment of osteolytic bone lesions associated with multiple myeloma or metastatic breast cancer; moderate to severe Paget's disease of bone

**USUAL DOSAGE** Drug must be diluted properly before administration and infused intravenously slowly (over at least 1 hour). Adults: I.V.:

Hypercalcemia of malignancy:

Moderate cancer-related hypercalcemia (corrected serum calcium: 12-13 mg/dL): 60-90 mg given as a slow infusion over 2-24 hours

Severe cancer-related hypercalcemia (corrected serum calcium: >13.5 mg/dL): 90 mg as a slow infusion over 2-24 hours

A period of 7 days should elapse before the use of second course; repeat infusions every 2-3 weeks have been suggested, however, could be administered every 2-3 months according to the degree and of severity of hypercalcemia and/or the type of malignancy

Osteolytic bone lesions with multiple myeloma: 90 mg in 500 mL $D_5W$, 0.45% NaCl or 0.9% NaCl administered over 4 hours on a monthly basis

Osteolytic bone lesions with metastatic breast cancer: 90 mg in 250 mL $D_5W$, 0.45% NaCl or 0.9% NaCl administered over 2 hours, repeated every 3-4 weeks

Paget's disease: 30 mg in 500 mL 0.45% NaCl, 0.9% NaCl or $D_5W$ administered over 4 hours for 3 consecutive days

**Dosing adjustment in renal impairment:** Adjustment is not necessary

**Dosage Forms Powder for inj, lyophilized, as disodium:** 30 mg, 60 mg, 90 mg

**Contraindications** Previous hypersensitivity to pamidronate or other biphosphonates

**Warnings/Precautions** Use caution in patients with renal impairment as nephropathy was seen in animal studies. However, in contrast to reports of renal failure with other biphosphonates, impairment of renal function has not been reported with pamidronate in studies to date. However, further experience is needed to assess the nephrotoxic potential with higher doses and prolonged administration. Use caution in patients who are pregnant or in the breast-feeding period; leukopenia has been observed with oral pamidronate and monitoring of white blood cell counts is suggested. Vein irritation and thrombophlebitis may occur with infusions. Has not been studied exclusively in the elderly; monitor serum electrolytes periodically since elderly are often receiving diuretics which can result in decreases in serum calcium, potassium, and magnesium.

**Pregnancy Risk Factor** C

**Adverse Reactions**

1% to 10%:

Central nervous system: Malaise, fever, convulsions

Endocrine & metabolic: Hypomagnesemia, hypocalcemia, hypokalemia, fluid overload, hypophosphatemia

Gastrointestinal: GI symptoms, nausea, diarrhea, constipation, anorexia

Hepatic: Abnormal hepatic function

Neuromuscular & skeletal: Bone pain

Respiratory: Dyspnea

(Continued)

## Pamidronate *(Continued)*

<1%: Pain, angioedema, skin rash, occult blood in stools, abnormal taste, leukopenia, increased risk of fractures, nephrotoxicity, hypersensitivity reactions

**Onset** Onset of effect: 24-48 hours; Maximum effect: 5-7 days

**Half-Life** Distribution half-life: ˙.6 hours; Urinary (elimination) half-life: 2.5 hours; Bone half-life: 300 days

**Special PA Issues**

**Patient Education:** This medication can only be administered I.V. Avoid foods high in calcium or vitamins with minerals during infusion or for 2-3 hours after completion. You may experience nausea or vomiting (small frequent meals and good mouth care may help); or recurrent bone pain (consult prescriber for analgesic). Report unusual muscle twitching or spasms, severe diarrhea/constipation, or acute bone pain.

**Monitoring Parameters:** Serum electrolytes, monitor for hypocalcemia for at least 2 weeks after therapy; serum calcium, phosphate, magnesium, potassium, serum creatinine, CBC with differential

**Reference Range:** Calcium (total): Adults: 9.0-11.0 mg/dL (SI: 2.05-2.54 mmol/L), may slightly decrease with aging; Phosphorus: 2.5-4.5 mg/dL (SI: 0.81-1.45 mmol/L)

- **Pamidronate Disodium** *see Pamidronate on previous page*
- **p-Aminoclonidine** *see Apraclonidine on page 76*
- **Pamprin IB® [OTC]** *see Ibuprofen on page 466*
- **Panadol® [OTC]** *see Acetaminophen on page 21*
- **Panasal® 5/500** *see Hydrocodone and Aspirin on page 450*
- **Pancrease®** *see Pancrelipase on this page*
- **Pancrease® MT 4** *see Pancrelipase on this page*
- **Pancrease® MT 10** *see Pancrelipase on this page*
- **Pancrease® MT 16** *see Pancrelipase on this page*
- **Pancrease® MT 20** *see Pancrelipase on this page*

## Pancrelipase *(pan kre LI pase)*

**Pharmacologic Class** Enzyme, Pancreatic; Pancreatic Enzyme

**U.S. Brand Names** Cotazym®; Cotazym-S®; Creon 10®; Creon 20®; Ilozyme®; Ku-Zyme® HP; Pancrease®; Pancrease® MT 4; Pancrease® MT 10; Pancrease® MT 16; Pancrease® MT 20; Protilase®; Ultrase® MT12; Ultrase® MT20; Viokase®; Zymase®

**Mechanism of Action** Replaces endogenous pancreatic enzymes to assist in digestion of protein, starch and fats

**Use** Replacement therapy in symptomatic treatment of malabsorption syndrome caused by pancreatic insufficiency

**USUAL DOSAGE** Oral:

Powder: Actual dose depends on the digestive requirements of the patient

Children <1 year: Start with ⅛ teaspoonful with feedings

Adults: 0.7 g with meals

Enteric coated microspheres and microtablets: The following dosage recommendations are only an approximation for initial dosages. The actual dosage will depend on the digestive requirements of the individual patient.

Children:

<1 year: 2000 units of lipase with meals

1-6 years: 4000-8000 units of lipase with meals and 4000 units with snacks

7-12 years: 4000-12,000 units of lipase with meals and snacks

Adults: 4000-16,000 units of lipase with meals and with snacks or 1-3 tablets/capsules before or with meals and snacks; in severe deficiencies, dose may be increased to 8 tablets/capsules

Occluded feeding tubes: One tablet of Viokase® crushed with one 325 mg tablet of sodium bicarbonate (to activate the Viokase®) in 5 mL of water can be instilled into the nasogastric tube and clamped for 5 minutes; then, flushed with 50 mL of tap water

**Dosage Forms Cap:** Cotazym®: Lipase 8000 units, protease 30,000 units, amylase 30,000 units, Ku-Zyme® HP: Lipase 8000 units, protease 30,000 units, amylase 30,000 units, Ultrase® MT12: Lipase 12,000 units, protease 39,000 units, amylase 39,000 units, Ultrase® MT20: Lipase 20,000 units, protease 65,000 units, amylase 65,000 units; **Enteric coated microspheres (Pancrease®):** Lipase 4000 units, protease 25,000 units, amylase 20,000 units; **Enteric coated microtab:** Pancrease® MT 4: Lipase 4500 units, protease 12,000 units, amylase 12,000 units, Pancrease® MT 10: Lipase 10,000 units, protease 30,000 units, amylase 30,000 units, Pancrease® MT 16: Lipase 16,000 units, protease 48,000 units, amylase 48,000 units, Pancrease® MT 20: Lipase 20,000 units, protease 44,000 units, amylase 56,000 units; **Enteric coated spheres:** Cotazym-S®: Lipase 5000 units, protease 20,000 units, amylase 20,000 units, Pancrelipase, Protilase®: Lipase 4000 units, protease 25,000 units, amylase 20,000 units, Zymase®: Lipase 12,000 units, protease 24,000 units, amylase 24,000 units; **Delayed release:** Creon® 10: Lipase 10,000 units, protease 37,500 units, amylase 33,200 units, Creon® 20: Lipase 20,000 units, protease 75,000 units, amylase 66,400 units; **Powder (Viokase®):** Lipase 16,800 units, protease 70,000 units, amylase 70,000 units per 0.7 g; **Tab:** Ilozyme®: Lipase 11,000 units, protease

30,000 units, amylase 30,000 units, Viokase®: Lipase 8000 units, protease 30,000 units, amylase 30,000 units

**Contraindications** Hypersensitivity to pancrelipase or any component, pork protein

**Warnings/Precautions** Pancrelipase is inactivated by acids; use microencapsulated products whenever possible, since these products permit better dissolution of enzymes in the duodenum and protect the enzyme preparations from acid degradation in the stomach

**Pregnancy Risk Factor** C

**Adverse Reactions**

1% to 10%: High doses:

Endocrine & metabolic: Hyperuricemia

Gastrointestinal: Nausea, cramps, constipation, diarrhea

Genitourinary: Hyperuricosuria

Ocular: Lacrimation

Respiratory: Sneezing, bronchospasm

<1%: Rash, shortness of breath, bronchospasm, irritation of the mouth

**Drug Interactions**

Decreased effect: Calcium carbonate, magnesium hydroxide

Increased effect: $H_2$-antagonists (eg, ranitidine, cimetidine)

**Special PA Issues**

**Patient Education:** Take before or with meals. Avoid taking with alkaline food. Do not chew, crush, or dissolve delayed release capsules; swallow whole. Do not inhale powder when preparing. You may experience some gastric discomfort. Report unusual joint pain or swelling, respiratory difficulty, or persistent GI upset.

# Pancuronium (paⁿ kyoo ROE nee um)

**Pharmacologic Class** Neuromuscular Blocker Agent, Nondepolarizing; Skeletal Muscle Relaxant

**U.S. Brand Names** Pavulon®

**Mechanism of Action** Blocks neural transmission at the myoneural junction by binding with cholinergic receptor sites

**Use** Drug of choice for neuromuscular blockade except in patients with renal failure, hepatic failure, or cardiovascular instability; produce skeletal muscle relaxation during surgery after induction of general anesthesia, increase pulmonary compliance during assisted respiration, facilitate endotracheal intubation, preferred muscle relaxant for neonatal cardiac patients, must provide artificial ventilation

**USUAL DOSAGE** Based on ideal body weight in obese patients. I.V.:

Infants >1 month, Children, and Adults: Initial: 0.04-0.1 mg/kg; maintenance dose: 0.02-0.1 mg/kg/dose every 30 minutes to 3 hours as needed

**Continuous I.V. infusions are not recommended due to case reports of prolonged paralysis**

**Dosing adjustment in renal impairment:** Elimination half-life is doubled, plasma clearance is reduced and rate of recovery is sometimes much slower

$Cl_{cr}$ 10-50 mL/minute: Administer 50% of normal dose

$Cl_{cr}$ <10 mL/minute: Do not use

**Dosing adjustment/comments in hepatic disease:** Elimination half-life is doubled, plasma clearance is doubled, recovery time is prolonged, volume of distribution is increased (50%) and results in a slower onset, higher total dosage and prolongation of neuromuscular blockade

Patients with liver disease may develop slow resistance to nondepolarizing muscle relaxant; large doses may be required and problems may arise in antagonism

**Dosage Forms Inj, as bromide:** 1 mg/mL (10 mL); 2 mg/mL (2 mL, 5 mL)

**Contraindications** Hypersensitivity to pancuronium, bromide, or any component

**Warnings/Precautions** Ventilation must be supported during neuromuscular blockade. Electrolyte imbalance alters blockade. Use with caution in patients with myasthenia gravis or other neuromuscular diseases, pre-existing pulmonary, hepatic, renal disease, and in the elderly.

**Pregnancy Risk Factor** C

**Adverse Reactions**

1% to 10%:

Cardiovascular: Elevation in pulse rate, elevated blood pressure, tachycardia, hypertension

Dermatologic: Rash, itching

Gastrointestinal: Excessive salivation

<1%: Skin flushing, edema, erythema, burning sensation along the vein, profound muscle weakness, wheezing, circulatory collapse, bronchospasm, hypersensitivity reaction

**Causes of prolonged neuromuscular blockade:**

Excessive drug administration

Cumulative drug effect, decreased metabolism/excretion (hepatic and/or renal impairment)

Accumulation of active metabolites

Electrolyte imbalance (hypokalemia, hypocalcemia, hypermagnesemia, hypernatremia)

(Continued)

## Pancuronium *(Continued)*

Hypothermia
Drug interactions
Increased sensitivity to muscle relaxants (eg, neuromuscular disorders such as myasthenia gravis or polymyositis)

### Drug Interactions

Increased toxicity: Magnesium sulfate, furosemide can increase or decrease neuromuscular blockade (dose-dependent)

#### Prolonged neuromuscular blockade:

Inhaled anesthetics
Local anesthetics
Calcium channel blockers
Antiarrhythmics (eg, quinidine or procainamide)
Antibiotics (eg, aminoglycosides, tetracyclines, vancomycin, clindamycin)
Immunosuppressants (eg, cyclosporine)

**Onset** 2-3 minutes

**Duration** 40-60 minutes

### Special PA Issues

**Monitoring Parameters:** Heart rate, blood pressure, assisted ventilation status; cardiac monitor, blood pressure monitor, and ventilator required

- ◆ **Pancuronium Bromide** *see Pancuronium on previous page*
- ◆ **Pandel®** *see Hydrocortisone on page 453*
- ◆ **Panmycin® Oral** *see Tetracycline on page 885*
- ◆ **Panretin®** *see Alitretinoin on page 41*
- ◆ **Panthoderm® [OTC]** *see Dexpanthenol on page 267*
- ◆ **Pantothenyl Alcohol** *see Dexpanthenol on page 267*

## Papaverine (pa PAV er een)

**Pharmacologic Class** Vasodilator

**U.S. Brand Names** Genabid®; Pavabid®; Pavatine®

**Mechanism of Action** Smooth muscle spasmolytic producing a generalized smooth muscle relaxation including: vasodilatation, gastrointestinal sphincter relaxation, bronchiolar muscle relaxation, and potentially a depressed myocardium (with large doses); muscle relaxation may occur due to inhibition or cyclic nucleotide phosphodiesterase, increasing cyclic AMP; muscle relaxation is unrelated to nerve innervation; papaverine increases cerebral blood flow in normal subjects; oxygen uptake is unaltered

**Use** Oral: Relief of peripheral and cerebral ischemia associated with arterial spasm and myocardial ischemia complicated by arrhythmias

**Investigational:** Parenteral: Various vascular spasms associated with muscle spasms as in myocardial infarction, angine, peripheral and pulmonary embolism, peripheral vascular disease, angiospastic states and visceral spasm (ureteral, biliary, and GI colic); testing for impotence

**USUAL DOSAGE** Adults: Oral, sustained release: 150-300 mg every 12 hours; in difficult cases: 150 mg every 8 hours

**Dosage Forms Cap, sustained release:** 150 mg; **Tab:** 30 mg, 60 mg, 100 mg, 150 mg, 200 mg, 300 mg; **Tab, timed release:** 200 mg

**Contraindications** Hypersensitivity to papaverine or its components

**Warnings/Precautions** Use with caution in patients with glaucoma; administer I.V. cautiously since apnea and arrhythmias may result; may, in large doses, depress A-V and intraventricular cardiac conduction leading to serious arrhythmias (eg, premature beats, paroxysmal tachycardia); chronic hepatitis noted with jaundice, eosinophilia, and abnormal LFTs

### Pregnancy Risk Factor C

**Adverse Reactions** <1% (oral forms unless stated otherwise): Flushing of the face, tachycardias, mild hypertension, arrhythmias with rapid I.V. use, vertigo, drowsiness, sedation, lethargy, headache, nausea, constipation, abdominal distress, anorexia, diarrhea, hepatic hypersensitivity, chronic hepatitis, apnea with rapid I.V. use

**Drug Interactions** CYP2D6 enzyme substrate

Decreased effect: Papaverine decreases the effects of levodopa
Increased toxicity: Additive effects with CNS depressants

**Onset** Oral: Rapid

**Half-Life** 0.5-1.5 hours

### Special PA Issues

**Patient Education:** Oral: Take as directed; do not alter dosage without consulting prescriber. Do not chew, crush, or dissolve extended release tablets. Avoid alcohol while taking this medication. May cause dizziness, confusion, or blurred vision (avoid driving or engaging in tasks that require alertness until response to drug is known). Increased fiber in diet, exercise, and adequate hydration (2-3 L/day of fluids unless instructed to restrict fluid intake) may help if you experience constipation. Report rapid heartbeat or palpitations, CNS depression, persistent sedation or lethargy, or acute headache.

- **Papaverine Hydrochloride** *see* Papaverine *on previous page*
- **Para-Aminosalicylate Sodium** *see* Aminosalicylate Sodium *on page 54*
- **Paracetamol** *see* Acetaminophen *on page 21*
- **Paraflex®** *see* Chlorzoxazone *on page 201*
- **Parafon Forte™ DSC** *see* Chlorzoxazone *on page 201*
- **Par Decon®** *see* Chlorpheniramine, Phenyltoloxamine, Phenylpropanolamine, and Phenylephrine *on page 196*

## Paregoric (par e GOR ik)

**Pharmacologic Class** Analgesic, Narcotic

**Mechanism of Action** Increases smooth muscle tone in GI tract, decreases motility and peristalsis, diminishes digestive secretions

**Use** Treatment of diarrhea or relief of pain; neonatal opiate withdrawal

**USUAL DOSAGE** Oral:

Neonatal opiate withdrawal: Instill 3-6 drops every 3-6 hours as needed, or initially 0.2 mL every 3 hours; increase dosage by approximately 0.05 mL every 3 hours until withdrawal symptoms are controlled; it is rare to exceed 0.7 mL/dose. Stabilize withdrawal symptoms for 3-5 days, then gradually decrease dosage over a 2- to 4-week period.

Children: 0.25-0.5 mL/kg 1-4 times/day

Adults: 5-10 mL 1-4 times/day

**Dosage Forms Liq:** 2 mg morphine equivalent/5 mL [equivalent to 20 mg opium powder] (5 mL, 60 mL, 473 mL, 4000 mL)

**Contraindications** Hypersensitivity to opium or any component; diarrhea caused by poisoning until the toxic material has been removed

**Warnings/Precautions** Use with caution in patients with respiratory, hepatic or renal dysfunction, severe prostatic hypertrophy, or history of narcotic abuse; opium shares the toxic potential of opiate agonists, and usual precautions of opiate agonist therapy should be observed; some preparations contain sulfites which may cause allergic reactions; infants <3 months of age are more susceptible to respiratory depression, use with caution and generally in reduced doses in this age group; tolerance or drug dependence may result from extended use

**Pregnancy Risk Factor** B (D when used long-term or in high doses)

**Adverse Reactions**

>10%:

Cardiovascular: Hypotension

Central nervous system: Drowsiness, dizziness

Gastrointestinal: Constipation

Neuromuscular & skeletal: Weakness

1% to 10%:

Central nervous system: Restlessness, headache, malaise

Genitourinary: Ureteral spasms, decreased urination

Miscellaneous: Histamine release

<1%: Peripheral vasodilation, insomnia, CNS depression, mental depression, increased intracranial pressure, anorexia, stomach cramps, nausea, vomiting, biliary tract spasm, urinary tract spasm, miosis, respiratory depression, physical and psychological dependence, increased LFTs

**Drug Interactions** Increased effect/toxicity with CNS depressants (eg, alcohol, narcotics, benzodiazepines, TCAs, MAO inhibitors, phenothiazine)

**Special PA Issues**

**Patient Education:** Take exactly as directed; do not increase dosage. May cause dependence with prolonged or excessive use. Avoid alcohol and all other prescription and OTC that may cause sedation (sleeping medications, some cough/cold remedies, antihistamines, etc). You may experience drowsiness, dizziness, or impaired judgment (use caution when driving or performing hazardous tasks) or postural hypotension (use caution when rising from sitting or lying position or when climbing stairs). You may experience nausea or loss of appetite (frequent small meals may help) or constipation (a laxative may be necessary). Report unresolved nausea, vomiting, respiratory difficulty (shortness of breath or decreased respirations), chest pain, or palpitations.

**Dietary Considerations:** Alcohol: Additive CNS effect, avoid use

- **Paremyd® Ophthalmic** *see* Hydroxyamphetamine and Tropicamide *on page 458*
- **Parenteral Multiple Vitamin** *see* Vitamins, Multiple *on page 964*
- **Parepectolin®** *see* Kaolin and Pectin With Opium *on page 505*
- **Par Glycerol®** *see* Iodinated Glycerol *on page 487*

## Paricalcitol (par eh CAL ci tol)

**Pharmacologic Class** Vitamin D Analog

**U.S. Brand Names** Zemplar™

**Mechanism of Action** Synthetic vitamin D analog which has been shown to reduce PTH serum concentrations

(Continued)

## Paricalcitol *(Continued)*

**Use** Prevention and treatmen of secondary hyperparathyroidism associated with chronic renal failure. Has been evaluated only in hemodialysis patients.

**USUAL DOSAGE** Adults: I.V.: 0.04-0.1 mcg/kg (2.8-7 mcg) given as a bolus dose no more frequently than every other day at any time during dialysis; doses as high as 0.24 mcg/kg (16.8 mcg) have been administered safely; usually start with 0.04 mcg/kg 3 times/week by I.V. bolus, increased by 0.04 mcg/kg every 2 weeks; the dose of paricalcitol should be adjusted based on serum PTH levels

### Serum PTH Levels

| PTH Level | Paricalcitol Dose |
|---|---|
| Same or increasing | Increase |
| Decreased by <30% | Increase |
| Decreased by <30% and <60% | Maintain |
| Decreased by >60% | Decrease |
| 1.5-3 times upper limit of normal | Maintain |

**Dosage Forms** Inj: 5 mcg/mL (1 mL, 2 mL, 5 mL)

**Contraindications** Should not be given to patients with evidence of vitamin D toxicity, hypercalcemia, or hypersensitivity to any of the ingredients of this product

**Warnings/Precautions** The most frequently reported adverse reactions with paricalcitol include nausea, vomiting, and edema. Chronic administration can place patients at risk of hypercalcemia, elevated calcium-phosphorus product and metastatic calcification; it should not be used in patients with evidence of hypercalcemia or vitamin D toxicity.

**Pregnancy Risk Factor** C

**Adverse Reactions** The three most frequently reported events in clinical studies were nausea, vomiting, and edema, which are commonly seen in hemodialysis patients.

>10%: Gastrointestinal: Nausea (13%)

1% to 10%:
Cardiovascular: Palpitations, peripheral edema (7%)
Central nervous system: Chills, malaise, fever, lightheadedness (5%)
Gastrointestinal: Vomiting (8%), GI bleeding (5%), xerostomia (3%)
Respiratory: Pneumonia (5%)
Miscellaneous: Flu-like symptoms, sepsis

**Drug Interactions** Phosphate or vitamin D-related compounds should not be taken concurrently; digitalis toxicity is potentiated by hypercalcemia

**Special PA Issues**

**Patient Education:** Take as directed; do not increase dosage without consulting prescriber. Adhere to diet as recommended (do not take any other phosphate or vitamin D related compounds while taking paricalcitol). You may experience nausea or vomiting (small frequent meals, chewing gums, or sucking on lozenges may help); swelling of extremities (elevate feet when sitting); lightheadedness or dizziness (use caution when driving or operating dangerous machinery). Report persistent fever, gastric disturbances, abdominal pain or blood in stool, chest pain or palpitations, or signs of respiratory infection or flu.

**Monitoring Parameters:** Serum calcium and phosphorus should be monitored closely (eg, twice weekly) during dose titration; monitor for signs and symptoms of vitamin D intoxication; serum PTH; in trials, a mean PTH level reduction of 30% was achieved within 6 weeks

♦ **Parkinson's Disease Management** *see* Chart *on page 1103*
♦ **Parlodel®** *see* Bromocriptine *on page 122*
♦ **Parnate®** *see* Tranylcypromine *on page 922*

## Paromomycin *(par oh moe MYE sin)*

**Pharmacologic Class** Amebicide

**U.S. Brand Names** Humatin®

**Mechanism of Action** Acts directly on ameba; has antibacterial activity against normal and pathogenic organisms in the GI tract; interferes with bacterial protein synthesis by binding to 30S ribosomal subunits

**Use** Treatment of acute and chronic intestinal amebiasis; preoperatively to suppress intestinal flora; tapeworm infestations; treatment of *Cryptosporidium*

**USUAL DOSAGE** Oral:
Intestinal amebiasis: Children and Adults: 25-35 mg/kg/day in 3 divided doses for 5-10 days
*Dientamoeba fragilis*: Children and Adults: 25-30 mg/kg/day in 3 divided doses for 7 days
*Cryptosporidium*: Adults with AIDS: 1.5-2.25 g/day in 3-6 divided doses for 10-14 days (occasionally courses of up to 4-8 weeks may be needed)

Tapeworm (fish, dog, bovine, porcine):
   Children: 11 mg/kg every 15 minutes for 4 doses
   Adults: 1 g every 15 minutes for 4 doses
Hepatic coma: Adults: 4 g/day in 2-4 divided doses for 5-6 days
Dwarf tapeworm: Children and Adults: 45 mg/kg/dose every day for 5-7 days

**Dosage Forms Cap, as sulfate:** 250 mg

**Contraindications** Intestinal obstruction, renal failure, known hypersensitivity to paromomycin or components

**Warnings/Precautions** Use with caution in patients with impaired renal function or possible or proven ulcerative bowel lesions

**Pregnancy Risk Factor** C

**Adverse Reactions**
1% to 10%: Gastrointestinal: Diarrhea, abdominal cramps, nausea, vomiting, heartburn
<1%: Headache, vertigo, exanthema, rash, pruritus, steatorrhea, secondary enterocolitis, eosinophilia, ototoxicity

**Drug Interactions**
Decreased effect of digoxin, vitamin A, and methotrexate
Increased effect of oral anticoagulants, neuromuscular blockers, and polypeptide antibiotics

**Special PA Issues**
   **Patient Education:** Take as directed, for full course of therapy. Do not skip doses. Maintain adequate hydration (2-3 L/day of fluids unless instructed to restrict fluid intake) and nutrition. If GI upset occurs, small frequent meals, frequent mouth care, and sucking on lozenges may help. Report unresolved or severe nausea or vomiting, dizziness, ringing in ears, or loss of hearing.

♦ **Paromomycin Sulfate** see Paromomycin on previous page

# Paroxetine (pa ROKS e teen)

**Pharmacologic Class** Antidepressant, Selective Serotonin Reuptake Inhibitor

**U.S. Brand Names** Paxil™; Paxil™ CR

**Mechanism of Action** Paroxetine is a selective serotonin reuptake inhibitor, chemically unrelated to tricyclic, tetracyclic, or other antidepressants; presumably, the inhibition of serotonin reuptake from brain synapse stimulated serotonin activity in the brain

**Use** Treatment of depression; treatment of panic disorder and obsessive-compulsive disorder

**USUAL DOSAGE** Adults: Oral:
Depression: 20 mg once daily (maximum: 60 mg/day), preferably in the morning; in elderly, debilitated, or patients with hepatic or renal impairment, start with 10 mg/day (maximum: 40 mg/day); adjust doses at 7-day intervals
Panic disorder and obsessive compulsive disorder: Recommended average daily dose: 40 mg, this dosage should be given after an adequate trial on 20 mg/day and then titrating upward

**Dosage Forms Tab:** 10 mg, 20 mg, 30 mg, 40 mg; **Tab, controlled release:** 12.5 mg, 25 mg

**Contraindications** Do not use within 14 days of MAO inhibitors

**Warnings/Precautions** Use cautiously in patients with a history of seizures, mania, renal disease, cardiac disease, suicidal patients, children, or during breast-feeding in lactating women

**Pregnancy Risk Factor** C

**Adverse Reactions**
>10%:
   Central nervous system: Headache, somnolence, dizziness, insomnia
   Gastrointestinal: Nausea, xerostomia, constipation, diarrhea
   Genitourinary: Ejaculatory disturbances
   Neuromuscular & skeletal: Weakness
   Miscellaneous: Diaphoresis
1% to 10%:
   Cardiovascular: Palpitations, vasodilation, postural hypotension
   Central nervous system: Nervousness, anxiety
   Endocrine & metabolic: Decreased libido
   Gastrointestinal: Anorexia, flatulence, vomiting
   Neuromuscular & skeletal: Tremor, paresthesia
<1%: Bradycardia, hypotension, migraine, akinesia, alopecia, amenorrhea, gastritis, anemia, leukopenia, arthritis, eye pain, ear pain, asthma, bruxism, thirst

**Drug Interactions** CYP2D6 enzyme substrate (minor); CYP1A2, 2D6, and 3A3/4 enzyme inhibitor

Decreased effect: Phenobarbital, phenytoin
Increased toxicity: Alcohol, cimetidine, MAO inhibitors (hyperpyrexic crisis); increased effect/toxicity of TCAs, fluoxetine, sertraline, phenothiazines, class 1C antiarrhythmics, warfarin

**Onset** Steady-state: ~10 days; therapeutic effects: >2 weeks

**Half-Life** 21 hours

(Continued)

## Paroxetine *(Continued)*

### Special PA Issues

**Patient Education:** Take exactly as directed (do not increase dose or frequency); may take 2-3 weeks to achieve desired results; may cause physical and/or psychological dependence. Take in the morning to reduce the incidence of insomnia. Avoid excessive alcohol, caffeine, and other prescription or OTC medications not approved by prescriber. Maintain adequate hydration (2-3 L/day of fluids unless instructed to restrict fluid intake). You may experience drowsiness, dizziness, or lightheadedness (use caution when driving or engaging in hazardous tasks until response to medication is known); nausea, vomiting, anorexia, or dry mouth (small frequent meals, frequent mouth care, or sucking lozenges may help); or orthostatic hypotension (use caution when climbing stairs or changing position from lying or sitting to standing). Report persistent insomnia or excessive daytime sedation; muscle cramping, tremors, weakness, or change in gait; chest pain, palpitations, or rapid heartbeat; vision changes or eye pain; difficulty breathing or breathlessness; abdominal pain or blood in stool; or worsening of condition.

**Monitoring Parameters:** Hepatic and renal function tests, blood pressure, heart rate

### Related Information

Antidepressant Agents *on page 998*

- ♦ **PAS** *see* Aminosalicylate Sodium *on page 54*
- ♦ **Pathocil®** *see* Dicloxacillin *on page 273*
- ♦ **Pavabid®** *see* Papaverine *on page 696*
- ♦ **Pavatine®** *see* Papaverine *on page 696*
- ♦ **Paveral Stanley Syrup With Codeine Phosphate** *see* Codeine *on page 232*
- ♦ **Pavulon®** *see* Pancuronium *on page 695*
- ♦ **Paxil™** *see* Paroxetine *on previous page*
- ♦ **Paxil™ CR** *see* Paroxetine *on previous page*
- ♦ **Paxipam®** *see* Halazepam *on page 433*
- ♦ **PBZ®** *see* Tripelennamine *on page 940*
- ♦ **PBZ-SR®** *see* Tripelennamine *on page 940*
- ♦ **PCA** *see* Procainamide *on page 759*
- ♦ **PCE®** *see* Erythromycin *on page 329*
- ♦ **PediaCare® Oral** *see* Pseudoephedrine *on page 780*
- ♦ **Pediacof®** *see* Chlorpheniramine, Phenylephrine, and Codeine *on page 196*
- ♦ **Pediaflor®** *see* Fluoride *on page 383*
- ♦ **Pediapred® Oral** *see* Prednisolone *on page 752*
- ♦ **PediaProfen™** *see* Ibuprofen *on page 466*
- ♦ **Pediatric Triban®** *see* Trimethobenzamide *on page 936*
- ♦ **Pediatrix** *see* Acetaminophen *on page 21*
- ♦ **Pediazole®** *see* Erythromycin and Sulfisoxazole *on page 330*
- ♦ **Pedi-Cort V® Creme** *see* Clioquinol and Hydrocortisone *on page 219*
- ♦ **PediOtic® Otic** *see* Neomycin, Polymyxin B, and Hydrocortisone *on page 645*
- ♦ **Pedituss®** *see* Chlorpheniramine, Phenylephrine, and Codeine *on page 196*
- ♦ **PedvaxHIB™** *see* Haemophilus b Conjugate Vaccine *on page 432*

## Pegademase Bovine *(peg A de mase BOE vine)*

**Pharmacologic Class** Enzyme, Replacement Therapy

**U.S. Brand Names** Adagen™

**Mechanism of Action** Adenosine deaminase is an enzyme that catalyzes the deamination of both adenosine and deoxyadenosine. Hereditary lack of adenosine deaminase activity results in severe combined immunodeficiency disease, a fatal disorder of infancy characterized by profound defects of both cellular and humoral immunity. It is estimated that 25% of patients with the autosomal recessive form of severe combined immunodeficiency lack adenosine deaminase.

**Use** Enzyme replacement therapy for adenosine deaminase (ADA) deficiency in patients with severe combined immunodeficiency disease (SCID) who can not benefit from bone marrow transplant; not a cure for SCID, unlike bone marrow transplants, injections must be used the rest of the child's life, therefore is not really an alternative

**USUAL DOSAGE** Children: I.M.: Dose given every 7 days, 10 units/kg the first dose, 15 units/kg the second dose, and 20 units/kg the third dose; maintenance dose: 20 units/kg/week is recommended depending on patient's ADA level; maximum single dose: 30 units/kg

**Dosage Forms Inj:** 250 units/mL (1.5 mL)

**Contraindications** Hypersensitivity to pegademase bovine; not to be used as preparatory or support therapy for bone marrow transplantation

**Warnings/Precautions** Use with caution in patients with thrombocytopenia

**Pregnancy Risk Factor** C

**Adverse Reactions** <1%: Headache, pain at injection site

**Drug Interactions** Decreased effect: Vidarabine

**Special PA Issues**
**Patient Education:** Not a cure for SCID; unlike bone marrow transplants, injections must be used the rest of the child's life; frequent blood tests are necessary to monitor effect and adjust the dose as needed

◆ Peglyte™ see Polyethylene Glycol-Electrolyte Solution *on page 736*

# Pemoline (PEM oh leen)
**Pharmacologic Class** Stimulant
**U.S. Brand Names** Cylert®
**Mechanism of Action** Blocks the reuptake mechanism of dopaminergic neurons, appears to act at the cerebral cortex and subcortical structures; CNS and respiratory stimulant with weak sympathomimetic effects; actions may be mediated via increase in CNS dopamine
**Use** Treatment of attention deficit/hyperactivity disorder (ADHD); narcolepsy
**USUAL DOSAGE** Children ≥6 years: Oral: Initial: 37.5 mg given once daily in the morning, increase by 18.75 mg/day at weekly intervals; usual effective dose range: 56.25-75 mg/day; maximum: 112.5 mg/day; dosage range: 0.5-3 mg/kg/24 hours; significant benefit may not be evident until third or fourth week of administration

**Dosing adjustment/comments in renal impairment:** $Cl_{cr}$ <50 mL/minute: Avoid use
**Dosage Forms Tab:** 18.75 mg, 37.5 mg, 75 mg; **Tab, chewable:** 37.5 mg
**Contraindications** Liver disease; hypersensitivity to pemoline or any component; children <6 years of age; Tourette's syndrome, psychoses
**Warnings/Precautions** Use with caution in patients with renal dysfunction, hypertension, or a history of abuse
**Pregnancy Risk Factor** B
**Adverse Reactions**
>10%:
Central nervous system: Insomnia
Gastrointestinal: Anorexia, weight loss
1% to 10%:
Central nervous system: Dizziness, drowsiness, mental depression
Dermatologic: Rash
Gastrointestinal: Stomach pain, nausea
<1%: Seizures, precipitation of Tourette's syndrome, hallucination, headache, movement disorders, growth reaction, diarrhea, increased liver enzymes (usually reversible upon discontinuation), hepatitis, jaundice
**Drug Interactions**
Decreased effect of insulin
Increased effect/toxicity with CNS depressants, CNS stimulants, sympathomimetics
**Onset** Peak effect: 4 hours
**Duration** 8 hours
**Half-Life** 12 hours
**Special PA Issues**
**Patient Education:** Take exactly as directed; do not change dosage or discontinue without consulting prescriber. Response may some time. Avoid alcohol, caffeine, or other stimulants. Maintain adequate fluid intake (2-3 L/day). You may experience nausea, decreased appetite, or altered taste sensation (small frequent meals may help maintain adequate nutrition); drowsiness, dizziness, or mental depression, especially during early therapy (use caution when driving or engaging in hazardous activities). Report unresolved rapid heartbeat; excessive agitation, nervousness, insomnia, tremors, dizziness, or seizures; skin rash or irritation; altered gait or movement; unusual mouth movements or vocalizations (Tourette's syndrome); or yellowing of skin or eyes, dark urine, or pale stools.
**Dietary Considerations:** Alcohol: Additive CNS effect, avoid use
**Monitoring Parameters:** Liver enzymes

# Penciclovir (pen SYE kloe veer)
**Pharmacologic Class** Antiviral Agent
**U.S. Brand Names** Denavir™
**Mechanism of Action** In cells infected with HSV-1 or HSV-2, viral thymidine kinase phosphorylates penciclovir to a monophosphate form which, in turn, is converted to penciclovir triphosphate by cellular kinases. Penciclovir triphosphate inhibits HSV polymerase competitively with deoxyguanosine triphosphate. Consequently, herpes viral DNA synthesis and, therefore, replication are selectively inhibited
**Use** Topical treatment of herpes simplex labialis (cold sores); potentially used for Epstein-Barr virus infections
**USUAL DOSAGE** Apply cream at the first sign or symptom of cold sore (eg, tingling, swelling); apply every 2 hours during waking hours for 4 days
**Dosage Forms Crm:** 1% [10 mg/g] (2 g)
**Contraindications** Previous and significant adverse reactions to famciclovir; hypersensitivity to the product or any of its components
(Continued)

## Penciclovir *(Continued)*

**Warnings/Precautions** Penciclovir should only be used on herpes labialis on the lips and face; because no data are available, application to mucous membranes is not recommended. Avoid application n or near eyes since it may cause irritation. The effect of penciclovir has not been established in immunocompromised patients.

**Pregnancy Risk Factor** B

**Adverse Reactions**

Central nervous system: Headache (5.3%)

Dermatologic: Mild erythema (50%), local anesthesia (0.9%)

**Half-Life** 2 hours

**Special PA Issues**

**Patient Education:** This is not a cure for herpes (recurrences tend to appear within 3 months of original infection), nor will this medication reduce the risk of transmission to others when lesions are present. For external use only. Wash hands before and after application. Apply this film over affected areas at first sign of cold sore. Avoid use of other topical creams, lotions, or ointments unless approved by prescriber. You may experience headache, mild rash, or taste disturbances.

**Monitoring Parameters:** Reduction in virus shedding, negative cultures for herpes virus; resolution of pain and healing of cold sore lesion

♦ **Penecort®** *see* Hydrocortisone *on page 453*

♦ **Penetrex™** *see* Enoxacin *on page 318*

## Penicillamine *(pen i SIL ε meen)*

**Pharmacologic Class** Chelating Agent

**U.S. Brand Names** Cuprimine®; Depen®

**Mechanism of Action** Chelates with lead, copper, mercury and other heavy metals to form stable, soluble complexes that are excreted in urine; depresses circulating IgM rheumatoid factor, depresses T-cell but not B-cell activity; combines with cystine to form a compound which is more soluble, thus cystine calculi are prevented

**Use** Treatment of Wilson's disease, cystinuria, adjunct in the treatment of rheumatoid arthritis; lead, mercury, copper, and possibly gold poisoning. (Note: Oral DMSA is preferable for lead or mercury poisoning); primary biliary cirrhosis; as adjunctive therapy following initial treatment with calcium EDTA or BAL

**USUAL DOSAGE** Oral:

Rheumatoid arthritis:

Children: Initial: 3 mg/kg/day (≤250 mg/day) for 3 months, then 6 mg/kg/day (≤500 mg/day) in divided doses twice daily for 3 months to a maximum of 10 mg/kg/day in 3-4 divided doses

Adults: 125-250 mg/day, may increase dose at 1- to 3-month intervals up to 1-1.5 g/day

Wilson's disease (doses titrated to maintain urinary copper excretion >1 mg/day):

Infants <6 months: 250 mg/dose once daily

Children <12 years: 250 mg/dose 2-3 times/day

Adults: 250 mg 4 times/day

Cystinuria:

Children: 30 mg/kg/day in 4 divided doses

Adults: 1-4 g/day in divided doses every 6 hours

Lead poisoning (continue until blood lead level is <60 µg/dL): Children and Adults: 25-35 mg/kg/d, administered in 3-4 divided doses; initiating treatment at 25% of this dose and gradually increasing to the full dose over 2-3 weeks may minimize adverse reactions

Primary biliary cirrhosis: 250 mg/day to start, increase by 250 mg every 2 weeks up to a maintenance dose of 1 g/day, usually given 250 mg 4 times/day

Arsenic poisoning: Children: 100 mg/kg/day in divided doses every 6 hours for 5 days; maximum: 1 g/day

**Dosing adjustment/comments in renal impairment:** $Cl_{cr}$ <50 mL/minute: Avoid use

**Dosage Forms** Cap: 125 mg, 250 mg; Tab: 250 mg

**Contraindications** Hypersensitivity to penicillamine or components; renal insufficiency; patients with previous penicillamine-related aplastic anemia or agranulocytosis; concomitant administration with other hematopoietic-depressant drugs (eg, gold, immunosuppressants, antimalarials, phenylbutazone)

**Warnings/Precautions** Cross-sensitivity with penicillin is possible; therefore, should be used cautiously in patients with a history of penicillin allergy. Patients on penicillamine for Wilson's disease or cystinuria should receive pyridoxine supplementation 25 mg/day; once instituted for Wilson's disease or cystinuria, continue treatment on a daily basis; interruptions of even a few days have been followed by hypersensitivity with reinstitution of therapy. Penicillamine has been associated with fatalities due to agranulocytosis, aplastic anemia, thrombocytopenia, Goodpasture's syndrome, and myasthenia gravis; patients should be warned to report promptly any symptoms suggesting toxicity; approximately 33% of patients will experience an allergic reaction; since toxicity may be dose related, it is recommended not to exceed 750 mg/day in elderly.

**Pregnancy Risk Factor** D

## Adverse Reactions

>10%:

Dermatologic: Rash, urticaria, itching (44% to 50%)

Gastrointestinal: Hypogeusia (25% to 33%)

Neuromuscular & skeletal: Arthralgia

1% to 10%:

Cardiovascular: Edema of the face, feet, or lower legs

Central nervous system: Fever, chills

Gastrointestinal: Weight gain, sore throat

Genitourinary: Bloody or cloudy urine

Hematologic: Aplastic or hemolytic anemia, leukopenia (2%), thrombocytopenia (4%)

Miscellaneous: White spots on lips or mouth, positive ANA

<1%: Fatigue, toxic epidermal necrolysis, pemphigus, increased friability of the skin, iron deficiency, nausea, vomiting, anorexia, pancreatitis, cholestatic jaundice, hepatitis, myasthenia gravis syndrome, weakness, optic neuritis, tinnitus, nephrotic syndrome, coughing, wheezing, SLE-like syndrome, spitting of blood allergic reactions, lymphadenopathy

## Drug Interactions

Decreased effect with iron and zinc salts, antacids (magnesium, calcium, aluminum) and food

Decreased effect/levels of digoxin

Increased effect of gold, antimalarials, immunosuppressants, phenylbutazone (hematologic, renal toxicity)

## Half-Life 1.7-3.2 hours

## Special PA Issues

**Patient Education:** Take this medication exactly as directed; do not increase dose without consulting prescriber. Capsules may be opened and contents mixed in 15-30 mL of chilled fruit juice or puree; do not take with milk or milk products. Avoid alcohol or excess intake of vitamin A. It is preferable to take penicillamine on empty stomach (1 hour before or 2 hours after meals). Maintain adequate hydration (2-3 L/day of fluids unless instructed to restrict fluid intake).

Wilson's disease: Avoid chocolate, shellfish, nuts, mushrooms, liver, broccoli, molasses.

Lead poisoning: Decrease dietary calcium.

Cystinuria: Take with large amounts of water.

You may experience anorexia, nausea, vomiting (frequent small meals, frequent oral care, sucking on lozenges, or chewing gum may help). Report persistent fever or chills, unhealed sores, white spots or sores in mouth or vaginal area, extreme fatigue, or signs of infection; breathlessness, difficulty breathing, or unusual cough; unusual bruising/bleeding; blood in urine, stool, mouth, or vomitus; swollen face or extremities; skin rash or itching; muscle pain or cramping; or pain on urination.

**Monitoring Parameters:** Urinalysis, CBC with differential, platelet count, liver function tests; weekly measurements of urinary and blood concentration of the intoxicating metal is indicated (3 months has been tolerated)

CBC: WBC <3500/mm$^3$, neutrophils <2000/mm$^3$ or monocytes >500/mm$^3$ indicate need to stop therapy immediately; quantitative 24-hour urine protein at 1- to 2-week intervals initially (first 2-3 months); urinalysis, LFTs occasionally; platelet counts <100,000/mm$^3$ indicate need to stop therapy until numbers of platelets increase

# Penicillin G Benzathine and Procaine Combined

(pen i SIL in jee BENZ a theen & PROE kane KOM bined)

**Pharmacologic Class** Antibiotic, Penicillin

**U.S. Brand Names** Bicillin® C-R; Bicillin® C-R 900/300

**Mechanism of Action** Inhibits bacterial cell wall synthesis by binding to one or more of the penicillin binding proteins (PBPs); which in turn inhibits the final transpeptidation step of peptidoglycan synthesis in bacterial cell walls, thus inhibiting cell wall biosynthesis. Bacteria eventually lyse due to ongoing activity of cell wall autolytic enzymes (autolysins and murein hydrolases) while cell wall assembly is arrested.

**Use** May be used in specific situations in the treatment of streptococcal infections

**USUAL DOSAGE** I.M.:

Children:

<30 lb: 600,000 units in a single dose

30-60 lb: 900,000 units to 1.2 million units in a single dose

Children >60 lb and Adults: 2.4 million units in a single dose

**Dosage Forms Inj:** 300,000 units [150,000 units each of penicillin g benzathine and penicillin g procaine] (10 mL), 600,000 units [300,000 units each penicillin g benzathine and penicillin g procaine] (1 mL), 1,200,000 units [600,000 units each penicillin g benzathine and penicillin g procaine] (2 mL), 2,400,000 units [1,200,000 units each penicillin g benzathine and penicillin g procaine] (4 mL); **Inj:** Penicillin g benzathine 900,000 units and penicillin g procaine 300,000 units per dose (2 mL)

**Contraindications** Known hypersensitivity to penicillin or any component

(Continued)

## Penicillin G Benzathine and Procaine Combined *(Continued)*

**Warnings/Precautions** Use with caution in patients with impaired renal function, impaired cardiac function or seizure disorder

**Pregnancy Risk Factor** B

**Drug Interactions** Probenecid, tetracyclines, methotrexate, aminoglycosides

**Special PA Issues**

**Monitoring Parameters:** Observe for signs and symptoms for anaphylaxis during first dose

## Penicillin G Benzathine, Parenteral (pen i SIL in jee BENZ a theen)

**Pharmacologic Class** Antibiotic, Penicillin

**U.S. Brand Names** Bicillin® L-A; Permapen®

**Mechanism of Action** Interferes with bacterial cell wall synthesis during active multiplication, causing cell wall death and resultant bactericidal activity against susceptible bacteria

**Use** Active against some gram-positive organisms, few gram-negative organisms such as *Neisseria gonorrhoeae*, and some anaerobes and spirochetes; used in the treatment of syphilis; used only for the treatment of mild to moderately severe infections caused by organisms susceptible to low concentrations of penicillin G or for prophylaxis of infections caused by these organisms

**USUAL DOSAGE** I.M.: Administer undiluted injection; higher doses result in more sustained rather than higher levels. Use a penicillin G benzathine-penicillin G procaine combination to achieve early peak levels in acute infections.

Infants and Children:

Group A streptococcal upper respiratory infection: 25,000-50,000 units/kg as a single dose; maximum: 1.2 million units

Prophylaxis of recurrent rheumatic fever: 25,000-50,000 units/kg every 3-4 weeks; maximum: 1.2 million units/dose

Early syphilis: 50,000 units/kg as a single injection; maximum: 2.4 million units

Syphilis of more than 1-year duration: 50,000 units/kg every week for 3 doses; maximum: 2.4 million units/dose

Adults:

Group A streptococcal upper respiratory infection: 1.2 million units as a single dose

Prophylaxis of recurrent rheumatic fever: 1.2 million units every 3-4 weeks or 600,000 units twice monthly

Early syphilis: 2.4 million units as a single dose in 2 injection sites

Syphilis of more than 1-year duration: 2.4 million units in 2 injection sites once weekly for 3 doses

Not indicated as single drug therapy for neurosyphilis, but may be given 1 time/week for 3 weeks following I.V. treatment (refer to penicillin G monograph for dosing)

**Dosage Forms** Inj: 300,000 units/mL (10 mL), 600,000 units/mL (1 mL, 2 mL, 4 mL)

**Contraindications** Known hypersensitivity to penicillin or any component

**Warnings/Precautions** Use with caution in patients with impaired renal function, seizure disorder, or history of hypersensitivity to other beta-lactams; CDC and AAP do not currently recommend the use of penicillin G benzathine to treat congenital syphilis or neurosyphilis due to reported treatment failures and lack of published clinical data on its efficacy

**Pregnancy Risk Factor** B

**Adverse Reactions**

1% to 10%: Local: Pain

<1%: Convulsions, confusion, drowsiness, fever, rash, electrolyte imbalance, hemolytic anemia, positive Coombs' reaction, thrombophlebitis, myoclonus, acute interstitial nephritis, Jarisch-Herxheimer reaction, hypersensitivity reactions, anaphylaxis

**Drug Interactions**

Decreased effect: Tetracyclines may decrease penicillin effectiveness; decreased oral contraceptive effect is possible

Increased effect:

Probenecid may increase penicillin levels

Aminoglycosides → synergistic efficacy; heparin and parenteral penicillins may result in increased bleeding

**Special PA Issues**

**Patient Education:** Take as directed, for full course of therapy. Maintain adequate hydration (2-3 L/day of fluids unless instructed to restrict fluid intake). If begin treated for sexually transmitted disease partner will also need to be treated. Small frequent meals or sucking on lozenges may reduce nausea or dry mouth. Important to maintain good oral and vaginal hygiene to reduce incidence of opportunistic infection. If diabetic, drug may cause false tests with Clinitest® urine glucose monitoring; use of glucose oxidase methods (Clinistix®) or serum glucose monitoring is preferable. This drug may interfere with oral contraceptives; an alternate form of birth control should be used. Report persistent diarrhea, fever, chills, unhealed sores, bloody urine or stool, muscle pain, mouth sores, or difficulty breathing.

**Monitoring Parameters:** Observe for signs and symptoms of anaphylaxis during first dose

## Penicillin G, Parenteral, Aqueous

(pen i SIL in jee, pa REN ter al, AYE kwee us)

**Pharmacologic Class** Antibiotic, Penicillin

**U.S. Brand Names** Pfizerpen®

**Mechanism of Action** Interferes with bacterial cell wall synthesis during active multiplication, causing cell wall death and resultant bactericidal activity against susceptible bacteria

**Use** Active against some gram-positive organisms, generally not *Staphylococcus aureus*; some gram-negative organisms such as *Neisseria gonorrhoeae*, and some anaerobes and spirochetes

**USUAL DOSAGE** I.M., I.V.:

Infants:

>7 days, >2000 g: 100,000 units/kg/day in divided doses every 6 hours

>7 days, <2000 g: 75,000 units/kg/day in divided doses every 8 hours

<7 days, >2000 g: 50,000 units/kg/day in divided doses every 8 hours

<7 days, <2000 g: 50,000 units/kg/day in divided doses every 12 hours

Infants and Children (sodium salt is preferred in children): 100,000-250,000 units/kg/day in divided doses every 4 hours

Severe infections: Up to 400,000 units/kg/day in divided doses every 4 hours; maximum dose: 24 million units/day

Adults: 2-24 million units/day in divided doses every 4 hours depending on sensitivity of the organism and severity of the infection

Congenital syphilis:

Newborns: 50,000 units/kg/day I.V. every 8-12 hours for 10-14 days

Infants: 50,000 units/kg every 4-6 hours for 10-14 days

Disseminated gonococcal infections or gonococcus ophthalmia (if organism proven sensitive): 100,000 units/kg/day in 2 equal doses (4 equal doses/day for infants >1 week)

Gonococcal meningitis: 150,000 units/kg in 2 equal doses (4 doses/day for infants >1 week)

**Dosing interval in renal impairment:**

Cl$_{cr}$ 30-50 mL/minute: Administer every 6 hours

Cl$_{cr}$ 10-30 mL/minute: Administer every 8 hours

Cl$_{cr}$ <10 mL/minute: Administer every 12 hours

Hemodialysis: Moderately dialyzable (20% to 50%)

Continuous arteriovenous or venovenous hemodiafiltration (CAVH) effects: Dose as for Cl$_{cr}$ 10-50 mL/minute

**Dosage Forms** Penicillin g potassium: **Inj:** Frozen premixed: 1 million units, 2 million units, 3 million units, Powder: 1 million units, 5 million units, 10 million units, 20 million units; Penicillin g sodium: **Inj:** 5 million units

**Contraindications** Known hypersensitivity to penicillin or any component

**Warnings/Precautions** Avoid intra-arterial administration or injection into or near major peripheral nerves or blood vessels since such injections may cause severe and/or permanent neurovascular damage; use with caution in patients with renal impairment (dosage reduction required), pre-existing seizure disorders, or with a history of hypersensitivity to cephalosporins

**Pregnancy Risk Factor** B

**Adverse Reactions** <1%: Convulsions, confusion, drowsiness, fever, rash, electrolyte imbalance, hemolytic anemia, positive Coombs' reaction, thrombophlebitis, myoclonus, acute interstitial nephritis, Jarisch-Herxheimer reaction, hypersensitivity reactions, anaphylaxis

**Drug Interactions**

Decreased effect: Tetracyclines may decrease penicillin effectiveness; decreased oral contraceptive effect is possible

Increased effect:

Probenecid may increase penicillin levels

Aminoglycosides may result in synergistic efficacy; heparin and parenteral penicillins may result in increased bleeding

**Half-Life** Normal renal function: 20-50 minutes; End-stage renal disease: 3.3-5.1 hours

**Special PA Issues**

**Patient Education:** This medication will be administered I.V. or I.M. Maintain adequate hydration (2-3 L/day of fluids unless instructed to restrict fluid intake). If being treated for sexually transmitted disease, partner will also need to be treated. Small frequent meals or sucking on lozenges may reduce nausea or dry mouth. Important to maintain good oral and vaginal hygiene to reduce incidence of opportunistic infection. If diabetic, drug may cause false tests with Clinitest® urine glucose monitoring; use of glucose oxidase methods (Clinistix®) or serum glucose monitoring is preferable. This drug may interfere with oral contraceptives; an alternate form of birth control should be used. Report persistent diarrhea, fever, chills, unhealed sores, bloody urine or stool, muscle pain, mouth sores, or difficulty breathing.

**Monitoring Parameters:** Observe for signs and symptoms of anaphylaxis during first dose

♦ **Penicillin G Potassium** *see* Penicillin G, Parenteral, Aqueous *on this page*

# Penicillin G Procaine (pen i SIL in jee PROE kane)

**Pharmacologic Class** Antibiotic, Penicillin

**U.S. Brand Names** Crysticillin® A.S.; Wycillin®

**Mechanism of Action** Inhibits bacterial cell wall synthesis by binding to one or more of the penicillin binding proteins (PBPs); which in turn inhibits the final transpeptidation step of peptidoglycan synthesis in bacterial cell walls, thus inhibiting cell wall biosynthesis. Bacteria eventually lyse due to ongoing activity of cell wall autolytic enzymes (autolysins and murein hydrolases) while cell wall assembly is arrested.

**Use** Moderately severe infections due to *Treponema pallidum* and other penicillin G-sensitive microorganisms that are susceptible to low but prolonged serum penicillin concentrations

**USUAL DOSAGE** I.M.:

Children: 25,000-50,000 units/kg/day in divided doses 1-2 times/day; not to exceed 4.8 million units/24 hours

Congenital syphilis: 50,000 units/kg/day for 10-14 days

Adults: 0.6-4.8 million units/day in divided doses every 12-24 hours

Endocarditis caused by susceptible viridans *Streptococcus* (when used in conjunction with an aminoglycoside): 1.2 million units every 6 hours for 2-4 weeks

Neurosyphilis: I.M.: 2-4 million units/day with 500 mg probenecid by mouth 4 times/day for 10-14 days; **penicillin G aqueous I.V. is the preferred agent**

Hemodialysis: Moderately dialyzable (20% to 50%)

**Dosage Forms Inj, susp:** 300,000 units/mL (10 mL), 500,000 units/mL (1.2 mL), 600,000 units/mL (1 mL, 2 mL, 4 mL)

**Contraindications** Known hypersensitivity to penicillin or any component; also contraindicated in patients hypersensitive to procaine

**Warnings/Precautions** May need to modify dosage in patients with severe renal impairment, seizure disorders, or history of hypersensitivity to cephalosporins; avoid I.V., intravascular, or intra-arterial administration of penicillin G procaine since severe and/or permanent neurovascular damage may occur

**Pregnancy Risk Factor** B

**Adverse Reactions**

>10%: Local: Pain at injection site

<1%: Myocardial depression vasodilation, conduction disturbances, CNS stimulation, seizures, confusion, drowsiness, hemolytic anemia, positive Coombs' reaction, sterile abscess at injection site, myoclonus, interstitial nephritis, pseudoanaphylactic reactions, Jarisch-Herxheimer reaction, hypersensitivity reactions

**Drug Interactions**

Decreased effect: Tetracyclines may decrease penicillin effectiveness; decreased oral contraceptive effect is possible

Increased effect:

Probenecid may increase penicillin levels

Aminoglycosides may result in synergistic efficacy; heparin and parenteral penicillins may result in increased bleeding

**Special PA Issues**

**Patient Education:** Take as directed, for full course of therapy. Maintain adequate hydration (2-3 L/day of fluids unless instructed to restrict fluid intake). If being treated for sexually transmitted disease partner will also need to be treated. Small frequent meals or sucking on lozenges may reduce nausea or dry mouth. Important to maintain good oral and vaginal hygiene to reduce incidence of opportunistic infection. If diabetic, drug may cause false tests with Clinitest® urine glucose monitoring; use of glucose oxidase methods (Clinistix®) or serum glucose monitoring is preferable. This drug may interfere with oral contraceptives; an alternate form of birth control should be used. Report persistent diarrhea, fever, chills, unhealed sores, bloody urine or stool, muscle pain, mouth sores, or difficulty breathing.

**Monitoring Parameters:** Periodic renal and hematologic function tests with prolonged therapy; fever, mental status, WBC count

♦ **Penicillin G Procaine and Benzathine Combined** see Penicillin G Benzathine and Procaine Combined on page 703

♦ **Penicillin G Sodium** see Penicillin G, Parenteral, Aqueous on previous page

# Penicillin V Potassium (pen i SIL in vee poe TASS ee um)

**Pharmacologic Class** Antibiotic, Penicillin

**U.S. Brand Names** Beepen-VK®; Betapen®-VK; Pen.Vee® K; Robicillin® VK; V-Cillin K®; Veetids®

**Mechanism of Action** Inhibits bacterial cell wall synthesis by binding to one or more of the penicillin binding proteins (PBPs); which in turn inhibits the final transpeptidation step of peptidoglycan synthesis in bacterial cell walls, thus inhibiting cell wall biosynthesis. Bacteria eventually lyse due to ongoing activity of cell wall autolytic enzymes (autolysins and murein hydrolases) while cell wall assembly is arrested.

**Use** Treatment of infections caused by susceptible organisms involving the respiratory tract, otitis media, sinusitis, skin, and urinary tract; prophylaxis in rheumatic fever

**USUAL DOSAGE** Oral:
Systemic infections:
Children <12 years: 25-50 mg/kg/day in divided doses every 6-8 hours; maximum dose: 3 g/day
Children ≥12 years and Adults: 125-500 mg every 6-8 hours
Prophylaxis of pneumococcal infections:
Children <5 years: 125 mg twice daily
Children ≥5 years and Adults: 250 mg twice daily
Prophylaxis of recurrent rheumatic fever:
Children <5 years: 125 mg twice daily
Children ≥5 years and Adults: 250 mg twice daily
**Dosing interval in renal impairment:** $Cl_{cr}$ <10 mL/minute: Administer 250 mg every 6 hours

**Dosage Forms** Powder for oral soln: 125 mg/5 mL (3 mL, 100 mL, 150 mL, 200 mL), 250 mg/5 mL (100 mL, 150 mL, 200 mL); **Tab:** 125 mg, 250 mg, 500 mg

**Contraindications** Known hypersensitivity to penicillin or any component

**Warnings/Precautions** Use with caution in patients with severe renal impairment (modify dosage), history of seizures, or hypersensitivity to cephalosporins

**Pregnancy Risk Factor** B

**Adverse Reactions**
>10%: Gastrointestinal: Mild diarrhea, vomiting, nausea, oral candidiasis
<1%: Convulsions, fever, hemolytic anemia, positive Coombs' reaction, acute interstitial nephritis, hypersensitivity reactions, anaphylaxis

**Drug Interactions**
Decreased effect: Tetracyclines may decrease penicillin effectiveness; decreased oral contraceptive effect is possible
Increased effect:
Probenecid may increase penicillin levels
Aminoglycosides may result in synergistic efficacy; heparin and parenteral penicillins may result in increased bleeding

**Half-Life** 0.5 hours; prolonged in patients with renal impairment

**Special PA Issues**
**Patient Education:** Take at regular intervals around-the-clock, preferably on an empty stomach (1 hour before or 2 hours after meals) with 8 oz of water. Take entire prescription; do not skip doses or discontinue without consulting prescriber. Small frequent meals or sucking on lozenges may reduce nausea or dry mouth. Important to maintain good oral and vaginal hygiene to reduce incidence of opportunistic infection. If diabetic, drug may cause false tests with Clinitest® urine glucose monitoring; use of glucose oxidase methods (Clinistix®) or serum glucose monitoring is preferable. This drug may interfere with oral contraceptives; an alternate form of birth control should be used. Report persistent diarrhea, fever, chills, unhealed sores, bloody urine or stool, muscle pain, mouth sores, and difficulty breathing.
**Dietary Considerations:** Food: Decreases drug absorption rate; decreases drug serum concentration. Take on an empty stomach 1 hour before or 2 hours after meals.
**Monitoring Parameters:** Periodic renal and hematologic function tests during prolonged therapy; monitor for signs of anaphylaxis during first dose

♦ **Penicilloyl-polylysine** *see* Benzylpenicilloyl-polylysine *on page 108*
♦ **Pentacarinat® Injection** *see* Pentamidine *on this page*
♦ **Pentam-300® Injection** *see* Pentamidine *on this page*

# Pentamidine (pen TAM i deen)

**Pharmacologic Class** Antibiotic, Miscellaneous
**U.S. Brand Names** NebuPent™ Inhalation; Pentacarinat® Injection; Pentam-300® Injection
**Mechanism of Action** Interferes with RNA/DNA, phospholipids and protein synthesis, through inhibition of oxidative phosphorylation and/or interference with incorporation of nucleotides and nucleic acids into RNA and DNA, in protozoa
**Use** Treatment and prevention of pneumonia caused by *Pneumocystis carinii*; treatment of trypanosomiasis and visceral leishmaniasis
**USUAL DOSAGE**
Children:
Treatment: I.M., I.V. (I.V. preferred): 4 mg/kg/day once daily for 10-14 days
Prevention:
I.M., I.V.: 4 mg/kg monthly or every 2 weeks
Inhalation (aerosolized pentamidine in children ≥5 years): 300 mg/dose given every 3-4 weeks via Respirgard® II inhaler (8 mg/kg dose has also been used in children <5 years)
Treatment of trypanosomiasis: I.V.: 4 mg/kg/day once daily for 10 days
Adults:
Treatment: I.M., I.V. (I.V. preferred): 4 mg/kg/day once daily for 14-21 days
Prevention: Inhalation: 300 mg every 4 weeks via Respirgard® II nebulizer
(Continued)

## Pentamidine *(Continued)*

Dialysis: Not removed by hemo or peritoneal dialysis or continuous arteriovenous or venovenous hemofiltration (CAVH/CAVHD); supplemental dosage is not necessary

**Dosing adjustment in renal impairment:** Adults: I.V.:

$Cl_{cr}$ 10-50 mL/minute: Administer 4 mg/kg every 24-36 hours

$Cl_{cr}$ <10 mL/minute: Administer 4 mg/kg every 48 hours

**Dosage Forms Inh:** 300 mg; **Powder for inj, lyophilized:** 300 mg

**Contraindications** Hypersensitivity to pentamidine isethionate or any component (inhalation and injection)

**Warnings/Precautions** Use with caution in patients with diabetes mellitus, renal or hepatic dysfunction; hypertension or hypotension; leukopenia, thrombocytopenia, asthma, hypo/hyperglycemia

**Pregnancy Risk Factor** C

**Adverse Reactions** Injection (I); Aerosol (A)

>10%:

Cardiovascular: Chest pain (A - 10% to 23%)

Central nervous system: Fatigue (A - 50% to 70%); dizziness (A - 31% to 47%)

Dermatologic: Rash (31% to 47%)

Endocrine & metabolic: Hyperkalemia

Gastrointestinal: Anorexia (A - 50% to 70%), nausea (A - 10% to 23%)

Local: Local reactions at injection site

Renal: Increased creatinine (I - 23%)

Respiratory: Wheezing (A - 10% to 23%), dyspnea (A - 50% to 70%), coughing (A - 31% to 47%), pharyngitis (10% to 23%)

1% to 10%:

Cardiovascular: Hypotension (I - 4%)

Central nervous system: Confusion/hallucinations (1% to 2%), headache (A - 1% to 5%)

Dermatologic: Rash (I - 3.3%)

Endocrine & metabolic: Hypoglycemia <25 mg/dL (I - 2.4%)

Gastrointestinal: Nausea/anorexia (I - 6%), diarrhea (A - 1% to 5%), vomiting

Hematologic: Severe leukopenia (I - 2.8%), thrombocytopenia <20,000/mm$^3$ (I - 1.7%), anemia (A - 1% to 5%)

Hepatic: Increased LFTs (I - 8.7%)

<1%: Hypotension <60 mm Hg systolic (I - 0.9%), tachycardia, arrhythmias, dizziness (I), fever, fatigue (I), hyperglycemia or hypoglycemia, hypocalcemia, pancreatitis, megaloblastic anemia, granulocytopenia, leukopenia, renal insufficiency, extrapulmonary pneumocystosis, irritation of the airway, pneumothorax, Jarisch-Herxheimer-like reaction, mild renal or hepatic injury

**Drug Interactions** CYP2C19 enzyme substrate

**Half-Life** 6.4-9.4 hours; may be prolonged in patients with severe renal impairment

**Special PA Issues**

**Patient Education:** I.V. or I.M. preparations must be given every day. For inhalant use as directed. Prepare solution and nebulizer as directed. Protect medication from light. You will be required to have frequent laboratory tests and blood pressure monitoring while taking this drug. PCP pneumonia may still occur despite pentamidine use. Maintain adequate hydration (2-3 L/day of fluids unless instructed to restrict fluid intake). Frequent mouth care or sucking on lozenges may relieve the metallic taste. Diabetics should check glucose levels frequently. You may experience dizziness or weakness with posture changes; rise or change position slowly. Report unusual confusion or hallucinations, chest pain, unusual bleeding, or rash.

**Monitoring Parameters:** Liver function tests, renal function tests, blood glucose, serum potassium and calcium, EKG, blood pressure

♦ **Pentamidine Isethionate** *see* Pentamidine *on previous page*

♦ **Pentamycetin®** *see* Chloramphenicol *on page 188*

♦ **Pentasa® Oral** *see* Mesalamine *on page 571*

## Pentazocine *(pen TAZ oh seen)*

**Pharmacologic Class** Analgesic, Narcotic

**U.S. Brand Names** Talwin®; Talwin® NX

**Mechanism of Action** Binds to opiate receptors in the CNS, causing inhibition of ascending pain pathways, altering the perception of and response to pain; produces generalized CNS depression; partial agonist-antagonist

**Use** Relief of moderate to severe pain; has also been used as a sedative prior to surgery and as a supplement to surgical anesthesia

**USUAL DOSAGE**

Children: I.M., S.C.:

5-8 years: 15 mg

8-14 years: 30 mg

Children >12 years and Adults: Oral: 50 mg every 3-4 hours; may increase to 100 mg/dose if needed, but should not exceed 600 mg/day

Adults:
    I.M., S.C.: 30-60 mg every 3-4 hours, not to exceed total daily dose of 360 mg
    I.V.: 30 mg every 3-4 hours
**Dosing adjustment in renal impairment:**
    $Cl_{cr}$ 10-50 mL/minute: Administer 75% of normal dose
    $Cl_{cr}$ <10 mL/minute: Administer 50% of normal dose
**Dosing adjustment in hepatic impairment:** Reduce dose or avoid use in patients with liver disease
**Dosage Forms Inj, as lactate:** 30 mg/mL (1 mL, 1.5 mL, 2 mL, 10 mL); **Tab:** Pentazocine hydrochloride 50 mg and naloxone hydrochloride 0.5 mg
**Contraindications** Hypersensitivity to pentazocine or any component, increased intracranial pressure (unless the patient is mechanically ventilated)
**Warnings/Precautions** Use with caution in seizure-prone patients, acute myocardial infarction, patients undergoing biliary tract surgery, patients with renal and hepatic dysfunction, head trauma, increased intracranial pressure, and patients with a history of prior opioid dependence or abuse; pentazocine may precipitate opiate withdrawal symptoms in patients who have been receiving opiates regularly; injection contains sulfites which may cause allergic reaction; tolerance or drug dependence may result from extended use
**Pregnancy Risk Factor** B (D if used for prolonged periods or in high doses at term)
**Adverse Reactions**
>10%:
    Central nervous system: Euphoria, drowsiness
    Gastrointestinal: Nausea, vomiting
    Neuromuscular & skeletal: Weakness
1% to 10%:
    Cardiovascular: Hypotension
    Central nervous system: Malaise, headache, restlessness, nightmares
    Dermatologic: Rash
    Gastrointestinal: Xerostomia
    Genitourinary: Ureteral spasm
    Ocular: Blurred vision
    Respiratory: Dyspnea
<1%: Insomnia, CNS depression, sedation, hallucinations, confusion, disorientation, seizures may occur in seizure-prone patients, increased intracranial pressure, palpitations, bradycardia, peripheral vasodilation, pruritus, antidiuretic hormone release, GI irritation, constipation, biliary tract spasm, urinary tract spasm, tissue damage and irritation with I.M./S.C. use, miosis, histamine release, physical and psychological dependence
**Drug Interactions** CYP2D6 enzyme substrate
May potentiate or reduce analgesic effect of opiate agonist, (eg, morphine) depending on patients tolerance to opiates can precipitate withdrawal in narcotic addicts
Increased effect/toxicity with tripelennamine (can be lethal), CNS depressants (phenothiazines, tranquilizers, anxiolytics, sedatives, hypnotics, or alcohol)
**Onset** Oral, I.M., S.C.: Within 15-30 minutes; I.V.: Within 2-3 minutes
**Duration** Oral: 4-5 hours; Parenteral: 2-3 hours
**Half-Life** 2-3 hours; increased with decreased hepatic function
**Special PA Issues**
    **Patient Education:** If self-administered, use exactly as directed (do not increase dose or frequency); may cause physical and/or psychological dependence. While using this medication, do not use alcohol and other prescription or OTC medications (especially sedatives, tranquilizers, antihistamines, or pain medications) without consulting prescriber. Maintain adequate hydration (2-3 L/day of fluids unless instructed to restrict fluid intake). May cause hypotension, dizziness, drowsiness, impaired coordination, or blurred vision (use caution when driving, climbing stairs, or changing position - rising from sitting or lying to standing, or when engaging in hazardous activities until response to medication is known); nausea, vomiting, loss of appetite, or dry mouth (frequent mouth care, small frequent meals, or sucking on lozenges may help); constipation (increased exercise, fluids, or dietary fruit and fiber may help - if constipation remains an unresolved problem, consult prescriber about use of stool softeners). Report persistent dizziness or headache; excessive fatigue or sedation; changes in mental status; changes in urinary elimination or pain on urination; weakness or trembling; blurred vision; or shortness of breath.
    **Dietary Considerations:** Alcohol: Additive CNS effect, avoid use
    **Monitoring Parameters:** Relief of pain, respiratory and mental status, blood pressure
**Related Information**
    Narcotic Agonists on page 1023

♦ **Pentazocine Hydrochloride** see Pentazocine on previous page
♦ **Pentazocine Lactate** see Pentazocine on previous page

# Pentoxifylline (pen toks I fi leen)
**Pharmacologic Class** Blood Viscosity Reducer Agent
**U.S. Brand Names** Trental®
(Continued)

## Pentoxifylline *(Continued)*

**Mechanism of Action** Mechanism of action remains unclear; is thought to reduce blood viscosity and improve blood flow by altering the rheology of red blood cells

**Use** Symptomatic management of peripheral vascular disease, mainly intermittent claudication

**Unapproved use:** AIDS patients with increased TNF, CVA, cerebrovascular diseases, diabetic atherosclerosis, diabetic neuropathy, gangrene, hemodialysis shunt thrombosis, vascular impotence, cerebral malaria, septic shock, sickle cell syndromes, and vasculitis

**USUAL DOSAGE** Adults: Oral: 400 mg 3 times/day with meals; may reduce to 400 mg twice daily if GI or CNS side effects occur

**Dosage Forms Tab, controlled release:** 400 mg

**Contraindications** Hypersensitivity to pentoxifylline or any component and other xanthine derivatives; patients with recent cerebral and/or retinal hemorrhage

**Warnings/Precautions** Use with caution in patients with renal impairment

**Pregnancy Risk Factor** C

**Adverse Reactions**

1% to 10%:
Central nervous system: Dizziness, headache
Gastrointestinal: Dyspepsia, nausea, vomiting
<1%: Mild hypotension, angina, agitation, blurred vision, earache

**Drug Interactions**

Increased effect/toxic potential with cimetidine (increased levels) and other H$_2$-antagonists, warfarin; increased effect of antihypertensives

Increased toxicity with theophylline

**Half-Life** Parent drug: 24-48 minutes; Metabolites: 60-96 minutes

**Special PA Issues**

**Patient Education:** Take as prescribed for full length of prescription. This may relieve pain of claudication, but additional therapy may be recommended. You may experience dizziness (use caution when driving); GI upset (small frequent meals may help). Report chest pain, persistent headache, nausea or vomiting.

- ◆ **Pen.Vee® K** *see* Penicillin V Potassium *on page 706*
- ◆ **Pen VK** *see* Penicillin V Potassium *on page 706*
- ◆ **Pepcid®** *see* Famotidine *on page 358*
- ◆ **Pepcid® AC Acid Controller [OTC]** *see* Famotidine *on page 358*
- ◆ **Pepcid® RPD** *see* Famotidine *on page 358*
- ◆ **Pepto-Bismol® [OTC]** *see* Bismuth *on page 116*
- ◆ **Pepto® Diarrhea Control [OTC]** *see* Loperamide *on page 540*
- ◆ **Peptol®** *see* Cimetidine *on page 208*
- ◆ **Percocet®** *see* Oxycodone and Acetaminophen *on page 688*
- ◆ **Percocet®-Demi** *see* Oxycodone and Acetaminophen *on page 688*
- ◆ **Percodan®** *see* Oxycodone and Aspirin *on page 688*
- ◆ **Percodan®-Demi** *see* Oxycodone and Aspirin *on page 688*
- ◆ **Percolone™** *see* Oxycodone *on page 687*
- ◆ **Perdiem® Plain [OTC]** *see* Psyllium *on page 781*

## Pergolide *(PER go lide)*

**Pharmacologic Class** Anti-Parkinson's Agent (Dopamine Agonist); Ergot Derivative

**U.S. Brand Names** Permax®

**Mechanism of Action** Pergolide is a semisynthetic ergot alkaloid similar to bromocriptine but stated to be more potent and longer-acting; it is a centrally-active dopamine agonist stimulating both D$_1$ and D$_2$ receptors

**Use** Adjunctive treatment to levodopa/carbidopa in the management of Parkinson's Disease

**USUAL DOSAGE** When adding pergolide to levodopa/carbidopa, the dose of the latter can usually and should be decreased. Patients no longer responsive to bromocriptine may benefit by being switched to pergolide.

Adults: Oral: Start with 0.05 mg/day for 2 days, then increase dosage by 0.1 or 0.15 mg/day every 3 days over next 12 days, increase dose by 0.25 mg/day every 3 days until optimal therapeutic dose is achieved, up to 5 mg/day maximum; usual dosage range: 2-3 mg/day in 3 divided doses

**Dosage Forms Tab, as mesylate:** 0.05 mg, 0.25 mg, 1 mg

**Contraindications** Known hypersensitivity to pergolide mesylate or other ergot derivatives

**Warnings/Precautions** Symptomatic hypotension occurs in 10% of patients; use with caution in patients with a history of cardiac arrhythmias, hallucinations, or mental illness

**Pregnancy Risk Factor** B

**Adverse Reactions**

>10%:
Central nervous system: Dizziness, somnolence, insomnia, confusion, hallucinations, anxiety, dystonia

Gastrointestinal: Nausea, constipation
Neuromuscular & skeletal: Dyskinesia
Respiratory: Rhinitis
1% to 10%:
Cardiovascular: Myocardial infarction, postural hypotension, syncope, arrhythmias, peripheral edema, vasodilation, palpitations, chest pain
Central nervous system: Chills
Gastrointestinal: Diarrhea, abdominal pain, vomiting, xerostomia, anorexia, weight gain
Neuromuscular & skeletal: Weakness
Ocular: Abnormal vision
Respiratory: Dyspnea
Miscellaneous: Flu syndrome

**Drug Interactions**
Decreased effect: Dopamine antagonists, metoclopramide
Increased toxicity: Highly plasma protein bound drugs

**Special PA Issues**
**Patient Education:** Take exactly as directed (may be prescribed in conjunction with levodopa/carbidopa); do not change dosage or discontinue without consulting prescriber. Therapeutic effects may take several weeks or months to achieve and you may need frequent monitoring during first weeks of therapy. Take with meals if GI upset occurs, before meals if dry mouth occurs, after eating if drooling or if nausea occurs. Take at same time each day. Maintain adequate hydration (2-3 L/day of fluids unless instructed to restrict fluid intake); void before taking medication. Do not use alcohol and prescription or OTC sedatives or CNS depressants without consulting prescriber. You may experience drowsiness, dizziness, confusion, or vision changes (use caution when driving, climbing stairs, or engaging in hazardous tasks); orthostatic hypotension (use caution when changing position - rising to standing from sitting or lying); constipation (increased exercise, fluids, or dietary fruit and fiber may help); runny nose or flu-like symptoms (consult prescriber for appropriate relief); nausea, vomiting, loss of appetite, or stomach discomfort (small frequent meals, chewing gum, or sucking on lozenges may help); photosensitivity (avoid direct sunlight, wear protective clothing, use sunblock). Report unresolved constipation or vomiting; chest pain, palpitations, irregular heartbeat; ringing in ears; CNS changes (hallucination, loss of memory, seizures, acute headache, nervousness, etc); painful or difficult urination; increased muscle spasticity, rigidity, or involuntary movements; skin rash; or significant worsening of condition.

**Monitoring Parameters:** Blood pressure (both sitting/supine and standing), symptoms of parkinsonism, dyskinesias, mental status

♦ **Pergolide Mesylate** see Pergolide on previous page
♦ **Pergonal®** see Menotropins on page 567
♦ **Periactin®** see Cyproheptadine on page 247
♦ **Peridex® Oral Rinse** see Chlorhexidine Gluconate on page 190

# Perindopril Erbumine (per IN doe pril er BYOO meen)

**Pharmacologic Class** Angiotensin-Converting Enzyme (ACE) Inhibitors
**U.S. Brand Names** Aceon®
**Mechanism of Action** Competitive inhibitor of angiotensin-converting enzyme (ACE); prevents conversion of angiotensin I to angiotensin II, a potent vasoconstrictor; results in lower levels of angiotensin II which, in turn, causes an increase in plasma renin activity and a reduction in aldosterone secretion
**Use** Treatment of stage I or II hypertension and congestive heart failure
**USUAL DOSAGE** Adults: Oral:
Congestive heart failure: 4 mg once daily
Hypertension: Initial: 4 mg/day but may be titrated to response; usual range: 4-8 mg/day, maximum: 16 mg/day
**Dosing adjustment in renal impairment:**
$Cl_{cr}$ >60 mL/minute: 4 mg/day
$Cl_{cr}$ 30-60 mL/minute: 2 mg/day
$Cl_{cr}$ 15-29 mL/minute: 2 mg every other day
$Cl_{cr}$ <15 mL/minute: 2 mg on the day of dialysis
Hemodialysis: Perindopril and its metabolites are dialyzable
**Dosing adjustment in hepatic impairment:** None needed
**Dosing adjustment in geriatric patients:** Due to greater bioavailability and lower renal clearance of the drug in elderly subjects, dose reduction of 50% is recommended
**Dosage Forms Tab:** 2 mg, 4 mg, 8 mg
**Contraindications** Hypersensitivity to perindopril, perindoprilat, other ACE inhibitors, or any component; pregnancy; history of angioedema with other ACE inhibitors
**Warnings/Precautions** Use with caution and modify dosage in patients with renal impairment (especially renal artery stenosis), severe congestive heart failure, or with coadministered diuretic therapy, valvular stenosis, hyperkalemia (>5.7 mEq/L); experience in children is limited. Severe hypotension may occur in patients who are sodium and/or volume depleted; initiate lower doses and monitor closely when starting therapy in these patients.
(Continued)

## Perindopril Erbumine *(Continued)*

**Pregnancy Risk Factor** D (especially during 2nd and 3rd trimester)

**Pregnancy Implications** Breast-feeding/lactation: Only small amounts are excreted in breast milk

**Adverse Reactions**

1% to 10%:

Central nervous system: Headache, dizziness, mood and sleep disorders, fatigue

Dermatologic: Rash, pruritus

Gastrointestinal: Nausea, epigastric pain, diarrhea, vomiting

Neuromuscular & skeletal: Muscle cramps

Respiratory: Cough (incidence is greater in women, 3:1)

<1%: Hypotension, angioedema, psoriasis, hyperkalemia, taste disturbances, impotence, agranulocytosis for all ACE inhibitors (especially in patients with renal impairment or collagen vascular disease), possibly neutropenia, dry eyes, blurred vision, optic phosphenes, decreases in creatinine clearance in some elderly hypertensive patients or those with chronic renal failure, worsening of renal function in patients with bilateral renal artery stenosis, or furosemide therapy; proteinuria

**Drug Interactions** Increased toxicity: See Drug-Drug Interactions With ACEIs *on page 997*

**Onset** Peak concentrations: 1-2 hours

**Half-Life** Parent drug: 1.5-3 hours; Metabolite: 25-30 hours

**Special PA Issues**

**Patient Education:** This medication does not replace the to need to follow exercise and diet recommendations for hypertension. Take as directed; do not miss doses, alter dosage, or discontinue without consulting prescriber. Consult prescriber for appropriate diet. Change position slowly when rising from sitting or lying. May cause transient drowsiness; avoid driving or engaging in tasks that require alertness until response to drug is known. Small frequent meals may help reduce any nausea, vomiting, or epigastric pain. You may experience persistent cough; contact prescriber. Report unusual weight gain or swelling of ankles and hands; persistent fatigue; dry cough; difficulty breathing; palpitations; or swelling of face, eyes, or lips.

**Monitoring Parameters:** Serum creatinine, electrolytes, and WBC with differential initially and repeated at 2-week intervals for at least 90 days

**Related Information**

Drug-Drug Interactions With ACEIs *on page 997*

♦ **PerioChip®** *see* Chlorhexidine Gluconate *on page 190*

♦ **PerioGard®** *see* Chlorhexidine Gluconate *on page 190*

♦ **Periostat™** *see* Doxycycline *on page 306*

♦ **Permapen®** *see* Penicillin G Benzathine, Parenteral *on page 704*

♦ **Permax®** *see* Pergolide *on page 710*

## Permethrin *(per METH rin)*

**Pharmacologic Class** Antiparasitic Agent, Topical; Scabicidal Agent

**U.S. Brand Names** Elimite™ Cream; Nix™ Creme Rinse

**Mechanism of Action** Inhibits sodium ion influx through nerve cell membrane channels in parasites resulting in delayed repolarization and thus paralysis and death of the pest

**Use** Single application treatment of infestation with *Pediculus humanus capitis* (head louse) and its nits or *Sarcoptes scabiei* (scabies); indicated for prophylactic use during epidemics of lice

**USUAL DOSAGE** Topical: Children >2 months and Adults:

Head lice: After hair has been washed with shampoo, rinsed with water, and towel dried, apply a sufficient volume of topical liquid to saturate the hair and scalp. Leave on hair for 10 minutes before rinsing off with water; remove remaining nits; may repeat in 1 week if lice or nits still present.

Scabies: Apply cream from head to toe; leave on for 8-14 hours before washing off with water; for infants, also apply on the hairline, neck, scalp, temple, and forehead; may reapply in 1 week if live mites appear

Permethrin 5% cream was shown to be safe and effective when applied to an infant <1 month of age with neonatal scabies; time of application was limited to 6 hours before rinsing with soap and water

**Dosage Forms Crm:** 5% (60 g); **Creme rinse:** 1% (60 mL with comb)

**Contraindications** Known hypersensitivity to pyrethroid, pyrethrin, or chrysanthemums

**Warnings/Precautions** Treatment may temporarily exacerbate the symptoms of itching, redness, swelling; for external use only; use during pregnancy only if clearly needed

**Pregnancy Risk Factor** B

**Adverse Reactions** 1% to 10%:

Dermatologic: Pruritus, erythema, rash of the scalp

Local: Burning, stinging, tingling, numbness or scalp discomfort, edema

#### Special PA Issues
**Patient Education:** For external use only. Do not apply to face and avoid contact with eyes or mucous membrane. Clothing and bedding must be washed in hot water or dry cleaned to kill nits. May need to treat all members of household and all sexual contacts concurrently. Wash all combs and brushes with permethrin and thoroughly rinse.

**Administration:**
Cream rinse: Apply immediately after hair is shampooed and rinsed. Apply enough to saturate hair and scalp. Leave on hair for 10 minutes before rinsing with water. Remove nits with fine-tooth comb. May repeat in 1 week if lice or nits are still present.
Cream: Apply from neck to toes. Bathe to remove drug after 8-14 hours before washing off. Repeat in 7 days if lice or nits are still present. Report if condition persists or infection occurs.

♦ **Permitil® Oral** *see* Fluphenazine *on page 388*

## Perphenazine (per FEN a zeen)
**Pharmacologic Class** Antipsychotic Agent, Phenothiazine, Piperazine
**U.S. Brand Names** Trilafon®
**Mechanism of Action** Blocks postsynaptic mesolimbic dopaminergic receptors in the brain; exhibits a strong alpha-adrenergic blocking effect and depresses the release of hypothalamic and hypophyseal hormones
**Use** Management of manifestations of psychotic disorders, depressive neurosis, alcohol withdrawal, nausea and vomiting, nonpsychotic symptoms associated with dementia in elderly, Tourette's syndrome, Huntington's chorea, spasmodic torticollis and Reye's syndrome

#### USUAL DOSAGE
Children:
Psychoses: Oral:
1-6 years: 4-6 mg/day in divided doses
6-12 years: 6 mg/day in divided doses
>12 years: 4-16 mg 2-4 times/day
I.M.: 5 mg every 6 hours
Nausea/vomiting: I.M.: 5 mg every 6 hours
Adults:
Psychoses:
Oral: 4-16 mg 2-4 times/day not to exceed 64 mg/day
I.M.: 5 mg every 6 hours up to 15 mg/day in ambulatory patients and 30 mg/day in hospitalized patients
Nausea/vomiting:
Oral: 8-16 mg/day in divided doses up to 24 mg/day
I.M.: 5-10 mg every 6 hours as necessary up to 15 mg/day in ambulatory patients and 30 mg/day in hospitalized patients
I.V. (severe): 1 mg at 1- to 2-minute intervals up to a total of 5 mg
Hemodialysis: Not dialyzable (0% to 5%)
**Dosing adjustment in hepatic impairment:** Dosage reductions should be considered in patients with liver disease although no specific guidelines are available
**Dosage Forms Conc, oral:** 16 mg/5 mL (118 mL); **Inj:** 5 mg/mL (1 mL); **Tab:** 2 mg, 4 mg, 8 mg, 16 mg
**Contraindications** Hypersensitivity to perphenazine or any component, cross-sensitivity with other phenothiazines may exist; avoid use in patients with narrow-angle glaucoma, bone marrow suppression, severe liver or cardiac disease; subcortical brain damage; circulatory collapse; severe hypotension or hypertension
**Warnings/Precautions** Safety in children <6 months of age has not been established; use with caution in patients with cardiovascular disease or seizures, bone marrow suppression, severe liver or cardiac disease
**Pregnancy Risk Factor** C
**Adverse Reactions**
>10%:
Cardiovascular: Hypotension, orthostatic hypotension
Central nervous system: Pseudoparkinsonism, akathisia, dystonias, tardive dyskinesia (persistent), dizziness
Gastrointestinal: Constipation
Ocular: Pigmentary retinopathy
Respiratory: Nasal congestion
Miscellaneous: Diaphoresis (decreased)
1% to 10%:
Dermatologic: Increased sensitivity to sun, rash
Endocrine & metabolic: Changes in menstrual cycle, changes in libido, breast pain
Gastrointestinal: Weight gain, vomiting, stomach pain, nausea
Genitourinary: Dysuria, ejaculatory disturbances
Neuromuscular & skeletal: Trembling of fingers
(Continued)

## Perphenazine *(Continued)*

<1%: Neuroleptic malignant syndrome (NMS), impairment of temperature regulation, lowering of seizures threshold, discoloration of skin (blue-gray), galactorrhea, priapism, agranulocytosis, leukopenia, cholestatic jaundice, hepatotoxicity, cornea and lens changes

**Drug Interactions** CYP2D6 enzyme substrate; CYP2D6 enzyme inhibitor

Decreased effect: Anticholinergics, anticonvulsants; decreased effect of guanethidine, epinephrine

Increased toxicity: CNS depressants; increased effect/toxicity of anticonvulsants

**Half-Life** 9 hours

**Special PA Issues**

**Patient Education:** Use exactly as directed (do not increase dose or frequency); may cause physical and/or psychological dependence. It may take 2-3 weeks to achieve desired results; do not discontinue without consulting prescriber. Dilute oral concentration with milk, water, or citrus; do not dilute with liquids containing coffee, tea, or apple juice. Do not take within 2 hours of any antacid. Avoid excess alcohol or caffeine and other prescription or OTC medications not approved by prescriber. Maintain adequate hydration (2-3 L/day of fluids unless instructed to restrict fluid intake). Avoid skin contact with medication; may cause contact dermatitis (wash immediately with warm, soapy water). You may experience excess drowsiness, restlessness, dizziness, or blurred vision (use caution driving or when engaging in hazardous tasks until response to medication is known); dry mouth, nausea, vomiting (small frequent meals, frequent mouth care, or sucking lozenges may help); constipation (increased exercise, fluids, or dietary fruit and fiber may help); postural hypotension (use caution climbing stairs or when changing position from lying or sitting to standing); urinary retention (void before taking medication); or photosensitivity (use sunscreen, protective clothing, and avoid prolonged exposure to direct sunlight); or decreased perspiration (avoid strenuous exercise in hot environments). Report persistent CNS effects (eg, trembling fingers, altered gait or balance, excessive sedation, seizures, unusual movements, anxiety, abnormal thoughts, confusion, personality changes); chest pain, palpitations, rapid heartbeat, severe dizziness; unresolved urinary retention or changes in urinary pattern; menstrual pattern, change in libido, or ejaculatory difficulty; vision changes; skin rash or yellowing of skin; difficulty breathing; or worsening of condition.

**Dietary Considerations:** Alcohol: Additive CNS effect, avoid use

**Reference Range:** 2-6 nmol/L

**Related Information**

Antipsychotic Agents *on page 1001*

♦ **Persantine®** *see* Dipyridamole *on page 293*

♦ **Pethidine Hydrochloride** *see* Meperidine *on page 567*

♦ **PFA** *see* Foscarnet *on page 401*

♦ **Pfizerpen®** *see* Penicillin G, Parenteral, Aqueous *on page 705*

♦ **PGE₁** *see* Alprostadil *on page 45*

♦ **PGE₂** *see* Dinoprostone *on page 288*

♦ **PGI₂** *see* Epoprostenol *on page 324*

♦ **PGX** *see* Epoprostenol *on page 324*

♦ **Phanatuss® Cough Syrup [OTC]** *see* Guaifenesin and Dextromethorphan *on page 428*

♦ **Pharmacal®** *see* Calcium Carbonate *on page 139*

♦ **Pharmaflur®** *see* Fluoride *on page 383*

♦ **Phenadex® Senior [OTC]** *see* Guaifenesin and Dextromethorphan *on page 428*

♦ **Phenahist-TR®** *see* Chlorpheniramine, Phenylephrine, Phenylpropanolamine, and Belladonna Alkaloids *on page 196*

♦ **Phenameth® DM** *see* Promethazine and Dextromethorphan *on page 769*

♦ **Phenaphen® With Codeine** *see* Acetaminophen and Codeine *on page 22*

♦ **Phenazine®** *see* Promethazine *on page 768*

♦ **Phenazo** *see* Phenazopyridine *on this page*

♦ **Phenazodine®** *see* Phenazopyridine *on this page*

## Phenazopyridine *(fen az oh PEER i deen)*

**Pharmacologic Class** Analgesic, Urinary

**U.S. Brand Names** Azo-Standard® [OTC]; Baridium® [OTC]; Geridium®; Phenazodine®; Prodium® [OTC]; Pyridiate®; Pyridium®; Urodine®; Urogesic®

**Mechanism of Action** An azo dye which exerts local anesthetic or analgesic action on urinary tract mucosa through an unknown mechanism

**Use** Symptomatic relief of urinary burning, itching, frequency and urgency in association with urinary tract infection or following urologic procedures

**USUAL DOSAGE** Oral:

Children: 12 mg/kg/day in 3 divided doses administered after meals for 2 days

Adults: 100-200 mg 3 times/day after meals for 2 days when used concomitantly with an antibacterial agent

**Dosing interval in renal impairment:**
  $Cl_{cr}$ 50-80 mL/minute: Administer every 8-16 hours
  $Cl_{cr}$ <50 mL/minute: Avoid use

**Dosage Forms Tab:** Azo-Standard®, Prodium®: 95 mg, Baridium®, Geridium®, Pyridiate®, Pyridium®, Urodine®, Urogesic®: 100 mg, Geridium®, Phenazodine®, Pyridium®, Urodine®: 200 mg

**Contraindications** Hypersensitivity to phenazopyridine or any component; kidney or liver disease

**Warnings/Precautions** Does not treat infection, acts only as an analgesic; drug should be discontinued if skin or sclera develop a yellow color; use with caution in patients with renal impairment. Use of this agent in the elderly is limited since accumulation of phenazopyridine can occur in patients with renal insufficiency. It should not be used in patients with a $Cl_{cr}$ <50 mL/minute.

**Pregnancy Risk Factor** B

**Adverse Reactions**
  1% to 10%:
    Central nervous system: Headache, dizziness
    Gastrointestinal: Stomach cramps
    <1%: Vertigo, skin pigmentation, rash, methemoglobinemia, hemolytic anemia, hepatitis, acute renal failure

**Special PA Issues**
  **Patient Education:** Take prescribed dose after meals. Urine may turn red-orange (normal but will stain fabric). Report persistent headache, dizziness, or stomach cramping.

- **Phenazopyridine Hydrochloride** *see* Phenazopyridine *on previous page*
- **Phenchlor® S.H.A.** *see* Chlorpheniramine, Phenylephrine, Phenylpropanolamine, and Belladonna Alkaloids *on page 196*
- **Phendry® Oral [OTC]** *see* Diphenhydramine *on page 289*

# Phenelzine (FEN el zeen)

**Pharmacologic Class** Antidepressant, Monoamine Oxidase Inhibitor

**U.S. Brand Names** Nardil®

**Mechanism of Action** Thought to act by increasing endogenous concentrations of epinephrine, norepinephrine, dopamine and serotonin through inhibition of the enzyme (monoamine oxidase) responsible for the breakdown of these neurotransmitters

**Use** Symptomatic treatment of atypical, nonendogenous or neurotic depression. The MAO inhibitors are usually reserved for patients who do not tolerate or respond to the traditional "cyclic" or "second generation" antidepressants. The brain activity of monoamine oxidase increases with age and even more so in patients with Alzheimer's disease. Therefore, the MAO inhibitors may have an increased role in patients with Alzheimer's disease who are depressed. Phenelzine is less stimulating than tranylcypromine.

**USUAL DOSAGE** Oral:
  Adults: 15 mg 3 times/day; may increase to 60-90 mg/day during early phase of treatment, then reduce to dose for maintenance therapy slowly after maximum benefit is obtained; takes 2-4 weeks for a significant response to occur
  Elderly: Initial: 7.5 mg/day; increase by 7.5-15 mg/day every 3-4 days as tolerated; usual therapeutic dose: 15-60 mg/day in 3-4 divided doses

**Dosage Forms Tab, as sulfate:** 15 mg

**Contraindications** Pheochromocytoma, hepatic or renal disease, cerebrovascular defect, cardiovascular disease, hypersensitivity to phenelzine or any component, do not use within 5 weeks of fluoxetine or 2 weeks of sertraline or paroxetine discontinuance

**Warnings/Precautions** Safety in children <16 years of age has not been established; use with caution in patients who are hyperactive, hyperexcitable, or who have glaucoma; avoid use of meperidine within 2 weeks of phenelzine use. Hypertensive crisis may occur with tyramine. See See Tyramine-Containing Foods in Appendix *on page 1148*

The MAO inhibitors are effective and generally well tolerated by older patients. It is the potential interactions with tyramine or tryptophan-containing foods and other drugs, and their effects on blood pressure that have limited their use.

**Pregnancy Risk Factor** C

**Adverse Reactions**
  >10%:
    Cardiovascular: Orthostatic hypotension
    Central nervous system: Drowsiness
    Endocrine & metabolic: Decreased sexual ability
    Neuromuscular & skeletal: Trembling, weakness
    Ocular: Blurred vision
  1% to 10%:
    Cardiovascular: Tachycardia, peripheral edema
    Central nervous system: Nervousness, chills
    Gastrointestinal: Diarrhea, anorexia, xerostomia, constipation
    <1%: Parkinsonism syndrome, leukopenia, hepatitis
  (Continued)

## Phenelzine *(Continued)*

### Drug Interactions

Increased effect/toxicity of barbiturates, psychotropics, rauwolfia alkaloids, CNS depressants

Increased toxicity with disulfiram (seizures), fluoxetine and other serotonin active agents (increased cardiac effect), tricyclic antidepressants (increased cardiovascular instability), meperidine (increased cardiovascular instability), phenothiazine (hypertensive crisis), sympathomimetics (hypertensive crisis), levodopa (hypertensive crisis), tyramine-containing foods (increased blood pressure), dextroamphetamine

**Onset** Within 2-4 weeks

**Duration** May continue to have a therapeutic effect and interactions 2 weeks after discontinuing therapy

### Special PA Issues

**Patient Education:** Take exactly as directed (do not increase dose or frequency); may take 2-3 weeks to achieve desired results; may cause physical and/or psychological dependence. Avoid excessive alcohol, caffeine, and other prescription or OTC medications not approved by prescriber. Avoid tyramine-containing foods (eg, pickles, aged cheese, wine). Maintain adequate hydration (2-3 L/day of fluids unless instructed to restrict fluid intake). You may experience postural hypotension (use caution when climbing stairs or changing position from lying or sitting to standing); drowsiness, lightheadedness, dizziness (use caution when driving or engaging in hazardous tasks until response to medication is known); anorexia, dry mouth (small frequent meals, frequent mouth care, or sucking lozenges may help); constipation (increased exercise, fluids, or dietary fruit and fiber may help); or diarrhea (buttermilk, yogurt, or boiled milk may help). Diabetic patients should monitor serum glucose closely (Nardil® may effect glucose levels). Report persistent insomnia; chest pain, palpitations, irregular or rapid heartbeat, or swelling of extremities; muscle cramping, tremors, or altered gait; blurred vision or eye pain; yellowing of eyes or skin; pale stools/dark urine; or worsening of condition.

**Dietary Considerations:**
Alcohol: Additive CNS effect, avoid use
Food: Avoid tyramine-containing foods

**Monitoring Parameters:** Blood pressure, heart rate, diet, weight, mood (if depressive symptoms)

### Related Information

Antidepressant Agents *on page 998*
Tyramine-Containing Foods *on page 1148*

♦ **Phenelzine Sulfate** *see Phenelzine on previous page*

♦ **Phenerbel-S®** *see Belladonna, Phenobarbital, and Ergotamine Tartrate on page 103*

♦ **Phenergan®** *see Promethazine on page 768*

♦ **Phenergan® VC Syrup** *see Promethazine and Phenylephrine on page 769*

♦ **Phenergan® VC With Codeine** *see Promethazine, Phenylephrine, and Codeine on page 769*

♦ **Phenergan® With Codeine** *see Promethazine and Codeine on page 769*

♦ **Phenergan® With Dextromethorphan** *see Promethazine and Dextromethorphan on page 769*

♦ **Phenhist® Expectorant** *see Guaifenesin, Pseudoephedrine, and Codeine on page 429*

## Pheniramine, Phenylpropanolamine, and Pyrilamine
*(fen EER a meen, fen il proe pa NOLE a meen, & peer IL a meen)*

**Pharmacologic Class** Antihistamine/Decongestant Combination

**U.S. Brand Names** Triaminic® Oral Infant Drops

**Dosage Forms Drops:** Pheniramine maleate 10 mg, phenylpropanolamine hydrochloride 20 mg, and pyrilamine maleate 10 mg per mL (15 mL)

♦ **Phenoxine® [OTC]** *see Phenylpropanolamine on page 720*

♦ **Phenoxymethyl Penicillin** *see Penicillin V Potassium on page 706*

## Phentermine *(FEN ter meen)*

**Pharmacologic Class** Anorexiant

**U.S. Brand Names** Adipex-P®; Fastin®; Ionamin®; Zantryl®

**Mechanism of Action** Phentermine is structurally similar to dextroamphetamine and is comparable to dextroamphetamine as an appetite suppressant, but is generally associated with a lower incidence and severity of CNS side effects. Phentermine, like other anorexiants, stimulates the hypothalamus to result in decreased appetite; anorexiant effects are most likely mediated via norepinephrine and dopamine metabolism. However, other CNS effects or metabolic effects may be involved.

**Use** Short-term adjunct in exogenous obesity in patients with an initial body mass index (BMI) ≥30 kg/m² or a BMI ≥27 kg/m² when other risk factors are present (eg, hypertension, diabetes, hyperlipidemia)

**Body Mass Index (BMI), kg/m$^2$**
**Height (feet, inches)**

| Weight (pounds) | 5'0' | 5'3' | 5'6' | 5'9' | 6'0' | 6'3' |
|---|---|---|---|---|---|---|
| 140 | 27 | 25 | 23 | 21 | 19 | 18 |
| 150 | 29 | 27 | 24 | 22 | 20 | 19 |
| 160 | 31 | 28 | 26 | 24 | 22 | 20 |
| 170 | 33 | 30 | 28 | 25 | 23 | 21 |
| 180 | 35 | 32 | 29 | 27 | 25 | 23 |
| 190 | 37 | 34 | 31 | 28 | 26 | 24 |
| 200 | 39 | 36 | 32 | 30 | 27 | 25 |
| 210 | 41 | 37 | 34 | 31 | 29 | 26 |
| 220 | 43 | 39 | 36 | 33 | 30 | 28 |
| 230 | 45 | 41 | 37 | 34 | 31 | 29 |
| 240 | 47 | 43 | 39 | 36 | 33 | 30 |
| 250 | 49 | 44 | 40 | 37 | 34 | 31 |

**USUAL DOSAGE** Oral:

Children 3-15 years: 5-15 mg/day for 4 weeks

Adults: 8 mg 3 times/day 30 minutes before meals or food or 15-37.5 mg/day before breakfast or 10-14 hours before retiring

**Dosage Forms Cap, as hydrochloride:** 15 mg, 18.75 mg, 30 mg, 37.5 mg; **Cap, resin complex, as hydrochloride:** 15 mg, 30 mg; **Tab, as hydrochloride:** 8 mg, 37.5 mg

**Contraindications** Known hypersensitivity to phentermine

**Warnings/Precautions** Do not use in children ≤16 years of age. Use with caution in patients with diabetes mellitus, cardiovascular disease, nephritis, angina pectoris, hypertension, glaucoma, patients with a history of drug abuse. **Primary pulmonary hypertension (PPH),** a rare and frequently fatal pulmonary disease, has been reported to occur in patients receiving a combination of phentermine and fenfluramine or dexfenfluramine. The possibility of an association between PPH and the use of phentermine alone cannot be ruled out.

**Pregnancy Risk Factor** C

**Adverse Reactions**

>10%:

Cardiovascular: Hypertension

Central nervous system: Euphoria, nervousness, insomnia

1% to 10%:

Central nervous system: Confusion, mental depression, restlessness

Gastrointestinal: Nausea, vomiting, constipation

Endocrine & metabolic: Changes in libido

Neuromuscular & skeletal: Tremor

Ocular: Blurred vision

<1%: Tachycardia, arrhythmias, insomnia, restlessness, nervousness, depression, headache, alopecia, nausea, vomiting, diarrhea, abdominal cramps, dysuria, polyuria, myalgia, tremor, dyspnea, diaphoresis (increased)

**Drug Interactions**

Decreased effect of guanethidine; decreased effect with CNS depressants

Increased effect/toxicity with MAO inhibitors (hypertensive crisis), sympathomimetics, CNS stimulants

**Half-Life** 20 hours

**Special PA Issues**

**Patient Education:** Take during day to avoid insomnia; do not discontinue abruptly, may cause physical and psychological dependence with prolonged use

**Monitoring Parameters:** CNS

♦ **Phentermine Hydrochloride** *see* Phentermine *on previous page*

# Phentolamine (fen TOLE a meen)

**Pharmacologic Class** Alpha$_1$ Blockers

**U.S. Brand Names** Regitine®

**Mechanism of Action** Competitively blocks alpha-adrenergic receptors to produce brief antagonism of circulating epinephrine and norepinephrine to reduce hypertension caused by alpha effects of these catecholamines; also has a positive inotropic and chronotropic effect on the heart

**Use** Diagnosis of pheochromocytoma and treatment of hypertension associated with pheochromocytoma or other caused by excess sympathomimetic amines; as treatment of dermal necrosis after extravasation of drugs with alpha-adrenergic effects (norepinephrine, dopamine, epinephrine, dobutamine)

(Continued)

## Phentolamine *(Continued)*

### USUAL DOSAGE

Treatment of alpha-adrenergic drug extravasation: S.C.:

Children: 0.1-0.2 mg/kg diluted in 10 mL 0.9% sodium chloride infiltrated into area of extravasation within 12 hours

Adults: Infiltrate area with small amount of solution made by diluting 5-10 mg in 10 mL 0.9% sodium chloride within 12 hours of extravasation

If dose is effective, normal skin color should return to the blanched area within 1 hour

Diagnosis of pheochromocytoma: I.M., I.V.:

Children: 0.05-0.1 mg/kg/dose, maximum single dose: 5 mg

Adults: 5 mg

Surgery for pheochromocytoma: Hypertension: I.M., I.V.:

Children: 0.05-0.1 mg/kg/dose given 1-2 hours before procedure; repeat as needed every 2-4 hours until hypertension is controlled; maximum single dose: 5 mg

Adults: 5 mg given 1-2 hours before procedure and repeated as needed every 2-4 hours

Hypertensive crisis: Adults 5-20 mg

**Dosage Forms** Inj, as mesylate: 5 mg/mL (1 mL)

**Contraindications** Hypersensitivity to phentolamine or any component; renal impairment; coronary or cerebral arteriosclerosis

**Warnings/Precautions** Myocardial infarction, cerebrovascular spasm and cerebrovascular occlusion have occurred following administration; use with caution in patients with gastritis or peptic ulcer, tachycardia, or a history of cardiac arrhythmias

### Pregnancy Risk Factor C

### Adverse Reactions

>10%:

Cardiovascular: Hypotension, tachycardia, arrhythmias, reflex tachycardia, anginal pain, orthostatic hypotension

Gastrointestinal: Nausea, vomiting, diarrhea, exacerbation of peptic ulcer, abdominal pain

Respiratory: Nasal congestion

1% to 10%:

Cardiovascular: Flushing of face, syncope

Central nervous system: Dizziness

Neuromuscular & skeletal: Weakness

Respiratory: Nasal congestion

<1%: Myocardial infarction, severe headache

### Drug Interactions

Decreased effect: Epinephrine, ephedrine

Increased toxicity: Ethanol (disulfiram reaction)

**Onset** I.M.: Within 15-20 minutes; I.V.: Immediate

**Duration** I.M.: 30-45 minutes; I.V.: 15-30 minutes

**Half-Life** 19 minutes

### Special PA Issues

**Patient Education:** Immediately report pain at infusion site. Report any dizziness, feelings of faintness, or palpitations. Do not change position rapidly; rise slowly or ask for assistance.

**Monitoring Parameters:** Blood pressure, heart rate

♦ **Phentolamine Mesylate** *see* Phentolamine *on previous page*

♦ **Phenylalanine Mustard** *see* Melphalan *on page 565*

♦ **Phenylazo Diamino Pyridine Hydrochloride** *see* Phenazopyridine *on page 714*

♦ **Phenyldrine® [OTC]** *see* Phenylpropanolamine *on page 720*

## Phenylephrine *(fen il EF rin)*

**Pharmacologic Class** Alpha/Beta Agonist; Ophthalmic Agent, Antiglaucoma; Ophthalmic Agent, Mydriatic

**U.S. Brand Names** AK-Dilate® Ophthalmic Solution; AK-Nefrin® Ophthalmic Solution; Alconefrin® Nasal Solution [OTC]; Doktors® Nasal Solution [OTC]; I-Phrine® Ophthalmic Solution; Isopto® Frin Ophthalmic Solution; Mydfrin® Ophthalmic Solution; Neo-Synephrine® Nasal Solution [OTC]; Neo-Synephrine® Ophthalmic Solution; Nostril® Nasal Solution [OTC]; Prefrin™ Ophthalmic Solution; Relief® Ophthalmic Solution; Rhinall® Nasal Solution [OTC]; Sinarest® Nasal Solution [OTC]; St. Joseph® Measured Dose Nasal Solution [OTC]; Vicks® Sinex® Nasal Solution [OTC]

**Mechanism of Action** Potent, direct-acting alpha-adrenergic stimulator with weak beta-adrenergic activity; causes vasoconstriction of the arterioles of the nasal mucosa and conjunctiva; activates the dilator muscle of the pupil to cause contraction; produces vasoconstriction of arterioles in the body; produces systemic arterial vasoconstriction

**Use** Treatment of hypotension, vascular failure in shock; as a vasoconstrictor in regional analgesia; symptomatic relief of nasal and nasopharyngeal mucosal congestion; as a mydriatic in ophthalmic procedures and treatment of wide-angle glaucoma; supraventricular tachycardia

**USUAL DOSAGE**
Ophthalmic procedures:
Infants <1 year: Instill 1 drop of 2.5% 15-30 minutes before procedures
Children and Adults: Instill 1 drop of 2.5% or 10% solution, may repeat in 10-60 minutes as needed
Nasal decongestant: (therapy should not exceed 5 continuous days)
Children:
2-6 years: Instill 1 drop every 2-4 hours of 0.125% solution as needed
6-12 years: Instill 1-2 sprays or instill 1-2 drops every 4 hours of 0.25% solution as needed
Children >12 years and Adults: Instill 1-2 sprays or instill 1-2 drops every 4 hours of 0.25% to 0.5% solution as needed; 1% solution may be used in adult in cases of extreme nasal congestion; do not use nasal solutions more than 3 days
Hypotension/shock:
Children:
I.M., S.C.: 0.1 mg/kg/dose every 1-2 hours as needed (maximum: 5 mg)
I.V. bolus: 5-20 mcg/kg/dose every 10-15 minutes as needed
I.V. infusion: 0.1-0.5 mcg/kg/minute
Adults:
I.M., S.C.: 2-5 mg/dose every 1-2 hours as needed (initial dose should not exceed 5 mg)
I.V. bolus: 0.1-0.5 mg/dose every 10-15 minutes as needed (initial dose should not exceed 0.5 mg)
I.V. infusion: 10 mg in 250 mL $D_5W$ or NS (1:25,000 dilution) (40 mcg/mL); start at 100-180 mcg/minute (2-5 mL/minute; 50-90 drops/minute) initially; when blood pressure is stabilized, maintenance rate: 40-60 mcg/minute (20-30 drops/minute)
Paroxysmal supraventricular tachycardia: I.V.:
Children: 5-10 mcg/kg/dose over 20-30 seconds
Adults: 0.25-0.5 mg/dose over 20-30 seconds

**Dosage Forms Inj (Neo-Synephrine®):** 1% [10 mg/mL] (1 mL); **Nasal soln: Drops:** Neo-Synephrine®: 0.125% (15 mL), Alconefrin® 12: 0.16% (30 mL), Alconefrin® 25, Neo-Synephrine®, Children's Nostril®, Rhinall®: 0.25% (15 mL, 30 mL, 40 mL), Alconefrin®, Neo-Synephrine®: 0.5% (15 mL, 30 mL); **Spr:** Alconefrin® 25, Neo-Synephrine®, Rhinall®: 0.25% (15 mL, 30 mL, 40 mL), Neo-Synephrine®, Nostril®, Sinex®: 0.5% (15 mL, 30 mL), Neo-Synephrine®: 1% (15 mL); **Ophth soln:** AK-Nefrin®, Isopto® Frin, Prefrin™ Liquifilm®, Relief®: 0.12% (0.3 mL, 15 mL, 20 mL), AK-Dilate®, Mydfrin®, Neo-Synephrine®, Phenoptic®: 2.5% (2 mL, 3 mL, 5 mL, 15 mL), AK-Dilate®, Neo-Synephrine®, Neo-Synephrine® Viscous: 10% (1 mL, 2 mL, 5 mL, 15 mL VIsc)

**Contraindications** Pheochromocytoma, severe hypertension, bradycardia, ventricular tachyarrhythmias; hypersensitivity to phenylephrine or any component; narrow-angle glaucoma (ophthalmic preparation), acute pancreatitis, hepatitis, peripheral or mesenteric vascular thrombosis, myocardial disease, severe coronary disease

**Warnings/Precautions** Injection may contain sulfites which may cause allergic reaction in some patients; do not use if solution turns brown or contains a precipitate; use with extreme caution in elderly patients, patients with hyperthyroidism, bradycardia, partial heart block, myocardial disease, or severe arteriosclerosis; infuse into large veins to help prevent extravasation which may cause severe necrosis; the 10% ophthalmic solution has caused increased blood pressure in elderly patients and its use should, therefore, be avoided

**Pregnancy Risk Factor** C

**Adverse Reactions**
Nasal:
>10%: Burning, rebound congestion, sneezing
1% to 10%: Stinging, dryness
Ophthalmic:
>10%: Transient stinging
1% to 10%:
Central nervous system: Headache, browache
Ocular: Blurred vision, photophobia, lacrimation
Systemic:
>10%: Neuromuscular & skeletal: Tremor
1% to 10%:
Cardiovascular: Peripheral vasoconstriction hypertension, angina, reflex bradycardia, arrhythmias
Central nervous system: Restlessness, excitability

**Drug Interactions**
Decreased effect: With alpha- and beta-adrenergic blocking agents
Increased effect: With oxytocic drugs
Increased toxicity: With sympathomimetics, tachycardia or arrhythmias may occur; with MAO inhibitors, actions may be potentiated

**Onset** I.M., S.C.: Within 10-15 minutes; I.V.: Immediate
**Duration** I.M.: 30 minutes to 2 hours; I.V.: 15-30 minutes; S.C.: 1 hour
**Half-Life** 2.5 hours
(Continued)

## Phenylephrine *(Continued)*

### Special PA Issues
**Patient Education:**

Nasal decongestant: Do not use for more than 5 days in a row. Clear nose as much as possible before use. Tilt head back and instill recommended dose of drops or spray. Do not blow nose for 5-10 minutes. You may experience transient stinging or burning.

Ophthalmic: Open eye, look at ceiling, and instill prescribed amount of solution. Close eye and roll eye in all directions, and apply gentle pressure to inner corner of eye for 1-2 minutes after instillation. Do not let tip of applicator touch eye or contaminate tip of applicator. Temporary stinging or blurred vision may occur. Report persistent pain, burning, double vision, severe headache, or if condition worsens.

**Monitoring Parameters:** Blood pressure, heart rate, arterial blood gases, central venous pressure

## Phenylephrine and Scopolamine (fen il EF rin & skoe POL a meen)
**Pharmacologic Class** Anticholinergic/Adrenergic Agonist

**U.S. Brand Names** Murocoll-2® Ophthalmic

**Dosage Forms Soln, ophth:** Phenylephrine hydrochloride 10% and scopolamine hydrobromide 0.3% (7.5 mL)

♦ **Phenylephrine Hydrochloride** see Phenylephrine on page 718

♦ **Phenylisohydantoin** see Pemoline on page 701

## Phenylpropanolamine (fen il proe pa NOLE a meen)
**Pharmacologic Class** Alpha/Beta Agonist

**U.S. Brand Names** Acutrim® 16 Hours [OTC]; Acutrim® II, Maximum Strength [OTC]; Acutrim® Late Day [OTC]; Control® [OTC]; Dexatrim® Pre-Meal [OTC]; Maximum Strength Dex-A-Diet® [OTC]; Maximum Strength Dexatrim® [OTC]; Phenoxine® [OTC]; Phenyldrine® [OTC]; Prolamine® [OTC]; Propagest® [OTC]; Rhindecon®; Unitrol® [OTC]

**Mechanism of Action** Releases tissue stores of epinephrine and thereby produces an alpha- and beta-adrenergic stimulation; this causes vasoconstriction and nasal mucosa blanching; also appears to depress central appetite centers

**Use** Anorexiant; nasal decongestant

### USUAL DOSAGE Oral:
Children: Decongestant:

2-6 years: 6.25 mg every 4 hours

6-12 years: 12.5 mg every 4 hours not to exceed 75 mg/day

Adults:

Decongestant: 25 mg every 4 hours or 50 mg every 8 hours, not to exceed 150 mg/day

Anorexic: 25 mg 3 times/day 30 minutes before meals or 75 mg (timed release) once daily in the morning

Precision release: 75 mg after breakfast

**Dosage Forms Cap:** 37.5 mg; **Cap, timed release:** 25 mg, 75 mg; **Tab:** 25 mg, 50 mg; **Tab:** Precision release: 75 mg, Timed release: 75 mg

**Contraindications** Known hypersensitivity to drug

**Warnings/Precautions** Use with caution in patients with high blood pressure, tachyarrhythmias, pheochromocytoma, bradycardia, cardiac disease, arteriosclerosis; do not use for more than 3 weeks for weight loss

**Pregnancy Risk Factor** C

### Adverse Reactions
>10%: Cardiovascular: Hypertension, palpitations

1% to 10%:

Central nervous system: Insomnia, restlessness, dizziness

Gastrointestinal: Xerostomia, nausea

<1%: Tightness in chest, bradycardia, arrhythmias, angina, severe headache, anxiety, nervousness, restlessness, dysuria

### Drug Interactions
Decreased effect of antihypertensives

Increased effect/toxicity with MAO inhibitors (hypertensive crisis), beta-blockers (increased pressor effects)

**Duration** Up to 24 hours (timed release)

**Half-Life** 4.6-6.6 hours

### Special PA Issues
**Patient Education:** Nasal decongestant: Do not use for longer than recommended (4-5 days in a row). Anorexiant: Do not use for longer than 3 weeks. With timed release form, take early in day; do not chew or crush. Do not use more often, or in greater dose than prescribed. You may experience dizziness or blurred vision (use caution when driving or engaging in hazardous activities). With nasal use you may experience burning or stinging (this will resolve). Report rapid heartbeat, chest pain, palpitations; persistent vomiting; excessive nervousness, trembling, or insomnia; difficult or painful urination; unresolved burning or stinging (eyes or nose); or acute headache.

**Monitoring Parameters:** Blood pressure, heart rate

♦ **Phenylpropanolamine Hydrochloride** *see* Phenylpropanolamine *on previous page*

## Phenyltoloxamine, Phenylpropanolamine, and Acetaminophen
(fen il tol OKS a meen, fen il proe pa NOLE a meen, & a seet a MIN oh fen)

**Pharmacologic Class** Antihistamine/Decongestant/Analgesic

**U.S. Brand Names** Sinubid®

**Dosage Forms Tab:** Phenyltoloxamine citrate 22 mg, phenylpropanolamine hydrochloride 25 mg, and acetaminophen 325 mg

## Phenyltoloxamine, Phenylpropanolamine, Pyrilamine, and Pheniramine
(fen il tol OKS a meen, fen il proe pa NOLE a meen, peer IL a meen, & fen IR a meen)

**Pharmacologic Class** Cold Preparation

**U.S. Brand Names** Poly-Histine-D® Capsule

**Dosage Forms Cap:** Phenyltoloxamine citrate 16 mg, phenylpropanolamine hydrochloride 50 mg, pyrilamine maleate 16 mg, and pheniramine maleate 16 mg

## Phenytoin (FEN i toyn)

**Pharmacologic Class** Antiarrhythmic Agent, Class I-B; Anticonvulsant, Hydantoin

**U.S. Brand Names** Dilantin®; Diphenylan Sodium®

**Mechanism of Action** Stabilizes neuronal membranes and decreases seizure activity by increasing efflux or decreasing influx of sodium ions across cell membranes in the motor cortex during generation of nerve impulses; prolongs effective refractory period and suppresses ventricular pacemaker automaticity, shortens action potential in the heart

**Use** Management of generalized tonic-clonic (grand mal), simple partial and complex partial seizures; prevention of seizures following head trauma/neurosurgery; ventricular arrhythmias, including those associated with digitalis intoxication, prolonged Q-T interval and surgical repair of congenital heart diseases in children; also used for epidermolysis bullosa

**USUAL DOSAGE**

Status epilepticus: I.V.:

Infants and Children: Loading dose: 15-20 mg/kg in a single or divided dose; maintenance dose: Initial: 5 mg/kg/day in 2 divided doses, usual doses:

6 months to 3 years: 8-10 mg/kg/day

4-6 years: 7.5-9 mg/kg/day

7-9 years: 7-8 mg/kg/day

10-16 years: 6-7 mg/kg/day, some patients may require every 8 hours dosing

Adults: Loading dose: 15-20 mg/kg in a single or divided dose, followed by 100-150 mg/ dose at 30-minute intervals up to a maximum of 1500 mg/24 hours; maintenance dose: 300 mg/day or 5-6 mg/kg/day in 3 divided doses or 1-2 divided doses using extended release

Anticonvulsant: Children and Adults: Oral:

Loading dose: 15-20 mg/kg; based on phenytoin serum concentrations and recent dosing history; administer oral loading dose in 3 divided doses given every 2-4 hours to decrease GI adverse effects and to ensure complete oral absorption; maintenance dose: same as I.V.

**Dosing adjustment/comments in renal impairment or hepatic disease:** Safe in usual doses in mild liver disease; clearance may be substantially reduced in cirrhosis and plasma level monitoring with dose adjustment advisable. Free phenytoin levels should be monitored closely.

**Dosage Forms** Phenytoin sodium: **Cap, extended release:** 30 mg, 100 mg; **Cap, prompt:** 30 mg, 100 mg; **Inj:** 50 mg/mL (2 mL, 5 mL); **Susp, oral:** 125 mg/5 mL (5 mL, 240 mL); **Tab, chewable:** 50 mg

**Contraindications** Hypersensitivity to phenytoin, other hydantoins, or any component; heart block, sinus bradycardia

**Warnings/Precautions** May increase frequency of petit mal seizures; I.V. form may cause hypotension, skin necrosis at I.V. site; avoid I.V. administration in small veins; use with caution in patients with porphyria; discontinue if rash or lymphadenopathy occurs; use with caution in patients with hepatic dysfunction, sinus bradycardia, S-A block, A-V block, or hepatic impairment; elderly may have reduced hepatic clearance and low albumin levels, which will increase the free fraction of phenytoin in the serum and, therefore, the pharmacologic response

**Pregnancy Risk Factor** D

**Pregnancy Implications**

Clinical effects on the fetus: Crosses the placenta. Cardiac defects and multiple other malformations reported; characteristic pattern of malformations called "fetal hydantin syndrome"; hemorrhagic disease of newborn due to fetal vitamin K depletion, maternal folic acid deficiency may occur. Epilepsy itself, number of medications, genetic factors, or a combination of these probably influence the teratogenicity of anticonvulsant therapy. Benefit:risk ratio usually favors continued use during pregnancy and breast-feeding.

Breast-feeding/lactation: Crosses into breast milk

(Continued)

## Phenytoin *(Continued)*

Clinical effects on the infant: Methemoglobinemia, drowsiness and decreased sucking reported in 1 case. American Academy of Pediatrics considers **compatible** with breast-feeding.

**Adverse Reactions** I.V. effects: Hypotension, bradycardia, cardiac arrhythmias, cardiovascular collapse (especially with rapid I.V. use), venous irritation and pain, thrombophlebitis

**Effects not related to plasma phenytoin concentrations:** Hypertrichosis, gingival hypertrophy, thickening of facial features, carbohydrate intolerance, folic acid deficiency, peripheral neuropathy, vitamin D deficiency, osteomalacia, systemic lupus erythematosus

**Dose-related effects:** Nystagmus, blurred vision, diplopia, ataxia, slurred speech, dizziness, drowsiness, lethargy, coma, rash, fever, nausea, vomiting, gum tenderness, confusion, mood changes, folic acid depletion, osteomalacia, hyperglycemia

### Related to elevated concentrations:

>20 mcg/mL: Far lateral nystagmus
>30 mcg/mL: 45° lateral gaze nystagmus and ataxia
>40 mcg/mL: Decreased mentation
>100 mcg/mL: Death

>10%:
Central nervous system: Psychiatric changes, slurred speech, dizziness, drowsiness
Gastrointestinal: Constipation, nausea, vomiting, gingival hyperplasia
Neuromuscular & skeletal: Trembling

1% to 10%:
Central nervous system: Headache, insomnia
Dermatologic: Rash
Gastrointestinal: Anorexia, weight loss
Hematologic: Leukopenia
Hepatic: Hepatitis
Renal: Increase in serum creatinine

<1%: Hypotension, bradycardia, cardiac arrhythmias, cardiovascular collapse, confusion, fever, ataxia, thrombophlebitis, peripheral neuropathy, paresthesia, diplopia, nystagmus, blurred vision, SLE-like syndrome, lymphadenopathy, hepatitis, Stevens-Johnson syndrome, blood dyscrasias, dyskinesias, pseudolymphoma, lymphoma, venous irritation and pain

**Drug Interactions** CYP2C9 and 2C19 enzyme substrate; CYP1A2, 2B6, 2C, 2C9, 2C18, 2C19, 2D6, 3A3/4, and 3A5-7 enzyme inducer

Decreased effect: Phenytoin with rifampin, cisplatin, vinblastine, bleomycin, folic acid, theophylline, and continuous NG feedings. Phenytoin may decrease the effect of oral contraceptives, itraconazole, mebendazole, methadone, oral midazolam, valproic acid, cyclosporine, theophylline, doxycycline, quinidine, mexiletine, disopyramide.

Amiodarone or disulfiram decreases metabolism of phenytoin.

Increased toxicity: Isoniazid, chloramphenicol, or fluconazole may increase phenytoin serum concentrations. Valproic acid may increase, decrease or have no effect on phenytoin serum concentrations. Phenytoin may increase the effect of dopamine (enhanced hypotension), warfarin (enhanced anticoagulation), increase the rate of conversion of primidone to phenobarbital resulting in increased phenobarbital serum concentrations. Ticlopidine increases serum phenytoin concentrations to increase toxicity of phenytoin

**Onset** I.V.: within 30 minutes to 1 hour; onset of fosphenytoin may be more rapid due to more rapid infusion

**Half-Life** Oral: 22 hours (range: 7-42 hours); I.V.: 10-15 hours

### Special PA Issues

**Patient Education:** Take this drug as directed, with food. Do not change brands or discontinue without consulting prescriber. Do not crush or open extended capsules. Follow good oral hygiene practices and have frequent dental check-ups. If diabetic, monitor your serum glucose regularly as directed by prescriber; insulin dosage may need to be adjusted. You may experience dizziness, confusion, or vision changes; use caution when driving or engaging in hazardous tasks. If GI upset occurs, frequent small meals may help. Report rash; unresolved nausea or vomiting; slurring speech or coordination difficulties; swollen glands; swollen, sore, or bleeding gums; yellowish color to skin or eyes; change in color of urine or stool; unusual bleeding and/or bruising; erection problems; difficulty breathing; or palpitations.

### Dietary Considerations:

Alcohol: Additive CNS depression has been reported with hydantoins
Alcohol (acute use): Inhibits metabolism of phenytoin; avoid or limit use; watch for sedation
Alcohol (chronic use): Stimulates metabolism of phenytoin; avoid or limit use
Food:
Folic acid: Low erythrocyte and CSF folate concentrations. Phenytoin may decrease mucosal uptake of folic acid; to avoid folic acid deficiency and megaloblastic anemia, some clinicians recommend giving patients on anticonvulsants prophylactic doses of folic acid and cyanocobalamin.

Calcium: Hypocalcemia has been reported in patients taking prolonged high-dose therapy with an anticonvulsant. Phenytoin may decrease calcium absorption. Monitor calcium serum concentration and for bone disorders (eg, rickets, osteomalacia). Some clinicians have given an additional 4,000 Units/week of vitamin D (especially in those receiving poor nutrition and getting no sun exposure) to prevent hypocalcemia.

Fresh fruits containing vitamin C: Displaces drug from binding sites, resulting in increased urinary excretion of hydantoin. Educate patients regarding the potential for a decreased anticonvulsant effect of hydantoins with consumption of foods high in vitamin C.

Vitamin D: Phenytoin interferes with vitamin D metabolism and osteomalacia may result; may need to supplement with vitamin D

Glucose: Hyperglycemia and glycosuria may occur in patients receiving high-dose therapy. Monitor blood glucose concentration, especially in patients with impaired renal function.

Tube feedings: Tube feedings decrease phenytoin bioavailability; to avoid decreased serum levels with continuous NG feeds, hold feedings for 2 hours prior to and 2 hours after phenytoin administration, if possible. There is a variety of opinions on how to administer phenytoin with enteral feedings. BE CONSISTENT throughout therapy.

**Monitoring Parameters:** Blood pressure, vital signs (with I.V. use), plasma phenytoin level, CBC, liver function tests

**Reference Range:**

Timing of serum samples: Because it is slowly absorbed, peak blood levels may occur 4-8 hours after ingestion of an oral dose. The serum half-life varies with the dosage and the drug follows Michaelis-Menten kinetics. The average adult half-life is about 24 hours. Steady-state concentrations are reached in 5-10 days.

Neonates: 8-15 µg/mL total phenytoin; 1-2 µg/mL free phenytoin

Children and Adults: Toxicity is measured clinically, and some patients require levels outside the suggested therapeutic range

Toxic: 30-50 µg/mL;

**Lethal:** >100 µg/mL

Therapeutic range:

Total phenytoin: 10-20 µg/mL (children and adults), 8-15 µg/mL (neonates)

Concentrations of 5-10 µg/mL may be therapeutic for some patients but concentrations <5 µg/mL are not likely to be effective

50% of patients show decreased frequency of seizures at concentrations >10 µg/mL

86% of patients show decreased frequency of seizures at concentrations >15 µg/mL

Add another anticonvulsant if satisfactory therapeutic response is not achieved with a phenytoin concentration of 20 µg/mL

Free phenytoin: 1-2.5 µg/mL

Toxic: <30-50 µg/mL (SI: <120-200 µmol/L)

**Lethal:** >100 µg/mL (SI: >400 µmol/L)

**When to draw levels:** This is dependent on the disease state being treated and the clinical condition of the patient

**Key points:**

Slow absorption minimizes fluctuations between peak and trough concentrations, timing of sampling not crucial

Trough concentrations are generally recommended for routine monitoring. Daily levels are not necessary and may result in incorrect dosage adjustments. If it is determined essential to monitor free phenytoin concentrations, concomitant monitoring of total phenytoin concentrations is not necessary and expensive.

After a loading dose: Draw level within 48-96 hours

Rapid achievement: Draw within 2-3 days of therapy initiation to ensure that the patient's metabolism is not remarkably different from that which would be predicted by average literature-derived pharmacokinetic parameters; early levels should be used cautiously in design of new dosing regimens

Second concentration: Draw within 6-7 days with subsequent doses of phenytoin adjusted accordingly

### Adjustment of Serum Concentration in Patients With Low Serum Albumin

| Measured Total Phenytoin Concentration (mcg/mL) | Patient's Serum Albumin (g/dL) | | | |
|---|---|---|---|---|
| | 3.5 | 3 | 2.5 | 2 |
| | Adjusted Total Phenytoin Concentration (mcg/mL)* | | | |
| 5 | 6 | 7 | 8 | 10 |
| 10 | 13 | 14 | 17 | 20 |
| 15 | 19 | 21 | 25 | 30 |

*Adjusted concentration = measured total concentration + [(0.2 x albumin) + 0.1].

(Continued)

## Phenytoin *(Continued)*

If plasma concentrations have not changed over a 3- to 5-day period, monitoring interval may be increased to once weekly in the acute clinical setting

In stable patients requiring long-term therapy, generally monitor levels at 3- to 12-month intervals

### Adjustment of Serum Concentration in Patients With Renal Failure (Cl$_{cr}$ ≤10 mL/min)

| Measured Total Phenytoin Concentration (mcg/mL) | Patient's Serum Albumin (g/dL) | | | | |
|---|---|---|---|---|---|
| | 4 | 3.5 | 3 | 2.5 | 2 |
| | Adjusted Total Phenytoin Concentration (mcg/mL)* | | | | |
| 5 | 10 | 11 | 13 | 14 | 17 |
| 10 | 20 | 22 | 25 | 29 | 33 |
| 15 | 30 | 33 | 38 | 43 | 50 |

*Adjusted concentration = measured total concentration + [(0.1 x albumin) + 0.1].

- ♦ **Phenytoin Sodium** *see Phenytoin on page 721*
- ♦ **Phenytoin Sodium, Extended** *see Phenytoin on page 721*
- ♦ **Phenytoin Sodium, Prompt** *see Phenytoin on page 721*
- ♦ **Pherazine® VC w/ Codeine** *see Promethazine, Phenylephrine, and Codeine on page 769*
- ♦ **Pherazine® w/DM** *see Promethazine and Dextromethorphan on page 769*
- ♦ **Pherazine® With Codeine** *see Promethazine and Codeine on page 769*
- ♦ **Phillips'® Milk of Magnesia [OTC]** *see Magnesium Hydroxide on page 552*
- ♦ **pHisoHex®** *see Hexachlorophene on page 441*
- ♦ **Phos-Flur®** *see Fluoride on page 383*
- ♦ **PhosLo®** *see Calcium Acetate on page 138*
- ♦ **Phosphate, Potassium** *see Potassium Phosphate on page 745*
- ♦ **Phospholine Iodide® Ophthalmic** *see Echothiophate Iodide on page 311*
- ♦ **Phosphonoformate** *see Foscarnet on page 401*
- ♦ **Phosphonoformic Acid** *see Foscarnet on page 401*
- ♦ **Photofrin®** *see Porfimer on page 738*
- ♦ **Phrenilin®** *see Butalbital Compound on page 131*
- ♦ **Phrenilin® Forte** *see Butalbital Compound on page 131*
- ♦ **p-Hydroxyampicillin** *see Amoxicillin on page 61*
- ♦ **Phyllocontin®** *see Theophylline Salts on page 888*
- ♦ **Phylloquinone** *see Phytonadione on next page*

## Physostigmine *(fye zoe STIG meen)*

**Pharmacologic Class** Acetylcholinesterase Inhibitor (Central); Ophthalmic Agent, Antiglaucoma

**U.S. Brand Names** Antilirium®; Isopto® Eserine

**Mechanism of Action** Inhibits destruction of acetylcholine by acetylcholinesterase which facilitates transmission of impulses across myoneural junction and prolongs the central and peripheral effects of acetylcholine

**Use** Reverse toxic CNS effects caused by anticholinergic drugs; used as miotic in treatment of glaucoma

**USUAL DOSAGE**

Children: Anticholinergic drug overdose: Reserve for life-threatening situations only: I.V.: 0.01-0.03 mg/kg/dose, (maximum: 0.5 mg/minute); may repeat after 5-10 minutes to a maximum total dose of 2 mg or until response occurs or adverse cholinergic effects occur

Adults: Anticholinergic drug overdose:

I.M., I.V., S.C.: 0.5-2 mg to start, repeat every 20 minutes until response occurs or adverse effect occurs

Repeat 1-4 mg every 30-60 minutes as life-threatening signs (arrhythmias, seizures, deep coma) recur; maximum I.V. rate: 1 mg/minute

Ophthalmic:

Ointment: Instill a small quantity to lower fornix up to 3 times/day

Solution: Instill 1-2 drops into eye(s) up to 4 times/day

**Dosage Forms Inj, as salicylate:** 1 mg/mL (2 mL); **Oint, ophth, as sulfate:** 0.25% (3.5 g, 3.7 g)

**Contraindications** Hypersensitivity to physostigmine or any component; GI or GU obstruction; physostigmine therapy of drug intoxications should be used with extreme caution in patients with asthma, gangrene, severe cardiovascular disease, or mechanical obstruction of the GI tract or urogenital tract. In these patients, physostigmine should be used only to treat life-threatening conditions.

**Warnings/Precautions** Use with caution in patients with epilepsy, asthma, diabetes, gangrene, cardiovascular disease, bradycardia. Discontinue if excessive salivation or emesis, frequent urination or diarrhea occur. Reduce dosage if excessive sweating or nausea occurs. Administer I.V. slowly or at a controlled rate not faster than 1 mg/minute. Due to the possibility of hypersensitivity or overdose/cholinergic crisis, atropine should be readily available; ointment may delay corneal healing, may cause loss of dark adaptation; not intended as a first-line agent for anticholinergic toxicity or Parkinson's disease.

**Pregnancy Risk Factor** C

**Adverse Reactions**
Ophthalmic:
>10%:
Ocular: Lacrimation, marked miosis, blurred vision, eye pain
Miscellaneous: Diaphoresis
1% to 10%:
Central nervous system: Headache, browache
Dermatologic: Burning, redness
Systemic:
>10%:
Gastrointestinal: Nausea, salivation, diarrhea, stomach pains
Ocular: Lacrimation
Miscellaneous: Diaphoresis
1% to 10%:
Cardiovascular: Palpitations, bradycardia
Central nervous system: Restlessness, nervousness, hallucinations, seizures
Genitourinary: Frequent urge to urinate
Neuromuscular & skeletal: Muscle twitching
Ocular: Miosis
Respiratory: Dyspnea, bronchospasm, respiratory paralysis, pulmonary edema

**Drug Interactions** Increased toxicity: Bethanechol, methacholine, succinylcholine may increase neuromuscular blockade with systemic administration

**Onset** Ophthalmic instillation: Within 2 minutes; Parenteral: Within 5 minutes

**Duration** Ophthalmic: 12-48 hours; Parenteral: 0.5-5 hours

**Half-Life** 15-40 minutes

**Special PA Issues**
**Patient Education:** Systemic: Maintain adequate hydration (2-3 L/day of fluids unless instructed to restrict fluid intake). May cause dizziness, drowsiness, or hypotension (rise slowly from sitting or lying position and use caution when driving or climbing stairs); vomiting or loss of appetite (frequent small meals, frequent mouth care, or sucking lozenges may help); or diarrhea (boiled milk, yogurt, or buttermilk may help). Report persistent abdominal discomfort; significantly increased salivation, sweating, tearing, or urination; flushed skin; chest pain or palpitations; acute headache; unresolved diarrhea; excessive fatigue, insomnia, dizziness, or depression; increased muscle, joint, or body pain; vision changes or blurred vision; or shortness of breath or wheezing.

Ophthalmic: For ophthalmic use only. Wash hands before using. Tilt head back and look upward. Put drops of suspension or apply thin ribbon of ointment inside lower eyelid. Close eye and roll eyeball in all directions. Do not blink for 1/2 minute. Apply gentle pressure to inner corner of eye for 30 seconds. Do not use any other eye preparation for at least 10 minutes. Do not touch tip of applicator to eye or contaminate tip of applicator. Do not share medication with anyone else. Wear sunglasses when in sunlight; you may be more sensitive to bright light. Inform prescriber if condition worsens or fails to improve or if you experience eye pain, vision disturbances, or other adverse eye response; excess sweating; urinary frequency; severe headache; or skin rash, redness, or burning.

♦ **Physostigmine Salicylate** see Physostigmine on previous page

♦ **Physostigmine Sulfate** see Physostigmine on previous page

♦ **Phytomenadione** see Phytonadione on this page

# Phytonadione (fye toe na DYE one)

**Pharmacologic Class** Vitamin, Fat Soluble

**U.S. Brand Names** AquaMEPHYTON® Injection; Konakion® Injection; Mephyton® Oral

**Mechanism of Action** Promotes liver synthesis of clotting factors (II, VII, IX, X); however, the exact mechanism as to this stimulation is unknown. Menadiol is a water soluble form of vitamin K; phytonadione has a more rapid and prolonged effect than menadione; menadiol sodium diphosphate ($K_4$) is half as potent as menadione ($K_3$).

**Use** Prevention and treatment of hypoprothrombinemia caused by drug-induced or anticoagulant-induced vitamin K deficiency, hemorrhagic disease of the newborn; phytonadione is more effective and is preferred to other vitamin K preparations in the presence of impending hemorrhage; oral absorption depends on the presence of bile salts

**USUAL DOSAGE** I.V. route should be restricted for emergency use only
Minimum daily requirement: Not well established
Infants: 1-5 mcg/kg/day
Adults: 0.03 mcg/kg/day
(Continued)

## Phytonadione *(Continued)*

Hemorrhagic disease of the newborn:
    Prophylaxis: I.M.: 0.5-1 mg within 1 hour of birth
    Treatment: I.M., S.C.: 1-2 mg/dose/day
Oral anticoagulant overdose:
    Infants: I.M., S.C.: 1-2 mg/dose every 4-8 hours
    Children and Adults: Oral, I.M., I.V., S.C.: 2.5-10 mg/dose; rarely up to 25-50 mg has been used; may repeat in 6-8 hours if given by I.M., I.V., S.C. route; may repeat 12-48 hours after oral route
Vitamin K deficiency: Due to drugs, malabsorption or decreased synthesis of vitamin K
    Infants and Children:
        Oral: 2.5-5 mg/24 hours
        I.M., I.V.: 1-2 mg/dose as a single dose
    Adults:
        Oral: 5-25 mg/24 hours
        I.M., I.V.: 10 mg

**Dosage Forms Inj: Aqueous colloidal:** 2 mg/mL (0.5 mL); 10 mg/mL (1 mL, 2.5 mL, 5 mL); **Aqueous (I.M. only):** 2 mg/mL (0.5 mL); 10 mg/mL (1 mL); **Tab:** 5 mg

**Contraindications** Hypersensitivity to phytonadione or any component

**Warnings/Precautions** Severe reactions resembling anaphylaxis or hypersensitivity have occurred rarely during or immediately after I.V. administration (even with proper dilution and rate of administration); restrict I.V. administration for emergency use only; ineffective in hereditary hypoprothrombinemia, hypoprothrombinemia caused by severe liver disease; severe hemolytic anemia has been reported rarely in neonates following large doses (10-20 mg) of phytonadione

**Pregnancy Risk Factor** C

**Adverse Reactions** <1%: Transient flushing reaction, rarely hypotension, cyanosis, dizziness (rarely), pain, abnormal taste, GI upset (oral), hemolysis in neonates and in patients with G-6-PD deficiency, tenderness at injection site, dyspnea, diaphoresis, anaphylaxis, hypersensitivity reactions

**Drug Interactions** Decreased effect: Warfarin sodium, dicumarol, anisindione effects antagonized by phytonadione; mineral oil may decrease GI absorption of vitamin K

**Onset** Onset of increased coagulation factors: Oral: Within 6-12 hours; Parenteral: Within 1-2 hours; prothrombin may become normal after 12-14 hours

**Special PA Issues**
    **Patient Education:** Oral: Take only as directed; do not take more or more often than prescribed. Avoid excessive or increased intake of vitamin K containing food (eg, green leafy vegetables, dairy products, meats) unless recommended by prescriber. Avoid alcohol and any OTC or prescribed medications containing aspirin that are not approved by prescriber. Report bleeding gums; blood in urine, stool, or vomitus; unusual bruising or bleeding; or abdominal cramping.
    **Monitoring Parameters:** PT

♦ **Pilagan® Ophthalmic** *see Pilocarpine on this page*

♦ **Pilocar® Ophthalmic** *see Pilocarpine on this page*

## Pilocarpine *(pye loe KAF peen)*

**Pharmacologic Class** Cholinergic Agonist; Ophthalmic Agent, Antiglaucoma; Ophthalmic Agent, Miotic

**U.S. Brand Names** Adsorbocarpine® Ophthalmic; Akarpine® Ophthalmic; Isopto® Carpine Ophthalmic; Ocu-Carpine® Ophthalmic; Ocusert Pilo-20® Ophthalmic; Ocusert Pilo-40® Ophthalmic; Pilagan® Ophthalmic; Pilocar® Ophthalmic; Pilopine HS® Ophthalmic; Piloptic® Ophthalmic; Pilostat® Ophthalmic; Salagen® Oral

**Mechanism of Action** Directly stimulates cholinergic receptors in the eye causing miosis (by contraction of the iris sphincter), loss of accommodation (by constriction of ciliary muscle), and lowering of intraocular pressure (with decreased resistance to aqueous humor outflow)

**Use**
    Ophthalmic: Management of chronic simple glaucoma, chronic and acute angle-closure glaucoma; counter effects of cycloplegics
    Oral: Symptomatic treatment of xerostomia caused by salivary gland hypofunction resulting from radiotherapy for cancer of the head and neck

**USUAL DOSAGE** Adults:
    Ophthalmic:
        Nitrate solution: Shake well before using; instill 1-2 drops 2-4 times/day
        Hydrochloride solution:
            Instill 1-2 drops up to 6 times/day; adjust the concentration and frequency as required to control elevated intraocular pressure
            To counteract the mydriatic effects of sympathomimetic agents: Instill 1 drop of a 1% solution in the affected eye
        Gel: Instill 0.5" ribbon into lower conjunctival sac once daily at bedtime

Ocular systems: Systems are labeled in terms of mean rate of release of pilocarpine over 7 days; begin with 20 mcg/hour at night and adjust based on response

Oral: 5 mg 3 times/day, titration up to 10 mg 3 times/day may be considered for patients who have not responded adequately

**Dosage Forms** Ocular therapeutic system (Ocusert® Pilo): Releases 20 or 40 mcg per hour for 1 week (8s) **Tab:** 5 mg

Pilocarpine hydrochloride; **Gel, ophth (Pilopine HS®):** 4% (3.5 g); **Soln, ophth (Adsorbocarpine®, Akarpine®, Isopto®, Carpine, Pilagan®, Pilocar®, Piloptic®, Pilostat®):** 0.25% (15 mL), 0.5% (15 mL, 30 mL), 1% (1 mL, 2 mL, 15 mL, 30 mL), 2% (1 mL, 2 mL, 15 mL, 30 mL), 3% (15 mL, 30 mL), 4% (1 mL, 2 mL, 15 mL, 30 mL), 5% (15 mL), 6% (15 mL, 30 mL), 8% (2 mL), 10% (15 mL);

Pilocarpine nitrate: **Soln, ophth (Pilagan®):** 1% (15 mL), 2% (15 mL), 4% (15 mL)

**Contraindications** Acute inflammatory disease of anterior chamber, hypersensitivity to pilocarpine or any component

**Warnings/Precautions** Use with caution in patients with corneal abrasion, CHF, asthma, peptic ulcer, urinary tract obstruction, Parkinson's disease, or narrow-angle glaucoma

**Pregnancy Risk Factor** C

**Adverse Reactions**

>10%: Ocular: Blurred vision, miosis

1% to 10%:

Central nervous system: Headache

Genitourinary: Polyuria

Local: Stinging, burning

Ocular: Ciliary spasm, retinal detachment, browache, photophobia, acute iritis, lacrimation, conjunctival and ciliary congestion early in therapy

Miscellaneous: Hypersensitivity reactions

<1%: Hypertension, tachycardia, nausea, vomiting, diarrhea, salivation, diaphoresis

**Onset**

Ophthalmic instillation: Miosis: Within 10-30 minutes; Intraocular pressure reduction: 1 hour required

Ocusert® Pilo application: Miosis: 1.5-2 hours; Reduced intraocular pressure: Within 1.5-2 hours; miosis within 10-30 minutes

**Duration**

Ophthalmic instillation: Miosis: 4-8 hours; Intraocular pressure reduction: 4-12 hours

Ocusert® Pilo application: Reduced intraocular pressure: ~1 week

**Special PA Issues**

**Patient Education:** Use as often as recommended. Ophthalmic: Wash hands before using. Sit or lie down. Open eye, look at ceiling, and instill prescribed amount of solution. Do not blink for 30 seconds, close eye and roll eye in all directions, and apply gentle pressure to inner corner of eye for 1-2 minutes. Do not let tip of applicator touch eye or contaminate tip of applicator. Temporary stinging or blurred vision may occur. You may experience altered dark adaptation; use caution when driving at night or in poorly lit environments. Report persistent pain, redness, burning, double vision, or severe headache.

**Monitoring Parameters:** Intraocular pressure, funduscopic exam, visual field testing

# Pilocarpine and Epinephrine (pye loe KAR peen & ep i NEF rin)

**Pharmacologic Class** Ophthalmic Agent, Antiglaucoma; Ophthalmic Agent, Miotic

**U.S. Brand Names** E-Pilo-x® Ophthalmic; P₁E₁® Ophthalmic

**Dosage Forms Soln, ophth:** Epinephrine bitartrate 1% and pilocarpine hydrochloride 1%, 2%, 3%, 4%, 6% (15 mL)

♦ **Pilocarpine Hydrochloride** see Pilocarpine on previous page

♦ **Pilocarpine Nitrate** see Pilocarpine on previous page

♦ **Pilopine HS® Ophthalmic** see Pilocarpine on previous page

♦ **Piloptic® Ophthalmic** see Pilocarpine on previous page

♦ **Pilostat® Ophthalmic** see Pilocarpine on previous page

♦ **Pima®** see Potassium Iodide on page 744

♦ **Pimaricin** see Natamycin on page 639

# Pimozide (PI moe zide)

**Pharmacologic Class** Antipsychotic Agent, Diphenylbutylperidine

**U.S. Brand Names** Orap™

**Mechanism of Action** A potent centrally-acting dopamine-receptor antagonist resulting in its characteristic neuroleptic effects

**Use** Suppression of severe motor and phonic tics in patients with Tourette's disorder

**USUAL DOSAGE** Children >12 years and Adults: Oral: Initial: 1-2 mg/day, then increase dosage as needed every other day; range is usually 7-16 mg/day, maximum dose: 20 mg/day or 0.3 mg/kg/day should not be exceeded

**Dosing adjustment in hepatic impairment:** Reduction of dose is necessary in patients with liver disease

(Continued)

## Pimozide *(Continued)*

**Dosage Forms Tab:** 2 mg

**Contraindications** Simple tics other than Tourette's, history of cardiac dysrhythmias, known hypersensitivity to pimozide; use in patients receiving macrolide antibiotics such as clarithromycin, erythromycin, azithromycin, and dirithromycin

**Pregnancy Risk Factor** C

**Adverse Reactions**

>10%:

Cardiovascular: Tachycardia, orthostatic hypotension

Central nervous system: Akathisia, akinesia, extrapyramidal effects, drowsiness

Dermatologic: Rash

Endocrine & metabolic: Edema of the breasts

Gastrointestinal: Constipation, xerostomia

1% to 10%:

Cardiovascular: Facial edema

Central nervous system: Tardive dyskinesia, mental depression

Gastrointestinal: Diarrhea, anorexia

<1%: Neuroleptic malignant syndrome (NMS), blood dyscrasias, jaundice

**Drug Interactions** CYP3A3/4 enzyme substrate

Increased effect/toxicity of alfentanil, CNS depressants, guanabenz (increased sedation), MAO inhibitors

**Half-Life** 50 hours

**Special PA Issues**

**Patient Education:** Use exactly as directed (do not increase dose or frequency); may cause physical and/or psychological dependence. It may take 2-3 weeks to achieve desired results; do not discontinue without consulting prescriber. Avoid excess alcohol or caffeine and other prescription or OTC medications not approved by prescriber. Maintain adequate hydration (2-3 L/day of fluids unless instructed to restrict fluid intake). You may experience excess drowsiness, restlessness, dizziness, or blurred vision (use caution driving or when engaging in hazardous tasks until response to medication is known); or constipation, dry mouth, anorexia (increased exercise, fluids, or dietary fruit and fiber may help). Report persistent CNS effects (eg, trembling fingers, altered gait or balance, excessive sedation, seizures, unusual muscle or facial movements, anxiety, abnormal thoughts, confusion, personality changes); unresolved constipation or gastrointestinal effects; breast swelling (male and female) or decreased sexual ability; vision changes; difficulty breathing; unusual cough or flu-like symptoms; or worsening of condition.

**Related Information**

Antipsychotic Agents *on page 1001*

## Pindolol *(PIN doe lole)*

**Pharmacological Class** Beta Blocker (with Intrinsic Sympathomimetic Activity)

**U.S. Brand Names** Visken®

**Mechanism of Action** Blocks both beta$_1$- and beta$_2$-receptors and has mild intrinsic sympathomimetic activity; pindolol has negative inotropic and chronotropic effects and can significantly slow A-V nodal conduction

**Use** Management of hypertension

**Unlabeled use:** Ventricular arrhythmias/tachycardia, antipsychotic-induced akathisia, situational anxiety; aggressive behavior associated with dementia

**USUAL DOSAGE**

Adults: Initial: 5 mg twice daily, increase as necessary by 10 mg/day every 3-4 weeks; maximum daily dose: 60 mg

Elderly: Initial: 5 mg once daily, increase as necessary by 5 mg/day every 3-4 weeks

**Dosing adjustment in renal and hepatic impairment:** Reduction is necessary in severely impaired

**Dosage Forms Tab:** 5 mg, 10 mg

**Contraindications** Uncompensated congestive heart failure, cardiogenic shock, bradycardia or heart block, asthma, COPD; hypersensitivity to any component

**Warnings/Precautions** Use with caution in patients with inadequate myocardial function, undergoing anesthesia, bronchospastic disease, diabetes mellitus, hyperthyroidism, impaired hepatic function; abrupt withdrawal of the drug should be avoided (may exacerbate symptoms; discontinue over 1-2 weeks); do not use in pregnant or nursing women; may potentiate hypoglycemia in a diabetic patient and mask signs and symptoms

**Pregnancy Risk Factor** B

**Adverse Reactions**

>10%:

Central nervous system: Insomnia (10%)

Neuromuscular & skeletal: Back pain/myalgia (10%)

1% to 10%:

Cardiovascular: Chest pain (3%), edema (6%)

Central nervous system: Nightmares/vivid dreams (5%), dizziness (9%), fatigue (8%), nervousness (7%)

Dermatologic: Rash, itching (4%)
Gastrointestinal: Diarrhea, nausea (5%), vomiting, abdominal discomfort (4%)
Neuromuscular & skeletal: Weakness (4%), paresthesia (3%), arthralgia (7%)
Respiratory: Dyspnea (5%)
<1%: Bradycardia, CHF, palpitations, claudication, hypotension, confusion, mental depression, hallucinations, anxiety (<2%), impotence, thrombocytopenia, dry eyes, wheezing

**Drug Interactions** CYP2D6 enzyme substrate
Decreased effect of beta-blockers with aluminum salts, barbiturates, calcium salts, cholestyramine, colestipol, NSAIDs, penicillins (ampicillin), rifampin, salicylates and sulfinpyrazone due to decreased bioavailability and plasma levels
Beta-blockers may decrease the effect of sulfonylureas
Increased effect/toxicity of beta-blockers with calcium blockers (diltiazem, felodipine, nicardipine), contraceptives, flecainide, quinidine (in extensive metabolizers), ciprofloxacin
Beta-blockers may increase the effect/toxicity of flecainide, acetaminophen, clonidine (hypertensive crisis after or during withdrawal of either agent), epinephrine (initial hypertensive episode followed by bradycardia), nifedipine and verapamil lidocaine, ergots (peripheral ischemia), prazosin (postural hypotension)
Beta-blockers may affect the action or levels of ethanol, disopyramide, nondepolarizing muscle relaxants and theophylline although the effects are difficult to predict

**Duration** ~12 hours

**Half-Life** 2.5-4 hours; increased with renal insufficiency, age, and cirrhosis

**Special PA Issues**
**Patient Education:** Take as directed; do not discontinue without consulting prescriber. Avoid alcohol and do not take with antacids. You may experience nervousness, dizziness, or fatigue; use caution when driving or engaging in hazardous activities until response to treatment is known. Frequent small meals may reduce incidence of nausea; adequate fluids and fiber intake may reduce constipation. Diabetic patients should monitor serum glucose regularly. Report chest pain, rapid heartbeat or palpitations, difficulty breathing, sudden increase in weight, swelling in ankles or hands, persistent dizziness or fatigue, trembling, increased anxiety, or sleeplessness.
**Monitoring Parameters:** Blood pressure, standing and sitting/supine, pulse, respiratory function

**Related Information**
Beta-Blockers *on page 1002*

♦ **Pink Bismuth® [OTC]** *see* Bismuth *on page 116*
♦ **Pin-Rid® [OTC]** *see* Pyrantel Pamoate *on page 782*
♦ **Pin-X® [OTC]** *see* Pyrantel Pamoate *on page 782*
♦ **PIO** *see* Pemoline *on page 701*

# Piperacillin (pi PER a sil in)

**Pharmacologic Class** Antibiotic, Penicillin

**U.S. Brand Names** Pipracil®

**Mechanism of Action** Inhibits bacterial cell wall synthesis by binding to one or more of the penicillin binding proteins (PBPs); which in turn inhibits the final transpeptidation step of peptidoglycan synthesis in bacterial cell walls, thus inhibiting cell wall biosynthesis. Bacteria eventually lyse due to ongoing activity of cell wall autolytic enzymes (autolysins and murein hydrolases) while cell wall assembly is arrested.

**Use** Treatment of susceptible infections such as septicemia, acute and chronic respiratory tract infections, skin and soft tissue infections, and urinary tract infections due to susceptible strains of *Pseudomonas*, *Proteus*, and *Escherichia coli* and *Enterobacter*; active against some streptococci and some anaerobic bacteria

**USUAL DOSAGE**
Neonates: 100 mg/kg every 12 hours
Infants and Children: I.M., I.V.: 200-300 mg/kg/day in divided doses every 4-6 hours
Higher doses have been used in cystic fibrosis: 350-500 mg/kg/day in divided doses every 4-6 hours
Adults: I.M., I.V.:
Moderate infections (urinary tract infections): 2-3 g/dose every 6-12 hours; maximum: 2 g I.M./site
Serious infections: 3-4 g/dose every 4-6 hours; maximum: 24 g/24 hours
Uncomplicated gonorrhea: 2 g I.M. in a single dose accompanied by 1 g probenecid 30 minutes prior to injection
**Dosing adjustment in renal impairment:** Adults: I.V.:
$Cl_{cr}$ 20-40 mL/minute: Administer 3-4 g every 8 hours
$Cl_{cr}$ <20 mL/minute: Administer 3-4 g every 12 hours
Moderately dialyzable (20% to 50%)
Continuous arteriovenous or venovenous hemodiafiltration (CAVH) effects: Dose as for $Cl_{cr}$ 20-40 mL/minute

**Dosage Forms Powder for inj, as sodium:** 2 g, 3 g, 4 g, 40 g

**Contraindications** Hypersensitivity to piperacillin or any component or penicillins
(Continued)

## Piperacillin *(Continued)*

**Warnings/Precautions** Dosage modification required in patients with impaired renal function; history of seizure activity; use with caution in patients with a history of beta-lactam allergy

**Pregnancy Risk Factor** B

**Adverse Reactions** Percentage unknown: Convulsions, confusion, drowsiness, fever, rash, electrolyte imbalance, hemolytic anemia, positive Coombs' reaction, abnormal platelet aggregation and prolonged PT (high doses), thrombophlebitis, myoclonus, acute interstitial nephritis, hypersensitivity reactions, anaphylaxis, Jarisch-Herxheimer reaction

**Drug Interactions**

Decreased effect: Tetracyclines may decrease penicillin effectiveness; aminoglycosides → physical inactivation of aminoglycosides in the presence of high concentrations of piperacillin and potential toxicity n patients with mild to moderate renal dysfunction; decreased efficacy of oral contraceptives is possible

Increased effect:

Probenecid may increase penicillin levels

Neuromuscular blockers may increase duration of blockade

Aminoglycosides → synergistic efficacy

Heparin with high-dose parenteral penicillins may result in increased risk of bleeding

**Half-Life** Dose-dependent; prolonged with moderately severe renal or hepatic impairment: 36-80 minutes

**Special PA Issues**

**Patient Education:** This medication will be administered I.V. or I.M. Maintain adequate hydration (2-3 L/day of fluids unless instructed to restrict fluid intake). If being treated for sexually transmitted disease, partner will also need to be treated. Small frequent meals or sucking on lozenges may reduce nausea or dry mouth. Important to maintain good oral and vaginal hygiene to reduce incidence of opportunistic infection. Diabetics should use serum glucose testing while on this medication. If diabetic, drug may cause false tests with Clinitest® urine glucose monitoring; use of glucose oxidase methods (Clinistix®) or serum glucose monitoring is preferable. This drug may interfere with oral contraceptives; an alternate form of birth control should be used. Report persistent diarrhea, fever, chills, unhealed sores, bloody urine or stool, muscle pain, mouth sores, or difficulty breathing.

**Monitoring Parameters:** Observe for signs and symptoms for anaphylaxis during first dose

## Piperacillin and Tazobactam Sodium

(pi PER a sil in & ta zoe BAK tam SOW dee um)

**Pharmacologic Class** Antibiotic, Penicillin

**U.S. Brand Names** Zosyn™

**Mechanism of Action** Inhibits bacterial cell wall synthesis by binding to one or more of the penicillin binding proteins (PBPs); which in turn inhibits the final transpeptidation step of peptidoglycan synthesis in bacterial cell walls, thus inhibiting cell wall biosynthesis. Bacteria eventually lyse due to ongoing activity of cell wall autolytic enzymes (autolysins and murein hydrolases) while cell wall assembly is arrested. Tazobactam inhibits many beta-lactamases, including staphylococcal penicillinase and Richmond and Sykes types II, III, IV, and V, including extended spectrum enzymes; it has only limited activity against class I beta-lactamases other than class Ic types.

**Use** Treatment of infections of lower respiratory tract, urinary tract, skin and skin structures, gynecologic, bone and joint infections, and septicemia caused by susceptible organisms. Tazobactam expands activity of piperacillin to include beta-lactamase producing strains of *S. aureus*, *H. influenzae*, *Eacteroides*, and other gram-negative bacteria.

**USUAL DOSAGE**

Children <12 years: Not recommended due to lack of data

Children >12 years and Adults:

Severe infections: I.V.: Piperacillin/tazobactam 4/0.5 g every 8 hours or 3/0.375 g every 6 hours

Moderate infections: I.M.: Piperacillin/tazobactam 2/0.25 g every 6-8 hours; treatment should be continued for ≥7-10 days depending on severity of disease (Note: I.M. route not FDA-approved)

**Dosing interval in renal impairment:**

$Cl_{cr}$ 20-40 mL/minute: Administer 2/0.25 g every 6 hours

$Cl_{cr}$ <20 mL/minute: Administer 2/0.25 g every 8 hours

Hemodialysis: Administer 2/0.25 g every 8 hours with an additional dose of 0.75 g after each dialysis

Continuous arteriovenous or venovenous hemodiafiltration (CAVH) effects: Dose as for $Cl_{cr}$ 10-50 mL/minute

**Dosage Forms Inj:** Piperacillin sodium 2 g and tazobactam sodium 0.25 g, piperacillin sodium 3 g and tazobactam sodium 0.375 g, piperacillin sodium 4 g and tazobactam sodium 0.5 g

**Contraindications** Hypersensitivity to penicillins, beta-lactamase inhibitors, or any component

**Warnings/Precautions** Due to sodium load and to the adverse effects of high serum concentrations of penicillins, dosage modification is required in patients with impaired or underdeveloped renal function; use with caution in patients with seizures or in patients with history of beta-lactam allergy; safety and efficacy have not been established in children <12 years of age

**Pregnancy Risk Factor** B

**Pregnancy Implications** Breast-feeding/lactation: Use by the breast-feeding mother may result in diarrhea, candidiasis, or allergic response in the infant

**Adverse Reactions**

>10%: Gastrointestinal: Diarrhea (11.3%)

1% to 10%:

Cardiovascular: Hypertension (1.6%)

Central nervous system: Insomnia (6.7%), headache (7% to 8%), agitation (2%), fever (2.4%), dizziness (1.4%)

Dermatologic: Rash (4%), pruritus (3%)

Gastrointestinal: Constipation (7% to 8%), nausea (6.9%), vomiting/dyspepsia (3.3%)

Respiratory: Rhinitis/dyspnea (~1%)

Miscellaneous: Serum sickness-like reaction

<1%: Hypotension, edema, confusion, pseudomembranous colitis, bronchospasm

Several laboratory abnormalities have rarely been associated with piperacillin/tazobactam including reversible eosinophilia, and neutropenia (associated most often with prolonged therapy), positive direct Coombs' test, prolonged PT and PTT, transient elevations of LFT, increases in creatinine

**Drug Interactions**

Decreased effect: Tetracyclines may decrease penicillin effectiveness; aminoglycosides → physical inactivation of aminoglycosides in the presence of high concentrations of piperacillin and potential toxicity in patients with mild to moderate renal dysfunction; decreased efficacy of oral contraceptives is possible

Increased effect:

Probenecid may increase penicillin levels

Neuromuscular blockers may increase duration of blockade

Aminoglycosides → synergistic efficacy

Heparin with high-dose parenteral penicillins may result in increased risk of bleeding

**Half-Life** Piperacillin: 1 hour; Piperacillin (desethyl) metabolite: 1-1.5 hours; Tazobactam: 0.7-0.9 hour

**Special PA Issues**

**Patient Education:** This medication will be administered I.V. or I.M. Maintain adequate hydration (2-3 L/day of fluids unless instructed to restrict fluid intake). Small frequent meals or sucking on lozenges may reduce nausea or dry mouth. Important to maintain good oral and vaginal hygiene to reduce incidence of opportunistic infection. Diabetics should use serum glucose testing while receiving this medication. If diabetic, drug may cause false tests with Clinitest® urine glucose monitoring; use of glucose oxidase methods (Clinistix®) or serum glucose monitoring is preferable. This drug may interfere with oral contraceptives; an alternate form of birth control should be used. Report persistent diarrhea, fever, chills, unhealed sores, bloody urine or stool, muscle pain, mouth sores, or difficulty breathing, or skin rash.

**Monitoring Parameters:** LFTs, creatinine, BUN, CBC with differential, serum electrolytes, urinalysis, PT, PTT; monitor for signs of anaphylaxis during first dose

♦ **Piperacillin Sodium** *see* Piperacillin *on page 729*

# Piperazine (Pl per a zeen)

**Pharmacologic Class** Anthelmintic

**U.S. Brand Names** Vermizine®

**Mechanism of Action** Causes muscle paralysis of the roundworm by blocking the effects of acetylcholine at the neuromuscular junction

**Use** Treatment of pinworm and roundworm infections (used as an alternative to first-line agents, mebendazole, or pyrantel pamoate)

**USUAL DOSAGE** Oral:

Pinworms: Children and Adults: 65 mg/kg/day (not to exceed 2.5 g/day) as a single daily dose for 7 days; in severe infections, repeat course after a 1-week interval

Roundworms:

Children: 75 mg/kg/day as a single daily dose for 2 days; maximum: 3.5 g/day

Adults: 3.5 g/day for 2 days (in severe infections, repeat course, after a 1-week interval)

**Dosage Forms Syr:** 500 mg/5 mL (473 mL, 4000 mL); **Tab:** 250 mg

**Contraindications** Seizure disorders, liver or kidney impairment, hypersensitivity to piperazine or any component

**Warnings/Precautions** Use with caution in patients with anemia or malnutrition; avoid prolonged use especially in children

**Pregnancy Risk Factor** B

(Continued)

## Piperazine (Continued)

**Adverse Reactions** <1%: Dizziness, vertigo, weakness, seizures, EEG changes, headache, nausea, vomiting, diarrhea, hemolytic anemia, visual impairment, hypersensitivity reactions, bronchospasms

**Drug Interactions** Pyrantel pamoate (antagonistic mode of action)

**Special PA Issues**
  **Patient Education:** Take on empty stomach; if severe or persistent headache, loss of balance or coordination, dizziness, vomiting, diarrhea, or rash occurs, contact physician. If used for pinworm infections, all members of the family should be treated.
  **Monitoring Parameters:** Stool exam for worms and ova

◆ **Piperazine Estrone Sulfate** see Estropipate on page 339

◆ **Piper methysticum** see Kava on page 505

## Pipobroman (pi poe BROE man)

**Pharmacologic Class** Antineoplastic Agent, Alkylating Agent

**U.S. Brand Names** Vercyte®

**Mechanism of Action** An alkylating agent considered to be cell-cycle nonspecific and capable of killing tumor cells in any phase of the cell cycle. Alkylating agents form covalent cross-links with DNA thereby resulting in cytotoxic, mutagenic, and carcinogenic effects. The end result of the alkylation process results in the misreading of the DNA code and the inhibition of DNA, RNA, and protein synthesis in rapidly proliferating tumor cells.

**Use** Treat polycythemia vera; chronic myelocytic leukemia (in patients refractory to busulfan)

**USUAL DOSAGE** Children >15 years and Adults: Oral:
  Polycythemia: 1 mg/kg/day for 30 days; may increase to 1.5-3 mg/kg until hematocrit reduced to 50% to 55%; maintenance: 0.1-0.2 mg/kg/day
  Myelocytic leukemia: 1.5-2.5 mg/kg/day until WBC drops to 10,000/mm³ then start maintenance 7-175 mg/day; stop if WBC falls to <3000/mm³ or platelets fall to <150,000/mm³

**Dosage Forms** Tab: 25 mg

**Contraindications** Pre-existing bone marrow suppression, hypersensitivity to any component

**Warnings/Precautions** The U.S. Food and Drug Administration (FDA) currently recommends that procedures for proper handling and disposal of antineoplastic agents be considered; bone marrow suppression may not occur for 4 weeks

**Pregnancy Risk Factor** D

**Adverse Reactions** 1% to 10%:
  Dermatologic: Rash
  Gastrointestinal: Vomiting, diarrhea, nausea, abdominal cramps
  Hematologic: Leukopenia, thrombocytopenia, anemia

**Special PA Issues**
  **Patient Education:** Notify physician if nausea, vomiting, diarrhea, or rash become severe or if unusual bleeding or bruising, sore throat, or fatigue occur; contraceptives are recommended during therapy
  **Monitoring Parameters:** CBC, liver and renal function tests

◆ **Pipracil®** see Piperacillin on page 729

## Pirbuterol (peer BYOO ter ole)

**Pharmacologic Class** Beta₂ Agonist

**U.S. Brand Names** Maxair™ Autohaler™; Maxair™ Inhalation Aerosol

**Mechanism of Action** Pirbuterol is a beta₂-adrenergic agonist with a similar structure to albuterol, specifically a pyridine ring has been substituted for the benzene ring in albuterol. The increased beta₂ selectivity of pirbuterol results from the substitution of a tertiary butyl group on the nitrogen of the side chain, which additionally imparts resistance of pirbuterol to degradation by monoamine oxidase and provides a lengthened duration of action in comparison to the less selective previous beta-agonist agents.

**Use** Prevention and treatment of reversible bronchospasm including asthma

**USUAL DOSAGE** Children >12 years and Adults: 2 inhalations every 4-6 hours for prevention; two inhalations at an interval of at least 1-3 minutes, followed by a third inhalation in treatment of bronchospasm, not to exceed 12 inhalations/day

**Dosage Forms** Aero, oral, as acetate: 0.2 mg per actuation (25.6 g (300 inhalations)); Autohaler™: 0.2 mg per actuation (2.8 g (80 inhalations), 14 g (400 inhalations))

**Contraindications** Hypersensitivity to pirbuterol or albuterol

**Warnings/Precautions** Excessive use may result in tolerance; some adverse reactions may occur more frequently in children 2-5 years of age; use with caution in patients with hyperthyroidism, diabetes mellitus; cardiovascular disorders including coronary insufficiency or hypertension or sensitivity to sympathomimetic amines

**Pregnancy Risk Factor** C

**Adverse Reactions**
  >10%:
    Central nervous system: Nervousness, restlessness

Neuromuscular & skeletal: Trembling

1% to 10%:

Central nervous system: Headache, dizziness

Gastrointestinal: Taste changes, vomiting, nausea

<1%: Hypertension, arrhythmias, chest pain, insomnia, bruising, anorexia, numbness in hands, weakness, paradoxical bronchospasm

### Drug Interactions

Decreased effect with beta-blockers

Increased toxicity with other beta agonists, MAO inhibitors, TCAs

**Onset** Peak therapeutic effect: Inhalation: 0.5-1 hour

**Half-Life** 2-3 hours

### Special PA Issues

**Patient Education:** Use exactly as directed (see Administration below). Do not use more often than recommended. Maintain adequate hydration (2-3 L/day of fluids unless instructed to restrict fluid intake). You may experience nervousness, dizziness, or fatigue (use caution when driving or engaging in hazardous activities until response to treatment is known); or dry mouth, stomach upset (frequent small meals, frequent mouth care, chewing gum, or sucking hard candy may help). Report unresolved GI upset; dizziness or fatigue; vision changes; chest pain, rapid heartbeat, or palpitations; nervousness or insomnia; muscle cramping or tremor; or unusual cough.

**Administration:** Self-administered inhalation: Store canister upside down; do not freeze. Shake canister before using. Sit when using medication. Close eyes when administering pirbuterol to avoid spray getting into eyes. Exhale slowly and completely through nose; inhale deeply through mouth while administering aerosol. Hold breath for 1-3 seconds after inhalation. Wait at least 1 full minute between inhalations. Wash mouthpiece between use. If more than one inhalation medication is used, use bronchodilator first and wait 5 minutes between medications.

**Monitoring Parameters:** Respiratory rate, heart rate, and blood pressure

♦ **Pirbuterol Acetate** see Pirbuterol on previous page

## Piroxicam (peer OKS i kam)

**Pharmacologic Class** Nonsteroidal Anti-Inflammatory Agent (NSAID)

**U.S. Brand Names** Feldene®

**Mechanism of Action** Inhibits prostaglandin synthesis, acts on the hypothalamus heat-regulating center to reduce fever, blocks prostaglandin synthetase action which prevents formation of the platelet-aggregating substance thromboxane $A_2$; decreases pain receptor sensitivity. Other proposed mechanisms of action for salicylate anti-inflammatory action are lysosomal stabilization, kinin and leukotriene production, alteration of chemotactic factors, and inhibition of neutrophil activation. This latter mechanism may be the most significant pharmacologic action to reduce inflammation.

**Use** Management of inflammatory disorders; symptomatic treatment of acute and chronic rheumatoid arthritis, osteoarthritis, and ankylosing spondylitis; also used to treat sunburn

**USUAL DOSAGE** Oral:

Children: 0.2-0.3 mg/kg/day once daily; maximum dose: 15 mg/day

Adults: 10-20 mg/day once daily; although associated with increase in GI adverse effects, doses >20 mg/day have been used (ie, 30-40 mg/day)

**Dosage adjustment in hepatic impairment:** Reduction of dosage is necessary

**Dosage Forms Cap:** 10 mg, 20 mg

**Contraindications** Hypersensitivity to piroxicam, any component, aspirin or other nonsteroidal anti-inflammatory drugs (NSAIDs); active GI bleeding

**Warnings/Precautions** Use with caution in patients with impaired cardiac function, hypertension, impaired renal function, GI disease (bleeding or ulcers) and patients receiving anticoagulants; elderly have increased risk for adverse reactions to NSAIDs

**Pregnancy Risk Factor** B (D if used in the 3rd trimester)

### Adverse Reactions

>10%:

Central nervous system: Dizziness

Dermatologic: Rash

Gastrointestinal: Abdominal cramps, heartburn, indigestion, nausea

1% to 10%:

Central nervous system: Headache, nervousness

Dermatologic: Itching

Endocrine & metabolic: Fluid retention

Gastrointestinal: Vomiting

Otic: Tinnitus

<1%: Congestive heart failure, hypertension, arrhythmias, tachycardia, confusion, hallucinations, aseptic meningitis, mental depression, drowsiness, insomnia, urticaria, erythema multiforme, toxic epidermal necrolysis, Stevens-Johnson syndrome, angioedema, polydipsia, hot flashes, gastritis, GI ulceration, cystitis, polyuria, agranulocytosis, anemia, hemolytic anemia, bone marrow suppression, leukopenia, thrombocytopenia, hepatitis, (Continued)

## Piroxicam *(Continued)*

peripheral neuropathy, toxic amblyopia, blurred vision, conjunctivitis, dry eyes, decreased hearing, acute renal failure, allergic rhinitis, shortness of breath, epistaxis

**Drug Interactions** CYP2C9 and 2C18 enzyme substrate

Decreased effect of diuretics, beta-blockers; decreased effect with aspirin, antacids, cholestyramine

Increased effect/toxicity of lithium, warfarin, methotrexate (controversial)

**Onset** Onset of analgesia: Oral: Within 1 hour; Peak effect: 3-5 hours

**Half-Life** 45-50 hours

**Special PA Issues**

**Patient Education:** Take this medication exactly as directed; do not increase dose without consulting prescriber. Do not crush tablets or break capsules. Take with food or milk to reduce GI distress. Maintain adequate fluid intake (2-3 L/day). Do not use alcohol, aspirin, or aspirin-containing medication, and all other anti-inflammatory medications without consulting prescriber. You may experience drowsiness, dizziness, or nervousness (use caution when driving or performing hazardous tasks); anorexia, nausea, vomiting, flatulence, or heartburn (frequent small meals, frequent oral care, sucking on lozenges, or chewing gum may help); fluid retention (weigh yourself weekly and report unusual (3-5 lb/week) weight gain). GI bleeding, ulceration, or perforation can occur with or without pain; discontinue medication and contact prescriber if persistent abdominal pain or cramping, or blood in stool occurs. Report unusual swelling of extremities or unusual weight gain; breathlessness, difficulty breathing, or unusual cough; chest pain, rapid heartbeat, palpitations; unusual bruising/bleeding; blood in urine, stool, mouth, or vomitus; unusual fatigue; changes in urinary pattern (polyuria or anuria); skin rash or itching; or change in hearing or ringing in ears.

**Monitoring Parameters:** Occult blood loss, hemoglobin, hematocrit, and periodic renal and hepatic function tests; periodic ophthalmologic exams with chronic use

**Related Information**

Nonsteroidal Anti-Inflammatory Agents *on page 1026*

## Podophyllin and Salicylic Acid (po DOF fil um & sal i SIL ik AS id)

**Pharmacologic Class** Keratolytic Agent

**U.S. Brand Names** Verrex-C&M®

**Dosage Forms Soln, top:** Podophyllum 10% and salicylic acid 30% with penederm 0.5% (7.5 mL)

## Podophyllum Resin (po DOF fil um REZ in)

**Pharmacologic Class** Keratolytic Agent

**U.S. Brand Names** Pod-Ben-25®; Podocon-25™; Podofin®

**Mechanism of Action** Directly affects epithelial cell metabolism by arresting mitosis through binding to a protein subunit of spindle microtubules (tubulin)

**Use** Topical treatment of benign growths including external genital and perianal warts, papillomas, fibroids; compound benzoin tincture generally is used as the medium for topical application

**USUAL DOSAGE** Topical:

Children and Adults: 10% to 25% solution in compound benzoin tincture; apply drug to dry surface, use 1 drop at a time allowing drying between drops until area is covered; total volume should be limited to <0.5 mL per treatment session

Condylomata acuminatum: 25% solution is applied daily; use a 10% solution when applied to or near mucous membranes

Verrucae: 25% solution is applied 3-5 times/day directly to the wart

**Dosage Forms Liq, top:** 25% in benzoin tincture (5 mL, 7.5 mL, 30 mL)

**Contraindications** Not to be used on birthmarks, moles, or warts with hair growth; cervical, urethral, oral warts; not to be used by diabetic patient or patient with poor circulation; pregnant women

**Warnings/Precautions** Use of large amounts of drug should be avoided; avoid contact with the eyes as it can cause severe corneal damage; do not apply to moles, birthmarks, or unusual warts; to be applied by a physician only; for external use only; 25% solution should not be applied to or near mucous membranes

**Pregnancy Risk Factor** X

**Adverse Reactions**

1% to 10%:

Dermatologic: Pruritus

Gastrointestinal: Nausea, vomiting, abdominal pain, diarrhea

<1%: Confusion, lethargy, hallucinations, leukopenia, thrombocytopenia, hepatotoxicity, peripheral neuropathy, renal failure

**Special PA Issues**

**Patient Education:** Cover with occlusive dressing to prevent contact with unaffected skin. Wash off medication as instructed by professional who applied the treatment.

♦ **Polydine®** [OTC] *see* Povidone-Iodine *on page 747*

## Polyestradiol (pol i es tra DYE ole)

**Pharmacologic Class** Antineoplastic Agent, Miscellaneous; Estrogen Derivative

**Mechanism of Action** Estrogens exert their primary effects on the interphase DNA-protein complex (chromatin) by binding to a receptor (usually located in the cytoplasm of a target cell) and initiating translocation of the hormone-receptor complex to the nucleus

**Use** Palliative treatment of advanced, inoperable carcinoma of the prostate

**USUAL DOSAGE** Adults: Deep I.M.: 40 mg every 2-4 weeks or less frequently; maximum dose: 80 mg

**Dosage Forms** Powder for inj, as phosphate: 40 mg

**Contraindications** Known or suspected estrogen-dependent neoplasm, carcinoma of the breast, active thromboembolic disorders, hypersensitivity to estrogens or any component, pregnancy

**Warnings/Precautions** Use with caution in patients with migraine, diabetes, cardiac, or renal impairment

**Pregnancy Risk Factor** X

**Adverse Reactions**

>10%:

Cardiovascular: Peripheral edema

Endocrine & metabolic: Enlargement of breasts (female and male), breast tenderness

Gastrointestinal: Nausea, anorexia, bloating

1% to 10%:

Central nervous system: Headache

Endocrine & metabolic: Increased libido (female), decrease libido (male)

Gastrointestinal: Vomiting, diarrhea

<1%: Hypertension, thromboembolism, myocardial infarction, edema, depression, dizziness, anxiety, stroke, chloasma, melasma, rash, amenorrhea, alterations in frequency and flow of menses, decreased glucose tolerance, increased triglycerides and LDL, nausea, GI distress, cholestatic jaundice, intolerance to contact lenses, increased susceptibility to *Candida* infection, breast tumors

♦ **Polyestradiol Phosphate** *see* Polyestradiol *on this page*

## Polyethylene Glycol-Electrolyte Solution

(pol i ETH i leen GLY kol ee LEK troe lite soe LOO shun)

**Pharmacologic Class** Cathartic; Laxative, Bowel Evacuant

**U.S. Brand Names** Colovage®; Colyte®; GoLYTELY®; NuLytely®; OCL®

**Mechanism of Action** Induces catharsis by strong electrolyte and osmotic effects

**Use** Bowel cleansing prior to GI examination or following toxic ingestion

**USUAL DOSAGE** The recommended dose for adults is 4 L of solution prior to gastrointestinal examination, as ingestion of this dose produces a satisfactory preparation in >95% of patients. Ideally the patient should fast for approximately 3-4 hours prior to administration, but in no case should solid food be given for at least 2 hours before the solution is given. The solution is usually administered orally, but may be given via nasogastric tube to patients who are unwilling or unable to drink the solution.

Children: Oral: 25-40 mL/kg/hour for 4-10 hours

Adults:

Oral: At a rate of 240 mL (8 oz) every 10 minutes, until 4 liters are consumed or the rectal effluent is clear; rapid drinking of each portion is preferred to drinking small amounts continuously

Nasogastric tube: At a rate of 20-30 mL/minute (1.2-1.8 L/hour); the first bowel movement should occur approximately 1 hour after the start of administration

**Dosage Forms** Powder, for oral soln: PEG 3350 236 g, sodium sulfate 22.74 g, sodium bicarbonate 6.74 g, sodium chloride 5.86 g and potassium chloride 2.97 g (2000 mL, 4000 mL, 4800 mL, 6000 mL)

**Contraindications** Gastrointestinal obstruction, gastric retention, bowel perforation, toxic colitis, megacolon

**Warnings/Precautions** Safety and efficacy not established in children; do not add flavorings as additional ingredients before use; observe unconscious or semiconscious patients with impaired gag reflex or those who are otherwise prone to regurgitation or aspiration during administration; use with caution in ulcerative colitis, caution against the use of hot loop polypectomy

**Pregnancy Risk Factor** C

**Adverse Reactions**

>10%: Gastrointestinal: Nausea, abdominal fullness, bloating

1% to 10%: Gastrointestinal: Abdominal cramps, vomiting, anal irritation

<1%: Rash

**Drug Interactions** Oral medications should not be administered within 1 hour of start of therapy

**Onset** Oral: Within 1-2 hours

**Special PA Issues**

**Patient Education:** Chilled solution is often more palatable. Produces a watery stool which cleanses the bowel before examination. Prepare solution according to instructions on the bottle. For best results, no solid food should be consumed during the 3- to 4-hour period before drinking solution, but in no case should solid foods be eaten within 2 hours of taking. Drink 240 mL every 10 minutes. Rapid drinking of each portion is better than drinking small amounts continuously. The first bowel movement should occur approximately 1 hour after the start of administration. May experience some abdominal bloating and distention before bowel starts to move. If severe discomfort or distention occurs, stop drinking temporarily or drink each portion at longer intervals until these symptoms disappear. Continue drinking until the watery stool is clear and free of solid matter. This usually requires at least 3 L. It is best to drink all of the solutions. Discard any unused portion.

**Monitoring Parameters:** Electrolytes, serum glucose, BUN, urine osmolality

♦ **Polygam®** *see* Immune Globulin, Intravenous *on page 472*

♦ **Polygam® S/D** *see* Immune Globulin, Intravenous *on page 472*

♦ **Poly-Histine CS®** *see* Brompheniramine, Phenylpropanolamine, and Codeine *on page 123*

♦ **Poly-Histine-D® Capsule** *see* Phenyltoloxamine, Phenylpropanolamine, Pyrilamine, and Pheniramine *on page 721*

♦ **Polymox®** *see* Amoxicillin *on page 61*

## Polymyxin B (pol i MIKS in bee)

**Pharmacologic Class** Antibiotic, Irrigation; Antibiotic, Miscellaneous

**Mechanism of Action** Binds to phospholipids, alters permeability, and damages the bacterial cytoplasmic membrane permitting leakage of intracellular constituents

**Use**

Topical: Wound irrigation and bladder irrigation against *Pseudomonas aeruginosa*; used occasionally for gut decontamination

Parenteral use of polymyxin B has mainly been replaced by less toxic antibiotics; it is reserved for life-threatening infections caused by organisms resistant to the preferred drugs (eg, pseudomonal meningitis - intrathecal administration)

**USUAL DOSAGE**

Otic: 1-2 drops, 3-4 times/day; should be used sparingly to avoid accumulation of excess debris

Infants <2 years:

I.M.: Up to 40,000 units/kg/day divided every 6 hours (not routinely recommended due to pain at injection sites)

I.V.: Up to 40,000 units/kg/day by continuous I.V. infusion

Intrathecal: 20,000 units/day for 3-4 days, then 25,000 units every other day for at least 2 weeks after CSF cultures are negative and CSF (glucose) has returned to within normal limits

Children ≥2 years and Adults:

I.M.: 25,000-30,000 units/kg/day divided every 4-6 hours (not routinely recommended due to pain at injection sites)

I.V.: 15,000-25,000 units/kg/day divided every 12 hours or by continuous infusion

Intrathecal: 50,000 units/day for 3-4 days, then every other day for at least 2 weeks after CSF cultures are negative and CSF (glucose) has returned to within normal limits

Total daily dose should not exceed 2,000,000 units/day

Bladder irrigation: Continuous irrigant or rinse in the urinary bladder for up to 10 days using 20 mg (equal to 200,000 units) added to 1 L of normal saline; usually no more than 1 L of irrigant is used per day unless urine flow rate is high; administration rate is adjusted to patient's urine output

Topical irrigation or topical solution: 500,000 units/L of normal saline; topical irrigation should not exceed 2 million units/day in adults

Gut sterilization: Oral: 15,000-25,000 units/kg/day in divided doses every 6 hours

*Clostridium difficile* enteritis: Oral: 25,000 units every 6 hours for 10 days

Ophthalmic: A concentration of 0.1% to 0.25% is administered as 1-3 drops every hour, then increasing the interval as response indicates to 1-2 drops 4-6 times/day

**Dosing adjustment/interval in renal impairment:**

Cl$_{cr}$ 20-50 mL/minute: Administer 75% to 100% of normal dose every 12 hours

Cl$_{cr}$ 5-20 mL/minute: Administer 50% of normal dose every 12 hours

Cl$_{cr}$ <5 mL/minute: Administer 15% of normal dose every 12 hours

**Dosage Forms** Inj: 500,000 units (20 mL); **Soln, otic:** 10,000 units of polymyxin B per mL in combination with hydrocortisone 0.5% solution (eg, Otobiotic®); **Susp, otic:** 10,000 units of polymixin B per mL in combination with hydrocortisone 1% and neomycin sulfate 0.5% (eg, PediOtic®); also available in a variety of other combination products for ophthalmic and otic use

**Contraindications** Concurrent use of neuromuscular blockers

**Warnings/Precautions** Use with caution in patients with impaired renal function, (modify dosage); polymyxin B-induced nephrotoxicity may be manifested by albuminuria, cellular casts, and azotemia. Discontinue therapy with decreasing urinary output and increasing BUN; neurotoxic reactions are usually associated with high serum levels, often in patients *(Continued)*

## Polymyxin B *(Continued)*

with renal dysfunction. Avoid concurrent or sequential use of other nephrotoxic and neurotoxic drugs (eg, aminoglycosides). The drug's neurotoxicity can result in respiratory paralysis from neuromuscular blockade, especially when the drug is given soon after anesthesia or muscle relaxants. Polymyxin B sulfate is most toxic when given parenterally; avoid parenteral use whenever possible.

**Pregnancy Risk Factor** B

**Adverse Reactions** <1%: Facial flushing, neurotoxicity (irritability, drowsiness, ataxia, perioral paresthesia, numbness of the extremities, and blurring of vision); drug fever, urticarial rash, hypocalcemia, hyponatremia, hypokalemia, hypochloremia, pain at injection site, neuromuscular blockade, weakness, nephrotoxicity, respiratory arrest, anaphylactoid reaction, meningeal irritation with intrathecal administration

**Drug Interactions** Polymyxin may increase/prolong effect of neuromuscular blocking agents; aminoglycosides may increase polymyxin's risk of respiratory paralysis and renal dysfunction

**Half-Life** 4.5-6 hours, increased with reduced renal function

**Special PA Issues**

**Patient Education:**

Wound irrigation/bladder irrigation/gut sterilization: Immediately report numbness or tingling of mouth, tongue, or extremities; constant blurring of vision; increased nervousness; irritability; excessive drowsiness; or difficulty breathing.

Ophthalmic: Tilt head back and place medication into eye and close eyes. Apply light pressure over inner corner of the eye for 1 minute. Do not touch medicine dropper to eye or contaminate tip of dropper. Vision may be temporarily blurred; use caution when driving or engaging in hazardous tasks until vision clears. Report any adverse effects including respiratory difficulty, unusual numbness or tingling of mouth or tongue, increased nervousness or irritability, or excessive drowsiness.

**Monitoring Parameters:** Neurologic symptoms and signs of superinfection; renal function (decreasing urine output and increasing BUN may require discontinuance of therapy)

**Reference Range:** Serum concentrations >5 µg/mL are toxic in adults

## Polymyxin B and Hydrocortisone

(pol i MIKS in bee & hye droe KOR ti sone)

**Pharmacologic Class** Antibiotic/Corticosteroid, Otic

**U.S. Brand Names** Otobiotic® Otic

**Dosage Forms Soln, otic:** Polymyxin B sulfate 10,000 units and hydrocortisone 0.5% [5 mg/mL] per mL (10 mL, 15 mL)

♦ **Polymyxin B and Neomycin** *see* Neomycin and Polymyxin B *on page 643*

♦ **Polymyxin B Sulfate** *see* Polymyxin B *on previous page*

♦ **Poly-Pred® Ophthalmic Suspension** *see* Neomycin, Polymyxin B, and Prednisolone *on page 645*

♦ **Polysporin® Ophthalmic** *see* Bacitracin and Polymyxin B *on page 97*

♦ **Polysporin® Topical** *see* Bacitracin and Polymyxin B *on page 97*

♦ **Polytopic** *see* Bacitracin and Polymyxin B *on page 97*

♦ **Polytrim® Ophthalmic** *see* Trimethoprim and Polymyxin B *on page 938*

♦ **Poly-Vi-Flor®** *see* Vitamins, Multiple *on page 964*

♦ **Poly-Vi-Sol® [OTC]** *see* Vitamins, Multiple *on page 964*

♦ **Pontocaine®** *see* Tetracaine *on page 884*

♦ **Pontocaine® With Dextrose Injection** *see* Tetracaine and Dextrose *on page 885*

♦ **Poor Mans Treacle** *see* Garlic *on page 410*

♦ **Porcelana® [OTC]** *see* Hydroquinone *on page 457*

♦ **Porcelana® Sunscreen [OTC]** *see* Hydroquinone *on page 457*

## Porfimer (POR fi mer)

**Pharmacologic Class** Antineoplastic Agent, Miscellaneous

**U.S. Brand Names** Photofrin®

**Mechanism of Action** Photosensitizing agent used in the photodynamic therapy (PDT) of tumors: cytotoxic and antitumor actions of porfimer are light and oxygen dependent. Cellular damage caused by porfimer PDT is a consequence of the propagation of radical reactions.

**Use** Esophageal cancer: Photodynamic therapy (PDT) with porfimer for palliation of patients with completely obstructing esophageal cancer, or of patients with partially obstructing esophageal cancer who cannot be satisfactorily treated with Nd:YAG laser therapy

**USUAL DOSAGE** I.V. (refer to individual protocols):

Children: Safety and efficacy have not been established

Adults: I.V.: 2 mg/kg over 3-5 minutes

Photodynamic therapy is a two-stage process requiring administration of both drug and light. The first stage of PDT is the I.V. injection of porfimer. Illumination with laser light 40-50 hours following the injection with porfimer constitutes the second stage of therapy. A second laser light application may be given 90-120 hours after injection, preceded by gentle debridement of residual tumor.

Patients may receive a second course of PDT a minimum of 30 days after the initial therapy; up to three courses of PDT (each separated by a minimum of 30 days) can be given. Before each course of treatment, evaluate patients for the presence of a tracheoesophageal or bronchoesophageal fistula.

**Dosage Forms Powder for inj, as sodium:** 75 mg

**Contraindications** Porphyria or in patients with known allergies to porphyrins; existing tracheoesophageal or bronchoesophageal fistula; tumors eroding into a major blood vessel

**Warnings/Precautions** The U.S. Food and Drug Administration (FDA) currently recommends that procedures for proper handling and disposal of antineoplastic agents be considered. If the esophageal tumor is eroding into the trachea or bronchial tree, the likelihood of tracheoesophageal or bronchoesophageal fistula resulting from treatment is sufficiently high that PDT is not recommended. All patients who receive porfimer sodium will be photosensitive and must observe precautions to avoid exposure of skin and eyes to direct sunlight or bright indoor light for 30 days. The photosensitivity is due to residual drug which will be present in all parts of the skin. Exposure of the skin to ambient indoor light is, however, beneficial because the remaining drug will be inactivated gradually and safely through a photobleaching reaction. Patients should not stay in a darkened room during this period and should be encouraged to expose their skin to ambient indoor light. Ocular discomfort has been reported; for 30 days, when outdoors, patients should wear dark sunglasses which have an average white light transmittance of <4%.

**Pregnancy Risk Factor** C

**Adverse Reactions**
>10%:
Cardiovascular: Atrial fibrillation, chest pain
Central nervous system: Fever, pain, insomnia
Dermatologic: Photosensitivity reaction
Gastrointestinal: abdominal pain, constipation, dysphagia, nausea, vomiting
Hematologic: Anemia
Neuromuscular & skeletal: Back pain
Respiratory: Dyspnea, pharyngitis, pleural effusion, pneumonia, respiratory insufficiency
1% to 10%:
Cardiovascular: Hypertension, hypotension, edema, cardiac failure, tachycardia, chest pain (substernal)
Central nervous system: Anxiety, confusion
Endocrine & metabolic: Dehydration
Gastrointestinal: Diarrhea, dyspepsia, eructation, esophageal edema, esophageal tumor bleeding, esophageal stricture, esophagitis, hematemesis, melena, weight loss, anorexia
Genitourinary: Urinary tract infection
Neuromuscular & skeletal: Weakness
Respiratory: Coughing, tracheoesophageal fistula
Miscellaneous: Moniliasis, surgical complication

**Drug Interactions**
Decreased effect: Compounds that quench active oxygen species or scavenge radicals (eg, dimethyl sulfoxide, beta-carotene, ethanol, mannitol) would be expected to decrease PDT activity; allopurinol, calcium channel blockers and some prostaglandin synthesis inhibitors could interfere with porfimer; drugs that decrease clotting, vasoconstriction or platelet aggregation could decrease the efficacy of PDT; glucocorticoid hormones may decrease the efficacy of the treatment
Increased toxicity: Concomitant administration of other photosensitizing agents (eg, tetracyclines, sulfonamides, phenothiazines, sulfonylureas, thiazide diuretics, griseofulvin) could increase the photosensitivity reaction

**Half-Life** 250 hours

**Special PA Issues**
**Patient Education:** This medication can only be administered I.V. and will be followed by laser light therapy. Avoid any exposure to sunlight or bright indoor light for 30 days following therapy (cover skin with protective clothing and wear dark sunglasses with light transmittance <4% when outdoors - severe blistering, burning, and skin/eye damage can result). After 30 days, test small area of skin (not face) for remaining sensitivity. Retest sensitivity if traveling to a different geographic area with greater sunshine. Exposure to indoor normal light is beneficial since it will help dissipate photosensitivity gradually. Maintain adequate hydration (2-3 L/day of fluids unless instructed to restrict fluid intake); maintain good oral hygiene (use soft toothbrush or cotton applicators several times a day and rinse mouth frequently). Small frequent meals or sucking on lozenges may reduce nausea or vomiting. Report rapid heart rate, chest pain or palpitations, difficulty breathing or air hunger, persistent fever or chills, foul-smelling urine or burning on urination, swelling of extremities, increased anxiety, confusion, or hallucination.

♦ **Porfimer Sodium** *see* Porfimer *on previous page*
♦ **Pork NPH Iletin® II** *see* Insulin Preparations *on page 479*
♦ **Pork Regular Iletin® II** *see* Insulin Preparations *on page 479*

◆ **Potasalan**® see Potassium Chloride on page 742

# Potassium Acetate (poe TASS ee um AS e tate)

**Pharmacologic Class** Electrolyte Supplement, Parenteral; Potassium Salt

**Mechanism of Action** Potassium is the major cation of intracellular fluid and is essential for the conduction of nerve impulses in heart, brain, and skeletal muscle; contraction of cardiac, skeletal and smooth muscles; maintenance of normal renal function, acid-base balance, carbohydrate metabolism, and gastric secretion

**Use** Potassium deficiency; to avoid chloride when high concentration of potassium is needed, source of bicarbonate

**USUAL DOSAGE** I.V. doses should be incorporated into the patient's maintenance I.V. fluids, intermittent I.V. potassium administration should be reserved for severe depletion situations and requires EKG monitoring; doses listed as mEq of potassium

Treatment of hypokalemia: I.V.:
  Children: 2-5 mEq/kg/day
  Adults: 40-100 mEq/day
I.V. intermittent infusion (must be diluted prior to administration):
  Children: 0.5-1 mEq/kg/dose (maximum: 30 mEq/dose) to infuse at 0.3-0.5 mEq/kg/hour (maximum: 1 mEq/kg/hour)
  Adults: 5-10 mEq/dose (maximum: 40 mEq/dose) to infuse over 2-3 hours (maximum: 40 mEq over 1 hour)

**Note: Continuous cardiac monitor recommended for rates >0.5 mEq/hour**

### Potassium Dosage/Rate of Infusion Guidelines

| Serum Potassium | Maximum Infusion Rate | Maximum Concentration | Maximum 24-Hour Dose |
|---|---|---|---|
| >2.5 mEq/L | 10 mEq/h | 40 mEq/L | 200 mEq |
| <2.5 mEq/L | 40 mEq/h | 80 mEq/L | 400 mEq |

**Dosage Forms** Inj 2 mEq/mL (20 mL, 50 mL, 100 mL), 4 mEq/mL (50 mL)

**Contraindications** Severe renal impairment, hyperkalemia

**Warnings/Precautions** Use with caution in patients with renal disease, hyperkalemia, cardiac disease, metabolic alkalosis; must be administered in patients with adequate urine flow

**Pregnancy Risk Factor** C

**Adverse Reactions**
>10%: Gastrointestinal: Diarrhea, nausea, stomach pain, flatulence, vomiting (oral)
1% to 10%:
  Cardiovascular: Bradycardia
  Endocrine & metabolic: Hyperkalemia
  Neuromuscular & skeletal: Weakness
  Respiratory: Dyspnea
  Local: Local tissue necrosis with extravasation
<1%: Chest pain, mental confusion, alkalosis, abdominal pain, throat pain, phlebitis, paresthesias, paralysis

**Drug Interactions** Increased effect/levels with potassium-sparing diuretics, salt substitutes, ACE inhibitors

**Special PA Issues**
  **Patient Education:** This form of potassium may only be given I.V. Report immediately any burning or pain at infusion site, chest pain, palpitations, unusual weakness in muscles, tarry stools, or easy bruising.

# Potassium Acetate, Potassium Bicarbonate, and Potassium Citrate

(poe TASS ee um AS e tate, poe TASS ee um bye KAR bun ate, & poe TASS ee um SIT rate)

**Pharmacologic Class** Electrolyte Supplement, Oral

**U.S. Brand Names** Tri-K®

**Dosage Forms** Soln, oral: 45 mEq/15 mL from potassium acetate 1500 mg, potassium bicarbonate 1500 mg, and potassium citrate 1500 mg per 15 mL

# Potassium Acid Phosphate (poe TASS ee um AS id FOS fate)

**Pharmacologic Class** Potassium Salt; Urinary Acidifying Agent

**U.S. Brand Names** K-Phos® Original

**Mechanism of Action** The principal intracellular cation; involved in transmission of nerve impulses, muscle contractions, enzyme activity, and glucose utilization

**Use** Acidifies urine and lowers urinary calcium concentration; reduces odor and rash caused by ammoniacal urine; increases the antibacterial activity of methenamine

**USUAL DOSAGE** Adults: Oral: 1000 mg dissolved in 6-8 oz of water 4 times/day with meals and at bedtime; for best results, soak tablets in water for 2-5 minutes, then stir and swallow

**Dosage Forms Tab, sodium free:** 500 mg [potassium 3.67 mEq]

**Contraindications** Severe renal impairment, hyperkalemia, hyperphosphatemia, and infected magnesium ammonium phosphate stones

**Warnings/Precautions** Use with caution in patients receiving other potassium supplementation and in patients with renal insufficiency, or severe tissue breakdown (eg, chemotherapy or hemodialysis)

**Pregnancy Risk Factor** C

**Adverse Reactions**

>10%: Gastrointestinal: Diarrhea, nausea, stomach pain, flatulence, vomiting

1% to 10%:

Cardiovascular: Bradycardia

Endocrine & metabolic: Hyperkalemia

Local: Local tissue necrosis with extravasation

Neuromuscular & skeletal: Weakness

Respiratory: Dyspnea

<1%: Chest pain, arrhythmia, edema, mental confusion, tetany, pain of extremities, hyperphosphatemia, hypocalcemia, alkalosis, abdominal pain, weight gain, throat pain, decreased urine output, phlebitis, paresthesias, paralysis, bone pain, arthralgia, weakness of extremities, shortness of breath, thirst

**Drug Interactions**

Increased effect/levels with potassium-sparing diuretics, salt substitutes, salicylates, ACE inhibitors

Decreased effect with antacids containing magnesium, calcium or aluminum (bind phosphate and decreased its absorption)

**Special PA Issues**

**Patient Education:** Take as directed; do not take more than directed. Dissolve tablet in 4-6 oz of water or juice and stir before drinking, with or after meals (do not take on empty stomach). Take any antacids 2 hours before or after potassium. Consult prescriber about advisability of increasing dietary potassium. Report tingling of hands or feet; unresolved nausea or vomiting; chest pain or palpitations; persistent abdominal pain; feelings of weakness, dizziness, listlessness, confusion, acute muscle weakness or cramping; blood in stool or tarry stools; or easy bruising or unusual bleeding.

**Monitoring Parameters:** Serum potassium, sodium, phosphate, calcium; serum salicylates (if taking salicylates)

# Potassium Bicarbonate and Potassium Chloride, Effervescent

(poe TASS ee um bye KAR bun ate & poe TASS ee um KLOR ide, ef er VES ent)

**Pharmacologic Class** Electrolyte Supplement, Oral

**U.S. Brand Names** Klorvess® Effervescent; K/Lyte/CL®

**Dosage Forms Granules for oral soln, effervescent (Klorvess®):** 20 mEq per packet; **Tab for oral soln, effervescent, Klorvess®:** 20 mEq per packet, K/Lyte/Cl®: 25 mEq, 50 mEq per packet

# Potassium Bicarbonate and Potassium Citrate, Effervescent

(poe TASS ee um bye KAR bun ate & poe TASS ee um SIT rate, ef er VES ent)

**Pharmacologic Class** Potassium Salt

**U.S. Brand Names** Effer-K™; K-Ide®; Klor-Con®/EF; K-Lyte®; K-Vescent®

**Mechanism of Action** Needed for the conduction of nerve impulses in heart, brain, and skeletal muscle; contraction of cardiac, skeletal and smooth muscles; maintenance of normal renal function

**Use** Treatment or prevention of hypokalemia

**USUAL DOSAGE** Oral:

Children: 1-4 mEq/kg/24 hours in divided doses as required to maintain normal serum potassium

Adults:

Prevention: 16-24 mEq/day in 2-4 divided doses

Treatment: 40-100 mEq/day in 2-4 divided doses

**Dosage Forms Cap, extended release:** 8 mEq, 10 mEq; **Powder for oral soln:** 15 mEq/packet, 20 mEq/packet, 25 mEq/packet; **Tab, effervescent:** 25 mEq, 50 mEq

**Contraindications** Severe renal impairment, hyperkalemia

**Warnings/Precautions** Use with caution in patients with renal disease, cardiac disease

**Pregnancy Risk Factor** C

**Adverse Reactions**

>10%: Gastrointestinal: Diarrhea, nausea, stomach pain, flatulence, vomiting

1% to 10%:

Cardiovascular: Bradycardia

Endocrine & metabolic: Hyperkalemia

Local: Local tissue necrosis with extravasation

Neuromuscular & skeletal: Weakness

(Continued)

## Potassium Bicarbonate and Potassium Citrate, Effervescent
### *(Continued)*

Respiratory: Dyspnea

<1%: Chest pain, mental contusion, alkalosis, abdominal pain, throat pain, phlebitis, paresthesias, paralysis

**Drug Interactions** Increased effect/levels with potassium-sparing diuretics, salt substitutes, ACE inhibitors

**Special PA Issues**

**Patient Education:** Take as directed; do not take more than directed. Dissolve powder or soak tablet in 4-6 oz of water or juice and stir before drinking. Do not chew or crush extended release capsules. Do not take on an empty stomach; take with or after meals. Consult prescriber about increasing dietary potassium (eg, salt substitutes, orange juice, bananas, etc). Report tingling of hands or feet, unresolved nausea or vomiting, chest pain, palpitations, persistent abdominal pain, muscle cramping or weakness, tarry stools, easy bruising, or unusual bleeding.

**Monitoring Parameters:** Serum potassium

## Potassium Bicarbonate, Potassium Chloride, and Potassium Citrate
(poe TASS ee um bye KAR bun ate, poe TASS ee um KLOR ide & poe TASS ee um SIT rate)

**Pharmacologic Class** Electrolyte Supplement, Oral

**U.S. Brand Names** Kaochlor-Eff®

**Dosage Forms Tab for oral soln:** 20 mEq from potassium bicarbonate 1 g, potassium chloride 600 mg, and potassium citrate 220 mg

## Potassium Chloride (poe TASS ee um KLOR ide)

**Pharmacologic Class** Electrolyte Supplement, Oral; Electrolyte Supplement, Parenteral; Potassium Salt

**U.S. Brand Names** Cena-K®; Gen-K®; K+ 10®; Kaochlor®; Kaochlor® SF; Kaon-Cl®; Kaon Cl-10®; Kay Ciel®; K+ Care®; K-Dur® 10; K-Dur® 20; K-Lease®; K-Lor™; Klor-Con®; Klor-Con® 8; Klor-Con® 10; Klor-Con/25®; Klorvess®; Klotrix®; K-Lyte/Cl®; K-Norm®; K-Tab®; Micro-K® 10; Micro-K® Extencaps®; Micro-K® LS®; Potasalan®; Rum-K®; Slow-K®; Ten-K®

**Mechanism of Action** Potassium is the major cation of intracellular fluid and is essential for the conduction of nerve impulses in heart, brain, and skeletal muscle; contraction of cardiac, skeletal and smooth muscles; maintenance of normal renal function, acid-base balance, carbohydrate metabolism, and gastric secretion

**Use** Treatment or prevention of hypokalemia

**USUAL DOSAGE** I.V. doses should be incorporated into the patient's maintenance I.V. fluids; intermittent I.V. potassium administration should be reserved for severe depletion situations in patients undergoing EKG monitoring.

Normal daily requirements: Oral, I.V.:

Premature infants: 2-6 mEq/kg/24 hours

Term infants 0-24 hours: 0-2 mEq/kg/24 hours

Infants >24 hours: 1-2 mEq/kg/24 hours

Children: 2-3 mEq/kg/day

Adults: 40-80 mEq/day

Prevention during diuretic therapy: Oral:

Children: 1-2 mEq/kg/day in 1-2 divided doses

Adults: 20-40 mEq/day in 1-2 divided doses

Treatment of hypokalemia: Children:

Oral: 1-2 mEq/kg initially, then as needed based on frequently obtained lab values. If deficits are severe or ongoing losses are great, I.V. route should be considered.

I.V.: 1 mEq/kg over 1-2 hours initially, then repeated as needed based on frequently obtained lab values; severe depletion or ongoing losses may require >200% of normal limit needs

I.V. intermittent infusion: Dose should not exceed 1 mEq/kg/hour, or 40 mEq/hour; if it exceeds 0.5 mEq/kg/hour, physician should be at bedside and patient should have continuous EKG monitoring; usual pediatric maximum: 3 mEq/kg/day or 40 mEq/m$^2$/day

#### Potassium Dosage/Rate of Infusion Guidelines

| Serum Potassium | Maximum Infusion Rate | Maximum Concentration | Maximum 24-Hour Dose |
|---|---|---|---|
| >2.5 mEq/L | 10 mEq/h | 40 mEq/L | 200 mEq |
| <2.5 mEq/L | 40 mEq/h | 80 mEq/L | 400 mEq |

Treatment of hypokalemia: Adults:

I.V. intermittent infusion: 5-10 mEq/hour (continuous cardiac monitor recommended for rates >5 mEq/hour), not to exceed 40 mEq/hour; usual adult maximum per 24 hours: 400 mEq/day. See table.

Potassium >2.5 mEq/L:

Oral: 60-80 mEq/day plus additional amounts if needed

I.V.: 10 mEq over 1 hour with additional doses if needed

Potassium <2.5 mEq/L:

Oral: Up to 40-60 mEq initial dose, followed by further doses based on lab values

I.V.: Up to 40 mEq over 1 hour, with doses based on frequent lab monitoring; deficits at a plasma level of 2 mEq/L may be as high as 400-800 mEq of potassium

**Dosage Forms Cap, controlled release (microcapsulated):** 600 mg [8 mEq], 750 mg [10 mEq], Micro-K® Extencaps®: 600 mg [8 mEq], K-Lease®, K-Norm®, Micro-K® 10: 750 mg [10 mEq]; **Liq:** 10% [20 mEq/15 mL] (480 mL, 4000 mL), 20% [40 mEq/15 mL] (480 mL, 4000 mL), Cena-K®, Kaochlor®, Kaochlor® SF, Kay Ciel®, Klorvess®, Potasalan®: 10% [20 mEq/15 mL] (480 mL, 4000 mL), Rum-K®: 15% [30 mEq/15 mL] (480 mL, 4000 mL), Cena-K®, Kaon-Cl® 20%: 20% [40 mEq/15 mL]; **Crystals for oral susp, extended release (Micro-K® LS®):** 20 mEq per packet; **Powder:** 20 mEq per packet (30s, 100s), K+ Care®, K-Lor™: 15 mEq per packet (30s, 100s), Gen-K®, Kay Ciel®, K+ Care®, K-Lor®, Klor-Con®: 20 mEq per packet (30s, 100s), K+ Care®, Klor-Con/25®: 25 mEq per packet (30s, 100s), K-Lyte/Cl®: 25 mEq per dose (30s); **Inf, conc:** 0.1 mEq/mL, 0.2 mEq/mL, 0.3 mEq/mL, 0.4 mEq/mL; **Inj, conc:** 1.5 mEq/mL, 2 mEq/mL, 3 mEq/mL; **Tab, controlled release (micro-encapsulated),** K-Dur® 10, Ten-K®: 750 mg [10 mEq], K-Dur® 20: 1500 mg [20 mEq]; **Tab, controlled release (wax matrix):** 600 mg [8 mEq]; 750 mg [10 mEq], Kaon-Cl®: 500 mg [6.7 mEq], Klor-Con® 8, Slow-K®: 600 mg [8 mEq], K+ 10®, Kaon Cl-10®, Klor-Con® 10, Klotrix®, K-Tab®: 750 mg [10 mEq]

**Contraindications** Severe renal impairment, untreated Addison's disease, heat cramps, hyperkalemia, severe tissue trauma; solid oral dosage forms are contraindicated in patients in whom there is a structural, pathological, and/or pharmacologic cause for delay or arrest in passage through the GI tract; an oral liquid potassium preparation should be used in patients with esophageal compression or delayed gastric emptying time

**Warnings/Precautions** Use with caution in patients with cardiac disease, severe renal impairment, hyperkalemia

**Pregnancy Risk Factor** A

**Adverse Reactions**

>10%: Gastrointestinal: Diarrhea, nausea, stomach pain, flatulence, vomiting (oral)

1% to 10%:

Cardiovascular: Bradycardia

Endocrine & metabolic: Hyperkalemia

Local: Local tissue necrosis with extravasation, pain at the site of injection

Neuromuscular & skeletal: Weakness

Respiratory: Dyspnea

<1%: Chest pain, arrhythmias, heart block, hypotension, mental confusion, alkalosis, abdominal pain, throat pain, phlebitis, paresthesias, paralysis

**Drug Interactions** Increased effect/levels with potassium-sparing diuretics, salt substitutes, ACE inhibitors

**Special PA Issues**

**Patient Education:** Oral: Take as directed; do not take more than directed. Dissolve tablet or powder in 4-6 oz of water or juice and stir drinking. Do not chew or crush extended release capsules. Take potassium with or after meals (do not take on empty stomach). Take any antacids 2 hours before or after potassium. Consult prescriber about advisability of increasing dietary potassium. Report tingling of hands or feet; unresolved nausea or vomiting; chest pain or palpitations; persistent abdominal pain; feelings of weakness, dizziness, listlessness, confusion, acute muscle weakness or cramping; blood in stool or tarry stools; or easy bruising or unusual bleeding.

**Monitoring Parameters:** Serum potassium, glucose, chloride, pH, urine output (if indicated), cardiac monitor (if intermittent infusion or potassium infusion rates >0.25 mEq/kg/hour)

# Potassium Chloride and Potassium Gluconate

(poe TASS ee um KLOR ide & poe TASS ee um GLOO coe nate)

**Pharmacologic Class** Electrolyte Supplement, Oral

**U.S. Brand Names** Kolyum®

**Dosage Forms Soln, oral:** Potassium 20 mEq/15 mL

# Potassium Citrate and Citric Acid

(poe TASS ee um SIT rate & SI trik AS id)

**Pharmacologic Class** Alkalinizing Agent

**U.S. Brand Names** Polycitra®-K

**Dosage Forms Crystals for reconstitution:** Potassium citrate 3300 mg and citric acid 1002 mg per pk; **Soln, oral:** Potassium citrate 1100 mg and citric acid 334 mg per 5 mL

♦ **Potassium Citrate and Potassium Bicarbonate, Effervescent** see Potassium Bicarbonate and Potassium Citrate, Effervescent on page 741

# Potassium Citrate and Potassium Gluconate

(poe TASS ee um SIT rate & poe TASS ee um GLOO coe nate)

**Pharmacologic Class** Electrolyte Supplement, Oral

**U.S. Brand Names** Twin-K®

**Dosage Forms Soln, oral:** 20 mEq/5 mL from potassium citrate 170 mg and potassium gluconate 170 mg per 5 mL

# Potassium Gluconate (poe TASS ee um GLOO coe nate)

**Pharmacologic Class** Potassium Salt

**U.S. Brand Names** Kaon®; Kaylixir®; K-G®

**Mechanism of Action** Potassium is the major cation of intracellular fluid and is essential for the conduction of nerve impulses in heart, brain, and skeletal muscle; contraction of cardiac, skeletal and smooth muscles; maintenance of normal renal function, acid-base balance, carbohydrate metabolism, and gastric secretion

**Use** Treatment or prevention of hypokalemia

**USUAL DOSAGE** Oral (doses listed as mEq of potassium):

Normal daily requirement:

Children: 2-3 mEq/kg/day

Adults: 40-80 mEq/day

Prevention of hypokalemia during diuretic therapy:

Children: 1-2 mEq/kg/day in 1-2 divided doses

Adults: 16-24 mEq/day in 1-2 divided doses

Treatment of hypokalemia:

Children: 2-5 mEq/kg/day in 2-4 divided doses

Adults: 40-100 mEq/day in 2-4 divided doses

**Dosage Forms Elix:** 20 mEq/15 mL, K-G®, Kaon®, Kaylixir®: 20 mEq/15 mL; **Tab:** Glu-K®: 2 mEq, Kaon®: 5 mEq

**Contraindications** Severe renal impairment, untreated Addison's disease, heat cramps, hyperkalemia, severe tissue trauma; solid oral dosage forms are contraindicated in patients in whom there is a structural, pathological, and/or pharmacologic cause for delay or arrest in passage through the GI tract; an oral liquid potassium preparation should be used in patients with esophageal compression or delayed gastric emptying time

**Warnings/Precautions** Use with caution in patients with cardiac disease, severe renal impairment, hyperkalemia; patients must be on a cardiac monitor during intermittent infusions

**Pregnancy Risk Factor** A

**Adverse Reactions**

>10%: Gastrointestinal: Diarrhea, nausea, stomach pain, flatulence, vomiting (oral)

1% to 10%:

Cardiovascular: Bradycardia

Endocrine & metabolic: Hyperkalemia

Neuromuscular & skeletal: Weakness

Respiratory: Dyspnea

<1%: Chest pain, mental confusion, alkalosis, throat pain, phlebitis, paresthesias, paralysis

**Drug Interactions** Increased effect/levels with potassium-sparing diuretics, salt substitutes, ACE inhibitors; increased effect of digitalis

**Special PA Issues**

**Patient Education:** Take as directed; do not take more than directed. Elixir must be diluted in 4-6 oz of water or juice. Swallow tablet whole (do not crush or chew) with full glass of water or juice. Take with or after meals (do not take on an empty stomach). Take any antacids 2 hours before or after potassium. Consult prescriber about advisability of increasing dietary potassium. Report tingling of hands or feet; unresolved nausea or vomiting; chest pain or palpitations; persistent abdominal pain; feelings of weakness, dizziness, listlessness, confusion, acute muscle weakness or cramping; blood in stool or tarry stools; or easy bruising or unusual bleeding.

**Monitoring Parameters:** Serum potassium, chloride, glucose, pH, urine output (if indicated)

# Potassium Iodide (poe TASS ee um EYE oh dide)

**Pharmacologic Class** Antithyroid Agent; Cough Preparation; Expectorant

**U.S. Brand Names** Pima®; SSKI®; Thyro-Block®

**Mechanism of Action** Reduces viscosity of mucus by increasing respiratory tract secretions; inhibits secretion of thyroid hormone, fosters colloid accumulation in thyroid follicles

**Use** Facilitate bronchial drainage and cough; reduce thyroid vascularity prior to thyroidectomy and management of thyrotoxic crisis; block thyroidal uptake of radioactive isotopes of iodine in a radiation emergency

**USUAL DOSAGE** Oral:

Adults: RDA: 130 mcg

Expectorant:

Children: 60-250 mg every 6-8 hours; maximum single dose: 500 mg

Adults: 300-650 mg 2-3 times/day

Preoperative thyroidectomy: Children and Adults: 50-250 mg (1-5 drops SSKI®) 3 times/day or 0.1-0.3 mL (3-5 drops) of strong iodine (Lugol's solution) 3 times/day; administer for 10 days before surgery

Thyrotoxic crisis:

Infants <1 year: 150-250 mg (3-5 drops SSKI®) 3 times/day

Children and Adults: 300-500 mg (6-10 drops SSKI®) 3 times/day or 1 mL strong iodine (Lugol's solution) 3 times/day

Sporotrichosis:

Initial:

Preschool: 50 mg/dose 3 times/day

Children: 250 mg/dose 3 times/day

Adults: 500 mg/dose 3 times/day

Oral increase 50 mg/dose daily

Maximum dose:

Preschool: 500 mg/dose 3 times/day

Children and Adults: 1-2 g/dose 3 times/day

Continue treatment for 4-6 weeks after lesions have completely healed

**Dosage Forms Soln, oral:** SSKI®: 1 g/mL (30 mL, 240 mL, 473 mL), Lugol's solution, strong iodine: 100 mg/mL with iodine 50 mg/mL (120 mL); **Syr:** 325 mg/5 mL; **Tab:** 130 mg

**Contraindications** Known hypersensitivity to iodine; hyperkalemia, pulmonary tuberculosis, pulmonary edema, bronchitis, impaired renal function

**Warnings/Precautions** Prolonged use can lead to hypothyroidism; cystic fibrosis patients have an exaggerated response; can cause acne flare-ups, can cause dermatitis, some preparations may contain sodium bisulfite (allergy); use with caution in patients with a history of thyroid disease, patients with renal failure, or GI obstruction

**Pregnancy Risk Factor** D

**Adverse Reactions** 1% to 10%:

Central nervous system: Fever, headache

Dermatologic: Urticaria, acne, angioedema, cutaneous hemorrhage

Endocrine & metabolic: Goiter with hypothyroidism

Gastrointestinal: Metallic taste, GI upset, soreness of teeth and gums

Hematologic: Eosinophilia, hemorrhage (mucosal)

Neuromuscular & skeletal: Arthralgia

Respiratory: Rhinitis

Miscellaneous: Lymph node enlargement

**Drug Interactions** Increased toxicity: Lithium → additive hypothyroid effects

**Onset** 24-48 hours; Peak effect: 10-15 days after continuous therapy

**Special PA Issues**

**Patient Education:** Take after meals. Dilute in 6 oz of water, fruit juice, milk, or broth. Do not chew tablets; swallow whole. Do not exceed recommended dosage. You may experience a metallic taste. Discontinue use and report stomach pain, severe nausea or vomiting, black or tarry stools, or unresolved weakness.

**Monitoring Parameters:** Thyroid function tests

## Potassium Phosphate (poe TASS ee um FOS fate)

**Pharmacologic Class** Electrolyte Supplement, Oral; Electrolyte Supplement, Parenteral; Phosphate Salt; Potassium Salt

**U.S. Brand Names** Neutra-Phos®-K

**Use** Treatment and prevention of hypophosphatemia or hypokalemia

**USUAL DOSAGE** I.V. doses should be incorporated into the patient's maintenance I.V. fluids; intermittent I.V. infusion should be reserved for severe depletion situations in patients undergoing continuous EKG monitoring. It is difficult to determine total body phosphorus deficit; the following dosages are empiric guidelines:

Normal requirements elemental phosphorus: Oral:

0-6 months: 240 mg

6-12 months: 360 mg

1-10 years: 800 mg

>10 years: 1200 mg

Pregnancy lactation: Additional 400 mg/day

Adults: 800 mg

Treatment: It is difficult to provide concrete guidelines for the treatment of severe hypophosphatemia because the extent of total body deficits and response to therapy are difficult to predict. Aggressive doses of phosphate may result in a transient serum elevation followed by redistribution into intracellular compartments or bone tissue. It is recommended that repletion of severe hypophosphatemia (<1 mg/dL in adults) be done I.V. because large doses of oral phosphate may cause diarrhea and intestinal absorption may be unreliable

(Continued)

## Potassium Phosphate (Continued)

### Pediatric I.V. phosphate repletion:

Children: 0.25-0.5 mmol/kg **administer over 4-6 hours and repeat if symptomatic hypophosphatemia persists**; to assess the need for further phosphate administration, obtain serum inorganic phosphate after administration of the first dose and base further doses on serum levels and clinical status

### Adult I.V. phosphate repletion:

Initial dose: 0.08 mmol/kg if recent uncomplicated hypophosphatemia

Initial dose: 0.16 mmol/kg if prolonged hypophosphatemia with presumed total body deficits; increase dose by 25% to 50% if patient symptomatic with severe hypophosphatemia

**Do not exceed 0.24 mmol/kg/day; administer over 6 hours by I.V. infusion**

**With orders for I.V. phosphate, there is considerable confusion associated with the use of millimoles (mmol) versus milliequivalents (mEq) to express the phosphate requirement.** Because inorganic phosphate exists as monobasic and dibasic anions, with the mixture of valences dependent on pH, ordering by mEq amounts is unreliable and may lead to large dosing errors. In addition, I.V. phosphate is available in the sodium and potassium salt; therefore, the content of these cations must be considered when ordering phosphate. The most reliable method of ordering I.V. phosphate is by millimoles, then specifying the potassium or sodium salt. For example, an order for 15 mmol of phosphate as potassium phosphate in one liter of normal saline The dosing of phosphate should be 0.2-0.3 mmol/kg with a usual daily requirement of 30-60 mmol/day or 15 mmol of phosphate per liter of TPN or 15 mmol phosphate per 1000 calories of dextrose. Would also provide 22 mEq of potassium.

Maintenance:

I.V. solutions:

Children: 0.5-1.5 mmol/kg/24 hours I.V. or 2-3 mmol/kg/24 hours orally in divided doses

Adults: 15-30 mmol/24 hours I.V. or 50-150 mmol/24 hours orally in divided doses

Oral:

Children <4 years: 1 capsule (250 mg phosphorus/8 mmol) 4 times/day; dilute as instructed

Children >4 years and Adults: 1-2 capsules (250-500 mg phosphorus/8-16 mmol) 4 times/day; dilute as instructed

**Dosage Forms Cap:** Neutra-Phos®-K: Phosphorus 250 mg [8 mmol] and potassium 556 mg [14.25 mEq] per capsule; **Inj:** Potassium phosphate monobasic anhydrous 224 mg and potassium phosphate dibasic anhydrous 236 mg per mL, [phosphorus 3 mmol and potassium 4.4 mEq per mL] (15 mL); **Powder:** Neutra-Phos®-K: Phosphorus 250 mg [8 mmol] and potassium 556 mg [14.25 mEq] per packet

**Contraindications** Hyperphosphatemia, hyperkalemia, hypocalcemia, hypomagnesemia, renal failure

**Warnings/Precautions** Use with caution in patients with renal insufficiency, cardiac disease, metabolic alkalosis; admixture of phosphate and calcium in I.V. fluids can result in calcium phosphate precipitation

### Pregnancy Risk Factor C

### Adverse Reactions

>10%: Gastrointestinal: Diarrhea, nausea, stomach pain, flatulence, vomiting

1% to 10%:

Cardiovascular: Bradycardia

Endocrine & metabolic: Hyperkalemia

Neuromuscular & skeletal: Weakness

Respiratory: Dyspnea

<1%: Chest pain, mental confusion, alkalosis, hypocalcemia tetany (with large doses of phosphate), abdominal pain, throat pain, phlebitis, paresthesias, paralysis, acute renal failure

### Drug Interactions

Decreased effect/levels with aluminum and magnesium-containing antacids or sucralfate which can act as phosphate binders

Increased effect/levels with potassium-sparing diuretics, salt substitutes, or ACE-inhibitors; increased effect of digitalis

### Special PA Issues

**Patient Education:** Take as directed; do not take more than directed. Swallow tablet whole with full glass of water or juice and stir before sipping slowly, with or after meals (do not take on an empty stomach). Take any antacids 2 hours before or after potassium. Consult prescriber about advisability of increasing dietary potassium. Report tingling of hands or feet; unresolved nausea or vomiting; chest pain or palpitations; persistent abdominal pain; feelings of weakness, dizziness, listlessness, confusion, acute muscle weakness or cramping; blood in stool or tarry stools; or easy bruising or unusual bleeding.

**Monitoring Parameters:** Serum potassium, calcium, phosphate, sodium, cardiac monitor (when intermittent infusion or high-dose I.V. replacement needed)

## Potassium Phosphate and Sodium Phosphate
(poe TASS ee um FOS fate & SOW dee um FOS fate)

**Pharmacologic Class** Phosphate Salt; Potassium Salt

**U.S. Brand Names** K-Phos® Neutral; Neutra-Phos®; Uro-KP-Neutral®

**Use** Treatment of conditions associated with excessive renal phosphate loss or inadequate GI absorption of phosphate; to acidify the urine to lower calcium concentrations; to increase the antibacterial activity of methenamine; reduce odor and rash caused by ammonia in urine

**USUAL DOSAGE** All dosage forms to be mixed in 6-8 oz of water prior to administration

Children: 2-3 mmol phosphate/kg/24 hours given 4 times/day **or** 1 capsule 4 times/day

Adults: 1-2 capsules (250-500 mg phosphorus/8-16 mmol) 4 times/day after meals and at bedtime

**Dosage Forms Cap (Neutra-Phos®):** Phosphorus 8 mmol, potassium 14.25 mEq; **Powder, conc:** Phosphate 8 mmol, sodium 7.125 mEq, and potassium 7.125 mEq per 75 mL when reconstituted; **Tab:** Phosphate 8 mmol, sodium 13 mEq, and potassium 1.1 mEq (114 mg of phosphorus)

**Contraindications** Addison's disease, hyperkalemia, hyperphosphatemia, infected urolithiasis or struvite stone formation, patients with severely impaired renal function

**Warnings/Precautions** Use with caution in patients with renal disease, hyperkalemia, cardiac disease and metabolic alkalosis

**Pregnancy Risk Factor** C

**Adverse Reactions**

>10%: Gastrointestinal: Diarrhea, nausea, stomach pain, flatulence, vomiting

1% to 10%:

Cardiovascular: Bradycardia

Endocrine & metabolic: Hyperkalemia

Neuromuscular & skeletal: Weakness

Respiratory: Dyspnea

<1%: Arrhythmia, chest pain, edema, mental confusion, tetany (with large doses of phosphate), alkalosis, weight gain, throat pain, decreased urine output, phlebitis, paresthesias, paralysis, pain/weakness of extremities, bone pain, arthralgia, acute renal failure, shortness of breath, thirst

**Drug Interactions**

Decreased effect/levels with aluminum and magnesium-containing antacids or sucralfate which can act as phosphate binders

Increased effect/levels with potassium-sparing diuretics or ACE inhibitors; salicylates

**Special PA Issues**

**Patient Education:** Take as directed; do not take more than directed. Dissolve tablet or contents of capsule in 4-6 oz of water or juice. Take with or after meals (do not take on an empty stomach). Take any antacids 2 hours before or after medication. Consult prescriber about advisability of increasing dietary potassium. Report tingling of hands or feet; unresolved nausea or vomiting; chest pain or palpitations; persistent abdominal pain; feelings of weakness, dizziness, listlessness, confusion, acute muscle weakness or cramping; blood in stool or tarry stools; or easy bruising or unusual bleeding.

**Monitoring Parameters:** Serum potassium, sodium, calcium, phosphate, EKG

## Povidone-Iodine (POE vi done EYE oh dyne)

**Pharmacologic Class** Antibacterial, Topical; Antifungal Agent, Topical; Antiviral Agent, Topical; Shampoos

**U.S. Brand Names** ACU-dyne® [OTC]; Aerodine® [OTC]; Betadine® [OTC]; Betagan® [OTC]; Biodine [OTC]; Efodine® [OTC]; Iodex® [OTC]; Iodex-p® [OTC]; Isodine® [OTC]; Mallisol® [OTC]; Massengill® Medicated Douche w/Cepticin [OTC]; Minidyne® [OTC]; Operand® [OTC]; Polydine® [OTC]; Summer's Eve® Medicated Douche [OTC]; Yeast-Gard® Medicated Douche

**Mechanism of Action** Povidone-iodine is known to be a powerful broad spectrum germicidal agent effective against a wide range of bacteria, viruses, fungi, protozoa, and spores.

**Use** External antiseptic with broad microbicidal spectrum against bacteria, fungi, viruses, protozoa, and yeasts

**USUAL DOSAGE**

Shampoo: Apply 2 teaspoons to hair and scalp, lather and rinse; repeat application 2 times/week until improvement is noted, then shampoo weekly

Topical: Apply as needed for treatment and prevention of susceptible microbial infections

**Dosage Forms Aero:** 5% (90 mL); **Cleanser, top:** 7.5% (30 mL, 120 mL); **Conc: Whirlpool:** 10% (3840 mL), **Perineal wash:** 10% (240 mL); **Douche:** 10% [0.3% when reconstituted]; **Foam, top:** 10% (250 g); **Gel, vag:** 10% (3 oz); **Mouthwash:** 0.5% (180 mL); **Oint, top:** 10% (0.9 g foil packet, 0.94 g, 28 g, 480 g); **Pads, antiseptic gauze:** 10% (3" x 9", 5" x 9"); **Scrub, surg:** 7.5% (480 mL, 946 mL); **Shamp:** 7.5% (120 mL); **Soln: Ophth, sterile prep:** 5% (50 mL), **Swab aid:** 10% (100s), **Swabsticks, 4":** 10%, **Top:** 10% (240 mL, 480 mL, 946 mL); **Supp, vag:** 10%

**Contraindications** Hypersensitivity to iodine

**Warnings/Precautions** Highly toxic if ingested; sodium thiosulfate is the most effective chemical antidote; avoid contact with eyes

(Continued)

## Povidone-Iodine *(Continued)*

**Pregnancy Risk Factor** D

**Adverse Reactions**
1% to 10%:
Dermatologic: Rash, pruritus
Local: Local edema
<1%: Systemic absorption in extensive burns causing iododerma, metabolic acidosis, and renal impairment

**Special PA Issues**
**Patient Education:** Do not swallow; avoid contact with eyes

♦ **PPA** *see* Phenylpropanolamine *on page 720*

♦ **PPD** *see* Tuberculin Tests *on page 945*

♦ **PPL** *see* Benzylpenicilloyl-polylysine *on page 108*

♦ **P. quinquefolium L.** *see* Ginseng *on page 415*

♦ **Pramet® FA** *see* Vitamins, Multiple *on page 964*

♦ **Pramilet® FA** *see* Vitamins, Multiple *on page 964*

## Pramipexole *(pra mi PEX ole)*

**Pharmacologic Class** Anti-Parkinson's Agent (Dopamine Agonist)

**U.S. Brand Names** Mirapex®

**Mechanism of Action** Pramipexole is a nonergot dopamine agonist with specificity for the $D_2$ dopamine receptor, but has also been shown to bind to $D_3$ and $D_4$ receptors. By binding to these receptors, it is thought that pramipexole can stimulate dopamine activity on the nerves of the striatum and substantia nigra.

**Use** Treatment of the signs and symptoms of idiopathic Parkinson's Disease; has been evaluated for use in the treatment of depression with positive results

**USUAL DOSAGE** Adults: Oral: Initial: 0.375 mg/day given in 3 divided doses, increase gradually by 0.125 mg/dose every 5-7 days; range: 1.5-4.5 mg/day

**Dosage Forms Tab:** 0.125 mg, 0.25 mg, 1 mg, 1.5 mg

**Contraindications** Patients with known hypersensitivity to pramipexole or any of the product's ingredients

**Warnings/Precautions** Caution should be taken in patients with renal insufficiency and in patients with pre-existing dyskinesias. Pathologic degeneration and loss of photoreceptor cells were observed in the retinas of albino rats during studies, however, similar changes have not been observed in the retinas of pigmented rats, mice, monkeys, or minipigs. The significance of these data for humans remains unestablished.

**Pregnancy Risk Factor** C

**Adverse Reactions**
1% to 10%:
Cardiovascular: Edema, postural hypotension, syncope, tachycardia, chest pain
Central nervous system: Malaise, fever, dizziness, somnolence, insomnia, hallucinations, confusion, amnesia, dystonias, akathisia, thinking abnormalities, myoclonus, headache
Endocrine & metabolic: Decreased libido
Gastrointestinal: Nausea, constipation, anorexia, dysphagia, xerostomia
Genitourinary: Urinary frequency (up to 3%)
Neuromuscular & skeletal: Weakness, muscle twitching, leg cramps
Ocular: Vision abnormalities (3%)
<1%: Elevated liver transaminase levels

**Drug Interactions** Increased effect/toxicity: Cimetidine increases pramipexole AUC and half-life; levodopa levels are increased with concurrent use of pramipexole

**Half-Life** ~8 hours (12-14 hours in the elderly)

**Special PA Issues**
**Patient Education:** Do not take other medications, including over-the-counter products without consulting prescriber (especially important are other medicines that could make you sleepy such as sleeping pills, tranquilizers, some cold and allergy medicines, narcotic pain killers, or medicines that relax muscles). Avoid alcohol as this may increase the potential for drowsiness or sedation.

**Dietary Considerations:** Food intake does not affect the extent of drug absorption, although the time to maximal plasma concentration is delayed by 60 minutes when taken with a meal

**Monitoring Parameters:** Monitor for improvement in symptoms of Parkinson's disease (eg, mentation, behavior, daily living activities, motor examinations), blood pressure, body weight changes, and heart rate

♦ **Pramosone®** *see* Pramoxine and Hydrocortisone *on this page*

## Pramoxine and Hydrocortisone *(pra MOKS een & hye droe KOR ti sone)*

**Pharmacologic Class** Anesthetic/Corticosteroid

**U.S. Brand Names** Enzone®; Pramosone®; Proctofoam®-HC; Zone-A Forte®

**Dosage Forms Crm, top:** Pramoxine hydrochloride 1% and hydrocortisone acetate 0.5% (30 g), pramoxine hydrochloride 1% and hydrocortisone acetate 1%; **Foam, rectal:** Pramoxine hydrochloride 1% and hydrocortisone acetate 1% (10 g); **Lot, top:** Pramoxine hydrochloride 1% and hydrocortisone 0.25%, pramoxine hydrochloride 1% and hydrocortisone 2.5%, pramoxine hydrochloride 2.5% and hydrocortisone 1% (37.5 mL, 120 mL, 240 mL)

♦ **Pravachol®** *see* Pravastatin *on this page*

# Pravastatin (PRA va stat in)

**Pharmacologic Class** Antilipemic Agent (HMG-CoA Reductase Inhibitor)

**U.S. Brand Names** Pravachol®

**Mechanism of Action** Pravastatin is a competitive inhibitor of 3-hydroxy-3-methylglutaryl coenzyme A (HMG-CoA) reductase, which is the rate-limiting enzyme involved in *de novo* cholesterol synthesis.

**Use**

"Primary prevention" in hypercholesterolemic patients without clinically-evident coronary heart disease to reduce the risk of myocardial infarction, reduce the risk of undergoing myocardial revascularization procedures, reduce the risk of cardiovascular mortality with no increase in death from noncardiovascular causes

"Secondary prevention" in hypercholesterolemic patients with clinically-evident coronary artery disease, including prior myocardial infarction, to slow the progression of coronary atherosclerosis, and reduce the risk of acute coronary events

"Secondary prevention" in patients with previous myocardial infarction, and normal cholesterol levels; to reduce the risk of recurrent myocardial infarction; reduce the risk of undergoing myocardial revascularization procedures; and reduce the risk of stroke or transient ischemic attack (TI)

Adjunct to diet to reduce elevated total cholesterol, LDL-cholesterol, and triglyceride levels in patients with primary hypercholesterolemia and mixed dyslipidemia (Fredrickson type IIa and IIb)

**USUAL DOSAGE** Adults: Oral: 10-20 mg once daily at bedtime, may increase to 40 mg/day at bedtime

**Dosage Forms Tab, as sodium:** 10 mg, 20 mg, 40 mg

**Contraindications** Previous hypersensitivity, active liver disease, or persistent, unexplained liver function enzyme elevations; specifically contraindicated in pregnant or lactating females

**Warnings/Precautions** May elevate aminotransferases; LFTs should be performed before and every 4-6 weeks during the first 12-15 months of therapy and periodically thereafter; can also cause myalgia and rhabdomyolysis; use with caution in patients who consume large quantities of alcohol or who have a history of liver disease

**Pregnancy Risk Factor** X

**Adverse Reactions**

1% to 10%:

Central nervous system: Headache, dizziness

Dermatologic: Rash

Gastrointestinal: Flatulence, abdominal cramps, diarrhea, constipation, nausea, dyspepsia, heartburn

Neuromuscular & skeletal: Myalgia, increased CPK

<1%: Abnormal taste, lenticular opacities, blurred vision

**Drug Interactions** CYP3A3/4 enzyme substrate

Increased effect with cholestyramine

Increased toxicity with gemfibrozil, clofibrate

Concurrent use of erythromycin and HMG-CoA reductase inhibitors may result in rhabdomyolysis

**Onset** Several days

**Half-Life** ~77 hours for parent and metabolites

**Special PA Issues**

**Patient Education:** Take at bedtime since highest rate of cholesterol synthesis occurs between midnight and 5 AM. Do not change dosage without consulting prescriber. Maintain diet and exercise program as as prescribed. Have periodic ophthalmic exam while taking pravastatin (check for cataracts). You may experience mild GI disturbances (gas, diarrhea, constipation); inform prescriber if these are severe, or if you experience severe muscle pain or tenderness accompanied with malaise, blurred vision, or chest pain.

**Monitoring Parameters:** Creatine phosphokinase due to possibility of myopathy

**Related Information**

Lipid-Lowering Agents *on page 1022*

♦ **Pravastatin Sodium** *see* Pravastatin *on this page*

# Praziquantel (pray zi KWON tel)

**Pharmacologic Class** Anthelmintic

**U.S. Brand Names** Biltricide®

(Continued)

## Praziquantel *(Continued)*

**Mechanism of Action** Increases the cell permeability to calcium in schistosomes, causing strong contractions and paralysis of worm musculature leading to detachment of suckers from the blood vessel walls and to dislodgment

**Use** All stages of schistosomiasis caused by all *Schistosoma* species pathogenic to humans; clonorchiasis and opisthorchiasis

  **Unlabeled use:** Cysticercosis, flukes, and many intestinal tapeworms

**USUAL DOSAGE** Children >4 years and Adults: Oral:

  Schistosomiasis: 20 mg/kg/dose 2-3 times/day for 1 day at 4- to 6-hour intervals

  Flukes: 25 mg/kg/dose every 8 hours for 1-2 days

  Cysticercosis: 50 mg/kg/day divided every 8 hours for 14 days

  Tapeworms: 10-20 mg/kg as a single dose (25 mg/kg for *Hymenolepis nana*)

  Clonorchiasis/opisthorchiasis 3 doses of 25 mg/kg as a 1-day treatment

**Dosage Forms** Tab, tri-scored: 600 mg

**Contraindications** Ocular cysticercosis, known hypersensitivity to praziquantel

**Warnings/Precautions** Use caution in patients with severe hepatic disease; patients with cerebral cysticercosis require hospitalization

**Pregnancy Risk Factor** B

**Adverse Reactions**

  1% to 10%:

    Central nervous system: Dizziness, drowsiness, headache, malaise

    Gastrointestinal: Abdominal pain, loss of appetite, nausea, vomiting

    Miscellaneous: Diaphoresis

  <1%: CSF reaction syndrome in patients being treated for neurocysticercosis, fever, rash, urticaria, itching, diarrhea

**Drug Interactions** Hydantoins may decrease praziquantel levels causing treatment failures

**Half-Life** Parent drug: 0.8-1.5 hours; Metabolites: 4.5 hours

**Special PA Issues**

  **Patient Education:** Take as scheduled by prescriber; take full dose of therapy. Do not chew tablets; swallow during meals to avoid bitter taste that could cause vomiting. Small frequent meals or sucking on lozenges may help to reduce nausea. You may experience sleepiness or dizziness; use caution when driving or engaging in hazardous activities that require alertness until response to treatment is known.

## Prazosin *(PRA zoe sin)*

**Pharmacologic Class** Alpha₁ Blockers

**U.S. Brand Names** Minipress®

**Mechanism of Action** Competitively inhibits postsynaptic alpha-adrenergic receptors which results in vasodilation of veins and arterioles and a decrease in total peripheral resistance and blood pressure

**Use** Treatment of hypertension, severe refractory congestive heart failure (in conjunction with diuretics and cardiac glycosides); may reduce mortality in stable postmyocardial patients with left ventricular dysfunction (ejection fraction ≤40%)

  **Unlabeled use:** Symptoms of benign prostatic hypertrophy, Raynaud's vasospasm

**USUAL DOSAGE** Oral:

  Children: Initial: 5 mcg/kg/dose (to assess hypotensive effects); usual dosing interval: every 6 hours; increase dosage gradually up to maximum of 25 mcg/kg/dose every 6 hours

  Adults:

    CHF, hypertension: Initial: 1 mg/dose 2-3 times/day; usual maintenance dose: 3-15 mg/day in divided doses 2-4 times/day; maximum daily dose: 20 mg

    Hypertensive urgency: 10-20 mg once, may repeat in 30 minutes

    Raynaud's: 0.5-3 mg twice daily

    Benign prostatic hypertrophy: 2 mg twice daily

**Dosage Forms** Cap, as hydrochloride: 1 mg, 2 mg, 5 mg

**Contraindications** Hypersensitivity to prazosin or any component

**Warnings/Precautions** Marked orthostatic hypotension, syncope, and loss of consciousness may occur with first dose ("first dose phenomenon") occurs more often in patients receiving beta-blockers, diuretics, low sodium diets, or larger first doses (ie, >1 mg/dose in adults); avoid rapid increase in dose; use with caution in patients with renal impairment

**Pregnancy Risk Factor** C

**Adverse Reactions**

  >10%:

    Central nervous system: Dizziness (10.3%), lightheadedness

  1% to 10%:

    Cardiovascular: Edema, palpitations (5%)

    Central nervous system: Nervousness, drowsiness (7.6%), headache (7.8%), orthostatic hypotension

    Gastrointestinal: Xerostomia, nausea (5%)

    Genitourinary: Urinary incontinence

    Neuromuscular & skeletal: Weakness (7%)

<1%: Angina, nightmares, hypothermia, rash, sexual dysfunction, nausea, priapism, polyuria, dyspnea, nasal congestion

**Drug Interactions**

Decreased effect (antihypertensive) with NSAIDs (eg, indomethacin); clonidine's antihypertensive effect may be decreased

Increased effect (hypotensive) with diuretics and antihypertensive medications (especially beta-blockers); verapamil may increase serum prazosin levels and sensitivity to postural hypotension

**Onset** Onset of hypotensive effect: Within 2 hours; Maximum decrease: 2-4 hours

**Duration** 10-24 hours

**Half-Life** 2-4 hours; increased with congestive heart failure

**Special PA Issues**

**Patient Education:** Take as directed (first dose at bedtime). Do not skip dose or discontinue without consulting prescriber. Follow recommended diet and exercise program. Do not use alcohol or OTC medications which may affect blood pressure (eg, cough or cold remedies, diet pills, stay-awake medications) without consulting physician. You may experience drowsiness, dizziness, or impaired judgment (use caution when driving or engaging in tasks that require alertness until response is known); postural hypotension (use caution when rising from sitting or lying position or when climbing stairs); dry mouth or nausea (frequent mouth care or sucking lozenges may help); or urinary incontinence (void before taking medication). Report altered CNS status (eg, fatigue, lethargy, confusion, nervousness); sudden weight gain (weigh yourself in the same clothes at same time of day once a week); unusual or persistent swelling of ankles, feet, or extremities; palpitations or rapid heartbeat; difficulty breathing; or other persistent side effects.

**Dietary Considerations:** Alcohol: Avoid use

**Monitoring Parameters:** Blood pressure, standing and sitting/supine

## Prazosin and Polythiazide (PRA zoe sin & pol i THYE a zide)

**Pharmacologic Class** Antihypertensive Agent, Combination

**U.S. Brand Names** Minizide®

**Dosage Forms Cap:** 1: Prazosin 1 mg and polythiazide 0.5 mg, 2: Prazosin 2 mg and polythiazide 0.5 mg, 5: Prazosin 5 mg and polythiazide 0.5 mg

♦ **Prazosin Hydrochloride** see Prazosin on previous page

♦ **Precose®** see Acarbose on page 19

♦ **Predair®** see Prednisolone on next page

♦ **Predaject®** see Prednisolone on next page

♦ **Predalone T.B.A.®** see Prednisolone on next page

♦ **Predcor®** see Prednisolone on next page

♦ **Predcor-TBA®** see Prednisolone on next page

♦ **Pred Forte® Ophthalmic** see Prednisolone on next page

♦ **Pred-G® Ophthalmic** see Prednisolone and Gentamicin on page 753

♦ **Pred Mild® Ophthalmic** see Prednisolone on next page

## Prednicarbate (PRED ni kar bate)

**Pharmacologic Class** Corticosteroid, Topical

**U.S. Brand Names** Dermatop®

**Mechanism of Action** Paclitaxel exerts its effects on microtubules and their protein subunits, tubulin dimers. Microtubules serve as facilitators of intracellular transport and maintain the integrity and function of cells. Paclitaxel promotes microtubule assembly by enhancing the action of tubulin dimers, stabilizing existing microtubules, and inhibiting their disassembly. Maintaining microtubule assembly inhibits mitosis and cell death. The $G_2$- and M-phases of the cell cycle are affected. In addition, the drug can distort mitotic spindles, resulting in the breakage of chromosomes. Topical corticosteroids have anti-inflammatory, antipruritic, vasoconstrictive, and antiproliferative actions

**Use** Relief of the inflammatory and pruritic manifestations of corticosteroid-responsive dermatoses (medium potency topical corticosteroid)

**USUAL DOSAGE** Adults: Topical: Apply a thin film to affected area twice daily

**Dosage Forms Crm:** 0.1% (15 g, 60 g)

**Contraindications** Hypersensitivity to prednicarbate or any component; fungal, viral, or tubercular skin lesions, herpes simplex or zoster

**Warnings/Precautions** Systemic absorption of topical corticosteroids has produced reversible HPA axis suppression. This is more likely to occur when the preparation is used on large surface or denuded areas for prolonged periods of time or with an occlusive dressing.

**Pregnancy Risk Factor** C

**Adverse Reactions**

1% to 10%: Dermatologic: Skin atrophy, shininess, thinness, mild telangiectasia

<1%: Pruritus, edema, urticaria, burning, allergic contact dermatitis and rash, folliculitis, acneiform eruptions, hypopigmentation, perioral dermatitis, secondary infection, striae, miliaria, paresthesia

(Continued)

## Prednicarbate *(Continued)*

### Special PA Issues

**Patient Education:** For external use only. Use exactly as directed; do not overuse. Do not apply to open wounds or weeping areas. Before using, wash and dry area gently. Apply a thin film to affected area and rub in gently. If dressing is necessary, use a porous dressing. Avoid contact with eyes. Avoid exposing treated area to direct sunlight; sunburn can occur. Report increased swelling, redness, rash, itching, signs of infection, worsening of condition, or lack of healing.

**Monitoring Parameters:** Relief of symptoms

♦ **Prednicen-M®** *see* Prednisone *on page 754*

## Prednisolone (pred NIS oh lone)

**Pharmacologic Class** Corticosteroid, Ophthalmic; Corticosteroid, Parenteral

**U.S. Brand Names** AK-Pred® Ophthalmic; Articulose-50® Injection; Delta-Cortef® Oral; Econopred® Ophthalmic; Econopred® Plus Ophthalmic; Inflamase® Forte Ophthalmic; Inflamase® Mild Ophthalmic; Key-Pred® Injection; Key-Pred-SP® Injection; Metreton® Ophthalmic; Pediapred® Oral; Predair®; Predaject®; Predalone T.B.A.®; Predcor®; Predcor-TBA®; Pred Forte® Ophthalmic; Pred Mild® Ophthalmic; Prednisol® TBA Injection; Prelone® Oral

**Mechanism of Action** Decreases inflammation by suppression of migration of polymorpho-nuclear leukocytes and reversal of increased capillary permeability; suppresses the immune system by reducing activity and volume of the lymphatic system

**Use** Treatment of palpebral and bulbar conjunctivitis; corneal injury from chemical, radiation, thermal burns, or foreign body penetration; endocrine disorders, rheumatic disorders, collagen diseases, dermatologic diseases, allergic states, ophthalmic diseases, respiratory diseases, hematologic disorders, neoplastic diseases, edematous states, and gastrointes-tinal diseases; useful in patients with inability to activate prednisone (liver disease)

**USUAL DOSAGE** Dose depends upon condition being treated and response of patient; dosage for infants and children should be based on severity of the disease and response of the patient rather than on strict adherence to dosage indicated by age, weight, or body surface area. Consider alternate day therapy for long-term therapy. Discontinuation of long-term therapy requires gradual withdrawal by tapering the dose.

Children:

Acute asthma:

Oral: 1-2 mg/kg/day in divided doses 1-2 times/day for 3-5 days

I.V. (sodium phosphate salt): 2-4 mg/kg/day divided 3-4 times/day

Anti-inflammatory or immunosuppressive dose: Oral, I.V., I.M. (sodium phosphate salt): 0.1-2 mg/kg/day in divided doses 1-4 times/day

Nephrotic syndrome: Oral:

Initial (first 3 episodes): 2 mg/kg/day **or** 60 mg/m$^2$/day (maximum: 80 mg/day) in divided doses 3-4 times/day until urine is protein free for 3 consecutive days (maximum: 28 days); followed by 1-1.5 mg/kg/dose **or** 40 mg/m$^2$/dose given every other day for 4 weeks

Maintenance (long-term maintenance dose for frequent relapses): 0.5-1 mg/kg/dose given every other day for 3-6 months

Adults:

Oral, I.V., I.M. (sodium phosphate salt): 5-60 mg/day

Multiple sclerosis (sodium phosphate): Oral: 200 mg/day for 1 week followed by 80 mg every other day for 1 month

Rheumatoid arthritis: Oral: Initial: 5-7.5 mg/day; adjust dose as necessary

Elderly: Use lowest effective dose

**Dosing adjustment in hyperthyroidism:** Prednisolone dose may need to be increased to achieve adequate therapeutic effects

Hemodialysis: Slightly dialyzable (5% to 20%); administer dose posthemodialysis

Peritoneal dialysis: Supplemental dose is not necessary

Intra-articular, intralesional, soft-tissue administration:

Tebutate salt: 4-40 mg/dose

Sodium phosphate salt: 2-30 mg/dose

Ophthalmic suspension/solution: Children and Adults: Instill 1-2 drops into conjunctival sac every hour during day, every 2 hours at night until favorable response is obtained, then use 1 drop every 4 hours

**Dosage Forms Inj, as acetate (for I.M., intralesional, intra-articular, or soft tissue administration only):** 25 mg/mL (10 mL, 30 mL), 50 mg/mL (30 mL); **Inj, as sodium phosphate (for I.M., I.V., intra-articular, intralesional, or soft tissue administration):** 20 mg/mL (2 mL, 5 mL, 10 mL); **Inj, as tebutate (for intra-articular, intralesional, soft tissue administration only):** 20 mg/mL (1 mL, 5 mL, 10 mL); **Liq, oral, as sodium phosphate:** 5 mg/5 mL (120 mL); **Soln, ophth, as sodium phosphate:** 0.125% (5 mL, 10 mL, 15 mL), 1% (5 mL, 10 mL, 15 mL); **Susp, ophth, as acetate:** 0.12% (5 mL, 10 mL), 0.125% (5 mL, 10 mL, 15 mL), 1% (1 mL, 5 mL, 10 mL, 15 mL); **Syr:** 15 mg/5 mL (240 mL); **Tab:** 5 mg

**Contraindications** Acute superficial herpes simplex keratitis; systemic fungal infections; varicella; hypersensitivity to prednisolone or any component

**Warnings/Precautions** Use with caution in patients with hyperthyroidism, cirrhosis, nonspecific ulcerative colitis, hypertension, osteoporosis, thromboembolic tendencies, CHF, convulsive disorders, myasthenia gravis, thrombophlebitis, peptic ulcer, diabetes; acute adrenal insufficiency may occur with abrupt withdrawal after long-term therapy or with stress; young pediatric patients may be more susceptible to adrenal axis suppression from topical therapy. Because of the risk of adverse effects, systemic corticosteroids should be used cautiously in the elderly, in the smallest possible dose, and for the shortest possible time.

**Pregnancy Risk Factor** C

**Adverse Reactions**

>10%:

Central nervous system: Insomnia, nervousness

Gastrointestinal: Increased appetite, indigestion

1% to 10%:

Dermatologic: Hirsutism

Endocrine & metabolic: Diabetes mellitus

Neuromuscular & skeletal: Arthralgia

Ocular: Cataracts, glaucoma

Respiratory: Epistaxis

<1%: Edema, hypertension, vertigo, seizures, psychoses, pseudotumor cerebri, headache, mood swings, delirium, hallucinations, euphoria, acne, skin atrophy, bruising, hyperpigmentation, Cushing's syndrome, pituitary-adrenal axis suppression, growth suppression, glucose intolerance, hypokalemia, alkalosis, amenorrhea, sodium and water retention, hyperglycemia, peptic ulcer, nausea, vomiting, abdominal distention, ulcerative esophagitis, pancreatitis, muscle weakness, osteoporosis, fractures, muscle wasting, hypersensitivity reactions

**Drug Interactions** CYP3A enzyme substrate; inducer of cytochrome P-450 enzymes

Decreased effect:

Barbiturates, phenytoin, rifampin decrease corticosteroid effectiveness

Decreases salicylates

Decreases vaccines

Decreases toxoids effectiveness

**Duration** 18-36 hours

**Half-Life** I.V.: 3.6 hours Biological: 18-36 hours; End-stage renal disease: 3-5 hours

**Special PA Issues**

**Patient Education:** Take exactly as directed; do not increase dose or discontinue abruptly without consulting prescriber. Take oral medication with or after meals. Limit intake of caffeine or stimulants. Prescriber may recommend increased dietary vitamins, minerals, or iron. Diabetics should monitor glucose levels closely (antidiabetic medication may need to be adjusted). Inform prescriber if you are experiencing greater than normal levels of stress (medication may need adjustment). Some forms of this medication may cause GI upset (oral medication may be taken with meals to reduce GI upset; small frequent meals and frequent mouth care may reduce GI upset). You may be more susceptible to infection (avoid crowds and persons with contagious or infective conditions). Report promptly excessive nervousness or sleep disturbances; any signs of infection (sore throat, unhealed injuries); excessive growth of body hair or loss of skin color; changes in vision; excessive or sudden weight gain (>3 lb/week); swelling of face or extremities; difficulty breathing; muscle weakness; change in color of stools (tarry) or persistent abdominal pain; or worsening of condition or failure to improve.

Ophthalmic: For ophthalmic use only. Wash hands before using. Tilt head back and look upward. Put drops of suspension or apply thin ribbon of ointment inside lower eyelid. Close eye and roll eyeball in all directions. Do not blink for ½ minute. Apply gentle pressure to inner corner of eye for 30 seconds. Do not use any other eye preparation for at least 10 minutes. Do not touch tip of applicator to eye or contaminate tip of applicator. Do not share medication with anyone else. Wear sunglasses when in sunlight; you may be more sensitive to bright light. Inform prescriber if condition worsens or fails to improve or if you experience eye pain, disturbances of vision, or other adverse eye response.

**Monitoring Parameters:** Blood pressure, blood glucose, electrolytes

**Related Information**

Corticosteroids *on page 1007*

♦ **Prednisolone Acetate** *see* Prednisolone *on previous page*

♦ **Prednisolone Acetate, Ophthalmic** *see* Prednisolone *on previous page*

# Prednisolone and Gentamicin (pred NIS oh lone & jen ta MYE sin)

**Pharmacologic Class** Antibiotic/Corticosteroid, Ophthalmic

**U.S. Brand Names** Pred-G® Ophthalmic

**Dosage Forms Oint, ophth:** Prednisolone acetate 0.6% and gentamicin sulfate 0.3% (3.5 g); **Susp, ophth:** Prednisolone acetate 1% and gentamicin sulfate 0.3% (2 mL, 5 mL, 10 mL)

♦ **Prednisolone Sodium Phosphate** *see* Prednisolone *on previous page*

♦ **Prednisolone Sodium Phosphate, Ophthalmic** *see* Prednisolone *on previous page*

♦ **Prednisolone Tebutate** see Prednisolone on page 752

♦ **Prednisol® TBA Injection** see Prednisolone on page 752

# Prednisone (PRED ni sone)

**Pharmacologic Class** Corticosteroid, Oral

**U.S. Brand Names** Deltasone®; Liquid Pred®; Meticorten®; Orasone®; Prednicen-M®; Sterapred®

**Mechanism of Action** Decreases inflammation by suppression of migration of polymorphonuclear leukocytes and reversal of increased capillary permeability; suppresses the immune system by reducing activity and volume of the lymphatic system; suppresses adrenal function at high doses. Antitumor effects may be related to inhibition of glucose transport, phosphorylation, or induction of cell death in immature lymphocytes. Antiemetic effects are thought to occur due to blockade of cerebral innervation of the emetic center via inhibition of prostaglandin synthesis.

**Use** Treatment of a variety of diseases including adrenocortical insufficiency, hypercalcemia, rheumatic, and collagen disorders; dermatologic, ocular, respiratory, gastrointestinal, and neoplastic diseases; organ transplantation and a variety of diseases including those of hematologic, allergic, inflammatory, and autoimmune in origin; not available in injectable form, prednisolone must be used

**Investigational:** Prevention of postherpetic neuralgia and relief of acute pain in the early stages

**USUAL DOSAGE** Oral: Dose depends upon condition being treated and response of patient; dosage for infants and children should be based on severity of the disease and response of the patient rather than on strict adherence to dosage indicated by age, weight, or body surface area. Consider alternate day therapy for long-term therapy. Discontinuation of long-term therapy requires gradual withdrawal by tapering the dose.

Children:

Anti-inflammatory or immunosuppressive dose: 0.05-2 mg/kg/day divided 1-4 times/day

Acute asthma: 1-2 mg/kg/day in divided doses 1-2 times/day for 3-5 days

Alternatively (for 3- to 5-day "burst"):

<1 year: 10 mg every 12 hours

1-4 years: 20 mg every 12 hours

5-13 years: 30 mg every 12 hours

>13 years: 40 mg every 12 hours

Asthma long-term therapy (alternative dosing by age):

<1 year: 10 mg every other day

1-4 years: 20 mg every other day

5-13 years: 30 mg every other day

>13 years: 40 mg every other day

Nephrotic syndrome: Initial (first 3 episodes): 2 mg/kg/day **or** 60 mg/m²/day (maximum: 80 mg/day) in divided doses 3-4 times/day until urine is protein free for 3 consecutive days (maximum: 28 days); followed by 1-1.5 mg/kg/dose **or** 40 mg/m²/dose given every other day for 4 weeks

Maintenance dose (long-term maintenance dose for frequent relapses): 0.5-1 mg/kg/dose given every other day for 3-6 months

Children and Adults: Physiologic replacement: 4-5 mg/m²/day

Adults: 5-60 mg/day in divided doses 1-4 times/day

Elderly: Use the lowest effective dose

**Dosing adjustment in hepatic impairment:** Prednisone is inactive and must be metabolized by the liver to prednisolone. This conversion may be impaired in patients with liver disease, however, prednisolone levels are observed to be higher in patients with severe liver failure than in normal patients. Therefore, compensation for the inadequate conversion of prednisone to prednisolone occurs.

**Dosing adjustment in hyperthyroidism:** Prednisone dose may need to be increased to achieve adequate therapeutic effects

Hemodialysis: Supplemental dose is not necessary

Peritoneal dialysis: Supplemental dose is not necessary

**Dosage Forms Soln: Concentrate:** 5 mg/mL (5 mL, 30 mL); **Oral:** 5 mg/5 mL (10 mL, 20 mL, 500 mL); **Syr:** 5 mg/5 mL (120 mL, 240 mL); **Tab:** 1 mg, 2.5 mg, 5 mg, 10 mg, 20 mg, 50 mg

**Contraindications** Serious infections, except septic shock or tuberculous meningitis; systemic fungal infections; hypersensitivity to prednisone or any component; varicella

**Warnings/Precautions** Withdraw therapy with gradual tapering of dose, may retard bone growth; use with caution in patients with hypothyroidism, cirrhosis, hypertension, congestive heart failure, ulcerative colitis, thromboembolic disorders, and patients at increased risk for peptic ulcer disease. Because of the risk of adverse effects, systemic corticosteroids should be used cautiously in the elderly, in the smallest possible dose, and for the shortest possible time.

**Pregnancy Risk Factor** B

## Pregnancy Implications

Clinical effects on the fetus: Crosses the placenta. Immunosuppression reported in 1 infant exposed to high-dose prednisone plus azathioprine throughout gestation. One report of congenital cataracts. Available evidence suggests safe use during pregnancy.

Breast-feeding/lactation: Crosses into breast milk. No data on clinical effects on the infant. American Academy of Pediatrics considers **compatible** with breast-feeding.

## Adverse Reactions

>10%:

Central nervous system: Insomnia, nervousness

Gastrointestinal: Increased appetite, indigestion

1% to 10%:

Dermatologic: Hirsutism

Endocrine & metabolic: Diabetes mellitus

Ocular: Cataracts, glaucoma

Neuromuscular & skeletal: Arthralgia

Respiratory: Epistaxis

<1%: Edema, hypertension, vertigo, seizures, psychoses, pseudotumor cerebri, headache, mood swings, delirium, hallucinations, euphoria, acne, skin atrophy, bruising, hyperpigmentation, Cushing's syndrome, pituitary-adrenal axis suppression, growth suppression, glucose intolerance, hypokalemia, alkalosis, amenorrhea, sodium and water retention, hyperglycemia, peptic ulcer, nausea, vomiting, abdominal distention, ulcerative esophagitis, pancreatitis, muscle weakness, osteoporosis, fractures, muscle wasting, hypersensitivity reactions

## Drug Interactions CYP3A3/4 enzyme substrate

Decreased effect:

Barbiturates, phenytoin, rifampin decrease corticosteroid effectiveness

Decreases salicylates

Decreases vaccines

Decreases toxoids effectiveness

## Duration Propofol

## Half-Life Normal renal function: 2.5-3.5 hours

## Special PA Issues

**Patient Education:** Take exactly as directed. Do not take more than prescribed dose and do not discontinue abruptly; consult prescriber. Take with or after meals. Take once-a-day dose with food in the morning. Limit intake of caffeine or stimulants. Maintain adequate nutrition; consult prescriber for possibility of special dietary recommendations. If diabetic, monitor serum glucose closely and notify prescriber of changes; this medication can alter hypoglycemic requirements. Notify prescriber if you are experiencing higher than normal levels of stress; medication may need adjustment. Periodic ophthalmic examinations will be necessary with long-term use. You will be susceptible to infection; avoid crowds or infected persons or persons with contagious diseases. You may experience insomnia or nervousness; use caution when driving or engaging in tasks requiring alertness until response to medication is known. Report weakness, change in menstrual pattern, vision changes, signs of hyperglycemia, signs of infection (eg, fever, chills, mouth sores, perianal itching, vaginal discharge), other persistent side effects, or worsening of condition.

**Monitoring Parameters:** Blood pressure, blood glucose, electrolytes

## Related Information

Corticosteroids on page 1007

# Primaquine Phosphate (PRIM a kween FOS fate)

**Pharmacologic Class** Aminoquinoline (Antimalarial)

**Mechanism of Action** Eliminates the primary tissue exoerythrocytic forms of *P. falciparum*; disrupts mitochondria and binds to DNA

**Use** Provides radical cure of *P. vivax* or *P. ovale* malaria after a clinical attack has been confirmed by blood smear or serologic titer and postexposure prophylaxis

**USUAL DOSAGE** Oral:

Children: 0.3 mg base/kg/day once daily for 14 days (not to exceed 15 mg/day) or 0.9 mg base/kg once weekly for 8 weeks not to exceed 45 mg base/week

Adults: 15 mg/day (base) once daily for 14 days or 45 mg base once weekly for 8 weeks

CDC treatment recommendations: Begin therapy during last 2 weeks of, or following a course of, suppression with chloroquine or a comparable drug

**Dosage Forms Tab, as phosphate:** 26.3 mg [15 mg base]

**Contraindications** Acutely ill patients who have a tendency to develop granulocytopenia (rheumatoid arthritis, SLE); patients receiving other drugs capable of depressing the bone marrow (eg, quinacrine and primaquine)

**Warnings/Precautions** Use with caution in patients with G-6-PD deficiency, NADH methemoglobin reductase deficiency, acutely ill patients who have a tendency to develop granulocytopenia; patients receiving other drugs capable of depressing the bone marrow; do not exceed recommended dosage

**Pregnancy Risk Factor** C

**Adverse Reactions**

>10%:

Gastrointestinal: Abdominal pain, nausea, vomiting

Hematologic: Hemolytic anemia in G-6-PD deficiency

1% to 10%: Hematologic: Methemoglobinemia in NADH-methemoglobin reductase-deficient individuals

<1%: Arrhythmias, headache, pruritus, leukopenia, agranulocytosis, leukocytosis, interference with visual accommodation

**Drug Interactions** Quinacrine may potentiate the toxicity of antimalarial compounds which are structurally related to primaquine

**Half-Life** 3.7-9.6 hours

**Special PA Issues**

**Patient Education:** It is important to complete full course of therapy for full effect. May be taken with meals to decrease GI upset and bitter aftertaste. Avoid alcohol. You should have regular ophthalmic exams (every 4-6 months) if using this medication over extended periods. You may experience nausea, vomiting, or loss of appetite (small frequent meals, frequent mouth care, or sucking lozenges may help). Report persistent GI disturbance, chest pain or palpitation, unusual fatigue, easy bruising or bleeding, visual or hearing disturbances, changes in urine (darkening, tinged with red, decreased volume), or any other persistent adverse reactions.

**Monitoring Parameters:** Periodic CBC, visual color check of urine, glucose, electrolytes; if hemolysis suspected - CBC, haptoglobin, peripheral smear, urinalysis dipstick for occult blood

# Primidone (PRI mi done)

**Pharmacologic Class** Anticonvulsant, Miscellaneous

**U.S. Brand Names** Mysoline®

**Mechanism of Action** Decreases neuron excitability, raises seizure threshold similar to phenobarbital; primidone has two active metabolites, phenobarbital and phenylethylmalonamide (PEMA); PEMA may enhance the activity of phenobarbital

**Use** Management of grand mal, complex partial, and focal seizures

**Unlabeled use:** Benign familial tremor (essential tremor)

**USUAL DOSAGE** Oral:

Children <8 years: Initial: 50-125 mg/day given at bedtime; increase by 50-125 mg/day increments every 3-7 days; usual dose: 10-25 mg/kg/day in divided doses 3-4 times/day

Children >8 years and Adults: Initial: 125-250 mg/day at bedtime; increase by 125-250 mg/day every 3-7 days; usual dose: 750-1500 mg/day in divided doses 3-4 times/day with maximum dosage of 2 g/day

**Dosing interval in renal impairment:**

Cl$_{cr}$ 50-80 mL/minute: Administer every 8 hours

$Cl_{cr}$ 10-50 mL/minute: Administer every 8-12 hours

$Cl_{cr}$ <10 mL/minute: Administer every 12-24 hours

Hemodialysis: Moderately dializable (20% to 50%); administer dose postdialysis or administer supplemental 30% dose

**Dosage Forms Susp, oral:** 250 mg/5 mL (240 mL); **Tab:** 50 mg, 250 mg

**Contraindications** Hypersensitivity to primidone, phenobarbital, or any component; porphyria

**Warnings/Precautions** Use with caution in patients with renal or hepatic impairment, pulmonary insufficiency; abrupt withdrawal may precipitate status epilepticus

**Pregnancy Risk Factor** D

**Pregnancy Implications**

Clinical effects on the fetus: Crosses the placenta. Dysmorphic facial features; hemorrhagic disease of newborn due to fetal vitamin K depletion, maternal folic acid deficiency may occur. Epilepsy itself, number of medications, genetic factors, or a combination of these probably influence the teratogenicity of anticonvulsant therapy. Benefit:risk ratio usually favors continued use during pregnancy and breast-feeding.

Breast-feeding/lactation: Crosses into breast milk

Clinical effects on the infant: Sedation; feeding problems reported. American Academy of Pediatrics recommends USE WITH CAUTION.

**Adverse Reactions**

>10%: Central nervous system: Drowsiness, vertigo, ataxia, lethargy, behavior change, sedation, headache

1% to 10%:

Gastrointestinal: Nausea, vomiting, anorexia

Genitourinary: Impotence

<1%: Behavior change, rash, leukopenia, malignant lymphoma-like syndrome, megaloblastic anemia, diplopia, nystagmus, systemic lupus-like syndrome

**Drug Interactions** CYP1A2, 2B6, 2C, 2C8, 3A3/4, and 3A5-7 enzyme inducer

Decreased effect: Primidone may decrease serum concentrations of ethosuximide, valproic acid, griseofulvin; phenytoin may decrease primidone serum concentrations

Increased toxicity: Methylphenidate may increase primidone serum concentrations; valproic acid may increase phenobarbital concentrations derived from primidone

**Half-Life** Age dependent: Primidone: 10-12 hours; PEMA: 16 hours; Phenobarbital: 52-118 hours

**Special PA Issues**

**Patient Education:** Take exactly as directed (do not increase dose or frequency or discontinue without consulting prescriber); may cause physical and/or psychological dependence. While using this medication, do not use alcohol and other prescription or OTC medications (especially pain medications, sedatives, antihistamines, or hypnotics) without consulting prescriber. Maintain adequate hydration (2-3 L/day of fluids unless instructed to restrict fluid intake). You may experience drowsiness, dizziness, or blurred vision (use caution when driving or engaging in hazardous tasks); nausea, vomiting, or loss of appetite (small frequent meals, good mouth care, chewing gum, or sucking on lozenges may help); impotence (reversible). Wear identification of epileptic status and medications. Report behavioral or CNS changes (confusion, depression, increased sedation, excitation, headache, insomnia, or lethargy); muscle weakness, or tremors; unusual bruising or bleeding (mouth, urine, stool); worsening of seizure activity, or loss of seizure control.

**Dietary Considerations:**

Food:

Folic acid: Low erythrocyte and CSF folate concentrations. Megaloblastic anemia has been reported. To avoid folic acid deficiency and megaloblastic anemia, some clinicians recommend giving patients on anticonvulsants prophylactic doses of folic acid and cyanocobalamin.

Protein-deficient diets: Increases duration of action of primidone. Should not restrict or delete protein from diet unless discussed with physician. Be consistent with protein intake during primidone therapy.

Fresh fruits containing vitamin C: Displaces drug from binding sites, resulting in increased urinary excretion of primidone. Educate patients regarding the potential for decreased primidone effect with consumption of foods high in vitamin C.

**Monitoring Parameters:** Serum primidone and phenobarbital concentration, CBC, neurological status. Due to CNS effects, monitor closely when initiating drug in elderly. Monitor CBC at 6-month intervals to compare with baseline obtained at start of therapy. Since elderly metabolize phenobarbital at a slower rate than younger adults, it is suggested to measure both primidone and phenobarbital levels together.

**Reference Range:** Therapeutic: Children <5 years: 7-10 µg/mL (SI: 32-46 µmol/L); Adults: 5-12 µg/mL (SI: 23-55 µmol/L); toxic effects rarely present with levels <10 µg/mL (SI: 46 µmol/L) if phenobarbital concentrations are low. Dosage of primidone is adjusted with reference mostly to the phenobarbital level; Toxic: >15 µg/mL (SI: >69 µmol/L)

♦ **Principen®** *see* Ampicillin *on page 64*

♦ **Prinivil®** *see* Lisinopril *on page 535*

# Probenecid (proe BEN e sid)

**Pharmacologic Class** Uricosuric Agent

**U.S. Brand Names** Benemic®; Probalan®

**Mechanism of Action** Competitively inhibits the reabsorption of uric acid at the proximal convoluted tubule, thereby promoting its excretion and reducing serum uric acid levels; increases plasma levels of weak organic acids (penicillins, cephalosporins, or other beta-lactam antibiotics) by competitively inhibiting their renal tubular secretion

**Use** Prevention of gouty arthritis; hyperuricemia; prolongation of beta-lactam effect (ie, serum levels)

**USUAL DOSAGE** Oral:

Children:

<2 years: Not recommended

2-14 years: Prolong penicillin serum levels: 25 mg/kg starting dose, then 40 mg/kg/day given 4 times/day

Gonorrhea: <45 kg: 25 mg/kg x 1 (maximum: 1 g/dose) 30 minutes before penicillin, ampicillin or amoxicillin

Adults:

Hyperuricemia with gout: 250 mg twice daily for one week; increase to 250-500 mg/day; may increase by 500 mg/month, if needed, to maximum of 2-3 g/day (dosages may be increased by 500 mg every 6 months if serum urate concentrations are controlled)

Prolong penicillin serum levels: 500 mg 4 times/day

Gonorrhea: 1 g 30 minutes before penicillin, ampicillin, procaine, or amoxicillin

Pelvic inflammatory disease: Cefoxitin 2 g I.M. plus probenecid 1 g orally as a single dose

Neurosyphilis: Aqueous procaine penicillin 2.4 units/day I.M. plus probenecid 500 mg 4 times/day for 10-14 days

**Dosing adjustment in renal impairment:** Cl$_{cr}$ <50 mL/minute: Avoid use

**Dosage Forms Tab:** 500 mg

**Contraindications** Hypersensitivity to probenecid or any component; high-dose aspirin therapy; moderate to severe renal impairment; children <2 years of age

**Warnings/Precautions** Use with caution in patients with peptic ulcer; use extreme caution in the use of probenecid with penicillin in patients with renal insufficiency; probenecid may not be effective in patients with a creatinine clearance <30 to 50 mL/minute; may cause exacerbation of acute gouty attack

**Pregnancy Risk Factor** B

**Adverse Reactions**

>10%:

Central nervous system: Headache

Gastrointestinal: Anorexia, nausea, vomiting

Neuromuscular & skeletal: Gouty arthritis (acute)

1% to 10%:

Cardiovascular: Flushing of face

Central nervous system: Dizziness

Dermatologic: Rash, itching

Gastrointestinal: Sore gums

Genitourinary: Painful urination

Renal: Renal calculi

<1%: Leukopenia, hemolytic anemia, aplastic anemia, hepatic necrosis, urate nephropathy, nephrotic syndrome, anaphylaxis

**Drug Interactions**

Decreased effect:

Salicylates (high dose) may decrease uricosuria

Nitrofurantoin may decrease efficacy

Increased toxicity:

Increases methotrexate toxic potential; combination with diflunisal has resulted in 40% decrease in its clearance and as much as a 65% increase in plasma concentrations due to inhibition of diflunisal metabolism

Probenecid decreases clearance of beta-lactams such as penicillins and cephalosporins; increases levels/toxicity of acyclovir, thiopental, clofibrate, dyphylline, pantothenic acid, benzodiazepines, rifampin, sulfonamide, dapsone, sulfonylureas, and zidovudine

Avoid concomitant use with ketorolac (and other NSAIDs) since its half-life is increased twofold and levels and toxicity are significantly increased

Allopurinol readministration may be beneficial by increasing the uric acid lowering effect
Pharmacologic effects of penicillamine may be attenuated

**Onset** Effect on penicillin levels reached in about 2 hours

**Half-Life** Normal renal function: 6-12 hours and is dose dependent

**Special PA Issues**

    **Patient Education:** Take as directed; do not discontinue without consulting prescriber. May take 6-12 months to reduce gouty attacks (attacks may increase in frequency and severity for first few months of therapy). Take with food or antacids or alkaline ash foods (milk, nuts, beets, spinach, turnip greens). Maintain adequate hydration (2-3 L/day of fluids unless instructed to restrict fluid intake). Avoid aspirin, or aspirin-containing substances. Diabetics should use serum glucose monitoring. If you experience severe headache, contact prescriber for medication. You may experience dizziness or lightheadedness (use caution when driving, changing position, or engaging in tasks that require alertness); nausea, vomiting, indigestion, or loss of appetite (small frequent meals or sucking on lozenges may help). Report skin rash or itching, persistent headache, blood in urine or painful urination, excessive tiredness or easy bruising or bleeding, or sore gums.

    **Dietary Considerations:** Food: Drug may cause GI upset; take with food if GI upset. Drink plenty of fluids.

    **Monitoring Parameters:** Uric acid, renal function, CBC

# Procainamide (proe kane A mide)

**Pharmacologic Class** Antiarrhythmic Agent, Class I-A

**U.S. Brand Names** Procanbid™; Promine®; Pronestyl®; Rhythmin®

**Mechanism of Action** Decreases myocardial excitability and conduction velocity and may depress myocardial contractility, by increasing the electrical stimulation threshold of ventricle, HIS-Purkinje system and through direct cardiac effects

**Use** Treatment of ventricular tachycardia, premature ventricular contractions, paroxysmal atrial tachycardia, and atrial fibrillation; to prevent recurrence of ventricular tachycardia, paroxysmal supraventricular tachycardia, atrial fibrillation or flutter

**USUAL DOSAGE** Must be titrated to patient's response

    Children:

        Oral: 15-50 mg/kg/24 hours divided every 3-6 hours

        I.M.: 50 mg/kg/24 hours divided into doses of $\frac{1}{8}$ to $\frac{1}{4}$ every 3-6 hours in divided doses until oral therapy is possible

        I.V. (infusion requires use of an infusion pump):

        Load: 3-6 mg/kg/dose over 5 minutes not to exceed 100 mg/dose; may repeat every 5-10 minutes to maximum of 15 mg/kg/load

        Maintenance as continuous I.V. infusion: 20-80 mcg/kg/minute; maximum: 2 g/24 hours

    Adults:

        Oral: 250-500 mg/dose every 3-6 hours or 500 mg to 1 g every 6 hours sustained release; usual dose: 50 mg/kg/24 hours; maximum: 4 g/24 hours **(Note: Twice daily dosing approved for Procanbid™)**

        I.M.: 0.5-1 g every 4-8 hours until oral therapy is possible

        I.V. (infusion requires use of an infusion pump): Loading dose: 15-18 mg/kg administered as slow infusion over 25-30 minutes or 100-200 mg/dose repeated every 5 minutes as needed to a total dose of 1 g; maintenance dose: 1-6 mg/minute by continuous infusion

        Infusion dose: 2 g/250 mL $D_5$W/NS (I.V. infusion requires use of an infusion pump):

            1 mg/minute: 7 mL/hour

            2 mg/minute: 15 mL/hour

            3 mg/minute: 21 mL/hour

            4 mg/minute: 30 mL/hour

            5 mg/minute: 38 mL/hour

            6 mg/minute: 45 mL/hour

        Refractory ventricular fibrillation: 30 mg/minute, up to a total of 17 mg/kg; I.V. maintenance infusion: 1-4 mg/minute; monitor levels and do not exceed 3 mg/minute for >24 hours in adults with renal failure

        ACLS guidelines: I.V.: Infuse 20 mg/minute until arrhythmia is controlled, hypotension occurs, QRS complex widens by 50% of its original width, or total of 17 mg/kg is given

    **Dosing interval in renal impairment:**

        $Cl_{cr}$ 10-50 mL/minute: Administer every 6-12 hours

        $Cl_{cr}$ <10 mL/minute: Administer every 8-24 hours

    Dialysis:

        Procainamide: Moderately hemodialyzable (20% to 50%): 200 mg supplemental dose posthemodialysis is recommended

        N-acetylprocainamide: Not dialyzable (0% to 5%)

        Procainamide/N-acetylprocainamide: Not peritoneal dialyzable (0% to 5%)

        Procainamide/N-acetylprocainamide: Replace by blood level during continuous arteriovenous or venovenous hemofiltration (CAVH/CAVHD)

    **Dosing adjustment in hepatic impairment:** Reduce dose 50%

**Dosage Forms** Procainamide hydrochloride: **Cap:** 250 mg, 375 mg, 500 mg; **Inj:** 100 mg/mL (10 mL), 500 mg/mL (2 mL); **Tab:** 250 mg, 375 mg, 500 mg; **Tab, sustained release:** (Continued)

## Procainamide *(Continued)*

250 mg, 500 mg, 750 mg, 1000 mg; **Tab, sustained release (Procanbid™):** 500 mg, 1000 mg

**Contraindications** Complete heart block; second or third degree heart block without pacemaker; "torsade de pointes"; hypersensitivity to the drug or procaine, or related drugs; SLE; concurrent use of sparfloxacin. Due to results of the CAST study, procainamide and other antiarrhythmic drugs with potentially proarrhythmic effects should be reserved only for documented ventricular arrhythmias which are life-threatening.

**Warnings/Precautions** Use with caution in patients with marked A-V conduction disturbances, myasthenia gravis, bundle-branch block, or severe cardiac glycoside intoxication, ventricular arrhythmias with organic heart disease or coronary occlusion, CHF supraventricular tachyarrhythmias unless adequate measures are taken to prevent marked increases in ventricular rates; concurrent therapy with other class IA drugs may accumulate in patients with renal or hepatic dysfunction; some tablets contain tartrazine; injection may contain bisulfite (allergens). Long-term administration leads to the development of a positive antinuclear antibody (ANA) test in 50% of patients which may result in a lupus erythematosus-like syndrome (in 20% to 30% of patients); discontinue procainamide with SLE symptoms and choose an alternative agent; elderly have reduced clearance and frequent drug interactions. Potentially fatal blood dyscrasias have occurred with therapeutic doses; close monitoring is recommended during the first 3 months of therapy.

**Pregnancy Risk Factor** C

**Adverse Reactions**

Cardiovascular: Tachycardia, Q-T prolongation, hypotension, second degree heart block

Central nervous system: Dizziness, lightheadedness, confusion, hallucinations, mental depression, disorientation, fever, drug fever

Dermatologic: Rash

Gastrointestinal: Diarrhea (3% to 4%), nausea, vomiting, GI complaints

Hematologic: Hemolytic anemia, agranulocytosis, neutropenia, thrombocytopenia (0.5%), positive Coombs' test

Neuromuscular & skeletal: Arthralgia, myalgia

Respiratory: Pleural effusion

Miscellaneous: SLE-like syndrome (increased incidence with long-term therapy)

**Drug Interactions**

Increased plasma/NAPA concentrations with cimetidine, ranitidine, beta-blockers, amiodarone, trimethoprim, and quinidine

Increased procainamide levels with ofloxacin (21% increase in peak plasma concentrations and 24% increase in AUC) due to inhibition of tubular secretion of procainamide; contraindicated with sparfloxacin due to increased risk of cardiotoxicity

Increased effect of skeletal muscle relaxants, quinidine and lidocaine and neuromuscular blockers (succinylcholine); additive cardiodepressant action occurs with lidocaine

**Onset** I.M. 10-30 minutes

**Half-Life**

Procainamide: (Dependent upon hepatic acetylator, phenotype, cardiac function, and renal function): Adults: 2.5-4.7 hours; Anephric: 11 hours

NAPA: (Dependent upon renal function): Adults: 6-8 hours; Anephric: 42 hours

**Special PA Issues**

**Patient Education:** Oral: Take exactly as directed; do not take additional doses or discontinue without consulting prescriber. You will need regular cardiac check-ups and blood tests while taking this medication. You may experience dizziness, lightheadedness, or visual changes (use caution when driving or performing tasks that require alertness until response to drug is determined); loss of appetite (small frequent meals, frequent mouth care, or sucking lozenges may help); headaches (prescriber may recommend mild analgesic); or diarrhea (exercise, yogurt, or boiled milk may help - if persistent consult prescriber). Report chest pain, palpitation, or erratic heartbeat; increased weight or swelling of hands or feet; acute diarrhea; or unusual fatigue and tiredness.

**Monitoring Parameters:** EKG, blood pressure, CBC with differential, platelet count; cardiac monitor and blood pressure monitor required during I.V. administration

**Reference Range:**

Timing of serum samples: Draw trough just before next oral dose; draw 6-12 hours after I.V. infusion has started; half-life is 2.5-5 hours

Therapeutic levels: Procainamide: 4-10 µg/mL; NAPA 15-25 µg/mL; Combined: 10-30 µg/mL

Toxic concentration: Procainamide: >10-12 µg/mL

♦ **Procainamide Hydrochloride** *see* Procainamide *on previous page*

## Procaine *(PROE kane)*

**Pharmacologic Class** Local Anesthetic

**U.S. Brand Names** Novocain® Injection

**Mechanism of Action** Blocks both the initiation and conduction of nerve impulses by decreasing the neuronal membrane's permeability to sodium ions, which results in inhibition of depolarization with resultant blockade of conduction

**Use** Produces spinal anesthesia and epidural and peripheral nerve block by injection and infiltration methods

**USUAL DOSAGE** Dose varies with procedure, desired depth, and duration of anesthesia, desired muscle relaxation, vascularity of tissues, physical condition, and age of patient

**Dosage Forms Inj, as hydrochloride:** 1% [10 mg/mL] (2 mL, 6 mL, 30 mL, 100 mL); 2% [20 mg/mL] (30 mL, 100 mL); 10% (2 mL)

**Contraindications** Known hypersensitivity to procaine, PABA, parabens, or other ester local anesthetics

**Warnings/Precautions** Patients with cardiac diseases, hyperthyroidism, or other endocrine diseases may be more susceptible to toxic effects of local anesthetics; some preparations contain metabisulfite

**Pregnancy Risk Factor** C

**Adverse Reactions**
1% to 10%:
Local: Burning sensation at site of injection, tissue irritation, pain at injection site
<1%: Aseptic meningitis resulting in paralysis can occur, CNS stimulation followed by CNS depression, chills, discoloration of skin, nausea, vomiting, miosis, tinnitus, anaphylactoid reaction

**Drug Interactions**
Decreased effect of sulfonamides with the PABA metabolite of procaine, chloroprocaine, and tetracaine
Decreased/increased effect of vasopressors, ergot alkaloids, and MAO inhibitors on blood pressure when using anesthetic solutions with a vasoconstrictor

**Onset** Onset of effect: Injection: Within 2-5 minutes

**Duration** 0.5-1.5 hours (dependent upon patient, type of block, concentration, and method of anesthesia)

**Half-Life** 7.7 minutes

**Special PA Issues**
Patient Education: The purpose of this medication is to reduce pain sensation. Report local burning or pain at injection site.

♦ **Procaine Amide Hydrochloride** *see* Procainamide *on page 759*

♦ **Procaine Benzylpenicillin** *see* Penicillin G Procaine *on page 706*

♦ **Procaine Hydrochloride** *see* Procaine *on previous page*

♦ **Procaine Penicillin G** *see* Penicillin G Procaine *on page 706*

♦ **Pro-Cal-Sof® [OTC]** *see* Docusate *on page 298*

♦ **Procanbid™** *see* Procainamide *on page 759*

# Procarbazine (proe KAR ba zeen)

**Pharmacologic Class** Antineoplastic Agent, Alkylating Agent

**U.S. Brand Names** Matulane®

**Mechanism of Action** Mechanism of action is not clear, methylating of nucleic acids; inhibits DNA, RNA, and protein synthesis; may damage DNA directly and suppresses mitosis; metabolic activation required by host

**Use** Treatment of Hodgkin's disease, non-Hodgkin's lymphoma, brain tumor, bronchogenic carcinoma

**USUAL DOSAGE** Refer to individual protocols. Dose based on patient's ideal weight if the patient is obese or has abnormal fluid retention. Oral:

Children:
BMT aplastic anemia conditioning regimen: 12.5 mg/kg/dose every other day for 4 doses
Hodgkin's disease: MOPP/IC-MOPP regimens: 100 mg/m$^2$/day for 14 days and repeated every 4 weeks
Neuroblastoma and medulloblastoma: Doses as high as 100-200 mg/m$^2$/day once daily have been used
Adults: Initial: 2-4 mg/kg/day in single or divided doses for 7 days then increase dose to 4-6 mg/kg/day until response is obtained or leukocyte count decreased <4000/mm$^3$ or the platelet count decreased <100,000/mm$^3$; maintenance: 1-2 mg/kg/day
In MOPP, 100 mg/m$^2$/day on days 1-14 of a 28-day cycle
**Dosing in renal/hepatic impairment:** Use with caution, may result in increased toxicity

**Dosage Forms Cap, as hydrochloride:** 50 mg

**Contraindications** Hypersensitivity to procarbazine or any component, or pre-existing bone marrow aplasia, alcohol ingestion

**Warnings/Precautions** The U.S. Food and Drug Administration (FDA) currently recommends that procedures for proper handling and disposal of antineoplastic agents be considered; use with caution in patients with pre-existing renal or hepatic impairment; modify dosage in patients with renal or hepatic impairment, or marrow disorders; reduce dosage with serum creatinine >2 mg/dL or total bilirubin >3 mg/dL; procarbazine possesses MAO inhibitor activity. Procarbazine is a carcinogen which may cause acute leukemia; procarbazine may cause infertility.

**Pregnancy Risk Factor** D
(Continued)

## Procarbazine *(Continued)*

### Adverse Reactions

>10%:

Central nervous system: Mental depression, manic reactions, hallucinations, dizziness, headache, nervousness, insomnia, nightmares, ataxia, disorientation, confusion, seizure, CNS stimulation

Endocrine & metabolic: Amenorrhea

Gastrointestinal: Severe nausea and vomiting occur frequently and may be dose-limiting; anorexia, abdominal pain, stomatitis, dysphagia, diarrhea, and constipation; use a nonphenothiazine antiemetic, when possible

Emetic potential: Moderately high (60% to 90%)

Time course of nausea/vomiting: Onset: 24-27 hours; Duration: variable

Hematologic: Thrombocytopenia, hemolytic anemia

Myelosuppressive: May be dose-limiting toxicity; procarbazine should be discontinued if leukocyte count is <4000/mm³ or platelet count <100,000/mm³

WBC: Moderate

Platelets: Moderate

Onset (days): 14

Nadir (days): 21

Recovery (days): 28

Neuromuscular & skeletal: Weakness, paresthesia, neuropathies, decreased reflexes, foot drop, tremors

Ocular: Nystagmus

Respiratory: Pleural effusion, cough

1% to 10%:

Dermatologic: Alopecia, hyperpigmentation

Hepatic: Hepatotoxicity

Neuromuscular & skeletal: Peripheral neuropathy

<1%: Orthostatic hypotension, hypertensive crisis, irritability, somnolence, dermatitis, alopecia, pruritus, hypersensitivity rash, disulfiram-like reaction, cessation of menses, jaundice, arthralgia, myalgia, diplopia, photophobia, pneumonitis, hoarseness, secondary malignancy, allergic reactions, flu-like syndrome

### Drug Interactions Increased toxicity:

Procarbazine exhibits weak monoamine oxidase (MAO) inhibitor activity; foods containing high amounts of tyramine should, therefore, be avoided (ie, beer, yogurt, yeast, wine, cheese, pickled herring, chicken liver, and bananas). When a MAO inhibitor is given with food high in tyramine, a hypertensive crisis, intracranial bleeding, and headache have been reported.

Sympathomimetic amines (epinephrine and amphetamines) and antidepressants (tricyclics) should be used cautiously with procarbazine.

Barbiturates, narcotics, phenothiazines, and other CNS depressants can cause somnolence, ataxia, and other symptoms of CNS depression

Alcohol has caused a disulfiram-like reaction with procarbazine; may result in headache, respiratory difficulties, nausea, vomiting, sweating, thirst, hypotension, and flushing

### Half-Life 1 hour

### Special PA Issues

**Patient Education:** Take as directed. Maintain adequate hydration (2-3 L/day of fluids unless instructed to restrict fluid intake). Avoid aspirin and aspirin-containing substances. Avoid alcohol; may cause acute disulfiram reaction - flushing, headache, acute vomiting, chest and/or abdominal pain. Avoid tyramine-containing foods (aged cheese, chocolate, pickles, aged meat, wine, etc). You may experience mental depression, nervousness, insomnia, nightmares, dizziness, confusion, or lethargy (use caution when driving or engaging in hazardous activities); photosensitivity (avoid sunlight, wear protective clothing, or use sunblock). You may experience rash or hair loss (reversible), loss of libido, increased sensitivity to infection (avoid crowds and infected persons). Report persistent fever, chills, sore throat, unusual bleeding, blood in urine, stool, or vomitus, or stool, unresolved depression, mania, hallucinations, nightmares, disorientation, seizures, chest pain or palpitations, or difficulty breathing.

**Dietary Considerations:**

Alcohol: Avoid use, including alcohol-containing products

Food: Avoid foods with high tyramine content

**Monitoring Parameters:** CBC with differential, platelet and reticulocyte count, urinalysis, liver function test, renal function test.

### Related Information

Tyramine-Containing Foods *on page 1148*

♦ **Procarbazine Hydrochloride** *see* Procarbazine *on previous page*

♦ **Procardia®** *see* Nifedipine *on page 654*

♦ **Procardia XL®** *see* Nifedipine *on page 654*

♦ **Procetofene** *see* Fenofibrate *on page 360*

## Prochlorperazine (proe klor PER a zeen)

**Pharmacologic Class** Antipsychotic Agent, Phenothiazine, Piperazine

**U.S. Brand Names** Compazine®

**Mechanism of Action** Blocks postsynaptic mesolimbic dopaminergic $D_1$ and $D_2$ receptors in the brain, including the medullary chemoreceptor trigger zone; exhibits a strong alpha-adrenergic and anticholinergic blocking effect and depresses the release of hypothalamic and hypophyseal hormones; believed to depress the reticular activating system, thus affecting basal metabolism, body temperature, wakefulness, vasomotor tone and emesis

**Use** Management of nausea and vomiting; acute and chronic psychosis

### USUAL DOSAGE

Antiemetic: Children:

Oral, rectal:

>10 kg: 0.4 mg/kg/24 hours in 3-4 divided doses; **or**

9-14 kg: 2.5 mg every 12-24 hours as needed; maximum: 7.5 mg/day

14-18 kg: 2.5 mg every 8-12 hours as needed; maximum: 10 mg/day

18-39 kg: 2.5 mg every 8 hours or 5 mg every 12 hours as needed; maximum: 15 mg/day

I.M.: 0.1-0.15 mg/kg/dose; usual: 0.13 mg/kg/dose; change to oral as soon as possible

I.V.: Not recommended in children <10 kg or <2 years

Antiemetic: Adults:

Oral: 5-10 mg 3-4 times/day; usual maximum: 40 mg/day

I.M.: 5-10 mg every 3-4 hours; usual maximum: 40 mg/day

I.V.: 2.5-10 mg; maximum 10 mg/dose or 40 mg/day; may repeat dose every 3-4 hours as needed

Rectal: 25 mg twice daily

Antipsychotic:

Children 2-12 years:

Oral, rectal: 2.5 mg 2-3 times/day; increase dosage as needed to maximum daily dose of 20 mg for 2-5 years and 25 mg for 6-12 years

I.M.: 0.13 mg/kg/dose; change to oral as soon as possible

Adults:

Oral: 5-10 mg 3-4 times/day; doses up to 150 mg/day may be required in some patients for treatment of severe disturbances

I.M.: 10-20 mg every 4-6 hours may be required in some patients for treatment of severe disturbances; change to oral as soon as possible

Dementia behavior (nonpsychotic): Elderly: Initial: 2.5-5 mg 1-2 times/day; increase dose at 4- to 7-day intervals by 2.5-5 mg/day; increase dosing intervals (twice daily, 3 times/day, etc) as necessary to control response or side effects; maximum daily dose should probably not exceed 75 mg in elderly; gradual increases (titration) may prevent some side effects or decrease their severity

Hemodialysis: Not dialyzable (0% to 5%)

**Dosage Forms Supp, rectal:** 2.5 mg, 5 mg, 25 mg (12/box)

Prochlorperazine edisylate: **Inj:** 5 mg/mL (2 mL, 10 mL); **Syr:** 5 mg/5 mL (120 mL);

Prochlorperazine maleate: **Cap, sustained action:** 10 mg, 15 mg, 30 mg; **Tab:** 5 mg, 10 mg, 25 mg

**Contraindications** Hypersensitivity to prochlorperazine or any component; cross-sensitivity with other phenothiazines may exist; avoid use in patients with narrow-angle glaucoma; bone marrow suppression; severe liver or cardiac disease

**Warnings/Precautions** Injection contains sulfites which may cause allergic reactions; may impair ability to perform hazardous tasks requiring mental alertness or physical coordination; some products contain tartrazine dye, avoid use in sensitive individuals

Tardive dyskinesia: Prevalence rate may be 40% in elderly; development of the syndrome and the irreversible nature are proportional to duration and total cumulative dose over time. May be reversible if diagnosed early in therapy.

High incidence of extrapyramidal reactions, especially in children or the elderly, so reserve use in children <5 years of age to those who are unresponsive to other antiemetics; incidence of extrapyramidal reactions is increased with acute illnesses such as chicken pox, measles, CNS infections, gastroenteritis, and dehydration

Drug-induced **Parkinson's syndrome** occurs often. **Akathisia** is the most common extrapyramidal reaction in elderly.

Increased confusion, memory loss, psychotic behavior, and agitation frequently occur as a consequence of anticholinergic effects

**Lowers seizure threshold**, use cautiously in patients with seizure history

Orthostatic hypotension is due to alpha-receptor blockade, the elderly are at greater risk for orthostatic hypotension

Antipsychotic associated sedation in nonpsychotic patients is extremely unpleasant due to feelings of depersonalization, derealization, and dysphoria

Life-threatening arrhythmias have occurred at therapeutic doses of antipsychotics

**Pregnancy Risk Factor** C

(Continued)

## Prochlorperazine *(Continued)*

### Pregnancy Implications

Clinical effects on the fetus: Crosses the placenta. Isolated reports of congenital anomalies, however some included exposures to other drugs. Available evidence with use of occasional low doses suggests safe use during pregnancy.

Breast-feeding/lactation: No data available. American Academy of Pediatrics considers compatible with breast-feeding.

### Adverse Reactions

Incidence of extrapyramidal reactions are higher with prochlorperazine than chlorpromazine

Central nervous system: Sedation, drowsiness, restlessness, anxiety, extrapyramidal reactions, parkinsonian signs and symptoms, seizures, altered central temperature regulation

Dermatologic: Photosensitivity, hyperpigmentation, pruritus, rash

Endocrine & metabolic: Amenorrhea, gynecomastia

Gastrointestinal: Weight gain, GI upset

Miscellaneous: Anaphylactoid reactions

>10%:

Cardiovascular: Hypotension (especially with I.V. use), orthostatic hypotension, tachycardia, arrhythmias

Central nervous system: Pseudoparkinsonism, akathisia, tardive dyskinesia (persistent), dizziness, dystonias

Gastrointestinal: Xerostomia, constipation

Genitourinary: Urinary retention

Ocular: Pigmentary retinopathy, blurred vision

Respiratory: Nasal congestion

Miscellaneous: Diaphoresis (decreased)

1% to 10%:

Dermatologic: Increased sensitivity to sun, rash

Endocrine & metabolic: Changes in menstrual cycle, breast pain, changes in libido

Gastrointestinal: Nausea, vomiting, stomach pain

Genitourinary: Dysuria, ejaculatory disturbances

Neuromuscular & skeletal: Trembling of fingers

<1%: Neuroleptic malignant syndrome (NMS), impairment of temperature regulation, lowering of seizures threshold, discoloration of skin (blue–gray), galactorrhea, priapism, agranulocytosis, leukopenia, thrombocytopenia, cholestatic jaundice, hepatotoxicity, cornea and lens changes

### Drug Interactions

Increased toxicity: Additive effects with other CNS depressants; anticonvulsants; epinephrine may cause hypotension

### Onset

Oral: Within 30-40 minutes; I.M.: Within 10-20 minutes; Rectal: Within 60 minutes

### Duration

Persists longest with I.M. and oral extended-release doses (12 hours); shortest following rectal and immediate release oral administration (3-4 hours)

### Half-Life

23 hours

### Special PA Issues

Patient Education: Take exact amount as prescribed. Do not change brand names. Do not crush or chew tablets or capsules. Do not discontinue without consulting prescriber. Avoid alcohol or other sedatives or sleep-inducing drugs. Avoid skin contact with drug; wash immediately with warm soapy water. You may experience appetite changes; small frequent meals may help. Maintain adequate fluid intake (2-3 L/day). May cause dizziness, tremors, or visual disturbance (especially during early therapy); use caution when driving or engaging in hazardous activities. Do not change position rapidly (rise slowly). May cause photosensitivity reaction; avoid prolonged exposure to sunlight and use protective clothing and sunglasses. Report immediately any changes in gait or muscular tremors. Report unresolved changes in voiding or elimination (constipation or diarrhea), acute dizziness or unresolved sedation, any vision changes, palpitations, yellowing of skin or eyes, and changes in color of urine or stool (pink or red brown urine is expected).

- ♦ **Prochlorperazine Edisylate** *see* Prochlorperazine *on previous page*
- ♦ **Prochlorperazine Maleate** *see* Prochlorperazine *on previous page*
- ♦ **Procort®** [OTC] *see* Hydrocortisone *on page 453*
- ♦ **Procrit®** *see* Epoetin Alfa *on page 322*
- ♦ **Proctocort™** *see* Hydrocortisone *on page 453*
- ♦ **Proctofene** *see* Fenofibrate *on page 360*
- ♦ **Proctofoam®-HC** *see* Pramoxine and Hydrocortisone *on page 748*
- ♦ **Procyclid** *see* Procyclidine *on this page*

## Procyclidine *(proe SYE kli deen)*

**Pharmacologic Class** Anticholinergic Agent; Anti-Parkinson's Agent (Anticholinergic)

**U.S. Brand Names** Kemadrin®

**Mechanism of Action** Thought to act by blocking excess acetylcholine at cerebral synapses; many of its effects are due to its pharmacologic similarities with atropine

**Use** Relieves symptoms of parkinsonian syndrome and drug-induced extrapyramidal symptoms

**USUAL DOSAGE** Adults: Oral: 2.5 mg 3 times/day after meals; if tolerated, gradually increase dose, maximum of 20 mg/day if necessary

**Dosing adjustment in hepatic impairment:** Decrease dose to a twice daily dosing regimen

**Dosage Forms** Tab, as hydrochloride: 5 mg

**Contraindications** Angle-closure glaucoma; safe use in children not established

**Warnings/Precautions** Use with caution in hot weather or during exercise. Elderly patients frequently develop increased sensitivity and require strict dosage regulation - side effects may be more severe in elderly patients with atherosclerotic changes. Use with caution in patients with tachycardia, cardiac arrhythmias, hypertension, hypotension, prostatic hypertrophy (especially in the elderly) or any tendency toward urinary retention, liver or kidney disorders and obstructive disease of the GI or GU tract. When given in large doses or to susceptible patients, may cause weakness and inability to move particular muscle groups.

**Pregnancy Risk Factor** C

**Adverse Reactions**

>10%:
Dermatologic: Dry skin
Gastrointestinal: Constipation, xerostomia, dry throat
Respiratory: Dry nose
Miscellaneous: Diaphoresis (decreased)

1% to 10%:
Dermatologic: Increased sensitivity to light
Endocrine & metabolic: Decreased flow of breast milk
Gastrointestinal: Dysphagia

<1%: Orthostatic hypotension, ventricular fibrillation, tachycardia, palpitations, confusion, drowsiness, headache, loss of memory, fatigue, ataxia, rash, bloated feeling, nausea, vomiting, dysuria, weakness, increased intraocular pain, blurred vision

**Drug Interactions**
Decreased effect of psychotropics
Increased toxicity with phenothiazines, meperidine, TCAs

**Onset** Oral: Within 30-40 minutes

**Duration** 4-6 hours

**Special PA Issues**

**Patient Education:** Take exactly as directed (after meals); do not increase, decrease, or discontinue without consulting prescriber. Take at same time each day. Do not use alcohol and all prescription or OTC sedatives or CNS depressants without consulting prescriber. You may experience drowsiness, dizziness, confusion, and blurred vision (use caution when driving, climbing stairs, or engaging in hazardous tasks); increased susceptibility to heat stroke, decreased perspiration (use caution in hot weather - maintain adequate fluids and reduce exercise activity); constipation (increased exercise, fluids, or dietary fruit and fiber may help); dry skin or nasal passages (consult prescriber for appropriate relief). Report unresolved constipation, chest pain or palpitations, difficulty breathing, CNS changes (hallucination, loss of memory, nervousness, etc), painful or difficult urination, increased muscle spasticity or rigidity, skin rash, or significant worsening of condition.

**Dietary Considerations:** Alcohol: Avoid use

◆ **Procyclidine Hydrochloride** *see* Procyclidine *on previous page*

◆ **Prodium® Plain** *see* Psyllium *on page 781*

◆ **Prodium® [OTC]** *see* Phenazopyridine *on page 714*

◆ **Profasi® HP** *see* Chorionic Gonadotropin *on page 205*

◆ **Profenal®** *see* Suprofen *on page 867*

◆ **Progestasert®** *see* Progesterone *on this page*

# Progesterone (proe JES ter one)

**Pharmacologic Class** Progestin

**U.S. Brand Names** Crinone™ Vaginal Gel; Progestasert®

**Mechanism of Action** Natural steroid hormone that induces secretory changes in the endometrium, promotes mammary gland development, relaxes uterine smooth muscle, blocks follicular maturation and ovulation, and maintains pregnancy

**Use** Intrauterine contraception in women who have had at least 1 child, are in a stable, mutually monogamous relationship, and have no history of pelvic inflammatory disease; amenorrhea; functional uterine bleeding; replacement therapy

**USUAL DOSAGE** Adults:

Amenorrhea: I.M.: 5-10 mg/day for 6-8 consecutive days

Functional uterine bleeding: I.M.: 5-10 mg/day for 6 doses

Contraception: Female: Intrauterine device: Insert a single system into the uterine cavity; contraceptive effectiveness is retained for 1 year and system must be replaced 1 year after insertion

Replacement therapy: Gel: Administer 90 mg once daily in women who require progesterone supplementation

(Continued)

## Progesterone *(Continued)*

**Dosage Forms Gel, single use:** 8% (90 mg applicator); **Intrauterine system, reservoir:** 38 mg in silicone fluid

**Contraindications** Pregnancy, thrombophlebitis, undiagnosed vaginal bleeding, hypersensitivity to progesterone or any component, carcinoma of the breast, cerebral apoplexy

**Warnings/Precautions** Use with caution in patients with impaired liver function, depression, diabetes, and epilepsy; use of any progestin during the first 4 months of pregnancy is not recommended; monitor closely for loss of vision, proptosis, diplopia, migraine, and signs and symptoms of embolic disorders. Not a progestin of choice in the elderly for hormonal cycling.

**Pregnancy Risk Factor** X

**Adverse Reactions**

Intrauterine device:

>10%:

Cardiovascular: Edema

Endocrine & metabolic Breakthrough bleeding, spotting, changes in menstrual flow, amenorrhea

Gastrointestinal: Anorexia

Neuromuscular & skeletal: Weakness

1% to 10%:

Cardiovascular: Embolism, central thrombosis

Central nervous system: Mental depression, fever, insomnia

Dermatologic: Melasma or chloasma, allergic rash with or without pruritus

Endocrine: Changes in cervical erosion and secretions, increased breast tenderness

Gastrointestinal: Weight gain or loss

Hepatic: Cholestatic jaundice

Injection (I.M.):

>10% Local: Pain at injection site

1% to 10%: Local: Thrombophlebitis

**Drug Interactions** CYP3A3/4 enzyme substrate; CYP3A3/4 enzyme inducer

Decreased effect: Aminoglutethimide may decrease effect by increasing hepatic metabolism

**Duration** 24 hours

**Half-Life** 5 minutes

**Special PA Issues**

**Patient Education:** This drug can only be given I.M. on a daily basis for a specific number of days (or inserted vaginally to remain for 1 year as a contraceptive). It is important that you you have an annual physical assessment, Pap smear, and vision assessment while taking this medication. You may experience increased facial hair or loss of head hair (reversible); photosensitivity (use sunblock, wear protective clothing, and avoid excessive exposure to sunlight); loss of appetite (small frequent meals will help); constipation (increased fluids, exercise, dietary fiber, or stool softeners may help). Diabetics should use accurate serum glucose testing to identify any changes in glucose tolerance. Report immediately pain or muscle soreness; swelling, heat, or redness in calves; shortness of breath; sudden loss of vision; unresolved leg or foot swelling; change in menstrual pattern (unusual bleeding, amenorrhea, breakthrough spotting); breast tenderness that does not go away; acute abdominal cramping; signs of vaginal infection (drainage, pain, itching); or changes in CNS (eg, blurred vision, confusion, acute anxiety, or unresolved depression).

**Monitoring Parameters:** Before starting therapy, a physical exam including the breasts and pelvis are recommended, also a PAP smear; signs or symptoms of depression, glucose in diabetics

## Promazine *(PROE ma zeen)*

**Pharmacologic Class** Antipsychotic Agent, Phenothiazine, Aliphatic

**U.S. Brand Names** Sparine®

**Mechanism of Action** Blocks postsynaptic mesolimbic dopaminergic $D_1$ and $D_2$ receptors in the brain; exhibits a strong alpha-adrenergic blocking and anticholinergic effect, depresses the release of hypothalamic and hypophyseal hormones; believed to depress the reticular activating system thus affecting basal metabolism, body temperature, wakefulness, vasomotor tone, and emesis

**Use** Management of manifestations of psychotic disorders; depressive neurosis; alcohol withdrawal; nausea and vomiting; nonpsychotic symptoms associated with dementia in elderly, Tourette's syndrome; Huntington's chorea; spasmodic torticollis and Reye's syndrome

**USUAL DOSAGE** Oral, I.M.:

Children >12 years: Antipsychotic: 10-25 mg every 4-6 hours

Adults:

Psychosis: 10-200 mg every 4-6 hours not to exceed 1000 mg/day

Antiemetic: 25-50 mg every 4-6 hours as needed

Hemodialysis: Not dialyzable (0% to 5%)

**Dosage Forms** Promazine hydrochloride: **Inj:** 25 mg/mL (10 mL); 50 mg/mL (1 mL, 2 mL, 10 mL); **Tab:** 25 mg, 50 mg, 100 mg

**Contraindications** Hypersensitivity to promazine or any component; severe CNS depression, cross-sensitivity to other phenothiazines may exist; avoid use in patients with narrow-angle glaucoma, blood dyscrasias, severe liver or cardiac disease; subcortical brain damage; circulatory collapse; severe hypotension or hypertension

**Warnings/Precautions**

Tardive dyskinesia: Prevalence rate may be 40% in elderly; development of the syndrome and the irreversible nature are proportional to duration and total cumulative dose over time. May be reversible if diagnosed early in therapy.

Extrapyramidal reactions are more common in elderly with up to 50% developing these reactions after 60 years of age. These reactions may be more common in dementia patients.

Drug-induced **Parkinson's syndrome** occurs often. **Akathisia** is the most common extrapyramidal reaction in elderly.

Increased confusion, memory loss, psychotic behavior, and agitation frequently occur as a consequence of anticholinergic effects

Orthostatic hypotension is due to alpha-receptor blockade, the elderly are at greater risk for orthostatic hypotension

Antipsychotic associated sedation in nonpsychotic patients is extremely unpleasant due to feelings of depersonalization, derealization, and dysphoria

Life-threatening arrhythmias have occurred at therapeutic doses of antipsychotics; use with caution in patients with narrow-angle glaucoma, severe liver disease or severe cardiac disease

**Pregnancy Risk Factor** C

**Adverse Reactions**

>10%:

Cardiovascular: Hypotension, orthostatic hypotension

Central nervous system: Pseudoparkinsonism, akathisia, dystonias, tardive dyskinesia (persistent), dizziness

Gastrointestinal: Constipation

Ocular: Pigmentary retinopathy

Respiratory: Nasal congestion

Miscellaneous: Diaphoresis (decreased)

1% to 10%:

Dermatologic: Increased sensitivity to sun, rash

Endocrine & metabolic: Changes in menstrual cycle, changes in libido, breast pain

Gastrointestinal: Weight gain, nausea, vomiting, stomach pain

Genitourinary: Dysuria, ejaculatory disturbances

Neuromuscular & skeletal: Trembling of fingers

<1%: Neuroleptic malignant syndrome (NMS), impairment of temperature regulation, lowering of seizures threshold, discoloration of skin (blue-gray), pigmentary retinopathy, galactorrhea, priapism, agranulocytosis, leukopenia, cholestatic jaundice, hepatotoxicity, cornea and lens changes

**Half-Life** The specific pharmacokinetics of promazine are poorly established but probably resemble those of other phenothiazines. Most phenothiazines have long half-lives in the range of 24 hours or more.

**Special PA Issues**

**Patient Education:** Use exactly as directed (do not increase dose or frequency); may cause physical and/or psychological dependence. It may take 2-3 weeks to achieve desired results; do not discontinue without consulting prescriber. Dilute oral concentration with milk, water, or citrus juice; drink immediately after mixing. Do not take within 2 hours of any antacid. Avoid excess alcohol or caffeine and other prescription or OTC medications not approved by prescriber. Maintain adequate hydration (2-3 L/day of fluids unless instructed to restrict fluid intake). Avoid skin contact with medication; may cause contact dermatitis (wash immediately with warm, soapy water). You may experience excess drowsiness, restlessness, dizziness, or blurred vision (use caution driving or when

(Continued)

## Promazine *(Continued)*

engaging in hazardous tasks until response to medication is known); dry mouth, nausea, vomiting (small frequent meals, frequent mouth care, or sucking lozenges may help); constipation (increased exercise, fluids, or dietary fruit and fiber may help); postural hypotension (use caution climbing stairs or when changing position from lying or sitting to standing); urinary retention (void before taking medication); photosensitivity (use sunscreen, protective clothing, and avoid prolonged exposure to direct sunlight); or decreased perspiration (avoid strenuous exercise in hot environments). Report persistent CNS effects (eg, trembling fingers, altered gait or balance, excessive sedation, seizures, unusual muscle or skeletal movements, anxiety, abnormal thoughts, confusion, personality changes); chest pain, palpitations, rapid heartbeat, severe dizziness; unresolved urinary retention or changes in urinary pattern; menstrual pattern changes, change in libido or ejaculatory difficulty; vision changes; skin rash or yellowing of skin; difficulty breathing; or worsening of condition.

### Related Information

Antipsychotic Agents *on page 1001*

♦ **Promazine Hydrochloride** *see* Promazine *on page 766*

♦ **Prometa®** *see* Metaproterenol *on page 575*

## Promethazine *(proe METH a zeen)*

**Pharmacologic Class** Antiemetic

**U.S. Brand Names** Anergan®; Phenazine®; Phenergan®; Prorex®

**Mechanism of Action** Blocks postsynaptic mesolimbic dopaminergic receptors in the brain; exhibits a strong alpha-adrenergic blocking effect and depresses the release of hypothalamic and hypophyseal hormones; competes with histamine for the $H_1$-receptor; reduces stimuli to the brainstem reticular system

**Use** Symptomatic treatment of various allergic conditions, antiemetic, motion sickness, and as a sedative

### USUAL DOSAGE

Children:

Antihistamine: Oral, rectal: 0.1 mg/kg/dose every 6 hours during the day and 0.5 mg/kg/dose at bedtime as needed

Antiemetic: Oral, I.M., I.V., rectal: 0.25-1 mg/kg 4-6 times/day as needed

Motion sickness: Oral, rectal: 0.5 mg/kg/dose 30 minutes to 1 hour before departure, then every 12 hours as needed

Sedation: Oral, I.M., I.V., rectal: 0.5-1 mg/kg/dose every 6 hours as needed

Adults:

Antihistamine (including allergic reactions to blood or plasma):

Oral, rectal: 12.5 mg 3 times/day and 25 mg at bedtime

I.M., I.V.: 25 mg, may repeat in 2 hours when necessary; switch to oral route as soon as feasible

Antiemetic: Oral, I.M., I.V., rectal: 12.5-25 mg every 4 hours as needed

Motion sickness: Oral, rectal: 25 mg 30-60 minutes before departure, then every 12 hours as needed

Sedation: Oral, I.M., I.V., rectal: 25-50 mg/dose

Hemodialysis: Not dialyzable (0% to 5%)

**Dosage Forms** Promethazine hydrochloride: **Inj:** 25 mg/mL (1 mL, 10 mL), 50 mg/mL (1 mL, 10 mL); **Supp, rectal:** 12.5 mg, 25 mg, 50 mg; **Syr:** 6.25 mg/5 mL (5 mL, 120 mL, 240 mL, 480 mL, 4000 mL), 25 mg/5 mL (120 mL, 480 mL, 4000 mL); **Tab:** 12.5 mg, 25 mg, 50 mg

**Contraindications** Hypersensitivity to promethazine or any component; narrow-angle glaucoma

**Warnings/Precautions** Do not administer S.C. or intra-arterially, necrotic lesions may occur; injection may contain sulfites which may cause allergic reactions in some patients; use with caution in patients with cardiovascular disease, impaired liver function, asthma, sleep apnea, seizures. Rapid I.V. administration may produce a transient fall in blood pressure, rate of administration should not exceed 25 mg/minute; slow I.V. administration may produce a slightly elevated blood pressure. Because promethazine is a phenothiazine (and can, therefore, cause side effects such as extrapyramidal symptoms), it is not considered an antihistamine of choice in the elderly.

**Pregnancy Risk Factor** C

**Pregnancy Implications**

Clinical effects on the fetus: Crosses the placenta. Possible respiratory depression if drug is administered near time of delivery; behavioral changes, EEG alterations, impaired platelet aggregation reported with use during labor. Available evidence with use of occasional low doses suggests safe use during pregnancy.

Breast-feeding/lactation: No data available. American Academy of Pediatrics makes NO RECOMMENDATION.

### Adverse Reactions

Hematologic: Thrombocytopenia

Hepatic: Jaundice

>10%:
  Central nervous system: Slight to moderate drowsiness
  Respiratory: Thickening of bronchial secretions
1% to 10%:
  Central nervous system: Headache, fatigue, nervousness, dizziness
  Gastrointestinal: Xerostomia, abdominal pain, nausea, diarrhea, increased appetite, weight gain
  Neuromuscular & skeletal: Arthralgia
  Respiratory: Pharyngitis
<1%: Tachycardia, bradycardia, palpitations, hypotension, sedation (pronounced), confusion, excitation, extrapyramidal reactions with high doses, dystonia, faintness with I.V. administration, depression, insomnia, photosensitivity, rash, angioedema, urinary retention, hepatitis, tremor, paresthesia, myalgia, blurred vision, irregular respiration, bronchospasm, epistaxis, allergic reactions

**Drug Interactions** CYP2D6 enzyme substrate
  Increased toxicity: Epinephrine should not be used together with promethazine since blood pressure may decrease further; additive effects with other CNS depressants

**Onset** I.V.: Within 20 minutes (3-5 minutes with I.V. injection)

**Duration** 2-6 hours

**Special PA Issues**
  **Patient Education:** Take this drug as prescribed; do not increase dosage. Do not use alcohol or other CNS depressants or sleeping aids without consulting prescriber. May cause dizziness, drowsiness, or blurred vision (use caution when driving or engaging in hazardous activities until effect of medication is known); nausea, dry mouth, appetite disturbances (small frequent meals, frequent mouth care, or sucking on lozenges may help). Report unusual weight gain, unresolved nausea or diarrhea, chest pain or palpitations, excess sedation or stimulation, or sore throat or difficulty breathing.

# Promethazine and Codeine (proe METH a zeen & KOE deen)
**Pharmacologic Class** Antihistamine/Antitussive
**U.S. Brand Names** Phenergan® With Codeine; Pherazine® With Codeine; Prothazine-DC®
**Dosage Forms Syr:** Promethazine hydrochloride 6.25 mg and codeine phosphate 10 mg per 5 mL (120 mL, 180 mL, 473 mL)

# Promethazine and Dextromethorphan
(proe METH a zeen & deks troe meth OR fan)
**Pharmacologic Class** Antihistamine/Antitussive
**U.S. Brand Names** Phenameth® DM; Phenergan® With Dextromethorphan; Pherazine® w/ DM
**Dosage Forms Syr:** Promethazine hydrochloride 6.25 mg and dextromethorphan hydrobromide 15 mg per 5 mL with alcohol 7% (120 mL, 480 mL, 4000 mL)

# Promethazine and Phenylephrine (proe METH a zeen & fen il EF rin)
**Pharmacologic Class** Antihistamine/Decongestant Combination
**U.S. Brand Names** Phenergan® VC Syrup; Promethazine VC Plain Syrup; Promethazine VC Syrup; Prometh VC Plain Liquid
**Dosage Forms Liq:** Promethazine hydrochloride 6.25 mg and phenylephrine hydrochloride 5 mg per 5 mL (120 mL, 240 mL, 473 mL)

♦ **Promethazine Hydrochloride** see Promethazine on previous page

# Promethazine, Phenylephrine, and Codeine
(proe METH a zeen, fen il EF rin, & KOE deen)
**Pharmacologic Class** Antihistamine/Decongestant/Antitussive
**U.S. Brand Names** Phenergan® VC With Codeine; Pherazine® VC w/ Codeine; Promethist® With Codeine; Prometh® VC With Codeine
**Dosage Forms Liq:** Promethazine hydrochloride 6.25 mg, phenylephrine hydrochloride 5 mg, and codeine phosphate 10 mg per 5 mL with alcohol 7% (120 mL, 240 mL, 480 mL, 4000 mL)

♦ **Promethazine VC Plain Syrup** see Promethazine and Phenylephrine on this page
♦ **Promethazine VC Syrup** see Promethazine and Phenylephrine on this page
♦ **Promethist® With Codeine** see Promethazine, Phenylephrine, and Codeine on this page
♦ **Prometh VC Plain Liquid** see Promethazine and Phenylephrine on this page
♦ **Prometh® VC With Codeine** see Promethazine, Phenylephrine, and Codeine on this page
♦ **Promine®** see Procainamide on page 759
♦ **Pronestyl®** see Procainamide on page 759
♦ **Pronto® Shampoo [OTC]** see Pyrethrins on page 783
♦ **Propacet®** see Propoxyphene and Acetaminophen on page 774
♦ **Propaderm®** see Beclomethasone on page 101

## Propafenone (proe pa FEEN one)

**Pharmacologic Class** Antiarrhythmic Agent, Class I-C

**U.S. Brand Names** Rythmol®

**Mechanism of Action** Propafenone is a 1C antiarrhythmic agent which possesses local anesthetic properties, blocks the fast inward sodium current, and slows the rate of increase of the action potential. prolongs conduction and refractoriness in all areas of the myocardium, with a slightly more pronounced effect on intraventricular conduction; it prolongs effective refractory period, reduces spontaneous automaticity and exhibits some beta-blockade activity.

**Use** Life-threatening ventricular arrhythmias

**Unlabeled use:** Supraventricular tachycardias, including those patients with Wolff-Parkinson-White syndrome

**USUAL DOSAGE** Adults: Oral: 150 mg every 8 hours, increase at 3- to 4-day intervals up to 300 mg every 8 hours. **Note:** Patients who exhibit significant widening of QRS complex or second or third degree A-V block may need dose reduction.

**Dosing adjustment in hepatic impairment:** Reduction is necessary

**Dosage Forms Tab, as hydrochloride:** 150 mg, 225 mg, 300 mg

**Contraindications** Hypersensitivity to propafenone or any component; uncontrolled congestive heart failure; bronchospastic disorders; cardiogenic shock, conduction disorders (A-V block, sick-sinus syndrome), bradycardia

**Warnings/Precautions** Until evidence to the contrary, propafenone should be considered acceptable only for the treatment of life-threatening arrhythmias; propafenone may cause new or worsened arrhythmias, worsen CHF, decrease A-V conduction and alter pacemaker thresholds; use with caution in patients with recent myocardial infarction, congestive heart failure, hepatic or renal dysfunction; elderly may be at greater risk for toxicity

**Pregnancy Risk Factor** C

**Adverse Reactions**

>10%: Central nervous system: Dizziness (6.5%), drowsiness

1% to 10%:

Cardiovascular: A-V block (first (4.5%) and second (1.2%) degree), cardiac conduction disturbances (eg, bundle-branch block (1.2%)), palpitations (2% to 4%), congestive heart failure, angina (1.2%), bradycardia

Central nervous system: Headache (4.5%), anxiety (2%), loss of balance (1.2%)

Gastrointestinal: Abnormal taste (7.3%), constipation (4%), nausea (1.2%), vomiting (2.8%), abdominal pain, dyspepsia, anorexia (1.6%), flatulence (1.2%), diarrhea (1.2%), xerostomia (2%)

Ocular: Blurred vision (2%)

Respiratory: Dyspnea (2%)

<1%: New or worsened arrhythmias (proarrhythmic effect), bundle-branch block, abnormal speech, vision, or dreams; leukopenia, thrombocytopenia, agranulocytosis, paresthesias, numbness, (+) ANA titers

**Drug Interactions** CYP1A2, 2D6, 3A3/4 enzyme substrate; CYP2D6 enzyme inhibitor

Decreased levels with rifampin

Increased levels/toxicity with cimetidine, quinidine, and beta-blockers; avoid use with ritonavir due to increased risk of propafenone toxicity especially cardiotoxicity

Increased effect/levels of warfarin, beta-blockers metabolized by the liver, local anesthetics, cyclosporine, and digoxin **(Note:** Reduce dose of digoxin by 25%)

**Half-Life** After a single dose (100-300 mg): 2-8 hours; half-life after chronic dosing ranges from 10-32 hours

**Special PA Issues**

**Patient Education:** Take exactly as directed; do not take additional doses or discontinue without consulting prescriber. You will need regular cardiac check-ups and blood tests while taking this medication. You may experience dizziness, drowsiness, or visual changes (use caution when driving or performing tasks that require alertness until response to drug is determined; abnormal taste, nausea or vomiting, or loss of appetite (small frequent meals, frequent mouth care, or sucking lozenges may help); headaches (prescriber may recommend mild analgesic); or diarrhea (exercise, yogurt, or boiled milk may help - if persistent consult prescriber). Report chest pain, palpitation, or erratic heartbeat; difficulty breathing, increased weight or swelling of hands or feet; acute persistent diarrhea or constipation; or changes in vision.

**Monitoring Parameters:** EKG, blood pressure, pulse (particularly at initiation of therapy)

♦ **Propafenone Hydrochloride** see Propafenone on this page

♦ **Propagest® [OTC]** see Phenylpropanolamine on page 720

## Propantheline (proe PAN the leen)

**Pharmacologic Class** Anticholinergic Agent

**U.S. Brand Names** Pro-Banthine®

**Use** Adjunctive treatment of peptic ulcer, irritable bowel syndrome, pancreatitis, ureteral and urinary bladder spasm; reduce duodenal motility during diagnostic radiologic procedures

**USUAL DOSAGE** Oral:

Antisecretory:

Children: 1-2 mg/kg/day in 3-4 divided doses

Adults: 15 mg 3 times/day before meals or food and 30 mg at bedtime

Elderly: 7.5 mg 3 times/day before meals and at bedtime

Antispasmodic:

Children: 2-3 mg/kg/day in divided doses every 4-6 hours and at bedtime

Adults: 15 mg 3 times/day before meals or food and 30 mg at bedtime

**Dosage Forms Tab, as bromide:** 7.5 mg, 15 mg

**Contraindications** Narrow-angle glaucoma, known hypersensitivity to propantheline; ulcerative colitis; toxic megacolon; obstructive disease of the GI or urinary tract

**Pregnancy Risk Factor** C

**Onset** Oral: Within 30-45 minutes

**Duration** 4-6 hours

**Special PA Issues**

**Patient Education:** Take as directed; 30 minutes prior to meals and at bedtime. Always empty bladder before taking medication. Frequent mouth care and sips of water, chewing gum, or sucking on lozenges may reduce dry mouth. You may experience drowsiness, dizziness, or blurred vision; use caution when driving or engaging in hazardous tasks. You may be more sensitive to light (wear sunglasses in bright sunlight), impotence (temporary), decreased sweating and increased sensitivity to heat (avoid excessively hot environments). Report rash, eye pain or acute sensitivity to light, unresolved constipation (increased fluids and dietary fiber may help), palpitations, respiratory problems, difficulty swallowing, loss of sensation, or CNS changes.

## Proparacaine (proe PAR a kane)

**Pharmacologic Class** Local Anesthetic

**U.S. Brand Names** AK-Taine®; Alcaine®; I-Paracaine®; Ophthetic®

**Mechanism of Action** Prevents initiation and transmission of impulse at the nerve cell membrane by decreasing ion permeability through stabilizing

**Use** Anesthesia for tonometry, gonioscopy; suture removal from cornea; removal of corneal foreign body; cataract extraction, glaucoma surgery; short operative procedure involving the cornea and conjunctiva

**USUAL DOSAGE** Children and Adults:

Ophthalmic surgery: Instill 1 drop of 0.5% solution in eye every 5-10 minutes for 5-7 doses

Tonometry, gonioscopy, suture removal: Instill 1-2 drops of 0.5% solution in eye just prior to procedure

**Dosage Forms Ophth, soln, as hydrochloride:** 0.5% (2 mL, 15 mL)

**Contraindications** Known hypersensitivity to proparacaine

**Warnings/Precautions** Use with caution in patients with cardiac disease, hyperthyroidism; for typical ophthalmic use only; prolonged use not recommended

**Pregnancy Risk Factor** C

**Adverse Reactions**

1% to 10%: Local: Burning, stinging, redness

<1%: Arrhythmias, CNS depression, allergic contact dermatitis, irritation, sensitization, lacrimation, keratitis, iritis, erosion of the corneal epithelium, conjunctival congestion and hemorrhage, corneal opacification, blurred vision, diaphoresis (increased)

**Drug Interactions** Increased effect of phenylephrine, tropicamide

**Special PA Issues**

**Patient Education:** May slow wound healing; use sparingly, avoid touching or rubbing the eye until anesthesia has worn off

## Proparacaine and Fluorescein (proe PAR a kane & FLURE e seen)

**Pharmacologic Class** Diagnostic Agent, Ophthalmic Dye; Local Anesthetic

**U.S. Brand Names** Fluoracaine® Ophthalmic

**Mechanism of Action** Prevents initiation and transmission of impulse at the nerve cell membrane by decreasing ion permeability through stabilizing

**Use** Anesthesia for tonometry, gonioscopy; suture removal from cornea; removal of corneal foreign body; cataract extraction, glaucoma surgery

**USUAL DOSAGE**

Ophthalmic surgery: Children and Adults: Instill 1 drop in each eye every 5-10 minutes for 5-7 doses

Tonometry, gonioscopy, suture removal: Adults: Instill 1-2 drops in each eye just prior to procedure

**Dosage Forms Soln:** Proparacaine hydrochloride 0.5% and fluorescein sodium 0.25% (2 mL, 5 mL)

**Contraindications** Known hypersensitivity to proparacaine or fluorescein or any component or ester-type local anesthetics

**Warnings/Precautions** Use with caution in patients with cardiac disease, hyperthyroidism; for topical ophthalmic use only; prolonged use not recommended

**Pregnancy Risk Factor** C

(Continued)

## Proparacaine and Fluorescein *(Continued)*

### Adverse Reactions
1% to 10%: Local: Burning, stinging of eye

<1%: Allergic contact dermatitis, irritation, sensitization, erosion of the corneal epithelium, conjunctival congestion and hemorrhage, keratitis, iritis, corneal opacification

### Special PA Issues
**Patient Education:** May slow wound healing; use sparingly, avoid touching or rubbing the eye until anesthesia has worn off

♦ **Proparacaine Hydrochloride** *see* Proparacaine *on previous page*

♦ **Propecia®** *see* Finasteride *on page 371*

♦ **Prophylaxis for Patients Exposed to Common Communicable Diseases** *see* Chart *on page 1108*

♦ **Propine® Ophthalmic** *see* Dipivefrin *on page 292*

♦ **Pro-Piroxicam®** *see* Piroxicam *on page 733*

## Propofol *(PROE po fole)*

**Pharmacologic Class** General Anesthetic

**U.S. Brand Names** Diprivan®

**Mechanism of Action** Propofol is a hindered phenolic compound with intravenous general anesthetic properties. The drug is unrelated to any of the currently used barbiturate, opioid, benzodiazepine, arylcyclohexylamine, or imidazole intravenous anesthetic agents.

**Use** Induction or maintenance of anesthesia for inpatient or outpatient surgery; may be used (for patients >18 years of age who are intubated and mechanically ventilated) as an alternative to benzodiazepines for the treatment of agitation in the intensive care unit; pain should be treated with analgesic agents, propofol must be titrated separately from the analgesic agent; has demonstrated antiemetic properties in the postoperative setting

**USUAL DOSAGE** Dosage must be individualized based on total body weight and titrated to the desired clinical effect; however, as a general guideline:

No pediatric dose has been established; however, induction for children 1-12 years 2-2.8 mg/kg has been used

Induction: I.V.:

Adults ≤55 years, and/or ASA I or II patients: 2-2.5 mg/kg of body weight (approximately 40 mg every 10 seconds until onset of induction)

Elderly, debilitated, hypovolemic, and/or ASA III or IV patients: 1-1.5 mg/kg of body weight (approximately 20 mg every 10 seconds until onset of induction)

Maintenance: I.V. infusion:

Adults ≤55 years, and/or ASA I or II patients: 0.1-0.2 mg/kg of body weight/minute (6-12 mg/kg of body weight/hour)

Elderly, debilitated, hypovolemic, and/or ASA III or IV patients: 0.05-0.1 mg/kg of body weight/minute (3-6 mg/kg of body weight/hour)

I.V. intermittent: 25-50 mg increments, as needed

ICU sedation: Rapid bolus injection should be avoided. Bolus injection can result in hypotension, oxyhemoglobin desaturation, apnea, airway obstruction, and oxygen desaturation. The preferred route of administration is slow infusion. Doses are based on individual need and titrated to response.

Recommended starting dose: 5 mcg/kg/minute (0.3-0.6 mg/kg/hour) over 5-10 minutes may be used until the desired level of sedation is achieved; infusion rate should be increased by increments of 5-10 mcg/kg/minute (0.3-0.6 mg/kg/hour) until the desired level of sedation is achieved; most adult patients require maintenance rates of 5-50 mcg/kg/minute (0.3-3 mg/kg/hour) or higher

Adjustments in dose can occur at 3- to 5-minute intervals. An 80% reduction in dose should be considered in elderly, debilitated, and ASA III or IV patients. Once sedation is established, the dose should be decreased for the maintenance infusion period and adjusted to response.

**Dosage Forms Inj:** 10 mg/mL (20 mL, 50 mL, 100 mL)

### Contraindications

**Absolute contraindications:**

Patients with a hypersensitivity to propofol

Patients with a hypersensitivity to propofol's emulsion which contains soybean oil, egg phosphatide, and glycerol or any of the components

Patients who are not intubated or mechanically ventilated

Patients who are pregnant or nursing: Propofol is not recommended for obstetrics, including cesarian section deliveries. Propofol crosses the placenta and, therefore, may be associated with neonatal depression.

**Relative contraindications:**

Pediatric Intensive Care Unit patients: Safety and efficacy of propofol is not established

Patients with severe cardiac disease (ejection fraction <50%) or respiratory disease - propofol may have more profound adverse cardiovascular responses

Patients with a history of epilepsy or seizures

Patients with increased intracranial pressure or impaired cerebral circulation - substantial decreases in mean arterial pressure and subsequent decreases in cerebral perfusion pressure may occur

Patients with hyperlipidemia as evidenced by increased serum triglyceride levels or serum turbidity

Patients who are hypotensive, hypovolemic, or hemodynamically unstable

**Warnings/Precautions** Use slower rate of induction in the elderly; transient local pain may occur during I.V. injection; perioperative myoclonia has occurred; do not administer with blood or blood products through the same I.V. catheter; not for obstetrics, including cesarean section deliveries. Safety and effectiveness has not been established in children. Abrupt discontinuation prior to weaning or daily wake up assessments should be avoided. Abrupt discontinuation can result in rapid awakening, anxiety, agitation, and resistance to mechanical ventilation; not for use in neurosurgical anesthesia.

**Pregnancy Risk Factor** B

**Adverse Reactions**

>10%:

Cardiovascular: Hypotension, intravenous propofol produces a dose-related degree of hypotension and decrease in systemic vascular resistance which is not associated with a significant increase in heart rate or decrease in cardiac output

Local: Pain at injection site occurs at an incidence of 28.5% when administered into smaller veins of hand versus 6% when administered into antecubital veins

Respiratory: Apnea (incidence occurs in 50% to 84% of patients and may be dependent on premedication, speed of administration, dose and presence of hyperventilation and hyperoxia)

1% to 10%:

Anaphylaxis: Several cases of anaphylactic reactions have been reported with propofol

Central nervous system: Dizziness, fever, headache; although propofol has demonstrated anticonvulsant activity, several cases of propofol-induced seizures with opisthotonos have occurred

Gastrointestinal: Nausea, vomiting, abdominal cramps

Respiratory: Cough, apnea

Neuromuscular & skeletal: Twitching

Miscellaneous: Hiccups

**Drug Interactions**

Increased toxicity:

Neuromuscular blockers:

Atracurium: Anaphylactoid reactions (including bronchospasm) have been reported in patients who have received concomitant atracurium and propofol

Vecuronium: Propofol may potentiate the neuromuscular blockade of vecuronium

Central nervous system depressants: Additive CNS depression and respiratory depression may necessitate dosage reduction when used with: Anesthetics, benzodiazepines, opiates, ethanol, narcotics, phenothiazines

Decreased effect: Theophylline: May antagonize the effect of propofol, requiring dosage increases

**Onset** Rapid, 30 seconds

**Duration** 3-10 minutes

**Half-Life** Initial: 40 minutes; Terminal: 1-3 days

**Special PA Issues**

**Monitoring Parameters:** Cardiac monitor, blood pressure monitor, and ventilator required; serum triglyceride levels should be obtained prior to initiation of therapy (ICU setting) and every 3-7 days, thereafter

Vital signs: Blood pressure, heart rate, cardiac output, pulmonary capillary wedge pressure should be monitored

# Propoxyphene (proe POKS i feen)

**Pharmacologic Class** Analgesic, Narcotic

**U.S. Brand Names** Darvon®; Darvon-N®; Dolene®

**Mechanism of Action** Binds to opiate receptors in the CNS, causing inhibition of ascending pain pathways, altering the perception of and response to pain; produces generalized CNS depression

**Use** Management of mild to moderate pain

**USUAL DOSAGE** Oral:

Children: Doses for children are not well established; doses of the hydrochloride of 2-3 mg/kg/d divided every 6 hours have been used

Adults:

Hydrochloride: 65 mg every 3-4 hours as needed for pain; maximum: 390 mg/day

Napsylate: 100 mg every 4 hours as needed for pain; maximum: 600 mg/day

**Dosing comments in renal impairment:** Cl$_{cr}$ <10 mL/minute: Avoid use

Hemodialysis: Not dialyzable (0% to 5%)

**Dosing adjustment in hepatic impairment:** Reduced doses should be used

**Dosage Forms Cap, as hydrochloride:** 65 mg; **Tab, as napsylate:** 100 mg

**Contraindications** Hypersensitivity to propoxyphene or any component

(Continued)

## Propoxyphene *(Continued)*

**Warnings/Precautions** Administer with caution in patients dependent on opiates, substitution may result in acute opiate withdrawal symptoms, use with caution in patients with severe renal or hepatic dysfunction; when given in excessive doses, either alone or in combination with other CNS depressants or propoxyphene products, propoxyphene is a major cause of drug-related deaths; **do not exceed recommended dosage**; tolerance or drug dependence may result from extended use

**Pregnancy Risk Factor** C (D if used for prolonged periods)

**Adverse Reactions**

Percentage unknown: Increased liver enzymes, may increase LFTs; may decrease glucose, urinary 17-OHCS

>10%:

Cardiovascular: Hypotension

Central nervous system: Dizziness, lightheadedness, sedation, paradoxical excitement and insomnia, fatigue, drowsiness

Gastrointestinal: Nausea, vomiting, constipation

Neuromuscular & skeletal: Weakness

1% to 10%:

Central nervous system: Nervousness, headache, restlessness, malaise, confusion

Gastrointestinal: Anorexia, stomach cramps, xerostomia, biliary spasm

Genitourinary: Decreased urination, ureteral spasms

Respiratory: Dyspnea, shortness of breath

<1%: Mental depression hallucinations, paradoxical CNS stimulation, increased intracranial pressure, rash, urticaria, paralytic ileus, psychologic and physical dependence with prolonged use, histamine release

**Drug Interactions** CYP3A3/4 enzyme inhibitor

Decreased effect with charcoal, cigarette smoking

Increased toxicity: CNS depressants may potentiate pharmacologic effects; propoxyphene may inhibit the metabolism and increase the serum concentrations of carbamazepine, phenobarbital, MAO inhibitors, tricyclic antidepressants, and warfarin

**Onset** Onset of effect: Oral: Within 0.5-1 hour

**Duration** 4-6 hours

**Half-Life** Parent drug: 8-24 hours (mean: ~15 hours); Norpropoxyphene: 34 hours

**Special PA Issues**

**Patient Education:** Take as directed; do not take a larger dose or more often than prescribed. Do not use alcohol, other prescription or OTC sedatives, tranquilizers, antihistamines, or pain medications without consulting prescriber. May cause dizziness, drowsiness, or impaired judgment; avoid driving or engaging in hazardous activities. If you experience vomiting or loss of appetite, frequent mouth care, small frequent meals, or sucking on lozenges may help. Increased fluid intake, exercise, fiber in diet may help with constipation (if unresolved consult prescriber). Report unresolved nausea or vomiting, difficulty breathing or shortness of breath, or unusual weakness.

**Dietary Considerations:**

Alcohol: Additive CNS effects, avoid or limit alcohol; watch for sedation

Food: May decrease rate of absorption, but may slightly increase bioavailability

Glucose may cause hyperglycemia; monitor blood glucose concentrations

**Monitoring Parameters:** Pain relief, respiratory and mental status, blood pressure

**Reference Range:**

Therapeutic: Ranges published vary between laboratories and may not correlate with clinical effect

Therapeutic concentration: 0.1-0.4 µg/mL (SI: 0.3-1.2 µmol/L)

Toxic: >0.5 µg/mL (SI: >1.5 µmol/L)

**Related Information**

Narcotic Agonists *on page 1023*

## Propoxyphene and Acetaminophen

(proe POKS i feen & a seet a MIN oh fen)

**Pharmacologic Class** Analgesic, Narcotic

**U.S. Brand Names** Darvocet-N®; Darvocet-N® 100; Genagesic®; Propacet®; Wygesic®

**Dosage Forms Tab:** Darvocet-N®: Propoxyphene napsylate 50 mg and acetaminophen 325 mg, Darvocet-N® 100: Propoxyphene napsylate 100 mg and acetaminophen 650 m, Genagesic®, Wygesic®: Propoxyphene hydrochloride 65 mg and acetaminophen 650 mg

## Propoxyphene and Aspirin (proe POKS i feen & AS pir in)

**Pharmacologic Class** Analgesic, Narcotic

**U.S. Brand Names** Bexophene®; Darvon® Compound-65 Pulvules®

**Dosage Forms Cap:** Propoxyphene hydrochloride 65 mg and aspirin 389 mg with caffeine 32.4 mg; **Tab (Darvon-N® with A.S.A.):** Propoxyphene napsylate 100 mg and aspirin 325 mg

◆ **Propoxyphene Hydrochloride** *see* Propoxyphene *on previous page*

♦ **Propoxyphene Hydrochloride and Acetaminophen** see Propoxyphene and Acetaminophen on previous page

♦ **Propoxyphene Napsylate** see Propoxyphene on page 773

♦ **Propoxyphene Napsylate and Acetaminophen** see Propoxyphene and Acetaminophen on previous page

## Propranolol (proe PRAN oh lole)

**Pharmacologic Class** Antiarrhythmic Agent, Class II; Beta Blocker, Nonselective

**U.S. Brand Names** Betachron E-R®; Inderal®; Inderal® LA

**Mechanism of Action** Nonselective beta-adrenergic blocker (class II antiarrhythmic); competitively blocks response to beta$_1$- and beta$_2$-adrenergic stimulation which results in decreases in heart rate, myocardial contractility, blood pressure, and myocardial oxygen demand

**Use** Management of hypertension, angina pectoris, pheochromocytoma, essential tremor, tetralogy of Fallot cyanotic spells, and arrhythmias (such as atrial fibrillation and flutter, A-V nodal re-entrant tachycardias, and catecholamine-induced arrhythmias); prevention of myocardial infarction, migraine headache; symptomatic treatment of hypertrophic subaortic stenosis

**Unlabeled use:** Tremor due to Parkinson's disease, alcohol withdrawal, aggressive behavior, antipsychotic-induced akathisia, esophageal varices bleeding, anxiety, schizophrenia, acute panic, and gastric bleeding in portal hypertension

## USUAL DOSAGE

Tachyarrhythmias:

Oral:

Children: Initial: 0.5-1 mg/kg/day in divided doses every 6-8 hours; titrate dosage upward every 3-7 days; usual dose: 2-4 mg/kg/day; higher doses may be needed; do not exceed 16 mg/kg/day or 60 mg/day

Adults: 10-30 mg/dose every 6-8 hours

Elderly: Initial: 10 mg twice daily; increase dosage every 3-7 days; usual dosage range: 10-320 mg given in 2 divided doses

I.V.:

Children: 0.01-0.1 mg/kg slow IVP over 10 minutes; maximum dose: 1 mg

Adults: 1 mg/dose slow IVP; repeat every 5 minutes up to a total of 5 mg

Hypertension: Oral:

Children: Initial: 0.5-1 mg/kg/day in divided doses every 6-12 hours; increase gradually every 3-7 days; maximum: 2 mg/kg/24 hours

Adults: Initial: 40 mg twice daily; increase dosage every 3-7 days; usual dose: ≤320 mg divided in 2-3 doses/day; maximum daily dose: 640 mg

Migraine headache prophylaxis: Oral:

Children: 0.6-1.5 mg/kg/day or

≤35 kg: 10-20 mg 3 times/day

>35 kg: 20-40 mg 3 times/day

Adults: Initial: 80 mg/day divided every 6-8 hours; increase by 20-40 mg/dose every 3-4 weeks to a maximum of 160-240 mg/day given in divided doses every 6-8 hours; if satisfactory response not achieved within 6 weeks of starting therapy, drug should be withdrawn gradually over several weeks

Tetralogy spells: Children:

Oral: 1-2 mg/kg/day every 6 hours as needed, may increase by 1 mg/kg/day to a maximum of 5 mg/kg/day, or if refractory may increase slowly to a maximum of 10-15 mg/kg/day

I.V.: 0.15-0.25 mg/kg/dose slow IVP; may repeat in 15 minutes

Thyrotoxicosis:

Adolescents and Adults: Oral: 10-40 mg/dose every 6 hours

Adults: I.V.: 1-3 mg/dose slow IVP as a single dose

Adults: Oral:

Angina: 80-320 mg/day in doses divided 2-4 times/day

Pheochromocytoma: 30-60 mg/day in divided doses

Myocardial infarction prophylaxis: 180-240 mg/day in 3-4 divided doses

Hypertrophic subaortic stenosis: 20-40 mg 3-4 times/day

Essential tremor: 40 mg twice daily initially; maintenance doses: usually 120-320 mg/day

**Dosing adjustment in renal impairment:**

Cl$_{cr}$ 31-40 mL/minute: Administer every 24-36 hours or administer 50% of normal dose

Cl$_{cr}$ 10-30 mL/minute: Administer every 24-48 hours or administer 50% of normal dose

Cl$_{cr}$ <10 mL/minute: Administer every 40-60 hours or administer 25% of normal dose

Hemodialysis: Not dialyzable (0% to 5%); supplemental dose is not necessary

Peritoneal dialysis: Supplemental dose is not necessary

**Dosing adjustment/comments in hepatic disease:** Marked slowing of heart rate may occur in cirrhosis with conventional doses; low initial dose and regular heart rate monitoring

**Dosage Forms Cap, sustained action:** 60 mg, 80 mg, 120 mg, 160 mg; **Inj:** 1 mg/mL (1 mL); **Soln, oral (strawberry-mint flavor):** 4 mg/mL (5 mL, 500 mL); 8 mg/mL (5 mL, 500 mL); **Sol, oral, concentrate:** 80 mg/mL (30 mL); **Tab:** 10 mg, 20 mg, 40 mg, 60 mg, 80 mg (Continued)

## Propranolol *(Continued)*

**Contraindications** Uncompensated congestive heart failure, cardiogenic shock, brady-cardia or heart block, pulmonary edema, severe hyperactive airway disease or chronic obstructive lung disease, Raynaud's disease, hypersensitivity to beta-blockers

**Warnings/Precautions** Safety and efficacy in children have not been established; administer very cautiously to patients with CHF, asthma, diabetes mellitus, hyperthyroidism. Abrupt withdrawal of the drug should be avoided, drug should be discontinued over 1-2 weeks; do not use in pregnant or nursing women; may potentiate hypoglycemia in a diabetic patient and mask signs and symptoms.

### Pregnancy Risk Factor C

### Pregnancy Implications

Clinical effects on the fetus: Crosses the placenta. IUGR, hypoglycemia, bradycardia, respiratory depression, hyperbilirubinemia, polycythemia, polydactyly reported. IUGR probably related to maternal hypertension. Preterm labor has been reported. Available evidence suggests safe use during pregnancy and breast-feeding. Monitor breast-fed infant for symptoms of beta-blockade.

Breast-feeding/lactation: Crosses into breast milk. American Academy of Pediatrics considers **compatible** with breast-feeding.

### Adverse Reactions

>10%:

Cardiovascular: Bradycardia

Central nervous system: Mental depression

Endocrine & metabolic: Decreased sexual ability

1% to 10%:

Cardiovascular: Congestive heart failure, reduced peripheral circulation

Central nervous system: Confusion, hallucinations, dizziness, insomnia, fatigue

Dermatologic: Rash

Gastrointestinal: Diarrhea, nausea, vomiting, stomach discomfort

Neuromuscular & skeletal: Weakness

Respiratory: Wheezing

<1%: Chest pain, hypotension, impaired myocardial contractility, worsening of A-V conduction disturbances, nightmares, vivid dreams, lethargy, red, scaling, or crusted skin; hypoglycemia, hyperglycemia, GI distress, leukopenia, thrombocytopenia, agranulocytosis, bronchospasm, cold extremities

### Drug Interactions CYP1A2, 2C18, 2C19, and 2D6 enzyme substrate

Decreased effect:

Aluminum salts, barbiturates, calcium salts, cholestyramine, colestipol, NSAIDs, penicillins (ampicillin), rifampin, salicylates and sulfinpyrazone decrease effect of beta-blockers due to decreased bioavailability and plasma levels

Beta-blockers may decrease the effect of sulfonylureas

Ascorbic acid decreases propranolol $C_{p_{max}}$ and AUC and increases the $T_{max}$ significantly resulting in a greater decrease in the reduction of heart rate, possibly due to decreased absorption and first pass metabolism

Nefazodone decreased peak plasma levels and AUC of propranolol and increases time to reach steady state

Increased effect:

Increased effect/toxicity of beta-blockers with calcium blockers (diltiazem, felodipine, nicardipine), contraceptives, flecainide, haloperidol (hypotensive effects), $H_2$-antagonists (cimetidine, possibly ranitidine), hydralazine, loop diuretics, possibly MAO inhibitors, phenothiazines, propafenone, quinidine (in extensive metabolizers), ciprofloxacin, thyroid hormones (when hypothyroid patient is converted to euthyroid state)

Beta-blockers may increase the effect/toxicity of flecainide, haloperidol (hypotensive effects), hydralazine, phenothiazines, acetaminophen, anticoagulants (warfarin), benzodiazepines, clonidine (hypertensive crisis after or during withdrawal of either agent), epinephrine (initial hypertensive episode followed by bradycardia), nifedipine, verapamil, lidocaine, ergots (peripheral ischemia), prazosin (postural hypotension)

Beta-blockers may affect the action or levels of ethanol, disopyramide, nondepolarizing muscle relaxants and theophylline although the effects are difficult to predict

**Onset** Onset of beta blockade: Oral: Within 1-2 hours

**Duration** ~6 hours

**Half-Life** 4-6 hours

### Special PA Issues

**Patient Education:** Take exactly as directed; do not increase, decrease, or discontinue without consulting prescriber. Take at same time each day. Tablets may be crushed and taken with liquids. Do not alter dietary intake of protein or carbohydrates without consulting prescriber. You may experience orthostatic hypotension, dizziness, drowsiness, or blurred vision (use caution when driving, climbing stairs, or changing position - rising from sitting or lying to standing - or when engaging in hazardous activities until response to medication is known); nausea, vomiting, or stomach discomfort (small frequent meals, chewing gum, or sucking on lozenges may help); decreased sexual ability (reversible). If diabetic, monitor serum glucose closely. Report unusual swelling of extremities, difficulty breathing, unresolved cough, or unusual weight gain, cold extremities, persistent diarrhea, confusion, hallucinations, headache, nervousness, lack of improvement, or worsening of condition.

**Monitoring Parameters:** Blood pressure, EKG, heart rate, CNS and cardiac effects

**Reference Range:** Therapeutic: 50-100 ng/mL (SI: 190-390 nmol/L) at end of dose interval

**Related Information**

Beta-Blockers *on page 1002*

## Propranolol and Hydrochlorothiazide

(proe PRAN oh lole & hye droe klor oh THYE a zide)

**Pharmacologic Class** Antihypertensive Agent, Combination

**U.S. Brand Names** Inderide®

**Dosage Forms Cap, long-acting (Inderide® LA):** 80/50 Propranolol hydrochloride 80 mg and hydrochlorothiazide 50 mg, 120/50 Propranolol hydrochloride 120 mg and hydrochlorothiazide 50 mg, 160/50 Propranolol hydrochloride 160 mg and hydrochlorothiazide 50 mg; **Tab (Inderide®):** 40/25 Propranolol hydrochloride 40 mg and hydrochlorothiazide 25 mg, 80/25 Propranolol hydrochloride 80 mg and hydrochlorothiazide 25 mg

♦ **Propranolol Hydrochloride** *see* Propranolol *on page 775*

♦ **Propulsid®** *see* Cisapride *on page 211*

♦ **2-Propylpentanoic Acid** *see* Valproic Acid and Derivatives *on page 952*

## Propylthiouracil (proe pil thye oh YOOR a sil)

**Pharmacologic Class** Antithyroid Agent

**Mechanism of Action** Inhibits the synthesis of thyroid hormones by blocking the oxidation of iodine in the thyroid gland; blocks synthesis of thyroxine and triiodothyronine

**Use** Palliative treatment of hyperthyroidism as an adjunct to ameliorate hyperthyroidism in preparation for surgical treatment or radioactive iodine therapy and in the management of thyrotoxic crisis. The use of antithyroid thioamides is as effective in elderly as they are in younger adults; however, the expense, potential adverse effects, and inconvenience (compliance, monitoring) make them undesirable. The use of radioiodine, due to ease of administration and less concern for long-term side effects and reproduction problems, makes it a more appropriate therapy.

**USUAL DOSAGE** Oral: Administer in 3 equally divided doses at approximately 8-hour intervals. Adjust dosage to maintain $T_3$, $T_4$, and TSH levels in normal range; elevated $T_3$ may be sole indicator of inadequate treatment. Elevated TSH indicates excessive antithyroid treatment.

Children: Initial: 5-7 mg/kg/day **or** 150-200 mg/m$^2$/day in divided doses every 8 hours
  **or**
  6-10 years: 50-150 mg/day
  >10 years: 150-300 mg/day
  Maintenance: Determined by patient response **or** $1/3$ to $2/3$ of the initial dose in divided doses every 8-12 hours. This usually begins after 2 months on an effective initial dose.
Adults: Initial: 300 mg/day in divided doses every 8 hours. In patients with severe hyperthyroidism, very large goiters, or both, the initial dosage is usually 450 mg/day; an occasional patient will require 600-900 mg/day; maintenance: 100-150 mg/day in divided doses every 8-12 hours
Elderly: Use lower dose recommendations; Initial: 150-300 mg/day
Withdrawal of therapy: Therapy should be withdrawn gradually with evaluation of the patient every 4-6 weeks for the first 3 months then every 3 months for the first year after discontinuation of therapy to detect any reoccurrence of a hyperthyroid state.

**Dosing adjustment in renal impairment:** Adjustment is not necessary

**Dosage Forms Tab:** 50 mg

**Contraindications** Hypersensitivity to propylthiouracil or any component

**Warnings/Precautions** Use with caution in patients >40 years of age because PTU may cause hypoprothrombinemia and bleeding, use with extreme caution in patients receiving other drugs known to cause agranulocytosis; may cause agranulocytosis, thyroid hyperplasia, thyroid carcinoma (usage >1 year); breast-feeding (crosses breast milk)

**Pregnancy Risk Factor** D

**Adverse Reactions**

>10%:
  Central nervous system: Fever
  Dermatologic: Skin rash
  Hematologic: Leukopenia
1% to 10%:
  Central nervous system: Dizziness
  Gastrointestinal: Nausea, vomiting, loss of taste perception, stomach pain
  Hematologic: Agranulocytosis
  Miscellaneous: SLE-like syndrome
<1%: Edema, cutaneous vasculitis, drowsiness, vertigo, headache, drug fever, urticaria, pruritus, exfoliative dermatitis, alopecia, goiter, constipation, weight gain, swollen salivary

(Continued)

## Propylthiouracil *(Continued)*

glands, thrombocytopenia, bleeding, aplastic anemia, cholestatic jaundice, hepatitis, arthralgia, paresthesia, neuritis, nephritis

**Drug Interactions** Increased effect: Increases anticoagulant activity

**Onset** For significant therapeutic effects 24-36 hours are required. Peak effect: Remissions of hyperthyroidism do not usually occur before 4 months of continued therapy.

**Half-Life** 1.5-5 hours; End-stage renal disease: 8.5 hours

**Special PA Issues**

**Patient Education:** Take as directed, at the same time each day around-the-clock; do not miss doses or make up missed doses. This drug will need to be taken for an extended period of time to achieve appropriate results. You may experience nausea or vomiting (small frequent meals may help), dizziness or drowsiness (use caution when driving or engaging in hazardous activities). Report rash, fever, unusual bleeding or bruising, unresolved headache, yellowing of eyes or skin, or changes in color of urine or feces, unresolved malaise.

**Monitoring Parameters:** CBC with differential, prothrombin time, liver function tests, thyroid function tests (TSH, $T_3$, $T_4$); periodic blood counts are recommended chronic therapy

**Reference Range:** See table.

### Laboratory Ranges

| | Normal Values |
|---|---|
| Total $T_4$ | 5-12 µg/dL |
| Serum $T_3$ | 90-185 ng/dL |
| Free thyroxine index ($FT_4$I) | 6-10.5 |
| TSH | 0.5-4.0 µIU/mL |

- **Propyl-Thyracil®** *see* Propylthiouracil *on previous page*
- **2-Propylvaleric Acid** *see* Valproic Acid and Derivatives *on page 952*
- **Prorazin®** *see* Prochlorperazine *on page 763*
- **Prorex®** *see* Promethazine *on page 768*
- **Proscar®** *see* Finasteride *on page 371*
- **ProSom™** *see* Estazolam *on page 331*
- **Prostacyclin** *see* Epoprostenol *on page 324*
- **Prostaglandin E₁** *see* Alprostadil *on page 45*
- **Prostaglandin E₂** *see* Dinoprostone *on page 288*
- **Prostaphlin®** *see* Oxacillin *on page 682*
- **ProStep® Patch** *see* Nicotine *on page 653*
- **Prostigmin®** *see* Neostigmine *on page 646*
- **Prostin E₂® Vaginal Suppository** *see* Dinoprostone *on page 288*
- **Prostin VR Pediatric® Injection** *see* Alprostadil *on page 45*

## Protamine Sulfate *(PROE ta meen SUL fate)*

**Pharmacologic Class** Antidote

**Mechanism of Action** Combines with strongly acidic heparin to form a stable complex (salt) neutralizing the anticoagulant activity of both drugs

**Use** Treatment of heparin overdosage; neutralize heparin during surgery or dialysis procedures

**USUAL DOSAGE** Protamine dosage is determined by the dosage of heparin; 1 mg of protamine neutralizes 90 USP units of heparin (lung) and 115 USP units of heparin (intestinal); maximum dose: 50 mg

In the situation of heparin overdosage, since blood heparin concentrations decrease rapidly **after** administration, adjust the protamine dosage depending upon the duration of time since heparin administration as follows:

| Time Elapsed | Dose of Protamine (mg) to Neutralize 100 units of Heparin |
|---|---|
| Immediate | 1-1.5 |
| 30-60 min | 0.5-0.75 |
| >2 h | 0.25-0.375 |

If heparin administered by deep S.C. injection, use 1-1.5 mg protamine per 100 units heparin; this may be done by a portion of the dose (eg, 25-50 mg) given slowly I.V. followed by the remaining portion as a continuous infusion over 8-16 hours (the expected absorption time of the S.C. heparin dose)

**Dosage Forms Inj:** 10 mg/mL (5 mL, 10 mL, 25 mL)

**Contraindications** Hypersensitivity to protamine or any component

**Warnings/Precautions** May not be totally effective in some patients following cardiac surgery despite adequate doses; may cause hypersensitivity reaction in patients with a history of allergy to fish (have epinephrine 1:1000 available) and in patients sensitized to protamine (via protamine zinc insulin); too rapid administration can cause severe hypotensive and anaphylactoid-like reactions. Heparin rebound associated with anticoagulation and bleeding has been reported to occur occasionally; symptoms typically occur 8-9 hours after protamine administration, but may occur as long as 18 hours later.

**Pregnancy Risk Factor** C

**Adverse Reactions**
>10%:
Cardiovascular: Sudden fall in blood pressure, bradycardia
Respiratory: Dyspnea
1% to 10%: Hemorrhage
<1%: Hypotension, flushing, lassitude, nausea, vomiting, pulmonary hypertension, hypersensitivity reactions

**Onset** I.V. injection: Heparin neutralization occurs within 5 minutes

**Special PA Issues**
Patient Education: Report any difficulty breathing, rash or flushing, feeling of warmth, tingling or numbness, dizziness, or disorientation.
Monitoring Parameters: Coagulation test, APTT or ACT, cardiac monitor and blood pressure monitor required during administration

♦ **Prothazine-DC®** see Promethazine and Codeine on page 769

♦ **Protilase®** see Pancrelipase on page 694

♦ **Protostat® Oral** see Metronidazole on page 601

♦ **Pro-Trin®** see Co-Trimoxazole on page 238

## Protriptyline (proe TRIP ti leen)

**Pharmacologic Class** Antidepressant, Tricyclic (Secondary Amine)

**U.S. Brand Names** Vivactil®

**Mechanism of Action** Increases the synaptic concentration of serotonin and/or norepinephrine in the central nervous system by inhibition of their reuptake by the presynaptic neuronal membrane

**Use** Treatment of various forms of depression, often in conjunction with psychotherapy

**USUAL DOSAGE** Oral:
Adolescents: 15-20 mg/day
Adults: 15-60 mg in 3-4 divided doses
Elderly: 15-20 mg/day

**Dosage Forms Tab, as hydrochloride:** 5 mg, 10 mg

**Contraindications** Narrow-angle glaucoma, hypersensitivity to protriptyline or any component

**Warnings/Precautions** Use with caution in patients with cardiac conduction disturbances, history of hyperthyroid, seizure disorders, or decreased renal function; safe use of tricyclic antidepressants in children <12 years of age has not been established; protriptyline should not be abruptly discontinued in patients receiving high doses for prolonged periods

**Pregnancy Risk Factor** C

**Adverse Reactions**
>10%:
Central nervous system: Dizziness, drowsiness, headache
Gastrointestinal: Xerostomia, constipation, unpleasant taste, weight gain, increased appetite, nausea
Neuromuscular & skeletal: Weakness
1% to 10%:
Cardiovascular: Arrhythmias, hypotension
Central nervous system: Confusion, delirium, hallucinations, nervousness, restlessness, parkinsonian syndrome, insomnia
Gastrointestinal: Diarrhea, heartburn
Genitourinary: Dysuria, sexual dysfunction
Neuromuscular & skeletal: Fine muscle tremors
Ocular: Blurred vision, eye pain
Miscellaneous: Diaphoresis (excessive)
<1%: Anxiety, seizures, alopecia, photosensitivity, breast enlargement, galactorrhea, SIADH, trouble with gums, decreased lower esophageal sphincter tone may cause GE reflux, testicular edema, agranulocytosis, leukopenia, eosinophilia, cholestatic jaundice, increased liver enzymes, increased intraocular pressure, tinnitus, allergic reactions

**Drug Interactions**
Decreased effect of guanethidine; decreased effect with barbiturates, carbamazepine, phenytoin
(Continued)

## Protriptyline *(Continued)*

Increased toxicity of alcohol, MAO inhibitors, sympathomimetics, CNS depressants, anticholinergics (paralytic ileus and hyperpyrexia); increased toxicity with MAO inhibitors (hyperpyretic crisis, convulsions, and death), cimetidine (increased drug levels)

**Onset** Maximum antidepressant effect: 2 weeks of continuous therapy is commonly required

**Half-Life** 54-92 hours, averaging 74 hours

**Special PA Issues**

**Patient Education:** Take exactly as directed (do not increase dose or frequency); may take 2-3 weeks to achieve desired results; may cause physical and/or psychological dependence. Avoid excessive alcohol, caffeine, and other prescription or OTC medications not approved by prescriber. Maintain adequate hydration (2-3 L/day of fluids unless instructed to restrict fluid intake). You may experience drowsiness, lightheadedness, impaired coordination, dizziness, or blurred vision (use caution when driving or engaging in hazardous tasks until response to medication is known); nausea, vomiting, altered taste, dry mouth (small frequent meals, frequent mouth care, or sucking lozenges may help); constipation (increased exercise, fluids, or dietary fruit and fiber may help); diarrhea (buttermilk, yogurt, or boiled milk may help); increased appetite (monitor dietary intake to avoid excess weight gain); postural hypotension (use caution when climbing stairs or changing position from lying or sitting to standing); urinary retention (void before taking medication); or sexual dysfunction (reversible). Report persistent CNS effects (eg, insomnia, nervousness, restlessness, hallucinations, daytime sedation, impaired cognitive function); muscle cramping or tremors; chest pain, palpitations, rapid heartbeat, swelling of extremities, or severe dizziness; blurred vision or eye pain; yellowing of eyes or skin; pale stools/dark urine; or worsening of condition.

**Reference Range:** Therapeutic: 70-250 ng/mL (SI: 266-950 nmol/L); Toxic: >500 ng/mL (SI: >1900 nmol/L)

**Related Information**

Antidepressant Agents *on page 998*

- ◆ **Protriptyline Hydrochloride** *see Protriptyline on previous page*
- ◆ **Protropin® Injection** *see Human Growth Hormone on page 444*
- ◆ **Proventil®** *see Albuterol on page 34*
- ◆ **Proventil® HFA** *see Albuterol on page 34*
- ◆ **Provera®** *see Medroxyprogesterone Acetate on page 561*
- ◆ **Provigil®** *see Modafinil on page 613*
- ◆ **Provisc®** *see Sodium Hyaluronate on page 841*
- ◆ **Provocholine®** *see Methacholine on page 578*
- ◆ **Proxigel® Oral [OTC]** *see Carbamide Peroxide on page 150*
- ◆ **Proxymetacaine** *see Proparacaine on page 771*
- ◆ **Prozac®** *see Fluoxetine on page 386*
- ◆ **PRP-D** *see Haemophilus b Conjugate Vaccine on page 432*
- ◆ **Prymaccone** *see Primaquine Phosphate on page 756*
- ◆ **Pseudo-Car® DM** *see Carbinoxamine, Pseudoephedrine, and Dextromethorphan on page 153*

## Pseudoephedrine *(soo doe e FED rin)*

**Pharmacologic Class** Alpha/Beta Agonist

**U.S. Brand Names** Actifed® Allergy Tablet (Day) [OTC]; Afrin® Tablet [OTC]; Cenafed® [OTC]; Children's Silfedrine® [OTC]; Decofed® Syrup [OTC]; Drixoral® Non-Drowsy [OTC]; Efidac/24® [OTC]; Neofed® [OTC]; PediaCare® Oral; Sudafed® [OTC]; Sudafed® 12 Hour [OTC]; Sufedrin® [OTC]; Triaminic® AM Decongestant Formula [OTC]

**Mechanism of Action** Directly stimulates alpha-adrenergic receptors of respiratory mucosa causing vasoconstriction; directly stimulates beta-adrenergic receptors causing bronchial relaxation, increased heart rate and contractility

**Use** Temporary symptomatic relief of nasal congestion due to common cold, upper respiratory allergies, and sinusitis; also promotes nasal or sinus drainage

**USUAL DOSAGE** Oral:

Children:

<2 years: 4 mg/kg/day in divided doses every 6 hours

2-5 years: 15 mg every 6 hours; maximum: 60 mg/24 hours

6-12 years: 30 mg every 6 hours; maximum: 120 mg/24 hours

Adults: 30-60 mg every 4-6 hours, sustained release: 120 mg every 12 hours; maximum: 240 mg/24 hours

**Dosing adjustment in renal impairment:** Reduce dose

**Dosage Forms** Pseudoephedrine hydrochloride: **Cap:** 60 mg; **Cap, timed release:** 120 mg; **Drops, oral:** 7.5 mg/0.8 mL (15 mL); **Liq:** 15 mg/5 mL (120 mL), 30 mg/5 mL (120 mL, 240 mL, 473 mL); **Syr:** 15 mg/5 mL (118 mL); **Tab:** 30 mg, 60 mg; **Tab, timed release:** 120 mg Pseudoephedrine sulfate: **Extended release:** 120 mg, 240 mg

**Contraindications** Hypersensitivity to pseudoephedrine or any component; MAO inhibitor therapy

**Warnings/Precautions** Use with caution in patients >60 years of age; administer with caution to patients with hypertension, hyperthyroidism, diabetes mellitus, cardiovascular disease, ischemic heart disease, increased intraocular pressure, or prostatic hypertrophy. Elderly patients are more likely to experience adverse reactions to sympathomimetics. Overdosage may cause hallucinations, seizures, CNS depression, and death.

**Pregnancy Risk Factor** C

**Adverse Reactions**

>10%:

Cardiovascular: Tachycardia, palpitations, arrhythmias

Central nervous system: Nervousness, transient stimulation, insomnia, excitability, dizziness, drowsiness, headache

Neuromuscular & skeletal: Tremor

1% to 10%:

Central nervous system: Headache

Neuromuscular & skeletal: Weakness

Miscellaneous: Diaphoresis

<1%: Convulsions, hallucinations, nausea, vomiting, dysuria, shortness of breath, dyspnea

**Drug Interactions**

Decreased effect of methyldopa, reserpine

Increased toxicity: MAO inhibitors may increase blood pressure effects of pseudoephedrine; propranolol, sympathomimetic agents may increase toxicity

**Onset** Decongestant effect: Oral: 15-30 minutes

**Duration** 4-6 hours (up to 12 hours with extended release formulation administration)

**Half-Life** 9-16 hours

**Special PA Issues**

**Patient Education:** Take only as prescribed; do not exceed prescribed dose or frequency. Do not chew or crush timed release capsule. Maintain adequate hydration (2-3 L/day of fluids unless instructed to restrict fluid intake). You may experience nervousness, insomnia, dizziness, or drowsiness (use caution when driving or engaging in hazardous tasks until response to therapy is known). Report persistent CNS changes (dizziness, sedation, tremor, agitation, or convulsions); difficulty breathing; chest pain, palpitations, or rapid heartbeat; muscle tremor; or lack of improvement or worsening or condition.

- ♦ **Pseudoephedrine and Acrivastine** see Acrivastine and Pseudoephedrine on page 27
- ♦ **Pseudoephedrine Hydrochloride** see Pseudoephedrine on previous page
- ♦ **Pseudoephedrine Sulfate** see Pseudoephedrine on previous page
- ♦ **Pseudomonic Acid A** see Mupirocin on page 622
- ♦ **Psorcon™** see Diflorasone on page 278
- ♦ **Psorion® Cream** see Betamethasone on page 111

# Psyllium (SIL i yum)

**Pharmacologic Class** Laxative, Bulk-Producing

**U.S. Brand Names** Effer-Syllium® [OTC]; Fiberall® Powder [OTC]; Fiberall® Wafer [OTC]; Hydrocil® [OTC]; Konsyl-D® [OTC]; Konsyl® [OTC]; Metamucil® [OTC]; Metamucil® Instant Mix [OTC]; Modane® Bulk [OTC]; Perdiem® Plain [OTC]; Reguloid® [OTC]; Serutan® [OTC]; Syllact® [OTC]; V-Lax® [OTC]

**Mechanism of Action** Adsorbs water in the intestine to form a viscous liquid which promotes peristalsis and reduces transit time

**Use** Treatment of chronic atonic or spastic constipation and in constipation associated with rectal disorders; management of irritable bowel syndrome

**USUAL DOSAGE** Oral (administer at least 3 hours before or after drugs):

Children 6-11 years: (Approximately ½ adult dosage) ½ to 1 rounded teaspoonful in 4 oz glass of liquid 1-3 times/day

Adults: 1-2 rounded teaspoonfuls or 1-2 packets or 1-2 wafers in 8 oz glass of liquid 1-3 times/day

**Dosage Forms Granules:** 4.03 g per rounded teaspoon (100 g, 250 g), 2.5 g per rounded teaspoon; **Powder:** Psyllium 50% and dextrose 50% (6.5 g, 325 g, 420 g, 480 g, 500 g); **Powder: Effervescent:** 3 g/dose (270 g, 480 g), 3.4 g/dose (single-dose packets), Psyllium hydrophilic: 3.4 g per rounded teaspoon (210 g, 300 g, 420 g, 630 g); **Squares, chewable:** 1.7 g, 3.4 g; **Wafers:** 3.4 g

**Contraindications** Fecal impaction, GI obstruction, hypersensitivity to psyllium or any component

**Warnings/Precautions** May contain aspartame which is metabolized in the GI tract to phenylalanine which is contraindicated in individuals with phenylketonuria; use with caution in patients with esophageal strictures, ulcers, stenosis, or intestinal adhesions; elderly may have insufficient fluid intake which may predispose them to fecal impaction and bowel obstruction.

**Pregnancy Risk Factor** C

**Adverse Reactions** 1% to 10%:

Gastrointestinal: Esophageal or bowel obstruction, diarrhea, constipation, abdominal cramps

Respiratory: Bronchospasm

(Continued)

## Psyllium *(Continued)*

Miscellaneous: Anaphylaxis upon inhalation in susceptible individuals, rhinoconjunctivitis

**Drug Interactions** Decreased effect of warfarin, digitalis, potassium-sparing diuretics, salicylates, tetracyclines, nitrofurantoin

**Onset** 12-24 hour, but full effect may take 2-3 days; Peak effect: May take 2-3 days

**Special PA Issues**

**Patient Education:** Mix in large (8 oz or more) glass of water or juice and drink immediately. Mix carefully; do not inhale powder. Report unresolved or persistent constipation, watery diarrhea, or respiratory difficulty.

- ♦ **Psyllium Hydrophilic Mucilloid** *see* Psyllium *on previous page*
- ♦ **Pteroylglutamic Acid** *see* Folic Acid *on page 397*
- ♦ **P. trifolius L.** *see* Ginseng *on page 415*
- ♦ **PTU** *see* Propylthiouracil *on page 777*
- ♦ **Pulmicort®** *see* Budesonide *on page 124*
- ♦ **Pulmicort Turbuhaler®** *see* Budesonide *on page 124*
- ♦ **Purinol®** *see* Allopurinol *on page 42*
- ♦ **Purple Coneflower** *see* Echinacea *on page 310*
- ♦ **PVF® K** *see* Penicillin V Potassium *on page 706*
- ♦ **P-V-Tussin®** *see* Hydrocodone, Phenylephrine, Pyrilamine, Phenindamine, Chlorpheniramine, and Ammonium Chloride *on page 453*
- ♦ **P₂E₁® Ophthalmic** *see* Pilocarpine and Epinephrine *on page 727*

## Pyrantel Pamoate *(p RAN tel PAM oh ate)*

**Pharmacologic Class** Anthelmintic

**U.S. Brand Names** Antiminth® [OTC]; Pin-Rid® [OTC]; Pin-X® [OTC]; Reese's® Pinworm Medicine [OTC]

**Mechanism of Action** Causes the release of acetylcholine and inhibits cholinesterase; acts as a depolarizing neuromuscular blocker, paralyzing the helminths

**Use** Treatment of pinworms (*Enterobius vermicularis*), whipworms (*Trichuris trichiura*), roundworms (*Ascaris lumbricoides*), and hookworms (*Ancylostoma duodenale*)

**USUAL DOSAGE** Children and Adults (purgation is not required prior to use): Oral:
Roundworm, pinworm, or trichostrongyliasis: 11 mg/kg administered as a single dose; maximum dose: 1 g. **(Note:** For pinworm infection, dosage should be repeated in 2 weeks and all family members should be treated).

Hookworm: 11 mg/kg administered once daily for 3 days

**Dosage Forms Cap:** 180 mg; **Liq:** 50 mg/mL (30 mL); 144 mg/mL (30 mL); **Susp, oral (caramel-currant flavor)** 50 mg/mL (60 mL)

**Contraindications** Known hypersensitivity to pyrantel pamoate

**Warnings/Precautions** Use with caution in patients with liver impairment, anemia, malnutrition, or pregnancy. Since pinworm infections are easily spread to others, treat all family members in close contact with the patient.

**Pregnancy Risk Factor** C

**Adverse Reactions**

1% to 10%: Gastrointestinal: Anorexia, nausea, vomiting, abdominal cramps, diarrhea

<1%: Dizziness, drowsiness, insomnia, headache, rash, elevated liver enzymes, tenesmus, weakness

**Drug Interactions** Decreased effect with piperazine

**Special PA Issues**

**Patient Education:** May mix drug with milk or fruit juice; strict hygiene is essential to prevent reinfection

**Monitoring Parameters:** Stool for presence of eggs, worms, and occult blood, serum AST and ALT

## Pyrazinamide *(peer a ZIN a mide)*

**Pharmacologic Class** Antitubercular Agent

**Mechanism of Action** Converted to pyrazinoic acid in susceptible strains of *Mycobacterium* which lowers the pH of the environment; exact mechanism of action has not been elucidated

**Use** Adjunctive treatment of tuberculosis in combination with other antituberculosis agents

**USUAL DOSAGE** Oral (calculate dose on ideal body weight rather than total body weight):
**Note:** A four-drug regimen (isoniazid, rifampin, pyrazinamide, and either streptomycin or ethambutol) is preferred for the initial, empiric treatment of TB. When the drug susceptibility results are available, the regimen should be altered as appropriate.

Children and Adults:

Daily therapy: 15-30 mg/kg/day (maximum: 2 g/day)

Directly observed therapy (DOT): Twice weekly: 50-70 mg/kg (maximum: 4 g)

DOT: 3 times/week: 50-70 mg/kg (maximum: 3 g)

Elderly: Start with a lower daily dose (15 mg/kg) and increase as tolerated

**Dosing adjustment in renal impairment:** Cl<sub>cr</sub> $Cl_{cr}$ <50 mL/minute: Avoid use or reduce dose to 12-20 mg/kg/day

**Dosing adjustment in hepatic impairment:** Reduce dose

**Dosage Forms Tab:** 500 mg

**Contraindications** Severe hepatic damage; hypersensitivity to pyrazinamide or any component; acute gout

**Warnings/Precautions** Use with caution in patients with renal failure, chronic gout, diabetes mellitus, or porphyria

**Pregnancy Risk Factor** C

**Adverse Reactions**
1% to 10%:
Central nervous system: Malaise
Gastrointestinal: Nausea, vomiting, anorexia
Neuromuscular & skeletal: Arthralgia, myalgia
<1%: Fever, rash, itching, acne, photosensitivity, gout, dysuria, porphyria, thrombocytopenia, hepatotoxicity, interstitial nephritis

**Half-Life** 9-10 hours, increased with reduced renal or hepatic function; End-stage renal disease: 9 hours

**Special PA Issues**
**Patient Education:** Take with food for full length of therapy. Do not miss doses and do not discontinue without consulting prescriber. You will need regular medical follow-up while taking this medication. You may experience nausea or loss of appetite; small frequent meals, sucking on lozenges, or frequent mouth care may help. Report unusual fever, unresolved nausea or vomiting, change in color of urine, pale stools, easy bruising or bleeding, blood in urine or difficulty urinating, yellowing of skin or eyes, or extreme joint pain.

**Monitoring Parameters:** Periodic liver function tests, serum uric acid, sputum culture, chest x-ray 2-3 months into treatment and at completion

♦ **Pyrazinoic Acid Amide** see Pyrazinamide on previous page

# Pyrethrins (pye RE thrins)

**Pharmacologic Class** Antiparasitic Agent, Topical; Pediculocide; Shampoo, Pediculocide

**U.S. Brand Names** A-200™ Shampoo [OTC]; Barc™ Liquid [OTC]; End Lice® Liquid [OTC]; Lice-Enz® Shampoo [OTC]; Pronto® Shampoo [OTC]; Pyrinex® Pediculicide Shampoo [OTC]; Pyrinyl II® Liquid [OTC]; Pyrinyl Plus® Shampoo [OTC]; R & C® Shampoo [OTC]; RID® Shampoo [OTC]; Tisit® Blue Gel [OTC]; Tisit® Liquid [OTC]; Tisit® Shampoo [OTC]; Triple X® Liquid [OTC]

**Mechanism of Action** Pyrethrins are derived from flowers that belong to the chrysanthemum family. The mechanism of action on the neuronal membranes of lice is similar to that of DDT. Piperonyl butoxide is usually added to pyrethrin to enhance the product's activity by decreasing the metabolism of pyrethrins in arthropods.

**Use** Treatment of Pediculus humanus infestations (head lice, body lice, pubic lice and their eggs)

**USUAL DOSAGE** Application of pyrethrins: Topical:
Apply enough solution to completely wet infested area, including hair
Allow to remain on area for 10 minutes
Wash and rinse with large amounts of warm water
Use fine-toothed comb to remove lice and eggs from hair
Shampoo hair to restore body and luster
Treatment may be repeated if necessary once in a 24-hour period
Repeat treatment in 7-10 days to kill newly hatched lice

**Dosage Forms Gel, top:** 0.3% (30 g, 480 g); **Liq, top:** 0.18% (60 mL), 0.2% (60 mL, 120 mL), 0.3% (60 mL, 120 mL, 240 mL); **Shamp:** 0.3% (60 mL, 118 mL), 0.33% (60 mL, 120 mL)

**Contraindications** Known hypersensitivity to pyrethrins, ragweed, or chrysanthemums

**Warnings/Precautions** For external use only; do not use in eyelashes or eyebrows

**Pregnancy Risk Factor** C

**Adverse Reactions** 1% to 10%:
Dermatologic: Pruritus
Local: Burning, stinging, irritation with repeat use

**Special PA Issues**
**Patient Education:** For external use only; avoid touching eyes, mouth, or other mucous membranes; contact physician if irritation occurs or if condition does not improve in 2-3 days

♦ **Pyridiate®** see Phenazopyridine on page 714

♦ **Pyridium®** see Phenazopyridine on page 714

# Pyridostigmine (peer id oh STIG meen)

**Pharmacologic Class** Acetylcholinesterase Inhibitor (Central)

**U.S. Brand Names** Mestinon®; Mestinon Time-Span®; Regonol® Injection
(Continued)

## Pyridostigmine *(Continued)*

**Mechanism of Action** Inhibits destruction of acetylcholine by acetylcholinesterase which facilitates transmission of impulses across myoneural junction

**Use** Symptomatic treatment of myasthenia gravis; also used as an antidote for nondepolarizing neuromuscular blockers; not a cure; patient may develop resistance to the drug

**USUAL DOSAGE** Normally, sustained release dosage form is used at bedtime for patients who complain of morning weakness

Myasthenia gravis:
Oral:
Children: 7 mg/kg/day in 5-6 divided doses
Adults: Initial: 60 mg 3 times/day with maintenance dose ranging from 60 mg to 1.5 g/day; sustained release formulation should be dosed at least every 6 hours (usually 12-24 hours)
I.M., I.V.:
Children: 0.05-0.15 mg/kg/dose (maximum single dose: 10 mg)
Adults: 2 mg every 2-3 hours or 1/30th of oral dose
Reversal of nondepolarizing neuromuscular blocker: I.M., I.V.:
Children: 0.1-0.25 mg/kg/dose preceded by atropine
Adults: 10-20 mg preceded by atropine

**Dosage Forms Inj:** 5 mg/mL (2 mL, 5 mL); **Syr (raspberry flavor):** 60 mg/5 mL (480 mL); **Tab:** 60 mg; **Tab, sustained release:** 180 mg

**Contraindications** Hypersensitivity to pyridostigmine, bromides, or any component; GI or GU obstruction

**Warnings/Precautions** Use with caution in patients with epilepsy, asthma, bradycardia, hyperthyroidism, cardiac arrhythmias, or peptic ulcer; adequate facilities should be available for cardiopulmonary resuscitation when testing and adjusting dose for myasthenia gravis; have atropine and epinephrine ready to treat hypersensitivity reactions; overdosage may result in cholinergic crisis, this must be distinguished from myasthenic crisis; anticholinesterase insensitivity can develop for brief or prolonged periods

**Pregnancy Risk Factor** C

**Adverse Reactions**
>10%:
Gastrointestinal: Diarrhea, nausea, stomach cramps, mouth watering
Miscellaneous: Diaphoresis (increased)
1% to 10%:
Genitourinary: Urge to urinate
Ocular: Small pupils, lacrimation
Respiratory: Increased bronchial secretions
<1%: Bradycardia, A-V block, seizures, headache, dysphoria, drowsiness, thrombophlebitis, muscle spasms, weakness, miosis, diplopia, laryngospasm, respiratory paralysis, hypersensitivity, hyper-reactive cholinergic responses

**Drug Interactions**
Increased effect of depolarizing neuromuscular blockers (succinylcholine)
Increased toxicity with edrophonium

**Onset** Oral: 15-30 minutes; I.M.: 15-30 minutes; I.V.: 2-5 minutes

**Duration** Oral: Up to 6-8 hours (due to slow absorption); I.V.: 2-3 hours

**Special PA Issues**
**Patient Education:** This drug will not cure myasthenia gravis, but may help reduce symptoms. Use as directed; do not increase dose or discontinue without consulting prescriber. Take extended release tablets at bedtime; do not chew or crush extended release tablets. Maintain adequate hydration (2-3 L/day of fluids unless instructed to restrict fluid intake). May cause dizziness, drowsiness, or hypotension (rise slowly from sitting or lying position and use caution when driving or climbing stairs); vomiting or loss of appetite (frequent small meals, frequent mouth care, or sucking lozenges may help); or diarrhea (boiled milk, yogurt, or buttermilk may help). Report persistent abdominal discomfort; significantly increased salivation, sweating, tearing, or urination; flushed skin; chest pain or palpitations; acute headache; unresolved diarrhea; excessive fatigue, insomnia, dizziness, or depression; increased muscle, joint, or body pain; vision changes or blurred vision; or shortness of breath or wheezing.

♦ **Pyridostigmine Bromide** *see* Pyridostigmine *on previous page*

## Pyridoxine *(peer i DOKS een)*

**Pharmacologic Class** Antidote; Vitamin, Water Soluble

**U.S. Brand Names** Nestrex®

**Mechanism of Action** Precursor to pyridoxal, which functions in the metabolism of proteins, carbohydrates, and fats; pyridoxal also aids in the release of liver and muscle-stored glycogen and in the synthesis of GABA (within the central nervous system) and heme

**Use** Prevents and treats vitamin $B_6$ deficiency, pyridoxine-dependent seizures in infants, adjunct to treatment of acute toxicity from isoniazid, cycloserine, or hydralazine overdose

## USUAL DOSAGE
Recommended daily allowance (RDA):
Children:
1-3 years: 0.9 mg
4-6 years: 1.3 mg
7-10 years: 1.6 mg
Adults:
Male: 1.7-2.0 mg
Female: 1.4-1.6 mg
Pyridoxine-dependent Infants:
Oral: 2-100 mg/day
I.M., I.V., S.C.: 10-100 mg
Dietary deficiency: Oral:
Children: 5-25 mg/24 hours for 3 weeks, then 1.5-2.5 mg/day in multiple vitamin product
Adults: 10-20 mg/day for 3 weeks
Drug-induced neuritis (eg, isoniazid, hydralazine, penicillamine, cycloserine): Oral:
Children:
Treatment: 10-50 mg/24 hours
Prophylaxis: 1-2 mg/kg/24 hours
Adults:
Treatment: 100-200 mg/24 hours
Prophylaxis: 25-100 mg/24 hours
Treatment of seizures and/or coma from acute isoniazid toxicity, a dose of pyridoxine hydrochloride equal to the amount of INH ingested can be given I.M./I.V. in divided doses together with other anticonvulsants; if the amount INH ingested is not known, administer 5 g I.V. pyridoxine
Treatment of acute hydralazine toxicity, a pyridoxine dose of 25 mg/kg in divided doses I.M./ I.V. has been used

**Dosage Forms** Pyridoxine hydrochloride: **Inj:** 100 mg/mL (10 mL, 30 mL); **Tab:** 25 mg, 50 mg, 100 mg; **Tab, extended release:** 100 mg

**Contraindications** Hypersensitivity to pyridoxine or any component

**Warnings/Precautions** Dependence and withdrawal may occur with doses >200 mg/day

**Pregnancy Risk Factor** A (C if dose exceeds RDA recommendation)

## Pregnancy Implications
Clinical effects on the fetus: Crosses the placenta; available evidence suggests safe use during pregnancy and breast-feeding
Breast-feeding/lactation: Crosses into breast milk; possible inhibition of lactation at doses >600 mg/day. American Academy of Pediatrics considers **compatible** with breast-feeding

**Adverse Reactions** <1%: Sensory neuropathy, seizures have occurred following I.V. administration of very large doses, headache, nausea, decreased serum folic acid secretions, increased AST, paresthesia, allergic reactions have been reported

**Drug Interactions** Decreased serum levels of levodopa, phenobarbital, and phenytoin

**Half-Life** 15-20 days

## Special PA Issues
**Patient Education:** Take exactly as directed. Do not take more than recommended. Do not chew or crush extended release tablets. Do not exceed recommended intake of dietary B6 (eg, red meat, bananas, potatoes, yeast, lima beans, and whole grain cereals). You may experience burning or pain at injection site; notify prescriber if this persists.
**Reference Range:** Over 50 ng/mL (SI: 243 nmol/L) (varies considerably with method). A broad range is ~25-80 ng/mL (SI: 122-389 nmol/L). HPLC method for pyridoxal phosphate has normal range of 3.5-18 ng/mL (SI: 17-88 nmol/L).

♦ **Pyridoxine Hydrochloride** see Pyridoxine on previous page

# Pyrimethamine (peer i METH a meen)
**Pharmacologic Class** Antimalarial Agent
**U.S. Brand Names** Daraprim®
**Mechanism of Action** Inhibits parasitic dihydrofolate reductase, resulting in inhibition of vital tetrahydrofolic acid synthesis
**Use** Prophylaxis of malaria due to susceptible strains of plasmodia; used in conjunction with quinine and sulfadiazine for the treatment of uncomplicated attacks of chloroquine-resistant P. falciparum malaria; used in conjunction with fast-acting schizonticide to initiate transmission control and suppression cure; synergistic combination with sulfonamide in treatment of toxoplasmosis

## USUAL DOSAGE
Malaria chemoprophylaxis (for areas where chloroquine-resistant P. falciparum exists): Begin prophylaxis 2 weeks before entering endemic area:
Children: 0.5 mg/kg once weekly; not to exceed 25 mg/dose
**or**
Children:
<4 years: 6.25 mg once weekly
(Continued)

## Pyrimethamine *(Continued)*

4-10 years: 12.5 mg once weekly

Children >10 years and Adults: 25 mg once weekly

Dosage should be continued for all age groups for at least 6-10 weeks after leaving endemic areas

Chloroquine-resistant *P. falciparum* malaria (when used in conjunction with quinine and sulfadiazine):

Children:

<10 kg: 6.25 mg/day once daily for 3 days

10-20 kg: 12.5 mg/day once daily for 3 days

20-40 kg: 25 mg/day once daily for 3 days

Adults: 25 mg twice daily for 3 days

Toxoplasmosis:

Infants for congenital toxoplasmosis: Oral: 1 mg/kg once daily for 6 months with sulfadiazine then every other month with sulfa, alternating with spiramycin.

Children: Loading dose: 2 mg/kg/day divided into 2 equal daily doses for 1-3 days (maximum: 100 mg/day) followed by 1 mg/kg/day divided into 2 doses for 4 weeks; maximum: 25 mg/day

With sulfadiazine or trisulfapyrimidines: 2 mg/kg/day divided every 12 hours for 3 days followed by 1 mg/kg/day once daily or divided twice daily for 4 weeks given with trisulfapyrimidines or sulfadiazine

Adults: 50-75 mg/day together with 1-4 g of a sulfonamide for 1-3 weeks depending on patient's tolerance and response, then reduce dose by 50% and continue for 4-5 weeks or 25-50 mg/day for 3-4 weeks

In HIV, life-long suppression is necessary to prevent relapse; leucovorin (5-10 mg/day) is given concurrently

**Dosage Forms Tab:** 25 mg

**Contraindications** Megaloblastic anemia secondary to folate deficiency; known hypersensitivity to pyrimethamine, chloroguanide; resistant malaria

**Warnings/Precautions** When used for more than 3-4 days, it may be advisable to administer leucovorin to prevent hematologic complications; monitor CBC and platelet counts every 2 weeks; use with caution in patients with impaired renal or hepatic function or with possible G-6-PD

**Pregnancy Risk Factor** C

**Adverse Reactions**

1% to 10%:

Gastrointestinal: Anorexia, abdominal cramps, vomiting

Hematologic: Megaloblastic anemia, leukopenia, thrombocytopenia, agranulocytosis

<1%: Insomnia, lightheadedness, fever, malaise, seizures, depression, rash, dermatitis, Stevens-Johnson syndrome, erythema multiforme, anaphylaxis, abnormal skin pigmentation, diarrhea, xerostomia, atrophic glossitis, pulmonary eosinophilia

**Drug Interactions**

Decreased effect: Pyrimethamine effectiveness decreased by acid

Increased effect: Sulfonamides (synergy), methotrexate, TMP/SMX may increase the risk of bone marrow suppression; mild hepatotoxicity with lorazepam

**Onset** Within 1 hour

**Half-Life** 80-95 hours

**Special PA Issues**

**Patient Education:** Take on schedule as directed and take full course of therapy. If used for prophylaxis, begin 2 weeks before traveling to endemic areas, continue during travel period, and for 6-10 weeks following return. Regular blood tests will be necessary during therapy. You may experience GI distress (frequent, small meals may help). You may experience dizziness, changes in mentation, insomnia, headache, or visual disturbances (use caution when driving or operating dangerous machinery). Report unresolved nausea or vomiting, anorexia, skin rash, fever, sore throat, unusual bleeding or bruising, yellowing of skin or eyes, and change in color of urine or stool.

**Monitoring Parameters:** CBC, including platelet counts

- ◆ **Pyrinex® Pediculicide Shampoo [OTC]** *see* Pyrethrins *on page 783*
- ◆ **Pyrinyl II® Liquid [OTC]** *see* Pyrethrins *on page 783*
- ◆ **Pyrinyl Plus® Shampoo [OTC]** *see* Pyrethrins *on page 783*
- ◆ **Pyronium®** *see* Phenazopyridine *on page 714*
- ◆ **Quaternium-18 Bentonite** *see* Bentoquatam *on page 104*
- ◆ **Queltuss®** *see* Guaifenesin and Dextromethorphan *on page 428*
- ◆ **Questran®** *see* Cholestyramine Resin *on page 202*
- ◆ **Questran® Light** *see* Cholestyramine Resin *on page 202*

## Quetiapine *(kwe TYE a peen)*

**Pharmacologic Class** Antipsychotic Agent, Dibenzothiazepine

**U.S. Brand Names** Seroquel®

**Mechanism of Action** Mechanism of action of quetiapine, as with other antipsychotic drugs, is unknown. However, it has been proposed that this drug's antipsychotic activity is mediated through a combination of dopamine type 2 ($D_2$) and serotonin type 2 (5-$HT_2$) antagonism. However, it is an antagonist at multiple neurotransmitter receptors in the brain: serotonin 5-$HT_{1A}$ and 5-$HT_2$, dopamine $D_1$ and $D_2$, histamine $H_1$, and adrenergic alpha$_1$- and alpha$_2$-receptors; but appears to have no appreciable affinity at cholinergic muscarinic and benzodiazepine receptors.

Antagonism at receptors other than dopamine and 5-$HT_2$ with similar receptor affinities may explain some of the other effects of quetiapine. The drug's antagonism of histamine $H_1$ receptors may explain the somnolence observed with it. The drug's antagonism of adrenergic alpha$_1$-receptors may explain the orthostatic hypotension observed with it.

**Use** Treatment of acute exacerbations of schizophrenia or other psychotic disorders. Like other atypical antipsychotics, quetiapine is probably best tried in cases for which typical antipsychotic drugs have proven ineffective.

**USUAL DOSAGE** Adults: Oral: 25-100 mg 2-3 times/day; usual starting dose: 25 mg twice daily and then increased in increments of 25-50 mg 2-3 times/day on the second or third day; by day 4, the dose should be in the range of 300-400 mg/day in 2-3 divided doses. Make further adjustments as needed at intervals of at least 2 days in adjustments of 25-50 mg twice daily. The usual maintenance range is 150-750 mg/day; maximum dose: 800 mg/day.

**Dosing comments in geriatric patients:** 40% lower mean oral clearance of quetiapine in adults >65 years of age; higher plasma levels expected and, therefore, dosage adjustment may be needed

**Dosing comments in hepatic insufficiency:** 30% lower mean oral clearance of quetiapine than normal subjects; higher plasma levels expected in hepatically impaired subjects; dosage adjustment may be needed

**Dosage Forms Tab, as fumarate:** 25 mg, 100 mg, 200 mg

**Contraindications** Known hypersensitivity to this drug or any of its ingredients

**Warnings/Precautions** May induce orthostatic hypotension associated with dizziness, tachycardia, and, in some cases, syncope, especially during the initial dose titration period. Should be used with particular caution in patients with known cardiovascular disease (history of MI or ischemic heart disease, heart failure, or conduction abnormalities), cerebrovascular disease, or conditions that predispose to hypotension. Development of cataracts has been observed in animal studies, therefore, lens examinations should be made upon initiation of therapy and every 6 months thereafter.

Neuroleptic malignant syndrome (NMS) is a potentially fatal symptom complex that has been reported in association with administration of antipsychotic drugs. Clinical manifestations of NMS are hyperpyrexia, muscle rigidity, altered mental status, and evidence of autonomic instability (irregular pulse or blood pressure, tachycardia, diaphoresis, and cardiac dysrhythmia). Management of NMS should include immediate discontinuation of antipsychotic drugs and other drugs not essential to concurrent therapy, intensive symptomatic treatment and medication monitoring, and treatment of any concomitant medical problems for which specific treatment are available.

Tardive dyskinesia; caution in patients with a history of seizures, decreases in total free thyroxine, pre-existing hyperprolactinemia, elevations of liver enzymes, cholesterol levels and/or triglyceride increases.

**Pregnancy Risk Factor** C

**Adverse Reactions**

Cardiovascular: Postural hypotension (4% to 14%)

Central nervous system: Agitation (6% to 28%), somnolence (6% to 39%), headache (5% to 31%), insomnia (4% to 15%), dizziness (2% to 11%)

Gastrointestinal: Xerostomia (8% to 19%)

Hepatic: Serum ALT increases (5% to 17%)

Miscellaneous: <2%: Tachycardia, dyspepsia, constipation, weight gain, increases in total cholesterol and triglycerides; hypothyroidism developed in a small number of patients. Treatment-related extrapyramidal symptoms were not observed in animal studies and lens changes have been observed in patients receiving long-term therapy.

**Drug Interactions** CYP2D6 and 3A3/4enzyme substrate

Caution with other centrally acting drugs; avoid alcohol. May enhance effects of antihypertensive agents; may antagonize levodopa, dopamine agonists. Increased clearance when given with phenytoin or thioridazine, caution with other liver enzyme inducers (carbamazepine, barbiturates, rifampin, glucocorticoids); although data is not yet available, caution is advised with inhibitors of cytochrome P-450 (eg, ketoconazole, erythromycin); reduces the clearance of lorazepam.

**Half-Life** 6 hours

**Special PA Issues**

**Patient Education:** Use exactly as directed (do not increase dose or frequency); may cause physical and/or psychological dependence. It may take 2-3 weeks to achieve desired results; do not discontinue without consulting prescriber. Avoid excess alcohol or caffeine and other prescription or OTC medications not approved by prescriber. Maintain adequate hydration (2-3 L/day of fluids unless instructed to restrict fluid intake). You may
(Continued)

## Quetiapine *(Continued)*

experience excess drowsiness, restlessness, dizziness, or blurred vision (use caution driving or when engaging in hazardous tasks until response to medication is known); mouth sores or GI upset (small frequent meals, frequent mouth care, or sucking lozenges may help); constipation (increased exercise, fluids, or dietary fruit and fiber may help); or postural hypotension (use caution climbing stairs or when changing position from lying or sitting to standing). Report persistent CNS effects (eg, somnolence, agitation, insomnia); severe dizziness; vision changes; difficulty breathing; or worsening of condition.

**Dietary Considerations:** In healthy volunteers, administration of quetiapine with food resulted in an increase in the peak serum concentration and AUC (each by ~150%) compared to the fasting state. The clinical relevance of these data requires qualification in further studies.

**Monitoring Parameters:** Patients should have eyes checked every 6 months for cataracts while on this medication

### Related Information

Antipsychotic Agents *on page 1001*

- ◆ **Quetiapine Fumarate** *see Quetiapine on page 786*
- ◆ **Quibron®** *see Theophylline and Guaifenesin on page 888*
- ◆ **Quibron®-T** *see Theophylline Salts on page 888*
- ◆ **Quibron®-T/SR** *see Theophylline Salts on page 888*
- ◆ **Quiess®** *see Hydroxyzine on page 462*
- ◆ **Quinaglute® Dura-Tabs®** *see Quinidine on next page*
- ◆ **Quinalan®** *see Quinidine on next page*

## Quinapril *(KWIN a pril)*

**Pharmacologic Class** Angiotensin-Converting Enzyme (ACE) Inhibitors

**U.S. Brand Names** Accupril®

**Mechanism of Action** Competitive inhibitor of angiotensin-converting enzyme (ACE); prevents conversion of angiotensin I to angiotensin II, a potent vasoconstrictor; results in lower levels of angiotensin II which causes an increase in plasma renin activity and a reduction in aldosterone secretion; a CNS mechanism may also be involved in hypotensive effect as angiotensin II increases adrenergic outflow from CNS; vasoactive kallikreins may be decreased in conversion to active hormones by ACE inhibitors, thus reducing blood pressure

**Use** Management of hypertension and treatment of congestive heart failure; increase circulation in Raynaud's phenomenon; idiopathic edema; believed to improve survival in heart failure

**Unlabeled use:** Hypertensive crisis, diabetic nephropathy, rheumatoid arthritis, diagnosis of anatomic renal artery stenosis, hypertension secondary to scleroderma renal crisis, diagnosis of aldosteronism, Bartter's syndrome, postmyocardial infarction for prevention of ventricular failure

### USUAL DOSAGE

Adults: Oral: Initial: 10 mg once daily, adjust according to blood pressure response at peak and trough blood levels in general, the normal dosage range is 20-80 mg/day for hypertension and 20-40 mg/day for edema in single or divided doses

Elderly: Initial: 2.5-5 mg/day; increase dosage at increments of 2.5-5 mg at 1- to 2-week intervals

**Dosing adjustment in renal impairment:**
$Cl_{cr}$ >60 mL/minute: Administer 10 mg/day
$Cl_{cr}$ 30-60 mL/minute: 5 mg/day
$Cl_{cr}$ 10-30 mL/minute: 2.5 mg/day

**Dosing comments in hepatic impairment:** In patients with alcoholic cirrhosis, hydrolysis of quinapril to quinaprilat is impaired; however, the subsequent elimination of quinaprilat is unaltered

**Dosage Forms Tab, as hydrochloride:** 5 mg, 10 mg, 20 mg, 40 mg

**Contraindications** Hypersensitivity to quinapril or history of angioedema induced by other ACE inhibitors

**Warnings/Precautions** Use with caution in patients with renal insufficiency, autoimmune disease, renal artery stenosis; excessive hypotension may be more likely in volume-depleted patients, the elderly, and following the first dose (first dose phenomenon); quinapril should be discontinued if laryngeal stridor or angioedema of the face, tongue, or glottis is observed

**Pregnancy Risk Factor** C (1st trimester); D (2nd and 3rd trimester)

### Adverse Reactions

1% to 10%:
Cardiovascular: Hypotension
Central nervous system: Dizziness (3.9%), headache (5.6%), fatigue (2.6%)
Gastrointestinal: Vomiting/nausea (1.4%)
Renal: Increased BUN/serum creatinine (transient)
Respiratory: Upper respiratory symptoms, cough (2%)

<1%: Chest discomfort, flushing, myocardial infarction, angina pectoris, orthostatic hypotension, rhythm disturbances, tachycardia, peripheral edema, vasculitis, palpitations, syncope, fever, malaise, depression, somnolence, insomnia, urticaria, pruritus, angioedema, gout, pancreatitis, abdominal pain, anorexia, constipation, flatulence, xerostomia, neutropenia, bone marrow suppression, hepatitis, arthralgia, shoulder pain, blurred vision, bronchitis, sinusitis, pharyngeal pain, diaphoresis

**Drug Interactions** See Drug-Drug Interactions With ACEIs *on page 997*

**Onset** 1 hour

**Duration** 24 hours

**Half-Life** Quinapril: 0.8 hours; Quinaprilat: 2 hours

**Special PA Issues**

    **Patient Education:** Take exactly as directed - 1 hour before or 2 hours after meals. Do not change dosage or stop taking without consulting prescriber. Follow prescribed diet. You may experience dizziness, fainting, or lightheadedness (use caution when driving or performing hazardous tasks and use caution when changing position eg, rising from sitting or lying) until response to therapy is established. You may experience nausea or vomiting or changes in taste perception (small frequent meals, frequent mouth care, or sucking on lozenges may reduce these effects). Report sore throat or unusual cough; persistent dizziness or fatigue; respiratory difficulty; chest pains or irregular heartbeat; unresolved nausea or vomiting.

**Related Information**

    ACE Inhibitors *on page 995*

    Heart Failure: Management of Patients with Left Ventricular Systolic Dysfunction *on page 1064*

    Drug-Drug Interactions With ACEIs *on page 997*

♦ **Quinapril Hydrochloride** *see* Quinapril *on previous page*

♦ **Quinidex® Extentabs®** *see* Quinidine *on this page*

## Quinidine (KWIN i deen)

**Pharmacologic Class** Antiarrhythmic Agent, Class I-A

**U.S. Brand Names** Cardioquin®; Quinaglute® Dura-Tabs®; Quinalan®; Quinidex® Extentabs®; Quinora®

**Mechanism of Action** Class 1A antiarrhythmic agent; depresses phase O of the action potential; decreases myocardial excitability and conduction velocity, and myocardial contractility by decreasing sodium influx during depolarization and potassium efflux in repolarization; also reduces calcium transport across cell membrane

**Use** Prophylaxis after cardioversion of atrial fibrillation and/or flutter to maintain normal sinus rhythm; also used to prevent reoccurrence of paroxysmal supraventricular tachycardia, paroxysmal A-V junctional rhythm, paroxysmal ventricular tachycardia, paroxysmal atrial fibrillation, and atrial or ventricular premature contractions; also has activity against *Plasmodium falciparum* malaria

**USUAL DOSAGE Dosage expressed in terms of the salt: 267 mg of quinidine gluconate = 200 mg of quinidine sulfate**

    Children: Test dose for idiosyncratic reaction (sulfate, oral or gluconate, I.M.): 2 mg/kg or 60 mg/m$^2$

        Oral (quinidine sulfate): 15-60 mg/kg/day in 4-5 divided doses or 6 mg/kg every 4-6 hours; usual 30 mg/kg/day or 900 mg/m$^2$/day given in 5 daily doses

        I.V. **not** recommended (quinidine gluconate): 2-10 mg/kg/dose given at a rate ≤10 mg/minute every 3-6 hours as needed

    Adults: Test dose: Oral, I.M.: 200 mg administered several hours before full dosage (to determine possibility of idiosyncratic reaction)

        Oral (for malaria):

            Sulfate: 100-600 mg/dose every 4-6 hours; begin at 200 mg/dose and titrate to desired effect (maximum daily dose: 3-4 g)

            Gluconate: 324-972 mg every 8-12 hours

        I.M.: 400 mg/dose every 2-6 hours; initial dose: 600 mg (gluconate)

        I.V.: 200-400 mg/dose diluted and given at a rate ≤10 mg/minute; may require as much as 500-750 mg

    **Dosing adjustment in renal impairment:** Cl$_{cr}$ <10 mL/minute: Administer 75% of normal dose

    Hemodialysis: Slightly hemodialyzable (5% to 20%); 200 mg supplemental dose posthemodialysis is recommended

    Peritoneal dialysis: Not dialyzable (0% to 5%)

    **Dosing adjustment/comments in hepatic impairment:** Larger loading dose may be indicated, reduce maintenance doses by 50% and monitor serum levels closely

**Dosage Forms** Quinidine gluconate: **Inj:** 80 mg/mL (10 mL); **Tab, sustained release:** 324 mg

    Quinidine polygalacturonate: **Tab:** 275 mg

    Quinidine sulfate: **Tab:** 200 mg, 300 mg; **Tab, sustained action:** 300 mg

**Contraindications** Patients with complete A-V block with an A-V junctional or idioventricular pacemaker; patients with intraventricular conduction defects (marked widening of QRS (Continued)

## Quinidine *(Continued)*

complex); patients with cardiac-glycoside induced A-V conduction disorders; hypersensitivity to the drug or cinchona derivatives; concurrent use of sparfloxacin or ritonavir

**Warnings/Precautions** Use with caution in patients with myocardial depression, sick-sinus syndrome, incomplete A-V block, hepatic and/or renal insufficiency, myasthenia gravis; hemolysis may occur in patients with G-6-PD (glucose-6-phosphate dehydrogenase) deficiency; quinidine-induced hepatotoxicity, including granulomatous hepatitis can occur, increased serum AST and alkaline phosphatase concentrations, and jaundice may occur; use with caution in nursing women and elderly

**Pregnancy Risk Factor** C

**Adverse Reactions**

>10%: Gastrointestinal: Bitter taste, diarrhea, anorexia, nausea, vomiting, stomach cramping

1% to 10%:

Cardiovascular: Hypotension, syncope

Central nervous system: Lightheadedness, severe headache

Dermatologic: Rash

Ocular: Blurred vision

Otic: Tinnitus

Respiratory: Wheezing

<1%: Tachycardia, heart block, ventricular fibrillation, vascular collapse, confusion, delirium, fever, vertigo, angioedema, anemia, thrombocytopenic purpura, blood dyscrasias, impaired hearing, respiratory depression, pneumonitis, bronchospasm

**Drug Interactions** CYP3A3/4 and 3A5-7 enzyme substrate; CYP2D6 and 3A3/4 enzyme inhibitor

Decreased effect: Phenobarbital, phenytoin, and rifampin may decrease quinidine serum concentrations (rifampin may decrease quinidine half-life by 50%, probably by inducing the CYP3A isozyme)

Increased toxicity:

Quinidine potentiates nondepolarizing and depolarizing muscle relaxants; quinidine may increase plasma concentration of digoxin, procainamide, propafenone, tricyclic antidepressants, closely monitor digoxin concentrations, digoxin dosage may need to be reduced (by one-half) when quinidine is initiated; quinidine may enhance coumarin anticoagulants

Beta-blockers + quinidine may increase bradycardia

Verapamil, amiodarone, alkalinizing agents, and cimetidine may increase quinidine serum concentrations

Avoid use with sparfloxacin due to increased risk of cardiotoxicity

Contraindicated with ritonavir due to increased risk of quinidine toxicity, especially cardiotoxicity

Increased disopyramide or decreased quinidine levels can occur when administered concurrently

**Half-Life** 6-8 hours; increased half-life with elderly, cirrhosis, and congestive heart failure

**Special PA Issues**

**Patient Education:** Take exactly as directed, around-the-clock; do not take additional doses or discontinue without consulting prescriber. Do not crush, chew, or break sustained release capsules. You will need regular cardiac check-ups and blood tests while taking this medication. You may experience dizziness, drowsiness, or visual changes (use caution when driving or performing tasks that require alertness until response to drug is determined); abnormal taste, nausea or vomiting, or loss of appetite (small frequent meals, frequent mouth care, or sucking lozenges may help); headaches (prescriber may recommend mild analgesic); or diarrhea (exercise, yogurt, or boiled milk may help - if persistent consult prescriber). Report chest pain, palpitation, or erratic heartbeat; difficulty breathing or wheezing; CNS changes (confusion, delirium, fever, consistent dizziness); skin rash; sense of fullness or ringing in ears; or changes in vision.

**Monitoring Parameters:** Cardiac monitor required during I.V. administration; CBC, liver and renal function tests should be routinely performed during long-term administration

**Reference Range:** Therapeutic: 2-5 µg/mL (SI: 6.2-15.4 µmol/L). Patient dependent therapeutic response occurs at levels of 3-6 µg/mL (SI: 9.2-18.5 µmol/L). Optimal therapeutic level is method dependent; >6 µg/mL (SI: >18 µmol/L).

♦ **Quinidine Gluconate** *see* Quinidine *on previous page*

♦ **Quinidine Polygalacturonate** *see* Quinidine *on previous page*

♦ **Quinidine Sulfate** *see* Quinidine *on previous page*

## Quinine (KWYE nine)

**Pharmacologic Class** Antimalarial Agent

**U.S. Brand Names** Formula Q®

**Mechanism of Action** Depresses oxygen uptake and carbohydrate metabolism; intercalates into DNA, disrupting the parasite's replication and transcription; affects calcium distribution within muscle fibers and decreases the excitability of the motor end-plate region; cardiovascular effects similar to quinidine

**Use** In conjunction with other antimalarial agents, suppression or treatment of chloroquine-resistant *P. falciparum* malaria; treatment of *Babesia microti* infection in conjunction with clindamycin; prevention and treatment of nocturnal recumbency leg muscle cramps

**USUAL DOSAGE** Oral:

Children:

Treatment of chloroquine-resistant malaria: 25-30 mg/kg/day in divided doses every 8 hours for 5-7 days in conjunction with another agent

Babesiosis: 25 mg/kg/day divided every 8 hours for 7 days

Adults:

Treatment of chloroquine-resistant malaria: 260-650 mg every 8 hours for 6-12 days in conjunction with another agent

Suppression of malaria: 325 mg twice daily and continued for 6 weeks after exposure

Babesiosis: 650 mg every 6-8 hours for 7 days

Leg cramps: 200-300 mg at bedtime

**Dosing interval/adjustment in renal impairment:**

$Cl_{cr}$ 10-50 mL/minute: Administer every 8-12 hours or 75% of normal dose

$Cl_{cr}$ <10 mL/minute: Administer every 24 hours or 30% to 50% of normal dose

Dialysis: Removed by hemodialysis

Peritoneal dialysis: Not effectively removed

Continuous arteriovenous or venovenous hemodiafiltration (CAVH) effects: Dose for $Cl_{cr}$ 10-50 mL/minute

**Dosage Forms Cap:** 64.8 mg, 65 mg, 200 mg, 300 mg, 325 mg; **Tab:** 162.5 mg, 260 mg

**Contraindications** Tinnitus, optic neuritis, G-6-PD deficiency, hypersensitivity to quinine or any component, history of black water fever, and thrombocytopenia with quinine or quinidine

**Warnings/Precautions** Use with caution in patients with cardiac arrhythmias (quinine has quinidine-like activity) and in patients with myasthenia gravis

**Pregnancy Risk Factor** X

**Adverse Reactions**

Percentage unknown: Cinchonism (risk of cinchonism is directly related to dose and duration of therapy): Severe headache, nausea, vomiting, diarrhea, blurred vision, tinnitus

<1%: Flushing of the skin, anginal symptoms, fever, rash, pruritus, hypoglycemia, epigastric pain, hemolysis in G-6-PD deficiency, thrombocytopenia, hepatitis, nightblindness, diplopia, optic atrophy, impaired hearing, hypersensitivity reactions

**Drug Interactions** CYP3A3/4 enzyme substrate; CYP3A3/4 enzyme inhibitor

Decreased effect: Phenobarbital, phenytoin, aluminum salt antacids, and rifampin may decrease quinine serum concentrations

Increased toxicity:

To avoid risk of seizures and cardiac arrest, delay mefloquine dosing at least 12 hours after last dose of quinine

Beta-blockers + quinine may increase bradycardia

Quinine may enhance coumarin anticoagulants and potentiate nondepolarizing and depolarizing muscle relaxants

Quinine may inhibit metabolism of astemizole resulting in toxic levels and potentially life-threatening cardiotoxicity

Quinine may increase plasma concentration of digoxin by as much as twofold; closely monitor digoxin concentrations and decrease digoxin dose with initiation of quinine by $\frac{1}{2}$

Verapamil, amiodarone, urinary alkalinizing agents, and cimetidine may increase quinine serum concentrations

**Half-Life** 8-14 hours

**Special PA Issues**

**Patient Education:** Take on schedule as directed, with full 8 oz of water. Do not chew or crush sustained release tablets. You will need to return for follow-up blood tests. You may experience GI distress (taking medication with food, and frequent small meals may help). You may experience dizziness, changes in mentation, insomnia, headache, or visual disturbances (use caution when driving or operating dangerous machinery). Report persistent sore throat, fever, chills, flu-like signs, ringing in ears, vision disturbances, or unusual bruising or bleeding. Seek emergency help for palpitations or chest pain.

**Reference Range:** Toxic: >10 µg/mL

♦ **Quinine Sulfate** *see* Quinine *on previous page*

♦ **Quinol** *see* Hydroquinone *on page 457*

♦ **Quinora®** *see* Quinidine *on page 789*

♦ **Quinsana Plus® [OTC]** *see* Tolnaftate *on page 915*

♦ **QYS®** *see* Hydroxyzine *on page 462*

# Rabies Immune Globulin (Human)

(RAY beez i MYUN GLOB yoo lin, HYU man)

**Pharmacologic Class** Immune Globulin

**U.S. Brand Names** Hyperab®; Imogam®

(Continued)

## Rabies Immune Globulin (Human) *(Continued)*

**Mechanism of Action** Rabies immune globulin is a solution of globulins dried from the plasma or serum of selected adult human donors who have been immunized with rabies vaccine and have developed high titers of rabies antibody. It generally contains 10% to 18% of protein of which not less than 80% is monomeric immunoglobulin G.

**Use** Part of postexposure prophylaxis of persons with rabies exposure who lack a history of pre-exposure or postexposure prophylaxis with rabies vaccine or a recently documented neutralizing antibody response to previous rabies vaccination; although it is preferable to administer RIG with the first dose of vaccine, it can be given up to 8 days after vaccination

**USUAL DOSAGE** Children and Adults: I.M.: 20 units/kg in a single dose (RIG should always be administered as part of rabies vaccine (HDCV)) regimen (as soon as possible after the first dose of vaccine, up to 8 days); infiltrate ½ of the dose locally around the wound; administer the remainder I M.

**Note:** Persons known to have an adequate titer or who have been completely immunized with rabies vaccine should not receive RIG, only booster doses of HDCV

**Dosage Forms Inj:** 150 units/mL (2 mL, 10 mL)

**Contraindications** Inadvertent I.V. administration; allergy to thimerosal or any component

**Warnings/Precautions** Use with caution in individuals with thrombocytopenia, bleeding disorders, or prior allergic reactions to immune globulins

**Pregnancy Risk Factor** C

**Adverse Reactions**
1% to 10%:
Central nervous system Fever (mild)
Local: Soreness at injection site
<1%: Urticaria, angioedema, stiffness, soreness of muscles, anaphylactic shock

**Drug Interactions** Decreased effect: Live virus vaccines (eg, MMR, rabies) may have delayed or diminished antibody response with immune globulin administration; should not be administered within 3 months unless antibody titers dictate as appropriate

♦ **Racemic Amphetamine Sulfate** *see Amphetamine on page 64*

♦ **Radiostol®** *see Ergocalciferol on page 326*

♦ **Radix** *see Valerian on page 951*

## Raloxifene (ral OX i feen)

**Pharmacologic Class** Selective Estrogen Receptor Modulator (SERM)

**U.S. Brand Names** Evista®

**Mechanism of Action** A selective estrogen receptor modulator, meaning that it affects some of the same receptors that estrogen does, but not all, and in some instances, it antagonizes or blocks estrogen; it acts like estrogen to prevent bone loss and improve lipid profiles, but it has the potential to block some estrogen effects such as those that lead to breast cancer and uterine cancer

**Use** Prevention of osteoporosis in postmenopausal women

**USUAL DOSAGE** Adults: Female: Oral: 60 mg/day which may be administered any time of the day without regard to meals

**Dosage Forms Tab, as hydrochloride:** 60 mg

**Contraindications** Pregnancy; prior hypersensitivity to raloxifene; active thromboembolic disorder; not intended for use in premenopausal women

**Warnings/Precautions** History of venous thromboembolism/pulmonary embolism; patients with cardiovascular disease; history of cervical/uterine carcinoma; renal/hepatic insufficiency (however, pharmacokinetic data are lacking); concurrent use of estrogens

**Pregnancy Risk Factor** X

**Pregnancy Implications** Raloxifene should not be used by pregnant women or by women planning to become pregnant in the immediate future

**Adverse Reactions** ≥2%:
Cardiovascular: Chest pain
Central nervous system: Migraine, depression, insomnia, fever
Dermatologic: Rash
Endocrine & metabolic: Hot flashes
Gastrointestinal: Nausea, dyspepsia, vomiting, flatulence, gastroenteritis, weight gain
Genitourinary: Vaginitis, urinary tract infection, cystitis, leukorrhea
Neuromuscular & skeletal: Leg cramps, arthralgia, myalgia, arthritis
Respiratory: Sinusitis, pharyngitis, cough, pneumonia, laryngitis
Miscellaneous: Infection, flu syndrome, diaphoresis

**Drug Interactions** Decreased effects: Ampicillin and cholestyramine decreases raloxifene absorption

**Half-Life** 28-32.5 hours

**Special PA Issues**
**Patient Education:** May be taken at any time of day without regard to meals. This medication is given to reduce incidence of osteoporosis; it will not reduce hot flashes or flushing. You may experience flu-like symptoms at beginning of therapy (these may resolve with use). Mild analgesics may reduce joint pain. Rest and cool environment may

reduce hot flashes. Report fever; acute migraine; insomnia or emotional depression; unusual weight gain; unresolved gastric distress; urinary infection or vaginal burning or itching; chest pain; or swelling, warmth, or pain in calves.

**Monitoring Parameters:** Radiologic evaluation of bone mineral density (BMD) is the best measure of the treatment of osteoporosis; to monitor for the potential toxicities of raloxifene, complete blood counts should be evaluated periodically.

# Ramipril (ra MI pril)

**Pharmacologic Class** Angiotensin-Converting Enzyme (ACE) Inhibitors

**U.S. Brand Names** Altace™

**Mechanism of Action** Ramipril is an angiotensin-converting enzyme (ACE) inhibitor which prevents the formation of angiotensin II from angiotensin I and exhibits pharmacologic effects that are similar to captopril. Ramipril must undergo enzymatic saponification by esterases in the liver to its biologically active metabolite, ramiprilat. The pharmacodynamic effects of ramipril result from the high-affinity, competitive, reversible binding of ramiprilat to angiotensin-converting enzyme thus preventing the formation of the potent vasoconstrictor angiotensin II. This isomerized enzyme-inhibitor complex has a slow rate of dissociation, which results in high potency and a long duration of action; a CNS mechanism may also be involved in the hypotensive effect as angiotensin II increases adrenergic outflow from CNS; vasoactive kallikreins may be decreased in conversion to active hormones by ACE inhibitors, thus reducing blood pressure

**Use** Treatment of hypertension, alone or in combination with thiazide diuretics; treatment of congestive heart failure within the first few days after myocardial infarction (**Note:** This indication is based on a study involving 2006 patients; a decrease by 26% in all-cause mortality was observed when ramipril was administered 3-10 days after a myocardial infarction)

**USUAL DOSAGE** Adults: Oral:

Hypertension: 2.5-5 mg once daily, maximum: 20 mg/day

Heart failure postmyocardial infarction: Initial: 2.5 mg twice daily titrated upward, if possible, to 5 mg twice daily

**Note:** The dose of any concomitant diuretic should be reduced; if the diuretic cannot be discontinued, initiate therapy with 1.25 mg; after the initial dose, the patient should be monitored carefully until blood pressure has stabilized

**Dosing adjustment in renal impairment:**

$Cl_{cr}$ <40 mL/minute: Administer 25% of normal dose

Renal failure and hypertension: 1.25 mg once daily, titrated upward as possible

Renal failure and heart failure: 1.25 mg once daily, increasing to 1.25 mg twice daily up to 2.5 mg twice daily as tolerated

**Dosage Forms Cap:** 1.25 mg, 2.5 mg, 5 mg, 10 mg

**Contraindications** Hypersensitivity to ramipril or ramiprilat, or history of angioedema with any other angiotensin-converting enzyme inhibitors

**Warnings/Precautions** Use with caution and modify dosage in patients with renal impairment (especially renal artery stenosis), severe congestive heart failure; severe hypotension may occur in the elderly and patients who are sodium and/or volume depleted, initiate lower doses and monitor closely when starting therapy in these patients; should be discontinued if laryngeal stridor or angioedema of the face, tongue, or glottis is observed

**Pregnancy Risk Factor** C (1st trimester); D (2nd and 3rd trimester)

**Adverse Reactions**

>10% Respiratory: Cough (12%)

<1%: Hypotension, syncope, arrhythmia, angina, palpitations, myocardial infarction, headache, dizziness, fatigue, insomnia, drowsiness, depression, malaise, nervousness, vertigo, amnesia, convulsions, rash, pruritus, alopecia, photosensitivity, angioedema rash, dermatitis, hyperkalemia (small increase in patients with renal dysfunction), abdominal pain (rarely occurs but may with enzyme changes which suggest pancreatitis), vomiting, nausea, diarrhea, dysgeusia, anorexia, constipation, dyspepsia, xerostomia, dysphagia, increased salivation, weight gain, impotence, neutropenia, eosinophilia, decreased hemoglobin (rare), muscle cramps, myalgia, arthritis, arthralgia, paresthesia, tremor, neuralgia, neuropathy, tinnitus, proteinuria, transient increases BUN/serum creatinine, epistaxis, dyspnea, flu-like symptoms, diaphoresis

## Drug-Drug Interactions With ACEIs

| Precipitant Drug | Drug (Category) and Effect | Description |
|---|---|---|
| Ramipril | Lithium: increased | Increased serum lithium levels and symptoms of toxicity may occur. |
| Ramipril | Potassium preps/ potassium-sparing diuretics increased | Coadministration may result in elevated potassium levels. |
| Rampiril | Diuretics | Additive hypotensive effects, especially with initiation of therapy or increased dose |

(Continued)

## Ramipril *(Continued)*

**Drug Interactions** See table

**Onset** 1-2 hours

**Duration** 24 hours

**Half-Life** Ramiprilat: >50 hou s

**Special PA Issues**

**Patient Education:** Take as directed, 1 hour before or 2 hours after meals. Do not change dosage or stop taking without consulting prescriber. Do not change amount of dietary salt without advice or consult of prescriber. You may experience some changes in taste perception. You may experience dizziness, fainting, or lightheadedness (use caution when driving or performing hazardous tasks and use caution when changing position - rising from sitting or lying) until response to therapy is established. Report sore throat; fever; rash; swelling of face, hands, feet, or legs; respiratory difficulty; chest pains or irregular heartbeat; unusual cough; persistent vomiting, diarrhea, sweating, or perspiration; or flu-like symptoms.

**Related Information**

ACE Inhibitors *on page 995*

Heart Failure: Management of Patients with Left Ventricular Systolic Dysfunction *on page 1064*

## Ranitidine Bismuth Citrate *(ra NI ti deen BIZ muth SIT rate)*

**Pharmacologic Class** Histamine $H_2$ Antagonist

**U.S. Brand Names** Tritec®

**Mechanism of Action** As a complex of ranitidine and bismuth citrate, gastric acid secretion is inhibited by histamine-blocking activity at the parietal cell and the structural integrity of *H. pylori* organisms is disrupted; additionally bismuth reduces the adherence of *H. pylori* to epithelial cells of the stomach and may exert a cytoprotectant effect, inhibiting pepsin, as well. Adequate eradication of *Helicobacter pylori* is achieved with the combination of clarithromycin.

**Use** In combination with clarithromycin for the treatment of active duodenal ulcer associated with *H. pylori* infection; not to be used as monotherapy

**USUAL DOSAGE** Adults: Oral: 400 mg twice daily for 4 weeks with clarithromycin 500 mg 2 times/day for first 2 week

**Dosing adjustment in renal impairment:** Not recommended with $Cl_{cr}$ <25 mL/minute

**Dosing adjustment in hepatic impairment:** No dosage change necessary

**Note:** Most patients not eradicated of *H. pylori* following an adequate course of therapy that includes clarithromycin will have clarithromycin-resistant isolates and should be treated with an alternative multiple drug regimen

**Dosage Forms Tab:** 400 mg (ranitidine 162 mg, trivalent bismuth 128 mg, and citrate 110 mg)

**Contraindications** Hypersensitivity to ranitidine or bismuth compounds or components; acute porphyria

**Warnings/Precautions** Avoid use in patients with $Cl_{cr}$ <25 mL/minute; do not use for maintenance therapy or for >16 weeks/year

**Pregnancy Risk Factor** C

**Adverse Reactions**

>1%:

Central nervous system: Headache (14%), dizziness (1% to 2%)

Gastrointestinal: Diarrhea (5%), nausea/vomiting (3%), constipation (2%), abdominal pain, gastric upset (<10%), darkening of the tongue and/or stool (60% to 70%), taste disturbance (11%)

Miscellaneous: Flu-like symptoms (2%)

<1%: Rash, pruritus, anemia, thrombocytopenia, elevated LFTs

**Drug Interactions** See individual monographs

Increased effect: Optimal antimicrobial effects of ranitidine bismuth citrate occur when the drug is taken with food

**Half-Life** Bismuth: 11-28 days; Ranitidine: 3 hours; Complex: 5-8 days

**Special PA Issues**

**Patient Education:** Take as directed, with food. Do not supplement therapy with OTC medications. This drug may cause darkening of tongue or stool and may change your taste sensation. Report unresolved headache (prescriber may recommend something for relief), dizziness, diarrhea, constipation (prescriber may recommend something for relief), weakness, or loss of appetite.

**Dietary Considerations:** May be taken without regard to food

**Monitoring Parameters:** (13) C-urea breath tests to detect *H. pylori*, endoscopic evidence of ulcer healing, CBCs, LFTs, renal function tests

## Ranitidine Hydrochloride *(ra NI ti deen hye droe KLOR ide)*

**Pharmacologic Class** Histamine $H_2$ Antagonist

**U.S. Brand Names** Zantac®; Zantac® 75 [OTC]

**Mechanism of Action** Competitive inhibition of histamine at $H_2$-receptors of the gastric parietal cells, which inhibits gastric acid secretion, gastric volume and hydrogen ion concentration reduced

**Use** Short-term treatment of active duodenal ulcers and benign gastric ulcers; long-term prophylaxis of duodenal ulcer and gastric hypersecretory states, gastroesophageal reflux, recurrent postoperative ulcer, upper GI bleeding, prevention of acid-aspiration pneumonitis during surgery, and prevention of stress-induced ulcers; causes fewer interactions than cimetidine

**USUAL DOSAGE** Giving oral dose at 6 PM may be better than 10 PM bedtime, the highest acid production usually starts at approximately 7 PM, thus giving at 6 PM controls acid secretion better

Children:

Oral: 1.25-2.5 mg/kg/dose every 12 hours; maximum: 300 mg/day

I.M., I.V.: 0.75-1.5 mg/kg/dose every 6-8 hours, maximum daily dose: 400 mg

Continuous infusion: 0.1-0.25 mg/kg/hour (preferred for stress ulcer prophylaxis in patients with concurrent maintenance I.V.s or TPNs)

Adults:

Short-term treatment of ulceration: 150 mg/dose twice daily or 300 mg at bedtime
Prophylaxis of recurrent duodenal ulcer: Oral: 150 mg at bedtime
Gastric hypersecretory conditions:

Oral: 150 mg twice daily, up to 600mg/day

I.M., I.V.: 50 mg/dose every 6-8 hours (dose not to exceed 400 mg/day)

I.V.: 50 mg/dose IVPB every 6-8 hours (dose not to exceed 400 mg/day)

**or**

Continuous I.V. infusion: Initial: 50 mg IVPB, followed by 6.25 mg/hour titrated to gastric pH >4.0 for prophylaxis or >7.0 for treatment; **continuous I.V. infusion is preferred in patients with active bleeding**

Gastric hypersecretory conditions: Doses up to 2.5 mg/kg/hour (220 mg/hour) have been used

**Dosing adjustment in renal impairment:**

$Cl_{cr}$ 10-50 mL/minute: Administer at 75% of normal dose or administer every 18-24 hours
$Cl_{cr}$ <10 mL/minute: Administer at 50% of normal dose or administer every 18-24 hours
Hemodialysis: Slightly dialyzable (5% to 20%)

**Dosing adjustment/comments in hepatic disease:** Unchanged

**Dosage Forms** Ranitidine hydrochloride: **Cap (GELdose™):** 150 mg, 300 mg; **Granules, effervescent (EFFERdose™):** 150 mg; **Inf, preservative free, in NaCl 0.45%:** 1 mg/mL (50 mL); **Inj:** 25 mg/mL (2 mL, 10 mL, 40 mL); **Syr (peppermint flavor):** 15 mg/mL (473 mL); **Tab:** 75 mg [OTC]; 150 mg, 300 mg; **Tab, effervescent (EFFERdose™):** 150 mg

**Contraindications** Hypersensitivity to ranitidine or any component

**Warnings/Precautions** Use with caution in children <12 years of age; use with caution in patients with liver and renal impairment; dosage modification required in patients with renal impairment; long-term therapy may cause vitamin $B_{12}$ deficiency

**Pregnancy Risk Factor** B

**Adverse Reactions**

Endocrine & metabolic: Gynecomastia

Hepatic: Hepatitis

Neuromuscular & skeletal: Arthralgia

1% to 10%:

Central nervous system: Dizziness, sedation, malaise, headache, drowsiness

Dermatologic: Rash

Gastrointestinal: Constipation, nausea, vomiting, diarrhea

<1%: Bradycardia, tachycardia, fever, confusion, thrombocytopenia, neutropenia, agranulocytosis, bronchospasm

**Drug Interactions** CYP2D6 and 3A3/4 enzyme inhibitor

Decreased effect: Variable effects on warfarin; antacids may decrease absorption of ranitidine; ketoconazole and itraconazole absorptions are decreased; may produce altered serum levels of procainamide and ferrous sulfate; decreased effect of nondepolarizing muscle relaxants, cefpodoxime, cyanocobalamin (decreased absorption), diazepam, oxaprozin

Decreased toxicity of atropine

Increased toxicity of cyclosporine (increased serum creatinine), gentamicin (neuromuscular blockade), glipizide, glyburide, midazolam (increased concentrations), metoprolol, pentoxifylline, phenytoin, quinidine

**Onset** 1-2 hours

**Duration** 8-12 hours

**Half-Life** Adults: 2-2.5 hours; End-stage renal disease: 6-9 hours

**Special PA Issues**

**Patient Education:** Take exactly as directed (at meals and bedtime); do not increase dose - may take several days before you notice relief. If antacids are approved by prescriber, allow 1 hour between antacid and ranitidine. Avoid OTC medications, especially cold or cough medication and aspirin or anything containing aspirin. Follow diet as (Continued)

## Ranitidine Hydrochloride *(Continued)*

prescriber recommends. You may experience constipation or diarrhea (request assistance from prescriber); nausea or vomiting (frequent small meals, frequent mouth care, or sucking on lozenges may help); impotence or loss of libido (reversible when drug is discontinued); drowsiness, dizziness, or fatigue (use caution when driving or engaging in hazardous activities). Report skin rash, fever, sore throat, tarry stools, changes in CNS, muscle or joint pain, yellowing of skin or eyes, and change in color of urine or stool.

**Monitoring Parameters:** AST, ALT, serum creatinine; when used to prevent stress-related GI bleeding, measure the intragastric pH and try to maintain pH >4; signs and symptoms of peptic ulcer disease, occult blood with GI bleeding, monitor renal function to correct dose; monitor for side effects

- ◆ **Raxar®** *see* Grepafloxacin *on page 426*
- ◆ **RBC** *see* Ranitidine Bismuth Citrate *on page 794*
- ◆ **R & C® Shampoo [OTC]** *see* Pyrethrins *on page 783*
- ◆ **Rea-Lo® [OTC]** *see* Urea *on page 947*
- ◆ **Rebetol®** *see* Ribavirin *on page 801*
- ◆ **Rebetron™** *see* Interferon Alfa-2b and Ribavirin Combination Pack *on page 484*
- ◆ **Recombinant Human Follicle Stimulating Hormone** *see* Follitropins *on page 397*
- ◆ **Recombinant Human Interleukin-11** *see* Oprelvekin *on page 678*
- ◆ **Recombinant Human Platelet-Derived Growth Factor B** *see* Becaplermin *on page 100*
- ◆ **Recombinant Interleukin-11** *see* Oprelvekin *on page 678*
- ◆ **Recombinant plasminogen activator** *see* Reteplase *on page 799*
- ◆ **Redisol®** *see* Cyanocobalamin *on page 242*
- ◆ **Redoxon®** *see* Ascorbic Acid *on page 79*
- ◆ **Redutemp® [OTC]** *see* Acetaminophen *on page 21*
- ◆ **Red Valerian** *see* Valerian *on page 951*
- ◆ **Reese's® Pinworm Medicine [OTC]** *see* Pyrantel Pamoate *on page 782*
- ◆ **Reference Values for Adults** *see* Chart *on page 1035*
- ◆ **Regitine®** *see* Phentolamine *on page 717*
- ◆ **Reglan®** *see* Metoclopramide *on page 597*
- ◆ **Regonol® Injection** *see* Pyridostigmine *on page 783*
- ◆ **Regranex®** *see* Becaplermin *on page 100*
- ◆ **Regular (Concentrated) Iletin® II U-500** *see* Insulin Preparations *on page 479*
- ◆ **Regular Iletin® I** *see* Insulin Preparations *on page 479*
- ◆ **Regular Insulin** *see* Insulin Preparations *on page 479*
- ◆ **Regular Purified Pork Insulin** *see* Insulin Preparations *on page 479*
- ◆ **Regular Strength Bayer® Enteric 500 Aspirin [OTC]** *see* Aspirin *on page 80*
- ◆ **Regulax SS® [OTC]** *see* Docusate *on page 298*
- ◆ **Regulex®** *see* Docusate *on page 298*
- ◆ **Reguloid® [OTC]** *see* Psyllium *on page 781*
- ◆ **Rela®** *see* Carisoprodol *on page 154*
- ◆ **Relafen®** *see* Nabumetone *on page 626*
- ◆ **Relaxadon®** *see* Hyoscyamine, Atropine, Scopolamine, and Phenobarbital *on page 464*
- ◆ **Relief® Ophthalmic Solution** *see* Phenylephrine *on page 718*
- ◆ **Remeron®** *see* Mirtazapine *on page 611*
- ◆ **Remicade™** *see* Infliximab *on page 478*

## Remifentanil *(rem i FEN ta nil)*

**Pharmacologic Class** Analgesic, Narcotic

**U.S. Brand Names** Ultiva™

**Mechanism of Action** Binds with stereospecific mu-opioid receptors at many sites within the CNS, increases pain threshold, alters pain reception, inhibits ascending pain pathways

**Use** Analgesic for use during general anesthesia for continued analgesia

**USUAL DOSAGE** Adults: I.V. continuous infusion:

During induction: 0.5-1 mcg/kg/minute

During maintenance:

With nitrous oxide (66%): 0.4 mcg/kg/minute (range: 0.1-2 mcg/kg/min)

With isoflurane: 0.25 mcg/kg/minute (range: 0.05-2 mcg/kg/min)

With propofol: 0.25 mcg/kg/minute (range: 0.05-2 mcg/kg/min)

Continuation as an analgesic in immediate postoperative period: 0.1 mcg/kg/minute (range: 0.025-0.2 mcg/kg/min)

**Dosage Forms Powder for inj, lyophilized:** 1 mg/3 mL vial, 2 mg/5 mL vial, 5 mg/10 mL vial

**Contraindications** Not for intrathecal or epidural administration, due to the presence of glycine in the formulation, it is also contraindicated in patients with a known hypersensitivity to remifentanil, fentanyl or fentanyl analogs; interruption of an infusion will result in offset of effects within 5-10 minutes; the discontinuation of remifentanil infusion should be preceded by the establishment of adequate postoperative analgesia orders, especially for patients in whom postoperative pain is anticipated

**Warnings/Precautions** Remifentanil is not recommended as the sole agent in general anesthesia, because the loss of consciousness cannot be assured and due to the high incidence of apnea, hypotension, tachycardia and muscle rigidity; it should be administered by individuals specifically trained in the use of anesthetic agents and should not be used in diagnostic or therapeutic procedures outside the monitored anesthesia setting; resuscitative and intubation equipment should be readily available

**Pregnancy Risk Factor** C

**Adverse Reactions**
>10%: Gastrointestinal: Nausea, vomiting
1% to 10%:
Cardiovascular: Hypotension, bradycardia, tachycardia, hypertension
Central nervous system: Dizziness, headache, agitation, fever
Dermatologic: Pruritus
Ocular: Visual disturbances
Respiratory: Respiratory depression, apnea, hypoxia
Miscellaneous: Shivering, postoperative pain

**Special PA Issues**
**Monitoring Parameters:** Respiratory and cardiovascular status, blood pressure, heart rate

**Related Information**
Narcotic Agonists *on page 1023*

- ◆ **Renagel®** *see Sevelamer on page 831*
- ◆ **Renal Function Tests** *see Chart on page 993*
- ◆ **Renedil®** *see Felodipine on page 359*
- ◆ **Renova™** *see Tretinoin, Topical on page 927*
- ◆ **Rentamine®** *see Chlorpheniramine, Ephedrine, Phenylephrine, and Carbetapentane on page 195*
- ◆ **Repan®** *see Butalbital Compound on page 131*
- ◆ **Reposans-10® Oral** *see Chlordiazepoxide on page 189*
- ◆ **Repronex™** *see Menotropins on page 567*
- ◆ **Requip™** *see Ropinirole on page 815*
- ◆ **Resa®** *see Reserpine on this page*
- ◆ **Rescaps-D® S.R. Capsule** *see Caramiphen and Phenylpropanolamine on page 148*
- ◆ **Rescriptor®** *see Delavirdine on page 257*
- ◆ **Resectisol® Irrigation Solution** *see Mannitol on page 557*

# Reserpine (re SER peen)

**Pharmacologic Class** Rauwolfia Alkaloid
**U.S. Brand Names** Resa®; Serpalan®; Serpasil®; Serpatabs®
**Mechanism of Action** Reduces blood pressure via depletion of sympathetic biogenic amines (norepinephrine and dopamine); this also commonly results in sedative effects
**Use** Management of mild to moderate hypertension
**Unlabeled use:** Management of tardive dyskinesia
**USUAL DOSAGE** Oral (full antihypertensive effects may take as long as 3 weeks):
Children: 0.01-0.02 mg/kg/24 hours divided every 12 hours; maximum dose: 0.25 mg/day (not recommended in children)
Adults:
Hypertension: 0.1-0.25 mg/day in 1-2 doses; initial: 0.5 mg/day for 1-2 weeks; maintenance: reduce to 0.1-0.25 mg/day
Psychiatric: Initial: 0.5 mg/day; usual range: 0.1-1 mg
Elderly: Initial: 0.05 mg once daily, increasing by 0.05 mg every week as necessary
**Dosing adjustment in renal impairment:** $Cl_{cr}$ <10 mL/minute: Avoid use
Dialysis: Not removed by hemo or peritoneal dialysis; supplemental dose is not necessary
**Dosage Forms** Tab: 0.1 mg, 0.25 mg
**Contraindications** Any ulcerative condition, mental depression, hypersensitivity to reserpine or any component
**Warnings/Precautions** Discontinue reserpine 7 days before electroshock therapy; use with caution in patients with impaired renal function or peptic ulcer disease, gallstones, and the elderly; at high doses, significant mental depression may occur; some products may contain tartrazine
**Pregnancy Risk Factor** C
**Adverse Reactions**
Cardiovascular: Peripheral edema, arrhythmias, bradycardia, chest pain, hypotension
Central nervous system: Dizziness, headache, drowsiness, fatigue, mental depression, parkinsonism
Dermatologic: Rash
Endocrine & metabolic: Sodium and water retention
(Continued)

## Reserpine *(Continued)*

Gastrointestinal: Anorexia, diarrhea, xerostomia, nausea, vomiting, black stools, increased gastric acid secretion

Genitourinary: Impotence, dysuria

Neuromuscular & skeletal: Trembling of hands/fingers

Respiratory: Nasal congestion

Miscellaneous: Bloody vomit

**Drug Interactions**

Decreased effect of indirect-acting sympathomimetics (ie, ephedrine, tyramine, amphetamines)

Increased effect/toxicity of MAO inhibitors (avoid use or use extreme caution), direct-acting sympathomimetics (ie, epinephrine, isoproterenol, phenylephrine, metaraminol), and tricyclic antidepressants; cardiac arrhythmias have occurred with digoxin

**Onset** Onset of antihypertensive effect: Within 3-6 days

**Duration** 2-6 weeks

**Half-Life** 50-100 hours

**Special PA Issues**

**Patient Education:** Take as directed; do not discontinue without consulting prescriber. May take up to 2 weeks to see effects of therapy. Avoid alcohol and maintain recommended diet. You may experience nervousness, dizziness, or fatigue; use caution when driving or engaging in hazardous activities until response to treatment is known. Rise slowly from sitting or lying position until response to therapy is known. Small frequent meals or sucking on lozenges may reduce nausea or loss of appetite; adequate dietary fruit, fluids, and fiber may reduce constipation. You may experience nasal stuffiness; avoid OTC medications, and consult prescriber. You may experience impotence; will resolve when medication is discontinued. Report chest pain, rapid heartbeat or palpitations, difficulty breathing, sudden increase in weight, swelling in ankles or hands, black tarry stools; or unusual feelings of depression.

**Monitoring Parameters:** Blood pressure, standing and sitting/supine

♦ **Respa-DM®** *see* Guaifenesin and Dextromethorphan *on page 428*

♦ **Respa-GF®** *see* Guaifenesin *on page 427*

♦ **Respbid®** *see* Theophylline Salts *on page 888*

♦ **RespiGam™** *see* Respiratory Syncytial Virus Immune Globulin (Intravenous) *on this page*

# Respiratory Syncytial Virus Immune Globulin (Intravenous)

(RES peer rah tor ee sin SISH al VYE rus i MYUN GLOB yoo lin in tra VEE nus)

**Pharmacologic Class** Immune Globulin

**U.S. Brand Names** RespiGam™

**Mechanism of Action** RSV-IGIV is a sterile liquid immunoglobulin G containing neutralizing antibody to respiratory syncytial virus. It is effective in reducing the incidence and duration of RSV hospitalization and the severity of RSV illness in high risk infants.

**Use** Prevention of serious lower respiratory infection caused by respiratory syncytial virus (RSV) in children <24 months of age with bronchopulmonary dysplasia (BPD) or a history of premature birth (≤35 weeks gestation)

**USUAL DOSAGE** I.V.: 750 mg/kg/month according to the following infusion schedule: 1.5 mL/kg/hour for 15 minutes, then at 3 mL/kg/hour for the next 15 minutes if the clinical condition does not contraindicate a higher rate, and finally, administer at 6 mL/kg/hour until completion of dose

**Dosage Forms** Inj: 2500 mg RSV immunoglobulin/50 mL vial

**Contraindications** Selective IgA deficiency; history of severe prior reaction to any immunoglobulin preparation

**Warnings/Precautions** Use caution to avoid fluid overload in patients, particularly infants with bronchopulmonary dysplasia (BPD), when administering RSV-IGIV; hypersensitivity including anaphylaxis or angioneurotic edema may occur; keep epinephrine 1:1000 readily available during infusion; rare occurrences of aseptic meningitis syndrome have been associated with IGIV treatment, particularly with high doses; observe carefully for signs and symptoms of such and treat promptly

**Pregnancy Risk Factor** C

**Adverse Reactions**

1% to 10%:

Dermatologic: Rash (1%)

Cardiovascular: Tachycardia (1%), hypertension (1%), hypotension

Central nervous system: Fever (6%)

Endocrine & metabolic: Fluid overload (1%)

Gastrointestinal: Vomiting (2%), diarrhea (1%), gastroenteritis (1%)

Local: Injection site inflammation (1%)

Respiratory: Respiratory distress (2%), wheezing (2%), rales, hypoxia (1%), tachypnea (1%)

<1%: Edema, pallor, heart murmur, cyanosis, flushing, palpitations, chest tightness, dizziness, anxiety, eczema, pruritus, abdominal cramps, myalgia, arthralgia, cough, rhinorrhea, dyspnea

**Drug Interactions**

Decreased toxicity: Antibodies present in IVIG preparations may interfere with the immune response to live virus vaccines (eg, MMR); reimmunization is recommended if such vaccines are administered within 10 months following RSV-IVIG treatment; additionally, it is advised that booster doses of oral polio, DPT, and HIB be considered 3-4 months after the last dose of RSV-IVIG in order to ensure immunity

**Special PA Issues**

**Monitoring Parameters:** Monitor for symptoms of allergic reaction; check vital signs, cardiopulmonary status after each rate increase and thereafter at 30-minute intervals until 30 minutes following completion of the infusion

♦ **Restoril®** see Temazepam on page 876

♦ **Retavase™** see Reteplase on this page

# Reteplase (RE ta plase)

**Pharmacologic Class** Thrombolytic Agent

**U.S. Brand Names** Retavase™

**Mechanism of Action** Reteplase is a nonglycosylated form of tPA produced by recombinant DNA technology using *E. coli*; it initiates local fibrinolysis by binding to fibrin in a thrombus (clot) and converts entrapped plasminogen to plasmin

**Use** Improvement of ventricular function following acute myocardial infarction, for the reduction of the incidence of CHF and the reduction of mortality associated with acute myocardial infarction

**USUAL DOSAGE**

Children: Not recommended

Adults: 10 units I.V. over 2 minutes, followed by a second dose 30 minutes later of 10 units I.V. over 2 minutes

Withhold second dose if serious bleeding or anaphylaxis occurs

**Dosage Forms Powder for inj, lyophilized:** 10.8 units [reteplase 18.8 mg]

**Contraindications** Active internal bleeding, history of cerebrovascular accident, recent intracranial or intraspinal surgery or trauma, intracranial neoplasm, arteriovenous malformations or aneurysm, known bleeding diathesis, severe uncontrolled hypertension, history of severe allergic reactions to reteplase, alteplase, anistreplase or streptokinase

**Pregnancy Risk Factor** C

**Adverse Reactions**

>10%:

Cardiovascular: Hypotension, arrhythmias, trauma arrhythmias

Hematologic: Bleeding

1% to 10%: Hematologic: Anemia, genitourinary bleeding, gastrointestinal bleeding, injection site bleeding

<1%: Intracranial hemorrhage, allergic reactions, anaphylaxis

**Drug Interactions** Increased effect: Anticoagulants, aspirin, ticlopidine, dipyridamole, abciximab and heparin are at least additive

**Onset** 30-90 minutes

**Half-Life** In serum, 13-16 minutes

**Special PA Issues**

**Patient Education:** This medication can only be administered I.V. You will have a tendency to bleed easily following this medication; use caution to prevent injury (use electric razor, use soft toothbrush, use caution with sharps). If bleeding occurs, apply pressure to bleeding spot until bleeding stops completely. Report unusual bruising or bleeding (eg, blood in urine, stool, or vomitus; bleeding gums; vaginal bleeding; nosebleeds); dizziness or changes in vision; back pain; skin rash; swelling of face, mouth, or throat; or difficulty breathing.

**Monitoring Parameters:** Monitor for signs of bleeding (hematuria, GI bleeding, gingival bleeding)

♦ **Retin-A™ Micro Topical** see Tretinoin, Topical on page 927

♦ **Retin-A™ Topical** see Tretinoin, Topical on page 927

♦ **Retinoic Acid** see Tretinoin, Topical on page 927

♦ **Retisol-A®** see Tretinoin, Topical on page 927

♦ **Retrovir®** see Zidovudine on page 972

♦ **Reversol® Injection** see Edrophonium on page 313

♦ **Revex®** see Nalmefene on page 632

♦ **Rēv-Eyes™** see Dapiprazole on page 255

♦ **ReVia®** see Naltrexone on page 634

♦ **Revitalose-C-1000®** see Ascorbic Acid on page 79

♦ **Rezine®** see Hydroxyzine on page 462

♦ **Rezulin®** see Troglitazone on page 941

- **rFSH-alpha** see Follitropins on page 397
- **rFSH-beta** see Follitropins on page 397
- **R-Gen®** see Iodinated Glycerol on page 487
- **rGM-CSF** see Sargramostim on page 822
- **Rheumatrex®** see Methotrexate on page 585
- **rhFSH-alpha** see Follitropins on page 397
- **rhFSH-beta** see Follitropins on page 397
- **rhIL-11** see Oprelvekin on page 678
- **Rhinalar®** see Flunisolide on page 379
- **Rhinall® Nasal Solution [OTC]** see Phenylephrine on page 718
- **Rhinaris®-F** see Flunisolide on page 379
- **Rhinatate® Tablet** see Chlorpheniramine, Pyrilamine, and Phenylephrine on page 197
- **Rhindecon®** see Phenylpropanclamine on page 720
- **Rhinocort®** see Budesonide on page 124
- **Rhinosyn-DMX® [OTC]** see Guaifenesin and Dextromethorphan on page 428

## Rh$_o$(D) Immune Globulin (Intramuscular)

(ar aych oh (dee) i MYUN GLOB yoo lin)

**Pharmacologic Class** Immune Globulin

**U.S. Brand Names** Gamulin® Rh; HypRho®-D; HypRho®-D Mini-Dose; MICRhoGAM™; Mini-Gamulin® Rh; RhoGAM™

**Mechanism of Action** Suppresses the immune response and antibody formation of Rh-negative individuals to Rh-positive red blood cells

**Use** Prevention of isoimmunization in Rh-negative individuals exposed to Rh-positive blood during delivery of an Rh-positive infant, as a result of an abortion, following amniocentesis or abdominal trauma, or following a transfusion accident; prevention of hemolytic disease of the newborn if there is a subsequent pregnancy with an Rh-positive fetus

**USUAL DOSAGE** Adults (administered I.M. to mothers **not** to infant) I.M.:

Obstetrical usage: 1 vial (300 mcg) prevents maternal sensitization if fetal packed red blood cell volume that has entered the circulation is <15 mL; if it is more, give additional vials. The number of vials = RBC volume of the calculated fetomaternal hemorrhage divided by 15 mL

Postpartum prophylaxis: 300 mcg within 72 hours of delivery

Antepartum prophylaxis: 300 mcg at approximately 26-28 weeks gestation; followed by 300 mcg within 72 hours of delivery if infant is Rh-positive

Following miscarriage, abortion, or termination of ectopic pregnancy at up to 13 weeks of gestation: 50 mcg ideally within 3 hours, but may be given up to 72 hours after; if pregnancy has been terminated at 13 or more weeks of gestation, administer 300 mcg

**Dosage Forms Inj:** Each package contains one single dose 300 mcg of Rh$_o$ (D) immune globulin; **Inj, microdose:** Each package contains one single dose of microdose, 50 mcg of Rh$_o$ (D) immune globulin

**Contraindications** Rh$_o$(D)-positive patient; known hypersensitivity to immune globulins or to thimerosal; transfusion of Rh$_o$(D)-positive blood in previous 3 months; prior sensitization to Rh$_o$(D)

**Warnings/Precautions** Use with caution in patients with thrombocytopenia or bleeding disorders, patients with IgA deficiency; do not inject I.V.; do not administer to neonates

**Pregnancy Risk Factor** C

**Adverse Reactions** <1%: Lethargy, splenomegaly, elevated bilirubin, pain at the injection site, myalgia, temperature elevation

**Special PA Issues**

**Patient Education:** Acetaminophen may be taken to ease minor discomfort after vaccination

## Rh$_o$(D) Immune Globulin (Intravenous-Human)

(ar aych oh (dee) i MYUN GLOB yoo lin in tra VEE nus HYU man)

**Pharmacologic Class** Immune Globulin

**U.S. Brand Names** WinRho SD®

**Mechanism of Action** The Rh$_o$(D) antigen is responsible for most cases of Rh sensitization, which occurs when Rh-positive fetal RBCs enter the maternal circulation of an Rh-negative woman. Injection of anti-D globulin results in opsonization of the fetal RBCs, which are then phagocytized in the spleen, preventing immunization of the mother. Injection of anti-D into an Rh-positive patient with ITP coats the patient's own D-positive RBCs with antibody and, as they are cleared by the spleen, they saturate the capacity of the spleen to clear antibody-coated cells, sparing antibody-coated platelets. Other proposed mechanisms involve the generation of cytokines following the interaction between antibody-coated RBCs and macrophages.

**Use**

Prevention of Rh isoimmunization in nonsensitized Rh$_o$(D) antigen-negative women within 72 hours after spontaneous or induced abortion, amniocentesis, chorionic villus sampling, ruptured tubal pregnancy, abdominal trauma, transplacental hemorrhage, or in the normal course of pregnancy unless the blood type of the fetus or father is known to be $Rh_o(D)$ antigen-negative.

Suppression of Rh isoimmunization in $Rh_o(D)$ antigen-negative female children and female adults in their childbearing years transfused with $Rh_o(D)$ antigen-positive RBCs or blood components containing $Rh_o(D)$ antigen-positive RBCs

Treatment of idiopathic thrombocytopenic purpura (ITP) in nonsplenectomized $Rh_o(D)$ antigen-positive patients

## USUAL DOSAGE

Prevention of Rh isoimmunization: I.V.: 1500 units (300 mcg) at 28 weeks gestation or immediately after amniocentesis if before 34 weeks gestation or after chorionic villus sampling; repeat this dose every 12 weeks during the pregnancy. Administer 600 units (120 mcg) at delivery (within 72 hours) and after invasive intrauterine procedures such as abortion, amniocentesis, or any other manipulation if at >34 weeks gestation. **Note:** If the Rh status of the baby is not known at 72 hours, administer $Rh_o(D)$ immune globulin to the mother at 72 hours after delivery. If >72 hours have elapsed, do not withhold $Rh_o(D)$ immune globulin, but administer as soon as possible, up to 28 days after delivery.

I.M.: Reconstitute vial with 1.25 mL and administer as above

Transfusion: Administer within 72 hours after exposure for treatment of incompatible blood transfusions or massive fetal hemorrhage as follows:

I.V.: 3000 units (600 mcg) every 8 hours until the total dose is administered (45 units [9 mcg] of Rh-positive blood/mL blood; 90 units [18 mcg] Rh-positive red cells/mL cells)

I.M.: 6000 units [1200 mcg] every 12 hours until the total dose is administered (60 units [12 mcg] of Rh-positive blood/mL blood; 120 units [24 mcg] Rh-positive red cells/mL cells)

Treatment of ITP: I.V.: Initial: 25-50 mcg/kg depending on the patient's Hgb concentration; maintenance: 25-60 mcg/kg depending on the clinical response

**Dosage Forms** Inj: 600 units [120 mcg], 1500 units [300 mcg]

**Contraindications** Hypersensitivity to immune globulin or any component, IgA deficiency

**Warnings/Precautions** Anaphylactic hypersensitivity reactions can occur; studies indicate that there is no discernible risk of transmitting HIV or hepatitis B; do not administer by S.C. route; use only the I.V. route when treating ITP

**Pregnancy Risk Factor** C

**Adverse Reactions** 1% to 10%:

Central nervous system: Headache (2%), fever (1%), chills (<2%)

Hematologic: Hemolysis (Hgb decrease of >2 g/dL in 5% to 10% of ITP patients)

Local: Slight edema and pain at the injection site

**Drug Interactions** Increased toxicity: Live virus, vaccines (measles, mumps, rubella); do not administer within 3 months after administration of these vaccines

♦ **Rhodis™** see Ketoprofen on page 507

♦ **Rhodis-EC™** see Ketoprofen on page 507

♦ **RhoGAM™** see $Rh_o(D)$ Immune Globulin (Intramuscular) on previous page

♦ **RhoIGIV** see $Rh_o(D)$ Immune Globulin (Intravenous-Human) on previous page

♦ **Rhoprolene** see Betamethasone on page 111

♦ **Rhoprosone** see Betamethasone on page 111

♦ **Rhotral** see Acebutolol on page 20

♦ **Rhotrimine®** see Trimipramine on page 938

♦ **rHuEPO-α** see Epoetin Alfa on page 322

♦ **Rhulicaine® [OTC]** see Benzocaine on page 105

♦ **Rhythmin®** see Procainamide on page 759

## Ribavirin (rye ba VYE rin)

**Pharmacologic Class** Antiviral Agent

**U.S. Brand Names** Rebetol®; Virazole® Aerosol

**Mechanism of Action** Inhibits replication of RNA and DNA viruses; inhibits influenza virus RNA polymerase activity and inhibits the initiation and elongation of RNA fragments resulting in inhibition of viral protein synthesis

**Use** Inhalation: Treatment of patients with respiratory syncytial virus (RSV) infections; may also be used in other viral infections including influenza A and B and adenovirus; specially indicated for treatment of severe lower respiratory tract RSV infections in patients with an underlying compromising condition (prematurity, bronchopulmonary dysplasia and other chronic lung conditions, congenital heart disease, immunodeficiency, immunosuppression), and recent transplant recipients

Oral capsules: The combination therapy of oral ribavirin with interferon alfa-2b, recombinant (Intron® A) injection is indicated for the treatment of chronic hepatitis C in patients with compensated liver disease who have relapsed after alpha interferon therapy.

**USUAL DOSAGE** Infants, Children, and Adults:

Aerosol inhalation: Use with Viratek® small particle aerosol generator (SPAG-2) at a concentration of 20 mg/mL (6 g reconstituted with 300 mL of sterile water without preservatives)

Aerosol only: 12-18 hours/day for 3 days, up to 7 days in length

(Continued)

## Ribavirin *(Continued)*

**Dosage Forms Cap:** 200 mg (available only in Rebetron combination package); **Powder for aero:** 6 g (100 mL)

**Contraindications** Females of childbearing age; hypersensitivity to ribavirin; patients with autoimmune hepatitis

**Warnings/Precautions** Use with caution in patients requiring assisted ventilation because precipitation of the drug in the respiratory equipment may interfere with safe and effective patient ventilation; monitor carefully in patients with COPD and asthma for deterioration of respiratory function. Ribavirin is potentially mutagenic, tumor-promoting, and gonadotoxic. Anemia has been observed in patients receiving the interferon/ribavirin combination. Severe psychiatric events have also occurred including depression and suicidal behavior during combination therapy; avoid use in patients with a psychiatric history.

**Pregnancy Risk Factor** X

**Adverse Reactions**

Inhalation:

1% to 10%:

Central nervous system: Fatigue, headache, insomnia

Gastrointestinal: Nausea, anorexia

Hematologic: Anemia

<1%: Hypotension, cardiac arrest, digitalis toxicity, rash, skin irritation, conjunctivitis, mild bronchospasm, worsening of respiratory function, apnea

**Note:** Incidence of adverse effects in healthcare workers approximate 51% headache; 32% conjunctivitis; 10% to 20% rhinitis, nausea, rash, dizziness, pharyngitis, and lacrimation

Oral: (All adverse reactions are documented while receiving combination therapy with interferon alpha-2b)

>10%:

Cardiovascular: Chest pain

Central nervous system: Dizziness, headache, fatigue, fever, insomnia, irritability, depression, emotional lability, impaired concentration

Dermatologic: Alopecia, rash, pruritus

Gastrointestinal: Nausea, anorexia, dyspepsia, vomiting

Hematologic: Decreased hemoglobin and WBC

Neuromuscular & skeletal: Myalgia, arthralgia, musculoskeletal pain, astenia, rigors

Respiratory: Dyspnea, sinusitis

Miscellaneous: Flu-like syndrome

1% to 10%:

Central nervous system: Nervousness

Endocrine & metabolic: Thyroid function test abnormalities

Gastrointestinal: Taste perversion

**Drug Interactions** Decreased effect of zidovudine

**Half-Life** 24 hours, much longer in the erythrocyte (16-40 days), which can be used as a marker for intracellular metabolism

**Special PA Issues**

**Patient Education:** Take as directed, for full course of therapy; do not discontinue even if feeling better. Use aerosol device as instructed. Maintain adequate fluid intake and report any swelling of ankles or feet, difficulty breathing, persistent lethargy, acute headache, insomnia, severe nausea or anorexia, confusion, fever, chills, sore throat, easy bruising or bleeding, mouth sores, or worsening of respiratory condition.

**Monitoring Parameters:** Respiratory function, CBC, reticulocyte count, I & O

## Riboflavin *(RYE boe flay vin)*

**Pharmacologic Class** Vitamin, Water Soluble

**U.S. Brand Names** Riobin®

**Mechanism of Action** Component of flavoprotein enzymes that work together, which are necessary for normal tissue respiration; also needed for activation of pyridoxine and conversion of tryptophan to niacin

**Use** Prevent riboflavin deficiency and treat ariboflavinosis

**USUAL DOSAGE** Oral:

Riboflavin deficiency:

Children: 2.5-10 mg/day in divided doses

Adults: 5-30 mg/day in divided doses

Recommended daily allowance:

Children: 0.4-1.8 mg

Adults: 1.2-1.7 mg

**Dosage Forms Tab:** 25 mg, 50 mg, 100 mg

**Warnings/Precautions** Riboflavin deficiency often occurs in the presence of other B vitamin deficiencies

**Pregnancy Risk Factor** A (C if dose exceeds RDA recommendation)

**Drug Interactions** Decreased absorption with probenecid

**Half-Life** Biologic: 66-84 minutes

**Special PA Issues**
**Patient Education:** Take with food. Large doses may cause bright yellow or orange urine.

♦ **Rid-A-Pain®** [OTC] *see* Benzocaine *on page 105*

♦ **Ridaura®** *see* Auranofin *on page 89*

♦ **Ridene** *see* Nicardipine *on page 651*

♦ **Ridenol®** [OTC] *see* Acetaminophen *on page 21*

♦ **RID® Shampoo** [OTC] *see* Pyrethrins *on page 783*

# Rifabutin (rif a BYOO tin)

**Pharmacologic Class** Antibiotic, Miscellaneous; Antitubercular Agent
**U.S. Brand Names** Mycobutin®
**Mechanism of Action** Inhibits DNA-dependent RNA polymerase at the beta subunit which prevents chain initiation
**Use** Prevention of disseminated *Mycobacterium avium* complex (MAC) in patients with advanced HIV infection; also utilized in multiple drug regimens for treatment of MAC
**USUAL DOSAGE** Oral:
 Children: Efficacy and safety of rifabutin have not been established in children; a limited number of HIV-positive children with MAC have been given rifabutin for MAC prophylaxis; doses of 5 mg/kg/day have been useful
 Adults: 300 mg once daily; for patients who experience gastrointestinal upset, rifabutin can be administered 150 mg twice daily with food
**Dosage Forms Cap:** 150 mg
**Contraindications** Hypersensitivity to rifabutin or any other rifamycins; rifabutin is contraindicated in patients with a WBC <1000/mm³ or a platelet count <50,000/mm³; concurrent use with ritonavir
**Warnings/Precautions** Rifabutin as a single agent must not be administered to patients with active tuberculosis since its use may lead to the development of tuberculosis that is resistant to both rifabutin and rifampin; rifabutin should be discontinued in patients with AST >500 units/L or if total bilirubin is >3 mg/dL. Use with caution in patients with liver impairment; modification of dosage should be considered in patients with renal impairment.
**Pregnancy Risk Factor** B
**Adverse Reactions**
 >10%:
  Dermatologic: Rash (11%)
  Genitourinary: Discolored urine (30%)
  Hematologic: Neutropenia (25%), leukopenia (17%)
 1% to 10%:
  Central nervous system: Headache (3%)
  Gastrointestinal: Vomiting/nausea (3%), abdominal pain (4%), diarrhea (3%), anorexia (2%), flatulence (2%), eructation (3%)
  Hematologic: Anemia, thrombocytopenia (5%)
  Hepatic: Increased AST/ALT (7% to 9%)
  Neuromuscular & skeletal: Myalgia
 <1%: Chest pain, fever, insomnia, dyspepsia, taste perversion, uveitis
**Drug Interactions** CYP3A3/4 enzyme inducer
 Decreased plasma concentration (due to induction of liver enzymes) of verapamil, methadone, digoxin, cyclosporine, corticosteroids, oral anticoagulants, theophylline, barbiturates, chloramphenicol, ketoconazole, oral contraceptives, quinidine, halothane, protease inhibitors, non-nucleoside reverse transcriptase inhibitors, and perhaps clarithromycin
 Increased concentration by indinavir; reduce to ½ standard dose when used with indinavir
 Increased risk of rifabutin-induced hematologic and ocular toxicity (uveitis) with concurrent administration of drug that inhibits CYP450 enzymes such as protease inhibitors, erythromycin, clarithromycin, ketoconazole, and itraconazole
**Half-Life** 45 hours (range: 16-69 hours)
**Special PA Issues**
 **Patient Education:** May take with food if GI upset occurs. Will discolor urine, stool, saliva, tears, sweat, and other body fluid a red-brown color. Stains on clothing or contact lenses are permanent. Report skin rash, vomiting, fever, chills, flu-like symptoms, dark urine or pale stools, unusual bleeding or bruising, or unusual confusion, depression, or fatigue.
 **Monitoring Parameters:** Periodic liver function tests, CBC with differential, platelet count

♦ **Rifadin®** *see* Rifampin *on this page*

♦ **Rifadin® Injection** *see* Rifampin *on this page*

♦ **Rifadin® Oral** *see* Rifampin *on this page*

♦ **Rifamate®** *see* Rifampin and Isoniazid *on page 805*

♦ **Rifampicin** *see* Rifampin *on this page*

# Rifampin (RIF am pin)

**Pharmacologic Class** Antibiotic, Miscellaneous; Antitubercular Agent
**U.S. Brand Names** Rifadin® Injection; Rifadin® Oral; Rimactane® Oral
(Continued)

# Rifampin *(Continued)*

**Mechanism of Action** Inhibits bacterial RNA synthesis by binding to the beta subunit of DNA-dependent RNA polymerase, blocking RNA transcription

**Use** Management of active tuberculosis in combination with other agents; eliminate meningococci from asymptomatic carriers; prophylaxis of *Haemophilus influenzae* type b infection; used in combination with other anti-infectives in the treatment of staphylococcal infections

**USUAL DOSAGE** Oral (I.V. infusion dose is the same as for the oral route):

**Tuberculosis therapy:**

**Note:** A four-drug regimen (isoniazid, rifampin, pyrazinamide, and either streptomycin or ethambutol) is preferred for the initial, empiric treatment of TB. When the drug susceptibility results are available, the regimen should be altered as appropriate.

Infants and Children <12 years:

Daily therapy: 10-20 mg/kg/day usually as a single dose (maximum: 600 mg/day)

Directly observed therapy (DOT): Twice weekly: 10-20 mg/kg (maximum: 600 mg); 3 times/week: 10-20 mg/kg (maximum: 600 mg)

Adults:

Daily therapy: 10 mg/kg/day (maximum: 600 mg/day)

Directly observed therapy (DOT): Twice weekly: 10 mg/kg (maximum: 600 mg); 3 times/week: 10 mg/kg (maximum: 600 mg)

**H. influenzae prophylaxis:**

Infants and Children: 20 mg/kg/day every 24 hours for 4 days, not to exceed 600 mg/dose

Adults: 600 mg every 24 hours for 4 days

**Meningococcal prophylaxis:**

<1 month: 10 mg/kg/day in divided doses every 12 hours for 2 days

Infants and Children: 20 mg/kg/day in divided doses every 12 hours for 2 days

Adults: 600 mg every 12 hours for 2 days

**Nasal carriers of *Staphylococcus aureus*:**

Children: 15 mg/kg/day divided every 12 hours for 5-10 days in combination with other antibiotics

Adults: 600 mg/day for 5-10 days in combination with other antibiotics

**Synergy for *Staphylococcus aureus* infections:** Adults: 300-600 mg twice daily with other antibiotics

**Dosing adjustment in hepatic impairment:** Dose reductions may be necessary to reduce hepatotoxicity

**Dosage Forms Cap:** 150 mg, 300 mg; **Powder for inj:** 600 mg (contains a sulfite)

**Contraindications** Hypersensitivity to any rifamycins or any component

**Warnings/Precautions** Use with caution and modify dosage in patients with liver impairment; observe for hyperbilirubinemia; discontinue therapy if this in conjunction with clinical symptoms or any signs of significant hepatocellular damage develop; since rifampin has enzyme-inducing properties, porphyria exacerbation is possible; use with caution in patients with porphyria; do not use or meningococcal disease, only for short-term treatment of asymptomatic carrier states

Monitor for compliance and effects including hypersensitivity, decreased thrombocytopenia in patients on intermittent therapy; urine, feces, saliva, sweat, tears, and CSF may be discolored to red/orange; do not administer I.V. form via I.M. or S.C. routes; restart infusion at another site if extravasation occurs; remove soft contact lenses during therapy since permanent staining may occur; regimens of 600 mg once or twice weekly have been associated with a high incidence of adverse reactions including a flu-like syndrome

**Pregnancy Risk Factor** C

**Pregnancy Implications** Clinical effects on the fetus: Teratogenicity has occurred in rodents given many times the adult human dose

**Adverse Reactions**

Percentage unknown: Flushing, edema headache, drowsiness, dizziness, confusion, numbness, behavioral changes pruritus, urticaria, pemphigoid reaction, eosinophilia, leukopenia, hemolysis, hemolytic anemia, thrombocytopenia (especially with high-dose therapy), hepatitis (rare), ataxia, myalgia, weakness, osteomalacia, visual changes, exudative conjunctivitis

1% to 10%:

Dermatologic: Rash (1% to 5%)

Gastrointestinal: (1% to 2%): Epigastric distress, anorexia, nausea, vomiting, diarrhea, cramps, pseudomembranous colitis, pancreatitis

Hepatic: Increased LFTs (up to 14%)

**Drug Interactions** CYP3A3/4 enzyme substrate; CYP1A2, 2C9, 2C18, 2C19, 2D6, 3A3/4, and 3A5-7 enzyme inducer

Decreased effect: Rifampin induces liver enzymes which may decrease the plasma concentration of calcium channel blockers (verapamil, diltiazem, nifedipine), methadone, digitalis, cyclosporine, corticosteroids, oral anticoagulants, haloperidol, theophylline, barbiturates, chloramphenicol, imidazole antifungals, oral or systemic hormonal contraceptives, acetaminophen, benzodiazepines, hydantoins, sulfa drugs, enalapril, beta-blockers, chloramphenicol, clofibrate, dapsone, antiarrhythmics (disopyramide, mexiletine, quinidine, tocainide), diazepam, doxycycline, fluoroquinolones, levothyroxine, nortriptyline, progestins, tacrolimus, zidovudine, protease inhibitors, and non-nucleoside reverse transcriptase inhibitors

Coadministration with INH or halothane may result in additive hepatotoxicity; probenecid and co-trimoxazole may increase rifampin levels while antacids may decrease its absorption

**Half-Life** 3-4 hours, prolonged with hepatic impairment; End-stage renal disease: 1.8-11 hours

**Special PA Issues**

**Patient Education:** Best to take on empty stomach (1 hour before or 2 hours after meals), however, may be taken with food if GI upset occurs. Will discolor urine, stool, saliva, tears, sweat, and other body fluid a red-brown color. Stains on clothing or contact lenses are permanent. Report vomiting, fever, chills, flu-like symptoms, dark urine or pale stools, or unusual bleeding or bruising.

**Dietary Considerations:** Food: Rifampin is best taken on an empty stomach since food decreases the extent of absorption

**Monitoring Parameters:** Periodic (baseline and every 2-4 weeks during therapy) monitoring of liver function (AST, ALT, bilirubin BSD), CBC; hepatic status and mental status, sputum culture, chest x-ray 2-3 months into treatment

# Rifampin and Isoniazid (RIF am pin & eye soe NYE a zid)
**Pharmacologic Class** Antibiotic, Miscellaneous
**U.S. Brand Names** Rifamate®
**Dosage Forms Cap:** Rifampin 300 mg and isoniazid 150 mg

# Rifampin, Isoniazid, and Pyrazinamide
(RIF am pin, eye soe NYE a zid, & peer a ZIN a mide)
**Pharmacologic Class** Antibiotic, Miscellaneous
**U.S. Brand Names** Rifater®
**Dosage Forms Tab:** Rifampin 120 mg, isoniazid 50 mg, and pyrazinamide 300 mg

# Rifapentine (RIF a pen teen)
**Pharmacologic Class** Antitubercular Agent
**U.S. Brand Names** Priftin®
**Mechanism of Action** Inhibits DNA-dependent RNA polymerase in susceptible strains of *Mycobacterium tuberculosis* (but not in mammalian cells). Rifapentine is bactericidal against both intracellular and extracellular MTB organisms. MTB resistant to other rifamycins including rifampin are likely to be resistant to rifapentine. Cross-resistance does not appear between rifapentine and other nonrifamycin antimycobacterial agents.

**Use** Treatment of pulmonary tuberculosis (indication is based on the 6-month follow-up treatment outcome observed in controlled clinical trial). Rifapentine must always be used in conjunction with at least one other antituberculosis drug to which the isolate is susceptible; it may also be necessary to add a third agent (either streptomycin or ethambutol) until susceptibility is known.

**USUAL DOSAGE**

Children: No dosing information available

Adults: **Rifapentine should not be used alone**; initial phase should include a 3- to 4-drug regimen

Intensive phase of short-term therapy: 600 mg (four 150 mg tablets) given weekly (every 72 hours); following the intensive phase, treatment should continue with rifapentine 600 mg once weekly for 4 months in combination with INH or appropriate agent for susceptible organisms

**Dosage adjustment in renal or hepatic impairment:** Unknown

**Dosage Forms Tab, film-coated:** 150 mg

**Contraindications** Patients with a history of hypersensitivity to rifapentine, rifampin, rifabutin, and any rifamycin analog

**Warnings/Precautions** Compliance with dosing regimen is absolutely necessary for successful drug therapy. patients with abnormal liver tests and/or liver disease should only be given rifapentine when absolutely necessary and under strict medical supervision. Monitoring of liver function tests should be carried out prior to therapy and then every 2-4 weeks during therapy if signs of liver disease occur or worsen, rifapentine should be discontinued. Pseudomembranous colitis has been reported to occur with various antibiotics including other rifamycins. If this is suspected, rifapentine should be stopped and the patient treated with specific and supportive treatment. Experience in treating TB in HIV-infected patients is limited.

Rifapentine may produce a red-orange discoloration of body tissues/fluids including skin, teeth, tongue, urine, feces, saliva, sputum, tears, sweat, and cerebral spinal fluid. Contact lenses may become permanently stained. All patients treated with rifapentine should have baseline measurements of liver function tests and enzymes, bilirubin, and a complete blood count. patients should be seen monthly and specifically questioned regarding symptoms associated with adverse reactions. Routine laboratory monitoring in people with normal baseline measurements is generally not necessary.

(Continued)

## Rifapentine *(Continued)*

### Pregnancy Risk Factor C

**Pregnancy Implications** Has been shown to be teratogenic in rats and rabbits. Rat offspring showed cleft palates, right aortic arch, and delayed ossification and increased number of ribs. Rabbits displayed ovarian agenesis, pes varus, arhinia, microphthalmia, and irregularities of the ossified facial tissues. Rat studies also show decreased fetal weight, increased number of stillborns, and decreased gestational survival. No adequate well-controlled studies in pregnant women are available. Rifapentine should be used during pregnancy only if the potential benefits justifies the potential risk to the fetus.

### Adverse Reactions

>10%: Endocrine & metabolic: Hyperuricemia (most likely due to pyrazinamide from initiation phase combination therapy)

1% to 10%:

Cardiovascular: Hypertension

Central nervous system: Headache, dizziness

Dermatologic: Rash, pruritus, acne

Gastrointestinal: Anorexia, nausea, vomiting, dyspepsia, diarrhea

Hematologic: Neutropenia, lymphopenia, anemia, leukopenia, thrombocytosis

Hepatic: Increased ALT/AST

Neuromuscular & skeletal: Arthralgia, pain

Renal: Pyuria, proteinuria, hematuria, urinary casts

Respiratory: Hemoptysis

<1%: Peripheral edema, aggressive reaction, fatigue, urticaria, skin discoloration, hyperkalemia, hypovolemia, increased alkaline phosphatase, increased LDH, constipation, esophagitis, gastritis, pancreatitis, thrombocytopenia, neutrophilia, leukocytosis, purpura, hematoma, bilirubinemia, hepatitis, gout, arthrosis

**Drug Interactions** CYP3A4 and 2C8/9 inducer. Rifapentine may increase the metabolism of coadministered drugs that are metabolized by these enzymes. Enzymes are induced within 4 days after the first dose and returned to baseline 14 days after discontinuation of rifapentine. The magnitude of enzyme induction is dose and frequency dependent. Rifampin has been shown to accelerate the metabolism and may reduce activity of the following drugs (therefore, rifapentine may also do the same): Phenytoin, disopyramide, mexiletine, quinidine, tocainide, chloramphenicol, clarithromycin, dapsone, doxycycline, fluoroquinolones, warfarin, fluconazole, itraconazole, ketoconazole, barbiturates, benzodiazepines, beta-blockers, diltiazem, nifedipine, verapamil, corticosteroids, cardiac glycoside preparations, clofibrate, oral or other systemic hormonal contraceptives, haloperidol, HIV protease inhibitors, sulfonylureas, cyclosporine, tacrolimus, levothyroxine, methadone, progestins, quinine, delavirdine, zidovudine, sildenafil, theophylline, amitriptyline, and nortriptyline.

Rifapentine should be used with extreme caution, if at all, in patients who are also taking protease inhibitors

Patients using oral or other systemic hormonal contraceptives should be advised to change to nonhormonal methods of birth control when receiving concomitant rifapentine.

Rifapentine metabolism is mediated by esterase activity, therefore, there is minimal potential for rifapentine metabolism to be affected by other drug therapy.

**Half-Life** Rifapentine: 14-17 hours; 25-desacetyl rifapentine: 13 hours

### Special PA Issues

**Patient Education:** Best to take on empty stomach (1 hour before or 2 hours after meals); however, may be taken with food if GI upset occurs. Follow recommended dosing schedule exactly; do not increase dose or skip doses. You will need to be monitored on a regular basis while taking this medication. This medication will stain urine, stool, saliva, tears, sweat, and other body fluids a red-brown color. Stains on clothing or contact lenses are permanent. Report vomiting; fever, chills or flu-like symptoms; muscle weakness or unusual fatigue; dark urine, pale stools, or unusual bleeding or bruising; yellowing skin or eyes; skin rash; swelling of extremities; chest pain or palpitations; or persistent gastrointestinal upset.

**Dietary Considerations:** Food increases AUC and maximum serum concentration by 43% and 44% respectively as compared to fasting conditions

**Monitoring Parameters:** Patients with pre-existing hepatic problems should have liver function tests monitored every 2-4 weeks during therapy

♦ **Rifater®** *see* Rifampin, Isoniazid and Pyrazinamide *on previous page*
♦ **rIFN-A** *see* Interferon Alfa-2a *on page 481*
♦ **rIFN-b** *see* Interferon Beta-1a *on page 486*
♦ **RIG** *see* Rabies Immune Globulin (Human) *on page 791*
♦ **rIL-11** *see* Oprelvekin *on page 678*
♦ **Rilutek®** *see* Riluzole *on this page*

## Riluzole *(RIL yoo zole)*

**Pharmacologic Class** Glutamate Inhibitor

**U.S. Brand Names** Rilutek®

**Mechanism of Action** Inhibitory effect on glutamate release, inactivation of voltage-dependent sodium channels; and ability to interfere with intracellular events that follow transmitter binding at excitatory amino acid receptors

**Use** Amyotrophic lateral sclerosis (ALS): Treatment of patients with ALS; riluzole can extend survival or time to tracheostomy

**USUAL DOSAGE** Adults: Oral: 50 mg every 12 hours; no increased benefit can be expected from higher daily doses, but adverse events are increased

**Dosage adjustment in smoking:** Cigarette smoking is known to induce CYP 1A2; patients who smoke cigarettes would be expected to eliminate riluzole faster. There is no information, however, on the effect of, or need for, dosage adjustment in these patients.

**Dosage adjustment in special populations:** Females and Japanese patients may possess a lower metabolic capacity to eliminate riluzole compared with male and Caucasian subjects, respectively

**Dosage adjustment in renal impairment:** Use with caution in patients with concomitant renal insufficiency

**Dosage adjustment in hepatic impairment:** Use with caution in patients with current evidence or history of abnormal liver function indicated by significant abnormalities in serum transaminase, bilirubin or GGT levels. Baseline elevations of several LFTs (especially elevated bilirubin) should preclude use of riluzole.

**Dosage Forms Tab:** 50 mg

**Contraindications** Severe hypersensitivity reactions to riluzole or any of the tablet components

**Warnings/Precautions** Among 4000 patients given riluzole for ALS, there were 3 cases of marked neutropenia (ANC <500/mm$^3$), all seen within the first 2 months of treatment. Use with caution in patients with concomitant renal insufficiency. Use with caution in patients with current evidence or history of abnormal liver function. Monitor liver chemistries.

**Pregnancy Risk Factor** C

**Adverse Reactions** >10%:
Gastrointestinal: Nausea, abdominal pain, constipation
Hepatic: Increased ALT

**Drug Interactions** CYP1A2 enzyme substrate
Decreased effect: Drugs that induce CYP 1A2 (eg, cigarette smoke, charbroiled food, rifampin, omeprazole) could increase the rate of riluzole elimination
Increased toxicity: Inhibitors of CYP 1A2 (eg, caffeine, theophylline, amitriptyline, quinolones) could decrease the rate of riluzole elimination

**Half-Life** 12 hours

**Special PA Issues**
**Patient Education:** This drug will not cure or stop disease but it may slow progression. Take as directed, at same time each day, preferably on an empty stomach (1 hour before or 2 hours after meals). Avoid alcohol. You may experience increased spasticity, dizziness or sleepiness; use caution when driving or engaging in tests that require alertness until response to medication is known. Small frequent meals, frequent mouth care, or sucking on lozenges may reduce nausea, vomiting, or anorexia. Report fever; severe vomiting, diarrhea, or constipation; change in color of urine or stool; yellowing of skin or eyes; acute back pain or muscle pain; or worsening of condition.

**Monitoring Parameters:** Monitor serum aminotransferases including ALT levels before and during therapy. Evaluate serum ALT levels every month during the first 3 months of therapy, every 3 months during the remainder of the first year and periodically thereafter. Evaluate ALT levels more frequently in patients who develop elevations. Maximum increases in serum ALT usually occurred within 3 months after the start of therapy and were usually transient when <5 x ULN (upper limits of normal).

In trials, if ALT levels were <5 x ULN, treatment continued and ALT levels usually returned to below 2 x ULN within 2-6 months. Treatment in studies was discontinued, however, if ALT levels exceed 5 x ULN, so that there is no experience with continued treatment of ALS patients once ALT values exceed 5 x ULN.

If a decision is made to continue treatment in patients when the ALT exceeds 5 x ULN, frequent monitoring (at least weekly) of complete liver function is recommended. Discontinue treatment if ALT exceeds 10 x ULN or if clinical jaundice develops.

♦ **Rimactane®** see Rifampin on page 803
♦ **Rimactane® Oral** see Rifampin on page 803

# Rimantadine (ri MAN ta deen)

**Pharmacologic Class** Antiviral Agent

**U.S. Brand Names** Flumadine®

**Mechanism of Action** Exerts its inhibitory effect on three antigenic subtypes of influenza A virus (H1N1, H2N2, H3N2) early in the viral replicative cycle, possibly inhibiting the uncoating process; it has no activity against influenza B virus and is two- to eightfold more active than amantadine

**Use** Prophylaxis (adults and children >1 year) and treatment (adults) of influenza A viral infection
(Continued)

## Rimantadine *(Continued)*

**USUAL DOSAGE** Oral:
Prophylaxis:
Children <10 years: 5 mg/kg once daily; maximum: 150 mg
Children >10 years and Adults: 100 mg twice daily; decrease to 100 mg/day in elderly or in patients with severe hepatic or renal impairment ($Cl_{cr}$ ≤10 mL/minute)
Treatment: Adults: 100 mg twice daily; decrease to 100 mg/day in elderly or in patients with severe hepatic or renal impairment ($Cl_{cr}$ ≤10 mL/minute)

**Dosage Forms Syr:** 50 mg/5 mL (60 mL, 240 mL, 480 mL); **Tab:** 100 mg

**Contraindications** Hypersensitivity to drugs of the adamantine class, including rimantadine and amantadine

**Warnings/Precautions** Use with caution in patients with renal and hepatic dysfunction; avoid use, if possible, in patients with recurrent and eczematoid dermatitis, uncontrolled psychosis, or severe psychoneurosis. An increase in seizure incidence may occur in patients with seizure disorders; discontinue drug if seizures occur; consider the development of resistance during rimantadine treatment of the index case as likely if failure of rimantadine prophylaxis among family contact occurs and if index case is a child; viruses exhibit cross-resistance between amantadine and rimantadine.

**Pregnancy Risk Factor** C

**Pregnancy Implications**
Clinical effects on the fetus: Embryotoxic in high dose rat studies
Breast-feeding/lactation: Avoid use in nursing mothers due to potential adverse effect in infants; rimantadine is concentrated in milk

**Adverse Reactions** 1% to 10%:
Cardiovascular: Orthostatic hypotension, edema
Central nervous system: Dizziness (1.9%), confusion, headache (1.4%), insomnia (2.1%), difficulty in concentrating, anxiety (1.3%), restlessness, irritability, hallucinations; incidence of CNS side effects may be less than that associated with amantadine
Gastrointestinal: Nausea (2.8%), vomiting (1.7%), xerostomia (1.5%), abdominal pain (1.4%), anorexia (1.6%)
Genitourinary: Urinary retention

**Drug Interactions**
Acetaminophen: Reduction in AUC and peak concentration of rimantadine
Aspirin: Peak plasma and AUC concentrations of rimantadine are reduced
Cimetidine: Rimantadine clearance is decreased (~16%)

**Half-Life** 25.4 hours (increased in the elderly)

**Special PA Issues**
**Patient Education:** Take as directed, for full course of therapy. Use caution when changing position (rising from sitting or lying) until response is known. Report CNS changes (eg, confusion, insomnia, anxiety, restlessness, irritability, hallucinations), difficulty urinating, or severe nausea or vomiting.
**Monitoring Parameters:** Monitor for CNS or GI effects in elderly or patients with renal or hepatic impairment

♦ **Rimantadine Hydrochloride** *see* Rimantadine *on previous page*

## Rimexolone (ri MEKS oh lone)

**Pharmacologic Class** Corticosteroid, Ophthalmic

**U.S. Brand Names** Vexol® Ophthalmic Suspension

**Mechanism of Action** Decreases inflammation by suppression of migration of polymorphonuclear leukocytes and reversal of increased capillary permeability

**Use** Treatment of inflammation after ocular surgery and the treatment of anterior uveitis

**USUAL DOSAGE** Adults: Ophthalmic: Instill 1 drop in conjunctival sac 2-4 times/day up to every 4 hours; may use every 1-2 hours during first 1-2 days

**Dosage Forms Susp, ophth:** 1% (5 mL, 10 mL)

**Contraindications** Fungal, viral, or untreated pus-forming bacterial ocular infections; hypersensitivity to any component

**Warnings/Precautions** Prolonged use has been associated with the development of corneal or scleral perforation and posterior subcapsular cataracts; may mask or enhance the establishment of acute purulent untreated infections of the eye; effectiveness and safety have not been established in children

**Pregnancy Risk Factor** C

**Adverse Reactions**
1% to 10%: Ocular: Temporary mild blurred vision
<1%: Stinging, burning eyes, corneal thinning, increased intraocular pressure, glaucoma, damage to the optic nerve, defects in visual activity, cataracts, secondary ocular infection

**Half-Life** 1-2 hours

**Special PA Issues**
**Patient Education:** For ophthalmic use only. Shake well before using. Apply prescribed amount as often as directed. Wash hands before using and do not let tip of applicator touch eye or contaminate tip of applicator. Tilt head back and look upward. Gently pull

down lower lid and put drop(s) in inner corner of eye. Close eye and roll eyeball in all directions. Do not blink for ½ minute. Apply gentle pressure to inner corner of eye for 30 seconds. Wipe away excess from skin around eye. Do not use any other eye preparation for at least 10 minutes. Do not touch tip of applicator to eye or contaminate tip of applicator. Do not share medication with anyone else. May cause sensitivity to bright light (dark glasses may help); temporary stinging or blurred vision may occur. Inform prescriber if you experience eye pain, redness, burning, watering, dryness, double vision, puffiness around eye, vision disturbances, or other adverse eye response; worsening of condition or lack of improvement.

**Monitoring Parameters:** Intraocular pressure and periodic examination of lens (with prolonged use)

♦ **Riobin**® *see* Riboflavin *on page 802*

♦ **Riphenidate** *see* Methylphenidate *on page 592*

# Risedronate (ris ED roe nate)

**Pharmacologic Class** Bisphosphonate Derivative

**U.S. Brand Names** Actonel®

**Mechanism of Action** A bisphosphonate which inhibits bone resorption via actions on osteoclasts or on osteoclast precursors; decreases the rate of bone resorption direction, leading to an indirect decrease in bone formation

**Use** Paget's disease of the bone

**Unlabeled use:** Osteoporosis in postmenopausal women

**USUAL DOSAGE** Oral:

Adults (patients with Paget's disease should receive supplemental calcium and vitamin D if dietary intake is inadequate):

Paget's disease of bone: 30 mg once daily for 2 months

Elderly: No dosage adjustment is necessary

**Dosage adjustment in renal impairment:** $Cl_{cr}$ <30 mL/minute: **Not** recommended

**Dosage Forms Tab:** 30 mg

**Contraindications** Hypersensitivity to risedronate, bisphosphonates, or any component; hypocalcemia; abnormalities of the esophagus which delay esophageal emptying such as stricture or achalasia; inability to stand or sit upright for at least 30 minutes

**Warnings/Precautions** Use caution in patients with renal impairment; concomitant hormone replacement therapy with alendronate for osteoporosis in postmenopausal women is not recommended; hypocalcemia must be corrected before therapy initiation with alendronate; ensure adequate calcium and vitamin D intake to provide for enhanced needs in patients with Paget's disease in whom the pretreatment rate of bone turnover may be greatly elevated.

**Pregnancy Risk Factor** C

**Adverse Reactions**

>10%:

Dermatological: Rash

Gastrointestinal: Abdominal pain, diarrhea

Neuromuscular & skeletal: Arthralgia

1% to 10%:

Cardiovascular: Chest pain

Central nervous system: Headache, dizziness

Gastrointestinal: Belching, colitis, constipation, nausea

Neuromuscular & skeletal: Bone pain, leg cramps, myasthenia

Respiratory: Bronchitis, rales/rhinitis

**Drug Interactions** Decreased effect: Calcium supplements and antacids interfere with the absorption of risedronate

**Onset** May require weeks

**Half-Life** Terminal: 220 hours

**Special PA Issues**

**Patient Education:** In order to be effective, this drug must be taken exactly as prescribed. The expected benefits of risedronate may only be obtained when each tablet is taken with plain water the first thing in the morning and at least 30 minutes before the first food, beverage, or medication of the day. Wait >30 minutes to improve alendronate absorption. Even dosing with orange juice or coffee markedly reduces the absorption of risedronate.

Take alendronate with a full glass of water (6-8 oz 180-240 mL) and do not lie down (stay fully upright sitting or standing) for at least 30 minutes following administration to facilitate delivery to the stomach and reduce the potential for esophageal irritation.

Take supplemental calcium and vitamin D if dietary intake is inadequate. Consider weight-bearing exercise along with the modification of certain behavioral factors, such as excessive cigarette smoking or alcohol consumption if these factors exist.

You may experience headache (request analgesic); skin rash; or abdominal pain, diarrhea, or constipation (report if persistent). Report unresolved muscle or bone pain or leg cramps; acute abdominal pain; chest pain, palpitations, or swollen extremities; disturbed vision or excessively dry eyes; ringing in the ears; or persistent flu-like symptoms.

(Continued)

## Risedronate *(Continued)*

**Monitoring Parameters:** Alkaline phosphatase should be periodically measured; serum calcium, phosphorus, and possibly potassium due to its drug class; use of absorptiometry may assist in noting benefit in osteoporosis; monitor pain and fracture rate

**Reference Range:** Calcium (total): Adults: 9.0-11.0 mg/dL (2.05-2.54 mmol/L), may slightly decrease with aging; phosphorus: 2.5-4.5 mg/dL (0.81-1.45 mmol/L)

♦ **Risedronate Sodium** *see Risedronate on previous page*

♦ **Risperdal®** *see Risperidone on this page*

## Risperidone (ris PER i done)

**Pharmacologic Class** Antipsychotic Agent, Benzisoxazole

**U.S. Brand Names** Risperdal®

**Mechanism of Action** Risperidone is a benzisoxazole derivative, mixed serotonin-dopamine antagonist; binds to 5-HT$_2$-receptors in the CNS and in the periphery with a very high affinity; binds to dopamine-D$_2$ receptors with less affinity. The binding affinity to the dopamine-D$_2$ receptor is 20 times lower than the 5-HT$_2$ affinity. The addition of serotonin antagonism to dopamine antagonism (classic neuroleptic mechanism) is thought to improve negative symptoms of psychoses and reduce the incidence of extrapyramidal side effects.

**Use** Management of psychotic disorders (eg, schizophrenia); nonpsychotic symptoms associated with dementia in elderly

**USUAL DOSAGE** Recommended starting dose: 1 mg twice daily; slowly increase to the optimum range of 4-6 mg/day; daily dosages >6 mg does not appear to confer any additional benefit, and the incidence of extrapyramidal reactions is higher than with lower doses

**Dosing adjustment in renal, hepatic impairment, and elderly:** Starting dose of 0.5 mg twice daily is advisable

**Dosage Forms Soln, oral:** 1 mg/mL (100 mL); **Tab:** 1 mg, 2 mg, 3 mg, 4 mg

**Contraindications** Known hypersensitivity to any component of the product

**Adverse Reactions**

1% to 10%:

Cardiovascular: Hypotension (especially orthostatic), tachycardia, arrhythmias, abnormal T waves with prolonged ventricular repolarization; EKG changes, syncope

Central nervous system: Sedation (occurs at daily doses ≥20 mg/day), headache, dizziness, restlessness, anxiety, extrapyramidal reactions, dystonic reactions, pseudoparkinson signs and symptoms, tardive dyskinesia, neuroleptic malignant syndrome, altered central temperature regulation

Dermatologic: Photosensitivity (rare)

Endocrine & metabolic: Amenorrhea, galactorrhea, gynecomastia sexual dysfunction (up to 60%)

Gastrointestinal: Constipation, adynamic ileus, GI upset, xerostomia (problem for denture user), nausea and anorexia, weight gain

Genitourinary: Urinary retention, overflow incontinence, priapism

Hematologic: Agranulocytosis, leukopenia (usually in patients with large doses for prolonged periods)

Hepatic: Cholestatic jaundice

Ocular: Blurred vision, retinal pigmentation, decreased visual acuity (may be irreversible)

<1%: Seizures

**Drug Interactions** CYP2D6 enzyme substrate; CYP2D6 inhibitor (weak)

Increased toxicity: Quinidine, warfarin

May antagonize effects of levodopa; carbamazepine decreases risperidone serum concentrations; clozapine decreases clearance of risperidone

**Half-Life** 24 hours (risperidone and its active metabolite)

**Special PA Issues**

**Patient Education:** Use exactly as directed (do not increase dose or frequency); may cause physical and/or psychological dependence. It may take 2-3 weeks to achieve desired results; do not discontinue without consulting prescriber. Dilute solution with water, milk, orange or grapefruit juice; do not dilute with beverages containing caffeine, tannin, or pactinate (eg, coffee, colas, tea, or apple juice). Avoid excess alcohol or caffeine and other prescription or OTC medications not approved by prescriber. Maintain adequate hydration (2-3 L/day of fluids unless instructed to restrict fluid intake). You may experience excess sedation, drowsiness, restlessness, dizziness, or blurred vision (use caution driving or when engaging in hazardous tasks until response to medication is known); dry mouth, nausea or GI upset (small frequent meals, frequent mouth care, or sucking lozenges may help); postural hypotension (use caution climbing stairs or when changing position from lying or sitting to standing); or urinary retention (void before taking medication). Report persistent CNS effects (eg, trembling fingers, altered gait or balance, excessive sedation, seizures, unusual muscle or skeletal movements, anxiety, abnormal thoughts, confusion, personality changes); chest pain, palpitations, rapid heartbeat, severe dizziness; swelling or pain in breasts (male and female), altered menstrual pattern, sexual dysfunction; pain or difficulty on urination; vision changes; skin rash or yellowing of skin; difficulty breathing; or worsening of condition.

**Related Information**

Antipsychotic Agents *on page 1001*

♦ **Ritalin®** *see* Methylphenidate *on page 592*

♦ **Ritalin-SR®** *see* Methylphenidate *on page 592*

# Ritodrine (RI toe dreen)

**Pharmacologic Class** Beta₂ Agonist

**U.S. Brand Names** Pre-Par®; Yutopar®

**Mechanism of Action** Tocolysis due to its uterine beta₂-adrenergic receptor stimulating effects; this agent's beta₂ effects can also cause bronchial relaxation and vascular smooth muscle stimulation

**Use** Inhibits uterine contraction in preterm labor

**USUAL DOSAGE** Adults: I.V.: 50-100 mcg/minute; increase by 50 mcg/minute every 10 minutes; continue for 12 hours after contractions have stopped

Hemodialysis: Removed by hemodialysis

**Dosage Forms Inf:** 0.3 mL (500 mL): **Inj:** 10 mg/mL (5 mL), 15 mg/mL (10 mL)

**Contraindications** Do not use before 20th week of pregnancy, cardiac arrhythmias, pheochromocytoma

**Warnings/Precautions** Monitor hydration status and blood glucose concentrations; fatal maternal pulmonary edema has been reported, sometimes after delivery; fluid overload must be avoided, hydration levels should be monitored closely; if pulmonary edema occurs, the drug should be discontinued; use with caution in patients with moderate pre-eclampsia, diabetes, or migraine; some products may contain sulfites; maternal deaths have been reported in patients treated with ritodrine and concurrent corticosteroids (pulmonary edema)

**Pregnancy Risk Factor** B

**Adverse Reactions**

>10%:

Cardiovascular: Increases in maternal and fetal heart rates and maternal hypertension, palpitations

Endocrine & metabolic: Temporary hyperglycemia

Gastrointestinal: Nausea, vomiting

Neuromuscular & skeletal: Tremor

1% to 10%:

Cardiovascular: Chest pain

Central nervous system: Nervousness, anxiety, restlessness

<1%: Ketoacidosis, impaired LFTs, anaphylactic shock

**Drug Interactions**

Decreased effect with beta-blockers

Increased effect/toxicity with meperidine, sympathomimetics, diazoxide, magnesium, betamethasone (pulmonary edema), potassium-depleting diuretics, general anesthetics

**Half-Life** 15 hours

**Special PA Issues**

**Patient Education:**

I.V.: Remain in left lateral position during infusion; do not get out of bed. Report rapid heartbeat, dizziness, difficulty breathing, nervousness or restlessness, skin itching or rash.

Oral: Take as directed and follow instruction of prescriber for physical activity. Report palpitations or chest pain, acute nausea or vomiting, difficulty breathing, skin irritation or rash, abdominal cramping, vaginal discharge, or other signs of labor.

**Monitoring Parameters:** Hematocrit, serum potassium, glucose, colloidal osmotic pressure, heart rate, and uterine contractions

♦ **Ritodrine Hydrochloride** *see* Ritodrine *on this page*

# Ritonavir (rye TON a veer)

**Pharmacologic Class** Antiretroviral Agent, Protease Inhibitor

**U.S. Brand Names** Norvir®

**Mechanism of Action** Ritonavir inhibits HIV protease and renders the enzyme incapable of processing of polyprotein precursor which leads to production of noninfectious immature HIV particles

**Use** In combination with other antiretroviral agents; treatment of HIV infection when therapy is warranted

**USUAL DOSAGE** Oral:

Children: 250 mg/m² twice daily; titrate dose upward to 400 mg/m² twice daily (maximum: 600 mg twice daily)

Adults: 600 mg twice daily; dose escalation tends to avoid nausea that many patients experience upon initiation of full dosing. Escalate the dose as follows: 300 mg twice daily for 1 day, 400 mg twice daily for 2 days, 500 mg twice daily for 1 day, then 600 mg twice daily. Ritonavir may be better tolerated when used in combination with other antiretrovirals by initiating the drug alone and subsequently adding the second agent within 2 weeks.

If used in combination with saquinavir, dose is 400 mg twice daily

(Continued)

## Ritonavir *(Continued)*

**Dosing adjustment in renal impairment:** None necessary

**Dosing adjustment in hepatic impairment:** Not determined; caution advised with severe impairment

**Dosage Forms Cap:** 100 mg; **Soln:** 80 mg/mL (240 mL)

**Contraindications** Patients with known hypersensitivity to ritonavir or any ingredients; see contraindicated medications table below

### Contraindicated Medications and Potential Alternatives*

| Contraindicated Medications† | | | Potential Alternatives‡ (these alternatives may not be therapeutically equivalent) | | |
|---|---|---|---|---|---|
| Drug Class | Generic Name | Brand Name | Generic Name | Brand Name | Exposed Patients |
| Analgesic | Meperidine | Demerol® | Acetaminophen | Tylenol® | N=135 |
| | Piroxicam | Feldene® | Aspirin | | N=43 |
| | Propoxyphene | Darvon® | Oxycodone | Percodan® | N=23 |
| Cardiovascular (antiarrythmic) | Amiodarone Flecainide Propafenone Quinidine | Cordarone® Tambocor® Rythmol® | Very limited clinical experience | | |
| Antimycobacterial | Rifabutin | Mycobutin® | Clarithromycin Ethambutol | Biaxin® Myambutol® | N=156§ N=66 |
| Cardiovascular (calcium channel blocker) | Bepridil | Vascor® | Very limited clinical experience | | |
| Cold and allergy (antihistamine) | Astemizole Terfenadine | Hismanal® Seldane® | Loratadine | Clarifin® | N=36 |
| Ergot alkaloid (vasoconstrictor) | Dihydro-ergotamine Ergotamine | D.H.E. 45® various | Very limited clinical experience | | |
| Gastrointestinal | Cisapride | Propulsid® | Very limited clinical experience | | |
| Psychotropic (antidepressant) | Bupropion | Wellbutrin® | Desipramine | Norpramin® | ¶ |
| Psychotropic (neuroleptic) | Clozapine Pimozide | Clozaril® Orap™ | Very limited clinical experience | | |
| Psychotropic (sedative-hypnotic) | Alprazolam Clorazepate Diazepam Estazolam Flurazepam Midazolam Triazolam Zolpidem | Xanax® Tranxene® Valium® ProSom™ Dalmane® Versed® Halcion® Ambien® | Temazepam Lorazepam | Restoril® Ativan® | N=40 N=33 |

* During clinical trials, Norvir® was given to patients concomitantly taking a variety of medications. These medications were not evaluated in drug interaction studies. The number of Norvir®-treated patients exposed to each drug is provided in the last column.

† See Contraindications in the drug monograph.

‡ See Warnings/Precautions and Drug Interactions in the drug monograph.

§ Also evaluated in drug interaction study (N=22). See Results of Drug Interaction Studies table.

¶ No clinical experience with combination. Only evaluated in drug interaction study (N=14). See Results of Drug Interaction Studies table.

**Warnings/Precautions** Use caution in patients with hepatic insufficiency; safety and efficacy have not been established in children <16 years of age; use caution with benzodiazepines, antiarrhythmics (flecainide, encainide, bepridil, amiodarone, quinidine) and certain analgesics (meperidine, piroxicam, propoxyphene)

**Pregnancy Risk Factor** B

**Pregnancy Implications**

Clinical effects on the fetus: Administer during pregnancy only if benefits to mother outweigh risks to the fetus

Breast-feeding/lactation: HIV-infected mothers are discouraged from breast-feeding to decrease postnatal transmission of HIV

**Adverse Reactions** Protease inhibitors cause dyslipidemia which includes elevated cholesterol and triglycerides and a redistribution of body fat centrally to cause "protease paunch", buffalo hump, facial atrophy, and breast enlargement. These agents also cause hyperglycemia.

>10%:

Gastrointestinal: Diarrhea, nausea, vomiting, taste perversion

Endocrine & metabolic: Increased triglycerides

Hematologic: Anemia, decreased WBCs

Hepatic: Increased GGT

Neuromuscular & skeletal: Weakness

1% to 10%:

Cardiovascular: Vasodilation

Central nervous system: Fever, headache, malaise, dizziness, insomnia, somnolence, thinking abnormally

Dermatologic: Rash

Endocrine & metabolic: Hyperlipidemia, increased uric acid, increased glucose

Gastrointestinal: Abdominal pain, anorexia, constipation, dyspepsia, flatulence, local throat irritation

Hematologic: Neutropenia, eosinophilia, neutrophilia, prolonged PT, leukocytosis

Hepatic: Increased LFTs

Neuromuscular & skeletal: Increased CPK, myalgia, paresthesia

Respiratory: Pharyngitis

Miscellaneous: Diaphoresis, increased potassium, increased calcium,

**Drug Interactions** CYP1A2, 2A6, 2C9, 2C19, 2E1, and 3A3/4 enzyme substrate, CYP2D6 enzyme substrate (minor); CYP1A2 and 2D6 enzyme inducer; CYP2A6, 2C9, 1A2, 2C19, 2D6, 2E1, and 3A3/4 inhibitor

### Results of Drug Interaction Studies

| Co-administered Drug | Finding |
|---|---|
| Amiodarone | Increased risk of amiodarone toxicity, including cardiotoxicity |
| Astemizole | Increased risk of toxicity |
| Benzodiazepines | Increased risk of prolonged sedation and respiratory depression |
| Bepridil | Increased risk of bepridil toxicity, including cardiotoxicity |
| Bupropion | Increased risk of bupropion toxicity, including seizures |
| Cisapride | Increased risk of cardiotoxicity |
| Clarithromycin | 77% increase in clarithromycin AUC; no dosage reduction is necessary in patients with normal renal function; for patients with Cl_cr from 30-60 mL/minute, decrease dose by 50%; for patients with Cl_cr<30 mL/minute, decrease dose by 75% |
| Clozapine | Increased risk of clozapine toxicity, including agranulocytosis, EKG changes, and seizures |
| Desipramine | 145% increase in desipramine AUC; dosage reduction should be considered |
| Didanosine (ddL) | 13% decrease in didanosine AUC; no dosage adjustment is necessary |
| Ethinyl estradiol | 40% decrease in ethinyl estradiol AUC; increase ethinyl estradiol dose or substitute with another contraceptive |
| Flecainide | Increased risk of flecainide toxicity, including cardiotoxicity |
| Fluconazole | 15% increase in ritonavir AUC |
| Meperidine | Increased risk of meperidine toxicity, including CNS side effects, seizures, and cardiac arrhythmias |
| Nevirapine | Efficacy of ritonavir may be decreased |
| Piroxicam | Increased risk of piroxicam |
| Propafenone | Increased risk of propafenone, including cardiotoxicity |
| Propoxyphene | Increased risk of propoxyphene toxicity, including respiratory depression |
| Quinidine | Increased risk of quinidine toxicity, including cardiotoxicity |
| Rifabutin | Efficacy of ritonavir may be decreased while the risk of rifabutin-induced hematologic toxicity may be increased |
| Saquinavir | Greater than 20-fold increase in saquinavir AUC |
| Sulfamethoxazole | 20% decrease is sulfamethoxazole AUC; no dosage adjustment is necessary |
| Terfenadine | Increased risk of cardiotoxicity |
| Theophylline | 43% decrease in theophylline AUC; increase in theophylline dose may be required |
| Zidovudine (AZT) | 25% decrease in zidovudine AUC; no dosage adjustment is necessary |
| Zolpidem | Increased risk of prolonged sedation and respiratory depression |

**Half-Life** 3-5 hours

**Special PA Issues**

**Patient Education:** Take with food. Mix liquid formulation with chocolate milk or liquid nutritional supplement. You may experience headache or confusion; if these persist notify prescriber. Diarrhea may be moderate to severe. Notify prescriber if problematic. Report swelling, numbness of tongue, mouth, lips, unresolved vomiting, fever, chills, or extreme fatigue.

**Monitoring Parameters:** Triglycerides, cholesterol, LFTs, CPK, uric acid, basic HIV monitoring, viral load, and CD4 count, glucose

♦ **Rivastatin** *see* Cerivastatin *on page 182*

♦ **Rivotril®** *see* Clonazepam *on page 224*

# Rizatriptan (rye za TRIP tan)

**Pharmacologic Class** Serotonin 5-HT$_{1D}$ Receptor Agonist

**U.S. Brand Names** Maxalt®; Maxalt-MLT™

**Mechanism of Action** Selective agonist for serotonin (5-HT$_{1D}$ receptor) in cranial arteries to cause vasoconstriction and reduce sterile inflammation associated with antidromic neuronal transmission correlating with relief of migraine

**Use** Acute treatment of migraine with or without aura

**USUAL DOSAGE** Oral: 5-10 mg, repeat after 2 hours if significant relief is not attained; maximum: 30 mg in a 24-hour period (Use 5 mg dose in patients receiving propranolol with a maximum of 15 mg in 24 hours)

**Dosage Forms Tab, as benzoate:** Maxalt®: 5 mg, 10 mg, Maxalt-MLT™ (orally disintegrating): 5 mg, 10 mg

**Contraindications** Prior hypersensitivity to rizatriptan; documented ischemic heart disease or Prinzmetal's angina; uncontrolled hypertension; basilar or hemiplegic migraine; during or within 2 weeks of MAO inhibitors

**Warnings/Precautions** Use only in patients with a clear diagnosis of migraine; use with caution in elderly or patients with hepatic or renal impairment, history of hypersensitivity to sumatriptan or adverse effects from sumatriptan, and in patients at risk of coronary artery disease. Do not use with ergotamines. May increase blood pressure transiently; may cause coronary vasospasm (less than sumatriptan); avoid in patients with signs/symptoms suggestive of reduced arterial flow (ischemic bowel, Raynaud's) which could be exacerbated by vasospasm. Phenylketonurics (tablets contain phenylalanine).

Patients who experience sensations of chest pain/pressure/tightness or symptoms suggestive of angina following dosing should be evaluated for coronary artery disease or Prinzmetal's angina before receiving additional doses.

Caution in dialysis patients or hepatically impaired. Reconsider diagnosis of migraine if no response to initial dose. Long-term effects on vision have not been evaluated.

**Pregnancy Risk Factor** C

**Adverse Reactions**

1% to 10%:

Cardiovascular: Systolic/diastolic blood pressure increases (5-10 mm Hg), chest pain (5%)

Central nervous system: Dizziness, drowsiness, fatigue (13% to 30% - dose related)

Dermatologic: Skin flushing

Endocrine & metabolic: Mild increase in growth hormone, hot flashes

Gastrointestinal: Nausea, vomiting, abdominal pain, dry mouth (<5%)

Respiratory: Dyspnea

<1%:

Cardiovascular: Syncope, facial edema, tachycardia, palpitation, bradycardia

Central nervous system: Chills, hangover, decreased mental activity, neurological/psychiatric abnormalities

Dermatologic: Pruritus

Neuromuscular & skeletal: Neck pain/stiffness, muscle weakness, myalgia, arthralgia

Ocular: Blurred vision, dry eyes, eye pain

Otic: Tinnitus

Renal: Polyuria

Respiratory: Nasopharyngeal irritation

Miscellaneous: Heat sensitivity, diaphoresis

**Drug Interactions**

Use within 24 hours of another selective 5-HT$_1$ agonist or ergot-containing drug should be avoided due to possible additive vasoconstriction

Propranolol: Plasma concentration of rizatriptan increased 70%

SSRIs: Rarely, concurrent use results in weakness and incoordination; monitor closely

MAO inhibitors and nonselective MAO inhibitors increase concentration of rizatriptan

**Onset** Within 30 minutes

**Duration** 14-16 hours

**Half-Life** 2-3 hours

**Special PA Issues**

**Patient Education:** Administration of orally disintegrating tablets: Do not open blister pack before using. Open with dry hands. Do not crush, chew, or swallow tablet; allow to dissolve on tongue. Take as prescribed; do not increase dosing schedule. May repeat one time after 2 hours, if first dose is ineffective. Do not ever take more than two doses without consulting prescriber. You may experience dizziness or drowsiness (use caution when driving, climbing stairs, or engaging in tasks that require alertness); skin flushing or hot flashes (cool clothes or a cool environment may help); mild abdominal discomfort or nausea or vomiting. Report severe dizziness, acute headache, chest pain or palpitation, stiff or painful neck or facial swelling, muscle weakness or pain, changes in mental acuity, blurred vision, eye pain, or excessive perspiration or urination.

**Dietary Considerations:** Food delays the absorption

**Monitoring Parameters:** Headache severity, signs/symptoms suggestive of angina; consider monitoring blood pressure, heart rate, and/or EKG with first dose in patients with likelihood of unrecognized coronary disease, such as patients with significant hypertension, hypercholesterolemia, obese patients, diabetics, smokers with other risk factors or strong family history of coronary artery disease

## Ropinirole (roe PIN i role)

**Pharmacologic Class** Anti-Parkinson's Agent (Dopamine Agonist)

**U.S. Brand Names** Requip™

**Mechanism of Action** Ropinirole has a high relative *in vitro* specificity and full intrinsic activity at the $D_2$ and $D_3$ dopamine receptor subtypes, binding with higher affinity to $D_3$ than to $D_2$ or $D_4$ receptor subtypes. Although precise mechanism of action of ropinirole is unknown, it is believed to be due to stimulation of postsynaptic dopamine $D_2$-type receptors within the caudate-putamen in the brain.

**Use** Treatment of idiopathic Parkinson's disease; in patients with early Parkinson's disease who were not receiving concomitant levodopa therapy as well as in patients with advanced disease on concomitant levodopa

**USUAL DOSAGE** Adults: Oral: Dosage should be increased to achieve a maximum therapeutic effect, balanced against the principle side effects of nausea, dizziness, somnolence, and dyskinesia

Recommended starting dose: 0.25 mg 3 times/day; based on individual patient response, the dosage should be titrated with weekly increments as described below:
  Week 1: 0.25 mg 3 times/day; total daily dose: 0.75 mg
  Week 2: 0.5 mg 3 times/day; total daily dose: 1.5 mg
  Week 3: 0.75 mg 3 times/day; total daily dose: 2.25 mg
  Week 4: 1 mg 3 times/day; total daily dose: 3 mg
After week 4, if necessary, daily dosage may be increased by 1.5 mg/day on a weekly basis up to a dose of 9 mg/day, and then by up to 3 mg/day weekly to a total of 24 mg/day

**Dosage Forms Tab, as hydrochloride:** 0.25 mg, 0.5 mg, 1 mg, 2 mg, 5 mg

**Contraindications** Hypersensitivity to ropinirole

**Warnings/Precautions** Syncope, sometimes associated with bradycardia, was observed in association with ropinirole in both early Parkinson's disease (without L-dopa) patients and (Continued)

## Ropinirole *(Continued)*

advanced Parkinson's disease (with L-dopa) patients. Dopamine agonists appear to impair the systemic regulation of blood pressure resulting in postural hypotension, especially during dose escalation. Parkinson's disease patients appear to have an impaired capacity to respond to a postural challenge. Parkinson's patients being treated with dopaminergic agonists ordinarily require careful monitoring for signs and symptoms of postural hypotension, especially during dose escalation, and should be informed of this risk. In patients with Parkinson's disease who were not treated with L-dopa, 5.2% of those treated with ropinirole reported hallucinations as compared to 1.4% on a placebo.

**Pregnancy Risk Factor** C

**Adverse Reactions**

**Early Parkinson's disease:**

Cardiovascular: Syncope, dependent/leg edema, orthostatic symptoms

Central nervous system: Dizziness, somnolence (40% vs 6% with placebo), headache, fatigue, pain, confusion, hallucinations

Gastrointestinal: Nausea (60% vs 22% with placebo), dyspepsia, constipation, abdominal pain

Genitourinary: Urinary tract infections

Neuromuscular & skeletal: Weakness

Ocular: Abnormal vision

Respiratory: Pharyngitis

Miscellaneous: Viral infection, diaphoresis (increased)

**Advanced Parkinson's disease (with levodopa):**

Cardiovascular: Hypotension (2%), syncope (3%)

Central nervous system: Dizziness (26% vs 16% with placebo), aggravated parkinsonism, somnolence (40%), headache (17% vs 12% with placebo), insomnia, hallucinations, confusion (9% vs 2% with placebo), pain (5% vs 3% with placebo), paresis (3%), amnesia (5%), anxiety (6%), abnormal dreaming (3%)

Gastrointestinal: Nausea (30% vs 18% with placebo), abdominal pain (9% vs 8% with placebo), vomiting (7% vs 4% with placebo), constipation (6%), diarrhea (5%), dysphagia (2%), flatulence (2%), increased salivation (2%), xerostomia, weight loss (2%)

Genitourinary: Urinary tract infections

Neuromuscular & skeletal: Dyskinesias (34% vs 13% with placebo), falls (10% vs 7% with placebo), hypokinesia (5%), paresthesia (5%), tremor (6%), arthralgia (7%), arthritis (3)

Respiratory: Upper respiratory tract infection

Miscellaneous: Injury, increased diaphoresis (7%), viral infection

<1%: Hypoglycemia, increased LDH, hyperphosphatemia, hyperuricemia, diabetes mellitus, hypokalemia, hypercholesterolemia, hyperkalemia, acidosis, hyponatremia, dehydration, hypochloremia, weight increase, increased alkaline phosphatase, increased CPK, elevated BUN, glycosuria, thirst, increased lactate dehydrogenase (LDH)

**Drug Interactions** Ropinirole is metabolized by CYP1A2 so there is the potential for interaction when given with inhibitors or inducers of this enzyme

Ciprofloxacin increased C max and AUC of ropinirole

Estrogens decreased clearance of ropinirole

Decreased effect: Dopamine antagonists (phenothiazine, haloperidol, metoclopramide)

**Special PA Issues**

**Patient Education:** Ropinirole can be taken with or without food. Hallucinations can occur and elderly are at a higher risk than younger patients with Parkinson's disease. Postural hypotension may develop with or without symptoms such as dizziness, nausea, syncope, and sometimes sweating. Hypotension and/or orthostatic symptoms may occur more frequently during initial therapy or with an increase in dose at any time. Use caution when rising rapidly after sitting or lying down, especially after having done so for prolonged periods and especially at the initiation of treatment with ropinirole. Because of additive sedative effects, caution should be used when taking CNS depressants (eg, benzodiazepines, antipsychotics, antidepressants) in combination with ropinirole.

♦ **Ropinirole Hydrochloride** *see* Ropinirole *on previous page*

## Ropivacaine *(roe PIV a kane)*

**Pharmacologic Class** Local Anesthetic

**U.S. Brand Names** Naropin™

**Mechanism of Action** Blocks both the initiation and conduction of nerve impulses by decreasing the neuronal membrane's permeability to sodium ions, which results in inhibition of depolarization with resultant blockade of conduction

**Use** Local anesthetic (injectable for use in surgery, postoperative pain management, and obstetrical procedures when local or regional anesthesia is needed. It can be administered via local infiltration, epidural block and epidural infusion, or intermittent bolus.

**USUAL DOSAGE** Dose varies with procedure, onset and depth of anesthesia desired, vascularity of tissues, duration of anesthesia, and condition of patient

Adults:

Lumbar epidural for surgery: 15-30 mL of 0.5% to 1%

Lumbar epidural block for cesarean section: 20-30 mL of 0.5%
Thoracic epidural block for postoperative pain relief: 5-15 mL of 0.5%
Major nerve block: 35-50 mL dose of 0.5% (175-250 mg)
Field block: 1-40 mL dose of 0.5% (5-200 mg)
Lumbar epidural for labor pain: Initial: 10-20 mL 0.2%; continuous infusion dose: 6-14 mL/hour of 0.2% with incremental injections of 10-15 mL/hour of 0.2% solution

**Dosage Forms Inf, as hydrochloride:** 2 mg/mL (100 mL, 200 mL); **Inj, as hydrochloride (single dose):** 2 mg/mL (20 mL), 5 mg/mL (30 mL), 7.5 mg/mL (10 mL, 20 mL), 10 mg/mL (10 mL, 20 mL)

**Contraindications** Hypersensitivity to amide-type local anesthetics (eg, bupivacaine, mepivacaine, lidocaine), septicemia, severe hypotension and for spinal anesthesia, in the presence of complete heart block

**Warnings/Precautions** Use with caution in patients with liver disease, cardiovascular disease, neurological or psychiatric disorders; it is not recommended for use in emergency situations where rapid administration is necessary

**Pregnancy Risk Factor** B

**Adverse Reactions**
>10% (dose and route related):
Cardiovascular: Hypotension, bradycardia
Gastrointestinal: Nausea, vomiting
Neuromuscular & skeletal: Back pain
Miscellaneous: Shivering
1% to 10% (dose related):
Cardiovascular: Hypertension, tachycardia
Central nervous system: Headache, dizziness, anxiety, lightheadedness
Neuromuscular & skeletal: Hypoesthesia, paresthesia, circumoral paresthesia
Otic: Tinnitus
Respiratory: Apnea

**Drug Interactions** CYP2D6 enzyme substrate
Increased effect: Other local anesthetics or agents structurally related to the amide-type anesthetics
Increased toxicity (possible but not yet reported): Drugs that decrease cytochrome P-450 1A enzyme function

♦ **Ropivacaine Hydrochloride** see Ropivacaine on previous page

♦ **Rosin Rose** see St Johns Wort on page 852

♦ **RotaShield®** see Rotavirus Vaccine on this page

# Rotavirus Vaccine (RO ta vye rus vak SEEN)

**Pharmacologic Class** Vaccine

**U.S. Brand Names** RotaShield®

**Mechanism of Action** The live virus vaccine stimulates production of IgG and IgA antibodies which cross-react with human serotypes. The four serotypes which cause the majority of infections in humans are neutralized by these antibodies.

**Use** Prevention of gastroenteritis caused by the rotavirus serotypes responsible for the majority of disease in infants and children in the U.S. (serotypes G 1,2,3 and 4)

**USUAL DOSAGE For oral administration only**
Children: Three 2.5 mL doses are administered. The recommended schedule for immunization is at 2, 4, and 6 months of age. The first dose may be administered as early as 6 weeks of age, with subsequent doses at least 3 weeks apart. The third dose has been administered to infants up to 33 weeks of age with no increase in adverse reactions. Initiation of vaccination after the age of 6 months is not currently recommended due to an increased risk of fever. RotaShield® does not diminish the efficacy of OPV, DTP, or Hib when administered concurrently. Repeat dosing of vaccine is not recommended if an infant should regurgitate a dose.
Adults: Not approved for administration to adults

**Dosage Forms Powder, lyophilized, for oral soln:** 2.5 mL diluent (Dispette®); specialized diluent contains citric acid and sodium bicarbonate

**Contraindications** Known hypersensitivity to any component of the vaccine (due to the method of preparation, rotavirus vaccine may include small amounts of an aminoglycoside antibiotic, monosodium glutamate, and amphotericin B). Contraindicated in patients with ongoing diarrhea or vomiting.

Immunocompromised patients may shed virus for prolonged periods. RotaShield® is contraindicated in patients with known or suspected immune deficiency states, or in patients receiving therapy with agents which may compromise immune function (alkylating agents, antimetabolites, radiation, or high-dose systemic corticosteroids). Use of steroids when administered topically, via inhalation aerosol, or by intra-articular, tendon, or bursal injection does not contraindicate therapy. Although antibodies to rotavirus may be present in breast milk, there is no evidence that the efficacy of the rotavirus vaccine is diminished when administered to breast-fed infants.

**Warnings/Precautions** Vaccine administration may be delayed due to current or recent severe to moderate febrile illness. Minor illness with or without low-grade fever is not (Continued)

## Rotavirus Vaccine *(Continued)*

generally a contraindication. Do not administer parenterally. Do not administer to immuno-compromised infants. Administer with caution to patients with possible latex allergy. Close association with immunosuppressed or other high-risk individuals should be avoided whenever possible for up to 4 weeks after administration. Data concerning administration to premature infants are insufficient to establish safety or efficacy. Prior to administration, the physician should take all known precautions for prevention of allergic or other reactions. A careful history for possible sensitivity should be taken and agents to control immediate allergic reactions, including epinephrine (1:1000), should be readily available.

**Pregnancy Risk Factor** C

**Adverse Reactions**

>10%: Central nervous system: Fever (>38°C to <39°C) (11% to 21%), decreased appetite (11% to 17%), irritability (36% to 41%), decreased activity (10% to 20%)

1% to 10%: Central nervous system: Fever (≥39°C) (1% to 2%)

The incidence of fever is greater when administered to infants >6 months of age. The highest incidence of adverse effects was associated with the first dose of the vaccine. By the third dose, there were no significant differences in the incidence of adverse effects between vaccine and placebo.

**Drug Interactions** No drug interactions have been reported. No data have been reported with respect to administration of orally or intravenously administered immune globulin-containing products.

**Special PA Issues**

**Patient Education:** Parents must be instructed as to the importance of completing the vaccination sequence

- ◆ **Roubac®** *see* Co-Trimoxazole *on page 238*
- ◆ **Rowasa® Rectal** *see* Mesalamine *on page 571*
- ◆ **Roxanol™ Oral** *see* Morphine Sulfate *on page 619*
- ◆ **Roxanol Rescudose®** *see* Morphine Sulfate *on page 619*
- ◆ **Roxanol SR™ Oral** *see* Morphine Sulfate *on page 619*
- ◆ **Roxicet® 5/500** *see* Oxycodone and Acetaminophen *on page 688*
- ◆ **Roxicodone™** *see* Oxycodone *on page 687*
- ◆ **Roxilox®** *see* Oxycodone and Acetaminophen *on page 688*
- ◆ **Roxiprin®** *see* Oxycodone and Aspirin *on page 688*
- ◆ **RP54274** *see* Riluzole *on page 806*
- ◆ **r-PA** *see* Reteplase *on page 799*
- ◆ **rPDGF-BB** *see* Becaplermin *on page 100*
- ◆ **RSV-IGIV** *see* Respiratory Syncytial Virus Immune Globulin (Intravenous) *on page 798*
- ◆ **R-Tannamine® Tablet** *see* Chlorpheniramine, Pyrilamine, and Phenylephrine *on page 197*
- ◆ **R-Tannate® Tablet** *see* Chlorpheniramine, Pyrilamine, and Phenylephrine *on page 197*
- ◆ **RTCA** *see* Ribavirin *on page 801*
- ◆ **Rubramin®** *see* Cyanocobalamin *on page 242*
- ◆ **Rubramin-PC®** *see* Cyanocobalamin *on page 242*
- ◆ **Rum-K®** *see* Potassium Chloride *on page 742*
- ◆ **Rustic Treacle** *see* Garlic *on page 410*
- ◆ **Ru-Tuss®** *see* Chlorpheniramine Phenylephrine, Phenylpropanolamine, and Belladonna Alkaloids *on page 196*
- ◆ **Ru-Tuss® Liquid** *see* Chlorpheniramine and Phenylephrine *on page 195*
- ◆ **Ru-Vert-M®** *see* Meclizine *on page 559*
- ◆ **Ryna-C® Liquid** *see* Chlorpheniramine, Pseudoephedrine, and Codeine *on page 197*
- ◆ **Rynacrom®** *see* Cromolyn Sodium *on page 240*
- ◆ **Ryna-CX®** *see* Guaifenesin, Pseudoephedrine, and Codeine *on page 429*
- ◆ **Rynatan® Pediatric Suspension** *see* Chlorpheniramine, Pyrilamine, and Phenylephrine *on page 197*
- ◆ **Rynatan® Tablet** *see* Chlorpheniramine, Pyrilamine, and Phenylephrine *on page 197*
- ◆ **Rynatuss® Pediatric Suspension** *see* Chlorpheniramine, Ephedrine, Phenylephrine, and Carbetapentane *on page 195*
- ◆ **Rythmol®** *see* Propafenone *on page 770*
- ◆ *Sabal serrulata* *see* Saw Palmetto *on page 824*
- ◆ *Sabaslis serrulatae* *see* Saw Palmetto *on page 824*
- ◆ **Sabulin** *see* Albuterol *on page 34*
- ◆ **Safe Tussin® 30 [OTC]** *see* Guaifenesin and Dextromethorphan *on page 428*
- ◆ **Saizen® Injection** *see* Human Growth Hormone *on page 444*
- ◆ **Salagen® Oral** *see* Pilocarpine *on page 726*
- ◆ **Salazopyrin®** *see* Sulfasalazine *on page 862*
- ◆ **Salazopyrin EN-Tabs®** *see* Sulfasalazine *on page 862*
- ◆ **Salbutamol** *see* Albuterol *on page 34*

- **Saleto-200®** [OTC] *see* Ibuprofen *on page 466*
- **Saleto-400®** *see* Ibuprofen *on page 466*
- **Salflex®** *see* Salsalate *on next page*
- **Salgesic®** *see* Salsalate *on next page*
- **Salicylazosulfapyridine** *see* Sulfasalazine *on page 862*

## Salicylic Acid and Lactic Acid (sal i SIL ik AS id & LAK tik AS id)
**Pharmacologic Class** Keratolytic Agent
**U.S. Brand Names** Duofilm® Solution
**Dosage Forms Soln, top:** Salicylic acid 16.7% and lactic acid 16.7% in flexible collodion (15 mL)

## Salicylic Acid and Propylene Glycol
(sal i SIL ik AS id & PROE pi leen GLYE cole)
**Pharmacologic Class** Keratolytic Agent
**U.S. Brand Names** Keralyt® Gel
**Dosage Forms Gel, top:** Salicylic acid 6% and propylene glycol 60% in ethyl alcohol 19.4% with hydroxypropyl methylcellulose and water (30 g)

- **Salicylsalicylic Acid** *see* Salsalate *on next page*
- **SalineX®** [OTC] *see* Sodium Chloride *on page 839*

## Salmeterol (sal ME te role)
**Pharmacologic Class** Beta$_2$ Agonist
**U.S. Brand Names** Serevent®; Serevent® Diskus®
**Mechanism of Action** Relaxes bronchial smooth muscle by selective action on beta$_2$-receptors with little effect on heart rate; because salmeterol acts locally in the lung, therapeutic effect is not predicted by plasma levels
**Use** Maintenance treatment of asthma and in prevention of bronchospasm in patients >12 years of age with reversible obstructive airway disease, including patients with symptoms of nocturnal asthma, who require regular treatment with inhaled, short-acting beta$_2$ agonists; prevention of exercise-induced bronchospasm; treatment of COPD-induced bronchospasm
**USUAL DOSAGE**
Inhalation: 42 mcg (2 puffs) twice daily (12 hours apart) for maintenance and prevention of symptoms of asthma
Prevention of exercise-induced asthma: 42 mcg (2 puffs) 30-60 minutes prior to exercise; additional doses should not be used for 12 hours
COPD: Adults: For maintenance treatment of bronchospasm associated with COPD (including chronic bronchitis and emphysema): 2 inhalations (42 mcg) twice daily (morning and evening - 12 hours apart); do not use a spacer with the inhalation powder
**Dosage Forms Aero, oral, as xinafoate:** 21 mcg/spray [60 inhalations] (6.5 g), [120 inhalations] (13 g); **Powder, diskus inhaler:** 50 mcg/inhalation
**Contraindications** Hypersensitivity to salmeterol, adrenergic amines or any ingredients; need for acute bronchodilation; within 2 weeks of MAO inhibitor use
**Warnings/Precautions** Salmeterol is not meant to relieve acute asthmatic symptoms. Acute episodes should be treated with short-acting beta$_2$ agonist. Do not increase the frequency of salmeterol. Cardiovascular effects are not common with salmeterol when used in recommended doses. All beta agonists may cause elevation in blood pressure, heart rate, and result in excitement (CNS). Use with caution in patients with prostatic hypertrophy, diabetes, cardiovascular disorders, convulsive disorders, thyrotoxicosis, or others who are sensitive to the effects of sympathomimetic amines. Paroxysmal bronchospasm (which can be fatal) has been reported with this and other inhaled agents. If this occurs, discontinue treatment. The elderly may be at greater risk of cardiovascular side effects; safety and efficacy have not been established in children <12 years of age.
**Pregnancy Risk Factor** C
**Adverse Reactions**
>10%:
Central nervous system: Headache
Respiratory: Pharyngitis
1% to 10%:
Cardiovascular: Tachycardia, palpitations, elevation or depression of blood pressure, cardiac arrhythmias
Central nervous system: Nervousness, CNS stimulation, hyperactivity, insomnia, malaise, dizziness
Gastrointestinal: GI upset, diarrhea, nausea
Neuromuscular & skeletal: Tremors (may be more common in the elderly), myalgias, back pain, arthralgia
Respiratory: Upper respiratory infection, cough, bronchitis
<1%: Immediate hypersensitivity reactions (rash, urticaria, bronchospasm)
**Drug Interactions** CYP3A3/4 enzyme substrate
Increased effect: Beta-adrenergic blockers (eg, propranolol)
Increased toxicity (cardiovascular): MAO inhibitors, tricyclic antidepressants
(Continued)

## Salmeterol (Continued)

**Onset** 5-20 minutes (average 10 minutes); Peak effect: 2-4 hours
**Duration** 12 hours
**Half-Life** 3-4 hours
**Special PA Issues**
    **Patient Education:** Use exactly as directed (see Administration below). Do not use more often than recommended (excessive use may result in tolerance, overdose may result in serious adverse effects) and do not discontinue without consulting prescriber. Do not use for acute attacks. Maintain adequate hydration (2-3 L/day of fluids unless instructed to restrict fluid intake). You may experience nervousness, dizziness, or fatigue (use caution when driving or engaging in hazardous activities until response to treatment is known); or dry mouth, stomach upset (frequent small meals, frequent mouth care, chewing gum, or sucking hard candy may help). Report unresolved GI upset; dizziness or fatigue; vision changes; chest pain, rapid heartbeat, or palpitations; insomnia; nervousness or hyperactivity; muscle cramping, tremors, or pain; unusual cough; or rash (hypersensitivity).

    **Administration:** Self-administered inhalation: Store canister upside down; do not freeze. Shake canister before using. Sit when using medication. Close eyes when administering salmeterol to avoid spray getting into eyes. Exhale slowly and completely through nose; inhale deeply through mouth while administering aerosol. Hold breath for 1-3 seconds after inhalation. Wait at least 1 full minute between inhalations. Wash mouthpiece between use. If more than one inhalation medication is used, use bronchodilator first and wait 5 minutes between medications.

    **Monitoring Parameters:** Pulmonary function tests, blood pressure, pulse, CNS stimulation

♦ **Salmeterol Xinafoate** see Salmeterol on previous page
♦ **Salmonine® Injection** see Calcitonin on page 136

## Salsalate (SAL sa late)

**Pharmacologic Class** Salicylate
**U.S. Brand Names** Argesic®-SA; Artha-G®; Disalcid®; Marthritic®; Mono-Gesic®; Salflex®; Salgesic®; Salsitab®
**Mechanism of Action** Inhibits prostaglandin synthesis, acts on the hypothalamus heat-regulating center to reduce fever, blocks prostaglandin synthetase action which prevents formation of the platelet-aggregating substance thromboxane $A_2$
**Use** Treatment of minor pain or fever; arthritis
**USUAL DOSAGE** Adults: Oral: 3 g/day in 2-3 divided doses
    **Dosing comments in renal impairment:** In patients with end-stage renal disease undergoing hemodialysis: 750 mg twice daily with an additional 500 mg after dialysis
**Dosage Forms Cap:** 500 mg; **Tab:** 500 mg, 750 mg
**Contraindications** GI ulcer or bleeding, known hypersensitivity to salsalate
**Warnings/Precautions** Use with caution in patients with platelet and bleeding disorders, renal dysfunction, erosive gastritis, or peptic ulcer disease, previous nonreaction does not guarantee future safe taking of medication; do not use aspirin in children <16 years of age for chickenpox or flu symptoms due to the association with Reye's syndrome
**Pregnancy Risk Factor** C
**Adverse Reactions**
    >10%: Gastrointestinal: Nausea, heartburn, stomach pains, dyspepsia
    1% to 10%:
        Central nervous system: Fatigue
        Dermatologic: Rash
        Gastrointestinal: Gastrointestinal ulceration
        Hematologic: Hemolytic anemia
        Neuromuscular & skeletal: Weakness
        Respiratory: Dyspnea
        Miscellaneous: Anaphylactic shock
    <1%: Insomnia, nervousness, jitters, leukopenia, thrombocytopenia, iron deficiency anemia, does not appear to inhibit platelet aggregation, occult bleeding, hepatotoxicity, impaired renal function, bronchospasm
**Drug Interactions**
    Decreased effect with urinary alkalinizers, antacids, corticosteroids; decreased effect of uricosurics, spironolactone
    Increased effect/toxicity of oral anticoagulants, hypoglycemics, methotrexate
**Onset** Therapeutic effects occur within 3-4 days of continuous dosing
**Half-Life** 7-8 hours
**Special PA Issues**
    **Patient Education:** Take this medication exactly as directed; do not increase dose without consulting prescriber. Do not crush tablets or break capsules. Take with food or milk to reduce GI distress. Maintain adequate fluid intake (2-3 L/day). Do not use alcohol, aspirin, or aspirin-containing medication, and all other anti-inflammatory medications without consulting prescriber. You may experience drowsiness (use caution when driving

or performing hazardous tasks); nausea or heartburn (frequent small meals, frequent oral care, sucking on lozenges, or chewing gum may help). GI bleeding, ulceration, or perforation can occur with or without pain; discontinue medication and contact prescriber if persistent abdominal pain or cramping, or blood in stool occurs. Report breathlessness or difficulty breathing; unusual bruising/bleeding; blood in urine, stool, mouth, or vomitus; unusual fatigue; skin rash or itching; change in urinary pattern; or change in hearing or ringing in ears.

- ♦ **Salsitab**® *see* Salsalate *on previous page*
- ♦ **Salt** *see* Sodium Chloride *on page 839*
- ♦ **Salt Poor Albumin** *see* Albumin *on page 34*
- ♦ **Sandimmune**® **Injection** *see* Cyclosporine *on page 245*
- ♦ **Sandimmune**® **Oral** *see* Cyclosporine *on page 245*
- ♦ **Sandoglobulin**® *see* Immune Globulin, Intravenous *on page 472*
- ♦ **Sandostatin**® *see* Octreotide Acetate *on page 671*
- ♦ **Sandostatin LAR**® **Depot** *see* Octreotide Acetate *on page 671*
- ♦ **Sang**® **CyA** *see* Cyclosporine *on page 245*
- ♦ **Sansert**® *see* Methysergide *on page 596*
- ♦ **Santyl**® *see* Collagenase *on page 235*

# Saquinavir (sa KWIN a veer)

**Pharmacologic Class** Antiretroviral Agent, Protease Inhibitor

**U.S. Brand Names** Fortovase®; Invirase®

**Mechanism of Action** As an inhibitor of HIV protease, saquinavir prevents the cleavage of viral polyprotein precursors which are needed to generate functional proteins in and maturation of HIV-infected cells

**Use** Treatment of HIV infection in selected patients; used in combination with other antiretroviral agents

**USUAL DOSAGE** Adults: Oral:

Fortovase®: Six 200 mg capsules (1200 mg) 3 times/day within 2 hours after a meal in combination with a nucleoside analog

Invirase®: Three 200 mg capsules (600 mg) 3 times/day within 2 hours after a full meal in combination with a nucleoside analog

Dose of either Fortovase® or Invirase® in combination with ritonavir: 400 mg twice daily

**Dosage Forms Cap (hard) as mesylate (Invirase®):** 200 mg; **Cap (soft) (Fortovase®):** 200 mg

**Contraindications** Hypersensitivity to saquinavir or any components; exposure to direct sunlight without sunscreen or protective clothing; coadministration with terfenadine, cisapride, astemizole, triazolam, midazolam, or ergot derivatives

**Warnings/Precautions** The indication for saquinavir for the treatment of HIV infection is based on changes in surrogate markers. At present, there are no results from controlled clinical trials evaluating its effect on patient survival or the clinical progression of HIV infection (ie, occurrence of opportunistic infections or malignancies); use caution in patients with hepatic insufficiency; safety and efficacy have not been established in children <16 years of age. May exacerbate pre-existing hepatic dysfunction; use with caution in patients with hepatitis B or C and in cirrhosis

**Pregnancy Risk Factor** B

**Pregnancy Implications**

Clinical effects on the fetus: Administer saquinavir during pregnancy only if benefits to the mother outweigh the risk to the fetus

Breast-feeding/lactation: HIV-infected mothers are discouraged from breast-feeding to decrease postnatal transmission of HIV

**Adverse Reactions** Protease inhibitors cause dyslipidemia which includes elevated cholesterol and triglycerides and a redistribution of body fat centrally to cause "protease paunch", buffalo hump, facial atrophy, and breast enlargement. These agents also cause hyperglycemia.

1% to 10%:

Dermatologic: Rash

Endocrine & metabolic: Hyperglycemia

Gastrointestinal: Diarrhea, abdominal discomfort, nausea, abdominal pain, buccal mucosa ulceration

Neuromuscular & skeletal: Paresthesia, weakness, increased CPK

<1%: Headache, confusion, seizures, ataxia, pain, Stevens-Johnson syndrome, hypoglycemia, hyper- and hypokalemia, low serum amylase, upper quadrant abdominal pain, acute myeloblastic leukemia, hemolytic anemia, thrombocytopenia, jaundice, ascites, bullous skin eruption, polyarthritis, portal hypertension, exacerbation of chronic liver disease, elevated LFTs, altered AST/ALT, bilirubin, Hgb, thrombophlebitis

**Drug Interactions** CYP3A3/4 enzyme substrate; CYP3A3/4 enzyme inhibitor

Decreased effect: Rifampin may decrease saquinavir's plasma levels and AUC by 40% to 80%; other enzyme inducers may induce saquinavir's metabolism (eg, phenobarbital, phenytoin, dexamethasone, carbamazepine); may decrease delavirdine concentrations

(Continued)

## Saquinavir *(Continued)*

Increased effect: Ketoconazole significantly increases plasma levels and AUC of saquinavir; as a known, although not potent inhibitor of the cytochrome P-450 system, saquinavir may decrease the metabolism of terfenadine and astemizole, as well as cisapride, ergot derivatives, midazolam, and triazolam (and result in rare but serious effects including cardiac arrhythmias); other drugs which may have increased adverse effects if coadministered with saquinavir include calcium channel blockers, clindamycin, dapsone, and quinidine. Both clarithromycin and saquinavir levels/effects may be increased with coadministration. Delavirdine may increase concentration; ritonavir may increase AUC >17-fold; concurrent administration of nelfinavir results in increase in nelfinavir (18%) and saquinavir (mean: 392%).

**Half-Life** 13 hours

**Special PA Issues**

**Patient Education:** Saquinavir is is not a cure for HIV nor has it been found to reduce transmission of HIV. Take as directed, with food. Diabetics will need to monitor glucose levels frequently while taking this medication; this medication may exacerbate diabetes and hyperglycemia. You may experience headache or confusion; if these persist notify prescriber. You may develop sensitivity to sunlight (wear protective clothing, use sunblock, or avoid direct sunlight); mouth sores (frequent oral care is necessary). Report persistent nausea, vomiting, abdominal pain, or diarrhea; skin rash or irritation; muscles weakness or tremors; easy bruising or bleeding; fever or chills; yellowing of eyes or skin; or dark urine or pale stools.

**Monitoring Parameters:** Monitor viral load, CD4 count, triglycerides, cholesterol, glucose

♦ **Saquinavir Mesylate** *see Saquinavir on previous page*

## Sargramostim *(sar GRAM oh stim)*

**Pharmacologic Class** Colony Stimulating Factor

**U.S. Brand Names** Leukine™

**Mechanism of Action** Stimulates proliferation, differentiation and functional activity of neutrophils, eosinophils, monocytes, and macrophages; see table.

| Proliferation/Differentiation | G-CSF (Filgrastim) | GM-CSF (Sargramostim) |
|---|---|---|
| Neutrophils | Yes | Yes |
| Eosinophils | No | Yes |
| Macrophages | No | Yes |
| Neutrophil migration | Enhanced | Inhibited |

**Use**

**Myeloid reconstitution after autologous bone marrow transplantation:**
Non-Hodgkin's lymphoma (NHL)
Acute lymphoblastic leukemia (ALL)
Hodgkin's lymphoma
Metastatic breast cancer

**Myeloid reconstitution after allogeneic bone marrow transplantation**
**Peripheral stem cell transplantation**
Metastatic breast cancer
Non-Hodgkin's lymphoma
Hodgkin's lymphoma
Multiple myeloma

**Acute myelogenous leukemia (AML)** following induction chemotherapy in older adults to shorten time to neutrophil recovery and to reduce the incidence of severe and life-threatening infections and infections resulting in death

**Bone marrow transplant (allogeneic or autologous) failure or engraftment delay**
Safety and efficacy of GM-CSF given simultaneously with cytotoxic chemotherapy have not been established. Concurrent treatment may increase myelosuppression.

**USUAL DOSAGE**

Children and Adults: I.V. infusion over ≥2 hours or S.C.
Existing clinical data suggest that starting GM-CSF between 24 and 72 hours subsequent to chemotherapy may provide optimal neutrophil recover; continue therapy until the occurrence of an absolute neutrophil count of 10,000/μL after the neutrophil nadir

**The available data suggest that rounding the dose to the nearest vial size may enhance patient convenience and reduce costs without clinical detriment**

**Myeloid reconstitution after peripheral stem cell, allogeneic or autologous bone marrow transplant:** I.V.: 250 mcg/m²/day for 21 days to begin 2-4 hours after the marrow infusion on day 0 of autologous bone marrow transplant or ≥24 hours after chemotherapy or 12 hours after last dose of radiotherapy

If a severe adverse reaction occurs, reduce or temporarily discontinue the dose until the reaction abates

If blast cells appear or progression of the underlying disease occurs, disrupt treatment
Interrupt or reduce the dose by half if ANC is >20,000 cells/mm³
Patients should not receive sargramostim until the postmarrow infusion ANC is <500 cells/mm³

**Neutrophil recovery following chemotherapy in AML:** I.V.: 250 mg/m²/day over a 4-hour period starting ~day 11 or 4 days following the completion of induction chemotherapy, if day 10 bone marrow is hypoblastic with <5% blasts

If a second cycle of chemotherapy is necessary, administer ~4 days after the completion of chemotherapy if the bone marrow is hypoblastic with <5% blasts
Continue sargramostim until ANC is >1500 cells/mm³ for consecutive days or a maximum of 42 days
Discontinue sargramostim immediately if leukemic regrowth occurs
If a severe adverse reaction occurs, reduce the dose by 50% or temporarily discontinue the dose until the reaction abates

**Mobilization of peripheral blood progenitor cells:** I.V.: 250 mcg/m²/day over 24 hours or S.C. once daily

Continue the same dose through the period of PBPC collection
The optimal schedule for PBPC collection has not been established (usually begun by day 5 and performed daily until protocol specified targets are achieved)
If WBC >50,000 cells/mm³, reduce the dose by 50%
If adequate numbers of progenitor cells are not collected, consider other mobilization therapy

**Postperipheral blood progenitor cell transplantation:** I.V.: 250 mcg/m²/day over 24 hours or S.C. once daily beginning immediately following infusion of progenitor cells and continuing until ANC is >1500 for 3 consecutive days is attained

**BMT failure or engraftment delay:** I.V.: 250 mcg/m²/day for 14 days as a 2-hour infusion

The dose can be repeated after 7 days off therapy if engraftment has not occurred
If engraftment still has not occurred, a third course of 500 mcg/m²/day for 14 days may be tried after another 7 days off therapy; if there is still no improvement, it is unlikely that further dose escalation will be beneficial
If a severe adverse reaction occurs, reduce or temporarily discontinue the dose until the reaction abates
If blast cells appear or disease progression occurs, discontinue treatment

**Dosage Forms** Inj: 250 mcg, 500 mcg

**Contraindications** GM-CSF is contraindicated in the following instances:

Patients with excessive myeloid blasts (>10%) in the bone marrow or peripheral blood
Patients with known hypersensitivity to GM-CSF, yeast-derived products, or any known component of the product

**Warnings/Precautions** Simultaneous administration with cytotoxic chemotherapy or radiotherapy or administration 24 hours preceding or following chemotherapy is recommended. Use with caution in patients with pre-existing cardiac problems, hypoxia, fluid retention, pulmonary infiltrates or congestive heart failure, renal or hepatic impairment.

Rapid increase in peripheral blood counts: If ANC >20,000/mm³ or platelets >500,000/mm³, decrease dose by 50% or discontinue drug (counts will fall to normal within 3-7 days after discontinuing drug)

Growth factor potential: Use with caution with myeloid malignancies. Precaution should be exercised in the usage of GM-CSF in any malignancy with myeloid characteristics. GM-CSF can potentially act as a growth factor for any tumor type, particularly myeloid malignancies. Tumors of nonhematopoietic origin may have surface receptors for GM-CSF.

There is a "first-dose effect" (refer to Adverse Reactions for details) which is rarely seen with the first dose and does not usually occur with subsequent doses.

**Pregnancy Risk Factor** C

**Pregnancy Implications** Clinical effects to the fetus: Animal reproduction studies have not been conducted. It is not known whether sargramostim can cause fetal harm when administered to a pregnant woman or can affect reproductive capability. Sargramostim should be given to a pregnant woman only if clearly needed.

**Adverse Reactions**

>10%:

"First-dose" effects: Fever, hypotension, tachycardia, rigors, flushing, nausea, vomiting, dyspnea
Central nervous system: Neutropenic fever
Dermatologic: Alopecia
Endocrine & metabolic: Polydipsia
Gastrointestinal: Nausea, vomiting, diarrhea, stomatitis, GI hemorrhage, mucositis
Neuromuscular & skeletal: Bone pain, myalgia

1% to 10%:

Cardiovascular: Chest pain, peripheral edema, capillary leak syndrome
Central nervous system: Headache
Dermatologic: Rash
Endocrine & metabolic: Fluid retention
Gastrointestinal: Anorexia, sore throat, stomatitis, constipation

(Continued)

## Sargramostim *(Continued)*

    Hematologic: Leukocytosis
    Local: Pain at injection site
    Neuromuscular & skeletal: Weakness
    Respiratory: Dyspnea, cough
    <1%: Hypotension, flushing, pericardial effusion, transient supraventricular arrhythmias, pericarditis, malaise, fever, headache, thrombophlebitis, rigors, anaphylactic reaction

**Drug Interactions**
    Increased toxicity: Lithium, corticosteroids may potentiate myeloproliferative effects

**Onset** Increase in WBC in 7-14 days

**Duration** WBC will return to baseline within 1 week after discontinuing drug.

**Half-Life** 2 hours

**Special PA Issues**
    **Patient Education:** You may experience bone pain (request analgesic), nausea and vomiting (small frequent meals may help), hair loss (reversible). Report fever, chills, unhealed sores, severe bone pain, difficulty breathing, swelling or pain at infusion site. Avoid crowds or exposure to infected persons; you will be susceptible to infection.
    **Monitoring Parameters:** Vital signs, weight, CBC with differential, platelets, renal/liver function tests, especially with previous dysfunction, WBC with differential, pulmonary function
    **Reference Range:** Excessive leukocytosis: ANC >20,000/mm$^3$ or WBC >50,000 cells/mm$^3$

♦ **S.A.S™** *see* Sulfasalazine *on page 862*

♦ **Sassafras albidum** *see* Sassafras Oil *on this page*

## Sassafras Oil

    **Mechanism of Action** Contains safrole (up to 80%) which inhibits liver microsomal enzymes; its metabolite may cause hepatic tumors
    **Use** Banned by FDA in food since 1960; has been used as a mild counterirritant on the skin (ie, for lice or insect bites); should not be ingested
    **USUAL DOSAGE** Sassafras tea can contain as much as 200 mg (3 mg/kg) of safrole
    Lethal dose: ~5 mL
    Toxic dose: 0.66 mg/kg is considered to be toxic to humans based on rodent studies
    **Adverse Reactions** (Primarily related to sassafras oil and safrole)
    Cardiovascular: Tachycardia, flushing, hypotension, sinus tachycardia
    Central nervous system: Anxiety, hallucinations, vertigo, aphasia
    Dermatologic: Contact dermatitis
    Gastrointestinal: Vomiting
    Hepatic: Fatty changes of the liver, hepatic necrosis
    Ocular: Mydriasis
    Miscellaneous: Diaphoresis

    Little documentation of adverse effects due to ingestion of herbal tea

    **Special PA Issues**
    **Patient Education:** Considered unsafe by the FDA

## Saw Palmetto

    **Mechanism of Action** Liposterolic extract of the berries may inhibit the enzymes 5α-reductase, along with cyclo-oxygenase and 5-lipoxygenase, thus exhibiting antiandrogen and anti-inflammatory effects; does not reduce prostatic enlargement but may help increase urinary flow (not FDA approved)
    **Use** Benign prostatic hyperplasia
    **USUAL DOSAGE** Adults: Dried fruit: 0.5-1 g 3 times/day
    **Contraindications** Pregnancy and breast-feeding
    **Pregnancy Implications** Do not use
    **Adverse Reactions**
    Central nervous system: Headache
    Endocrine & metabolic: Gynecomastia
    Gastrointestinal: Stomach problems (in rare cases) per Commission E

♦ **Scabene®** *see* Lindane *on page 534*

♦ **Scalpicin®** *see* Hydrocortisone *on page 453*

♦ **Sclavo-PPD Solution®** *see* Tuberculin Tests *on page 945*

♦ **Sclavo Test-PPD®** *see* Tuberculin Tests *on page 945*

♦ **Scopace™ Tablet** *see* Scopolamine *on this page*

## Scopolamine *(skoe POL a meen)*

    **Pharmacologic Class** Anticholinergic Agent
    **U.S. Brand Names** Isopto® Hyoscine Ophthalmic; Scopace™ Tablet; Transderm Scop® Patch

**Mechanism of Action** Blocks the action of acetylcholine at parasympathetic sites in smooth muscle, secretory glands and the CNS; increases cardiac output, dries secretions, antagonizes histamine and serotonin

**Use** Preoperative medication to produce amnesia and decrease salivary and respiratory secretions; to produce cycloplegia and mydriasis; treatment of iridocyclitis; prevention of motion sickness; prevention of nausea/vomiting associated with anesthesia or opiate analgesia (patch); symptomatic treatment of postencephalitic parkinsonism and paralysis agitans (oral); inhibits excessive motility and hypertonus of the gastrointestinal tract in such conditions as the irritable colon syndrome, mild dysentery, diverticulitis, pylorospasm, and cardiospasm; it may also prevent motion sickness (oral)

## USUAL DOSAGE

Preoperatively:

Children: I.M., S.C.: 6 mcg/kg/dose (maximum: 0.3 mg/dose) or 0.2 mg/m$^2$ may be repeated every 6-8 hours **or** alternatively:

4-7 months: 0.1 mg

7 months to 3 years: 0.15 mg

3-8 years: 0.2 mg

8-12 years: 0.3 mg

Adults:

I.M., I.V., S.C.: 0.3-0.65 mg; may be repeated every 4-6 hours

Transdermal patch: Apply 2.5 cm$^2$ patch to hairless area behind ear the night before surgery (the patch should be applied no sooner than 1 hour before surgery for best results)

Motion sickness: Transdermal: Children >12 years and Adults: Apply 1 disc behind the ear at least 4 hours prior to exposure and every 3 days as needed; effective if applied as soon as 2-3 hours before anticipated need, best if 12 hours before

Ophthalmic:

Refraction:

Children: Instill 1 drop of 0.25% to eye(s) twice daily for 2 days before procedure

Adults: Instill 1-2 drops of 0.25% to eye(s) 1 hour before procedure

Iridocyclitis:

Children: Instill 1 drop of 0.25% to eye(s) up to 3 times/day

Adults: Instill 1-2 drops of 0.25% to eye(s) up to 4 times/day

Oral: 0.4 to 0.8 mg as a range; the dosage may be cautiously increased in parkinsonism and spastic states.

**Dosage Forms Disc, transdermal:** 1.5 mg/disc (4's); **Inj, as hydrobromide:** 0.3 mg/mL (1 mL), 0.4 mg/mL (0.5 mL, 1 mL), 0.86 mg/mL (0.5 mL), 1 mg/mL (1 mL); **Soln, ophth, as hydrobromide:** 0.25% (5 mL, 15 mL); **Tab:** 0.4 mg

**Contraindications** Hypersensitivity to scopolamine or any component; narrow-angle glaucoma; acute hemorrhage, gastrointestinal or genitourinary obstruction, thyrotoxicosis, tachycardia secondary to cardiac insufficiency, paralytic ileus

**Warnings/Precautions** Use with caution with hepatic or renal impairment since adverse CNS effects occur more often in these patients; use with caution in infants and children since they may be more susceptible to adverse effects of scopolamine; use with caution in patients with GI obstruction; anticholinergic agents are not well tolerated in the elderly and their use should be avoided when possible

## Pregnancy Risk Factor C

## Adverse Reactions

Ophthalmic:

>10%: Ocular: Blurred vision, photophobia

1% to 10%:

Ocular: Local irritation, increased intraocular pressure

Respiratory: Congestion

<1%: Vascular congestion, edema, drowsiness, eczematoid dermatitis, follicular conjunctivitis, exudate

Systemic:

>10%:

Dermatologic: Dry skin

Gastrointestinal: Constipation, xerostomia, dry throat

Local: Irritation at injection site

Respiratory: Dry nose

Miscellaneous: Diaphoresis (decreased)

1% to 10%:

Dermatologic: Increased sensitivity to light

Endocrine & metabolic: Decreased flow of breast milk

Gastrointestinal: Dysphagia

<1%: Orthostatic hypotension, ventricular fibrillation, tachycardia, palpitations, confusion, drowsiness, headache, loss of memory, ataxia, fatigue, rash, bloated feeling, nausea, vomiting, dysuria, weakness, increased intraocular pain, blurred vision

**Note:** Systemic adverse effects have been reported following ophthalmic administration

## Drug Interactions

Decreased effect of acetaminophen, levodopa, ketoconazole, digoxin, riboflavin, potassium chloride in wax matrix preparations

(Continued)

## Scopolamine *(Continued)*

Increased toxicity: Additive adverse effects with other anticholinergic agents; GI absorption of the following drugs may be affected: acetaminophen, levodopa, ketoconazole, digoxin, riboflavin, potassium chloride wax-matrix preparations

**Onset** Onset of effect: Oral, I.M.: 0.5-1 hour; I.V.: 10 minutes

**Duration** Oral, I.M.: 4-6 hours; I.V.: 2 hours; Transdermal: 3 days

**Special PA Issues**

**Patient Education:** Take as directed (see Administration). You may experience drowsiness, confusion, impaired judgment, or vision changes (use caution when driving or engaging in hazardous activity until response to medication is known); dry mouth, nausea, or vomiting (small frequent meals or sucking on lozenges may help); orthostatic hypotension (use caution when climbing stairs and when rising from lying or sitting position); constipation (increased exercise, fluid, or dietary fiber may reduce constipation, if not effective consult prescriber); increased sensitivity to heat and decreased perspiration (avoid extremes of heat, reduce exercise in hot weather); decreased milk if breastfeeding. Report hot, dry, flushed skin; blurred vision or vision changes; difficulty swallowing; chest pain, palpitations, or rapid heartbeat; painful or difficult urination; increased confusion, depression, or loss of memory; rapid or difficult respirations; muscle weakness or tremors; or eye pain.

**Administration:**

Transdermal: Apply patch behind ear the day before traveling. Wash hands before applying and avoid contact with the eyes. Do not remove for 3 days.

Ophthalmic: Instill as often as recommended. Wash hands before using. Sit or lie down, open eye, look at ceiling and instill prescribed amount of solution. Do not blink for 30 seconds, close eye and roll eye in all directions, and apply gentle pressure to inner corner of eye for 1-2 minutes. Do not let tip of applicator touch eye or contaminate tip of applicator. Temporary stinging or blurred vision may occur.

♦ **Scopolamine Hydrobromide** *see* Scopolamine *on page 824*

♦ **Scot-Tussin® [OTC]** *see* Guaifenesin *on page 427*

♦ **Scot-Tussin® Senior Clear [OTC]** *see* Guaifenesin and Dextromethorphan *on page 428*

♦ **Scurvy Root, American Coneflower** *see* Echinacea *on page 310*

♦ **SeaMist® [OTC]** *see* Sodium Chloride *on page 839*

♦ **Sebizon® Topical Lotion** *see* Sulfacetamide Sodium *on page 858*

♦ **Secran®** *see* Vitamins, Multiple *on page 964*

♦ **Sectral®** *see* Acebutolol *on page 20*

♦ **Sedapap-10®** *see* Butalbital Compound *on page 131*

♦ **Selax®** *see* Docusate *on page 298*

## Selegiline *(seh LEDGE ah leen)*

**Pharmacologic Class** Antidepressant, Monoamine Oxidase Inhibitor; Anti-Parkinson's Agent (Monoamine Oxidase Inhibitor)

**U.S. Brand Names** Eldepryl®

**Mechanism of Action** Potent monoamine oxidase (MAO) type-B inhibitor; MAO-B plays a major role in the metabolism of dopamine; selegiline may also increase dopaminergic activity by interfering with dopamine reuptake at the synapse

**Use** Adjunct in the management of parkinsonian patients in which levodopa/carbidopa therapy is deteriorating

**Unlabeled use:** Early Parkinson's disease

**Investigational:** Alzheimer's disease

Selegiline is also being studied in Alzheimer's disease. Small studies have shown some improvement in behavioral and cognitive performance in patients, however, further study is needed.

**USUAL DOSAGE** Oral:

Adults: 5 mg twice daily with breakfast and lunch or 10 mg in the morning

Elderly: Initial: 5 mg in the morning, may increase to a total of 10 mg/day

**Dosage Forms Cap, as hydrochloride (Eldepryl®):** 5 mg; **Tab:** 5 mg

**Contraindications** Known hypersensitivity to selegiline, concomitant use of meperidine

**Warnings/Precautions** Increased risk of nonselective MAO inhibition occurs with doses >10 mg/day; is a monoamine oxidase inhibitor type "B", there should **not** be a problem with tyramine-containing products as long as the typical doses are employed

**Pregnancy Risk Factor** C

**Adverse Reactions**

>10%:

Central nervous system: Mood changes, dizziness

Gastrointestinal: Nausea, vomiting, xerostomia, abdominal pain

Neuromuscular & skeletal: Dyskinesias

1% to 10%:

Cardiovascular: Orthostatic hypotension, arrhythmias, hypertension

Central nervous system: Hallucinations, confusion, depression, insomnia, agitation, loss of balance

Neuromuscular & skeletal: Increased involuntary movements, bradykinesia, muscle twitches

Miscellaneous: Bruxism

**Drug Interactions** CYP2D6 enzyme substrate

Increased toxicity: Meperidine in combination with selegiline has caused agitation, delirium, and death; it may be prudent to avoid other opioids as well; fluoxetine increases pressor effect

**Onset** Onset of therapeutic effects: Within 1 hour

**Duration** 24-72 hours

**Half-Life** 9 minutes

**Special PA Issues**

**Patient Education:** Take exactly as directed (may be prescribed in conjunction with levodopa/carbidopa); do not change dosage or discontinue without consulting prescriber. Therapeutic effects may take several weeks or months to achieve and you may need frequent monitoring during first weeks of therapy. Take with meals if GI upset occurs, before meals if dry mouth occurs, after eating if drooling or if nausea occurs. Take at same time each day. Avoid tyramine-containing foods (low potential for reaction). Maintain adequate hydration (2-3 L/day of fluids unless instructed to restrict fluid intake); void before taking medication. Do not use alcohol and prescription or OTC sedatives or CNS depressants without consulting prescriber. You may experience drowsiness, dizziness, confusion, or vision changes (use caution when driving, climbing stairs, or engaging in hazardous tasks); orthostatic hypotension (use caution when changing position - rising to standing from sitting or lying); constipation (increased exercise, fluids, or dietary fruit and fiber may help); runny nose or flu-like symptoms (consult prescriber for appropriate relief); nausea, vomiting, loss of appetite, or stomach discomfort (small frequent meals, chewing gum, or sucking on lozenges may help). Report unresolved constipation or vomiting; chest pain, palpitations, irregular heartbeat; CNS changes (hallucination, loss of memory, seizures, acute headache, nervousness, etc); painful or difficult urination; increased muscle spasticity, rigidity, or involuntary movements; skin rash; or significant worsening of condition.

**Monitoring Parameters:** Blood pressure, symptoms of parkinsonism

**Related Information**

Tyramine-Containing Foods *on page 1148*

♦ **Selegiline Hydrochloride** *see Selegiline on previous page*

# Selenium (se LEE nee um)

**Pharmacologic Class** Trace Element, Parenteral

**U.S. Brand Names** Sele-Pak®; Selepen®

**Mechanism of Action** Part of glutathione peroxidase which protects cell components from oxidative damage due to peroxidases produced in cellular metabolism

**Use** Trace metal supplement

**USUAL DOSAGE** I.V. in TPN solutions:

Children: 3 mcg/kg/day

Adults:

Metabolically stable: 20-40 mcg/day

Deficiency from prolonged TPN support: 100 mcg/day for 24 and 21 days

**Dosage Forms** Inj: 40 mcg/mL (10 mL, 30 mL)

**Contraindications** Known hypersensitivity to selenium or any component

**Pregnancy Risk Factor** C

**Adverse Reactions** 1% to 10%:

Central nervous system: Lethargy

Dermatologic: Alopecia or hair discoloration

Gastrointestinal: Vomiting following long-term use on damaged skin; abdominal pain, garlic breath

Local: Irritation

Neuromuscular & skeletal: Tremor

Miscellaneous: Diaphoresis

# Selenium Sulfide (se LEE nee um SUL fide)

**Pharmacologic Class** Antiseborrheic Agent, Topical; Shampoos

**U.S. Brand Names** Exsel®; Head & Shoulders® Intensive Treatment [OTC]; Selsun®; Selsun Blue® [OTC]; Selsun Gold® for Women [OTC]

**Mechanism of Action** May block the enzymes involved in growth of epithelial tissue

**Use** Treatment of itching and flaking of the scalp associated with dandruff, to control scalp seborrheic dermatitis; treatment of tinea versicolor

**USUAL DOSAGE** Topical:

Dandruff, seborrhea: Massage 5-10 mL into wet scalp, leave on scalp 2-3 minutes, rinse thoroughly, and repeat application; shampoo twice weekly for 2 weeks initially, then use once every 1-4 weeks as indicated depending upon control

(Continued)

## Selenium Sulfide (Continued)

Tinea versicolor: Apply the 2.5% lotion to affected area and lather with small amounts of water; leave on skin for 10 minutes, then rinse thoroughly; apply every day for 7 days

**Dosage Forms** Lot: 2.5% (120 mL); **Shamp:** 1% (120 mL, 210 mL, 240 mL, 330 mL), 2.5% (120 mL)

**Contraindications** Known hypersensitivity to selenium or any component

**Warnings/Precautions** Do not use on damaged skin to avoid any systemic toxicity; avoid topical use in very young children; safety of topical in infants has not been established

**Pregnancy Risk Factor** C

**Adverse Reactions**

>10%: Dermatologic: Unusual dryness or oiliness of scalp

1% to 10%:

Central nervous system: Lethargy

Dermatologic: Alopecia or hair discoloration

Gastrointestinal: Vomiting following long-term use on damaged skin, abdominal pain, garlic breath

Local: Irritation

Neuromuscular & skeletal: Tremor

Miscellaneous: Diaphoresis

**Special PA Issues**

**Patient Education:** Topical formulations are for external use only; notify physician if condition persists or worsens; avoid contact with eyes; thoroughly rinse after application

♦ **Sele-Pak®** *see* Selenium *on previous page*

♦ **Selepen®** *see* Selenium *on previous page*

♦ **Selsun®** *see* Selenium Sulfide *on previous page*

♦ **Selsun Blue® [OTC]** *see* Selenium Sulfide *on previous page*

♦ **Selsun Gold® for Women [OTC]** *see* Selenium Sulfide *on previous page*

♦ **Semprex®-D** *see* Acrivastine and Pseudoephedrine *on page 27*

# Senna

**Mechanism of Action** Contains up to 3% anthraquinone glycosides which can cause colonic stimulation

**Use** Catharsis

**USUAL DOSAGE**

Sennosides:

Children >6 years: 20 mg at bedtime

Adults: 20-40 mg with water at bedtime

Senna granules: 2.5-5 mL (163-326 mg) at bedtime; maximum dose: 10 mL (652 mg)/day

Senna tablets:

Children >60 pounds: 1 tablet (187 mg) at bedtime; maximum daily dose: 2 tablets

Adults: 1-2 tablets (187-374 mg) at bedtime; maximum daily dose: 4 tablets (Note: Extra strength senna tablets contain 374 mg each)

Senna syrup:

Children

1 month to 1 year: 1.25-2.5 mL (55-109 mg) at bedtime up to 5 mL/day

1-5 years: 2.5-5 mL (109-218 mg) at bedtime, up to 10 mL/day

5-15 years: 5-10 mL (218-436 mg) at bedtime, up to 20 mL/day

Adults: 10-15 mL (436-654 mg); maximum daily dose: 30 mL (1308 mg)

Senna suppositories:

Children >60 pounds: 1/2 suppository (326 mg)

Adults: 1 suppository (652 mg) at bedtime; can repeat in 2 hours

Tea: 1/2 to 2 teaspoons of leaves (0.5-4 g of the herb)

**Contraindications** Per Commission E: Intestinal obstruction, acute intestinal inflammation (eg, Crohn's disease), colitis ulcerosa, appendicitis, abdominal pain of unknown origin, children <12 years, and pregnancy

**Adverse Reactions**

Cardiovascular: Palpitations

Central nervous system: Tetany, dizziness

Dermatologic: Finger clubbing (reversible)

Endocrine & metabolic: Hypokalemia

Gastrointestinal:Vomiting (with fresh plant leaves or pods), diarrhea, abdominal cramping, nausea, melanosis coli (reversible), cachexia

Genitourinary: red discoloration in alkaline urine (yellow-brown in acidic urine)

Hepatic: Hepatitis

Renal: Oliguria, proteinuria

Respiratory: Dyspnea

Per Commission E:

Endocrine & metabolic: Long-term use/abuse can cause electrolyte imbalance

Gastrointestinal: In single incidents, cramp-like discomforts of G.I. tract requiring a reduction in dosage

**Drug Interactions** Per Commission E: Potentiation of cardiac glycosides (with long-term use) is possible due to loss in potassium; effect on antiarrhythmics is possible; potassium deficiency can be increased by simultaneous application of thiazide diuretics, corticosteroids, and licorice root

- **Senna Alexandria** *see* Senna *on previous page*
- **Sensorcaine®** *see* Bupivacaine *on page 126*
- **Sensorcaine®-MPF** *see* Bupivacaine *on page 126*
- **Septa® Topical Ointment [OTC]** *see* Bacitracin, Neomycin, and Polymyxin B *on page 97*
- **Septisol®** *see* Hexachlorophene *on page 441*
- **Septra®** *see* Co-Trimoxazole *on page 238*
- **Septra® DS** *see* Co-Trimoxazole *on page 238*
- **Ser-Ap-Es®** *see* Hydralazine, Hydrochlorothiazide, and Reserpine *on page 447*
- **Serax®** *see* Oxazepam *on page 685*
- **Serenoa repens** *see* Saw Palmetto *on page 824*
- **Serentil®** *see* Mesoridazine *on page 572*
- **Serevent®** *see* Salmeterol *on page 819*
- **Serevent® Diskus®** *see* Salmeterol *on page 819*

# Sermorelin Acetate (ser moe REL in AS e tate )

**Pharmacologic Class** Diagnostic Agent, Pituitary Function

**U.S. Brand Names** Geref® Injection

**Use** For the evaluation of short children whose height is at least 2 standard deviations below the mean height for their chronological age and sex, presenting with low basal serum levels of IGF-1 and IGF-1-BP3. A single intravenous injection of sermorelin is indicated for evaluating the ability of the somatotroph of the pituitary gland to secrete growth hormone (GH). A normal plasma GH response demonstrates that the somatotroph is intact.

>Orphan drug: Sermorelin has been designated an orphan product for use in the treatment of growth hormone deficiencies, AIDS-associated catabolism or weight loss, and as an adjunct to gonadotropin on ovulation induction.

**USUAL DOSAGE** I.V.: As a single dose in the morning following an overnight fast:

>Children and Adults:
>><50 kg: Draw venous blood samples for GH determinations 15 minutes before and immediately prior to administration, then administer 1 mcg/kg followed by a 3 mL normal saline flush, draw blood samples again for GH determinations
>>>50 kg: Determine the number of ampuls needed based on a dose of 1 mcg/kg, draw venous blood samples for GH determinations 15 minutes before and immediately prior to administration, then administer 1 mcg/kg followed by a 3 mL normal saline flush, draw blood samples again for GH determinations

**Dosage Forms Powder for inj, lyophilized:** 50 mcg

**Contraindications** Known hypersensitivity to sermorelin acetate, mannitol, or albumin

**Warnings/Precautions** Not used for the diagnosis of acromegaly; subnormal GH response may cause obesity, hyperglycemia, and elevated plasma fatty acids

**Pregnancy Risk Factor** C

**Pregnancy Implications** Clinical effects on the fetus: Sermorelin has been shown to produce minor variations in fetuses of rats and rabbits when given in S.C. doses of 50, 150, and 500 mcg/kg. In the rat teratology study, external malformations (thin tail) were observed in the higher dose groups, and there was an increase in minor skeletal variants at the high dose. Some visceral malformations (hydroureter) were observed in all treatment groups, with the incidence greatest in the high-dose group. In rabbits, minor skeletal anomalies were significantly greater in the treated animals than in the controls. There are no adequate and well-controlled studies in pregnant women.

**Adverse Reactions** 1% to 10%:

>Cardiovascular: Tightness in the chest
>Central nervous system: Headache
>Dermatologic: Transient flushing of the face
>Gastrointestinal: Nausea, vomiting
>Local: Pain, redness, and/or swelling at the injection site

**Drug Interactions** The test should not be conducted in the presence of drugs that directly affect the pituitary secretion of somatotropin. These include preparations that contain or release somatostatin, insulin, glucocorticoids, or cyclo-oxygenase inhibitors such as ASA or indomethacin. Somatotropin levels may be transiently elevated by clonidine, levodopa, and insulin-induced hypoglycemia. Response to sermorelin may be blunted in patients who are receiving muscarinic antagonists (atropine) or who are hypothyroid or being treated with antithyroid medications such as propylthiouracil. Obesity, hyperglycemia, and elevated plasma fatty acids generally are associated with subnormal GH responses to sermorelin. Exogenous growth hormone therapy should be discontinued at least 1 week before administering the test.

(Continued)

## Sermorelin Acetate *(Continued)*

### Special PA Issues

**Reference Range:** Peak growth hormone levels of >7-10 mcg/L are rarely achieved upon provocation in patients with classic growth hormone deficiency; a marked growth hormone response in these patients (>10-12 mcg/L) is strongly suggestive of hypothalamic dysfunction, as opposed to pituitary dysfunction

♦ **Seromycin® Pulvules®** *see* Cycloserine *on page 244*

♦ **Serophene®** *see* Clomiphene *on page 222*

♦ **Seroquel®** *see* Quetiapine *on page 786*

♦ **Serostim® Injection** *see* Human Growth Hormone *on page 444*

♦ **Serpalan®** *see* Reserpine *on page 797*

♦ **Serpasil®** *see* Reserpine *on page 797*

♦ **Serpatabs®** *see* Reserpine *on page 797*

♦ **Sertan®** *see* Primidone *on page 756*

# Sertraline *(SER tra leen)*

**Pharmacologic Class** Antidepressant, Selective Serotonin Reuptake Inhibitor

**U.S. Brand Names** Zoloft™

**Mechanism of Action** Antidepressant with selective inhibitory effects on presynaptic serotonin (5-HT) reuptake

**Use** Treatment of major depression; also being studied for use in obesity and obsessive-compulsive disorder

**USUAL DOSAGE** Oral:

Adults: Start with 50 mg/day in the morning and increase by 50 mg/day increments every 2-3 days if tolerated to 100 mg/day; additional increases may be necessary; maximum dose: 200 mg/day. If somnolence is noted, administer at bedtime.

Elderly: Start treatment with 25 mg/day in the morning and increase by 25 mg/day increments every 2-3 days if tolerated to 75-100 mg/day; additional increases may be necessary; maximum dose: 200 mg/day

Hemodialysis: Not removed by hemodialysis

**Dosage comments in hepatic impairment:** Sertraline is extensively metabolized by the liver; caution should be used in patients with hepatic impairment

**Dosage Forms Tab, as hydrochloride:** 25 mg, 50 mg, 100 mg

**Contraindications** Hypersensitivity to sertraline or any component

**Warnings/Precautions** Do not use in combination with monoamine oxidase inhibitor or within 14 days of discontinuing treatment or initiating treatment with a monoamine oxidase inhibitor due to the risk of serotonin syndrome; use with caution in patients with pre-existing seizure disorders, patients in whom weight loss is undesirable, patients with recent myocardial infarction, unstable heart disease, hepatic or renal impairment, patients taking other psychotropic medications, agitated or hyperactive patients as drug may produce or activate mania or hypomania; because the risk of suicide is inherent in depression, patient should be closely monitored until depressive symptoms remit and prescriptions should be written for minimum quantities to reduce the risk of overdose

**Pregnancy Risk Factor** C

**Adverse Reactions** 1% to 10%: In clinical trials, dizziness and nausea were two most frequent side effects that led to discontinuation of therapy

Cardiovascular: Palpitations

Central nervous system: Insomnia, agitation, dizziness, headache, somnolence, nervousness, fatigue, pain

Dermatologic: Dermatological reactions

Endocrine & metabolic: Sexual dysfunction in men

Gastrointestinal: Xerostomia, diarrhea or loose stools, nausea, constipation

Genitourinary: Urinary disorders

Neuromuscular & skeletal: Tremors

Ocular: Visual difficulty

Otic: Tinnitus

Miscellaneous: Diaphoresis

**Drug Interactions** CYP3A3/4 enzyme substrate, CYP2D6 enzyme substrate (minor); CYP1A2 and 2D6 enzyme inhibitor (weak); CYP2C9, 2C18, 2C19 and 3A3/4 enzyme inhibitor

**All serotonin reuptake inhibitors are capable of inhibiting CYP2D6 isoenzyme enzyme system.** The drugs metabolized by this system include desipramine, dextromethorphan, encainide, haloperidol, imipramine, metoprolol, perphenazine, propafenone, and thioridazine

Increased toxicity:

MAO inhibitors and possibly with lithium or tricyclic antidepressants → **serotonin syndrome** serotonergic hyperstimulation with the following clinical features: mental status changes, restlessness, myoclonus, hyper-reflexia, diaphoresis, diarrhea, shivering, and tremor

May decrease metabolism/plasma clearance of some drugs (diazepam, tolbutamide) to result in increased duration and pharmacological effects

May displace highly plasma protein bound drugs from binding sites (eg, warfarin) to result in increased effect

**Onset** Steady-state: 7 days; therapeutic effect: >2 weeks

**Half-Life** Parent: 24 hours; Metabolites: 66 hours

**Special PA Issues**

**Patient Education:** Take exactly as directed (do not increase dose or frequency); may take 2-3 weeks to achieve desired results; may cause physical and/or psychological dependence. Take in the morning to reduce the incidence of insomnia. Avoid excessive alcohol, caffeine, and other prescription or OTC medications not approved by prescriber. Maintain adequate hydration (2-3 L/day of fluids unless instructed to restrict fluid intake). You may experience drowsiness, dizziness, or lightheadedness (use caution when driving or engaging in hazardous tasks until response to medication is known); nausea, vomiting, anorexia, or dry mouth (small frequent meals, frequent mouth care, or sucking lozenges may help); postural hypotension (use caution when climbing stairs or changing position from sitting or lying to standing); urinary pattern changes (void before taking medication); or male sexual dysfunction (reversible). Report persistent insomnia or daytime sedation, agitation, nervousness, fatigue; muscle cramping, tremors, weakness, or change in gait; chest pain, palpitations, or swelling of extremities; vision changes or eye pain; changes in hearing or ringing in ears; difficulty breathing or breathlessness; skin rash or irritation; or worsening of condition.

**Related Information**

Antidepressant Agents *on page 998*

♦ **Sertraline Hydrochloride** *see* Sertraline *on previous page*

♦ **Serutan® [OTC]** *see* Psyllium *on page 781*

♦ **Serzone®** *see* Nefazodone *on page 640*

# Sevelamer (se VEL a mer)

**Pharmacologic Class** Phosphate Binder

**U.S. Brand Names** Renagel®

**Mechanism of Action** Sevelamer (a polymeric compound) binds phosphate within the intestinal lumen, limiting absorption and decreasing serum phosphate concentrations without altering calcium, aluminum, or bicarbonate concentrations

**Use** Reduction of serum phosphorous in patients with end-stage renal disease

**USUAL DOSAGE** Adults: Oral: 2-4 capsules 3 times/day with meals; the initial dose may be based on serum phosphorous:

(Phosphorous: Initial Dose)

>6.0 mg/dL and <7.5 mg/dL: 2 capsules 3 times/day

>7.5 mg/dL and <9.0 mg/dL: 3 capsules 3 times/day

≥9.0 mg/dL: 4 capsules 3 times/day

Dosage should be adjusted based on serum phosphorous concentration, with a goal of lowering to <6.0 mg/dL; maximum daily dose studied was 30 capsules/day.

**Dosage Forms Cap:** 403 mg

**Contraindications** Hypersensitivity to sevelamer or any component of the formulation, hypophosphatemia, or bowel obstruction

**Warnings/Precautions** Use with caution in patients with gastrointestinal disorders including dysphagia, swallowing disorders, severe gastrointestinal motility disorders, or major gastrointestinal surgery. May cause reductions in vitamin D, E, K, and folic acid absorption. Long-term studies of carcinogenic potential have not been completed. Capsules should not be taken apart or chewed.

**Pregnancy Risk Factor** C

**Pregnancy Implications** It is not known whether sevelamer is excreted in human milk. Because sevelamer may cause a reduction in the absorption of some vitamins, it should be used with caution in pregnant and/or nursing women.

**Adverse Reactions**

>10%:

Cardiovascular: Hypotension (11%), thrombosis (10%)

Central nervous system: Headache (10%)

Endocrine and metabolic: Decreased absorption of vitamins D, E, K and folic acid

Gastrointestinal: Diarrhea (16%), dyspepsia (5% to 11%), vomiting (12%)

Neuromuscular and skeletal: Pain (13%)

Miscellaneous: Infection (15%)

1% to 10%:

Cardiovascular: Hypertension (9%)

Gastrointestinal: Nausea (7%), flatulence (4%), diarrhea (4%), constipation (2%)

Respiratory: Cough (4%)

**Drug Interactions** No formal drug interaction studies have been undertaken. Sevelamer may bind to some drugs in the gastrointestinal tract and decrease their absorption. When changes in absorption of oral medications may have significant clinical consequences (such (Continued)

## Sevelamer *(Continued)*

as antiarrhythmic and antiseizure medications), these medications should be taken at least 1 hour before or 3 hours after a dose of sevelamer.

### Special PA Issues

**Patient Education:** Take as directed, with meals. Do not break or chew capsule. You may experience headache or dizziness (use caution when driving or engaging in hazardous tasks until response to medication is known); upset stomach, nausea, or vomiting (frequent small meals, frequent mouth care, or sucking hard candy may help); diarrhea (yogurt or buttermilk may help); hypotension (use caution when rising from sitting or lying position or when climbing stairs or bending over); or mild neuromuscular pain or stiffness (mild analgesic may help). Report persistent adverse reactions.

**Monitoring Parameters:** Serum phosphorus

♦ **Sevelamer Hydrochloride** *see* Sevelamer *on previous page*

## Sibutramine (si BYOO tra meen)

**Pharmacologic Class** Anorexiant

**U.S. Brand Names** Meridia®

**Mechanism of Action** Blocks the neuronal reuptake of norepinephrine and, to a lesser extent, serotonin and dopamine

**Use** Management of obesity, including weight loss and maintenance of weight loss, and should be used in conjunction with a reduced calorie diet

### Body Mass Index (BMI), kg/m² Height (feet, inches)

| Weight (pounds) | 5'0" | 5'3" | 5'6" | 5'9" | 6'0" | 6'3" |
|---|---|---|---|---|---|---|
| 140 | 27 | 25 | 23 | 21 | 19 | 18 |
| 150 | 29 | 27 | 24 | 22 | 20 | 19 |
| 160 | 31 | 28 | 26 | 24 | 22 | 20 |
| 170 | 33 | 30 | 28 | 25 | 23 | 21 |
| 180 | 35 | 32 | 29 | 27 | 25 | 23 |
| 190 | 37 | 34 | 31 | 28 | 26 | 24 |
| 200 | 39 | 36 | 32 | 30 | 27 | 25 |
| 210 | 41 | 37 | 34 | 31 | 29 | 26 |
| 220 | 43 | 39 | 36 | 33 | 30 | 28 |
| 230 | 45 | 41 | 37 | 34 | 31 | 29 |
| 240 | 47 | 43 | 39 | 36 | 33 | 30 |
| 250 | 49 | 44 | 40 | 37 | 34 | 31 |

**USUAL DOSAGE** Adults ≥16 years: Initial: 10 mg once daily; after 4 weeks may titrate up to 15 mg once daily as needed and tolerated; doses >15 mg/day are not recommended

**Dosage Forms Cap, as hydrochloride:** 5 mg, 10 mg, 15 mg

**Contraindications** During or within 2 weeks of MAO inhibitors (eg, phenelzine, selegiline) or concomitant centrally-acting appetite suppressants. Use is not recommended in patients with anorexia nervosa; uncontrolled or poorly controlled hypertension, congestive heart failure, coronary heart disease conduction disorders (arrhythmias) or stroke.

**Warnings/Precautions** Use with caution in severe renal impairment or severe hepatic dysfunction, seizure disorder, hypertension, narrow-angle glaucoma, nursing mothers, elderly patients

**Pregnancy Risk Factor** C

**Adverse Reactions** ≥1%:

Cardiovascular: Hypertension, tachycardia, vasodilation, palpitations

Central nervous system: Insomnia, headache, migraine, dizziness, nervousness, depression, somnolence

Gastrointestinal: Xerostomia, GI upset, anorexia, constipation, increased appetite, nausea, vomiting

Ocular: Mydriasis

**Drug Interactions** CYP3A3/4 enzyme substrate

Caution with other CNS active agents, avoid concurrent use with other serotonergic agents such as venlafaxine, selective serotonin reuptake inhibitors (eg, fluoxetine, fluvoxamine, paroxetine, sertraline), sumatriptan, dihydroergotamine, lithium, tryptophan, some opioid/analgesics (eg, dextromethorphan, tramadol). Other drugs that can raise the blood pressure can worsen the possibility of sibutramine-associated cardiovascular complications (eg, decongestants, centrally acting weight loss products, amphetamines, and amphetamine-like compounds). Possible interaction with ketoconazole, erythromycin, and other agents metabolized by the CYP3A4 enzyme system.

**Special PA Issues**

**Patient Education:** Take exactly as directed (do not increase dose or frequency without consulting prescriber). Take with or without meals; if gastric distress occurs, may be taken with meals (do not take at bedtime). Avoid alcohol, caffeine, or OTC medications that act as stimulants. You may experience restlessness, dizziness, sleepiness (use caution when driving or engaging in hazardous activities); experience insomnia (taking medication early in morning may help, warm milk and quiet environment at bedtime may help); increased appetite, nausea or vomiting (small frequent meals, frequent mouth care may help); constipation (increased exercise, dietary fiber, fruit, or fluid may help); diarrhea (buttermilk, boiled milk, or yogurt may help); or altered menstrual periods (reversible). Report chest pain, palpitations, or irregular heartbeat; excessive nervousness, excitation, or sleepiness; back pain, muscle weakness, or tremors; CNS changes (acute headache, aggressiveness, restlessness, excitation, sleep disturbances); menstrual pattern changes; rash; blurred vision; runny nose, sinusitis, cough, or difficulty breathing.

**Dietary Considerations:** Avoid concurrent excess alcohol ingestion; sibutramine, as an appetite suppressant, is the most effective when combined with a low calorie diet and behavior modification counseling

**Monitoring Parameters:** Do initial blood pressure and heart rate evaluation and then monitor regularly during therapy. If patient has sustained increases in either blood pressure or pulse rate, consider discontinuing or reducing the dose of the drug.

♦ **Sibutramine Hydrochloride** *see* Sibutramine *on previous page*

♦ **Siladryl® Oral [OTC]** *see* Diphenhydramine *on page 289*

# Sildenafil (sil DEN a fil)

**Pharmacologic Class** Phosphodiesterase Enzyme Inhibitor

**U.S. Brand Names** Viagra™

**Mechanism of Action** Does not directly cause penile erections, but affects the response to sexual stimulation. The physiologic mechanism of erection of the penis involves release of nitric oxide (NO) in the corpus cavernosum during sexual stimulation. NO then activates the enzyme guanylate cyclase, which results in increased levels of cyclic guanosine monophosphate (cGMP), producing smooth muscle relaxation and inflow of blood to the corpus cavernosum. Sildenafil enhances the effect of NO by inhibiting phosphodiesterase type 5 (PDE5), which is responsible for degradation of cGMP in the corpus cavernosum; when sexual stimulation causes local release of NO, inhibition of PDE5 by sildenafil causes increased levels of cGMP in the corpus cavernosum, resulting in smooth muscle relaxation and inflow of blood to the corpus cavernosum; at recommended doses, it has no effect in the absence of sexual stimulation.

**Use** Treatment of erectile dysfunction

**USUAL DOSAGE** Adults: Oral: For most patients, the recommended dose is 50 mg taken as needed, approximately 1 hour before sexual activity. However, sildenafil may be taken anywhere from 30 minutes to 4 hours before sexual activity. Based on effectiveness and tolerance, the dose may be increased to a maximum recommended dose of 100 mg or decreased to 25 mg. The maximum recommended dosing frequency is once daily.

**Dosage adjustment for patients >65 years of age, hepatic impairment (cirrhosis), severe renal impairment (creatinine clearance <30 mL/minute), or concomitant use of potent cytochrome P-450 3A4 inhibitors (erythromycin, ketoconazole, itraconazole):** Higher plasma levels have been associated which may result in increase in efficacy and adverse effects and a starting dose of 25 mg should be considered

**Dosage Forms** Tab, as citrate: 25 mg, 50 mg, 100 mg

**Contraindications** In patients with a known hypersensitivity to any component of the tablet; has been shown to potentiate the hypotensive effects of nitrates, and its administration to patients who are concurrently using organic nitrates in any form is contraindicated

**Warnings/Precautions** There is a degree of cardiac risk associated with sexual activity; therefore, physicians may wish to consider the cardiovascular status of their patients prior to initiating any treatment for erectile dysfunction. Agents for the treatment of erectile dysfunction should be used with caution in patients with anatomical deformation of the penis (angulation, cavernosal fibrosis, or Peyronie's disease), or in patients who have conditions which may predispose them to priapism (sickle cell anemia, multiple myeloma, leukemia). The safety and efficacy of sildenafil with other treatments for erectile dysfunction have not been studied and are, therefore, not recommended as combination therapy.

A minority of patients with retinitis pigmentosa have generic disorders of retinal phosphodiesterases. There is no safety information on the administration of sildenafil to these patients and sildenafil should be administered with caution.

**Pregnancy Risk Factor** B

**Adverse Reactions**

>10%:
  Central nervous system: Headache
  Cardiovascular: Flushing
1% to 10%:
  Central nervous system: Dizziness
  Dermatologic: Rash
(Continued)

## Sildenafil *(Continued)*

Gastrointestinal: Dyspepsia, diarrhea
Genitourinary: Urinary tract infection
Ocular: Abnormal vision
Respiratory: Nasal congestion

**Drug Interactions** CYP3A3/4 enzyme substrate (major); CYP2C9 enzyme substrate (minor)

Do not use with nitrates

Increased effect/toxicity: Cimetidine, erythromycin, ketoconazole, itraconazole, mibefradil
Decreased effect: Rifampin

**Onset** ~60 minutes

**Duration** 2-4 hours

**Special PA Issues**

**Patient Education:** Inform prescriber of all other medications you are taking; serious side effects can result when sildenafil is used with nitrates and some other medications. Do not combine sildenafil with other approaches to treating erectile dysfunction without consulting prescriber. Note that sildenafil provides no protection against sexually transmitted diseases, including HIV. You may experience headache, flushing, or abnormal vision (blurred or increased sensitivity to light); use caution when driving at night or in poorly lit environments. Report immediately acute allergic reactions, chest pain or palpitations, persistent dizziness, sign of urinary tract infection, rash, respiratory difficulties, genital swelling, or other adverse reactions.

- ♦ **Silphen® Cough [OTC]** *see* Diphenhydramine *on page 289*
- ♦ **Siltussin® [OTC]** *see* Guaifenesin *on page 427*
- ♦ **Siltussin DM® [OTC]** *see* Guaifenesin and Dextromethorphan *on page 428*
- ♦ **Silvadene®** *see* Silver Sulfadiazine *on next page*

## Silver Nitrate *(SIL ver NYE trate)*

**Pharmacologic Class** Antibiotic, Ophthalmic; Antibiotic, Topical; Cauterizing Agent, Topical; Topical Skin Product, Antibacterial

**U.S. Brand Names** Dey-Drop® Ophthalmic Solution

**Mechanism of Action** Free silver ions precipitate bacterial proteins by combining with chloride in tissue forming silver chloride; coagulates cellular protein to form an eschar; silver ions or salts or colloidal silver preparations can inhibit the growth of both gram-positive and gram-negative bacteria. This germicidal action is attributed to the precipitation of bacterial proteins by liberated silver ions. Silver nitrate coagulates cellular protein to form an eschar, and this mode of action is the postulated mechanism for control of benign hematuria, rhinitis, and recurrent pneumothorax.

**Use** Prevention of gonococcal ophthalmia neonatorum; cauterization of wounds and sluggish ulcers, removal of granulation tissue and warts; aseptic prophylaxis of burns

**USUAL DOSAGE**

Neonates: Ophthalmic: Instill 2 drops immediately after birth (no later than 1 hour after delivery) into conjunctival sac of each eye as a single dose, allow to sit for ≥30 seconds; do not irrigate eyes following instillation of eye drops

Children and Adults:
Ointment: Apply in an apertured pad on affected area or lesion for approximately 5 days
Sticks: Apply to mucous membranes and other moist skin surfaces only on area to be treated 2-3 times/week for 2-3 weeks
Topical solution: Apply a cotton applicator dipped in solution on the affected area 2-3 times/week for 2-3 weeks

**Dosage Forms Applicator, top:** 75% with potassium nitrate 25% (6"); **Oint, top:** 10% (30 g); **Soln: Ophth:** 1% (wax ampuls); **Top:** 10% (30 mL), 25% (30 mL), 50% (30 mL)

**Contraindications** Not for use on broken skin or cuts; hypersensitivity to silver nitrate or any component

**Warnings/Precautions** Do not use applicator sticks on the eyes; repeated applications of the ophthalmic solution into the eye can cause cauterization of the cornea and blindness

**Pregnancy Risk Factor** C

**Adverse Reactions**

>10%:
Dermatologic: Burning and skin irritation
Ocular: Chemical conjunctivitis

1% to 10%:
Dermatologic: Staining of the skin
Hematologic: Methemoglobinemia
Ocular: Cauterization of the cornea, blindness

**Drug Interactions** Decreased effect: Sulfacetamide preparations are **incompatible**

**Special PA Issues**

**Patient Education:** Use as directed; do not use more often than instructed. Store container in dry, dark place.

Ointment: Apply on pad to affected area for 4-5 days.

Sticks: Apply to mucous membranes and other moist skin surfaces to be treated 2-3 times each week for 2-3 weeks.

Solution: Apply to affected area with cotton applicator dipped in solution 2-3 times each week for 2-3 weeks.

Handle with care; silver nitrate stains skin, clothing and utensils. Discontinue and contact prescriber if treated areas worsen or if redness, or irritation develops in surrounding area.

**Monitoring Parameters:** With prolonged use, monitor methemoglobin levels

# Silver Sulfadiazine (SIL ver sul fa DYE a zeen)

**Pharmacologic Class** Antibiotic, Topical

**U.S. Brand Names** Silvadene®; SSD® AF; SSD® Cream; Thermazene®

**Mechanism of Action** Acts upon the bacterial cell wall and cell membrane. Bactericidal for many gram-negative and gram-positive bacteria and is effective against yeast. Active against *Pseudomonas aeruginosa, Pseudomonas maltophilia, Enterobacter* species, *Klebsiella* species, *Serratia* species, *Escherichia coli, Proteus mirabilis, Morganella morganii, Providencia rettgeri, Proteus vulgaris, Providencia* species, *Citrobacter* species, *Acinetobacter calcoaceticus, Staphylococcus aureus, Staphylococcus epidermidis, Enterococcus* species, *Candida albicans, Corynebacterium diphtheriae,* and *Clostridium perfringens*

**Use** Prevention and treatment of infection in second and third degree burns

**USUAL DOSAGE** Children and Adults: Topical: Apply once or twice daily with a sterile-gloved hand; apply to a thickness of $1/16"$; burned area should be covered with cream at all times

**Dosage Forms** Crm, top: 1% [10 mg/g] (20 g, 50 g, 100 g, 400 g, 1000 g)

**Contraindications** Hypersensitivity to silver sulfadiazine or any component; premature infants or neonates <2 months of age because sulfonamides compete with bilirubin for protein binding sites which may displace bilirubin and cause kernicterus, pregnant women approaching or at term

**Warnings/Precautions** Use with caution in patients with G-6-PD deficiency, renal impairment, or history of allergy to other sulfonamides; sulfadiazine may accumulate in patients with impaired hepatic or renal function; fungal superinfection may occur; use of analgesic might be needed before application; systemic absorption is significant and adverse reactions may occur

**Pregnancy Risk Factor** B

**Adverse Reactions**

1% to 10%:

Dermatologic: Itching, rash, erythema multiforme, discoloration of skin

Hematologic: Hemolytic anemia, leukopenia, agranulocytosis, aplastic anemia

Hepatic: Hepatitis

Renal: Interstitial nephritis

Miscellaneous: Allergic reactions may be related to sulfa component

<1%: Photosensitivity

**Drug Interactions** Decreased effect: Topical proteolytic enzymes are inactivated

**Special PA Issues**

**Patient Education:** Usually applied by professional in burn care setting. Patient instruction should be appropriate to extent of burn, patient understanding, etc.

**Monitoring Parameters:** Serum electrolytes, urinalysis, renal function tests, CBC in patients with extensive burns on long-term treatment

♦ **Simron®** [OTC] *see* Ferrous Gluconate *on page 367*

♦ **Simulect®** *see* Basiliximab *on page 98*

# Simvastatin (SIM va stat in)

**Pharmacologic Class** Antilipemic Agent (HMG-CoA Reductase Inhibitor)

**U.S. Brand Names** Zocor®

**Mechanism of Action** Simvastatin is a methylated derivative of lovastatin that acts by competitively inhibiting 3-hydroxy-3-methylglutaryl-coenzyme A (HMG-CoA) reductase, the enzyme that catalyzes the rate-limiting step in cholesterol biosynthesis

**Use** "Secondary prevention" in patients with coronary heart disease and hypercholesterolemia to reduce the risk of total mortality by reducing coronary death; reduce the risk of nonfatal myocardial infarction; reduce the risk of undergoing myocardial revascularization procedures; and reduce the risk of stroke or transient ischemic attack

Adjunct to diet to reduce elevated total cholesterol, LDL-cholesterol, apo-B and triglyceride levels in patients with primary hypercholesterolemia (heterozygous, familial, and nonfamilial), and mixed dyslipidemia (Fredrickson types IIa and IIb)

**USUAL DOSAGE** Oral:

Adults:

Initial: 20 mg once daily in the evening; patients who require only a moderate reduction of LDL cholesterol may be started at 10 mg

Maintenance: Recommended dosing range: 5-80 mg/day as a single dose in the evening; doses should be individualized according to the baseline LDL-C levels, the recommended goal of therapy, and the patient's response

(Continued)

## Simvastatin *(Continued)*

Adjustments: Should be made at intervals of 4 weeks or more

Patients with homozygous familial hypercholesteremia: Adults: 40 mg in the evening or 80 mg/day in 3 divided doses of 20 mg, 20 mg, and an evening dose of 40 mg

Elderly: Maximum reductions in LDL-cholesterol may be achieved with daily dose of ≤20 mg

Patients who are concomitantly receiving cyclosporine: Initial: 5 mg, should not exceed 10 mg/day

Patients receiving concomitant fibrates or niacin: Dose should **not** exceed 10 mg/day

**Dosing adjustment/comments in renal impairment:** Because simvastatin does not undergo significant renal excretion, modification of dose should not be necessary in patients with mild to moderate renal insufficiency

Severe renal impairment: $Cl_{cr}$ <10 mL/minute: Initial: 5 mg/day with close monitoring

**Dosage Forms Tab:** 5 mg, 10 mg, 20 mg, 40 mg, 80 mg

**Contraindications** Previous hypersensitivity to simvastatin or lovastatin or other HMG-CoA reductase inhibitors; active liver disease or unexplained elevations of serum transaminases; pregnancy and lactation

**Pregnancy Risk Factor** X

**Adverse Reactions**

1% to 10%:

Central nervous system: Headache (3.5%)

Gastrointestinal: Flatulence (1.9%), abdominal cramps (3.2%), diarrhea (1.9%), constipation (2.3%), nausea/vomiting (1.3%), dyspepsia/heartburn (1.1%)

Neuromuscular & skeletal: Myalgia, weakness (1.6%), increased CPK

Respiratory: Upper respiratory infection (2.1%)

<1%: Abnormal taste, lenticular opacities, blurred vision

**Drug Interactions** CYP3A3/4 enzyme substrate

Increased effect of warfarin and digoxin possible with simvastatin or other HMG-CoA reductase inhibitors

Possibly increased toxicity of simvastatin with itraconazole since itraconazole increases lovastatin levels by as much as 20-fold

Concurrent use of erythromycin, gemfibrozil, cyclosporine, and niacin with HMG-CoA reductase inhibitors may result in rhabdomyolysis

Decreased antihyperlipidemic activity possible with rifampin, nicotinic acid (fluvastatin) and isradipine (lovastatin)

**Onset** >3 days; maximal effects after 2 weeks

**Special PA Issues**

**Patient Education:** Take this medication as directed, with meals, 1 hour prior to or after any other medications. You may experience nausea, flatulence, dyspepsia (small frequent meals may help), headache, muscle or joint pain (will probably lessen with continued use), and light sensitivity (use sunblock and wear protective clothing). Report severe and unresolved gastric upset, any vision changes, changes in color of urine or stool, yellowing of skin or eyes, and any unusual bruising.

**Monitoring Parameters:** Creatine phosphokinase levels due to possibility of myopathy; serum cholesterol (total and fractionated)

**Related Information**

Lipid-Lowering Agents *on page 1022*

- ♦ **Sinarest® Nasal Solution [OTC]** *see* Phenylephrine *on page 718*
- ♦ **Sinemet®** *see* Levodopa and Carbidopa *on page 525*
- ♦ **Sinemet® CR** *see* Levodopa and Carbidopa *on page 525*
- ♦ **Sinequan® Oral** *see* Doxepin *on page 304*
- ♦ **Singulair®** *see* Montelukast *on page 617*
- ♦ **Sinubid®** *see* Phenyltoloxamine, Phenylpropanolamine, and Acetaminophen *on page 721*
- ♦ **Sinumist®-SR Capsulets®** *see* Guaifenesin *on page 427*
- ♦ **Sinupan®** *see* Guaifenesin and Phenylephrine *on page 429*
- ♦ **Skelaxin®** *see* Metaxalone *on page 576*
- ♦ **Skelid®** *see* Tiludronate *on page 904*

## Skin Test Antigens, Multiple *(skin test AN tee gens, MUL ti pul)*

**Pharmacologic Class** Diagnostic Agent, Hypersensitivity Skin Testing

**U.S. Brand Names** Multitest CMI®

**Use** Detection of nonresponsiveness to antigens by means of delayed hypersensitivity skin testing

**USUAL DOSAGE** Select only test sites that permit sufficient surface area and subcutaneous tissue to allow adequate penetration of all eight points, avoid hairy areas. Press loaded unit into the skin with sufficient pressure to puncture the skin and allow adequate penetration of all points, maintain firm contact for at least 5 seconds, during application the device should not be "rocked" back and forth and side to side without removing any of the test heads from the skin sites.

If adequate pressure is applied it will be possible to observe:
1. The puncture marks of the nine tines on each of the eight test heads
2. An imprint of the circular platform surrounding each test head
3. Residual antigen and glycerin at each of the eight sites

If any of the above three criteria are not fully followed, the test results may not be reliable.

Reading should be done in good light, read the test sites at both 24 and 48 hours, the largest reaction recorded from the two readings at each test site should be used. If two readings are not possible, a single 48 hour is recommended. A positive reaction from any of the seven delayed hypersensitivity skin test antigens is **induration ≥2 mm** providing there is no induration at the negative control site. The size of the induration reactions with this test may be smaller than those obtained with other intradermal procedures.

**Dosage Forms** Individual carton containing one preloaded skin test antigen for cellular hypersensitivity

**Contraindications** Infected or inflamed skin, known hypersensitivity to skin test antigens; do not apply at sites involving acneiform, infected or inflamed skin; although severe systemic reactions are rare to diphtheria and tetanus antigens, persons known to have a history of systemic reactions should be tested with this test only after the test heads containing these antigens have been removed

**Warnings/Precautions** Epinephrine should be available is case of severe reactions. Safety and effectiveness in children <17 years of age have not been established; discard applicator after use, do not reuse.

**Pregnancy Risk Factor** C

**Adverse Reactions** 1% to ·10%: Local irritation

**Drug Interactions** Decreased effect: Drugs or procedures that suppress immunity such as corticosteroids, chemotherapeutic agents, antilymphocyte globulin and irradiation, may possibly cause a loss of reactivity

- **Sleep-eze 3® Oral [OTC]** *see* Diphenhydramine *on page 289*
- **Sleepinal® [OTC]** *see* Diphenhydramine *on page 289*
- **Sleepwell 2-nite® [OTC]** *see* Diphenhydramine *on page 289*
- **Slim-Mint® [OTC]** *see* Benzocaine *on page 105*
- **Slo-bid™** *see* Theophylline Salts *on page 888*
- **Slo-Niacin® [OTC]** *see* Niacin *on page 649*
- **Slo-Phyllin®** *see* Theophylline Salts *on page 888*
- **Slo-Phyllin® GG** *see* Theophylline and Guaifenesin *on page 888*
- **Slow FE® [OTC]** *see* Ferrous Sulfate *on page 367*
- **Slow-K®** *see* Potassium Chloride *on page 742*
- **Slow-Mag® (Chloride)** *see* Magnesium Salts (Other) *on page 554*
- **SMX-TMP** *see* Co-Trimoxazole *on page 238*
- **SMZ-TMP** *see* Co-Trimoxazole *on page 238*
- **Snakeroot** *see* Echinacea *on page 310*

## Sodium Acetate (SOW dee um AS e tate)

**Pharmacologic Class** Alkalinizing Agent, Parenteral; Electrolyte Supplement, Parenteral; Sodium Salt

**Use** Sodium source in large volume I.V. fluids to prevent or correct hyponatremia in patients with restricted intake; used to counter acidosis through conversion to bicarbonate

**USUAL DOSAGE** Sodium acetate is metabolized to bicarbonate on an equimolar basis outside the liver; administer in large volume I.V. fluids as a sodium source. Refer to Sodium Bicarbonate monograph.

Maintenance electrolyte requirements of sodium in parenteral nutrition solutions:
Daily requirements: 3-4 mEq/kg/24 hours or 25-40 mEq/1000 kcal/24 hours
Maximum: 100-150 mEq/24 hours

**Dosage Forms** Inj: 2 mEq/mL (20 mL, 50 mL, 100 mL), 4 mEq/mL (50 mL, 100 mL)

**Contraindications** Alkalosis, hypocalcemia, low sodium diets, edema, cirrhosis

**Warnings/Precautions** Avoid extravasation, use with caution in patients with hepatic failure

**Pregnancy Risk Factor** C

**Adverse Reactions**
Cardiovascular: Thrombosis, hypervolemia
Dermatologic: Chemical cellulitis at injection site (extravasation)
Endocrine & metabolic: Hypernatremia, dilution of serum electrolytes, overhydration, hypokalemia, metabolic alkalosis, hypocalcemia
Gastrointestinal: Gastric distension, flatulence
Local: Phlebitis
Respiratory: Pulmonary edema
Miscellaneous: Congestive conditions

- **Sodium Acid Carbonate** *see* Sodium Bicarbonate *on next page*

## Sodium Ascorbate (SOW dee um a SKOR bate)

**Pharmacologic Class** Urinary Acidifying Agent; Vitamin, Water Soluble

**U.S. Brand Names** Cenolate®

**Use** Prevention and treatment of scurvy and to acidify urine

**USUAL DOSAGE** Oral, I.V., S.C.:

Infants:

Daily protective requirement: 30 mg

Treatment: 100-300 mg/day (75-100 mg in premature infants)

Children:

Scurvy: 100-300 mg/day in divided doses for at least 2 weeks

Urinary acidification: 500 mg every 6-8 hours

Dietary supplement: 35-45 mg/day

Adults:

Scurvy: 100-250 mg 1-2 times/day for at least 2 weeks

Urinary acidification: 4-12 g/day in divided doses

Dietary supplement: 50-60 mg/day (RDA: 60 mg)

Prevention and treatment of cold: 1-3 g/day

**Dosage Forms Crystals:** 1020 mg per ¼ teaspoonful [ascorbic acid 900 mg]; **Inj:** 250 mg/mL [ascorbic acid 222 mg/mL] (30 mL), 562.5 mg/mL [ascorbic acid 500 mg/mL] (1 mL, 2 mL); **Tab:** 585 mg [ascorbic acid 500 mg]

**Contraindications** Large doses during pregnancy

**Pregnancy Risk Factor** C

## Sodium Bicarbonate (SOW dee um bye KAR bun ate)

**Pharmacologic Class** Alkalinizing Agent; Antacid; Electrolyte Supplement, Oral; Electrolyte Supplement, Parenteral

**U.S. Brand Names** Neut® Injection

**Mechanism of Action** Dissociates to provide bicarbonate ion which neutralizes hydrogen ion concentration and raises blood and urinary pH

**Use** Management of metabolic acidosis; gastric hyperacidity; as an alkalinization agent for the urine; treatment of hyperkalemia

**USUAL DOSAGE**

Cardiac arrest: **Routine use of NaHCO₃ is not recommended and should be given only after adequate alveolar ventilation has been established and effective cardiac compressions are provided**

Infants and Children: I.V.: 0.5-1 mEq/kg/dose repeated every 10 minutes or as indicated by arterial blood gases; rate of infusion should not exceed 10 mEq/minute; neonates and children <2 years of age should receive 4.2% (0.5 mEq/mL) solution

Adults: I.V.: Initial: 1 mEq/kg/dose one time; maintenance: 0.5 mEq/kg/dose every 10 minutes or as indicated by arterial blood gases

Metabolic acidosis: Dosage should be based on the following formula if blood gases and pH measurements are available:

Infants and Children:

$HCO_3^-(mEq) = 0.3 \times$ weight (kg) $\times$ base deficit (mEq/L) **or**

$HCO_3^-(mEq) = 0.5 \times$ weight (kg) $\times$ [24 - serum $HCO_3^-$ (mEq/L)]

Adults:

$HCO_3^-(mEq) = 0.2 \times$ weight (kg) $\times$ base deficit (mEq/L) **or**

$HCO_3^-(mEq) = 0.5 \times$ weight (kg) $\times$ [24 - serum $HCO_3^-$ (mEq/L)]

If acid-base status is not available: Dose for older Children and Adults: 2-5 mEq/kg I.V. infusion over 4-8 hours; subsequent doses should be based on patient's acid-base status

Chronic renal failure: Oral: Initiate when plasma $HCO_3^-$ <15 mEq/L

Children: 1-3 mEq/kg/day

Adults: Start with 20-36 mEq/day in divided doses, titrate to bicarbonate level of 18-20 mEq/L

Renal tubular acidosis: Oral:

Distal:

Children: 2-3 mEq/kg/day

Adults: 0.5-2 mEq/kg/day in 4-5 divided doses

Proximal: Children: Initial: 5-10 mEq/kg/day; maintenance: Increase as required to maintain serum bicarbonate in the normal range

Urine alkalinization: Oral:

Children: 1-10 mEq (84-840 mg)/kg/day in divided doses every 4-6 hours; dose should be titrated to desired urinary pH

Adults: Initial: 48 mEq (4 g), then 12-24 mEq (1-2 g) every 4 hours; dose should be titrated to desired urinary pH; doses up to 16 g/day (200 mEq) in patients <60 years and 8 g (100 mEq) in patients >60 years

Antacid: Adults: Oral: 325 mg to 2 g 1-4 times/day

**Dosage Forms Inj:** 4% [40 mg/mL = 2.4 mEq/5 mL] (5 mL), 4.2% [42 mg/mL = 5 mEq/10 mL] (10 mL), 7.5% [75 mg/mL = 8.92 mEq/10 mL] (10 mL, 50 mL), 8.4% [84 mg/mL = 10 mEq/10 mL] (10 mL, 50 mL); **Powder:** 120 g, 480 g; **Tab:** 300 mg [3.6 mEq], 325 mg [3.8 mEq], 520 mg [6.3 mEq], 600 mg [7.3 mEq], 650 mg [7.6 mEq]

**Contraindications** Alkalosis, hypernatremia, severe pulmonary edema, hypocalcemia, unknown abdominal pain

**Warnings/Precautions** Rapid administration in neonates and children <2 years of age has led to hypernatremia, decreased CSF pressure and intracranial hemorrhage. **Use of I.V. NaHCO₃ should be reserved for documented metabolic acidosis and for hyperkalemia-induced cardiac arrest.** Routine use in cardiac arrest is not recommended. Avoid extravasation, tissue necrosis can occur due to the hypertonicity of $NaHCO_3$. May cause sodium retention especially if renal function is impaired; not to be used in treatment of peptic ulcer; use with caution in patients with CHF, edema, cirrhosis, or renal failure. Not the antacid of choice for the elderly because of sodium content and potential for systemic alkalosis.

**Pregnancy Risk Factor** C

**Adverse Reactions**
Cardiovascular: Edema, cerebral hemorrhage, aggravation of congestive heart failure
Central nervous system: Tetany, intracranial acidosis
Endocrine & metabolic: Metabolic alkalosis, hypernatremia, hypokalemia, hypocalcemia, hyperosmolality
Gastrointestinal: Belching, gastric distension, flatulence (with oral)
Respiratory: Pulmonary edema
Miscellaneous: Increased affinity of hemoglobin for oxygen-reduced pH in myocardial tissue necrosis when extravasated; milk alkali syndrome (especially with renal dysfunction)

**Drug Interactions**
Decreased effect/levels of lithium, chlorpropamide, methotrexate, tetracyclines, and salicylates due to urinary alkalinization
Increased toxicity/levels of amphetamines, anorexiants, mecamylamine, ephedrine, pseudoephedrine, flecainide, quinidine, quinine due to urinary alkalinization

**Onset** Oral: Rapid; I.V.: 15 minutes

**Duration** Oral: 8-10 minutes; I.V.: 1-2 hours

**Special PA Issues**
**Patient Education:** Do not use for chronic gastric acidity. Take as directed. Chew tablets thoroughly and follow with a full glass of water, preferably on an empty stomach (2 hours before or after food). Take at least 2 hours before or after any other medications. Report CNS effects (eg, irritability, confusion); muscle rigidity or tremors; swelling of feet or ankles; difficulty breathing; chest pain or palpitations; respiratory changes; or tarry stools.

## Sodium Chloride (SOW dee um KLOR ide)

**Pharmacologic Class** Electrolyte Supplement, Oral; Electrolyte Supplement, Parenteral; Lubricant, Ocular; Sodium Salt

**U.S. Brand Names** Adsorbonac® Ophthalmic [OTC]; Afrin® Saline Mist [OTC]; AK-NaCl® [OTC]; Ayr® Saline [OTC]; Breathe Free® [OTC]; Dristan® Saline Spray [OTC]; HuMist® Nasal Mist [OTC]; Muro 128® Ophthalmic [OTC]; Muroptic-5® [OTC]; NāSal™ [OTC]; Nasal Moist® [OTC]; Ocean Nasal Mist [OTC]; Pretz® [OTC]; SalineX® [OTC]; SeaMist® [OTC]

**Mechanism of Action** Principal extracellular cation; functions in fluid and electrolyte balance, osmotic pressure control, and water distribution

**Use** Parenteral restoration of sodium ion in patients with restricted oral intake (especially hyponatremia states or low salt syndrome). In general, parenteral saline uses:
Normal saline: Restores water/sodium losses
Hypotonic sodium chloride: Hydrating solution
Hypertonic sodium chloride: For severe hyponatremia and hypochloremia
Bacteriostatic sodium chloride: Dilution or dissolving drugs for I.M./I.V./S.C. injections
Concentrated sodium chloride: Additive for parenteral fluid therapy
Pharmaceutical aid/diluent for infusion of compatible drug additives

**USUAL DOSAGE**
Newborn electrolyte requirement:
Premature: 2-8 mEq/kg/24 hours
Term:
0-48 hours: 0-2 mEq/kg/24 hours
>48 hours: 1-4 mEq/kg/24 hours
Children: I.V.: Hypertonic solutions (>0.9%) should only be used for the initial treatment of acute serious symptomatic hyponatremia; maintenance: 3-4 mEq/kg/day; maximum: 100-150 mEq/day; dosage varies widely depending on clinical condition
Replacement: Determined by laboratory determinations mEq
Sodium deficiency (mEq/kg) = [% dehydration (L/kg)/100 x 70 (mEq/L)] + [0.6 (L/kg) x (140 - serum sodium) (mEq/L)]
Nasal: Use as often as needed
Adults:
GU irrigant: 1-3 L/day by intermittent irrigation
Heat cramps: Oral: 0.5-1 g with full glass of water, up to 4.8 g/day
Replacement I.V.: Determined by laboratory determinations mEq
Sodium deficiency (mEq/kg) = [% dehydration (L/kg)/100 x 70 (mEq/L)] + [0.6 (L/kg) x (140 - serum sodium) (mEq/L)]
(Continued)

## Sodium Chloride *(Continued)*

To correct acute, serious hyponatremia: mEq sodium = [desired sodium (mEq/L) - actual sodium (mEq/L)] x [0.6 x wt (kg)]; for acute correction use 125 mEq/L as the desired serum sodium; acutey correct serum sodium in 5 mEq/L/dose increments; more gradual correction in increments of 10 mEq/L/day is indicated in the asymptomatic patient

Chloride maintenance electrolyte requirement in parenteral nutrition: 2-4 mEq/kg/24 hours or 25-40 mEq/1000 kcals/24 hours; maximum: 100-150 mEq/24 hours

Sodium maintenance electrolyte requirement in parenteral nutrition: 3-4 mEq/kg/24 hours or 25-40 mEq/1000 kcals/24 hours; maximum: 100-150 mEq/24 hours. See table.

### Approximate Deficits of Water and Electrolytes in Moderately Severe Dehydration

| Condition | Water (mL/kg) | Sodium (mEq/kg) |
|---|---|---|
| Fasting and thirsting | 100-120 | 5-7 |
| Diarrhea | | |
| isonatremic | 100-120 | 8-10 |
| hypernatremic | 100-120 | 2-4 |
| hyponatremic | 100-120 | 10-12 |
| Pyloric stenosis | 100-120 | 8-10 |
| Diabetic acidosis | 100-120 | 9-10 |

*A **negative** deficit indicates total body **excess** prior to treatment.

Adapted from Behrman RE, Kleigman RM, Nelson WE, et al, eds, *Nelson Textbook of Pediatrics*, 14th ed, WB Saunders Co, 1992.

Ophthalmic:
   Ointment: Apply once daily or more often
   Solution: Instill 1-2 drops into affected eye(s) every 3-4 hours
Abortifacient: 20% (250 mL) administered by transabdominal intra-amniotic instillation
**Dosage Forms Drops, nasal:** 0.9% with dropper; **Inj:** 0.2% (3 mL), 0.45% (3 mL, 5 mL, 500 mL, 1000 mL), 0.9% (1 mL, 2 mL, 3 mL, 4 mL, 5 mL, 10 mL, 20 mL, 25 mL, 30 mL, 50 mL, 100 mL, 130 mL, 150 mL, 250 mL, 500 mL, 1000 mL), 3% (500 mL), 5% (500 mL), 20% (250 mL), 23.4% (30 mL, 100 mL); **Inj: Admixtures:** 50 mEq (20 mL), 100 mEq (40 mL), 625 mEq (250 mL); **Bacteriostatic:** 0.9% (30 mL); **Concentrated:** 14.6% (20 mL, 40 mL, 200 mL), 23.4% (10 mL, 20 mL, 30 mL); **Irrigation:** 0.45% (500 mL, 1000 mL, 1500 mL), 0.9% (250 mL, 500 mL, 1000 mL, 1500 mL, 2000 mL, 3000 mL, 4000 mL); **Oint, ophth:** 5% (3.5 g); **Soln: Irrigation:** 0.9% (1000 mL, 2000 mL), **Nasal:** 0.4% (15 mL, 50 mL), 0.6% (15 mL), 0.65% (20 mL, 45 mL, 50 mL), **Ophth:** 2% (15 mL), 5% (15 mL, 30 mL), **Tab:** 650 mg, 1 g, 2.25 g; **Tab: Enteric coated:** 1 g, **Slow release:** 600 mg
**Contraindications** Hypertonic uterus, hypernatremia, fluid retention
**Warnings/Precautions** Use with caution in patients with congestive heart failure, renal insufficiency, liver cirrhosis, hypertension, edema; sodium toxicity is almost exclusively related to how fast a sodium deficit is corrected; both rate and magnitude are extremely important; do not use bacteriostatic sodium chloride in newborns since benzyl alcohol preservatives have been associated with toxicity
**Pregnancy Risk Factor** C
**Adverse Reactions**
   Cardiovascular: Thrombosis, hypervolemia
   Endocrine & metabolic: Hypernatremia, dilution of serum electrolytes, overhydration, hypokalemia
   Local: Phlebitis
   Respiratory: Pulmonary edema
   Miscellaneous: Congestive conditions, extravasation
**Drug Interactions** Decreased levels of lithium
**Special PA Issues**
   **Patient Education:** Blurred vision is common with ophthalmic ointment; may sting eyes when first applied
   **Monitoring Parameters:** Serum sodium, potassium, chloride, and bicarbonate levels; I & O, weight
   **Reference Range:** Serum/plasma sodium levels:
   Neonates: Full-term: 133-142 mEq/L; Premature: 132-140 mEq/L
   Children ≥2 months to Adults: 135-145 mEq/L

## Sodium Citrate and Citric Acid *(SOW dee um SIT rate & SI trik AS id)*
**Pharmacologic Class** Alkalinizing Agent
**U.S. Brand Names** Bicitra®; Cracit®
**Use** Treatment of metabolic acidosis; alkalinizing agent in conditions where long-term maintenance of an alkaline urine is desirable

**USUAL DOSAGE** Oral:

    Infants and Children: 2-3 mEq/kg/day in divided doses 3-4 times/day **or** 5-15 mL with water after meals and at bedtime

    Adults: 15-30 mL with water after meals and at bedtime

**Dosage Forms Soln, oral: Bicitra®:** Sodium citrate 500 mg and citric acid 334 mg per 5 mL (15 mL unit dose, 480 mL), **Oracit®:** Sodium citrate 490 mg and citric acid 640 mg per 5 mL, **Polycitra®:** Sodium citrate 500 mg and citric acid 334 mg with potassium citrate 550 mg per 5 mL

**Contraindications** Severe renal insufficiency, sodium-restricted diet

**Warnings/Precautions** Conversion to bicarbonate may be impaired in patients with hepatic failure, in shock, or who are severely ill

**Pregnancy Risk Factor** C

**Adverse Reactions**

    Central nervous system: Tetany

    Endocrine & metabolic: Metabolic alkalosis, hyperkalemia

    Gastrointestinal: Diarrhea, nausea, vomiting

**Drug Interactions**

    Decreased effect/levels of lithium, chlorpropamide, salicylates due to urinary alkalinization

    Increased toxicity/levels of amphetamines, ephedrine, pseudoephedrine, flecainide, quinidine, quinine due to urinary alkalinization

**Special PA Issues**

    **Patient Education:** Take as often as directed, preferably on an empty stomach (1 hour before or 2 hours after meals) and at least 2 hours before or after any other medications. Dilute with 4-6 oz of chilled water. You may experience diarrhea or nausea and vomiting; if severe, contact prescriber. Report changes in CNS status (eg, irritability, tremors, confusion), swelling of feet or ankles, difficulty breathing, palpitations, abdominal pain, or tarry stools.

# Sodium Citrate and Potassium Citrate Mixture

(SOW dee um SIT rate & poe TASS ee um SIT rate MIKS chur)

**Pharmacologic Class** Alkalinizing Agent

**U.S. Brand Names** Polycitra®

**Dosage Forms Syr:** Sodium citrate 500 mg, potassium citrate 550 mg, with citric acid 334 mg per 5 mL [sodium 1 mEq, potassium 1 mEq, bicarbonate 2 mEq]

♦ **Sodium Edetate** *see* Edetate Disodium *on page 312*

♦ **Sodium Etidronate** *see* Etidronate Disodium *on page 354*

♦ **Sodium Ferric Gluconate** *see* Ferric Gluconate *on page 365*

♦ **Sodium Fluoride** *see* Fluoride *on page 383*

# Sodium Hyaluronate (SOW dee um hye al yoor ON nate)

**Pharmacologic Class** Ophthalmic Agent, Viscoelastic

**U.S. Brand Names** AMO Vitrax®; Amvisc®; Amvisc® Plus; Healon®; Healon® GV; Provisc®

**Mechanism of Action** Functions as a tissue lubricant and is thought to play an important role in modulating the interactions between adjacent tissues. Sodium hyaluronate is a polysaccharide which is distributed widely in the extracellular matrix of connective tissue in man. (Vitreous and aqueous humor of the eye, synovial fluid, skin, and umbilical cord.) Sodium hyaluronate forms a viscoelastic solution in water (at physiological pH and ionic strength) which makes it suitable for aqueous and vitreous humor in ophthalmic surgery.

**Use** Surgical aid in cataract extraction, intraocular implantation, corneal transplant, glaucoma filtration, and retinal attachment surgery

**USUAL DOSAGE** Depends upon procedure (slowly introduce a sufficient quantity into eye)

**Dosage Forms Inj, intraocular:** Healon®: 10 mg/mL (0.4 mL, 0.55 mL, 0.85 mL, 2 mL), Amvisc®: 12 mg/mL (0.5 mL, 0.8 mL), Healon® GV: 14 mg/mL (0.55 mL, 0.85 mL), Amvisc® Plus: 16 mg/mL (0.5 mL, 8 mL), AMO Vitrax®: 30 mg/mL (0.65 mL)

**Contraindications** Hypersensitivity to hyaluronate

**Warnings/Precautions** Do not overfill the anterior chamber; carefully monitor intraocular pressure; risk of hypersensitivity exists

**Pregnancy Risk Factor** C

**Adverse Reactions** 1% to 10%: Ocular: Postoperative inflammatory reactions (iritis, hypopyon), corneal edema, corneal decompensation, transient postoperative increase in IOP

**Special PA Issues**

    **Monitoring Parameters:** Intraocular pressure

♦ **Sodium Hyaluronate-Chrondroitin Sulfate** *see* Chondroitin Sulfate-Sodium Hyaluronate *on page 204*

♦ **Sodium Hydrogen Carbonate** *see* Sodium Bicarbonate *on page 838*

# Sodium Hypochlorite Solution
(SOW dee um hye poe KLOR ite soe LOO shun)
**Pharmacologic Class** Disinfectant, Antibacterial (Topical)
**Use** Treatment of athlete's foot (0.5%); wound irrigation (0.5%); disinfect utensils and equipment (5%)
**USUAL DOSAGE** Topical irrigation
**Dosage Forms Soln:** 5% (4000 mL), Modified Dakin's solution: Full strength: 0.5% (1000 mL), Half strength: 0.25% (1000 mL), Quarter strength: 0.125% (1000 mL)
**Contraindications** Hypersensitivity
**Warnings/Precautions** For external use only; avoid eye or mucous membrane contact; do not use on open wounds
**Pregnancy Risk Factor** C
**Adverse Reactions** 1% to 10%: Dissolves blood clots, delays clotting, irritating to skin
**Special PA Issues**
**Patient Education:** Use exactly as directed; do not overuse. Avoid contact with eyes. Report worsening of condition or lack of healing.

♦ **Sodium Methicillin** see Methicillin on page 583
♦ **Sodium Nafcillin** see Nafcillin on page 630
♦ **Sodium Nitroferricyanide** see Nitroprusside on page 662
♦ **Sodium Nitroprusside** see Nitroprusside on page 662
♦ **Sodium P.A.S.** see Aminosalicylate Sodium on page 54

# Sodium Phenylacetate and Sodium Benzoate
(SOW dee um fen il AS e tate & SOW dee um BENZ oh ate)
**Pharmacologic Class** Ammonium Detoxicant
**U.S. Brand Names** Ucephan©
**Dosage Forms Soln:** Sodium phenylacetate 100 mg and sodium benzoate 100 mg per mL (100 mL)

# Sodium Phenylbutyrate (SOW dee um fen il BYOO ti rate)
**Pharmacologic Class** Urea Cycle Disorder (UCD) Treatment Agent
**U.S. Brand Names** Buphenyl©
**Mechanism of Action** Sodium phenylbutyrate is a prodrug that, when given orally, is rapidly converted to phenylacetate, which is in turn conjugated with glutamine to form the active compound phenylacetylglutamine; phenylacetylglutamine serves as a substitute for urea and is excreted in the urine whereby it carries with it 2 moles of nitrogen per mole of phenylacetylglutamine and can thereby assist in the clearance of nitrogenous waste in patients with urea cycle disorders
**Use** Adjunctive therapy in the chronic management of patients with urea cycle disorder involving deficiencies of carbamoylphosphate synthetase, ornithine transcarbamylase, or argininosuccinic acid synthetase
**USUAL DOSAGE**
Powder: Patients weighing <20 kg: 450-600 mg/kg/day or 9.9-13 g/m$^2$/day, administered in equally divided amounts with each meal or feeding, four to six times daily; safety and efficacy of doses >20 g/day has not been established
Tablet: Children >20 kg and Adults: 450-600 mg/kg/day or 9.9-13 g/m$^2$/day, administered in equally divided amounts with each meal; safety and efficacy of doses >20 g/day have not been established
**Dosage Forms Powder:** 3.2 g [sodium phenylbutyrate 3 g] per teaspoon (500 mL, 950 mL), 9.1 g [sodium phenylbutyrate 8.6 g] per **tablespoon** (500 mL, 950 mL); **Tab:** 500 mg
**Contraindications** Previous hypersensitivity to phenylbutyrate, severe hypertension, heart failure or renal dysfunction; phenylbutyrate is not indicated in the treatment of acute hyperammonemia
**Warnings/Precautions** Since no studies have been conducted in pregnant women, sodium phenylbutyrate should be used cautiously during pregnancy; each 1 gram of drug contains 125 mg of sodium and, therefore, should be used cautiously, if at all, in patients who must maintain a low sodium intake
**Adverse Reactions**
>10%: Endocrine & metabolic: Amenorrhea, menstrual dysfunction
1% to 10%:
Gastrointestinal: Anorexia, abnormal taste
Miscellaneous: Offensive body odor
**Special PA Issues**
**Patient Education:** It is important that patients understand and follow the dietary restrictions required when treating this disorder, the medication must be taken in strict accordance with the prescribed regimen and the patient should avoid altering the dosage without the prescriber's knowledge; the powder formulation has a very salty taste

♦ **Sodium Phosphate and Potassium Phosphate** see Potassium Phosphate and Sodium Phosphate on page 747

## Sodium Polystyrene Sulfonate (SOW dee um pol ee STYE reen SUL fon ate)
**Pharmacologic Class** Antidote

**U.S. Brand Names** Kayexalate®; SPS®

**Mechanism of Action** Removes potassium by exchanging sodium ions for potassium ions in the intestine before the resin is passed from the body; exchange capacity is 1 mEq/g *in vivo*, and *in vitro* capacity is 3.1 mEq/g, therefore, a wide range of exchange capacity exists such that close monitoring of serum electrolytes is necessary

**Use** Treatment of hyperkalemia

**USUAL DOSAGE**

Children:

Oral: 1 g/kg/dose every 6 hours

Rectal: 1 g/kg/dose every 2-6 hours (In small children and infants, employ lower doses t using the practical exchange ratio of 1 mEq K+/g of resin as the basis for calculation)

Adults:

Oral: 15 g (60 mL) 1-4 times/day

Rectal: 30-50 g every 6 hours

**Dosage Forms** Oral or rectal: **Powder for susp:** 454 g; **Susp:** 1.25 g/5 mL with sorbitol 33% and alcohol 0.3% (60 mL, 120 mL, 200 mL, 500 mL)

**Contraindications** Hypernatremia, hypersensitivity to any component

**Warnings/Precautions** Use with caution in patients with severe congestive heart failure, hypertension, edema, or renal failure; avoid using the commercially available liquid product in neonates due to the preservative content; large oral doses may cause fecal impaction (especially in elderly); enema will reduce the serum potassium faster than oral administration, but the oral route will result in a greater reduction over several hours.

**Pregnancy Risk Factor** C

**Adverse Reactions**

Endocrine & metabolic: Hypokalemia, hypocalcemia, hypomagnesemia, sodium retention

Gastrointestinal: Fecal impaction, constipation, loss of appetite, nausea, vomiting

**Drug Interactions** Systemic alkalosis and seizure has occurred after cation-exchange resins were administered with nonabsorbable cation-donating antacids and laxatives (eg, magnesium hydroxide, aluminum carbonate)

**Onset** Within 2-24 hours

**Special PA Issues**

**Patient Education:** Emergency instructions depend on patient's condition. You will be monitored for effects of this medication and frequent blood tests may be necessary. Oral: Take as directed. Mix well with a full glass of liquid (not orange juice). You may experience nausea or vomiting (small frequent meals, good mouth care, chewing gum, or sucking lozenges may help); or constipation or fecal impaction (increased dietary fluids and exercise may help). Report persistent constipation or gastrointestinal distress; chest pain or rapid heartbeat; or mental confusion or muscle weakness.

**Monitoring Parameters:** Serum electrolytes (potassium, sodium, calcium, magnesium), EKG

**Reference Range:** Serum potassium: Adults: 3.5-5.2 mEq/L

♦ **Sodium Sulamyd® Ophthalmic** *see* Sulfacetamide Sodium *on page 858*

♦ **Sodium Sulfacetamide** *see* Sulfacetamide Sodium *on page 858*

## Sodium Tetradecyl Sulfate (SOW dee um tetra DEK il)
**Pharmacologic Class** Sclerosing Agent

**U.S. Brand Names** Sotradecol®

**Mechanism of Action** Acts by irritation of the vein intimal endothelium

**Use** Treatment of small, uncomplicated varicose veins of the lower extremities; endoscopic sclerotherapy in the management of bleeding esophageal varices

**USUAL DOSAGE** I.V.: Test dose: 0.5 mL given several hours prior to administration of larger dose; 0.5-2 mL in each vein, maximum: 10 mL per treatment session; 3% solution reserved for large varices

**Dosage Forms Inj:** 1% [10 mg/mL] (2 mL); 3% [30 mg/mL] (2 mL)

**Contraindications** Arterial disease, thrombophlebitis, hypersensitivity to sodium tetradecyl or any component, valvular or deep vein incompetence, phlebitis, migraines, cellulitis, acute infections; bedridden patients; patients with uncontrolled systemic disease such as diabetes, toxic hyperthyroidism, tuberculosis, asthma, neoplasm, sepsis, blood dyscrasias, and acute respiratory or skin diseases

**Warnings/Precautions** Buerger's disease, peripheral arteriosclerosis, avoid extravasation; observe for hypersensitivity/anaphylactic reaction

**Pregnancy Risk Factor** C

**Adverse Reactions** Percentage unknown: Headache, urticaria; sloughing and tissue necrosis following extravasation; nausea, vomiting, mucosal lesions, esophageal perforation, discoloration at the site of injection, ulceration at the site, pain at injection site, pulmonary edema, asthma

**Drug Interactions** Chemically **incompatible** with heparin

(Continued)

## Sodium Tetradecyl Sulfate *(Continued)*

### Special PA Issues
**Patient Education:** Notify physician if chest pain, shortness of breath, or heat, pain, or tenderness in lower extremities

# Sodium Thiosulfate (SOW dee um thye oh SUL fate)

**Pharmacologic Class** Antidote; Antifungal Agent, Topical
**U.S. Brand Names** Tinver® Lotion
### Mechanism of Action
Cyanide toxicity: Increases the rate of detoxification of cyanide by the enzyme rhodanese by providing an extra sulfur
Cisplatin toxicity: Complexes with cisplatin to form a compound that is nontoxic to either normal or cancerous cells

### Use
Parenteral: Used alone or with sodium nitrite or amyl nitrite in cyanide poisoning or arsenic poisoning; reduce the risk of nephrotoxicity associated with cisplatin therapy
Topical: Treatment of tinea versicolor

### USUAL DOSAGE
Cyanide and nitroprusside antidote: I.V.:
Children <25 kg: 50 mg/kg after receiving 4.5-10 mg/kg sodium nitrite; a half dose of each may be repeated if necessary
Children >25 kg and Adults: 12.5 g after 300 mg of sodium nitrite; a half dose of each may be repeated if necessary
Cyanide poisoning: I.V.: Dose should be based on determination as with nitrite, at rate of 2.5-5 mL/minute to maximum of 50 mL. See table.

### Variation of Sodium Nitrite and Sodium Thiosulfate Dose With Hemoglobin Concentration*

| Hemoglobin (g/dL) | Initial Dose Sodium Nitrite (mg/kg) | Initial Dose Sodium Nitrite 3% (mL/kg) | Initial Dose Sodium Thiosulfate 25% (mL/kg) |
|---|---|---|---|
| 7 | 5.8 | 0.19 | 0.95 |
| 8 | 6.6 | 0.22 | 1.10 |
| 9 | 7.5 | 0.25 | 1.25 |
| 10 | 8.3 | 0.27 | 1.35 |
| 11 | 9.1 | 0.30 | 1.50 |
| 12 | 10.0 | 0.33 | 1.65 |
| 13 | 10.3 | 0.36 | 1.80 |
| 14 | 11.3 | 0.39 | 1.95 |

*Adapted from Berlin DM Jr, "The Treatment of Cyanide Poisoning in Children," *Pediatrics*, 1970, 46:793.

Cisplatin rescue should be given before or during cisplatin administration: I.V. infusion (in sterile water): 12 g/m² over 6 hours or 9 g/m² I.V. push followed by 1.2 g/m² continuous infusion for 6 hours
Arsenic poisoning: I.V.: 1 mL first day, 2 mL second day, 3 mL third day, 4 mL fourth day, 5 mL on alternate days thereafter
Children and Adults: Topical: 20% to 25% solution: Apply a thin layer to affected areas twice daily

**Dosage Forms** Inj: 100 mg/mL (10 mL), 250 mg/mL (50 mL); Lot: 25% with salicylic acid 1% and isopropyl alcohol 10% (120 mL, 180 mL)
**Contraindications** Hypersensitivity to any component
**Warnings/Precautions** Safety in pregnancy has not been established; discontinue topical use if irritation or sensitivity occurs; rapid I.V. infusion has caused transient hypotension and EKG changes in dogs; can increase risk of thiocyanate intoxication
**Pregnancy Risk Factor** C
**Adverse Reactions** 1% to 10%:
Cardiovascular: Hypotension
Central nervous system: Coma, CNS depression secondary to thiocyanate intoxication, psychosis, confusion
Dermatologic: Contact dermatitis, local irritation
Neuromuscular & skeletal: Weakness
Otic: Tinnitus
### Special PA Issues
**Patient Education:** Avoid topical application near the eyes, mouth, or other mucous membranes; notify physician if condition worsens or burning or irritation occurs; shake well before using
**Monitoring Parameters:** Monitor for signs of thiocyanate toxicity

♦ **Sodol®** *see* Carisoprodol *on page 154*
♦ **SoFlax™** *see* Docusate *on page 298*

- **Solaquin®** [OTC] *see* Hydroquinone *on page 457*
- **Solaquin Forte®** *see* Hydroquinone *on page 457*
- **Solarcaine®** [OTC] *see* Benzocaine *on page 105*
- **Solarcaine® Aloe Extra Burn Relief** [OTC] *see* Lidocaine *on page 531*
- **Solatene®** *see* Beta-Carotene *on page 111*
- **Solium®** *see* Chlordiazepoxide *on page 189*
- **Soluble Fluorescein** *see* Fluorescein Sodium *on page 382*
- **Solu-Cortef®** *see* Hydrocortisone *on page 453*
- **Solu-Medrol® Injection** *see* Methylprednisolone *on page 593*
- **Solurex L.A.®** *see* Dexamethasone *on page 264*
- **Soma®** *see* Carisoprodol *on page 154*
- **Soma® Compound** *see* Carisoprodol and Aspirin *on page 154*
- **Soma® Compound w/Codeine** *see* Carisoprodol, Aspirin, and Codeine *on page 154*
- **Somatrem** *see* Human Growth Hormone *on page 444*
- **Somatropin** *see* Human Growth Hormone *on page 444*
- **Sominex® Oral** [OTC] *see* Diphenhydramine *on page 289*
- **Somnol®** *see* Flurazepam *on page 390*
- **Som Pam®** *see* Flurazepam *on page 390*
- **Sopamycetin** *see* Chloramphenicol *on page 188*
- **Soprodol®** *see* Carisoprodol *on page 154*

## Sorbitol (SOR bi tole)

**Pharmacologic Class** Genitourinary Irrigant; Laxative, Miscellaneous

**Mechanism of Action** A polyalcoholic sugar with osmotic cathartic actions

**Use** Genitourinary irrigant in transurethral prostatic resection or other transurethral resection or other transurethral surgical procedures; diuretic; humectant; sweetening agent; hyperosmotic laxative; facilitate the passage of sodium polystyrene sulfonate through the intestinal tract

**USUAL DOSAGE** Hyperosmotic laxative (as single dose, at infrequent intervals):

Children 2-11 years:

Oral: 2 mL/kg (as 70% solution)

Rectal enema: 30-60 mL as 25% to 30% solution

Children >12 years and Adults:

Oral: 30-150 mL (as 70% solution)

Rectal enema: 120 mL as 25% to 30% solution

Adjunct to sodium polystyrene sulfonate: 15 mL as 70% solution orally until diarrhea occurs (10-20 mL/2 hours) or 20-100 mL as an oral vehicle for the sodium polystyrene sulfonate resin

When administered with charcoal:

Oral:

Children: 4.3 mL/kg of 35% sorbitol with 1 g/kg of activated charcoal

Adults: 4.3 mL/kg of 70% sorbitol with 1 g/kg of activated charcoal every 4 hours until first stool containing charcoal is passed

Topical: 3% to 3.3% as transurethral surgical procedure irrigation

**Dosage Forms Soln:** 70%; **Soln, genitourinary irrigation:** 3% (1500 mL, 3000 mL), 3.3% (2000 mL)

**Contraindications** Anuria

**Warnings/Precautions** Use with caution in patients with severe cardiopulmonary or renal impairment and in patients unable to metabolize sorbitol

**Adverse Reactions** 1% to 10%:

Cardiovascular: Edema

Endocrine & metabolic: Fluid and electrolyte losses, lactic acidosis

Gastrointestinal: Diarrhea, nausea, vomiting, abdominal discomfort, xerostomia

**Onset** About 0.25-1 hour

**Special PA Issues**

**Patient Education:** Cathartic: Use of cathartics on a regular basis will have adverse effects. Increased exercise, increased fluid intake, or increased dietary fruit and fiber may be effective in preventing and resolving constipation.

- **Sorbitrate®** *see* Isosorbide Dinitrate *on page 498*
- **Soridol®** *see* Carisoprodol *on page 154*
- **Sotacor®** *see* Sotalol *on this page*

## Sotalol (SOE ta lole)

**Pharmacologic Class** Antiarrhythmic Agent, Class II; Antiarrhythmic Agent, Class III; Beta Blocker, Beta₁ Selective

**U.S. Brand Names** Betapace®

(Continued)

## Sotalol *(Continued)*

### Mechanism of Action
Beta-blocker which contains both beta-adrenoreceptor-blocking (Vaughan Williams Class II) and cardiac action potential duration prolongation (Vaughan Williams Class III) properties

Class II effects: Increased sinus cycle length, slowed heart rate, decreased A-V nodal conduction, and increased A-V nodal refractoriness

Class III effects: Prolongation of the atrial and ventricular monophasic action potentials, and effective refractory prolongation of atrial muscle, ventricular muscle, and atrioventricular accessory pathways in both the antegrade and retrograde directions

Sotalol is a racemic mixture of *d*- and *l*-sotalol; both isomers have similar Class III antiarrhythmic effects while the *l*-isomer is responsible for virtually all of the beta-blocking activity

Sotalol has both beta₁- and beta₂-receptor blocking activity

The beta-blocking effect of sotalol is a noncardioselective [half maximal at about 80 mg/day and maximal at doses of 320-640 mg/day]. Significant beta-blockade occurs at oral doses as low as 25 mg/day.

The Class III effects are seen only at oral doses ≥160 mg/day

### Use
Treatment of documented ventricular arrhythmias, such as sustained ventricular tachycardia, that in the judgment of the physician are life-threatening

**Unlabeled use:** Supraventricular arrhythmias

### USUAL DOSAGE
Sotalol should be initiated and doses increased in a hospital with facilities for cardiac rhythm monitoring and assessment. Proarrhythmic events can occur after initiation of therapy and with each upward dosage adjustment.

Children: Oral: The safety and efficacy of sotalol in children have not been established
Supraventricular arrhythmias: 2-4 mg/kg/24 hours was given in 2 equal doses every 12 hours to 18 infants (≤2 months of age). All infants, except one with chaotic atrial tachycardia, were successfully controlled with sotalol. Ten infants discontinued therapy between the ages of 7-18 months when it was no longer necessary. Median duration of treatment was 12.8 months.

Adults: Oral:
Initial: 80 mg twice daily
Dose may be increased (gradually allowing 2-3 days between dosing increments in order to attain steady-state plasma concentrations and to allow monitoring of Q-T intervals) to 240-320 mg/day
Most patients respond to a total daily dose of 160-320 mg/day in 2-3 divided doses
Some patients, with life-threatening refractory ventricular arrhythmias, may require doses as high as 480-640 mg/day; however, these doses should only be prescribed when the potential benefit outweighs the increased of adverse events

Elderly patients: Age does not significantly alter the pharmacokinetics of sotalol, but impaired renal function in elderly patients can increase the terminal half-life, resulting in increased drug accumulation

**Dosing adjustment in renal impairment:**
Cl_cr >60 mL/minute: Administer every 12 hours
Cl_cr 30-60 mL/minute: Administer every 24 hours
Cl_cr 10-30 mL/minute: Administer every 36-48 hours
Cl_cr <10 mL/minute: Individualize dose
Dialysis: Hemodialysis would be expected to reduce sotalol plasma concentrations because sotalol is not bound to plasma proteins and does not undergo extensive metabolism; administer dose postdialysis or administer supplemental 80 mg dose; peritoneal dialysis does not remove sotalol; supplemental dose is not necessary

### Dosage Forms
Tab, as hydrochloride: 80 mg, 120 mg, 160 mg, 240 mg

### Contraindications
Bronchial asthma, sinus bradycardia, second and third degree A-V block (unless a functioning pacemaker is present), congenital or acquired long Q-T syndromes, cardiogenic shock, uncontrolled congestive heart failure, and previous evidence of hypersensitivity to sotalol; concurrent use with sparfloxacin

### Warnings/Precautions
Use with caution in patients with congestive heart failure, peripheral vascular disease, hypokalemia, hypomagnesemia, renal dysfunction, sick-sinus syndrome; abrupt withdrawal may result in return of life-threatening arrhythmias; sotalol can provoke new or worsening ventricular arrhythmias

### Pregnancy Risk Factor
B

### Pregnancy Implications
Clinical effects on the fetus: Although there are no adequate and well controlled studies in pregnant women, sotalol has been shown to cross the placenta, and is found in amniotic fluid. There has been a report of subnormal birth weight with sotalol, therefore, sotalol should be used during pregnancy only if the potential benefit outweighs the potential risk.

### Adverse Reactions
>10%:
Cardiovascular: Bradycardia (16%), chest pain (16%), palpitations (14%)
Central nervous system: Fatigue (20%), dizziness (20%)
Neuromuscular & skeletal: Weakness (13%)

Respiratory: Dyspnea (21%)

1% to 10%:

Cardiovascular: Congestive heart failure, reduced peripheral circulation (3%), edema (8%), abnormal EKG (7%), hypotension (6%), proarrhythmia (5%), syncope (5%)

Central nervous system: Mental confusion (6%), anxiety (4%), headache (8%), sleep problems (8%), depression (4%)

Dermatologic: Itching/rash (5%)

Endocrine & metabolic: Decreased sexual ability (3%)

Gastrointestinal: Diarrhea (7%), nausea/vomiting (10%), stomach discomfort (3% to 6%)

Hematologic: Bleeding (2%)

Neuromuscular & skeletal: Paresthesia (4%)

Ocular: Visual problems (5%)

Respiratory: Upper respiratory problems (5% to 8%), asthma (2%)

<1%: Raynaud's phenomenon, red, crusted skin, skin necrosis after extravasation; leukopenia, phlebitis, diaphoresis, cold extremities

**Drug Interactions**

Decreased effect of beta-blockers with aluminum salts, barbiturates, calcium salts, cholestyramine, colestipol, NSAIDs, penicillins (ampicillin), rifampin, salicylates and sulfinpyrazone due to decreased bioavailability and plasma levels

Beta-blockers may decrease the effect of sulfonylureas and beta agonists

Increased effect/toxicity of beta-blockers with calcium blockers (diltiazem, felodipine, nicardipine), contraceptives, flecainide, quinidine (in extensive metabolizers), ciprofloxacin

Beta-blockers may increase the effect/toxicity of digoxin, flecainide, and other antiarrhythmics (especially class Ia), haloperidol, phenothiazines, acetaminophen, clonidine (hypertensive crisis after or during withdrawal of either agent), epinephrine (initial hypertensive episode followed by bradycardia), nifedipine and verapamil, lidocaine, ergots (peripheral ischemia), prazosin (postural hypotension), and catecholamine-depleting agents (reserpine and guanethidine)

Beta-blockers may affect the action or levels of ethanol, disopyramide, nondepolarizing muscle relaxants and theophylline although the effects are difficult to predict

Avoid use of sotalol with sparfloxacin, terfenadine, and astemizole since risk of cardiotoxicity may be increased

**Onset** Rapid, 1-2 hours; Peak effect: 2.5-4 hours

**Duration** 8-16 hours

**Half-Life** 12 hours

**Special PA Issues**

**Patient Education:** Take exactly as directed; do not take additional doses or discontinue without consulting prescriber. You will need regular cardiac check-ups and blood tests while taking this medication. You may experience dizziness, drowsiness, or visual changes (use caution when driving or performing tasks that require alertness until response to drug is determined); orthostatic hypotension (use caution when climbing stairs or when changing position - rising from lying or sitting position); abnormal taste, nausea or vomiting, or loss of appetite (small frequent meals, frequent mouth care, or sucking lozenges may help); decreased sexual ability (reversible); or constipation (increased exercise, dietary fiber, fruit, or fluid may help). Report chest pain, palpitation, or erratic heartbeat; difficulty breathing or unusual cough; mental depression or persistent insomnia (hallucinations); or changes in vision.

**Monitoring Parameters:** Serum magnesium, potassium, EKG

**Related Information**

Beta-Blockers *on page 1002*

♦ **Sotalol Hydrochloride** *see* Sotalol *on page 845*

♦ **Sotradecol®** *see* Sodium Tetradecyl Sulfate *on page 843*

♦ **Soyacal®** *see* Fat Emulsion *on page 359*

♦ **SPA** *see* Albumin *on page 34*

♦ **Spancap® No. 1** *see* Dextroamphetamine *on page 268*

♦ **Span-FF® [OTC]** *see* Ferrous Fumarate *on page 366*

# Sparfloxacin (spar FLOKS a sin)

**Pharmacologic Class** Antibiotic, Quinolone

**U.S. Brand Names** Zagam®

**Mechanism of Action** Inhibits DNA-gyrase in susceptible organisms; inhibits relaxation of supercoiled DNA and promotes breakage of double-stranded DNA

**Use** Treatment of adults with community-acquired pneumonia caused by *C. pneumoniae, H. influenzae, H. parainfluenza, M. catarrhalis, M. pneumoniae* or *S. pneumoniae*; treatment of acute bacterial exacerbations of chronic bronchitis caused by *C. pneumoniae, E. cloacae, H. influenzae, H. parainfluenza, K. pneumoniae, M. catarrhalis, S. aureus* or *S. pneumoniae*

**USUAL DOSAGE** Adults: Oral:

Loading dose: 2 tablets (400 mg) on day 1

Maintenance: 1 tablet (200 mg) daily for 10 days total therapy (total 11 tablets)

**Dosing adjustment in renal impairment:** $Cl_{cr}$ <50 mL/minute: Administer 400 mg on day 1, then 200 mg every 48 hours for a total of 9 days of therapy (total 6 tablets)

(Continued)

## Sparfloxacin *(Continued)*

**Dosage Forms Tab:** 200 mg

**Contraindications** Hypersensitivity to sparfloxacin, any component, or other quinolones; a concurrent administration with drugs which increase the Q-T interval including: amiodarone, bepridil, bretylium, disopyramide, furosemide, procainamide, quinidine, sotalol, albuterol, astemizole, chloroquine, cisapride, halofantrine, phenothiazines, prednisone, terfenadine, and tricyclic antidepressants

**Warnings/Precautions** Not recommended in children <18 years of age, other quinolones have caused transient arthropathy in children; CNS stimulation may occur (tremor, restlessness, confusion, and very rarely hallucinations or seizures); use with caution in patients with known or suspected CNS disorder or renal dysfunction; prolonged use may result in superinfection; if an allergic reaction (itching, urticaria, dyspnea, pharyngeal or facial edema, loss of consciousness, tingling, cardiovascular collapse) occurs, discontinue the drug immediately; use caution to avoid possible photosensitivity reactions during and for several days following fluoroquinolone therapy; pseudomembranous colitis may occur and should be considered in patients who present with diarrhea

**Pregnancy Risk Factor** C

**Pregnancy Implications**

Clinical effects on the fetus: Avoid use in pregnant women unless the benefit justifies the potential risk to the fetus

Breast-feeding/lactation: Quinolones are known to distribute well into breast milk; consequently use during lactation should be avoided if possible

**Adverse Reactions**

>1%:

Central nervous system: Insomnia, agitation, sleep disorders, anxiety, delirium

Gastrointestinal: Diarrhea, abdominal pain, vomiting

Hematologic: Leukopenia, eosinophilia, anemia

Hepatic: Increased LFTs

<1%: Photosensitivity, rash, myalgia, arthralgia

**Drug Interactions**

Decreased effect: Decreased absorption with antacids containing aluminum, magnesium, and/or calcium and by products containing zinc and iron salts when administered concurrently; phenytoin serum levels may be reduced by quinolones; antineoplastic agents may also decrease serum levels of fluoroquinolones

Increased toxicity/serum levels: Quinolones cause increased levels of caffeine, warfarin, cyclosporine, and theophylline (although one study indicates that sparfloxacin may not affect theophylline metabolism), cimetidine and probenecid increase quinolone levels; an increased incidence of seizures may occur with foscarnet. Avoid use with drugs which increase Q-T interval as significant risk of cardiotoxicity may occur

**Half-Life** 16 hours

**Special PA Issues**

**Patient Education:** Take per recommended schedule around-the-clock. Maintain adequate hydration (2-3 L/day of fluids unless instructed to restrict fluid intake). Take complete prescription and do not skip doses; if dose is missed take as soon as possible, do not double doses. Do not take with antacids. You may experience dizziness, lightheadedness, anxiety, insomnia, or confusion; use caution when driving or engaging in tasks that require alertness. Small frequent meals and frequent mouth care may reduce nausea, vomiting, or taste disturbances. You may experience photosensitivity; use sunblock, wear appropriate clothing, and avoid direct sun. Report palpitations or chest pain; persistent diarrhea or GI disturbances or abdominal pain; muscle tremor or pain; pain, inflammation, or rupture of tendon; yellowing of eyes or skin, easy bruising or bleeding; unusual fatigue; fever, chills, signs of infection; or worsening of condition.

**Monitoring Parameters:** Evaluation of organ system functions (renal, hepatic, ophthalmologic, and hematopoietic) is recommended periodically during therapy; the possibility of crystalluria should be assessed; WBC and signs and symptoms of infection

♦ **Sparine®** *see* Promazine *on page 766*

♦ **Spaslin®** *see* Hyoscyamine, Atropine, Scopolamine, and Phenobarbital *on page 464*

♦ **Spasmolin®** *see* Hyoscyamine, Atropine, Scopolamine, and Phenobarbital *on page 464*

♦ **Spasmophen®** *see* Hyoscyamine, Atropine, Scopolamine, and Phenobarbital *on page 464*

♦ **Spasquid®** *see* Hyoscyamine, Atropine, Scopolamine, and Phenobarbital *on page 464*

♦ **Spec-T® [OTC]** *see* Benzocaine *on page 105*

♦ **Spectam®** *see* Spectinomycin *on this page*

♦ **Spectazole™ Topical** *see* Econazole *on page 311*

## Spectinomycin *(spek ti noe MYE sin)*

**Pharmacologic Class** Antibiotic, Miscellaneous

**U.S. Brand Names** Spectam®; Trobicin®

**Mechanism of Action** A bacteriostatic antibiotic that selectively binds to the 30s subunits of ribosomes, and thereby inhibiting bacterial protein synthesis

**Use** Treatment of uncomplicated gonorrhea

**USUAL DOSAGE** I.M.:

Children:

<45 kg: 40 mg/kg/dose 1 time (ceftriaxone preferred)

≥45 kg: See adult dose

Children >8 years who are allergic to PCNS/cephalosporins may be treated with oral tetracycline

Adults:

Uncomplicated urethral endocervical or rectal gonorrhea: 2 g deep I.M. or 4 g where antibiotic resistance is prevalent 1 time; 4 g (10 mL) dose should be given as two 5 mL injections, followed by doxycycline 100 mg twice daily for 7 days

Disseminated gonococcal infection: 2 g every 12 hours

**Dosing adjustment in renal impairment:** None necessary

Hemodialysis: 50% removed by hemodialysis

**Dosage Forms Inj, as hydrochloride:** 2 g, 4 g

**Contraindications** Hypersensitivity to spectinomycin or any component

**Pregnancy Risk Factor** B

**Adverse Reactions** <1%: Dizziness, headache, chills, urticaria, rash, pruritus, nausea, vomiting, pain at injection site

**Duration** Up to 8 hours

**Half-Life** 1.7 hours

**Special PA Issues**

**Patient Education:** This medication can only be administered I.M. You will need to return for follow-up blood tests.

♦ **Spectinomycin Hydrochloride** see Spectinomycin on previous page

♦ **Spectrobid®** see Bacampicillin on page 95

# Spironolactone (speer on oh LAK tone)

**Pharmacologic Class** Diuretic, Potassium Sparing

**U.S. Brand Names** Aldactone®

**Mechanism of Action** Competes with aldosterone for receptor sites in the distal renal tubules, increasing sodium chloride and water excretion while conserving potassium and hydrogen ions; may block the effect of aldosterone on arteriolar smooth muscle as well

**Use** Management of edema associated with excessive aldosterone excretion; hypertension; primary hyperaldosteronism; hypokalemia; treatment of hirsutism; cirrhosis of liver accompanied by edema or ascites

**USUAL DOSAGE** Administration with food increases absorption. To reduce delay in onset of effect, a loading dose of 2 or 3 times the daily dose may be administered on the first day of therapy. Oral:

Neonates: Diuretic: 1-3 mg/kg/day divided every 12-24 hours

Children:

Diuretic, hypertension: 1.5-3.5 mg/kg/day or 60 mg/m$^2$/day in divided doses every 6-24 hours

Diagnosis of primary aldosteronism: 125-375 mg/m$^2$/day in divided doses

Vaso-occlusive disease: 7.5 mg/kg/day in divided doses twice daily (not FDA approved)

Adults:

Edema, hypertension, hypokalemia: 25-200 mg/day in 1-2 divided doses

Diagnosis of primary aldosteronism: 100-400 mg/day in 1-2 divided doses

Hirsutism in women: 50-200 mg/day in 1-2 divided doses

Elderly: Initial: 25-50 mg/day in 1-2 divided doses, increasing by 25-50 mg every 5 days as needed

**Dosing interval in renal impairment:**

Cl$_{cr}$ 10-50 mL/minute: Administer every 12-24 hours

Cl$_{cr}$ <10 mL/minute: Avoid use

**Dosage Forms Tab:** 25 mg, 50 mg, 100 mg

**Contraindications** Hypersensitivity to spironolactone or any components, hyperkalemia, renal failure, anuria, patients receiving other potassium-sparing diuretics or potassium supplements

**Warnings/Precautions** Use with caution in patients with dehydration, hepatic disease, hyponatremia, renal sufficiency; it is recommended the drug may be discontinued several days prior to adrenal vein catheterization; shown to be tumorigenic in toxicity studies using rats at 25-250 times the usual human dose

**Pregnancy Risk Factor** D

**Pregnancy Implications**

Clinical effects on the fetus: No data available on crossing the placenta. 1 report of oral cleft. Generally, use of diuretics during pregnancy is avoided due to risk of decreased placental perfusion.

Breast-feeding/lactation: Crosses into breast milk. American Academy of Pediatrics considers **compatible** with breast-feeding.

**Adverse Reactions**

Cardiovascular: Arrhythmia

(Continued)

## Spironolactone *(Continued)*

Central nervous system: Confusion, nervousness, dizziness, drowsiness, lack of energy, unusual fatigue, headache, fever, chills, ataxia

Dermatologic: Skin rash

Endocrine & metabolic: Hyperkalemia, breast tenderness in females, deepening of voice in females, enlargement of breast in males, inability to achieve or maintain an erection, increased hair growth in females, decreased sexual ability, menstrual changes

Gastrointestinal: Diarrhea, nausea, vomiting, stomach cramps, dryness of mouth

Genitourinary: Painful urination, dysuria

Neuromuscular & skeletal: Weakness, numbness or paresthesia in hands, feet, or lips; lower back or side pain

Respiratory: Shortness of breath, dyspnea, cough or hoarseness

Miscellaneous: Increased thirst, diaphoresis

### Drug Interactions

Decreased effect: Effects of anticoagulants may be decreased; diuretic effect of spironolactone may be decreased by salicylates

Increased toxicity: Potassium, potassium-sparing diuretics (eg, triamterene), indomethacin, angiotensin-converting enzymes inhibitors may increase serum potassium levels

Variable effects of digoxin have occurred with concurrent dosing

### Half-Life 78-84 minutes

### Special PA Issues

**Patient Education:** Take as directed, with meals or milk. This diuretic does not cause potassium loss; avoid excessive potassium intake (eg, salt substitutes, low-salt foods, bananas, nuts). Weigh yourself weekly at same time, in the same clothes, and report weight loss more than 5 lb/week. You may experience dizziness, drowsiness, headache; use caution when driving or engaging in tasks that require alertness. Small frequent meals, frequent mouth care, or sucking on lozenges may reduce dry mouth, nausea, or vomiting. You may experience decreased sexual ability (reversible with discontinuing of medication). Report mental confusion; clumsiness; persistent fatigue, chills, numbness, or muscle weakness in hands, feet, or face; acute persistent diarrhea; breast tenderness or increased body hair in females; breast enlargement or inability to achieve erection in males; chest pain, rapid heartbeat or palpitations; or difficulty breathing.

**Monitoring Parameters:** Blood pressure, serum electrolytes (potassium, sodium), renal function, I & O ratios and daily weight throughout therapy

### Related Information

Heart Failure: Management of Patients with Left Ventricular Systolic Dysfunction *on page 1064*

♦ **Sporanox®** *see* Itraconazole *on page 501*

♦ **SPS®** *see* Sodium Polystyrene Sulfonate *on page 843*

♦ **S-P-T** *see* Thyroid *on page 897*

♦ **SRC® Expectorant** *see* Hydrocodone, Pseudoephedrine, and Guaifenesin *on page 453*

♦ **SSD® AF** *see* Silver Sulfadiazine *on page 835*

♦ **SSD® Cream** *see* Silver Sulfadiazine *on page 835*

♦ **SSKI®** *see* Potassium Iodide *or page 744*

♦ **Stadol®** *see* Butorphanol *on page 133*

♦ **Stadol® NS** *see* Butorphanol *on page 133*

♦ **Stagesic®** *see* Hydrocodone and Acetaminophen *on page 449*

♦ **Stahist®** *see* Chlorpheniramine, Phenylephrine, Phenylpropanolamine, and Belladonna Alkaloids *on page 196*

♦ **Stannous Fluoride** *see* Fluoride *on page 383*

## Stanozolol *(stan OH zoe lole)*

**Pharmacologic Class** Anabolic Steroid

**U.S. Brand Names** Winstrol®

**Mechanism of Action** Synthetic testosterone derivative with similar androgenic and anabolic actions

**Use** Prophylactic use against hereditary angioedema

### USUAL DOSAGE

Children: Acute attacks:

<6 years: 1 mg/day

6-12 years: 2 mg/day

Adults: Oral: Initial: 2 mg 3 times/day, may then reduce to a maintenance dose of 2 mg/day or 2 mg every other day after 1-3 months

**Dosing adjustment in hepatic impairment:** Stanozolol is **not** recommended for patients with severe liver dysfunction

**Dosage Forms Tab:** 2 mg

**Contraindications** Nephrosis, carcinoma of breast or prostate, pregnancy, hypersensitivity to any component

**Warnings/Precautions** May stunt bone growth in children; anabolic steroids may cause peliosis hepatis, liver cell tumors, and blood lipid changes with increased risk of arteriosclerosis; monitor diabetic patients carefully; use with caution in elderly patients, they may be at greater risk for prostatic hypertrophy; use with caution in patients with cardiac, renal, or hepatic disease or epilepsy

**Pregnancy Risk Factor** X

**Adverse Reactions**
**Male:**
Postpubertal:
>10%:
Dermatologic: Acne
Endocrine & metabolic: Gynecomastia
Genitourinary: Bladder irritability, priapism
1% to 10%:
Central nervous system: Insomnia, chills
Endocrine & metabolic: Decreased libido, hepatic dysfunction,
Gastrointestinal: Nausea, diarrhea
Genitourinary: Prostatic hypertrophy (elderly)
Hematologic: Iron deficiency anemia, suppression of clotting factors
<1%: Hepatic necrosis, hepatocellular carcinoma
Prepubertal:
>10%:
Dermatologic: Acne
Endocrine & metabolic: Virilism
1% to 10%:
Central nervous system: Chills, insomnia, factors
Dermatologic: Hyperpigmentation
Gastrointestinal: Diarrhea, nausea
Hematologic: Iron deficiency anemia, suppression of clotting
<1%: Hepatic necrosis, hepatocellular carcinoma

**Female:**
>10%: Endocrine & metabolic: Virilism
1% to 10%:
Central nervous system: Chills, insomnia
Endocrine & metabolic: Hypercalcemia
Gastrointestinal: Nausea, diarrhea
Hematologic: Iron deficiency anemia, suppression of clotting factors
Hepatic: Hepatic dysfunction
<1%: Hepatic necrosis, hepatocellular carcinoma

**Drug Interactions** Increased toxicity: ACTH, adrenal steroids may increase risk of edema and acne; stanozolol enhances the hypoprothrombinemic effects of oral anticoagulants; enhances the hypoglycemic effects of insulin and sulfonylureas (oral hypoglycemics)

**Special PA Issues**
**Patient Education:** These drugs do not enhance athletic ability. Take as prescribed. A high protein, high caloric diet is suggested. Restrict salt intake. Glucose tolerance may be altered in diabetics. Monitor blood glucose or sugar in urine closely. Report swelling of ankles, skin color changes, severe nausea and vomiting, body hair growth, hoarseness, deepening of voice, acne, or menstrual irregularities in women.

- ♦ **Staphcillin®** *see* Methicillin *on page 583*
- ♦ **Statex®** *see* Morphine Sulfate *on page 619*

# Stavudine (STAV yoo deen)

**Pharmacologic Class** Antiretroviral Agent, Reverse Transcriptase Inhibitor (Nucleoside)
**U.S. Brand Names** Zerit®
**Mechanism of Action** Stavudine is a thymidine analog which interferes with HIV viral DNA dependent DNA polymerase resulting in inhibition of viral replication; nucleoside reverse transcriptase inhibitor
**Use** Treatment of adults with HIV infection in combination with other antiretroviral agents
**USUAL DOSAGE** Oral:
Children: 2 mg/kg/day
Adults:
≥60 kg: 40 mg every 12 hours
<60 kg: 30 mg every 12 hours
Dose may be cut in half if symptoms of peripheral neuropathy occur
**Dosing adjustment in renal impairment:**
Cl$_{cr}$ >50 mL/minute:
≥60 kg: 40 mg every 12 hours
<60 kg: 30 mg every 12 hours
Cl$_{cr}$ 26-50 mL/minute:
≥60 kg: 20 mg every 12 hours
<60 kg: 15 mg every 12 hours
(Continued)

## Stavudine *(Continued)*

Hemodialysis:
≥60 kg: 20 mg every 24 hours
<60 kg: 15 mg every 24 hours

**Dosage Forms Cap:** 15 mg, 20 mg, 30 mg, 40 mg; **Powder for oral soln:** 1 mg/mL (200 mL)

**Contraindications** Hypersensitivity to stavudine

**Warnings/Precautions** Use with caution in patients who demonstrate previous hypersensitivity to zidovudine, didanosine, zalcitabine, pre-existing bone marrow suppression, renal insufficiency, or peripheral neuropathy. Peripheral neuropathy may be the dose-limiting side effect. Zidovudine should not be used in combination with stavudine. Potentially fatal lactic acidosis and hepatomegaly have been reported, use with caution in patients at risk of hepatic disease

**Pregnancy Risk Factor** C

**Pregnancy Implications**

Clinical effects on the fetus: Administer during pregnancy only if benefits to mother outweigh risks to the fetus

Breast-feeding/lactation: HIV-infected mothers are discouraged from breast-feeding to decrease potential transmission of HIV

**Adverse Reactions** All adverse reactions reported below were similar to comparative agent, zidovudine, except for peripheral neuropathy, which was greater for stavudine.

>10%:
Central nervous system: Headache, chills/fever, malaise, insomnia, anxiety, depression, pain
Dermatologic: Rash
Gastrointestinal: Nausea, vomiting, diarrhea, pancreatitis, abdominal pain
Neuromuscular & skeletal: Peripheral neuropathy (15% to 21%)
1% to 10%:
Hematologic: Neutropenia, thrombocytopenia
Hepatic: Increased hepatic transaminases, increased bilirubin
Neuromuscular & skeletal: Myalgia, back pain, weakness
<1%: Lactic acidosis, hepatomegaly, hepatic failure, anemia, pancreatitis

**Half-Life** 1-1.6 hours

**Special PA Issues**

**Patient Education:** This medication does not cure HIV. Use appropriate precautions to prevent transmission to others. Take as directed, around-the-clock, and take for full length of prescription. Maintain adequate hydration (2-3 L/day of fluids unless instructed to restrict fluid intake) and nutrition. Frequent small meals, frequent mouth care, or sucking on lozenges may reduce nausea or vomiting. Buttermilk or yogurt may help reduce diarrhea. Report immediately any tingling, unusual pain, or numbness in extremities. Report fever, chills, unusual fatigue or acute depression, acute abdominal or back pain, persistent muscle pain or weakness, or unusual bruising or bleeding.

**Monitoring Parameters:** Monitor liver function tests and signs and symptoms of peripheral neuropathy; monitor viral load and CD4 count

♦ **S-T Cort®** *see* Hydrocortisone *on page 453*

♦ **Stelazine®** *see* Trifluoperazine *on page 934*

♦ **Stemetil®** *see* Prochlorperazine *on page 763*

♦ **Sterapred®** *see* Prednisone *on page 754*

♦ **Stieva-A®** *see* Tretinoin, Topical *on page 927*

♦ **Stieva-A® Forte** *see* Tretinoin, Topical *on page 927*

♦ **Stilbestrol** *see* Diethylstilbestrol *on page 277*

♦ **Stilphostrol®** *see* Diethylstilbestrol *on page 277*

♦ **Stimate® Nasal** *see* Desmopressin Acetate *on page 261*

♦ **Stinking Rose** *see* Garlic *on page 410*

# St Johns Wort

**Mechanism of Action** Active ingredients are xanthones flavonoids (hypericin) which can act as monoamine oxidase inhibitors, although *in vitro* activity is minimal; majority of activity appears to be related to GABA modulation; may be related to dopamine, serotonin norepinephrine modulation also

**Use** Mild to moderate depression; also used traditionally for treatment of stress, anxiety, insomnia; used topically for vitiligo; also a popular drug for AIDS patients due to possible antiretroviral activity; used topically for wound healing

Per Commission E: Psychovegetative disorders, depressive moods, anxiety and/or nervous unrest; oily preparations for dyspeptic complaints; oily preparations externally for treatment of post-therapy of acute and contused injuries, myalgia, first degree burns

**USUAL DOSAGE** Based on hypericin extract content

Oral: 300 mg 3 times daily (not to be used longer than 8 weeks)

Herb: 2-4 g 3 times daily

Liquid extract: 2-4 mL 3 times/day

Tincture: 2-4 mL 3 times/day

Topical: Crushed leaves and flowers are applied to affected area after cleansing with soap and water

Per Commission E: 2-4 g drug (dried herb) or 0.2-1 mg of total hypericin in other forms of drug application

**Contraindications** Endogenous depression, pregnancy, children <2 years of age (not confirmed in animal models, *in vitro* only).

**Warnings/Precautions** May be photosensitizing

**Pregnancy Implications** Do not use

**Adverse Reactions**

Cardiovascular: Sinus tachycardia

Dermatologic: Photosensitization is possible, especially in fair-skinned persons (per Commission E)

Gastrointestinal: Stomach pains, abdominal pain

**Drug Interactions** Avoid amphetamines or other stimulants; use with caution in patients taking MAO inhibitors, levodopa, and 5-hydroxytryptophan; avoid tyramine-containing foods due to presence of hypercin although human data of this potential drug interaction is lacking; avoid concurrent use with SSRI or other antidepressants

- ◆ **St Joseph® Adult Chewable Aspirin [OTC]** *see* Aspirin *on page 80*
- ◆ **St. Joseph® Measured Dose Nasal Solution [OTC]** *see* Phenylephrine *on page 718*
- ◆ **Stop® [OTC]** *see* Fluoride *on page 383*
- ◆ **Streptase®** *see* Streptokinase *on this page*

# Streptokinase (strep toe KYE nase)

**Pharmacologic Class** Thrombolytic Agent

**U.S. Brand Names** Kabikinase®; Streptase®

**Mechanism of Action** Activates the conversion of plasminogen to plasmin by forming a complex, exposing plasminogen-activating site, and cleaving a peptide bond that converts plasminogen to plasmin; plasmin degrades fibrin, fibrinogen and other procoagulant proteins into soluble fragments; effective both outside and within the formed thrombus/embolus

**Use** Thrombolytic agent used in treatment of recent severe or massive deep vein thrombosis, pulmonary emboli, myocardial infarction, and occluded arteriovenous cannulas

**USUAL DOSAGE** I.V.:

Children: Safety and efficacy not established; limited studies have used 3500-4000 units/kg over 30 minutes followed by 1000-1500 units/kg/hour

Clotted catheter: 25,000 units, clamp for 2 hours then aspirate contents and flush with normal saline

Adults: Antibodies to streptokinase remain for at least 3-6 months after initial dose: Administration requires the use of an infusion pump

An intradermal skin test of 100 units has been suggested to predict allergic response to streptokinase. If a positive reaction is not seen after 15-20 minutes, a therapeutic dose may be administered.

Guidelines for acute myocardial infarction (AMI): 1.5 million units over 60 minutes

Administration:

Dilute two 750,000 unit vials of streptokinase with 5 mL dextrose 5% in water ($D_5W$) each, gently swirl to dissolve

Add this dose of the 1.5 million units to 150 mL $D_5W$

This should be infused over 60 minutes; an in-line filter ≥0.45 micron should be used

Monitor for the first few hours for signs of anaphylaxis or allergic reaction. **Infusion should be slowed if lowering of 25 mm Hg in blood pressure or terminated if asthmatic symptoms appear**.

Begin heparin 5000-10,000 unit bolus followed by 1000 units/hour approximately 3-4 hours after completion of streptokinase infusion or when PTT is <100 seconds

Guidelines for acute pulmonary embolism (APE): 3 million unit dose over 24 hours

Administration:

Dilute four 750,000 unit vials of streptokinase with 5 mL dextrose 5% in water ($D_5W$) each, gently swirl to dissolve

Add this dose of 3 million units to 250 mL $D_5W$, an in-line filter ≥0.45 micron should be used

Administer 250,000 units (23 mL) over 30 minutes followed by 100,000 units/hour (9 mL/hour) for 24 hours

Monitor for the first few hours for signs of anaphylaxis or allergic reaction. **Infusion should be slowed if blood pressure is lowered by 25 mm Hg or if asthmatic symptoms appear**.

Begin heparin 1000 units/hour about 3-4 hours after completion of streptokinase infusion or when PTT is <100 seconds

Monitor PT, PTT, and fibrinogen levels during therapy

Thromboses: 250,000 units to start, then 100,000 units/hour for 24-72 hours depending on location

(Continued)

## Streptokinase *(Continued)*

Cannula occlusion: 250,000 units into cannula, clamp for 2 hours, then aspirate contents and flush with normal saline

**Dosage Forms Powder for inj:** 250,000 units (5 mL, 6.5 mL), 600,000 units (5 mL), 750,000 units (6 mL, 6.5 mL), 1,500,000 units (6.5 mL, 10 mL, 50 mL)

**Contraindications** Hypersensitivity to streptokinase or any component; recent streptococcal infection within the last 6 months; any internal bleeding; brain carcinoma; pregnancy; cerebrovascular accident or transient ischemic attack, gastrointestinal bleeding, trauma or surgery, prolonged external cardiac massage, intracranial or intraspinal surgery or trauma within 1 month; arteriovenous malformation or aneurysm; bleeding diathesis; severe hepatic or renal disease; subacute bacterial endocarditis; pericarditis; hemostatic defects; suspected aortic dissection. severe uncontrolled hypertension (BP systolic ≥180 mm Hg, BP diastolic ≥110 mm Hg)

**Warnings/Precautions** Avoid I.M. injections; use with caution in patients with a history of cardiac arrhythmias, major surgery within last 10 days, recent trauma, or severe hypertension; antibodies to streptokinase remain for 3-6 months after initial dose, use another thrombolytic enzyme (ie, alteplase) if thrombolytic therapy is indicated in patients with prior streptokinase therapy

**Pregnancy Risk Factor** C

**Adverse Reactions**

>10%:

Cardiovascular: Hypotension, arrhythmias, trauma arrhythmias

Dermatologic: Angioneurotic edema

Hematologic: Surface bleeding, internal bleeding, cerebral hemorrhage

Ocular: Periorbital swelling

Respiratory: Bronchospasm

<1%: Flushing, headache, chills, fever, rash, itching, nausea, vomiting, anemia, musculoskeletal pain, eye hemorrhage, epistaxis, diaphoresis, anaphylaxis

**Drug Interactions**

Decreased effect: Antifibrinolytic agents (aminocaproic acid) may decrease effectiveness

Increased toxicity: Anticoagulants, antiplatelet agents may increase risk of bleeding

**Onset** Activation of plasminogen occurs almost immediately

**Duration** Fibrinolytic effects last only a few hours, while anticoagulant effects can persist for 12-24 hours.

**Half-Life** 83 minutes

**Special PA Issues**

**Patient Education:** Bedrest is required. Avoid even slight injury. Report any sign of unusual bleeding.

**Monitoring Parameters:** Blood pressure, PT, APTT, platelet count, hematocrit, fibrinogen concentration, signs of bleeding

**Reference Range:**

Partial thromboplastin time (PTT) activated: 20.4-33.2 seconds

Prothrombin time (PT): 10.9-13.7 seconds (same as control)

Fibrinogen: 200-400 mg/dL

## Streptomycin *(strep toe MYE sin)*

**Pharmacologic Class** Antibiotic, Aminoglycoside; Antitubercular Agent

**Mechanism of Action** Inhibits bacterial protein synthesis by binding directly to the 30S ribosomal subunits causing faulty peptide sequence to form in the protein chain

**Use** Part of combination therapy of active tuberculosis; used in combination with other agents for treatment of streptococcal or enterococcal endocarditis, mycobacterial infections, plague, tularemia, and brucellosis

**USUAL DOSAGE**

Children:

Daily therapy: 20-30 mg/kg/day (maximum: 1 g/day)

Directly observed therapy (DOT): Twice weekly: 25-30 mg/kg (maximum: 1.5 g)

DOT: 3 times/week: 25-30 mg/kg (maximum: 1 g)

Adults:

Daily therapy: 15 mg/kg/day (maximum: 1 g)

Directly observed therapy (DOT): Twice weekly: 25-30 mg/kg (maximum: 1.5 g)

DOT: 3 times/week: 25-30 mg/kg (maximum: 1 g)

Enterococcal endocarditis 1 g every 12 hours for 2 weeks, 500 mg every 12 hours for 4 weeks in combination with penicillin

Streptococcal endocarditis 1 g every 12 hours for 1 week, 500 mg every 12 hours for 1 week

Tularemia: 1-2 g/day in divided doses for 7-10 days or until patient is afebrile for 5-7 days

Plague: 2-4 g/day in divided doses until the patient is afebrile for at least 3 days

Elderly: 10 mg/kg/day, not to exceed 750 mg/day; dosing interval should be adjusted for renal function; some authors suggest not to give more than 5 days/week or give as 20-25 mg/kg/dose twice weekly

**Dosing interval in renal impairment:**
Cl$_{cr}$ 10-50 mL/minute: Administer every 24-72 hours
Cl$_{cr}$ <10 mL/minute: Administer every 72-96 hours
Removed by hemo and peritoneal dialysis: Administer dose postdialysis
**Dosage Forms** Inj, as sulfate: 400 mg/mL (2.5 mL)
**Contraindications** Hypersensitivity to streptomycin or any component
**Warnings/Precautions** Use with caution in patients with pre-existing vertigo, tinnitus, hearing loss, neuromuscular disorders, or renal impairment; modify dosage in patients with renal impairment; aminoglycosides are associated with significant nephrotoxicity or ototoxicity; the ototoxicity is directly proportional to the amount of drug given and the duration of treatment; tinnitus or vertigo are indications of vestibular injury and impending bilateral irreversible damage; renal damage is usually reversible
**Pregnancy Risk Factor** D
**Adverse Reactions**
1% to 10%:
Central nervous system: Neurotoxicity
Renal: Nephrotoxicity
Otic: Ototoxicity (auditory), ototoxicity (vestibular)
<1%: Skin rash, drug fever, headache, paresthesia, tremor, nausea, vomiting, eosinophilia, arthralgia, anemia, hypotension, difficulty in breathing, drowsiness, weakness
**Drug Interactions**
Increased/prolonged effect: Depolarizing and nondepolarizing neuromuscular blocking agents
Increased toxicity: Concurrent use of amphotericin may increase nephrotoxicity
**Half-Life** 2-4.7 hours, prolonged with renal impairment
**Special PA Issues**
**Patient Education:** This medication can only be given by intramuscular injection. Therapy for TB or HIV will generally last several months. Do not discontinue even if you are feeling better. Maintain adequate hydration (2-3 L/day of fluids unless instructed to restrict fluid intake). You may experience headache or dizziness (use caution when driving or engaging in tasks that require alertness); nausea, vomiting, or loss of appetite (frequent small meals, frequent mouth care, or sucking on lozenges may help). Report immediately any rash, joint or back pain, or difficulty breathing; swelling of extremities or weight gain greater than 5 lb/week; fever, chills, mouth sores, vaginal itching or drainage, or foul-smelling stool; change in hearing, ringing or sense of fullness in ears; numbness, loss of sensation, clumsiness, change in strength, or altered gait.
**Monitoring Parameters:** Hearing (audiogram), BUN, creatinine; serum concentration of the drug should be monitored in all patients; eighth cranial nerve damage is usually preceded by high-pitched tinnitus, roaring noises, sense of fullness in ears, or impaired hearing and may persist for weeks after drug is discontinued
**Reference Range:** Therapeutic: Peak: 20-30 µg/mL; Trough: <5 µg/mL; Toxic: Peak: >50 µg/mL; Trough: >10 µg/mL

♦ **Stresstabs® 600 Advanced Formula Tablets [OTC]** *see* Vitamins, Multiple *on page 964*

♦ **Stromectol®** *see* Ivermectin *on page 503*

♦ **Strong Iodine Solution** *see* Potassium Iodide *on page 744*

# Strontium-89 (STRON shee um atey nine)

**Pharmacologic Class** Radiopharmaceutical
**U.S. Brand Names** Metastron®
**Use** Relief of bone pain in patients with skeletal metastases
**USUAL DOSAGE** Adults: I.V.: 148 megabecquerel (4 millicurie) administered by slow I.V. injection over 1-2 minutes or 1.5-2.2 megabecquerel (40-60 microcurie)/kg; repeated doses are generally not recommended at intervals <90 days; measure the patient dose by a suitable radioactivity calibration system immediately prior to administration
**Dosage Forms** Inj, as chloride: 10.9-22.6 mg/mL [148 megabecquerel, 4 millicurie] (10 mL)
**Contraindications** Patients with a history of hypersensitivity to any strontium-containing compounds, or any other component; pregnancy, lactation
**Warnings/Precautions** Use caution in patients with bone marrow compromise; incontinent patients may require urinary catheterization. Body fluids may remain radioactive up to one week after injection. Not indicated for use in patients with cancer not involving bone and should be used with caution in patients whose platelet counts fall <60,000 or whose white blood cell counts fall <2400. A small number of patients have experienced a transient increase in bone pain at 36-72 hours postdose; this reaction is generally mild and self-limiting. It should be handled cautiously, in a similar manner to other radioactive drugs. Appropriate safety measures to minimize radiation to personnel should be instituted.
**Pregnancy Risk Factor** D
**Adverse Reactions** Most severe reactions of marrow toxicity can be managed by conventional means
(Continued)

## Strontium-89 *(Continued)*

Percentage unknown:
    Cardiovascular: Flushing (most common after rapid injection)
    Central nervous system: Fever and chills (rare)
    Hematologic: Thrombocytopenia, leukopenia
    Neuromuscular & skeletal: An increase in bone pain may occur (10% to 20% of patients)

**Special PA Issues**
  **Patient Education:** Eat and drink normally, there is no need to avoid alcohol or caffeine unless already advised to do so; may be advised to take analgesics until Metastron® begins to become effective; the effect lasts for several months, if pain returns before that, notify medical personnel
  **Monitoring Parameters** Routine blood tests

♦ **Strontium-89 Chloride** *see* Strontium-89 *on previous page*
♦ **Stuartnatal® 1 + 1** *see* Vitamins, Multiple *on page 964*
♦ **Stuart Prenatal® [OTC]** *see* Vitamins, Multiple *on page 964*
♦ **Sublimaze® Injection** *see* Fentanyl *on page 362*

## Sucralfate *(soo KRAL fate)*

**Pharmacologic Class** Gastrointestinal Agent, Miscellaneous
**U.S. Brand Names** Carafate®
**Mechanism of Action** Forms a complex by binding with positively charged proteins in exudates, forming a viscous paste-like, adhesive substance. This selectively forms a protective coating that protects the lining against peptic acid, pepsin, and bile salts.
**Use** Short-term management of duodenal ulcers
  **Unlabeled use:** Gastric ulcers; maintenance of duodenal ulcers; suspension may be used topically for treatment of stomatitis due to cancer chemotherapy and other causes of esophageal and gastric erosions; GERD, esophagitis; treatment of NSAID mucosal damage; prevention of stress ulcers; postsclerotherapy for esophageal variceal bleeding
**USUAL DOSAGE** Oral:
  Children: Dose not established, doses of 40-80 mg/kg/day divided every 6 hours have been used
  Stomatitis: 2.5-5 mL (1 g/10 mL suspension), swish and spit or swish and swallow 4 times/day
  Adults:
    Stress ulcer prophylaxis: 1 g 4 times/day
    Stress ulcer treatment: 1 g every 4 hours
    Duodenal ulcer:
      Treatment: 1 g 4 times/day on an empty stomach and at bedtime for 4-8 weeks, or alternatively 2 g twice daily; treatment is recommended for 4-8 weeks in adults, the elderly may require 12 weeks
      Maintenance: Prophylaxis: 1 g twice daily
    Stomatitis: 1 g/10 mL suspension, swish and spit or swish and swallow 4 times/day
  **Dosage comment in renal impairment:** Aluminum salt is minimally absorbed (<5%), however, may accumulate in renal failure
**Dosage Forms Susp, oral:** 1 g/10 mL (420 mL); **Tab:** 1 g
**Contraindications** Hypersensitivity to sucralfate or any component
**Warnings/Precautions** Successful therapy with sucralfate should not be expected to alter the posthealing frequency of recurrence or the severity of duodenal ulceration; use with caution in patients with chronic renal failure who have an impaired excretion of absorbed aluminum. Because of the potential for sucralfate to alter the absorption of some drugs, separate administration (take other medication 2 hours before sucralfate) should be considered when alterations in bioavailability are believed to be critical
**Pregnancy Risk Factor** B
**Pregnancy Implications**
  Clinical effects on the fetus: No data available; available evidence suggests safe use during pregnancy and breast-feeding
  Breast-feeding/lactation: No data available. American Academy of Pediatrics has NO RECOMMENDATION.
**Adverse Reactions**
  1% to 10%: Gastrointestinal: Constipation
  <1%: Dizziness, sleepiness, vertigo, insomnia, rash, pruritus, diarrhea, nausea, vomiting, gastric discomfort, indigestion, xerostomia, back pain
**Drug Interactions** Decreased effect: Digoxin, phenytoin (hydantoins), warfarin, ketoconazole, quinidine, ciprofloxacin, norfloxacin (quinolones), tetracycline, theophylline; because of the potential for sucralfate to alter the absorption of some drugs, separate administration (take other medications 2 hours before sucralfate) should be considered when alterations in bioavailability are believed to be critical

  **Note:** When given with aluminum-containing antacids, may increase serum/body aluminum concentrations (see Warnings/Precautions)
**Onset** Paste formation and ulcer adhesion occur within 1-2 hours.

**Duration** Up to 6 hours

**Special PA Issues**

    **Patient Education:** Take recommended dose before meals or on an empty stomach. Take any other medications at least 2 hours before taking sucralfate. Do not take antacids within 30 minutes of taking sucralfate. May cause constipation; increased exercise, increased dietary fiber, fruit or fluids, or mild stool softener may be helpful. If constipation or gastric distress persists, consult prescriber.

♦ **Sucrets®** [OTC] *see* Dyclonine *on page 310*

♦ **Sudafed®** [OTC] *see* Pseudoephedrine *on page 780*

♦ **Sudafed® 12 Hour** [OTC] *see* Pseudoephedrine *on page 780*

♦ **Sufedrin®** [OTC] *see* Pseudoephedrine *on page 780*

♦ **Sular®** *see* Nisoldipine *on page 658*

♦ **Sulbactam and Ampicillin** *see* Ampicillin and Sulbactam *on page 66*

## Sulconazole (sul KON a zole)

**Pharmacologic Class** Antifungal Agent, Topical

**U.S. Brand Names** Exelderm®

**Mechanism of Action** Substituted imidazole derivative which inhibits metabolic reactions necessary for the synthesis of ergosterol, an essential membrane component. The end result is usually fungistatic; however, sulconazole may act as a fungicide in *Candida albicans* and parapsilosis during certain growth phases.

**Use** Treatment of superficial fungal infections of the skin, including tinea cruris (jock itch), tinea corporis (ringworm), tinea versicolor, and possibly tinea pedis (athlete's foot - cream only)

**USUAL DOSAGE** Adults: Topical: Apply a small amount to the affected area and gently massage once or twice daily for 3 weeks (tinea cruris, tinea corporis, tinea versicolor) to 4 weeks (tinea pedis).

**Dosage Forms Crm:** 1% (15 g, 30 g, 60 g); **Soln, top:** 1% (30 mL)

**Contraindications** Known hypersensitivity to sulconazole

**Warnings/Precautions** Use with caution in nursing mothers; for external use only

**Pregnancy Risk Factor** C

**Adverse Reactions** 1% to 10%:

    Dermatologic: Itching

    Local: Burning, stinging, redness

**Special PA Issues**

    **Patient Education:** For external use only; avoid contact with eyes; if burning or irritation develops, notify physician

**Related Information**

    Antifungal Agents, Topical *on page 1000*

♦ **Sulconazole Nitrate** *see* Sulconazole *on this page*

♦ **Sulcrate®** *see* Sucralfate *on previous page*

♦ **Sulcrate® Suspension Plus** *see* Sucralfate *on previous page*

♦ **Sulf-10®** Ophthalmic *see* Sulfacetamide Sodium *on next page*

## Sulfabenzamide, Sulfacetamide, and Sulfathiazole

(sul fa BENZ a mide, sul fa SEE ta mide & sul fa THYE a zole)

**Pharmacologic Class** Antibiotic, Vaginal

**U.S. Brand Names** Femguard®; Gyne-Sulf®; Sulfa-Gyn®; Sulfa-Trip®; Sultrin™; Trysul®; Vagilia®; V.V.S.®

**Mechanism of Action** Interferes with microbial folic acid synthesis and growth via inhibition of para-aminobenzoic acid metabolism

**Use** Treatment of *Haemophilus vaginalis* vaginitis

**USUAL DOSAGE** Adults:

    Cream: Insert one applicatorful in vagina twice daily for 4-6 days; dosage may then be decreased to ½ to ¼ of an applicatorful twice daily

    Tablet: Insert one intravaginally twice daily for 10 days

**Dosage Forms Crm, vag:** Sulfabenzamide 3.7%, sulfacetamide 2.86%, and sulfathiazole 3.42% (78 g with applicator, 90 g, 120 g); **Tab, vag:** Sulfabenzamide 184 mg, sulfacetamide 143.75 mg, and sulfathiazole 172.5 mg (20 tabs/box with vaginal applicator)

**Contraindications** Hypersensitivity to sulfabenzamide, sulfacetamide, sulfathiazole or any component, renal dysfunction

**Warnings/Precautions** Associated with Stevens-Johnson syndrome; if local irritation or systemic toxicity develops, discontinue therapy

**Pregnancy Risk Factor** C

**Adverse Reactions**

    >10%: Local: Irritation, pruritus, urticaria

    <1%: Allergic reactions, Stevens-Johnson syndrome

    (Continued)

## Sulfabenzamide, Sulfacetamide, and Sulfathiazole *(Continued)*
### Special PA Issues
**Patient Education:** This medication is to be inserted into vagina; do not ingest tablets. Complete full course of therapy. Wash hands before inserting applicator gently into vagina and releasing cream or tablet. Wash hands and applicator with soap and water following each application. Discontinue and notify prescriber immediately if burning, irritation, or signs of allergic reaction occur.

## Sulfacetamide Sodium (sul fa SEE ta mide SOW dee um)
**Pharmacologic Class** Antibiotic, Ophthalmic; Antibiotic, Sulfonamide Derivative

**U.S. Brand Names** AK-Sulf® Ophthalmic; Bleph®-10 Ophthalmic; Cetamide® Ophthalmic; Isopto® Cetamide® Ophthalmic; Klaron® Lotion; Ocusulf-10® Ophthalmic; Sebizon® Topical Lotion; Sodium Sulamyd® Ophthalmic; Sulf-10® Ophthalmic

**Mechanism of Action** Interferes with bacterial growth by inhibiting bacterial folic acid synthesis through competitive antagonism of PABA

**Use** Treatment and prophylaxis of conjunctivitis due to susceptible organisms; corneal ulcers; adjunctive treatment with systemic sulfonamides for therapy of trachoma; topical application in scaling dermatosis (seborrheic); bacterial infections of the skin

### USUAL DOSAGE
Children >2 months and Adults: Ophthalmic:
Ointment: Apply to lower conjunctival sac 1-4 times/day and at bedtime
Solution: Instill 1-3 drops several times daily up to every 2-3 hours in lower conjunctival sac during waking hours and less frequently at night
Children >12 years and Adults: Topical:
Seborrheic dermatitis: Apply at bedtime and allow to remain overnight; in severe cases, may apply twice daily
Secondary cutaneous bacterial infections: Apply 2-4 times/day until infection clears

**Dosage Forms Lot:** 10% (85 g); **Oint, ophth:** 10% (3.5 g); **Soln, ophth:** 10% (1 mL, 2 mL, 2.5 mL, 5 mL, 15 mL), 15% (5 mL, 15 mL), 30% (15 mL)

**Contraindications** Hypersensitivity to sulfacetamide or any component, sulfonamides; infants <2 months of age

**Warnings/Precautions** Inactivated by purulent exudates containing PABA; use with caution in severe dry eye; ointment may retard corneal epithelial healing; sulfite in some products may cause hypersensitivity reactions; cross-sensitivity may occur with previous exposure to other sulfonamices given by other routes

**Pregnancy Risk Factor** C

### Adverse Reactions
1% to 10%: Local: Irritation, stinging, burning
<1%: Headache, Stevens-Johnson syndrome, exfoliative dermatitis, toxic epidermal necrolysis, blurred vision, browache, hypersensitivity reactions

**Drug Interactions** Decreased effect: Silver, gentamicin (antagonism)

**Half-Life** 7-13 hours

### Special PA Issues
**Patient Education:** Use as directed. Complete full course of therapy even if condition appears improved.

Topical: For topical use only. Apply a thin film of ointment to affected area as often as directed. Do not cover with occlusive dressing. Report increased skin redness, irritation, or development of open sores; or if condition worsens or does not improve.

Ophthalmic: For ophthalmic use only. Store at room temperature. Shake before using. Apply prescribed amount as often as directed. Wash hands before using and do not let tip of applicator touch eye or contaminate tip of applicator. Tilt head back and look upward. Gently pull down lower lid and put drop(s) in inner corner of eye. Close eye and roll eyeball in all directions. Do not blink for ½ minute. Apply gentle pressure to inner corner of eye for 30 seconds. Wipe away excess from skin around eye. Do not use any other eye preparation for at least 10 minutes. Do not touch tip of applicator to eye or contaminate tip of applicator. Do not share medication with anyone else. May cause sensitivity to bright light (dark glasses may help); temporary stinging or blurred vision may occur. Inform prescriber if you experience eye pain, redness, burning, watering, dryness, double vision, puffiness around eye, vision disturbances, or other adverse eye response; worsening of condition or lack of improvement within 3-4 days.

**Monitoring Parameters:** Response to therapy

## Sulfacetamide Sodium and Fluorometholone
(sul fa SEE ta mide SOW dee um & flure oh METH oh lone)
**Pharmacologic Class** Antibiotic/Corticosteroid, Ophthalmic

**U.S. Brand Names** FML-S® Ophthalmic Suspension

**Dosage Forms Susp, ophth:** Sulfacetamide sodium 10% and fluorometholone 0.1% (5 mL, 10 mL)

## Sulfacetamide Sodium and Phenylephrine
(sul fa SEE ta mide SOW dee um & fen il EF rin)

**Pharmacologic Class** Antibiotic, Ophthalmic

**U.S. Brand Names** Vasosulf® Ophthalmic

**Dosage Forms Soln, ophth:** Sulfacetamide sodium 15% and phenylephrine hydrochloride 0.125% (5 mL, 15 mL)

## Sulfacetamide Sodium and Prednisolone
(sul fa SEE ta mide SOW dee um & pred NIS oh lone)

**Pharmacologic Class** Antibiotic, Ophthalmic; Corticosteroid, Ophthalmic

**U.S. Brand Names** AK-Cide® Ophthalmic; Blephamide® Ophthalmic; Cetapred® Ophthalmic; Isopto® Cetapred® Ophthalmic; Metimyd® Ophthalmic; Vasocidin® Ophthalmic

**Dosage Forms Oint, ophth:** AK-Cide®, Metimyd®, Vasocidin®: Sulfacetamide sodium 10% and prednisolone acetate 0.5% (3.5 g), Blephamide®: Sulfacetamide sodium 10% and prednisolone acetate 0.2% (3.5 g), Cetapred®: Sulfacetamide sodium 10% and prednisolone acetate 0.25% (3.5 g); **Susp, ophth:** Sulfacetamide sodium 10% and prednisolone sodium phosphate 0.25% (5 mL), AK-Cide®, Metimyd®: Sulfacetamide sodium 10% and prednisolone acetate 0.5% (5 mL), Blephamide®: Sulfacetamide sodium 10% and prednisolone acetate 0.2% (2.5 mL, 5 mL, 10 mL), Isopto® Cetapred®: Sulfacetamide sodium 10% and prednisolone acetate 0.25% (5 mL, 15 mL), Vasocidin®: Sulfacetamide sodium 10% and prednisolone sodium phosphate: 0.25% (5 mL, 10 mL)

♦ **Sulfacet-R® Topical** *see* Sulfur and Sulfacetamide Sodium *on page 865*

## Sulfadiazine (sul fa DYE a zeen)

**Pharmacologic Class** Antibiotic, Sulfonamide Derivative

**U.S. Brand Names** Microsulfon®

**Mechanism of Action** Interferes with bacterial growth by inhibiting bacterial folic acid synthesis through competitive antagonism of PABA

**Use** Treatment of urinary tract infections and nocardiosis, rheumatic fever prophylaxis; adjunctive treatment in toxoplasmosis; uncomplicated attack of malaria

**USUAL DOSAGE** Oral:

Congenital toxoplasmosis:

Newborns and Children <2 months: 100 mg/kg/day divided every 6 hours in conjunction with pyrimethamine 1 mg/kg/day once daily and supplemental folinic acid 5 mg every 3 days for 6 months

Children >2 months: 25-50 mg/kg/dose 4 times/day

Toxoplasmosis:

Children >2 months: Loading dose: 75 mg/kg; maintenance dose: 120-150 mg/kg/day, maximum dose: 6 g/day; divided every 4-6 hours in conjunction with pyrimethamine 2 mg/kg/day divided every 12 hours for 3 days followed by 1 mg/kg/day once daily (maximum: 25 mg/day) with supplemental folinic acid

Adults: 2-4 g/day divided every 4-8 hours in conjunction with pyrimethamine 25 mg/day and with supplemental folinic acid

Prevention of recurrent attacks of rheumatic fever:

>30 kg: 1 g/day

<30 kg: 0.5 g/day

**Dosage Forms Tab:** 500 mg

**Contraindications** Porphyria, hypersensitivity to any sulfa drug or any component, pregnancy at term, children <2 months of age unless indicated for the treatment of congenital toxoplasmosis, sunscreens containing PABA, nursing mothers

**Warnings/Precautions** Use with caution in patients with impaired hepatic function or impaired renal function, G-6-PD deficiency; dosage modification required in patients with renal impairment; fluid intake should be maintained ≥1500 mL/day, or administer sodium bicarbonate to keep urine alkaline; more likely to cause crystalluria because it is less soluble than other sulfonamides

**Pregnancy Risk Factor** B (D at term)

**Adverse Reactions**

>10%:

Central nervous system: Fever, dizziness, headache

Dermatologic: Itching, rash, photosensitivity

Gastrointestinal: Anorexia, nausea, vomiting, diarrhea

1% to 10%:

Dermatologic: Lyell's syndrome, Stevens-Johnson syndrome

Hematologic: Granulocytopenia, leukopenia, thrombocytopenia, aplastic anemia, hemolytic anemia

Hepatic: Hepatitis

<1%: Thyroid function disturbance, crystalluria, jaundice, interstitial nephritis, acute nephropathy, hematuria, serum sickness-like reactions

**Drug Interactions** Decreased effect with PABA or PABA metabolites of drugs (eg, procaine, proparacaine, tetracaine, sunscreens); increased effect of oral anticoagulants and oral hypoglycemic agents

(Continued)

## Sulfadiazine *(Continued)*

**Half-Life** 10 hours

**Special PA Issues**

**Patient Education:** Take as directed, at regular intervals around-the-clock. Take 1 hour before or 2 hours after meals with full glass of water. Complete full course of therapy even if you are feeling better. Avoid aspirin or aspirin-containing products and avoid large quantities of vitamin C. It is very important to maintain adequate hydration (2-3 L/day of fluids unless instructed to restrict fluid intake) to prevent kidney damage. You may experience dizziness or headache (use caution when driving or engaging in hazardous tasks); photosensitivity (use sunblock, wear protective clothing and dark eye protection, or avoid direct sunlight); nausea, vomiting, or loss of appetite (small frequent meals, frequent mouth care, or sucking on lozenges may help). Report skin rash, persistent diarrhea, persistent or severe sore throat, fever, vaginal itching or discharge, unusual bruising or bleeding, fatigue, persistent headache or abdominal pain, or difficulty breathing.

## Sulfadiazine, Sulfamethazine, and Sulfamerazine

(sul fa DYE a zeen sul fa METH a zeen & sul fa MER a zeen)

**Pharmacologic Class** Antibiotic, Sulfonamide Derivative

**Mechanism of Action** Interferes with microbial folic acid synthesis and growth via inhibition of para-aminobenzoic acid metabolism

**Use** Treatment of toxoplasmosis and other susceptible organisms, however, other agents are preferred

**USUAL DOSAGE** Adults: Oral: 2-4 g to start, then 2-4 g/day in 3-6 divided doses

**Dosage Forms Tab:** Sulfadiazine 167 mg, sulfamethazine 167 mg, and sulfamerazine 167 mg

**Contraindications** Porphyria, known hypersensitivity to any sulfa drug or any component

**Pregnancy Risk Factor** B (D at term)

**Special PA Issues**

**Patient Education:** Drink plenty of fluids

## Sulfadoxine and Pyrimethamine (sul fa DOKS een & peer i METH a meen)

**Pharmacologic Class** Antimalarial Agent

**Mechanism of Action** Sulfadoxine interferes with bacterial folic acid synthesis and growth via competitive inhibition of para-aminiobenzoic acid; pyrimethamine inhibits microbial dihydrofolate reductase, resulting in inhibition of tetrahydrofolic acid synthesis

**Use** Treatment of *Plasmodium falciparum* malaria in patients in whom chloroquine resistance is suspected; malaria prophylaxis for travelers to areas where chloroquine-resistant malaria is endemic

**USUAL DOSAGE** Children and Adults: Oral:

Treatment of acute attack of malaria: A single dose of the following number of Fansidar® tablets is used in sequence with quinine or alone:

2-11 months: 1/4 tablet

1-3 years: 1/2 tablet

4-8 years: 1 tablet

9-14 years: 2 tablets

>14 years: 2-3 tablets

Malaria prophylaxis:

The first dose of Fansidar® should be taken 1-2 days before departure to an endemic area (CDC recommends that therapy be initiated 1-2 weeks before such travel), administration should be continued during the stay and for 4-6 weeks after return. Dose = pyrimethamine 0.5 mg/kg/dose and sulfadoxine 10 mg/kg/dose up to a maximum of 25 mg pyrimethamine and 500 mg sulfadoxine/dose weekly.

2-11 months: 1/8 tablet weekly or 1/4 tablet once every 2 weeks

1-3 years: 1/4 tablet once weekly or 1/2 tablet once every 2 weeks

4-8 years: 1/2 tablet once weekly or 1 tablet once every 2 weeks

9-14 years: 3/4 tablet once weekly or 1 1/2 tablets once every 2 weeks

>14 years: 1 tablet once weekly or 2 tablets once every 2 weeks

**Dosage Forms Tab:** Sulfadoxine 500 mg and pyrimethamine 25 mg

**Contraindications** Known hypersensitivity to any sulfa drug, pyrimethamine, or any component; porphyria, megaloblastic anemia, severe renal insufficiency; children <2 months of age due to competition with bilirubin for protein binding sites

**Warnings/Precautions** Use with caution in patients with renal or hepatic impairment, patients with possible folate deficiency, and patients with seizure disorders, increased adverse reactions are seen in patients also receiving chloroquine; fatalities associated with sulfonamides, although rare have occurred due to severe reactions including Stevens-Johnson syndrome, toxic epidermal necrolysis, hepatic necrosis, agranulocytosis, aplastic anemia and other blood dyscrasias; discontinue use at first sign of rash or any sign of adverse reaction; hemolysis occurs in patients with G-6-PD deficiency; leucovorin should be administered to reverse signs and symptoms of folic acid deficiency

**Pregnancy Risk Factor** C

#### Adverse Reactions

>10%:
    Central nervous system: Ataxia, seizures, headache
    Dermatologic: Photosensitivity
    Gastrointestinal: Atrophic glossitis, vomiting, gastritis
    Hematologic: Megaloblastic anemia, leukopenia, thrombocytopenia, pancytopenia
    Neuromuscular & skeletal: Tremors
    Miscellaneous: Hypersensitivity

1% to 10%:
    Dermatologic: Stevens-Johnson syndrome
    Hepatic: Hepatitis

<1%: Erythema multiforme, toxic epidermal necrolysis, rash, thyroid function dysfunction, anorexia, glossitis, crystalluria, hepatic necrosis, respiratory failure

#### Drug Interactions

Decreased effect with PABA or PABA metabolites of local anesthetics
Increased toxicity with methotrexate, other sulfonamides, co-trimoxazole

#### Special PA Issues

**Patient Education:** Begin prophylaxis at least 2 days before departure; drink plenty of fluids; avoid prolonged exposure to the sun; notify physician if rash, sore throat, pallor, or glossitis occurs

**Monitoring Parameters:** CBC, including platelet counts, and urinalysis should be performed periodically

♦ **Sulfa-Gyn®** *see* Sulfabenzamide, Sulfacetamide, and Sulfathiazole *on page 857*

♦ **Sulfalax®** [OTC] *see* Docusate *on page 298*

## Sulfamethoxazole (sul fa meth OKS a zole)

**Pharmacologic Class** Antibiotic, Sulfonamide Derivative

**U.S. Brand Names** Gantanol®; Urobak®

**Mechanism of Action** Interferes with bacterial growth by inhibiting bacterial folic acid synthesis through competitive antagonism of PABA

**Use** Treatment of urinary tract infections, nocardiosis, toxoplasmosis, acute otitis media, and acute exacerbations of chronic bronchitis due to susceptible organisms

**USUAL DOSAGE** Oral:
Children >2 months: 50-60 mg/kg as single dose followed by 50-60 mg/kg/day divided every 12 hours; maximum: 3 g/24 hours or 75 mg/kg/day
Adults: Initial: 2 g, then 1 g 2-3 times/day; maximum: 3 g/24 hours

**Dosing adjustment/interval in renal impairment:**
$Cl_{cr}$ 10-50 mL/minute: Administer every 12-24 hours
$Cl_{cr}$ <10 mL/minute: Administer every 24 hours
Hemodialysis: Moderately dialyzable (20% to 50%)

**Dosage Forms Susp, oral (cherry flavor):** 500 mg/5 mL (480 mL); **Tab:** 500 mg

**Contraindications** Porphyria, hypersensitivity to any sulfa drug or any component, pregnancy during 3rd trimester, children <2 months of age unless indicated for the treatment of congenital toxoplasmosis, sunscreens containing PABA

**Warnings/Precautions** Maintain adequate fluid intake to prevent crystalluria; use with caution in patients with renal or hepatic impairment, and patients with G-6-PD deficiency; should not be used for group A beta-hemolytic streptococcal infections

**Pregnancy Risk Factor** B (D at term)

#### Adverse Reactions

>10%:
    Central nervous system: Fever, dizziness, headache
    Dermatologic: Itching, rash, photosensitivity
    Gastrointestinal: Anorexia, nausea, vomiting, diarrhea

1% to 10%:
    Dermatologic: Lyell's syndrome, Stevens-Johnson syndrome
    Hematologic: Granulocytopenia, leukopenia, thrombocytopenia, aplastic anemia, hemolytic anemia
    Hepatic: Hepatitis

<1%: Vasculitis, thyroid function disturbance, crystalluria, jaundice, hematuria, acute nephropathy, interstitial nephritis, serum sickness-like reactions

#### Drug Interactions

Decreased effect with PABA or PABA metabolites of drugs (ie, procaine, proparacaine, tetracaine); cyclosporine levels may be decreased
Increased effect/toxicity of oral anticoagulants, oral hypoglycemic agents, hydantoins, uricosuric agents, methotrexate when administered with sulfonamides
Increased toxicity of sulfonamides with diuretics, indomethacin, methenamine, probenecid, and salicylates

**Half-Life** 9-12 hours, prolonged with renal impairment

#### Special PA Issues

**Patient Education:** Take as directed, at regular intervals around-the-clock. Take 1 hour before or 2 hours after meals with a full glass of water. Take full course of therapy even if
(Continued)

## Sulfamethoxazole *(Continued)*

you feeling better. Avoid aspirin or aspirin-containing products and avoid large quantities of vitamin C. It is very important to maintain adequate hydration (2-3 L/day of fluids unless instructed to restrict fluid intake) to prevent kidney damage. You may experience dizziness or headache (use caution when driving or engaging in hazardous tasks); photosensitivity (use sunblock, wear protective clothing and dark eye protection, or avoid direct sunlight); nausea, vomiting, or loss of appetite (small frequent meals, frequent mouth care, or sucking on lozenges may help). Report skin rash, persistent diarrhea, persistent or severe sore throat, fever, vaginal itching or discharge, unusual bruising or bleeding, fatigue, persistent headache or abdominal pain, or difficulty breathing.

**Monitoring Parameters:** Monitor urine output

## Sulfamethoxazole and Phenazopyridine

(sul fa meth OKS a zole & fen az oh PEER i deen)

**Pharmacologic Class** Antibiotic, Sulfonamide Derivative

**Dosage Forms Tab:** Sulfamethoxazole 500 mg and phenazopyridine 100 mg

♦ **Sulfamethoxazole and Trimethoprim** *see* Co-Trimoxazole *on page 238*

♦ **Sulfamylon® Topical** *see* Mafenide *on page 551*

## Sulfanilamide (sul fa NIL a mide)

**Pharmacologic Class** Antifungal Agent, Vaginal

**U.S. Brand Names** AVC™ Cream; AVC™ Suppository; Vagitrol®

**Mechanism of Action** Interferes with microbial folic acid synthesis and growth via inhibition of para-aminiobenzoic acid metabolism; exerts a bacteriostatic action

**Use** Treatment of vulvovaginitis caused by *Candida albicans*

**USUAL DOSAGE** Adults: Female: Insert one applicatorful intravaginally once or twice daily continued through 1 complete menstrual cycle or insert one suppository intravaginally once or twice daily for 30 days

**Dosage Forms Crm, vag (AVC™, Vagitrol®):** 15% [150 mg/g] (120 g with applicator); **Supp, vag (AVC™):** 1.05 g (16s)

**Contraindications** Hypersensitivity to sulfanilamide or any component

**Warnings/Precautions** Since sulfonamides may be absorbed from vaginal mucosa, the same precaution for oral sulfonamides apply (eg, blood dyscrasias); if a rash develops, terminate therapy immediately. Use vaginal applicators very cautiously after the 7th month of pregnancy.

**Pregnancy Risk Factor** C; kernicterus possible in nursing newborn, avoid breast-feeding if possible

**Adverse Reactions** Percentage unknown: Rarely, systemic reactions occur; increased discomfort, burning, allergic reactions, Stevens-Johnson syndrome (infrequent)

**Special PA Issues**

**Patient Education:** Complete full course of therapy as directed. Insert vaginally as directed by prescriber or see package insert. You may be sensitive to direct sunlight (wear protective clothing, use sunblock, and avoid excessive exposure to direct sunlight). Sexual partner may experience irritation of penis; best to refrain from intercourse during period of treatment. Report persistent vaginal burning, itching, or irritation; rash; yellowing of eyes or skin, dark urine, or pale stool; unresolved nausea or vomiting; or painful urination.

## Sulfasalazine (sul fa SAL a zeen)

**Pharmacologic Class** 5-Aminosalicylic Acid Derivative

**U.S. Brand Names** Azulfidine®; Azulfidine® EN-tabs®

**Mechanism of Action** Acts locally in the colon to decrease the inflammatory response and systemically interferes with secretion by inhibiting prostaglandin synthesis

**Use** Management of ulcerative colitis; enteric coated tablets are used for for rheumatoid arthritis in patients who inadequately respond to analgesics and NSAIDs

**USUAL DOSAGE** Oral:

Children >2 years: Initial: 40-60 mg/kg/day in 3-6 divided doses; maintenance dose: 20-30 mg/kg/day in 4 divided doses

Adults: Initial: 1 g 3-4 times/day, 2 g/day maintenance in divided doses; may initiate therapy with 0.5-1 g/day enteric-coated tablets

**Dosing interval in renal impairment:**

$Cl_{cr}$ 10-30 mL/minute: Administer twice daily

$Cl_{cr}$ <10 mL/minute: Administer once daily

**Dosing adjustment in hepatic impairment:** Avoid use

**Dosage Forms Susp, oral:** 250 mg/5 mL (473 mL); **Tab:** 500 mg; **Tab, enteric coated:** 500 mg

**Contraindications** Hypersensitivity to sulfasalazine, sulfa drugs, or any component; porphyria, GI or GU obstruction; hypersensitivity to salicylates; children <2 years of age

**Warnings/Precautions** Use with caution in patients with renal impairment; impaired hepatic function or urinary obstruction, blood dyscrasias severe allergies or asthma, or G-6-PD deficiency; may cause folate deficiency (consider providing 1 mg/day folate supplement)

**Pregnancy Risk Factor** B (D at term)

**Adverse Reactions**

>10%:

Central nervous system: Dizziness, headache (33%)

Dermatologic: Photosensitivity

Gastrointestinal: Anorexia, nausea, vomiting, diarrhea (33%)

Genitourinary: Reversible oligospermia (33%)

<3%:

Dermatologic: Urticaria/pruritus (<3%)

Hematologic: Hemolytic anemia (<3%), Heinz body anemia (<3%)

<0.1%: Lyell's syndrome, Stevens-Johnson syndrome, thyroid function disturbance, crystalluria, granulocytopenia, leukopenia, thrombocytopenia, aplastic anemia, jaundice, interstitial nephritis, acute nephropathy, hematuria, serum sickness-like reactions

**Drug Interactions**

Decreased effect of iron, digoxin, folic acid, and like other sulfa drugs PABA or PABA metabolites of drugs (ie, procaine, proparacaine, tetracaine)

Increased effect of oral anticoagulants, methotrexate, and oral hypoglycemic agents as with other sulfa drugs

**Half-Life** 5.7-10 hours

**Special PA Issues**

**Patient Education:** Do not crush, chew, or dissolve coated tablets. Shake suspension well before use. Do not take on an empty stomach or with antacids. Maintain adequate hydration (2-3 L/day of fluids unless instructed to restrict fluid intake) to prevent kidney damage. Increased dietary iron may be recommended. You may experience nervousness or dizziness (use caution when driving or engaging in hazardous activities until response to treatment is known). You may experience photosensitivity (wear protective clothing, use sunblock, or avoid direct sunlight). Orange-yellow color of urine, sweat, tears is normal and will stain contact lenses and clothing. Report rash, persistent nausea or anorexia, or lack of improvement in symptoms (after 1-2 months).

♦ **Sulfatrim®** *see* Co-Trimoxazole *on page 238*

♦ **Sulfa-Trip®** *see* Sulfabenzamide, Sulfacetamide, and Sulfathiazole *on page 857*

# Sulfinpyrazone (sul fin PEER a zone)

**Pharmacologic Class** Uricosuric Agent

**U.S. Brand Names** Anturane®

**Mechanism of Action** Acts by increasing the urinary excretion of uric acid, thereby decreasing blood urate levels; this effect is therapeutically useful in treating patients with acute intermittent gout, chronic tophaceous gout, and acts to promote resorption of tophi; also has antithrombic and platelet inhibitory effects

**Use** Treatment of chronic gouty arthritis and intermittent gouty arthritis

**Unlabeled use:** To decrease the incidence of sudden death postmyocardial infarction

**USUAL DOSAGE** Adults: Oral: 100-200 mg twice daily; maximum daily dose: 800 mg

**Dosing adjustment in renal impairment:** $Cl_{cr}$ <50 mL/minute: Avoid use

**Dosage Forms Cap:** 200 mg; **Tab:** 100 mg

**Contraindications** Active peptic ulcers, hypersensitivity to sulfinpyrazone, phenylbutazone, or other pyrazoles, GI inflammation, blood dyscrasias

**Warnings/Precautions** Safety and efficacy not established in children <18 years of age, use with caution in patients with impaired renal function and urolithiasis

**Pregnancy Risk Factor** C

**Adverse Reactions**

Cardiovascular: Flushing

Central nervous system: Dizziness, headache

Dermatologic: Dermatitis, rash

Gastrointestinal: Nausea, vomiting, stomach pain

Hematologic: Anemia, leukopenia, increased bleeding time (decreased platelet aggregation)

Hepatic: Hepatic necrosis

Genitourinary: Polyuria

Renal: Nephrotic syndrome, uric acid stones

**Drug Interactions** CYP2C and 3A3/4 enzyme inducer; CYP2C9 enzyme inhibitor

Decreased effect/levels of theophylline, verapamil; decreased uricosuric activity with salicylates, niacins

Increased effect of oral anticoagulants

Risk of acetaminophen hepatotoxicity is increased, but therapeutic effects may be reduced

**Half-Life** 2.7-6 hours

**Special PA Issues**

**Patient Education:** Take as directed, with meals or antacids and a full glass of water. Avoid aspirin or acetaminophen products and avoid large quantities of vitamin C. It is very

(Continued)

## Sulfinpyrazone *(Continued)*

important to maintain adequate hydration (2-3 L/day of fluids unless instructed to restrict fluid intake) to prevent kidney damage. You may experience nausea or vomiting (small frequent meals, frequent mouth care, or sucking on lozenges may help). Report skin rash, persistent stomach pain, painful urination or bloody urine, unusual bruising or bleeding, fatigue, or yellowing of eyes or skin.

**Monitoring Parameters:** Serum and urinary uric acid, CBC

## Sulfisoxazole (sul fi SOKS a zole)

**Pharmacologic Class** Antibiotic, Sulfonamide Derivative

**Mechanism of Action** Interferes with bacterial growth by inhibiting bacterial folic acid synthesis through competitive antagonism of PABA

**Use** Treatment of urinary tract infections, otitis media, *Chlamydia*; nocardiosis; treatment of acute pelvic inflammatory disease in prepubertal children; often used in combination with trimethoprim

**USUAL DOSAGE** Not for use in patients <2 months of age:

Children >2 months: Oral: Initial: 75 mg/kg, followed by 120-150 mg/kg/day in divided doses every 4-6 hours; not to exceed 6 g/day

Pelvic inflammatory disease: 100 mg/kg/day in divided doses every 6 hours; used in combination with ceftriaxone

*Chlamydia trachomatis*: 100 mg/kg/day in divided doses every 6 hours

Adults: Oral: Initial: 2-4 g, then 4-8 g/day in divided doses every 4-6 hours

Pelvic inflammatory disease: 500 mg every 6 hours for 21 days; used in combination with ceftriaxone

*Chlamydia trachomatis*: 500 mg every 6 hours for 10 days

Dosing interval in renal impairment:

$Cl_{cr}$ 10-50 mL/minute: Administer every 8-12 hours

$Cl_{cr}$ <10 mL/minute: Administer every 12-24 hours

Hemodialysis: >50% removed by hemodialysis

Children and Adults: Ophthalmic:

Solution: Instill 1-2 drops to affected eye every 2-3 hours

Ointment: Apply small amount to affected eye 1-3 times/day and at bedtime

**Dosage Forms Susp, oral, pediatric, as acetyl (raspberry flavor):** 500 mg/5 mL (480 mL); **Tab:** 500 mg

**Contraindications** Hypersensitivity to any sulfa drug or any component, porphyria, pregnancy during 3rd trimester, infants <2 months of age (sulfas compete with bilirubin for protein binding sites), patients with urinary obstruction, sunscreens containing PABA

**Warnings/Precautions** Use with caution in patients with G-6-PD deficiency (hemolysis may occur), hepatic or renal impairment; dosage modification required in patients with renal impairment; risk of crystalluria should be considered in patients with impaired renal function

**Pregnancy Risk Factor** B (D at term)

**Adverse Reactions**

>10%:

Central nervous system: Fever, dizziness, headache

Dermatologic: Itching, rash, photosensitivity

Gastrointestinal: Anorexia, nausea, vomiting, diarrhea

1% to 10%:

Dermatologic: Lyell's syndrome, Stevens-Johnson syndrome

Hematologic: Granulocytopenia, leukopenia, thrombocytopenia, aplastic anemia, hemolytic anemia

Hepatic: Hepatitis

<1%: Vasculitis, thyroid function disturbance, crystalluria, jaundice, hematuria, acute nephropathy, interstitial nephritis, serum sickness-like reactions

**Drug Interactions**

Decreased effect with PABA or PABA metabolites of drugs (ie, procaine, proparacaine, tetracaine); cyclosporine levels may be decreased

Increased effect/toxicity of oral anticoagulants, oral hypoglycemic agents, hydantoins, uricosuric agents, methotrexate when administered with sulfonamides

Increased toxicity of sulfonamides with diuretics, indomethacin, methenamine, probenecid, and salicylates

**Half-Life** 4-7 hours, prolonged with renal impairment

**Special PA Issues**

**Patient Education:** Take as directed, at regular intervals around-the-clock. Take 1 hour before or 2 hours after meals with a full glass of water. Take full course of therapy even if you are feeling better. Avoid aspirin or aspirin-containing products and avoid large quantities of vitamin C. It is very important to maintain adequate hydration (2-3 L/day of fluids unless instructed to restrict fluid intake) to prevent kidney damage. You may experience dizziness or headache (use caution when driving or engaging in hazardous tasks); photosensitivity (use sunblock, wear protective clothing or dark eye protection, or avoid direct sunlight); nausea, vomiting, or loss of appetite (small frequent meals, frequent mouth care, or sucking on lozenges may help). Diabetics: Drug may cause false tests with

Clinitest® urine glucose monitoring; use of glucose oxidase methods (Clinistix®) or serum glucose monitoring is preferable. Report persistent nausea, vomiting, diarrhea, or abdominal pain; skin rash; persistent or severe sore throat, mouth sores, fever, or vaginal itching or discharge; unusual bruising or bleeding; fatigue; or difficulty breathing.

Ophthalmic: Instill as often as recommended. Wash hands before using. Sit or lie down, open eye, look at ceiling, and instill prescribed amount of solution. Ointment: Pull lower lid down gently and instill thin ribbon of ointment inside lid. Close eye and roll eye in all directions, and apply gentle pressure to inner corner of eye for 1-2 minutes. Do not let tip of applicator touch eye or contaminate tip of applicator. Temporary stinging or blurred vision may occur. Report persistent pain, redness, burning, double vision, severe headache, or respiratory congestion.

**Monitoring Parameters:** CBC, urinalysis, renal function tests, temperature

♦ **Sulfisoxazole Acetyl** *see* Sulfisoxazole *on previous page*

♦ **Sulfisoxazole and Erythromycin** *see* Erythromycin and Sulfisoxazole *on page 330*

# Sulfisoxazole and Phenazopyridine
(sul fi SOKS a zole & fen az oh PEER i deen)
**Pharmacologic Class** Antibiotic, Sulfonamide Derivative; Local Anesthetic
**U.S. Brand Names** Azo-Sulfisoxazole
**Dosage Forms Tab:** Sulfisoxazole 500 mg and phenazopyridine 50 mg

♦ **Sulfizole®** *see* Sulfisoxazole *on previous page*

♦ **Sulfonamide Derivatives** *see* Chart *on page 1027*

# Sulfur and Sulfacetamide Sodium
(SUL fur & sul fa SEE ta mide SOW dee um)
**Pharmacologic Class** Antiseborrheic Agent, Topical
**U.S. Brand Names** Novacet® Topical; Sulfacet-R® Topical
**Dosage Forms Lot, top:** Sulfur colloid 5% and sulfacetamide sodium 10% (30 mL)

# Sulindac (sul IN dak)
**Pharmacologic Class** Nonsteroidal Anti-Inflammatory Agent (NSAID)
**U.S. Brand Names** Clinoril®
**Mechanism of Action** Inhibits prostaglandin synthesis by decreasing the activity of the enzyme, cyclo-oxygenase, which results in decreased formation of prostaglandin precursors
**Use** Management of inflammatory disease, rheumatoid disorders; acute gouty arthritis; structurally similar to indomethacin but acts like aspirin; safest NSAID for use in mild renal impairment
**USUAL DOSAGE** Maximum therapeutic response may not be realized for up to 3 weeks
Oral:
Children: Dose not established
Adults: 150-200 mg twice daily or 300-400 mg once daily; not to exceed 400 mg/day
**Dosing adjustment in hepatic impairment:** Dose reduction is necessary
**Dosage Forms Tab:** 150 mg, 200 mg
**Contraindications** Hypersensitivity to sulindac, any component, aspirin or other nonsteroidal anti-inflammatory drugs (NSAIDs)
**Warnings/Precautions** Use with caution in patients with peptic ulcer disease, GI bleeding, bleeding abnormalities, impaired renal or hepatic function, congestive heart failure, hypertension, and patients receiving anticoagulants
**Pregnancy Risk Factor** B (D at term)
**Adverse Reactions**
>10%:
Central nervous system: Dizziness
Dermatologic: Rash
Gastrointestinal: Abdominal cramps, heartburn, indigestion, nausea
1% to 10%:
Central nervous system: Headache, nervousness
Dermatologic: Itching
Endocrine & metabolic: Fluid retention
Gastrointestinal: Vomiting
Otic: Tinnitus
<1%: Congestive heart failure, hypertension, arrhythmias tachycardia, confusion, hallucinations, aseptic meningitis, mental depression, drowsiness, insomnia, urticaria, erythema multiforme, toxic epidermal necrolysis, Stevens-Johnson syndrome, angioedema, polydipsia, hot flashes, gastritis, GI ulceration, cystitis, polyuria, agranulocytosis, anemia, hemolytic anemia, bone marrow suppression, leukopenia, thrombocytopenia, hepatitis, peripheral neuropathy, toxic amblyopia, blurred vision, conjunctivitis, dry eyes, decreased hearing, acute renal failure, allergic rhinitis, shortness of breath, epistaxis
**Drug Interactions**
Decreased effect of diuretics, beta-blockers, hydralazine, captopril
(Continued)

## Sulindac *(Continued)*

Increased toxicity with probenecid, NSAIDs; increased toxicity of digoxin, methotrexate, lithium, aminoglycosides antibiotics (reported in neonates), cyclosporine (increased nephrotoxicity), potassium-sparing diuretics (hyperkalemia), anticoagulants

**Onset** Analgesic: ~1 hour

**Duration** 12-24 hours

**Half-Life** Parent drug: 7 hours; Active metabolite: 18 hours

**Special PA Issues**

**Patient Education:** Take this medication exactly as directed; do not increase dose without consulting prescriber. Take with food or milk to reduce GI distress. Maintain adequate fluid intake (2-3 L/day). Do not use alcohol, aspirin, or aspirin-containing medication, and all other anti-inflammatory medications without consulting prescriber. You may experience dizziness, nervousness, or headache (use caution when driving or performing hazardous tasks); nausea, vomiting, or heartburn (frequent small meals, frequent oral care, sucking on lozenges, or chewing gum may help); constipation (increased exercise, fluids, or dietary fruit and fiber may help). GI bleeding, ulceration, or perforation can occur with or without pain; discontinue medication and contact prescriber if persistent abdominal pain or cramping, or blood in stool occurs. Report breathlessness or difficulty breathing; unusual bruising/bleeding; blood in urine, stool, mouth, or vomitus; unusual fatigue; skin rash or itching; change in urinary pattern; or change in hearing or ringing in ears.

**Dietary Considerations:** Food: May decrease the rate but not the extent of oral absorption. Drug may cause GI upset, bleeding, ulceration, perforation; take with food or milk to minimize GI upset.

**Monitoring Parameters:** Liver enzymes, BUN, serum creatinine, CBC, blood pressure

**Related Information**

Nonsteroidal Anti-Inflammatory Agents *on page 1026*

♦ **Sulphafurazole** *see* Sulfisoxazole *on page 864*

♦ **Sultrin**™ *see* Sulfabenzamide, Sulfacetamide, and Sulfathiazole *on page 857*

## Sumatriptan Succinate (SOO ma trip tan SUKS i nate)

**Pharmacologic Class** Serotonin 5-HT$_{1D}$ Receptor Agonist

**U.S. Brand Names** Imitrex®

**Mechanism of Action** Selective agonist for serotonin (5-HT$_{1D}$ receptor) in cranial arteries to cause vasoconstriction and reduces sterile inflammation associated with antidromic neuronal transmission correlating with relief of migraine

**Use** Acute treatment of migraine with or without aura

Sumatriptan injection: Acute treatment of cluster headache episodes

**USUAL DOSAGE** Adults:

Oral: 25 mg (taken with fluids); maximum recommended dose is 100 mg. If a satisfactory response has not been obtained at 2 hours, a second dose of up to 100 mg may be given. Efficacy of this second dose has not been examined. If a headache returns, additional doses may be taken at intervals of at least 2 hours up to a daily maximum of 300 mg. There is no evidence that an initial dose of 100 mg provides substantially greater relief than 25 mg.

Intranasal: A single dose of 5, 10 or 20 mg administered in one nostril. A 10 mg dose may be achieved by administering a single 5 mg dose in each nostril. If headache returns, the dose maybe be repeated once after 2 hours not to exceed a total daily dose of 40 mg. The safety of treating an average of >4 headaches in a 30-day period has not been established.

S.C.: 6 mg; a second injection may be administered at least 1 hour after the initial dose, but not more than 2 injections in a 24-hour period. If side effects are dose-limiting, lower doses may be used.

**Dosage Forms Inj:** 12 mg/mL (0.5 mL, 2 mL); **Spray, nasal:** 5 mg (100 mcL), 20 mg (100 mcL); **Tab:** 25 mg, 50 mg

**Contraindications** Intravenous administration; use in patients with ischemic heart disease or Prinzmetal angina, patients with signs or symptoms of ischemic heart disease, uncontrolled HTN; use with ergotamine derivatives (within 24 hours of); use in 24 hours of another 5-HT$_1$ agonist; concurrent administration or within 2 weeks of discontinuing an MAOI; hypersensitivity to any component; management of hemiplegic or basilar migraine

**Warnings/Precautions**

Sumatriptan is indicated only in patient populations with a clear diagnosis of migraine or cluster headache

Cardiac events (coronary artery vasospasm, transient ischemia, myocardial infarction, ventricular tachycardia/fibrillation, cardiac arrest and death) have been reported with 5-HT$_1$ agonist administration. Significant elevation in blood pressure, including hypertensive crisis, has also been reported on rare occasions in patients with and without a history of hypertension. Vasospasm-related reactions have been reported other than coronary artery vasospasm. Peripheral vascular ischemia and colonic ischemia with abdominal pain and bloody diarrhea have occurred.

**Pregnancy Risk Factor** C

**Adverse Reactions**
>10%:
Central nervous system: Dizziness
Endocrine & metabolic: Hot flashes
Local: Injection site reaction
Neuromuscular & skeletal: Paresthesia
1% to 10%:
Cardiovascular: Tightness in chest
Central nervous system: Drowsiness, headache
Dermatologic: Burning sensation
Gastrointestinal: Abdominal discomfort, mouth discomfort
Neuromuscular & skeletal: Myalgia, numbness, weakness, neck pain, jaw discomfort
Miscellaneous: Diaphoresis
<1%: Rashes, polydipsia, dehydration, dysmenorrhea, dysuria, renal calculus, dyspnea, thirst, hiccups

**Drug Interactions** Increased toxicity: Ergot-containing drugs, MAOIs, SSRIs can lead to symptoms of hyper-reflexia, weakness, and incoordination

**Onset** Within 30 minutes

**Half-Life** After S.C. administration: Distribution: 15 minutes; Terminal: 115 minutes

**Special PA Issues**
**Patient Education:** Take at first sign of migraine attack. This drug is to be used to reduce your migraine, not to prevent or reduce number of attacks. Oral: If headache returns or is not fully resolved after first dose, the dose may be repeated after 2 hours. **Do not exceed 300 mg in 24 hours.** S.C.: If headache returns or is not fully resolved after first dose, the dose may be repeated after 1 hour. **Do not exceed two injections in 24 hours. Do not take within 24 hours of any other migraine medication without first consulting prescriber.** You may experience some dizziness (use caution); hot flashes (cool room may help); nausea or vomiting (frequent small meals or sucking on lozenges may help); pain at injection site (lasts about 1 hour, will resolve); or excess sweating (will resolve). Report chest tightness or pain; excessive drowsiness; acute abdominal pain; skin rash or burning sensation; muscle weakness, soreness, or numbness; or respiratory difficulty.

♦ **Summer's Eve® Medicated Douche [OTC]** see Povidone-Iodine on page 747
♦ **Sumycin® Oral** see Tetracycline on page 885
♦ **Supeudol®** see Oxycodone on page 687
♦ **Supprelin™ Injection** see Histrelin on page 442
♦ **Suprax®** see Cefixime on page 163

# Suprofen (soo PROE fen)

**Pharmacologic Class** Nonsteroidal Anti-Inflammatory Agent (NSAID)

**U.S. Brand Names** Profenal®

**Mechanism of Action** Inhibits prostaglandin synthesis, acts on the hypothalamus heat-regulating center to reduce fever, blocks prostaglandin synthetase action which prevents formation of the platelet-aggregating substance thromboxane $A_2$; decreases pain receptor sensitivity.

**Use** Inhibition of intraoperative miosis

**USUAL DOSAGE** Adults: On day of surgery, instill 2 drops in conjunctival sac at 3, 2, and 1 hour prior to surgery; or 2 drops in sac every 4 hours, while awake, the day preceding surgery

**Dosage Forms** Soln, ophth: 1% (2.5 mL)

**Contraindications** Previous hypersensitivity or intolerance to suprofen; epithelial herpes simplex keratitis; history of hypersensitivity reactions to aspirin or other nonsteroidal anti-inflammatory agents

**Warnings/Precautions** Use with caution in patients sensitive to acetylsalicylic acid and other NSAIDs; some systemic absorption occurs; use with caution in patients with bleeding tendencies; perform ophthalmic evaluation for those who develop eye complaints during therapy (blurred vision, diminished vision, changes in color vision, retinal changes)

**Pregnancy Risk Factor** C

**Adverse Reactions**
1% to 10%: Topical: Transient burning or stinging, redness, iritis
<1%: Chemosis, photophobia, discomfort, pain, punctate epithelial staining

**Drug Interactions** Decreased effect: When used concurrently with suprofen, acetylcholine chloride and carbachol may be ineffective

**Special PA Issues**
**Patient Education:** Avoid aspirin and aspirin-containing products while taking this medication; get instructions on administration of eye drops

♦ **Surfak® [OTC]** see Docusate on page 298
♦ **Surmontil®** see Trimipramine on page 938
♦ **Survanta®** see Beractant on page 110
♦ **Susano®** see Hyoscyamine, Atropine, Scopolamine, and Phenobarbital on page 464

## Tacrine (TAK reen)

**Pharmacologic Class** Acetylcholinesterase Inhibitor (Central)

**U.S. Brand Names** Cognex®

**Use** Treatment of mild to moderate dementia of the Alzheimer's type

**USUAL DOSAGE** Adults: Initial: 10 mg 4 times/day; may increase by 40 mg/day adjusted every 6 weeks; maximum: 160 mg/day; best administered separate from meal times; see table.

### Dose Adjustment Based Upon Transaminase Elevations

| ALT | Regimen |
|---|---|
| ≤3 x ULN* | Continue titration |
| >3 to ≤5 x ULN | Decrease dose by 40 mg/day, resume when ALT returns to normal |
| >5 x ULN | Stop treatment, may rechallenge upon return of ALT to normal |

*ULN = upper limit of normal.

Patients with clinical jaundice confirmed by elevated total bilirubin (>3 mg/dL) should not be rechallenged with tacrine

**Dosage Forms Cap, as hydrochloride:** 10 mg, 20 mg, 30 mg, 40 mg

**Contraindications** Patients previously treated with the drug who developed jaundice and in those who are hypersensitive to tacrine or acridine derivatives

**Warnings/Precautions** The use of tacrine has been associated with elevations in serum transaminases; serum transaminases (specifically ALT) must be monitored throughout therapy; use extreme caution in patients with current evidence of a history of abnormal liver function tests; use caution in patients with bladder outlet obstruction, asthma, and sick-sinus syndrome (tacrine may cause bradycardia). Also, patients with cardiovascular disease, asthma, or peptic ulcer should use cautiously.

**Pregnancy Risk Factor** C

**Drug Interactions** CYP1A2 enzyme substrate; CYP1A2 inhibitor

Increased effect of theophylline, cimetidine, succinylcholine, cholinesterase inhibitors, or cholinergic agonists

**Onset** May require weeks of treatment

**Half-Life** 2-4 hours

**Special PA Issues**

**Patient Education:** This medication will not cure the disease, but may help reduce symptoms. Use as directed; do not increase dose or discontinue without consulting prescriber. Maintain adequate hydration (2-3 L/day of fluids unless instructed to restrict fluid intake). May cause dizziness, sedation, or hypotension (rise slowly from sitting or lying position and use caution when driving or climbing stairs); vomiting or loss of appetite (frequent small meals, frequent mouth care, or sucking lozenges may help); or diarrhea (boiled milk, yogurt, or buttermilk may help). Report persistent abdominal discomfort; significantly increased salivation, sweating, tearing, or urination; flushed skin; chest pain or palpitations; acute headache; unresolved diarrhea; excessive fatigue, insomnia, dizziness, or depression; increased muscle, joint, or body pain; vision changes or blurred vision; shortness of breath or wheezing; or signs of jaundice (yellowing of eyes or skin, dark colored urine or light colored stool, abdominal pain, or easy fatigue).

**Monitoring Parameters:** ALT (SGPT) levels and other liver enzymes weekly for at least the first 18 weeks, then monitor once every 3 months

**Reference Range:** In clinical trials, serum concentrations >20 ng/mL were associated with a much higher risk of development of symptomatic adverse effects

♦ **Tacrine Hydrochloride** *see* Tacrine *on previous page*

# Tacrolimus (ta KROE li mus)

**Pharmacologic Class** Immunosuppressant Agent

**U.S. Brand Names** Prograf®

**Mechanism of Action** Binds to 40 FK binding protein resulting in inhibition of calcium-dependent signal transduction pathway in T cells, thereby blocking the secretion of IL-2 and other cytokines

**Use** Potent immunosuppressive drug used in liver, kidney, heart, lung, small bowel transplant recipients; immunosuppressive drug for peripheral stem cell/bone marrow transplantation

**USUAL DOSAGE**

Children: Patients without pre-existing renal or hepatic dysfunction have required and tolerated higher doses than adults to achieve similar blood concentrations. It is recommended that therapy be initiated at high end of the recommended adult I.V. and oral dosing ranges.

Oral: 0.3 mg/kg/day divided every 12 hours; children generally require higher maintenance dosages on a mg/kg basis than adults

I.V. continuous infusion: 0.05-0.15 mg/kg/day

Adults:

Oral (usually 3-4 times the I.V. dose): 0.15-0.30 mg/kg/day in two divided doses administered every 12 hours and given 8-12 hours after discontinuation of the I.V. infusion. Lower tacrolimus doses may be sufficient as maintenance therapy.

**Solid organ transplantation:** Oral: 0.15-0.30 mg/kg/day in two divided doses administered every 12 hours; lower tacrolimus doses may be sufficient as maintenance therapy

**Peripheral stem cell/bone marrow transplantation:** Oral (usually ~2-3 times the intravenous dose): 0.06-0.09 mg/kg/day (maximum: 0.12 mg/kg/day) in two divided doses administered every 12 hours and given 8-12 hours after discontinuation of the intravenous infusion; adjust doses based on trough serum concentrations

I.V.:

**Solid organ transplantation:** Initial (given at least 6 hours after transplantation): 0.05-0.10 mg/kg/day; corticosteroid therapy is advised to enhance immunosuppression. Patients should be switched to oral therapy as soon as possible (within 2-3 days).

**Peripheral stem cell/bone marrow transplantation:** Initial: 0.03 mg/kg/day as a continuous intravenous infusion

**Dosing adjustment in renal impairment:** Evidence suggests that lower doses should be used; patients should receive doses at the lowest value of the recommended I.V. and oral dosing ranges; further reductions in dose below these ranges may be required

Tacrolimus therapy should usually be delayed up to 48 hours or longer in patients with postoperative oliguria

Hemodialysis: Not removed by hemodialysis; supplemental dose is not necessary

Peritoneal dialysis: Significant drug removal is unlikely based on physiochemical characteristics

**Dosing adjustment in hepatic impairment:** Use of tacrolimus in liver transplant recipients experiencing post-transplant hepatic impairment may be associated with increased risk of developing renal insufficiency related to high whole blood levels of tacrolimus. The presence of moderate-to-severe hepatic dysfunction (serum bilirubin >2 mg/dL) appears to affect the metabolism of FK506. The half-life of the drug was prolonged and the clearance reduced after I.V. administration. The bioavailability of FK506 was also increased after oral administration. The higher plasma concentrations as determined by ELISA, in patients with severe hepatic dysfunction are probably due to the accumulation of FK506

(Continued)

## Tacrolimus *(Continued)*

metabolites of lower activity. These patients should be monitored closely and dosage adjustments should be considered. Some evidence indicates that lower doses could be used in these patients. See table.

### Dosing Tacrolimus

| Condition | Tacrolimus |
|---|---|
| Switch from I.V. to oral therapy | Threefold increase in dose |
| T-tube clamping | No change in dose |
| Pediatric patients | About 2 times higher dose compared to adults |
| Liver dysfunction | Decrease I.V. dose; decrease oral dose |
| Renal dysfunction | Does not affect kinetics; decrease dose to decrease levels if renal dysfunction is related to the drug |
| Dialysis | Not removed |
| Inhibitors of hepatic metabolism | Decrease dose |
| Inducers of hepatic metabolism | Monitor drug level; increase dose |

**Dosage Forms Cap:** 1 mg, 5 mg; **Inj, with alcohol and surfactant:** 5 mg/mL (1 mL)

**Contraindications** Hypersensitivity to tacrolimus or any component; hypersensitivity to HCO-60 polyoxyl 60 hydrogenated castor oil (used in the parenteral dosage formulation) is a contraindication to parenteral tacrolimus therapy

**Warnings/Precautions** Increased susceptibility to infection and the possible development of lymphoma may occur after administration of tacrolimus; it should not be administered simultaneously with cyclosporine; since the pharmacokinetics show great inter- and intrapatient variability over time, monitoring of serum concentrations (trough for oral therapy) is essential to prevent organ rejection and reduce drug-related toxicity; tonic clonic seizures may have been triggered by tacrolimus. Injection contains small volume of ethanol.

**Pregnancy Risk Factor** C

**Pregnancy Implications**

Tacrolimus crosses the placenta and reaches concentrations four times greater than maternal plasma concentrations

Tacrolimus concentrations in breast milk are equivalent to plasma concentrations; breast-feeding is not advised while therapy is ongoing

### Drug Interactions With Tacrolimus

| Drugs Which May INCREASE Tacrolimus Blood Levels | | |
|---|---|---|
| Calcium Channel Blockers | Antibiotic/Antifungal Agents | Other Drugs |
| Diltiazem<br>Nicardipine<br>Verapamil | Clotrimazole<br>Erythromycin<br>Fluconazole<br>Itraconazole<br>Ketoconazole | Bromocriptine<br>Cimetidine<br>Clarithromycin<br>Cyclosporine<br>Danazol<br>Methylprednisolone<br>Metoclopramide<br>Grapefruit juice |
| Drugs Which May DECREASE Tacrolimus Blood Levels | | |
| Anticonvulsants | Antibiotics | |
| Carbamazepine<br>Phenobarbital<br>Phenytoin | Rifabutin<br>Rifampin | |

### Adverse Reactions

>10%:

Cardiovascular: Hypertension, peripheral edema

Central nervous system: Headache, insomnia, pain, fever

Dermatologic: Pruritus

Endocrine & metabolic: Hypo-/hyperkalemia, hyperglycemia, hypomagnesemia

Gastrointestinal: Diarrhea, nausea, anorexia, vomiting, abdominal pain

Hematologic: Anemia, leukocytosis

Hepatic: LFT abnormalities, ascites

Neuromuscular & skeletal: Tremors, paresthesias, back pain, weakness

Renal: Nephrotoxicity, increased BUN/creatinine

Respiratory: Pleural effusion, atelectasis, dyspnea

Miscellaneous: Infection

1% to 10%:

Central nervous system: Seizures

Dermatologic: Rash

Endocrine & metabolic: Hyperphosphatemia, hyperuricemia, pancreatitis

Gastrointestinal: Constipation

Genitourinary: Urinary tract infection

Hematologic: Thrombocytopenia

Neuromuscular & skeletal: Myoclonus

Renal: Oliguria

<1%: Hypertrophic cardiomyopathy, arthralgia, myalgia, hemolytic uremic syndrome, anaphylaxis, expressive aphasia, photophobia, secondary malignancy

**Drug Interactions** CYP3A3/4 enzyme substrate

Decreased effect: Separate administration of antacids and Carafate® from tacrolimus by at least 2 hours

Increased effect: Cyclosporine is associated with synergistic immunosuppression and increased nephrotoxicity

Increased toxicity: Nephrotoxic antibiotics, NSAIDs and amphotericin B potentially increase nephrotoxicity

See table.

**Half-Life** 12 hours (range: 4-40 hours)

**Special PA Issues**

**Patient Education:** Take as directed, preferably 30 minutes hour before or 30 minutes after meals. Do not take within 2 hours before or after antacids. Do not alter dose and do not discontinue without consulting prescriber. Maintain adequate hydration (2-3 L/day of fluids unless instructed to restrict fluid intake) during entire course of therapy. You will be susceptible to infection (avoid crowds and people with infections or contagious diseases). If you are diabetic, monitor glucose levels closely (may alter glucose levels). You may experience nausea, vomiting, loss of appetite (frequent small meals, frequent mouth care may help); diarrhea (boiled milk, yogurt, or buttermilk may help); constipation (increased exercise or dietary fruit, fluid, or fiber may help, if not consult prescriber); muscle or back pain (mild analgesics may be recommended). Report chest pain; acute headache or dizziness; symptoms of respiratory infection, cough, or difficulty breathing; unresolved gastrointestinal effects; fatigue, chills, fever, unhealed sores, white plaques in mouth, irritation in genital area; unusual bruising or bleeding; pain or irritation on urination or change in urinary patterns; rash or skin irritation; or other unusual effects related to this medication.

**Monitoring Parameters:** Renal function, hepatic function, serum electrolytes, glucose and blood pressure, hypersensitivity indicators, neurological responses, and other clinical parameters; monitoring of serum concentrations (trough for oral therapy); measure 3 times/week for first few weeks, then gradually decrease frequency as patient stabilizes

**Reference Range:**

**Whole blood:** Trough level: 7-20 ng/mL (ELISA). Plasma levels are generally 0.02-0.2 times whole blood levels; increased precision with whole blood levels.

**Plasma:** Trough level: 0.5-2 ng/mL (ELISA, plasma, extracted at 37°C) for all transplant procedures (liver, heart, lung, kidney, small bowel) whole blood measurements produce concentration 5-40 times higher than those in serum due to high binding to RBCs (therapeutic range: 5-10 ng/mL, although levels >20 mg/mL may be desirable for short periods to prevent rejection)

♦ **Tagamet®** *see* Cimetidine *on page 208*

♦ **Tagamet® HB [OTC]** *see* Cimetidine *on page 208*

♦ **Talwin®** *see* Pentazocine *on page 708*

♦ **Talwin® NX** *see* Pentazocine *on page 708*

♦ **Tambocor™** *see* Flecainide *on page 373*

♦ **Tamofen®** *see* Tamoxifen *on this page*

♦ **Tamone®** *see* Tamoxifen *on this page*

# Tamoxifen (ta MOKS i fen)

**Pharmacologic Class** Antineoplastic Agent, Miscellaneous

**U.S. Brand Names** Nolvadex®

**Mechanism of Action** Competitively binds to estrogen receptors on tumors and other tissue targets, producing a nuclear complex that decreases DNA synthesis and inhibits estrogen effects; nonsteroidal agent with potent antiestrogenic properties which compete with estrogen for binding sites in breast and other tissues; cells accumulate in the $G_0$ and $G_1$ phases; therefore, tamoxifen is cytostatic rather than cytocidal.

**Use** Palliative or adjunctive treatment of advanced breast cancer; reduce the incidence of breast cancer in women at high risk (taking into account age, number of first-degree relatives with breast cancer, previous breast biopsies, age at first live birth, age at first menstrual period, and a history of lobular carcinoma *in situ*)

**Unlabeled use:** Treatment of mastalgia, gynecomastia, male breast cancer, and pancreatic carcinoma. Studies have shown tamoxifen to be effective in the treatment of primary breast cancer in elderly women. Comparative studies with other antineoplastic agents in elderly women with breast cancer had more favorable survival rates with tamoxifen. Initiation of hormone therapy rather than chemotherapy is justified for elderly patients with metastatic breast cancer who are responsive.

(Continued)

## Tamoxifen *(Continued)*

**USUAL DOSAGE** Oral (refer to individual protocols):
Adults: 10-20 mg twice daily in the morning and evening
High-dose therapy is under investigation

**Dosage Forms Tab, as citrate:** 10 mg, 20 mg

**Contraindications** Hypersensitivity to tamoxifen

**Warnings/Precautions** Use with caution in patients with leukopenia, thrombocytopenia, or hyperlipidemias; ovulation may be induced; "hot flashes" may be countered by Bellergal-S® tablets; decreased visual acuity, retinopathy, and corneal changes have been reported with use for more than 1 year at doses above recommended; hypercalcemia in patients with bone metastasis; hepatocellular carcinomas have been reported in animal studies; endometrial hyperplasia and polyps have occurred

**Pregnancy Risk Factor** D

**Adverse Reactions**

>10%:

Cardiovascular: Flushing

Dermatologic: Skin rash

Gastrointestinal: Little to mild nausea (10%), vomiting, weight gain

Hematologic: Myelosuppressive: Transient thrombocytopenia occurs in ~24% of patients receiving 10-20 mg/day; platelet counts return to normal within several weeks in spite of continued administration; leukopenia has also been reported and does resolve during continued therapy; anemia has also been reported

WBC: Rare

Platelets: None

Hepatic: Hepatotoxicity

Neuromuscular & skeletal: Increased bone and tumor pain and local disease flare shortly after starting therapy; this will subside rapidly, but patients should be aware of this since many may discontinue the drug due to the side effects

1% to 10%:

Cardiovascular: Thromboembolism: Tamoxifen has been associated with the occurrence of venous thrombosis and pulmonary embolism; arterial thrombosis has also been described in a few case reports

Central nervous system: Lightheadedness, depression, dizziness, headache, lassitude, mental confusion

Dermatologic: Rash

Endocrine & metabolic: Hypercalcemia may occur in patients with bone metastases; galactorrhea and vitamin deficiency, menstrual irregularities

Genitourinary: Vaginal bleeding or discharge, endometriosis, priapism, possible endometrial cancer

Neuromuscular & skeletal: Weakness

Ocular: Ophthalmologic effects (visual acuity changes, cataracts, or retinopathy), corneal opacities

**Drug Interactions** CYP1A2, 2A6, 2B6, 2C, 2D6, 2E1, and 3A3/4 enzyme substrate

Increased toxicity: Allopurinol results in exacerbation of allopurinol-induced hepatotoxicity; cyclosporine may result in increase in cyclosporine serum levels; warfarin results in significant enhancement of the anticoagulant effects of warfarin

**Half-Life** 7 days

**Special PA Issues**

**Patient Education:** Take as directed, morning and night and maintain adequate hydration (2-3 L/day of fluids unless instructed to restrict fluid intake). You may experience menstrual irregularities, vaginal bleeding, hot flashes, hair loss, loss of libido (these will subside when treatment is completed). Bone pain may indicate a good therapeutic responses (consult prescriber for mild analgesics). For nausea, vomiting small, frequent meals, chewing gum, or sucking on lozenges may help. You may experience photosensitivity (avoid direct sunlight, wear protective clothing, or use sunblock). Report unusual bleeding or bruising, severe weakness, sedation, mental changes, swelling or pain in calves, difficulty breathing, or any changes in vision.

**Monitoring Parameters:** Monitor WBC and platelet counts, tumor

♦ **Tamoxifen Citrate** *see* Tamoxifen *on previous page*

## Tamsulosin *(tam SOO loe sin)*

**Pharmacologic Class** Alpha₁ Blockers

**U.S. Brand Names** Flomax®

**Mechanism of Action** An antagonist of alpha$_{1A}$ adrenoceptors in the prostate. Three subtypes identified: alpha$_{1A}$, alpha$_{1B}$, alpha$_{1D}$ have distribution that differs between human organs and tissue. Approximately 70% of the alpha₁-receptors in human prostate are of alpha$_{1A}$ subtype. The symptoms associated with benign prostatic hyperplasia (BPH) are related to bladder outlet obstruction, which is comprised of two underlying components: static and dynamic. Static is related to an increase in prostate size, partially caused by a proliferation of smooth muscle cells in the prostatic stroma. Severity of BPH symptoms and the degree of urethral obstruction do not correlate well with the size of the prostate.

Dynamic is a function of an increase in smooth muscle tone in the prostate and bladder neck leading to constriction of the bladder outlet. Smooth muscle tone is mediated by the sympathetic nervous stimulation of alpha$_1$ adrenoceptors, which are abundant in the prostate, prostatic capsule, prostatic urethra, and bladder neck. Blockade of these adrenoceptors can cause smooth muscles in the bladder neck and prostate to relax, resulting in an improvement in urine flow rate and a reduction in symptoms of BPH.

**Use** Treatment of signs and symptoms of benign prostatic hyperplasia (BPH)

**USUAL DOSAGE** Oral: Adults: 0.4 mg once daily approximately 30 minutes after the same meal each day

**Dosage Forms Cap, as hydrochloride:** 0.4 mg

**Warnings/Precautions** Not intended for use as an antihypertensive drug; may cause orthostasis (ie, postural hypotension, dizziness, vertigo); patients should avoid situations where injury could result if syncope occurs; rule out the presence of carcinoma of prostate before beginning tamsulosin therapy

**Pregnancy Risk Factor** C

**Adverse Reactions**

Central nervous system: Headache, dizziness (0.4 mg: 14.9%; 0.8 mg: 17.1%), somnolence (0.4 mg: 3.0%; 0.8 mg: 4.3%), insomnia

Endocrine & metabolic: Decreased libido

Gastrointestinal: Diarrhea, nausea, tooth disorder

Genitourinary: Ejaculation disturbances

Neuromuscular & skeletal: Back pain, chest pain, asthenia

Ocular: Amblyopia

Respiratory: Rhinitis, pharyngitis, increased cough, sinusitis

Miscellaneous: Infections, allergic-type reactions such as skin rash, pruritus, angioedema, and urticaria have been reported upon drug rechallenge

**Drug Interactions** Use caution with concomitant administration of warfarin and tamsulosin; no dosage adjustments necessary if administered with atenolol, enalapril, or Procardia XL®; cimetidine resulted in a significant decrease (26%) in the clearance of tamsulosin which resulted in a moderate increase in tamsulosin AUC (44%); therefore, use with caution when used in combination with cimetidine (especially doses >0.4 mg); do not use in combination with other alpha-adrenergic blocking agents

**Half-Life** Healthy volunteers: 9-13 hours; target population: 14-15 hours

**Special PA Issues**

**Patient Education:** Take as directed 30 minutes, after same meal each day. Do not skip dose or discontinue without consulting prescriber. You may experience drowsiness, dizziness, or impaired judgment (use caution when driving or engaging in tasks that require alertness until response is known); postural hypotension (use caution when rising from sitting or lying position or when climbing stairs); nausea (frequent mouth care or sucking lozenges may help); urinary incontinence (void before taking medication); ejaculatory disturbance (reversible, may resolve with continued use); diarrhea (boiled milk or yogurt may help); palpitations or rapid heartbeat; difficulty breathing, unusual cough, or sore throat; or other persistent side effects.

**Dietary Considerations:** The time to maximum concentration ($T_{max}$) is reached by 4-5 hours under fasting conditions and by 6-7 hours when administered with food. Taking it under fasted conditions results in a 30% increase in bioavailability and 40% to 70% increase in peak concentrations ($C_{max}$) compared to fed conditions.

## Tazarotene (taz AR oh teen)

**Pharmacologic Class** Keratolytic Agent

**U.S. Brand Names** Tazorac®

**Mechanism of Action** Synthetic, acetylenic retinoid which modulates differentiation and proliferation of epithelial tissue and exerts some degree of anti-inflammatory and immunological activity

(Continued)

## Tazarotene *(Continued)*

**Use** Topical treatment of facial acne vulgaris; topical treatment of stable plaque psoriasis of up to 20% body surface area involvement

**USUAL DOSAGE** Children >12 years and Adults: Topical:

Acne: Cleanse the face gently. After the skin is dry, apply a thin film of tazarotene (2 mg/cm$^2$) once daily, in the evening, to the skin where the acne lesions appear. Use enough to cover the entire affected area. Tazarotene was investigated ≤12 weeks during clinical trials for acne.

Psoriasis: Apply tazarotene once daily, in the evening, to psoriatic lesions using enough (2 mg/cm$^2$) to cover only the lesion with a thin film to no more than 20% of body surface area. If a bath or shower is taken prior to application, dry the skin before applying the gel. Because unaffected skin may be more susceptible to irritation, avoid application of tazarotene to these areas. Tazarotene was investigated for up to 12 months during clinical trials for psoriasis.

**Dosage Forms** Gel: 0.05% (30 g, 100 g), 0.1% (30 g, 100 g)

**Contraindications** Hypersensitivity to tazarotene and other retinoids or vitamin A derivatives (isotretinoin, tretinoin, etretinate); pregnancy

**Warnings/Precautions** Use with caution in patients who are breast-feeding. Use with caution in patients with eczema or open wounds (increased irritation and absorption may occur). Because of heightened burning susceptibility, exposure to sunlight should be avoided unless deemed medically necessary, and in such cases, exposure should be minimized during use of tazarotene. Administer with caution if the patient is also taking drugs known to be photosensitizers (thiazides, tetracyclines, fluoroquinolones, phenothiazines, sulfonamides) because of the increased possibility of augmented photosensitivity. Patients should be warned to use sunscreens (SPF minimum of 15) and protective clothing when using tazarotene. Application may cause a transitory feeling of burning or stinging. For external use only; avoid contact with eyes, eyelids, and mouth. The safety of use over >20% of body surface area has not been established.

**Pregnancy Risk Factor** X

**Adverse Reactions**

>10%: Local: Pruritus, burning/stinging, erythema, worsening of psoriasis, irritation, skin pain

1% to 10%: Dermatologic: Rash, desquamation, irritant contact dermatitis, skin inflammation, fissure, bleeding, dry skin, skin discoloration

**Special PA Issues**

**Patient Education:** Do not take this medication if you have had an allergic reaction to tazarotene. Do not use tazarotene if you are pregnant or planning to become pregnant. Tazarotene may cause birth defects or be harmful to an unborn baby if used during pregnancy. This may be more likely if the medicine is used on large areas of skin.

Your physician will tell you how much medicine to use and how often. Do not use more of the medication than your physician ordered. Using too much of the medication can cause red, peeling, or irritated skin. Wash your hands before and after using this medication (unless treating psoriasis lesions on your hands). Use this medication on your skin only. Do not put the medication in your eyes, eyelids, or in your mouth. If you do get the medication in your eyes, rinse them with large amounts of cool water. Tell your physician if you have eye pain or redness that does not go away.

Acne patients: Gently wash and dry your face. Apply a thin layer of medication to cover the acne. Your acne should start to clear up in about 4 weeks.

Psoriasis patients: If using the medication after bathing or showering, make sure your skin is completely dry before applying the medication. Apply a thin layer to lesions.

Wash off any medication that gets on skin areas that do not need to be treated. The medication can irritate skin that does not need treatment. Do not bandage or cover the treated skin. Ask your physician or pharmacist before taking any other medication, including over-the-counter products. Talk with your physician or pharmacist before using medicated cosmetics or shampoos, abrasive soaps or cleansers, products with alcohol, spice, or lime in them, other acne medicines, hair removal products, or products that dry your skin.

This medication may make your skin sensitive to sunlight and cause a rash or sunburn. Avoid spending long periods of time in direct sunlight and protect your skin with clothing and a strong sunscreen when you are outdoors. Do not use a sunlamp or tanning booth. Call your physician if you have blistering or crusting skin, severe redness, pain, or swelling on the areas that you use the medication.

**Monitoring Parameters:** Disease severity in plaque psoriasis during therapy (reduction in erythema, scaling, induration); routine blood chemistries (including transaminases) are suggested during long-term topical therapy

◆ **Tazicef®** *see* Ceftazidime *on page 172*

◆ **Tazidime®** *see* Ceftazidime *on page 172*

◆ **Tazorac®** *see* Tazarotene *on previous page*

◆ **3TC** *see* Lamivudine *on page 513*

## Telmisartan (Continued)

May increase serum digoxin levels (increased peak levels by a median of 49% and trough levels by 20%)

Has been associated with slight reductions in warfarin serum concentrations; however, this was not associated with a change in INR

**Onset** 1-2 hours
**Duration** Up to 24 hours
**Half-Life** Terminal: ~24 hours

**Special PA Issues**
**Patient Education:** Take exactly as directed. Do not miss doses, alter dosage, or discontinue without consulting prescriber. Do not alter salt or potassium intake without consulting prescriber. Monitor blood pressure on a regular basis as recommended by prescriber; at same time each day. You may experience postural hypotension (change position slowly when rising from sitting or lying, when climbing stairs, or bending over); or transient nervousness, headache, insomnia (use caution when driving or engaging in hazardous tasks until response to medication is known). Report unusual weight gain or swelling of ankles and hands; swelling of face, lips, throat, or tongue; persistent fatigue; dry cough or difficulty breathing; palpitations or chest pain; CNS changes; gastrointestinal disturbances; muscle or bone pain, cramping, or tremors; change in urinary pattern; or changes in hearing or vision.

**Dietary Considerations:** May be administered without regard to food

**Monitoring Parameters:** Supine blood pressure, electrolytes, serum creatinine, BUN, urinalysis, symptomatic hypotension, and tachycardia

## Temazepam (te MAZ e pam)
**Pharmacologic Class** Benzodiazepine

**U.S. Brand Names** Restoril®

**Mechanism of Action** Benzodiazepine anxiolytic sedative that produces CNS depression at the subcortical level, except at high doses, whereby it works at the cortical level; causes minimal change in REM sleep patterns

**Use** Treatment of anxiety and as an adjunct in the treatment of depression; also may be used in the management of panic attacks; transient insomnia and sleep latency

**USUAL DOSAGE** Adults: Oral: 15-30 mg at bedtime; 15 mg in elderly or debilitated patients

**Dosage Forms** Cap: 7.5 mg, 15 mg, 30 mg

**Contraindications** Hypersensitivity to temazepam or any component, severe uncontrolled pain, pre-existing CNS depression, or narrow-angle glaucoma; not to be used in pregnancy or lactation

**Warnings/Precautions** Safety and efficacy in children <18 years of age have not been established; do not use in pregnant women; may cause drug dependency; avoid abrupt discontinuance in patients with prolonged therapy or seizure disorders; use with caution in patients receiving other CNS depressants, in patients with hepatic dysfunction, and the elderly

**Pregnancy Risk Factor X**

**Adverse Reactions**
<10%:
Cardiovascular: Tachycardia, chest pain
Central nervous system: Drowsiness, fatigue, ataxia, lightheadedness, memory impairment, insomnia, anxiety, depression, headache
Dermatologic: Rash
Endocrine & metabolic: Decreased libido
Gastrointestinal: Xerostomia, constipation, diarrhea, decreased salivation, nausea, vomiting, increased or decreased appetite
Neuromuscular & skeletal: Dysarthria
Ocular: Blurred vision
Miscellaneous: Diaphoresis
1% to 10%:
Cardiovascular: Syncope, hypotension
Central nervous system: Confusion, nervousness, dizziness, akathisia
Dermatologic: Dermatitis
Gastrointestinal: Increased salivation, weight gain or loss
Otic: Tinnitus
Neuromuscular & skeletal: Rigidity, tremor, muscle cramps
Respiratory: Nasal congestion, hyperventilation
<1%: Menstrual irregularities, blood dyscrasias, reflex slowing, drug dependence

**Drug Interactions** CYP3A3/4 enzyme substrate
Increased effect of CNS depressants

**Half-Life** 9.5-12.4 hours

**Special PA Issues**
**Patient Education:** Use exactly as directed (do not increase dose or frequency or discontinue without consulting prescriber); may cause physical and/or psychological dependence. May take with food to decrease GI upset. While using this medication, do

- **TCN** see Tetracycline on page 885
- **Td** see Diphtheria and Tetanus Toxoid on page 291
- **Tebamide®** see Trimethobenzamide on page 936
- **Tebrazid** see Pyrazinamide on page 782
- **Teczem®** see Enalapril and Diltiazem on page 318
- **Tedral®** see Theophylline, Ephedrine, and Phenobarbital on page 888
- **Tegison®** see Etretinate on page 356
- **Tegopen®** see Cloxacillin on page 229
- **Tegretol®** see Carbamazepine on page 148
- **Tegretol®-XR** see Carbamazepine on page 148
- **Tegrin®-HC [OTC]** see Hydrocortisone on page 453
- **Teladar®** see Betamethasone on page 111

## Telmisartan (tel mi SAR tan)

**Pharmacologic Class** Angiotensin II Antagonists

**U.S. Brand Names** Micardis®

**Mechanism of Action** Angiotensin II acts as a vasoconstrictor. In addition to causing direct vasoconstriction, angiotensin II also stimulates the release of aldosterone. Once aldosterone is released, sodium as well as water are reabsorbed. The end result is an elevation in blood pressure. Telmisartan is a nonpeptide AT1 angiotensin II receptor antagonist. This binding prevents angiotensin II from binding to the receptor thereby blocking the vasoconstriction and the aldosterone secreting effects of angiotensin II.

**Use** Alone or in combination with other antihypertensive agents in treating essential hypertension

**USUAL DOSAGE** Adults: Oral: Initial: 40 mg once daily; may be administered with or without food; usual maintenance dose range: 20-80 mg/day

Patients with volume depletion: Should be initiated on a lower dosage with close supervision or the condition should be corrected prior to initiating therapy or the use of an alternative AT II antagonist during initiation of therapy's warranted

Dosing in the elderly: No initial dose adjustment is required

Dosing in hepatic/biliary impairment: Supervise patient closely

Dosing in renal impairment: No initial dosing adjustment is necessary; patients on dialysis may develop orthostatic hypotension

**Dosage Forms** Tab: 40 mg, 80 mg

**Contraindications** Hypersensitivity to telmisartan or any component (telmisartan, sodium hydroxide, meglumine, povidone, sorbitol, magnesium stearate); sensitivity to other A-II receptor antagonists; pregnancy

**Warnings/Precautions** Avoid use or use smaller dose if volume-depleted patients. Drugs which alter renin-angiotensin system have been associated with deterioration in renal function, including oliguria, acute renal failure, and progressive azotemia. Use with caution in patients with renal artery stenosis (unilateral or bilateral) to avoid decrease in renal function; use caution in patients with pre-existing renal insufficiency (may decrease renal perfusion); the major route of elimination for telmisartan is via biliary elimination and as a result, patients with biliary obstruction can be expected to have reduced clearance and, therefore, telmisartan should be used with caution.

**Pregnancy Risk Factor** C (1st trimester); D (2nd and 3rd trimester)

**Pregnancy Implications** Avoid use in the nursing mother, if possible, since telmisartan may be excreted in breast milk. The drug should be discontinued as soon as possible when pregnancy is detected. Drugs which act directly on renin-angiotensin can cause fetal and neonatal morbidity and death.

**Adverse Reactions**
1% to 10%:
Cardiovascular: Hypertension (1%), chest pain (1%), peripheral edema (1%)
Central nervous system: Headache (1%), dizziness (1%), pain (1%), fatigue (1%)
Gastrointestinal: Diarrhea (3%, compared to 2% with placebo), dyspepsia (1%), nausea (1%), abdominal pain (1%)
Genitourinary: Urinary tract infection (7%, compared to 6% with placebo)
Neuromuscular & skeletal: Back pain (3%, compared to 1% with placebo), myalgia (1%)
Respiratory: Upper respiratory infection (7%, compared to 6% with placebo), sinusitis (3%, compared to 2% with placebo), pharyngitis (1%, cough (1.6%, same as placebo)
Miscellaneous: Flu-like syndrome (1%)
<1%: Angioedema, allergic reaction, elevate liver enzymes, decreased hemoglobin, increased creatinine/BUN, impotence, sweating, flushing, fever, malaise, palpitations, angina, tachycardia, abnormal EKG, insomnia, anxiety, nervousness, migraine, vertigo, depression, somnolence, paresthesias, involuntary muscle contractions, constipation, flatulence, dry mouth, hemorrhoids, gastroenteritis, toothache, gout, hypercholesterolemia, diabetes mellitus, arthralgias, leg cramps, anxiety, depression, nervousness, infection, asthma, bronchitis, rhinitis, dyspnea, epistaxis, dermatitis, rash, eczema, pruritus, micturition frequency, cystitis, cerebrovascular disorder, abnormal vision, conjunctivitis, tinnitus, earache

**Drug Interactions** Not metabolized by cytochrome P-450

(Continued)

not use alcohol or other prescription or OTC medications (especially, pain medications, sedatives, antihistamines, or hypnotics) without consulting prescriber. Maintain adequate hydration (2-3 L/day of fluids unless instructed to restrict fluid intake). You may experience drowsiness, dizziness, lightheadedness, or blurred vision (use caution when driving or engaging in hazardous tasks); or dry mouth or gastrointestinal discomfort (small frequent meals, good mouth care, chewing gum, or sucking lozenges may help). Report CNS changes (confusion, depression, increased sedation, excitation, headache, abnormal thinking, insomnia, or nightmares, memory impairment, impaired coordination); muscle pain or weakness; difficulty breathing; persistent dizziness, chest pain, or palpitations; alterations in normal gait; vision changes; or ineffectiveness of medication.

**Dietary Considerations:** Alcohol: Additive CNS effect, avoid use

**Monitoring Parameters:** Respiratory and cardiovascular status

**Reference Range:** Therapeutic: 26 ng/mL after 24 hours

## Terazosin (ter AY zoe sin)

**Pharmacologic Class** Alpha₁ Blockers

**U.S. Brand Names** Hytrin®

**Mechanism of Action** Alpha₁-specific blocking agent with minimal alpha₂ effects; this allows peripheral postsynaptic blockade, with the resultant decrease in arterial tone, while preserving the negative feedback loop which is mediated by the peripheral presynaptic alpha₂-receptors; terazosin relaxes the smooth muscle of the bladder neck, thus reducing bladder outlet obstruction

**Use** Management of mild to moderate hypertension; used alone or in combination with other agents such as diuretics or beta-blockers; benign prostate hypertrophy

**USUAL DOSAGE** Adults: Oral:

Hypertension: Initial: 1 mg at bedtime; slowly increase dose to achieve desired blood pressure, up to 20 mg/day; usual dose: 1-5 mg/day

Dosage reduction may be needed when adding a diuretic or other antihypertensive agent; if drug is discontinued for greater than several days, consider beginning with initial dose and retitrate as needed; dosage may be given on a twice daily regimen if response is diminished at 24 hours and hypotensive is observed at 2-4 hours following a dose

Benign prostatic hypertrophy: Initial: 1 mg at bedtime, increasing as needed; most patients require 10 mg day; if no response after 4-6 weeks of 10 mg/day, may increase to 20 mg/ day

**Dosage Forms Cap:** 1 mg, 2 mg, 5 mg, 10 mg; **Tab:** 1 mg, 2 mg, 5 mg, 10 mg

**Contraindications** Hypersensitivity to terazosin, other alpha-adrenergic antagonists, or any component

**Warnings/Precautions** Marked orthostatic hypotension, syncope, and loss of consciousness may occur with first dose ("first dose phenomenon"). This reaction is more likely to occur in patients receiving beta-blockers, diuretics, low sodium diets, or first doses >1 mg/ dose in adults; avoid rapid increase in dose; use with caution in patients with renal impairment.

**Pregnancy Risk Factor** C

**Adverse Reactions**

>10%:

Central nervous system: Dizziness (9% to 19%), headache (5% to 16%)

Neuromuscular & skeletal: Weakness (7.4% to 11.3%)

1% to 10%:

Cardiovascular: Peripheral edema (5.5%), palpitations (0.9% to 4.3%), postural hypotension (0.6% to 3.9%), tachycardia (1.9%)

Central nervous system: Fatigue, nervousness (2.3%)

Gastrointestinal: Xerostomia, nausea (4.4%), vomiting (1%), diarrhea/constipation (1%), abdominal pain (1%), flatulence (1%)

Neuromuscular & skeletal: Paresthesia (2.9%)

Respiratory: Dyspnea (1.7% to 3.1%), nasal congestion (1.9% to 5.9%)

<1%: Angina (~1%), syncope, depression, insomnia, rash, sexual dysfunction, decreased libido, priapism, polyuria, arthritis, myalgia, blurred vision, conjunctivitis, tinnitus, bronchospasm, epistaxis, pharyngitis, flu-like symptoms

(Continued)

## Terazosin *(Continued)*

### Drug Interactions
Decreased antihypertensive response with NSAIDs and alpha$_1$-blockers; decreased clonidine effects

Increased hypotensive effect with diuretics and antihypertensive medications (especially beta-blockers)

**Onset** 1-2 hours

**Half-Life** 9.2-12 hours

### Special PA Issues
**Patient Education:** Take as directed, at bedtime. Do not skip dose or discontinue without consulting prescriber. Follow recommended diet and exercise program. Do not use alcohol or OTC medications which may affect blood pressure (eg, cough or cold remedies, diet pills, stay-awake medications) without consulting physician. You may experience drowsiness, dizziness, or impaired judgment (use caution when driving or engaging in tasks that require alertness until response is known); postural hypotension (use caution when rising from sitting or lying position or when climbing stairs); dry mouth or nausea (frequent mouth care or sucking lozenges may help); urinary incontinence (void before taking medication); or sexual dysfunction (reversible, may resolve with continued use). Report altered CNS status (eg, fatigue, lethargy, confusion, nervousness); sudden weight gain (weigh yourself in the same clothes at same time of day once a week); unusual or persistent swelling of ankles, feet, or extremities; palpitations or rapid heartbeat; difficulty breathing; muscle weakness; or other persistent side effects.

**Monitoring Parameters:** Standing and sitting/supine blood pressure, especially following the initial dose at 2-4 hours following the dose and thereafter at the trough point to ensure adequate control throughout the dosing interval; urinary symptoms

## Terbinafine *(TER bin a feen)*

**Pharmacologic Class** Antifungal Agent, Oral; Antifungal Agent, Topical

**U.S. Brand Names** Daskil®; Lamisil®

**Mechanism of Action** Synthetic alkylamine derivative which inhibits squalene epoxidase, a key enzyme in sterol biosynthesis in fungi. This results in a deficiency in ergosterol within the fungal cell wall and results in fungal cell death.

**Use** Active against most strains of *Trichophyton mentagrophytes*, *Trichophyton rubrum*; may be effective for infections of *Microsporum gypseum* and *M. nanum*, *Trichophyton verrucosum*, *Epidermophyton floccosum*, *Candida albicans*, and *Scopulariopsis brevicaulis*

Oral: Onychomycosis of the toenail or fingernail due to susceptible dermatophytes

Topical: Antifungal for the treatment of tinea pedis (athlete's foot), tinea cruris (jock itch), and tinea corporis (ringworm)

**Unlabeled use:** Topical: Cutaneous candidiasis and pityriasis versicolor

### USUAL DOSAGE Adults:
Oral:

Superficial mycoses: Fingernail: 250 mg/day for up to 6 weeks; toenail: 250 mg/day for 12 weeks; doses may be given in two divided doses

Systemic mycosis: 250-500 mg/day for up to 16 months

Topical:

Athlete's foot: Apply to affected area twice daily for at least 1 week, not to exceed 4 weeks

Ringworm and jock itch: Apply to affected area once or twice daily for at least 1 week, not to exceed 4 weeks

**Dosing adjustment in renal impairment**: Although specific guidelines are not available, dose reduction in significant renal insufficiency (GFR <50 mL/minute) is recommended

**Dosage Forms Crm:** 1% (15 g, 30 g); **Tab:** 250 mg

**Contraindications** Hypersensitivity to terbinafine, naftifine or any component; pre-existing liver or renal disease (≤50 mL/minute GFR)

**Warnings/Precautions** While rare, the following complications have been reported and may require discontinuation of therapy: Changes in the ocular lens and retina, pancytopenia, neutropenia, Stevens-Johnson syndrome, toxic epidermal necrolysis. Discontinue if symptoms or signs of hepatobiliary dysfunction or cholestatic hepatitis develop. If irritation/sensitivity develop with topical use, discontinue therapy.

### Pregnancy Risk Factor B

### Pregnancy Implications
Clinical effects on the fetus: Avoid use in pregnancy since treatment of onychomycosis is postponable

Breast-feeding/lactation: Although minimal concentrations of terbinafine cross into breast milk after topical use, oral or topical treatment during lactation should be avoided

### Adverse Reactions
Oral:

1% to 10%:

Central nervous system: Headache, dizziness, vertigo

Dermatologic: Rash, pruritus, and alopecia with oral therapy; irritation, burning, contact dermatitis, pruritus, and dryness with topical product

Gastrointestinal: Nausea, diarrhea, dyspepsia, abdominal pain, appetite decrease, taste disturbance

Hematologic: Neutropenia, lymphocytopenia

Hepatic: Cholestasis, jaundice, hepatitis, liver enzyme elevations

Ocular: Visual disturbance

Miscellaneous: Allergic reaction

Topical:

1% to 10%:

Dermatologic: Pruritus, contact dermatitis

Local: Irritation, stinging

**Drug Interactions**

Decreased effect: Cyclosporine clearance is increased (~15%) with concomitant terbinafine; rifampin increases terbinafine clearance (100%)

Increased effect: Terbinafine clearance is decreased by cimetidine (33%) and terfenadine (16%); caffeine clearance is decreased by terfenadine (19%)

**Special PA Issues**

**Patient Education:** Topical: Avoid contact with eyes, nose, or mouth during treatment with cream; nursing mothers should not use on breast tissue; advise physician if eyes or skin becomes yellow or if irritation, itching, or burning develops. Do not use occlusive dressings concurrent with therapy. Full clinical effect may require several months due to the time required for a new nail to grow.

**Monitoring Parameters:** CBC and LFTs at baseline and repeated if use is for >6 weeks

**Related Information**

Antifungal Agents, Topical *on page 1000*

♦ **Terbinafine Hydrochloride** *see* Terbinafine *on previous page*

# Terbutaline (ter BYOO ta leen)

**Pharmacologic Class** Beta$_2$ Agonist

**U.S. Brand Names** Brethaire® Inhalation Aerosol; Brethine® Injection; Brethine® Oral; Bricanyl® Injection; Bricanyl® Oral

**Mechanism of Action** Relaxes bronchial smooth muscle by action on beta$_2$-receptors with less effect on heart rate

**Use** Bronchodilator in reversible airway obstruction and bronchial asthma

**USUAL DOSAGE**

Children <12 years:

Oral: Initial: 0.05 mg/kg/dose 3 times/day, increased gradually as required; maximum: 0.15 mg/kg/dose 3-4 times/day or a total of 5 mg/24 hours

S.C.: 0.005-0.01 mg/kg/dose to a maximum of 0.3 mg/dose every 15-20 minutes for 3 doses

Nebulization: 0.01-0.03 mg/kg/dose every 4-6 hours

Inhalation: 1-2 inhalations every 4-6 hours

Children >12 years and Adults:

Oral:

12-15 years: 2.5 mg every 6 hours 3 times/day; not to exceed 7.5 mg in 24 hours

>15 years: 5 mg/dose every 6 hours 3 times/day; if side effects occur, reduce dose to 2.5 mg every 6 hours; not to exceed 15 mg in 24 hours

S.C.: 0.25 mg/dose repeated in 15-30 minutes for one time only; a total dose of 0.5 mg should not be exceeded within a 4-hour period

Nebulization: 0.01-0.03 mg/kg/dose every 4-6 hours

Inhalation: 2 inhalations every 4-6 hours; wait 1 minute between inhalations

**Dosing adjustment/comments in renal impairment:**

Cl$_{cr}$ 10-50 mL/minute: Administer at 50% of normal dose

Cl$_{cr}$ <10 mL/minute: Avoid use

**Dosage Forms Aero, oral:** 0.2 mg/actuation (10.5 g); **Inj:** 1 mg/mL (1 mL); **Tab:** 2.5 mg, 5 mg

**Contraindications** Hypersensitivity to terbutaline or any component, cardiac arrhythmias associated with tachycardia, tachycardia caused by digitalis intoxication

**Warnings/Precautions** Excessive or prolonged use may lead to tolerance; paradoxical bronchoconstriction may occur with excessive use; if it occurs, discontinue terbutaline immediately

**Pregnancy Risk Factor** B

**Adverse Reactions**

>10%:

Central nervous system: Nervousness, restlessness

Neuromuscular & skeletal: Trembling

1% to 10%:

Cardiovascular: Tachycardia, hypertension

Central nervous system: Dizziness, drowsiness, headache, insomnia

Gastrointestinal: Xerostomia, nausea, vomiting, bad taste in mouth

Neuromuscular & skeletal: Muscle cramps, weakness

Miscellaneous: Diaphoresis

<1%: Chest pain, arrhythmias, paradoxical bronchospasm

(Continued)

## Terbutaline *(Continued)*

### Drug Interactions
Decreased effect with beta-blockers
Increased toxicity with MAO inhibitors, TCAs

**Onset** Oral: 30-45 minutes; S.C.: Within 6-15 minutes

**Half-Life** 11-16 hours

### Special PA Issues

**Patient Education:** Use exactly as directed (see Administration below). Do not use more often than recommended (excessive use may result in tolerance, overdose may result in serious adverse effects) and do not discontinue without consulting prescriber. Maintain adequate hydration (2-3 L/day of fluids unless instructed to restrict fluid intake). You may experience nervousness, dizziness, or fatigue (use caution when driving or engaging in hazardous activities until response to treatment is known); or dry mouth, stomach upset (frequent small meals, frequent mouth care, chewing gum, or sucking hard candy may help). Report unresolved GI upset; dizziness or fatigue; vision changes; chest pain, rapid heartbeat, or palpitations; insomnia, nervousness, or hyperactivity; muscle cramping, tremors, or pain; unusual cough; or rash (hypersensitivity).

Preterm labor: Notify prescriber immediately if labor resumes or adverse side effects are noted.

**Administration:** Self-administered inhalation: Store canister upside down; do not freeze. Shake canister before using. Sit when using medication. Close eyes when administering terbutaline to avoid spray getting into eyes. Exhale slowly and completely through nose; inhale deeply through mouth while administering aerosol. Hold breath for 1-3 seconds after inhalation. Wait at least 1 full minute between inhalations. Wash mouthpiece between use. If more than one inhalation medication is used, use bronchodilator first and wait 5 minutes between medications.

**Monitoring Parameters:** Serum potassium, heart rate, blood pressure, respiratory rate

♦ **Terbutaline Sulfate** *see Terbutaline on previous page*

## Terconazole *(ter KONE e zole)*

**Pharmacologic Class** Antifungal Agent, Vaginal

**U.S. Brand Names** Terazol® Vaginal

**Mechanism of Action** Triazole ketal antifungal agent; involves inhibition of fungal cytochrome P-450. Specifically terconazole inhibits cytochrome P-450-dependent 14-alpha-demethylase which results in accumulation of membrane disturbing 14-alpha-demethyl-sterols and ergosterol depletion.

**Use** Local treatment of vulvovaginal candidiasis

**USUAL DOSAGE** Adults: Female: Insert 1 applicatorful intravaginally at bedtime for 7 consecutive days

**Dosage Forms Crm, vag:** 0.4% (45 g); 0.8% (20 g); **Supp, vag:** 80 mg (3s)

**Contraindications** Known hypersensitivity to terconazole or components of the vaginal cream or suppository

**Warnings/Precautions** Should be discontinued if sensitization or irritation occurs. Microbiological studies (KOH smear and/or cultures) should be repeated in patients not responding to terconazole in order to confirm the diagnosis and rule out other other pathogens.

**Pregnancy Risk Factor** C

**Adverse Reactions** 1% to 10%: Genitourinary: Vulvar/vaginal burning

### Special PA Issues

**Patient Education:** Complete full course of therapy as directed. Insert vaginally as directed by prescriber or see package insert. Sexual partner may experience irritation of penis; best to refrain from intercourse during period of treatment. Report persistent vaginal burning, itching, irritation, or discharge.

## Terpin Hydrate and Codeine *(TER pin HYE drate & KOE deen)*

**Pharmacologic Class** Expectorant

**Dosage Forms Elix:** Terpin hydrate 85 mg and codeine 10 mg per 5 mL with alcohol 42.5%

♦ **Terra-Cortril® Ophthalmic Suspension** *see Oxytetracycline and Hydrocortisone on page 691*

♦ **Terramycin® I.M. Injection** *see Oxytetracycline on page 690*

♦ **Terramycin® Ophthalmic Ointment** *see Oxytetracycline and Polymyxin B on page 691*

♦ **Terramycin® Oral** *see Oxytetracycline on page 690*

♦ **Terramycin® w/Polymyxin B Ophthalmic Ointment** *see Oxytetracycline and Polymyxin B on page 691*

♦ **Teslac®** *see Testolactone on next page*

♦ **Tessalon® Perles** *see Benzonatate on page 106*

♦ **Testex®** *see Testosterone on next page*

♦ **Testoderm® Transdermal System** *see Testosterone on next page*

## Testolactone (tes toe LAK tone)

**Pharmacologic Class** Androgen

**U.S. Brand Names** Teslac®

**Mechanism of Action** Testolactone is a synthetic testosterone derivative without significant androgen activity. The drug inhibits steroid aromatase activity, thereby blocking the production of estradiol and estrone from androgen precursors such as testosterone and androstenedione. Unfortunately, the enzymatic block provided by testolactone is transient and is usually limited to a period of 3 months.

**Use** Palliative treatment of advanced disseminated breast carcinoma

**USUAL DOSAGE** Adults: Female: Oral: 250 mg 4 times/day for at least 3 months; desired response may take as long as 3 months

**Dosage Forms Tab:** 50 mg

**Contraindications** In men for the treatment of breast cancer; known hypersensitivity to testolactone

**Warnings/Precautions** The U.S. Food and Drug Administration (FDA) currently recommends that procedures for proper handling and disposal of antineoplastic agents be considered. Use with caution in hepatic, renal, or cardiac disease; prolonged use may cause drug-induced hepatic disease; history or porphyria.

**Pregnancy Risk Factor** C

**Adverse Reactions** 1% to 10%:

Cardiovascular: Edema

Dermatologic: Maculopapular rash

Endocrine & metabolic: Hypercalcemia,

Gastrointestinal: Anorexia, diarrhea, nausea, edema of the tongue

Neuromuscular & skeletal: Paresthesias, peripheral neuropathies

**Special PA Issues**

**Patient Education:** Take as directed; do not stop without consulting prescriber. Effectiveness of therapy may take as long as 3 months. Maintain adequate fluid intake (2-3 L/day) to reduce incidence of hypercalcemia. Maintain diet and exercise program recommended by prescriber (passive exercises may help maintain mobility). Report numbness of toes, fingers, or face; persistent insomnia, nausea, or vomiting; swelling of extremities; or weight gain >5 lb/week.

**Monitoring Parameters:** Plasma calcium levels

♦ Testopel® Pellet *see* Testosterone *on this page*

## Testosterone (tes TOS ter one)

**Pharmacologic Class** Androgen

**U.S. Brand Names** Androderm® Transdermal System; Andro-L.A.® Injection; Andropository® Injection; Delatest® Injection; Delatestryl® Injection; depAndro® Injection; Depotest® Injection; Depo®-Testosterone Injection; Duratest® Injection; Durathate® Injection; Everone® Injection; Histerone® Injection; Testex®; Testoderm® Transdermal System; Testopel® Pellet

**Mechanism of Action** Principal endogenous androgen responsible for promoting the growth and development of the male sex organs and maintaining secondary sex characteristics in androgen-deficient males

**Use** Androgen replacement therapy in the treatment of delayed male puberty; postpartum breast pain and engorgement; inoperable breast cancer; male hypogonadism

**USUAL DOSAGE**

Children: I.M.:

Male hypogonadism:

Initiation of pubertal growth: 40-50 mg/m²/dose (cypionate or enanthate ester) monthly until the growth rate falls to prepubertal levels

Terminal growth phase: 100 mg/m²/dose (cypionate or enanthate ester) monthly until growth ceases

Maintenance virilizing dose: 100 mg/m²/dose (cypionate or enanthate ester) twice monthly

Delayed puberty: 40-50 mg/m²/dose monthly (cypionate or enanthate ester) for 6 months

Adults: Inoperable breast cancer: I.M.: 200-400 mg every 2-4 weeks

Male: Short-acting formulations: Testosterone Aqueous/Testosterone Propionate (in oil): I.M.:

Androgen replacement therapy: 10-50 mg 2-3 times/week

Male hypogonadism: 40-50 mg/m²/dose monthly until the growth rate falls to prepubertal levels (~5 cm/year); during terminal growth phase: 100 mg/m²/dose monthly until growth ceases; maintenance virilizing dose: 100 mg/m²/dose twice monthly or 50-400 mg/dose every 2-4 weeks

Male: Long-acting formulations: Testosterone enthanate (in oil)/testosterone cypionate (in oil): I.M.:

Male hypogonadism: 50-400 mg every 2-4 weeks

Male with delayed puberty: 50-200 mg every 2-4 weeks for a limited duration

(Continued)

## Testosterone *(Continued)*

Male ≥18 years: Transdermal: Primary hypogonadism **or** hypogonadotropic hypogonadism:

Testoderm®: Apply 6 mg patch daily to scrotum (if scrotum is inadequate, use a 4 mg daily system)

Testoderm-TSS®: Apply 5 mg patch daily to clean, dry area of skin on the arm, back or upper buttocks

**Do not apply Testoderm-TSS® to the scrotum**

Androderm®: Apply 2 systems nightly to clean, dry area on the back, abdomen, upper arms or thighs for 24 hours for a total of 5 mg/day

**Dosing adjustment/comments in hepatic disease:** Reduce dose

**Dosage Forms Inj: Aqueous susp:** 25 mg/mL (10 mL, 30 mL), 50 mg/mL (10 mL, 30 mL), 100 mg/mL (10 mL, 30 mL); **In oil, as cypionate:** 100 mg/mL (1 mL, 10 mL), 200 mg/mL (1 mL, 10 mL); **In oil, as enanthate:** 100 mg/mL (5 mL, 10 mL), 200 mg/mL (5 mL, 10 mL); **In oil, as propionate:** 50 mg/mL (10 mL, 30 mL), 100 mg/mL (10 mL, 30 mL); **Pellet:** 75 mg (1 pellet per vial); **Transdermal system:** 2.5 mg/day; 4 mg/day, 5 mg/day, 6 mg/day

**Contraindications** Severe renal or cardiac disease, benign prostatic hypertrophy with obstruction, undiagnosed genital bleeding, males with carcinoma of the breast or prostate; hypersensitivity to testosterone or any component; pregnancy

**Warnings/Precautions** Perform radiographic examination of the hand and wrist every 6 months to determine the rate of bone maturation; may accelerate bone maturation without producing compensating gain in linear growth; has both androgenic and anabolic activity, the anabolic action may enhance hypoglycemia

**Pregnancy Risk Factor** X

**Adverse Reactions**

>10%:

Dermatologic: Acne

Endocrine & metabolic: Menstrual problems (amenorrhea), virilism, breast soreness

Genitourinary: Epididymitis, priapism, bladder irritability

1% to 10%:

Cardiovascular: Flushing, edema

Central nervous system: Excitation, aggressive behavior, sleeplessness, anxiety, mental depression, headache

Dermatologic: Hirsutism (increase in pubic hair growth)

Gastrointestinal: Nausea, vomiting, GI irritation

Genitourinary: Prostatic hypertrophy, prostatic carcinoma, impotence, testicular atrophy

Hepatic: Hepatic dysfunction

<1%: Gynecomastia, hypercalcemia, hypoglycemia, leukopenia, suppression of clotting factors, polycythemia, cholestatic hepatitis, hepatic necrosis, hypersensitivity reactions

**Drug Interactions** CYP3A3/4 and 3A5-7 enzyme substrate

Increased toxicity: Effects of oral anticoagulants may be enhanced

**Duration** Based upon the route of administration and which testosterone ester is used; cypionate and enanthate esters have the longest duration, up to 2-4 weeks after I.M. administration.

**Half-Life** 10-100 minutes

**Special PA Issues**

**Patient Education:** Breast cancer: This drug must be administered I.M., usually once or twice a month. Maintain adequate fluid intake (2-3 L/day) and nutrition (frequent small meals may help). Diabetic patients should monitor glucose regularly (medication may alter glucose tolerance) and report changes so antidiabetic medication can be adjusted if necessary. Report swelling of extremities (ankles, feet, fingers), weight gain (>5 lb/week), respiratory difficulty, persistent nausea or vomiting. Females should report menstrual irregularities or abnormal hair growth and males penile pain, persistent erection, or difficulty urinating.

**Monitoring Parameters:** Periodic liver function tests, radiologic examination of wrist and hand every 6 months (when using in prepubertal children)

**Reference Range:** Testosterone, urine: Male: 100-1500 ng/24 hours; Female: 100-500 ng/24 hours

- ♦ **Testosterone Cypionate** *see* Testosterone *on previous page*
- ♦ **Testosterone Enanthate** *see* Testosterone *on previous page*
- ♦ **Testosterone Propionate** *see* Testosterone *on previous page*
- ♦ **Testred®** *see* Methyltestosterone *on page 595*
- ♦ **Tetanus and Diphtheria Toxoid** *see* Diphtheria and Tetanus Toxoid *on page 291*

## Tetanus Antitoxin *(TET a nus an tee TOKS in)*

**Pharmacologic Class** Antitoxin

**Mechanism of Action** Provides passive immunization; solution of concentrated globulins containing antitoxic antibodies obtained from horse serum after immunization against tetanus toxin

**Use** Tetanus prophylaxis or treatment of active tetanus only when tetanus immune globulin (TIG) is not available; tetanus immune globulin (Hyper-Tet®) is the preferred tetanus immunoglobulin for the treatment of active tetanus; may be given concomitantly with tetanus toxoid adsorbed when immediate treatment is required, but active immunization is desirable

**USUAL DOSAGE**

Prophylaxis: I.M., S.C.:

Children <30 kg: 1500 units

Children and Adults ≥30 kg: 3000-5000 units

Treatment: Children and Adults: Inject 10,000-40,000 units into wound; administer 40,000-100,000 units

**Dosage Forms Inj, equine:** Not less than 400 units/mL (12.5 mL, 50 mL)

**Contraindications** Patients sensitive to equine-derived preparations

**Warnings/Precautions** Tetanus antitoxin is not the same as tetanus immune globulin; sensitivity testing should be conducted in all individuals regardless of clinical history; have epinephrine 1:1000 available

**Pregnancy Risk Factor** D

**Adverse Reactions** Skin eruptions, erythema, urticaria, local pain, numbness, arthralgia, serum sickness may develop up to several weeks after injection in 10% of patients, anaphylaxis

# Tetanus Immune Globulin (Human)

(TET a nus i MYUN GLOB yoo lin HYU man)

**Pharmacologic Class** Immune Globulin

**U.S. Brand Names** Hyper-Tet®

**Mechanism of Action** Passive immunity toward tetanus

**Use** Passive immunization against tetanus; tetanus immune globulin is preferred over tetanus antitoxin for treatment of active tetanus; part of the management of an unclean, wound in a person whose history of previous receipt of tetanus toxoid is unknown or who has received less than three doses of tetanus toxoid; elderly may require TIG more often than younger patients with tetanus infection due to declining antibody titers with age

**USUAL DOSAGE** I.M.:

Prophylaxis of tetanus:

Children: 4 units/kg; some recommend administering 250 units to small children

Adults: 250 units

Treatment of tetanus:

Children: 500-3000 units; some should infiltrate locally around the wound

Adults: 3000-6000 units

**Dosage Forms Inj:** 250 units/mL

**Contraindications** Hypersensitivity to tetanus immune globulin, thimerosal, or any immune globulin product or component; patients with IgA deficiency; I.V. administration

**Warnings/Precautions** Have epinephrine 1:1000 available for anaphylactic reactions; do not administer I.V.

**Pregnancy Risk Factor** C

**Adverse Reactions**

>10%: Local: Pain, tenderness, erythema at injection site

1% to 10%:

Central nervous system: Fever (mild)

Dermatologic: Urticaria, angioedema

Neuromuscular & skeletal: Muscle stiffness

Miscellaneous: Anaphylaxis reaction

<1%: Sensitization to repeated injections

**Drug Interactions** Never administer tetanus toxoid and TIG in same syringe (toxoid will be neutralized); toxoid may be given at a separate site; concomitant administration with Td may decrease its immune response, especially in individuals with low prevaccination antibody titers

# Tetanus Toxoid, Adsorbed (TET a nus TOKS oyd, ad SORBED)

**Pharmacologic Class** Toxoid

**Mechanism of Action** Tetanus toxoid preparations contain the toxin produced by virulent tetanus bacilli (detoxified growth products of *Clostridium tetani*). The toxin has been modified by treatment with formaldehyde so that it has lost toxicity but still retains ability to act as antigen and produce active immunity; the aluminum salt, a mineral adjuvant, delays the rate of absorption and prolongs and enhances its properties; duration ~10 years

**Use** Selective induction of active immunity against tetanus in selected patients. **Note:** Tetanus and diphtheria toxoids for adult use (Td) is the preferred immunizing agent for most adults and for children after their seventh birthday. Young children should receive trivalent DTwP or DTaP (diphtheria/tetanus/pertussis - whole cell or acellular), as part of their childhood immunization program, unless pertussis is contraindicated, then TD is warranted.

**USUAL DOSAGE** Adults: I.M.:

Primary immunization: 0.5 mL; repeat 0.5 mL at 4-8 weeks after first dose and at 6-12 months after second dose

Routine booster doses are recommended only every 5-10 years

(Continued)

# Tetanus Toxoid, Adsorbed *(Continued)*

**Dosage Forms** Inj, adsorbed: Tetanus 5 Lf units per 0.5 mL dose (0.5 mL, 5 mL); Tetanus 10 Lf units per 0.5 mL dose (0.5 mL, 5 mL)

**Contraindications** Hypersensitivity to tetanus toxoid or any component (may use the fluid tetanus toxoid to immunize the rare patient who is hypersensitive to aluminum adjuvant); avoid use with chloramphenicol or if neurological signs or symptoms occurred after prior administration; poliomyelitis outbreaks require deferral of immunizations; acute respiratory infections or other active infections may dictate deferral of administration of routine primary immunizing but not emergency doses

**Warnings/Precautions** Not equivalent to tetanus toxoid fluid; the tetanus toxoid adsorbed is the preferred toxoid for immunization and Td, TD or DTaP/DTwP are the preferred adsorbed forms; avoid injection into a blood vessel; have epinephrine (1:1000) available; not for use in treatment of tetanus infection nor for immediate prophylaxis of unimmunized individuals; immunosuppressive therapy or other immunodeficiencies may diminish antibody response, however it is recommended for routine immunization of symptomatic and asymptomatic HIV-infected patients; deferral of immunization until immunosuppression is discontinued or administration of an additional dose >1 month after treatment is recommended; allergic reactions may occur; epinephrine 1:1000 must be available; use in pediatrics should be deferred until >1 year of age when a history of a CNS disorder is present; elderly may not mount adequate antibody titers following immunization

**Pregnancy Risk Factor** C

**Adverse Reactions**
>10%: Local: Induration/redness at injection site
1% to 10%:
    Central nervous system: Chills, fever
    Local: Sterile abscess at injection site
    Miscellaneous: Allergic reaction
<1%: Fever >103°F, malaise, neurological disturbances, blistering at injection site, Arthustype hypersensitivity reactions

**Drug Interactions** Decreased response: If primary immunization is started in individuals receiving an immunosuppressive agent or corticosteroids, serologic testing may be needed to ensure adequate antibody response; concurrent use of TIG and tetanus toxoid may delay the development of active immunity by several days

**Special PA Issues**
**Patient Education:** A nodule may be palpable at the injection site for a few weeks. DT, Td and T vaccines cause few problems; they may cause mild fever or soreness, swelling, and redness where the shot was given. These problems usually last 1-2 days, but this does not happen nearly as often as with DTP vaccine. Sometimes, adults who get these vaccines can have a lot of soreness and swelling where the shot was given.

# Tetanus Toxoid, Fluid *(TET a nus TOKS oyd FLOO id)*

**Pharmacologic Class** Toxoid

**Mechanism of Action** Tetanus toxoid preparations contain the toxin produced by virulent tetanus bacilli (detoxified growth products of *Clostridium tetani*). The toxin has been modified by treatment with formaldehyde so that is has lost toxicity but still retains ability to act as antigen and produce active immunity.

**Use** Detection of delayed hypersensitivity and assessment of cell-mediated immunity; active immunization against tetanus in the rare adult or child who is allergic to the aluminum adjuvant (a product containing adsorbed tetanus toxoid is preferred)

**USUAL DOSAGE**
Anergy testing: Intradermal: 0.1 mL
Primary immunization (**Note:** Td, TD, DTaP/DTwP are recommended): Adults: Inject 3 doses of 0.5 mL I.M. or S.C. at 4- to 8-week intervals; administer fourth dose 6-12 months after third dose
Booster doses: I.M., S.C.: 0.5 mL every 10 years

**Dosage Forms** Inj, fluid: Tetanus 4 Lf units per 0.5 mL dose (7.5 mL); Tetanus 5 Lf units per 0.5 mL dose (0.5 mL, 7.5 mL)

**Contraindications** Hypersensitivity to tetanus toxoid or any product components

**Warnings/Precautions** Epinephrine 1:1000 should be readily available; skin test responsiveness may be delayed or reduced in elderly patients

**Pregnancy Risk Factor** C

**Adverse Reactions** Percentage unknown: Very hypersensitive persons may develop a local reaction at the injection site; urticaria, anaphylactic reactions, shock and death are possible

**Drug Interactions** Increased effect: Cimetidine may augment delayed hypersensitivity responses to skin test antigens

♦ **Tetanus Toxoid Plain** *see* Tetanus Toxoid, Fluid *on this page*

# Tetracaine *(TET ra kane)*

**Pharmacologic Class** Local Anesthetic
**U.S. Brand Names** Pontocaine®

**Mechanism of Action** Ester local anesthetic blocks both the initiation and conduction of nerve impulses by decreasing the neuronal membrane's permeability to sodium ions, which results in inhibition of depolarization with resultant blockade of conduction

**Use** Spinal anesthesia; local anesthesia in the eye for various diagnostic and examination purposes; topically applied to nose and throat for various diagnostic procedures; **approximately 10 times more potent than procaine**

**USUAL DOSAGE** Maximum adult dose: 50 mg

Children: Safety and efficacy have not been established

Adults:

Ophthalmic (not for prolonged use):

Ointment: Apply ½" to 1" to lower conjunctival fornix

Solution: Instill 1-2 drops

Spinal anesthesia:

High, medium, low, and saddle blocks: 0.2% to 0.3% solution

Prolonged (2-3 hours): 1% solution

Subarachnoid injection: 5-20 mg

Saddle block: 2-5 mg; a 1% solution should be diluted with equal volume of CSF before administration

Topical mucous membranes (2% solution): Apply as needed; dose should not exceed 20 mg

Topical for skin: Ointment/cream: Apply to affected areas as needed

**Dosage Forms Crm, as hydrochloride:** 1% (28 g); **Inj, as hydrochloride:** 1% [10 mg/mL] (2 mL); **Inj, as hydrochloride, with dextrose 6%:** 0.2% [2 mg/mL] (2 mL), 0.3% [3 mg/mL] (5 mL); **Oint, as hydrochloride: Ophth:** 0.5% [5 mg/mL] (3.75 g); **Top:** 0.5% [5 mg/mL] (28 g); **Powder for inj, as hydrochloride:** 20 mg; **Soln, as hydrochloride: Ophth:** 0.5% [5 mg/mL] (1 mL, 2 mL, 15 mL, 59 mL); **Top:** 2% [20 mg/mL] (30 mL, 118 mL)

**Contraindications** Hypersensitivity to tetracaine or any component; ophthalmic secondary bacterial infection, patients with liver disease, CNS disease, meningitis (if used for epidural or spinal anesthesia), myasthenia gravis

**Warnings/Precautions** No pediatric dosage recommendations; ophthalmic preparations may delay wound healing; use with caution in patients with cardiac disease and hyperthyroidism

**Pregnancy Risk Factor** C

**Adverse Reactions**

1% to 10%: Dermatologic: Contact dermatitis, burning, stinging, angioedema

<1%: Tenderness, urticaria, urethritis, methemoglobinemia in infants

**Drug Interactions** Decreased effect: Aminosalicylic acid, sulfonamides effects may be antagonized

**Onset** Onset of anesthetic effect:

Ophthalmic instillation: Within 60 seconds

Topical or spinal injection: Within 3-8 minutes after applied to mucous membranes or when saddle block administered for spinal anesthesia

**Duration** Topical: 1.5-3 hours

**Special PA Issues**

**Patient Education:** Topical or ophthalmic anesthesia effects may last for some time following use; you will need to observe appropriate safety precautions to prevent injury (eg, do not rub or touch your eye, scratch your nose, or eat or drink (depending on use) until all sensation returns).

Ophthalmic: May cause temporary rash or stinging when used. Report any ringing in ears, feeling of weakness or faintness, chest pain or palpitation, or increased restlessness.

## Tetracaine and Dextrose (TET ra kane & DEKS trose)

**Pharmacologic Class** Local Anesthetic

**U.S. Brand Names** Pontocaine® With Dextrose Injection

**Dosage Forms Inj:** Tetracaine hydrochloride 0.2% and dextrose 6% (2 mL); tetracaine hydrochloride 0.3% and dextrose 6% (5 mL)

♦ **Tetracaine Hydrochloride** see Tetracaine on previous page

♦ **Tetracap® Oral** see Tetracycline on this page

♦ **Tetracosactide** see Cosyntropin on page 238

## Tetracycline (tet ra SYE kleen)

**Pharmacologic Class** Antibiotic, Ophthalmic; Antibiotic, Tetracycline Derivative; Antibiotic, Topical

**U.S. Brand Names** Achromycin® Ophthalmic; Achromycin® Topical; Nor-tet® Oral; Panmycin® Oral; Sumycin® Oral; Tetracap® Oral; Topicycline® Topical

**Mechanism of Action** Inhibits bacterial protein synthesis by binding with the 30S and possibly the 50S ribosomal subunit(s) of susceptible bacteria; may also cause alterations in the cytoplasmic membrane

**Use** Treatment of susceptible bacterial infections of both gram-positive and gram-negative organisms; also infections due to *Mycoplasma*, *Chlamydia*, and *Rickettsia*; indicated for
(Continued)

## Tetracycline *(Continued)*

acne, exacerbations of chronic bronchitis, and treatment of gonorrhea and syphilis in patients that are allergic to penicillin; used concomitantly with metronidazole, bismuth subsalicylate and an $H_2$-antagonist for the treatment of duodenal ulcer disease induced by *H. pylori*

### USUAL DOSAGE

Children >8 years: Oral: 25-50 mg/kg/day in divided doses every 6 hours

Children >8 years and Adults:

Ophthalmic:

Ointment: Instill every 2-12 hours

Suspension: Instill 1-2 drops 2-4 times/day or more often as needed

Topical: Apply to affected areas 1-4 times/day

Adults: Oral: 250-500 mg/dose every 6 hours

*Helicobacter pylori:* Clinically effective treatment regimens include triple therapy with amoxicillin or tetracycline, metronidazole, and bismuth subsalicylate; amoxicillin, metronidazole, and $H_2$-receptor antagonist; or double therapy with amoxicillin and omeprazole. Adult dose: 850 mg 3 times/day to 500 mg 4 times/day

**Dosing interval in renal impairment:**

$Cl_{cr}$ 50-80 mL/minute: Administer every 8-12 hours

$Cl_{cr}$ 10-50 mL/minute: Administer every 12-24 hours

$Cl_{cr}$ <10 mL/minute: Administer every 24 hours

Dialysis: Slightly dialyzable (5% to 20%) via hemo- and peritoneal dialysis nor via continuous arteriovenous or venovenous hemofiltration (CAVH/CAVHD); no supplemental dosage necessary

**Dosing adjustment in hepatic impairment:** Avoid use or maximum dose is 1 g/day

**Dosage Forms Cap:** 100 mg, 250 mg, 500 mg; **Oint: Ophth:** 1% [10 mg/mL] (3.5 g); **Top:** 3% [30 mg/mL] (14.2 g, 30 g); **Soln, top:** 2.2 mg/mL (70 mL); **Susp: Ophth:** 1% [10 mg/mL] (0.5 mL, 1 mL, 4 mL); **Oral:** 125 mg/5 mL (60 mL, 480 mL); **Tab:** 250 mg, 500 mg

**Contraindications** Hypersensitivity to tetracycline or any component; do not administer to children ≤8 years of age

**Warnings/Precautions** Use of tetracyclines during tooth development may cause permanent discoloration of the teeth and enamel, hypoplasia and retardation of skeletal development and bone growth with risk being the greatest for children <4 years and those receiving high doses; use with caution in patients with renal or hepatic impairment (eg, elderly) and in pregnancy; dosage modification required in patients with renal impairment since it may increase BUN as an antianabolic agent; pseudotumor cerebri has been reported with tetracycline use (usually resolves with discontinuation); outdated drug can cause nephropathy; superinfection possible; use protective measure to avoid photosensitivity

**Pregnancy Risk Factor** D; B (topical)

**Pregnancy Implications** Breast-feeding/lactation: Excreted in breast milk; avoid use if possible in lactating mothers

### Adverse Reactions

>10%: Discoloration of teeth and enamel hypoplasia (young children)

1% to 10%:

Dermatologic: Photosensitivity

Gastrointestinal: Nausea, diarrhea

<1%: Pericarditis, increased intracranial pressure, bulging fontanels in infants, pseudotumor cerebri, dermatologic effects, pruritus, pigmentation of nails, exfoliative dermatitis, diabetes insipidus syndrome, vomiting, esophagitis, anorexia, abdominal cramps, antibiotic-associated pseudomembranous colitis, staphylococcal enterocolitis, hepatotoxicity, thrombophlebitis, paresthesia, acute renal failure, azotemia, renal damage, superinfections, anaphylaxis, hypersensitivity reactions, candidal superinfection

### Drug Interactions

Decreased effect: Calcium, magnesium or aluminum-containing antacids, oral contraceptives, iron, zinc, sodium bicarbonate, penicillins, cimetidine may decrease tetracycline absorption

Although no clinical evidence exists, may bind with bismuth or calcium carbonate, an excipient in bismuth subsalicylate, during treatment for *H. pylori*

Increased toxicity: Methoxyflurane anesthesia when concurrent with tetracycline may cause fatal nephrotoxicity; warfarin with tetracyclines may result in increased anticoagulation; tetracyclines may rarely increase digoxin serum levels

**Half-Life** Normal renal function: 8-11 hours; End-stage renal disease: 57-108 hours

### Special PA Issues

**Patient Education:** Take this medication exactly as directed. Take all of the prescription even if you see an improvement in your condition. Do not use more or more often than recommended.

Oral: Preferable to take on an empty stomach (1 hour before or 2 hours after meals). Take at regularly scheduled times, around-the-clock. Avoid antacids, iron, or dairy products within 2 hours of taking tetracycline. You may experience photosensitivity (use sunblock, wear protective clothing, avoid exposure to direct sunlight); dizziness or lightheadedness (use caution when driving or engaging in hazardous tasks); nausea/vomiting (frequent small meals, frequent mouth care, sucking on lozenges may help). Effect of oral contraceptives may be reduced; use barrier contraception. Report rash or intense itching, yellowing of skin or eyes, change in color of urine or stools, fever or chills, dark urine, pale stools, vaginal itching or discharge, foul-smelling stools, excessive thirst or urination, acute headache, unresolved diarrhea, difficulty breathing, condition does not improve, or worsening of condition.

Ophthalmic: Sit down, tilt head back, instill solution or drops inside lower eyelid, and roll eyeball in all directions. Close eye and apply gentle pressure to inner corner of eye for 30 seconds. Do not touch tip of applicator to eye or any contaminated surface. May experience temporary stinging or blurred vision. Inform prescriber if condition worsens or does not improve in 3-4 days.

Topical: Wash area and pat dry (unless contraindicated). Avoid getting in mouth or eyes. You may experience temporary stinging or burning which will resolve quickly. Treated skin may turn yellow; this will wash off. May stain clothing (permanent). Report rash. Inform prescriber if condition worsens or does not improve in a few days.

**Dietary Considerations:** Food: Dairy products decrease effect of tetracycline

**Monitoring Parameters:** Renal, hepatic, and hematologic function test, temperature, WBC, cultures and sensitivity, appetite, mental status

- ◆ **Tetracycline Hydrochloride** *see* Tetracycline *on page 885*
- ◆ **Tetrahydroaminoacrine** *see* Tacrine *on page 868*
- ◆ **Tetrahydrocannabinol** *see* Dronabinol *on page 307*
- ◆ **T-Gen®** *see* Trimethobenzamide *on page 936*
- ◆ **T-Gesic®** *see* Hydrocodone and Acetaminophen *on page 449*
- ◆ **THA** *see* Tacrine *on page 868*
- ◆ **Thalidomid®** *see* Thalidomide *on this page*

## Thalidomide (tha LI doe mide)

**Pharmacologic Class** Immunosuppressant Agent

**U.S. Brand Names** Thalidomid®

**Mechanism of Action** A derivative of glutethimide; mode of action for immunosuppression is unclear; inhibition of neutrophil chemotaxis and decreased monocyte phagocytosis may occur; may cause 50% to 80% reduction of tumor necrosis factor - alpha

**Use** Treatment of erythema nodosum leprosum

**Orphan status:** Crohn's disease

**Investigational:** Treatment or prevention of graft-versus-host reactions after bone marrow transplantation; in aphthous ulceration in HIV-positive patients; Langerhans cell histocytosis, Behçet's syndrome; hypnotic agent; also may be effective in rheumatoid arthritis, discoid lupus, and erythema multiforme; useful in type 2 lepra reactions, but not type 1; can assist in healing mouth ulcers in AIDS patients

## USUAL DOSAGE

Leprosy: Up to 400 mg/day; usual maintenance dose: 50-100 mg/day

Behçet's syndrome: 100-400 mg/day

Graft-vs-host reactions:

Children: 3 mg/kg 4 times/day

Adults: 100-1600 mg/day; usual initial dose: 200 mg 4 times/day for use up to 700 days

AIDS-related aphthous stomatitis: 200 mg twice daily for 5 days, then 200 mg/day for up to 8 weeks

Discoid lupus erythematosus: 100-400 mg/day; maintenance dose: 25-50 mg

**Contraindications** Pregnancy or women in childbearing years, neuropathy (peripheral), thalidomide hypersensitivity

**Warnings/Precautions** Liver, hepatic, neurological disorders, constipation, congestive heart failure, hypertension

**Pregnancy Risk Factor** X

**Pregnancy Implications** Embryotoxic with limb defects noted from the 27th to 40th gestational day of exposure; all cases of phocomelia occur from the 27th to 42nd gestational day; fetal cardiac, gastrointestinal, and genitourinary tract abnormalities have also been described

**Adverse Reactions** Percentage unknown: Tachycardia, sinus tachycardia, dizziness, headache, irritability, lethargy, fever, edema, alopecia, pruritus, amenorrhea, sexual dysfunction, nausea, vomiting, xerostomia, constipation, leukopenia, sensory neuropathy (peripheral) (after prolonged therapy due to neuronal degeneration), clonus, myoclonus

**Half-Life** 8.7 hours

## Special PA Issues

**Patient Education:** You will be given oral and written instructions about the necessity of using two methods of contraception and and the necessity of keeping return visits for pregnancy testing. You may experience sleepiness, dizziness, lack of concentration (use caution when driving, climbing stairs, or engaging in tasks that require alertness); nausea or vomiting or loss of appetite (small, frequent meals, chewing gum, or sucking on lozenges may help); constipation or diarrhea; oral thrush (frequent mouth care is necessary); sexual dysfunction (reversible). Report any of the above if persistent or severe. (Continued)

## Thalidomide *(Continued)*

> Report chest pain or palpitations or swelling of extremities; back, neck, or muscle pain or stiffness; skin rash or eruptions; increased nervousness, anxiety, or insomnia; or any other symptom of adverse reactions.
> **Reference Range:** Therapeutic plasma thalidomide levels in graft-vs-host reactions are 5-8 µg/mL, although it has been suggested that lower plasma levels (0.5-1.5 µg/mL) may be therapeutic; peak serum thalidomide level after a 200 mg dose: 1.2 µg/mL

♦ **Thalitone®** *see Chlorthalidone on page 200*

♦ **THC** *see Dronabinol on page 307*

♦ **Theo-24®** *see Theophylline Salts on this page*

♦ **Theobid®** *see Theophylline Salts on this page*

♦ **Theochron®** *see Theophylline Salts on this page*

♦ **Theoclear® L.A.** *see Theophylline Salts on this page*

♦ **Theo-Dur®** *see Theophylline Salts on this page*

♦ **Theo-Dur® Sprinkle** *see Theophylline Salts on this page*

♦ **Theolair™** *see Theophylline Salts on this page*

♦ **Theon®** *see Theophylline Salts on this page*

♦ **Theophylline** *see Theophylline Salts on this page*


## Theophylline and Guaifenesin *(thee OF i lin & gwye FEN e sin)*

**Pharmacologic Class** Theophylline Derivative

**U.S. Brand Names** Bronchial®; Glycerol-T®; Quibron®; Slo-Phyllin® GG

**Dosage Forms Cap:** Theophylline 150 mg and guaifenesin 90 mg, theophylline 300 mg and guaifenesin 180 mg; **Elix:** Theophylline 150 mg and guaifenesin 90 mg per 15 mL (480 mL)


## Theophylline, Ephedrine, and Hydroxyzine

*(thee OF i lin, e FED rin, & hye DROKS i zeen)*

**Pharmacologic Class** Theophylline Derivative

**U.S. Brand Names** Hydrophed®; Marax®

**Dosage Forms Syr, dye free:** Theophylline 32.5 mg, ephedrine 6.25 mg, and hydroxyzine 2.5 mg per 5 mL; **Tab:** Theophylline 130 mg, ephedrine 25 mg, and hydroxyzine 10 mg


## Theophylline, Ephedrine, and Phenobarbital

*(thee OF i lin, e FED rin, & fee noe BAR bi tal)*

**Pharmacologic Class** Theophylline Derivative

**U.S. Brand Names** Tedral®

**Dosage Forms Susp:** Theophylline 65 mg, ephedrine sulfate 12 mg, and phenobarbital 4 mg per 5 mL; **Tab:** Theophylline 118 mg, ephedrine sulfate 25 mg, and phenobarbital 11 mg; theophylline 130 mg, ephedrine sulfate 24 mg, and phenobarbital 8 mg


## Theophylline Salts *(thee OFF i lin salts)*

**Pharmacologic Class** Theophylline Derivative

**U.S. Brand Names** Aerolate®; Aerolate III®; Aerolate JR®; Aerolate SR®; Aminophyllin™; Aquaphyllin®; Asmalix®; Bronkodyl®; Choledyl®; Constant-T®; Duraphyl™; Elixophyllin®; Elixophyllin® SR; LaBID®; Phyllocontin®; Quibron®-T; Quibron®-T/SR; Respbid®; Slo-bid™; Slo-Phyllin®; Sustaire®; Theo-24®; Theobid®; Theochron®; Theoclear® L.A.; Theo-Dur®; Theo-Dur® Sprinkle; Theolair™; Theon®; Theospan®-SR; Theovent®; Truphylline®

**Mechanism of Action** Causes bronchodilatation, diuresis, CNS and cardiac stimulation, and gastric acid secretion by blocking phosphodiesterase which increases tissue concentrations of cyclic adenine monophosphate (cAMP) which in turn promotes catecholamine stimulation of lipolysis, glycogenolysis, and gluconeogenesis and induces release of epinephrine from adrenal medulla cells

**Use** Bronchodilator in reversible airway obstruction due to asthma, chronic bronchitis, and emphysema; for neonatal apnea/bradycardia

**USUAL DOSAGE** Use ideal body weight for obese patients

Neonates:

**Apnea of prematurity:** Oral, I.V.: Loading dose: 4 mg/kg (theophylline); 5 mg/kg (aminophylline)

There appears to be a delay in theophylline elimination in infants <1 year of age, especially neonates; both the initial dose and maintenance dosage should be conservative

I.V.: Initial: Maintenance infusion rates:
Neonates:
≤24 days: 0.08 mg/kg/hour theophylline
>24 days: 0.12 mg/kg/hour theophylline
Infants 6-52 weeks: 0.008 (age in weeks) + 0.21 mg/kg/hour theophylline

Children >1 year and Adults:
**Treatment of acute bronchospasm**: I.V.: Loading dose (in patients not currently receiving aminophylline or theophylline): 6 mg/kg (based on aminophylline) given I.V. over 20-30 minutes; administration rate should not exceed 25 mg/minute (aminophylline). See table.

### Approximate I.V. Theophylline Dosage for Treatment of Acute Bronchospasm

| Group | Dosage for Next 12 h* | Dosage After 12 h* |
|---|---|---|
| Infants 6 wk - 6 mo | 0.5 mg/kg/h | |
| Children 6 mo - 1 y | 0.6-0.7 mg/kg/h | |
| Children 1-9 y | 0.95 mg/kg/h (1.2 mg/kg/h) | 0.79 mg/kg/h (1 mg/kg/h) |
| Children 9-16 y and young adult smokers | 0.79 mg/kg/h (1 mg/kg/h) | 0.63 mg/kg/h (0.8 mg/kg/h) |
| Healthy, nonsmoking adults | 0.55 mg/kg/h (0.7 mg/kg/h) | 0.39 mg/kg/h (0.5 mg/kg/h) |
| Older patients and patients with cor pulmonale | 0.47 mg/kg/h (0.6 mg/kg/h) | 0.24 mg/kg/h (0.3 mg/kg/h) |
| Patients with congestive heart failure or liver failure | 0.39 mg/kg/h (0.5 mg/kg/h) | 0.08-0.16 mg/kg/h (0.1-0.2 mg/kg/h) |

*Equivalent hydrous aminophylline dosage indicated in parentheses.

**Approximate I.V. maintenance dosages are based upon continuous infusions**; bolus dosing (often used in children <6 months of age) may be determined by multiplying the hourly infusion rate by 24 hours and dividing by the desired number of doses/day; see table.

### Maintenance Dose for Acute Symptoms

| Population Group | Oral Theophylline (mg/kg/day) | I.V. Aminophylline |
|---|---|---|
| Premature infant or newborn - 6 wk (for apnea/bradycardia) | 4 | 5 mg/kg/day |
| 6 wk - 6 mo | 10 | 12 mg/kg/day or continuous I.V. infusion* |
| Infants 6 mo - 1 y | 12-18 | 15 mg/kg/day or continuous I.V. infusion* |
| Children 1-9 y | 20-24 | 1 mg/kg/h |
| Children 9-12 y, and adolescent daily smokers of cigarettes or marijuana, and otherwise healthy adult smokers <50 y | 16 | 0.9 mg/kg/h |
| Adolescents 12-16 y (nonsmokers) | 13 | 0.7 mg/kg/h |
| Otherwise healthy nonsmoking adults (including elderly patients) | 10 (not to exceed 900 mg/day) | 0.5 mg/kg/h |
| Cardiac decompensation, cor pulmonale and/or liver dysfunction | 5 (not to exceed 400 mg/day) | 0.25 mg/kg/h |

*For continuous I.V. infusion divide total daily dose by 24 = mg/kg/h.

Dosage should be adjusted according to serum level measurements during the first 12- to 24-hour period; see table.

### Dosage Adjustment After Serum Theophylline Measurement

| Serum Theophylline | | Guidelines |
|---|---|---|
| Within normal limits | 10-20 mcg/mL | Maintain dosage if tolerated. Recheck serum theophylline concentration at 6- to 12-month intervals.* |
| Too high | 20-25 mcg/mL | Decrease doses by about 10%. Recheck serum theophylline concentration after 3 days and then at 6- to 12-month intervals.* |
| | 25-30 mcg/mL | Skip next dose and decrease subsequent doses by about 25%. Recheck serum theophylline. |
| | >30 mcg/mL | Skip next 2 doses and decrease subsequent doses by 50%. Recheck serum theophylline. |
| Too low | 7.5-10 mcg/mL | Increase dose by about 25%.† Recheck serum theophylline concentration after 3 days and then at 6- to 12-month intervals.* |
| | 5-7.5 mcg/mL | Increase dose by about 25% to the nearest dose increment† and recheck serum theophylline for guidance in further dosage adjustment (another increase will probably be needed, but this provides a safety check). |

*Finer adjustments in dosage may be needed for some patients.

†Dividing the daily dose into 3 doses administered at 8-hour intervals may be indicated if symptoms occur repeatedly at the end of a dosing interval.

From Weinberger M and Hendeles L, "Practical Guide to Using Theophylline," *J Resp Dis*, 1981,2:12-27.

**Oral theophylline:** Initial dosage recommendation: Loading dose (to achieve a serum level of about 10 mcg/mL; loading doses should be given using a rapidly absorbed oral product **not** a sustained release product):

If no theophylline has been administered in the previous 24 hours: 4-6 mg/kg theophylline

If theophylline has been administered in the previous 24 hours: administer ½ loading dose or 2-3 mg/kg theophylline can be given in emergencies when serum levels are not available

On the average, for every 1 mg/kg theophylline given, blood levels will rise 2 mcg/mL

Ideally, defer the loading dose if a serum theophylline concentration can be obtained rapidly. However, if this is not possible, exercise clinical judgment. If the patient is not experiencing theophylline toxicity, this is unlikely to result in dangerous adverse effects.

### Oral Theophylline Dosage for Bronchial Asthma*

| Age | Initial 3 Days | Second 3 Days | Steady-State Maintenance |
|---|---|---|---|
| <1 y | 0.2 x (age in weeks) + 5 | | 0.3 x (age in weeks) + 8 |
| 1-9 y | 16 up to a maximum of 400 mg/24 h | 20 | 22 |
| 9-12 y | 16 up to a maximum of 400 mg/24 h | 16 up to a maximum of 600 mg/24 h | 20 up to a maximum of 800 mg/24 h |
| 12-16 y | 16 up to a maximum of 400 mg/24 h | 16 up to a maximum of 600 mg/24 h | 18 up to a maximum of 900 mg/24 h |
| Adults | 400 mg/24 h | 600 mg/24 h | 900 mg/24 h |

*Dose in mg/kg/24 hours of theophylline.

**Increasing dose:** The dosage may be increased in approximately 25% increments at 2- to 3-day intervals so long as the drug is tolerated or until the maximum dose is reached (Continued)

**Maintenance dose:** In newborns and infants, a fast-release oral product can be used. The total daily dose can be divided every 12 hours in newborns and every 6-8 hours in infants. In children and healthy adults, a slow-release product can be used. The total daily dose can be divided every 8-12 hours.

These recommendations, based on mean clearance rates for age or risk factors, were calculated to achieve a serum level of 10 mcg/mL (5 mcg/mL for newborns with apnea/bradycardia)

Dosage should be adjusted according to serum level

**Oral oxtriphylline:**

Children 1-9 years: 6.2 mg/kg/dose every 6 hours

Children 9-16 years and Adult smokers: 4.7 mg/kg/dose every 6 hours

Adult nonsmokers: 4.7 mg/kg/dose every 8 hours

Dose should be further adjusted based on serum levels

**Dosing adjustment/comments in hepatic disease:** Higher incidence of toxic effects including seizures in cirrhosis; plasma levels should be monitored closely during long-term administration in cirrhosis and during acute hepatitis, with dose adjustment as necessary

Hemodialysis: Administer dose posthemodialysis or administer supplemental 50% dose

Peritoneal dialysis: Supplemental dose is not necessary

Continuous arteriovenous or venovenous hemodiafiltration (CAVH/CAVHD) effects: Supplemental dose is not necessary

## Dosage Forms

Aminophylline (79% theophylline): **Inj:** 25 mg/mL (10 mL, 20 mL); 250 mg (equivalent to 187 mg theophylline) per 10 mL, 500 mg (equivalent to 394 mg theophylline) per 20 mL; **Liq, oral:** 105 mg (equivalent to 90 mg theophylline) per 5 mL (240 mL, 500 mL); **Supp, rectal:** 250 mg (equivalent to 198 mg theophylline), 500 mg (equivalent to 395 mg theophylline); **Tab:** 100 mg (equivalent to 79 mg theophylline), 200 mg (equivalent to 158 mg theophylline); **Tab, cont release:** 225 mg (equivalent to 178 mg theophylline)

Oxtriphylline (64% theophylline): **Elix:** 100 mg (equivalent to 64 mg theophylline)/5 mL (5 mL, 10 mL, 473 mL); **Syr:** 50 mg (equivalent to 32 mg theophylline)/5 mL (473 mL); **Tab:** 100 mg (equivalent to 64 mg theophylline); 200 mg (equivalent to 127 mg theophylline); **Tab, sustained release:** 400 mg (equivalent to 254 mg theophylline); 600 mg (equivalent to 382 mg theophylline)

Theophylline: **Cap: Immediate release:** 100 mg, 200 mg, **Sustained release (8-12 hours):** 50 mg, 60 mg, 65 mg, 75 mg, 100 mg, 125 mg, 130 mg, 200 mg, 250 mg, 260 mg, 300 mg, **Timed release (12 hours):** 50 mg, 75 mg, 125 mg, 130 mg, 200 mg, 250 mg, 260 mg, **Timed release (24 hours):** 100 mg, 200 mg, 300 mg; **Inj:** Theophylline in 5% dextrose: 200 mg/container (50 mL, 100 mL), 400 mg/container (100 mL, 250 mL, 500 mL, 1000 mL), 800 mg/container (250 mL, 500 mL, 1000 mL); **Elix, oral:** 80 mg/15 mL (15 mL, 30 mL, 500 mL, 4000 mL); **Soln, oral:** 80 mg/15 mL (15 mL, 18.75 mL, 30 mL, 120 mL, 500 mL, 4000 mL), 150 mg/15 mL (480 mL); **Syr, oral:** 80 mg/15 mL (5 mL, 15 mL, 30 mL, 120 mL, 500 mL, 4000 mL), 150 mg/15 mL (480 mL); **Tab: Immediate release:** 100 mg, 125 mg, 200 mg, 250 mg, 300 mg, **Timed release (8-12 hours):** 100 mg, 200 mg, 250 mg, 300 mg, 500 mg, **Timed release (8-24 hours):** 100 mg, 200 mg, 300 mg, 450 mg, **Timed release (12-24 hours):** 100 mg, 200 mg, 300 mg, **Timed release (24 hours):** 400 mg

**Contraindications** Uncontrolled arrhythmias, hyperthyroidism, peptic ulcers, uncontrolled seizure disorders, hypersensitivity to xanthines or any component

**Warnings/Precautions** Use with caution in patients with peptic ulcer, hyperthyroidism, hypertension, tachyarrhythmias, and patients with compromised cardiac function; do not inject I.V. solution faster than 25 mg/minute; elderly, acutely ill, and patients with severe respiratory problems, pulmonary edema, or liver dysfunction are at greater risk of toxicity because of reduced drug clearance

Although there is a great intersubject variability for half-lives of methylxanthines (2-10 hours), elderly as a group have slower hepatic clearance. Therefore, use lower initial doses and monitor closely for response and adverse reactions. Additionally, elderly are at greater risk for toxicity due to concomitant disease (eg, CHF, arrhythmias), and drug use (eg, cimetidine, ciprofloxacin, etc).

**Pregnancy Risk Factor** C

**Pregnancy Implications**

Clinical effects on the fetus: Crosses the placenta. Transient tachycardia, irritability, vomiting in newborn especially if maternal serum concentrations >20 mcg/mL. Apneic spells attributed to withdrawal in newborn exposed throughout gestation period. Available evidence suggests safe use during pregnancy.

Breast-feeding/lactation: Crosses into breast milk

Clinical effects on the infant: Irritability reported in infants. American Academy of Pediatrics considers **compatible** with breast-feeding.

**Adverse Reactions** See table.

**Uncommon at serum theophylline concentrations ≤20 mcg/mL**

1% to 10%:

Cardiovascular: Tachycardia

Central nervous system: Nervousness, restlessness

(Continued)

# Theophylline Salts (Continued)

Gastrointestinal: Nausea, vomiting

<1%: Allergic reactions, insomnia, irritability, seizures, rash, gastric irritation, tremor

| Theophylline Serum Levels (mcg/mL)* | Adverse Reactions |
|---|---|
| 15-25 | GI upset, diarrhea, N/V, abdominal pain, nervousness, headache, insomnia, agitation, dizziness, muscle cramp, tremor |
| 25-35 | Tachycardia, occasional PVC |
| >35 | Ventricular tachycardia, frequent PVC, seizure |

*Adverse effects do not necessarily occur according to serum levels. Arrhythmia and seizure can occur without seeing the other adverse effects.

**Drug Interactions** CYP1A2 and 3A3/4 enzyme substrate, CYP2E enzyme substrate (minor) Cytochrome P-450 1A2 enzyme substrate and cytochrome P-450 2E1 enzyme substrate (minor)

Decreased effect/increased toxicity: Changes in diet may affect the elimination of theophylline; charcoal-broiled foods may increase elimination, reducing half-life by 50%; see table for factors affecting serum levels.

### Factors Reported to Affect Theophylline Serum Levels

| Decreased Theophylline Level | Increased Theophylline Level |
|---|---|
| Aminoglutethimide | Allopurinol (>600 mg/d) |
| Barbiturates | Beta-blockers |
| Carbamazepine | Calcium channel blockers |
| Charcoal | Carbamazepine |
| High protein/low carbohydrate diet | CHF |
| Hydantoins | Cimetidine |
| Isoniazid | Ciprofloxacin |
| I.V. isoproterenol | Cor pulmonale |
| Ketoconazole | Corticosteroids |
| Loop diuretics | Disulfiram |
| Phenobarbital | Ephedrine |
| Phenytoin | Erythromycin |
| Rifampin | Fever/viral illness |
| Smoking (cigarettes, marijuana) | Hepatic cirrhosis |
| Sulfinpyrazone | Influenza virus vaccine |
| Sympathomimetics | Interferon |
| | Isoniazid |
| | Loop diuretics |
| | Macrolides |
| | Mexiletine |
| | Oral contraceptives |
| | Propranolol |
| | Quinolones |
| | Thiabendazole |
| | Thyroid hormones |
| | Troleandomycin |

**Onset** Oral: 1-2 hours; I.V.: <30 minutes

**Half-Life** Variable; dependent on age, liver function, cardiac function, lung disease, and smoking history; range: 4-30 hours

**Special PA Issues**

**Patient Education:** Oral preparations should be taken with a full glass of water; capsule forms may be opened and sprinkled on soft foods; do not chew beads; notify physician if nausea, vomiting, severe GI pain, restlessness, or irregular heartbeat occurs; do not drink or eat large quantities of caffeine-containing beverages or food (colas, coffee, chocolate); remain in bed for 15-20 minutes after inserting suppository; do not chew or crush enteric coated or sustained release products; take at regular intervals; notify physician if insomnia, nervousness, irritability, palpitations, seizures occur; do not change brands or doses without consulting physician

**Monitoring Parameters:** Heart rate, CNS effects (insomnia, irritability); respiratory rate (COPD patients often have resting controlled respiratory rates in low 20s), serum theophylline level, arterial or capillary blood gases (if applicable)

**Reference Range:**

Sample size: 0.5-1 mL serum (red top tube)
Saliva levels are approximately equal to 60% of plasma levels

Therapeutic levels: 10-20 μg/mL
Neonatal apnea 6-13 μg/mL

Pregnancy: 3-12 µg/mL
Toxic concentration: >20 µg/mL

Timing of serum samples: If toxicity is suspected, draw a level any time during a continuous I.V. infusion, or 2 hours after an oral dose; if lack of therapeutic is effected, draw a trough immediately before the next oral dose; see table.

### Guidelines for Drawing Theophylline Serum Levels

| Dosage Form | Time to Draw Level |
| --- | --- |
| I.V. bolus | 30 min after end of 30 min infusion |
| I.V. continuous infusion | 12-24 h after initiation of infusion |
| P.O. liquid, fast-release tab | Peak: 1 h postdose after at least 1 day of therapy<br>Trough: Just before a dose after at least one day of therapy |
| P.O. slow-release product | Peak: 4 h postdose after at least 1 day of therapy<br>Trough: Just before a dose after at least one day of therapy |

- ♦ **Theospan®-SR** see Theophylline Salts on page 888
- ♦ **Theovent®** see Theophylline Salts on page 888
- ♦ **Therabid® [OTC]** see Vitamins, Multiple on page 964
- ♦ **Thera-Flur®** see Fluoride on page 383
- ♦ **Thera-Flur-N®** see Fluoride on page 383
- ♦ **Theragran® [OTC]** see Vitamins, Multiple on page 964
- ♦ **Theragran® Hematinic®** see Vitamins, Multiple on page 964
- ♦ **Theragran® Liquid [OTC]** see Vitamins, Multiple on page 964
- ♦ **Theragran-M® [OTC]** see Vitamins, Multiple on page 964
- ♦ **Therapeutic Multivitamins** see Vitamins, Multiple on page 964
- ♦ **Thermazene®** see Silver Sulfadiazine on page 835

## Thiabendazole (thye a BEN da zole)
**Pharmacologic Class** Anthelmintic
**U.S. Brand Names** Mintezol®
**Mechanism of Action** Inhibits helminth-specific mitochondrial fumarate reductase
**Use** Treatment of strongyloidiasis, cutaneous larva migrans, visceral larva migrans, dracunculiasis, trichinosis, and mixed helminthic infections
**USUAL DOSAGE** Purgation is not required prior to use; drinking of fruit juice aids in expulsion of worms by removing the mucous to which the intestinal tapeworms attach themselves.

  Children and Adults: Oral: 50 mg/kg/day divided every 12 hours (if >68 kg: 1.5 g/dose); maximum dose: 3 g/day
    Strongyloidiasis, ascariasis, uncinariasis, trichuriasis: For 2 consecutive days
    Cutaneous larva migrans: For 2-5 consecutive days
    Visceral larva migrans: For 5-7 consecutive days
    Trichinosis: For 2-4 consecutive days
    Dracunculosis: 50-75 mg/kg/day divided every 12 hours for 3 days
  **Dosing comments in renal/hepatic impairment:** Use with caution
**Dosage Forms Susp, oral:** 500 mg/5 mL (120 mL); **Tab, chewable (orange flavor):** 500 mg
**Contraindications** Known hypersensitivity to thiabendazole
**Warnings/Precautions** Use with caution in patients with renal or hepatic impairment, malnutrition or anemia, or dehydration
**Pregnancy Risk Factor** C
**Adverse Reactions**
  >10%:
    Central nervous system: Seizures, hallucinations, delirium, dizziness, drowsiness, headache
    Gastrointestinal: Anorexia, diarrhea, nausea, vomiting, drying of mucous membranes
    Neuromuscular & skeletal: Numbness
    Otic: Tinnitus
  1% to 10%: Dermatologic: Rash, Stevens-Johnson syndrome
  <1%: Chills, malodor of urine, leukopenia, hepatotoxicity, blurred or yellow vision, nephrotoxicity, lymphadenopathy, hypersensitivity reactions
**Drug Interactions** Increased levels of theophylline and other xanthines
**Special PA Issues**
  **Patient Education:** Take exactly as directed, for full course of medication. Tablets may be chewed, swallowed whole, or crushed and mixed with food. Increase dietary intake of fruit juices. All family members and close friends should also be treated. To reduce possibility of reinfection, wash hands and scrub nails carefully with soap and hot water before handling food, before eating, and before and after toileting. Keep hands out of mouth. Disinfect toilet daily and launder bed lines, undergarments, and nightclothes daily
(Continued)

## Thiabendazole *(Continued)*

with hot water and soap. May cause unusual odor in urine (normal); dizziness or drowsiness (use caution when driving or engaging in hazardous tasks); nausea or vomiting (frequent small meals, frequent mouth care, or sucking on lozenges may help). Report delirium, hallucination, or other acute CNS disturbances; unresolved diarrhea or vomiting; tingling or numbness of extremities; or skin rash.

♦ **Thiamazole** *see* Methimazole *on page 584*

♦ **Thiamilate®** *see* Thiamine *on this page*

## Thiamine *(THYE a min)*

**Pharmacologic Class** Vitamin, Water Soluble
**U.S. Brand Names** Thiamilate®
**Mechanism of Action** An essential coenzyme in carbohydrate metabolism by combining with adenosine triphosphate to form thiamine pyrophosphate
**Use** Treatment of thiamine deficiency including beriberi, Wernicke's encephalopathy syndrome, and peripheral neuritis associated with pellagra, alcoholic patients with altered sensorium; various genetic metabolic disorders

**USUAL DOSAGE**
Recommended daily allowance:
    <6 months: 0.3 mg
    6 months to 1 year: 0.4 mg
    1-3 years: 0.7 mg
    4-6 years: 0.9 mg
    7-10 years: 1 mg
    11-14 years: 1.1-1.3 mg
    >14 years: 1-1.5 mg
Thiamine deficiency (beriberi):
    Children: 10-25 mg/dose I.M. or I.V. daily (if critically ill), or 10-50 mg/dose orally every day for 2 weeks, then 5-10 mg/dose orally daily for 1 month
    Adults: 5-30 mg/dose I.M. or I.V. 3 times/day (if critically ill); then orally 5-30 mg/day in single or divided doses 3 times/day for 1 month
Wernicke's encephalopathy: Adults: Initial: 100 mg I.V., then 50-100 mg/day I.M. or I.V. until consuming a regular, balanced diet
Dietary supplement (depends on caloric or carbohydrate content of the diet):
    Infants: 0.3-0.5 mg/day
    Children: 0.5-1 mg/day
    Adults: 1-2 mg/day
    **Note:** The above doses can be found in multivitamin preparations
Metabolic disorders: Oral: Adults: 10-20 mg/day (dosages up to 4 g/day in divided doses have been used)
**Dosage Forms** Thiamine hydrochloride: **Inj:** 100 mg/mL (1 mL, 2 mL, 10 mL, 30 mL); 200 mg/mL (30 mL); **Tab:** 50 mg, 100 mg, 250 mg, 500 mg; **Tab, enteric coated:** 20 mg
**Contraindications** Hypersensitivity to thiamine or any component
**Warnings/Precautions** Use with caution with parenteral route (especially I.V.) of administration
**Pregnancy Risk Factor** A (C if dose exceeds RDA recommendation)
**Adverse Reactions** <1%: Cardiovascular collapse and death, warmth, rash, angioedema, paresthesia
**Special PA Issues**
**Patient Education:** Take exactly as directed; do not discontinue without consulting prescriber (deficiency state can occur in as little as 3 weeks). Follow dietary instructions (dietary sources include legumes, pork, beef, whole grains, yeast, fresh vegetables).
    **Reference Range:** Therapeutic: 1.6-4 mg/dL

♦ **Thiamine Hydrochloride** *see* Thiamine *on this page*

♦ **Thiaminium Chloride Hydrochloride** *see* Thiamine *on this page*

## Thiethylperazine *(thye eth il PER a zeen)*

**Pharmacologic Class** Antiemetic
**U.S. Brand Names** Norzine®; Torecan®
**Mechanism of Action** Blocks postsynaptic mesolimbic dopaminergic receptors in the brain; exhibits a strong alpha-adrenergic blocking effect and depresses the release of hypothalamic and hypophyseal hormones; acts directly on chemoreceptor trigger zone and vomiting center
**Use** Relief of nausea and vomiting
    **Unlabeled use:** Treatment of vertigo
**USUAL DOSAGE** Children >12 years and Adults:
    Oral, I.M., rectal: 10 mg 1-3 times/day as needed
    I.V. and S.C. routes of administration are not recommended
    Hemodialysis: Not dialyzable (0% to 5%)
    **Dosing comments in hepatic impairment:** Use with caution

**Dosage Forms** Thiethylperazine maleate: **Inj:** 5 mg/mL (2 mL); **Supp, rectal:** 10 mg; **Tab:** 10 mg

**Contraindications** Comatose states, hypersensitivity to thiethylperazine or any component; pregnancy, cross-sensitivity to other phenothiazines may exist

**Warnings/Precautions** Reduce or discontinue if extrapyramidal effects occur; safety and efficacy in children <12 years of age have not been established; postural hypotension may occur after I.M. injection; the injectable form contains sulfite which may cause allergic reactions in some patients; use caution in patients with narrow-angle glaucoma

**Pregnancy Risk Factor** X

**Adverse Reactions**

>10%:

Central nervous system: Drowsiness, dizziness

Gastrointestinal: Xerostomia

Respiratory: Dry nose

1% to 10%:

Cardiovascular: Tachycardia, orthostatic hypotension

Central nervous system: Confusion, convulsions, extrapyramidal effects, tardive dyskinesia, fever, headache

Hematologic: Agranulocytosis

Hepatic: Cholestatic jaundice

Otic: Tinnitus

**Drug Interactions** Increased effect/toxicity with CNS depressants (eg, anesthetics, opiates, tranquilizers, alcohol), lithium, atropine, epinephrine, MAO inhibitors, TCAs

**Onset** Onset of antiemetic effect: Within 30 minutes

**Duration** ~4 hours

**Special PA Issues**

**Patient Education:** Take as directed; do not use more than recommended. Do not use alcohol and prescription or OTC depressant without consulting prescriber. May cause drowsiness, dizziness, stupor (use caution when driving or engaging in hazardous tasks); dry mouth (frequent oral care and sucking on lozenges may help); photosensitivity (use sunblock, wear protective clothing and eyewear, or avoid exposure to direct sunlight); postural hypotension (rise slowly from sitting or lying position and use caution when climbing stairs). Report abnormal or involuntary muscle movements or twitching or facial tics, acute drowsiness or restlessness, excessive fatigue or dizziness.

♦ **Thiethylperazine Maleate** *see* Thiethylperazine *on previous page*

# Thioridazine (thye oh RID a zeen)

**Pharmacologic Class** Antipsychotic Agent, Phenothiazine, Piperidine

**U.S. Brand Names** Mellaril®; Mellaril-S®

**Mechanism of Action** Blocks postsynaptic mesolimbic dopaminergic receptors in the brain; exhibits a strong alpha-adrenergic blocking effect and depresses the release of hypothalamic and hypophyseal hormones

**Use** Management of manifestations of psychotic disorders; depressive neurosis; alcohol withdrawal; dementia in elderly; behavioral problems in children

**USUAL DOSAGE** Oral:

Children >2 years: Range: 0.5-3 mg/kg/day in 2-3 divided doses; usual: 1 mg/kg/day; maximum: 3 mg/kg/day

Behavior problems: Initial: 10 mg 2-3 times/day, increase gradually

Severe psychoses: Initial: 25 mg 2-3 times/day, increase gradually

Adults:

Psychoses: Initial: 50-100 mg 3 times/day with gradual increments as needed and tolerated; maximum: 800 mg/day in 2-4 divided doses; if >65 years, initial dose: 10 mg 3 times/day

Depressive disorders, dementia: Initial: 25 mg 3 times/day; maintenance dose: 20-200 mg/day

Hemodialysis: Not dialyzable (0% to 5%)

**Dosage Forms** Thioridazine hydrochloride: **Conc, oral, as hydrochloride:** 30 mg/mL (120 mL); 100 mg/mL (3.4 mL, 120 mL); **Susp, oral, as hydrochloride:** 25 mg/5 mL (480 mL); 100 mg/5 mL (480 mL); **Tab, as hydrochloride:** 10 mg, 15 mg, 25 mg, 50 mg, 100 mg, 150 mg, 200 mg

**Contraindications** Severe CNS depression, hypersensitivity to thioridazine or any component; cross-sensitivity to other phenothiazines may exist

**Warnings/Precautions** Oral formulations may cause stomach upset; may cause thermoregulatory changes; use caution in patients with narrow-angle glaucoma, severe liver or cardiac disease; doses of 1 g/day frequently cause pigmentary retinopathy

**Pregnancy Risk Factor** C

**Adverse Reactions**

>10%:

Central nervous system: Pseudoparkinsonism, akathisia, dystonias, tardive dyskinesia (persistent), dizziness

Cardiovascular: Hypotension, orthostatic hypotension

(Continued)

## Thioridazine *(Continued)*

Gastrointestinal: Constipation
Ocular: Pigmentary retinopathy
Respiratory: Nasal congestion
Miscellaneous: Diaphoresis (decreased)

1% to 10%:

Dermatologic: Increased sensitivity to sun, rash
Endocrine & metabolic: Changes in menstrual cycle, changes in libido, breast pain
Gastrointestinal: Weight gain, nausea, vomiting, stomach pain
Genitourinary: Dysuria, ejaculatory disturbances
Neuromuscular & skeletal: Trembling of fingers

<1%: Neuroleptic malignant syndrome (NMS), impairment of temperature regulation, lowering of seizures threshold, discoloration of skin (blue-gray), galactorrhea, priapism, agranulocytosis, leukopenia, cholestatic jaundice, hepatotoxicity, cornea and lens changes

**Drug Interactions** CYP1A2 and 2D6 enzyme substrate; CYP2D6 enzyme inhibitor

Decreased effect with anticholinergics
Decreased effect of guanethidine
Increased toxicity with CNS depressants, epinephrine (hypotension), lithium (rare), TCA (cardiotoxicity), propranolol, pindolol

**Duration** 4-5 days

**Half-Life** 21-25 hours

**Special PA Issues**

**Patient Education:** Use exactly as directed (do not increase dose or frequency); may cause physical and/or psychological dependence. Do not discontinue without consulting prescriber. Tablets/capsules may be taken with food. Mix oral solution with 2-4 oz of liquid (eg, juice, milk, water, pudding). Do not take within 2 hours of any antacid. Store away from light. Avoid excess alcohol or caffeine and other prescription or OTC medications not approved by prescriber. Maintain adequate hydration (2-3 L/day of fluids unless instructed to restrict fluid intake). Avoid skin contact with liquid medication; may cause contact dermatitis (wash immediately with warm, soapy water). May turn urine red-brown (normal). You may experience excess drowsiness, lightheadedness, dizziness, or blurred vision (use caution driving or when engaging in hazardous tasks until response to medication is known); nausea, vomiting, or dry mouth (small frequent meals, frequent mouth care, or sucking lozenges may help); constipation (increased exercise, fluids, or dietary fruit and fiber may help); postural hypotension (use caution climbing stairs or when changing position from lying or sitting to standing); urinary retention (void before taking medication); ejaculatory dysfunction (reversible); decreased perspiration (avoid strenuous exercise in hot environments); photosensitivity (use sunscreen, protective clothing, and avoid prolonged exposure to direct sunlight). Report persistent CNS effects (eg, trembling fingers, altered gait or balance, excessive sedation, seizures, unusual movements, anxiety, abnormal thoughts, confusion, personality changes); chest pain, palpitations, rapid heartbeat, severe dizziness; unresolved urinary retention or changes in urinary pattern; altered menstrual pattern, change in libido, swelling or pain in breasts (male or female); vision changes; skin rash, irritation, or changes in color of skin (gray-blue); or worsening of condition.

**Dietary Considerations:** Alcohol: Additive CNS effect, avoid use

**Monitoring Parameters:** For patients on prolonged therapy: CBC, ophthalmologic exam, blood pressure, liver function tests

**Reference Range:** Therapeutic: 1.0-1.5 µg/mL (SI: 2.7-4.1 µmol/L); Toxic: >10 µg/mL (SI: >27 µmol/L)

**Related Information**

Antipsychotic Agents *on page 1001*

♦ **Thioridazine Hydrochloride** *see* Thioridazine *on previous page*

## Thiothixene *(thye oh THIKS een)*

**Pharmacologic Class** Antipsychotic Agent, Thioxanthene Derivative

**U.S. Brand Names** Navane®

**Mechanism of Action** Elicits antipsychotic activity by postsynaptic blockade of CNS dopamine receptors resulting in inhibition of dopamine-mediated effects; also has alpha-adrenergic blocking activity

**Use** Management of psychotic disorders

**USUAL DOSAGE**

Children <12 years: Oral: 0.25 mg/kg/24 hours in divided doses (dose not well established)

Children >12 years and Adults: Mild to moderate psychosis:

Oral: 2 mg 3 times/day, up to 20-30 mg/day; more severe psychosis: Initial: 5 mg 2 times/day, may increase gradually, if necessary; maximum: 60 mg/day

I.M.: 4 mg 2-4 times/day, increase dose gradually; usual: 16-20 mg/day; maximum: 30 mg/day; change to oral dose as soon as able

Hemodialysis: Not dialyzable (0% to 5%)

**Dosage Forms Cap:** 1 mg, 2 mg, 5 mg, 10 mg, 20 mg; **Conc, as hydrochloride:** 5 mg/mL
**Contraindications** Hypersensitivity to thiothixene or any component; cross-sensitivity with other phenothiazines may exist, lactation
**Warnings/Precautions** Watch for hypotension when administering I.M. or I.V.; safety in children <6 months of age has not been established; use with caution in patients with narrow-angle glaucoma, bone marrow suppression, severe liver or cardiac disease, seizures

**Pregnancy Risk Factor** C
**Adverse Reactions**
>10%:
Cardiovascular: Hypotension, orthostatic hypotension
Central nervous system: Pseudoparkinsonism, akathisia, dystonias, tardive dyskinesia (persistent), dizziness
Gastrointestinal: Constipation
Respiratory: Nasal congestion
Miscellaneous: Diaphoresis (decreased)
1% to 10%:
Dermatologic: Increased sensitivity to sun, rash
Endocrine & metabolic: Changes in menstrual cycle, changes in libido, breast pain
Gastrointestinal: Weight gain, nausea, vomiting, stomach pain
Genitourinary: Dysuria, ejaculatory disturbances
Neuromuscular & skeletal: Trembling of fingers
Ocular: Pigmentary retinopathy
<1%: Neuroleptic malignant syndrome (NMS), impairment of temperature regulation, lowering of seizures threshold, discoloration of skin (blue-gray), galactorrhea, priapism, agranulocytosis, leukopenia, cholestatic jaundice, hepatotoxicity, cornea and lens changes

**Drug Interactions** CYP1A2 enzyme substrate
Decreased effect of guanethidine
Increased toxicity with CNS depressants, anticholinergics, alcohol
**Half-Life** >24 hours with chronic use
**Special PA Issues**
**Patient Education:** Use exactly as directed (do not increase dose or frequency); may cause physical and/or psychological dependence. Do not discontinue without consulting prescriber. Tablets/capsules may be taken with food. Mix oral solution with 2-4 oz of liquid (eg, juice, milk, water, pudding). Do not take within 2 hours of any antacid. Avoid excess alcohol or caffeine and other prescription or OTC medications not approved by prescriber. Maintain adequate hydration (2-3 L/day of fluids unless instructed to restrict fluid intake). May turn urine red-brown (normal). You may experience excess drowsiness, lightheadedness, dizziness, or blurred vision (use caution driving or when engaging in hazardous tasks until response to medication is known); nausea or vomiting (small frequent meals, frequent mouth care, or sucking lozenges may help); constipation (increased exercise, fluids, or dietary fruit and fiber may help); postural hypotension (use caution climbing stairs or when changing position from lying or sitting to standing); urinary retention (void before taking medication); ejaculatory dysfunction (reversible); decreased perspiration (avoid strenuous exercise in hot environments); photosensitivity (use sunscreen, protective clothing, and avoid prolonged exposure to direct sunlight). Report persistent CNS effects (eg, trembling fingers, altered gait or balance, excessive sedation, seizures, unusual movements, anxiety, abnormal thoughts, confusion, personality changes); chest pain, palpitations, rapid heartbeat, severe dizziness; unresolved urinary retention or changes in urinary pattern; altered menstrual pattern, change in libido, swelling or pain in breasts (male or female); vision changes; skin rash, irritation, or changes in color of skin (gray-blue); or worsening of condition.
**Dietary Considerations:** Alcohol: Additive CNS effect, avoid use
**Monitoring Parameters:** Liver function tests; for patients on prolonged therapy: CBC, ophthalmologic exam
**Related Information**
Antipsychotic Agents *on page 1001*

◆ **Thorazine®** *see* Chlorpromazine *on page 197*
◆ **Thymoglobulin®** *see* Antithymocyte Globulin (Rabbit) *on page 73*
◆ **Thyrar®** *see* Thyroid *on this page*
◆ **Thyro-Block®** *see* Potassium Iodide *on page 744*
◆ **Thyrogen®** *see* Thyrotropin Alpha *on page 899*

# Thyroid (THYE royd)
**Pharmacologic Class** Thyroid Product
**U.S. Brand Names** Armour® Thyroid; S-P-T; Thyrar®; Thyroid Strong®
**Mechanism of Action** The primary active compound is $T_3$ (triiodothyronine), which may be converted from $T_4$ (thyroxine) and then circulates throughout the body to influence growth and maturation of various tissues; exact mechanism of action is unknown; however, it is believed the thyroid hormone exerts its many metabolic effects through control of DNA
(Continued)

## Thyroid *(Continued)*

transcription and protein synthesis; involved in normal metabolism, growth, and development; promotes gluconeogenesis, increases utilization and mobilization of glycogen stores and stimulates protein synthesis, increases basal metabolic rate

**Use** Replacement or supplemental therapy in hypothyroidism; pituitary TSH suppressants (thyroid nodules, thyroiditis, multinodular goiter, thyroid cancer), thyrotoxicosis, diagnostic suppression tests

**USUAL DOSAGE** Oral:

Children: See table

### Recommended Pediatric Dosage for Congenital Hypothyroidism

| Age | Daily Dose (mg) | Daily Dose/kg (mg) |
|---|---|---|
| 0-6 mo | 15-30 | 4.8-6 |
| 6-12 mo | 30-45 | 3.6-4.8 |
| 1-5 y | 45-60 | 3-3.6 |
| 6-12 y | 60-90 | 2.4-3 |
| >12 y | >90 | 1.2-1.8 |

Adults: Initial: 30 mg (15 mg in patients with long-standing myxedema especially if cardiovascular involvement); increase with 15 mg increments every 2-4 weeks. Maintenance dose: Usually 60-120 mg/day; monitor TSH and clinical symptoms.

Thyroid cancer: Requires larger amounts than replacement therapy

**Dosage Forms Cap, pork source in soybean oil (S-P-T):** 60 mg, 120 mg, 180 mg, 300 mg; **Tab:** Armour® Thyroid: 15 mg, 30 mg, 60 mg, 90 mg, 120 mg, 180 mg, 240 mg, 300 mg, Thyrar® (bovine source): 30 mg, 60 mg, 120 mg, Thyroid Strong® (60 mg is equivalent to 90 mg thyroid USP): Regular: 30 mg, 60 mg, 120 mg, Sugar coated: 30 mg, 60 mg, 120 mg, 180 mg, Thyroid USP: 15 mg, 30 mg, 60 mg, 120 mg, 180 mg, 300 mg

**Contraindications** Recent myocardial infarction or thyrotoxicosis, uncomplicated by hypothyroidism; uncorrected adrenal insufficiency, hypersensitivity to active or extraneous constituents

**Warnings/Precautions** Ineffective for weight reduction; high doses may produce serious or even life-threatening toxic effects particularly when used with some anorectic drugs; use cautiously in patients with pre-existing cardiovascular disease (angina, CHD), elderly since they may be more likely to have compromised cardiovascular function. Chronic hypothyroidism predisposes patients to coronary artery disease. Desiccated thyroid contains variable amounts of $T_3$, $T_4$, and other triiodothyronine compounds which are more likely to cause cardiac signs and symptoms due to fluctuating levels; should avoid use in elderly for this reason; drug of choice is levothyroxine in the minds of many clinicians.

**Pregnancy Risk Factor** A

**Adverse Reactions** <1%: Palpitations, tachycardia, cardiac arrhythmias, chest pain, nervousness, headache, insomnia, fever, ataxia, alopecia, changes in menstrual cycle, weight loss, increased appetite, diarrhea, abdominal cramps, vomiting, constipation, excessive bone loss with overtreatment (excess thyroid replacement), tremor, hand tremors, myalgia, shortness of breath, heat intolerance, diaphoresis

**Drug Interactions**

Decreased effect:

Beta-blocker effect is decreased when patients become euthyroid

Thyroid hormones increase the therapeutic need for oral hypoglycemics or insulin

Estrogens increase TBG, thereby decreasing effect of thyroid replacement

Cholestyramine and colestipol decrease the effect of orally administered thyroid replacement

Serum digitalis concentrations are reduced in hyperthyroidism or when hypothyroid patients are converted to a euthyroid state

Theophylline levels decrease when hypothyroid patients converted to a euthyroid state

Increased toxicity: Thyroid may potentiate the hypoprothrombinemic effect of oral anticoagulants

**Half-Life** Liothyronine: 1-2 days; Thyroxine: 6-7 days

**Special PA Issues**

**Patient Education:** Thyroid replacement therapy is generally for life. Take as directed, in the morning before breakfast. Do not change brands and do not discontinue without consulting prescriber. Consult prescriber if drastically increasing or decreasing intake of goitrogenic food (eg, asparagus, cabbage, peas, turnip greens, broccoli, spinach, Brussels sprouts, lettuce, soybeans). Report chest pain, rapid heart rate, palpitations, heat intolerance, excessive sweating, increased nervousness, agitation, or lethargy.

**Monitoring Parameters:** $T_4$, TSH, heart rate, blood pressure, clinical signs of hypo- and hyperthyroidism; TSH is the most reliable guide for evaluating adequacy of thyroid replacement dosage. TSH may be elevated during the first few months of thyroid replacement despite patients being clinically euthyroid. In cases where $T_4$ remains low and TSH is within normal limits, an evaluation of "free" (unbound) $T_4$ is needed to evaluate further increase in dosage.

**Reference Range:**
TSH: 0.4-10 (for those ≥80 years) mIU/L
$T_4$: 4-12 µg/dL (51-154 nmol/L)
$T_3$ (RIA) (total $T_3$): 80-230 ng/dL (1.2-3.5 nmol/L)
$T_4$ free (free $T_4$): 0.7-1.8 ng/dL (9-23 pmol/L)

♦ **Thyroid Extract** see Thyroid on page 897
♦ **Thyroid Stimulating Hormone** see Thyrotropin on this page
♦ **Thyroid Strong®** see Thyroid on page 897
♦ **Thyrotropic Hormone** see Thyrotropin on this page

# Thyrotropin (thye roe TROE pin)
**Pharmacologic Class** Diagnostic Agent, Hypothyroidism; Diagnostic Agent, Thyroid Function
**U.S. Brand Names** Thytropar®
**Mechanism of Action** Stimulates formation and secretion of thyroid hormone, increases uptake of iodine by thyroid gland
**Use** Diagnostic aid to differentiate thyroid failure; diagnosis of decreased thyroid reserve, to differentiate between primary and secondary hypothyroidism and between primary hypothyroidism and euthyroidism in patients receiving thyroid replacement
**USUAL DOSAGE** Adults: I.M., S.C.: 10 units/day for 1-3 days; follow by a radioiodine study 24 hours past last injection, no response in thyroid failure, substantial response in pituitary failure
**Dosage Forms Inj:** 10 units
**Contraindications** Coronary thrombosis, untreated Addison's disease, hypersensitivity to thyrotropin or any component
**Warnings/Precautions** Use with caution in patients with angina pectoris or cardiac failure, patients with hypopituitarism, adrenal cortical suppression as may be seen with corticosteroid therapy; may cause thyroid hyperplasia
**Pregnancy Risk Factor** C
**Adverse Reactions** <1%: Tachycardia, fever, headache, menstrual irregularities, nausea, vomiting, increased bowel motility, anaphylaxis with repeated administration
**Half-Life** 35 minutes, dependent upon thyroid state
**Special PA Issues**
**Patient Education:** You will receive this medication for 3 days prior to the radiologic studies. You may experience some nausea or vomiting. Report dizziness, faintness, palpitations, or any respiratory difficulties.

# Thyrotropin Alpha (thye roe TROE pin AL fa)
**Pharmacologic Class** Diagnostic Agent
**U.S. Brand Names** Thyrogen®
**Mechanism of Action** An exogenous source of human TSH that offers an additional diagnostic tool in the follow-up of patients with a history of well-differentiated thyroid cancer. Binding of thyrotropin alpha to TSH receptors on normal thyroid epithelial cells or on well-differentiated thyroid cancer tissue stimulates iodine uptake and organification and synthesis and secretion of thyroglobulin, triiodothyronine, and thyroxine.
**Use** As an adjunctive diagnostic tool for serum thyroglobulin (Tg) testing with or without radioiodine imaging in the follow-up of patients with well-differentiated thyroid cancer

Potential clinical uses:
1. Patients with an undetectable Tg on thyroid hormone suppressive therapy to exclude the diagnosis of residual or recurrent thyroid cancer
2. Patients requiring serum Tg testing and radioiodine imaging who are unwilling to undergo thyroid hormone withdrawal testing and whose treating physician believes that use of a less sensitive test is justified
3. Patients who are either unable to mount an adequate endogenous TSH response to thyroid hormone withdrawal or in whom withdrawal is medically contraindicated

**USUAL DOSAGE** Children >16 years and Adults: I.M.: 0.9 mg every 24 hours for 2 doses or every 72 hours for 3 doses. For radioiodine imaging, radioiodine administration should be given 24 hours following the final Thyrogen® injection. Scanning should be performed 48 hours after radioiodine administration (72 hours after the final injection of Thyrogen®).
**Dosage Forms Kits** containing two 1.1 mg vials (>4 int. units) of thyrogen® and two 10 mL vials of sterile water for injection
**Contraindications** Hypersensitivity to any component
**Warnings/Precautions** Caution should be exercised when administered to patients who have been previously treated with bovine TSH and, in particular, to those patients who have experienced hypersensitivity reactions to bovine TSH
(Continued)

## Thyrotropin Alpha *(Continued)*

Considerations in the use of thyrogen:

1. There remains a meaningful risk of a diagnosis of thyroid cancer or of an underestimating the extent of disease when thyrogen-stimulated Tg testing is performed and in combination with radioiodine imaging
2. Thyrogen® Tg levels are generally lower than, and do not correlate with, Tg levels after thyroid hormone withdrawal
3. Newly detectable Tg level or a Tg level rising over time after Thyrogen® or a high index of suspicion of metastatic disease, even in the setting of a negative or low-stage Thyrogen® radioiodine scan, should prompt further evaluation such as thyroid hormone withdrawal to definitively establish the location and extent of thyroid cancer.
4. Decision to perform a Thyrogen® radioiodine scan in conjunction with a Thyrogen® serum Tg test and whether or when to withdraw a patient from thyroid hormones are complex. Pertinent factors in this decision include the sensitivity of the Tg assay used, the Thyrogen® Tg level obtained, and the index of suspicion of recurrent or persistent local or metastatic disease.
5. Thyrogen® is not recommended to stimulate radioiodine uptake for the purposes of ablative radiotherapy of thyroid cancer
6. The signs and symptoms of hypothyroidism which accompany thyroid hormone withdrawal are avoided with Thyrogen® use

**Pregnancy Risk Factor** C
**Adverse Reactions**

1% to 10%:

Central nervous system: Headache, chills, fever, flu-like syndrome, dizziness
Gastrointestinal: Nausea, vomiting
Neuromuscular & skeletal: Weakness, paresthesia

♦ **Thytropar®** *see* Thyrotropin *on previous page*

♦ **Tiabendazole** *see* Thiabendazole *on page 893*

## Tiagabine *(tye AG a bene)*

**Pharmacologic Class** Anticonvulsant, Miscellaneous
**U.S. Brand Names** Gabitril®
**Mechanism of Action** The exact mechanism by which tiagabine exerts antiseizure activity is not definitively known; however, *in vitro* experiments demonstrate that it enhances the activity of gamma aminobutyric acid (GABA), the major neuroinhibitory transmitter in the nervous system. It is thought that binding to the GABA uptake carrier inhibits the uptake of GABA into presynaptic neurons, allowing an increased amount of GABA to be available to postsynaptic neurons. Based on *in vitro* studies, tiagabine does not inhibit the uptake of dopamine, norepinephrine, serotonin, glutamate, or choline.
**Use** Adjunctive therapy in adults and children ≥12 years of age in the treatment of partial seizures
**USUAL DOSAGE** Take with food; Oral:

Children 12-18 years: 4 mg once daily for 1 week; may increase to 8 mg daily in 2 divided doses for 1 week; then may increase by 4-8 mg weekly to response or up to 32 mg daily in 2-4 divided doses

Adults: 4 mg once daily for 1 week; may increase by 4-8 mg weekly to response or up to 56 mg daily in 2-4 divided doses

**Dosage Forms Tab, as hydrochloride:** 4 mg, 12 mg, 16 mg, 20 mg
**Contraindications** Patients who have demonstrated hypersensitivity to the drug or any of its ingredients
**Warnings/Precautions** Anticonvulsants should not be discontinued abruptly because of the possibility of increasing seizure frequency; tiagabine should be withdrawn gradually to minimize the potential of increased seizure frequency, unless safety concerns require a more rapid withdrawal
**Pregnancy Risk Factor** C
**Adverse Reactions** All adverse effects are dose-related

Central nervous system: Dizziness, headache, somnolence, CNS depression, memory disturbance, ataxia, emotional lability
Neuromuscular & skeletal: Tremors, weakness

**Drug Interactions** CYP2D6 and 3A3/4 enzyme substrate

The clearance of tiagabine is affected by the coadministration of hepatic enzyme-inducing antiepilepsy drugs; tiagabine is cleared more rapidly in patients who have been treated with carbamazepine, phenytoin, primidone, and phenobarbital than in patients who have not received these drugs

**Half-Life** Volunteers: 7-9 hours; in patients receiving enzyme-inducing drugs: 4-7 hours
**Special PA Issues**

Patient Education: Take exactly as directed (do not increase dose or frequency or discontinue without consulting prescriber). While using this medication, do not use alcohol and other prescription or OTC medications (especially pain medications, sedatives, antihistamines, or hypnotics) without consulting prescriber. Maintain adequate hydration (2-3 L/day of fluids unless instructed to restrict fluid intake). You may experience drowsiness, dizziness, disturbed concentration, or blurred vision (use caution when driving or engaging in hazardous tasks); nausea, vomiting, or loss of appetite (small frequent meals, good mouth care, chewing gum, or sucking on lozenges may help). Wear identification of epileptic status and medications. Report behavioral or CNS changes; skin rash; muscle cramping, weakness, tremors, changes in gait; vision difficulties; persistent GI distress (cramping, pain, vomiting); chest pain, irregular heartbeat, or palpitations; cough or difficulty breathing; worsening of seizure activity, or loss of seizure control.

**Monitoring Parameters:** A reduction in seizure frequency is indicative of therapeutic response to tiagabine in patients with partial seizures. Complete blood counts, renal function tests, liver function tests, and routine blood chemistry should be monitored periodically during therapy.

**Reference Range:** Maximal plasma level after a 24 mg/dose: 552 ng/mL

♦ **Tiamate®** see Diltiazem on page 286
♦ **Tiamol®** see Fluocinonide on page 381
♦ **Tiazac™** see Diltiazem on page 286
♦ **Ticar®** see Ticarcillin on this page

# Ticarcillin (tye kar SIL in)

**Pharmacologic Class** Antibiotic, Penicillin

**U.S. Brand Names** Ticar®

**Mechanism of Action** Inhibits bacterial cell wall synthesis by binding to one or more of the penicillin binding proteins (PBPs); which in turn inhibits the final transpeptidation step of peptidoglycan synthesis in bacterial cell walls, thus inhibiting cell wall biosynthesis. Bacteria eventually lyse due to ongoing activity of cell wall autolytic enzymes (autolysins and murein hydrolases) while cell wall assembly is arrested.

**Use** Treatment of susceptible infections such as septicemia, acute and chronic respiratory tract infections, skin and soft tissue infections, and urinary tract infections due to susceptible strains of Pseudomonas, and other gram-negative bacteria

**USUAL DOSAGE** Ticarcillin is generally given I.V., I.M. injection is only for the treatment of uncomplicated urinary tract infections and dose should not exceed 2 g/injection when administered I.M.

Neonates: I.M., I.V.:
  Postnatal age <7 days:
    <2000 g: 75 mg/kg/dose every 12 hours
    >2000 g: 75 mg/kg/dose every 8 hours
  Postnatal age >7 days:
    <1200 g: 75 mg/kg/dose every 12 hours
    1200-2000 g: 75 mg/kg/dose every 8 hours
    >2000 g: 75 mg/kg/dose every 6 hours
Infants and Children:
  Systemic infections: I.V.: 200-300 mg/kg/day in divided doses every 4-6 hours
  Urinary tract infections: I.M., I.V.: 50-100 mg/kg/day in divided doses every 6-8 hours
  Maximum dose: 24 g/day
Adults: I.M., I.V.: 1-4 g every 4-6 hours, usual dose: 3 g I.V. every 4-6 hours

**Dosing adjustment in renal impairment:** Adults:
  $Cl_{cr}$ 30-60 mL/minute: 2 g every 4 hours or 3 g every 8 hours
  $Cl_{cr}$ 10-30 mL/minute: 2 g every 8 hours or 3 g every 12 hours
  $Cl_{cr}$ <10 mL/minute: 2 g every 12 hours
Moderately dialyzable (20% to 50%)
Continuous arteriovenous or venovenous hemodiafiltration (CAVH) effects: Dose as for $Cl_{cr}$ 10-50 mL/minute

**Dosage Forms** Powder for inj, as disodium: 1 g, 3 g, 6 g, 20 g, 30 g

**Contraindications** Hypersensitivity to ticarcillin or any component or penicillins

**Warnings/Precautions** Due to sodium load and adverse effects (anemia, neuropsychological changes), use with caution and modify dosage in patients with renal impairment; serious and occasionally severe or fatal hypersensitivity (anaphylactoid) reactions have been reported in patients on penicillin therapy (especially with a history of beta-lactam hypersensitivity and/or a history of sensitivity to multiple allergens); use with caution in patients with seizures

**Pregnancy Risk Factor** B

**Adverse Reactions** Percentage unknown: Convulsions, confusion, drowsiness, fever, rash, electrolyte imbalance, hemolytic anemia, positive Coombs' reaction, eosinophilia, bleeding, thrombophlebitis, myoclonus, acute interstitial nephritis, hypersensitivity reactions, anaphylaxis, Jarisch-Herxheimer reaction

**Drug Interactions**

Decreased effect:
  Tetracyclines may decrease penicillin effectiveness
  Aminoglycosides → physical inactivation of aminoglycosides in the presence of high concentrations of ticarcillin
  Decreased effectiveness of oral contraceptives

(Continued)

## Ticarcillin *(Continued)*

Increased effect:

Probenecid may increase penicillin levels

Neuromuscular blockers may increase duration of blockade

Potential toxicity in patients with mild to moderate renal dysfunction

Aminoglycosides → synergistic efficacy

Increased bleeding risk with large I.V. doses and anticoagulants

**Half-Life** 1-1.3 hours, prolonged with renal impairment and/or hepatic impairment

**Special PA Issues**

**Patient Education:** This medication will be administered I.V. or I.M. Maintain adequate hydration (2-3 L/day of fluids unless instructed to restrict fluid intake). Small frequent meals or sucking on lozenges may reduce nausea or dry mouth. Maintain good oral and vaginal hygiene to reduce incidence of opportunistic infection. If diabetic, drug may cause false tests with Clinitest® urine glucose monitoring; use of glucose oxidase methods (Clinistix®) or serum glucose monitoring is preferable. This drug may interfere with oral contraceptives; an alternate form of birth control should be used. Report persistent diarrhea or abdominal pain (do not use antidiarrhea medication without consulting prescriber), fever, chills, unhealed sores, bloody urine or stool, muscle pain, mouth sores, difficulty breathing, or skin rash.

**Monitoring Parameters:** Serum electrolytes, bleeding time, and periodic tests of renal, hepatic, and hematologic function; monitor for signs of anaphylaxis during first dose

# Ticarcillin and Clavulanate Potassium

(tye kar SIL in & klav yoo LAN ate poe TASS ee um)

**Pharmacologic Class** Antibiotic, Penicillin

**U.S. Brand Names** Timentin®

**Mechanism of Action** Inhibits bacterial cell wall synthesis by binding to one or more of the penicillin binding proteins (PBPs); which in turn inhibits the final transpeptidation step of peptidoglycan synthesis in bacterial cell walls, thus inhibiting cell wall biosynthesis. Bacteria eventually lyse due to ongoing activity of cell wall autolytic enzymes (autolysins and murein hydrolases) while cell wall assembly is arrested.

**Use** Treatment of infections of lower respiratory tract, urinary tract, skin and skin structures, bone and joint, and septicemia caused by susceptible organisms. Clavulanate expands activity of ticarcillin to include beta-lactamase producing strains of *S. aureus, H. influenzae, Bacteroides* species, and some other gram-negative bacilli

**USUAL DOSAGE** I.V.:

Children and Adults <60 kg: 200-300 mg of ticarcillin component/kg/day in divided doses every 4-6 hours

Children >60 kg and Adults: 3.1 g (ticarcillin 3 g plus clavulanic acid 0.1 g) every 4-6 hours; maximum: 24 g/day

Urinary tract infections 3.1 g every 6-8 hours

**Dosing adjustment in renal impairment:**

$Cl_{cr}$ 30-60 mL/minute: Administer 2 g every 4 hours or 3.1 g every 8 hours

$Cl_{cr}$ 10-30 mL/minute: Administer 2 g every 8 hours or 3.1 g every 12 hours

$Cl_{cr}$ <10 mL/minute: Administer 2 g every 12 hours

Moderately dialyzable (20% to 50%)

Continuous arteriovenous or venovenous hemodiafiltration (CAVH) effects: Dose as for $Cl_{cr}$ 10-50 mL/minute

**Dosage Forms Inf, premixed (frozen):** Ticarcillin disodium 3 g and clavulanate potassium 0.1 g (100 mL); **Powder for inj:** Ticarcillin disodium 3 g and clavulanate potassium 0.1 g (3.1 g, 31 g)

**Contraindications** Known hypersensitivity to ticarcillin, clavulanate, or any penicillin

**Warnings/Precautions** Not approved for use in children <12 years of age; use with caution and modify dosage in patients with renal impairment; use with caution in patients with a history of allergy to cephalosporins and in patients with CHF due to high sodium load

**Pregnancy Risk Factor** 3

**Adverse Reactions** Percentage unknown: Convulsions, confusion, drowsiness, fever, rash, electrolyte imbalance, hemolytic anemia, positive Coombs' reaction, bleeding, thrombophlebitis, myoclonus, acute interstitial nephritis, hypersensitivity reactions, anaphylaxis, Jarisch-Herxheimer reaction

**Drug Interactions**

Decreased effect:

Tetracyclines may decrease penicillin effectiveness

Aminoglycosides → physical inactivation of aminoglycosides in the presence of high concentrations of ticarcillin

Decreased effectiveness of oral contraceptives

Increased effect:

Probenecid may increase penicillin levels

Neuromuscular blockers may increase duration of blockade

Potential toxicity in patients with with mild to moderate renal dysfunction

Aminoglycosides → synergistic efficacy

Increased bleeding risk with large I.V. doses and anticoagulants

**Half-Life**
Clavulanate: 66-90 minutes
Ticarcillin: 66-72 minutes in patients with normal renal function; clavulanic acid does not affect the clearance of ticarcillin
Renal failure: Ticarcillin: ~13 hours

**Special PA Issues**
**Patient Education:** This medication will be administered I.V. or I.M. Maintain adequate hydration (2-3 L/day of fluids unless instructed to restrict fluid intake). Small frequent meals or sucking on lozenges may reduce nausea or dry mouth. Maintain good oral and vaginal hygiene to reduce incidence of opportunistic infection. If diabetic, drug may cause false tests with Clinitest® urine glucose monitoring; use of glucose oxidase methods (Clinistix®) or serum glucose monitoring is preferable. This drug may interfere with oral contraceptives; an alternate form of birth control should be used. Report persistent diarrhea or abdominal pain (do not use antidiarrhea medication without consulting prescriber), fever, chills, unhealed sores, bloody urine or stool, muscle pain, mouth sores, difficulty breathing, or skin rash.

**Monitoring Parameters:** Observe signs and symptoms of anaphylaxis during first dose

◆ **Ticarcillin and Clavulanic Acid** *see* Ticarcillin and Clavulanate Potassium *on previous page*

◆ **Ticarcillin Disodium** *see* Ticarcillin *on page 901*

◆ **Ticlid®** *see* Ticlopidine *on this page*

# Ticlopidine (tye KLOE pi deen)

**Pharmacologic Class** Antiplatelet Agent

**U.S. Brand Names** Ticlid®

**Mechanism of Action** Ticlopidine is an inhibitor of platelet function with a mechanism which is different from other antiplatelet drugs. The drug significantly increases bleeding time. This effect may not be solely related to ticlopidine's effect on platelets. The prolongation of the bleeding time caused by ticlopidine is further increased by the addition of aspirin in *ex vivo* experiments. Although many metabolites of ticlopidine have been found, none have been shown to account for *in vivo* activity.

**Use** Platelet aggregation inhibitor that reduces the risk of thrombotic stroke in patients who have had a stroke or stroke precursors
**Unlabeled use:** Protection of aortocoronary bypass grafts, diabetic microangiopathy, ischemic heart disease, prevention of postoperative DVT, reduction of graft loss following renal transplant; reduction of postoperative reocclusion in patients receiving PTCA with stents

**USUAL DOSAGE** Adults: Oral: 1 tablet twice daily with food

**Dosage Forms** Tab, as hydrochloride: 250 mg

**Contraindications** Hypersensitivity to ticlopidine; active bleeding disorders; neutropenia or thrombocytopenia; severe liver impairment

**Warnings/Precautions** Patients predisposed to bleeding such as those with gastric or duodenal ulcers; patients with underlying hematologic disorders; patients receiving oral anticoagulant therapy or nonsteroidal anti-inflammatory agents (including aspirin); liver disease; patients undergoing lumbar puncture or surgical procedure. Ticlopidine should be discontinued if the absolute neutrophil count falls to <1200/mm$^3$ or if the platelet count falls to <80,000/mm$^3$. If possible, ticlopidine should be discontinued 10-14 days prior to surgery. Use caution when phenytoin or propranolol is used concurrently.

**Pregnancy Risk Factor** B

**Adverse Reactions**
>1%:
Dermatologic: Rash
Hematologic: Thrombotic thrombocytopenic purpura (TTP)
<1%: Bruising, diarrhea, nausea, vomiting, GI pain, neutropenia, thrombocytopenia, increased LFTs, tinnitus, hematuria, epistaxis

**Drug Interactions** CYP2C19 inhibitor
Decreased effect with antacids (decreased absorption), corticosteroids; decreased effect of digoxin, cyclosporine
Increased effect/toxicity of aspirin, anticoagulants, antipyrine, theophylline, cimetidine (increased levels), NSAIDs

**Onset** Within 6 hours; Peak: Achieved after 3-5 days of oral therapy; serum levels do not correlate with clinical antiplatelet activity.

**Half-Life** 24 hours

**Special PA Issues**
**Patient Education:** Take exact dosage prescribed, with food. Do not use aspirin or aspirin-containing medications and OTC medications without consulting prescriber. You may experience easy bleeding or bruising (use soft toothbrush or cotton swabs and frequent mouth care, use electric razor, avoid sharp knives or scissors). Report unusual bleeding or bruising or persistent fever or sore throat; blood in urine, stool, or vomitus; delayed healing of any wounds; skin rash; yellowing of skin or eyes; changes in color of urine of stool; pain or burning on urination; respiratory difficulty; or skin rash.
(Continued)

## Ticlopidine (Continued)

**Monitoring Parameters:** Signs of bleeding; CBC with differential every 2 weeks starting the second week through the third month of treatment; more frequent monitoring is recommended for patients whose absolute neutrophil counts have been consistently declining or are 30% less than baseline values. Liver function tests (alkaline phosphatase and transaminases) should be performed in the first 4 months of therapy if liver dysfunction is suspected.

♦ **Ticlopidine Hydrochloride** see Ticlopidine on previous page
♦ **Ticon®** see Trimethobenzamide on page 936
♦ **TIG** see Tetanus Immune Globulin (Human) on page 883
♦ **Tigan®** see Trimethobenzamide on page 936
♦ **Tilade® Inhalation Aerosol** see Nedocromil Sodium on page 639

## Tiludronate (tye LOO droe nate)

**Pharmacologic Class** Bisphosphonate Derivative
**U.S. Brand Names** Skelid®
**Mechanism of Action** Inhibition of normal and abnormal bone resorption. Inhibits osteoclasts through at least two mechanisms: disruption of the cytoskeletal ring structure, possibly by inhibition of protein-tyrosine-phosphatase, thus leading to the detachment of osteoclasts from the bone surface area and the inhibition of the osteoclast proton pump.
**Use** Treatment of Paget's disease of the bone (1) who have a level of serum alkaline phosphatase (SAP) at least twice the upper limit of normal, (2) or who are symptomatic, (3) or who are at risk for future complications of their disease
**USUAL DOSAGE** Tiludronate should be taken with 6-8 oz of plain water and not taken within 2 hours of food
Adults: Oral: 400 mg (2 tablets of tiludronic acid) daily for a period of 3 months; allow an interval of 3 months to assess response
**Dosing adjustment in renal impairment:** Cl$_{cr}$ <30 mL/minute: **Not recommended**
**Dosing adjustment in hepatic impairment:** Adjustment is not necessary
**Dosage Forms Tab, as disodium:** 240 mg [tiludronic acid 200 mg]; dosage is expressed in terms of tiludronic acid.
**Contraindications** Hypersensitivity to biphosphonates or any component of the product
**Warnings/Precautions** Not recommended in patients with severe renal impairment (Cl$_{cr}$ <30 mL/minute). Use with caution in patients with active upper GI problems (eg, dysphagia, symptomatic esophagea diseases, gastritis, duodenitis, ulcers).
**Pregnancy Risk Factor** C
**Adverse Reactions** 1% to 10%:
Cardiovascular: Flushing
Central nervous system: Vertigo, involuntary muscle contractions, anxiety, nervousness
Dermatologic: Pruritus, increased sweating, Stevens-Johnson type syndrome (rare)
Gastrointestinal: Xerostomia, gastritis
Genitourinary: Urinary tract infection
Neuromuscular & skeletal: Weakness, pathological fracture
Respiratory: Bronchitis
Miscellaneous: Increased diaphoresis
**Drug Interactions**
Decreased effect:
Calcium supplements, antacids interfere with the bioavailability (decreased 60%) when administered 1 hour before tiludronate
Aspirin decreases the bioavailability of tiludronate by up to 50% when taken 2 hours after tiludronate
Increased effect/toxicity: Indomethacin increases the bioavailability of tiludronate two- to fourfold
**Onset** Delayed, may require several weeks
**Half-Life** Healthy volunteers: 50 hours; Pagetic patients: 150 hours
**Special PA Issues**
**Patient Education:** In order to be effective this drug must be taken exactly as prescribed: Take 2 hours before or 2 hours after meals, aspirin, indomethacin, or calcium, magnesium, or aluminum containing medications such as antacids. Take with 6-8 oz. of water. Do not remove medication from foil strip until ready to be used. You may experience mild skin rash; abdominal pain, diarrhea, or constipation (report if persistent). Report unresolved muscle or bone pain or leg cramps; acute abdominal pain; chest pain, palpitations, or swollen extremities; disturbed vision or excessively dry eyes; ringing in the ears; persistent rash or skin disorder; unusual weakness or increased perspiration.
**Dietary Considerations:** In single-dose studies, the bioavailability of tiludronate was reduced by 90% when an oral dose was administered with, or 2 hours after, a standard breakfast compared to the same dose administered after an overnight fast and 4 hours before a standard breakfast; therefore, do not take within 2 hours of food

♦ **Tiludronate Disodium** see Tiludronate on this page
♦ **Timentin®** see Ticarcillin and Clavulanate Potassium on page 902

## Timolol (TYE moe lole)

**Pharmacologic Class** Beta Blocker, Nonselective; Ophthalmic Agent, Antiglaucoma

**U.S. Brand Names** Betimol® Ophthalmic; Blocadren® Oral; Timoptic® OcuDose®; Timoptic® Ophthalmic; Timoptic-XE® Ophthalmic

**Mechanism of Action** Blocks both beta$_1$- and beta$_2$-adrenergic receptors, reduces intraocular pressure by reducing aqueous humor production or possibly outflow; reduces blood pressure by blocking adrenergic receptors and decreasing sympathetic outflow, produces a negative chronotropic and inotropic activity through an unknown mechanism

**Use** Ophthalmic dosage form used to treat elevated intraocular pressure such as glaucoma or ocular hypertension; orally for treatment of hypertension and angina and reduce mortality following myocardial infarction and prophylaxis of migraine

### USUAL DOSAGE

Children and Adults: Ophthalmic: Initial: 0.25% solution, instill 1 drop twice daily; increase to 0.5% solution if response not adequate; decrease to 1 drop/day if controlled; do not exceed 1 drop twice daily of 0.5% solution

Adults: Oral:

Hypertension: Initial: 10 mg twice daily, increase gradually every 7 days, usual dosage: 20-40 mg/day in 2 divided doses; maximum: 60 mg/day

Prevention of myocardial infarction: 10 mg twice daily initiated within 1-4 weeks after infarction

Migraine headache: Initial: 10 mg twice daily, increase to maximum of 30 mg/day

**Dosage Forms** Timolol hemihydrate: **Soln, ophth (Betimol®):** 0.25% (2.5 mL, 5 mL, 10 mL, 15 mL), 0.5% (2.5 mL, 5 mL, 10 mL, 15 mL);

Timolol maleate: **Gel, ophth (Timoptic-XE®):** 0.25% (2.5 mL, 5 mL); 0.5% (2.5 mL, 5 mL); **Soln, ophth (Timoptic®):** 0.25% (2.5 mL, 5 mL, 10 mL, 15 mL), 0.5% (2.5 mL, 5 mL, 10 mL, 15 mL); **Soln, ophth, preservative free, single use (Timoptic® OcuDose®):** 0.25%, 0.5%; **Tab (Blocadren®):** 5 mg, 10 mg, 20 mg

**Contraindications** Uncompensated congestive heart failure, cardiogenic shock, bradycardia or heart block, severe chronic obstructive pulmonary disease, asthma, hypersensitivity to beta-blockers

**Warnings/Precautions** Some products contain sulfites which can cause allergic reactions; tachyphylaxis may develop; use with a miotic in angle-closure glaucoma; use with caution in patients with decreased renal or hepatic function (dosage adjustment required); severe CNS, cardiovascular and respiratory adverse effects have been seen following ophthalmic use; patients with a history of asthma, congestive heart failure, or bradycardia appear to be at a higher risk

### Pregnancy Risk Factor C

### Adverse Reactions

Ophthalmic:

1% to 10%:

Dermatologic: Alopecia

Ocular: Burning, stinging of eyes

<1%: Rash, blepharitis, conjunctivitis, keratitis, vision disturbances

Oral:

>10%: Endocrine & metabolic: Decreased sexual ability

1% to 10%:

Cardiovascular: Bradycardia, arrhythmia, reduced peripheral circulation

Central nervous system: Dizziness, fatigue

Dermatologic: Itching

Neuromuscular & skeletal: Weakness

Ocular: Burning eyes, stinging of eyes

Respiratory: Dyspnea

<1%: Chest pain, congestive heart failure, hallucinations, mental depression, anxiety, nightmares, skin rash, diarrhea, nausea, vomiting, stomach discomfort, numbness in toes and fingers, dry sore eyes

**Drug Interactions** CYP2D6 enzyme substrate

Decreased effect of beta-blockers with aluminum salts, barbiturates, calcium salts, cholestyramine, colestipol, NSAIDs, penicillins (ampicillin), rifampin, salicylates and sulfinpyrazone due to decreased bioavailability and plasma levels

Beta-blockers may decrease the effect of sulfonylureas

Increased effect/toxicity of beta-blockers with calcium blockers (diltiazem, felodipine, nicardipine), contraceptives, flecainide, propafenone (metoprolol, propranolol), quinidine (in extensive metabolizers), ciprofloxacin

Beta-blockers may increase the effect/toxicity of flecainide, phenothiazines, acetaminophen, clonidine (hypertensive crisis after or during withdrawal of either agent), epinephrine (initial hypertensive episode followed by bradycardia), nifedipine and verapamil lidocaine, ergots (peripheral ischemia), prazosin (postural hypotension)

Beta-blockers may affect the action or levels of ethanol, disopyramide, nondepolarizing muscle relaxants and theophylline although the effects are difficult to predict

**Onset** Onset of hypotensive effect: Oral: Within 15-45 minutes; Peak effect: Within 0.5-2.5 hours

**Duration** ~4 hours; intraocular effects persist for 24 hours after ophthalmic instillation

(Continued)

## Timolol (Continued)

**Half-Life** 2-2.7 hours; prolonged with reduced renal function

**Special PA Issues**

**Patient Education:**

Oral: Take exact dose prescribed; do not increase, decrease, or discontinue dosage without consulting prescriber. Take at same time each day. Does not replace recommended diet or exercise program. If diabetic, monitor serum glucose closely. May cause postural hypotension (use caution when rising from sitting or lying position or climbing stairs); dizziness, drowsiness, or blurred vision (use caution when driving or engaging in tasks requiring alertness until response to mediation is known); decreased sexual ability (reversible); or nausea or vomiting (small frequent meals or frequent mouth care may help). Report swelling of extremities, respiratory difficulty, or new cough; weight gain (>3 lb/week); unresolved diarrhea or vomiting; or cold blue extremities.

Ophthalmic: For ophthalmic use only. Apply prescribed amount as often as directed. Wash hands before using and do not touch tip of applicator to eye or contaminate tip of applicator. Tilt head back and look upward. Gently pull down lower lid and put drop(s) inside lower eyelid at inner corner. Close eye and roll eyeball in all directions. Do not blink for 1/2 minute. Apply gentle pressure to inner corner of eye for 30 seconds. Wipe away excess from skin around eye. Do not use any other eye preparation for at least 10 minutes. Do not share medication with anyone else. Temporary stinging or blurred vision may occur. Immediately report any adverse cardiac or CNS effects (usually signifies overdose). Report persistent eye pain, redness, burning, watering, dryness, double vision, puffiness around eye, vision disturbances, other adverse eye response, worsening of condition or lack of improvement. Inform prescriber if you are or intend to be pregnant. Consult prescriber if breast-feeding.

**Monitoring Parameters:** Blood pressure, apical and radial pulses, fluid I & O, daily weight, respirations, mental status, and circulation in extremities before and during therapy

**Related Information**

Beta-Blockers on page 1002

- ♦ **Timolol Hemihydrate** see Timolol on previous page
- ♦ **Timolol Maleate** see Timolol on previous page
- ♦ **Timoptic® OcuDose®** see Timolol on previous page
- ♦ **Timoptic® Ophthalmic** see Timolol on previous page
- ♦ **Timoptic-XE® Ophthalmic** see Timolol on previous page
- ♦ **Tinactin® [OTC]** see Tolnaftate on page 915
- ♦ **Tinactin® for Jock Itch [OTC]** see Tolnaftate on page 915
- ♦ **Tindal®** see Acetophenazine on page 25
- ♦ **Tine Test** see Tuberculin Tests on page 945
- ♦ **Tine Test PPD** see Tuberculin Tests on page 945
- ♦ **Ting® [OTC]** see Tolnaftate on page 915
- ♦ **Tinver® Lotion** see Sodium Thiosulfate on page 844

## Tioconazole (tye oh KONE a zole)

**Pharmacologic Class** Antifungal Agent, Vaginal

**U.S. Brand Names** Vagistat® Vaginal

**Mechanism of Action** A 1-substituted imidazole derivative with a broad antifungal spectrum against a wide variety of dermatophytes and yeasts, usually at a concentration ≤6.25 mg/L; has been demonstrated to be at least as active in vitro as other imidazole antifungals. In vitro, tioconazole has been demonstrated 2-8 times as potent as miconazole against common dermal pathogens including Trichophyton mentagrophytes, T. rubrum, T. erinacei, T. tonsurans, Microsporum canis, Microsporum gypseum, and Candida albicans. Both agents appear to be similarly effective against Epidermophyton floccosum.

**Use** Local treatment of vulvovaginal candidiasis

**USUAL DOSAGE** Adults: Vaginal: Insert 1 applicatorful in vagina, just prior to bedtime, as a single dose; therapy may extend to 7 days

**Dosage Forms Crm, vag:** 6.5% with applicator (4.6 g)

**Contraindications** Known hypersensitivity to tioconazole

**Warnings/Precautions** Not effective when applied to the scalp; may interact with condoms and vaginal contraceptive diaphragms; avoid these products for 3 days following treatment

**Pregnancy Risk Factor** C

**Adverse Reactions**

1% to 10%: Genitourinary: Vulvar/vaginal burning

<1%: Vulvar itching, soreness, edema, or discharge; polyuria

**Half-Life** 21-24 hours

**Special PA Issues**

**Patient Education:** Complete full course of therapy as directed. Insert vaginally as directed by prescriber or see package insert. Report persistent vaginal burning, itching, irritation, or discharge.

- ◆ **Tiotixene** *see* Thiothixene *on page 896*
- ◆ **Tisit® Blue Gel [OTC]** *see* Pyrethrins *on page 783*
- ◆ **Tisit® Liquid [OTC]** *see* Pyrethrins *on page 783*
- ◆ **Tisit® Shampoo [OTC]** *see* Pyrethrins *on page 783*
- ◆ **TMP** *see* Trimethoprim *on page 937*
- ◆ **TMP-SMX** *see* Co-Trimoxazole *on page 238*
- ◆ **TMP-SMZ** *see* Co-Trimoxazole *on page 238*
- ◆ **TOBI™ Inhalation Solution** *see* Tobramycin *on this page*
- ◆ **TobraDex® Ophthalmic** *see* Tobramycin and Dexamethasone *on page 909*

# Tobramycin (toe bra MYE sin)

**Pharmacologic Class** Antibiotic, Aminoglycoside; Antibiotic, Ophthalmic

**U.S. Brand Names** AKTob® Ophthalmic; Nebcin® Injection; TOBI™ Inhalation Solution; Tobrex® Ophthalmic

**Mechanism of Action** Interferes with bacterial protein synthesis by binding to 30S and 50S ribosomal subunits resulting in a defective bacterial cell membrane

**Use** Treatment of documented or suspected infections caused by susceptible gram-negative bacilli including *Pseudomonas aeruginosa*; topically used to treat superficial ophthalmic infections caused by susceptible bacteria

**USUAL DOSAGE** Individualization is critical because of the low therapeutic index.

**Use of ideal body weight (IBW) for determining the mg/kg/dose appears to be more accurate than dosing on the basis of total body weight (TBW).**

In morbid obesity, dosage requirement may best be estimated using a dosing weight of IBW + 0.4 (TBW - IBW).

Initial and periodic peak and trough plasma drug levels should be determined, particularly in critically ill patients with serious infections or in disease states known to significantly alter aminoglycoside pharmacokinetics (eg, cystic fibrosis, burns, or major surgery). Two to three serum level measurements should be obtained after the initial dose to measure the half-life in order to determine the frequency of subsequent doses.

Once daily dosing: Higher peak serum drug concentration to MIC ratios, demonstrated aminoglycoside postantibiotic effect, decreased renal cortex drug uptake, and improved cost-time efficiency are supportive reasons for the use of once daily dosing regimens for aminoglycosides. Current research indicates these regimens to be as effective for nonlife-threatening infections, with no higher incidence of nephrotoxicity, than those requiring multiple daily doses. Doses are determined by calculating the entire day's dose via usual multiple dose calculation techniques and administering this quantity as a single dose. Doses are then adjusted to maintain mean serum concentrations above the MIC(s) of the causative organism(s). (Example: 2.5-5 mg/kg as a single dose; expected $Cp_{max}$: 10-20 mcg/mL and $Cp_{min}$: <1 mcg/mL). Further research is needed for universal recommendation in all patient populations and gram-negative disease; exceptions may include those with known high clearance (eg, children, patients with cystic fibrosis, or burns who may require shorter dosage intervals) and patients with renal function impairment for whom longer than conventional dosage intervals are usually required.

Some clinicians suggest a daily dose of 4-7 mg/kg for all patients with normal renal function. This dose is at least as efficacious with similar, if not less, toxicity than conventional dosing.

Infants and Children <5 years: I.M., I.V.: 2.5 mg/kg/dose every 8 hours

Children >5 years: 1.5-2.5 mg/kg/dose every 8 hours

**Note:** Some patients may require larger or more frequent doses if serum levels document the need (ie, cystic fibrosis or febrile granulocytopenic patients).

Adults: I.M., I.V.:

Severe life-threatening infections: 2-2.5 mg/kg/dose

Urinary tract infection: 1.5 mg/kg/dose

Synergy (for gram-positive infections): 1 mg/kg/dose

Children and Adults: Ophthalmic: Instill 1-2 drops of solution every 4 hours; apply ointment 2-3 times/day; for severe infections apply ointment every 3-4 hours, or solution 2 drops every 30-60 minutes initially, then reduce to less frequent intervals

Inhalation:

Standard aerosolized tobramycin:

Children: 40-80 mg 2-3 times/day

Adults: 60-80 mg 3 times/day

High dose regimen: Children ≥6 years and Adults: 300 mg every 12 hours (do not administer doses less than 6 hours apart); administer in repeated cycles of 28 days on drug followed by 28 days off drug

**Dosing interval in renal impairment:**

$Cl_{cr}$ ≥60 mL/minute: Administer every 8 hours

(Continued)

# Tobramycin *(Continued)*

$Cl_{cr}$ 40-60 mL/minute: Administer every 12 hours

$Cl_{cr}$ 20-40 mL/minute: Administer every 24 hours

$Cl_{cr}$ 10-20 mL/minute: Administer every 48 hours

$Cl_{cr}$ <10 mL/minute: Administer every 72 hours

Hemodialysis: Dialyzable; 30% removal of aminoglycosides occurs during 4 hours of HD - administer dose after dialysis and follow levels

Continuous arteriovenous or venovenous hemofiltration (CAVH/CAVHD): Dose as for $Cl_{cr}$ 10-20 mL/minute and follow levels

Administration in CAPD fluid:

Gram-negative infection: 4-8 mg/L (4-8 mcg/mL) of CAPD fluid

Gram-positive infection (ie, synergy): 3-4 mg/L (3-4 mcg/mL) of CAPD fluid

Administration IVPB/I.M.: Dose as for $Cl_{cr}$ <10 mL/minute and follow levels

**Dosing adjustment/comments in hepatic disease:** Monitor plasma concentrations

**Dosage Forms Inj, (Nebcin®):** 10 mg/mL (2 mL), 40 mg/mL (1.5 mL, 2 mL); **Oint, ophth (Tobrex®):** 0.3% (3.5 g); **Powder for inj (Nebcin®):** 40 mg/mL (1.2 g vials); **Soln, ophth:** 0.3% (5 mL), AKTob®, Tobrex®: 0.3% (5 mL)

**Contraindications** Hypersensitivity to tobramycin or other aminoglycosides or components

**Warnings/Precautions** Use with caution in patients with renal impairment; pre-existing auditory or vestibular impairment; and in patients with neuromuscular disorders; dosage modification required in patients with impaired renal function; (I.M. & I.V.) Aminoglycosides are associated with significant nephrotoxicity or ototoxicity; the ototoxicity is directly proportional to the amount of drug given and the duration of treatment; tinnitus or vertigo are indications of vestibular injury; ototoxicity is often irreversible; renal damage is usually reversible

**Pregnancy Risk Factor** C

**Adverse Reactions**

1% to 10%:

Renal: Nephrotoxicity

Neuromuscular & skeletal: Neurotoxicity (neuromuscular blockade)

Otic: Ototoxicity (auditory), ototoxicity (vestibular)

<1%: Hypotension, drug fever, headache, drowsiness, rash, nausea, vomiting, eosinophilia, anemia, paresthesia, tremor, arthralgia, weakness, lacrimation, itching eyes, edema of the eyelid, keratitis, dyspnea

**Drug Interactions**

Increased effect: Extended spectrum penicillins (synergistic)

Increased toxicity:

Neuromuscular blockers increase neuromuscular blockade

Amphotericin B, cephalosporins, loop diuretics, and vancomycin may increase risk of nephrotoxicity

**Half-Life** 2-3 hours, directly dependent upon glomerular filtration rate; Adults with impaired renal function: 5-70 hours

**Special PA Issues**

**Patient Education:**

Systemic: Maintain adequate hydration (2-3 L/day of fluids unless instructed to restrict fluid intake). Report decreased urine output, swelling of extremities, difficulty breathing, vaginal itching or discharge, rash, diarrhea, oral thrush, unhealed wounds, dizziness, change in hearing acuity or ringing in ears, or worsening of condition.

Ophthalmic: Use as frequently as recommended; do not overuse. Sit down, tilt head back, instill solution or drops inside lower eyelid, and roll eyeball in all directions. Close eye and apply gentle pressure to inner corner of eye for 30 seconds. Do not touch tip of applicator to eye or any contaminated surface. May experience temporary stinging or blurred vision. Do not use any other eye preparation for 10 minutes. Inform prescriber if condition worsens or does not improve in 3-4 days.

**Dietary Considerations:** Calcium, magnesium, potassium: Renal wasting may cause hypocalcemia, hypomagnesemia, and/or hypokalemia

**Monitoring Parameters:** Urinalysis, urine output, BUN, serum creatinine, peak and trough plasma tobramycin levels; be alert to ototoxicity; hearing should be tested before and during treatment

**Reference Range:**

Timing of serum samples: Draw peak 30 minutes after 30-minute infusion has been completed or 1 hour following I.M. injection or beginning of infusion; draw trough immediately before next dose

Therapeutic levels:

Peak:

Serious infections: 6-8 µg/mL (SI: 12-17 mg/L)

Life-threatening infections: 8-10 µg/mL (SI: 17-21 mg/L)

Urinary tract infections: 4-6 µg/mL (SI: 7-12 mg/L)

Synergy against gram-positive organisms: 3-5 µg/mL

Trough:

Serious infections: 0.5-1 µg/mL

Life-threatening infections: 1-2 µg/mL

Monitor serum creatinine and urine output; obtain drug levels after the third dose unless otherwise directed

## Tobramycin and Dexamethasone (toe bra MYE sin & deks a METH a sone)
**Pharmacologic Class** Antibiotic, Ophthalmic; Corticosteroid, Ophthalmic
**U.S. Brand Names** TobraDex® Ophthalmic
**Dosage Forms Oint, ophth:** Tobramycin 0.3% and dexamethasone 0.1% (3.5 g); **Susp, ophth:** Tobramycin 0.3% and dexamethasone 0.1% (2.5 mL, 5 mL)

♦ **Tobramycin Sulfate** see Tobramycin on page 907

♦ **Tobrex® Ophthalmic** see Tobramycin on page 907

## Tocainide (toe KAY nide)
**Pharmacologic Class** Antiarrhythmic Agent, Class I-B
**U.S. Brand Names** Tonocard®
**Mechanism of Action** Class 1B antiarrhythmic agent; suppresses automaticity of conduction tissue, by increasing electrical stimulation threshold of ventricle, HIS-Purkinje system, and spontaneous depolarization of the ventricles during diastole by a direct action on the tissues; blocks both the initiation and conduction of nerve impulses by decreasing the neuronal membrane's permeability to sodium ions, which results in inhibition of depolarization with resultant blockade of conduction
**Use** Suppress and prevent symptomatic life-threatening ventricular arrhythmias
**Unlabeled use:** Trigeminal neuralgia
**USUAL DOSAGE** Adults: Oral: 1200-1800 mg/day in 3 divided doses, up to 2400 mg/day
**Dosage adjustment in renal impairment:** $Cl_{cr}$ <30 mL/minute: Administer 50% of normal dose or 600 mg once daily
Hemodialysis: Moderately dialyzable (20% to 50%)
**Dosage adjustment in hepatic impairment:** Maximum daily dose: 1200 mg
**Dosage Forms Tab, as hydrochloride:** 400 mg, 600 mg
**Contraindications** Second or third degree A-V block without a pacemaker, hypersensitivity to tocainide, amide-type anesthetics, or any component
**Warnings/Precautions** May exacerbate some arrhythmias (ie, atrial fibrillation/flutter); use with caution in CHF patients; administer with caution in patients with pre-existing bone marrow failure, cytopenia, severe renal or hepatic disease
**Pregnancy Risk Factor** C
**Adverse Reactions**
>10%:
Central nervous system: Dizziness (8% to 15%)
Gastrointestinal: Nausea (14% to 15%)
1% to 10%:
Cardiovascular: Tachycardia (3%), bradycardia/angina/palpitations (0.5% to 1.8%)
Central nervous system: Nervousness (0.5% to 1.5%), confusion (2% to 3%)
Dermatologic: Rash (0.5% to 8.4%)
Gastrointestinal: Vomiting, diarrhea (4% to 5%), anorexia (1% to 2%)
Neuromuscular & skeletal: Paresthesia (3.5% to 9%), tremor (2.9% to 8.4%)
Ocular: Blurred vision (~1.5%)
<1%: Ataxia, agranulocytosis, anemia, leukopenia, neutropenia, respiratory arrest, diaphoresis
**Drug Interactions**
Decreased plasma levels: Phenobarbital, phenytoin, rifampin, and other hepatic enzyme inducers, cimetidine and drugs which make the urine acidic
Increased toxicity/levels of caffeine and theophylline
Increased effects with metoprolol
**Half-Life** 11-14 hours, prolonged with renal and hepatic impairment with half-life increased to 23-27 hours
**Special PA Issues**
**Patient Education:** Take exactly as directed, with food. If dose is missed, take as soon as possible, do not double next dose. Do not discontinue without consulting prescriber. You will need regular cardiac check-ups while taking this medication. You may experience dizziness, nervousness, or visual changes (use caution when driving or engaging in tasks that require alertness until response to drug is determines); nausea or vomiting, or loss of appetite (frequent small meals, frequent mouth care, or sucking lozenges may help); mild muscle discomfort (analgesics may be recommended). Report chest pain, palpitations, or erratic heartbeat; difficulty breathing or unusual cough; mental confusion or depression; muscle tremor, weakness, or pain; or changes in vision.
**Reference Range:** Therapeutic: 5-12 µg/mL (SI: 22-52 µmol/L)

♦ **Tocainide Hydrochloride** see Tocainide on this page

♦ **Toesen®** see Oxytocin on page 691

♦ **Tofranil®** see Imipramine on page 469

♦ **Tofranil-PM®** see Imipramine on page 469

# Tolazamide (tole AZ a mide)

**Pharmacologic Class** Antidiabetic Agent (Sulfonylurea)

**U.S. Brand Names** Tolinase®

**Mechanism of Action** Stimulates insulin release from the pancreatic beta cells; reduces glucose output from the liver; insulin sensitivity is increased at peripheral target sites

**Use** Adjunct to diet for the management of mild to moderately severe, stable, noninsulin-dependent (type II) diabetes mellitus

**USUAL DOSAGE** Oral (doses >1000 mg/day normally do not improve diabetic control):

Adults:

Initial: 100-250 mg/day with breakfast or the first main meal of the day

Fasting blood sugar <200 mg/dL: 100 mg/day

Fasting blood sugar >200 mg/dL: 250 mg/day

Patient is malnourished, underweight, elderly, or not eating properly: 100 mg/day

Adjust dose in increments of 100-250 mg/day at weekly intervals to response. If >500 mg/day is required, give in divided doses twice daily; maximum daily dose: 1 g (doses >1 g/day are not likely to improve control)

**Conversion from insulin → tolazamide**

10 units day = 100 mg/day

20-40 units/day = 250 mg/day

>40 units/day = 250 mg/day and 50% of insulin dose

Doses >500 mg/day should be given in 2 divided doses

**Dosing adjustment in renal impairment:** Conservative initial and maintenance doses are recommended because tolazamide is metabolized to active metabolites, which are eliminated in the urine

**Dosing comments in hepatic impairment:** Conservative initial and maintenance doses and careful monitoring of blood glucose are recommended

**Dosage Forms Tab:** 100 mg, 250 mg, 500 mg

**Contraindications** Type I diabetes therapy (IDDM), hypersensitivity to sulfonylureas, diabetes complicated by ketoacidosis

**Warnings/Precautions** False-positive response has been reported in patients with liver disease, idiopathic hypoglycemia of infancy, severe malnutrition, acute pancreatitis, renal dysfunction. Transferring a patient from one sulfonylurea to another does not require a priming dose; doses >1000 mg/day normally do not improve diabetic control. Has not been studied in older patients; however, except for drug interactions, it appears to have a safe profile and decline in renal function does not affect its pharmacokinetics. How "tightly" an elderly patient's blood glucose should be controlled is controversial; however, a fasting blood sugar <150 mg/dL is now an acceptable end point. Such a decision should be based on the patient's functional and cognitive status, how well they recognize hypoglycemic or hyperglycemic symptoms, and how to respond to them and their other disease states.

**Pregnancy Risk Factor** D

**Adverse Reactions**

>10%:

Central nervous system: Headache, dizziness

Gastrointestinal: Anorexia, nausea, vomiting, diarrhea, constipation, heartburn, epigastric fullness

1% to 10%: Dermatologic: Rash, urticaria, photosensitivity

<1%: Hypoglycemia, aplastic anemia, hemolytic anemia, bone marrow suppression, thrombocytopenia, agranulocytosis, cholestatic jaundice, diuretic effect

**Drug Interactions**

Increased toxicity: Monitor patient closely; large number of drugs interact with sulfonylureas including salicylates, anticoagulants, $H_2$-antagonists, TCAs, MAO inhibitors, beta-blockers, thiazides

**Onset** Oral: Within 4-6 hours

**Duration** 10-24 hours

**Half-Life** 7 hours

**Special PA Issues**

**Patient Education:** Ideally, you will probably be referred to a diabetic educator for diabetic counseling. Eat regularly; do not skip meals. Carry a quick sugar source. Monitor serum glucose as directed. Do not alter dosage or discontinue current medications or introduce new medications without consulting prescriber. Avoid alcohol while taking this drug (disulfiram reactions). Report unresolved nausea or vomiting, constipation or diarrhea, headache, anorexia, sore throat, or skin rash. You may be sensitive to sun; avoid excessive exposure and use appropriate sunblock and clothing.

**Dietary Considerations:** Alcohol: Avoid use

**Monitoring Parameters:** Signs and symptoms of hypoglycemia, (fatigue, sweating, numbness of extremities); urine for glucose and ketones; fasting blood glucose; hemoglobin $A_{1c}$ or fructosamine

**Reference Range:** Target range:

Fasting blood glucose: Adults: 80-140 mg/dL; Geriatrics: 100-150 mg/dL

Glycosylated hemoglobin: <7%

**Related Information**
Hypoglycemic Drugs *on page 1020*

# Tolazoline (tole AZ oh leen)

**Pharmacologic Class** Alpha-Adrenergic Blocking Agent, Parenteral

**U.S. Brand Names** Priscoline®

**Mechanism of Action** Competitively blocks alpha-adrenergic receptors to produce brief antagonism of circulating epinephrine and norepinephrine; reduces hypertension caused by catecholamines and causes vascular smooth muscle relaxation (direct action); results in peripheral vasodilation and decreased peripheral resistance

**Use** Treatment of persistent pulmonary vasoconstriction and hypertension of the newborn (persistent fetal circulation), peripheral vasospastic disorders

**USUAL DOSAGE**
Neonates: Initial: I.V.: 1-2 mg/kg over 10-15 minutes via scalp vein or upper extremity; maintenance: 1-2 mg/kg/hour; use lower maintenance doses in patients with decreased renal function. Also used in neonates for acute vasospasm "cath toes" at 0.25 mg/kg/hour (no load); maximum dose: 6-8 mg/kg/hour.

**Dosing interval in renal impairment in newborns:** Urine output <0.9 mL/kg/hour: Decrease dose to 0.08 mg/kg/hour for every 1 mg/kg of loading dose

Adults: Peripheral vasospastic disorder: I.M., I.V., S.C.: 10-50 mg 4 times/day

**Dosage Forms Inj, as hydrochloride:** 25 mg/mL (4 mL)

**Contraindications** Hypersensitivity to tolazoline; known or suspected coronary artery disease

**Warnings/Precautions** Stimulates gastric secretion and may activate stress ulcers; therefore, use with caution in patients with gastritis, peptic ulcer; use with caution in patients with mitral stenosis

**Pregnancy Risk Factor** C

**Adverse Reactions**
Cardiovascular: Hypotension, peripheral vasodilation, tachycardia, hypertension, arrhythmias

Endocrine & metabolic: Hypochloremic alkalosis

Gastrointestinal: GI bleeding, abdominal pain, nausea, diarrhea

Hematologic: Thrombocytopenia, increased agranulocytosis, pancytopenia

Local: Burning at injection site

Neuromuscular & skeletal: Increased pilomotor activity

Ocular: Mydriasis

Renal: Acute renal failure, oliguria

Respiratory: Pulmonary hemorrhage

Miscellaneous: Increased secretions

**Drug Interactions**
Decreased effect (vasopressor) of epinephrine followed by a rebound increase in blood pressure

Increased toxicity: Disulfiram reaction may possibly be seen with concomitant ethanol use

**Special PA Issues**
**Patient Education:** Side effects decrease with continued therapy; avoid alcohol
**Dietary Considerations:** Alcohol: Avoid use
**Monitoring Parameters:** Vital signs, blood gases, cardiac monitor

♦ **Tolazoline Hydrochloride** *see* Tolazoline *on this page*

# Tolbutamide (tole BYOO ta mide)

**Pharmacologic Class** Antidiabetic Agent (Sulfonylurea)

**U.S. Brand Names** Orinase® Diagnostic Injection; Orinase® Oral

**Mechanism of Action** Stimulates insulin release from the pancreatic beta cells; reduces glucose output from the liver; insulin sensitivity is increased at peripheral target sites, suppression of glucagon may also contribute

**Use** Adjunct to diet for the management of mild to moderately severe, stable, noninsulin-dependent (type II) diabetes mellitus

**USUAL DOSAGE** Divided doses may increase gastrointestinal side effects
Adults:
Oral: Initial: 1-2 g/day as a single dose in the morning or in divided doses throughout the day. Total doses may be taken in the morning; however, divided doses may allow increased gastrointestinal tolerance. Maintenance dose: 0.25-3 g/day; however, a maintenance dose >2 g/day is seldom required.

I.V. bolus: 1 g over 2-3 minutes

Elderly: Oral: Initial: 250 mg 1-3 times/day; usual: 500-2000 mg; maximum: 3 g/day

**Dosing adjustment in renal impairment:** Adjustment is not necessary

Hemodialysis: Not dialyzable (0% to 5%)

**Dosing adjustment in hepatic impairment:** Reduction of dose may be necessary in patients with impaired liver function

(Continued)

## Tolbutamide (Continued)

**Dosage Forms Inj, diagnostic:** 1 g (20 mL); **Tab:** 250 mg, 500 mg

**Contraindications** Diabetes complicated by ketoacidosis, therapy of IDDM, hypersensitivity to sulfonylureas

**Warnings/Precautions** False-positive response has been reported in patients with liver disease, idiopathic hypoglycemia of infancy, severe malnutrition, acute pancreatitis. Because of its low potency and short duration, it is a useful agent in the elderly if drug interactions can be avoided. How "tightly" an elderly patient's blood glucose should be controlled is controversial; however, a fasting blood sugar <150 mg/dL is now an acceptable end point. Such a decision should be based on the patient's functional and cognitive status, how well they recognize hypoglycemic or hyperglycemic symptoms, and how to respond to them and their other disease states.

**Pregnancy Risk Factor** D

**Adverse Reactions**

>10%:

Central nervous system: Headache, dizziness

Gastrointestinal: Constipation, diarrhea, heartburn, anorexia, epigastric fullness

1% to 10%: Dermatologic: Rash, urticaria, photosensitivity

<1%: Venospasm, SIADH, disulfiram-type reactions, thrombocytopenia, agranulocytosis, hypoglycemia, leukopenia, aplastic anemia, hemolytic anemia, bone marrow suppression, cholestatic jaundice, thrombophlebitis, tinnitus, hypersensitivity reaction

**Drug Interactions** CYP2C8, 2C9, 2C18, and 2C19 enzyme substrate; CYP2C19 enzyme inhibitor

Increased effects with salicylates, probenecid, MAO inhibitors, chloramphenicol, insulin, phenylbutazone, antidepressants, metformin, H$_2$-antagonists, and others

Decreased effects:

Hypoglycemic effects may be decreased by beta-blockers, cholestyramine, hydantoins, thiazides, rifampin, and others

Ethanol may decrease the half-life of tolbutamide

**Onset** Peak hypoglycemic action: Oral: 1-3 hours; I.V.: 30 minutes

**Duration** Oral: 6-24 hours; I.V.: 3 hours

**Half-Life** Plasma: 4-25 hours; Elimination: 4-9 hours

**Special PA Issues**

**Patient Education:** Ideally, you will be referred to a diabetic educator for diabetic counseling. Eat regularly; do not skip meals. Carry a quick sugar source. Monitor serum glucose as directed. Do not alter dosage or discontinue current medications or introduce new medications without consulting prescriber. Avoid alcohol while taking this drug (disulfiram reactions). Report unresolved nausea or vomiting, constipation or diarrhea, headache, anorexia, sore throat, or skin rash. You may be sensitive to sun; avoid excessive exposure and use appropriate sunblock and clothing.

**Dietary Considerations:** Alcohol: Avoid use

**Monitoring Parameters:** Fasting blood glucose, hemoglobin A$_{1c}$ or fructosamine

**Reference Range:** Target range:

Fasting blood glucose: <120 mg/dL; Adults: 80-140 mg/dL; Geriatrics: 100-150 mg/dL

Glycosylated hemoglobin: <7%

**Related Information**

Hypoglycemic Drugs *on page 1020*

♦ **Tolbutamide Sodium** *see* Tolbutamide *on previous page*

## Tolcapone (TOLE ka pone)

**Pharmacologic Class** Anti-Parkinson's Agent (COMT Inhibitor)

**U.S. Brand Names** Tasmar®

**Mechanism of Action** A reversible inhibitor of catechol-O-methyltransferase (COMT). COMT is the major route of metabolism for levodopa. When tolcapone is taken with levodopa the pharmacokinetics are altered, resulting in more sustained levodopa serum levels compared to levodopa taken alone. The resulting levels of levodopa provide for increased concentrations available for absorption across the blood-brain barrier, thereby providing for increased CNS levels of dopamine, the active metabolite of levodopa.

**Use** An adjunct to levodopa/carbidopa for the treatment of signs and symptoms of Parkinson's disease

**USUAL DOSAGE** Oral: 100 mg 3 times/day always given as an adjunct to levodopa/carbidopa. The first dose of the day should be given with the first dose of the day of levodopa/carbidopa, and then administer the next 2 doses 6 and 12 hours later. Because increased liver enzymes occur more frequently with 200 mg 3 times/day, only increase to 200 mg if clinically justified.

**Note:** Many patients will require a decrease in levodopa dosage to avoid increased dopaminergic side effects

**Dosing adjustment in renal impairment:** Generally, no adjustment necessary; however, in patients with severe renal failure, treat with caution and do not exceed 100 mg 3 times/day

**Dosing adjustment in hepatic impairment:** Do not use if the patient has evidence of active liver disease or the AST or ALT are greater than the upper limit of normal

**Dosage Forms Tab:** 100 mg, 200 mg

**Contraindications** Hypersensitivity to tolcapone or other ingredients, including tolcapone, lactose monohydrate, cellulose, povidone, sodium starch glycolate, talc, and/or magnesium stearate; patients with liver disease or who had increased LFTs on tolcapone; patients with a history of nontraumatic rhabdomyolysis or hyperpyrexia and confusion possibly related to medication

**Warnings/Precautions Note:** Due to reports of fatal liver injury associated with use of this drug, the manufacturer is advising that tolcapone be reserved for use only in patients who do not have severe movement abnormalities and who do not respond to or who are not appropriate candidates for other available treatments. Before initiating therapy with tolcapone, the risks should be discussed with the patient, and the patient can provide written informed consent (form available from Roche).

It is not recommended that patients receive tolcapone concomitantly with nonselective MAO inhibitors (see Drug Interactions). Selegiline is a selective MAO-B inhibitor and can be taken with tolcapone.

Patients receiving tolcapone are predisposed to orthostatic hypotension, diarrhea (usually within the first 6-12 weeks of therapy), transient hallucinations (most commonly within the first 2 weeks of therapy), and new onset or worsened dyskinesia. Use with caution in patients with severe renal failure. Tolcapone is secreted into maternal milk in rats and may be excreted into human milk; until more is known, tolcapone should be considered **incompatible** with breast-feeding.

**Pregnancy Risk Factor** C

**Adverse Reactions** Patients receiving tolcapone are predisposed to orthostatic hypotension. Inform the patient and explain methods to manage the symptoms. Patients may experience diarrhea, most commonly 6-12 weeks after tolcapone is started. Diarrhea is sometimes associated with anorexia. Patients may experience hallucinations shortly after starting therapy, most commonly within the first 2 weeks. Hallucinations may diminish or resolve with a decrease in the levodopa dose. Hallucinations commonly accompany confusion and sometimes insomnia or excessive dreaming. Tolcapone may exacerbate or induce dyskinesia; lowering the levodopa dose may help. Use tolcapone with caution in patients with severe renal or hepatic failure.

>10%:
  Cardiovascular: Orthostasis
  Central nervous system: Sleep disorder, excessive dreaming, headache, dizziness, somnolence, confusion
  Gastrointestinal: Nausea, anorexia, diarrhea
  Neuromuscular & skeletal: Dyskinesia, dystonia, muscle cramps
1% to 10%:
  Cardiovascular: Hypotension, chest pain
  Central nervous system: Hallucination, syncope, fatigue
  Gastrointestinal: Vomiting, constipation, dry mouth, dyspepsia, abdominal pain, flatulence
  Genitourinary: Urine discoloration
  Neuromuscular & skeletal: Hyperkinesia, stiffness, arthritis
  Respiratory: Dyspnea
<1%: Fatal liver injury, bradycardia, coronary artery disorder, heart arrest, angina pectoris, myocardial infarct, myocardial ischemia, arteriosclerosis, thrombosis, hypertension, vasodilation, amnesia, extrapyramidal syndrome, manic reaction, cerebrovascular accident, psychosis, myoclonus, delirium, encephalopathy, meningitis, cellulitis, hypercholesteremia, gastrointestinal hemorrhage, colitis, duodenal ulcer, uterine hemorrhage, anemia, leukemia, thrombocytopenia, cholecystitis, neuralgia, hemiplegia, hematuria, bronchitis, epistaxis, hyperventilation, allergic reaction

**Drug Interactions** Theoretically, nonselective MAO inhibitors (phenelzine and tranylcypromine) taken with tolcapone may inhibit the major metabolic pathways of catecholamines, which may result in excessive adverse effects possibly due to levodopa accumulation. Concomitant therapy is not recommended.

**Half-Life** 2-3 hours

**Special PA Issues**

**Patient Education:** Take exactly as directed (may be prescribed in conjunction with levodopa/carbidopa); do not change dosage or discontinue without consulting prescriber. Therapeutic effects may take several weeks or months to achieve and you may need frequent monitoring during first weeks of therapy. Best to take 2 hours before or after a meal; however, may be taken with meals if GI upset occurs. Take at same time each day. Maintain adequate hydration (2-3 L/day of fluids unless instructed to restrict fluid intake). Do not use alcohol and prescription or OTC sedatives or CNS depressants without consulting prescriber. Urine or perspiration may appear darker. You may experience drowsiness, dizziness, confusion, or vision changes (use caution when driving, climbing stairs, or engaging in hazardous tasks); orthostatic hypotension (use caution when changing position - rising to standing from sitting or lying); increased susceptibility to heat stroke, decreased perspiration (use caution in hot weather - maintain adequate fluids and
(Continued)

## Tolcapone *(Continued)*

reduce exercise activity); constipation (increased exercise, fluids, or dietary fruit and fiber may help); dry skin or nasal passages (consult prescriber for appropriate relief); nausea, vomiting, loss of appetite, or stomach discomfort (small frequent meals, chewing gum, or sucking on lozenges may help). Report unresolved constipation or vomiting; chest pain or irregular heartbeat; difficulty breathing; acute headache or dizziness; CNS changes (hallucination, loss of memory, nervousness, etc); painful or difficult urination; abdominal pain or blood in stool; increased muscle spasticity, rigidity, or involuntary movements; skin rash; or significant worsening of condition.

**Dietary Considerations:** Tolcapone taken with food within 1 hour before or 2 hours after the dose decreases bioavailability by 10% to 20%

**Monitoring Parameters:** Blood pressure, symptoms of Parkinson's disease, liver enzymes at baseline and then every 2 weeks for the first year of therapy, every 4 weeks for the next 6 months, then every 8 weeks thereafter. If the dose is increased to 200 mg 3 times/day, reinitiate LFT monitoring at the previous frequency. Discontinue therapy if the ALT or AST exceeds the upper limit of normal or if the clinical signs and symptoms suggest the onset of liver failure.

- ◆ **Tolectin® 200** *see* Tolmetin *on this page*
- ◆ **Tolectin® 400** *see* Tolmetin *on this page*
- ◆ **Tolectin® DS** *see* Tolmetin *on this page*
- ◆ **Tolinase®** *see* Tolazamide *on page 910*

## Tolmetin *(TOLE met in)*

**Pharmacologic Class** Nonsteroidal Anti-Inflammatory Agent (NSAID)

**U.S. Brand Names** Tolectin® 200; Tolectin® 400; Tolectin® DS

**Mechanism of Action** Inhibits prostaglandin synthesis by decreasing the activity of the enzyme, cyclo-oxygenase, which results in decreased formation of prostaglandin precursors

**Use** Treatment of rheumatoid arthritis and osteoarthritis, juvenile rheumatoid arthritis

**USUAL DOSAGE** Oral:

Children ≥2 years:

Anti-inflammatory: Initial: 20 mg/kg/day in 3 divided doses, then 15-30 mg/kg/day in 3 divided doses

Analgesic: 5-7 mg/kg/dose every 6-8 hours

Adults: 400 mg 3 times/day; usual dose: 600 mg to 1.8 g/day; maximum: 2 g/day

**Dosage Forms Cap (Tolectin® DS):** 400 mg; **Tab (Tolectin®):** 200 mg, 600 mg

**Contraindications** Known hypersensitivity to tolmetin or any component, aspirin, or other nonsteroidal anti-inflammatory drugs (NSAIDs)

**Warnings/Precautions** Use with caution in patients with upper GI disease, impaired renal function, congestive heart failure, hypertension, and patients receiving anticoagulants; if GI upset occurs with tolmetin, take with antacids other than sodium bicarbonate

**Pregnancy Risk Factor** C (D at term)

**Adverse Reactions**

>10%:

Central nervous system: Dizziness

Dermatologic: Rash

Gastrointestinal: Abdominal cramps, heartburn, indigestion, nausea

1% to 10%:

Central nervous system: Headache, nervousness

Dermatologic: Itching

Endocrine & metabolic: Fluid retention

Gastrointestinal: Vomiting

Otic: Tinnitus

<1%: Congestive heart failure, hypertension, arrhythmias, tachycardia, confusion, hallucinations, aseptic meningitis, mental depression, drowsiness, insomnia, urticaria, erythema multiforme, toxic epidermal necrolysis, Stevens-Johnson syndrome, angioedema, polydipsia, hot flashes, gastritis, GI ulceration, cystitis, polyuria, agranulocytosis, anemia, hemolytic anemia, bone marrow suppression, leukopenia, thrombocytopenia, hepatitis, peripheral neuropathy, toxic amblyopia, blurred vision, conjunctivitis, dry eyes, decreased hearing, acute renal failure, allergic rhinitis, shortness of breath, epistaxis

**Drug Interactions**

Decreased effect with aspirin; decreased effect of thiazides, furosemide

Increased toxicity of digoxin, methotrexate, cyclosporine, lithium, insulin, sulfonylureas, potassium-sparing diuretics, aspirin

**Onset** Analgesic: 1-2 hours; Anti-inflammatory: Days - weeks

**Half-Life** Biphasic: rapid: 2 hours; slow: 5 hours

**Special PA Issues**

**Patient Education:** Take this medication exactly as directed; do not increase dose without consulting prescriber. Do not crush tablets or break capsules. Take with food or milk to reduce GI distress. Maintain adequate fluid intake (2-3 L/day). Do not use alcohol, aspirin, or aspirin-containing medication, and all other anti-inflammatory medications without consulting prescriber. You may experience dizziness, nervousness, or headache (use caution when driving or performing hazardous tasks); nausea, vomiting, or heartburn (frequent small meals, frequent oral care, sucking on lozenges, or chewing gum may help); constipation (increased exercise, fluids, or dietary fruit and fiber may help). GI bleeding, ulceration, or perforation can occur with or without pain; discontinue medication and contact prescriber if persistent abdominal pain or cramping, or blood in stool occurs. Report chest pain or palpitations; breathlessness or difficulty breathing; unusual bruising/bleeding; blood in urine, stool, mouth, or vomitus; unusual fatigue; skin rash or itching; unusual weight gain or swelling of extremities; change in urinary pattern; or change in vision or hearing or ringing in ears.

**Monitoring Parameters:** Occult blood loss, CBC, liver enzymes, BUN, serum creatinine, periodic liver function test

**Related Information**

Nonsteroidal Anti-Inflammatory Agents *on page 1026*

♦ **Tolmetin Sodium** *see* Tolmetin *on previous page*

# Tolnaftate (tole NAF tate)

**Pharmacologic Class** Antifungal Agent, Topical

**U.S. Brand Names** Absorbine® Antifungal [OTC]; Absorbine® Jock Itch [OTC]; Absorbine Jr.® Antifungal [OTC]; Aftate® for Athlete's Foot [OTC]; Aftate® for Jock Itch [OTC]; Blis-To-Sol® [OTC]; Breezee® Mist Antifungal [OTC]; Dr Scholl's Athlete's Foot [OTC]; Dr Scholl's Maximum Strength Tritin [OTC]; Genaspor® [OTC]; NP-27® [OTC]; Quinsana Plus® [OTC]; Tinactin® [OTC]; Tinactin® for Jock Itch [OTC]; Ting® [OTC]; Zeasorb-AF® Powder [OTC]

**Mechanism of Action** Distorts the hyphae and stunts mycelial growth in susceptible fungi

**Use** Treatment of tinea pedis, tinea cruris, tinea corporis, tinea manuum, tinea versicolor infections

**USUAL DOSAGE** Children and Adults: Topical: Wash and dry affected area; apply 1-3 drops of solution or a small amount of cream or powder and rub into the affected areas 2-3 times/day for 2-4 weeks

**Dosage Forms** Aero, top: Liq: 1% (59.2 mL, 90 mL, 120 mL); **Powder:** 1% (56.7 g, 100 g, 105 g, 150 g); **Crm:** 1% (15 g, 30 g); **Gel, top:** 1% (15 g); **Powder, top:** 1% (45 g, 90 g); **Soln, top:** 1% (10 mL)

**Contraindications** Known hypersensitivity to tolnaftate; nail and scalp infections

**Warnings/Precautions** Cream is not recommended for nail or scalp infections; keep from eyes; if no improvement within 4 weeks, treatment should be discontinued. Usually not effective alone for the treatment of infections involving hair follicles or nails.

**Pregnancy Risk Factor** C

**Adverse Reactions** 1% to 10%:

Dermatologic: Pruritus, contact dermatitis

Local: Irritation, stinging

**Special PA Issues**

**Patient Education:** Avoid contact with the eyes; apply to clean dry area; consult the physician if a skin irritation develops or if the skin infection worsens or does not improve after 10 days of therapy; does not stain skin or clothing

**Related Information**

Antifungal Agents, Topical *on page 1000*

# Tolterodine (tole TER oh dine)

**Pharmacologic Class** Anticholinergic Agent

**U.S. Brand Names** Detrol™

**Mechanism of Action** Tolterodine is a competitive antagonist of muscarinic receptors. In animal models, tolterodine demonstrates selectivity for urinary bladder receptors over salivary receptors. Urinary bladder contraction is mediated by muscarinic receptors. Tolterodine increases residual urine volume and decreases detrusor muscle pressure.

**Use** Treatment of patients with an overactive bladder with symptoms of urinary frequency, urgency, or urge incontinence

**USUAL DOSAGE** Adults: Oral: Initial: 2 mg twice daily; the dose may be lowered to 1 mg twice daily based on individual response and tolerability

Dosing adjustment in patients concurrently taking cytochrome P-450 3A4 inhibitors: 1 mg twice daily

**Dosing adjustment in renal impairment:** Use with caution

**Dosing adjustment in hepatic impairment:** Administer 1 mg twice daily

**Dosage Forms** Tab, as tartrate: 1 mg, 2 mg

**Contraindications** Urinary retention or gastric retention; uncontrolled narrow-angle glaucoma; demonstrated hypersensitivity to tolterodine or ingredients

**Warnings/Precautions** Caution in patients with bladder flow obstruction, pyloric stenosis or other GI obstruction, narrow-angle glaucoma (controlled), reduced hepatic/renal function

**Pregnancy Risk Factor** C

**Adverse Reactions**

>10%: Central nervous system: Headache

(Continued)

## Tolterodine *(Continued)*

1% to 10%:

Cardiovascular: Chest pain, hypertension (1.5%)

Central nervous system: Vertigo (8.6%), nervousness (1.1%), somnolence (3.0%)

Dermatologic: Pruritus (1.3%), rash (1.9%), dry skin (1.7%)

Gastrointestinal: Abdominal pain (7.6%), constipation (6.5%), diarrhea (4.0%), dyspepsia (5.9%), flatulence (1.3%), nausea (4.2%), vomiting (1.7%), weight gain (1.5%)

Genitourinary: Dysuria (2.5%), polyuria (1.1%), urinary retention (1.7%), urinary tract infection (5.5%)

Neuromuscular & skeletal: Back pain, falling (1.3%), paresthesia (1.1%)

Ocular: Vision abnormalities (4.7%), dry eyes (3.8%)

Respiratory: Bronchitis (2.1%), cough (2.1%), pharyngitis (1.5%), rhinitis (1.1%), sinusitis (1.1%), upper respiratory infection (5.9%)

Miscellaneous: Flu-like symptoms (4.4%), infection (2.1%)

**Drug Interactions** CYP3A3/4 substrate; CYP2D6 substrate

Increased toxicity: Macrolide antibiotics/azole antifungal agents may inhibit the metabolism of tolterodine. Doses of tolterodine >1 mg twice daily should not be exceeded.

Fluoxetine, which inhibits cytochrome P-450 2D6, increases concentration 4.8 times. Other drugs which inhibit this isoenzyme may also interact. Studies with inhibitors of cytochrome isoenzyme 3A4 have not been performed.

**Special PA Issues**

**Patient Education:** Take as directed, preferably with food. You may experience headache (a mild analgesic may help); dizziness, nervousness, or sleepiness (use caution when driving, climbing stairs, or engaging in tasks that require alertness); abdominal discomfort, diarrhea, constipation, nausea or vomiting (small frequent meals, increased exercise, adequate fluid intake may help). Report back pain, muscle spasms, alteration in gait, or numbness of extremities; unresolved or persistent constipation, diarrhea, or vomiting; or symptoms of upper respiratory infection or flu. Report immediately any chest pain or palpitations; difficulty urinating or pain on urination.

**Dietary Considerations:** Food increases bioavailability (~53% increase)

- ◆ **Tolu-Sed® DM [OTC]** *see* Guaifenesin and Dextromethorphan *on page 428*
- ◆ **Tonga** *see* Kava *on page 505*
- ◆ **Tonocard®** *see* Tocainide *on page 909*
- ◆ **Topactin®** *see* Fluocinonide *on page 381*
- ◆ **Topamax®** *see* Topiramate *on this page*
- ◆ **Topicort®** *see* Desoximetasone *on page 263*
- ◆ **Topicort®-LP** *see* Desoximetasone *on page 263*
- ◆ **Topicycline® Topical** *see* Tetracycline *on page 885*
- ◆ **Topilene** *see* Betamethasone *on page 111*

# Topiramate *(toe PYE ra mate)*

**Pharmacologic Class** Anticonvulsant, Miscellaneous

**U.S. Brand Names** Topamax®

**Mechanism of Action** Mechanism is not fully understood, it is thought to decrease seizure frequency by blocking sodium channels in neurons, enhancing GABA activity and by blocking glutamate activity

**Use** Adjunctive therapy for partial onset seizures in adults

Orphan drug: Topiramate has also been granted orphan drug status for the treatment of Lennox-Gastaut syndrome

**USUAL DOSAGE**

Adults: Initial: 50 mg/day; titrate by 50 mg/day at 1-week intervals to target dose of 200 mg twice daily; usual maximum dose: 1600 mg/day

**Dosing adjustment in renal impairment:** $Cl_{cr}$ <70 mL/minute: Administer 50% dose and titrate more slowly

**Dosing adjustment in hepatic impairment:** Clearance may be minimally reduced

**Dosage Forms Cap, sprinkle:** 15 mg, 25 mg; **Tab:** 25 mg, 100 mg, 200 mg

**Contraindications** Patients with a known hypersensitivity to any components of this drug

**Warnings/Precautions** Avoid abrupt withdrawal of topiramate therapy, it should be withdrawn slowly to minimize the potential of increased seizure frequency; the risk of kidney stones is about 2-4 times that of the untreated population, the risk of this event may be reduced by increasing fluid intake; use cautiously in patients with hepatic or renal impairment, during pregnancy or in nursing mothers.

**Pregnancy Risk Factor** C

**Pregnancy Implications** Breast-feeding/lactation: In studies of rats topiramate has been shown to be secreted in milk; however, it has not been studied in humans

**Adverse Reactions**

>10%:

Central nervous system: Fatigue, dizziness, ataxia, somnolence, psychomotor slowing, nervousness, memory difficulties, speech problems

Gastrointestinal: Nausea
Neuromuscular & skeletal: Paresthesia, tremor
Ocular: Nystagmus
Respiratory: Upper respiratory infections
1% to 10%:
Cardiovascular: Chest pain, edema
Central nervous system: Language problems, abnormal coordination, confusion, depression, difficulty concentrating, hypoesthesia
Endocrine & metabolic: Hot flashes
Gastrointestinal: Dyspepsia, abdominal pain, anorexia, constipation, xerostomia, gingivitis, weight loss
Neuromuscular & skeletal: Myalgia, weakness, back pain, leg pain, rigors
Otic: Decreased hearing
Renal: Nephrolithiasis
Respiratory: Pharyngitis, sinusitis, epistaxis
Miscellaneous: Flu-like symptoms

**Drug Interactions** CYP2C19 enzyme substrate; CYP2C19 enzyme inhibitor
Decreased effect: Phenytoin can decrease topiramate levels by as much as 48%, carbamazepine reduces it by 40% and valproic acid reduces topiramate by 14%; digoxin levels and norethindrone blood levels are decreased when coadministered with topiramate
Increased toxicity: Concomitant administration with other CNS depressants will increase its sedative effects; coadministration with other carbonic anhydrase inhibitors may increase the chance of nephrolithiasis

**Half-Life** Mean: 21 hours

**Special PA Issues**
**Patient Education:** Take exactly as directed; do not increase dose or frequency or discontinue without consulting prescriber. While using this medication, do not use alcohol and other prescription or OTC medications (especially pain medications, sedatives, antihistamines, or hypnotics) without consulting prescriber. Maintain adequate hydration (2-3 L/day of fluids unless instructed to restrict fluid intake). You may experience drowsiness, dizziness, disturbed concentration, memory changes, or blurred vision (use caution when driving or engaging in hazardous tasks); mouth sores, nausea, vomiting, or loss of appetite (small frequent meals, good mouth care, chewing gum, or sucking on lozenges may help). Wear identification of epileptic status and medications. Report behavioral or CNS changes; skin rash; muscle cramping, weakness, tremors, changes in gait; chest pain, irregular heartbeat, or palpitations; hearing loss; cough or difficulty breathing; worsening of seizure activity, or loss of seizure control.

- ♦ **Topisone** see Betamethasone on page 111
- ♦ **Toprol XL®** see Metoprolol on page 599
- ♦ **Topsyn®** see Fluocinonide on page 381
- ♦ **Toradol® Injection** see Ketorolac Tromethamine on page 508
- ♦ **Toradol® Oral** see Ketorolac Tromethamine on page 508
- ♦ **Torecan®** see Thiethylperazine on page 894

# Toremifene (TORE em i feen)
**Pharmacologic Class** Antineoplastic Agent, Miscellaneous
**U.S. Brand Names** Fareston®
**Mechanism of Action** Nonsteroidal, triphenylethylene derivative. Competitively binds to estrogen receptors on tumors and other tissue targets, producing a nuclear complex that decreases DNA synthesis and inhibits estrogen effects. Nonsteroidal agent with potent antiestrogenic properties which compete with estrogen for binding sites in breast and other tissues; cells accumulate in the $G_0$ and $G_1$ phases; therefore, tamoxifen is cytostatic rather than cytocidal.
**Use** Treatment of metastatic breast cancer in postmenopausal women with estrogen-receptor (ER) positive or ER unknown tumors
**USUAL DOSAGE** Refer to individual protocols
Adults: Oral: 60 mg once daily, generally continued until disease progression is observed
**Dosage adjustment in renal impairment:** No dosage adjustment necessary
**Dosage adjustment in hepatic impairment:** Toremifene is extensively metabolized in the liver and dosage adjustments may be indicated in patients with liver disease; however, no specific guidelines have been developed
**Dosage Forms** Tab, as citrate: 60 mg
**Contraindications** Hypersensitivity to toremifene
**Warnings/Precautions** Hypercalcemia and tumor flare have been reported in some breast cancer patients with bone metastases during the first weeks of treatment. Tumor flare is a syndrome of diffuse musculoskeletal pain and erythema with increased size of tumor lesions that later regress. It is often accompanied by hypercalcemia. Tumor flare does not imply treatment failure or represent tumor progression. Institute appropriate measures if hypercalcemia occurs, and if severe, discontinue treatment. Drugs that decrease renal calcium excretion (eg, thiazide diuretics) may increase the risk of hypercalcemia in patients receiving toremifene.
(Continued)

## Toremifene *(Continued)*

Patients with a history of thromboembolic disease should generally not be treated with toremifene

**Pregnancy Risk Factor** D

**Adverse Reactions**

>10%:

Endocrine & metabolic: Vaginal discharge, hot flashes

Gastrointestinal: Nausea

Miscellaneous: Diaphoresis

1% to 10%:

Cardiovascular: Thromboembolism: Tamoxifen has been associated with the occurrence of venous thrombosis and pulmonary embolism; arterial thrombosis has also been described in a few case reports; cardiac failure, myocardial infarction, edema

Central nervous system: Dizziness

Endocrine & metabolic: Hypercalcemia may occur in patients with bone metastases; galactorrhea and vitamin deficiency, menstrual irregularities

Gastrointestinal: Vomiting

Genitourinary: Vaginal bleeding or discharge, endometriosis, priapism, possible endometrial cancer

Ocular: Ophthalmologic effects (visual acuity changes, cataracts, or retinopathy), corneal opacities, dry eyes

**Drug Interactions** CYP3A3/4 enzyme substrate

Decreased effect: CYP 3A4 enzyme inducers: Phenobarbital, phenytoin and carbamazepine increase the rate of toremifene metabolism and lower the steady state concentration in serum

Increased toxicity:

CYP3A4-6 enzyme inhibitors (ketoconazole, erythromycin) inhibit the metabolism of toremifene

Warfarin results in significant enhancement of the anticoagulant effects of warfarin; has been speculated that a decrease in antitumor effect of tamoxifen may also occur due to alterations in the percentage of active tamoxifen metabolites

**Half-Life** ~5 days

**Special PA Issues**

**Patient Education:** Take as directed, without regard to food. You may experience an initial "flare" of this disease (increased bone pain and hot flashes) which will subside with continued use. You may experience nausea, vomiting, or loss of appetite (frequent mouth care, frequent small meals, chewing gum, or sucking on lozenges may help); dizziness (use caution when driving, climbing stairs, or engaging in tasks that require alertness); or loss of hair (will grow back). Report vomiting that occurs immediately after taking medication; chest pain, palpitations or swollen extremities; vaginal bleeding, hot flashes, or excessive perspiration; chest pain, unusual coughing, or difficulty breathing; or any changes in vision or dry eyes.

**Monitoring Parameters:** Obtain periodic complete blood counts, calcium levels, and liver function tests. Closely monitor patients with bone metastases for hypercalcemia during the first few weeks of treatment. Leukopenia and thrombocytopenia have been reported rarely; monitor leukocyte and platelet counts during treatment.

♦ **Toremifene Citrate** *see* Toremifene *on previous page*

♦ **Tornalate®** *see* Bitolterol *on page 118*

## Torsemide *(TOR se mide)*

**Pharmacologic Class** Diuretic, Loop

**U.S. Brand Names** Demadex®

**Mechanism of Action** Inhibits reabsorption of sodium and chloride in the ascending loop of Henle and distal renal tubule, interfering with the chloride-binding cotransport system, thus causing increased excretion of water, sodium, chloride, magnesium, and calcium; does not alter GFR, renal plasma flow, or acid-base balance

**Use** Management of edema associated with congestive heart failure and hepatic or renal disease; used alone or in combination with antihypertensives in treatment of hypertension; I.V. form is indicated when rapid onset is desired

**USUAL DOSAGE** Adults: Oral, I.V.:

Congestive heart failure: 10-20 mg once daily; may increase gradually for chronic treatment by doubling dose until the diuretic response is apparent (for acute treatment, I.V. dose may be repeated every 2 hours with double the dose as needed)

Chronic renal failure: 20 mg once daily; increase as described above

Hepatic cirrhosis: 5-10 mg once daily with an aldosterone antagonist or a potassium-sparing diuretic; increase as described above

Hypertension: 5 mg once daily; increase to 10 mg after 4-6 weeks if an adequate hypotensive response is not apparent; if still not effective, an additional antihypertensive agent may be added

**Dosage Forms Inj:** 10 mg/mL (2 mL, 5 mL); **Tab:** 5 mg, 10 mg, 20 mg, 100 mg

**Contraindications** Anuria; hypersensitivity to torsemide or any component, or other sulfonylureas; safety in children <18 years has not been established

**Warnings/Precautions** Excessive diuresis may result in dehydration, acute hypotensive or thromboembolic episodes and cardiovascular collapse; rapid injection, renal impairment, or excessively large doses may result in ototoxicity; SLE may be exacerbated; sudden alterations in electrolyte balance may precipitate hepatic encephalopathy and coma in patients with hepatic cirrhosis and ascites; monitor carefully for signs of fluid or electrolyte imbalances, especially hypokalemia in patients at risk for such (eg, digitalis therapy, history of ventricular arrhythmias, elderly, etc), hyperuricemia, hypomagnesemia, or hypocalcemia; use caution with exposure to ultraviolet light.

**Pregnancy Risk Factor** B

**Pregnancy Implications** Clinical effect on the fetus: A decrease in fetal weight, an increase in fetal resorption, and delayed fetal ossification has occurred in animal studies

**Adverse Reactions**
>10%: Cardiovascular: Orthostatic hypotension
1% to 10%:
   Central nervous system: Headache, dizziness, vertigo, pain
   Dermatologic: Photosensitivity, urticaria
   Endocrine & metabolic: Electrolyte imbalance, dehydration, hyperuricemia
   Gastrointestinal: Diarrhea, loss of appetite, stomach cramps, pancreatitis
   Ocular: Blurred vision
<1%: Rash, gout, pancreatitis, nausea, hepatic dysfunction, agranulocytosis, leukopenia, anemia, thrombocytopenia, redness at injection site, ototoxicity, nephrocalcinosis, prerenal azotemia, interstitial nephritis

**Drug Interactions** CYP2C9 enzyme substrate
Aminoglycosides: Ototoxicity may be increased; anticoagulant activity is enhanced
Beta-blockers: Plasma concentrations of beta-blockers may be increased with furosemide
Cisplatin: Ototoxicity may be increased
Digitalis: Arrhythmias may occur with diuretic-induced electrolyte disturbances
Lithium: Plasma concentrations of lithium may be increased
NSAIDs: Torsemide efficacy may be decreased
Probenecid: Torsemide action may be reduced
Salicylates: Diuretic action may be impaired in patients with cirrhosis and ascites
Sulfonylureas: Glucose tolerance may be decreased
Thiazides: Synergistic effects may result
Chloral hydrate: Transient diaphoresis, hot flashes, hypertension may occur

**Onset** Onset of diuresis: 30-60 minutes; Peak effect: 1-4 hours

**Duration** ~6 hours

**Half-Life** 2-4; 7-8 hours in cirrhosis (dose modification appears unnecessary)

**Special PA Issues**
   **Patient Education:** Take recommended dosage with food or milk at the same time each day (preferably not in the evening to avoid sleep interruption). Do not miss doses, alter dosage, or discontinue without consulting prescriber. Include orange juice or bananas (or other potassium-rich foods) in daily diet; do not take potassium supplements without consulting prescriber. Do not use alcohol or OTC medications without consulting prescriber. You may experience postural hypotension; change position slowly when rising from sitting or lying. May cause transient drowsiness, blurred vision, or dizziness; avoid driving or engaging in tasks that require alertness until response to drug is known. You may have reduced tolerance to heat (avoid strenuous activity in hot weather or excessively hot showers). Increased exercise and increased dietary fiber, fruit, and fluids may reduce constipation. Report unusual weight gain or loss (>5 lb/week), swelling of ankles and hands, persistent fatigue, unresolved constipation or diarrhea, weakness, fatigue, dizziness, vomiting, cramps, change in hearing, or chest pain or palpitations.

   **Monitoring Parameters:** Renal function, electrolytes, and fluid status (weight and I & O), blood pressure

♦ **Totacillin®** see Ampicillin on page 64

♦ **Totacillin®-N** see Ampicillin on page 64

♦ **Touro Ex®** see Guaifenesin on page 427

♦ **t-PA** see Alteplase on page 46

# Tramadol (TRA ma dole)

**Pharmacologic Class** Analgesic, Non-narcotic

**U.S. Brand Names** Ultram®

**Mechanism of Action** Binds to μ-opiate receptors in the CNS causing inhibition of ascending pain pathways, altering the perception of and response to pain; also inhibits the reuptake of norepinephrine and serotonin, which also modifies the ascending pain pathway

**Use** Relief of moderate to moderately severe pain

**USUAL DOSAGE** Adults: Oral: 50-100 mg every 4-6 hours, not to exceed 400 mg/day
   Initiation of low dose followed by titration in increments of 50 mg/day every 3 days to effective dose (not >400 mg/day) may minimize dizziness and vertigo
   (Continued)

# Tramadol *(Continued)*

**Dosage Forms** Tab, as hydrochloride: 50 mg

**Contraindications** Previous hypersensitivity to tramadol or any components; do not give to opioid-dependent patients; concurrent use of monoamine oxidase inhibitors; acute alcohol intoxication; concurrent use of centrally acting analgesics, opioids, or psychotropic drugs

**Warnings/Precautions** Elderly patients and patients with chronic respiratory disorders may be at greater risk of adverse events; liver disease; patients with myxedema, hypothyroidism, or hypoadrenalism should use tramadol with caution and at reduced dosages; not recommended during pregnancy or in nursing mothers; increased incidence of seizures may occur in patients receiving concurrent tricyclic antidepressants; tolerance or drug dependence may result from extended use

**Pregnancy Risk Factor** C

**Adverse Reactions**

>1%:
Central nervous system: Dizziness, headache, somnolence, stimulation, restlessness
Gastrointestinal: Nausea, diarrhea, constipation, vomiting, dyspepsia
Neuromuscular & skeletal: Weakness
Miscellaneous: Diaphoresis
<1%: Palpitations, seizures, respiratory depression, suicidal tendency

**Drug Interactions** CYP2D6 enzyme substrate
Decreased effects: Carbamazepine (decreases half-life by 33% to 50%)
Increased toxicity: Monoamine oxidase inhibitors and tricyclic antidepressants (seizures); quinidine (inhibits CYP2D6, thereby increases tramadol serum concentrations); cimetidine (tramadol half-life increased 20% to 25%)

**Onset** 1 hour

**Half-Life** 6.3-7.4 hours

**Special PA Issues**

**Patient Education:** If self-administered, use exactly as directed (do not increase dose or frequency); may cause physical and/or psychological dependence. Take with food or milk. While using this medication, do not use alcohol and other prescription or OTC medications (especially pain medications, sedatives, antihistamines, or cough preparations) without consulting prescriber. Maintain adequate hydration (2-3 L/day of fluids unless instructed to restrict fluid intake). You may experience drowsiness, dizziness, or blurred vision (use caution when driving or engaging in hazardous tasks); nausea, vomiting, or loss of appetite (small frequent meals, good mouth care, chewing gum, or sucking on lozenges may help); constipation (increased exercise, fluids, or dietary fruit and fiber may help). Report severe unresolved constipation; difficulty breathing or shortness of breath; excessive sedation or increased insomnia and restlessness; changes in urinary pattern or menstrual pattern; muscle weakness or tremors; or chest pain or palpitations.

**Monitoring Parameters:** Monitor patient for pain, respiratory rate, and look for signs of tolerance and, therefore, abuse potential; monitor blood pressure and pulse rate, especially in patients on higher doses

**Reference Range:** 100-300 ng/mL; however, serum level monitoring is not required

♦ **Tramadol Hydrochloride** *see* Tramadol *on previous page*

♦ **Trandate®** *see* Labetalol *on page 510*

# Trandolapril *(tran DOE la pril)*

**Pharmacologic Class** Angiotensin-Converting Enzyme (ACE) Inhibitors

**U.S. Brand Names** Mavik®

**Mechanism of Action** Trandolapril is an angiotensin-converting enzyme (ACE) inhibitor which prevents the formation of angiotensin II from angiotensin I. Trandolapril must undergo enzymatic hydrolysis, mainly in liver, to its biologically active metabolite, trandolaprilat. A CNS mechanism may also be involved in the hypotensive effect as angiotensin II increases adrenergic outflow from the CNS. Vasoactive kallikrein's may be decreased in conversion to active hormones by ACE inhibitors, thus, reducing blood pressure.

**Use** Treatment of hypertension (alone or in combination with other antihypertensive medications such as hydrochlorothiazide). For stable patients who have evidence of left-ventricular systolic dysfunction (identified by wall motion abnormalities) or who are symptomatic from CHF within the first few days after sustaining acute myocardial infarction. Administration to Caucasians decreases the risk of death (principally cardiovascular death) and decreases the risk of heart failure–related admissions.

**USUAL DOSAGE** Adults: Oral:

Hypertension: Initial dose in patients not receiving a diuretic: 1 mg/day (2 mg/day in black patients). Adjust dosage according to the blood pressure response. Make dosage adjustments at intervals of ≥1 week. Most patients have required dosages of 2-4 mg/day. There is a little experience with doses >8 mg/day. Patients inadequately treated with once daily dosing at 4 mg may be treated with twice daily dosing. If blood pressure is not adequately controlled with trandolapril monotherapy, a diuretic may be added.

Heart failure postmyocardial infarction or left-ventricular dysfunction postmyocardial infarction: Initial: 1 mg/day; titrate patients (as tolerated) towards the target dose of 4 mg/day. If a 4 mg dose is not tolerated, patients can continue therapy with the greatest tolerated dose.

**Dosing adjustment in renal impairment:** $Cl_{cr}$ ≤30 mL/minute: Recommended starting dose: 0.5 mg/day

**Dosing adjustment in hepatic impairment:** Cirrhosis: Recommended starting dose: 0.5 mg/day

**Dosage Forms Tab:** 1 mg, 2 mg, 4 mg

**Contraindications** Hypersensitivity to trandolapril, other ACE inhibitors, in patients with a history of angioedema related to previous treatment with an ACE inhibitor, or any component

**Warnings/Precautions** Neutropenia, agranulocytosis, angioedema, decreased renal function (hypertension, renal artery stenosis, CHF), hepatic dysfunction (elimination, activation), proteinuria, first-dose hypotension (hypovolemia, CHF, dehydrated patients at risk, eg, diuretic use, elderly), elderly (due to renal function changes); use with caution and modify dosage in patients with renal impairment; use with caution in patients with collagen vascular disease, CHF, hypovolemia, valvular stenosis, hyperkalemia (>5.7 mEq/L), anesthesia

Patients taking diuretics are at risk for developing hypotension on initial dosing; to prevent this, discontinue diuretics 2-3 days prior to initiating trandolapril; may restart diuretics if blood pressure is not controlled by trandolapril alone

**Pregnancy Risk Factor** C (1st trimester); D (2nd and 3rd trimesters)

**Adverse Reactions**
1% to 10%:
  Cardiovascular: Chest pain, hypotension, syncope
  Central nervous system: Fatigue
  Gastrointestinal: Dyspepsia
  Neuromuscular & skeletal: Myalgia
  Respiratory: Cough (1.9% to 35%)
≤1%: Palpitations, flushing, insomnia, sleep disturbances, vertigo, anxiety, pruritus, rash, angioedema, decreased libido, abdominal pain, vomiting, diarrhea, constipation, pancreatitis, urinary tract infection, impotence, paresthesia, muscle cramps, dyspnea, upper respiratory infection

**Drug Interactions**
ACE inhibitors (trandolapril) and potassium-sparing diuretics may have additive hyperkalemic effect

ACE inhibitors (trandolapril) and indomethacin or nonsteroidal anti-inflammatory agents may reduce antihypertensive response to ACE inhibitors (trandolapril)

Allopurinol and trandolapril → neutropenia

Antacids and ACE inhibitors may decrease absorption of ACE inhibitors

Phenothiazines and ACE inhibitors may increase ACE inhibitor effect

Probenecid and ACE inhibitors (trandolapril) may increase ACE inhibitors (trandolapril) levels

Rifampin and ACE inhibitors (trandolapril) may decrease ACE inhibitor effect

Digoxin and ACE inhibitors may increase serum digoxin levels

Lithium and ACE inhibitors may increase lithium serum levels

Tetracycline and ACE inhibitors (trandolapril) may decrease tetracycline absorption (up to 37%)

Food decreases trandolapril absorption; rate, but not extent, of ramipril and fosinopril is reduced by concomitant administration with food; food does not reduce absorption of enalapril, lisinopril, or benazepril; trandolapril has a decreased rate and extent (25% to 30%) of absorption when taken with a high fat meal

**Onset** 1-2 hours

**Duration** Trandolaprilat (active metabolite) is very lipophilic in comparison to other ACE inhibitors which may contribute to its prolonged duration of action (72 hours after a single dose)

**Half-Life** Parent: 6 hours; Active metabolite trandolaprilat: 10 hours

**Special PA Issues**
**Patient Education:** Take as directed, preferably 1 hour before or 2 hours after meals. Do not change dosage or stop taking without consulting prescriber. Follow diet recommended by prescriber. You may experience dizziness, fainting, or lightheadedness (use caution when driving or performing hazardous tasks) and use caution when changing position (rising from sitting or lying) until response to therapy is established. Report sore throat; fever; rash; swelling of hands, feet, or legs; respiratory difficulty; chest pains or irregular heartbeat; unusual cough; persistent vomiting, diarrhea, sweating, or perspiration; or flu-like symptoms. Do not get pregnant; use appropriate contraceptive measures.
**Monitoring Parameters:** Serum potassium, renal function, serum creatinine, BUN, CBC
**Related Information**
ACE Inhibitors *on page 995*

# Trandolapril and Verapamil (tran DOE la pril & ver AP a mil)
**Pharmacologic Class** Antihypertensive Agent, Combination
**U.S. Brand Names** Tarka®
(Continued)

# Trandolapril and Verapamil *(Continued)*

**Dosage Forms Tab:** Trandolapril 1 mg and verapamil hydrochloride 240 mg, Trandolapril 2 mg and verapamil hydrochloride 180 mg, Trandolapril 2 mg and verapamil hydrochloride 240 mg, Trandolapril 4 mg and verapamil hydrochloride 240 mg

♦ **Transamine Sulphate** *see* Tranylcypromine *on this page*

♦ **Transdermal-NTG® Patch** *see* Nitroglycerin *on page 660*

♦ **Transderm-Nitro® Patch** *see* Nitroglycerin *on page 660*

♦ **Transderm Scop® Patch** *see* Scopolamine *on page 824*

♦ ***trans*-Retinoic Acid** *see* Tretinoin, Topical *on page 927*

♦ **Tranxene®** *see* Clorazepate *on page 227*

# Tranylcypromine *(tran il SIP roe meen)*

**Pharmacologic Class** Antidepressant, Monoamine Oxidase Inhibitor

**U.S. Brand Names** Parnate®

**Mechanism of Action** Inhibits the enzymes monoamine oxidase A and B which are responsible for the intraneuronal metabolism of norepinephrine and serotonin and increasing their availability to postsynaptic neurons; decreased firing rate of the locus ceruleus, reducing norepinephrine concentration in the brain; agonist effects of serotonin

**Use** Symptomatic treatment of depressed patients refractory to or intolerant to tricyclic antidepressants or electroconvulsive therapy; has a more rapid onset of therapeutic effect than other MAO inhibitors, but causes more severe hypertensive reactions

**USUAL DOSAGE** Adults: Oral: 10 mg twice daily, increase by 10 mg increments at 1- to 3-week intervals; maximum: 60 mg/day

**Dosing comments in hepatic impairment:** Use with care and monitor plasma levels and patient response closely

**Dosage Forms Tab, as sulfate:** 10 mg

**Contraindications** Uncontrolled hypertension, known hypersensitivity to tranylcypromine, pheochromocytoma, cardiovascular disease, severe renal or hepatic impairment, pheochromocytoma

**Warnings/Precautions** Safety in children <16 years of age has not been established; use with caution in patients who are hyperactive, hyperexcitable, or who have glaucoma, suicidal tendencies, diabetes, elderly

**Pregnancy Risk Factor** C

**Adverse Reactions**

1% to 10%: Cardiovascular: Orthostatic hypotension

<1%: Edema, hypertensive crises, drowsiness, hyperexcitability, headache, rash, photosensitivity, xerostomia, constipation, urinary retention, hepatitis, blurred vision

**Drug Interactions** CYP2A6 and 2C19 enzyme inhibitor

Decreased effect of antihypertensives

Increased toxicity with disulfiram (seizures), fluoxetine and other serotonin-active agents (eg, paroxetine, sertraline), TCAs (cardiovascular instability), meperidine (cardiovascular instability), phenothiazine (hypertensive crisis), sympathomimetics (hypertensive crisis), sumatriptan (hypothetical), CNS depressants, levodopa (hypertensive crisis), tyramine-containing foods (eg, aged foods), dextroamphetamine (psychosis)

**Onset** 2-3 weeks of continued dosing are required to obtain full therapeutic effect

**Duration** May continue to have a therapeutic effect and interactions 2 weeks after discontinuing therapy

**Half-Life** 90-190 minutes

**Special PA Issues**

**Patient Education:** Take exactly as directed (do not increase dose or frequency); may take 2-3 weeks to achieve desired results; may cause physical and/or psychological dependence. Take in the morning to reduce the incidence of insomnia. Avoid excessive alcohol, caffeine, and other prescription or OTC medications not approved by prescriber. Avoid tyramine-containing foods (eg pickles, aged cheese, wine); see prescriber for complete list of foods to be avoided. Maintain adequate hydration (2-3 L/day of fluids unless instructed to restrict fluid intake). You may experience drowsiness, dizziness, or blurred vision (use caution when driving or engaging in hazardous tasks until response to medication is known; anorexia or dry mouth (small frequent meals, frequent mouth care, or sucking lozenges may help); constipation (increased exercise, fluids, or dietary fruit and fiber may help); diarrhea (buttermilk, yogurt, or boiled milk may help); orthostatic hypotension (use caution when climbing stairs or changing position from lying or sitting to standing); or altered sexual ability (reversible). Report persistent excessive sedation; muscle cramping, tremors, weakness, or change in gait; chest pain, palpitations, rapid heartbeat, or swelling of extremities; vision changes; or worsening of condition.

**Dietary Considerations:**

Alcohol: Avoid use

Food: Avoid tyramine-containing foods

**Monitoring Parameters:** Blood pressure, blood glucose
**Related Information**
Antidepressant Agents *on page 998*
Tyramine-Containing Foods *on page 1148*

♦ **Tranylcypromine Sulfate** *see* Tranylcypromine *on previous page*

# Trastuzumab (tras TU zoo mab)

**Pharmacologic Class** Antineoplastic Agent, Miscellaneous
**U.S. Brand Names** Herceptin®
**Mechanism of Action** Trastuzumab is a monoclonal antibody which binds to the extracellular domain of the human epidermal growth factor receptor 2 protein (HER2); it mediates antibody-dependent cellular cytotoxicity against cells which overproduce HER2
**Use**
Single agent for the treatment of patients with metastatic breast cancer whose tumors overexpress the HER2/neu protein and who have received one or more chemotherapy regimens for their metastatic disease
Combination therapy with paclitaxel for the treatment of patients with metastatic breast cancer whose tumors overexpress the HER2/neu protein and who have not received chemotherapy for their metastatic disease
Note: HER2/neu protein overexpression or amplification has been noted in ovarian, gastric, colorectal, endometrial, lung, bladder, prostate, and salivary gland tumors. It is not yet known whether trastuzumab may be effective in these other carcinomas which overexpress HER2/neu protein.
**USUAL DOSAGE** I.V. infusion:
Adults:
Initial loading dose: 4 mg/kg intravenous infusion over 90 minutes
Maintenance dose: 2 mg/kg intravenous infusion over 90 minutes (can be administered over 30 minutes if prior infusions are well tolerated) weekly until disease progression
**Dosing adjustment in renal impairment:** Data suggest that the disposition of trastuzumab is not altered based on age or serum creatinine (up to 2 mg/dL); however, no formal interaction studies have been performed
**Dosing adjustment in hepatic impairment:** No data is currently available
**Dosage Forms Powder for inj:** 440 mg
**Contraindications** None known
**Warnings/Precautions** Congestive heart failure associated with trastuzumab may be severe and has been associated with disabling cardiac failure, death, mural thrombus, and stroke. Left ventricular function should be evaluated in all patients prior to and during treatment with trastuzumab. Discontinuation should be strongly considered in patients who develop a clinically significant decrease in ejection fraction during therapy. Combination therapy which includes anthracyclines and cyclophosphamide increases the incidence and severity of cardiac dysfunction. Extreme caution should be used when treating patients with pre-existing cardiac disease or dysfunction, and in patients with previous exposure to anthracyclines. Advanced age may also predispose to cardiac toxicity. Hypersensitivity to hamster ovary cell proteins or any component of this product.
**Pregnancy Risk Factor** B
**Pregnancy Implications** It is not known whether trastuzumab is secreted in human milk; because many immunoglobulins are secreted in milk, and the potential for serious adverse reactions exists, patients should discontinue nursing during treatment and for 6 months after the last dose
**Adverse Reactions**
>10%:
Central nervous system: Pain (47%), fever (36%), chills (32%), headache (26%)
Dermatologic: Rash (18%)
Neuromuscular & skeletal: Weakness (42%), back pain (22%)
Gastrointestinal: Nausea (33%), diarrhea (25%), vomiting (23%), abdominal pain (22%), anorexia (14%)
Respiratory: Cough (26%), dyspnea (22%), rhinitis (14%), pharyngitis (12%)
Miscellaneous: Infection (20%)
1% to 10%:
Cardiovascular: Peripheral edema (10%), congestive heart failure (7%), tachycardia (5%)
Central nervous system: Insomnia (14%), dizziness (13%), paresthesia (9%), depression (6%), peripheral neuritis (2%), neuropathy (1%)
Dermatologic: Herpes simplex (2%), acne (2%)
Gastrointestinal: Nausea and vomiting (8%)
Genitourinary: Urinary tract infection (5%)
Hematologic: Anemia (4%), leukopenia (3%)
Neuromuscular & skeletal: Bone pain (7%), arthralgia (6%)
Respiratory: Sinusitis (9%)
Miscellaneous: Flu syndrome (10%), accidental injury (6%), allergic reaction (3%)
<1%: Vascular thrombosis, pericardia effusion, cardiac arrest, hypotension, hemorrhage, shock, arrhythmia, syncope, cellulitis, hypothyroidism, gastroenteritis, hematemesis, (Continued)

## Trastuzumab *(Continued)*

ileus, intestinal obstruction, colitis, esophageal ulcer, stomatitis, pancreatitis, pancytopenia, acute leukemia, coagulopathy, lymphangitis, ascites, hydrocephalus, hepatic failure, hepatitis, amblyopia, deafness, anaphylactoid reaction, radiation injury

**Drug Interactions** Increased effect: Paclitaxel may result in a decrease in clearance of trastuzumab, increasing serum concentrations

**Half-Life** Mean: 5.8 days (range: 1-32 days)

**Special PA Issues**

**Patient Education:** This medication can only be administered by infusion. Report immediately any adverse reactions during infusion (eg, chills, fever, headache, backache, or nausea/vomiting) so appropriate medication can be administered. You will be susceptible to infection (avoid crowds or exposure to persons with infections or contagious diseases). You may experience dizziness or weakness (use caution when driving or engaging in hazardous activities); nausea or vomiting (small frequent meals, frequent mouth care, or sucking lozenges may help); diarrhea (boiled milk, yogurt, or buttermilk may help); or headache, back or joint pain (mild analgesics may offer relief). Report persistent gastrointestinal effects; sore throat, runny nose, or difficulty breathing; chest pain, irregular heartbeat, palpitations, swelling of extremities, or unusual weight gain; muscle or joint weakness, numbness, or pain; skin rash or irritation; itching or pain on urination; unhealed sores, white plaques in mouth or genital area, unusual bruising or bleeding; or other unusual effects related to this medication.

**Monitoring Parameters:** Signs and symptoms of cardiac dysfunction

♦ **Trasylol®** *see* Aprotinin *on page 76*

## Trazodone *(TRAZ oh done)*

**Pharmacologic Class** Antidepressant, Serotonin Reuptake Inhibitor/Antagonist

**U.S. Brand Names** Desyrel®

**Mechanism of Action** Inhibits reuptake of serotonin and norepinephrine by the presynaptic neuronal membrane and desensitization of adenyl cyclase, down regulation of beta-adrenergic receptors, and down regulation of serotonin receptors

**Use** Treatment of depression

**USUAL DOSAGE** Oral: Therapeutic effects may take up to 4 weeks to occur; therapy is normally maintained for several months after optimum response is reached to prevent recurrence of depression

Children 6-18 years: Initial: 1.5-2 mg/kg/day in divided doses; increase gradually every 3-4 days as needed; maximum: 6 mg/kg/day in 3 divided doses

Adolescents: Initial: 25-50 mg/day; increase to 100-150 mg/day in divided doses

Adults: Initial: 150 mg/day in 3 divided doses (may increase by 50 mg/day every 3-7 days); maximum: 600 mg/day

Elderly: 25-50 mg at bedtime with 25-50 mg/day dose increase every 3 days for inpatients and weekly for outpatients, if tolerated; usual dose: 75-150 mg/day

**Dosage Forms** Tab, as hydrochloride: 50 mg, 100 mg, 150 mg, 300 mg

**Contraindications** Hypersensitivity to trazodone or any component

**Warnings/Precautions** Safety and efficacy in children <18 years of age have not been established; monitor closely and use with extreme caution in patients with cardiac disease or arrhythmias. Very sedating, but little anticholinergic effects; therapeutic effects may take up to 4 weeks to occur; therapy is normally maintained for several months after optimum response is reached to prevent recurrence of depression.

**Pregnancy Risk Factor** C

**Adverse Reactions**

>10%:

Central nervous system: Dizziness, headache, confusion

Gastrointestinal: Nausea, bad taste in mouth, xerostomia

Neuromuscular & skeletal: Muscle tremors

1% to 10%:

Gastrointestinal: Diarrhea, constipation

Neuromuscular & skeletal: Weakness

Ocular: Blurred vision

<1%: Hypotension, tachycardia, bradycardia, agitation, seizures, extrapyramidal reactions, rash, prolonged priapism, urinary retention, hepatitis

**Drug Interactions** CYP2D6 and 3A3/4 enzyme substrate

Decreased effect: Clonidine, methyldopa, anticoagulants

Increased toxicity: Fluoxetine; increased effect/toxicity of phenytoin, CNS depressants, MAO inhibitors; digoxin serum levels increase

**Onset** Therapeutic effects take 1-3 weeks to appear

**Half-Life** 4-7.5 hours, 2 compartment kinetics

**Special PA Issues**

**Patient Education:** Take exactly as directed (do not increase dose or frequency); may take 2-4 weeks to achieve desired results; may cause physical and/or psychological dependence. Take after meals. Avoid excessive alcohol, caffeine, and other prescription or OTC medications not approved by prescriber. Maintain adequate hydration (2-3 L/day of fluids unless instructed to restrict fluid intake). You may experience drowsiness, light-headedness, dizziness (use caution when driving or engaging in hazardous tasks until response to medication is known); postural hypotension (use caution when climbing stairs or changing position from lying or sitting to standing); nausea, dry mouth (small frequent meals, frequent mouth care, or sucking lozenges may help); constipation (increased exercise, fluids, or dietary fruit and fiber may help); or diarrhea (buttermilk, yogurt, or boiled milk may help). Report persistent dizziness or headache; muscle cramping, tremors, or altered gait; blurred vision or eye pain; chest pain or irregular heartbeat; or worsening of condition.

**Dietary Considerations:** Alcohol: Avoid use

**Reference Range: Plasma levels do not always correlate with clinical effectiveness**
Therapeutic: 0.5-2.5 µg/mL
Potentially toxic: >2.5 µg/mL
Toxic: >4 µg/mL

**Related Information**
Antidepressant Agents *on page 998*

♦ **Trazodone Hydrochloride** *see* Trazodone *on previous page*
♦ **Treatment of Sexually Transmitted Diseases** *see* Chart *on page 1145*
♦ **Trecator®-SC** *see* Ethionamide *on page 352*
♦ **Tremytoine®** *see* Phenytoin *on page 721*
♦ **Trendar® [OTC]** *see* Ibuprofen *on page 466*
♦ **Trental®** *see* Pentoxifylline *on page 709*

# Tretinoin, Oral (TRET i noyn, oral)

**Pharmacologic Class** Antineoplastic Agent, Miscellaneous

**U.S. Brand Names** Vesanoid®

**Mechanism of Action** Retinoid that induces maturation of acute promyelocytic leukemia (APL) cells in cultures; induces cytodifferentiation and decreased proliferation of APL cells

**Use** Acute promyelocytic leukemia (APL): Induction of remission in patients with APL, French American British (FAB) classification M3 (including the M3 variant), characterized by the presence of the t(15;17) translocation or the presence of the PML/RARα gene who are refractory to or who have relapsed from anthracycline chemotherapy, or for whom anthra-cycline-based chemotherapy is contraindicated. Tretinoin is for the induction of remission only. All patients should receive an accepted form of remission consolidation or mainte-nance therapy for APL after completion of induction therapy with tretinoin.

**USUAL DOSAGE** Oral:
Children: There are limited clinical data on the pediatric use of tretinoin. Of 15 pediatric patients (age range: 1-16 years) treated with tretinoin, the incidence of complete remis-sion was 67%. Safety and efficacy in pediatric patients <1 year of age have not been established. Some pediatric patients experience severe headache and pseudotumor cerebri, requiring analgesic treatment and lumbar puncture for relief. Increased caution is recommended. Consider dose reduction in children experiencing serious or intolerable toxicity; however, the efficacy and safety of tretinoin at doses <45 mg/m$^2$/day have not been evaluated.

Adults: 45 mg/m$^2$/day administered as two evenly divided doses until complete remission is documented. Discontinue therapy 30 days after achievement of complete remission or after 90 days of treatment, whichever occurs first. If after initiation of treatment the presence of the t(15;17) translocation is not confirmed by cytogenetics or by polymerase chain reaction studies and the patient has not responded to tretinoin, consider alternative therapy.

Note: Tretinoin is for the induction of remission only. Optimal consolidation or maintenance regimens have not been determined. All patients should therefore receive a standard consolidation or maintenance chemotherapy regimen for APL after induction therapy with tretinoin unless otherwise contraindicated.

**Dosage Forms Cap:** 10 mg

**Contraindications** Sensitivity to parabens, vitamin A, or other retinoids

**Warnings/Precautions** Patients with acute promyelocytic leukemia (APL) are at high risk and can have severe adverse reactions to tretinoin. Administer under the supervision of a physician who is experienced in the management of patients with acute leukemia and in a facility with laboratory and supportive services sufficient to monitor drug tolerance and to protect and maintain a patient compromised by drug toxicity, including respiratory compro-mise.

About 25% of patients with APL, who have been treated with tretinoin, have experienced a syndrome called the retinoic acid-APL (RA-APL) syndrome which is characterized by fever, dyspnea, weight gain, radiographic pulmonary infiltrates and pleural or pericardial effusions. This syndrome has occasionally been accompanied by impaired myocardial contractility and episodic hypotension. It has been observed with or without concomitant leukocytosis. Endotracheal intubation and mechanical ventilation have been required in some cases due to progressive hypoxemia, and several patients have expired with multiorgan failure. The
(Continued)

# Tretinoin, Oral *(Continued)*

syndrome usually occurs during the first month of treatment, with some cases reported following the first dose.

Management of the syndrome has not been defined, but high-dose steroids given at the first suspicion of RA-APL syndrome appear to reduce morbidity and mortality. At the first signs suggestive of the syndrome, immediately initiate high-dose steroids (dexamethasone 10 mg I.V.) every 12 hours for 3 days or until resolution of symptoms, regardless of the leukocyte count. The majority of patients do not require termination of tretinoin therapy during treatment of the RA-APL syndrome.

During treatment, ~40% of patients will develop rapidly evolving leukocytosis. Rapidly evolving leukocytosis is associated with a higher risk of life-threatening complications.

If signs and symptoms of the RA-APL syndrome are present together with leukocytosis, initiate treatment with high-dose steroids immediately. Consider adding full-dose chemotherapy (including an anthracycline, if not contraindicated) to the tretinoin therapy on day 1 or 2 for patients presenting with a WBC count of >5 x $10^9$/L or immediately, for patients presenting with a WBC count of <5 x $10^9$/L, if the WBC count reaches ≥6 x $10^9$/L by day 5, or ≥10 x $10^9$/L by day 10 or ≥15 x $10^9$/L by day 28.

**Not to be used in women of childbearing potential** unless the woman is capable of complying with effective contraceptive measures; therapy is normally begun on the second or third day of next normal menstrual period; two reliable methods of effective contraception must be used during therapy and for 1 month after discontinuation of therapy, unless abstinence is the chosen method. Within one week prior to the institution of tretinoin therapy, the patient should have blood or urine collected for a serum or urine pregnancy test with a sensitivity of at least 50 mIU/L. When possible, delay tretinoin therapy until a negative result from this test is obtained. When a delay is not possible, place the patient on two reliable forms of contraception. Repeat pregnancy testing and contraception counseling monthly throughout the period of treatment.

Initiation of therapy with tretinoin may be based on the morphological diagnosis of APL. Confirm the diagnosis of APL by detection of the t(15;17) genetic marker by cytogenetic studies. If these are negative, PML/RARα fusion should be sought using molecular diagnostic techniques. The response rate of other AML subtypes to tretinoin has not been demonstrated.

Retinoids have been associated with pseudotumor cerebri (benign intracranial hypertension), especially in children. Early signs and symptoms include papilledema, headache, nausea, vomiting and visual disturbances.

Up to 60% of patients experienced hypercholesterolemia or hypertriglyceridemia, which were reversible upon completion of treatment.

Elevated liver function test results occur in 50% to 60% of patients during treatment. Carefully monitor liver function test results during treatment and give consideration to a temporary withdrawal of tretinoin if test results reach >5 times the upper limit of normal.

**Pregnancy Risk Factor** D

**Adverse Reactions** Virtually all patients experience some drug-related toxicity, especially headache, fever, weakness and fatigue. These adverse effects are seldom permanent or irreversible nor do they usually require therapy interruption

>10%:

- Cardiovascular: Arrhythmias, flushing, hypotension, hypertension, peripheral edema, chest discomfort, edema
- Central nervous system: Dizziness, anxiety, insomnia, depression, confusion, malaise, pain
- Dermatologic: Burning, redness, cheilitis, inflammation of lips, dry skin, pruritus, photosensitivity
- Endocrine & metabolic: Increased serum concentration of triglycerides
- Gastrointestinal: GI hemorrhage, abdominal pain, other GI disorders, diarrhea, constipation, dyspepsia, abdominal distention, weight gain or loss, anorexia, xerostomia
- Hematologic: Hemorrhage, disseminated intravascular coagulation
- Local: Phlebitis, injection site reactions
- Neuromuscular & skeletal: Bone pain, arthralgia, myalgia, paresthesia
- Ocular: Itching of eye
- Renal: Renal insufficiency
- Respiratory: Upper respiratory tract disorders, dyspnea, respiratory insufficiency, pleural effusion, pneumonia, rales, expiratory wheezing, dry nose
- Miscellaneous: Infections, shivering

1% to 10%:

- Cardiovascular: Cardiac failure, cardiac arrest, myocardial infarction, enlarged heart, heart murmur, ischemia, stroke, myocarditis, pericarditis, pulmonary hypertension, secondary cardiomyopathy, cerebral hemorrhage, pallor
- Central nervous system: Intracranial hypertension, agitation, hallucination, agnosia, aphasia, cerebellar edema, cerebellar disorders, convulsions, coma, CNS depression,

encephalopathy, hypotaxia, no light reflex, neurologic reaction, spinal cord disorder, unconsciousness, dementia, forgetfulness, somnolence, slow speech, hypothermia

Dermatologic: Skin peeling on hands or soles of feet, rash, cellulitis

Endocrine & metabolic: Fluid imbalance, acidosis

Gastrointestinal: Hepatosplenomegaly, ulcer, unspecified liver disorder

Genitourinary: Dysuria, polyuria, enlarged prostate

Hepatic: Ascites, hepatitis

Neuromuscular & skeletal: Tremor, leg weakness, hyporeflexia, dysarthria, facial paralysis, hemiplegia, flank pain, asterixis, abnormal gait

Ocular: Dry eyes, photophobia

Renal: Acute renal failure, renal tubular necrosis

Respiratory: Lower respiratory tract disorders, pulmonary infiltration, bronchial asthma, pulmonary/larynx edema, unspecified pulmonary disease

Miscellaneous: Face edema, lymph disorders

<1%: Mood changes, pseudomotor cerebri, alopecia, pruritus, hyperuricemia, xerostomia, anorexia, nausea, vomiting, inflammatory bowel syndrome, bleeding of gums, increase in erythrocyte sedimentation rate, decrease in hemoglobin and hematocrit, hepatitis, conjunctivitis, corneal opacities, optic neuritis, cataracts

**Drug Interactions** CYP3A3/4 enzyme substrate

Metabolized by the hepatic cytochrome P-450 system; therefore, all drugs that induce or inhibit this system would be expected to interact with tretinoin CYP2C9 substrate

Increased toxicity: Ketoconazole increases the mean plasma AUC of tretinoin

**Half-Life** Parent drug: 0.5-2 hours

**Special PA Issues**

**Patient Education:** Take with food. Do not crush, chew, or dissolve capsules. You will need frequent blood tests while taking this medication. Maintain adequate hydration (2-3 L/day of fluids unless instructed to restrict fluid intake), avoid alcohol and foods containing vitamin A, and foods with high fat content. You may experience lethargy, dizziness, visual changes, confusion, anxiety (avoid driving or engaging in hazardous tasks). For nausea and vomiting, loss of appetite, or dry mouth small, frequent meals, chewing gum, or sucking on lozenges may help. You may experience photosensitivity (avoid direct sunlight, wear protective clothing, or use sunblock). You may experience dry, itchy, skin, and dry or irritated eyes (avoid contact lenses). Report persistent vomiting or diarrhea, difficulty breathing, unusual bleeding or bruising, acute GI pain, bone pain, or vision changes immediately.

**Dietary Considerations:** Absorption of retinoids has been shown to be enhanced when taken with food

**Monitoring Parameters:** Monitor the patient's hematologic profile, coagulation profile, liver function test results and triglyceride and cholesterol levels frequently

# Tretinoin, Topical (TRET i noyn, TOP i kal)

**Pharmacologic Class** Retinoic Acid Derivative

**U.S. Brand Names** Avita®; Renova™; Retin-A™ Micro Topical; Retin-A™ Topical

**Mechanism of Action** Keratinocytes in the sebaceous follicle become less adherent which allows for easy removal; inhibits microcomedone formation and eliminates lesions already present

**Use** Treatment of acne vulgaris, photodamaged skin, and some skin cancers

**USUAL DOSAGE** Children >12 years and Adults: Topical: Begin therapy with a weaker formulation of tretinoin (0.025% cream or 0.01% gel) and increase the concentration as tolerated; apply once daily before retiring or on alternate days; if stinging or irritation develop, decrease frequency of application

**Dosage Forms Crm:** Retin-A™: 0.025% (20 g, 45 g), 0.05% (20 g, 45 g), 0.1% (20 g, 45 g), Avita®: 0.025% (20 g, 45 g); **Gel, top:** Retin-A™: 0.01% (15 g, 45 g), 0.025% (15 g, 45 g), Retin-A™ Micro: 0.1% (20 g, 45 g); **Liq, top (Retin-A™):** 0.05% (28 mL)

**Contraindications** Hypersensitivity to tretinoin or any component; sunburn

**Warnings/Precautions** Use with caution in patients with eczema; avoid excessive exposure to sunlight and sunlamps; avoid contact with abraded skin, mucous membranes, eyes, mouth, angles of the nose

**Pregnancy Risk Factor** C

**Pregnancy Implications** Clinical effects on the fetus: Oral tretinoin is teratogenic and fetotoxic in rats at doses 1000 and 500 times the topical human dose, respectively; however, tretinoin does not appear to be teratogenic when used topically since it is rapidly metabolized by the skin

**Adverse Reactions** 1% to 10%:

Cardiovascular: Edema

Dermatologic: Excessive dryness, erythema, scaling of the skin, hyperpigmentation or hypopigmentation, photosensitivity, initial acne flare-up

Local: Stinging, blistering

**Drug Interactions** CYP3A3/4 enzyme substrate

Increased toxicity: Sulfur, benzoyl peroxide, salicylic acid, resorcinol (potentiates adverse reactions seen with tretinoin)

(Continued)

## Tretinoin, Topical *(Continued)*

### Special PA Issues

**Patient Education:** For once a day use, do not overuse. Avoid increased intake of vitamin A. Thoroughly wash hands before applying. Wash area to be treated at least 30 minutes before applying. Do not wash face more frequently than 2-3 times a day. Avoid using topical preparations that contain alcohol or harsh chemicals during treatment. You may experience increased sensitivity to sunlight; protect skin with sunblock, wear protective clothing, or avoid direct sunlight. Stop treatment and inform prescriber if rash, skin irritation, redness, scaling, or excessive dryness occurs.

♦ **Triacet**™ *see* Triamcinolone *on this page*

♦ **Triacin-C**® *see* Triprolidine, Pseudoephedrine, and Codeine *on page 941*

♦ **Triaconazole** *see* Terconazole *on page 880*

♦ **Triadapin**® *see* Doxepin *on page 304*

♦ **Triam-A**® *see* Triamcinolone *on this page*

## Triamcinolone (trye am SIN oh lone)

**Pharmacologic Class** Corticosteroid, Adrenal; Corticosteroid, Oral Inhaler; Corticosteroid, Nasal; Corticosteroid, Parenteral

**U.S. Brand Names** Amcort®; Aristocort®; Aristocort® A; Aristocort® Forte; Aristocort® Intralesional; Aristospan® Intra-Articular; Aristospan® Intralesional; Atolone®; Azmacort™; Delta-Tritex®; Flutex®; Kenacort®; Kenaject-40®; Kenalog®; Kenalog-10®; Kenalog-40®; Kenalog® H; Kenalog® in Orabase®; Kenonel®; Nasacort®; Nasacort® AQ; Tac™-3; Tac™-40; Triacet™; Triam-A®; Triam Forte®; Triderm®; Tri-Kort®; Trilog®; Trilone®; Tristoject®

**Mechanism of Action** Decreases inflammation by suppression of migration of polymorphonuclear leukocytes and reversal of increased capillary permeability; suppresses the immune system by reducing activity and volume of the lymphatic system; suppresses adrenal function at high doses

### Use

Inhalation: Control of bronchial asthma and related bronchospastic conditions.

Systemic: Adrenocortical insufficiency, rheumatic disorders, allergic states, respiratory diseases, systemic lupus erythematosus, and other diseases requiring anti-inflammatory or immunosuppressive effects

Topical: Inflammatory dermatoses responsive to steroids

**USUAL DOSAGE** In general, single I.M. dose of 4-7 times oral dose will control patient from 4-7 days up to 3-4 weeks

Children 6-12 years:

Oral inhalation: 1-2 inhalations 3-4 times/day, not to exceed 12 inhalations/day

I.M. (acetonide or hexacetonide): 0.03-0.2 mg/kg at 1- to 7-day intervals

Intra-articular, intrabursal, or tendon-sheath injection: 2.5-15 mg, repeated as needed

Children >12 years and Adults:

Intranasal: 2 sprays in each nostril once daily; may increase after 4-7 days up to 4 sprays once daily or 1 spray 4 times/day in each nostril

Topical: Apply a thin film 2-3 times/day

Oral: 4-48 mg/day

I.M. (acetonide or hexacetonide): 60 mg (of 40 mg/mL), additional 20-100 mg doses (usual: 40-80 mg) may be given when signs and symptoms recur, best at 6-week intervals to minimize HPA suppression

Intra-articular (hexacetonide): 2-20 mg every 3-4 weeks

Intralesional (diacetate or acetonide - use 10 mg/mL): 1 mg/injection site, may be repeated one or more times/week depending upon patient's response; maximum: 30 mg at any one time; may use multiple injections if they are more than 1 cm apart

Intra-articular, intrasynovial, and soft-tissue (diacetate or acetonide - use 10 mg/mL or 40 mg/mL) 2.5-40 mg depending upon location, size of joints, and degree of inflammation; repeat when signs and symptoms recur

### Triamcinolone Dosing

| | Acetonide | Diacetate | Hexacetonide |
|---|---|---|---|
| Intrasynovial | 2.5-40 mg | 5-40 mg | |
| Intralesional | 2.5-40 mg | 5-48 mg | Up to 0.5 mg/sq inch affected area |
| Sublesional | 1-30 mg | | |
| Systemic I.M. | 2.5-60 mg/d | ~40 mg/wk | 20-100 mg |
| Intra-articular | | 5-40 mg | 2-20 mg average |
| large joints | 5-15 mg | | 10-20 mg |
| small joints | 2.5-5 mg | | 2-6 mg |
| Tendon sheaths | 10-40 mg | | |
| Intradermal | 1 mg/site | | |

Sublesionally (as acetonide): Up to 1 mg per injection site and may be repeated one or more times weekly; multiple sites may be injected if they are 1 cm or more apart, not to exceed 30 mg

See table.

Oral inhalation: 2 inhalations 3-4 times/day, not to exceed 16 inhalations/day

**Dosage Forms Aero: Oral inh:** 100 mcg/metered spray (2 oz); **Nasal:** 55 mcg per actuation (15 mL); **Oint, oral:** 0.1% (5 g); **Syr:** 2 mg/5 mL (120 mL), 4 mg/5 mL (120 mL); **Tab:** 1 mg, 2 mg, 4 mg, 8 mg

Triamcinolone acetonide: **Aero, top:** 0.2 mg/2 second spray (23 g, 63 g); **Crm:** 0.025% (15 g, 60 g, 80 g, 240 g, 454 g), 0.1% (15 g, 30 g, 60 g, 80 g, 90 g, 120 g, 240 g), 0.5% (15 g, 20 g, 30 g, 240 g); **Inj:** 10 mg/mL (5 mL); 40 mg/mL (1 mL, 5 mL, 10 mL); **Lot:** 0.025% (60 mL), 0.1% (15 mL, 60 mL); **Oint, top:** 0.025% (15 g, 30 g, 60 g, 80 g, 120 g, 454 g), 0.1% (15 g, 30 g, 60 g, 80 g, 120 g, 240 g, 454 g), 0.5% (15 g, 20 g, 30 g, 240 g); **Spray, nasal:** 55 mcg per actuation in aqueous base (16.5 g)

Triamcinolone diacetate: **Inj:** 25 mg/mL (5 mL), 40 mg/mL (1 mL, 5 mL, 10 mL)

Triamcinolone hexacetonide: **Inj:** 5 mg/mL (5 mL), 20 mg/mL (1 mL, 5 mL)

**Contraindications** Known hypersensitivity to triamcinolone; systemic fungal infections; serious infections (except septic shock or tuberculous meningitis); primary treatment of status asthmaticus

**Warnings/Precautions** Fatalities have occurred due to adrenal insufficiency in asthmatic patients during and after transfer from systemic corticosteroids to aerosol steroids; several months may be required for recovery from this syndrome; during this period, aerosol steroids do **not** provide the increased systemic steroid requirement needed to treat patients having trauma, surgery or infections; avoid using higher than recommended dose

Use with caution in patients with hypothyroidism, cirrhosis, nonspecific ulcerative colitis and patients at increased risk for peptic ulcer disease; do not use occlusive dressings on weeping or exudative lesions and general caution with occlusive dressings should be observed; discontinue if skin irritation or contact dermatitis should occur; do not use in patients with decreased skin circulation; avoid the use of high potency steroids on the face

Because of the risk of adverse effects, systemic corticosteroids should be used cautiously in the elderly, in the smallest possible dose, and for the shortest possible time. Azmacort™ (metered dose inhaler) comes with its own spacer device attached and may be easier to use in older patients. Controlled clinical studies have shown that inhaled and intranasal corticosteroids may cause a reduction in growth velocity in pediatric patients. Growth velocity provides a means of comparing the rate of growth among children of the same age.

In studies involving inhaled corticosteroids, the average reduction in growth velocity was approximately 1 cm (about 1/3 of an inch) per year. It appears that the reduction is related to dose and how long the child takes the drug.

FDA's Pulmonary and Allergy Drugs and Metabolic and Endocrine Drugs advisory committees discussed this issue at a July 1998 meeting. They recommended that the agency develop class-wide labeling to inform healthcare providers so they would understand this potential side effect and monitor growth routinely in pediatric patients who are treated with inhaled corticosteroids, intranasal corticosteroids or both.

Long-term effects of this reduction in growth velocity on final adult height are unknown. Likewise, it also has not yet been determined whether patients' growth will "catch up" if treatment in discontinued. Drug manufacturers will continue to monitor these drugs to learn more about long-term effects. Children are prescribed inhaled corticosteroids to treat asthma. Intranasal corticosteroids are generally used to prevent and treat allergy-related nasal symptoms.

Patients are advised not to stop using their inhaled or intranasal corticosteroids without first speaking to their healthcare providers about the benefits of these drugs compared to their risks.

**Pregnancy Risk Factor** C

**Pregnancy Implications**

Clinical effects on the fetus: No data on crossing the placenta or effect on fetus

Breast-feeding/lactation: No data on crossing into breast milk or clinical effects on the infant

**Adverse Reactions**

>10%:

Central nervous system: Insomnia, nervousness

Gastrointestinal: Increased appetite, indigestion

1% to 10%:

Ocular: Cataracts

Endocrine & metabolic: Diabetes mellitus hirsutism

Neuromuscular & skeletal: Arthralgia

Respiratory: Epistaxis

<1%: Fatigue, seizures, mood swings, headache, delirium, hallucinations, euphoria, itching, hypertrichosis, skin atrophy, hyperpigmentation, hypopigmentation, acne, bruising, amenorrhea, sodium and water retention, Cushing's syndrome, hyperglycemia, bone growth suppression, oral candidiasis, dry throat, xerostomia, peptic ulcer, abdominal distention, (Continued)

# Triamcinolone *(Continued)*

ulcerative esophagitis, pancreatitis, burning, osteoporosis, muscle wasting, hoarseness, wheezing, cough, hypersensitivity reactions

**Drug Interactions**

Decreased effect: Barbiturates, phenytoin, rifampin ↑ metabolism of triamcinolone; vaccine and toxoid effects may be reduced

Increased toxicity: Salicylates may increase risk of GI ulceration

**Duration** Oral: 8-12 hours

**Half-Life** Biologic: 18-36 hours

**Special PA Issues**

**Patient Education:** Take exactly as directed; do not increase dose or discontinue abruptly without consulting prescriber. Take oral medication with or after meals. Limit intake of caffeine or stimulants. Prescriber may recommend increased dietary vitamins, minerals, or iron. Diabetics should monitor glucose levels closely (antidiabetic medication may need to be adjusted). Inform prescriber if you are experiencing greater than normal levels of stress (medication may need adjustment). Some forms of this medication may cause GI upset (oral medication may be taken with meals to reduce GI upset; small frequent meals and frequent mouth care may reduce GI upset). You may be more susceptible to infection (avoid crowds and persons with contagious or infective conditions). Report promptly excessive nervousness or sleep disturbances; any signs of infection (sore throat, unhealed injuries); excessive growth of body hair or loss of skin color; changes in vision; excessive or sudden weight gain (>3 lb/week); swelling of face or extremities; difficulty breathing; muscle weakness; change in color of stools (tarry) or persistent abdominal pain; or worsening of condition or failure to improve.

Topical: For external use only. Not for eyes or mucous membranes or open wounds. Apply in very thin layer to occlusive dressing. Apply dressing to area being treated. Avoid prolonged or excessive use around sensitive tissues, genital, or rectal areas. Inform prescriber if condition worsens (swelling, redness, irritation, pain, open sores) or fails to improve.

Aerosol: Not for use during acute asthmatic attack. Follow directions that accompany product. Rinse mouth and throat after use to prevent candidiasis. Do not use intranasal product if you have a nasal infection, nasal injury, or recent nasal surgery. If using two products, consult prescriber in which order to use the two products. Inform prescriber if condition worsens or does not improve.

**Related Information**

Corticosteroids *on page 1007*
Asthma Therapy Guidelines *on page 1049*

# Triamterene *(trye AM ter een)*

**Pharmacologic Class** Diuretic, Potassium Sparing

**U.S. Brand Names** Dyrenium®

**Mechanism of Action** Interferes with potassium/sodium exchange (active transport) in the distal tubule, cortical collecting tubule and collecting duct by inhibiting sodium, potassium-ATPase; decreases calcium excretion; increases magnesium loss

**Use** Alone or in combination with other diuretics to treat edema and hypertension; decreases potassium excretion caused by kaliuretic diuretics

**USUAL DOSAGE** Adults: Oral: 100-300 mg/day in 1-2 divided doses; maximum dose: 300 mg/day

**Dosing comments in renal impairment:** $Cl_{cr}$ <10 mL/minute: Avoid use

**Dosing adjustment in hepatic impairment:** Dose reduction is recommended in patients with cirrhosis

**Dosage Forms Cap:** 50 mg, 100 mg

**Contraindications** Hyperkalemia, renal impairment, diabetes, hypersensitivity to triamterene or any component; do not administer to patients receiving spironolactone, amiloride, or potassium supplementation unless the patient has documented evidence of hypokalemia unresponsive to either agent alone

**Warnings/Precautions** Use with caution in patients with severe hepatic encephalopathy, patients with diabetes, renal dysfunction, a history of renal stones, or those receiving potassium supplements, potassium-containing medications, blood or ACE inhibitors

**Pregnancy Risk Factor** B

**Pregnancy Implications**

Clinical effects on the fetus: No data available. Generally, use of diuretics during pregnancy is avoided due to risk of decreased placental perfusion.

Breast-feeding/lactation: No data available

**Adverse Reactions**

1% to 10%:

Cardiovascular: Hypotension, edema, congestive heart failure, bradycardia

Central nervous system: Dizziness, headache, fatigue

Dermatologic: Rash

Gastrointestinal: Constipation, nausea

Respiratory: Dyspnea

<1%: Flushing, hyperkalemia, dehydration, hyponatremia, gynecomastia, hyperchloremic metabolic acidosis, postmenopausal bleeding, inability to achieve or maintain an erection

**Drug Interactions**

Increased risk of hyperkalemia if given together with amiloride, spironolactone, angiotensin-converting enzyme (ACE) inhibitors; use of indomethacin may result in renal failure; avoid concurrent use if possible; cimetidine may increase bioavailability and decrease clearance of triamterene

Increased toxicity of amantadine (possibly by decreasing its renal excretion)

**Onset** Diuresis occurs within 2-4 hours

**Duration** 7-9 hours

**Special PA Issues**

**Patient Education:** Take as directed, preferably after meals. This diuretic does not cause potassium loss; avoid excessive potassium intake (eg, salt substitutes, low-salt foods, bananas, nuts). Weigh yourself daily at the same time, in the same clothes, and report weight loss greater than 5 lb/week. Urine may appear blue (normal). You may experience dizziness, drowsiness, headache (use caution when driving or engaging in tasks that require alertness); nausea (small frequent meals, frequent mouth care, or sucking on lozenges may help); decreased sexual ability (reversible with discontinuing of medication); or postural hypotension (change position slowly when rising from sitting or lying). Report persistent fatigue, muscle weakness, paresthesia, confusion, anorexia, headaches, lethargy, hyper-reflexia, seizures, swelling of extremities or respiratory difficulty (eg, chest pain, rapid heartbeat or palpitations).

**Monitoring Parameters:** Blood pressure, serum electrolytes (especially potassium), renal function, weight, I & O

**Related Information**

Heart Failure: Management of Patients with Left Ventricular Systolic Dysfunction *on page 1064*

♦ **Triapin®** *see* Butalbital Compound *on page 131*

♦ **Triavil®** *see* Amitriptyline and Perphenazine *on page 59*

## Triazolam (trye AY zoe lam)

**Pharmacologic Class** Benzodiazepine

**U.S. Brand Names** Halcion®

**Mechanism of Action** Depresses all levels of the CNS, including the limbic and reticular formation, probably through the increased action of gamma-aminobutyric acid (GABA), which is a major inhibitory neurotransmitter in the brain

**Use** Short-term treatment of insomnia

**USUAL DOSAGE** Onset of action is rapid, patient should be in bed when taking medication

Oral:

Children <18 years: Dosage not established

Adults: 0.125-0.25 mg at bedtime

**Dosing adjustment/comments in hepatic impairment:** Reduce dose or avoid use in cirrhosis

**Dosage Forms Tab:** 0.125 mg, 0.25 mg

**Contraindications** Hypersensitivity to triazolam, or any component, cross-sensitivity with other benzodiazepines may occur; severe uncontrolled pain; pre-existing CNS depression; narrow-angle glaucoma; not to be used in pregnancy or lactation

**Warnings/Precautions** May cause drug dependency; avoid abrupt discontinuance in patients with prolonged therapy or seizure disorders; not considered a drug of choice in the elderly

**Pregnancy Risk Factor** X

**Adverse Reactions**

>10%:

Cardiovascular: Tachycardia, chest pain

Central nervous system: Drowsiness, fatigue, ataxia, lightheadedness, memory impairment, insomnia, anxiety, depression, headache

(Continued)

## Triazolam *(Continued)*

Dermatologic: Rash
Endocrine & metabolic: Decreased libido
Gastrointestinal: Xerostomia, decreased salivation, constipation, nausea, vomiting, diarrhea, increased or decreased appetite
Neuromuscular & skeletal: Dysarthria
Ocular: Blurred vision
Miscellaneous: Diaphoresis
1% to 10%:
Cardiovascular: Syncope, hypotension
Central nervous system: Confusion, nervousness, dizziness, akathisia
Dermatologic: Dermatitis
Gastrointestinal: Weight gain or loss, increased salivation, muscle cramps
Neuromuscular & skeletal: Rigidity, tremor
Otic: Tinnitus
Respiratory: Nasal congestion, hyperventilation
<1%: Menstrual irregularities, blood dyscrasias, reflex slowing, drug dependence

**Drug Interactions** CYP3A3/4 and 3A5-7 enzyme substrate

Decreased effect with phenytoin, phenobarbital
Increased effect/toxicity with CNS depressants, cimetidine, erythromycin, nefazodone

**Onset** Onset of hypnotic effect: Within 15-30 minutes

**Duration** 6-7 hours

**Half-Life** 1.7-5 hours

**Special PA Issues**

· **Patient Education:** Take exactly as directed (do not increase dose or frequency); may take 2-3 weeks to achieve desired results; may cause physical and/or psychological dependence. Do not use excessive alcohol or other prescription or OTC medications (especially pain medications, sedatives, antihistamines, or hypnotics) without consulting prescriber. Maintain adequate hydration (2-3 L/day of fluids unless instructed to restrict fluid intake). You may experience drowsiness, lightheadedness, impaired coordination, dizziness, or blurred vision (use caution when driving or engaging in hazardous tasks until response to medication is known); nausea, vomiting, or dry mouth (small frequent meals, good mouth care, chewing gum, or sucking lozenges may help); constipation (increased exercise, fluids, or dietary fruit and fiber may help); altered sexual drive or ability (reversible); or photosensitivity (use sunscreen, protective clothing, and avoid extended exposure to direct sunlight). Report persistent CNS effects (eg, memory impairment, confusion, depression, increased sedation, excitation, headache, agitation, insomnia or nightmares, dizziness, fatigue, impaired coordination, changes in personality, or changes in cognition); changes in urinary pattern; muscle cramping, weakness, tremors, or rigidity; ringing in ears or visual disturbances; chest pain, palpitations, or rapid heartbeat; excessive perspiration; excessive GI symptoms (cramping, constipation, vomiting, anorexia); or worsening of condition.

**Dietary Considerations:** Alcohol: Additive CNS effect, avoid use

**Monitoring Parameters:** Respiratory and cardiovascular status

♦ **Triban®** *see* Trimethobenzamide *on page 936*

♦ **Tribavirin** *see* Ribavirin *on page 801*

## Trichlormethiazide (trye klor meth EYE a zide)

**Pharmacologic Class** Diuretic, Thiazide

**U.S. Brand Names** Metahydrin®; Naqua®

**Mechanism of Action** The diuretic mechanism of action of the thiazides is primarily inhibition of sodium, chloride, and water reabsorption in the renal distal tubules, thereby producing diuresis with a resultant reduction in plasma volume. The antihypertensive mechanism of action of the thiazides is unknown. It is known that doses of thiazides produce greater reduction in blood pressure than equivalent diuretic doses of loop diuretics. There has been speculation that the thiazides may have some influence on vascular tone mediated through sodium depletion, but this remains to be proven.

**Use** Management of mild to moderate hypertension; treatment of edema in congestive heart failure and nephrotic syndrome

**USUAL DOSAGE** Adults: Oral: 1-4 mg/day; initially doses may be given twice daily
**Dosage adjustment in renal impairment:** Reduced dosage is necessary

**Dosage Forms Tab:** 2 mg, 4 mg

**Contraindications** Hypersensitivity to trichlormethiazide, other thiazides and sulfonamides, or any component

**Warnings/Precautions** Use with caution in renal disease, hepatic disease, gout, lupus erythematosus, diabetes mellitus; some products may contain tartrazine

**Pregnancy Risk Factor** D

**Adverse Reactions**
1% to 10%:
Endocrine & metabolic: Hypokalemia

Respiratory: Dyspnea (<5%)

<1%: Hypotension, photosensitivity, lichenoid dermatitis, fluid and electrolyte imbalances (hypocalcemia, hypomagnesemia, hyponatremia); hyperglycemia, rarely blood dyscrasias, prerenal azotemia

**Drug Interactions**
Decreased effect:
Thiazides may decrease the effect of anticoagulants, antigout agents, sulfonylureas
Bile acid sequestrants, methenamine, and NSAIDs may decrease the effect of the thiazides
Increased effect: Thiazides may increase the toxicity of allopurinol, anesthetics, antineoplastics, calcium salts, diazoxide, digitalis, lithium, loop diuretics, methyldopa, nondepolarizing muscle relaxants, vitamin D; amphotericin B and anticholinergics may increase the toxicity of thiazides

**Special PA Issues**
**Patient Education:** May be taken with food or milk; take early in day to avoid nocturia; take the last dose of multiple doses no later than 6 PM unless instructed otherwise. A few people who take this medication become more sensitive to sunlight and may experience skin rash, redness, itching, or severe sunburn, especially if sun block SPF ≥15 is not used on exposed skin areas.

- **Trichloroacetaldehyde Monohydrate** see Chloral Hydrate on page 186
- **TriCor™** see Fenofibrate on page 360
- **Tricosal®** see Choline Magnesium Trisalicylate on page 202
- **Tri-Cyclen®** see Ethinyl Estradiol and Norgestimate on page 350
- **Triderm®** see Triamcinolone on page 928
- **Tridesilon® Topical** see Desonide on page 262
- **Tridil® Injection** see Nitroglycerin on page 660

## Trientine (TRYE en teen)

**Pharmacologic Class** Chelating Agent

**U.S. Brand Names** Syprine®

**Mechanism of Action** Trientine hydrochloride is an oral chelating agent structurally dissimilar from penicillamine and other available chelating agents; an effective oral chelator of copper used to induce adequate cupriuresis

**Use** Treatment of Wilson's disease in patients intolerant to penicillamine

**USUAL DOSAGE** Oral (administer on an empty stomach):
Children <12 years: 500-750 mg/day in divided doses 2-4 times/day; maximum: 1.5 g/day
Adults: 750-1250 mg/day in divided doses 2-4 times/day; maximum dose: 2 g/day

**Dosage Forms Cap, as hydrochloride:** 250 mg

**Contraindications** Rheumatoid arthritis, biliary cirrhosis, cystinuria, known hypersensitivity to trientine

**Warnings/Precautions** May cause iron deficiency anemia; monitor closely; use with caution in patients with reactive airway disease

**Pregnancy Risk Factor** C

**Adverse Reactions** Percentage unknown: Malaise, iron deficiency, heartburn, epigastric pain, anemia, tenderness, thickening and fissuring of skin, muscle cramps, systemic lupus erythematosus (SLE)

**Drug Interactions** Decreased effect with iron and possibly other mineral supplements

**Special PA Issues**
**Patient Education:** Take 1 hour before or 2 hours after meals and at least 1 hour apart from any drug, food, or milk; do not chew capsule, swallow whole followed by a full glass of water; notify physician of any fever or skin changes; any skin exposed to the contents of a capsule should be promptly washed with water

- **Trientine Hydrochloride** see Trientine on this page

## Triethanolamine Polypeptide Oleate-Condensate

(trye eth a NOLE a meen pol i PEP tide OH lee ate-KON den sate)

**Pharmacologic Class** Otic Agent, Cerumenolytic

**U.S. Brand Names** Cerumenex® Otic

**Mechanism of Action** Emulsifies and disperses accumulated cerumen

**Use** Removal of ear wax (cerumen)

**USUAL DOSAGE** Children and Adults: Otic: Fill ear canal, insert cotton plug; allow to remain 15-30 minutes; flush ear with lukewarm water as a single treatment; if a second application is needed for unusually hard impactions, repeat the procedure

**Dosage Forms Soln, otic:** 6 mL, 12 mL

**Contraindications** Perforated tympanic membrane or otitis media, hypersensitivity to product or any component

**Warnings/Precautions** Avoid undue exposure to peridural skin during administration and the flushing out of ear canal; discontinue if sensitization or irritation occurs

**Pregnancy Risk Factor** C
(Continued)

## Triethanolamine Polypeptide Oleate-Condensate *(Continued)*

**Adverse Reactions** <1%: Mild erythema and pruritus, severe eczematoid reactions, localized dermatitis

**Onset** Produces slight disintegration of very hard ear wax by 24 hours.

**Special PA Issues**

**Patient Education:** For external use only. Warm container in hand or mildly warm water, lie on side with affected ear up, hold the ear lobe up and back, instill in ear without inserting dropper into ear, and remain in that position for 15-20 minutes. Flush ear with lukewarm water. If a second application is needed, repeat the procedure.

**Monitoring Parameters:** Evaluate hearing before and after instillation of medication

♦ **Trifed-C®** *see* Triprolidine, Pseudoephedrine, and Codeine *on page 941*

## Trifluoperazine *(trye floo oh PER a zeen)*

**Pharmacologic Class** Antipsychotic Agent, Phenothiazine, Piperazine

**U.S. Brand Names** Stelazine®

**Mechanism of Action** Blocks postsynaptic mesolimbic dopaminergic receptors in the brain; exhibits a strong alpha-adrenergic blocking effect and depresses the release of hypothalamic and hypophyseal hormones

**Use** Treatment of psychoses and management of nonpsychotic anxiety

**USUAL DOSAGE**

Children 6-12 years: Psychoses:

Oral: Hospitalized or well supervised patients: Initial: 1 mg 1-2 times/day, gradually increase until symptoms are controlled or adverse effects become troublesome; maximum: 15 mg/day

I.M.: 1 mg twice daily

Adults:

Psychoses:

Outpatients: Oral: 1-2 mg twice daily

Hospitalized or well supervised patients: Initial: 2-5 mg twice daily with optimum response in the 15-20 mg/day range; do not exceed 40 mg/day

I.M.: 1-2 mg every 4-6 hours as needed up to 10 mg/24 hours maximum

Nonpsychotic anxiety: Oral: 1-2 mg twice daily; maximum: 6 mg/day; therapy for anxiety should not exceed 12 weeks; do not exceed 6 mg/day for longer than 12 weeks when treating anxiety; agitation, jitteriness, or insomnia may be confused with original neurotic or psychotic symptoms

Hemodialysis: Not dialyzable (0% to 5%)

**Dosage Forms** Trifluoperazine hydrochloride: **Conc, oral:** 10 mg/mL (60 mL); **Inj:** 2 mg/mL (10 mL); **Tab:** 1 mg, 2 mg, 5 mg, 10 mg

**Contraindications** Hypersensitivity to trifluoperazine or any component, cross-sensitivity with other phenothiazines may exist, coma, circulatory collapse, history of blood dyscrasias

**Warnings/Precautions** Safety in children <6 months of age has not been established; use with caution in patients with cardiovascular disease, seizures, hepatic dysfunction, narrow-angle glaucoma, or bone marrow suppression; watch for hypotension when administering I.M. or I.V.; use with caution in patients with myasthenia gravis or Parkinson's disease

**Pregnancy Risk Factor** C

**Adverse Reactions**

>10%:

Cardiovascular: Hypotension, orthostatic hypotension

Central nervous system: Pseudoparkinsonism, akathisia, dystonias, tardive dyskinesia (persistent), dizziness

Gastrointestinal: Constipation

Ocular: Pigmentary retinopathy

Respiratory: Nasal congestion

Miscellaneous: Diaphoresis (decreased)

1% to 10%:

Genitourinary: Dysuria, ejaculatory disturbances

Dermatologic: Increased sensitivity to sun, rash

Endocrine & metabolic: Changes in menstrual cycle, changes in libido, breast pain

Gastrointestinal: Weight gain, nausea, vomiting, stomach pain

Neuromuscular & skeletal: Trembling of fingers

<1%: Neuroleptic malignant syndrome (NMS), impairment of temperature regulation, lowering of seizures threshold, discoloration of skin (blue-gray), galactorrhea, priapism, agranulocytosis, leukopenia, cholestatic jaundice, hepatotoxicity, cornea and lens changes

**Drug Interactions** CYP1A2 enzyme substrate

Decreased effect of anticonvulsants (increases requirements), guanethidine, anticoagulants; decreased effect with anticholinergics

Increased effect/toxicity with CNS depressants, metrizamide (increases seizures), propranolol, lithium (rare encephalopathy)

**Half-Life** >24 hours with chronic use

**Special PA Issues**

**Patient Education:** Use exactly as directed (do not increase dose or frequency); may cause physical and/or psychological dependence. Do not discontinue without consulting prescriber. Tablets/capsules may be taken with food. Mix oral solution with 2-4 oz of liquid (eg, juice, milk, water, pudding). Do not take within 2 hours of any antacid. Avoid excess alcohol or caffeine and other prescription or OTC medications not approved by prescriber. Maintain adequate hydration (2-3 L/day of fluids unless instructed to restrict fluid intake). Avoid skin contact with liquid medication; may cause contact dermatitis (wash immediately with warm, soapy water). You may experience excess drowsiness, lightheadedness, dizziness, or blurred vision (use caution driving or when engaging in hazardous tasks until response to medication is known); nausea or vomiting (small frequent meals, frequent mouth care, or sucking lozenges may help); constipation (increased exercise, fluids, or dietary fruit and fiber may help); postural hypotension (use caution climbing stairs or when changing position from lying or sitting to standing); urinary retention (void before taking medication); ejaculatory dysfunction (reversible); decreased perspiration (avoid strenuous exercise in hot environments); photosensitivity (use sunscreen, protective clothing, and avoid prolonged exposure to direct sunlight). Report persistent CNS effects (eg, trembling fingers, altered gait or balance, excessive sedation, seizures, unusual movements, anxiety, abnormal thoughts, confusion, personality changes); chest pain, palpitations, rapid heartbeat, severe dizziness; unresolved urinary retention or changes in urinary pattern; altered menstrual pattern, changes in libido, swelling or pain in breasts (male or female); vision changes; skin rash, irritation, or changes in color of skin (gray-blue); or worsening of condition.

**Reference Range:** Therapeutic response and blood levels have not been established

**Related Information**

Antipsychotic Agents *on page 1001*

♦ **Trifluoperazine Hydrochloride** *see* Trifluoperazine *on previous page*

♦ **Trifluorothymidine** *see* Trifluridine *on this page*

# Trifluridine (trye FLURE i deen)

**Pharmacologic Class** Antiviral Agent, Ophthalmic

**U.S. Brand Names** Viroptic® Ophthalmic

**Mechanism of Action** Interferes with viral replication by incorporating into viral DNA in place of thymidine, inhibiting thymidylate synthetase resulting in the formation of defective proteins

**Use** Treatment of primary keratoconjunctivitis and recurrent epithelial keratitis caused by herpes simplex virus types I and II

**USUAL DOSAGE** Adults: Instill 1 drop into affected eye every 2 hours while awake, to a maximum of 9 drops/day, until re-epithelialization of corneal ulcer occurs; then use 1 drop every 4 hours for another 7 days; do **not** exceed 21 days of treatment; if improvement has not taken place in 7-14 days, consider another form of therapy

**Dosage Forms** Soln, ophth: 1% (7.5 mL)

**Contraindications** Known hypersensitivity to trifluridine or any component

**Warnings/Precautions** Mild local irritation of conjunctival and cornea may occur when instilled but usually transient effects

**Pregnancy Risk Factor** C

**Adverse Reactions**

1% to 10%: Local: Burning, stinging

<1%: Hyperemia, palpebral edema, epithelial keratopathy, keratitis, stromal edema, increased intraocular pressure, hypersensitivity reactions

**Special PA Issues**

**Patient Education:** For ophthalmic use only. Store in refrigerator; do not use discolored solution. Apply prescribed amount as often as directed. Wash hands before using and do not let tip of applicator touch eye or contaminate tip of applicator. Tilt head back and look upward. Gently pull down lower lid and put drop(s) in inner corner of eye. Close eye and roll eyeball in all directions. Do not blink for ½ minute. Apply gentle pressure to inner corner of eye for 30 seconds. Wipe away excess from skin around eye. Do not use any other eye preparation for at least 10 minutes. Do not touch tip of applicator to eye or contaminate tip of applicator. Do not share medication with anyone else. May cause sensitivity to bright light (dark glasses may help); temporary stinging or blurred vision may occur. Inform prescriber if you experience eye pain, redness, burning, watering, dryness, double vision, puffiness around eye, vision disturbances, or other adverse eye response; worsening of condition or lack of improvement within 7-14 days.

♦ **Trihexy®** *see* Trihexyphenidyl *on this page*

♦ **Trihexyphen®** *see* Trihexyphenidyl *on this page*

# Trihexyphenidyl (trye heks ee FEN i dil)

**Pharmacologic Class** Anticholinergic Agent; Anti-Parkinson's Agent (Anticholinergic)

**U.S. Brand Names** Artane®; Trihexy®

**Mechanism of Action** Thought to act by blocking excess acetylcholine at cerebral synapses; many of its effects are due to its pharmacologic similarities with atropine

(Continued)

## Trihexyphenidyl *(Continued)*

**Use** Adjunctive treatment of Parkinson's disease; also used in treatment of drug-induced extrapyramidal effects and acute dystonic reactions

**USUAL DOSAGE** Adults: Oral: Initial: 1-2 mg/day, increase by 2 mg increments at intervals of 3-5 days; usual dose: 5-15 mg/day in 3-4 divided doses

**Dosage Forms** Trihexyphenidyl hydrochloride: **Cap, sustained release:** 5 mg; **Elix:** 2 mg/5 mL (480 mL); **Tab:** 2 mg, 5 mg

**Contraindications** Hypersensitivity to trihexyphenidyl or any component, patients with narrow-angle glaucoma; pyloric or duodenal obstruction, stenosing peptic ulcers; bladder neck obstructions; achalasia; myasthenia gravis

**Warnings/Precautions** Use with caution in hot weather or during exercise. Elderly patients require strict dosage regulation. Use with caution in patients with tachycardia, cardiac arrhythmias, hypertension, hypotension, prostatic hypertrophy or any tendency toward urinary retention, liver or kidney disorders, and obstructive disease of the GI or GU tract. May exacerbate mental symptoms when used to treat extrapyramidal reactions When given in large doses or to susceptible patients, may cause weakness.

**Pregnancy Risk Factor** C

**Adverse Reactions**

>10%:
Dermatologic: Dry skin
Gastrointestinal: Constipation, xerostomia, dry throat
Respiratory: Dry nose
Miscellaneous: Diaphoresis (decreased)

1% to 10%:
Dermatologic: Increased sensitivity to light
Endocrine & metabolic Decreased flow of breast milk
Gastrointestinal: Dysphagia

<1%: Orthostatic hypotension, ventricular fibrillation, tachycardia, palpitations, confusion, drowsiness, headache loss of memory, fatigue, ataxia, rash, bloated feeling, nausea, vomiting, dysuria, weakness, increased intraocular pain, blurred vision

**Drug Interactions**

Decreased effect of levodopa
Increased toxicity with narcotic analgesics, phenothiazines, TCAs, quinidine, levodopa; anticholinergics

**Onset** Peak effect: Within 1 hour

**Half-Life** 3.3-4.1 hours

**Special PA Issues**

**Patient Education:** Take exactly as directed; with meals if GI upset occurs, before meals if dry mouth occurs, after eating if drooling or if nausea occurs. Take at same time each day. Maintain adequate hydration (2-3 L/day of fluids unless instructed to restrict fluid intake); void before taking medication. Do not use alcohol and all prescription or OTC sedatives or CNS depressants without consulting prescriber. You may experience drowsiness, confusion, or vision changes (use caution when driving, climbing stairs, or engaging in hazardous tasks); increased susceptibility to heat stroke, decreased perspiration (use caution in hot weather - maintain adequate fluids and reduce exercise activity); constipation (increased exercise, fluids, or dietary fruit and fiber may help); dry skin or nasal passages (consult prescriber for appropriate relief). Report unresolved constipation, chest pain or palpitations, difficulty breathing, CNS changes (hallucination, loss of memory, nervousness etc), painful or difficult urination, increased muscle spasticity or rigidity, skin rash, or significant worsening of condition.

**Dietary Considerations:** Alcohol: Additive CNS effect, avoid use

**Monitoring Parameters:** IOP monitoring and gonioscopic evaluations should be performed periodically

## Trimethobenzamide *(trye meth oh BEN za mide)*

**Pharmacologic Class** Anticholinergic Agent; Antiemetic

**U.S. Brand Names** Arrestin®; Pediatric Triban®; Tebamide®; T-Gen®; Ticon®; Tigan®; Triban®; Trimazide®

**Mechanism of Action** Acts centrally to inhibit the medullary chemoreceptor trigger zone

**Use** Control of nausea and vomiting (especially for long-term antiemetic therapy); less effective than phenothiazines but may be associated with fewer side effects

**USUAL DOSAGE** Rectal use is contraindicated in neonates and premature infants

Children:

Rectal: <14 kg: 100 mg 3-4 times/day

Oral, rectal: 14-40 kg: 100-200 mg 3-4 times/day

Adults:

Oral: 250 mg 3-4 times/day

I.M., rectal: 200 mg 3-4 times/day

**Dosage Forms** Trimethobenzamide hydrochloride: **Cap:** 100 mg, 250 mg; **Inj:** 100 mg/mL (2 mL, 20 mL); **Supp, rectal:** 100 mg, 200 mg

**Contraindications** Hypersensitivity to trimethobenzamide, benzocaine, or any component; injection contraindicated in children and suppositories are contraindicated in premature infants or neonates

**Warnings/Precautions** May mask emesis due to Reye's syndrome or mimic CNS effects of Reye's syndrome in patients with emesis of other etiologies; use in patients with acute vomiting should be avoided

**Pregnancy Risk Factor** C

**Adverse Reactions**

>10%: Central nervous system: Drowsiness

1% to 10%:

Cardiovascular: Hypotension

Central nervous system: Dizziness, headache

Gastrointestinal: Diarrhea

Neuromuscular & skeletal: Muscle cramps

<1%: Mental depression, convulsions, opisthotonus, hypersensitivity skin reactions, blood dyscrasias, hepatic impairment

**Drug Interactions** Antagonism of oral anticoagulants may occur

**Onset** Onset of antiemetic effect: Oral: Within 10-40 minutes; I.M.: Within 15-35 minutes

**Duration** 3-4 hours

**Special PA Issues**

**Patient Education:** Avoid use of alcohol or other CNS depressants. May cause drowsiness, impaired judgment, or coordination. Do not drive or perform activities requiring alertness. Report any restlessness or involuntary movements to prescriber.

♦ **Trimethobenzamide Hydrochloride** *see* Trimethobenzamide *on previous page*

# Trimethoprim (trye METH oh prim)

**Pharmacologic Class** Antibiotic, Miscellaneous

**U.S. Brand Names** Proloprim®; Trimpex®

**Mechanism of Action** Inhibits folic acid reduction to tetrahydrofolate, and thereby inhibits microbial growth

**Use** Treatment of urinary tract infections due to susceptible strains of *E. coli*, *P. mirabilis*, *K. pneumoniae*, *Enterobacter* sp and coagulase-negative *Staphylococcus* including *S. saprophyticus*; acute otitis media in children; acute exacerbations of chronic bronchitis in adults; in combination with other agents for treatment of toxoplasmosis, *Pneumocystis carinii*; treatment of superficial ocular infections involving the conjunctiva and cornea

**USUAL DOSAGE** Oral:

Children: 4 mg/kg/day in divided doses every 12 hours

Adults: 100 mg every 12 hours or 200 mg every 24 hours; in the treatment of *Pneumocystis carinii* pneumonia; dose may be as high as 15-20 mg/kg/day in 3-4 divided doses

**Dosing interval in renal impairment:** $Cl_{cr}$ 15-30 mL/minute: Administer 50 mg every 12 hours

Hemodialysis: Moderately dialyzable (20% to 50%)

**Dosage Forms Tab:** 100 mg, 200 mg

**Contraindications** Hypersensitivity to trimethoprim or any component, megaloblastic anemia due to folate deficiency

**Warnings/Precautions** Use with caution in patients with impaired renal or hepatic function or with possible folate deficiency

**Pregnancy Risk Factor** C

**Adverse Reactions**

1% to 10%:

Dermatologic: Rash (3% to 7%), pruritus

Hematologic: Megaloblastic anemia (with chronic high doses)

<1%: Fever, exfoliative dermatitis, nausea, vomiting, epigastric distress, thrombocytopenia, neutropenia, leukopenia, hyperkalemia, cholestatic jaundice, increased LFTs, elevated BUN/serum creatinine

**Drug Interactions** Increased effect/toxicity/levels of phenytoin; increased myelosuppression with methotrexate; may increase levels of digoxin

**Half-Life** 8-14 hours, prolonged with renal impairment

(Continued)

## Trimethoprim *(Continued)*

### Special PA Issues

**Patient Education:** Take as directed and take full course of drug. Do not crush or chew tablets. Maintain adequate hydration (2-3 L/day of fluids unless instructed to restrict fluid intake). Take with milk or food to reduce GI upset. Report, skin rash, fever, sore throat, unusual bleeding or bruising, or feelings of extreme fatigue.

**Reference Range:** Therapeutic: Peak: 5-15 mg/L; Trough: 2-8 mg/L

## Trimethoprim and Polymyxin B (trye METH oh prim & pol i MIKS in bee)

**Pharmacologic Class** Antibiotic, Ophthalmic

**U.S. Brand Names** Polytrim® Ophthalmic

**Dosage Forms Soln, ophth:** Trimethoprim sulfate 1 mg and polymyxin B sulfate 10,000 units per mL (10 mL)

♦ **Trimethoprim and Sulfamethoxazole** *see* Co-Trimoxazole *on page 238*

♦ **Trimethylpsoralen** *see* Trioxsalen *on next page*

## Trimetrexate Glucuronate (tri me TREKS ate gloo KYOOR oh nate)

**Pharmacologic Class** Antineoplastic Agent, Miscellaneous

**U.S. Brand Names** Neutrexin® Injection

**Mechanism of Action** Exerts an antimicrobial effect through potent inhibition of the enzyme dihydrofolate reductase (DHFR)

**Use** Alternative therapy for the treatment of moderate-to-severe *Pneumocystis carinii* pneumonia (PCP) in immunocompromised patients, including patients with acquired immunodeficiency syndrome (AIDS), who are intolerant of, or are refractory to, co-trimoxazole therapy or for whom co-trimoxazole and pentamidine are contraindicated. **Concurrent folinic acid (leucovorin) must always be administered.**

**USUAL DOSAGE** Adults: I.V.: 45 mg/m$^2$ once daily over 60 minutes for 21 days; it is necessary to reduce the dose in patients with liver dysfunction, although no specific recommendations exist; concurrent folinic acid 20 mg/m$^2$ every 6 hours orally or I.V. for 24 days

**Dosage Forms Powder for inj:** 25 mg

**Contraindications** Previous hypersensitivity to trimetrexate or methotrexate, severe existing myelosuppression

**Warnings/Precautions** Must be administered with concurrent leucovorin to avoid potentially serious or life-threatening toxicities; leucovorin therapy must extend for 72 hours past the last dose of trimetrexate; use with caution in patients with mild myelosuppression, severe hepatic or renal dysfunction, hypoproteinemia, hypoalbuminemia, or previous extensive myelosuppressive therapies

**Pregnancy Risk Factor** D

**Adverse Reactions** 1% to 10%:

Central nervous system: Seizures, fever

Dermatologic: Rash

Gastrointestinal: Stomatitis, nausea, vomiting

Hematologic: Neutropenia, thrombocytopenia, anemia

Hepatic: Elevated LFTs

Neuromuscular & skeletal: Peripheral neuropathy

Renal: Increased serum creatinine

Miscellaneous: Flu-like illness, hypersensitivity reactions

**Drug Interactions**

Decreased effect of pneumococcal vaccine

Increased toxicity (infection rates) of yellow fever vaccine

**Half-Life** 15-17 hours

**Special PA Issues**

**Patient Education:** This medication can only be administered I.V. Frequent blood tests will be required to assess effectiveness of therapy. Avoid aspirin, and aspirin-containing medication unless approved by prescriber. Report persistent fever, chills, joint pain, numbness or tingling of extremities, vomiting or nausea, acute abdominal pain, mouth sores, increased bruising or bleeding, blood in urine or stool, changes in sensorium (eg, confusion, hallucinations, seizures), increased difficulty breathing, or acute persistent malaise or weakness.

**Monitoring Parameters:** Check and record patient's temperature daily; absolute neutrophil counts (ANC), platelet count, renal function tests (serum creatinine, BUN), hepatic function tests (ALT, AST, alkaline phosphatase)

## Trimipramine (trye MI pra meen)

**Pharmacologic Class** Antidepressant, Tricyclic (Tertiary Amine)

**U.S. Brand Names** Surmontil®

**Mechanism of Action** Increases the synaptic concentration of serotonin and/or norepinephrine in the central nervous system by inhibition of their reuptake by the presynaptic neuronal membrane

**Use** Treatment of various forms of depression, often in conjunction with psychotherapy

**USUAL DOSAGE** Adults: Oral: 50-150 mg/day as a single bedtime dose up to a maximum of 200 mg/day outpatient and 300 mg/day inpatient

**Dosage Forms** Cap, as maleate: 25 mg, 50 mg, 100 mg

**Contraindications** Narrow-angle glaucoma; avoid use during pregnancy and lactation

**Warnings/Precautions** Use with caution in patients with cardiovascular disease, conduction disturbances, seizure disorders, urinary retention, hyperthyroidism or those receiving thyroid replacement; avoid use during lactation; use with caution in pregnancy; do not discontinue abruptly in patients receiving chronic high-dose therapy

**Pregnancy Risk Factor** C

**Adverse Reactions**

>10%:

Central nervous system: Dizziness, drowsiness, headache

Gastrointestinal: Xerostomia, constipation, increased appetite, nausea, unpleasant taste, weight gain

Neuromuscular & skeletal: Weakness

1% to 10%:

Cardiovascular: Arrhythmias, hypotension

Central nervous system: Confusion, delirium, hallucinations, nervousness, restlessness, parkinsonian syndrome, insomnia

Endocrine & metabolic: Sexual dysfunction

Gastrointestinal: Diarrhea, heartburn

Genitourinary: Dysuria

Neuromuscular & skeletal: Fine muscle tremors

Ocular: Blurred vision, eye pain

Miscellaneous: Diaphoresis (excessive)

<1%: Anxiety, seizures, alopecia, photosensitivity, breast enlargement, galactorrhea, SIADH, trouble with gums, decreased lower esophageal sphincter tone may cause GE reflux, testicular edema, agranulocytosis, leukopenia, eosinophilia, cholestatic jaundice, increased liver enzymes, increased intraocular pressure, tinnitus, allergic reactions

**Drug Interactions** CYP2D6 enzyme substrate

Decreased effect of guanethidine, clonidine; decreased effect with barbiturates, carbamazepine, phenytoin

Increased effect/toxicity with MAO inhibitors (hyperpyretic crises), CNS depressants, alcohol (CNS depression), methylphenidate (increased levels), cimetidine (decreased clearance), anticholinergics

**Onset** Oral: Therapeutic effects require >2 weeks

**Half-Life** 20-26 hours

**Special PA Issues**

**Patient Education:** Take exactly as directed (do not increase dose or frequency); may take 2-3 weeks to achieve desired results; may cause physical and/or psychological dependence. Take at bedtime. Avoid excessive alcohol, caffeine, and other prescription or OTC medications not approved by prescriber. Maintain adequate hydration (2-3 L/day of fluids unless instructed to restrict fluid intake). You may experience drowsiness, lightheadedness, dizziness, or blurred vision (use caution when driving or engaging in hazardous tasks until response to medication is known); nausea, altered taste, dry mouth (small frequent meals, frequent mouth care, or sucking lozenges may help); constipation (increased exercise, fluids, or dietary fruit and fiber may help); diarrhea (buttermilk, yogurt, or boiled milk may help); increased appetite (monitor dietary intake to avoid excess weight gain); postural hypotension (use caution when climbing stairs or changing position from lying or sitting to standing); urinary retention (void before taking medication); or sexual dysfunction (reversible). Report persistent CNS effects (eg, insomnia, restlessness, fatigue, anxiety, impaired cognitive function, seizures); muscle cramping or tremors; chest pain, palpitations, rapid heartbeat, swelling of extremities, or severe dizziness; unresolved urinary retention; vision changes or eye pain; yellowing of eyes or skin; pale stools/dark urine; or worsening of condition.

**Dietary Considerations:** Alcohol: Avoid use

**Monitoring Parameters:** Blood pressure and pulse rate prior to and during initial therapy; evaluate mental status; monitor weight

**Related Information**

Antidepressant Agents *on page 998*

♦ **Trimipramine Maleate** *see* Trimipramine *on previous page*

♦ **Trimox®** *see* Amoxicillin *on page 61*

♦ **Trimpex®** *see* Trimethoprim *on page 937*

♦ **Trinalin®** *see* Azatadine and Pseudoephedrine *on page 90*

♦ **Tri-Norinyl®** *see* Ethinyl Estradiol and Norethindrone *on page 348*

♦ **Triotann® Tablet** *see* Chlorpheniramine, Pyrilamine, and Phenylephrine *on page 197*

# Trioxsalen (trye OKS a len)

**Pharmacologic Class** Psoralen

**U.S. Brand Names** Trisoralen®

(Continued)

## Trioxsalen *(Continued)*

**Mechanism of Action** Psoralens are thought to form covalent bonds with pyrimidine bases in DNA which inhibit the synthesis of DNA. This reaction involves excitation of the trioxsalen molecule by radiation in the long-wave ultraviolet light (UVA) resulting in transference of energy to the trioxsalen molecule producing an excited state. Binding of trioxsalen to DNA occurs only in the presence of ultraviolet light. The increase in skin pigmentation produced by trioxsalen and UVA radiation involves multiple changes in melanocytes and interaction between melanocytes and keratinocytes. In general, melanogenesis is stimulated but the size and distribution of melanocytes is unchanged.

**Use** In conjunction with controlled exposure to ultraviolet light or sunlight for repigmentation of idiopathic vitiligo; increasing tolerance to sunlight with albinism; enhance pigmentation

**USUAL DOSAGE** Children >12 years and Adults: Oral: 10 mg/day as a single dose, 2-4 hours before controlled exposure to UVA (for 15-35 minutes) or sunlight; do not continue for longer than 14 days

**Dosage Forms** Tab: 5 mg

**Contraindications** Hypersensitivity to psoralens, melanoma, a history of melanoma, or other diseases associated with photosensitivity; porphyria, acute lupus erythematosus; patients <12 years of age

**Warnings/Precautions** Serious burns from UVA or sunlight can occur if dosage or exposure schedules are exceeded; patients must wear protective eye wear to prevent cataracts; use with caution in patients with severe hepatic or cardiovascular disease

**Pregnancy Risk Factor** C

**Adverse Reactions**
>10%:
Dermatologic: Itching
Gastrointestinal: Nausea
1% to 10%:
Central nervous system: Dizziness, headache, mental depression, insomnia, nervousness
Dermatologic: Severe burns from excessive sunlight or ultraviolet exposure
Gastrointestinal: Gastric discomfort

**Onset** Peak photosensitivity: 2 hours

**Duration** Skin sensitivity to light remains for 8-12 hours

**Half-Life** ~2 hours

**Special PA Issues**
**Patient Education:** This medication is used in conjunction with specific ultraviolet treatment. Follow prescriber's directions exactly for oral medication which can be taken with food or milk to reduce nausea. Avoid use of any other skin treatments unless approved by prescriber. You must wear protective eyewear during treatments. Control exposure to direct sunlight as per prescriber's instructions. If sunlight cannot be avoided, use sunblock (consult prescriber for specific SPF level), wear protective clothing, and wraparound protective eyewear. Consult prescriber immediately if burning, blistering, or skin irritation occur.

## Tripelennamine *(tri pel EN a meen)*

**Pharmacologic Class** Antihistamine

**U.S. Brand Names** PBZ®; PBZ-SR®

**Mechanism of Action** Competes with histamine for $H_1$-receptor sites on effector cells in the gastrointestinal tract, blood vessels, and respiratory tract

**Use** Perennial and seasonal allergic rhinitis and other allergic symptoms including urticaria

**USUAL DOSAGE** Oral:
Infants and Children: 5 mg/kg/day in 4-6 divided doses, up to 300 mg/day maximum
Adults: 25-50 mg every 4-6 hours, extended release tablets 100 mg morning and evening up to 100 mg every 8 hours

**Dosage Forms** Tripelennamine hydrochloride: **Tab:** 25 mg, 50 mg; **Tab, extended release:** 100 mg

**Contraindications** Hypersensitivity to tripelennamine or any component

**Warnings/Precautions** Use with caution in patients with narrow-angle glaucoma, bladder neck obstruction, symptomatic prostate hypertrophy, asthmatic attacks, and stenosing peptic ulcer

**Pregnancy Risk Factor** B

**Adverse Reactions**
>10%:
Central nervous system: Slight to moderate drowsiness
Respiratory: Thickening of bronchial secretions
1% to 10%:
Central nervous system: Headache, fatigue, nervousness, dizziness
Gastrointestinal: Appetite increase, weight gain, nausea, diarrhea, abdominal pain, xerostomia
Neuromuscular & skeletal: Arthralgia
Respiratory: Pharyngitis

**<1%:** Edema, palpitations, hypotension, depression, sedation, paradoxical excitement, insomnia, angioedema, photosensitivity, rash, urinary retention, hepatitis, myalgia, paresthesia, tremor, blurred vision, bronchospasm, epistaxis

**Drug Interactions** Increased effect/toxicity with alcohol, CNS depressants, MAO inhibitors

**Onset** Onset of antihistaminic effect: Within 15-30 minutes

**Duration** 4-6 hours (up to 8 hours with PBZ-SR®)

**Special PA Issues**

> **Patient Education:** Take as directed; do not exceed recommended dose. Avoid use of other depressants, alcohol, or sleep-inducing medications unless approved by prescriber. You may experience drowsiness or dizziness (use caution when driving or engaging in hazardous activity until response to medication is known); or dry mouth, nausea, or abdominal discomfort (frequent small meals, frequent mouth care, chewing gum, or sucking hard candy may help). Report persistent dizziness, sedation, or agitation; chest pain, rapid heartbeat, or palpitations; difficulty breathing; changes in urinary pattern; yellowing of skin or eyes; dark urine or pale stool; or lack of improvement or worsening or condition.

> **Dietary Considerations:** Alcohol: Additive CNS effect, avoid use

- ♦ **Tripelennamine Citrate** see Tripelennamine on previous page
- ♦ **Tripelennamine Hydrochloride** see Tripelennamine on previous page
- ♦ **Triphasil®** see Ethinyl Estradiol and Levonorgestrel on page 347
- ♦ **Tri-Phen-Chlor®** see Chlorpheniramine, Phenyltoloxamine, Phenylpropanolamine, and Phenylephrine on page 196
- ♦ **Triple Antibiotic® Topical** see Bacitracin, Neomycin, and Polymyxin B on page 97
- ♦ **Triple Sulfa** see Sulfabenzamide, Sulfacetamide, and Sulfathiazole on page 857
- ·♦ **Triple X® Liquid [OTC]** see Pyrethrins on page 783

# Triprolidine, Pseudoephedrine, and Codeine
(trye PROE li deen, soo doe e FED rin, & KOE deen)

**Pharmacologic Class** Antihistamine/Decongestant/Antitussive

**U.S. Brand Names** Actagen-C®; Allerfrin® w/Codeine; Aprodine® w/C; Triacin-C®; Trifed-C®

**Dosage Forms** Syr: Triprolidine hydrochloride 1.25 mg, pseudoephedrine hydrochloride 30 mg, and codeine phosphate 10 mg per 5 mL with alcohol 4.3%

- ♦ **Triptil®** see Protriptyline on page 779
- ♦ **Trisoralen®** see Trioxsalen on page 939
- ♦ **Tri-Statin® II Topical** see Nystatin and Triamcinolone on page 670
- ♦ **Tristoject®** see Triamcinolone on page 928
- ♦ **Trisulfa®** see Co-Trimoxazole on page 238
- ♦ **Trisulfapyrimidines** see Sulfadiazine, Sulfamethazine, and Sulfamerazine on page 860
- ♦ **Trisulfa-S®** see Co-Trimoxazole on page 238
- ♦ **Tri-Tannate Plus®** see Chlorpheniramine, Ephedrine, Phenylephrine, and Carbetapentane on page 195
- ♦ **Tri-Tannate® Tablet** see Chlorpheniramine, Pyrilamine, and Phenylephrine on page 197
- ♦ **Tritec®** see Ranitidine Bismuth Citrate on page 794
- ♦ **Tri-Vi-Flor®** see Vitamins, Multiple on page 964
- ♦ **Trobicin®** see Spectinomycin on page 848
- ♦ **Trocaine® [OTC]** see Benzocaine on page 105

# Troglitazone (TROE gli to zone)

**Pharmacologic Class** Antidiabetic Agent (Thiazolidinedione)

**U.S. Brand Names** Rezulin®

**Mechanism of Action** Thiazolidinedione antidiabetic agent that lowers blood glucose by improving target cell response to insulin, without increasing pancreatic insulin secretion. It has a unique mechanism of action that is dependent on the presence of insulin for activity. Troglitazone decreases hepatic glucose output and increases insulin-dependent glucose disposal in skeletal muscle and possible liver and adipose tissue.

**Use** Type II diabetes: For use in patients with type II diabetes currently on insulin therapy whose hyperglycemia is inadequately controlled (Hb $A_{1c}$ >8.5%) despite insulin therapy >30 units/day given as multiple injections.

> Management of type II diabetes should include diet control. Caloric restriction, weight loss and exercise are essential for the proper treatment of the diabetic patient. This is important not only the primary treatment of type II diabetes but in maintaining the efficacy of drug therapy. Prior to initiation of troglitazone therapy, investigate secondary causes of poor glycemic control (eg, infection or poor injection technique).

> Either monotherapy or combination therapy with sulfonylureas, for patients with type II diabetes

**Investigational:** A study showed troglitazone may be beneficial in the productive and metabolic consequences of polycystic ovary syndrome (PCOS) (400 mg/day) and less essential hypertension with NIDDM, but more studies are needed.

(Continued)

## Troglitazone *(Continued)*

**USUAL DOSAGE** Oral (take with meals):

Adults:

Combination therapy with insulin: Continue the current insulin dose upon initiation of troglitazone therapy

Initiate therapy at 200 mg once daily in patients on insulin therapy. For patients not responding adequately, increase the dose after 2-4 weeks. The usual dose is 400 mg/day; maximum recommended dose: 600 mg/day.

It is recommended that the insulin dose be decreased by 10% to 25% when fasting plasma glucose concentrations decrease to <120 mg/dL in patients receiving concomitant insulin and troglitazone. Individualize further adjustments based on glucose-lowering response.

Monotherapy: Initial: 400 mg once daily with a meal. For patients not responding to 400 mg/day, the troglitazone dose should be increased to 600 mg after 1 month. For patients not responding adequately to 600 mg after 1 month, troglitazone should be discontinued and alternate therapeutic options should be pursued.

Elderly: Steady-state pharmacokinetics of troglitazone and metabolites in healthy elderly subjects were comparable to those seen in young adults

**Dosing adjustment/comments in renal impairment:** Dose adjustment is not necessary

**Dosing adjustment in hepatic impairment:** Troglitazone should **not** be initiated if the patient exhibits clinical evidence of active liver disease or increased serum transaminase levels (ALT >1.5 times the upper limit of normal).

**Dosage Forms Tab:** 200 mg, 400 mg

**Contraindications** Hypersensitivity to troglitazone or any component

**Warnings/Precautions** Patients with New York Heart Association (NYHA) Class III and IV cardiac status were not studied during clinical trials. Heart enlargement without microscopic changes has been observed in rodents at exposures exceeding 14 times the AUC of the 400 mg human dose. Caution is advised during the administration of troglitazone to patients with NYHA Class III or IV cardiac status.

A total of 150 adverse event reports postmarketing have been reported to the FDA including 3 deaths from liver failure linked to the use of troglitazone. Approximately 600,000 patients in the U.S. and 200,000 patients in Japan have been treated with troglitazone.

Patients on troglitazone who develop jaundice or whose laboratory results indicate liver injury should stop taking the drug. Approximately 2% of patients can expect to stop taking the drug because of elevated liver enzymes.

Because of its mechanism of action, troglitazone is active only in the presence of insulin. Therefore, do not use in type I diabetes or for the treatment of diabetic ketoacidosis.

Patients receiving troglitazone in combination with insulin may be at risk for hypoglycemia, and a reduction in the dose of insulin may be necessary. Hypoglycemia has not been observed during the administration of troglitazone as monotherapy and would not be expected based on the mechanism of action.

Across all clinical studies, hemoglobin declined by 3% to 4% in troglitazone-treated patients compared with 1% to 2% with placebo. White blood cell counts also declined slightly in troglitazone-treated patients compared with those treated with placebo. These changes occurred within the first 4-8 weeks of therapy. Levels stabilized and remained unchanged for ≤2 years of continuing therapy. These changes may be due to the dilutional effects of increased plasma volume and have not been associated with any significant hematologic clinical effects.

**Pregnancy Risk Factor** B

**Adverse Reactions**

>10%:

Central nervous system: Headache, pain

Miscellaneous: Infection

1% to 10%:

Cardiovascular: Peripheral edema

Central nervous system: Dizziness

Gastrointestinal: Nausea, diarrhea, pharyngitis

Genitourinary: Urinary tract infection

Neuromuscular & skeletal: Neck pain, weakness

Respiratory: Rhinitis

**Drug Interactions** CYP3A3/4 enzyme substrate; CYP3A3/4 enzyme inducer; CYP2C9, 2C19, and 3A3/4 enzyme inhibitor

Decreased effects:

Cholestyramine: Concomitant administration of cholestyramine with troglitazone reduces the absorption of troglitazone by 70%; COADMINISTRATION OF CHOLESTYRAMINE AND TROGLITAZONE IS NOT RECOMMENDED.

Oral contraceptives: Administration of troglitazone with an oral contraceptive containing ethinyl estradiol and norethindrone reduced the plasma concentrations of both by 30%. These changes could result in loss of contraception.

Terfenadine: Coadministration of troglitazone with terfenadine decreases plasma concentrations of terfenadine and its active metabolite by 50% to 70% and may reduce the effectiveness of terfenadine

Increased toxicity:

Sulfonylureas (glyburide): Coadministration of troglitazone with glyburide may further decrease plasma glucose levels

**Onset** Generally requires >3 weeks

**Half-Life** 16-34 hours

**Special PA Issues**

**Patient Education:** Take with meals. Follow directions of prescriber. If dose is missed at the usual meal, take it with next meal. Do not double dose if daily dose is missed completely. Monitor urine or serum glucose as recommended by prescriber. More frequent monitoring is required during periods of stress, trauma, surgery, pregnancy, increased activity or exercise. Avoid alcohol. Report chest pain, rapid heartbeat or palpitations, abdominal pain, fever, rash, hypoglycemia reactions, yellowing of skin or eyes, dark urine or light stool, or unusual fatigue or nausea/vomiting.

**Monitoring Parameters:** Urine for glucose and ketones, fasting blood glucose, hemoglobin $A_{1c}$, and fructosamine. **Serum transaminase levels should be monitored at the start of therapy, monthly for the first 8 months of treatment, every other month for the remainder of the first year, and periodically thereafter.** Additionally, liver function tests should be performed on any patient on troglitazone who develops symptoms of liver dysfunction, such as nausea, vomiting, abdominal pain, fatigue, loss of appetite, or dark urine.

**Reference Range:** Target range: Adults: Fasting blood glucose: <120 mg/dL; Glycosylated hemoglobin: <7%

**Related Information**

Hypoglycemic Drugs *on page 1020*

♦ **Tropicacyl®** *see* Tropicamide *on this page*

# Tropicamide (troe PIK a mide)

**Pharmacologic Class** Ophthalmic Agent, Mydriatic

**U.S. Brand Names** Mydriacyl®; Opticyl®; Tropicacyl®

**Mechanism of Action** Prevents the sphincter muscle of the iris and the muscle of the ciliary body from responding to cholinergic stimulation

**Use** Short-acting mydriatic used in diagnostic procedures; as well as preoperatively and postoperatively; treatment of some cases of acute iritis, iridocyclitis, and keratitis

**USUAL DOSAGE** Children and Adults (individuals with heavily pigmented eyes may require larger doses):

Cycloplegia: Instill 1-2 drops (1%); may repeat in 5 minutes

Exam must be performed within 30 minutes after the repeat dose; if the patient is not examined within 20-30 minutes, instill an additional drop

Mydriasis: Instill 1-2 drops (0.5%) 15-20 minutes before exam; may repeat every 30 minutes as needed

**Dosage Forms Soln, ophth:** 0.5% (2 mL, 15 mL), 1% (2 mL, 3 mL, 15 mL)

**Contraindications** Glaucoma, hypersensitivity to tropicamide or any component

**Warnings/Precautions** Use with caution in infants and children since tropicamide may cause potentially dangerous CNS disturbances; tropicamide may cause an increase in intraocular pressure

**Pregnancy Risk Factor** C

**Adverse Reactions** 1% to 10%:

Cardiovascular: Tachycardia, vascular congestion, edema

Central nervous system: Parasympathetic stimulations, drowsiness, headache

Dermatologic: Eczematoid dermatitis

Gastrointestinal: Xerostomia

Local: Transient stinging

Ocular: Blurred vision, photophobia with or without corneal staining, increased intraocular pressure, follicular conjunctivitis

**Special PA Issues**

**Patient Education:** If irritation persists or increases, discontinue use, may cause blurred vision and increased light sensitivity

**Monitoring Parameters:** Ophthalmic exam

# Trovafloxacin (TROE va flox a sin)

**Pharmacologic Class** Antibiotic, Quinolone

**U.S. Brand Names** Trovan™

**Mechanism of Action** Inhibits DNA-gyrase in susceptible organisms; inhibits relaxation of supercoiled DNA and promotes breakage of double-stranded DNA

**Use** Treatment of nosocomial pneumonia, community-acquired pneumonia, acute exacerbation of chronic bronchitis, acute sinusitis, intra-abdominal infections, gynecologic/pelvic infections, skin and skin structure infections, urinary tract infections, pelvic inflammatory disease, cervicitis, and gonorrhea.

(Continued)

## Trovafloxacin *(Continued)*

Trovafloxacin is active against most aerobic gram-negative bacilli including *Pseudomonas aeruginosa* and many gram-positive cocci including staphylococcal sp and streptococcal sp (including *S. pneumoniae*). Trovafloxacin also has activity against many anaerobes including *Bacteroides fragilis*.

**USUAL DOSAGE** Adults:

Nosocomial pneumonia: I.V.: 300 mg single dose followed by 200 mg/day orally for a total duration of 10-14 days

Community-acquired pneumonia: Oral, I.V.: 200 mg/day for 7-14 days

Acute bacterial exacerbation of chronic bronchitis: Oral: 100 mg/day for 7-10 days

Acute sinusitis: Oral: 200 mg/day for 10 days

Complicated intra-abdominal infections, including postsurgical infections/gynecologic and pelvic infections: I.V.: 300 mg as a single dose followed by 200 mg orally for a total duration of 7-14 days

Surgical prophylaxis (elective colorectal surgery, elective and abdominal and vaginal hysterectomy): Oral, I.V.: 200 mg as a single dose within 30 minutes to 4 hours before surgery

Skin and skin structure infections: Oral: 100 mg/day for 7-10 days

Skin and skin structure infections, complicated, including diabetic foot infections: Oral, I.V.: 200 mg/day for 10-14 days

Uncomplicated UTI (cystitis): Oral: 100 mg/day for 3 days

Chronic bacterial prostatitis: Oral: 200 mg/day for 28 days

Uncomplicated urethral gonorrhea in males; endocervical/rectal gonorrhea in females: Oral: 100 mg single dose

Cervicitis caused by *Chlamydia trachomatis*: Oral: 200 mg/day for 5 days

Pelvic inflammatory disease (mild to moderate): Oral: 200 mg for 14 days

**Dosage adjustment in renal impairment:** No adjustment is necessary

**Dosage adjustment for hemodialysis:** None required; trovafloxacin not sufficiently removed by hemodialysis

**Dosage adjustment in hepatic impairment:**

Mild to moderate cirrhosis:

Initial dose for normal hepatic function: 300 mg I.V.; 200 mg I.V. or oral; 100 mg oral
Reduced dose: 200 mg I.V.; 100 mg I.V. or oral; 100 mg oral

Severe cirrhosis: No data available

**Dosage Forms Inj, as mesylate (alatrofloxacin):** 5 mg/mL (40 mL, 60 mL); **Tab, as mesylate (trovafloxacin):** 100 mg, 200 mg

**Contraindications** History of hypersensitivity to trovafloxacin, alatrofloxacin, quinolone antimicrobial agents or any other components of these products

**Warnings/Precautions** May alter GI flora resulting in pseudomembranous colitis due to *Clostridium difficile*; use with caution in patients with seizure disorders or severe cerebral atherosclerosis; discontinue if skin rash or pain, inflammation, or rupture of a tendon; photosensitivity; CNS stimulation may occur which may lead to tremor, restlessness, confusion, hallucinations, paranoia, depression, nightmares, insomnia, or lightheadedness. May cause liver enzyme abnormalities, hepatitis, or liver failure

**Pregnancy Risk Factor** C

**Adverse Reactions** <10%:

Central nervous system: Dizziness, lightheadedness, headache

Dermatologic: Rash, pruritus

Gastrointestinal: Nausea, vomiting, diarrhea, abdominal pain

Genitourinary: Vaginitis

Hepatic: Increased LFTs

Local: Injection site reaction, pain, or inflammation

<1%: Anaphylaxis, hepatic necrosis, pancreatitis, Stevens-Johnson syndrome

**Drug Interactions** Decreased effect of oral trovafloxacin:

Antacids containing magnesium or aluminum, sucralfate, citric acid buffered with sodium citrate, and metal cations: Administer oral trovafloxacin doses at least 2 hours before or 2 hours after

Morphine: Administer I.V. morphine at least 2 hours after oral trovafloxacin in the fasting state and at least 4 hours after oral trovafloxacin when taken with food

**Half-Life** 9.1-12.7 hours

**Special PA Issues**

**Patient Education:** Take per recommended schedule. Dizziness may be reduced if taken at bedtime with food. Avoid antacids and milk products 2 hours before or 2 hours after trovafloxacin. Maintain adequate hydration (2-3 L/day of fluids unless instructed to restrict fluid intake). Take complete prescription; do not skip doses. If dose is missed, take as soon as possible; do not double doses. You may experience dizziness, lightheadedness, or headache (use caution when driving or engaging in tasks that require alertness); nausea (small frequent meals and frequent mouth care may help); photosensitivity (use sunscreen, appropriate clothing, or avoid direct sun exposure). Report immediately any CNS disturbances such as hallucinations, tremor, confusion, or seizures; palpitations, chest pain or tightness; or difficulty breathing or swallowing. Report persistent diarrhea or abdominal pain; muscle tremor or pain; pain, inflammation, or rupture of tendon; unusual fatigue; fever, chills, or signs of infection; rash; or worsening of condition.

**Dietary Considerations:** Dairy products such as milk and yogurt reduce the absorption of oral trovafloxacin - avoid concurrent use. The bioavailability may also be decreased by enteral feedings.

**Monitoring Parameters:** Periodic assessment of liver function tests should be considered

♦ **Trovan™** *see* Trovafloxacin *on page 943*

♦ **Truphylline®** *see* Theophylline Salts *on page 888*

♦ **Trusopt®** *see* Dorzolamide *on page 302*

## Trypsin, Balsam Peru, and Castor Oil
(TRIP sin, BAL sam pe RUE, & KAS tor oyl)

**Pharmacologic Class** Protectant, Topical

**U.S. Brand Names** Granulex

**Dosage Forms Aero, top:** Trypsin 0.1 mg, balsam Peru 72.5 mg, and castor oil 650 mg per 0.82 mL (60 g, 120 g)

♦ **Trysul®** *see* Sulfabenzamide, Sulfacetamide, and Sulfathiazole *on page 857*

♦ **TSH** *see* Thyrotropin Alpha *on page 899*

♦ **TSH** *see* Thyrotropin *on page 899*

♦ **TST** *see* Tuberculin Tests *on this page*

♦ **Tubasal®** *see* Aminosalicylate Sodium *on page 54*

♦ **Tuberculin Purified Protein Derivative** *see* Tuberculin Tests *on this page*

♦ **Tuberculin Skin Test** *see* Tuberculin Tests *on this page*

## Tuberculin Tests (too BER kyoo lin tests)

**Pharmacologic Class** Diagnostic Agent, Skin Test

**U.S. Brand Names** Aplisol®; Aplitest®; Sclavo-PPD Solution®; Sclavo Test-PPD®; Tine Test PPD; Tubersol®

**Mechanism of Action** Tuberculosis results in individuals becoming sensitized to certain antigenic components of the *M. tuberculosis* organism. Culture extracts called tuberculins are contained in tuberculin skin test preparations. Upon intracutaneous injection of these culture extracts, a classic delayed (cellular) hypersensitivity reaction occurs. This reaction is characteristic of a delayed course (peak occurs >24 hours after injection, induration of the skin secondary to cell infiltration, and occasional vesiculation and necrosis). Delayed hypersensitivity reactions to tuberculin may indicate infection with a variety of nontuberculosis mycobacteria, or vaccination with the live attenuated mycobacterial strain of *M. bovis* vaccine, BCG, in addition to previous natural infection with *M. tuberculosis*.

**Use** Skin test in diagnosis of tuberculosis, cell-mediated immunodeficiencies

**USUAL DOSAGE** Children and Adults: Intradermal: 0.1 mL about 4" below elbow; use ¼" to ½" or 26- or 27-gauge needle; significant reactions are ≥5 mm in diameter

Interpretation of induration of tuberculin skin test injections: Positive: ≥10 mm; inconclusive: 5-9 mm; negative: <5 mm

Interpretation of induration of Tine test injections: Positive: >2 mm and vesiculation present; inconclusive: <2 mm (give patient Mantoux test of 5 TU/0.1 mL - base decisions on results of Mantoux test); negative: <2 mm or erythema of any size (no need for retesting unless person is a contact of a patient with tuberculosis or there is clinical evidence suggestive of the disease)

**Dosage Forms Inj:** First test strength: 1 TU/0.1 mL (1 mL); Intermediate test strength: 5 TU/0.1 mL (1 mL, 5 mL, 10 mL); Second test strength: 250 TU/0.1 mL (1 mL); **Tine:** 5 TU each test

**Contraindications** 250 TU strength should not be used for initial testing

**Warnings/Precautions** Do not administer I.V. or S.C.; epinephrine (1:1000) should be available to treat possible allergic reactions

**Pregnancy Risk Factor** C

**Adverse Reactions** 1% to 10%:
Dermatologic: Ulceration, vesiculation
Local: Pain at injection site
Miscellaneous: Necrosis

**Drug Interactions** Decreased effect: Reaction may be suppressed in patients receiving systemic corticosteroids, aminocaproic acid, or within 4-6 weeks following immunization with live or inactivated viral vaccines

**Special PA Issues**
**Patient Education:** Return to physician for reaction interpretation at 48-72 hours

♦ **Tuberculosis** *see* Chart *on page 1111*

♦ **Tubersol®** *see* Tuberculin Tests *on this page*

♦ **Tumeric Root** *see* Golden Seal *on page 421*

♦ **Tums®** [OTC] *see* Calcium Carbonate *on page 139*

♦ **Tums® E-X Extra Strength Tablet** [OTC] *see* Calcium Carbonate *on page 139*

- **Tums® Extra Strength Liquid [OTC]** *see* Calcium Carbonate *on page 139*
- **Tusibron® [OTC]** *see* Guaifenesin *on page 427*
- **Tusibron-DM® [OTC]** *see* Guaifenesin and Dextromethorphan *on page 428*
- **Tussafed® Drops** *see* Carbinoxamine, Pseudoephedrine, and Dextromethorphan *on page 153*
- **Tussafin® Expectorant** *see* Hydrocodone, Pseudoephedrine, and Guaifenesin *on page 453*
- **Tuss-Allergine® Modified T.D. Capsule** *see* Caramiphen and Phenylpropanolamine *on page 148*
- **Tussar® SF Syrup** *see* Guaifenesin, Pseudoephedrine, and Codeine *on page 429*
- **Tuss-DM® [OTC]** *see* Guaifenesin and Dextromethorphan *on page 428*
- **Tussigon®** *see* Hydrocodone and Homatropine *on page 451*
- **Tussionex®** *see* Hydrocodone and Chlorpheniramine *on page 451*
- **Tussi-Organidin® DM NR** *see* Guaifenesin and Dextromethorphan *on page 428*
- **Tussi-Organidin® NR** *see* Guaifenesin and Codeine *on page 428*
- **Tussogest® Extended Release Capsule** *see* Caramiphen and Phenylpropanolamine *on page 148*
- **Tusstat® Syrup** *see* Diphenhydramine *on page 289*
- **Twilite® Oral [OTC]** *see* Diphenhydramine *on page 289*
- **Twin-K®** *see* Potassium Citrate and Potassium Gluconate *on page 744*
- **Two-Dyne®** *see* Butalbital Compound *on page 131*
- **Tylenol® [OTC]** *see* Acetaminophen *on page 21*
- **Tylenol® Extended Relief [OTC]** *see* Acetaminophen *on page 21*
- **Tylenol® With Codeine** *see* Acetaminophen and Codeine *on page 22*
- **Tylox®** *see* Oxycodone and Acetaminophen *on page 688*
- **Tyramine-Containing Foods** *see* Chart *on page 1148*
- **Tyrodone® Liquid** *see* Hydrocodone and Pseudoephedrine *on page 453*
- **U-90152S** *see* Delavirdine *on page 257*
- **UAD® Otic** *see* Neomycin, Polymyxin B, and Hydrocortisone *on page 645*
- **UCB-P071** *see* Cetirizine *on page 183*
- **Ucephan®** *see* Sodium Phenylacetate and Sodium Benzoate *on page 842*
- **U-Cort™** *see* Hydrocortisone *on page 453*
- **Ultiva™** *see* Remifentanil *on page 796*
- **Ultracef®** *see* Cefadroxil *on page 159*
- **Ultram®** *see* Tramadol *on page 919*
- **Ultra Mide® Topical** *see* Urea *on next page*
- **Ultraquin™** *see* Hydroquinone *on page 457*
- **Ultrase® MT12** *see* Pancrelipase *on page 694*
- **Ultrase® MT20** *see* Pancrelipase *on page 694*
- **Ultravate™ Topical** *see* Halobetasol *on page 434*
- **Unasyn®** *see* Ampicillin and Sulbactam *on page 66*
- **Unguentine® [OTC]** *see* Benzocaine *on page 105*
- **Uni-Ace® [OTC]** *see* Acetaminophen *on page 21*
- **Uni-Bent® Cough Syrup** *see* Diphenhydramine *on page 289*
- **Unicap® [OTC]** *see* Vitamins, Multiple *on page 964*
- **Uni-Decon®** *see* Chlorpheniramine, Phenyltoloxamine, Phenylpropanolamine, and Phenylephrine *on page 196*
- **Unipen® Injection** *see* Nafcillin *on page 630*
- **Unipen® Oral** *see* Nafcillin *on page 630*
- **Uni-Pro® [OTC]** *see* Ibuprofen *on page 466*
- **Uniretic™** *see* Moexipril and Hydrochlorothiazide *on page 616*
- **Unitrol® [OTC]** *see* Phenylpropanolamine *on page 720*
- **Uni-Tussin® [OTC]** *see* Guaifenesin *on page 427*
- **Uni-tussin® DM [OTC]** *see* Guaifenesin and Dextromethorphan *on page 428*
- **Univasc®** *see* Moexipril *on page 615*
- **Unna's Boot** *see* Zinc Gelatin *on page 975*
- **Unna's Paste** *see* Zinc Gelatin *on page 975*
- **Urabeth®** *see* Bethanechol *on page 114*

# Uracil Mustard (YOOR a sil MUS tard)
**Pharmacologic Class** Antineoplastic Agent, Alkylating Agent

**Mechanism of Action** Polyfunctional alkylating agent. The basic reaction of uracil mustard, like that of any alkylating agent, is the replacement of the hydrogen in a reacting chemical with an alkyl group; cell cycle-phase nonspecific antineoplastic agent; exact site of drug action within the cell is not known, but the nucleoproteins of the cell nucleus are believed to be involved.

**Use** Palliative treatment in symptomatic chronic lymphocytic leukemia; non-Hodgkin's lymphomas, chronic myelocytic leukemia, mycosis fungoides, thrombocytosis, polycythemia vera, ovarian carcinoma

**USUAL DOSAGE** Oral (do not administer until 2-3 weeks after maximum effect of any previous x-ray or cytotoxic drug therapy of the bone marrow is obtained):

Children: 0.3 mg/kg in a single weekly dose for 4 weeks
Adults: 0.15 mg/kg in a single weekly dose for 4 weeks
Thrombocytosis: 1-2 mg/day for 14 days

**Dosage Forms Cap:** 1 mg

**Contraindications** Severe leukopenia, thrombocytopenia, aplastic anemia; in patients whose bone marrow is infiltrated with malignant cells; hypersensitivity to any component; pregnancy

**Warnings/Precautions** The U.S. Food and Drug Administration (FDA) currently recommends that procedures for proper handling and disposal of antineoplastic agents be considered. Impaired kidney or liver function. The drug should be discontinued if intractable vomiting or diarrhea, precipitous falls in leukocyte or platelet count, or myocardial ischemia occurs. Use with caution in patients who have had high-dose pelvic radiation or previous use of alkylating agents. Patient should be hospitalized during initial course of therapy; may impair fertility in men and women; use with caution in patients with pre-existing marrow suppression.

**Pregnancy Risk Factor** X

**Adverse Reactions**
>10%:
Gastrointestinal: Nausea, vomiting, diarrhea
Hematologic: Myelosuppressive; leukopenia and thrombocytopenia nadir: 2-4 weeks, anemia
1% to 10%:
Central nervous system: Mental depression, nervousness
Dermatologic: Hyperpigmentation, alopecia
Endocrine & metabolic: Hyperuricemia
<1%: Pruritus, stomatitis, hepatotoxicity

**Special PA Issues**
**Patient Education:** This drug may take weeks or months for effectiveness to become apparent. Do not discontinue without consulting prescriber. Maintain adequate hydration (2-3 L/day of fluids unless instructed to restrict fluid intake). For nausea or vomiting, loss of appetite, or dry mouth, small frequent meals, chewing gum, or sucking on lozenges may help. You may experience hair loss (reversible); diarrhea (if persistent, consult prescriber); nervousness, irritability, shakiness, amenorrhea, altered sperm production (usually reversible). Report persistent nausea or vomiting, fever, sore throat, chills, unusual bleeding or bruising, consistent feelings of tiredness or weakness, or yellowing of skin or eyes.

♦ **Urasal®** see Methenamine on page 582

# Urea (yoor EE a)

**Pharmacologic Class** Diuretic, Osmotic; Keratolytic Agent; Topical Skin Product
**U.S. Brand Names** Amino-Cerv™ Vaginal Cream; Aquacare® Topical [OTC]; Carmol® Topical [OTC]; Gormel® Creme [OTC]; Lanaphilic® Topical [OTC]; Nutraplus® Topical [OTC]; Rea-Lo® [OTC]; Ultra Mide® Topical; Ureacin®-20 Topical [OTC]; Ureacin®-40; Ureaphil® Injection
**Mechanism of Action** Elevates plasma osmolality by inhibiting tubular reabsorption of water, thus enhancing the flow of water into extracellular fluid
**Use** Reduces intracranial pressure and intraocular pressure; topically promotes hydration and removal of excess keratin in hyperkeratotic conditions and dry skin; mild cervicitis
**USUAL DOSAGE**
Children: I.V. slow infusion:
<2 years: 0.1-0.5 g/kg
>2 years: 0.5-1.5 g/kg
Adults:
I.V. infusion: 1-1.5 g/kg by slow infusion (1-2½ hours); maximum: 120 g/24 hours
Topical: Apply 1-3 times/day
Vaginal: Insert 1 applicatorful in vagina at bedtime for 2-4 weeks
**Dosage Forms Crm: Top:** 2% [20 mg/mL] (75 g), 10% [100 mg/mL] (75 g, 90 g, 454 g), 20% [200 mg/mL] (45 g, 75 g, 90 g, 454 g), 30% [300 mg/mL] (60 g, 454 g), 40% (30 g); **Vag:** 8.34% [83.4 mg/g] (82.5 g); **Inj:** 40 g/150 mL; **Lot:** 2% (240 mL), 10% (180 mL, 240 mL, 480 mL), 15% (120 mL, 480 mL), 25% (180 mL)
**Contraindications** Severely impaired renal function, hepatic failure; active intracranial bleeding, sickle cell anemia, topical use in viral skin disease
**Warnings/Precautions** Urea should not be used near the eyes; use with caution if applied to face, broken, or inflamed skin; use with caution in patients with mild hepatic or renal impairment
**Pregnancy Risk Factor** C
(Continued)

# Urea (Continued)

## Adverse Reactions

Central nervous system: Headache

Endocrine & metabolic: Electrolyte imbalance

Gastrointestinal: Nausea, vomiting

Local: Transient stinging, local irritation, tissue necrosis from extravasation of I.V. preparation

**Drug Interactions** Decreased effect/toxicity/levels of lithium

**Onset** I.V.: Maximum effects within 1-2 hours

**Duration** I.V.: 3-6 hours (diuresis can continue for up to 10 hours)

**Half-Life** 1 hour

## Special PA Issues

### Patient Education:

Topical: For external use only. Best effect is obtained when applied to skin while still wet or moist after washing or bathing. Do not apply to broken, inflamed, or infected skin. Do not use near eyes. Report skin redness, irritation, or worsening of condition.

Vaginal: Wash hands before using. Insert full applicator into vagina gently and expel cream at bedtime. Wash applicator with soap and water following use. Remain lying down for 30 minutes following administration. Report if condition worsens or does not improve.

# Urea and Hydrocortisone (yoor EE a & hye droe KOR ti sone)

**Pharmacologic Class** Corticosteroid, Topical

**U.S. Brand Names** Carmol-HC® Topical

**Dosage Forms Crm, top:** Urea 10% and hydrocortisone acetate 1% in a water-washable vanishing cream base (30 g)

♦ **Ureacin®-20 Topical [OTC]** see Urea on previous page

♦ **Ureacin®-40** see Urea on previous page

♦ **Urea Peroxide** see Carbamide Peroxide on page 150

♦ **Ureaphil® Injection** see Urea on previous page

♦ **Urecholine®** see Bethanechol on page 114

♦ **Uremol™** see Urea on previous page

♦ **Urex®** see Methenamine on page 582

♦ **Uridon®** see Chlorthalidone on page 200

♦ **Urisec®** see Urea on previous page

♦ **Urispas®** see Flavoxate on page 372

♦ **Uri-Tet® Oral** see Oxytetracycline on page 690

♦ **Uritol®** see Furosemide on page 405

♦ **Urobak®** see Sulfamethoxazole on page 861

♦ **Urodine®** see Phenazopyridine on page 714

♦ **Urofollitropin** see Follitropins on page 397

♦ **Urogesic®** see Phenazopyridine on page 714

# Urokinase (yoor oh KIN ase)

**Pharmacologic Class** Thrombolytic Agent

**U.S. Brand Names** Abbokinase® Injection

**Mechanism of Action** Promotes thrombolysis by directly activating plasminogen to plasmin, which degrades fibrin, fibrinogen, and other procoagulant plasma proteins

**Use** Thrombolytic agent used in treatment of recent severe or massive deep vein thrombosis, pulmonary emboli, myocardial infarction, and occluded arteriovenous cannulas; not useful on thrombi over 1 week old

## USUAL DOSAGE

Children and Adults: Deep vein thrombosis: I.V.: Loading: 4400 units/kg over 10 minutes, then 4400 units/kg/hour for 12 hours

Adults:

Myocardial infarction: Intracoronary: 750,000 units over 2 hours (6000 units/minute over up to 2 hours)

Occluded I.V. catheters:

5000 units (use only Abbokinase® Open Cath) in each lumen over 1-2 minutes, leave in lumen for 1-4 hours, then aspirate; may repeat with 10,000 units in each lumen if 5000 units fails to clear the catheter; **do not infuse into the patient;** volume to instill into catheter is equal to the volume of the catheter

I.V. infusion: 200 units/kg/hour in each lumen for 12-48 hours at a rate of at least 20 mL/hour

Dialysis patients: 5000 units is administered in each lumen over 1-2 minutes; leave urokinase in lumen for 1-2 days, then aspirate

Clot lysis (large vessel thrombi): Loading: I.V.: 4400 units/kg over 10 minutes, increase to 6000 units/kg/hour; maintenance: 4400-6000 units/kg/hour adjusted to achieve clot lysis or patency of affected vessel; doses up to 50,000 units/kg/hour have been used.

**Note:** Therapy should be initiated as soon as possible after diagnosis of thrombi and continued until clot is dissolved (usually 24-72 hours).

Acute pulmonary embolism: Three treatment alternatives: 3 million unit dosage

Alternative 1: 12-hour infusion: 4400 units/kg (2000 units/lb) bolus over 10 minutes followed by 4400 units/kg/hour (2000 units/lb); begin heparin 1000 units/hour approximately 3-4 hours after completion of urokinase infusion or when PTT is <100 seconds

Alternative 2: 2-hour infusion: 1 million unit bolus over 10 minutes followed by 2 million units over 110 minutes; begin heparin 1000 units/hour approximately 3-4 hours after completion of urokinase infusion or when PTT is <100 seconds

Alternative 3: Bolus dose only: 15,000 units/kg over 10 minutes; begin heparin 1000 units/hour approximately 3-4 hours after completion of urokinase infusion or when PTT is <100 seconds

**Dosage Forms Powder for inj:** 250,000 units (5 mL); **Powder for inj, catheter clear:** 5000 units (1 mL)

**Contraindications** Active internal bleeding, history of a cerebrovascular accident, recent intracranial or intraspinal surgery (within prior two months), recent trauma including cardiopulmonary resuscitation, intracranial neoplasm, AV malformation or aneurysm, known bleeding diathesis, or severe uncontrolled arterial hypertension; hypersensitivity to urokinase or any component

**Warnings/Precautions** Use with caution in patients with recent (within 10 days) major surgery, obstetrical delivery, organ biopsy, previous puncture of noncompressible vessels, recent serious GI bleeding, high likelihood of left heart thrombus (eg, mitral stenosis with A-fib), subacute bacterial endocarditis, hemostatic defects including those secondary to severe hepatic or renal disease, pregnancy, cerebrovascular disease, diabetic hemorrhagic retinopathy, or any other condition in which bleeding might constitute a significant hazard or be particularly difficult to manage because of its location

The FDA is recommending (1/25/99) that Abbokinase® be reserved for only those situations where a physician has considered the alternatives and has determined that the use of urokinase is critical to the care of a specific patient in a specific situation; Abbokinase® is produced from primary cultures of kidney cells harvested postmortem from human neonates. Products manufactured from human source materials have the potential to transmit infectious agents. While some procedures to help control such risks in products of human source are in place, recent manufacturing inspections revealed deficiencies in some of the procedures used by Abbott and its supplier of the human neonatal kidney cells that could increase the risk of transmitting infectious agents. In considering this risk, the prescriber should be aware of the following information regarding currently available lots of urokinase; the kidney cells used in the manufacture of this product were harvested postmortem from human neonates from a population at high risk for a variety of infectious diseases, including tropical diseases. The screening of potential donors did not include the questioning of the mothers to determine infectious disease status or specific risk factors for infectious diseases; neither the mothers nor the neonate donors were tested for hepatitis C virus (HCV) infection; Abbott has recently instituted a test for HCV in the kidney cells used in the manufacture of Abbokinase® and negative test results have been obtained for currently available lots; however, Abbott has not validated this test; prior to use in the manufacture of Abbokinase®, the human kidney cells were harvested, stored and handled in a manner which may have permitted contamination with infectious agents; the FDA is not aware of any cases of infectious diseases that can be attributed to the use of Abbokinase®; however, the likelihood that cases of infectious diseases caused by Abbokinase®, if any, would have been recognized as such and reported to FDA is probably very low; therefore, the actual risk to patients of developing an infectious disease as a result of using Abbokinase® is unknown; for each setting in which the use of Abbokinase® is being contemplated, we encourage you to consider the appropriateness of other treatment options; FDA approved indications for Abbokinase® are: pulmonary embolism, coronary artery thrombosis, and I.V. catheter clearance; it should also be noted that the FDA has not approved the use of Abbokinase® for clearance of peripheral venous and arterial obstructions or for clearance of arterio-venous cannulas; other thrombolytic products on the U.S. market with well-described experience in multiple indications include Streptase® (Streptokinase), Kabikinase® (Streptokinase), Activase® (Alteplase), Eminase® (Anistreplase), and Retavase™ (Reteplase). We encourage all physicians to consider the appropriateness of other treatment options

**Pregnancy Risk Factor** B

**Adverse Reactions**

>10%:

Cardiovascular: Hypotension, arrhythmias

Hematologic: Bleeding, especially at sites of percutaneous trauma

Ocular: Periorbital swelling

Respiratory: Dyspnea

<1%: Headache, chills, rash, nausea, vomiting, anemia, eye hemorrhage, bronchospasm, epistaxis, diaphoresis, anaphylaxis

**Drug Interactions** Increased toxicity (increased bleeding) with anticoagulants, antiplatelet drugs, aspirin, indomethacin, dextran

**Onset** I.V.: Fibrinolysis occurs rapidly

(Continued)

## Urokinase *(Continued)*

**Duration** 4 or more hours

**Half-Life** 10-20 minutes

**Special PA Issues**

**Patient Education:** You will require frequent blood tests. Report any signs of unusual bleeding. Use electric razor and soft toothbrush.

**Monitoring Parameters:** CBC, reticulocyte count, platelet count, DIC panel (fibrinogen, plasminogen, FDP, D-dimer, PT, PTT), thrombosis panel (AT-III, protein C), urinalysis, ACT

♦ **Uro-KP-Neutral®** *see* Potassium Phosphate and Sodium Phosphate *on page 747*

♦ **Urolene Blue®** *see* Methylene Blue *on page 591*

♦ **Urozide®** *see* Hydrochlorothiazide *on page 447*

♦ **Ursodeoxycholic Acid** *see* Ursodiol *on this page*

## Ursodiol *(ER soe dye ole)*

**Pharmacologic Class** Gallstone Dissolution Agent

**U.S. Brand Names** Actigall™

**Mechanism of Action** Decreases the cholesterol content of bile and bile stones by reducing the secretion of cholesterol from the liver and the fractional reabsorption of cholesterol by the intestines

**Use** Gallbladder stone dissolution

**USUAL DOSAGE** Adults: Oral: 8-10 mg/kg/day in 2-3 divided doses; use beyond 24 months is not established; obtain ultrasound images at 6-month intervals for the first year of therapy; 30% of patients have stone recurrence after dissolution

**Dosage Forms Cap:** 300 mg

**Contraindications** Not to be used with cholesterol, radiopaque, bile pigment stones, or stones >20 mm in diameter; allergy to bile acids

**Warnings/Precautions** Gallbladder stone dissolution may take several months of therapy; complete dissolution may not occur and recurrence of stones within 5 years has been observed in 50% of patients; use with caution in patients with a nonvisualizing gallbladder and those with chronic liver disease; not recommended for children

**Pregnancy Risk Factor** B

**Adverse Reactions**

1% to 10%: Gastrointestinal: Diarrhea

<1%: Fatigue, headache, pruritus, rash, nausea, vomiting, dyspepsia, metallic taste, abdominal pain, biliary pain, constipation

**Drug Interactions** Decreased effect with aluminum-containing antacids, cholestyramine, colestipol, clofibrate, oral contraceptives (estrogens)

**Half-Life** 100 hours

**Special PA Issues**

**Patient Education:** Frequent blood work will be necessary to follow drug effects. Drug will need to be taken for 1-3 months after stone is dissolved. Stones may recur. Report any persistent nausea, vomiting, abdominal pain, or yellowing of skin or eyes.

**Monitoring Parameters:** ALT, AST, sonogram

♦ **Uvadex®** *see* Methoxsalen *on page 589*

♦ **Vagilia®** *see* Sulfabenzamide, Sulfacetamide, and Sulfathiazole *on page 857*

♦ **Vagistat® Vaginal** *see* Tioconazole *on page 906*

♦ **Vagitrol®** *see* Sulfanilamide *on page 862*

## Valacyclovir *(val ay SYE kloe veer)*

**Pharmacologic Class** Antiviral Agent, Ophthalmic

**U.S. Brand Names** Valtrex®

**Mechanism of Action** Valacyclovir is rapidly and nearly completely converted to acyclovir by intestinal and hepatic metabolism. Acyclovir is converted to acyclovir monophosphate by virus-specific thymidine kinase then further converted to acyclovir triphosphate by other cellular enzymes. Acyclovir triphosphate inhibits DNA synthesis and viral replication by competing with deoxyguanosine triphosphate for viral DNA polymerase and being incorporated into viral DNA.

**Use** Treatment of herpes zoster (shingles) in immunocompetent patients; episodic treatment or prophylaxis of recurrent genital herpes in immunocompetent patients; for first episode genital herpes

**USUAL DOSAGE** Oral: Adults:

Shingles: 1 g 3 times/day for 7 days

Genital herpes:

Episodic treatment: 500 mg twice daily for 5 days

Prophylaxis: 500-1000 mg once daily

**Dosing interval in renal impairment:**

$Cl_{cr}$ 30-49 mL/minute: 1 g every 12 hours

$Cl_{cr}$ 10-29 mL/minute: 1 g every 24 hours

$Cl_{cr}$ <10 mL/minute: 500 mg every 24 hours

Hemodialysis: 33% removed during 4-hour session

**Dosage Forms Caplet:** 500 mg

**Contraindications** Hypersensitivity to the drug or any component

**Warnings/Precautions** Thrombotic thrombocytopenic purpura/hemolytic uremic syndrome has occurred in immunocompromised patients; use caution and adjust the dose in elderly patients or those with renal insufficiency; safety and efficacy in children have not been established

**Pregnancy Risk Factor** B

**Pregnancy Implications**

Clinical effects on the fetus: Teratogenicity registry, thus far, has shown no increased rate of birth defects than that of the general population; however, the registry is small and use during pregnancy is only warranted if the potential benefit to the mother justifies the risk of the fetus

Breast-feeding/lactation: Avoid use in breast-feeding, if possible, since the drug distributes in high concentrations in breast milk

**Adverse Reactions**

>10%:

Central nervous system: Headache (13% to 17%)

Gastrointestinal: Nausea (8% to 16%)

1% to 10%:

Central nervous system: Dizziness (2% to 4%)

Dermatologic: Pruritus

Gastrointestinal: Diarrhea (4% to 5%), constipation (1% to 5%), abdominal pain (2% to 3%), anorexia (≤3%), vomiting (≤7%)

Neuromuscular & skeletal: Weakness (2% to 4%)

Ocular: Photophobia

**Drug Interactions** Decreased toxicity: Cimetidine and/or probenecid has decreased the rate but not the extent of valacyclovir conversion to acyclovir

**Half-Life**

Normal renal function: 2.5-3.3 hours (acyclovir); ~30 minutes (valacyclovir)

End-stage renal disease: 14 hours removed partially by hemodialysis, half-life during dialysis: 4 hours; liver disease may decrease rate but not extent of conversion to acyclovir (half-life not affected)

**Special PA Issues**

Patient Education: Begin use as soon as possible following development of signs of herpes zoster. Take with plenty of fluids. May take without regard to meals.

Monitoring Parameters: Urinalysis, BUN, serum creatinine, liver enzymes, and CBC

♦ **Valergen® Injection** see Estradiol on page 332

# Valerian

**Mechanism of Action** Most pharmacologic activity located in fresh root or dried rhizome; the plant contains essential oils (valerenic acid and valenol, valepotriates, and alkaloids <0.2% concentration) which may affect neurotransmitter levels (serotonin, GABA, and norepinephrine); also has antispasmodic properties

**Use** Herbal medicine use as a sleep-promoting agent and minor tranquilizer (similar to benzodiazepines); used in anxiety, panic attacks, intestinal cramps, headaches

Per Commission E: Restlessness, sleep disorders based on nervous conditions

**USUAL DOSAGE** Adults:

Sedative: 1-3 g (1-3 mL of tincture)

Sleep aid: 1-3 mL of tincture at bedtime

Dried root: 0.3-1 g

**Adverse Reactions**

Cardiovascular: Cardiac disturbances (unspecified)

Central nervous system: Lightheadedness, restlessness, fatigue

Gastrointestinal: Nausea

Neuromuscular & skeletal: Tremor

Ocular: Blurred vision

**Drug Interactions** Not synergistic with alcohol; potentiation of other CNS depressants is possible

♦ *Valeriana edulis* see Valerian on this page
♦ *Valeriana wallichi* see Valerian on this page
♦ **Valertest No.1® Injection** see Estradiol and Testosterone on page 334
♦ **Valisone®** see Betamethasone on page 111
♦ **Valium® Injection** see Diazepam on page 269
♦ **Valium® Oral** see Diazepam on page 269
♦ **Valpin® 50** see Anisotropine on page 70
♦ **Valproate Semisodium** see Valproic Acid and Derivatives on next page
♦ **Valproate Sodium** see Valproic Acid and Derivatives on next page
♦ **Valproic Acid** see Valproic Acid and Derivatives on next page

## Valproic Acid and Derivatives (val PROE ik AS id & dah RIV ah tives)

**Pharmacologic Class** Anticonvulsant, Miscellaneous

**U.S. Brand Names** Depacon®; Depakene®; Depakote®

**Mechanism of Action** Causes increased availability of gamma-aminobutyric acid (GABA), an inhibitory neurotransmitter, to brain neurons or may enhance the action of GABA or mimic its action at postsynaptic receptor sites

**Use** Management of simple and complex absence seizures; mixed seizure types; myoclonic and generalized tonic-clonic (grand mal) seizures; may be effective in partial seizures, infantile spasms, bipolar disorder; prevention of migraine headaches

**USUAL DOSAGE** Children and Adults:

Oral: Initial: 10-15 mg/kg/day in 1-3 divided doses; increase by 5-10 mg/kg/day at weekly intervals until therapeutic levels are achieved; maintenance: 30-60 mg/kg/day in 2-3 divided doses

Children receiving more than 1 anticonvulsant (ie, polytherapy) may require doses up to 100 mg/kg/day in 3-4 divided doses

I.V.: Administer as a 60 minute infusion (≤20 mg/min) with the same frequency as oral products; switch patient to oral products as soon as possible

Rectal: Dilute syrup 1:1 with water for use as a retention enema; loading dose: 17-20 mg/kg one time; maintenance: 10-15 mg/kg/dose every 8 hours

Not dialyzable (0% to 5%)

**Dosing adjustment/comments in hepatic impairment:** Reduce dose

**Dosage Forms** Divalproex sodium: **Cap, sprinkle (Depakote® Sprinkle®):** 125 mg; **Tab, delayed release, as divalproex sodium (Depakote®):** 125 mg, 250 mg, 500 mg;

Valproic acid: **Cap (Depakene®):** 250 mg

Valproate sodium: **Inj (Depacon®):** 100 mg/mL (5 mL); **Syr (Depakene®):** 250 mg/5 mL (5 mL, 50 mL, 480 mL)

**Contraindications** Hypersensitivity to valproic acid or derivatives or any component; hepatic dysfunction

**Warnings/Precautions** Hepatic failure resulting in fatalities has occurred in patients; children <2 years of age are at considerable risk; monitor patients closely for appearance of malaise, weakness, facial edema, anorexia, jaundice, and vomiting; may cause severe thrombocytopenia, bleeding; hepatotoxicity has been reported after 3 days to 6 months of therapy; tremors may indicate overdosage; use with caution in patients receiving other anticonvulsants

**Pregnancy Risk Factor** D

**Pregnancy Implications**

Clinical effects on the fetus: Crosses the placenta. Neural tube, cardiac, facial (characteristic pattern of dysmorphic facial features), skeletal, multiple other defects reported. Epilepsy itself, number of medications, genetic factors, or a combination of these probably influence the teratogenicity of anticonvulsant therapy. Risk of neural tube defects with use during first 30 days of pregnancy warrants discontinuation prior to pregnancy and through this period of possible.

Breast-feeding/lactation: Crosses into breast milk. American Academy of Pediatrics considers compatible with breast-feeding.

**Adverse Reactions**

1% to 10%:

Endocrine & metabolic: Change in menstrual cycle

Gastrointestinal: Abdominal cramps, anorexia, diarrhea, nausea, vomiting, weight gain

<1%: Drowsiness, ataxia, irritability, confusion, restlessness, hyperactivity, headache, malaise, alopecia, erythema multiforme, hyperammonemia, pancreatitis, thrombocytopenia, prolongation of bleeding time, transient increased liver enzymes, liver failure, tremor, nystagmus, spots before eyes

**Drug Interactions** CYP2C19 enzyme substrate; CYP2C9 and 2D6 enzyme inhibitor, CYP3A3/4 enzyme inhibitor (weak)

Decreased effects of phenytoin

Decreased effects with carbamazepine, lamotrigine, possibly clonazepam (increased absence seizures have been reported)

Increased effects/toxicity of diazepam, CNS depressants, alcohol

Increased effects/toxicity with aspirin (increase valproic acid levels)

**Half-Life** 8-17 hours

**Special PA Issues**

**Patient Education:** When used to treat generalized seizures, patient instructions are determined by patient's condition and ability to understand.

Oral: Take as directed; do not alter dose or timing of medication. Do not increase dose or take more than recommended. Do not crush or chew capsule or enteric-coated pill. While using this medication, do not use alcohol and other prescription or OTC medications (especially pain medications, sedatives, antihistamines, or hypnotics) without consulting prescriber. Maintain adequate hydration (2-3 L/day of fluids unless instructed to restrict fluid intake). Diabetics should monitor serum glucose closely (valproic acid will alter results of urine ketones). Report alterations in menstrual cycle; abdominal cramps, unresolved diarrhea, vomiting, or constipation; skin rash; unusual bruising or bleeding; blood in urine, stool or vomitus; malaise; weakness; facial swelling; yellowing of skin or eyes; excessive sedation; or restlessness.

**Dietary Considerations:**

Alcohol: Additive CNS depression, avoid or limit alcohol

Food:

Valproic acid may cause GI upset; take with large amount of water or food to decrease GI upset. May need to split doses to avoid GI upset.

Food may delay but does not affect the extent of absorption

Coated particles of divalproex sodium may be mixed with semisolid food (eg, apple-sauce or pudding) in patients having difficulty swallowing; particles should be swallowed and not chewed

Valproate sodium oral solution will generate valproic acid in carbonated beverages and may cause mouth and throat irritation; do not mix valproate sodium oral solution with carbonated beverages

Milk: No effect on absorption; may take with milk

Sodium: SIADH and water intoxication; monitor fluid status. May need to restrict fluid.

**Monitoring Parameters:** Liver enzymes, CBC with platelets

**Reference Range:** Therapeutic: 50-100 µg/mL (SI: 350-690 µmol/L); Toxic: >200 µg/mL (SI: >1390 µmol/L). Seizure control may improve at levels >100 µg/mL (SI: 690 µmol/L), but toxicity may occur at levels of 100-150 µg/mL (SI: 690-1040 µmol/L).

# Valsartan (val SAR tan)

**Pharmacologic Class** Angiotensin II Antagonists

**U.S. Brand Names** Diovan™

**Mechanism of Action** As a prodrug, valsartan produces direct antagonism of the angiotensin II (AT2) receptors, unlike the angiotensin-converting enzyme inhibitors. It displaces angiotensin II from the AT1 receptor and produces its blood pressure lowering effects by antagonizing AT1-induced vasoconstriction, aldosterone release, catecholamine release, arginine vasopressin release, water intake, and hypertrophic responses. This action results in more efficient blockade of the cardiovascular effects of angiotensin II and fewer side effects than the ACE inhibitors.

**Use** Alone or in combination with other antihypertensive agents in treating essential hypertension; may have an advantage over losartan due to minimal metabolism requirements and consequent use in mild to moderate hepatic impairment

**USUAL DOSAGE** Adults: 80 mg/day; may be increased to 160 mg if needed (maximal effects observed in 4-6 weeks)

**Dosing adjustment in renal impairment:** No dosage adjustment necessary if $Cl_{cr}$ >10 mL/minute

**Dosing adjustment in hepatic impairment** (mild - moderate): ≤80 mg/day

Dialysis: Not significantly removed

**Dosage Forms Cap:** 80 mg, 160 mg

**Contraindications** Hypersensitivity to valsartan or any components, pregnancy, severe hepatic insufficiency, biliary cirrhosis or biliary obstruction, primary hyperaldosteronism, bilateral renal artery stenosis

**Warnings/Precautions** Use extreme caution with concurrent administration of potassium-sparing diuretics or potassium supplements, in patients with mild to moderate hepatic dysfunction (adjust dose), in those who may be sodium/water depleted (eg, on high-dose diuretics), and in the elderly; avoid use in patients with congestive heart failure, unilateral renal artery stenosis, aortic/mitral valve stenosis, coronary artery disease, or hypertrophic cardiomyopathy, if possible

**Pregnancy Risk Factor** C (1st trimester); D (2nd and 3rd trimesters)

**Pregnancy Implications** Breast-feeding/lactation: Although no human data exist, valsartan is known to be excreted in animal breast milk and should be avoided in lactating mothers if possible

**Adverse Reactions** Similar incidence to placebo; independent of race, age, and gender

>1%:

Central nervous system: Headache, dizziness, drowsiness, ataxia

Endocrine & metabolic: Decreased libido

Gastrointestinal: Diarrhea, abdominal pain, nausea, abnormal taste

Genitourinary: Polyuria

Hematologic: Neutropenia

Hepatic: Increased LFTs

Neuromuscular & skeletal: Arthralgia

Respiratory: Cough, upper respiratory infection, rhinitis, sinusitis, pharyngitis

<1%: Anemia, increased Cr

**Drug Interactions**

Decreased effect: Phenobarbital, ketoconazole, troleandomycin, sulfaphenazole

Increased effect: Cimetidine, moxonidine

**Half-Life** 9 hours

(Continued)

## Valsartan *(Continued)*

### Special PA Issues

**Patient Education:** Take as directed; do not change dosage or stop taking without consulting prescriber. Follow prescribed dietary regimen. You may experience dizziness, fainting, or lightheadedness (use caution when driving or performing hazardous tasks and use caution when changing position - rising from sitting or lying) until response to therapy is established. You may experience decreased libido and some arthralgia. Report immediately any swelling of face, lips, throat, tongue, or difficulty breathing. Report sore throat; fever; rash; swelling of hands, feet, or legs; respiratory difficulty; chest pains or irregular heartbeat; unusual cough; persistent vomiting, diarrhea, sweating, or perspiration; or flu-like symptoms.

**Monitoring Parameters:** Baseline and periodic electrolyte panels, renal and liver function tests, urinalysis; symptoms of hypotension or hypersensivity

## Valsartan and Hydrochlorothiazide

(val SAR tan & hye droe klor oh THYE a zide)

**Pharmacologic Class** Antihypertensive Agent, Combination

**U.S. Brand Names** Diovan™ HCT

**Dosage Forms Tab:** Valsartan 80 mg and hydrochlorothiazide 12.5 mg; valsartan 160 mg and hydrochlorothiazide 12.5 mg

♦ **Valtrex®** *see* Valacyclovir *on page 950*

♦ **Vamate®** *see* Hydroxyzine *on page 462*

♦ **Vancenase® AQ Inhaler** *see* Beclomethasone *on page 101*

♦ **Vancenase® Nasal Inhaler** *see* Beclomethasone *on page 101*

♦ **Vanceril® Oral Inhaler** *see* Beclomethasone *on page 101*

♦ **Vancocin®** *see* Vancomycin *on this page*

♦ **Vancocin® CP** *see* Vancomycin *on this page*

♦ **Vancoled®** *see* Vancomycin *on this page*

## Vancomycin (van koe MYE sin)

**Pharmacologic Class** Antibiotic, Miscellaneous

**U.S. Brand Names** Lyphocin®; Vancocin®; Vancoled®

**Mechanism of Action** Inhibits bacterial cell wall synthesis by blocking glycopeptide polymerization through binding tightly to D-alanyl-D-alanine portion of cell wall precursor

**Use** Treatment of patients with infections caused by staphylococcal species and streptococcal species; used orally for staphylococcal enterocolitis or for antibiotic-associated pseudomembranous colitis produced by *C. difficile*

**USUAL DOSAGE** Initial dosage recommendation: I.V.:

Neonates:

Postnatal age ≤7 days:

<1200 g: 15 mg/kg/dose every 24 hours

1200-2000 g: 10 mg/kg/dose every 12 hours

>2000 g: 15 mg/kg/dose every 12 hours

Postnatal age >7 days:

<1200 g: 15 mg/kg/dose every 24 hours

≥1200 g: 10 mg/kg/dose divided every 8 hours

Infants >1 month and Children:

40 mg/kg/day in divided doses every 6 hours

Prophylaxis for bacterial endocarditis:

Dental, oral, or upper respiratory tract surgery: 20 mg/kg 1 hour prior to the procedure

GI/GU procedure: 20 mg/kg plus gentamicin 2 mg/kg 1 hour prior to surgery

Infants >1 month and Children with staphylococcal central nervous system infection: 60 mg/kg/day in divided doses every 6 hours

Adults:

With normal renal function: 1 g **or** 10-15 mg/kg/dose every 12 hours

Prophylaxis for bacterial endocarditis:

Dental, oral, or upper respiratory tract surgery: 1 g 1 hour before surgery

GI/GU procedure: 1 g plus 1.5 mg/kg gentamicin 1 hour prior to surgery

**Dosing interval in renal impairment (vancomycin levels should be monitored in patients with any renal impairment):**

$Cl_{cr}$ >60 mL/minute: Start with 1 g or 10-15 mg/kg/dose every 12 hours

$Cl_{cr}$ 40-60 mL/minute: Start with 1 g or 10-15 mg/kg/dose every 24 hours

$Cl_{cr}$ <40 mL/minute: Will need longer intervals; determine by serum concentration monitoring

Hemodialysis: Not dialyzable (0% to 5%); generally not removed; exception minimal-moderate removal by some of the newer high-flux filters; dose may need to be administered more frequently; monitor serum concentrations

Continuous ambulatory peritoneal dialysis (CAPD): Not significantly removed; administration via CAPD fluid: 15-30 mg/L (15-30 mcg/mL) of CAPD fluid

Continuous arteriovenous hemofiltration: Dose similar to $Cl_{cr}$ of approximately 10-15 mL/minute

**Antibiotic lock technique (for catheter infections):** 2 mg/mL in SWI/NS or $D_5W$; instill 3-5 mL into catheter port as a flush solution instead of heparin lock (**Note:** Do not mix with any other solutions)

**Intrathecal:** Vancomycin is available as a powder for injection and may be diluted to 1-5 mg/mL concentration in preservative-free 0.9% sodium chloride for administration into the CSF

Neonates: 5-10 mg/day

Children: 5-20 mg/day

Adults: Up to 20 mg/day

Oral: Pseudomembranous colitis produced by *C. difficile*:

Neonates: 10 mg/kg/day in divided doses

Children: 40 mg/kg/day in divided doses, added to fluids

Adults: 125 mg 4 times/day for 10 days

**Dosage Forms Cap:** 125 mg, 250 mg; **Powder for oral soln:** 1 g, 10 g; **Powder for inj:** 500 mg, 1 g, 2 g, 5 g, 10 g

**Contraindications** Hypersensitivity to vancomycin or any component; avoid in patients with previous severe hearing loss

**Warnings/Precautions** Use with caution in patients with renal impairment or those receiving other nephrotoxic or ototoxic drugs; dosage modification required in patients with impaired renal function (especially elderly)

**Pregnancy Risk Factor** C

**Adverse Reactions**

Oral:

>10%: Gastrointestinal: Bitter taste, nausea, vomiting

1% to 10%:

Central nervous system: Chills, drug fever

Hematologic: Eosinophilia

<1%: Vasculitis, thrombocytopenia, ototoxicity, renal failure, interstitial nephritis

Parenteral:

>10%:

Cardiovascular: Hypotension accompanied by flushing

Dermatologic: Erythematous rash on face and upper body (red neck or red man syndrome - infusion rate related)

1% to 10%:

Central nervous system: Chills, drug fever

Dermatologic: Rash

Hematologic: Eosinophilia, reversible neutropenia

<1%: Vasculitis, Stevens-Johnson syndrome, ototoxicity (especially with large doses), thrombocytopenia, renal failure (especially with renal dysfunction or pre-existing hearing loss)

**Drug Interactions** Increased toxicity: Anesthetic agents; other ototoxic or nephrotoxic agents

**Half-Life** Half-life (biphasic): Terminal: Adults: 5-11 hours, prolonged significantly with reduced renal function; End-stage renal disease: 200-250 hours

**Special PA Issues**

**Patient Education:** Complete full course of therapy. Report pain at infusion site, decrease in urine output, sudden weight gain, dizziness, fullness or ringing in ears with I.V. use. Nausea or vomiting with oral use.

**Monitoring Parameters:** Periodic renal function tests, urinalysis, serum vancomycin concentrations, WBC, audiogram

**Reference Range:**

Timing of serum samples: Draw peak 1 hour after 1-hour infusion has completed; draw trough just before next dose

Therapeutic levels: Peak: 25-40 µg/mL; Trough: 5-12 µg/mL

Toxic: >80 µg/mL (SI: >54 µmol/L)

♦ **Vancomycin Hydrochloride** *see* Vancomycin *on previous page*

♦ **Vanoxide-HC®** *see* Benzoyl Peroxide and Hydrocortisone *on page 107*

♦ **Vansil™** *see* Oxamniquine *on page 682*

♦ **Vantin®** *see* Cefpodoxime *on page 170*

♦ **Vapocet®** *see* Hydrocodone and Acetaminophen *on page 449*

♦ **Vapo-Iso®** *see* Isoproterenol *on page 496*

# Varicella-Zoster Immune Globulin (Human)

(var i SEL a- ZOS ter i MYUN GLOB yoo lin HYU man)

**Pharmacologic Class** Immune Globulin

**Mechanism of Action** The exact mechanism has not been clarified but the antibodies in varicella-zoster immune globulin most likely neutralize the varicella-zoster virus and prevent its pathological actions

(Continued)

## Varicella-Zoster Immune Globulin (Human) *(Continued)*

**Use** Passive immunization of susceptible immunodeficient patients after exposure to varicella; most effective if begun within 96 hours of exposure; there is no evidence VZIG modifies established varicella-zoster infections.

### Restrict administration to those patients meeting the following criteria:

Neoplastic disease (eg, leukemia or lymphoma)

Congenital or acquired immunodeficiency

Immunosuppressive therapy with steroids, antimetabolites or other immunosuppressive treatment regimens

Newborn of mother who had onset of chickenpox within 5 days before delivery or within 48 hours after delivery

Premature (≥28 weeks gestation) whose mother has no history of chickenpox

Premature (<28 weeks gestation or ≤1000 g VZIG) regardless of maternal history

### One of the following types of exposure to chickenpox or zoster patient(s) may warrant administration:

Continuous household contact

Playmate contact (>1 hour play indoors)

Hospital contact (in same 2-4 bedroom or adjacent beds in a large ward or prolonged face-to-face contact with an infectious staff member or patient)

Susceptible to varicella-zoster

Age <15 years; administer to immunocompromised adolescents and adults and to other older patients on an individual basis

An acceptable alternative to VZIG prophylaxis is to treat varicella, if it occurs, with high-dose I.V. acyclovir

Age is the most important risk factor for reactivation of varicella zoster; persons <50 years of age have incidence of 2.5 cases per 1000, whereas those 60-79 have 6.5 cases per 1000 and those >80 years have 10 cases per 1000

**USUAL DOSAGE** High risk susceptible patients who are exposed again more than 3 weeks after a prior dose of VZIG should receive another full dose; there is no evidence VZIG modifies established varicella-zoster infections.

I.M.: Administer by deep injection in the gluteal muscle or in another large muscle mass. Inject 125 units/10 kg (22 lb); maximum dose: 625 units (5 vials); minimum dose: 125 units; do not administer fractional doses. Do not inject I.V. See table.

### VZIG Dose Based on Weight

| Weight of Patient | | Dose | |
|---|---|---|---|
| kg | lb | Units | No. of Vials |
| 0-10 | 0-22 | 125 | 1 |
| 10.1-20 | 22.1-44 | 250 | 2 |
| 20.1-30 | 44.1-66 | 375 | 3 |
| 30.1-40 | 66.1-88 | 500 | 4 |
| >40 | >88 | 625 | 5 |

**Dosage Forms Inj:** 125 units of antibody in single dose vials

**Contraindications Not** for prophylactic use in immunodeficient patients with history of varicella, unless patient's immunosuppression is associated with bone marrow transplantation; **not** recommended for nonimmunodeficient patients, including pregnant women, because the severity of chickenpox is much less than in immunosuppressed patients; allergic response to gamma globulin or anti-immunoglobulin; sensitivity to thimerosal; persons with IgA deficiency; do not administer to patients with thrombocytopenia or coagulopathies

**Warnings/Precautions** VZIG is not indicated for prophylaxis or therapy of normal adults who are exposed to or who develop varicella; it is not indicated for treatment of herpes zoster. Do not inject I.V.

**Pregnancy Risk Factor** C

### Adverse Reactions

1% to 10%: Local: Discomfort at the site of injection (pain, redness, edema)

<1%: Malaise, headache, rash, angioedema, GI symptoms, respiratory symptom, anaphylactic shock

**Drug Interactions** Decreased effect: Live virus vaccines (do not administer within 3 months of immune globulin administration)

♦ **Vascor®** *see* Bepridil *on page 109*

♦ **Vaseretic® 10-25** *see* Enalapril and Hydrochlorothiazide *on page 318*

♦ **Vasocidin® Ophthalmic** *see* Sulfacetamide Sodium and Prednisolone *on page 859*

♦ **VasoClear® [OTC]** *see* Naphazoline *on page 635*

♦ **Vasocon Regular®** *see* Naphazoline *on page 635*

## Vasopressin (vay soe PRES in)

**Pharmacologic Class** Antidiuretic Hormone Analog; Hormone, Posterior Pituitary

**U.S. Brand Names** Pitressin® Injection

**Mechanism of Action** Increases cyclic adenosine monophosphate (cAMP) which increases water permeability at the renal tubule resulting in decreased urine volume and increased osmolality; causes peristalsis by directly stimulating the smooth muscle in the GI tract

**Use** Treatment of diabetes insipidus; prevention and treatment of postoperative abdominal distention; differential diagnosis of diabetes insipidus

**Unlabeled use:** Adjunct in the treatment of GI hemorrhage and esophageal varices

**USUAL DOSAGE**

Diabetes insipidus (highly variable dosage; titrated based on serum and urine sodium and osmolality in addition to fluid balance and urine output):

I.M., S.C.:

Children: 2.5-10 units 2-4 times/day as needed

Adults: 5-10 units 2-4 times/day as needed (dosage range 5-60 units/day)

Continuous I.V. infusion: Children and Adults: 0.5 milliunit/kg/hour (0.0005 unit/kg/hour); double dosage as needed every 30 minutes to a maximum of 0.01 unit/kg/hour

Intranasal: Administer on cotton pledget or nasal spray

Abdominal distention (aqueous): Adults: I.M.: 5 mg stat, 10 mg every 3-4 hours

GI hemorrhage: I.V. infusion: Dilute aqueous in NS or $D_5W$ to 0.1-1 unit/mL

Children: Initial: 0.002-0.005 units/kg/minute; titrate dose as needed; maximum: 0.01 unit/kg/minute; continue at same dosage (if bleeding stops) for 12 hours, then taper off over 24-48 hours

Adults: Initial: 0.2-0.4 unit/minute, then titrate dose as needed, if bleeding stops; continue at same dose for 12 hours, taper off over 24-48 hours

**Dosing adjustment in hepatic impairment:** Some patients respond to much lower doses with cirrhosis

**Dosage Forms Inj, aqueous:** 20 pressor units/mL (0.5 mL, 1 mL)

**Contraindications** Hypersensitivity to vasopressin or any component

**Warnings/Precautions** Use with caution in patients with seizure disorders, migraine, asthma, vascular disease, renal disease, cardiac disease; chronic nephritis with nitrogen retention. Goiter with cardiac complications, arteriosclerosis; I.V. infiltration may lead to severe vasoconstriction and localized tissue necrosis; also, gangrene of extremities, tongue, and ischemic colitis. Elderly patients should be cautioned not to increase their fluid intake beyond that sufficient to satisfy their thirst in order to avoid water intoxication and hyponatremia; under experimental conditions, the elderly have shown to have a decreased responsiveness to vasopressin with respect to its effects on water homeostasis

**Pregnancy Risk Factor** B

**Adverse Reactions**

1% to 10%:

Cardiovascular: Increased blood pressure, bradycardia, arrhythmias, venous thrombosis, vasoconstriction with higher doses, angina

Central nervous system: Pounding in the head, fever, vertigo

Dermatologic: Urticaria, circumoral pallor

Gastrointestinal: Flatulence, abdominal cramps, nausea, vomiting

Neuromuscular & skeletal: Tremor

Miscellaneous: Diaphoresis

<1%: Myocardial infarction, water intoxication, allergic reaction

**Drug Interactions**

Decreased effect: Lithium, epinephrine, demeclocycline, heparin, and alcohol block antidiuretic activity to varying degrees

Increased effect: Chlorpropamide, phenformin, urea and fludrocortisone potentiate antidiuretic response

**Onset** Nasal: 1 hour

**Duration** Nasal: 3-8 hours; Parenteral: I.M., S.C.: 2-8 hours

**Half-Life** Nasal: 15 minutes; Parenteral: 10-20 minutes

**Special PA Issues**

Patient Education: Side effects such as abdominal cramps and nausea may be reduced by drinking a glass of water with each dose. Avoid alcohol use.

Monitoring Parameters: Serum and urine sodium, urine output, fluid input and output, urine specific gravity, urine and serum osmolality

Reference Range: Plasma: 0-2 pg/mL (SI: 0-2 ng/L) if osmolality <285 mOsm/L; 2-12 pg/mL (SI: 2-12 ng/L) if osmolality >290 mOsm/L

♦ **Vasopressin Tannate** see Vasopressin on this page

♦ **Vasosulf® Ophthalmic** see Sulfacetamide Sodium and Phenylephrine on page 859

♦ **Vasotec®** see Enalapril on page 316

♦ **Vasotec® I.V.** see Enalapril on page 316

♦ **Vasoxyl®** see Methoxamine on page 589

♦ **V-Cillin K®** see Penicillin V Potassium on page 706

- ♦ **Veetids®** see Penicillin V Potassium on page 706
- ♦ **Velosef®** see Cephradine on page 181
- ♦ **Velosulin® Human** see Insulin Preparations on page 479
- ♦ **Velvelan®** see Urea on page 947

# Venlafaxine (VEN la faks een)

**Pharmacologic Class** Antidepressant, Serotonin/Norepinephrine Reuptake Inhibitor

**U.S. Brand Names** Effexor®; Effexor® XR

**Mechanism of Action** Venlafaxine and its active metabolite o-desmethylvenlafaxine (ODV) are potent inhibitors of neuronal serotonin and norepinephrine reuptake and weak inhibitors of dopamine reuptake; causes beta-receptor down regulation and reduces adenylcyclase coupled beta-adrenergic systems in the brain

**Use** Treatment of depression in adults

**Unapproved use:** Obsessive-compulsive disorder

**USUAL DOSAGE** Adults: Oral:

Immediate-release tablets: 75 mg/day, administered in 2 or 3 divided doses, taken with food; dose may be increased in 75 mg/day increments at intervals of at least 4 days, up to 225-375 mg/day

Extended-release capsules: 75 mg once daily taken with food; for some new patients, it may be desirable to start at 37.5 mg/day for 4-7 days before increasing to 75 mg once daily; dose may be increased by up to 75 mg/day increments every 4 days as tolerated, up to a maximum of 225 mg/day

**Dosing adjustment in renal impairment:** Cl$_{cr}$ 10-70 mL/minute: Decrease dose by 25%; decrease total daily dose by 50% if dialysis patients; dialysis patients should receive dosing after completion of dialysis

**Dosing adjustment in moderate hepatic impairment:** Reduce total daily dosage by 50%

**Dosage Forms Tab:** 25 mg, 37.5 mg, 50 mg, 75 mg, 100 mg

**Contraindications** Do not use concomitantly with MAO inhibitors, contraindicated in patients with hypersensitivity to venlafaxine or other components

**Warnings/Precautions** Venlafaxine is associated with sustained increases in blood pressure (10-15 mm Hg SDBP); venlafaxine may actuate mania or hypomania and seizures. Concurrent therapy with a monoamine oxidase inhibitor may result in serious or fatal reactions; at least 14 days should elapse between treatment with an MAO inhibitor and venlafaxine. Patients with cardiovascular disorders or a recent myocardial infarction probably should only receive venlafaxine if the benefits of therapy outweigh the risks.

**Pregnancy Risk Factor** C

**Adverse Reactions**

≥10%:

Central nervous system: Headache, somnolence, dizziness, insomnia, nervousness

Gastrointestinal: Nausea, xerostomia, constipation

Genitourinary: Abnormal ejaculation

Neuromuscular & skeletal: Weakness, neck pain

Miscellaneous: Diaphoresis

1% to 10%:

Cardiovascular: Palpitations, hypertension, sinus tachycardia

Central nervous system: Anxiety

Gastrointestinal: Weight loss, anorexia, vomiting, diarrhea, dysphagia

Genitourinary: Impotence

Neuromuscular & skeletal: Tremor

Ocular: Blurred vision

<1%: Seizures, ear pain

**Drug Interactions** CYP2D6, 2E1, and 3A3/4 enzyme substrate; CYP2D6 enzyme inhibitor (weak)

Increased toxicity: Cimetidine MAO inhibitors (hyperpyrexic crisis); TCAs, fluoxetine, sertraline, phenothiazine, class 1C antiarrhythmics, warfarin; venlafaxine is a weak inhibitor of CYP2D6, which is responsible for metabolizing antipsychotics, antiarrhythmics, TCAs, and beta-blockers. Therefore, interactions with these agents are possible, however, less likely than with more potent enzyme inhibitors such as the SSRIs.

**Onset** Therapeutic effects: >2 weeks

**Half-Life** Active metabolite: 11-13 hours; Venlafaxine: 3-7 hours

**Special PA Issues**

**Patient Education:** Take exactly as directed (do not increase dose or frequency); may take 2-3 weeks to achieve desired results; may cause physical and/or psychological dependence. Take with food. Avoid excessive alcohol, caffeine, and other prescription or OTC medications not approved by prescriber. Maintain adequate hydration (2-3 L/day of fluids unless instructed to restrict fluid intake). You may experience excess drowsiness, lightheadedness, dizziness, or blurred vision (use caution when driving or engaging in hazardous tasks until response to medication is known); nausea, vomiting, anorexia, altered taste, dry mouth (small frequent meals, frequent mouth care, or sucking lozenges may help); constipation (increased exercise, fluids, or dietary fruit and fiber may help); diarrhea (buttermilk, yogurt, or boiled milk may help); postural hypotension (use caution when climbing stairs or changing position from lying or sitting to standing); urinary retention (void before taking medication); or sexual dysfunction (reversible). Report persistent CNS effects (eg, insomnia, restlessness, fatigue, anxiety, abnormal thoughts, confusion, personality changes, impaired cognitive function); muscle cramping or tremors; chest pain, palpitations, rapid heartbeat, swelling of extremities, or severe dizziness; unresolved urinary retention; vision changes or eye pain; hearing changes or ringing in ears; skin rash or irritation; or worsening of condition.

**Dietary Considerations:**
Alcohol: Additive CNS effect, avoid use
Food: May be taken without regard to food

**Monitoring Parameters:** Blood pressure should be regularly monitored, especially in patients with a high baseline blood pressure

**Reference Range:** Peak serum level of 163 ng/mL (325 ng/mL of ODV metabolite) obtained after a 150 mg oral dose

**Related Information**
Antidepressant Agents on page 998

♦ **Venoglobulin®-I** see Immune Globulin, Intravenous on page 472
♦ **Venoglobulin®-S** see Immune Globulin, Intravenous on page 472
♦ **Ventolin®** see Albuterol on page 34
♦ **Ventolin® Rotocaps®** see Albuterol on page 34

## Verapamil (ver AP a mil)

**Pharmacologic Class** Antiarrhythmic Agent, Class IV; Calcium Channel Blocker

**U.S. Brand Names** Calan®; Calan® SR; Covera-HS®; Isoptin®; Isoptin® SR; Verelan®

**Mechanism of Action** Inhibits calcium ion from entering the "slow channels" or select voltage-sensitive areas of vascular smooth muscle and myocardium during depolarization; produces a relaxation of coronary vascular smooth muscle and coronary vasodilation; increases myocardial oxygen delivery in patients with vasospastic angina; slows automaticity and conduction of A-V node.

**Use** Orally used for treatment of angina pectoris (vasospastic, chronic stable, unstable) and hypertension; I.V. for supraventricular tachyarrhythmias (PSVT, atrial fibrillation, atrial flutter); only Covera-HS® is approved for both hypertension and angina as a sustained release product

**USUAL DOSAGE**
Children: SVT:
I.V.:
<1 year: 0.1-0.2 mg/kg over 2 minutes; repeat every 30 minutes as needed
1-15 years: 0.1-0.3 mg/kg over 2 minutes; maximum: 5 mg/dose, may repeat dose in 15 minutes if adequate response not achieved; maximum for second dose: 10 mg/dose
Oral (dose not well established):
1-5 years: 4-8 mg/kg/day in 3 divided doses **or** 40-80 mg every 8 hours
>5 years: 80 mg every 6-8 hours
Adults:
SVT: I.V.: 5-10 mg (approximately 0.075-0.15 mg/kg), second dose of 10 mg (~0.15 mg/kg) may be given 15-30 minutes after the initial dose if patient tolerates, but does not respond to initial dose
Angina: Oral: Initial dose: 80-120 mg 3 times/day (elderly or small stature: 40 mg 3 times/day); range: 240-480 mg/day in 3-4 divided doses
Hypertension: 80 mg 3 times/day or 240 mg/day (sustained release); range: 240-480 mg/day; 120 mg/day in the elderly or small patients (no evidence of additional benefit in doses >360 mg/day)
**Note:** One time per day dosing is recommended at bedtime with Covera-HS®

**Dosing adjustment in renal impairment:** Cl$_{cr}$ <10 mL/minute: Administer at 50% to 75% of normal dose

Dialysis: Not dialyzable (0% to 5 %) via hemo or peritoneal dialysis; supplemental dose is not necessary

**Dosing adjustment/comments in hepatic disease:** Reduce dose in cirrhosis, reduce dose to 20% to 50% of normal and monitor EKG

**Dosage Forms** Verapamil hydrochloride: **Cap, sustained release (Verelan®):** 120 mg, 180 mg, 240 mg, 360 mg; **Inj:** 2.5 mg/mL (2 mL, 4 mL), Isoptin®: 2.5 mg/mL (2 mL, 4 mL); **Tab:** 40 mg, 80 mg, 120 mg, Calan®, Isoptin®: 40 mg, 80 mg, 120 mg; **Tab sustained release:** 180 mg, 240 mg, Calan® SR, Isoptin® SR: 120 mg, 180 mg, 240 mg, Covera-HS®: 180 mg, 240 mg

**Contraindications** Sinus bradycardia; advanced heart block; ventricular tachycardia; cardiogenic shock; hypersensitivity to verapamil or any component; atrial fibrillation or flutter associated with accessory conduction pathways

**Warnings/Precautions** Use with caution in sick-sinus syndrome, severe left ventricular dysfunction, hepatic or renal impairment, hypertrophic cardiomyopathy (especially obstructive), abrupt withdrawal may cause increased duration and frequency of chest pain; avoid I.V. use in neonates and young infants due to severe apnea, bradycardia, or hypotensive (Continued)

959

## Verapamil *(Continued)*

reactions; elderly may experience more constipation and hypotension. Monitor EKG and blood pressure closely in patients receiving I.V. therapy particularly in patients with supraventricular tachycardia.

**Pregnancy Risk Factor** C

**Pregnancy Implications**

Clinical effects on the fetus: Use in pregnancy only when clearly needed and when the benefits outweigh the potential hazard to the fetus. Crosses the placenta. 1 report of suspected heart block when used to control fetal supraventricular tachycardia. May exhibit tocolytic effects.

Breast-feeding/lactation: Crosses into breast milk. American Academy of Pediatrics considers **compatible** with breast-feeding.

**Adverse Reactions** O (oral); I.V. (intravenous):

1% to 10%:

Cardiovascular: Bradycardia; first, second, or third degree A-V block; congestive heart failure (1.8%), hypotension (O - 2.5%; I.V. - 1.5%), peripheral edema (2.1%)

Central nervous system: Dizziness/lightheadedness (O - 3.5%; I.V. - 1.2%), fatigue, headache (O - 2.2%; I.V. - 1.2%)

Dermatologic: Rash (1.2%)

Gastrointestinal: Constipation (7.3%), nausea (O - 2.7%; I.V. - 0.9%)

Neuromuscular & skeletal: Weakness

<1%: Chest pain, hypotension (excessive), tachycardia, flushing, galactorrhea, gingival hyperplasia

**Drug Interactions** CYP1A2 and 3A3/4 enzyme substrate; CYP3A3/4 inhibitor

Decreased effect: Phenobarbital, hydantoins, vitamin D, sulfinpyrazone, and rifampin may decrease verapamil serum concentrations by increased hepatic metabolism

Increased effect of quinidine with verapamil

Increased toxicity:

Verapamil and alcohol may increase blood alcohol levels and prolong its effects

Verapamil and amiodarone may increase cardiotoxicity

Verapamil and aspirin may cause bruising

Verapamil and cimetidine may cause increased bioavailability of verapamil

Verapamil and beta-blockers may cause increased cardiac depressant effects on A-V conduction

Verapamil and carbamazepine may cause increased carbamazepine levels

Verapamil and cyclosporine may cause increased cyclosporine levels

Verapamil and digoxin may cause increased digoxin levels

Verapamil and doxorubicin may cause increased doxorubicin levels

Verapamil and lithium has reportedly increased the patient's sensitivity to the effects of lithium (neurotoxicity)

Verapamil and theophylline may cause increased pharmacologic actions of theophylline secondary to decreased clearance of theophylline

Verapamil and vecuronium may cause increased vecuronium levels

Dantrolene and verapamil may result in hyperkalemia and myocardial depression

Disopyramide: Avoid combination with disopyramide, discontinue disopyramide 48 hours before starting therapy, do not restart until 24 hours after verapamil has been discontinued

**Onset** Oral (nonsustained tablets): Peak effect: 2 hours; I.V.: Peak effect: 1-5 minutes

**Duration** Oral (nonsustained tablets): 6-8 hours; I.V.: 10-20 minutes

**Half-Life** Single dose: 2-8 hours, increased up to 12 hours with multiple dosing; increased half-life with hepatic cirrhosis

**Special PA Issues**

Patient Education: Oral: Take as directed, around-the-clock. Do not alter dosage or discontinue therapy without consulting prescriber. Do not crush or chew extended release form. Avoid (or limit) alcohol and caffeine. You may experience dizziness or lightheadedness (use caution when driving or engaging in tasks that require alertness); nausea or vomiting (small frequent meals, frequent mouth care, or sucking lozenges may help); constipation (increased exercise, dietary fiber, fruit, or fluids may help); diarrhea (buttermilk, boiled milk, or yogurt may help). Report chest pain, palpitations, or irregular heartbeat; unusual cough, difficulty breathing, or swelling of extremities (feet/ankles); muscle tremors or weakness; confusion or acute lethargy; or skin irritation or rash.

**Monitoring Parameters:** Monitor blood pressure closely

**Reference Range:** Therapeutic: 50-200 ng/mL (SI: 100-410 nmol/L) for parent; under normal conditions norverapamil concentration is the same as parent drug. Toxic: >90 µg/mL

**Related Information**

Calcium Channel Blocking Agents *on page 1004*

♦ **Verapamil Hydrochloride** *see* Verapamil *on previous page*

♦ **Verazinc® [OTC]** *see* Zinc Supplements *on page 975*

♦ **Vercyte®** *see* Pipobroman *on page 732*

- **Verelan®** *see* Verapamil *on page 959*
- **Vergon®** **[OTC]** *see* Meclizine *on page 559*
- **Vermizine®** *see* Piperazine *on page 731*
- **Vermox®** *see* Mebendazole *on page 559*
- **Verrex-C&M®** *see* Podophyllin and Salicylic Acid *on page 735*
- **Versed®** *see* Midazolam *on page 606*
- **Vesanoid®** *see* Tretinoin, Oral *on page 925*
- **Vexol® Ophthalmic Suspension** *see* Rimexolone *on page 808*
- **Viagra™** *see* Sildenafil *on page 833*
- **Vibazine®** *see* Buclizine *on page 123*
- **Vibramycin®** *see* Doxycycline *on page 306*
- **Vibramycin® IV** *see* Doxycycline *on page 306*
- **Vibra-Tabs®** *see* Doxycycline *on page 306*
- **Vicks® 44E [OTC]** *see* Guaifenesin and Dextromethorphan *on page 428*
- **Vicks® Children's Chloraseptic® [OTC]** *see* Benzocaine *on page 105*
- **Vicks® Chloraseptic® Sore Throat [OTC]** *see* Benzocaine *on page 105*
- **Vicks® Pediatric Formula 44E [OTC]** *see* Guaifenesin and Dextromethorphan *on page 428*
- **Vicks® Sinex® Nasal Solution [OTC]** *see* Phenylephrine *on page 718*
- **Vicodin®** *see* Hydrocodone and Acetaminophen *on page 449*
- **Vicodin® ES** *see* Hydrocodone and Acetaminophen *on page 449*
- **Vicodin® HP** *see* Hydrocodone and Acetaminophen *on page 449*
- **Vicon Forte®** *see* Vitamins, Multiple *on page 964*
- **Vicon® Plus [OTC]** *see* Vitamins, Multiple *on page 964*
- **Vicoprofen®** *see* Hydrocodone and Ibuprofen *on page 452*

## Vidarabine (vye DARE a been)

**Pharmacologic Class** Antiviral Agent, Ophthalmic

**U.S. Brand Names** Vira-A® Ophthalmic

**Mechanism of Action** Inhibits viral DNA synthesis by blocking DNA polymerase

**Use** Treatment of acute keratoconjunctivitis and epithelial keratitis due to herpes simplex virus type 1 and 2; superficial keratitis caused by herpes simplex virus which has not responded to topical idoxuridine, or when toxic or hypersensitivity reactions to idoxuridine have occurred

**USUAL DOSAGE** Children and Adults: Ophthalmic: Keratoconjunctivitis: Instill ½" of ointment in lower conjunctival sac 5 times/day every 3 hours while awake until complete re-epithelialization has occurred, then twice daily for an additional 7 days

**Dosage Forms Oint, ophth, as monohydrate:** 3% [30 mg/mL = 28 mg/mL base] (3.5 g)

**Contraindications** Hypersensitivity to vidarabine or any component; sterile trophic ulcers

**Warnings/Precautions** Not effective against RNA virus, adenoviral ocular infections, bacterial fungal or chlamydial infections of the cornea, or trophic ulcers; temporary visual haze may be produced; neoplasia has occurred with I.M. vidarabine-treated animals; although *in vitro* studies have been inconclusive, they have shown mutagenesis

**Pregnancy Risk Factor** C

**Adverse Reactions** Percentage unknown: Burning eyes, lacrimation, keratitis, photophobia, foreign body sensation, uveitis

**Special PA Issues**

**Patient Education:** For ophthalmic use only. Store in refrigerator. Apply prescribed amount as often as directed. Wash hands before using and do not let tip of applicator touch eye or contaminate tip of applicator. Tilt head back and look upward. Gently pull down lower lid and put drop(s) in inner corner of eye. Close eye and roll eyeball in all directions. Do not blink for ½ minute. Apply gentle pressure to inner corner of eye for 30 seconds. Wipe away excess from skin around eye. Do not use any other eye preparation for at least 10 minutes. Do not touch tip of applicator to eye or contaminate tip of applicator. Do not share medication with anyone else. May cause sensitivity to bright light (dark glasses may help); temporary stinging or blurred vision may occur. Inform prescriber if you experience eye pain, redness, burning, watering, dryness, double vision, puffiness around eye, vision disturbances, or other adverse eye response; worsening of condition or lack of improvement within 7-14 days.

- **Vidarabine Monohydrate** *see* Vidarabine *on this page*
- **Vi-Daylin® [OTC]** *see* Vitamins, Multiple *on page 964*
- **Vi-Daylin/F®** *see* Vitamins, Multiple *on page 964*
- **Videx®** *see* Didanosine *on page 274*
- **Vioform® [OTC]** *see* Clioquinol *on page 219*
- **Viokase®** *see* Pancrelipase *on page 694*
- **Viosterol** *see* Ergocalciferol *on page 326*
- **Vira-A® Ophthalmic** *see* Vidarabine *on this page*

- **Viracept®** *see* Nelfinavir *on page 641*
- **Viramune®** *see* Nevirapine *on page 648*
- **Virazole® Aerosol** *see* Ribavirin *on page 801*
- **Virilon®** *see* Methyltestosterone *on page 595*
- **Viroptic® Ophthalmic** *see* Trifluridine *on page 935*
- **Viscoat®** *see* Chondroitin Sulfate-Sodium Hyaluronate *on page 204*
- **Visken®** *see* Pindolol *on page 728*
- **Vistacon-50®** *see* Hydroxyzine *on page 462*
- **Vistaject-25®** *see* Hydroxyzine *on page 462*
- **Vistaject-50®** *see* Hydroxyzine *on page 462*
- **Vistaquel®** *see* Hydroxyzine *on page 462*
- **Vistaril®** *see* Hydroxyzine *on page 462*
- **Vistazine®** *see* Hydroxyzine *on page 462*
- **Vistide®** *see* Cidofovir *on page 206*
- **Vita-C® [OTC]** *see* Ascorbic Acid *on page 79*

## Vitamin A (VYE ta min aye)

**Pharmacologic Class** Vitamin, Fat Soluble

**U.S. Brand Names** Aquasol A®; Del-Vi-A®; Palmitate-A® 5000 [OTC]

**Mechanism of Action** Needed for bone development, growth, visual adaptation to darkness, testicular and ovarian function, and as a cofactor in many biochemical processes

**Use** Treatment and prevention of vitamin A deficiency

**USUAL DOSAGE**

RDA:

<1 year: 375 mcg

1-3 years: 400 mcg

4-6 years: 500 mcg*

7-10 years: 700 mcg*

>10 years: 800-1000 mcg*

Male: 1000 mcg

Female: 800 mcg

* mcg retinol equivalent (0.3 mcg retinol = 1 unit vitamin A)

Vitamin A supplementation in measles (recommendation of the World Health Organization): Children: Oral: Administer as a single dose; repeat the next day and at 4 weeks for children with ophthalmologic evidence of vitamin A deficiency:

6 months to 1 year: 100,000 units

>1 year: 200,000 units

**Note:** Use of vitamin A in measles is recommended only for patients 6 months to 2 years of age hospitalized with measles and its complications **or** patients >6 months of age who have any of the following risk factors and who are not already receiving vitamin A: immunodeficiency, ophthalmologic evidence of vitamin A deficiency including night blindness, Bitot's spots or evidence of xerophthalmia, impaired intestinal absorption, moderate to severe malnutrition including that associated with eating disorders, or recent immigration from areas where high mortality rates from measles have been observed

**Note:** Monitor patients closely; dosages >25,000 units/kg have been associated with toxicity

Severe deficiency with xerophthalmia: Oral:

Children 1-8 years: 5000-10,000 units/kg/day for 5 days or until recovery occurs

Children >8 years and Adults: 500,000 units/day for 3 days, then 50,000 units/day for 14 days, then 10,000-20,000 units/day for 2 months

Deficiency (without corneal changes): Oral:

Infants <1 year: 100,000 units every 4-6 months

Children 1-8 years: 200,000 units every 4-6 months

Children >8 years and Adults: 100,000 units/day for 3 days then 50,000 units/day for 14 days

Malabsorption syndrome (prophylaxis): Children >8 years and Adults: Oral: 10,000-50,000 units/day of water miscible product

Dietary supplement: Oral:

Infants up to 6 months: 1500 units/day

Children:

6 months to 3 years: 1500-2000 units/day

4-6 years: 2500 units/day

7-10 years: 3300-3500 units/day

Children >10 years and Adults: 4000-5000 units/day

**Dosage Forms Cap:** 10,000 units [OTC], 25,000 units, 50,000 units; **Drops, oral (water miscible) [OTC]:** 5000 units/0.1 mL (30 mL); **Inj:** 50,000 units/mL (2 mL); **Tab [OTC]:** 5000 units

**Contraindications** Hypervitaminosis A, hypersensitivity to vitamin A or any component; pregnancy if dose exceeds RDA recommendations

**Warnings/Precautions** Evaluate other sources of vitamin A while receiving this product; patients receiving >25,000 units/day should be closely monitored for toxicity

**Pregnancy Risk Factor** A (X if dose exceeds RDA recommendation)

**Pregnancy Implications** Clinical effect on the fetus: Excessive use of vitamin A shortly before and during pregnancy could be harmful to babies

**Adverse Reactions** 1% to 10%:

Central nervous system: Irritability, vertigo, lethargy, malaise, fever, headache

Dermatologic: Drying or cracking of skin

Endocrine & metabolic: Hypercalcemia

Gastrointestinal: Weight loss

Ocular: Visual changes

Miscellaneous: Hypervitaminosis A

**Drug Interactions**

Decreased effect: Cholestyramine decreases absorption of vitamin A; neomycin and mineral oil may also interfere with vitamin A absorption

Increased toxicity: Retinoids may have additive adverse effects

**Special PA Issues**

**Patient Education:** Take exactly as directed; do not take more than the recommended dose. Take with meals. Do not use mineral oil or other vitamin A supplements without consulting prescriber. Report persistent nausea, vomiting, or loss of appetite; excessively dry skin or lips; headache or CNS irritability; loss of hair; or changes in vision.

**Reference Range:** 1 RE = 1 retinol equivalent; 1 RE = 1 µg retinol or 6 µg beta-carotene; Normal levels of Vitamin A in serum = 80-300 units/mL

- ◆ **Vitamin A Acid** see Tretinoin, Topical on page 927
- ◆ **Vitamin B₁** see Thiamine on page 894
- ◆ **Vitamin B₂** see Riboflavin on page 802
- ◆ **Vitamin B₃** see Niacinamide on page 650
- ◆ **Vitamin B₃** see Niacin on page 649
- ◆ **Vitamin B₆** see Pyridoxine on page 784
- ◆ **Vitamin B₁₂** see Cyanocobalamin on page 242

# Vitamin B Complex With Vitamin C and Folic Acid

(VYE ta min bee KOM pleks with VYE ta min see & FOE lik AS id)

**Pharmacologic Class** Vitamin, Water Soluble

**U.S. Brand Names** Berocca®; Nephrocaps®

**Dosage Forms Cap**

- ◆ **Vitamin C** see Ascorbic Acid on page 79
- ◆ **Vitamin D₂** see Ergocalciferol on page 326

# Vitamin E (VYE ta min ee)

**Pharmacologic Class** Vitamin, Fat Soluble

**U.S. Brand Names** Amino-Opti-E® [OTC]; Aquasol E® [OTC]; E-Complex-600® [OTC]; E-Vitamin® [OTC]; Vita-Plus® E Softgels® [OTC]; Vitec® [OTC]; Vite E® Creme [OTC]

**Mechanism of Action** Prevents oxidation of vitamin A and C; protects polyunsaturated fatty acids in membranes from attack by free radicals and protects red blood cells against hemolysis

**Use** Prevention and treatment hemolytic anemia secondary to vitamin E deficiency, dietary supplement

**Investigational:** To reduce the risk of bronchopulmonary dysplasia or retrolental fibroplasia in infants exposed to high concentrations of oxygen

**USUAL DOSAGE** One unit of vitamin E = 1 mg dl-alpha-tocopherol acetate. Oral:

Vitamin E deficiency:

Children (with malabsorption syndrome): 1 unit/kg/day of water miscible vitamin E (to raise plasma tocopherol concentrations to the normal range within 2 months and to maintain normal plasma concentrations)

Adults: 60-75 units/day

Prevention of vitamin E deficiency: Adults: 30 units/day

Prevention of retinopathy of prematurity or BPD secondary to O₂ therapy: (American Academy of Pediatrics considers this use investigational and routine use is not recommended)

Retinopathy prophylaxis: 15-30 units/kg/day to maintain plasma levels between 1.5-2 µg/mL (may need as high as 100 units/kg/day)

Cystic fibrosis, beta-thalassemia, sickle cell anemia may require higher daily maintenance doses:

Cystic fibrosis: 100-400 units/day

Beta-thalassemia: 750 units/day

Sickle cell: 450 units/day

Recommended daily allowance:

Premature infants ≤3 months: 17 mg (25 units)

(Continued)

## Vitamin E *(Continued)*

Infants:
≤6 months: 3 mg (4.5 units)
6-12 months: 4 mg (6 units)
Children:
1-3 years: 6 mg (9 units)
4-10 years: 7 mg (10.5 units)
Children >11 years and Adults:
Male: 10 mg (15 units)
Female: 8 mg (12 units)
Topical: Apply a thin layer over affected area

**Dosage Forms Cap:** 100 units, 200 units, 330 mg, 400 units, 500 units, 600 units, 1000 units; **Cap, water miscible:** 73.5 mg, 147 mg, 165 mg, 330 mg, 400 units; **Crm:** 50 mg/g (15 g, 30 g, 60 g, 75 g, 120 g, 454 g); **Drops, oral:** 50 mg/mL (12 mL, 30 mL); **Liq, top:** 10 mL, 15 mL, 30 mL, 60 mL; **Lot:** 120 mL; **Oil:** 15 mL, 30 mL, 60 mL; **Oint, top:** 30 mg/g (45 g, 60 g); **Tab:** 200 units, 400 units

**Contraindications** Hypersensitivity to drug or any components; I.V. route

**Warnings/Precautions** May induce vitamin K deficiency; necrotizing enterocolitis has been associated with oral administration of large dosages (eg, >200 units/day) of a hyperosmolar vitamin E preparation in low birth weight infants

**Pregnancy Risk Factor** A (C if dose exceeds RDA recommendation)

**Adverse Reactions** <1%: Headache, fatigue, contact dermatitis with topical preparation, nausea, diarrhea, intestinal cramps, weakness, blurred vision, gonadal dysfunction

**Drug Interactions**
Decreased absorption with mineral oil
Delayed absorption of iron
Increased effect of oral anticoagulants

**Special PA Issues**

**Patient Education:** Take exactly as directed; do not take more than the recommended dose. Do not use mineral oil or other vitamin E supplements without consulting prescriber. Report persistent nausea, vomiting, or cramping; or gonadal dysfunction.

**Reference Range:** Therapeutic: 0.8-1.5 mg/dL (SI: 19-35 μmol/L), some method variation

♦ **Vitamin G** *see* Riboflavin *on page 802*

♦ **Vitamin K₁** *see* Phytonadione *on page 725*

♦ **Vitamin, Multiple, Prenatal** *see* Vitamins, Multiple *on this page*

♦ **Vitamin, Multiple, Therapeutic** *see* Vitamins, Multiple *on this page*

♦ **Vitamin, Multiple With Iron** *see* Vitamins, Multiple *on this page*

# Vitamins, Multiple *(VYE ta mins, MUL ti pul)*

**Pharmacologic Class** Vitamin

**U.S. Brand Names** Adeflor®; Allbee® With C; Becotin® Pulvules®; Cefol® Filmtab®; Chromagen® OB [OTC]; Eldercaps® [OTC]; Filibon® [OTC]; Florvite®; Iberet-Folic-500®; LKV-Drops® [OTC]; Mega-B® [OTC]; Multi Vit® Drops [OTC]; M.V.I.®; M.V.I.®-12; M.V.I.® Concentrate; M.V.I.® Pediatric; Natabec® [OTC]; Natabec® FA [OTC]; Natabec® Rx; Natalins® [OTC]; Natalins Rx; NeoVadrin® [OTC]; Niferex®-PN; Poly-Vi-Flor®; Poly-Vi-Sol® [OTC]; Pramet® FA; Pramilet® FA; Prenavite® [OTC]; Secran®; Stresstabs® 600 Advanced Formula Tablets [OTC]; Stuartnatal® 1 + 1; Stuart Prenatal® [OTC]; Therabid® [OTC]; Theragran® [OTC]; Theragran® Hematinic®; Theragran® Liquid [OTC]; Theragran-M® [OTC]; Tri-Vi-Flor®; Unicap® [OTC]; Vicon Forte®; Vicon® Plus [OTC]; Vi-Daylin® [OTC]; Vi-Daylin/F®

**Use** Dietary supplement

**USUAL DOSAGE**

Infants 1.5-3 kg: I.V.: 3.25 mL/24 hours (M.V.I.® Pediatric)
Children:
Oral:
≤2 years: Drops: 1 mL/day (premature infants may get 0.5-1 mL/day)
>2 years: Chew 1 tablet/day
≥4 years: 5 mL/day liquid
I.V.: >3 kg and <11 years: 5 mL/24 hours (M.V.I.® Pediatric)
Adults:
Oral: 1 tablet/day or 5 mL/day liquid
I.V.: 5 mL of vials 1 and 2 (M.V.I.®-12)/one TPN bag/day
I.V. solutions: 10 mL/24 hours (M.V.I.®-12)

**Dosage Forms** See Multivitamins table.

**Contraindications** Hypersensitivity to product components

**Warnings/Precautions** RDA values are not requirements, but are recommended daily intakes of certain essential nutrients; periodic dental exams should be performed to check for dental fluorosis; use with caution in patients with severe renal or liver failure

**Pregnancy Risk Factor** A (C if used in doses above RDA recommendation)

## Multivitamin Products

| Product | Content Given Per | A IU | D IU | E IU | C mg | FA mg | $B_1$ mg | $B_2$ mg | $B_3$ mg | $B_6$ mg | $B_{12}$ mcg | Other |
|---|---|---|---|---|---|---|---|---|---|---|---|---|
| Theragran® | 5 mL liquid | 10,000 | 400 | | 200 | | 10 | 10 | 100 | 4.1 | 5 | $B_5$ 21.4 mg |
| Vi-Daylin® | 1 mL drops | 1500 | 400 | 4.1 | 35 | | 0.5 | 0.6 | 8 | 0.4 | 1.5 | Alcohol <0.5% |
| Vi-Daylin® Iron | 1 mL | 1500 | 400 | 4.1 | 35 | | 0.5 | 0.6 | 8 | 0.4 | | Fe 10 mg |
| Albee® with C | tablet | | | | 300 | | 15 | 10.2 | | 5 | | Niacinamide 50 mg, pantothenic acid 10 mg |
| Vitamin B complex | tablet | | | | | 400 mcg | 1.5 | 1.7 | | 2 | 6 | Niacinamide 20 mg |
| Hexavitamin | cap/tab | 5000 | 400 | | 75 | | 2 | 3 | 20 | | | |
| Iberet-Folic-500® | tablet | | | | 500 | 0.8 | 6 | 6 | 30 | 5 | 25 | $B_5$ 10 mg, Fe 105 mg |
| Stuartnatal® 1+1 | tablet | 4000 | 400 | 11 | 120 | 1 | 1.5 | 3 | 20 | 10 | 12 | Cu, Zn 25 mg, Fe 65 mg, Ca 200 mg |
| Theragran-M® | tablet | 5000 | 400 | 30 | 90 | 0.4 | 3 | 3.4 | 30 | 3 | 9 | Cl, Cr, I, K, $B_5$ 10 mg, Mg, Mn, Mo, P, Se, Zn 15 mg, Fe 27 mg, biotin 30 mcg, beta-carotene 1250 IU |
| Vi-Daylin® | tablet | 2500 | 400 | 15 | 60 | 0.3 | 1.05 | 1.2 | 13.5 | 1.05 | 4.5 | $B_5$ 15 mg, biotin 60 mcg |
| M.V.I.®-12 injection | 5 mL | 3300 | 200 | 10 | 100 | 0.4 | 3 | 3.6 | 40 | 4 | 5 | |
| M.V.I.®-12 unit vial | 20 mL | | | | | | | | | | | |
| M.V.I.® pediatric powder | 5 mL | 2300 | 400 | 7 | 80 | 0.14 | 1.2 | 1.4 | 17 | 1 | 1 | $B_5$ 5 mg, biotin 20 mcg, vitamin K 200 mcg |

## Vitamins, Multiple (Continued)

**Adverse Reactions** 1% to 10%: Hypervitaminosis; refer to individual vitamin entries for individual reactions

**Special PA Issues**

**Patient Education:** Do not take more than the recommended dose.

**Reference Range:** Recommended daily allowances are published by Food and Nutrition Board, National Research Council - National Academy of Sciences and are revised periodically. RDA quantities apply only to healthy persons and are not intended to cover therapeutic nutrition requirements in disease or other abnormal states (ie, metabolic disorders, weight reduction, chronic disease, drug therapy).

- ◆ **Vita-Plus® E Softgels® [OTC]** see Vitamin E on page 963
- ◆ **Vitec® [OTC]** see Vitamin E on page 963
- ◆ **Vite E® Creme [OTC]** see Vitamin E on page 963
- ◆ **Vito Reins®** see Phenazopyridine on page 714
- ◆ **Vitrasert®** see Ganciclovir on page 408
- ◆ **Vitravene™** see Fomivirsen on page 400
- ◆ **Vivactil®** see Protriptyline on page 779
- ◆ **Vivelle® Transdermal** see Estradiol on page 332
- ◆ **Vivol®** see Diazepam on page 269
- ◆ **V-Lax® [OTC]** see Psyllium on page 781
- ◆ **Volmax®** see Albuterol on page 34
- ◆ **Voltaren® Ophthalmic** see Diclofenac on page 271
- ◆ **Voltaren® Oral** see Diclofenac on page 271
- ◆ **Voltaren Rapide®** see Diclofenac on page 271
- ◆ **Voltaren-XR® Oral** see Diclofenac on page 271
- ◆ **VōSol®** see Acetic Acid on page 25
- ◆ **VōSol® HC Otic** see Acetic Acid, Propylene Glycol Diacetate, and Hydrocortisone on page 25
- ◆ **V.V.S.®** see Sulfabenzamide, Sulfacetamide, and Sulfathiazole on page 857
- ◆ **Vytone® Topical** see Iodoquinol and Hydrocortisone on page 488
- ◆ **VZIG** see Varicella-Zoster Immune Globulin (Human) on page 955

## Warfarin (WAR far in)

**Pharmacologic Class** Anticoagulant

**U.S. Brand Names** Coumadin®

**Mechanism of Action** Interferes with hepatic synthesis of vitamin K-dependent coagulation factors (II, VII, IX, X)

**Use** Prophylaxis and treatment of venous thrombosis, pulmonary embolism and thromboembolic disorders; atrial fibrillation with risk of embolism and as an adjunct in the prophylaxis of systemic embolism after myocardial infarction

**Unlabeled use:** Prevention of recurrent transient ischemic attacks and to reduce risk of recurrent myocardial infarction

**USUAL DOSAGE**

Oral:

Infants and Children: 0.05-0.34 mg/kg/day; infants <12 months of age may require doses at or near the high end of this range; consistent anticoagulation may be difficult to maintain in children <5 years of age

Adults: 5-15 mg/day for 2-5 days, then adjust dose according to results of prothrombin time; usual maintenance dose ranges from 2-10 mg/day

I.V. (administer as a slow bolus injection): 2-5 mg/day

**Dosing adjustment/comments in hepatic disease:** Monitor effect at usual doses; the response to oral anticoagulants may be markedly enhanced in obstructive jaundice (due to reduced vitamin K absorption) and also in hepatitis and cirrhosis (due to decreased production of vitamin K-dependent clotting factors); prothrombin index should be closely monitored

**Dosage Forms** Warfarin sodium: **Powder for inj, lyophilized:** 2 mg, 5 mg; **Tab:** 1 mg, 2 mg, 2.5 mg, 3 mg, 4 mg, 5 mg, 6 mg, 7.5 mg, 10 mg

**Contraindications** Hypersensitivity to warfarin or any component; severe liver or kidney disease; open wounds; uncontrolled bleeding; GI ulcers; neurosurgical procedures; malignant hypertension, pregnancy

**Warnings/Precautions**

Do not switch brands once desired therapeutic response has been achieved

Use with caution in patients with active tuberculosis or diabetes

Concomitant use with vitamin K may decrease anticoagulant effect; monitor carefully

Concomitant use with NSAIDs or aspirin may cause severe GI irritation and also increase the risk of bleeding due to impaired platelet function

Salicylates may further increase warfarin's effect by displacing it from plasma protein binding sites

Patients with protein C or S deficiency are at increased risk of skin necrosis syndrome

Before committing an elderly patient to long-term anticoagulation therapy, their risk for bleeding complications secondary to falls, drug interactions, living situation, and cognitive status should be considered. The risk for bleeding complications decreases with the duration of therapy and may increase with advancing age.

If a patient is to undergo an invasive surgical procedure (dental to actual minor/major surgery), warfarin should be stopped 3 days before the scheduled surgery date and the INR/PT should be checked prior to the procedure

## Pregnancy Risk Factor D

## Pregnancy Implications

Clinical effects on the fetus: Oral anticoagulants cross the placenta and produce fetal abnormalities. Warfarin should not be used during pregnancy because of significant risks. Adjusted-dose heparin can be given safely throughout pregnancy in patients with venous thromboembolism.

Breast-feeding/lactation: Warfarin does not pass into breast milk and can be given to nursing mothers

## Adverse Reactions

1% to 10%:

Dermatologic: Skin lesions, alopecia, skin necrosis

Gastrointestinal: Anorexia, nausea, vomiting, stomach cramps, diarrhea

Hematologic: Hemorrhage, leukopenia, unrecognized bleeding sites (eg, colon cancer) may be uncovered by anticoagulation

Respiratory: Hemoptysis

<1%: Fever, rash, anorexia, agranulocytosis, hepatotoxicity, renal damage, mouth ulcers, discolored toes (blue or purple)

**Drug Interactions** CYP1A2 enzyme substrate (minor), CYP2C8, 2C9, 2C18, 2C19, and 3A3/4 enzyme substrate; CYP2C9 enzyme inhibitor

### Decreased Anticoagulant Effects

| Induction of Enzymes | | Increased Procoagulant Factors | Decreased Drug Absorption | Other |
|---|---|---|---|---|
| Barbiturates Carbamazepine Glutethimide Griseofulvin | Nafcillin Phenytoin Rifampin | Estrogens Oral contraceptives Vitamin K (including nutritional supplements) | Aluminum hydroxide Cholestyramine* Colestipol* | Ethchlorvynol Griseofulvin Spironolactone† Sucralfate |

Decreased anticoagulant effect may occur when these drugs are administered with oral anticoagulants.

*Cholestyramine and colestipol may increase the anticoagulant effect by binding vitamin K in the gut; yet, the decreased drug absorption appears to be of more concern.

†Diuretic-induced hemoconcentration with subsequent concentration of clotting factors has been reported to decrease the effects of oral anticoagulants.

### Enhanced Anticoagulant Effects

| Decrease Vitamin K | Displace Anticoagulant | Inhibit Metabolism | Other |
|---|---|---|---|
| Oral antibiotics Can ↑ or ↓ INR Check INR 3 days after patient begins antibiotics to see the INR value and adjust the warfarin dose accordingly | Chloral hydrate Clofibrate Diazoxide Ethacrynic acid Miconazole Nalidixic acid Phenylbutazone Salicylates Sulfonamides Sulfonylureas Triclofos | Alcohol (acute ingestion)* Allopurinol Amiodarone Chloramphenicol Chlorpropamide Cimetidine Co-trimoxazole Disulfiram Metronidazole Phenylbutazone Phenytoin Propoxyphene Sulfinpyrazone Sulfonamides Tolbutamide | Acetaminophen Anabolic steroids Clofibrate Danazol Erythromycin Gemfibrozil Glucagon Influenza vaccine Ketoconazole Propranolol Ranitidine Sulindac Thyroid drugs |

* The hypoprothrombinemic effect of oral anticoagulants has been reported to be both increased and decreased during chronic and excessive alcohol ingestion. Data are insufficient to predict the direction of this interaction in alcoholic patients.

# Warfarin *(Continued)*

## Increased Bleeding Tendency

| Inhibit Platelet Aggregation | Inhibit Procoagulant Factors | Ulcerogenic Drugs |
|---|---|---|
| Cephalosporins | Antimetabolites | Adrenal corticosteroids |
| Dipyridamole | Quinidine | Indomethacin |
| Indomethacin | Quinine | Oxyphenbutazone |
| Oxyphenbutazone | Salicylates | Phenylbutazone |
| Penicillin, parenteral | | Potassium products |
| Phenylbutazone | | Salicylates |
| Salicylates | | |
| Sulfinpyrazone | | |

Use of these agents with oral anticoagulants may increase the chances of hemorrhage.

**Onset** INR may increase within 36-72 hours; full therapeutic effect is not established until 5-7 days

**Half-Life** 3-5 days, highly variable among individuals

## Special PA Issues

**Patient Education:** Medication should be taken as directed. If dose is missed, take as soon as remembered that day. Do not double doses. Report any signs of bleeding or excessive bruising from brushing your teeth or from injuries. Report red/brown urine or black, tarry stools. Report sore throat, fever, chills, severe headaches, or unexpected pregnancy. Wear MediAlert® ID Tag identifying drug usage. Avoid hazardous activities. Avoid injury, skin breaks, or invasive procedures including I.M. injections if possible. Use soft toothbrush, safety razor, and use care in cutting nails.

Many things can change your response to this drug (eg, change of diet, illness with fever, other medications). Do not take any medications that your prescriber is unaware of. Be sure of food and drugs to avoid. A balanced diet with a consistent vitamin K is essential. Avoid large amounts of alfalfa, avocado, broccoli, asparagus, Brussels sprouts, cabbage, cauliflower, fish oils, green teas, kale, lettuce, liver, omega 3 fatty acids, soy protein, soybean oil, spinach, papain, turnip greens, and watercress. Avoid fried or boiled onions, herbal teas, and remedies such as tonka beans, melilot, and woodruff; these may increase the effect of warfarin.

## Dietary Considerations:

Alcohol: Chronic use of alcohol inhibits warfarin metabolism; avoid or limit use

Food:

Vitamin K: Foods high in vitamin K (eg, beef liver, pork liver, green tea and leafy green vegetables) inhibit anticoagulant effect. Do not change dietary habits once stabilized on warfarin therapy; a balanced diet with a consistent intake of vitamin K is essential; avoid large amounts of alfalfa, asparagus, broccoli, Brussels sprouts, cabbage, cauliflower, green teas, kale, lettuce, spinach, turnip greens, watercress. It is recommended that the diet contain a CONSISTENT vitamin K content of 70-140 mcg/day. Check with physician before changing diet.

Vitamin E: May increase warfarin effect; do not change dietary habits or vitamin supplements once stabilized on warfarin therapy

**Monitoring Parameters:** Prothrombin time, hematocrit, INR

## Reference Range:

Therapeutic: 2-5 µg/mL (SI: 6.5-16.2 µmol/L)

Prothrombin time should be 1½ to 2 times the control or INR should be ↑ 2 to 3 times based upon indication

Normal prothrombin time: 10-13 seconds

## INR Ranges Based Upon Indication

| Diagnosis | Desired INR Range |
|---|---|
| Atrial fibrillation | 2.0-3.0 |
| Venous thromboembolism (DVT, PE) | 2.0-3.0 |
| TIA and stroke | 2.0-3.0 |
| Bioprosthetic heart valve | 2.0-3.0 |
| Acute myocardial infarction with risk factors* | 2.5-3.5 |
| Mechanical heart valve (bileaflet, tilting disk) | 2.5-3.5 |
| Mechanical heart valve (caged ball, caged disk) | 3.0-4.0 |

*Anterior Q-wave infarction, severe left-ventricular dysfunction, mural thrombus on 2D echo, atrial fibrillation, history of systemic or pulmonary embolism, congestive heart failure

Warfarin levels are not used for monitoring degree of anticoagulation. They may be useful if a patient with unexplained coagulopathy is using the drug surreptitiously or if it is unclear whether clinical resistance is due to true drug resistance or lack of drug intake. Normal prothrombin time (PT): 10.9-12.9 seconds. Healthy premature newborns have prolonged coagulation test screening results (eg, PT, APTT, TT) which return to normal adult values at approximately 6 months of age. Healthy prematures, however, do not develop spontaneous hemorrhage or thrombotic complications because of a balance between procoagulants and inhibitors

The World Health Organization (WHO), in cooperation with other regulatory-advisory bodies, has developed system of standardizing the reporting of PT values through the determination of the International Normalized Ratio (INR). The INR involves the standardization of the PT by the generation of two pieces of information: the PT ratio and the International Sensitivity Index (ISI)

Therapeutic ranges are now available or being developed to assist practicing physicians in their treatment of patients with a wide variety of thrombotic disorders

**Related Information**
Anticoagulant Therapy *on page 1040*

♦ **Warfarin Sodium** *see* Warfarin *on page 966*
♦ **Warfilone®** *see* Warfarin *on page 966*
♦ **Wellbutrin®** *see* Bupropion *on page 128*

♦ **Wellbutrin® SR** *see* Bupropion *on page 128*
♦ **Wellcovorin®** *see* Leucovorin *on page 520*
♦ **Westcort®** *see* Hydrocortisone *on page 453*

♦ **Whitehorn** *see* Hawthorn *on page 438*
♦ **Wigraine®** *see* Ergotamine *on page 328*
♦ **Wild Quinine** *see* Feverfew *on page 368*

♦ **Wimpred** *see* Prednisone *on page 754*
♦ **40 Winks® [OTC]** *see* Diphenhydramine *on page 289*
♦ **WinRho SD®** *see* Rh₀(D) Immune Globulin (Intravenous-Human) *on page 800*

♦ **Winstrol®** *see* Stanozolol *on page 850*
♦ **Wycillin®** *see* Penicillin G Procaine *on page 706*
♦ **Wydase® Injection** *see* Hyaluronidase *on page 445*
♦ **Wygesic®** *see* Propoxyphene and Acetaminophen *on page 774*

♦ **Wymox®** *see* Amoxicillin *on page 61*
♦ **Wytensin®** *see* Guanabenz *on page 429*
♦ **Xalatan®** *see* Latanoprost *on page 516*

♦ **Xanax®** *see* Alprazolam *on page 43*
♦ **Xenical®** *see* Orlistat *on page 679*
♦ **Xylocaine®** *see* Lidocaine *on page 531*

♦ **Xylocaine® With Epinephrine** *see* Lidocaine and Epinephrine *on page 532*
♦ **Xylocard®** *see* Lidocaine *on page 531*
♦ **Yeast-Gard® Medicated Douche** *see* Povidone-Iodine *on page 747*

♦ **Yellow Indian Paint** *see* Golden Seal *on page 421*
♦ **Yellow Root** *see* Golden Seal *on page 421*

♦ **Yodoxin®** *see* Iodoquinol *on page 487*
♦ **Yutopar®** *see* Ritodrine *on page 811*

# Zafirlukast (za FIR loo kast)
**Pharmacologic Class** Leukotriene Receptor Antagonist
**U.S. Brand Names** Accolate®
**Mechanism of Action** Zafirlukast is a selectively and competitive leukotriene-receptor antagonist (LTRA) of leukotriene D4 and E4 (LTD4 and LTE4), components of slow-reacting substance of anaphylaxis (SRSA). Cysteinyl leukotriene production and receptor occupation have been correlated with the pathophysiology of asthma, including airway (Continued)

## Zafirlukast *(Continued)*

edema, smooth muscle constriction and altered cellular activity associated with the inflammatory process, which contribute to the signs and symptoms of asthma.

**Use** Prophylaxis and chronic treatment of asthma in adults and children ≥12 years of age

**USUAL DOSAGE** Oral:

Children <12 years: Safety and effectiveness has not been established

Adults: 20 mg twice daily

Elderly: The mean dose (mg/kg) normalized AUC and $C_{max}$ increase and plasma clearance decreases with increasing age. In patients >65 years of age, there is an 2-3 fold greater $C_{max}$ and AUC compared to younger adults.

**Dosing adjustment in renal impairment:** There are no apparent differences in the pharmacokinetics between renally impaired patients and normal subjects.

**Dosing adjustment in hepatic impairment:** In patients with hepatic impairment (ie, biopsy-proven cirrhosis), there is a 50% to 60% greater $C_{max}$ and AUC compared to normal subjects.

**Dosage Forms Tab:** 20 mg

**Contraindications** Hypersensitivity to zafirlukast or any of its inactive ingredients

**Warnings/Precautions** The clearance of zafirlukast is reduced in patients with stable alcoholic cirrhosis such that the $C_{max}$ and AUC are approximately 50% to 60% greater than those of normal adults.

Zafirlukast is not indicated for use in the reversal of bronchospasm in acute asthma attacks, including status asthmaticus. Therapy with zafirlukast can be continued during acute exacerbations of asthma.

An increased proportion of zafirlukast patients >55 years old reported infections as compared to placebo-treated patients. these infections were mostly mild or moderate in intensity and predominantly affected the respiratory tract. Infections occurred equally in both sexes, were dose-proportional to total milligrams of zafirlukast exposure and were associated with coadministration of inhaled corticosteroids.

Although the frequency of hepatic transaminase elevations was comparable between zafirlukast and placebo-treated patients, a single case of symptomatic hepatitis and hyperbilirubinemia, without other attributable cause, occurred in patient who had received 40 mg/day of zafirlukast for 100 days. In this patient, the liver enzymes returned to normal within 3 months of stopping zafirlukast.

**Pregnancy Risk Factor** B

**Pregnancy Implications**

Clinical effects on the fetus: At 2,000 mg/kg/day in rats, maternal toxicity and deaths were seen with increased incidence of early fetal resorption. Spontaneous abortions occurred in cynomolgus monkeys at a maternally toxic dose of 2,000 mg/kg/day orally. There are no adequate and well controlled trials in pregnant women.

Breast-feeding/lactation: Zafirlukast is excreted in breast milk; do not administer to nursing women

**Adverse Reactions**

>10%: Central nervous system: Headache (12.9%)

1% to 10%:

Central nervous system: Dizziness, pain, fever

Gastrointestinal: Nausea, diarrhea, abdominal pain, vomiting, dyspepsia

Neuromuscular & skeletal: Myalgia, weakness

**Drug Interactions** CYP2C9 enzyme substrate; CYP2C9 and 3A3/4 enzyme inhibitor

Decreased effect:

Erythromycin: Coadministration of a single dose of zafirlukast with erythromycin to steady state results in decreased mean plasma levels of zafirlukast by 40% due to a decrease in zafirlukast bioavailability.

Terfenadine: Coadministration of zafirlukast with terfenadine to steady state results in a decrease in the mean $C_{max}$ (66%) and AUC (54%) of zafirlukast. No effect of zafirlukast on terfenadine plasma concentrations or EKG parameters was seen.

Theophylline: Coadministration of zafirlukast at steady state with a single dose of liquid theophylline preparations results in decreased mean plasma levels of zafirlukast by 30%, but no effects on plasma theophylline levels were observed.

Increased effect: Aspirin: Coadministration of zafirlukast with aspirin results in mean increased plasma levels of zafirlukast by 45%

Increased toxicity: Warfarin: Coadministration of zafirlukast with warfarin results in a clinically significant increase in prothrombin time (PT). Closely monitor prothrombin times of patients on oral warfarin anticoagulant therapy and zafirlukast, and adjust anticoagulant dose accordingly.

**Onset** Peak concentrations: 3 hours

**Half-Life** 10 hours

**Special PA Issues**

**Patient Education:** Do not use during acute bronchospasm. Take regularly as prescribed, even during symptom-free periods. Do not take more than recommended or discontinue use without consulting prescriber. Do not stop taking other antiasthmatic medications unless instructed by prescriber. Avoid aspirin or aspirin-containing medications unless approved by prescriber. You may experience headache, drowsiness, dizziness, or blurred vision (use caution when driving or engaging in hazardous tasks until response to medication is known); gastric upset, nausea, or vomiting (small frequent meals, good mouth care, chewing gum, or sucking lozenges may help). Report persistent CNS or GI symptoms; muscle or back pain; weakness, fever, chills; yellowing of skin or eyes; dark urine, or pale stool; skin rash; or worsening of condition.

♦ **Zagam®** *see* Sparfloxacin *on page 847*

# Zalcitabine (zal SITE a been)

**Pharmacologic Class** Antiretroviral Agent, Reverse Transcriptase Inhibitor (Nucleoside)
**U.S. Brand Names** Hivid®
**Mechanism of Action** Purine nucleoside analogue, zalcitabine or 2',3'-dideoxycytidine (ddC) is converted to active metabolite ddCTP; lack the presence of the 3'-hydroxyl group necessary for phosphodiester linkages during DNA replication. As a result viral replication is prematurely terminated. ddCTP acts as a competitor for binding sites on the HIV-RNA dependent DNA polymerase (reverse transcriptase) to further contribute to inhibition of viral replication.
**Use** In combination with at least two other antiretrovirals in the treatment of patients with HIV infection; it is not recommended that zalcitabine be given in combination with didanosine, stavudine, or lamivudine due to overlapping toxicities, virologic interactions, or lack of clinical data

**USUAL DOSAGE** Oral:
Children <13 years: Safety and efficacy have not been established
Adults: Daily dose: 0.75 mg every 8 hours
**Dosing adjustment in renal impairment:** Adults:
$Cl_{cr}$ 10-40 mL/minute: 0.75 mg every 12 hours
$Cl_{cr}$ <10 mL/minute: 0.75 mg every 24 hours
Moderately dialyzable (20% to 50%)

**Dosage Forms** Tab: 0.375 mg, 0.75 mg

**Contraindications** Hypersensitivity to zalcitabine or any component

**Warnings/Precautions** Careful monitoring of pancreatic enzymes and liver function tests in patients with a history of pancreatitis, increased amylase, those on parenteral nutrition or with a history of ethanol abuse; discontinue use immediately if pancreatitis is suspected; lactic acidosis and severe hepatomegaly and failure have rarely occurred with zalcitabine resulting in fatality; some cases may possibly be related to underlying hepatitis B; use with caution in patients on digitalis, congestive heart failure, renal failure, hyperphosphatemia; zalcitabine can cause severe peripheral neuropathy; avoid use, if possible, in patients with pre-existing neuropathy

**Pregnancy Risk Factor** C
**Pregnancy Implications**
Clinical effects on the fetus: Administer during pregnancy only if benefits to mother outweigh risks to the fetus
Breast-feeding/lactation: HIV-infected mothers are discouraged from breast-feeding to decrease potential transmission of HIV

**Adverse Reactions**
>10%:
Central nervous system: Fever (5% to 17%), malaise (2% to 13%)
Neuromuscular & skeletal: Peripheral neuropathy (28.3%)
1% to 10%:
Central nervous system: Headache (2.1%), dizziness (1.1%), myalgia (1% to 6%), foot pain, fatigue (3.8%), seizures (1.3%)
Endocrine & metabolic: Hypoglycemia (1.8% to 6.3%), hyponatremia (3.5%), hyperglycemia (1% to 6%)
Hematologic: Anemia (occurs as early as 2-4 weeks), granulocytopenia (usually after 6-8 weeks)
Dermatologic: Rash (2% to 11%), pruritus (3% to 5%)
Gastrointestinal: Nausea (3%), dysphagia (1% to 4%), anorexia (3.9%), abdominal pain (3% to 8%), vomiting (1% to 3%), diarrhea (0.4% to 9.5%), weight loss, oral ulcers (3% to 7%), increased amylase (3% to 8%)
Hepatic: Abnormal hepatic function (8.9%), hyperbilirubinemia (2% to 5%)
Respiratory: Pharyngitis (1.8%), cough (6.3%), nasal discharge (3.5%)
<1%: Edema, hypertension, palpitations, syncope, atrial fibrillation, tachycardia, heart racing, chest pain, night sweats, pain, hypocalcemia, constipation, pancreatitis, jaundice, hepatitis, hepatomegaly, hepatic failure, myositis, weakness, epistaxis

**Drug Interactions**
Decreased effect: Magnesium/aluminum-containing antacids and metoclopramide may reduce zalcitabine absorption
Increased toxicity:
Amphotericin, foscarnet, cimetidine, probenecid, and aminoglycosides may potentiate the risk of developing peripheral neuropathy or other toxicities associated with zalcitabine by interfering with the renal elimination of zalcitabine

(Continued)

## Zalcitabine *(Continued)*

Other drugs associated with peripheral neuropathy which should be avoided, if possible, include chloramphenicol, cisplatin, dapsone, disulfiram, ethionamide, glutethimide, didanosine, gold, hydralazine, iodoquinol, isoniazid, metronidazole, nitrofurantoin, phenytoin, ribavirin, and vincristine

It is not recommended that zalcitabine be given in combination with didanosine, stavudine, or lamivudine due to overlapping toxicities, virologic interactions, or lack of clinical data

**Half-Life** 2.9 hours

**Special PA Issues**

**Patient Education:** Zalcitabine is not a cure for AIDS, nor has it been found to reduce transmission of AIDS. Take as directed, preferably on an empty stomach (1 hour before or 2 hours after meals). Take around-the-clock; do not take with other medications. You may experience headache or insomnia; if these persist notify prescriber. Report chest pain, palpitations, or rapid heartbeat; swelling of extremities; weight gain or loss >5 lb/week; signs of infection (eg, fever, chills, sore throat, burning urination, fatigue); unusual bleeding (eg, tarry stools, easy bruising, or blood in stool, urine, or mouth); pain, tingling, or numbness of toes or fingers; skin rash or irritation; or muscles weakness or tremors.

**Dietary Considerations:** Food: Extent and rate of absorption may be decreased with food

**Monitoring Parameters:** Renal function, viral load, liver function tests, CD4 counts, CBC, serum amylase, triglycerides, calcium

- **Zantac®** *see* Ranitidine Hydrochloride *on page 794*
- **Zantac® 75 [OTC]** *see* Ranitidine Hydrochloride *on page 794*
- **Zantryl®** *see* Phentermine *on page 716*
- **Zapex®** *see* Oxazepam *on page 685*
- **Zarontin®** *see* Ethosuximide *on page 353*
- **Zaroxolyn®** *see* Metolazone *on page 598*
- **Zeasorb-AF® Powder [OTC]** *see* Tolnaftate *on page 915*
- **Zeasorb-AF® Powder [OTC]** *see* Miconazole *on page 604*
- **Zebeta®** *see* Bisoprolol *on page 117*
- **Zefazone®** *see* Cefmetazole *on page 164*
- **Zemplar™** *see* Paricalcitol *on page 697*
- **Zenapax®** *see* Dacliximab *on page 250*
- **Zerit®** *see* Stavudine *on page 851*
- **Zestoretic®** *see* Lisinopril and Hydrochlorothiazide *on page 536*
- **Zestril®** *see* Lisinopril *on page 535*
- **Ziac™** *see* Bisoprolol and Hydrochlorothiazide *on page 118*
- **Ziagen®** *see* Abacavir *on page 18*

## Zidovudine (zye DOE vyoo deen)

**Pharmacologic Class** Antiretroviral Agent, Reverse Transcriptase Inhibitor (Nucleoside)

**U.S. Brand Names** Retrovir®

**Mechanism of Action** Zidovudine is a thymidine analog which interferes with the HIV viral RNA dependent DNA polymerase resulting in inhibition of viral replication; nucleoside reverse transcriptase inhibitor

**Use** Management of patients with HIV infections in combination with at least two other antiretroviral agents; for prevention of maternal/fetal HIV transmission as monotherapy

**USUAL DOSAGE**

Prevention of maternal-fetal HIV transmission:

Neonatal: Oral: 2 mg/kg/dose every 6 hours for 6 weeks beginning 8-12 hours after birth; infants unable to receive oral dosing may receive 1.5 mg/kg I.V. infused over 30 minutes every 6 hours

Maternal (>14 weeks gestation): Oral: 100 mg 5 times/day with the start of labor; during labor and delivery, administer zidovudine I.V. at 2 mg/kg over 1 hour followed by a continuous I.V. infusion of 1 mg/kg/hour until the umbilical cord is clamped

Children 3 months to 12 years for HIV infection:

Oral: 160 mg/m²/dose every 8 hours; dosage range: 90 mg/m²/dose to 180 mg/m²/dose every 6-8 hours; some Working Group members use a dose of 180 mg/m² every 12 hours when using in drug combinations with other antiretroviral compounds, but data on this dosing in children is limited

I.V. continuous infusion: 20 mg/m²/hour

I.V. intermittent infusion: 120 mg/m²/dose every 6 hours

Adults:

Oral: 300 mg twice daily or 200 mg 3 times/day

I.V.: 1-2 mg/kg/dose (infused over 1 hour) administered every 4 hours around-the-clock (6 doses/day)

Prevention of HIV following needlesticks: 200 mg 3 times/day plus lamivudine 150 mg twice daily; a protease inhibitor (eg, indinavir) may be added for high risk exposures; begin therapy within 2 hours of exposure if possible

˙**Patients should receive I.V. therapy only until oral therapy can be administered**

**Dosing interval in renal impairment:** $Cl_{cr}$ <10 mL/minute: May require minor dose adjustment

Hemodialysis: At least partially removed by hemo- and peritoneal dialysis; administer dose after hemodialysis or administer 100 mg supplemental dose; during CAPD, dose as for $Cl_{cr}$ <10 mL/minute

Continuous arteriovenous or venovenous hemodiafiltration (CAVH) effects: Administer 100 mg every 8 hours

**Dosing adjustment in hepatic impairment:** Reduce dose by 50% or double dosing interval in patients with cirrhosis

**Dosage Forms Cap:** 100 mg; **Inj:** 10 mg/mL (20 mL); **Syr (strawberry flavor):** 50 mg/5 mL (240 mL); **Tab:** 300 mg

**Contraindications** Life-threatening hypersensitivity to zidovudine or any component

**Warnings/Precautions** Often associated with hematologic toxicity including granulocytopenia and severe anemia requiring transfusions; zidovudine has been shown to be carcinogenic in rats and mice

**Pregnancy Risk Factor** C

**Pregnancy Implications**

Clinical effect on the fetus: Administer during pregnancy only if benefits to mother outweigh risks to the fetus

Breast-feeding/lactation: HIV-infected mothers are discouraged from breast-feeding to decrease potential transmission of HIV

**Adverse Reactions**

>10%:

Central nervous system: Severe headache (42%), fever (16%)

Dermatologic: Rash (17%)

Gastrointestinal: Nausea (46% to 61%), anorexia (11%), diarrhea (17%), pain (20%), vomiting (6% to 25%)

Hematologic: Anemia (23% in children), leukopenia, granulocytopenia (39% in children)

Neuromuscular & skeletal: Weakness (19%)

1% to 10%:

Central nervous system: Malaise (8%), dizziness (6%), insomnia (5%), somnolence (8%)

Dermatologic: Hyperpigmentation of nails (bluish-brown)

Gastrointestinal: Dyspepsia (5%)

Hematologic: Changes in platelet count

Neuromuscular & skeletal: Paresthesia (6%)

<1%: Neurotoxicity, confusion, mania, seizures, bone marrow suppression, granulocytopenia, thrombocytopenia, pancytopenia, hepatotoxicity, cholestatic jaundice, tenderness, myopathy

**Drug Interactions**

Decreased effect: Acetaminophen may decrease AUC of zidovudine as can the rifamycins

Increased toxicity: Coadministration with drugs that are nephrotoxic (amphotericin b), cytotoxic (flucytosine, Adriamycin®, vincristine, vinblastine, doxorubicin, interferon), inhibit glucuronidation or excretion (acetaminophen, cimetidine, indomethacin, lorazepam, probenecid, aspirin), or interfere with RBC/WBC number or function (acyclovir, ganciclovir, pentamidine, dapsone); although the AUC was unaffected, the rate of absorption and peak plasma concentrations were increased significantly when zidovudine was administered with clarithromycin (n=18); valproic acid increased AZT's AUC by 80% and decreased clearance by 38% (believed due to inhibition first pass metabolism); fluconazole may increase zidovudine's AUC and half-life, concomitant interferon alfa may increase hematologic toxicities and phenytoin, trimethoprim, and interferon beta-1b may increase zidovudine levels

**Half-Life** Terminal: 60 minutes

**Special PA Issues**

**Patient Education:** Zidovudine is not a cure for AIDS, nor has it been found to reduce transmission of AIDS. Take as directed, preferably on an empty stomach (1 hour before or 2 hours after meals). Take around-the-clock; do not take with other medications. Take precautions to avoid transmission to others. You may experience headache or insomnia; if these persist notify prescriber. Report unresolved nausea or vomiting; signs of infection (eg, fever, chills, sore throat, burning urination, flu-like symptoms, fatigue); unusual bleeding (eg, tarry stools, easy bruising, or blood in stool, urine, or mouth); pain, tingling, or numbness of toes or fingers; skin rash or irritation; or muscles weakness or tremors.

**Dietary Considerations:** Food: Administration with a fatty meal decreased zidovudine's AUC and peak plasma concentration

**Monitoring Parameters:** Monitor CBC and platelet count at least every 2 weeks, MCV, serum creatinine kinase, viral load, and CD4 cell count; observe for appearance of opportunistic infections

# Zidovudine and Lamivudine (zye DOE vyoo deen & la MI vyoo deen)

**Pharmacologic Class** Antiretroviral Agent, Reverse Transcriptase Inhibitor (Nucleoside)

**U.S. Brand Names** Combivir®

(Continued)

## Zidovudine and Lamivudine *(Continued)*

**Dosage Forms Tab:** Zidovudine 300 mg and lamivudine 150 mg

♦ **Zilactin-B® Medicated [OTC]** *see* Benzocaine *on page 105*

♦ **Zilactin-L® [OTC]** *see* Lidocaine *on page 531*

## Zileuton *(zye LOO ton)*

**Pharmacologic Class** 5-Lipoxygenase Inhibitor

**U.S. Brand Names** Zyflo™

**Mechanism of Action** Specific inhibitor of 5-lipoxygenase and thus inhibits leukotriene (LTB1, LTC1, LTD1 and LTE1) formation. Leukotrienes are substances that induce numerous biological effects including augmentation of neutrophil and eosinophil migration, neutrophil and monocyte aggregation, leukocyte adhesion, increased capillary permeability and smooth muscle contraction.

**Use** Prophylaxis and chronic treatment of asthma in adults and children ≥12 years of age

**USUAL DOSAGE** Oral:

Adults: 600 mg 4 times/day with meals and at bedtime

Elderly: Zileuton pharmacokinetics were similar in healthy elderly subjects (>65 years) compared with healthy younger adults (18-40 years)

**Dosing adjustment in renal impairment:** Dosing adjustment is not necessary in renal impairment or renal failure (even during dialysis)

**Dosing adjustment in hepatic impairment:** Contraindicated in patients with active liver disease

**Dosage Forms Tab:** 600 mg

**Contraindications** Active liver disease or transaminase elevations greater than or equal to three times the upper limit of normal (≥3 x ULN), hypersensitivity to zileuton or any of its active ingredients

**Warnings/Precautions** Elevations of one or more liver function tests may occur during therapy. These laboratory abnormalities may progress, remain unchanged or resolve with continued therapy. Use with caution in patients who consume substantial quantities of alcohol or have a past history of liver disease. Zileuton is not indicated for use in the reversal of bronchospasm in acute asthma attacks, including status asthmaticus. Zileuton can be continued during acute exacerbations of asthma.

**Pregnancy Risk Factor** C

**Pregnancy Implications**

Clinical effects on the fetus: Developmental studies indicated adverse effects (reduced body weight and increased skeletal variations ) in rats at an oral dose of 300 mg/kg/day. There are no adequate and well controlled studies in pregnant women.

Breast-feeding/lactation: Zileuton and its metabolites are excreted in rat milk; it is not known if zileuton is excreted in breast milk

**Adverse Reactions**

>10%:

Central nervous system: Headache (24.6%)

Hepatic: Increased ALT (12%)

1% to 10%:

Cardiovascular: Chest pain

Central nervous system: Pain, dizziness, fever, insomnia, malaise, nervousness, somnolence

Gastrointestinal: Dyspepsia, nausea, abdominal pain, constipation, flatulence

Hematologic: Low white blood cell count

Neuromuscular & skeletal: Myalgia, arthralgia, weakness

Ocular: Conjunctivitis

**Drug Interactions** CYP1A2, 2C9, and 3A3/4 enzyme substrate; CYP1A2 and 3A3/4 inhibitor

Increased toxicity:

Propranolol: Doubling of propranolol AUC and consequent increased beta-blocker activity

Terfenadine: Decrease in clearance of terfenadine leading to increase in AUC

Theophylline: Doubling of serum theophylline concentrations - reduce theophylline dose and monitor serum theophylline concentrations closely.

Warfarin: Clinically significant increases in prothrombin time (PT) - monitor PT closely

**Onset** Peak concentrations: 1-2 hours

**Half-Life** 2.5 hours

**Special PA Issues**

**Patient Education:** This medication is not for an acute asthmatic attack; in acute attack, follow instructions of prescriber. Do not stop other asthma medication unless advised by prescriber. Take with meals and at bedtime on a continuous bases; do not discontinue even if feeling better (this medication may help reduce incidence of acute attacks). Avoid alcohol and other medications unless approved by your prescriber. You may experience mild headache (mild analgesic may help); fatigue or dizziness (use caution when driving); or nausea or heartburn (frequent mouth care, sucking on lozenges, or chewing gum may help). Report persistent headache, chest pain, rapid heartbeat, or palpitations; skin rash or itching; unusual bleeding (eg, tarry stools, easy bruising, or blood in stool, urine, or mouth); skin rash or irritation; muscle weakness or tremors; redness, irritation, or infections of the eye; or worsening of asthmatic condition.

**Monitoring Parameters:** Evaluate hepatic transaminases at initiation of and during therapy with zileuton. Monitor serum ALT before treatment begins, once-a-month for the first 3 months, every 2-3 months for the remainder of the first year, and periodically thereafter for patients receiving long-term zileuton therapy. If symptoms of liver dysfunction (right upper quadrant pain, nausea, fatigue, lethargy, pruritus, jaundice or "flu-like" symptoms) develop or transaminase elevations >5 times the ULN occur, discontinue therapy and follow transaminase levels until normal.

♦ **Zinacef® Injection** *see* Cefuroxime *on page 176*

♦ **Zinca-Pak®** *see* Zinc Supplements *on this page*

♦ **Zincate®** *see* Zinc Supplements *on this page*

♦ **Zinc Chloride** *see* Zinc Supplements *on this page*

# Zinc Gelatin (zingk JEL ah tin)
**Pharmacologic Class** Topical Skin Product
**U.S. Brand Names** Gelucast®
**Use** As a protectant and to support varicosities and similar lesions of the lower limbs
**USUAL DOSAGE** Apply externally as an occlusive boot
**Dosage Forms Bandage:** 3" x 10 yards, 4" x 10 yards
**Contraindications** Hypersensitivity to any component
**Adverse Reactions** 1% to 10%: Local: Irritation

♦ **Zinc Gelatin Boot** *see* Zinc Gelatin *on this page*

♦ **Zinc Gluconate** *see* Zinc Supplements *on this page*

♦ **Zinc Sulfate** *see* Zinc Supplements *on this page*

# Zinc Supplements (zink SUP la ments)
**Pharmacologic Class** Mineral, Oral; Mineral, Parenteral; Trace Element
**U.S. Brand Names** Eye-Sed® [OTC]; Orazinc® [OTC]; Verazinc® [OTC]; Zinca-Pak®; Zincate®
**Mechanism of Action** Provides for normal growth and tissue repair, is a cofactor for more than 70 enzymes; ophthalmic astringent and weak antiseptic due to precipitation of protein and clearing mucus from outer surface of the eye
**Use** Cofactor for replacement therapy to different enzymes helps maintain normal growth rates, normal skin hydration and senses of taste and smell; zinc supplement (oral and parenteral); may improve wound healing in those who are deficient. May be useful to promote wound healing in patients with pressure sores.
**USUAL DOSAGE** Clinical response may not occur for up to 6-8 weeks
Zinc sulfate:
RDA: Oral:
Birth to 6 months: 3 mg elemental zinc/day
6-12 months: 5 mg elemental zinc/day
1-10 years: 10 mg elemental zinc/day (44 mg zinc sulfate)
≥11 years: 15 mg elemental zinc/day (65 mg zinc sulfate)
Zinc deficiency: Oral:
Infants and Children: 0.5-1 mg elemental zinc/kg/day divided 1-3 times/day; somewhat larger quantities may be needed if there is impaired intestinal absorption or an excessive loss of zinc
Adults: 110-220 mg zinc sulfate (25-50 mg elemental zinc)/dose 3 times/day
Parenteral: TPN: I.V. infusion (chloride or sulfate): Supplemental to I.V. solutions (clinical response may not occur for up to 6-8 weeks):
Premature Infants <1500 g, up to 3 kg: 300 mcg/kg/day
Full-term Infants and Children ≤5 years: 100 mcg/kg/day
**or**
Premature Infants: 400 mcg/kg/day
Term <3 months: 250 mcg/kg/day
Term >3 months: 100 mcg/kg/day
Children: 50 mcg/kg/day
Adults:
Stable with fluid loss from small bowel: 12.2 mg zinc/liter TPN or 17.1 mg zinc/kg (added to 1000 mL I.V. fluids) of stool or ileostomy output
Metabolically stable: 2.5-4 mg/day, add 2 mg/day for acute catabolic states
**Dosage Forms**
Zinc carbonate, complex: **Liq:** 15 mg/mL (30 mL)
Zinc chloride: **Inj:** 1 mg/mL (10 mL)
Zinc gluconate (14.3% zinc): **Tab:** 10 mg (elemental zinc 1.4 mg), 15 mg (elemental zinc 2 mg), 50 mg (elemental zinc 7 mg), 78 mg (elemental zinc 11 mg)
Zinc sulfate (23% zinc): **Cap:** 110 mg (elemental zinc 25 mg), 220 mg (elemental zinc 50 mg); **Inj:** 1 mg/mL (10 mL, 30 mL), 4 mg/mL (10 mL), 5 mg/mL (5 mL, 10 mL); **Tab:** 66 mg (elemental zinc 15 mg), 110 mg (elemental zinc 25 mg), 200 mg (elemental zinc 45 mg)
(Continued)

## Zinc Supplements *(Continued)*

**Contraindications** Hypersensitivity to any component

**Warnings/Precautions** Do not take undiluted by direct injection into a peripheral vein because of potential for phlebitis, tissue irritation, and potential to increase renal loss of minerals from a bolus injection; administration of zinc in absence of copper may decrease plasma levels; excessive dose may increase HDL and impair immune system function

**Pregnancy Risk Factor** C

**Adverse Reactions** <1%: Hypotension, indigestion, nausea, vomiting, neutropenia, leukopenia, jaundice, pulmonary edema

**Drug Interactions**

Decreased effect: Decreased penicillamine, decreased tetracycline effect reduced, iron decreased uptake of zinc, bran products, dairy products reduce absorption of zinc

**Special PA Issues**

**Patient Education:** Take as directed; do not take more than recommended. Take with food; however, avoid foods high in calcium, phosphorous, or phytate. Stop medication and contact prescriber if you develop severe nausea or vomiting or acute indigestion; easy bruising or bleeding; persistent dizziness; or unusual respiratory difficulty.

**Dietary Considerations:** Food: Avoid foods high in calcium or phosphorus

**Monitoring Parameters:** Patients on TPN therapy should have periodic serum copper and serum zinc levels, skin integrity

**Reference Range:**

Serum: 50-150 µg/dL (<20 µg/dL as solid test with dermatitis followed by alopecia)
Therapeutic: 66-110 µg/dL (SI: 10-16.8 µmol/L)

- **Zingiber officinale** *see* Ginger *on page 414*

- **Zithromax™** *see* Azithromycin *on page 93*

- **Zocor®** *see* Simvastatin *on page 835*

- **Zofran®** *see* Ondansetron *on page 675*

- **Zoladex® Implant** *see* Goserelin *on page 423*

- **Zolicef®** *see* Cefazolin *on page 161*

## Zolmitriptan (zohl mi TRIP tan)

**Pharmacologic Class** Serotonin 5-HT$_{1D}$ Receptor Agonist

**U.S. Brand Names** Zomig®

**Mechanism of Action** Selective agonist for serotonin (5-HT$_{1B}$ and 5-HT$_{1D}$ receptors) in cranial arteries to cause vasoconstriction and reduce sterile inflammation associated with antidromic neuronal transmission correlating with relief of migraine

**Use** Acute treatment of migraine with or without auras

**USUAL DOSAGE** Adults:

Oral: Initial recommended dose: 2.5 mg or lower (achieved by manually breaking a 2.5 mg tablet in half). If the headache returns, the dose may be repeated after 2 hours, not to exceed 10 mg within a 24-hour period. Response is greater following the 2.5 or 5 mg dose compared with 1 mg, with little added benefit and increased side effects associated with the 5 mg dose.

**Dosage adjustment in hepatic impairment:** Administer with caution in patients with liver disease, generally using doses <2.5 mg. Patients with moderate-to-severe hepatic impairment may have decreased clearance of zolmitriptan, and significant elevation in blood pressure was observed in some patients.

**Dosage Forms** Tab: 2.5 mg, 5 mg

**Contraindications**

Use in patients with ischemic heart disease or Prinzmetal angina, patients with signs or symptoms of ischemic heart disease, uncontrolled hypertension; use in patients with symptomatic Wolff-Parkinson-White syndrome or arrhythmias associated with other cardiac accessory conduction pathway disorders

Use with ergotamine derivatives (within 24 hours of); use within 24 hours of another 5-HT$_1$ agonist; concurrent administration or within 2 weeks of discontinuing an MAOI; hypersensitivity to any component; management of hemiplegic or basilar migraine

**Warnings/Precautions** Zolmitriptan is indicated only in patient populations with a clear diagnosis of migraine. Cardiac events (coronary artery vasospasm, transient ischemia, myocardial infarction, ventricular tachycardia/fibrillation, cardiac arrest, and death) have been reported with 5-HT$_1$ agonist administration. Significant elevation in blood pressure, including hypertensive crisis, has also been reported on rare occasions in patients with and without a history of hypertension. Vasospasm-related reactions have been reported other than coronary artery vasospasm. Peripheral vascular ischemia and colonic ischemia with abdominal pain and bloody diarrhea have occurred. Use with caution in patients with hepatic impairment.

**Pregnancy Risk Factor** C

**Adverse Reactions**

>10%:

Central nervous system: Dizziness

Endocrine & metabolic: Hot flashes

Neuromuscular & skeletal: Paresthesia

1% to 10%:

Cardiovascular: Tightness in chest

Central nervous system: Drowsiness, headache

Dermatologic: Burning sensation

Gastrointestinal: Abdominal discomfort, mouth discomfort

Neuromuscular & skeletal: Myalgia, numbness, weakness, neck pain, jaw discomfort

Miscellaneous: Diaphoresis

<1%: Rashes, polydipsia, dehydration, dysmenorrhea, dysuria, renal calculus, dyspnea, thirst, hiccups

**Drug Interactions** Increased toxicity: Ergot-containing drugs, MAOIs, cimetidine, oral contraceptives, SSRIs

**Onset** Within 30 minutes to 1 hour

**Half-Life** 3 hours

**Special PA Issues**

**Patient Education:** This drug is to be used to reduce your migraine, not to prevent or reduce number of attacks. If first dose brings relief, second dose may be taken anytime after 2 hours if migraine returns. If you have no relief with first dose, do not take a second dose without consulting prescriber. Do not exceed 10 mg in 24 hours. You may experience some dizziness or drowsiness; use caution when driving or engaging in tasks that require alertness. Frequent mouth care and sucking on lozenges may relieve dry mouth. Report immediately any chest pain, heart throbbing or tightness in throat; swelling of eyelids, face, or lips; skin rash or hives; easy bruising; blood in urine, stool, or vomitus; pain or itching with urination; or pain, warmth, or numbness in extremities.

♦ **Zoloft™** see Sertraline on page 830

# Zolpidem (zole Pl dem)

**Pharmacologic Class** Hypnotic, Miscellaneous

**U.S. Brand Names** Ambien™

**Mechanism of Action** Structurally dissimilar to benzodiazepine, however, has much or all of its actions explained by its effects on benzodiazepine (BZD) receptors, especially the omega-1 receptor; retains hypnotic and much of the anxiolytic properties of the BZD, but has reduced effects on skeletal muscle and seizure threshold.

**Use** Short-term treatment of insomnia

**USUAL DOSAGE** Duration of therapy should be limited to 7-10 days

Adults: Oral: 10 mg immediately before bedtime; maximum dose: 10 mg

Elderly: 5 mg immediately before bedtime

Hemodialysis: Not dialyzable

**Dosing adjustment in hepatic impairment:** Decrease dose to 5 mg

**Dosage Forms** Tab, as tartrate: 5 mg, 10 mg

**Contraindications** Lactation

**Warnings/Precautions** Closely monitor elderly or debilitated patients for impaired cognitive or motor performance; not recommended for use in children <18 years of age

**Pregnancy Risk Factor** B

**Adverse Reactions**

1% to 10%:

Central nervous system: Headache, drowsiness, dizziness

Gastrointestinal: Nausea, diarrhea

Neuromuscular & skeletal: Myalgia

<1%: Amnesia, confusion, vomiting, falls, tremor

**Drug Interactions** CYP3A3/4 enzyme substrate

Increased effect/toxicity with alcohol, CNS depressants

**Onset** 30 minutes

**Duration** 6-8 hours

**Half-Life** 2-2.6 hours, in cirrhosis increased to 9.9 hours

**Special PA Issues**

**Patient Education:** Use exactly as directed (do not increase dose or frequency or discontinue without consulting prescriber); may cause physical and/or psychological dependence. While using this medication, do not use alcohol or other prescription or OTC medications (especially, pain medications, sedatives, antihistamines, or hypnotics) without consulting prescriber. Maintain adequate hydration (2-3 L/day of fluids unless instructed to restrict fluid intake). You may experience drowsiness, dizziness, or blurred vision (use caution when driving or engaging in hazardous tasks); nausea (small frequent meals, good mouth care, chewing gum, or sucking lozenges may help); or diarrhea (buttermilk, boiled milk, yogurt may help). Report CNS changes (confusion, depression, increased sedation, excitation, headache, abnormal thinking, insomnia, or nightmares); muscle pain or weakness; difficulty breathing; chest pain or palpitations; or ineffectiveness of medication.

(Continued)

## Zolpidem *(Continued)*

**Dietary Considerations:** Alcohol: Additive CNS effect, avoid use
**Monitoring Parameters:** Respiratory, cardiac and mental status
**Reference Range:** 80-150 ng/mL

- **Zolpidem Tartrate** *see* Zolpidem *on previous page*
- **Zomig®** *see* Zolmitriptan *on page 976*
- **Zonalon® Topical Cream** *see* Doxepin *on page 304*
- **Zone-A Forte®** *see* Pramoxine and Hydrocortisone *on page 748*
- **ZORprin®** *see* Aspirin *on page 80*
- **Zosyn™** *see* Piperacillin and Tazobactam Sodium *on page 730*
- **Zovia®** *see* Ethinyl Estradiol and Ethynodiol Diacetate *on page 345*
- **Zovirax®** *see* Acyclovir *on page 28*
- **Zyban™** *see* Bupropion *on page 128*
- **Zydone®** *see* Hydrocodone and Acetaminophen *on page 449*
- **Zyflo™** *see* Zileuton *on page 974*
- **Zyloprim®** *see* Allopurinol *on page 42*
- **Zymase®** *see* Pancrelipase *on page 694*
- **Zyprexa™** *see* Olanzapine *on page 673*
- **Zyrtec®** *see* Cetirizine *on page 183*

# APPENDIX
# TABLE OF CONTENTS

**Miscellaneous**

# MILLIEQUIVALENT AND MILLIMOLE CALCULATIONS & CONVERSIONS

## DEFINITIONS & CALCULATIONS

**Definitions**

| | | |
|---|---|---|
| mole | = | gram molecular weight of a substance (aka molar weight) |
| millimole (mM) | = | milligram molecular weight of a substance (a millimole is 1/1000 of a mole) |
| equivalent weight | = | gram weight of a substance which will combine with or replace one gram (one mole) of hydrogen; an equivalent weight can be determined by dividing the molar weight of a substance by its ionic valence |
| milliequivalent (mEq) | = | milligram weight of a substance which will combine with or replace one milligram (one millimole) of hydrogen (a milliequivalent is 1/1000 of an equivalent) |

**Calculations**

$$\text{moles} = \frac{\text{weight of a substance (grams)}}{\text{molecular weight of that substance (grams)}}$$

$$\text{millimoles} = \frac{\text{weight of a substance (milligrams)}}{\text{molecular weight of that substance (milligrams)}}$$

$$\text{equivalents} = \text{moles x valence of ion}$$

$$\text{milliequivalents} = \text{millimoles x valence of ion}$$

$$\text{moles} = \frac{\text{equivalents}}{\text{valence of ion}}$$

$$\text{millimoles} = \frac{\text{milliequivalents}}{\text{valence of ion}}$$

$$\text{millimoles} = \text{moles x 1000}$$

$$\text{milliequivalents} = \text{equivalents x 1000}$$

**Note:** Use of equivalents and milliequivalents is valid only for those substances which have fixed ionic valences (eg, sodium, potassium, calcium, chlorine, magnesium bromine, etc). For substances with variable ionic valences (eg, phosphorous), a reliable equivalent value cannot be determined. In these instances, one should calculate millimoles (which are fixed and reliable) rather than milliequivalents.

## MILLIEQUIVALENT CONVERSIONS

To convert mg/100 mL to mEq/L the following formula may be used:

$$\frac{(\text{mg/100 mL}) \times 10 \times \text{valence}}{\text{atomic weight}} = \text{mEq/L}$$

To convert mEq/L to mg/100 mL the following formula may be used:

$$\frac{(\text{mEq/L}) \times \text{atomic weight}}{10 \times \text{valence}} = \text{mg/100 mL}$$

To convert mEq/L to volume of percent of a gas the following formula may be used:

$$\frac{(\text{mEq/L}) \times 22.4}{10} = \text{volume percent}$$

## MILLIEQUIVALENT AND MILLIMOLE CALCULATIONS & CONVERSIONS *(Continued)*

### Valences and Atomic Weights of Selected Ions

| Substance | Electrolyte | Valence | Molecular Wt |
|---|---|---|---|
| Calcium | $Ca^{++}$ | 2 | 40 |
| Chloride | $Cl^-$ | 1 | 35.5 |
| Magnesium | $Mg^{++}$ | 2 | 24 |
| Phosphate | $HPO_4^{--}$ (80%) | 1.8 | 96* |
| pH = 7.4 | $H_2PO_4^-$ (20%) | 1.8 | 96* |
| Potassium | $K^+$ | 1 | 39 |
| Sodium | $Na^+$ | 1 | 23 |
| Sulfate | $SO_4^{--}$ | 2 | 96* |

*The molecular weight of phosphorus only is 31, and sulfur only is 32.

### Approximate Milliequivalents — Weights of Selected Ions

| Salt | mEq/g Salt | Mg Salt/mEq |
|---|---|---|
| Calcium carbonate ($CaCO_3$) | 20 | 50 |
| Calcium chloride ($CaCl_2 - 2H_2O$) | 14 | 73 |
| Calcium gluconate (Ca gluconate$_2 - 1H_2O$) | 4 | 224 |
| Calcium lactate (Ca lactate$_2 - 5H_2O$) | 6 | 154 |
| Magnesium sulfate ($MgSO_4$) | 16 | 60 |
| Magnesium sulfate ($MgSO_4 - 7H_2O$) | 8 | 123 |
| Potassium acetate (K acetate) | 10 | 98 |
| Potassium chloride (KCl) | 13 | 75 |
| Potassium citrate ($K_3$ citrate $- 1H_2O$) | 9 | 108 |
| Potassium iodide (KI) | 6 | 166 |
| Sodium bicarbonate ($NaHCO_3$) | 12 | 84 |
| Sodium chloride (NaCl) | 17 | 58 |
| Sodium citrate ($Na_3$ citrate $- 2H_2O$) | 10 | 98 |
| Sodium iodine (NaI) | 7 | 150 |
| Sodium lactate (Na lactate) | 9 | 112 |

## CORRECTED SODIUM

Corrected $Na^+$ = measured $Na^+$ + [1.5 x (glucose − 150 divided by 100)]

**Note:** Do not correct for glucose <150.

## WATER DEFICIT

Water deficit = 0.6 x body weight [1 − (140 divided by $Na^+$)]

**Note: Body weight** is estimated weight in kg when fully hydrated; **$Na^+$** is serum or plasma sodium. Use corrected $Na^+$ if necessary. Consult medical references for recommendations for replacement of deficit.

## TOTAL SERUM CALCIUM CORRECTED FOR ALBUMIN LEVEL

[(Normal albumin − patient's albumin) x 0.8] + patient's measured total calcium

## ACID-BASE ASSESSMENT

**Henderson-Hasselbalch Equation**

$$pH = 6.1 + log (HCO_3^-/ (0.03) (pCO_2))$$

## Alveolar Gas Equation

$PIO_2$ = $FiO_2$ x (total atmospheric pressure – vapor pressure of $H_2O$ at 37°C)

= $FiO_2$ x (760 mm Hg – 47 mm Hg)

$PAO_2$ = $PIO_2 - PACO_2 / R$

Alveolar/arterial oxygen gradient = $PAO_2 - PaO_2$

Normal ranges:

| | |
|---|---|
| Children | 15-20 mm Hg |
| Adults | 20-25 mm Hg |

where:

$PIO_2$ = Oxygen partial pressure of inspired gas (mm Hg) (150 mm Hg in room air at sea level)

$FiO_2$ = Fractional pressure of oxygen in inspired gas (0.21 in room air)

$PAO_2$ = Alveolar oxygen partial pressure

$PACO_2$ = Alveolar carbon dioxide partial pressure

$PaO_2$ = Arterial oxygen partial pressure

R = Respiratory exchange quotient (typically 0.8, increases with high carbohydrate diet, decreases with high fat diet)

## Acid-Base Disorders

Acute metabolic acidosis (<12 h duration):
$$PaCO_2 \text{ expected} = 1.5 (HCO_3^-) + 8 \pm 2$$
or
expected change in $pCO = (1-1.5)$ x change in $HCO_3^-$

Acute metabolic alkalosis (<12 h duration):
expected change in $pCO_2 = (0.5-1)$ x change in $HCO_3^-$

Acute respiratory acidosis (<6 h duration):
expected change in $HCO_3^- = 0.1$ x $pCO_2$

Acute respiratory acidosis (>6 h duration):
expected change in $HCO_3^- = 0.4$ x change in $pCO_2$

Acute respiratory alkalosis (<6 h duration):
expected change in $HCO_3^- = 0.2$ x change in $pCO_2$

Acute respiratory alkalosis (>6 h duration):
expected change in $HCO_3^- = 0.5$ x change in $pCO_2$

# ACID-BASE EQUATION

$H^+$ (in mEq/L) = (24 x $PaCO_2$) divided by $HCO_3^-$

# Aa GRADIENT

Aa gradient $[(713)(FiO_2 - (PaCO_2 \text{ divided by } 0.8))] - PaO_2$

| | | |
|---|---|---|
| Aa gradient | = | alveolar-arterial oxygen gradient |
| $FiO_2$ | = | inspired oxygen (expressed as a fraction) |
| $PaCO_2$ | = | arterial partial pressure carbon dioxide (mm Hg) |
| $PaO_2$ | = | arterial partial pressure oxygen (mm Hg) |

## MILLIEQUIVALENT AND MILLIMOLE CALCULATIONS & CONVERSIONS *(Continued)*

## OSMOLALITY

**Definition:** The summed concentrations of all osmotically active solute particles.

Predicted serum osmolality =

2 Na$^+$ + glucose (mg/dL) / 18 + BUN (mg/dL) / 2.8

The normal range of serum osmolality is 285-295 mOsm/L.

Differential diagnosis of increased serum osmolal gap (>10 mOsm/L)

Medications and toxins

Alcohols (ethanol, methanol, isopropanol, glycerol, ethylene glycol)

Mannitol

Paraldehyde

**Calculated Osm**

Osmolal gap = measured Osm – calculated Osm

0 to +10: Normal

>10: Abnormal

<0: Probable lab or calculation error

**For drugs causing increased osmolar gap, see "Toxicology Information" section in this Appendix.**

## BICARBONATE DEFICIT

HCO$_3^-$ deficit = (0.4 x wt in kg) x (HCO$_3^-$ desired – HCO$_3^-$ measured)

**Note:** In clinical practice, the calculated quantity may differ markedly from the actual amount of bicarbonate needed or that which may be safely administered.

## ANION GAP

**Definition:** The difference in concentration between unmeasured cation and anion equivalents in serum.

Anion gap = Na$^+$ – Cl$^-$ – HCO$_3^-$

(The normal anion gap is 10-14 mEq/L)

### Differential Diagnosis of Increased Anion Gap Acidosis

Organic anions

Lactate (sepsis, hypovolemia, seizures, large tumor burden)

Pyruvate

Uremia

Ketoacidosis (β-hydroxybutyrate and acetoacetate)

Amino acids and their metabolites

Other organic acids

Inorganic anions

Hyperphosphatemia

Sulfates

Nitrates

**Differential Diagnosis of Decreased Anion Gap**

Organic cations

Hypergammaglobulinemia

Inorganic cations

Hyperkalemia
Hypercalcemia
Hypermagnesemia

Medications and toxins

Lithium

Hypoalbuminemia

# RETICULOCYTE INDEX

(% retic divided by 2) x (patient's Hct divided by normal Hct) or (% retic divided by 2) x (patient's Hgb divided by normal Hgb)

Normal index: 1.0
Good marrow response: 2.0-6.0

# BODY SURFACE AREA OF ADULTS AND CHILDREN

### Calculating Body Surface Area in Children

In a child of average size, find weight and corresponding surface area on the boxed scale to the left; or, use the nomogram to the right. Lay a straightedge on the correct height and weight points for the child, then read the intersecting point on the surface area scale.

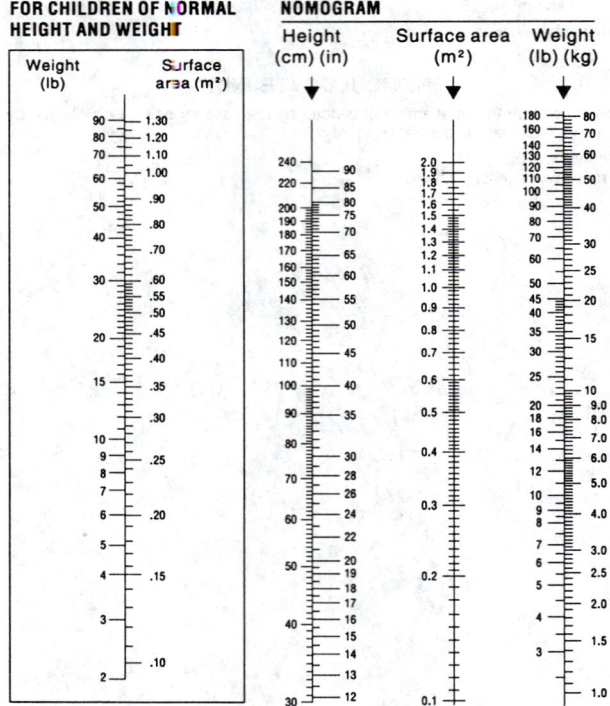

## BODY SURFACE AREA FORMULA
### (Adult and Pediatric)

$$\text{BSA (m}^2) = \sqrt{\frac{\text{Ht (in) x Wt (lb)}}{3131}} \quad \text{or, in metric: BSA (m}^2) = \sqrt{\frac{\text{Ht (cm) x Wt (kg)}}{3600}}$$

References

Lam TK and Leung D⁻, "More on Simplified Calculation of Body Surface Area," *N Engl J Med*, 1988, 318(17):1130 (Letter).

Mosteller RD, "Simplified Calculation of Body Surface Area", *N Engl J Med*, 1987, 317(17):1098 (Letter).

# IDEAL BODY WEIGHT CALCULATION

**Adults (18 years and older) (IBW is in kg)**

IBW (male) = 50 + (2.3 x height in inches over 5 feet)

IBW (female) = 45.5 + (2.3 x height in inches over 5 feet)

**Children (IBW is in kg; height is in cm)**

a.  1-18 years

IBW $= \dfrac{(\text{height}^2 \times 1.65)}{1000}$

b.  5 feet and taller

IBW (male) = 39 + (2.27 x height in inches over 5 feet)

IBW (female) = 42.2 + (2.27 x height in inches over 5 feet)

# BODY MASS INDEX CHART

The Body Mass Index (BMI) shown below is a practical marker to assess obesity and an indicator of optimal weight for health. BMI is a relationship between height and weight. Overweight adults (18 years or older) with a BMI ≥25 are at risk for comorbid disease.

## Height (Feet and Inches)

| Weight (Pounds) | 5'0" | 5'1" | 5'2" | 5'3" | 5'4" | 5'5" | 5'6" | 5'7" | 5'8" | 5'9" | 5'10" | 5'11" | 6'0" | 6'1" | 6'2" | 6'3" | 6'4" |
|---|---|---|---|---|---|---|---|---|---|---|---|---|---|---|---|---|---|
| 100 | 20 | 19 | 18 | 18 | 17 | 17 | 16 | 16 | 15 | 15 | 14 | 14 | 14 | 13 | 13 | 12 | 12 |
| 105 | 21 | 20 | 19 | 19 | 18 | 17 | 17 | 16 | 16 | 15 | 15 | 15 | 14 | 14 | 13 | 13 | 13 |
| 110 | 21 | 21 | 20 | 19 | 19 | 18 | 18 | 17 | 17 | 16 | 16 | 15 | 15 | 15 | 14 | 14 | 13 |
| 115 | 22 | 22 | 21 | 20 | 20 | 19 | 19 | 18 | 17 | 17 | 17 | 16 | 16 | 15 | 15 | 14 | 14 |
| 120 | 23 | 23 | 22 | 21 | 21 | 20 | 19 | 19 | 18 | 18 | 17 | 17 | 16 | 16 | 15 | 15 | 15 |
| 125 | 24 | 24 | 23 | 22 | 21 | 21 | 20 | 20 | 19 | 18 | 18 | 17 | 17 | 16 | 16 | 16 | 15 |
| 130 | 25 | 25 | 24 | 23 | 22 | 22 | 21 | 20 | 20 | 19 | 19 | 18 | 18 | 17 | 17 | 16 | 16 |
| 135 | 26 | 26 | 25 | 24 | 23 | 22 | 22 | 21 | 21 | 20 | 19 | 19 | 18 | 18 | 17 | 17 | 16 |
| 140 | 27 | 26 | 26 | 25 | 24 | 23 | 23 | 22 | 21 | 21 | 20 | 20 | 19 | 18 | 18 | 17 | 17 |
| 145 | 28 | 27 | 27 | 26 | 25 | 24 | 23 | 23 | 22 | 21 | 21 | 20 | 20 | 19 | 19 | 18 | 18 |
| 150 | 29 | 28 | 27 | 27 | 26 | 25 | 24 | 23 | 23 | 22 | 22 | 21 | 20 | 20 | 19 | 19 | 18 |
| 155 | 30 | 29 | 28 | 27 | 27 | 26 | 25 | 24 | 24 | 23 | 22 | 22 | 21 | 20 | 20 | 19 | 19 |
| 160 | 31 | 30 | 29 | 28 | 27 | 27 | 26 | 25 | 24 | 24 | 23 | 22 | 22 | 21 | 21 | 20 | 19 |
| 165 | 32 | 31 | 30 | 29 | 28 | 27 | 27 | 26 | 25 | 24 | 24 | 23 | 22 | 22 | 21 | 21 | 20 |
| 170 | 33 | 32 | 31 | 30 | 29 | 28 | 27 | 27 | 26 | 25 | 24 | 24 | 23 | 22 | 22 | 21 | 21 |
| 175 | 34 | 33 | 32 | 31 | 30 | 29 | 28 | 27 | 27 | 26 | 25 | 24 | 24 | 23 | 22 | 22 | 21 |
| 180 | 35 | 34 | 33 | 32 | 31 | 30 | 29 | 28 | 27 | 27 | 26 | 25 | 24 | 24 | 23 | 22 | 22 |
| 185 | 36 | 35 | 34 | 33 | 32 | 31 | 30 | 29 | 28 | 27 | 27 | 26 | 25 | 24 | 24 | 23 | 23 |
| 190 | 37 | 36 | 35 | 34 | 33 | 32 | 31 | 30 | 29 | 28 | 27 | 26 | 26 | 25 | 24 | 24 | 23 |
| 195 | 38 | 37 | 36 | 35 | 33 | 32 | 31 | 31 | 30 | 29 | 28 | 27 | 26 | 26 | 25 | 24 | 24 |
| 200 | 39 | 38 | 37 | 36 | 34 | 33 | 32 | 31 | 30 | 30 | 29 | 28 | 27 | 26 | 26 | 25 | 24 |
| 205 | 40 | 39 | 37 | 36 | 35 | 34 | 33 | 32 | 31 | 30 | 29 | 29 | 28 | 27 | 26 | 26 | 25 |
| 210 | 41 | 40 | 38 | 37 | 36 | 35 | 34 | 33 | 32 | 31 | 29 | 29 | 28 | 28 | 27 | 26 | 26 |
| 215 | 42 | 41 | 39 | 38 | 37 | 36 | 35 | 34 | 33 | 32 | 30 | 30 | 29 | 28 | 28 | 27 | 26 |
| 220 | 43 | 42 | 40 | 39 | 38 | 37 | 36 | 34 | 33 | 32 | 31 | 31 | 30 | 29 | 28 | 27 | 27 |
| 225 | 44 | 43 | 41 | 40 | 39 | 37 | 36 | 35 | 34 | 33 | 32 | 31 | 31 | 30 | 29 | 28 | 27 |
| 230 | 45 | 43 | 42 | 41 | 39 | 38 | 37 | 36 | 35 | 34 | 32 | 32 | 31 | 30 | 30 | 29 | 28 |
| 235 | 46 | 44 | 43 | 42 | 40 | 38 | 38 | 37 | 36 | 35 | 33 | 33 | 32 | 31 | 30 | 29 | 29 |
| 240 | 47 | 45 | 44 | 43 | 41 | 40 | 39 | 38 | 36 | 35 | 34 | 33 | 33 | 32 | 31 | 30 | 29 |
| 245 | 48 | 46 | 45 | 43 | 42 | 41 | 40 | 39 | 37 | 36 | 34 | 34 | 33 | 32 | 31 | 31 | 30 |
| 250 | 49 | 47 | 46 | 44 | 43 | 42 | 40 | 39 | 38 | 37 | 35 | 35 | 34 | 33 | 32 | 31 | 30 |

☐ Underweight  ☐ Weight Appropriate  ☐ Overweight  ■ Obese

# APOTHECARY/METRIC EQUIVALENTS

## Approximate Liquid Measures

Basic equivalent: 1 fluid ounce = 30 mL

Examples:

| | | | |
|---|---|---|---|
| 1 gallon | 3800 mL | 1 gallon | 128 fluid ounces |
| 1 quart | 960 mL | 1 quart | 32 fluid ounces |
| 1 pint | 480 mL | 1 pint | 16 fluid ounces |
| 8 fluid oz | 240 mL | 15 minims | 1 mL |
| 4 fluid oz | 120 mL | 10 minims | 0.6 mL |

## Approximate Household Equivalents

| | | | |
|---|---|---|---|
| 1 teaspoonful | 5 mL | 1 tablespoonful | 15 mL |

## Weights

Basic equivalents:

| | | | |
|---|---|---|---|
| 1 oz | 30 g | 15 gr | 1 g |

Examples:

| | | | |
|---|---|---|---|
| 4 oz | 120 g | 1 gr | 60 mg |
| 2 oz | 60 g | 1/100 gr | 600 mcg |
| 10 gr | 600 mg | 1/150 gr | 400 mcg |
| 7½ gr | 500 mg | 1/200 gr | 300 mcg |
| 16 oz | 1 lb | | |

## Metric Conversions

Basic equivalents:

| | | | |
|---|---|---|---|
| 1 g | 1000 mg | 1 mg | 1000 mcg |

Examples:

| | | | |
|---|---|---|---|
| 5 g | 5000 mg | 5 mg | 5000 mcg |
| 0.5 g | 500 mg | 0.5 g | 500 mcg |
| 0.05 g | 50 mg | 0.05 mg | 50 mcg |

## Exact Equivalents

| | | | | | |
|---|---|---|---|---|---|
| 1 g | = | 15.43 gr | 0.1 mg | = | 1/600 gr |
| 1 mL | = | 16.23 minims | 0.12 mg | = | 1/500 gr |
| 1 minim | = | 0.06 mL | 0.15 mg | = | 1/400 gr |
| 1 gr | = | 64.8 mg | 0.2 mg | = | 1/300 gr |
| 1 pint (pt) | = | 473.2 mL | 0.3 mg | = | 1/200 gr |
| 1 oz | = | 28.35 g | 0.4 mg | = | 1/150 gr |
| 1 lb | = | 453.6 g | 0.5 mg | = | 1/120 gr |
| 1 kg | = | 2.2 lbs | 0.6 mg | = | 1/100 gr |
| 1 qt | = | 946.4 mL | 0.8 mg | = | 1/80 gr |
| | | | 1 mg | = | 1/65 gr |

## Solids*

| | | |
|---|---|---|
| ¼ grain | = | 15 mg |
| ½ grain | = | 30 mg |
| 1 grain | = | 60 mg |
| 1½ grains | = | 90 mg |
| 5 grains | = | 300 mg |
| 10 grains | = | 600 mg |

*Use exact equivalents for compounding and calculations requiring a high degree of accuracy.

# LIVER DISEASE

## Pugh's Modification of Child's Classification for Severity

| Parameter | Points for Increasing Abnormality | | |
|---|---|---|---|
| | 1 | 2 | 3 |
| Encephalopathy | None | 1 or 2 | 3 or 4 |
| Ascites | Absent | Slight | Moderate |
| Bilirubin (mg/dL) | <2.9 | 2.9-5.8 | >5.8 |
| Albumin (g/dL) | >3.5 | 2.8-3.5 | <2.8 |
| Prothrombin time (seconds over control) | 1-4 | 4-6 | >6 |

Scores:

**Mild hepatic impairment** = <6 points.
**Moderate hepatic impairment** = 6-10 points.
**Severe hepatic impairment** = >10 points.

## Considerations for Drug Dose Adjustment

| Extent of Change in Drug Dose | Conditions or Requirements to Be Satisfied |
|---|---|
| No or minor change | Mild liver disease |
| | Extensive elimination of drug by kidneys and no renal dysfunction |
| | Elimination by pathways of metabolism spared by liver disease |
| | Drug is enzyme-limited and given acutely |
| | Drug is flow/enzyme-sensitive and only given acutely by I.V. route |
| | No alteration in drug sensitivity |
| Decrease in dose up to 25% | Elimination by the liver does not exceed 40% of the dose; no renal dysfunction |
| | Drug is flow-limited and given by I.V. route, with no large change in protein binding |
| | Drug is flow/enzyme-limited and given acutely by oral route |
| | Drug has a large therapeutic ratio |
| >25% decrease in dose | Drug metabolism is affected by liver disease; drug administered chronically |
| | Drug has a narrow therapeutic range; protein binding altered significantly |
| | Drug is flow-limited and given orally |
| | Drug is eliminated by kidneys and renal function severely affected |
| | Altered sensitivity to drug due to liver disease |

## Reference

Arns PA, Wedlund PJ, and Branch RA, "Adjustment of Medications in Liver Failure," *The Pharmacologic Approach to the Critically Ill Patient*, 2nd ed, Chernow B, ed, Baltimore, MD: Williams & Wilkins, 1988, 85-111.

# CREATININE CLEARANCE ESTIMATING METHODS IN PATIENTS WITH STABLE RENAL FUNCTION

These formulas provide an acceptable estimate of the patient's creatinine clearance **except** in the following instances.

- Patient's serum creatinine is changing rapidly (either up or down).

- Patients are markedly emaciated.

In above situations, certain assumptions have to be made.

- In patients with rapidly rising serum creatinines (ie, >0.5-0.7 mg/dL/day), it is best to assume that the patient's creatinine clearance is probably <10 mL/minute.

- In emaciated patients, although their actual creatinine clearance is less than their calculated creatinine clearance (because of decreased creatinine production), it is not possible to easily predict how much less.

## Infants

**Estimation of creatinine clearance using serum creatinine and body length** (to be used when an adequate timed specimen cannot be obtained). **Note:** This formula may not provide an accurate estimation of creatinine clearance for infants younger than 6 months of age and for patients with severe starvation or muscle wasting.

$Cl_{cr} = K \times L/S_{cr}$

where:

| | | |
|---|---|---|
| $Cl_{cr}$ | = | creatinine clearance in mL/minute/1.73 m² |
| K | = | constant of proportionality that is age specific |

| Age | K |
|---|---|
| Low birth weight ≤1 y | 0.33 |
| Full-term ≤1 y | 0.45 |
| 2-12 y | 0.55 |
| 13-21 y female | 0.55 |
| 13-21 y male | 0.70 |

| | | |
|---|---|---|
| L | = | length in cm |
| $S_{cr}$ | = | serum creatinine concentration in mg/dL |

### Reference

Schwartz GJ, Brion LP, and Spitzer A, "The Use of Plasma Creatinine Concentration for Estimating Glomerular Filtration Rate in Infants, Children and Adolescents," *Ped Clin N Amer*, 1987, 34:571-90.

## Children (1-18 years)

Method 1: (Traub SL, Johnson CE, *Am J Hosp Pharm*, 1980, 37:195-201)

$$Cl_{cr} = \frac{0.48 \times (height) \times BSA}{S_{cr} \times 1.73}$$

where:

| | | |
|---|---|---|
| BSA | = | body surface area in m² |
| $Cl_{cr}$ | = | creatinine clearance in mL/min |
| $S_{cr}$ | = | serum creatinine in mg/dL |
| Height | = | in cm |

# CREATININE CLEARANCE ESTIMATING
## METHODS IN PATIENTS WITH STABLE RENAL FUNCTION
*(Continued)*

<u>Method 2</u>: Nomogram (Traub SL and Johnson CE, *Am J Hosp Pharm*, 1980, 37:195-201)

### Children 1-18 Years

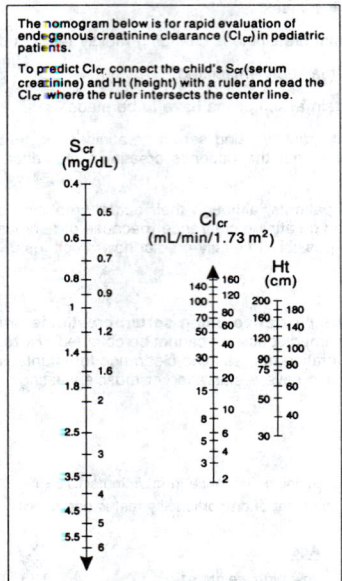

The nomogram below is for rapid evaluation of endogenous creatinine clearance ($Cl_{cr}$) in pediatric patients.

To predict $Cl_{cr}$ connect the child's $S_{cr}$ (serum creatinine) and Ht (height) with a ruler and read the $Cl_{cr}$ where the ruler intersects the center line.

$S_{cr}$ (mg/dL)

$Cl_{cr}$ (mL/min/1.73 m²)

Ht (cm)

## Adults (18 years and older)

<u>Method</u>: (Cockroft DW and Gault MH, *Nephron*, 1976, 16:31-41)

Estimated creatinine clearance ($Cl_{cr}$) (mL/min):

$$Male = \frac{(140 - age)\ IBW\ (kg)}{72 \times S_{cr}}$$

$$Female = estimated\ Cl_{cr}\ male \times 0.85$$

**Note:** The use of the patient's ideal body weight (IBW) is recommended for the above formula except when the patient's actual body weight is less than ideal. Use of the IBW is especially important in obese patients.

# RENAL FUNCTION TESTS

**Endogenous creatinine clearance vs age** (timed collection)

Creatinine clearance (mL/min/1.73 m$^2$) = $(Cr_uV/Cr_sT)$ (1.73/A)

where:

| | | |
|---|---|---|
| $Cr_u$ | = | urine creatinine concentration (mg/dL) |
| V | = | total urine collected during sampling period (mL) |
| $Cr_s$ | = | serum creatinine concentration (mg/dL) |
| T | = | duration of sampling period (min) (24 h = 1440 min) |
| A | = | body surface area (m$^2$) |

Age-specific normal values

| | |
|---|---|
| 5-7 d | 50.6 ± 5.8 mL/min/1.73 m$^2$ |
| 1-2 mo | 64.6 ± 5.8 mL/min/1.73 m$^2$ |
| 5-8 mo | 87.7 ± 11.9 mL/min/1.73 m$^2$ |
| 9-12 mo | 86.9 ± 8.4 mL/min/1.73 m$^2$ |
| ≥18 mo | |
| male | 124 ± 26 mL/min/1.73 m$^2$ |
| female | 109 ± 13.5 mL/min/1.73 m$^2$ |
| Adults | |
| male | 105 ± 14 mL/min/1.73 m$^2$ |
| female | 95 ± 18 mL/min/1.73 m$^2$ |

**Note:** In patients with renal failure (creatinine clearance <25 mL/min), creatinine clearance may be elevated over GFR because of tubular secretion of creatinine.

## Calculation of Creatinine Clearance From a 24-Hour Urine Collection

Equation 1:

$$Cl_{cr} = \frac{U \times V}{P}$$

where:

| | | |
|---|---|---|
| $Cl_{cr}$ | = | creatinine clearance |
| U | = | urine concentration of creatinine |
| V | = | total urine volume in the collection |
| P | = | plasma creatinine concentration |

Equation 2:

$$Cl_{cr} = \frac{\text{(total urine volume [mL]) x (urine Cr concentration [mg/dL])}}{\text{(serum creatinine [mg/dL]) x (time of urine collection [minutes])}}$$

Occasionally, a patient will have a 12- or 24-hour urine collection done for direct calculation of creatinine clearance. Although a urine collection for 24 hours is best, it is difficult to do since many urine collections occur for a much shorter period. A 24-hour urine collection is the desired duration of urine collection because the urine excretion of creatinine is diurnal and thus the measured creatinine clearance will vary throughout the day as the creatinine in the urine varies. When the urine collection is less than 24 hours, the total excreted creatinine will be affected by the time of the day during which the collection is performed. A 24-hour urine collection is sufficient to be able to accurately average the diurnal creatinine excretion variations. If a patient has 24 hours of urine collected for creatinine clearance, equation 1 can be used for calculating the creatinine clearance. To use equation 1 to calculate the creatinine clearance, it will be necessary to know the duration of urine collection, the urine collection volume, the urine creatinine concentration, and the serum creatinine value that reflects the urine collection period. In most cases, a serum creatinine concentration is drawn anytime during the day, but it is best to have the value drawn halfway through the collection period.

## RENAL FUNCTION TESTS *(Continued)*

### Amylase/Creatinine Clearance Ratio*

$$\frac{Amylase_u \times creatinine_p}{Amylase_p \times creatinine_u} \times 100$$

u = urine; p = plasma

### Serum BUN/Serum Creatinine Ratio

Serum BUN (mg/dL:serum creatinine (mg/dL))

Normal BUN:creatinine ratio is 10-15

BUN:creatinine ratio >20 suggests prerenal azotemia (also seen with high urea-generation states such as GI bleeding)

BUN:creatinine ratio <5 may be seen with disorders affecting urea biosynthesis such as urea cycle enzyme deficiencies and with hepatitis.

### Fractional Sodium Excretion

Fractional sodium secretion (FENa) = $Na_u Cr_s/Na_s Cr_u \times 100\%$

where:

$Na_u$ = urine sodium (mEq/L)
$Na_s$ = serum sodium (mEq/L)
$Cr_u$ = urine creatinine (mg/dL)
$Cr_s$ = serum creatinine (mg/dL)

FENa <1% suggests prerenal failure

FENa >2% suggest intrinsic renal failure
(for newborns, normal FENa is approximately 2.5%)

**Note:** Disease states associated with a falsely elevated FENa include severe volume depletion (>10%), early acute tubular necrosis and volume depletion in chronic renal disease. Disorders associated with a lowered FENa include acute glomerulonephritis, hemoglobinuric or myoglobinuric renal failure, nonoliguric acute tubular necrosis and acute urinary tract obstruction. In addition, FENa may be <1% in patients with acute renal failure **and** a second condition predisposing to sodium retention (eg, burns, congestive heart failure, nephrotic syndrome).

### Urine Calcium/Urine Creatinine Ratio (spot sample)

Urine calcium (mg/dL): urine creatinine (mg/dL)

Normal values <0.21 (mean values 0.08 males, 0.06 females)

Premature infants show wide variability of calcium:creatinine ratio, and tend to have lower thresholds for calcium loss than older children. Prematures without nephrolithiasis had mean Ca:Cr ratio of $0.75 \pm 0.76$. Infants with nephrolithiasis had mean Ca:Cr ratio of $1.32 \pm 1.03$ (Jacinto, et al, *Pediatrics*, vol 81, p 31.)

### Urine Protein/Urine Creatinine Ratio (spot sample)

| $P_u/Cr_u$ | Total Protein Excretion $(mg/m^2/d)$ |
|---|---|
| 0.1 | 80 |
| 1 | 800 |
| 10 | 8000 |

where:

$P_u$ = urine protein concentration (mg/dL)
$Cr_u$ = urine creatinine concentration (mg/dL)

# ACE INHIBITORS

## ACE Inhibitors Comparison*

| | Benazepril (Lotensin®) | Captopril (Capoten®) | Enalapril (Vasotec®) | Enalaprilat (Vasotec®) | Fosinopril (Monopril®) | Lisinopril (Prinivil®, Zestril®) | Moexipril (Univasc®) | Quinapril (Accupril®) | Ramipril (Altace™) | Trandolapril (Mavik®) |
|---|---|---|---|---|---|---|---|---|---|---|
| Route | P.O. | P.O. | P.O. | I.V. | P.O. | P.O. | P.O. | P.O. | P.O. | P.O. |
| Dosage forms (mg) | 5 10 20 40 | 12.5 25 50 100 | 2.5 5 10 20 | 1.25 mg/mL | 10 20 | 2.5 5.0 10 20 40 | 7.5 15 | 5 10 20 40 | 1.25 2.5 5 10 | 1 2 4 |
| Usual starting dose (mg) | 10 | 12.5-25 | 5 | 1.25 mg/mL | 10 | 5 | 7.5 | 10 | 2.5 | 1-2 |
| Dosing interval | qd | tid | qd | q6h over 5 min | qd | qd | qd | qd | qd | qd |
| **Indications and starting dose** | | | | | | | | | | |
| HTN | 10 mg qd 5 mg qd# | 12.5-25 mg bid-tid | 5 mg qd 2.5 mg qd# | x | 10 mg qd | 10 mg qd 5 mg qd# | 7.5 mg qd 3.75 mg qd• | 10 mg qd 5 mg qd# | 2.5 mg qd 1.25 mg qd• | 1 mg nonblack patient 2 mg black patient |
| CHF | | 12.5-25 mg tid | 2.5 mg qd-bid | | 10 mg qd | 5 mg qd | | 5 mg bid¶ 2.5 mg bid## | 2.5 mg bid 1.25 mg qd• | |
| Protein binding | >95% | 25%-30% | | 50%-60% | ~95% | — | ~50% | <97% | ~73% ramipril 56% ramiprilat | 80% |
| Active metabolites | Benazeprilat | | Enalaprilat | Enalaprilat | Fosinoprilat | | Moexiprilat | Quinaprilat | Ramiprilat | Trandolaprilat |
| Half-life normal renal function (h) | 10-11† | <2 | 1.3 | 11 | 12‡ | 12 | 2-9 (moexiprilat) | 2 | 13-17 | 6-10 |
| Half-life impaired renal function (h) | Prolonged | 3.5-32 | No data | Prolonged | Prolonged | Prolonged | Prolonged | Prolonged | Prolonged | Prolonged |
| **Elimination** | | | | | | | | | | |
| Total | No data | >95% | 94% urine and feces | No data | 50% urine 50% feces | No data | 13% urine 53% feces | 60% urine 37% feces | 60% urine 40% feces | 33% urine 66% feces |
| Unchanged | Trace | 40%-50% urine | 54% urine (40% enalapril) | >90% urine | Negligible | 100% urine§ | 1% urine 1% feces | Trace | <2§ | - |
| **Incidence of side effects (%)** | | | | | | | | | | |
| Cough | 1.9-3.4 | 0.5-2 | 1.3-2.2 | 11 | 2.2 | 2.9-4.5 | 6.1 | 2 | 12 | 1.9 |
| Angioedema | 0.5 | 0.1 | 0.2 | | ≤1 | 0.1 | <1 | 0.1 | 0.3 | <1 |

## ACE INHIBITORS *(Continued)*

### ACE Inhibitors Comparison*

| | Benazepril (Lotensin®) | Captopril (Capoten®) | Enalapril (Vasotec®) | Enalaprilat (Vasotec®) | Fosinopril (Monopril®) | Lisinopril (Prinvil®, Zestril®) | Moexipril (Univasc®) | Quinapril (Accupril®) | Ramipril (Altace™) | Trandolapril (Mavik®) |
|---|---|---|---|---|---|---|---|---|---|---|
| Rash | x | 4-7 | 1.3-1.4 | | ≤1 | 1.5 | 1.6 | x | x | <1 |
| Headache | 5 | 0.5-2 | 1.8-5.2 | | 3.2 | 5.3 | >1 | 5.6 | 5.4 | 1.3 |
| Dizziness | 3.3 | 0.5-2 | 4.3-7.9 | | 1.6 | 6.3 | 4.3 | 3.9 | 2.2 | <1 |
| Chest pain | | 1 | 2.1 | | ≤1 | 1.3 | >1 | x | <1 | <1 |
| Hypotension | 0.3 | x | 6.7 | | ≤1 | 1.2-5 | 0.5 | x | 0.5 | <1 |
| Diarrhea | | 0.5-2 | 1.4-2.1 | | 1.5 | 3.2 | 3.1 | | | 1 |

*All doses listed are oral and assume patient is **not** on a diuretic. See specific drug monograph for dosing concurrently with diuretics to avoid adverse reactions.

†Half-life accumulates after multiple dosing.

‡Fosinoprilat, after I.V. administration.

§Time frame undefined.

¶CL$_{cr}$ 30-60 mL/min.

#CL$_{cr}$ 10-30 mL/min.

•CL$_{cr}$ <40 mL/min.

x — reported, no incidence given.

## Drug-Drug Interactions With ACEIs

| Precipitant Drug | Drug (Category) and Effect | Description |
|---|---|---|
| Antacids | ACEIs: decreased | Decreased bioavailability of ACEIs. May be more likely with captopril. Separate administration times by 1-2 hours. |
| NSAIDs (indomethacin) | ACEIs: decreased | Reduced hypotensive effects of ACEIs. More prominent in low renin or volume dependent hypertensive patients. |
| ACEIs | Allopurinol: increased | Higher risk of hypersensitivity reaction possible when given concurrently. Three case reports of Stevens-Johnson syndrome with captopril. |
| ACEIs | Digoxin: increased | Increased plasma digoxin levels. |
| ACEIs | Lithium: increased | Increased serum lithium levels and symptoms of toxicity may occur. |
| ACEIs | Potassium preps/ potassium-sparing diuretics increased | Coadministration may result in elevated potassium levels. |
| Rifampin | Enalapril decreased | Effects decreased by rifampin |
| ACEIs | Probenecid | Increased captopril levels and decreased clearance have occurred |
| ACEIs | Diuretics | Additive hypotensive effects |

# ANTIDEPRESSANT AGENTS

| Drug | Class | Anticholinergic Side Effects | Cardiac Arrhythmia | Sedation | Orthostatic Hypotension | Time to Reach Steady State (d) | Half-life (h) | Dosage Range* (mg/d) |
|---|---|---|---|---|---|---|---|---|
| Amitriptyline (Elavil®) | TCA | ++++ | +++ | ++++ | ++ | 4-10 | 31-46 | 50-300 |
| Amoxapine (Asendin®) | TCA | +++ | ++ | ++ | + | 2-7 | 8 | 50-600 |
| Bupropion (Wellbutrin®) | Amino ketone | ++ | + | ++ | + | 1.5-5 | 8-24 | 200-450 |
| Citalopram (Celexa®) | SRI | 0 | 0 | 0 | 0 | 5-10 | 24-48 | 20-60 |
| Clomipramine (Anafranil®) | TCA | +++ | +++ | +++ | ++ | 7-14 | 19-37 | 25-250 |
| Desipramine (Norpramin®) | TCA | + | ++ | + | + | 2-11 | 12-24 | 25-300 |
| Doxepin (Sinequan®) | TCA | ++ | ++ | +++ | ++ | 2-8 | 8-24 | 25-300 |
| Fluoxetine (Prozac®) | SRI | 0/+ | 0 | 0/+ | 0/+ | 28-35 | 48-216 | 20-80 |
| Fluvoxamine (Luvox®) | SRI | + | 0 | − | + | 4-7 | 15 | 50-300 |
| Imipramine (Tofranil®) | TCA | ++ | +++ | ++ | +++ | 2-5 | 11-25 | 30-300 |
| Maprotiline (Ludiomil®) | Tetracyclic | ++ | ++ | ++ | + | 6-10 | 21-25 | 50-225 |
| Mirtazapine (Remeron®) | Tetracyclic | ++ | + | ++++ | + | 5 | 20-40 | 15-45 |
| Nefazodone (Serzone®) | Phenylpiperazine | + | + | + | + | 4-5 | 2-4 | 50-600 |
| Nortriptyline (Pamelor®, Aventyl®) | TCA | ++ | ++ | ++ | + | 4-19 | 18-44 | 30-100 |
| Paroxetine (Paxil®) | SRI | 0 | 0 | 0/+ | 0 | ~10 | 10-24 | 10-50 |
| Phenelzine (Nardil®) | MAO inhibitor | + | − | + | + | — | 2.4-2.8 | 45-90 |
| Protriptyline (Vivactil®) | TCA | +++ | +++ | + | + | 14-19 | 67-89 | 15-60 |

| Drug | Class | Anticholinergic Side Effects | Cardiac Arrhythmia | Sedation | Orthostatic Hypotension | Time to Reach Steady State (d) | Half-life (h) | Dosage Range[a] (mg/d) |
|---|---|---|---|---|---|---|---|---|
| Sertraline (Zoloft®) | SRI | 0 | 0 | + | 0 | 7 | 26 to >100 | 50-200 |
| Tranylcypromine (Parnate®) | MAO inhibitor | + | — | + | 0 | — | — | 30-60 |
| Trazodone (Desyrel®) | Triazalopyridine | + | + | ++ | ++ | 3-7 | 4-9 | 150-600 |
| Trimipramine (Surmontil®) | TCA | ++ | +++ | +++ | ++ | 2-6 | 7-30 | 50-300 |
| Venlafaxine (Effexor®) | Phenylethylamine | 0 | + | 0 | 0 | 3-4 | 5-11 | 75-375 |

TCA = tricyclic antidepressant.

SRI = serotonin reuptake inhibitor.

[a]This dosage range represents manufacturer guidelines and must be individualized for age, indication, and concurrent disease states.

# ANTIFUNGAL AGENTS, TOPICAL

| Generic (Brand) Name(s) | Comments |
| --- | --- |
| Butenafine (Mentax®) | Topical treatment of tinea pedis (athlete's foot) tinea cruris (jock itch). Apply once daily for 4 weeks. |
| Clioquinol (Vioform®) OTC | Topically used in the treatment of tinea pedis (athlete's foot), tinea cruris (jock itch), and skin infections caused by dermatophytic fungi (ringworm).<br>Apply 2-3 times daily. Do not use for longer than 7 days. |
| Ciclopirox (Loprox®) | Treatment of tinea pedis (athlete's foot), tinea cruris (jock itch), tinea corporis (ringworm), cutaneous candidiasis, and tinea versicolor (pityriasis).<br>Apply twice daily. Gently massage into affected area. If no improvement after 4 weeks, re-evaluate diagnosis. |
| Haloprogin (Halotex®) | Topical treatment of tinea pedis (athlete's foot), tinea cruris (jock itch), tinea corporis (ringworm), tinea manuum caused by *Trichophyton rubrum, Trichophyton tonsurans, Trichophyton mentagrophytes, Microsporum canis*, or *Epidermophyton floccosum*.. Topical treatment of *Malassezia furfur*. Apply liberally twice daily for 2-3 weeks. Intertriginous areas may require up to 4 weeks of treatment. |
| Naftifine (Naftin®) | Topical treatment of tinea cruris (jock itch), tinea corporis (ringworm), and tinea pedis (athlete's foot. Apply cream once daily and gel twice daily (morning and evening) for up to 4 weeks. |
| Oxiconazole (Oxistat®) | Treatment of tinea pedis (athlete's foot), tinea cruris (jock itch), and tinea corporis (ringworm). Apply once or twice daily to affected areas for 2 weeks for tinea corporis/tinea cruris and up to 1 month for tinea pedis. |
| Sulconazole (Exelderm®) | Treatment of superficial fungal infections of the skin, including tinea cruris (jock itch), tinea corporis (ringworm), tinea versicolor, and possible tinea pedis (athlete's foot – cream only). For tinea cruris, tinea corporis, and tinea versicolor, apply a small amount to the affected area and gently massage once or twice daily for 3 weeks (4 weeks for tinea pedis). |
| Terbinafine (Lamisil®) | Topical antifungal for the treatment of tinea pedis (athlete's foot), tinea cruris (jock itch), and tinea corporis (ringworm). **Unlabeled use:** Cutaneous candidiasis and pityriasis versicolor. For athlete's foot, apply to affected area twice daily for at least 1 week, not to exceed 4 weeks. For ringworm and jock itch, apply to affected area once or twice daily for at least 1 week, not to exceed 4 weeks. |
| Tolnaftate (Absorbine® Antifungal; Absorbine® Jock Itch; Absorbine Jr.® Antifungal; Aftate® for Athlete's Foot; Aftate® for Jock Itch; Blis-To-Sol®; Breezee® Mist Antifungal; Dr Scholl's® Athlete's Foot; Dr Scholl's® Maximum Strength Tritin; Genaspor®; NP-27®; Quinsana Plus®; Tinactin®; Tinactin® for Jock Itch; Ting®; Pitrex® (Canadian); Tinaderm® (Mexican)) | Treatment of tinea pedis (athlete's foot), tinea cruris (jock itch), tinea corporis (ringworm), tinea manuum, and tinea versicolor infections. Wash and dry affected area. Apply 1-2 drops of solution or small amount of cream or powder and rub into affected areas twice daily for 2-4 weeks. |
| Undecylenic acid and derivatives (Caldesene® Topical; Cruex® Topical; Fungoid® Topical Solution; Merlenate® Topical; Pedi-Dri® Topical; Pedi-Pro® Topical; Undoguent® Topical) | Treat athlete's foot (tinea pedis), ringworm (except nails and scalp), prickly heat, jock itch (tinea cruris), diaper rash, and other minor skin irritations due to superficial dermatophytes. Cleanse the affected area and apply as needed twice daily for 2-4 weeks. |

# ANTIPSYCHOTIC AGENTS

| Antipsychotic Agent | I.M./P.O. Potency | Equivalent Dosages (approx) (mg) | Usual Adult Daily Maintenance Dose (mg) | Sedation (Incidence) | Extrapyramidal Side Effects | Anticholinergic Side Effects | Cardiovascular Side Effects | Comments |
|---|---|---|---|---|---|---|---|---|
| Acetophenazine (Tindal®) | | 20 | 60-120 | Moderate | High | Low | Low | |
| Chlorpromazine (Thorazine®) | 4:1 | 100 | 200-1000 | High | Moderate | Moderate | Moderate/high | |
| Chlorprothixine* (Taractan®) | | 100 | 75-600 | High | Moderate | Moderate | Moderate | |
| Clozapine (Clozaril®) | | 50 | 75-900 | High | Very Low | High | High | <1% incidence of agranulocytosis; weekly-biweekly CBC required |
| Fluphenazine (Prolixin®, Permitil®) | 2:1 | 2 | 0.5-40 | Low | High | Low | Low | |
| Haloperidol (Haldol®) | 2:1 | 2 | 1-15 | Low | High | Low | Low | |
| Loxapine (Loxitane®) | | 10 | 25-250 | Moderate | Moderate | Low | Low | |
| Mesoridazine (Serentil®) | 3:1 | 50 | 30-400 | High | Low | High | Moderate | |
| Molindone (Moban®) | | 15 | 15-225 | Low | Moderate | Low | Low | May cause less weight gain |
| Olanzapine (Zyprexa™) | | 2 | 5-20 | Moderate/High | Low | Moderate/High | Moderate/High | |
| Perphenazine (Trilafon®) | | 10 | 16-64 | Low | Moderate | Low | Low | |
| Pimozide (Orap™) | | 2 | 1-20 | Moderate | High | Moderate | Low | Contraindicated with macrolide antibiotics |
| Promazine (Sparine®) | | 200 | 40-1000 | Moderate | Moderate | High | Moderate | |
| Quetiapine (Seroquel®) | | N/A | 75-750 | Moderate | Very Low | Moderate | Moderate | |
| Risperidone (Risperdal®) | | 1 | 1-16 | Low/Moderate | Low | Low | Low | Target dose: 4-6 mg/d |
| Thioridazine (Mellaril®) | | 100 | 200-800 | High | Low | High | Moderate/high | May cause irreversible retinitis; pigmentosis at doses >800 mg/d |
| Thiothixene (Navane®) | 4:1 | 4 | 5-40 | Low | High | Low | Low/moderate | |
| Trifluoperazine (Stelazine®) | | 5 | 2-40 | Low | High | Low | Low | |

NA = not available

*Withdrawn from market

# BETA-BLOCKERS

| Agent | Adrenergic Receptor Blocking Activity | Lipid Solubility | Protein Bound (%) | Half-Life (h) | Bioavailability (%) | Primary (Secondary) Route of Elimination | Indications | Usual Dosage |
|---|---|---|---|---|---|---|---|---|
| Acebutolol (Sectral®) | beta₁ | Low | 15-25 | 3-4 | 40 7-fold* | Hepatic (renal) | Hypertension, arrhythmias | P.O.: 400-1200 mg/d |
| Atenolol (Tenormin®) | beta₁ | Low | <5-10 | 6-9† | 50-60 4-fold* | Renal (hepatic) | Hypertension, angina pectoris, acute MI | P.O.: 50-200 mg/d; I.V.: 5 mg x 2 doses |
| Betaxolol (Kerlone®) | beta₁ | Low | 50-55 | 14-22 | 84-94 | Hepatic (renal) | Hypertension | P.O.: 10-20 mg/d |
| Bisoprolol (Zebeta®) | beta₁ | Low | 26-33 | 9-12 | 80 | Renal (hepatic) | Hypertension | P.O.: 2.5-5 mg |
| Carteolol (Cartrol®) | beta₁, beta₂ | Low | 20-30 | 6 | 80-85 | Renal | Hypertension | P.O.: 2.5-10 mg/d |
| Carvedilol (Coreg™) | | | | 7-10 | 25-35 | Bile into feces | Hypertension | P.O.: 6.25 mg twice daily |
| Esmolol (Brevibloc®) | beta₁ | Low | 55 | 0.15 | NA 5-fold* | Red blood cell | Supraventricular tachycardia, sinus tachycardia | I.V. infusion: 25-300 mcg/kg/min |
| Labetalol (Trandate®, Normodyne®) | alpha₁, beta₁, beta₂ | Moderate | 50 | 5.5-8 | 18-30 10-fold* | Renal (hepatic) | Hypertension | P.O.: 200-2400 mg/d; I.V.: 20-80 mg at 10-min intervals up to a maximum of 300 mg or continuous infusion of 2 mg/min |
| Metoprolol (Lopressor®) | beta₁ | Moderate | 10-12 | 3-7 | 50 10-fold* | Hepatic/renal | Hypertension, angina pectoris, acute MI | P.O.: 100-450 mg/d; I.V.: Post-MI 15 mg Angina: 15 mg then 2-5 mg/h Arrhythmias: 0.2 mg/kg |
| Nadolol (Corgard®) | beta₁, beta₂ | Low | 25-30 | 20-24 | 30 5-8 fold* | Renal | Hypertension, angina pectoris | P.O.: 40-320 mg/d |
| Penbutolol (Levatol™) | beta₁, beta₂ | High | 80-98 | 5 | ≈100 | Hepatic (renal) | Hypertension | P.O.: 20-80 mg/d |
| Pindolol (Visken®) | beta₁, beta₂ | Moderate | 57 | 3-4† | 90 4-fold* | Hepatic (renal) | Hypertension | P.O.: 20-60 mg/d |
| Propranolol (Inderal®, various) | beta₁, beta₂ | High | 90 | 3-5† | 30 20-fold* | Hepatic | Hypertension, angina pectoris, arrhythmias | P.O.: 40-480 mg/d; I.V.: Reflex tachycardia 1-10 mg |
| Propranolol long-acting (Inderal-LA®) | beta₁, beta₂ | High | 90 | 9-18 | 20-30 fold* | Hepatic | Hypertrophic subaortic stenosis, prophylaxis (post-MI) | P.O.: 180-240 mg/d |

| Agent | Adrenergic Receptor Blocking Activity | Lipid Solubility | Protein Bound (%) | Half-Life (h) | Bioavailability (%) | Primary (Secondary) Route of Elimination | Indications | Usual Dosage |
|---|---|---|---|---|---|---|---|---|
| Sotalol (Betapace®) | beta₁ beta₂ | Low | 0 | 12 | 90-100 | Renal | Ventricular arrhythmias/ tachyarrhythmias | P.O. 160-320 mg/d |
| Timolol (Blocadren®) | beta₁ beta₂ | Low to moderate | <10 | 4 | 75 7-fold* | Hepatic (renal) | Hypertension, prophylaxis (post-MI) | P.O.: 20-60 mg/d P.O.: 20 mg/d |

Dosage is based on 70 kg adult with normal hepatic and renal function

Note: All beta₁-selective agents will inhibit beta₂ receptors at higher doses.

*Interpatient variations in plasma levels.

†Half-life increased to 16-27 h in creatinine clearance of 15-35 mL/min and >27 h in creatinine clearances <15 mL/min.

# CALCIUM CHANNEL BLOCKING AGENTS

| | Amlodipine | Bepridil | Diltiazem | Felodipine | Isradipine | Nicardipine | Nifedipine | Nisoldipine | Verapamil |
|---|---|---|---|---|---|---|---|---|---|
| Bioavailability (%) | 60-65 | 59 | 40 | 15 | 15-24 | 35 | 60-75 | 5 | 20-35 |
| Protein binding (%) | 95-98 | >99 | 77-85 | 99 | 95 | 95 | 95 | >99 | 83-92 |
| Half-life | 35-50 h | 24 h | 3.5-6 h (5-7 h in sustained released preparations) | 10-16 h | 8 h | 2-4 h | 2-5 h | 7-12 h | Oral: One dose: 2.8-7.4 h; Rep dose: 4.5-12 h; I.V. (biphasic) Short phase: 4 min; Long phase: 2-5 h |
| Onset of action | — | 60 min | Oral: 60 min | 2-5 h | 120 min | 20 min | Oral: 10-20 min | — | Oral: 30 min; I.V.: 1-5 min |
| Peak | 6-12 h | 2-3 h | Oral: 2-3 h | 2-4 h | 1.5 h | 0.5-2 h | Oral: 0.5-6 h | 6-12 h | Oral: 1-2.2 h; Oral, ext release: 5-7 h; I.V.: 2 h |
| Duration of action | 24 h | — | Ext release: 12 h; Tablet: 6-8 h | 24 h | — | 8 h | 12-24 h | — | Oral, ext release: 24 h; Tablet: 8-10 h; I.V.: 2 h |
| Elimination | Renal; fecal | Renal | Biliary/renal: 96%-98% (2%-4% unchanged) | Renal: 70%; Biliary: 30% | Renal | Renal: 60% Biliary/fecal 35% | Renal: 80% Biliary/fecal 20% | Renal | Renal: 70% Biliary/fecal: 9%-16% |
| Solubility in water | — | — | Yes | — | — | Slightly | No | — | Yes |
| Maximum tolerated dosage (adult) | 250 mg | — | 12 g | — | — | 600 mg (standard) 2160 mg (sustained) | 900 mg | — | 16 g (standard) 9.6 g (sustained) |
| Therapeutic dose | 5-10 mg/day | 200-400 mg/day | 30-60 mg tid or qid for standard 180-400 mg daily for sustained release | 2-10 mg/day | 5-20 mg/day | 20-40 mg tid for standard 30-60 mg bid for sustained release | 10-40 mg tid or qid for standard 90-180 mg once daily for sustained release | 20-60 mg/day | 80-160 mg qid for standard 120-240 mg once daily for sustained release |

| Actions | Amlodipine | Bepridil | Diltiazem | Felodipine | Isradipine | Nicardipine | Nifedipine | Nisoldipine | Verapamil |
|---|---|---|---|---|---|---|---|---|---|
| contractility | 0 | ↓ | ↓ | 0/↑ | 0 | ↓ | ↑ | 0 | ↓↓ |
| heart rate | 0 | ↓ | ↓ | ↑ | +/- | ↑ | ↑ | +/- | ↓ |
| cardiac output | 0 | 0 | ↑ | ↑ | ↑ | ↑↑ | ↑ | 0 | ↓↑ |
| peripheral vascular resistance | ↓↑ | ↓ | ↓ | ↓↑ | ↓↑ | ↓↑ | ↓↑ | ↓↑ | ↓↑ |

++ = most frequent

+ = less frequent

- = rare

0 = no effect

## CALCIUM CHANNEL BLOCKING AGENTS *(Continued)*

### Calcium Channel Blockers & Gingival Hyperplasia

| Generic Preparation | FDA Approval | Cases Cited in Literature | Common Name | Manufacturer |
|---|---|---|---|---|
| Amlodipine | 1992 | 4 | Norvasc® | Pfizer |
| Bepridil | 1993 | 0 | Vascor® | McNeil |
| Diltiazem | 1982 | >20 | Cardizem®; Dilacor® | Marion Merrell Dow; Rorer |
| Felodipine | 1992 | 1 | Plendil® | Merck Sharpe Dome |
| Isradipine | 1991 | 0 | DynaCirc® | Sandoz |
| Nicardipine | 1989 | 0 | Cardene® | Syntex |
| Nifedipine | 1982 | >120 | Adalat®; Procardia® | Miles; Pfizer |
| Nimodipine | 1989 | 0 | Nimotop® | Miles |
| Nitrendipine | — | 1 | Baypress® | Miles |
| Verapamil | 1982 | 7 | Calan®; Isoptin®; Verelan® | GD Searle; Knoll; Lederle; Wyeth-Ayerst |

### Some General Observations of CCB-Induced GH

Most of the reported cases listed in the Calcium Channel Blockers and Gingival Hyperplasia table have involved patients >50 years of age taking CCBs chronically for postmyocardial infarction syndrome, angina pain, essential hypertension, and Raynaud's syndrome. Nifedipine-induced GH has appeared between 1 and 9 months after a daily dose of 30-100 mg, verapamil-induced GH has appeared at 11 months or more after a daily dose of 240-360 mg, and diltiazem-induced GH has appeared between 1 and 24 months after a daily dose of 60-135 mg. As with phenytoin, there does not seem to be a dose-dependent effect of CCBs on the severity of the hyperplastic syndrome. Discontinuance of the CCB usually results in complete disappearance or marked regression of symptoms, with symptoms reappearing upon remedication. The time required after drug discontinuance for marked regression of GH has been 1 week. Complete disappearance of all symptoms usually takes 2 months. If gingivectomy is performed and the drug retained or resumed, the hyperplasia will usually recur. Only when the medication is discontinued or a switch to a non-CCB occurs will the gingivectomy usually be successful. One study of Nishikawa[1], et al, showed that if nifedipine could not be discontinued, hyperplasia did not recur after gingivectomy when extensive plaque control was carried out. If the CCB is changed to another class of cardiovascular agent, the gingival hyperplasia will probably regress and disappear. A switch to another CCB, however, will probably result in continued hyperplasia. For example, Giustiniani[2], et al, reported disappearance of symptoms within 15 days after discontinuance of verapamil, with the reoccurrence of symptoms after resumption with diltiazem. The reader is referred to the review of 1991[3] for descriptive clinical and histological findings of CCB-induced GH, and to Johnson's article for photographic description.[4]

### Footnotes

1. Nishikawa SI, Tada H, Hamasaki A, et al, "Nifedipine-Induced Gingival Hyperplasia: A Clinical and *in Vitro* Study," *J Periodontal*, 1991, 62(1):30-5.
2. Giustiniani S, Robestelli della Cuna F, and Marienei M, "Hyperplastic Gingivitis During Diltiazem Therapy," *Int J Cardiol*, 1987, 15(2):247-9.
3. Wynn RL, "Calcium Channel Blockers and Gingival Hyperplasia," *Gen Dent*, 1991, 240-3.
4. Johnson RP, "Nifedipine-Induced Gingival Overgrowth," *Ann Pharmacother*, 1997, 31:935.

# CORTICOSTEROIDS

## Corticosteroids, Systemic Equivalencies

| Glucocorticoid | Pregnancy Category | Approximate Equivalent Dose (mg) | Routes of Administration | Relative Anti-Inflammatory Potency | Relative Mineralocorticoid Potency | Protein Binding (%) | Half-life | |
|---|---|---|---|---|---|---|---|---|
| | | | | | | | Plasma (min) | Biologic (h) |
| **Short-Acting** | | | | | | | | |
| Cortisone | D | 25 | P.O., I.M. | 0.8 | 2 | 90 | 30 | 8-12 |
| Hydrocortisone | C | 20 | I.M., I.V. | 1 | 2 | 90 | 80-118 | 8-12 |
| **Intermediate-Acting** | | | | | | | | |
| Methylprednisolone* | — | 4 | P.O., I.M., I.V. | 5 | 0 | — | 78-188 | 18-36 |
| Prednisolone | B | 5 | P.O., I.M., I.V., intra-articular, intradermal, soft tissue injection | 4 | 1 | 90-95 | 115-212 | 18-36 |
| Prednisone | B | 5 | P.O. | 4 | 1 | 70 | 60 | 18-36 |
| Triamcinolone* | C | 4 | P.O., I.M., intra-articular, intradermal, intrasynovial, soft tissue injection | 5 | 0 | — | 200+ | 18-36 |
| **Long-Acting** | | | | | | | | |
| Betamethasone | C | 0.6-0.75 | P.O., I.M., intra-articular, intradermal, intrasynovial, soft tissue injection | 25 | 0 | 64 | 300+ | 36-54 |
| Dexamethasone | C | 0.75 | P.O., I.M., I.V., intra-articular, intradermal, soft tissue injection | 25-30 | 0 | — | 110-210 | 36-54 |
| **Mineralocorticoids** | | | | | | | | |
| Fludrocortisone | C | — | P.O. | 10 | 125 | 42 | 210+ | 18-36 |

*May contain propylene glycol as an excipient in injectable forms.

## CORTICOSTEROIDS *(Continued)*

### Corticosteroids, Topical

| Steroid | | Vehicle |
|---------|---|---------|
| **Very High Potency** | | |
| 0.05% | Augmented betamethasone dipropionate | Ointment |
| 0.05% | Clobetasol propionate | Cream, ointment |
| 0.05% | Diflorasone diacetate | Gel, ointment |
| 0.05% | Halobetasol propionate | Cream, ointment |
| **High Potency** | | |
| 0.1% | Amcinonide | Cream, ointment |
| 0.05% | Betamethasone dipropionate | Cream, ointment, lotion |
| 0.25% | Desoximetasone | Cream, ointment |
| 0.2% | Fluocinolone | Cream |
| 0.05% | Fluocinonide | Cream, ointment |
| 0.1% | Halcinonide | Cream, ointment, solution |
| 0.5% | Triamcinolone acetonide | Cream, ointment |
| **Intermediate Potency** | | |
| 0.025% | Betamethasone benzoate | Cream, gel, lotion |
| 0.1% | Betamethasone valerate | Cream, ointment, lotion |
| 0.05% | Desoximetasone | Cream |
| 0.025% | Fluocinolone acetonide | Cream, ointment |
| 0.05% | Flurandrenolide | Cream, ointment, lotion |
| 0.05% | Fluticasone propionate | Cream |
| 0.025% | Halcinonide | Cream, ointment |
| 0.1% | Mometasone furoate | Cream, ointment, lotion |
| 0.1% | Triamcinolone acetonide | Cream, ointment |
| **Low Potency** | | |
| 0.01% | Betamethasone valerate | Cream |
| 0.1% | Clocortolone† | Cream |
| 0.01% | Fluocinolone acetonide | Cream, solution, shampoo, oil |
| 0.025% | Flurandrenolide | Cream, ointment |
| 0.2% | Hydrocortisone valerate† | Cream |
| 0.025% | Triamcinolone acetonide | Cream, ointment |
| **Lowest Potency** (may be ineffective for some indications) | | |
| 0.05% | Alclometasone | Cream, ointment |
| 0.1% | Betamethasone | Cream |
| 0.2% | Betamethasone | Cream |
| 0.05% | Desonide† | Cream, ointment, lotion |
| 0.04% | Dexamethasone | Aerosol |
| 0.1% | Dexamethasone | Cream |
| 1% | Hydrocortisone† | Cream, ointment, lotion |
| 2.5% | Hydrocortisone† | Cream, ointment |
| 0.25% | Methylprednisolone acetate† | Ointment |
| 1% | Methylprednisolone acetate† | Ointment |

†Fluorinated.

# CYTOCHROME P-450 ENZYMES AND DRUG METABOLISM

## Background

There are five distinct groups of drug metabolizing which account for the majority of drug metabolism in humans. These enzymes "families", known as isoenzymes, are localized primarily in the liver. The nomenclature of this system has been standardized. Isoenzyme families are identified as a cytochrom (CYP prefix), followed by their numerical designation (eg, 1A2).

Enzymes may be inhibited (slowing metabolism through this pathway) or induced (increased in activity or number). Individual drugs metabolized by a specific enzyme are identified as substrates for the isoenzyme. Considerable effort has been expended in recent years to classify drugs metabolized by this system as either an inhibitor, inducer, or substrate of a specific isoenzyme. It should be noted that a drug may demonstrate complex activity within this scheme, acting as an inhibitor of one isoenzyme while serving as a substrate for another.

By recognizing that a substrate's metabolism may be dramatically altered by concurrent therapy with either an inducer or inhibitor, potential interactions may be identified and addressed. For example, a drug which inhibits CYP1A2 is likely to block metabolism of theophylline (a substrate for this isoenzyme). Because of this interaction, the dose of theophylline required to maintain a consistent level in the patient should be reduced when an inhibitor is added. Failure to make this adjustment may lead to supratherapeutic theophylline concentrations and potential toxicity.

This approach does have limitations. For example, the metabolism of specific drugs may have primary and secondary pathways. The contribution of secondary pathways to the overall metabolism may limit the impact of any given inhibitor. In addition, there may be up to a tenfold variation in the concentration of an isoenzyme across the broad population. In fact, a complete absence of an isoenzyme may occur in some genetic subgroups. Finally, the relative potency of inhibition, relative to the affinity of the enzyme for its substrate, demonstrates a high degree of variability. These issues make it difficult to anticipate whether a theoretical interaction will have a clinically relevant impact in a specific patient.

The details of this enzyme system continue to be investigated, and information is expanding daily. However, to be complete, it should be noted that other enzyme systems also influence a drug's pharmacokinetic profile. For example, a key enzyme system regulating the absorption of drugs is the p-glycoprotein system. Recent evidence suggests that some interaction originally attributed to the cytochrome system may, in fact, have been the result of inhibition of this system.

The following tables represent an attempt to detail the available information with respect to isoenzyme activities. Within certain limits, they may be used to identify potential interactions. Of particular note, an effort has been made in each drug monograph to identify involvement of a particular isoenzyme in the drug's metabolism. These tables are intended to supplement the limited space available to list drug interactions in the monograph. Consequently, they may be used to define a greater range of both actual and potential drug interactions.

## CYTOCHROME P-450 ENZYMES AND DRUG METABOLISM
*(Continued)*

### CYTOCHROME P-450 ENZYMES AND RESPECTIVE METABOLIZED DRUGS

---

### CYTOCHROME P-450 1A2 (CYP 1A2)

---

#### Substrates

Acetaminophen
Acetanilid
Aminophylline
Amitriptyline (demethylation)
Antipyrine
Betaxolol
Caffeine
Chlorpromazine
Clomipramine (demethylation)
Clozapine
Cyclobenzaprine (demethylation)
Desipramine (demethylation)
Diazepam
Estradiol
Fluvoxamine
Grepafloxacin
Haloperidol
Imipramine (demethylation)
Levopromazine
Maprotiline
Methadone
Metoclopramide
Mirtazapine (hydroxylation)
Nortriptyline
Olanzapine (demethylation, hydroxylation)
Ondansetron
Phenacetin
Phenothiazines
Propafenone
Propranolol
Riluzole
Ritonavir
Ropinirole
Ropivacaine
Tacrine
Tamoxifen
Theophylline
Thioridazine
Thiothixene
Trifluoperazine
Verapamil
Warfarin (R-warfarin, minor pathway)
Zileuton
Zopiclone

#### Inducers

Carbamazepine
Charbroiled foods
Cigarette smoke
Cruciferous vegetables (cabbage, brussels sprouts, broccoli, cauliflower)
Nicotine
Omeprazole
Phenobarbital
Phenytoin
Primidone
Rifampin
Ritonavir

#### Inhibitors

Anastrozole
Cimetidine
Ciprofloxacin
Citalopram (weak)
Clarithromycin
Diethyldithiocarbamate
Diltiazem
Enoxacin
Erythromycin
Ethinyl estradiol
Fluvoxamine
Fluoxetine (high dose)
Grapefruit juice
Isoniazid
Ketoconazole
Levofloxacin
Mexiletine
Mibefradil
Norfloxacin
Paroxetine (high dose)
Ritonavir
Sertraline (weak)
Tacrine
Tertiary TCAs
Zileuton

## CYTOCHROME P-450 2A6 (CYP 2A6)

### Substrates

Letrozole
Montelukast
Nicotine

Ritonavir
Tamoxifen

### Inducers

Barbiturates

### Inhibitors

Diethyldithiocarbamate
Letrozole

Ritonavir
Tranylcypromine

## CYTOCHROME P-450 2B6 (CYP 2B6)

### Substrates

Antipyrine
Bupropion (hydroxylation)
Cyclophosphamide
Ifosfamide

Nicotine

Orphenadrine

Tamoxifen

### Inducers

Phenobarbital
Phenytoin

Primidone

### Inhibitors

Diethyldithiocarbamate

Orphenadrine

## CYTOCHROME P-450 2C (CYP2C)
## (Specific isozyme has not been identified)

### Substrates

Antipyrine
Carvedilol
Clozapine (minor)
Mestranol

Mephobarbital

Tamoxifen

Ticrynafen

### Inducers

Carbamazepine
Phenobarbital
Phenytoin

Primidone
Sulfinpyrazone

### Inhibitors

Isoniazid
Ketoconazole

Ketoprofen

## CYTOCHROME P-450 ENZYMES AND DRUG METABOLISM
*(Continued)*

---

### CYTOCHROME P-450 2C8 (CYP 2C8)

#### Substrates

| | |
|---|---|
| Carbamazepine | Omeprazole |
| Diazepam | Paclitaxel |
| Diclofenac | Retinoic acid |
| Ibuprofen | Tolbutamide |
| Mephobarbital | Warfarin (S-warfarin) |
| Naproxen (5-hydroxylation) | |

#### Inducers

| | |
|---|---|
| Phenobarbital | Primidone |

#### Inhibitors

| | |
|---|---|
| Anastrozole | Omeprazole |

---

### CYTOCHROME P-450 2C9 (CYP 2C9)

#### Substrates

| | |
|---|---|
| Amitriptyline (demethylation) | Mirtazapine |
| Clomipramine | Montelukast |
| Dapsone | Naproxen (5-hydroxylation) |
| Diazepam | Omeprazole |
| Diclofenac | Phenytoin |
| Flurbiprofen | Piroxicam |
| Fluvastatin | Ritonavir |
| Glimepiride | Sildenafil citrate |
| Hexobarbital | Tenoxicam |
| Ibuprofen | Tetrahydrocannabinol |
| Imipramine (demethylation) | Tolbutamide |
| Indomethacin | Torsemide |
| Irbesartan | Warfarin (S-warfarin) |
| Losartan | Zafirlukast (hydroxylation) |
| Mefenamic acid | Zileuton |
| Metronidazole | |

#### Inducers

| | |
|---|---|
| Carbamazepine | Phenobarbital |
| Fluconazole | Phenytoin |
| Fluoxetine | Rifampin |

#### Inhibitors

| | |
|---|---|
| Amiodarone | Metronidazole |
| Anastrozole | Omeprazole |
| Chloramphenicol | Phenylbutazone |
| Cimetidine | Ritonavir |
| Diclofenac | Sertraline |
| Disulfiram | Sulfamethoxazole-trimethoprim |
| Flurbiprofen | Sulfaphenazole |
| Fluoxetine | Sulfinpyrazone |
| Fluvastatin | Sulfonamides |
| Fluvoxamine (potent) | Troglitazone |
| Isoniazid | Valproic acid |
| Ketoconazole (weak) | Warfarin (R-warfarin) |
| Ketoprofen | Zafirlukast |

## CYTOCHROME P-450 2C18 (CYP 2C18)

### Substrates

Amitriptyline
Clomipramine
Dronabinol
Imipramine
Naproxen
Omeprazole

Piroxicam
Proguanil
Propranolol
Retinoic acid
Tolbutamide
Warfarin

### Inducers

Carbamazepine
Phenobarbital

Phenytoin
Rifampin

### Inhibitors

Cimetidine
Fluconazole
Fluoxetine
Fluvastatin

Ketoconazole (weak)
Isoniazid
Sertraline

## CYTOCHROME P-450 2C19 (CYP 2C19)

### Substrates

Amitriptyline (demethylation)
Barbiturates
Carisoprodol
Citalopram
Clomipramine (demethylation)
Desmethyldiazepam
Diazepam (N-demethylation, minor
   pathway)
Divalproex sodium
Hexobarbital
Imipramine (demethylation)
Lansoprazole
Mephenytoin

Mephobarbital
Moclobemide
Olanzapine (minor)
Omeprazole
Pentamidine
Phenytoin
Proguanil
Propranolol
Ritonavir
Tolbutamide
Topiramate
Valproic acid
Warfarin (R-warfarin)

### Inducers

Carbamazepine
Phenobarbital

Phenytoin
Rifampin

### Inhibitors

Cimetidine
Citalopram (weak)
Felbamate
Fluconazole
Fluoxetine
Fluvastatin
Fluvoxamine
Isoniazid
Ketoconazole (weak)
Letrozole

Omeprazole
Proguanil
Ritonavir
Sertraline
Teniposide
Tolbutamide
Topiramate
Tranylcypromine
Troglitazone

## CYTOCHROME P-450 ENZYMES AND DRUG METABOLISM
*(Continued)*

---

### CYTOCHROME P-450 2D6 (CYP 2D6)

#### Substrates

Amitriptyline (hydroxylation)
Amphetamine
Betaxolol
Bisoprolol
Brofaromine
Bufurolol
Bupropion
Captopril
Carvedilol
Chlorpheniramine
Chlorpromazine
Cinnarizine
Clomipramine (hydroxylation)
Clozapine (minor pathway)
Codeine (hydroxylation, o-demethylation)
Cyclobenzaprine (hydroxylation)
Cyclophosphamide
Debrisoquin
Delavirdine
Desipramine
Dexfenfluramine
Dextromethorphan (o-demethylation)
Dihydrocodeine
Diphenhydramine
Dolasetron
Donepezil
Doxepin
Encainide
Fenfluramine
Flecainide
Fluoxetine (minor pathway)
Fluphenazine
Halofantrine
Haloperidol (minor pathway)
Hydrocodone
Hydrocortisone
Hydroxyamphetamine
Imipramine (hydroxylation)
Labetalol
Loratadine
Maprotiline
m-Chlorophenylpiperazine (m-CPP)
Meperidine
Methadone

Methamphetamine
Metoclopramide
Metoprolol
Mexiletine
Mianserin
Mirtazapine (hydroxylation)
Molindone
Morphine
Nortriptyline (hydroxylation)
Olanzapine (minor, hydroxymethylation)
Ondansetron
Orphenadrine
Oxycodone
Papaverine
Paroxetine (minor pathway)
Penbutolol
Pentazocine
Perhexiline
Perphenazine
Phenformin
Pindolol
Promethazine
Propafenone
Propranolol
Quetiapine
Remoxipride
Risperidone
Ritonavir (minor)
Ropivacaine
Selegiline
Sertindole
Sertraline (minor pathway)
Sparteine
Tamoxifen
Thioridazine
Tiagabine
Timolol
Tolterodine
Tramadol
Trazodone
Trimipramine
Tropisetron
Venlafaxine (o-desmethylation)
Yohimbine

#### Inducers

Carbamazepine
Phenobarbital
Phenytoin

Rifampin
Ritonavir

#### Inhibitors

Amiodarone
Chloroquine
Chlorpromazine
Cimetidine
Citalopram
Clomipramine
Codeine
Delavirdine

Desipramine
Dextropropoxyphene
Diltiazem
Doxorubicin
Fluoxetine
Fluphenazine
Fluvoxamine
Haloperidol

Labetalol
Lobeline
Lomustine
Methadone
Mibefradil
Moclobemide
Norfluoxetine
Paroxetine
Perphenazine
Propafenone
Quinacrine
Quinidine

Ranitidine
Risperidone (weak)
Ritonavir
Sertindole
Sertraline (weak)
Thioridazine
Valproic acid
Venlafaxine (weak)
Vinblastine
Vincristine
Vinorelbine
Yohimbine

## CYTOCHROME P-450 2E1 (CYP 2E1)

### Substrates

Acetaminophen
Acetone
Aniline
Benzene
Caffeine
Chlorzoxazone
Clozapine
Dapsone
Dextromethorphan
Enflurane
Ethanol
Halothane

Isoflurane
Isoniazid
Methoxyflurane
Nitrosamine
Ondansetron
Phenol
Ritonavir
Sevoflurane
Styrene
Tamoxifen
Theophylline
Venlafaxine

### Inducers

Ethanol

Isoniazid

### Inhibitors

Diethyldithiocarbamate (disulfiram metabolite)
Dimethyl sulfoxide

Disulfiram
Ritonavir

## CYTOCHROME P-450 3A3/4 (CYP 3A3/4)

### Substrates

Acetaminophen
Alfentanil
Alprazolam**
Amiodarone
Amitriptyline (minor)
Amlodipine
Anastrozole
Androsterone
Antipyrine
Astemizole**
Atorvastatin
Benzphetamine
Bepridil
Budesonide
Bupropion (minor)
Buspirone
Busulfan
Bromazepam
Bromocriptine
Busulfan
Caffeine
Cannabinoids
Carbamazepine

Cerivastatin
Chlorpromazine
Cimetidine
Cisapride**
Citalopram
Clarithromycin
Clindamycin
Clomipramine
Clonazepam
Clozapine
Cocaine
Codeine (demethylation)
Cortisol
Cortisone
Cyclobenzaprine (demethylation)
Cyclophosphamide
Cyclosporine
Dapsone
Dehydroepiandrostendione
Delavirdine
Desmethyldiazepam
Dexamethasone

## CYTOCHROME P-450 ENZYMES AND DRUG METABOLISM
(Continued)

Dextromethorphan (minor,
  N-demethylation)
Diazepam (minor; hydroxylation,
  N-demethylation)
Digitoxin
Diltiazem
Disopyramide
Docetaxel
Dolasetron
Donepezil
Doxorubicin
Doxycycline
Dronabinol
Enalapril
Erythromycin
Estradiol
Ethinyl estradiol
Ethosuximide
Etoposide
Felodipine
Fentanyl
Fexofenadine
Finasteride
Fluoxetine
Flutamide
Glyburide
Granisetron
Halofantrine
Hydrocortisone
Hydroxyarginine
Ifosfamide
Imipramine
Indinavir
Isradipine
Itraconazole
Ketoconazole
Lansoprazole (minor)
Letrozole
Lidocaine
Loratadine
Losartan
Lovastatin
Methadone
Mibefradil
Miconazole
Midazolam
Mifepristone
Mirtazapine (N-demethylation)
Montelukast
Navelbine
Nefazodone
Nelfinavir**
Nevirapine
Nicardipine
Nifedipine
Niludipine
Nimodipine

Nisoldipine
Nitrendipine
Omeprazole (sulfonation)
Ondansetron
Oral contraceptives
Orphenadrine
Paclitaxel
Pimozide**
Pravastatin
Prednisone
Progesterone
Proguanil
Propafenone
Quercetin
Quetiapine
Quinidine
Quinine
Repaglinide
Retinoic acid
Rifampin
Ritonavir**
Salmeterol
Saquinavir
Sertindole
Sertraline
Sibutramine##
Sildenafil citrate
Simvastatin
Sufentanil
Tacrolimus
Tamoxifen
Temazepam
Teniposide
Terfenadine**
Testosterone
Tetrahydrocannabinol
Theophylline
Tiagabine
Tolterodine
Toremifene
Trazodone
Tretinoin
Triazolam**
Troglitazone
Troleandomycin
Venlafaxine (N-demethylation)
Verapamil
Vinblastine
Vincristine
Warfarin (R-warfarin)
Yohimbine
Zatoestron
Zileuton
Ziprasidone
Zolpidem**
Zonisamide

### Inducers

Carbamazepine
Dexamethasone
Ethosuximide
Glucocorticoids
Griseofulvin
Nafcillin

Nelfinavir
Nevirapine
Phenobarbital
Phenylbutazone
Phenytoin
Primidone

Progesterone
Rifabutin
Rifampin

Sulfadimidine
Sulfinpyrazone
Troglitazone

## Inhibitors

Amiodarone
Anastrozole
Azithromycin
Cannabinoids
Cimetidine
Clarithromycin**
Clotrimazole
Cyclosporine
Danazol
Delavirdine
Dexamethasone
Diethyldithiocarbamate
Diltiazem
Dirithromycin
Disulfiram
Erythromycin**
Ethinyl estradiol
Fluconazole (weak)
Fluoxetine
Fluvoxamine**
Gestodene
Grapefruit juice
Indinavir
Isoniazid
Itraconazole**
Ketoconazole**

Metronidazole
Mibefradil**
Miconazole (moderate)
Nefazodone**
Nelfinavir
Nevirapine
Norfloxacin
Norfluoxetine
Omeprazole (weak)
Oxiconazole
Paroxetine (weak)
Propoxyphene
Quinidine
Quinine**
Ranitidine
Ritonavir**
Saquinavir
Sertindole
Sertraline
Troglitazone
Troleandomycin
Valproic acid (weak)
Verapamil
Zafirlukast
Zileuton

**\*\*Contraindications:**
Terfenadine, astemizole, cisapride, and triazolam contraindicated with nefazodone
Pimozide contraindicated with macrolide antibiotics
Alprazolam and triazolam contraindicated with ketoconazole and itraconazole
Terfenadine, astemizole, and cisapride contraindicated with fluvoxamine
Terfenadine contraindicated with mibefradil, ketoconazole, erythromycin, clarithromycin, troleandomycin
Ritonavir contraindicated with triazolam, zolpidem, astemizole, rifabutin, quinine, clarithromycin, troleandomycin
Mibefradil contraindicated with astemizole
Nelfinavir contraindicated with rifabutin

##Do not use with SSRIs, sumatriptan, lithium, meperidine, fentanyl, dextromethorphan, or pentazocine within 2 weeks of a MAOI.

---

# CYTOCHROME P-450 3A5-7 (CYP 3A5-7)

## Substrates

Cortisol
Ethinyl estradiol
Lovastatin
Nifedipine
Quinidine

Terfenadine
Testosterone
Triazolam
Vinblastine
Vincristine

## Inducers

Phenobarbital
Phenytoin

Primidone
Rifampin

## Inhibitors

Clotrimazole
Ketoconazole
Metronidazole

Miconazole
Troleandomycin

# CYTOCHROME P-450 ENZYMES AND DRUG METABOLISM
*(Continued)*

## References

Baker GB, Urichuk CJ, and Coutts RT, "Drug Metabolism and Metabolic Drug-Drug Interactions in Psychiatry," *Child Adolescent Psychopharm News (Suppl).*

DeVane CL, "Pharmacogenetics and Drug Metabolism of Newer Antidepressant Agents," *J Clin Psychiatry,* 1994, 55(Suppl 12):38-45.

*Drug Interactions Analysis and Management. Cytochrome (CYP) 450 Isozyme Drug Interactions,* Vancouver, WA: Applied Therapeutics, Inc, 523-7.

Ereshefsky L, "Drug-Drug Interactions Involving Antidepressants: Focus on Venlafaxine," *J Clin Psychopharmacol,* 1996, 16(3 Suppl 2):375-535.

Ereshefsky L, *Psychiatr Annal,* 1996, 26:342-50.

Fleishaker JC and Hulst LK, "A Pharmacokinetic and Pharmacodynamic Evaluation of the Combined Administration of Alprazolam and Fluvoxamine," *Eur J Clin Pharmacol,* 1994, 46(1):35-9.

Flockhart DA, et al, *Clin Pharmacol Ther,* 1996, 59:189.

Ketter TA, Flockhart DA, Post RM, et al, "The Emerging Role of Cytochrome P-450 3A in Psychopharmacology," *J Clin Psychopharmacol,* 1995, 15(6):387-98.

Michalets EL, "Update: Clinically Significant Cytochrome P-450 Drug Interactions," *Pharmacotherapy,* 1998, 18(1):84-112.

Nemeroff CB, DeVane CL, and Pollock BG, "Newer Antidepressants and the Cytochrome P450 System," *Am J Psychiatry,* 1996, 153(3):311-20.

Pollock BG, "Recent Developments in Drug Metabolism of Relevance to Psychiatrists," *Harv Rev Psychiatry,* 1994, 2(4):204-13.

Richelson E, "Pharmacokinetic Drug Interactions of New Antidepressants: A Review of the Effects on the Metabolism of Other Drugs," *Mayo Clin Proc,* 1997, 72(9):835-47.

Riesenman C, "Antidepressant Drug Interactions and the Cytochrome P450 System: A Critical Appraisal," *Pharmacotherapy,* 1995, 15(6 Pt 2):84S-99S.

Schmider J, Greenblatt DJ, von Moltke LL, et al, "Relationship of *In Vitro* Data on Drug Metabolism to *In Vivo* Pharmacokinetics and Drug Interactions: Implications for Diazepam Disposition in Humans," *J Clin Psychopharmacol,* 1996, 16(4):267-72.

Slaughter RL, *Pharm Times,* 1996, 7:6-16.

Watkins PB, "Role of Cytochrome P450 in Drug Metabolism and Hepatotoxicity," *Semin Liver Dis,* 1990, 10(4):235-50.

# HALLUCINOGENIC DRUGS

## Principal Pharmacological Properties of Hallucinogenic Drugs

| Drug; Chemical Structure | Duration of Acute Effect (h) | pKa | Route of Metabolism/ Excretion | Half-Life | Protein Binding (%) | V$_d$ (L/kg) | Urine Screen Positive for | Duration of Psychotropic Effects | Doses of Abuse | Fatal Dose |
|---|---|---|---|---|---|---|---|---|---|---|
| Phencyclidine (PCP); arylcyclohexylamine | 4–6 | 8.5 | Hepatic/urine | 1 h | 65 | 6.2–0.3 | 2 wk | Up to 1 mo | 1–9 mg | 1 mg/kg |
| Cocaine; tropane alkaloid | 0.5 | 5.6 | Plasma hydrolysis* | 48–75 min | 9–90 | 1.2–1.9 | 4 days (benzoyl-ecgonine) | ≤5–7 d | 20–200 mg (intranasally) | 1–1.2 g |
| Cannabis; monoterpenoid | 0.5–3 | 10.6 | Hepatic hydroxylation | 25–57 h | 97–99 | 10 | Up to 4 d | ≤6 h | 5–15 mg THC | |
| LSD; indole alkylamine | 0.7–8 | 7.8 | Hepatic hydroxylation | 2.5 h | | 0.27 | 120 h | May last for days | 100–300 mcg | 0.2 mg/kg |
| Psilocybin; tryptamine | 0.5–6 | | | | | | Not detected | 12 h | 20–100 mushrooms | 5–15 mg of psilocybin |
| Mescaline; phenylalkylamine | 4.6 | Not known | Hepatic/urine† | 6 h | None | Not known | | 12 h | 5 mg/kg | 20 mg/kg |
| Morphine; alkaloid/ derivative of opium | 4–5 | 8.05 | Glucuronidation/ urine | 1.9–3.1 h | 35 | 3.2 | 48 h | ≤6 h | 2–20 mg | Variable – dependent on tolerance, nontolerant fatal dose is 120 mg orally or 30 mg parenterally |
| Heroin; diacetylmorphine | 3.4 | 7.6 | Hepatic‡ | 3–20 min | 40 | 25 | ~40 h | ≤6 h | 2.2 mg | Variable – dependent on tolerance |
| Amphetamine; β-(phenylisopropyl)-amine | Variable | 9.93 | Hepatic§ | 12 h¶ | 16–20 | 3–6 | 2–4 d | Delusions may remain for months | 100–1000 mg/d | Variable – dependent on tolerance |

*By serum cholinesterase.
†60% excreted unchanged.
‡Converted to morphine.
§Converted to phenylacetone.
¶Urine pH-dependent.

Reprinted with permission from Leikin JB, Krantz AJ, Zell-Kanter M, et al, "Clinical Features and Management of Intoxication Due to Hallucinogenic Drugs," *Med Toxicol Adverse Drug Exp*, 1989, 4(6):328.

# HYPOGLYCEMIC DRUGS

## Contraindications to Therapy and Potential Adverse Effects of Oral Antidiabetic Agents

| | Sulfonylureas/ Meglitinide | Metformin | Acarbose/ Miglitol | Troglitazone |
|---|---|---|---|---|
| **CONTRAINDICATIONS** | | | | |
| Insulin dependency | A | A | A* | |
| Pregnancy/lactation | A | A | A | |
| Hypersensitivity to the agent | A | A | A | A |
| Hepatic impairment | R | A | R | |
| Renal impairment | R | A | R | |
| Congestive heart failure | | A | | R |
| Chronic lung disease | | A | | |
| Peripheral vascular disease | | A | | |
| Steroid-induced diabetes | R | R | | |
| Inflammatory bowel disease | | A | A | |
| Major recurrent illness | R | A | | |
| Surgery | R | A | | |
| Alcoholism | R | A | | |
| **ADVERSE EFFECTS** | | | | |
| Hypoglycemia | Yes | No | No | N |
| Body weight gain | Yes | No | No | N |
| Hypersensitivity | Yes | No | No | |
| Drug interactions | Yes | No | No | Y |
| Lactic acidosis | No | Yes | No | |
| Gastrointestinal disturbances | No | Yes | No | N |

*Can be used in conjunction with insulin. A = absolute; R = relative.

## Comparative Pharmacokinetics

| Drug | Duration of Action (h) | Dose and Frequency (mg) | Metabolism |
|---|---|---|---|
| **Sulfonylureas – First Generation Agents** | | | |
| Acetohexamide | 12-24 | 250-1500 bid | Hepatic (60%) with active metabolite |
| Chlorpropamide | 24-72 | 100-500 qd | Renal excretion (30%) and hepatic metabolism with active metabolites |
| Tolazamide | 10-24 | 100-1000 qd or bid | Hepatic with active metabolites |
| Tolbutamide | 6-24 | 500-3000 qd-tid | Hepatic |
| **Sulfonylureas – Second Generation Agents** | | | |
| Glimepiride | 24 | 1-4 mg qd | Hepatic |
| Glipizide | 12-24 | 2.5-40 qd or bid | Hepatic |
| Glipizide GITS | 24 | 5-10 qd | Hepatic |
| Glyburide | 16-24 | 1.25-20 qd or bid | Hepatic with active metabolites |
| **Thiazolidinedione** | | | |
| Troglitazone | 8 wk | 200-600 mg qd | Hepatic |
| **Meglitinides** | | | |
| Repaglinide | <4 hours (single dose) | 0.4-4 mg administered with meals 2, 3, or 4 times/day | Hepatic to inactive metabolites |

# LAXATIVES, CLASSIFICATION AND PROPERTIES

| Laxative | Onset of Action | Site of Action | Mechanism of Action |
|---|---|---|---|
| **Saline** | | | |
| Magnesium citrate (Citroma®) Magnesium hydroxide (Milk of Magnesia) | 30 min to 3 h | Small and large intestine | Attract/retain water in intestinal lumen increasing intraluminal pressure; cholecystokinin release |
| Sodium phosphate/ biphosphate enema (Fleet® Enema) | 2-15 min | Colon | |
| **Irritant/Stimulant** | | | |
| Cascara Casanthranol Senna (Senokot®) | 6-10 h | Colon | Direct action on intestinal mucosa; stimulate myenteric plexus; alter water and electrolyte secretion |
| Bisacodyl (Dulcolax®) tablets, suppositories | 15 min to 1 h | Colon | |
| Castor oil | 2-6 h | Small intestine | |
| Cascara aromatic fluid extract | 6-10 h | Colon | |
| **Bulk-Producing** | | | |
| Methylcellulose Psyllium (Metamucil®) Malt soup extract (Maltsupex®) Calcium polycarbophil (Mitrolan®, FiberCon®) | 12-24 h (up to 72 h) | Small and large intestine | Holds water in stool; mechanical distention; malt soup extract reduces fecal pH |
| **Lubricant** | | | |
| Mineral oil | 6-8 h | Colon | Lubricates intestine; retards colonic absorption of fecal water; softens stool |
| **Surfactants/Stool Softener** | | | |
| Docusate sodium (Colace®) Docusate calcium (Surfak®) Docusate potassium (Dialose®) | 24-72 h | Small and large intestine | Detergent activity; facilitates admixture of fat and water to soften stool |
| **Miscellaneous and Combination Laxatives** | | | |
| Glycerin suppository | 15-30 min | Colon | Local irritation; hyperosmotic action |
| Lactulose (Cephulac®) | 24-48 h | Colon | Delivers osmotically active molecules to colon |
| Docusate/casanthranol (Peri-Colace®) | 8-12 h | Small and large intestine | Casanthranol – mild stimulant; docusate – stool softener |

# LIPID-LOWERING AGENTS

## Possible Effects on Lipoproteins

| Drug | Total Cholesterol (%) | LDLC (%) | HDLC (%) | TG (%) |
|------|----------------------|----------|----------|--------|
| Bile-acid resins | ↓20-25 | ↓20-35 | → | ↑5-20 |
| Fibric acid derivatives | ↓10 | ↓10 (↑) | ↑10-25 | ↓40-55 |
| HMG-CoA RI (statins) | ↓15-45 | ↓20-60 | ↑2-15 | ↓7-37 |
| Nicotinic acid | ↓25 | ↓20 | ↑20 | ↓40 |

## Comparative Dosages of Agents Used to Treat Hyperlipidemia

| Antilipemic Agent* | Usual Total Daily Dose | Average Dosing Interval |
|--------------------|------------------------|-------------------------|
| **HMG-CoA Reductase Inhibitors** | | |
| Atorvastatin | 10-80 mg | qd |
| Cerivastatin | 0.2-0.3 mg | qd |
| Fluvastatin | 20-40 mg | qd hs |
| Lovastatin | 20-40 mg | qd hs |
| Pravastatin | 20-40 mg | qd hs |
| Simvastatin | 10-20 mg | qd hs |
| **Fibric Acid Derivatives** | | |
| Clofibrate | 2000 mg | qid |
| Gemfibrozil | 1200 mg | bid |
| **Miscellaneous Agents** | | |
| Niacin | 6 g | tid |
| **Bile Acid Sequestrants** | | |
| Colestipol | 30 g | bid |
| Cholestyramine | 24 g | tid-qid |

Dosage is based on 70 kg adult with normal hepatic and renal function.

## Antihyperlipidemic Drugs: Effects

| Drug | Effects on Serum Lipids | | | Total Cholesterol % | Side Effects/Monitoring Notes |
|------|------|------|------|------|------|
| | LDL % | HDL % | TRIG % | | |
| Atorvastatin (Lipitor®) | 40-60 ↓ | 5-8 ↑ | 19-37 ↓ | 25-45 ↓ | GI, hepatic dysfunction, myositis; monitor LFTs, CPK if muscle pain. |
| Cerivastatin (Baycol®) | 25-28 ↓ | 10 ↑ | 11-13 ↓ | 17-20 ↓ | GI, hepatic dysfunction, myositis; monitor LFTs, CPK if muscle pain. |
| Colestipol (Colestid®) or Cholestyramine (Prevalite®) | 15-30 ↓ | 3-5 ↑ | No change ↑ | 17 ↓ | Possible increased TG, dose-dependent upper/lower GI distress; may inhibit absorption of coadministered drugs |
| Fluvastatin (Lescol®) | 22-35 ↓ | — | — | — | GI, hepatic dysfunction, myositis; monitor LFTs, CPK if muscle pain. |
| Gemfibrozil (Lopid®) | 0-15 ↓ | 10-15 ↑ | 20-50 ↓ | | GI rashes, hepatic dysfunction, gallstones; potentiates warfarin; monitor LFTs |
| Lovastatin (Mevacor®) | 20-40 ↓ | 5-15 ↑ | 10-20 ↓ | 27-34 ↓ | GI, hepatic dysfunction, myositis; monitor LFTs, CPK if muscle pain. |
| Niacin | 10-25 ↓ | 15-30 ↑ | 20-50 ↓ | | Flushing, upper GI distress, hepatic dysfunction, hyperglycemia, increased uric acid |
| Niacin, sustained release | 10-25 ↓ | 15-30 ↑ | 20-50 ↓ | | Monitor LFTs, FBS; use with caution in patients with PUD, diabetes, history of liver disease, or gout. |
| Pravastatin (Pravachol®) | 22-34 ↓ | 7-12 ↑ | 15-24 ↓ | 16-25 ↓ | GI, hepatic dysfunction, myositis; monitor LFTs, CPK if muscle pain. |
| Simvastatin (Zocor®) | 30-40 ↓ | 5-15 ↑ | 10-20 ↓ | 17-28 ↓ | GI, hepatic dysfunction, myositis; monitor LFTs, CPK if muscle pain. |

# NARCOTIC AGONISTS

Comparative Pharmacokinetics

| Drug | Onset (min) | Peak (h) | Duration (h) | Half-Life (h) | Average Dosing Interval (h) | | Equianalgesic Doses* (mg) | |
|---|---|---|---|---|---|---|---|---|
| | | | | | Median | Range | I.M. | Oral |
| Alfentanil | Immediate | ND | ND | 1-2 | — | — | ND | NA |
| Buprenorphine | 15 | 1 | 4-8 | 2-3 | — | — | 0.4 | — |
| Butorphanol | I.M.: 30-60 / I.V.: 4-5 | 0.5-1 | 3-5 | 2.5-3.5 | 3 | (3-6) | 2 | — |
| Codeine | P.O.: 30-60 / I.M.: 10-30 | 0.5-1 | 4-6 | 3-4 | 3 | (3-6) | 120 | 200 |
| Fentanyl | I.M.: 7-15 / I.V.: Immediate | ND | 1-2 | 1.5-6 | 1 | (0.5-2) | 0.1 | NA |
| Hydrocodone | ND | ND | 4-8 | 3.3-4.4 | 6 | (4-8) | ND | ND |
| Hydromorphone | P.O.: 15-30 | 0.5-1 | 4-6 | 2-4 | 4 | (3-6) | 1.5 | 7.5 |
| Levorphanol | P.O.: 10-60 | 0.5-1 | 4-8 | 12-16 | 6 | (6-24) | 2 | 4 |
| Meperidine | P.O./I.M./S.C.: 10-15 / I.V.: ≤5 | 0.5-1 | 2-4 | 3-4 | 3 | (2-4) | 75 | 300 |
| Methadone | P.O.: 30-60 / I.V.: 10-20 | 0.5-1 | 4-6 (acute) / >8 (chronic) | 15-30 | 8 | (6-12) | 10 | 20 |
| Morphine | P.O.: 15-60 / I.V.: ≤5 | P.O./I.M./S.C.: 0.5-1 / I.V.: 0.3 | 3-6 | 2-4 | 4 | (3-6) | 10 | 60† (acute) / 30 (chronic) |
| Nalbuphine | I.M.: 30 / I.V.: 1-3 | 1 | 3-6 | 5 | | — | 10 | — |
| Naloxone‡ | 2-5 | 0.5-2 | 0.5-1 | 0.5-1.5 | | — | — | — |
| Oxycodone | P.O.: 10-15 | 0.5-1 | 4-6 | 3-4 | 4 | (3-6) | NA | 30 |
| Oxymorphone | 5-15 | 0.5-1 | 3-6 | | | | 1 | 10§ |
| Pentazocine | 15-20 | 0.25-1 | 3-4 | 2-3 | 3 | (3-6) | | |

**NARCOTIC AGONISTS** *(Continued)*

## Comparative Pharmacokinetics *(continued)*

| Drug | Onset (min) | Peak (h) | Duration (h) | Half-Life (h) | Average Dosing Interval (h) | | Equianalgesic Doses* (mg) | |
|---|---|---|---|---|---|---|---|---|
| | | | | | Median | Range | I.M. | Oral |
| Propoxyphene | P.O.: 30-60 | 2-2.5 | 4-6 | 3.5-15 | 6 | (4-8) | ND | 130†-200# |
| Remifentanil | 1-3 | <0.3 | 0.1-0.2 | 0.15-0.3 | — | — | ND | ND |
| Sufentanil | 1.3-3 | ND | ND | 2.5-3 | — | — | 0.02 | NA |

ND = no data available. NA = not applicable.

*Based on acute, short-term use. Chronic administration may alter pharmacokinetics and decrease the oral:parenteral dose ratio. The morphine oral:parenteral ratio decreases to ~ 1.5-2.5:1 upon chronic dosing.

†Extensive survey data suggest that the relative potency of I.M.:P.O. morphine of 1:6 changes to 1:2-3 with chronic dosing.

‡Narcotic antagonist

§Rectal.

¶HCl salt.

#Napsylate salt.

## Comparative Pharmacology

| Drug | Analgesic | Antitussive | Constipation | Respiratory Depression | Sedation | Emesis |
|---|---|---|---|---|---|---|
| **Phenanthrenes** | | | | | | |
| Codeine | + | +++ | + | + | + | + |
| Hydrocodone | + | +++ | | + | | |
| Hydromorphone | ++ | +++ | + | ++ | + | + |
| Levorphanol | ++ | ++ | ++ | ++ | ++ | + |
| Morphine Sulfate | ++ | +++ | ++ | ++ | ++ | ++ |
| Oxycodone | ++ | +++ | ++ | ++ | ++ | |
| Oxymorphone | ++ | + | ++ | +++ | | +++ |
| **Phenylpiperidines** | | | | | | |
| Alfentanil | ++ | | | | | |
| Fentanyl | ++ | | | + | | + |
| Meperidine | ++ | + | + | ++ | + | |
| Sufentanil | +++ | | | | | |
| **Diphenylheptanes** | | | | | | |
| Methadone | ++ | ++ | ++ | ++ | + | + |
| Propoxyphene | + | | | + | + | + |
| **Agonist/Antagonist** | | | | | | |
| Buprenorphine | ++ | N/A | +++ | +++ | ++ | ++ |
| Butorphanol | ++ | N/A | +++ | +++ | ++ | + |
| Dezocine | ++ | | + | ++ | + | ++ |
| Nalbuphine | ++ | N/A | +++ | +++ | ++ | ++ |
| Pentazocine | ++ | N/A | + | ++ | ++ or stimulation | ++ |

# NONSTEROIDAL ANTI-INFLAMMATORY AGENTS

## Comparative Dosages and Pharmacokinetics

| Drug | Maximum Recommended Daily Dose (mg) | Time to Peak Levels (h)* | Half-life (h) |
|---|---|---|---|
| **Propionic Acids** | | | |
| Fenoprofen (Nalfon®) | 3200 | 1-2 | 2-3 |
| Flurbiprofen (Ansaid®) | 300 | 1.5 | 5.7 |
| Ibuprofen | 3200 | 1-2 | 1.8-2.5 |
| Ketoprofen (Orudis®) | 300 | 0.5-2 | 2-4 |
| Naproxen (Naprosyn®) | 1500 | 2-4 | 12-15 |
| Naproxen sodium (Anaprox®) | 1375 | 1-2 | 12-13 |
| Oxaprozin | 1800 | 3-5 | 42-50 |
| **Acetic Acids** | | | |
| Diclofenac sodium delayed release (Voltaren®) | 225 | 2-3 | 1-2 |
| Diclofenac potassium immediate release (Cataflam®) | 200 | 1 | 1-2 |
| Etodolac (Lodine®) | 1200 | 1-2 | 7.3 |
| Indomethacin (Indocin®) | 200 | 1-2 | 4.5 |
| Indomethacin SR | 150 | 2-4 | 4.5-6 |
| Ketorolac (Toradol®) | I.M.: 120† P.O.: 40 | 0.5-1 | 3.8-8.6 |
| Sulindac (Clinoril®) | 400 | 2-4 | 7.8 (16.4)‡ |
| Tolmetin (Tolectin®) | 2000 | 0.5-1 | 1-1.5 |
| **Fenamates (Anthranilic Acids)** | | | |
| Meclofenamate (Meclomen®) | 400 | 0.5-1 | 2 (3.3)§ |
| Mefenamic acid (Ponstel®) | 1000 | 2-4 | 2-4 |
| **Nonacidic Agent** | | | |
| Nabumetone (Relafen®) | 2000 | 3-6 | 24 |
| **Oxicam** | | | |
| Piroxicam (Feldene®) | 20 | 3-5 | 30-86 |

Dosage is based on 70 kg adult with normal hepatic and renal function.

*Food decreases the rate of absorption and may delay the time to peak levels.

†150 mg on the first day.

‡Half-life of active sulfide metabolite.

§Half-life with multiple doses.

# SULFONAMIDE DERIVATIVES

The following table lists commonly prescribed drugs which are either sulfonamide derivatives or are structurally similar to sulfonamides. Please note that the list may not be all inclusive.

## Commonly Prescribed Drugs

| Classification | Specific Drugs |
|---|---|
| Antimicrobial Agents | Mafenide acetate (Sulfamylon®)<br>Silver sulfadiazine (Silvadene®)<br>Sodium sulfacetamide (Sodium Sulamyd®)<br>Sulfadiazine<br>Sulfamethizole<br>Sulfamethoxazole (ie, Bactrim™ and co-trimoxazole)<br>Sulfisoxazole (Gantrisin®) |
| Diuretics, Carbonic Anhydrase Inhibitors | Acetazolamide (Diamox®)<br>Dichlorphenamide (Daranide®)<br>Methazolamide (Neptazane®) |
| Diuretics, Loop | Bumetanide (Bumex®)<br>Furosemide (Lasix®)<br>Torsemide (Demadex®) |
| Diuretics, Thiazide | Bendroflumethiazide<br>Benzthiazide<br>Chlorothiazide (Diuril®)<br>Chlorthalidone (Hygroton®)<br>Cyclothiazide (Anhydron®)<br>Hydrochlorothiazide (Dyazide®, HydroDIURIL®, Maxzide®)<br>Hydroflumethiazide<br>Indapamide (Lozol®)<br>Methyclothiazide (Enduron®)<br>Metolazone (Diulo®, Zaroxolyn®)<br>Polythiazide<br>Quinethazone<br>Trichlormethiazide |
| Hypoglycemic Agents, Oral | Acetohexamide (Dymelor®)<br>Chlorpropamide (Diabinese®)<br>Glipizide (Glucotrol®)<br>Glyburide (DiaBeta®, Micronase®)<br>Tolazamide (Tolinase®)<br>Tolbutamide (Orinase®) |
| Other Agents | Sulfasalazine (Azulfidine®) |

# ANTIMICROBIAL DRUGS OF CHOICE

The following table lists the antimicrobial drugs of choice for various infecting organisms. This table is reprinted with permission from *The Medical Letter*, 1998, 40(1023): 37-42. Users should not assume that all antibiotics which are appropriate for a given organism are listed or that those not listed are inappropriate. The infection caused by the organism may encompass varying degrees of severity, and since the antibiotics listed may not be appropriate for the differing degrees of severity, or because of other patient-related factors, it cannot be assumed that the antibiotics listed for any specific organism are interchangeable. This table should not be used by itself without first referring to *The Medical Letter*, an infectious disease manual, or the infectious disease department. Therefore, only use this table as a tool for obtaining more information about the therapies available.

| Infecting Organism | Drug of First Choice | Alternative Drugs |
|---|---|---|
| **Gram-Positive Cocci** | | |
| *Enterococcus[1] | | |
|   endocarditis or other severe infection | Penicillin G or ampicillin + gentamicin or streptomycin | Vancomycin + gentamicin or streptomycin; quinupristin/dalfopristin[2] |
|   uncomplicated urinary tract infection | Ampicillin or amoxicillin | Nitrofurantoin; a fluoroquinolone[3]; fosfomycin |
| *Staphylococcus aureus or epidermidis | | |
|   nonpenicillinase-producing | Penicillin G or V[4] | A cephalosporin[5,6]; vancomycin; imipenem or meropenem; clindamycin; a fluoroquinolone[3] |
|   penicillinase-producing | A penicillinase-resistant penicillin[7] | A cephalosporin[5,6]; vancomycin; amoxicillin/clavulanic acid; ticarcillin/clavulanic acid; piperacillin/tazobactam; ampicillin/sulbactam; imipenem or meropenem; clindamycin; a fluoroquinolone[3] |
|   methicillin-resistant[8] | Vancomycin ± gentamicin ± rifampin | Trimethoprim-sulfamethoxazole; a fluoroquinolone[3]; minocycline[9] |
| *Streptococcus pyogenes* (group A) and groups C and G[10] | Penicillin G or V[4] | Clindamycin; erythromycin; a cephalosporin[5,6]; vancomycin; clarithromycin[11]; azithromycin |
| *Streptococcus*, group B | Penicillin G or ampicillin | A cephalosporin[5,6]; vancomycin; erythromycin |
| *Streptococcus*, viridans group[1] | Penicillin G ± gentamicin | A cephalosporin[5,6]; vancomycin |
| *Streptococcus bovis*[1] | Penicillin G | A cephalosporin[5,6]; vancomycin |
| *Streptococcus*, anaerobic or *Peptostreptococcus* | Penicillin G | Clindamycin; a cephalosporin[5,6]; vancomycin |
| *Streptococcus pneumoniae*[12] (pneumococcus), penicillin-susceptible (MIC <0.1 mcg/mL) | Penicillin G or V[4] | A cephalosporin[5,6]; erythromycin; azithromycin; clarithromycin[11]; a fluoroquinolone; meropenem; imipenem; trimethoprim-sulfamethoxazole; clindamycin; a tetracycline[9] |
| Penicillin-intermediate resistance (MIC 0.1-1 mcg/mL) | Penicillin G I.V. (12 million units/day for adults) or ceftriaxone or cefotaxime | Levofloxacin, grepafloxacin or trovafloxacin; vancomycin |
| Penicillin-high level resistance (MIC ≥2 mcg/mL) | Meningitis: Vancomycin + ceftriaxone or cefotaxime ± rifampin | Meropenem; imipenem |
| | Other infections: Vancomycin + ceftriaxone or cefotaxime; or levofloxacin, grepafloxacin, or trovafloxacin | Quinupristin/dalfopristin[2] |

| Infecting Organism | Drug of First Choice | Alternative Drugs |
|---|---|---|
| **Gram-Negative Cocci** | | |
| *Moraxella (Branhamella) catarrhalis* | Trimethoprim-sulfamethoxazole | Amoxicillin/clavulanic acid; erythromycin; a tetracycline[9]; cefuroxime[6]; cefotaxime[5]; ceftizoxime[5]; ceftriaxone[6]; cefuroxime axetil[5]; cefixime[6]; cefpodoxime[5]; a fluoroquinolone[3]; clarithromycin[11]; azithromycin |
| *Neisseria gonorrhoeae* (gonococcus)[13] | Ceftriaxone[5] or cefixime[5] or ciprofloxacin[3] or ofloxacin[3] | Cefotaxime[5]; spectinomycin; penicillin G |
| *Neisseria meningitidis*[14] (meningococcus) | Penicillin G | Cefotaxime[5]; ceftizoxime[5]; ceftriaxone[5]; chloramphenicol[15]; a sulfonamide[16]; a fluoroquinolone[3] |
| **Gram-Positive Bacilli** | | |
| *Bacillus anthracis* (anthrax) | Penicillin G | Erythromycin; a tetracycline[9] |
| *Bacillus cereus, subtilis* | Vancomycin | Imipenem or meropenem; clindamycin |
| *Clostridium perfringens*[17] | Penicillin G | Clindamycin; metronidazole; imipenem or meropenem; chloramphenicol[15] |
| *Clostridium tetani*[18] | Penicillin G | A tetracycline[9] |
| *Clostridium difficile*[19] | Metronidazole | Vancomycin (oral) |
| *Corynebacterium diphtheriae*[20] | Erythromycin | Penicillin G |
| *Corynebacterium*, JK group | Vancomycin | Penicillin G + gentamicin; erythromycin |
| *Erysipelothrix rhusiopethiae* | Penicillin G | Erythromycin, a cephalosporin[5,6]; a fluoroquinolone[3] |
| *Listeria monocytogenes* | Ampicillin ± gentamicin | Trimethoprim-sulfamethoxazole |
| **Enteric Gram-Negative Bacilli** | | |
| *Bacteroides* | Metronidazole or clindamycin | Imipenem or meropenem; amoxicillin/clavulanic acid; ticarcillin/clavulanic acid; piperacillin/tazobactam; cefoxitin[5]; cefotetan[5]; ampicillin/sulbactam; chloramphenicol[15]; cefmetazole[5]; trovafloxacin; penicillin G |
| *Campylobacter fetus* | Imipenem or meropenem | Gentamicin |
| *Campylobacter jejuni* | Fluoroquinolone[3] or erythromycin | A tetracycline[9]; gentamicin |
| *Citrobacter freundi* | Imipenem or meropenem[21] | A fluoroquinolone[3]; amikacin; tetracycline[9]; trimethoprim-sulfamethoxazole; cefotaxime[5,21]; ceftizoxime[5,21]; ceftriazone[5,21]; cefepime[5,21]; or ceftazidime[5,21] |
| *Enterobacter* | Imipenem or meropenem[21] | Gentamicin, tobramycin, or amikacin; trimethoprim-sulfamethoxazole; ciprofloxacin[22]; ticarcillin[23]; mezlocillin[23] or piperacillin[23]; aztreonam[21]; cefotaxime[5,21]; ceftizoxime[5,21]; ceftriaxone[5,21]; cefepime[5,21]; or ceftazidime[5,21] |
| *Escherichia coli*[24] | Cefotaxime, ceftizoxime, ceftriaxone, cefepime, or ceftazidime[5,21] | Ampicillin ± gentamicin, tobramycin or amikacin; carbenicillin[23]; ticarcillin[23]; mezlocillin[23] or piperacillin[23]; gentamicin, tobramycin, or amikacin; amoxicillin/clavulanic acid[21]; ticarcillin/clavulanic acid[23]; piperacillin/tazobactam[23]; ampicillin/sulbactam[21]; trimethoprim/sulfamethoxazole; imipenem or meropenem[21]; aztreonam[21]; fluoroquinolone[3]; another cephalosporin[5,6] |
| *Helicobacter pylori*[25] | Tetracycline hydrochloride[9] + metronidazole + bismuth subsalicylate | Tetracycline hydrochloride + clarithromycin[11] + bismuth subsalicylate; amoxicillin + metronidazole + bismuth subsalicylate; amoxicillin + clarithromycin[11] |

# ANTIMICROBIAL DRUGS OF CHOICE (Continued)

| Infecting Organism | Drug of First Choice | Alternative Drugs |
|---|---|---|
| *Klebsiella pneumoniae[24] | Cefotaxime, ceftizoxime, ceftriaxone, cefepime, or ceftazidime[5,21] | Imipenem or meropenem[21]; gentamicin, tobramycin, or amikacin; amoxicillin/clavulanic acid[21]; ticarcillin/clavulanic acid[23]; piperacillin; tazobactam[23]; ampicillin/sulbactam[21]; trimethoprim-sulfamethoxazole; aztreonam[21]; a fluoroquinolone[3]; mezlocillin[23] or piperacillin[23]; another cephalosporin[5,6] |
| *Proteus mirabilis[24] | Ampicillin[26] | A cephalosporin[6,21]; ticarcillin[23]; mezlocillin[23] or piperacillin[23]; gentamicin, tobramycin, or amikacin; trimethoprim-sulfamethoxazole; imipenem or meropenem[21]; aztreonam[21]; a fluoroquinolone[3]; chloramphenicol[15] |
| Proteus, indole-positive (including Providencia rettgeri, Morganella morganii, and Proteus vulgaris) | Cefotaxime, ceftizoxime, ceftriaxone, cefepime, or ceftazidime[5,21] | Imipenem or meropenem[21]; gentamicin, tobramycin, or amikacin; carbenicillin[23]; ticarcillin[23]; mezlocillin[23] or piperacillin[23]; amoxicillin/clavulanic acid[21]; ticarcillin/clavulanic acid[23]; piperacillin/tazobactam[23]; ampicillin/sulbactam[21]; aztreonam[21]; trimethoprim-sulfamethoxazole; a fluoroquinolone[3] |
| *Providencia stuartii | Cefotaxime, ceftizoxime, ceftriaxone, cefepime, or ceftazidime[5,21] | Imipenem or meropenem[21]; ticarcillin/clavulanic acid[23]; piperacillin/tazobactam[23]; gentamicin, tobramycin, or amikacin; carbenicillin[23]; ticarcillin[23], mezlocillin[23], or piperacillin[23]; aztreonam[21]; trimethoprim-sulfamethoxazole; fluoroquinolone[3] |
| *Salmonella typhi[27] | A fluoroquinolone[3] or ceftriaxone[5] | Chloramphenicol[15]; trimethoprim-sulfamethoxazole; ampicillin; amoxicillin |
| *other Salmonella[28] | Cefotaxime[5] or ceftriaxone[5] or a fluoroquinolone[3] | Ampicillin or amoxicillin; trimethoprim-sulfamethoxazole; chloramphenicol[15] |
| *Serratia | Cefotaxime, ceftizoxime, ceftriaxone, cefepime, or ceftazidime[5,29] | Gentamicin or amikacin; imipenem or meropenem[29]; aztreonam[29]; trimethoprim-sulfamethoxazole; carbenicillin[30], ticarcillin[30], mezlocillin[30] or piperacillin[30]; a fluoroquinolone[3] |
| *Shigella | A fluoroquinolone[3] | Azithromycin; trimethoprim-sulfamethoxazole; ampicillin; ceftriaxone[5] |
| *Yersinia enterocolitica | Trimethoprim-sulfamethoxazole | A fluoroquinolone[3]; gentamicin, tobramycin, or amikacin; cefotaxime or ceftizoxime[5] |

## Other Gram-Negative Bacilli

| | | |
|---|---|---|
| *Acinetobacter | Imipenem or meropenem[21] | Amikacin, tobramycin, or gentamicin; ciprofloxacin[22]; trimethoprim-sulfamethoxazole; ticarcillin[23], mezlocillin[23], or piperacillin[23]; ceftazidime[21]; minocycline[9]; doxycycline[9] |
| *Aeromonas | Trimethoprim-sulfamethoxazole | Gentamicin or tobramycin; imipenem; a fluoroquinolone[3] |
| Bartonella | | |
| Agent of bacillary angiomatosis (Bartonella henselae or quintana)[31] | Erythromycin | Doxycycline[9]; azithromycin |
| Cat scratch bacillus (Bartonella henselae)[31,32] | Ciprofloxacin[22] | Trimethoprim-sulfamethoxazole; gentamicin; rifampin; azithromycin |
| Bordetella pertussis (whooping cough) | Erythromycin | Trimethoprim-sulfamethoxazole |
| *Brucella | A tetracycline[9] + streptomycin or gentamicin | A tetracycline[9] + rifampin; chloramphenicol[15] ± streptomycin; trimethoprim-sulfamethoxazole ± gentamicin; rifampin + a tetracycline[9] |

| Infecting Organism | Drug of First Choice | Alternative Drugs |
|---|---|---|
| *Burkholderia capacia | Trimethoprim-sulfamethoxazole | Ceftazidime[5]; chloramphenicol[15] |
| Calymmatobacterium granulomatis (granuloma inguinale) | Trimethoprim-sulfamethoxazole | Doxycycline[9] or ciprofloxacin ± gentamicin |
| Capnocytophaga canimorsus (DF-2)[33] | Penicillin G | Cefotaxime[5]; ceftizoxime[5]; ceftriaxone[5]; imipenem or meropenem; vancomycin; a fluoroquinolone[3]; clindamycin |
| *Eikenella corrodens | Ampicillin | An erythromycin; a tetracycline[9]; amoxicillin/clavulanic acid; ampicillin/sulbactam; ceftriaxone[5] |
| *Francisella tularensis (tularemia) | Streptomycin | Gentamicin; a tetracycline[9]; chloramphenicol[16] |
| *Fusobacterium | Penicillin G | Metronidazole; clindamycin; cefoxitin[5]; chloramphenicol[15] |
| Gardnerella vaginalis (bacterial vaginosis) | Oral metronidazole[34] | Topical clindamycin or metronidazole; oral clindamycin |
| *Haemophilus ducreyi (chancroid) | Azithromycin or ceftriaxone | Ciprofloxacin[22] or erythromycin |
| *Haemophilus influenzae | | |
| meningitis, epiglottitis, arthritis, and other serious infections | Cefotaxime or ceftriaxone[5] | Cefuroxime[5] (but not for meningitis); chloramphenicol[15]; meropenem |
| upper respiratory infections and bronchitis | Trimethoprim-sulfamethoxazole | Cefuroxime[5]; amoxicillin/clavulanic acid; cefuroxime axetil[5]; cefpodoxime[5]; cefaclor[5]; cefotaxime[5]; ceftizoxime[5]; ceftriaxone[5]; cefixime[5]; a tetracycline[9]; clarithromycin[11]; azithromycin; a fluoroquinolone[3]; ampicillin or amoxicillin |
| Legionella species[35] | Erythromycin or clarithromycin[11] or azithromycin[11] or a fluoroquinolone[3] ± rifampin | Doxycycline[9] ± rifampin; trimethoprim-sulfamethoxazole |
| Leptotrichia buccalis | Penicillin G | A tetracycline[9]; clindamycin; erythromycin |
| Pasteurella multocida | Penicillin G | A tetracycline[9]; a cephalosporin[5,6]; amoxicillin/clavulanic acid; ampicillin/sulbactam |
| *Pseudomonas aeruginosa | | |
| urinary tract infection | Ciprofloxacin[22] | Carbenicillin, ticarcillin, piperacillin, or mezlocillin; ceftazidime[5]; cefepime[5]; imipenem or meropenem; aztreonam; tobramycin; gentamicin; amikacin |
| other infections | Ticarcillin, mezlocillin, or piperacillin + tobramycin, gentamicin, or amikacin[36] | Ceftazidime[5], imipenem, meropenem, aztreonam, cefepime[5] + tobramycin, gentamicin, or amikacin; ciprofloxacin[22]; trovafloxacin[22] |
| Pseudomonas mallei (glanders) | Streptomycin + a tetracycline[9] | Streptomycin + chloramphenicol[15] |
| *Pseudomonas pseudomallei (melioidosis) | Ceftazidime[5] | Chloramphenicol[15] + doxycycline[9] + trimethoprim-sulfamethoxazole; amoxicillin/clavulanic acid; imipenem or meropenem |
| Spirillum minus (rat bite fever) | Penicillin G | A tetracycline[9]; streptomycin |
| *Stenotrophomonas maltophilia (Pseudomonas maltophilia) | Trimethoprim-sulfamethoxazole | Minocycline[9]; ceftazidime; [5] a fluoroquinolone[3] |
| Streptobacillus moniliformis (rat bite fever, Haverhill fever) | Penicillin G | A tetracycline[9]; streptomycin |
| Vibrio cholerae (cholera)[37] | A tetracycline[9] | A fluoroquinolone[3]; trimethoprim-sulfamethoxazole |
| Vibrio vulnificus | A tetracycline[9] | Cefotaxime[6] |
| Yersinia pestis (plague) | Streptomycin ± a tetracycline[9] | Chloramphenicol[15]; gentamicin; trimethoprim-sulfamethoxazole |

## ANTIMICROBIAL DRUGS OF CHOICE *(Continued)*

| Infecting Organism | Drug of First Choice | Alternative Drugs |
|---|---|---|
| **Acid-Fast Bacilli** | | |
| *Mycobacterium tuberculosis | Isoniazid + rifampin + pyrazinamide ± ethambutol or streptomycin[15] | Ciprofloxacin, ofloxacin, or levofloxacin[22]; cycloserine[15]; capreomycin[15] or kanamycin[15] or amikacin[15]; ethionamide[15]; clofazimine[15]; aminosalicylic acid[15] |
| *Mycobacterium kansasii | Isoniazid + rifampin ± ethambutol or streptomycin[15] | Clarithromycin[11]; ethionamide[15]; cycloserine[15] |
| *Mycobacterium avium complex | Clarithromycin[11] or azithromycin + one or more of the following: ethambutol; rifabutin; ciprofloxacin[22] | Rifampin; amikacin[15] |
| prophylaxis | Clarithromycin[11] | Rifabutin |
| *Mycobacterium fortuitum complex | Amikacin + doxycycline[9] | Cefoxitin[5]; rifampin; a sulfonamide |
| Mycobacterium marinum (balnei)[38] | Minocycline[9] | Trimethoprim-sulfamethoxazole; rifampin; clarithromycin[11]; doxycycline[9] |
| Mycobacterium leprae (leprosy) | Dapsone + rifampin ± clofazimine | Minocycline[9]; ofloxacin[22,39]; sparfloxacin; clarithromycin[11,40] |
| **Actinomycetes** | | |
| Actinomyces israelii (actinomycosis) | Penicillin G | A tetracycline[9]; erythromycin; clindamycin |
| Nocardia | Trimethoprim-sulfamethoxazole | Sulfisoxazole; amikacin[15]; a tetracycline[9]; imipenem or meropenem; cycloserine[15] |
| *Rhodococcus equi | Vancomycin ± a fluoroquinolone[3], rifampin, imipenem or meropenem or amikacin | Erythromycin |
| Tropheryma whippelii[41] (agent of Whipple's disease) | Trimethoprim-sulfamethoxazole | Penicillin G; a tetracycline[9] |
| **Chlamydiae** | | |
| Chlamydia psittaci (psittacosis, ornithosis) | A tetracycline[9] | Chloramphenicol[15] |
| Chlamydia trachomatis | | |
| (trachoma) | Azithromycin | A tetracycline[9] (topical plus oral); a sulfonamide (topical plus oral) |
| (inclusion conjunctivitis) | Erythromycin (oral or I.V.) | A sulfonamide |
| (pneumonia) | Erythromycin | A sulfonamide |
| (urethritis, cervicitis) | Azithromycin or doxycycline[9] | Erythromycin; ofloxacin[22]; amoxicillin |
| (lymphogranuloma venereum) | A tetracycline[9] | Erythromycin |
| Chlamydia pneumoniae (TWAR strain) | A tetracycline[9] | Erythromycin; clarithromycin[11]; azithromycin; a fluoroquinolone[22] |
| **Ehrlichia** | | |
| Ehrlichia chaffeensis | A tetracycline[9] | Chloramphenicol[15] |
| Agent of human granulocytic ehrlichiosis[42] | A tetracycline[9] | |
| **Mycoplasma** | | |
| Mycoplasma pneumoniae | Erythromycin or a tetracycline[9] or clarithromycin[11] or azithromycin | A fluoroquinolone[3] |
| Ureaplasma urealyticum | Erythromycin | A tetracycline[9]; clarithromycin[11]; azithromycin; ofloxacin[22] |

| Infecting Organism | Drug of First Choice | Alternative Drugs |
|---|---|---|
| **Rickettsia** — Rocky Mountain spotted fever, endemic typhus (murine), epidemic typhus (louseborne), scrub typhus, trench fever, Q fever | A tetracycline[9] | Chloramphenicol[15]; a fluoroquinolone[3] |
| **Spirochetes** | | |
| *Borrelia burgdorferi* (Lyme disease)[43] | Doxycycline[9] or amoxicillin or cefuroxime axetil[5] | Ceftriaxone[5]; cefotaxime[5]; penicillin G; azithromycin; clarithromycin[11] |
| *Borrelia recurrentis* (relapsing fever) | A tetracycline[9] | Penicillin G |
| *Treponema pallidum* (syphilis) | Penicillin G[4] | A tetracycline[9]; ceftriaxone[5] |
| *Treponema pertenue* (yaws) | Penicillin G | A tetracycline[9] |

*Resistance may be a problem; susceptibility tests should be performed.

1. Disk sensitivity testing may not provide adequate information; beta-lactamase assays, "E" tests, and dilution tests for susceptibility should be used in serious infections.

2. An investigational drug in the U.S.A. (*Synercid®*) available through Rhone-Poulenc Rorer (610-454-3071).

3. Among the fluoroquinolones, levofloxacin, sparfloxacin, grepafloxacin, and trovafloxacin have the greatest *in vitro* activity against *S. pneumoniae*, including penicillin and cephalosporin-resistant strains. Levofloxacin, sparfloxacin, grepafloxacin, and trovafloxacin also have good activity against many strains of *S. aureus*, but resistance has become frequent among methicillin-resistant strains. Ciprofloxacin and trovafloxacin have the greatest activity against *Pseudomonas aeruginosa*. Trovafloxacin is the most active against anaerobes. Sparfloxacin has a substantial incidence of photosensitivity reactions. For urinary tract infections, norfloxacin, lomefloxacin, or enoxacin can be used. Ciprofloxacin, ofloxacin, levofloxacin, and trovafloxacin are available for intravenous use. None of these agents are recommended for children or pregnant women.

4. Penicillin V (or amoxicillin) is preferred for oral treatment of infections caused by non-penicillinase-producing staphylococci and other gram-positive cocci. For initial therapy of severe infections, penicillin G, administered parenterally, is first choice. For somewhat longer action in less severe infections due to group A streptococci, pneumococci, or *Treponema pallidum*, procaine penicillin G, an intramuscular formulation, is given once or twice daily. Benzathine penicillin G, a slowly absorbed preparation, is usually given in a single monthly injection for prophylaxis of rheumatic fever, once for treatment of group A streptococcal pharyngitis and once or more for treatment of syphilis.

5. The cephalosporins have been used as alternatives to penicillin in patients allergic to penicillins, but such patients may also have allergic reactions to cephalosporins.

6. For parenteral treatment of staphylococcal or nonenterococcal streptococcal infections, a first-generation cephalosporin such as cephalothin or cefazolin can be used. For oral therapy, cephalexin or cephradine can be used. The second-generation cephalosporins cefamandole, cefprozil, cefuroxime axetil, cefonicid, cefotetan, cefmetazole, cefoxitin, and loracarbef are more active than the first-generation drugs against gram-negative bacteria. Cefuroxime is active against ampicillin-resistant strains of *H. influenzae*. Cefoxitin, cefotetan, and cefmetazole are the most active of the cephalosporins against *B. fragilis*, but cefotetan and cefmetazole have been associated with prothrombin deficiency. The third-generation cephalosporins cefotaxime, cefoperazone, ceftizoxime, ceftriaxone, and ceftazidime, and the fourth-generation cefepime have greater activity than the second-generation drugs against enteric gram-negative bacilli. Ceftazidime has poor activity against many gram-positive cocci and anaerobes, and ceftizoxime has poor activity against penicillin-resistant *S. pneumoniae* (Hess DW and Bonczar T, *J Antimicrob Chemother*, 1996, 38:293). Cefepime has *in vitro* activity against gram-positive cocci similar to cefotaxime and ceftriaxone and somewhat greater activity against enteric gram-negative bacilli. The activity of cefepime against *Pseudomonas aeruginosa* is similar to that of ceftazidime. Cefixime, cefpodoxime, and cefibuten are oral cephalosporins with more activity than second-generation cephalosporins against facultative gram-negative bacilli; they have no useful activity against anaerobes or *Pseudomonas aeruginosa* and cefixime and ceftibuten have no useful activity against staphylococci. With the exception of cefoperazone (which, like cefamandole, can cause bleeding), ceftazidime and cefepime, the activity of all currently available cephalosporins against *Pseudomonas aeruginosa* is poor or inconsistent.

7. For oral use against penicillinase-producing staphylococci, cloxacillin or dicloxacillin is preferred; for severe infections, a parenteral formulation of nafcillin or oxacillin should be used. Ampicillin, amoxicillin, bacampicillin, carbenicillin, ticarcillin, mezlocillin, and piperacillin are not effective against penicillinase-producing staphylococci. The combination of clavulanic acid with amoxicillin or ticarcillin, sulbactam with ampicillin, and tazobactam with piperacillin are active against these organisms.

8. Many strains of coagulase-positive staphylococci and coagulase-negative staphylococci are resistant to penicillinase-resistant penicillins; those strains are also resistant to cephalosporins, imipenem, and meropenem.

9. Tetracyclines are generally not recommended for pregnant women or children younger than 8 years old.

10. For serious soft-tissue infection due to group A streptococci, clindamycin may be more effective than penicillin. Group A streptococci may, however, be resistant to clindamycin; therefore, some *Medical Letter* consultants suggest using both clindamycin and penicillin to treat serious soft-tissue infections. Group A streptococci may also be resistant to erythromycin, azithromycin, and clarithromycin.

11. Not recommended for use in pregnancy.

12. Some strains of *S. pneumoniae* are resistant to erythromycin, clindamycin, trimethoprim-sulfamethoxazole, clarithromycin, azithromycin and chloramphenicol. Nearly all strains tested so far are

## ANTIMICROBIAL DRUGS OF CHOICE *(Continued)*

susceptible to some of the newer fluoroquinolones (levofloxacin, sparfloxacin, grepafloxacin, and trovafloxacin) and quinupristin/dalfopristin.

13. Patients with gonorrhea should be treated presumptively for coinfection with *C. trachomatis* with azithromycin or doxycycline.

14. Rare strains of *N. meningitidis* are resistant or relatively resistant to penicillin. Rifampin or a fluoroquinolone is recommended for prophylaxis after close contact with infected patients.

15. Because of the possibility of serious adverse effects, this drug should be used only for severe infections when less hazardous drugs are ineffective.

16. Sulfonamide-resistant strains are frequent in the U.S.; sulfonamides should be used only when susceptibility is established by susceptibility tests.

17. Debridement is primary. Large doses of penicillin G are required. Hyperbaric oxygen therapy may be a useful adjunct to surgical debridement in management of the spreading, necrotic type.

18. For prophylaxis, a tetanus toxoid booster and, for some patients, tetanus immune globulin (human) are required.

19. In order to decrease the emergence of vancomycin-resistant enterococci in hospitals, many clinicians now recommend use of metronidazole first in treatment of most patients with *C. difficile* colitis, with oral vancomycin used only for seriously ill patients or those who do not respond to metronidazole (Wenisch C, *Clin Infect Dis*, 1996, 22:813).

20. Antitoxin is primary; antimicrobials are used only to halt further toxin production and to prevent the carrier state.

21. In severely ill patients, most *Medical Letter* consultants would add gentamicin, tobramycin, or amikacin.

22. Usually not recommended for use in children or pregnant women.

23. In severely ill patients, most *Medical Letter* consultants would add gentamicin, tobramycin, or amikacin (but see footnote 36)

24. For an acute, uncomplicated urinary tract infection, before the infecting organism is known, the drug of first choice is trimethoprim-sulfamethoxazole.

25. Eradication of *H. pylori* with various antibacterial combinations, given concurrently with an $H_2$-receptor blocker or proton pump inhibitor, has led to rapid healing of active peptic ulcers and low recurrence rates (*Medical Letter*, 1997, 39:1).

26. Large doses (6 g or more/day) are usually necessary for systemic infections. In severely ill patients, some *Medical Letter* consultants would add gentamicin, tobramycin, or amikacin.

27. A fluoroquinolone or amoxicillin is the drug of choice for *S. typhi* carriers.

28. Most cases of *Salmonella* gastroenteritis subside spontaneously without antimicrobial therapy.

29. In severely ill patients, most *Medical Letter* consultants would add gentamicin or amikacin.

30. In severely ill patients, most *Medical Letter* consultants would add gentamicin or amikacin (but see footnote 36).

31. Schwartzman W, *Annu Rev Med*, 1996, 47:365.

32. Role of antibiotics is not clear (Chia JKS, et al, *Clin Infect Dis*, 1998, 26:193).

33. Pera C, et al, *Clin Infect Dis*, 1998, 23:71.

34. Metronidazole is effective for bacterial vaginosis even though it is not usually active against *Gardnerella in vitro*.

35. Stout JE and Yu VL, *N Eng J Med*, 1997, 337:682.

36. Neither gentamicin, tobramycin, netilmicin, or amikacin should be mixed in the same bottle with carbenicillin, ticarcillin, mezlocillin, or piperacillin for intravenous administration. When used in high doses or in patients with renal impairment, these penicillins may inactivate the aminoglycosides.

37. Antibiotic therapy is an adjunct to and not a substitute for prompt fluid and electrolyte replacement.

38. Most infections are self-limited without drug treatment (American Thoracic Society, *Am H Respir Crit Care Med*, 1997, 156:S17.

39. Ji B, et al, *Antimicrob Agents Chemother*, 1997, 41:1953.

40. Gelber RH, Ji B, et al, *Antimicrob Agents Chemother*, 1997, 41:1618.

41. Durand DV, et al, *Medicine*, 1997, 76:170.

42. Jacobs RF and Schalzo GE, *J Pediatr*, 1997, 131:184.

43. For treatment of erythema migrans, facial nerve palsy, mild cardiac disease, and some cases of arthritis, oral therapy is satisfactory; for more serious neurologic or cardiac disease or arthritis, parenteral therapy with ceftriaxone, cefotaxime, or penicillin G is recommended (*Medical Letter*, 1997, 39:47).

# REFERENCE VALUES FOR ADULTS

### Automated Chemistry (CHEMISTRY A)

| Test | Values | Remarks |
|---|---|---|
| **SERUM PLASMA** | | |
| Acetone | Negative | |
| Albumin | 3.2-5 g/dL | |
| Alcohol, ethyl | Negative | |
| Aldolase | 1.2-7.6 IU/L | |
| Ammonia | 20-70 mcg/dL | Specimen to be placed on ice as soon as collected |
| Amylase | 30-110 units/L | |
| Bilirubin, direct | 0-0.3 mg/dL | |
| Bilirubin, total | 0.1-1.2 mg/dL | |
| Calcium | 8.6-10.3 mg/dL | |
| Calcium, ionized | 2.24-2.46 mEq/L | |
| Chloride | 95-108 mEq/L | |
| Cholesterol, total | ≤220 mg/dL | Fasted blood required – normal value affected by dietary habits. This reference range is for a general adult population |
| HDL cholesterol | 40-60 mg/dL | Fasted blood required – normal value affected by dietary habits |
| LDL cholesterol | 65-170 mg/dL | LDLC calculated by Friewald formula... which has certain inaccuracies and is invalid at trig levels >300 mg/dL |
| $CO_2$ | 23-30 mEq/L | |
| Creatine kinase (CK) isoenzymes | | |
| CK-BB | 0% | |
| CK-MB | 0%-3.9% | |
| CK-MM | 96%-100% | |

CK-MB levels must be both ≥4% and 10 IU/L to meet diagnostic criteria for CK-MB positive result consistent with myocardial injury.

| Test | Values | Remarks |
|---|---|---|
| Creatine phosphokinase (CPK) | 8-150 IU/L | |
| Creatinine | 0.5-1.4 mg/dL | |
| Ferritin | 13-300 ng/mL | |
| Folate | 3.6-20 ng/dL | |
| GGT (gamma-glutamyltranspeptidase) | | |
| male | 11-63 IU/L | |
| female | 8-35 IU/L | |
| GLDH | To be determined | |
| Glucose (2-h postprandial) | Up to 140 mg/dL | |
| Glucose, fasting | 60-110 mg/dL | |
| Glucose, nonfasting (2-h postprandial) | 60-140 mg/dL | |
| Hemoglobin $A_{1c}$ | 8 | |
| Hemoglobin, plasma free | <2.5 mg/100 mL | |
| Hemoglobin, total glycosylated (Hb $A_1$) | 4%-8% | |
| Iron | 65-150 mcg/dL | |
| Iron binding capacity, total (TIBC) | 250–420 mcg/dL | |

# REFERENCE VALUES FOR ADULTS *(Continued)*

## Automated Chemistry (CHEMISTRY A) *(continued)*

| Test | Values | Remarks |
|---|---|---|
| Lactic acid | 0.7-2.1 mEq/L | Specimen to be kept on ice and sent to lab as soon as possible |
| Lactate dehydrogenase (LDH) | 56-194 IU/L | |
| Lactate dehydrogenase (LDH) isoenzymes | | |
| $LD_1$ | 20%-34% | |
| $LD_2$ | 29%-41% | |
| $LD_3$ | 15%-25% | |
| $LD_4$ | 1%-12% | |
| $LD_5$ | 1%-15% | |

Flipped $LD_1/LD_2$ ratios (>1 may be consistent with myocardial injury) particularly when considered in combination with a recent CK-MB positive result

| | | |
|---|---|---|
| Lipase | 23-208 units/L | |
| Magnesium | 1.6-2.5 mg/dL | Increased by slight hemolysis |
| Osmolality | 289-308 mOsm/kg | |
| Phosphatase, alkaline | | |
| adults 25-60 y | 33-131 IU/L | |
| adults 61 y or older | 51-153 IU/L | |
| infancy-adolescence | Values range up to 3-5 times higher than adults | |
| Phosphate, inorganic | 2.8-4.2 mg/dL | |
| Potassium | 3.5-5.2 mEq/L | Increased by slight hemolysis |
| Prealbumin | >15 mg/dL | |
| Protein, total | 6.5-7.9 g/dL | |
| SGOT (AST) | <35 IU/L | |
| SGPT (ALT) | <35 IU/L | |
| Sodium | 134-149 mEq/L | |
| Transferrin | >200 mg/dL | |
| Triglycerides | 45-155 mg/dL | Fasted blood required |
| Urea nitrogen (BUN) | 7-20 mg/dL | |
| Uric acid | | |
| male | 2.0-8.0 mg/dL | |
| female | 2.0-7.5 mg/dL | |

### CEREBROSPINAL FLUID

| | | |
|---|---|---|
| Glucose | 50-70 mg/dL | |
| Protein | | |
| adults and children | 15-45 mg/dL | CSF obtained by lumbar puncture |
| newborn infants | 60-90 mg/dL | |

On CSF obtained by cisternal puncture: About 25 mg/dL

On CSF obtained by ventricular puncture: About 10 mg/dL

**Note:** Bloody specimen gives erroneously high value due to contamination with blood proteins

## Automated Chemistry (CHEMISTRY A) *(continued)*

| Test | Values | Remarks |
|------|--------|---------|
| **URINE** | | |
| **(24-hour specimen is required for all these tests unless specified)** | | |
| Amylase | 32-641 units/L | The value is in units/L and **not** calculated for total volume |
| Amylase, fluid (random samples) | | Interpretation of value left for physician, depends on the nature of fluid |
| Calcium | Depends upon dietary intake | |
| Creatine | | |
|   male | 150 mg/24 h | Higher value on children and during pregnancy |
|   female | 250 mg/24 h | |
| Creatinine | 1000-2000 mg/24 h | |
| Creatinine clearance (endogenous) | | |
|   male | 85-125 mL/min | A blood sample must accompany urine specimen |
|   female | 75-115 mL/min | |
| Glucose | 1 g/24 h | |
| 5-hydroxyindoleacetic acid | 2-8 mg/24 h | |
| Iron | 0.15 mg/24 h | Acid washed container required |
| Magnesium | 146-209 mg/24 h | |
| Osmolality | 500-800 mOsm/kg | With normal fluid intake |
| Oxalate | 10-40 mg/24 h | |
| Phosphate | 400-1300 mg/24 h | |
| Potassium | 25-120 mEq/24 h | Varies with diet; the interpretation of urine electrolytes and osmolality should be left for the physician |
| Sodium | 40-220 mEq/24 h | |
| Porphobilinogen, qualitative | Negative | |
| Porphyrins, qualitative | Negative | |
| Proteins | 0.05-0.1 g/24 h | |
| Salicylate | Negative | |
| Urea clearance | 60-95 mL/min | A blood sample must accompany specimen |
| Urea N | 10-40 g/24 h | Dependent on protein intake |
| Uric acid | 250-750 mg/24 h | Dependent on diet and therapy |
| Urobilinogen | 0.5-3.5 mg/24 h | For qualitative determination on random urine, send sample to urinalysis section in Hematology Lab |
| Xylose absorption test | | |
|   children | 16%-33% of ingested xylose | |
|   adults | >4 g in 5 h | |
| **FECES** | | |
| Fat, 3-day collection | <5 g/d | Value depends on fat intake of 100 g/d for 3 days preceding and during collection |
| **GASTRIC ACIDITY** | | |
| Acidity, total, 12 h | 10-60 mEq/L | Titrated at pH 7 |

# REFERENCE VALUES FOR ADULTS *(Continued)*

## BLOOD GASES

|  | Arterial | Capillary | Venous |
|---|---|---|---|
| pH | 7.35-7.45 | 7.35-7.45 | 7.32-7.42 |
| $pCO_2$ (mm Hg) | 35-45 | 35-45 | 38-52 |
| $pO_2$ (mm Hg) | 70-100 | 60-80 | 24-48 |
| $HCO_3$ (mEq/L) | 19-25 | 19-25 | 19-25 |
| $TCO_2$ (mEq/L) | 19-29 | 19-29 | 23-33 |
| $O_2$ saturation (%) | 90-95 | 90-95 | 40-70 |
| Base excess (mEq/L) | -5 to +5 | -5 to +5 | -5 to +5 |

## HEMATOLOGY

### Complete Blood Count

| Age | Hgb (g/dL) | Hct (%) | RBC (mill/mm³) | RDW |
|---|---|---|---|---|
| 0-3 d | 15.0-20.0 | 45-61 | 4.0-5.9 | <18 |
| 1-2 wk | 12.5-18.5 | 39-57 | 3.6-5.5 | <17 |
| 1-6 mo | 10.0-13.0 | 29-42 | 3.1-4.3 | <16.5 |
| 7 mo to 2 y | 10.5-13.0 | 33-38 | 3.7-4.9 | <16 |
| 2-5 y | 11.5-13.0 | 34-39 | 3.9-5.0 | <15 |
| 5-8 y | 11.5-14.5 | 35-42 | 4.0-4.9 | <15 |
| 13-18 y | 12.0-15.2 | 36-47 | 4.5-5.1 | <14.5 |
| Adult male | 13.5-16.5 | 41-50 | 4.5-5.5 | <14.5 |
| Adult female | 12.0-15.0 | 36-44 | 4.0-4.9 | <14.5 |

| Age | MCV (fL) | MCH (pg) | MCHC (%) | PLTS (x 10³/mm³) |
|---|---|---|---|---|
| 0-3 d | 95-115 | 31-37 | 29-37 | 250-450 |
| 1-2 wk | 86-110 | 28-36 | 28-38 | 250-450 |
| 1-6 mo | 74-96 | 25-35 | 30-36 | 300-700 |
| 7 mo to 2 y | 70-84 | 23-30 | 31-37 | 250-600 |
| 2-5 y | 75-87 | 24-30 | 31-37 | 250-550 |
| 5-8 y | 77-95 | 25-33 | 31-37 | 250-550 |
| 13-18 y | 78-96 | 25-35 | 31-37 | 150-550 |
| Adult male | 80-100 | 26-34 | 31-37 | 150-450 |
| Adult female | 80-100 | 26-34 | 31-37 | 150-450 |

## WBC and Diff

| Age | WBC (x 10³/mm³) | Segs | Bands | Lymphs | Monos |
|---|---|---|---|---|---|
| 0-3 d | 9.0-35.0 | 32-62 | 10-18 | 19-29 | 5-7 |
| 1-2 wk | 5.0-20.0 | 14-34 | 6-14 | 36-45 | 6-10 |
| 1-6 mo | 6.0-17.5 | 13-33 | 4-12 | 41-71 | 4-7 |
| 7 mo to 2 y | 6.0-17.0 | 15-35 | 5-11 | 45-76 | 3-6 |
| 2-5 y | 5.5-15.5 | 23-45 | 5-11 | 35-65 | 3-6 |
| 5-8 y | 5.0-14.5 | 32-54 | 5-11 | 28-48 | 3-6 |
| 13-18 y | 4.5-13.0 | 34-64 | 5-11 | 25-45 | 3-6 |
| Adults | 4.5-11.0 | 35-66 | 5-11 | 24-44 | 3-6 |

| Age | Eosinophils | Basophils | Atypical Lymphs | No. of NRBCs |
|---|---|---|---|---|
| 0-3 d | 0-2 | 0-1 | 0-8 | 0-2 |
| 1-2 wk | 0-2 | 0-1 | 0-8 | 0 |
| 1-6 mo | 0-3 | 0-1 | 0-8 | 0 |
| 7 mo to 2 y | 0-3 | 0-1 | 0-8 | 0 |
| 2-5 y | 0-3 | 0-1 | 0-8 | 0 |
| 5-8 y | 0-3 | 0-1 | 0-8 | 0 |
| 13-18 y | 0-3 | 0-1 | 0-8 | 0 |
| Adults | 0-3 | 0-1 | 0-8 | 0 |

Segs = segmented neutrophils          Lymphs = lymphocytes
Bands = band neutrophils          Monos = monocytes

## Erythrocyte Sedimentation Rates and Reticulocyte Counts

Sedimentation rate, Westergren          Children  0-20 mm/hour
                                        Adult male  0-15 mm/hour
                                        Adult female  0-20 mm/hour

Sedimentation rate, Wintrobe          Children  0-13 mm/hour
                                      Adult male  0-10 mm/hour
                                      Adult female  0-15 mm/hour

Reticulocyte count          Newborns  2%-6%
                            1-6 mo  0%-2.8%
                            Adults  0.5%-1.5%

# ANTICOAGULANT THERAPY

This information, for the use of heparin and warfarin in adults, was obtained from a review of current literature. This information is intended to optimize therapeutic anticoagulation by minimizing patient bleeding risks, decreasing the time required for titration to achieve a desired level of anticoagulation, and promoting efficient use of laboratory tests.

## Initiation of Intravenous Heparin Therapy Treatment of Venous Thrombosis and Pulmonary Embolism[1]

| Monitoring | Dosing |
|---|---|
| Check baseline aPTT, PT/INR, CBC | Bolus 80 units/kg I.V.<br>Initial drip 18 units/kg/hour I.V. |
| Check CBC with platelet count every 3 days, aPTT 6 hours post bolus and 6 hours after each dosing adjustment. When two consecutive aPTTs are therapeutic, monitor aPTT every 24 hours and readjust heparin drip as needed. | Refer to nomogram below |

| aPTT*(s) | Dosing |
|---|---|
| <35 | 80 units/kg bolus, increase drip 4 units/kg/hour |
| 35-45 | 40 units/kg bolus, increase drip 2 units/kg/hour |
| 46-70 | No change |
| 71-90 | Reduce drip by 2 units/kg/hour |
| >90 | Stop infusion 1 hour, reduce drip by 3 units/kg/hour |

aPTT — activated partial thromboplastin time; PT/INR — prothrombin time/International Normalized Ratio; CBC — complete blood count and platelet count; s — seconds; kg — kilogram

*It is recommended that each lab perform an *in vitro* heparin titration curve to establish the therapeutic range for a specific aPTT reagent which is equivalent to a heparin concentration of 0.2-0.4 units/mL. Thus, the therapeutic range will vary depending upon the aPTT reagent in use.

## Intensity of Anticoagulation With Coumadin® (Warfarin Sodium)[2]

| Indication | INR | |
|---|---|---|
| | Target | Range |
| Prophylaxis of venous thrombosis | 2.5 | 2.0-3.0 |
| Treatment of venous thrombosis | 2.5 | 2.0-3.0 |
| Treatment of pulmonary embolism | 2.5 | 2.0-3.0 |
| Prevention of systemic embolism† | | |
| Tissue heart valves | 2.5 | 2.0-3.0 |
| Atrial fibrillation* | 2.5 | 2.0-3.0 |
| Recurrent systemic embolism | 2.5 | 2.0-3.0† |
| Mechanical prosthetic valves | 3.0 | 2.5-3.5 |
| Postmyocardial infarction | 3.0 | 2.5-3.5 |

*See treatment algorithm for thromboembolic stroke prevention.

†In cases where the risk of thromboembolism is great, a higher PT/INR may be required, such as in patients with recurrent systemic embolism.

## INITIATION OF ORAL ANTICOAGULATION WITH COUMADIN®

The dosing of Coumadin® must be individualized according to the patient's response to the drug as indicated by the PT/INR. Use of a large loading dose may increase the incidence of hemorrhagic and other complications, does not offer more rapid protection against thrombus formation, and is not recommended. Low initiation doses (eg, 2-5 mg/day) are recommended for elderly and/or debilitated patients and patients with potential for increased responsiveness to Coumadin®.

**Step 1:** Obtain baseline PT/INR

Begin therapy with Coumadin® (warfarin sodium) with a dose of 2-5 mg per day with dosage adjustment based on the results of PT/INR determinations.

**For patients on heparin:** Since the anticoagulant effect of Coumadin® is delayed, heparin is preferred initially for rapid anticoagulation. Conversion to Coumadin® may begin concomitantly with heparin therapy or may be delayed 3-6 days. When Coumadin® has produced the desired therapeutic range, INR, or prothrombin time, heparin may be discontinued.

**Step 2: Day that the PT/INR is stabilized in the therapeutic range:** Check PT/INR daily. Adjust warfarin dose based on the results of PT/INR determinations.

**Patients stabilized in the therapeutic range:** Intervals between subsequent PT/INR determinations should be based upon the physician's judgment of the patient's reliability and response to Coumadin® in order to maintain the individual within the therapeutic range. Acceptable intervals for PT/INR determinations are normally with the range of 1-4 weeks after a stable dosage has been determined. Most patients are satisfactorily maintained on Coumadin® at a dose of 2-10 mg daily.

## MONITORING — THE INTERNATIONAL NORMALIZED RATIO (INR)

Because PT results are very dependent on the thromboplastin reagent used, a system of standardizing the prothrombin time in oral anticoagulant therapy was introduced by the World Health Organization in 1983. It is based upon determination of an INR, which is equivalent to the PT ratio one would obtain if a sensitive reference thromboplastin were used for the PT.

- Thromboplastin sensitivity is determined by the manufacturer and is expressed as an International Sensitivity Index (ISI)

- The INR can be calculated as **INR = (Observed PT ratio)$^{ISI}$**

- The calculation of the INR from the PT ratio is usually performed by the laboratory

### Reminder

- Be aware of potential drug interactions and other factors that may affect INR (refer to prescribing information for Coumadin®)

- Patient/staff education about Coumadin® is an important part of therapy. Effective therapeutic levels with minimal complications are in part dependent upon cooperative and well-instructed patients who communicate effectively with their physician. Various Coumadin® patient educational guides are available to health professionals on request.

## DRUG INTERACTIONS WITH COUMADIN®

Numerous factors, alone or in combination, including travel, changes in diet, environment, physical state, and medication may influence response of the patient to anticoagulants. It is generally good practice to monitor the patient's response with additional PT/INR determinations in the period immediately after discharge from the hospital, and whenever other medications are initiated, discontinued, or taken irregularly. The following factors are listed for reference; however, other factors may also affect the anticoagulant response.

The following factors, alone or in combination, may be responsible for **increased** PT/INR response.

**Exogenous Factors**
Potential drug interactions with Coumadin® (warfarin sodium) are listed below by drug class. For specific drugs in these classes that have been reported to interact, see full prescribing information for Coumadin®.

adrenergic stimulants, central
alcohol abuse reduction preparations
analgesics
anesthetics, inhalation
antiarrhythmics†
antibiotics†
    aminoglycosides (oral)
    cephalosporins, parenteral
    macrolides
    metronidazole
    miscellaneous
        penicillins (intravenous high-
           dose)
        quinolones (fluoroquinolones)
        sulfonamides, long-acting
        tetracyclines

anticoagulants
anticonvulsants†
antidepressants†
antimalarial agents
antineoplastics†
antiparasitic/antimicrobials
antiplatelet drugs/effects
antithyroid drugs†
beta-adrenergic blockers
bromelains
cholelitholytic agents
diabetes agents, oral
diuretics†
fungal medications, systemic†
gastrointestinal, ulcerative colitis agents
gout treatment agents

# ANTICOAGULANT THERAPY *(Continued)*

hemorrheologic agents
hepatotoxic drugs
hyperglycemic agents
hypertensive emergency agents
hypnotics†
hypolipidemics†
monoamine oxidase inhibitors
narcotics, prolonged
NSAIDs
psychostimulants
pyrazolones

salicylates
steroids, adrenocortical†
steroids, anabolic (17-alkyl testosterone
   derivatives)
thrombolytics
thyroid drugs†
tuberculosis agents†
uricosuric agents
vaccines
vitamin E

**Also:** Other medications affecting blood elements which may modify hemostasis, dietary deficiencies, prolonged hot weather, unreliable PT/INR determinations.

†Increased and decreased PT/INR responses have been reported.

The following factors, alone or in combination, may be responsible for **decreased** PT/INR response.

**Exogenous Factors**

Potential drug interactions with Coumadin® (warfarin sodium) are listed below by drug class. For specific drugs in these classes that have been reported to interact, see full prescribing information for Coumadin®.

adrenal cortical steroid inhibitors
antacids
antianxiety agents
antiarrhythmics†
antibiotics†
anticonvulsants†
antidepressants†
antihistamines
antineoplastics†
antipsychotic medications
antithyroid drugs†
barbiturates

diuretics†
enteral nutritional supplements
fungal medications, systemic†
gastric acidity and peptic ulcer agents†
hypnotics†
hypolipidemics†
immunosuppressives
oral contraceptives, estrogen-containing
steroids, adrenocortical†
thyroid drugs†
tuberculosis agents†
vitamin K

**Also:** Diet high in vitamin K and unreliable PT/INR determinations

†Increased and decreased PT/INR responses have been reported.

Because a patient may be exposed to a combination of the above factors, the net effect of Coumadin® on PT/INR response may be unpredictable. More frequent PT/INR monitoring is therefore advisable. Medications of unknown interaction with coumarins are best regarded with caution. When these medications are started or stopped, more frequent PT/INR monitoring is advisable.

It has been reported that concomitant administration of warfarin and ticlopidine may be associated with cholestatic hepatitis.

**Effect on other drugs:** Coumarins may also affect the action of other drugs. Hypoglycemic agents (chlorpropamide and tolbutamide) and anticonvulsants (phenytoin and phenobarbital) may accumulate in the body as a result of interference with either their metabolism or excretion.

## THERAPY WITH COUMADIN® (Warfarin Sodium)

Coumadin® is indicated for the prophylaxis and/or treatment of venous thrombosis and its extension, and pulmonary embolism.

Coumadin® is indicated for the prophylaxis and/or treatment of the thromboembolic complications associated with atrial fibrillation and/or cardiac valve replacement.

Coumadin® is indicated to reduce the risk of death, recurrent myocardial infarction, and thromboembolic events such as stroke or systemic embolization after myocardial infarction.

The benefits of oral anticoagulant therapy in reducing the occurrence of thromboembolic events in patients with atrial fibrillation has been confirmed by a number of major clinical trials.[3-9] A pooled analysis of five major clinical trials demonstrated a 68% risk reduction of thromboembolic stroke in patients receiving warfarin (INR 2.0-3.0). The annual rate of major hemorrhage was 1.0% for the control group and 1.3% for the warfarin group.[10]

Coumadin® is contraindicated in:

- patients where the risk of hemorrhage outweighs the potential clinical benefits of therapy
- pregnancy
- alcoholism/drug abuse
- unsupervised dementia/psychosis

### Treatment Algorithm for Thromboembolic Stroke Prevention in Patients with Atrial Fibrillation

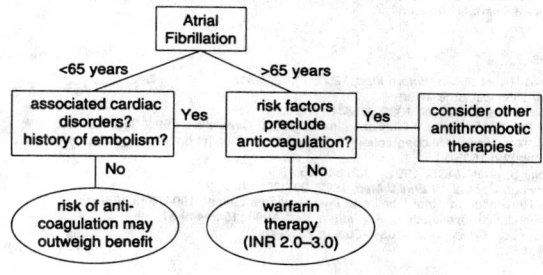

### Managing Prolongations of the INR
### American College of CHEST Physicians
### Consensus Conference Recommendations

| INR | Symptoms | Recommendation |
|---|---|---|
| Above therapeutic range but <6 | No bleeding and rapid reversal not indicated for reasons of surgical intervention | Omit next few doses of warfarin and commence at a lower dose when INR is in therapeutic range. |
| 6-10 | No bleeding or when rapid reversal in required for elective surgery | Administer subcutaneously 1.0-2.0 mg vitamin $K_1$*; expect reduction in INR in 8 hours, many patients will be in therapeutic range in 24 hours. If INR still too high in 24 hours, an additional dose of 0.5 mg can be given. Resume warfarin at lower dose when INR returns to the desired range. |
| >10 | No bleeding | Administer subcutaneously 3.0 mg vitamin $K_1$; expect reduction in INR in 6 hours; check INR in 6 hours and repeat vitamin $K_1$ if necessary. |
| >20 | Serious bleeding or major warfarin overdose | Administer subcutaneously 10.0 mg vitamin $K_1$ and supplement with fresh plasma transfusion or prothrombin complex concentrate depending on the urgency of the situation. Check INR every 6 hours; vitamin $K_1$ may have to be repeated every 12 hours. |
|  | Life-threatening bleeding/ serious warfarin overdose | Administer subcutaneously prothrombin complex concentrate supplemented with 10 mg vitamin $K_1$ to be repeated as necessary depending on the INR. It is not usually necessary to give vitamin $K_1$ for the immediate reversal if prothrombin complex concentrates containing factor VII are used. |

## ANTICOAGULANT THERAPY *(Continued)*

### Managing Prolongations of the INR
### American College of CHEST Physicians
### Consensus Conference Recommendations *(continued)*

| INR | Symptoms | Recommendation |
|-----|----------|----------------|
| Use of high doses of vitamin K₁ (10.0-15.0) may cause resistance to warfarin for up to a week. Heparin can be given until the patient becomes responsive to warfarin. | | |

*Please see recommendations accompanying vitamin K₁ preparations prior to use. A risk of hepatitis and other viral diseases is associated with the use of these blood products. See Full Prescribing Information for Coumadin® (warfarin sodium).

### Footnotes

1. Raschke RA, et al, *Ann Intern Med*, 1993, 119:874-81.
2. COUMADIN® package insert
3. Petersen P, et al, *Lancet*, 1989, 1(8631):175-9.
4. Stroke Prevention in Atrial Fibrillation Investigators, *Circulation*, 1991, 84(2):527-39.
5. The Boston Area Anticoagulation Trial for Atrial Fibrillation Investigators, *N Engl J Med*, 1990, 323(22):1505-11.
6. Connolly S, et al, *JACC*, 1991, 18(2):349-55.
7. Ezekowitz MD, et al, *N Engl J Med*, 1992, 327(20):1406-12.
8. Stroke Prevention in Atrial Fibrillation Investigations, *Lancet*, 1994, 343:687-91.
9. Atrial Fibrillation Investigators, *Ann Intern Med*, 1994, 154:1449-57.
10. Hirsh J, et al, *Chest*, 1995, 108(4-Suppl): 231S-46S.

# ANTIDEPRESSANT MEDICATIONS

The under diagnosis and under treatment of depression in nursing homes has been documented in a *Journal of the American Medical Association* paper entitled "Depression and Mortality in the Nursing home" (*JAMA*, February 27, 1991, 265(8)). HCFA continues to support the accurate identification and treatment of depression in nursing homes.

The surveyor should not urge a facility to use behavioral monitoring charts (eg, documenting quantitatively (number of episodes) and objectively (eg, withdrawn behavior such as staying in their room, refusal to speak, etc)) when antidepressant drugs are used in nursing homes. Such charts are promoted in the interpretative guidelines for antipsychotic and benzodiazepine and other anxiolytic/sedative drugs, but **not** for antidepressant drugs. These charts may be helpful for monitoring the effects of antidepressant drugs in nursing homes, but they may place additional paperwork burden on the facility and thus act as a deterrent to the appropriate diagnosis and treatment of this condition.

The following is a list of commonly used antidepressant drugs.

| Generic Name | Brand Name |
| --- | --- |
| Amitriptyline* | Elavil® |
| Amoxapine | Asendin® |
| Bupropion | Wellbutrin® |
| Butriptyline* | Evadene® |
| Citalopram* | Celexa® |
| Clomipramine* | Anafranil® |
| Desipramine | Norpramin® |
| Dibenzepin* | Noveril® |
| Doxepin* | Sinequan® |
| Fluoxetine | Prozac® |
| Fluvoxamine | Luvox® |
| Imipramine* | Tofranil |
| Isocarboxazid* | Marplan® |
| Maprotiline | Ludiomil® |
| Mirtazapine | Remeron® |
| Nefazodone | Serzone® |
| Nortriptyline | Aventyl®, Pamelor® |
| Paroxetine | Paxil™ |
| Phenelzine* | Nardil® |
| Protriptyline | Vivactil® |
| Sertraline | Zoloft™ |
| Tranylcypromine* | Parnate® |
| Trazodone | Desyrel® |
| Trimipramine* | Surmontil® |
| Venlafaxine | Effexor® |

*These are not necessarily drugs of choice for depression in the elderly. They are listed here only in the event of their potential use.

# ANTIPSYCHOTIC MEDICATIONS

Appropriate indications for use of antipsychotic medications are outlined in the Health Care Finance Administration's Omnibus Reconciliation Act (OBRA) of 1987. These regulations require that antipsychotics be used to treat specific conditions (listed below) and not solely for behavior control.

**Approved indications include:**

- acute psychotic episode
- atypical psychosis
- brief reactive psychosis
- delusional disorder
- Huntington's disease
- psychotic mood disorder (including manic depression and depression with psychotic features)
- schizo-affective disorder
- schizophrenia
- schizophrenic form disorder
- Tourette's disease
- short-term (7 days) for hiccups, nausea, vomiting, or pruritus
- organic mental syndrome with psychotic or agitated features:
  - behaviors are quantitatively and objectively documented
  - behaviors must be **persistent**
  - behaviors are not caused by preventable reasons
  - patient presents a danger to self or others
  - continuous crying or screaming if this impairs functional status
  - psychotic symptoms (hallucinations, paranoia, delusions) which cause resident distress or impaired functional capacity

"Clinically contraindicated" means that a resident with a "specific condition" who has had a history of recurrence of psychotic symptoms (eg, delusions, hallucinations) which have been stabilized with a maintenance dose of an antipsychotic drug without incurring significant side effects (eg, tardive dyskinesia) **should not receive gradual dose reductions**. In residents with organic mental syndromes (eg, dementia, delirium), "clinically contraindicated" means that a gradual dose reduction has been attempted **twice** in 1 year and that attempt resulted in the return of symptoms for which the drug was prescribed to a degree that a cessation in the gradual dose reduction, or a return to previous dose levels was necessary.

If the medication is being used outside the guidelines, the physician must provide justification why the continued use of the drug and the dose of the drug is clinically appropriate.

Antipsychotics should not be used if one or more of the following is/are the **only** indication:

- wandering
- poor self care
- restlessness
- impaired memory
- anxiety
- depression (without psychotic features)
- insomnia
- unsociability
- indifference to surroundings
- fidgeting
- nervousness
- uncooperativeness
- agitated behaviors which do **not** represent danger to the resident or others

Selection of an antipsychotic agent should be based on the side effect profile since all antipsychotic agents are equally effective at equivalent doses. Coadministration of two or more antipsychotics does not have any pharmacological basis or clinical advantage and increases the potential for side effects. See Antipsychotic Agents table in Comparative Drug Charts.

## DOSING GUIDELINES

1. Daily dosages should be equal to or less than those listed below, unless documentation exists to support the need for higher doses to maintain or improve functional status.

| Generic | Brand | Daily Dose for Patients With Organic Mental Syndrome |
|---------|-------|------------------------------------------------------|
| Acetophenazine | Tindal® | 20 mg |
| Chlorpromazine | Thorazine® | 75 mg |
| Clozapine | Clozaril® | 50 mg |
| Fluphenazine | Prolixin® | 4 mg |
| Haloperidol | Haldol® | 4 mg |
| Loxapine | Loxitane® | 10 mg |
| Mesoridazine | Serentil® | 25 mg |
| Molindone | Moban® | 10 mg |
| Olanzapine | Zyprexa® | 5 mg |
| Perphenazine | Trilafon® | 8 mg |
| Pimozide | Orap™ | 4 mg |
| Prochlorperazine | Compazine® | 10 mg |
| Promazine | Sparine® | 150 mg |
| Quetiapine | Seroquel® | 100 mg |
| Risperidone | Risperdal® | 2 mg |
| Thioridazine | Mellaril® | 75 mg |
| Thiothixene | Navane® | 7 mg |
| Trifluoperazine | Stelazine® | 8 mg |

2. The dose of prochlorperazine may be exceeded for short-term (up to 7 days) for treatment of nausea and vomiting. Residents with nausea and vomiting secondary to cancer or cancer chemotherapy can also be treated with higher doses for longer periods of time.

3. The residents must receive adequate monitoring for significant side effects such as tardive dyskinesia, postural hypotension, cognitive-behavioral impairment, akathisia, and parkinsonism.

4. Gradual dosage reductions are to be attempted twice in 1 year if prescribed for OMS. If symptoms for which the drug has been prescribed return and both reduction attempts have proven unsuccessful, the physician may indicate further reductions are clinically contraindicated.

5. "Clinically contraindicated" means that a resident **need not undergo** a "gradual dose reduction" or "behavioral interventions" if:

   - The resident has a "specific condition" and has a history of recurrence of psychotic symptoms (eg, delusions, hallucinations), which have been stabilized with a maintenance dose of an antipsychotic drug without incurring significant side effects.

   - The resident has organic mental syndrome (now called "delirium, dementia, and amnestic and other cognitive disorders" by DSM IV) and has had a gradual dose reduction attempted **twice** in 1 year and that attempt resulted in the return of symptoms for which the drug was prescribed to a degree that a cessation in the gradual dose reduction, or a return to previous dose reduction was necessary.

   - The resident's physician provides a justification why the continued use of the drug and the dose of the drug is clinically appropriate. This justification should include: a) a diagnosis, but not simply a diagnostic label or code, but the description of symptoms, b) a discussion of the differential psychiatric and medical diagnosis (eg, why the resident's behavioral symptom is thought to be a result of a dementia with associated psychosis and/or agitated behaviors, and not the result of an unrecognized painful medical condition or a psychosocial or environmental stressor), c) a description of the justification for the choice of a particular treatment, or treatments, and d) a discussion of why the present dose is necessary to manage the symptoms of the resident. This information need

## ANTIPSYCHOTIC MEDICATIONS *(Continued)*

not necessarily be in the physician's progress notes, but must be a part of the resident's clinical record.

Examples of evidence that would support a justification of why a drug is being used outside these guidelines but in the best interests of the resident may include, but are not limited to the following.

1. A physician's note indicating for example, that the dosage, duration, indication, and monitoring are clinically appropriate, **and the reasons why they are clinically appropriate**; this note should demonstrate that the physician has carefully considered the risk/benefit to the resident in using drugs outside the guidelines.

2. A medical or psychiatric consultation or evaluation (eg, Geriatric Depression Scale) that confirms the physician's judgment that use of a drug outside the guidelines is in the best interest of the resident.

3. Physician, nursing, or other health professional documentation indicating that the resident is being monitored for adverse consequences or complications of the drug therapy.

4. Documentation confirming that previous attempts at dosage reduction have been unsuccessful.

5. Documentation (including MDS documentation) showing resident's subjective or objective improvement, or maintenance of function while taking the medication.

6. Documentation showing that a resident's decline or deterioration is evaluated by the interdisciplinary team to determine whether a particular drug, or a particular dose, or duration of therapy, may be the cause.

7. Documentation showing why the resident's age, weight, or other factors would require a unique drug dose or drug duration, indication, or monitoring.

8. Other evidence you may deem appropriate.

# ASTHMA

## NATIONAL ASTHMA EDUCATION AND PREVENTION PROGRAM

### EXPERT PANEL REPORT II:
### GUIDELINES FOR THE DIAGNOSIS AND MANAGEMENT OF ASTHMA

#### February 1997

#### Stepwise Approach for Managing Asthma in Adults and Children >5 Years of Age: Classify Severity

### Goals of Asthma Treatment

- Prevent chronic and troublesome symptoms (eg, coughing or breathlessness in the night, in the early morning, or after exertion)

- Maintain (near) "normal" pulmonary function

- Maintain normal activity levels (including exercise and other physical activity)

- Prevent recurrent exacerbations of asthma and minimize the need for emergency department visits or hospitalizations

- Provide optimal pharmacotherapy with minimal or no adverse effects

- Meet patients' and families' expectations of and satisfaction with asthma care

### Clinical Features Before Treatment*

| Symptoms** | Nighttime Symptoms | Lung Function |
|---|---|---|
| **STEP 4: Severe Persistent** | | |
| •Continual symptoms<br>•Limited physical activity<br>•Frequent exacerbations | Frequent | •$FEV_1$/PEF ≤60% predicted<br>•PEF variability >30% |
| **STEP 3: Moderate Persistent** | | |
| •Daily symptoms<br>•Daily use of inhaled short-acting beta₂-agonist<br>•Exacerbations affect activity<br>•Exacerbations ≥2 times/week; may last days | >1 time/week | •$FEV_1$/PEF >60% - 80% predicted<br>•PEF variability >30% |
| **STEP 2: Mild Persistent** | | |
| •Symptoms >2 times/week but <1 time/day<br>•Exacerbations may affect activity | >2 times/month | •$FEV_1$/PEF ≥80% predicted<br>•PEF variability 20% - 30% |
| **STEP 1: Mild Intermittent** | | |
| •Symptoms ≤2 times/week<br>•Asymptomatic and normal PEF between exacerbations<br>•Exacerbations brief (from a few hours to a few days); intensity may vary | ≤2 times/month | •$FEV_1$/PEF ≥80% predicted<br>•PEF variability ≤20% |

*The presence of one of the features of severity is sufficient to place a patient in that category. An individual should be assigned to the most severe grade in which any feature occurs. The characteristics noted in this figure are general and may overlap because asthma is highly variable. Furthermore, an individual's classification may change over time.

**Patients at any level of severity can have mild, moderate, or severe exacerbations. Some patients with intermittent asthma experience severe and life-threatening exacerbations separated by long periods of normal lung function and no symptoms.

# ASTHMA *(Continued)*

## Stepwise Approach for Managing Asthma in Adults and Children >5 Years of Age: Treatment

(Preferred treatments are in **bold** print)

| Long-Term Control | Quick Relief | Education |
|---|---|---|
| **STEP 4: Severe Persistent** | | |
| Daily medications:<br>• **Anti-inflammatory: Inhaled corticosteroid (high dose)** AND<br>• Long-acting bronchodilator: Either **long-acting inhaled beta₂-agonist**, sustained-release theophylline, or long-acting beta₂-agonist tablets AND<br>• Corticosteroid tablets or syrup long term (2 mg/kg/day, generally do not exceed 60 mg per day). | • Short-acting bronchodilator: **Inhaled beta₂-agonists** as needed for symptoms.<br>• Intensity of treatment will depend on severity of exacerbation; see "Managing Exacerbations"<br>• Use of short-acting inhaled beta₂-agonists on a daily basis, or increasing use, indicates the need for additional long-term control therapy. | Steps 2 and 3 actions plus:<br>• Refer to individual education/counseling |
| **STEP 3: Moderate Persistent** | | |
| Daily medication:<br>• Either<br>— **Anti-inflammatory: Inhaled corticosteroid (medium dose)** OR<br>— **Inhaled corticosteroid (low-medium dose)** and add a long-acting bronchodilator, especially for nighttime symptoms: Either **long-acting inhaled beta₂-agonist**, sustained-release theophylline, or long-acting beta₂-agonist tablets.<br>• If needed<br>— Anti-inflammatory: **Inhaled corticosteroids (medium-high dose) AND**<br>— **Long-acting bronchodilator,** especially for nighttime symptoms; either **long-acting inhaled beta₂-agonist,** sustained-release theophylline, or long-acting beta₂-agonist tablets. | • Short-acting bronchodilator: **Inhaled beta₂-agonists** as needed for symptoms.<br>• Intensity of treatment will depend on severity of exacerbation; see "Managing Exacerbations."<br>• Use of short-acting inhaled beta₂-agonists on a daily basis, or increasing use, indicates the need for additional long-term control therapy. | Step 1 actions plus:<br>• Teach self-monitoring<br>• Refer to group education if available<br>• Review and update self-management plan |
| **STEP 2: Mild Persistent** | | |
| One daily medication:<br>• **Anti-inflammatory:** Either **inhaled corticosteroid (low doses)** or **cromolyn or nedocromil** (children usually begin with a trial of cromolyn or nedocromil).<br>• Sustained-release theophylline to serum concentration of 5-15 mcg/mL is an alternative, but not preferred, therapy. Zafirlukast or zileuton may also be considered for patients ≥12 years of age, although their position in therapy is not fully established. | • Short-acting bronchodilator: **Inhaled beta₂-agonists** as needed for symptoms.<br>• Intensity of treatment will depend on severity of exacerbation; see "Managing Exacerbations."<br>•Use of short-acting inhaled beta₂-agonists on a daily basis, or increasing use, indicates the need for additional long-term control therapy. | Step 1 actions plus:<br>• Teach self-monitoring<br>• Refer to group education if available<br>• Review and update self-management plan |
| **STEP 1: Mild Intermittent** | | |
| No daily medication needed. | • Short-acting bronchodilator: **Inhaled beta₂-agonists** as needed for symptoms.<br>• Intensity of treatment will depend on severity of exacerbation; see "Managing Exacerbations"<br>• Use of short-acting inhaled beta₂-agonists more than 2 times/week may indicate the need to initiate long-term control therapy | • Teach basic facts about asthma<br>•Teach inhaler/spacer/holding chamber technique<br>• Discuss roles of medications<br>•Develop self-management plan<br>•Develop action plan for when and how to take rescue actions, especially for patients with a history of severe exacerbations<br>• Discuss appropriate environmental control measures to avoid exposure to known allergens and irritants |

**↓ Step down**
Review treatment every 1-6 months; a gradual stepwise reduction in treatment may be possible.

**↑Step up**
If control is not maintained, consider step up. First, review patient medication technique, adherence, and environmental control (avoidance of allergens or other factors that contribute to asthma severity.)

**Notes:**

- **The stepwise approach presents general guidelines to assist clinical decision making; it is not intended to be a specific prescription. Asthma is highly variable; clinicians should tailor specific medication plans to the needs and circumstances of individual patients.**

- Gain control as quickly as possible; then decrease treatment to the least medication necessary to maintain control. Gaining control may be accomplished by either starting treatment at the step most appropriate to the initial severity of the condition or starting at a higher level of therapy (eg, a course of systemic corticosteroids or higher dose of inhaled corticosteroids).

- A rescue course of systemic corticosteroids may be needed at any time and at any step.

- Some patients with intermittent asthma experience severe and life-threatening exacerbations separated by long periods of normal lung function and no symptoms. This may be especially common with exacerbations provoked by respiratory infections. A short course of systemic corticosteroids is recommended.

- At each step, patients should control their environment to avoid or control factors that make their asthma worse (eg, allergens, irritants); this requires specific diagnosis and education.

## ASTHMA *(Continued)*

### Stepwise Approach for Managing Infants and Young Children (≤5 Years of Age) With Acute or Chronic Asthma Symptoms

| Long-Term Control | Quick Relief |
|---|---|
| **STEP 4: Severe Persistent** | |
| Daily anti-inflammatory medicine<br>• High-dose inhaled corticosteroid with spacer/holding chamber and face mask<br>• If needed, add systemic corticosteroids 2 mg/kg/day and reduce to lowest daily or alternate-day dose that stabilizes symptoms | •Bronchodilator as needed for symptoms (see step 1) up to 3 times/day |
| **STEP 3: Moderate Persistent** | |
| Daily anti-inflammatory medication. Either:<br>• Medium-dose inhaled corticosteroid with spacer/holding chamber and face mask<br>OR<br>Once control is established:<br>• Medium-dose inhaled corticosteroid and nedocromil<br>OR<br>• Medium-dose inhaled corticosteroid and long-acting bronchodilator (theophylline) | • Bronchodilator as needed for symptoms (see step 1) up to 3 times/day |
| **STEP 2: Mild Persistent** | |
| Daily anti-inflammatory medication. Either:<br>• Cromolyn (nebulizer is preferred; or MDI) or nedocromil (MDI only) tid-qid<br>• Infants and young children usually begin with a trial of cromolyn or nedocromil<br>OR<br>• Low-dose inhaled corticosteroid with spacer/holding chamber and face mask | • Bronchodilator as needed for symptoms (see step 1) |
| **STEP 1: Mild Intermittent** | |
| No daily medication needed | • Bronchodilator as needed for symptoms <2 times/week. Intensity of treatment will depend upon severity of exacerbation (see "Managing Exacerbations"). Either:<br>— Inhaled short-acting beta$_2$-agonist by nebulizer or face mask and spacer/holding chamber<br>OR<br>— Oral beta$_2$-agonist for symptoms<br>• With viral respiratory infection:<br>— Bronchodilator q4-6h up to 24 hours (longer with physician consult) but, in general, repeat no more than once every 6 weeks<br>— Consider systemic corticosteroid if current exacerbation is severe<br>OR<br>Patient has history of previous severe exacerbations |

↓ **Step Down**
Review treatment every 1-6 months. If control is sustained for at least 3 months, a gradual stepwise reduction in treatment may be possible.

↑ **Step Up**
If control is not achieved, consider step up. But first: review patient medication technique, adherence, and environmental control (avoidance of allergens or other precipitant factors)

**Notes:**

- **The stepwise approach presents guidelines to assist clinical decision making. Asthma is highly variable; clinicians should tailor specific medication plans to the needs and circumstances of individual patients.**

- Gain control as quickly as possible; then decrease treatment to the least medication necessary to maintain control. Gaining control may be accomplished by either starting treatment at the step most appropriate to the initial severity of their condition or by starting at a higher level of therapy (eg, a course of systemic corticosteroids or higher dose of inhaled corticosteroids).

- A rescue course of systemic corticosteroid (prednisolone) may be needed at any time and step.

- In general, use of short-acting beta$_2$-agonist on a daily basis indicates the need for additional long-term control therapy.

- It is important to remember that there are very few studies on asthma therapy for infants.

- Consultation with an asthma specialist is recommended for patients with moderate or severe persistent asthma in this age group. Consultation should be considered for all patients with mild persistent asthma.

## Management of Asthma Exacerbations: Home Treatment*

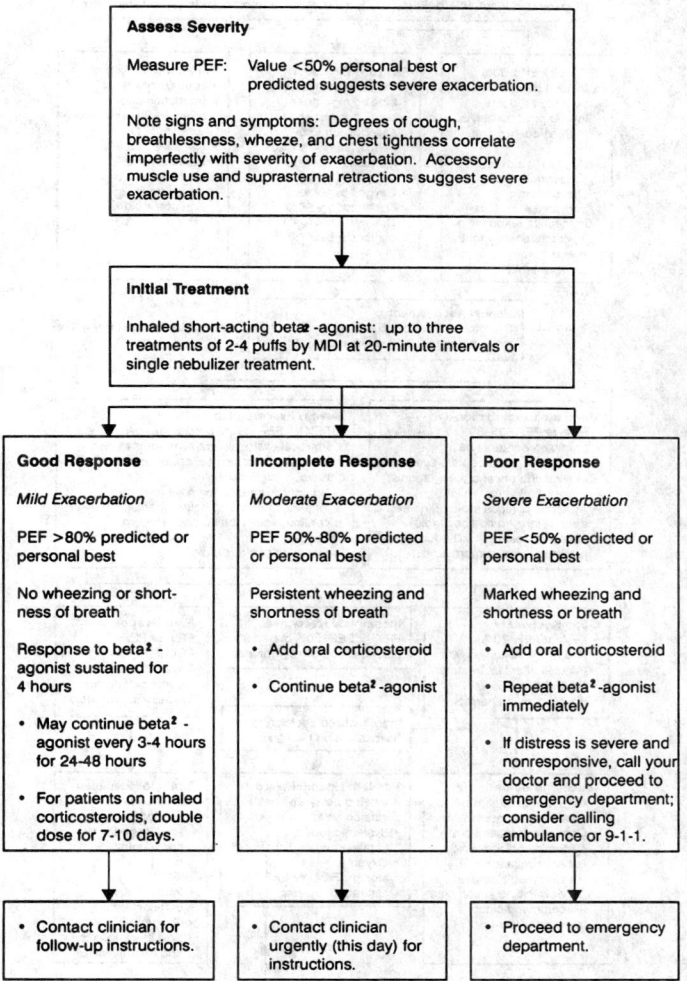

**Assess Severity**

Measure PEF: Value <50% personal best or predicted suggests severe exacerbation.

Note signs and symptoms: Degrees of cough, breathlessness, wheeze, and chest tightness correlate imperfectly with severity of exacerbation. Accessory muscle use and suprasternal retractions suggest severe exacerbation.

**Initial Treatment**

Inhaled short-acting beta$_2$-agonist: up to three treatments of 2-4 puffs by MDI at 20-minute intervals or single nebulizer treatment.

**Good Response**

*Mild Exacerbation*

PEF >80% predicted or personal best

No wheezing or short-ness of breath

Response to beta$_2$-agonist sustained for 4 hours

- May continue beta$_2$-agonist every 3-4 hours for 24-48 hours

- For patients on inhaled corticosteroids, double dose for 7-10 days.

- Contact clinician for follow-up instructions.

**Incomplete Response**

*Moderate Exacerbation*

PEF 50%-80% predicted or personal best

Persistent wheezing and shortness of breath

- Add oral corticosteroid

- Continue beta$_2$-agonist

- Contact clinician urgently (this day) for instructions.

**Poor Response**

*Severe Exacerbation*

PEF <50% predicted or personal best

Marked wheezing and shortness or breath

- Add oral corticosteroid

- Repeat beta$_2$-agonist immediately

- If distress is severe and nonresponsive, call your doctor and proceed to emergency department; consider calling ambulance or 9-1-1.

- Proceed to emergency department.

*Patients required.at high risk of asthma-related death should receive immediate clinical attention after initial treatment. Additional therapy may be required.

## ASTHMA *(Continued)*

### Management of Asthma Exacerbations: Emergency Department and Hospital-Based Care

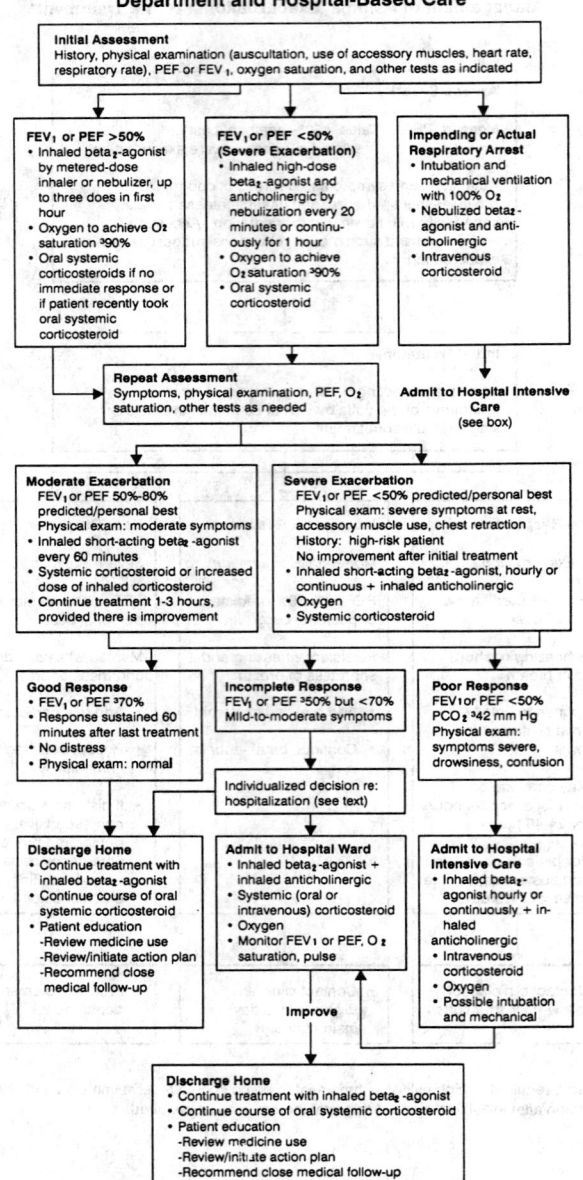

**Initial Assessment**
History, physical examination (auscultation, use of accessory muscles, heart rate, respiratory rate), PEF or FEV₁, oxygen saturation, and other tests as indicated

---

**FEV₁ or PEF >50%**
- Inhaled beta₂-agonist by metered-dose inhaler or nebulizer, up to three does in first hour
- Oxygen to achieve O₂ saturation ≥90%
- Oral systemic corticosteroids if no immediate response or if patient recently took oral systemic corticosteroid

**FEV₁ or PEF <50% (Severe Exacerbation)**
- Inhaled high-dose beta₂-agonist and anticholinergic by nebulization every 20 minutes or continuously for 1 hour
- Oxygen to achieve O₂ saturation ≥90%
- Oral systemic corticosteroid

**Impending or Actual Respiratory Arrest**
- Intubation and mechanical ventilation with 100% O₂
- Nebulized beta₂-agonist and anticholinergic
- Intravenous corticosteroid

---

**Repeat Assessment**
Symptoms, physical examination, PEF, O₂ saturation, other tests as needed

**Admit to Hospital Intensive Care**
(see box)

---

**Moderate Exacerbation**
FEV₁ or PEF 50%-80% predicted/personal best
Physical exam: moderate symptoms
- Inhaled short-acting beta₂-agonist every 60 minutes
- Systemic corticosteroid or increased dose of inhaled corticosteroid
- Continue treatment 1-3 hours, provided there is improvement

**Severe Exacerbation**
FEV₁ or PEF <50% predicted/personal best
Physical exam: severe symptoms at rest, accessory muscle use, chest retraction
History: high-risk patient
No improvement after initial treatment
- Inhaled short-acting beta₂-agonist, hourly or continuous + inhaled anticholinergic
- Oxygen
- Systemic corticosteroid

---

**Good Response**
- FEV₁ or PEF ≥70%
- Response sustained 60 minutes after last treatment
- No distress
- Physical exam: normal

**Incomplete Response**
FEV₁ or PEF ≥50% but <70%
Mild-to-moderate symptoms

**Poor Response**
FEV₁ or PEF <50%
PCO₂ ≥42 mm Hg
Physical exam: symptoms severe, drowsiness, confusion

---

Individualized decision re: hospitalization (see text)

---

**Discharge Home**
- Continue treatment with inhaled beta₂-agonist
- Continue course of oral systemic corticosteroid
- Patient education
  - Review medicine use
  - Review/initiate action plan
  - Recommend close medical follow-up

**Admit to Hospital Ward**
- Inhaled beta₂-agonist + inhaled anticholinergic
- Systemic (oral or intravenous) corticosteroid
- Oxygen
- Monitor FEV₁ or PEF, O₂ saturation, pulse

**Improve**

**Admit to Hospital Intensive Care**
- Inhaled beta₂-agonist hourly or continuously + inhaled anticholinergic
- Intravenous corticosteroid
- Oxygen
- Possible intubation and mechanical

---

**Discharge Home**
- Continue treatment with inhaled beta₂-agonist
- Continue course of oral systemic corticosteroid
- Patient education
  - Review medicine use
  - Review/initiate action plan
  - Recommend close medical follow-up

## ESTIMATED COMPARATIVE DAILY DOSAGES FOR INHALED CORTICOSTEROIDS

### Adults

| Drug | Low Dose | Medium Dose | High Dose |
|---|---|---|---|
| Beclomethasone dipropionate | 168-504 mcg | 504-840 mcg | >840 mcg |
| 42 mcg/puff | (4-12 puffs — 42 mcg) | (12-20 puffs — 42 mcg) | (>20 puffs — 42 mcg) |
| 84 mcg/puff | (2-6 puffs — 84 mcg) | (6-10 puffs — 84 mcg) | (>10 puffs — 84 mcg) |
| Budesonide Turbuhaler | 200-400 mcg | 400-600 mcg | >600 mcg |
| 200 mcg/dose | (1-2 inhalations) | (2-3 inhalations) | (>3 inhalations) |
| Flunisolide | 500-1000 mcg | 1000-2000 mcg | >2000 mcg |
| 250 mcg/puff | (2-4 puffs) | (4-8 puffs) | (>8 puffs) |
| Fluticasone | 88-264 mcg | 264-660 mcg | >660 mcg |
| MDI: 44, 110, 220 mcg/puff | (2-6 puffs — 44 mcg) | (2-6 puffs — 110 mcg) | (>6 puffs — 110 mcg) |
| | or | | or |
| | (2 puffs — 110 mcg) | | (>3 puffs — 220 mcg) |
| DPI: 50, 100, 250 mcg/dose | (2-6 inhalations — 50 mcg) | (3-6 inhalations — 100 mcg) | (>6 inhalations — 100 mcg) |
| Triamcinolone acetonide | 400-1000 mcg | 1000-2000 mcg | >2000 mcg |
| 100 mcg/puff | (4-10 puffs) | (10-20 puffs) | (>20 puffs) |

### Children

| Drug | Low Dose | Medium Dose | High Dose |
|---|---|---|---|
| Beclomethasone dipropionate | 84-336 mcg | 336-672 mcg | >672 mcg |
| 42 mcg/puff | (2-8 puffs) | (8-16 puffs) | (>16 puffs) |
| 84 mcg/puff | | | |
| Budesonide Turbuhaler | 100-200 mcg | 200-400 mcg | >400 mcg |
| 200 mcg/dose | | (1-2 inhalations — 200 mcg) | (>2 inhalations — 200 mcg) |
| Flunisolide | 500-750 mcg | 1000-1250 mcg | >1250 mcg |
| 250 mcg/puff | (2-3 puffs) | (4-5 puffs) | (>5 puffs) |
| Fluticasone | 88-176 mcg | 176-440 mcg | >440 mcg |
| MDI: 44, 110, 220 mcg/puff | (2-4 puffs — 44 mcg) | (4-10 puffs — 44 mcg) | (>4 puffs — 110 mcg) |
| | | or | |
| | | (2-4 puffs — 110 mcg) | |
| DPI: 50, 100, 250 mcg/dose | (2-4 inhalations — 50 mcg) | (2-4 inhalations — 100 mcg) | (>4 inhalations — 100 mcg) |
| Triamcinolone acetonide | 400-800 mcg | 800-1200 mcg | >1200 mcg |
| 100 mcg/puff | (4-8 puffs) | (8-12 puffs) | (>12 puffs) |

Notes:

- **The most important determinant of appropriate dosing is the clinician's judgment of the patient's response to therapy.** The clinician must monitor the patient's response on several clinical parameters and adjust the dose accordingly. The stepwise approach to therapy emphasizes that once control of asthma is achieved, the dose of mediation should be carefully titrated to the minimum dose required to maintain control, thus reducing the potential for adverse effect.
- The reference point for the range in the dosages for children is data on the safety on inhaled corticosteroids in children, which, in general, suggest that the dose ranges are equivalent to beclomethasone dipropionate 200-400 mcg/day (low dose), 400-800 mcg/day (medium dose), and >800 mcg/day (high dose).
- Some dosages may be outside package labeling.
- Metered-dose inhaler (MDI) dosages are expressed as the actuator dose (the amount of drug leaving the actuator and delivered to the patient), which is the labeling required in the United States. This is different from the dosage expressed as the valve dose (the amount of drug leaving the valve, all of which is not available to the patient), which is used in many European countries and in some of the scientific literature. Dry powder inhaler (DPI) doses (eg, Turbuhaler) are expressed as the amount of drug in the inhaler following activation.

## ASTHMA *(Continued)*

### ESTIMATED CLINICAL COMPARABILITY OF DOSES FOR INHALED CORTICOSTEROIDS

Data from *in vitro* and in clinical trials suggest that the different inhaled corticosteroid preparations are not equivalent on a per puff or microgram basis. However, it is not entirely clear what implications these differences have for dosing recommendations in clinical practice because there are few data directly comparing the preparations. Relative dosing for clinical comparability is affected by differences in topical potency, clinical effects at different doses, delivery device, and bioavailability. The Expert Panel developed recommended dose ranges for different preparations based on available data and the following assumptions and cautions about estimating relative doses needed to achieve comparable clinical effect.

- **Relative topical potency using human skin blanching**

  - The standard test for determining relative topical anti-inflammatory potency is the topical vasoconstriction (MacKenzie skin blanching) test.

  - The MacKenzie topical skin blanching test correlates with binding affinities and binding half-lives for human lung corticosteroid receptors (see table below) (Dahlberg, et al, 1984; Hogger and Rohdewald 1994).

  - The relationship between relative topical anti-inflammatory effect and clinical comparability in asthma management is not certain. However, recent clinical trials suggest that different in vitro measures of anti-inflammatory effect is not certain. However, recent clinical trials suggest that different in vitro measures of anti-inflammatory effect correlate with clinical efficacy (Barnes and Pedersen 1993; Johnson 1996; Kamada, et al, 1996; Ebden, et al, 1986; Leblanc, et al, 1994; Gustafsson, et al, 1993; Lundback, et al, 1993; Barnes, et al, 1993; Fabbri, et al, 1993; Langdon and Capsey, 1994; Ayres, et al, 1995; Rafferty, et al, 1985; Bjorkander, et al, 1982, Stiksa, et al, 1982; Willey, et al, 1982.)

| Medication | Topical Potency (Skin Blanching)* | Corticosteroid Receptor Binding Half-Life | Receptor Binding Affinity |
|---|---|---|---|
| Beclomethasone dipropionate (BDP) | 600 | 7.5 hours | 13.5 |
| Budesonide (BUD) | 980 | 5.1 hours | 9.4 |
| Flunisolide (FLU) | 330 | 3.5 hours | 1.8 |
| Fluticasone propionate (FP) | 1200 | 10.5 hours | 18.0 |
| Triamcinolone acetonide (TAA) | 330 | 3.9 hours | 3.6 |

*Numbers are assigned in reference to dexamethasone, which has a value of "1" in the MacKenzie test.

- **Relative doses to achieve similar clinical effects**

  - Clinical effects are evaluated by a number of outcome parameters (eg, changes in spirometry, peak flow rates, symptom scores, quick-relief beta$_2$-agonist use, frequency of exacerbations, airway responsiveness).

  - The daily dose and duration of treatment may affect these outcome parameters differently (eg, symptoms and peak flow may improve at lower doses and over a shorter treatment time than bronchial reactivity) (van Essen-Zandvliet, et al, 1992; Haahtela, et al, 1991)

  - Delivery systems influence comparability. For example, the delivery device for budesonide (Turbuhaler) delivers approximately twice the amount of drug to the airway as the MDI, thus enhancing the clinical effect (Thorsson, et al, 1994); Agertoft and Pedersen, 1993).

  - Individual patients may respond differently to different preparations, as noted by clinical experience.

  - Clinical trials comparing effects in reducing symptoms and improving peak expiratory flow demonstrate:

  - BDP and BUD achieved comparable effects at similar microgram doses by MDI (Bjorkander, et al, 1982; Ebden, et al, 1986; Rafferty, et al, 1985).

  - BDP achieved effects similar to twice the dose of TAA on a microgram basis.

# COMMUNITY-ACQUIRED PNEUMONIA IN ADULTS

## GUIDELINES FOR MANAGEMENT

Adapted from the Guidelines From the Infectious Diseases Society of America, *Clinical Infectious Diseases*, 1998, 26:811-38.

### Algorithm

The table below is the prediction model for identification of patient risk for persons with community-acquired pneumonia. This model may be used to help guide the initial decision

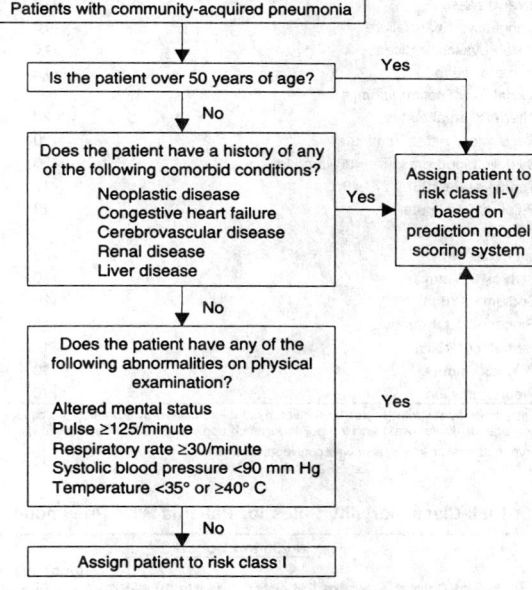

**Stratification of Risk Score**

| Risk | Risk class | Based on Algorithm |
|------|-----------|--------------------|
| | I | |
| Low | II | ≤ 70 total points |
| | III | 71-90 total points |
| Moderate | IV | 91-130 total points |
| High | V | > 130 total points |

on site of care; however, its use may not be appropriate for all patients with this illness and, therefore, should be applied in conjunction with physician judgment.

# COMMUNITY-ACQUIRED PNEUMONIA IN ADULTS *(Continued)*

## Scoring System

| Patient Characteristic | Points Assigned[1] |
|---|---|
| Demographic factors | |
| Age: Male | age (in years) |
| Female | age (in years) -10 |
| Nursing home resident | +10 |
| Comorbid illnesses | |
| Neoplastic disease | +30 |
| Liver disease | +20 |
| Congestive heart failure | +10 |
| Cerebrovascular disease | +10 |
| Renal disease | +10 |
| Physical examination findings | |
| Altered mental status | +20 |
| Respiratory rate ≥30/minute | +20 |
| Systolic blood pressure <90 mm Hg | +20 |
| Temperature <35°C or ≥40°C | +15 |
| Pulse ≥125/minute | +10 |
| Laboratory findings | |
| pH <7.35 | +30 |
| BUN >10.7 mmol/L | +20 |
| Sodium <130 mEq/L | +20 |
| Glucose >13.9 mmol/L | +10 |
| Hematocrit <30% | +10 |
| $PO_2$ <60 mm Hg[2] | +10 |
| Pleural effusion | +10 |

[1] A risk score (reset point score) for a given patient is obtained by summing the patient age in years (age -10 for females) and the points for each applicable patient characteristic.

[2] Oxygen saturation <90% also was considered normal.

## Risk-Class Mortality Rates for Patients With Pneumonia

| Risk Class | No. of Points | Validation Cohort | | Recommendations for Site of Care |
|---|---|---|---|---|
| | | No. of Patients | Mortality (%) | |
| I | No predictors | 3,034 | 0.1 | Outpatient |
| II | ≤70 | 5,778 | 0.6 | Outpatient |
| III | 71-90 | 6,790 | 2.8 | Inpatient (briefly) |
| IV | 91-130 | 13,104 | 8.2 | Inpatient |
| V | >130 | 9,333 | 29.2 | Inpatient |

**Epidemiological and Underlying Conditions Related to Specific Pathogens in Selected Patients With Community-Acquired Pneumonia**

| Conditions | Commonly Encountered Pathogens |
| --- | --- |
| Alcoholism | *Streptococcus pneumoniae*, anaerobes, gram-negative bacilli |
| COPD/smoker | *S. pneumoniae, Haemophilus influenzae, Moraxella catarrhalis, Legionella* species |
| Nursing home residency | *S. pneumoniae*, gram-negative bacilli, *H. influenzae, Staphylococcus aureus*, anaerobes, *Chlamydia pneumoniae* |
| Poor dental hygiene | Anaerobes |
| Epidemic Legionnaires' disease | *Legionella* species |
| Exposure to bats or soil enriched with bird droppings | *Histoplasma capsulatum* |
| Exposure to birds | *Chlamydia psittaci* |
| Exposure to rabbits | *Francisella tularensis* |
| HIV infection (early stage) | *S. pneumoniae, H. influenzae, Mycobacterium tuberculosis* |
| Travel to the southwestern United States | *Coccidioides immiris* |
| Exposure to farm animals or parturient cats | *Caxiella burnetii** |
| Influenza active in community | Influenza, *S. pneumoniae, S. aureus, Streptococcus pyogenes, H. influenzae* |
| Suspected large-volume aspiration | Anaerobes, chemical pneumonitis |
| Structural disease of the lung (bronchiectasis or cystic fibrosis) | *Pseudomonas aeruginosa, Burkholderia (Pseudomonas) cepacia*, or *S. aureus* |
| Injection drug use | *S. aureus*, anaerobes, *M. tuberculosis* |
| Airway obstruction | Anaerobes |

*Agent of Q fever

COPD = chronic obstructive pulmonary disease.

## COMMUNITY-ACQUIRED PNEUMONIA IN ADULTS *(Continued)*

### Flow Chart Approach to Treating Outpatients and Inpatients with Community-Acquired Pneumonia

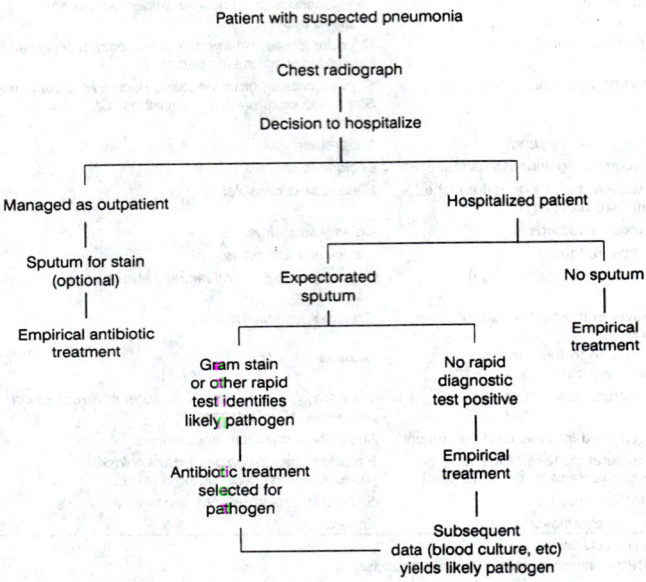

### Community-Acquired Pneumonia

**Possible reasons for failure of empirical treatment in patients with community-acquired pneumonia.**

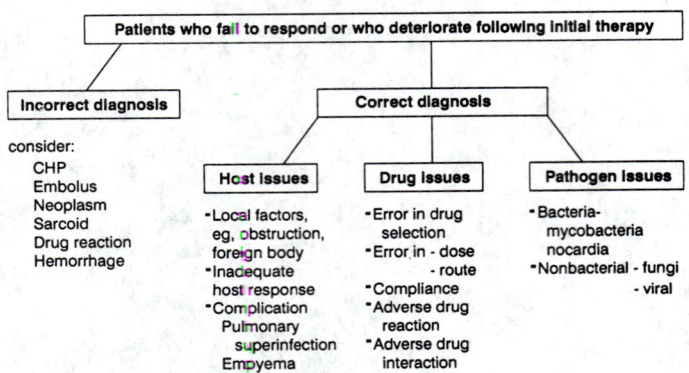

## Treatment of Pneumonia According to Pathogen

| Pathogen | Preferred Antimicrobial | Alternative Antimicrobial |
|---|---|---|
| *Streptococcus pneumoniae* | | |
| Penicillin susceptible (MIC, <0.1 mcg/mL) | Penicillin G or penicillin V, amoxicillin | Cephalosporins,* macrolides,† clindamycin, fluoroquinolones,‡ doxycycline |
| Intermediately penicillin resistant (MIC, 0.1-1 mcg/mL) | Parenteral penicillin G, ceftriaxone or cefotaxime, amoxicillin, fluoroquinolones,‡ other agents based on *in vitro* susceptibility test results | Clindamycin, doxycycline, oral cephalosporins* |
| Highly penicillin-resistant¤ (MIC, ≥2 mcg/mL) | Agents based on *in vitro* susceptibility results, fluoroquinolones,‡ vancomycin | |
| Empirical selection | Fluoroquinolones,‡ selection based on susceptibility test results in community§ | Clindamycin, doxycycline, vancomycin |
| | Penicillin¶ | Cephalosporins,* macrolides,† amoxicillin, clindamycin |
| *Haemophilus influenzae* | Second- or third-generation cephalosporins, doxycycline, beta-lactam - beta-lactamase inhibitor, fluoroquinolones‡ | Azithromycin, TMP-SMZ |
| *Moraxella catarrhalis* | Second- or third-generation cephalosporins, TMP-SMZ, amoxicillin/clavulanate | Macrolides,† fluoroquinolones,‡ beta-lactam - beta-lactamase inhibitor |
| Anaerobes | Clindamycin, penicillin plus metronidazole, beta-lactam - beta-lactamase inhibitor | Penicillin G or penicillin V, ampicillin/amoxicillin with or without metronidazole |
| *Staphylococcus aureus*¤ | | |
| Methicillin-susceptible | Nafcillin/oxacillin with or without rifampin or gentamicin¤ | Cefazolin or cefuroxime, vancomycin, clindamycin, TMP-SMZ, fluoroquinolones‡ |
| Methicillin-resistant | Vancomycin with or without rifampin or gentamicin | Requires *in vitro* testing; TMP-SMZ |
| Enterobacteriaceae (coliforms: *Escherichia coli, Klebsiella, Proteus, Enterobacter*)¤ | Third-generation cephalosporin with or without an aminoglycoside, carbapenems** | Aztreonam, beta-lactam - beta-lactamase inhibitor, fluoroquinolones‡ |
| *Pseudomonas aeruginosa*¤ | Aminoglycoside plus antipseudomonal beta-lactam: ticarcillin, piperacillin, mezlocillin, cefazidime, cefepime, aztreonam, or carbapenems** | Aminoglycoside plus ciprofloxacin, ciprofloxacin plus antipseudomonal beta-lactam |
| *Legionella* species | Macrolides† with or without rifampin, fluoroquinolones‡ | Doxycycline with or without rifampin |
| *Mycoplasma pneumoniae* | Doxycycline, macrolides,† fluoroquinolones‡ | |
| *Chlamydia pneumoniae* | Doxycycline, macrolides,† fluoroquinolones‡ | |
| *Chlamydia psittaci* | Doxycycline | Erythromycin, chloramphenicol |
| *Nocardia* species | Sulfonamide with or without minocycline or amikacin, TMP-SMZ | Imipenem with or without amikacin, doxycycline, or minocycline |
| *Coxiella burnetii*# | Tetracycline | Chloramphenicol |
| Influenza A | Amantadine or rimantadine | |
| Hantavirus | None†† | |

**Note:** TMP-SMZ = trimethoprim-sulfamethoxazole
*Intravenous: Cefazolin, cefuroxime, cefotaxime, ceftriaxone; oral: cefpodoxime, cefprozil, cefuroxime
†Erythromycin, clarithromycin, or azithromycin
‡Levofloxacin, sparfloxacin, grepafloxacin, trovafloxacin, or another fluoroquinolone with enhanced activity against *S. pneumoniae*; ciprofloxacin is appropriate for *Legionella* species, fluoroquinolone-susceptible *S. aureus*, and most gram-negative bacilli.
¤*In vitro* susceptibility tests are required for optimal treatment; for *Enterobacter* species, the preferred antibiotics are fluoroquinolones and carbapenems.
§High rates of high-level penicillin resistance, susceptibility of community strains unknown, and/or patient is seriously ill
¶Low rates of penicillin resistance in community and patient is at low risk for infection with resistant *S. pneumoniae*
**Imipenem and meropenem

# COMMUNITY-ACQUIRED PNEUMONIA IN ADULTS *(Continued)*

#Agent of Q fever
††Provide supportive care

## Empirical Antibiotic Selection for Patients With Community-Acquired Pneumonia

Outpatients

Generally preferred: Macrolides,* fluoroquinolones,† or doxycycline

Modifying factors

  Suspected penicillin-resistant *Streptococcus pneumoniae*: Fluoroquinolones†

  Young adult (>17–40 y): Doxycycline

  Hospitalized patients

    General medical ward

    Generally preferred: Beta-lactam‡ with or without a macrolide* or a fluoroquinolone† (alone)

  Alternatives: Cefuroxime with or without a macrolide* or azithromycin (alone)

Hospitalized in the intensive care unit for serious pneumonia

Generally preferred: Erythromycin, azithromycin, or a fluoroquinolone† plus cefotaxime, ceftriaxone, or a beta-lactam - beta-lactamase inhibitor¤

Modifying factors

Structural disease of the lung: Antipseudomonal penicillin, a carbapenem, or cefepime plus a macrolide* or a fluoroquinolone† plus an aminoglycoside

Penicillin allergy: A fluoroquinolone† with or without clindamycin

Suspected aspiration: A fluoroquinolone plus either clindamycin or metronidazole or a beta-lactam - beta-lactamase inhibitor¤

*Azithromycin, clarithromycin, or erythromycin

†Levofloxacin, sparfloxacin, grepafloxacin, trovafloxacin, or another fluoroquinolone with enhanced activity against *S. pneumoniae*

‡Cefotaxime, ceftriaxone, or a beta-lactam - beta-lactamase inhibitor

¤Ampicillin/sulbactam, or ticarcillin/clavulanate, or piperacillin/tazobactam (for structural disease of the lung, ticarcillin/clavulanate or piperacillin)

# DIABETES MELLITUS TREATMENT

## INSULIN-DEPENDENT DIABETES MELLITUS

Treatment goals that emphasize glycemic control have been recommended by the American Diabetes Association (see table).

### Glycemic Control for People With Diabetes

| Biochemical Index | Nondiabetic | Goal | Action Suggested |
|---|---|---|---|
| Preprandial glucose | <115 | 80-120 | <80<br>>140 |
| Bedtime glucose (mg/dL) | <120 | 100-140 | <100<br>>160 |
| Hb $A_{1C}$ (%) | <8 | <7 | >8 |

These values are for nonpregnant individuals. Action suggested depends on individual patient circumstances, Hb $A_{1C}$ referenced to a nondiabetic range of 4% to 6% (mean 5%, SD 0.5%).

## NONINSULIN-DEPENDENT DIABETES MELLITUS

### Pharmacological Therapy of NIDDM - Consensus Statement

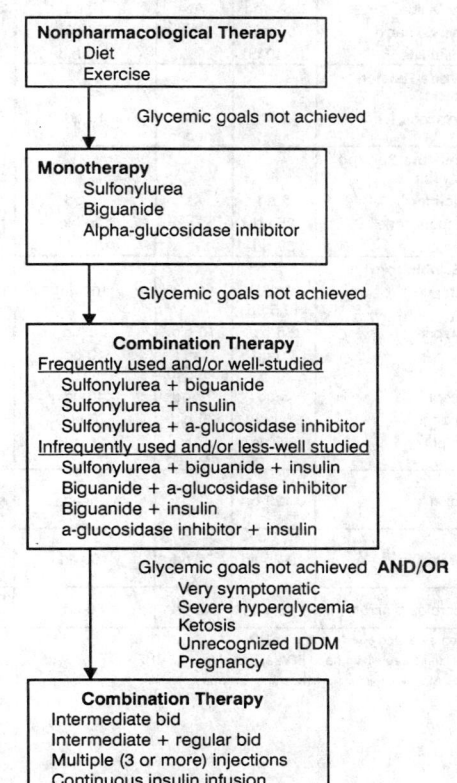

**Nonpharmacological Therapy**
  Diet
  Exercise

*Glycemic goals not achieved*

**Monotherapy**
  Sulfonylurea
  Biguanide
  Alpha-glucosidase inhibitor

*Glycemic goals not achieved*

**Combination Therapy**
Frequently used and/or well-studied
  Sulfonylurea + biguanide
  Sulfonylurea + insulin
  Sulfonylurea + a-glucosidase inhibitor
Infrequently used and/or less-well studied
  Sulfonylurea + biguanide + insulin
  Biguanide + a-glucosidase inhibitor
  Biguanide + insulin
  a-glucosidase inhibitor + insulin

*Glycemic goals not achieved* **AND/OR**
            Very symptomatic
            Severe hyperglycemia
            Ketosis
            Unrecognized IDDM
            Pregnancy

**Combination Therapy**
Intermediate bid
Intermediate + regular bid
Multiple (3 or more) injections
Continuous insulin infusion

# HEART FAILURE: MANAGEMENT OF PATIENTS WITH LEFT VENTRICULAR SYSTOLIC DYSFUNCTION

Adapted from U.S. Department of Health & Human Services, the Agency for Healthcare Policy and Research (ACHPR) Publication No. 94-0613, June, 1994

## Medications Commonly Used for Heart Failure

| Drug | Initial Dose (mg) | Target Dose (mg) | Recommended Maximal Dose (mg) | Major Adverse Reactions |
|---|---|---|---|---|
| **Thiazide Diuretics** Chlorthalidone Hydrochlorothiazide | 25 qd | As needed | 50 qd | Postural hypotension, hypokalemia, hyperglycemia, hyperuricemia, rash; rare severe reaction includes pancreatitis, bone marrow suppression, and anaphylaxis |
| **Loop Diuretics** Bumetanide Ethacrynic acid Furosemide | 0.5–1 qd 50 qd 10–40 qd | As needed | 10 qd 200 bid 240 bid | Same as thiazide diuretics |
| **Thiazide-Related Diuretic** Metolazone | 2.5* | As needed | 10 qd | Same as thiazide diuretics |
| **Potassium-Sparing Diuretics** Amiloride Spironolactone Triamterene | 5 qd 25 qd 50 qd | As needed | 40 qd 100 bid 100 bid | Hyperkalemia (especially if administered with ACE inhibitor), rash, gynecomastia (spironolactone only) |
| **ACE Inhibitors†** Captopril | 6.25–12.5 tid | 50 tid | 100 tid | Hypotension, hyperkalemia, renal insufficiency, cough, skin rash, angioedema, neutropenia |
| Enalapril | 2.5 bid | 10 bid | 20 bid | |
| Fosinopril | 10 qd | As needed | 40 qd | |
| Lisinopril | 5 qd | 20 qd | 40 qd | |
| Quinapril | 5 bid | 20 bid | 20 bid | |
| Ramipril | 2.5 qd | As needed | 20 qd | |
| Digoxin | 0.125 qd | As needed | As needed | Cardiotoxicity, confusion, nausea, anorexia, visual disturbances |
| Hydralazine | 10–25 tid | 75 tid | 100 tid | Headache, nausea, dizziness, tachycardia. lupus-like syndrome |
| Isosorbide dinitrate | 10 tid | 40 tid | 80 tid | Headache, hypotension, flushing |

*Given as a single test dose initially.

†ACE inhibitors which have FDA approval to treat CHF.

**Note:** ACE = angiotensin-converting enzyme.

# *HELICOBACTER PYLORI* TREATMENT

## Multiple Drug Regimens for the Treatment of *H. pylori* Infection

| Drug | Dosages* | Duration of Therapy |
|---|---|---|
| **Regimen 1†** | | |
| Bismuth subsalicylate (Pepto-Bismol®) | Two 262 mg tablets 4 times/day | 2 weeks |
| *plus* | | |
| Metronidazole (Flagyl®) | 250 mg 3 or 4 times/day | 2 weeks |
| *plus* | | |
| Tetracycline (various) or amoxicillin (Amoxil®, others) | 250-500 mg 4 times/day | 2 weeks |
| *plus* | | |
| Histamine $H_2$-receptor antagonist | Full dose‡ at bedtime | 4-6 weeks |
| **Regimen 2** | | |
| Metronidazole (Flagyl®) | 500 mg 3 times/day | 12-14 days |
| *plus* | | |
| Arnoxicillin (Amoxil®, others) | 750 mg 3 times/day | 12-14 days |
| *plus* | | |
| Histamine $H_2$-receptor antagonist | Full dose† at bedtime | 6-10 weeks |
| **Regimen 3** | | |
| Bismuth subsalicylate (Pepto-Bismol®) | Two 262 mg tablets 4 times/day | 2 weeks |
| *plus* | | |
| Tetracycline (various) | 500 mg 4 times/day | 2 weeks |
| *plus* | | |
| Clarithromycin (Biaxin™) | 500 mg 3 times/day | 2 weeks |
| *plus* | | |
| Histamine $H_2$-receptor antagonist | Full dose† after evening meal | 6 weeks |
| **Regimen 4** | | |
| Omeprazole (Prilosec™) | 20 mg twice daily | 2 weeks |
| *plus* | | |
| Amoxicillin (Amoxil®, others) | 1 g twice daily or 500 mg 4 times/day | 2 weeks |
| **Regimen 5** | | |
| Omeprazole (Prilosec™) | 20 mg twice daily | 2 weeks |
| *plus* | | |
| Clarithromycin (Biaxin™) | 250 mg twice a day or 500 mg 2 or 3 times/day | 2 weeks |
| *or* | | |
| Lansoprazole (Prevacid®) | 30 mg/day | |
| *plus* | | |
| Amoxicillin (Amoxil®) | 1 g twice daily | |
| *plus* | | |
| Clarithromycin (Biaxin™) | 500 mg twice daily | |
| **Regimen 6** | | |
| Ranitidine bismuth citrate (Tritec™) | 400 mg twice daily | 4 weeks |
| *plus* | | |
| Clarithromycin (Biaxin™) | 500 mg 3 times/day | 2 weeks |

*All therapies are oral and begin concurrently.

†Marketed as Helidac®, a packet containing 262.4 mg bismuth subsalicylate, 250 mg metronidazole and 500 mg tetracycline; an $H_2$-antagonist must be purchased separately.

‡Full dose refers to the dosage used to treat acute ulcers, not to the maintenance dose.

# HYPERLIPIDEMIA

(*JAMA*, 1993, 269(23), 3015-23)

### Risk Status Based on Presence of CHD Risk Factors Other Than Low-Density Lipoprotein Cholesterol*

**Positive Risk Factors**

Male ≥45 y

Female ≥55 y or premature menopause without estrogen replacement therapy

Family history of premature CHD (definite myocardial infarction or sudden death before 55 y of age in father or other male first-degree relative, or before 65 y of age in mother or other female first-degree relative)

Current cigarette smoking

Hypertension (blood pressure ≥140/90 mm Hg†, or taking antihypertensive medication)

Low HDL cholesterol (<35 mg/dL† [0.9 mmol/L])

Diabetes mellitus

**Negative Risk Factor‡**

High HDL cholesterol (≥60 mg/dL [1.6 mmol/L])

*High risk, defined as a net of two or more coronary heart disease (CHD) risk factors, leads to more vigorous intervention, shown in Figures 1 and 2. Age (defined differently for men and women) is treated as a risk factor because rates of CHD are higher in the elderly than in the young, and in men than in women of the same age. Obesity is not listed as a risk factor because it operates through other risk factors that are included (hypertension, hyperlipidemia, decreased high-density lipoprotein [HDL] cholesterol, and diabetes mellitus), but it should be considered a target for intervention. Physical inactivity is similarly not listed as a risk factor, but it too should be considered a target for intervention, and physical activity is recommended as desirable for everyone. High risk due to coronary or peripheral atherosclerosis is addressed directly in Figure 3.

†Confirmed by measurements on several occasions.

‡If the HDL cholesterol level is ≥60 mg/dL (1.6 mmol/L), subtract one risk factor (because high HDL cholesterol levels decrease CHD risk)

### Initial Classification Based on Total Cholesterol and HDL Cholesterol Levels*

| Cholesterol Level | | Initial Classification |
|---|---|---|
| **Total Cholesterol** | | |
| <200 mg/dL | (5.2 mmol/L) | Desirable blood cholesterol |
| 200-239 mg/dL | (5.2-6.2 mmol/L) | Borderline-high blood cholesterol |
| ≥240 mg/dL | (6.2 mmol/L) | High blood cholesterol |
| **HDL Cholesterol** | | |
| <35 mg/dL | (0.9 mmol/L) | Low HDL cholesterol |

*HDL indicated high-density lipoprotein.

## Summary of the Second Report of the National Cholesterol Education Program (NCEP) Expert Panel on Detection, Evaluation, and Treatment of High Blood Cholesterol in Adults (Adult Treatment Panel II)

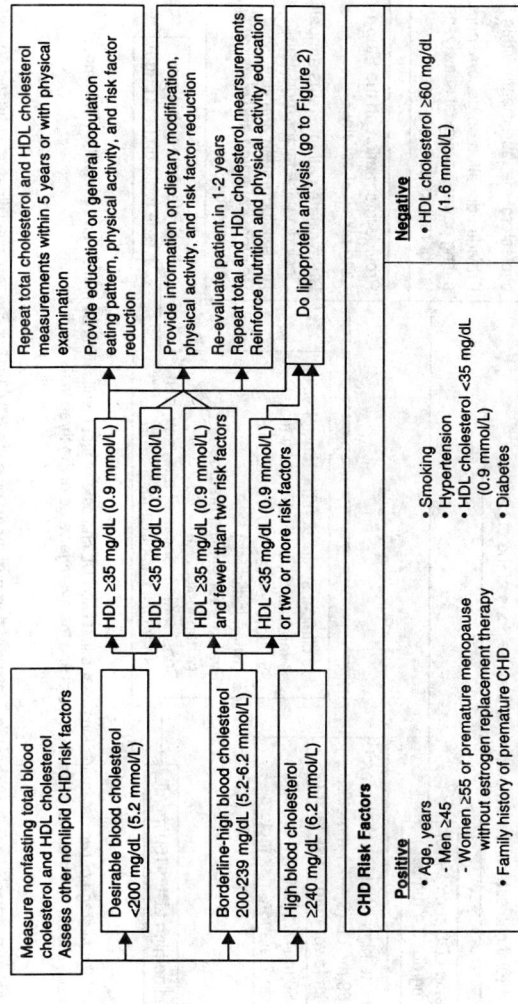

**Fig. 1** - Primary prevention in adults without evidence of coronary heart disease (CHD). Initial classification is based on total cholesterol and high-density lipoprotein (HDL) cholesterol levels.

## HYPERLIPIDEMIA (Continued)

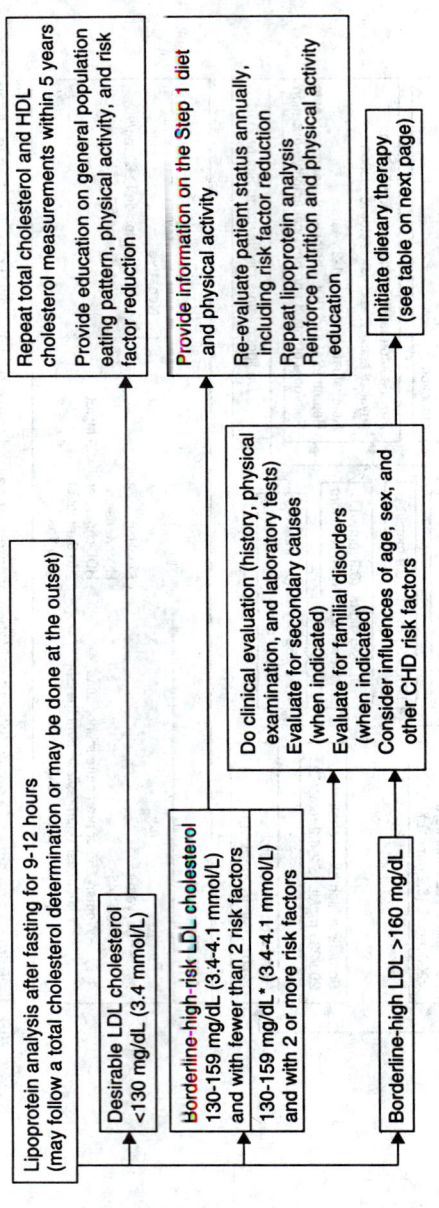

Lipoprotein analysis after fasting for 9-12 hours
(may follow a total cholesterol determination or may be done at the outset)

**Desirable LDL cholesterol**
<130 mg/dL (3.4 mmol/L)
→ Repeat total cholesterol and HDL cholesterol measurements within 5 years
Provide education on general population eating pattern, physical activity, and risk factor reduction

**Borderline-high-risk LDL cholesterol**
130-159 mg/dL (3.4-4.1 mmol/L) and with fewer than 2 risk factors
→ Provide information on the Step 1 diet and physical activity
Re-evaluate patient status annually, including risk factor reduction
Repeat lipoprotein analysis
Reinforce nutrition and physical activity education

130-159 mg/dL* (3.4-4.1 mmol/L) and with 2 or more risk factors

**Borderline-high LDL >160 mg/dL**
→ Do clinical evaluation (history, physical examination, and laboratory tests)
Evaluate for secondary causes (when indicated)
Evaluate for familial disorders (when indicated)
Consider influences of age, sex, and other CHD risk factors
→ Initiate dietary therapy (see table on next page)

* On the basis of the average of two determinations. If the first two LDL cholesterol test results differ by more than 30 mg/dL (0.7 mmol/L), a third test result should be obtained within 1-8 weeks and the average value of the three tests used.

**Fig. 2 -** Primary prevention in adults **without** evidence of coronary heart disease (CHD). Subsequent classification is based on low-density lipoprotein (LDL) cholesterol level.

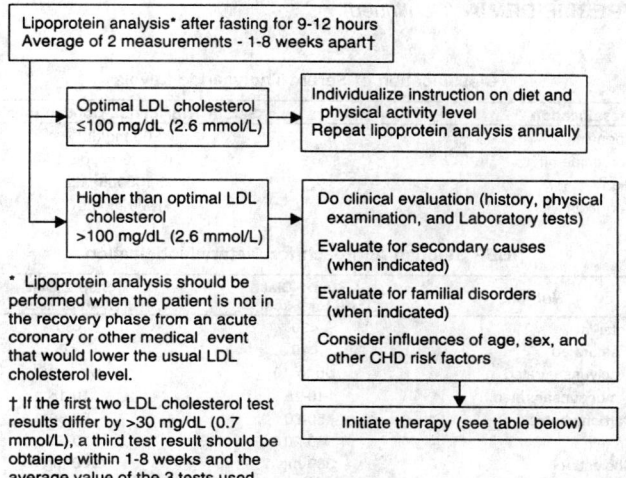

Lipoprotein analysis* after fasting for 9-12 hours
Average of 2 measurements - 1-8 weeks apart†

Optimal LDL cholesterol
≤100 mg/dL (2.6 mmol/L) → Individualize instruction on diet and physical activity level
Repeat lipoprotein analysis annually

Higher than optimal LDL cholesterol
>100 mg/dL (2.6 mmol/L) → Do clinical evaluation (history, physical examination, and Laboratory tests)

Evaluate for secondary causes (when indicated)

Evaluate for familial disorders (when indicated)

Consider influences of age, sex, and other CHD risk factors

* Lipoprotein analysis should be performed when the patient is not in the recovery phase from an acute coronary or other medical event that would lower the usual LDL cholesterol level.

† If the first two LDL cholesterol test results differ by >30 mg/dL (0.7 mmol/L), a third test result should be obtained within 1-8 weeks and the average value of the 3 tests used.

Initiate therapy (see table below)

**Fig. 3 -** Secondary prevention in adults **with** evidence of coronary heart disease (CHD). Classification is based on low-density lipoprotein (LDL) cholesterol level.

## Treatment Decisions Based on LDL Cholesterol Level*

| Patient Category | Initiation Level | LDL Goal |
|---|---|---|
| **Dietary Therapy** | | |
| Without CHD and with fewer than two risk factors | ≥160 mg/dL (4.1 mmol/L) | <160 mg/dL (4.1 mmol/L) |
| Without CHD and with two or more risk factors | ≥130 mg/dL (3.4 mmol/L) | <130 mg/dL (3.4 mmol/L) |
| With CHD | >100 mg/dL (2.6 mmol/L) | ≤100 mg/dL (2.6 mmol/L) |
| **Drug Treatment** | | |
| Without CHD and with fewer than two risk factors | ≥190 mg/dL (4.9 mmol/L) | <160 mg/dL (4.1 mmol/L) |
| Without CHD and with two or more risk factors | ≥160 mg/dL (4.1 mmol/L) | <130 mg/dL (3.4 mmol/L) |
| With CHD | ≥130 mg/dL (3.4 mmol/L) | ≤100 mg/dL (2.6 mmol/L) |

*LDL: low-density lipoprotein; CHD: coronary heart disease

## HYPERLIPIDEMIA *(Continued)*

### Class fication of Serum Triglyceride Levels

| Classification | Serum Triglyceride Concentration |
|---|---|
| Normal | ≤200 mg/dL |
| Borderline-high | 200-400 mg/dL |
| High | 400-1000 mg/dL |
| Very high | >1000 mg/dL |

### NCEP Stepped Approach for Dietary Modification

| Nutrient | Step 1 Diet (% total kcal) | Step 2 Diet (% total kcal) |
|---|---|---|
| Total fat | <30 | <30 |
| saturated | <10 | <7 |
| polyunsaturated | Up to 10 | Up to 10 |
| monounsaturated | 10-15 | 10-15 |
| Carbohydrates | 50-60 | 50-60 |
| Protein | 10-20 | 10-20 |
| Cholesterol | <300 mg/d | <200 mg/d |
| Total calories | qs to maintain desirable wt | qs to maintain desirable wt |

# HYPERTENSION

**The Sixth Report of the Joint National Committee on Prevention, Detection, Evaluation, and Treatment of High Blood Pressure**

| Category | Systolic (mm Hg) | | Diastolic (mm Hg) |
|---|---|---|---|
| Optimal | <120 | and | <80 |
| Normal | <130 | and | <85 |
| High normal | 130-139 | or | 85-89 |
| Hypertension† | | | |
| Stage 1 | 140-159 | or | 90-99 |
| Stage 2 | 160-179 | or | 100-109 |
| Stage 3 | ≥180 | or | ≥110 |

Not taking antihypertensive drugs and not acutely ill. When systolic and diastolic blood pressures fall into different categories, the higher category should be selected to classify the individual's blood pressure status. For example, 160/92 mm Hg should be classified as stage 2 hypertension, and 174/120 mm Hg should be classified as stage 3 hypertension. Isolated systolic hypertension is defined as SBP ≥140 mm Hg and DBP <90 mm Hg and staged appropriately (eg, 170/82 mm Hg is defined as stage 2 isolated systolic hypertension). In addition to classifying stages of hypertension on the basis of average blood pressure levels, the clinician should specify presence or absence of target-organ disease and additional risk factors. This specificity is important for risk classification and management. Optimal blood pressure with respect to cardiovascular risk is <120/80 mm Hg. However, unusually low readings should be evaluated for clinical significance.

†Based on the average of two or more readings taken at each of two or more visits after an initial screening.

| Age (years) | Girls' SBP/DBP | | Boys' SBP/DBP | |
|---|---|---|---|---|
| | 50th Percentile for Height | 75th Percentile for Height | 50th Percentile for Height | 75th Percentile for Height |
| 1 | 104/58 | 105/59 | 102/57 | 104/58 |
| 6 | 111/73 | 112/73 | 114/74 | 115/75 |
| 12 | 123/80 | 124/81 | 123/81 | 125/82 |
| 17 | 129/84 | 130/85 | 136/87 | 138/88 |

Adapted from the report by the NHBPEP Working Group on Hypertension Control in Children and Adolescents. SBP indicates systolic blood pressure; DBP, diastolic blood pressure.

## Manifestations of Target-Organ Disease

| Organ System | Manifestations |
|---|---|
| Cardiac | Clinical, electrocardiographic, or radiologic evidence of coronary artery disease; left ventricular hypertrophy or "strain" by electrocardiography or left ventricular hypertrophy by echocardiography; left ventricular dysfunction or cardiac failure |
| Cerebrovascular | Transient ischemic attack or stroke |
| Peripheral vascular | Absence of 1 or more major pulses in extremities (except for dorsalis pedis) with or without intermittent claudication; aneurysm |
| Renal | Serum creatinine ≥130 μmol/L (1.5 mg/dL); proteinuria (1+ or greater); microalbuminuria |
| Retinopathy | Hemorrhages or exudates, with or without papilledema |

## HYPERTENSION *(Continued)*

### Recommendations for Follow-up Based on Initial Set of Blood Pressure Measurements for Adults

**Initial Screening Blood Pressure (mm Hg)***

| Systolic | Diastolic | Follow-up Recommended† |
|---|---|---|
| <130 | <85 | Recheck in 2 years |
| 130-139 | 85-89 | Recheck in 1 year‡ |
| 140-159 | 90-99 | Confirm within 2 months‡ |
| 160-179 | 100-109 | Evaluate or refer to source of care within 1 months |
| ≥180 | ≥110 | Evaluate or refer to source of care immediately or within 1 week depending on clinical situation |

*If the systolic and diastolic categories are different, follow recommendation for the shorter time follow-up (eg, 160/86 mm Hg should be evaluated or referred to source of care within 1 month).

†Provide advice about lifestyle modifications.

‡Modify the scheduling of follow-up according to reliable information about past blood pressure measurements, other cardiovascular risk factors, or target organ disease.

### Major Risk Factors

Smoking
Dyslipidemia
Diabetes mellitus
Age >60 years
Sex (men and postmenopausal women)
Family history of cardiovascular disease; women <65 years or men <55 years

### Target Organ Damage/Clinical Cardiovascular Disease

Heart diseases
- Left ventricular hypertrophy
- Angina/prior myocardial infarction
- Prior coronary revascularization
- Heart failure

Stroke or transient ischemic attack
Nephropathy
Peripheral arterial disease
Retinopathy

| Blood Pressure Stages (mm Hg) | Risk Group A (No Risk Factors, No TOD/CCD)* | Risk Group B (At least 1 Risk Factor, Not Including Diabetes; No TOD/CCD) | Risk Group C (TOD/CCD and/or Diabetes, With or Without Other Risk Factors) |
|---|---|---|---|
| High-normal (130-139/85-89) | Lifestyle modification | Lifestyle modification | Drug therapy† |
| Stage 1 (140-159/90-99) | Lifestyle modification (up to 12 months) | Lifestyle modification‡ (up to 6 months) | Drug therapy |
| State 2 and 3 (≥160/≥100) | Drug therapy | Drug therapy | Drug therapy |

For example, a patient with diabetes and a blood pressure of 142/94 mm Hg plus left ventricular hypertrophy should be classified as having stage 1 hypertension with target organ disease (left ventricular hypertrophy) and with another major risk factor (diabetes), this patient would be categorized as stage 1, Risk group C and recommended for immediate initiation of pharmacologic treatment.

*Lifestyle modification should be adjunctive therapy for all patients recommended for pharmacologic therapy.

TOD/CCD indicates target organ disease/clinical cardiovascular disease

†For those with heart failure, renal insufficiency, or diabetes.

‡For patients with multiple risk factors, clinicians should consider drugs as initial therapy plus lifestyle modifications.

## Risk Group A

Risk group A includes patients with high-normal blood pressure or state 1, 2, or 3 hypertension who do not have clinical cardiovascular disease, target organ damage, or other risk factors. Persons with stage 1 hypertension in risk group A are candidates for a longer trial (up to 1 year) of vigorous lifestyle modification with vigilant blood pressure monitoring. If goal blood pressure is not achieved, pharmacologic therapy should be added. For those with stage 2 or stage 3 hypertension, drug therapy is warranted.

## Risk Group B

Risk group B includes patients with hypertension who do not have clinical cardiovascular disease or target organ damage, but have one or more of the risk factors shown in the table above but not diabetes mellitus. This group contains the large majority of patients with high blood pressure. If multiple risk factors are present, clinicians should consider antihypertensive drugs as initial therapy. Lifestyle modification and management of reversible risk factors should be strongly recommended.

## Risk Group C

Risk group C includes patients with hypertension who have clinically manifested cardiovascular disease or target organ damage, as delineated in the above table. It is the clinical opinion of the JNC VI executive committee that some patients who have high-normal blood pressure as well as renal insufficiency, heart failure, or diabetes mellitus should be considered for prompt pharmacologic therapy. Appropriate lifestyle modifications always should be recommended as adjunct treatment.

- Lose weight if overweight.
- Limit alcohol intake to no more than 1 oz (30 mL) ethanol (eg, 24 oz [720 mL] beer, 10 oz [300 mL] wine, or 2 oz "60 mL" 100-proof whiskey) per day or 0.5 oz (15 mL) ethanol per day for women and lighter weight people.
- Increase aerobic physical activity (30-45 minutes most days of the week).
- Reduce sodium intake to no more than 100 mmol/day (2.4 g sodium or 6 g sodium chloride).
- Maintain adequate intake of dietary potassium (approximately 90 mmol/day).
- Maintain adequate intake of dietary calcium and magnesium for general health.
- Stop smoking and reduce intake of dietary saturated fat and cholesterol for overall cardiovascular health.

# HYPERTENSION (Continued)

| Indication | Drug Therapy |
|---|---|
| **Compelling Indications Unless Contraindicated** | |
| Diabetes mellitus (type 1) with proteinuria | ACE I |
| Heart failure | ACE I, diuretics |
| Isolated systolic hypertension (older patients) | Diuretics (preferred), CA (long-acting DHP) |
| Myocardial infarction | Beta-blockers (non-ISA), ACE I (with systolic dysfunction) |
| **May Have Favorable Effects on Comorbid Conditions** | |
| Angina | Beta-blockers, CA |
| Atrial tachycardia and fibrillation | Beta-blockers, CA (non-DHP) |
| Cyclosporine-induced hypertension (caution with the dose of cyclosporine) | CA |
| Diabetes mellitus (types 1 and 2) with proteinuria | ACE I (preferred), CA |
| Diabetes mellitus (type 2) | Low-dose diuretics |
| Dyslipidemia | Alpha-blockers |
| Essential tremor | Beta-blockers (non-CS) |
| Heart failure | Carvedilol, losartan potassium |
| Hyperthyroidism | Beta-blockers |
| Migraine | Beta-blockers (non-CS), CA (non-DHP) |
| Myocardial infarction | Diltiazem hydrochloride, verapamil hydrochloride |
| Osteoporosis | Thiazides |
| Preoperative hypertension | Beta-blockers |
| Prostatism (BPH) | Alpha-blockers |
| Renal insufficiency (caution in renovascular hypertension and creatinine ≥265.2 mmol/L [3 mg/dL]) | ACE I |
| **May Have Unfavorable Effects on Comorbid Conditions\*** | |
| Bronchospastic disease | Beta-blockers† |
| Depression | Beta-blockers, central alpha-agonists, reserpine† |
| Diabetes mellitus (types 1 and 2) | Beta-blockers, high-dose diuretics |
| Dyslipidemia | Beta-blockers (non-ISA), diuretics (high-dose) |
| Gout | Diuretics |
| 2° or 3° heart block | Beta-blockers†, CA (non-DHP)† |
| Heart failure | Beta-blockers (except carvedilol), CA (except amlodipine besylate, felodipine) |
| Liver disease | Labetalol hydrochloride, methyldopa† |
| Peripheral vascular disease | Beta-blockers |
| Pregnancy | ACE I†, angiotensin II receptor blockers† |
| Renal insufficiency | Potassium-sparing agents |
| Renovascular disease | ACE I, angiotensin II receptor blockers |

ACE I indicates angiotensin-converting enzyme inhibitors; BPH, benign prostatic hyperplasia; CA, calcium antagonists; DHP, dihydropyridine; ISA, intrinsic sympathomimetic activity; MI, myocardial infarction; and non-CS, noncardioselective.

Conditions and drugs are listed in alphabetical order.

*These drugs may be used with special monitoring unless contraindicated.

†Contraindicated.

The report of the NHBPEP Working Group on High Blood Pressure in Pregnancy permits continuation of drug therapy in women with chronic hypertension (except for ACE inhibitors). In addition, angiotensin II receptor blockers should not be used during pregnancy. In women with chronic hypertension with diastolic levels of 100 mm Hg or greater (lower when end organ damage or underlying renal disease is present) and in women with acute hypertension when levels are 105 mm Hg or greater, the following agents are suggested.

| Suggested Drug | Comments |
|---|---|
| Central alpha-agonists | Methyldopa (C) is the drug of choice recommended by the NHBPEP Working Group. |
| Beta-blockers | Atenolol (C) and metoprolol (C) appear to be safe and effective in late pregnancy. Labetalol (C) also appears to be effective (alpha- and beta-blockers). |
| Calcium antagonists | Potential synergism with magnesium sulfate may lead to precipitous hypotension. (C) |
| ACE inhibitors, angiotensin II receptor blockers | Fetal abnormalities, including death, can be caused, and these drugs should not be used in pregnancy. (D) |
| Diuretics | Diuretics (C) are recommended for chronic hypertension if prescribed before gestation or if patients appear to be salt-sensitive. They are not recommended in pre-eclampsia. |
| Direct vasodilators | Hydralazine (C) is the parenteral drug of choice based on its long history of safety and efficacy. (C) |

Adapted from Sibai and Lindheimer. There are several other antihypertensive drugs for which there are very limited data. The U.S. Food and Drug Administration classifies pregnancy risk as follows: C, adverse effects in animals; no controlled trials in humans; use if risk appears justified; D, positive evidence of fetal risk. ACE indicates angiotensin-converting enzyme.

## HYPERTENSION *(Continued)*

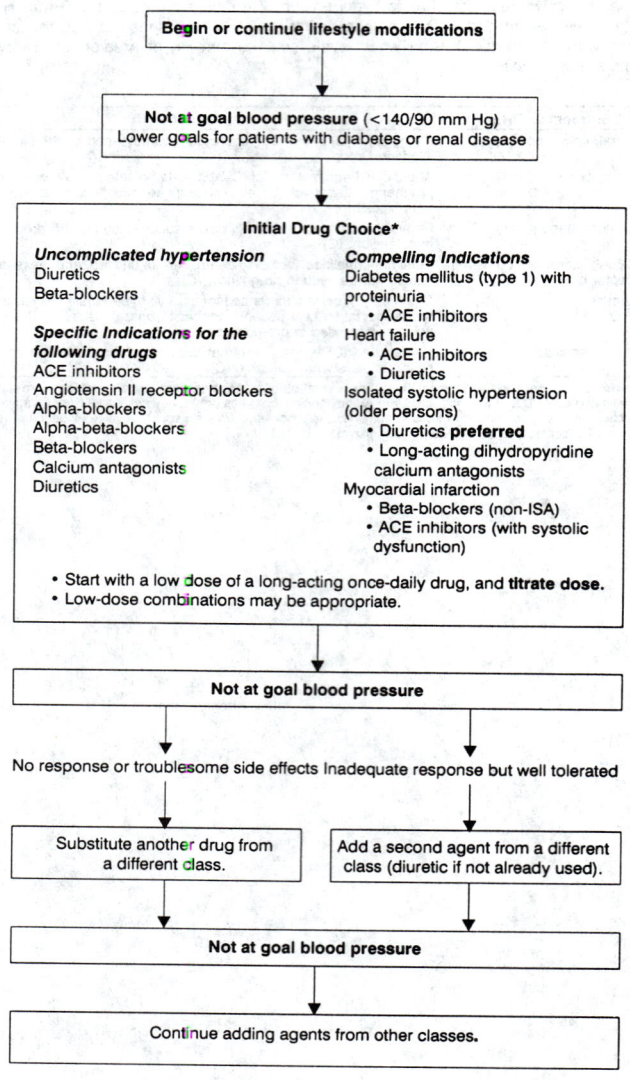

Begin or continue lifestyle modifications

**Not at goal blood pressure** (<140/90 mm Hg)
Lower goals for patients with diabetes or renal disease

### Initial Drug Choice*

***Uncomplicated hypertension***
Diuretics
Beta-blockers

***Specific Indications for the
following drugs***
ACE inhibitors
Angiotensin II receptor blockers
Alpha-blockers
Alpha-beta-blockers
Beta-blockers
Calcium antagonists
Diuretics

***Compelling Indications***
Diabetes mellitus (type 1) with
proteinuria
  • ACE inhibitors
Heart failure
  • ACE inhibitors
  • Diuretics
Isolated systolic hypertension
(older persons)
  • Diuretics **preferred**
  • Long-acting dihydropyridine
    calcium antagonists
Myocardial infarction
  • Beta-blockers (non-ISA)
  • ACE inhibitors (with systolic
    dysfunction)

• Start with a low dose of a long-acting once-daily drug, and **titrate dose.**
• Low-dose combinations may be appropriate.

**Not at goal blood pressure**

No response or troublesome side effects    Inadequate response but well tolerated

Substitute another drug from
a different class.

Add a second agent from a different
class (diuretic if not already used).

**Not at goal blood pressure**

Continue adding agents from other classes.

* Unless contraindicated. ACE indicates angiotensin-converting enzyme; ISA,
  intrinsic sympathomimetic activity. Based on randomized controlled trials.

## General Treatment Principles in the Treatment of Hypertensive Emergencies

| Principle | Considerations |
|---|---|
| Admit the patient to the hospital, preferably in the intensive care unit. Monitor vital signs appropriately. | Establish intravenous access and place patient on a cardiac monitor. Place a femoral intra-arterial line and pulmonary arterial catheter, if indicated, to assess cardiopulmonary function and intravascular volume status. |
| Perform rapid but thorough history and physical examination. | Determine cause of, or precipitating factors to, hypertensive crisis if possible (remember to obtain a medication history including Rx, OTC, and illicit drugs). Obtain details regarding any prior history of hypertension (severity, duration, treatment), as well as other coexisting illnesses. Assess the extent of hypertensive end organ damage. Determine if a hypertensive urgency or emergency exists. |
| Determine goal blood pressure based on premorbid level, duration, severity and rapidity of increase of blood pressure, concomitant medical conditions, race, and age. | Acute decreases in blood pressure to normal or subnormal levels during the initial treatment period may reduce perfusion to the brain, heart, and kidneys, and must be avoided except in specific instances (ie, dissecting aortic aneurysm). Gradually establish a normal (or reasonable) blood pressure over the next 1-2 weeks. |
| Select an appropriate antihypertensive regimen depending on the individual patient and clinical setting. | Initiate a controlled decrease in blood pressure. Avoid concomitant administration of multiple agents that may cause precipitous falls in blood pressure. Select the agent with the best hemodynamic profile based on the primary treatment goal. Avoid diuretics and sodium restriction during the initial treatment period unless there is a clear clinical indication (ie, CHF, pulmonary edema). Avoid sedating antihypertensives in patients with hypertensive encephalopathy, CVA, or other CNS disorders in whom mental status must be monitored. Use caution with direct vasodilating agents that induce reflex tachycardia or increase cardiac output in patients with coronary heart disease, history of angina or myocardial infarction, or dissecting aortic aneurysm. Preferably choose an agent that does not adversely affect glomerular filtration rate or renal blood flow. Preferably choose agents that have favorable effects on cerebral blood flow and its autoregulation, especially patients with hypertensive encephalopathy or CVAs. Select the most efficacious agent with the fewest adverse effects based on the underlying cause of the hypertensive crisis and other individual patient factors. |
| Initiate a chronic antihypertensive regimen after the patient's blood pressure is stabilized | Begin oral antihypertensive therapy once goal blood pressure is achieved before gradually tapering parenteral medications. Select the best oral regimen based on cost, ease of administration, adverse effect profile, and concomitant medical conditions. |

## HYPERTENSION (Continued)

### Oral Agents Used in the Treatment of Hypertensive Urgencies and Emergencies

| Drug | Dose | Onset | Cautions |
|------|------|-------|----------|
| Captopril* | P.O.: 25 mg, repeat as required | 15-30 min | Hypotension, renal failure in bilateral renal artery stenosis |
| Clonidine | P.O.: 0.1-0.2 mg, repeated every hour as needed to a total dose of 0.6 mg | 30-60 min | Hypotension, drowsiness, dry mouth |
| Labetalol | P.O.: 200-400 mg, repeat every 2-3 h | 30 min to 2 h | Bronchoconstriction, heart block, orthostatic hypotension |

*There is no clearly defined clinical advantage in the use of sublingual over oral routes of administration with these agents.

### Recommendations for the Use of Intravenous Antihypertensive Drugs in Selected Hypertensive Emergencies

| Condition | Agent(s) of Choice | Agent(s) to Avoid or Use With Caution | General Treatment Principle |
|-----------|--------------------|--------------------------------------|----------------------------|
| Hypertensive encephalopathy | Nitroprusside, labetalol, diazoxide | Methyldopa, reserpine | Avoid drugs with CNS sedating effects |
| Acute intracranial or subarachnoid hemorrhage | Nicardipine*, nitroprusside, trimethaphan | Beta-blockers | Careful titration with a short-acting agent |
| Cerebral infarction | Nicardipine*, nitroprusside, labetalol, trimethaphan | Beta-blockers, minoxidil, diazoxide | Careful titration with a short-acting agent. Avoid agents that may decrease cerebral blood flow. |
| Head trauma | Esmolol, labetalol | Methyldopa, reserpine, nitroprusside, nitroglycerin, hydralazine | Avoid drugs with CNS sedating effects, or those that may increase intracranial pressure |
| Acute myocardial infarction, myocardial ischemia | Nitroglycerin, nicardipine* (calcium channel blockers), labetalol | Hydralazine, diazoxide, minoxidil | Avoid drugs which cause reflex tachycardia and increased myocardial oxygen consumption |
| Acute pulmonary edema | Nitroprusside, nitroglycerin, loop diuretics | Beta-blockers (labetalol), minoxidil, methyldopa | Avoid drugs which may cause sodium and water retention and edema exacerbation |
| Renal dysfunction | Hydralazine, calcium channel blockers | Nitroprusside, ACE inhibitors, beta-blockers (labetalol) | Avoid drugs with increased toxicity in renal failure and those that may cause decreased renal blood flow. |
| Eclampsia | Hydralazine, labetalol, nitroprusside† | Trimethaphan, diuretics, diazoxide (diazoxide may cause cessation of labor) | Avoid drugs that may cause adverse fetal effects, compromise placental circulation, or decrease cardiac output. |
| Pheochromo-cytoma | Phentolamine, nitroprusside, beta-blockers (eg, esmolol) only after alpha blockade (phentolamine) | Beta-blockers in the absence of alpha blockade, methyldopa, minoxidil | Use drugs of proven efficacy and specificity. Unopposed beta blockade may exacerbate hypertension. |

## Recommendations for the Use of Intravenous Antihypertensive Drugs in Selected Hypertensive Emergencies *(continued)*

| Condition | Agent(s) of Choice | Agent(s) to Avoid or Use With Caution | General Treatment Principle |
|---|---|---|---|
| Dissecting aortic aneurysm | Nitroprusside and beta blockade, trimethaphan | Hydralazine, diazoxide, minoxidil | Avoid drugs which may increase cardiac output. |
| Postoperative hypertension | Nitroprusside, nicardipine*, labetalol | Trimethaphan | Avoid drugs which may exacerbate postoperative ileus. |

*The use of nicardipine in these situations is by the recommendation of the author based on a review of the literature.

†Reserve nitroprusside for eclamptic patients with life-threatening hypertension unresponsive to other agents due to the potential risk to the fetus (cyanide and thiocyanate metabolites may cross the placenta).

# HYPERTENSION *(Continued)*

| Drug | Dose* | Onset of Action | Duration of Action | Adverse Effects† | Special Indications |
|------|-------|-----------------|--------------------|-----------------|--------------------|
| **Vasodilators** | | | | | |
| Sodium nitroprusside | 0.25-10 mcg/kg/min as I.V. infusion‡ (maximum dose for 10 minutes only) | Immediate | 1-2 min | Nausea, vomiting, muscle twitching, sweating, thiocyanate and cyanide intoxication | Most hypertensive emergencies; caution with high intracranial pressure or azotemia |
| Nicardipine hydrochloride | 5-15 mg/hl.V. | 5-10 min | 1-4 h | Tachycardia, headache, flushing, local phlebitis | Most hypertensive emergencies except acute heart failure; caution with coronary ischemia |
| Fenoldopam mesylate | 0.1-0.3 mcg/kg/min I.V. infusion | <5 min | 30 min | Tachycardia, headache, nausea, flushing | Most hypertensive emergencies; caution with glaucoma |
| Nitroglycerin | 5-100 mcg/min as I.V. infusion‡ | 2-5 min | 3-5 min | Headache, vomiting, methemoglobinemia, tolerance with prolonged use | Coronary ischemia |
| Enalaprilat | 1.25-5 mg every 6 hours I.V. | 15-30 min | 6 h | Precipitous fall in pressure in high-renin states; response variable | Acute left ventricular failure; avoid in acute myocardial infarction |
| Hydralazine hydrochloride | 10-20 mg I.V.<br>10-50 mg I.M. | 10-20 min<br>20-30 min | 3-8 h | Tachycardia, flushing, headache, vomiting, aggravation of angina | Eclampsia |
| Diazoxide | 50-100 mg I.V. bolus repeated, or 15-30 mg/min infusion | 2-4 min | 6-12 h | Nausea, flushing, tachycardia, chest pain | Now obsolete; when no intensive monitoring available |
| **Adrenergic Inhibitors** | | | | | |
| Labetalol hydrochloride | 20-80 mg I.V. bolus every 10 minutes; 0.5-2 mg/min I.V. infusion | 5-10 min | 3-6 h | Vomiting, scalp tingling, burning in throat, dizziness, nausea, heart block, orthostatic hypotension | Most hypertensive emergencies except acute heart failure |
| Esmolol hydrochloride | 250-500 mcg/kg/min for 1 minute, then 50-100 mcg/kg/min for 4 minutes; may repeat sequence | 1-2 min | 10-20 min | Hypotension, nausea | Aortic dissection, perioperative |
| Phentolamine | 5-15 mg I.V. | 1-2 min | 3-10 min | Tachycardia, flushing, headache | Catecholamine excess |

I.V. indicates intravenous; I.M., intramuscular

*These doses may vary from those in the *Physicians' Desk Reference* (51st edition).

†Hypotension may occur with all agents.

‡Require special delivery system.

# IMMUNIZATION RECOMMENDATIONS

## Standards for Pediatric Immunization Practices

| | |
|---|---|
| Standard 1. | Immunization services are readily available. |
| Standard 2. | There are no barriers or unnecessary prerequisites to the receipt of vaccines. |
| Standard 3. | Immunization services are available free or for a minimal fee. |
| Standard 4. | Providers utilize all clinical encounters to screen and, when indicated, immunize children. |
| Standard 5. | Providers educate parents and guardians about immunizations in general terms. |
| Standard 6. | Providers question parents or guardians about contraindications and, before immunizing a child, inform them in specific terms about the risks and benefits of the immunizations their child is to receive. |
| Standard 7. | Providers follow only true contraindications. |
| Standard 8. | Providers administer simultaneously all vaccine doses for which a child is eligible at the time of each visit. |
| Standard 9. | Providers use accurate and complete recording procedures. |
| Standard 10. | Providers co-schedule immunization appointments in conjunction with appointments for other child health services. |
| Standard 11. | Providers report adverse events following immunization promptly, accurately, and completely. |
| Standard 12. | Providers operate a tracking system. |
| Standard 13. | Providers adhere to appropriate procedures for vaccine management. |
| Standard 14. | Providers conduct semiannual audits to assess immunization coverage levels and to review immunization records in the patient populations they serve. |
| Standard 15. | Providers maintain up-to-date, easily retrievable medical protocols at all locations where vaccines are administered. |
| Standard 16. | Providers operate with patient-oriented and community-based approaches. |
| Standard 17. | Vaccines are administered by properly trained individuals. |
| Standard 18. | Providers receive ongoing education and training on current immunization recommendations. |

Recommended by the National Vaccine Advisory Committee, April 1992.

Approved by the United States Public Health Service, May 1992.

Endorsed by the American Academy of Pediatrics, May 1992.

The Standards represent the consensus of the National Vaccine Advisory Committee (NVAC) and of a broad group of medical and public health experts about what constitutes the most desirable immunization practices. It is recognized by the NVAC that not all of the current immunization practices of public and private providers are in compliance with the Standards. Nevertheless, the Standards are expected to be useful as a means of helping providers to identify needed changes, to obtain resources if necessary, and to actually implement the desirable immunization practices in the future.

## IMMUNIZATION RECOMMENDATIONS *(Continued)*

### Recommended Childhood Immunization Schedule
### United States, January - December 1999

Vaccines [1] are listed under the routinely recommended ages. Bars indicate range of recommended ages for immunization. Any dose not given at the recommended age should be given as a "catch up" immunization at any subsequent visit when indicated and feasible.
Ovals indicate vaccines to be given if previously recommended doses were missed or given earlier than the recommended minimum age.

| Age ▶ Vaccine ▼ | Birth | 1 mo | 2 mos | 4 mos | 6 mos | 12 mos | 15 mos | 18 mos | 4-6 yrs | 11-12 yrs | 14-16 yrs |
|---|---|---|---|---|---|---|---|---|---|---|---|
| Hepatitis B[2] | Hep B | Hep B | | | Hep B | | | | | Hep B | |
| Diphtheria, Tetanus, Pertussis[3] | | | DTaP | DTaP | DTaP | | DTaP[3] | | DTaP | Td | |
| H. influenzae type b[4] | | | Hib | Hib | Hib | Hib | | | | | |
| Polio[5] | | | IPV | IPV | Polio[5] | | | | Polio | | |
| Rotavirus[6] | | | Rv[6] | Rv[6] | Rv[6] | | | | | | |
| Measles, Mumps, Rubella[7] | | | | | | MMR | | | MMR[7] | MMR[7] | |
| Varicella[8] | | | | | | Var | | | | Var[8] | |

[1] This schedule indicates the recommended ages for routine administration of currently licensed childhood vaccines. Combination vaccines may be used whenever any components of the combination are indicated and its other components are not contraindicated. Providers should consult the manufacturers' package inserts for detailed recommendations.

[2] Infants born to HBsAg-negative mothers should receive the 2nd dose of hepatitis B vaccine at least 1 month after the 1st dose. The 3rd dose should be administered at least 4 months after the 1st dose and at least 2 months after the 2nd dose, but not before 6 months of age for infants.

Infants born to HBsAg-positive mothers should receive hepatitis B vaccine and 0.5 mL hepatitis B immune globulin (HBIG) within 12 hours of birth at separate sites. The 2nd dose is recommended at 1-2 months of age and the 3rd dose at 6 months of age.

Infants born to mothers whose HBsAg status is unknown should receive hepatitis B vaccine within 12 hours of birth. Maternal blood should be drawn at the time of delivery to determine the mother's HBsAg status; if the HBsAg test is positive, the infant should receive HBIG as soon as possible (no later than 1 week of age).
All children and adolescents (through 18 years of age) who have not been immunized against hepatitis B may begin the series during any visit. Special efforts should be made to immunize children who were born in or whose parents were born in areas of the world with moderate or high endemicity of HBV infection.

[3] DTaP (diphtheria and tetanus toxoids and acellular pertussis vaccine) is the preferred vaccine for all doses in the immunization series, including completion of the series in children who have received 1 or more doses of whole-cell DTP vaccine. Whole-cell DTP is an acceptable alternative to DTaP. The 4$^{th}$ dose (DTP or DTaP) may be administered as early as 12 months of age, provided 6 months have elapsed since the 3rd dose and if the child is unlikely to return at age 15-18 months. Td (tetanus and diphtheria toxoids) is recommended at 11-12 years of age if at least 5 years have elapsed since the last dose of DTP, DTaP, or DT. Subsequent routine Td boosters are recommended every 10 years.

[4] Three *H. influenzae* type b (Hib) conjugate vaccines are licensed for infant use. If PRP-OMP (PedvaxHIB and COMVAX [Merck]) is administered at 2 and 4 months of age, a dose at 6 months is not required. Because clinical studies in infants have demonstrated that using some combination products may induce a lower immune response to the Hib vaccine component, DTaP/Hib combination products should not be used for primary immunization in infants at 2, 4, or 6 months of age, unless FDA-approved for these ages.

*(continued)*

[5] Two poliovirus vaccines currently are licensed in the United States: Inactivated poliovirus vaccine (IPV) and oral poliovirus vaccine (OPV). The ACIP, AAP, and AAFP now recommend that the first two doses of poliovirus vaccine should be IPV. The ACIP continues to recommend a sequential schedule of two doses of IPV administered at ages 2 and 4 months, followed by two doses of OPV at 12-18 months and 4-6 years. Use of IPV for all doses also is acceptable and is recommended for immunocompromised persons and their household contacts. OPV is no longer recommended for the first two doses of the schedule and is acceptable only for special circumstances such as: Children of parents who do not accept the recommended number of injections, late initiation of immunization which would require an unacceptable number of injections, and imminent travel to polio-endemic areas. OPV remains the vaccine of choice for mass immunization campaigns to control outbreaks due to wild poliovirus.

[6] Rotavirus vaccine (*Rv*) is italicized to indicate: 1) Health care providers may require time and resources to incorporate this new vaccine into practice; and 2) the AAFP feels that the decision to use rotavirus vaccine should be made by the parent or guardian in consultation with their physician or other health care provider. The first dose of Rv vaccine should not be administered before 6 weeks of age, and the minimum interval between doses is 3 weeks. The Rv vaccine series should not be initiated at 7 months of age or older, and all doses should be completed by the first birthday.

[7] The 2nd dose of measles, mumps, and rubella vaccine (MMR) is recommended routinely at 4-6 years of age but may be administered during any visit, provided at least 4 weeks have elapsed since receipt of the 1st dose and that both doses are administered beginning at or after 12 months of age. Those who have not previously received the second dose should complete the schedule by the 11- to 12-year-old visit.

[8] Varicella vaccine is recommended at any visit on or after the first birthday for susceptible children, ie, those who lack a reliable history of chickenpox (as judged by a health care provider) and who have not been immunized. Susceptible persons 13 years of age or older should receive 2 doses, given at least 4 weeks apart.

Adapted from Advisory Committee on Immunization Practices (ACIP), the American Academy of Pediatrics (AAP), and the American Academy of Family Physicians (AAFP).

## IMMUNIZATION RECOMMENDATIONS *(Continued)*

### RECOMMENDATIONS OF THE ADVISORY COMMITTEE ON IMMUNIZATION PRACTICES (ACIP)

#### Recommended Poliovirus Vaccination Schedules for Children

| Vaccine | Child's Age | | | |
|---|---|---|---|---|
| | 2 mo | 4 mo | 12-18 mo | 4-6 y |
| Sequential IPV*/OPV*/OPV† | IPV | IPV | OPV | OPV |
| OPV* | OPV | OPV | OPV‡ | OPV |
| IPV† | IPV | IPV | IPV | OPV |

*Inactivated poliovirus vaccine.

†Live, oral poliovirus vaccine.

‡For children who receive only OPV, the third dose of OPV may be administered as early as 6 months of age.

Adapted from *MMWR Morb Mortal Wkly Rep*, "Poliomyelitis Prevention in the United States: Introduction of a Sequential Vaccination Schedule of Inactivated Poliovirus Vaccine Followed by Oral Poliovirus Vaccine" 1997, 46(RR-3).

#### Recommendations for Measles Vaccination*

| Category | Recommendations |
|---|---|
| Unvaccinated, no history of measles (12-15 mo) | A 2-dose schedule (with MMR) is recommended if born after 1956. The first dose is recommended at 12-15 mo; the second is recommended at 4-6 y |
| Children 12 mo in areas of recurrent measles transmission | Vaccinate; a second dose is indicated at 4-6 y (at school entry) |
| Children 6-11 mo in epidemic situations† | Vaccinate (with monovalent measles vaccine or, if not available, MMR); revaccination (with MMR) at 12-15 mo is necessary and a third dose is indicated at 4-6 y |
| Children 11-12 y who have received 1 dose of measles vaccine at ≥12 mo | Revaccinate (1 dose) |
| Students in college and other posthigh school institutions who have received 1 dose of measles vaccine at ≥12 mo | Revaccinate (1 dose) |
| History of vaccination before the first birthday | Consider susceptible and vaccinate (2 doses) |
| Unknown vaccine, 1963-1967 | Consider susceptible and vaccinate (2 doses) |
| Further attenuated or unknown vaccine given with IG | Consider susceptible and vaccinate (2 doses) |
| Egg allergy | Vaccinate; no reactions likely |
| Neomycin allergy, nonanaphylactic | Vaccinate; no reactions likely |
| Tuberculosis | Vaccinate; vaccine does not exacerbate infection |
| Measles exposure | Vaccinate or give IG, depending on circumstances |
| HIV-infected | Vaccinate (2 doses) unless severely compromised |
| Immunoglobulin or blood product received | Vaccinate at the appropriate interval |

*See text for details. MMR indicates measles-mumps-rubella vaccine; IG, immune globulin.

†See Outbreak Control.

Adapted from "Report of the Committee on Infectious Diseases," *1997 Red Book*®, 24th ed.

## Recommended Immunization Schedules for Children Not Immunized in the First Year of Life*

| Recommended Time/Age | Immunization(s)[1,2,3] | Comments |
|---|---|---|
| **Younger Than 7 Years** | | |
| First visit | DTaP (or DTP), Hib, HBV, MMR, OPV[3] | If indicated, tuberculin testing may be done at same visit. |
| | | If child is ≥5 y of age, Hib is not indicated in most circumstances. |
| Interval after first visit | | |
| 1 mo (4 wk) | DTaP (or DTP), HBV, Var[4] | The second dose of OPV may be given if accelerated poliomyelitis vaccination is necessary, such as for travelers to areas where polio is endemic. |
| 2 mo | DTaP (or DTP), Hib, OPV[3] | Second dose of Hib is indicated only if the first dose was received when <15 mo. |
| ≥8 mo | DTaP (or DTP), HBV, OPV[3] | OPV and HBV are not given if the third doses were given earlier. |
| Age 4-6 y (at or before school entry) | DTaP (or DTP), OPV,[3] MMR[5] | DTaP (or DTP) is not necessary if the fourth dose was given after the fourth birthday; OPV is not necessary if the third dose was given after the fourth birthday. |
| Age 11-12 y | See Childhood Immunization Schedule | |
| **7-12 Years** | | |
| First visit | HBV, MMR, Td, OPV[3] | |
| Interval after first visit | | |
| 2 mo (8 wk) | HBV, MMR,[5] Var,[4] Td, OPV[3] | OPV also may be given 1 mo after the first visit if accelerated poliomyelitis vaccination is necessary. |
| 8-14 mo | HBV,[6] Td, OPV[3] | OPV is not given if the third dose was given earlier. |
| Age 11-12 y | See Childhood Immunization Schedule | |

*Table is not completely consistent with all package inserts. For products used, also consult manufacturer's package insert for instructions on storage, handling, dosage, and administration. Biologics prepared by different manufacturers may vary, and package inserts of the same manufacturer may change from time to time. Therefore, the physician should be aware of the contents of the current package insert. Vaccine abbreviations: HBV indicates hepatitis B virus vaccine; Var, varicella vaccine; DTP, diphtheria and tetanus toxoids and pertussis vaccine; DTaP, diphtheria and tetanus toxoids and acellular pertussis vaccine; Hib, *Haemophilus influenzae* type b conjugate vaccine; OPV, oral poliovirus vaccine; IPV, inactivated poliovirus vaccine; MMR, live measles-mumps-rubella vaccine; Td, adult tetanus toxoid (full dose) and diphtheria toxoid (reduced dose), for children ≥7 years and adults.

[1] If all needed vaccines cannot be administered simultaneously, priority should be given to protecting the child against those diseases that pose the greatest immediate risk. In the United States, these diseases for children <2 years usually are measles and *Haemophilus influenzae* type b infection; for children >7 years, they are measles, mumps, and rubella. Before 13 years of age, immunity against hepatitis B and varicella should be ensured.

[2] DTaP, HBV, Hib, MMR, and Var can be given simultaneously at separate sites if failure of the patient to return for future immunizations is a concern.

[3] IPV is also acceptable. However, for infants and children starting vaccination late (ie, after 6 months of age), OPV is preferred in order to complete an accelerated schedule with a minimum number of injections.

[4] Varicella vaccine can be administered to susceptible children any time after 12 months of age. Unvaccinated children who lack a reliable history of chickenpox should be vaccinated before their 13th birthday.

[5] Minimal interval between doses of MMR is 1 month (4 weeks).

[6] HBV may be given earlier in a 0-, 2-, and 4-month schedule.

Adapted from "Report of the Committee on Infectious Diseases," *1997 Red Book*®, 24th ed.

# IMMUNIZATION RECOMMENDATIONS *(Continued)*

## Minimum Age for Initial Vaccination and Minimum Interval Between Vaccine Doses, by Type of Vaccine

| Vaccine | Minimum *Age* for First Dose* | Minimum *Interval* From Dose 1 to 2* | Minimum *Interval* From Dose 2 to 3* | Minimum *Interval* From Dose 3 to 4* |
|---|---|---|---|---|
| DTP (DT)† | 6 wk‡ | 4 wk | 4 wk | 6 mo |
| Combined DTP-Hib | 6 wk | 1 mo | 1 mo | 6 mo |
| DTaP* | 6 wk | | | 6 mo |
| Hib (primary series) | | | | |
| HbOC | 6 wk | 1 mo | 1 mo | § |
| PRP-T | 6 wk | 1 mo | 1 mo | § |
| PRP-OMP | 6 wk | 1 mo | § | |
| OPV | | | 6 wk | |
| IPV¶ | 6 wk | 4 wk | 6 mo# | |
| MMR | 12 mo• | 1 mo | | |
| Hepatitis B | Birth | 1 mo | 2 mo♦ | |
| Varicella-zoster | 12 mo | 4 wk | | |

DTP = diphtheria-tetanus-pertussis.

DTaP = diphtheria-tetanus-acellular pertussis.

Hib = *Haemophilus influenzae* type b conjugate.

IPV = inactivated poliovirus vaccine.

MMR = measles-mumps-rubella.

OPV = poliovirus vaccine, live oral, trivalent.

Modified from *MMWR Morb Mortal Wkly Rep*, 1994, 43(RR-1).

*These minimum acceptable ages and intervals may not correspond with the optimal recommended ages and intervals for vaccination. See tables for the current recommended routine and accelerated vaccination schedules.

†DTaP can be used in place of the fourth (and fifth) dose of DTP for children who are at least 15 months of age. Children who have received all four primary vaccination doses before their fourth birthday should receive a fifth dose of DTP (DT) or DTaP at 4-6 years of age before entering kindergarten or elementary school **and** at least 6 months after the fourth dose. The total number of doses of diphtheria and tetanus toxoids should not exceed six each before the seventh birthday.

‡The American Academy of Pediatrics permits DTP to be administered as early as 4 weeks of age in areas with high endemicity and during outbreaks.

§The booster dose of Hib vaccine which is recommended following the primary vaccination series should be administered no earlier than 12 months of age **and** at least 2 months after the previous dose of Hib vaccine.

¶See text to differentiate conventional inactivated poliovirus vaccine from enhanced-potency IPV.

#For unvaccinated adults at increased risk of exposure to poliovirus with <3 months but >2 months available before protection is needed, three doses of IPV should be administered at least 1 month apart.

•Although the age for measles vaccination may be as young as 6 months in outbreak areas where cases are occurring in children <1 year of age, children initially vaccinated before the first birthday should be revaccinated at 12-15 months of age and an additional dose of vaccine should be administered at the time of school entry or according to local policy. Doses of MMR or other measles-containing vaccines should be separated by at least 1 month.

♦This final dose is recommended no earlier than 4 months of age.

## Recommended Immunization Schedule For HIV-Infected Children[1]

| Age ▶<br>Vaccine ▼ | Birth | 1 mo | 2 mo | 4 mo | 6 mo | 12 mo | 15 mo | 18 mo | 24 mo | 4-6 y | 11-12 y | 14-16 y |
|---|---|---|---|---|---|---|---|---|---|---|---|---|
| ◀— Recommendations for these vaccines are the same as those for immunocompetent children ◀— | | | | | | | | | | | | |
| Hepatitis B[2] | HepB-1 | | | | | | | | | | | |
| | | Hep B-2 | | Hep B-3 | | | | | | | Hep B[3] | |
| Diphtheria, Tetanus, Pertussis[4] | | | DTaP or DTP | DTaP or DTP | DTaP or DTP | | DTaP or DTP[4] | | | DTaP or DTP | Td | |
| Haemophilus influenzae type b[5] | | | Hib | Hib | Hib | Hib | | | | | | |
| ◀— Recommendations for these vaccines differ from those for immunocompetent children ◀— | | | | | | | | | | | | |
| Polio[6] | | | IPV | IPV | | IPV | | | | IPV | | |
| Measles, Mumps, Rubella[7] | | | | | | MMR | | | MMR | | | |
| Influenza[8] | | | | | | Influenza (a dose is required every year) | | | | | | |
| Streptococcus pneumoniae[9] | | | | | | | | | pneumo-coccal | | | |
| Varicella | | | | | | CONTRAINDICATED in **all** HIV-infected persons | | | | | | |

Note: Modified from the immunization schedule for immunocompetent children. This schedule also applies to children born to HIV-infected mothers whose HIV infection status has not been determined. Once a child is known not to be HIV-infected, the schedule for immunocompetent children applies. This schedule indicates the recommended age for routine administration of currently licensed childhood vaccines. Some combination vaccines are available and may be used whenever administration of all components of the vaccine is indicated. Providers should consult the manufacturers' package inserts for detailed recommendations.

1 Vaccines are listed under the routinely recommended ages. [Bars] indicate range of acceptable ages for vaccination. [Shaded bars] indicate catch-up vaccination: at 11-12 years of age, hepatitis B vaccine should be administered to children not previously vaccinated.

2 **Infants born to HB$_s$Ag-negative mothers** should receive 2.5 mcg of Merch vaccine (Recombivax HB®) or 10 mcg of Smith Kline Beecham (SB) vaccine (Engerix-B®). The 2nd dose should be administered >1 mo after the 1st dose.

**Infants born to HB$_s$Ag-positive mothers** should receive 0.5 mL of hepatitis B immune globulin (HBIG) within 12 h of birth and either 5 mcg of Merck vaccine (Recombivax HB®) or 10 mcg of SB vaccine (Engerix-B®) at a separate site. The 2nd dose is recommended at 1-2 months of age and the 3rd dose at 6 months of age.

**Infants born to mothers whose HB$_s$Ag status is unknown** should receive either 5 mcg of Merck vaccine (Recombivax HB®) or 10 mcg of SB vaccine (Engerix-B®) within 12 hours of birth. The 2nd dose of vaccine is recommended at 1 month of age and the 3rd dose at 6 months of age. Blood should be drawn at the time of delivery to determine the mother's HB$_s$Ag status; if it is positive, the infant should receive HBIG as soon as possible (no later than 1 week of age). The dosage and timing of subsequent vaccine doses should be based upon the mother's HB$_s$Ag status.

3 Children and adolescents who have not been vaccinated against hepatitis B in infancy may begin the series during any childhood visit. Those who have not previously received 3 doses of hepatitis B vaccine should initiate or complete the series during the 11- to 12-year-old visit. The 2nd dose should be administered at least 1 month after the 1st dose and at least 2 months after the 2nd dose.

4 DTaP (diphtheria and tetanus toxoids and acellular pertussis vaccine) is the preferred vaccine for all doses in the vaccination series, including completion of the series in children who have received >1 dose of whole-cell DTP vaccine. Whole-cell DTP is an acceptable alternative to DTaP. The 4th dose of DTaP may be administered as early as 12 months of age, provided 6 months have elapsed since the 3rd dose, and if the child is considered unlikely to return at 15-18 months of age. Td (tetanus and diphtheria toxoids, absorbed for adult use) is recommended at 11-12 years of age if at least 5 years have elapsed since the last dose of DTP, DTaP, or DT. Subsequent routine Td boosters are recommended every 10 years.

5 Three *H. influenzae* type b (Hib) conjugate vaccines are licensed for infant use. If PRP-OMP (PedvaxHIB® [Merck]) is administered at 2 and 4 months of age, a dose at 6 months is not required. After the primary series has been completed, any Hib conjugate vaccine may be used as a booster.

6 Inactivated poliovirus vaccine (IPV) is the only polio vaccine recommended for HIV-infected persons and their household contacts. Although the third dose of IPV is generally administered at 12-18 months, the 3rd dose of IPV has been approved to be administered as early as 6 months of age. Oral poliovirus vaccine (OPV) should NOT be administered to HIV-infected persons or their household contacts.

7 MMR should not be administered to severely immunocompromised children. HIV-infected children without severe immunosuppression should routinely receive their first dose of MMR as soon as possible upon reaching the first birthday. Consideration should be given to administering the 2nd dose of MMR vaccine as soon as 1 month (ie, minimum 28 days) after the 1st dose, rather than waiting until school entry.

8 Influenza virus vaccine should be administered to all HIV-infected children >6 months of age each year. Children 6 months to 8 years of age who are receiving influenza vaccine for the first time should receive 2 doses of split virus vaccine separated by at least 1 month. In subsequent years, a single dose should be administered each year. The dose of vaccine for children aged 6-35 months is 0.25 mL; the dose for children ≥3 years of age is 0.5 mL.

9 The 23-valent pneumococcal vaccine should be administered to HIV-infected children at 24 months of age. Revaccination should generally be offered to HIV-infected children vaccinated 3-5 years (children ≤10 years of age) or >5 years (children >10 years of age) earlier.

Adapted from the American Academy of Pediatrics and American Academy of Family Practice Physicians, Advisory Committee on Immunization Practices and the Centers for Disease Control.

## IMMUNIZATION RECOMMENDATIONS *(Continued)*

### Licensed Vaccines and Toxoids Available in the United States, by Type and Recommended Routes of Administration

| | Type | Route |
|---|---|---|
| Adenovirus* | Live virus | Oral |
| Anthrax† | Inactivated bacteria | Subcutaneous |
| *Bacillus* of Calmette and Guerin (BCG) | Live bacteria | Intradermal/percutaneous |
| Cholera | Inactivated bacteria | Subcutaneous, intramuscular, or intradermal‡ |
| Diphtheria-tetanus-pertussis (DTP) | Toxoids and inactivated whole bacteria | Intramuscular |
| DTP-*Haemophilus influenzae* type b conjugate (DTP-Hib) | Toxoids, inactivated whole bacteria, and bacterial polysaccharide conjugated to protein | Intramuscular |
| Diphtheria-tetanus-acellular pertussis (DTaP) | Toxoids and inactivated bacterial components | Intramuscular |
| Hepatitis A | Inactivated virus | Intramuscular |
| Hepatitis B | Purified viral antigen | Intramuscular |
| *Haemophilus influenzae* type b conjugate (Hib)§ | Bacterial polysaccharide conjugated to protein | Intramuscular |
| Influenza | Inactivated virus or viral components | Intramuscular |
| Japanese encephalitis | Inactivated virus | Subcutaneous |
| Measles | Live virus | Subcutaneous |
| Measles-mumps-rubella (MMR) | Live virus | Subcutaneous |
| Meningococcal | Bacterial polysaccharides of serotypes A/C/Y/W-135 | Subcutaneous |
| Mumps | Live virus | Subcutaneous |
| Pertussis† | Inactivated whole bacteria | Intramuscular |
| Plague | Inactivated bacteria | Intramuscular |
| Pneumococcal | Bacterial polysaccharides of 23 pneumococcal types | Intramuscular or subcutaneous |
| Poliovirus vaccine | | |
|   Inactivated (IPV) | Inactivated viruses of all 3 serotypes | Subcutaneous |
|   Oral (OPV) | Live viruses of all 3 serotypes | Oral |
| Rabies | Inactivated virus | Intramuscular or intradermal¶ |
| Rubella | Live virus | Subcutaneous |
| Tetanus | Inactivated toxin (toxoid) | Intramuscular# |
| Tetanus-diphtheria (Td or DT)• | Inactivated toxins (toxoids) | Intramuscular# |
| Typhoid | | |
|   Parenteral | Inactivated bacteria | Subcutaneous♦ |
|   Ty21a oral | Live bacteria | Oral |
| Varicella | Live virus | Subcutaneous |
| Yellow fever | Live virus | Subcutaneous |

Modified from *MMWR Morb Mortal Wkly Rep*, 1994, 43(RR-1).

*Available only to the U.S. Armed Forces.

†Distributed by the Division of Biologic Products, Michigan Department of Public Health.

‡The intradermal dose is lower than the subcutaneous dose.

§The recommended schedule for infants depends on the vaccine manufacturer; consult the package insert and ACIP recommendations for specific products.

¶The intradermal dose of rabies vaccine, human diploid cell (HDCV), is lower than the intramuscular dose and is used only for pre-exposure vaccination. **Rabies vaccine, adsorbed (RVA) should not be used intradermally.**

#Preparations with adjuvants should be administered intramuscularly.

•Td-tetanus and diphtheria toxoids for use among persons ≥7 years of age. Td contains the same amount of tetanus toxoid as DTP or DT, but contains a smaller dose of diphtheria toxoid. DT = tetanus and diphtheria toxoids for use among children <7 years of age.

♦Booster doses may be administered intradermally unless vaccine that is acetone-killed and dried is used.

## Immune Globulins and Antitoxins* Available in the United States, by Type of Antibodies and Indications for Use

| Immunobiologic | Type | Indication(s) |
|---|---|---|
| Botulinum antitoxin | Specific equine antibodies | Treatment of botulism |
| Cytomegalovirus immune globulin, intravenous (CMV-IGIV) | Specific human antibodies | Prophylaxis for bone marrow and kidney transplant recipients |
| Diphtheria antitoxin | Specific equine antibodies | Treatment of respiratory diphtheria |
| Immune globulin (IG) | Pooled human antibodies | Hepatitis A pre- and postexposure prophylaxis; measles postexposure prophylaxis |
| Immune globulin, intravenous (IGIV) | Pooled human antibodies | Replacement therapy for antibody deficiency disorders; immune thrombocytopenic purpura (ITP); hypogammaglobulinemia in chronic lymphocytic leukemia; Kawasaki disease |
| Hepatitis B immune globulin (HBIG) | Specific human antibodies | Hepatitis B postexposure prophylaxis |
| Rabies immune globulin (HRIG)† | Specific human antibodies | Rabies postexposure management of persons not previously immunized with rabies vaccine |
| Tetanus immune globulin (TIG) | Specific human antibodies | Tetanus treatment; postexposure prophylaxis of persons not adequately immunized with tetanus toxoid |
| Vaccinia immune globulin (VIG) | Specific human antibodies | Treatment of eczema vaccinatum, vaccinia necrosum, and ocular vaccinia |
| Varicella-zoster immune globulin (VZIG) | Specific human antibodies | Postexposure prophylaxis of susceptible immunocompromised persons, certain susceptible pregnant women, and perinatally exposed newborn infants |

Modified from *MMWR Morb Mortal Wkly Rep*, 1994, 43(RR-1).

*Immune globulin preparations and antitoxins are administered intramuscularly unless otherwise indicated.

†HRIG is administered around the wounds in addition to the intramuscular injection.

# IMMUNIZATION RECOMMENDATIONS *(Continued)*

### Suggested Intervals Between Administration of Immune Globulin Preparations for Various Indications and Vaccines Containing Live Measles Virus*

| Indication | Dose (including mg IgG/kg) | Time Interval (mo) Before Measles Vaccination |
|---|---|---|
| Tetanus (TIG) prophylaxis | I.M.: 250 units (10 mg IgG/kg) | 3 |
| Hepatitis A (IG) prophylaxis | | |
| Contact prophylaxis | I.M.: 0.02 mL/kg (3.3 mg IgG/kg) | 3 |
| International travel | I.M.: 0.06 mL/kg (10 mg IgG/kg) | 3 |
| Hepatitis B prophylaxis (HBIG) | I.M.: 0.06 mL/kg (10 mg IgG/kg) | 3 |
| Rabies immune globulin (HRIG) | I.M.: 20 IU/kg (22 mg IgG/kg) | 4 |
| Varicella prophylaxis (VZIG) | I.M.: 125 units/10 kg (20-40 mg IgG/kg) (max: 625 units) | 5 |
| Measles prophylaxis (IG) Standard (ie, nonimmunocompromised contact) | I.M.: 0.25 mL/kg (40 mg IgG/kg) | 5 |
| Immunocompromised contact | I.M.: 0.50 mL/kg (80 mg IgG/kg) | 6 |
| Blood transfusion | | |
| RBCs, washed | I.V.: 10 mL/kg (negligible IgG/kg) | 0 |
| RBCs, adenine-saline added | I.V.: 10 mL/kg (10 mg IgG/kg) | 3 |
| Packed RBCs (Hct 65%)† | I.V.: 10 mL/kg (60 mg IgG/kg) | 6 |
| Whole blood cells (Hct 35%-50%)† | I.V.: 10 mL/kg (80-100 mg IgG/kg) | 6 |
| Plasma/platelet products | I.V.: 10 mL/kg (160 mg IgG/kg) | 7 |
| Replacement therapy for immune deficiencies | I.V.: 300-400 mg/kg (as IGIV)‡ | 8 |
| Treatment of | | |
| Immune thrombocytopenic purpura§ | I.V.: 400 mg/kg (as IGIV) | 8 |
| Immune thrombocytopenic purpura§ | I.V.: 1000 mg/kg (as IGIV) | 10 |
| Kawasaki disease | I.V.: 2 g/kg (as IGIV) | 11 |

*This table is not intended for determining the correct indications and dosage for the use of immune globulin preparations. Unvaccinated persons may not be fully protected against measles during the entire suggested time interval, and additional doses of immune globulin and/or measles vaccine may be indicated after measles exposure. The concentration of measles antibody in a particular immune globulin preparation can vary by lot. The rate of antibody clearance after receipt of an immune globulin preparation also can vary. The recommended time intervals are extrapolated from an estimated half-life of 30 days of passively acquired antibody and an observed interference with the immune response to measles vaccine for 5 months after a dose of 80 mg IgG/kg.

†Assumes a serum IgG concentration of 16 mg/mL.

‡Measles vaccination is recommended for most HIV-infected children who do not have evidence of severe immunosuppression, but it is contraindicated for patients who have congenital disorders of the immune system.

§Formerly referred to as idiopathic thrombocytopenic purpura.

Modified from *MMWR Morb Mortal Wkly Rep*, 1996, 45(RR-12).

## HAEMOPHILUS INFLUENZAE VACCINATION

### Recommendations for Haemophilus influenzae Type b Conjugate Vaccination in Children Immunized Beginning at 2-6 Months of Age

| Vaccine Product at Initiation* | Total No. of Doses to Be Administered | Currently Recommended Vaccine Regimens |
|---|---|---|
| HbOC or PRP-T | 4 | 3 doses at 2-month intervals<br>When feasible, same vaccine for doses 1-3<br>Fourth dose at 12-15 months of age<br>Any conjugate vaccine for dose 4 |
| PRP-OMP | 3 | 2 doses at 2-month intervals<br>When feasible, same vaccine for doses 1 and 2<br>Third dose at 12-15 months of age<br>Any conjugate vaccine for dose 3† |

Adapted from "Report of the Committee on Infectious Diseases," *1994 Red Book*®, 23rd ed, Montvale, NJ: Medical Economics Co, Inc.

*See text. The HbOC, PRP-T, or PRP-OMP should be given in a separate syringe and at a separate site from other immunizations unless specific combinations are approved by the FDA. HbOC is also available as a combination vaccine with DTP (HbOC-DTP). This combination can be used in infants scheduled to receive separate injections of DTP and HbOC. PRP-T may be reconstituted with DTP, made by Connaught Laboratories; other licensed formulations of DTP may not be used for this purpose.

†The safety and efficacy of PRP-OMP, PRP-D, PRP-T, and HbOC are likely to be equivalent in children 12 months and older.

### Recommendations for Haemophilus influenzae Type b Conjugate Vaccination in Children in Whom Initial Vaccination Is Delayed Until 7 Months of Age or Older

| Age at Initiation of Immunization (mo) | Vaccine Product at Initiation | Total No. of Doses to Be Administered | Currently Recommended Vaccine Regimens* |
|---|---|---|---|
| 7-11 | HbOC, PRP-T, or PRP-OMP | 3 | 2 doses at 2-month intervals†<br>When feasible, same vaccine for doses 1 and 2<br>Third dose at 12-18 months, given at least 2 months after dose 2<br>Any conjugate vaccine for dose 3‡ |
| 12-14 | HbOC, PRP-T, PRP-OMP, or PRP-D | 2 | 2-month interval between doses†<br>Any conjugate vaccine for dose 2‡ |
| 15-59 | HbOC, PRP-T, PRP-OMP, or PRP-D | 1 | Any conjugate vaccine |
| 60 and older§ | HbOC, PRP-T, PRP-OMP, or PRP-D | 1 or 2¶ | Any conjugate vaccine |

Adapted from "Report of the Committee on Infectious Diseases," *1994 Red Book*®, 23rd ed, Montvale, NJ: Medical Economics Co, Inc.

*See text. HbOC, PRP-T, or PRP-OMP should be given in a separate syringe and at a separate site from other immunizations unless specific combinations are approved by the FDA. HbOC is also available as a combination vaccine with DTP (HbOC-DTP). This combination can be used in infants scheduled to receive separate injections of DTP and HbOC. PRP-T may be reconstituted with DTP, made by Connaught Laboratories; other licensed formulations of DTP may not be used for this purpose. In children 15 months or older eligible to receive DTaP (containing acellular pertussis vaccine), however, separate injections of conjugate vaccine and DTaP are acceptable because of the lower rate of febrile, minor local and systemic reactions associated with DTaP.

†For "catch up," a minimum of a 1-month interval between doses may be used.

‡The safety and efficacy of PRP-OMP, PRP-D, PRP-T, and HbOC are likely to be equivalent for use as a booster dose in children 12 months or older.

§Only for children with chronic illness known to be associated with an increased risk for *H. influenzae* type b disease (see text).

¶Two doses separated by 2 months are recommended by some experts for children with certain underlying diseases associated with increased risk of disease and impaired antibody responses to *H. influenzae* type b conjugate vaccination (see text).

# IMMUNIZATION RECOMMENDATIONS *(Continued)*

## Recommendations for *Haemophilus influenzae* Type b Conjugate Vaccination in Children With a Lapse in Vaccination

| Age at Presentation (mo) | Previous Vaccination History | Recommended Regimen |
|---|---|---|
| 7-11 | 1 dose* | 1 dose of conjugate at 7-11 months, with a booster dose given at least 2 months later, at 12-15 months† |
| | 2 doses of HbOC or PRP-T | Same as above |
| 12-14 | 2 doses before 12 months* | A single dose of any licensed conjugate‡ |
| | 1 dose before 12 months* | 2 additional doses of any licensed conjugate, separated by 2 months‡ |
| 15-59 | Any incomplete schedule | A single dose of any licensed conjugate‡ |

Adapted from "Report of the Committee on Infectious Diseases," *1994 Red Book*®, 23rd ed, Montvale, NJ: Medical Economics Co, Inc.

*PRP-OMP, PRP-T, or HbOC. HbOC is also available as a combination vaccine with DTP (HbOC-DTP), which may be used in infants scheduled to receive separate injections of DTP and HbOC. PRP-T may be reconstituted with DTP, made by Connaught Laboratories; other licensed formulations of DTP may not be used for this purpose. In children 15 months or older eligible to receive DTaP (containing acellular pertussis), however, separate injections of conjugate vaccine and DTaP may be given because of the lower rate of febrile, minor local and systemic reactions associated with DTaP.

†For the dose given at 7-11 months, when feasible, the same vaccine should be given as was used for the dose given at 2-6 months. For the dose given at 12-15 months, any licensed conjugate can be used.

‡The Academy considers that safety and efficacy of PRP-OMP, PRP-D, PRP-T, or HbOC are likely to be equivalent when used in children ≥12 months of age.

# POSTEXPOSURE PROPHYLAXIS FOR HEPATITIS B*

| Exposure | Hepatitis B Immune Globulin | Hepatitis B Vaccine |
|---|---|---|
| Perinatal | 0.5 mL I.M. within 12 h of birth | 0.5 mL† I.M. within 12 h of birth (no later than 7 d), and at 1 and 6 mo‡; test for HB$_s$Ag and anti-HB$_s$ at 12-15 mo |
| Sexual | 0.06 mL/kg I.M. within 14 d of sexual contact; a second dose should be given if the index patient remains HB$_s$Ag-positive after 3 mo and hepatitis B vaccine was not given initially | 1 mL I.M. at 0, 1, and 6 mo for homosexual and bisexual men and regular sexual contacts of persons with acute and chronic hepatitis B |
| **Percutaneous; exposed person unvaccinated** | | |
| Source known HB$_s$Ag-positive | 0.06 mL/kg I.M. within 24 h | 1 mL I.M. within 7 d, and at 1 and 6 mo§ |
| Source known, HB$_s$Ag status not known | Test source for HB$_s$Ag; if source is positive, give exposed person 0.06 mL/kg I.M. once within 7 d | 1 mL I.M. within 7 d, and at 1 and 6 mo§ |
| Source not tested or unknown | Nothing required | 1 mL I.M. within 7 d, and at 1 and 6 mo |
| **Percutaneous; exposed person vaccinated** | | |
| Source known HB$_s$Ag-positive | Test exposed person for anti-HB$_s$¶. If titer is protective, nothing is required; if titer is not protective, give 0.06 mL/kg within 24 h | Review vaccination status# |

# POSTEXPOSURE PROPHYLAXIS FOR HEPATITIS B* *(continued)*

| Exposure | Hepatitis B Immune Globulin | Hepatitis B Vaccine |
|---|---|---|
| Source known, HB$_s$Ag status not known | Test source for HB$_s$Ag and exposed person for anti-HB$_s$. If source is HB$_s$Ag-negative, or if source is HB$_s$Ag-positive but anti-HB$_s$ titer is protective, nothing is required. If source is HB$_s$Ag-positive and anti-HB$_s$ titer is not protective or if exposed person is a known nonresponder, give 0.06 mL/kg I.M. within 24 h. A second dose of hepatitis B immune globulin can be given 1 mo later if a booster dose of hepatitis B vaccine is not given. | Review vaccination status# |
| Source not tested or unknown | Test exposed person for anti-HB$_s$. If anti-HB$_s$ titer is protective, nothing is required. If anti-HB$_s$ titer is not protective, 0.06 mL/kg may be given along with a booster dose of hepatitis B vaccine | Review vaccination status# |

*HB$_s$Ag = hepatitis B surface antigen; anti-HB$_s$ = antibody to hepatitis B surface antigen; I.M. = intramuscularly; SRU = standard ratio units.

†Each 0.5 mL dose of plasma-derived hepatitis B vaccine contains 10 μg of HB$_s$Ag; each 0.5 mL dose of recombinant hepatitis B vaccine contains 5 μg (Merck Sharp & Dohme) or 10 μg (SmithKline Beecham) of HB$_s$Ag.

‡If hepatitis B immune globulin and hepatitis B vaccine are given simultaneously, they should be given at separate sites.

§If hepatitis B vaccine is not given, a second dose of hepatitis B immune globulin should be given 1 month later.

¶Anti-HB$_s$ titers <10 SRU by radioimmunoassay or negative by enzyme immunoassay indicate lack of protection. Testing the exposed person for anti-HB$_s$ is not necessary if a protective level of antibody has been shown within the previous 24 months.

#If the exposed person has not completed a three-dose series of hepatitis B vaccine, the series should be completed. Test the exposed person for anti-HB$_s$. If the antibody level is protective, nothing is required. If an adequate antibody response in the past is shown on retesting to have declined to an inadequate level, a booster dose (1 mL) of hepatitis B vaccine should be given. If the exposed person has inadequate antibody or is a known nonresponder to vaccination, a booster dose can be given along with one dose of hepatitis B immune globulin.

## IMMUNIZATION RECOMMENDATIONS *(Continued)*

# PREVENTION OF HEPATITIS A THROUGH ACTIVE OR PASSIVE IMMUNIZATION

**Recommendations of the Advisory Committee on Immunization Practices (ACIP)**

### PROPHYLAXIS AGAINST HEPATITIS A VIRUS INFECTION

#### Recommended Doses of Immune Globulin (IG) for Hepatitis A Pre-exposure and Postexposure Prophylaxis

| Setting | Duration of Coverage | IG Dose* |
|---|---|---|
| Pre-exposure | Short-term (1-2 months) | 0.02 mL/kg |
| | Long-term (3-5 months) | 0.06 mL/kg† |
| Postexposure | — | 0.02 mL/kg |

*IG should be administered by intramuscular injection into either the deltoid or gluteal muscle. For children <24 months of age, IG can be administered in the anterolateral thigh muscle.

†Repeat every 5 months if continued exposure to HAV occurs.

#### Recommended Dosages of Havrix®*

| Vaccinee's Age (y) | Dose (EL.U.)† | Volume (mL) | No. Doses | Schedule (mo)‡ |
|---|---|---|---|---|
| 2-18 | 720 | 0.5 | 2 | 0, 6-12 |
| >18 | 1440 | 1.0 | 2 | 0, 6-12 |

*Hepatitis A vaccine, inactivated, SmithKline Beecham Biologicals.

†ELISA units.

‡0 months represents timing of the initial dose; subsequent numbers represent months after the initial dose.

#### Recommended Dosages of VAQTA®*

| Vaccinee's Age (y) | Dose (units) | Volume (mL) | No. Doses | Schedule (mo)† |
|---|---|---|---|---|
| 2-17 | 25 | 0.5 | 2 | 0, 6-18 |
| >17 | 50 | 1.0 | 2 | 0, 6 |

*Hepatitis A vaccine, inactivated, Merck & Company, Inc.

†0 months represents timing of the initial dose; subsequent numbers represent months after the initial dose.

From *MMWR Morb Mortal Wkly Rep*, 1996, 45(RR-15).

# RECOMMENDATIONS FOR TRAVELERS

## Recommended Immunizations for Travelers to Developing Countries*

| Immunizations | Length of Travel[1] | | |
| --- | --- | --- | --- |
| | Brief, <2 wk | Intermediate, 2 wk - 3 mo | Long-term Residential, >3 mo |
| Review and complete age-appropriate childhood schedule | + | + | + |
| • DTaP (or DTP) may be given at 4 wk intervals[2] | | | |
| • Poliovirus vaccine may be given at 4-8 wk intervals[2] | | | |
| • Measles: extra dose given if 6-11 mo old at 1st dose | | | |
| • Varicella | | | |
| • Hepatitis B[3] | | | |
| Yellow fever[4] | + | + | + |
| Typhoid fever[5] | ± | + | + |
| Meningococcal meningitis[6] | ± | ± | ± |
| Rabies[7] | + | + | + |
| Japanese encephalitis[4] | − | ± | + |

*See disease-specific chapters for details. For further sources of information, see text.

[1] + indicates recommended; ± consider; and −, not recommended.

[2] If necessary to complete the recommended schedule before departure.

[3] If insufficient time to complete 6-month primary series, accelerated series can be given (see *Red Book* for details).

[4] For endemic regions see *Health Information for International Travel*, page 2 of *Red Book*.

[5] Indicated for travelers who will consume food at nontourist facilities.

[6] For endemic regions of central Africa and during local epidemics.

[7] Indicated for persons with high risk of wild animal exposure and for spelunkers.

Adapted from "Report of the Committee on Infectious Diseases," *1997 Red Book*, 24th ed.

## Recommendations for Pre-exposure Immunoprophylaxis of Hepatitis A Infection for Travelers*

| Age (y) | Likely Exposure (mo) | Recommended Prophylaxis |
| --- | --- | --- |
| <2 | <3 | IG 0.02 mL/kg† |
| | 3-5 | IG 0.06 mL/kg† |
| | Long term | IG 0.06 mL/kg at departure and every 5 mo thereafter† |
| ≥2 | <3‡ | HAV vaccine§¶ |
| | | **or** |
| | | IG 0.02 mL/kg† |
| | 3-5‡ | HAV vaccine§¶ |
| | | **or** |
| | | IG 0.06 mL/kg† |
| | | HAV vaccine§¶ |

*HAV, hepatitis A virus; IG, immune globulin.

†IG should be administered deep into a large muscle mass. Ordinarily no more than 5 mL should be administered in one site in an adult or large child; lesser amounts (max: 3 mL) should be given to small children and infants.

‡Vaccine is preferable, but IG is an acceptable alternative.

§To ensure protection in travelers whose departure is imminent, IG also may be given (see text).

¶Dose and schedule of HAV vaccine as recommended according to age.

Adapted from "Report of the Committee on Infectious Diseases," *1997 Red Book*, 24th ed.

## IMMUNIZATION RECOMMENDATIONS *(Continued)*

### Vaccine Advice for Travelers

| Vaccine | Indication | Dose | Comments |
|---|---|---|---|
| Cholera | The risk to tourists is very low | Refer to product labeling | The currently licensed parenteral vaccine (prepared from killed bacteria) has limited effectiveness, often causes reactions, and is generally not recommended for travelers |
| Hepatitis B vaccine | Not ordinarily recommended for foreign travel, except for medical personnel whose work could require handling of body fluids, or for people who expect to have sexual contacts, receive medical or dental care, or stay for >6 months in areas such as Southeast Asia or sub-Saharan Africa, where hepatitis B is highly endemic | I.M.: 3 doses over 2-6 (preferable) months | Hepatitis B vaccine is less effective when injected into the gluteal area, and should be injected into the deltoid muscle |
| Japanese encephalitis vaccine | Travelers who anticipate spending a month or longer in rural rice-growing areas where they will be heavily exposed to mosquitoes. Countries where the disease may be a problem include Bangladesh, Cambodia, China, India, Indonesia, Korea, Laos, Malaysia, Meaner (Burma), Nepal, Pakistan, the Philippines, Singapore, Sri Lanka, Taiwan, Thailand, Vietnam, and eastern areas of Russia. | Primary series of 3 doses given over 2-4 (preferable) weeks. | Formalin-activated, purified mouse-brain-derived vaccine |
| Measles vaccine | People born after 1956 who have not received 2 doses of measles vaccine (after their first birthday) and do not have a physician-documented history of infection or laboratory evidence of immunity should receive before traveling anywhere | Single dose of measles (or measles-mumps-rubella) vaccine at least 2 weeks before or 3 months after immune globulin | |
| Meningococcal vaccine | Only for tourists traveling to areas where epidemics are occurring. Epidemics occur frequently in sub-Saharan Africa from December to June, and also in northern India and Nepal. Saudi Arabia requires a certificate of immunization for pilgrims to Mecca. | Single dose | |

## Vaccine Advice for Travelers *(continued)*

| Vaccine | Indication | Dose | Comments |
|---|---|---|---|
| Polio vaccine | Adult travelers to tropical or developing countries who have not previously been immunized against polio | Adults: If protection is needed within 4 weeks, a single dose of enhanced inactivated polio vaccine (eIPV) or trivalent (live) oral polio vaccine (OPV) is recommended. Travelers who have previously completed a primary series should receive a booster of OPT or eIPV. | OPV rarely can cause vaccine-induced polio, particularly in previously unimmunized adults |
| Rabies vaccine | Travelers with an occupational risk of exposure or those traveling for extended periods in endemic areas | 3 injections of vaccine over 3-4 weeks | |
| Tetanus and diphtheria toxoids | Tetanus-diphtheria toxoid (Td) booster every 10 years. Especially for travelers going to developing countries and to Russia and the Ukraine, where a large outbreak of diphtheria has been occurring in recent years. | | |

## IMMUNIZATION RECOMMENDATIONS *(Continued)*

### Vaccine Advice for Travelers *(continued)*

| Vaccine | Indication | Dose | Comments |
|---|---|---|---|
| Typhoid vaccine | Travel to rural areas of tropical countries, where typhoid tends to endemic, or to any area where an outbreak was occurring | P.O.: One capsule every other day for a total of 4 capsules, beginning at least 2 weeks before departure<br>Parenteral:<br>AKD and HP: Adults and children ≥10 y: Two doses of 0.5 mL S.C. administered at ≥4-week intervals<br>Children <10 y: Two doses of 0.25 mL S.C. administered at ≥4 week intervals<br>Vi: Adults and children ≥2 y: I.M.: 0.5 mL single dose | Killed bacteria parenteral vaccine is not fully protective and causes 1-2 days of pain at the site of injection sometimes accompanied by fever, malaise, and headache.<br>Live oral vaccine reported to provide equally effective, longer than parenteral vaccine and have less adverse effects.<br>Antibiotics should be avoided, if possible, for 1 week before and 3 weeks after oral typhoid vaccine. |
| Yellow fever vaccine | Travelers to rural areas in the yellow fever endemic zones, which include most of tropical South America and most of Africa between 15°N and 15°S.<br>Some countries in Africa require a certificate of yellow fever vaccination from all entering travelers. Other countries in Africa, South America, and Asia require evidence of vaccination from travelers coming from infected or endemic areas. | Boosters are given every 10 years. | Attenuated live virus vaccine. Need to administer 10 days prior to entry in countries requiring yellow fever vaccination certification. |

More than one vaccine can be given at the same time.
Immunocompromised or pregnant patients generally should not receive live virus vaccines, but measles vaccine is recommended for HIV-infected patients.

## Prevention of Malaria*

| Drug† | Adult Dosage | Pediatric Dosage |
|---|---|---|
| **Chloroquine-Sensitive Areas** | | |
| Chloroquine phosphate | P.O.: 300 mg base (500 mg salt), once/week beginning 1 week before exposure, and continuing for 4 weeks after last exposure | 5 mg/kg base (8.3 mg/kg salt) once/week (max: 300 mg base) |
| **Chloroquine-Resistant Areas** | | |
| Mefloquine‡ | P.O.: 250 mg salt (228 mg base), once/week, beginning 1 week before travel and continuing for 4 weeks after last exposure | 15-19 kg: $1/4$ tablet/wk<br>20-30 kg: $1/2$ tablet/wk<br>31-45 kg: $3/4$ tablet/wk<br>>45 kg: 1 tablet/wk |
| *Alternatives* | | |
| Doxycycline§ | 100 mg/d, starting 1-2 days before exposure and continuing for 4 weeks after last exposure | >8 y: P.O.: 2 mg/kg/d (max: 100 mg/d) |
| **or** | | |
| Chloroquine phosphate | Same as above | Same as above |
| **with or without** | | |
| Proguanil# | 200 mg daily during exposure and for 4 weeks after last exposure | <2 y: 50 mg/d<br>2-6 y: 100 mg/d<br>7-10 y: 150 mg/d<br>>10 y: 200 mg/d |
| **plus** | | |
| Pyrimethamine-sulfadoxine (Fansidar®) for presumptive treatment¶ | Carry a single dose (3 tablets) for self-treatment of febrile illness when medical care is not immediately available | Used as for adults in the following doses:<br><1 y: $1/4$ tablet<br>1-3 y: $1/2$ tablet<br>4-8 y: 1 tablet<br>9-14 y: 2 tablets<br>>14 y: 3 tablets |

*Currently, no drug regimen guarantees protection against malaria. Travelers to countries with risk of malaria should be advised to avoid mosquito bites by using personal protective measures (see text).

†All drugs should be continued for 4 weeks after last exposure.

‡Mefloquine is not licensed by the Food and Drug Administration for children weighing <15 kg, but recent recommendations from the Centers for Disease Control and Prevention allow use of the drug to be considered in children without weight restrictions when travel to chloroquine-resistant *P. falciparum* areas cannot be avoided. Mefloquine is **contraindicated** for use by travelers with a known hypersensitivity to mefloquine and travelers with a history of epilepsy or severe psychiatric disorders. A review of available data suggests that a mefloquine may be administered to persons concurrently receiving β-blockers if they have no underlying arrhythmia. However, mefloquine is not recommended for persons with cardiac conduction abnormalities until additional data are available. Caution may be advised for persons involved in tasks requiring fine coordination and spatial discrimination, such as airline pilots. Quinidine or quinine may exacerbate the known side effects or mefloquine; patients not responding to mefloquine therapy or failing mefloquine prophylaxis should be closely monitored if they are treated with quinidine or quinine.

§Physicians who prescribe doxycycline as malaria chemoprophylaxis should advise patients to limit the exposure to direct sunlight to minimize the possibility of photosensitivity reaction. Use of doxycycline is contraindicated in pregnant women and usually in children <8 years. Physicians must weight the benefits of doxycycline therapy against the possibility of dental staining in children <8 years (see Antimicrobial and Related Therapy).

#Proguanil (chloroguanide hydrochloride) is not available in the United States but is widely available overseas. It is recommended primarily for use in Africa south of the Sahara. Failures in prophylaxis with chloroquine and chloroguanide have been reported commonly, however, as they are only 40% to 60% effective.

¶Use of Fansidar®, which contains 25 mg pyrimethamine and 500 mg sulfadoxine per tablet, is contraindicated in patients with a history of sulfonamide or pyrimethamine intolerance, in infants <2 months, and in pregnant women at term. Resistance to pyrimethamine-sulfadoxine has been reported from Southeast Asia and the Amazon Basin and therefore should not be used for treatment of malaria acquired in these area.

Adapted from "Report of the Committee on Infectious Diseases," *1997 Red Book®*, 24th ed.

# OSTEOPOROSIS MANAGEMENT QUICK REFERENCE

## Prevalence

Osteoporosis effects 25 million Americans of which 80% are women. 27% of American women >80 years of age have osteopenia and 70% of American women >80 years of age have osteoporosis.

## Consequences

1.3 million bone fractures annually (low impact/nontraumatic) and pain, pulmonary insufficiency, decreased quality of life, and economic costs; >250,000 hip fractures per year with a 20% mortality rate

## Risk Factors

Advanced age, female, chronic renal disease, hyperparathyroidism, Cushing's disease, hypogonadism/anorexia, hyperprolactinemia, cancer, large and prolonged dose heparin or glucocorticoids, anticonvulsants, hyperthyroidism (current or history, or excessive thyroid supplements), sedentary, excessive exercise, early menopause, oophorectomy without hormone replacement, excessive aluminum-containing antacid, smoking, methotrexate.

## Diagnosis/Monitoring

DXA bone density, history of fracture (low impact or nontraumatic), compressed vertebrae, decreased height, hump-back appearance. Osteomark™ urine assay measures bone breakdown fragments and may help assess therapy response earlier than DXA but diagnostic value is uncertain as Osteomark™ doesn't reveal extent of bone loss. Bone markers may be tested to evaluate effectiveness of antiresorptive urine therapy.

## Osteoporosis Prevention

1.  Adequate dietary calcium (eg, dairy products)

2.  Vitamin D (eg, fortified dairy products, cod, fatty fish)

3.  Weight-bearing exercise (eg, walking) as tolerated

4.  Calcium supplement of 1000-1500 mg elemental calcium daily (divided in 500 mg increments); women >65 years on estrogen replacement therapy supplement 1000 mg elemental calcium; women >65 not receiving estrogens and men >55 years supplement 1500 mg elemental calcium. To minimize constipation add fiber and start with 500 mg/day for several months, then increase to 500 mg twice daily taken at different times than fiber. Chewable and liquid products are available. Calcium carbonate is given with food to enhance bioavailability. Calcium citrate may be given without regards to meals.

    *   Contraindications: Hypercalcemia, ventricular fibrillation
    *   Side effects: Constipation, anorexia
    *   Drug interactions: Fiber, tetracycline, iron supplement, minerals

5.  Vitamin D Supplement: 400-800 units daily (often satisfied by 1-2 multivitamins or fortified milk) in addition to calcium or a combined calcium and vitamin D supplement and/or >15 minutes direct sunlight/day. Some elderly, especially with significant renal or liver disease can't metabolize (activate) vitamin D and require calcitriol 0.25 mcg orally twice daily or adjusted per serum calcium level, the active form of vitamin D; can check 1,25 OH vitamin D level to confirm need for calcitriol.

    *   Contraindications: Hypercalcemia (weakness, headache, drowsiness, nausea, diarrhea), hypercalciuria and renal stones
    *   Side effects (uncommon): Hypercalcemia (see above)
    *   Monitor 24-hour urine and serum calcium if using >1000 units/day

6.  Estrogen: Especially useful if bone density <80% of average plus symptoms of estrogen deficiency or cardiac disease. Bone density increases over 1-2 years then plateaus. This is considered 1st line therapy unless contraindicated due to medicinal history (see below) or patient preference to avoid HRT (hormone replacement therapy).

- Contraindications: Pregnancy, breast or estrogen-dependent cancer, undiagnosed abnormal genital bleeding, active thrombophlebitis, or history of thromboembolism during previous estrogen or oral contraceptive therapy or pregnancy. Pretreatment mammogram, gynecological exam are advised along with routine breast exam because of a possibly increased risk of breast cancer with long-term use.

- Dose: Conjugated estrogen of 0.625 mg/day or its equivalent (continuous therapy preferred).

- Side effects: Vaginal spotting/bleeding, nausea, vomiting, breast tenderness/enlargement, amenorrheic with extended use.

  Initiate therapy slowly (side effects are more common and severe in women without estrogen for many years). Administer with medroxyprogesterone acetate (MPA) 2.5-5 mg daily in women with uterus (unopposed estrogen can cause endometrial cancer). MPA can increase vaginal bleeding, increase weight, edema, mood changes.

- Drug Interactions: May increase corticosteroid effect, monitor for need to decrease corticosteroid dose.

## Osteoporosis Treatment

1. Calcium, vitamin D, exercise, and estrogen: As above

2. Alendronate (Fosamax®): Consider if patient is intolerant of, or refuses estrogen or it is contraindicated, especially if severe osteoporosis (ie, ≥2.5 standard deviations below average young adult bone density, T-score, or history of low impact or nontraumatic fracture). Increasing bone density of hip and spine observed for at least 3 years (ie, no plateau as seen with estrogen).

   - Contraindications: Hypocalcemia, not advised if existing gastrointestinal disorders (eg, esophageal disorders such as reflux, sensitive stomach).

   - Dose: 10 mg once daily (treatment dose for osteoporosis; not recommended if creatinine clearance <35 mL/minute) before breakfast on an empty stomach with 6-8 ounces tap water (not mineral water, coffee, or juice) and remain upright or raise head of bed for bedridden patients at least 30 degree angle for at least 30 minutes (otherwise may cause ulcerative esophagitis) before eating or drinking. Osteopenia: 5 mg per day for prevention.

   Therapy with calcium and vitamin D is advised, but must be given at a different time of day than alendronate.

   - Side effects (well tolerated): Difficulty swallowing, heartburn, abdominal discomfort, nausea (GI side effects increase with aspirin products), arthralgia/myalgia, constipation, diarrhea, headache, esophagitis.

   - Drug interactions: None known to date.

3. Etidronate: Not FDA approved for postmenopausal osteoporosis and can decrease the quality of bone formation, therefore, change to alendronate.

4. Calcitonin (nasal; Miacalcin®): Indicated if estrogen refused, intolerant, or contraindicated. Potential analgesic effect.

   - Contraindications: Hypersensitivity to salmon protein or gelatin diluent; 1 spray (200 units) into 1 nostril daily (alternate right and left nostril daily); 5 days on and 2 days off is also effective; alternate day administration not effective. If used only for pain, can decrease dose once pain is controlled.

   - Side effects (few): Nasal dryness and irritation (periodically inspect); adequate dietary or supplemental calcium + vitamin D is essential.

   Subcutaneous route (100 units daily): Many side effects (eg, nausea, flushing, anorexia) and the discomfort/inconvenience of injection.

5. Fall prevention: Minimize psychoactive and cardiovascular drugs (monitor BP for orthostasis), give diuretics early in the day, environmental safety check.

## OSTEOPOROSIS MANAGEMENT QUICK REFERENCE (Continued)

| | % Elemental Calcium | Elemental Calcium |
|---|---|---|
| Calcium gluconate (various) | 9 | 500 mg = 45 mg |
| Calcium glubionate (Neo-Calglucon®) | 6.5 | 1.8 g = 115 g/5 mL |
| Calcium lactate (various) | 13 | 325 mg = 42.25 mg |
| Calcium citrate (Citrical®) | 21 | 950 mg = 200 mg |
| Effervescent tabs (Citrical Liquitab®) | | 2376 mg = 500 mg |
| Calcium acetate | | |
| Phos-Ex 250® | 25 | 1000 mg = 250 mg |
| Phos-Lo® | | 667 mg = 169 mg |
| Tricalcium phosphate (Posture®) | 39 | 1565.2 mg = 600 mg |
| Calcium carbonate | | |
| Tums® | 40 | 1.2 g = 500 mg |
| Oscal-500® oral suspension | | 1.2 g/5 mL = 500 mg |
| Caltrate 600® | | 1.5 g = 600 mg |

### References

Ashworth L, "Focus on Alendronate. A Nonhormonal Option for the Treatment of Osteoporosis in Postmenopausal Women," *Formulary*, 1996, 31:23-30.

Johnson SR, "Should Older Women Use Estrogen Replacement," *J Am Geriatr Soc*, 1996, 44:89-90.

Liberman UA, Weiss SR, and Broci J, "Effect of Oral Alendronate on Bone-Mineral Density and the Incidence of Fracture in Postmenopausal Osteoporosis," *N Engl J Med*, 1995, 333:1437-43.

"New Drugs for Osteoporosis," *Med Lett Drugs Ther*, 1996, 38:1-3.

NIH Consensus Development Panel on Optimal Calcium Intake, *JAMA*, 1994, 272:1942-8.

PCA Osteoporosis Prevention and Treatment Video-Teleconference (March 1, April 2 and 3, 1996).

# PARKINSON'S DISEASE MANAGEMENT

**Management of Parkinson's Disease**

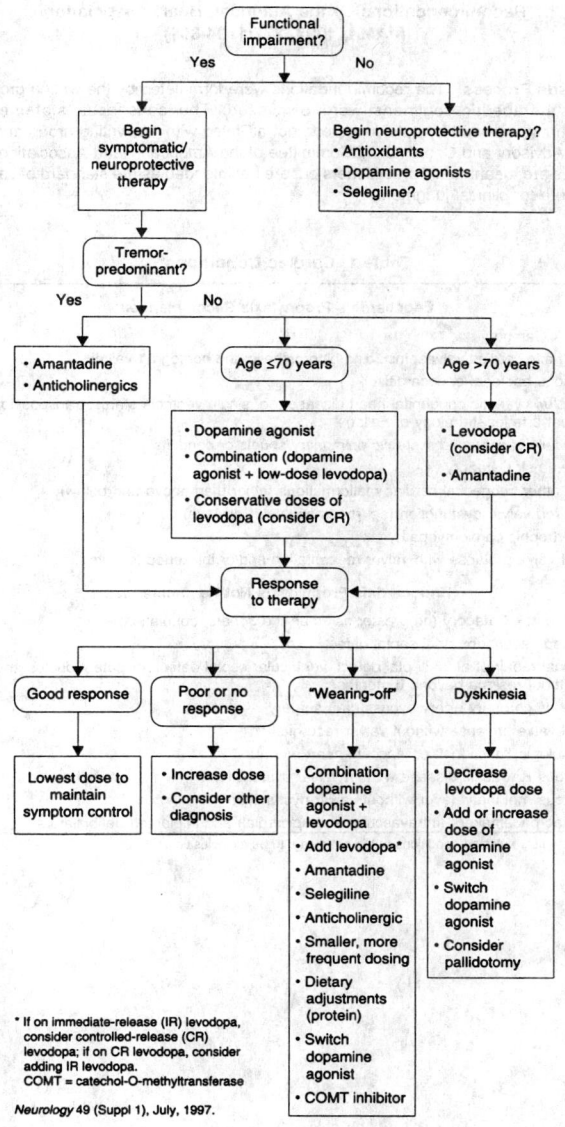

* If on immediate-release (IR) levodopa, consider controlled-release (CR) levodopa; if on CR levodopa, consider adding IR levodopa.
COMT = catechol-O-methyltransferase

*Neurology* 49 (Suppl 1), July, 1997.

# PREVENTION OF BACTERIAL ENDOCARDITIS

### Recommendations by the American Heart Association
### (*JAMA*, 1997, 277:1794-801)

**Consensus Process** - The recommendations were formulated by the writing group after specific therapeutic regimens were discussed. The consensus statement was subsequently reviewed by outside experts not affiliated with the writing group and by the Science Advisory and Coordinating Committee of the American Heart Association. These guidelines are meant to aid practitioners but are not intended as the standard of care or as a substitute for clinical judgment.

### Table 1. Cardiac Conditions*

#### Endocarditis Prophylaxis Recommended

High-risk Category

    Prosthetic cardiac valves including bioprosthetic and homograft valves

    Previous bacterial endocarditis

    Complex cyanotic congenital heart disease (eg, single ventricle states, transposition of the great arteries, tetralogy of Fallot)

    Surgically constructed systemic pulmonary shunts or conduits

Moderate-risk Category

    Most other congenital cardiac malformations (other than above and below)

    Acquired valvar dysfunction (eg, rheumatic heart disease)

    Hypertrophic cardiomyopathy

    Mitral valve prolapse with valvar regurgitation and/or thickened leaflets

#### Endocarditis Prophylaxis Not Recommended

Negligible-risk Category (no greater risk than the general population)

    Isolated secundum atrial septal defect

    Surgical repair of atrial septal defect, ventricular septal defect, or patent ductus arteriosus (without residua beyond 6 months)

    Previous coronary artery bypass graft surgery

    Mitral valve prolapse without valvar regurgitation†

    Physiologic, functional, or innocent heart murmurs

    Previous Kawasaki disease without valvar dysfunction

    Previous rheumatic fever without valvar dysfunction

    Cardiac pacemakers (intravascular and epicardial) and implanted defibrillators

*This table lists selected conditions but is not meant to be all-inclusive.

**Patient With Suspected Mitral Valve Prolapse**

## Table 2. Dental Procedures and Endocarditis Prophylaxis

### Endocarditis Prophylaxis Recommended*

Dental extractions

Periodontal procedures including surgery, scaling and root planing, probing, and recall maintenance

Dental implant placement and reimplantation of avulsed teeth

Endodontic (root canal) instrumentation or surgery only beyond the apex

Subgingival placement of antibiotic fibers or strips

Initial placement of orthodontic bands but not brackets

Intraligamentary local anesthetic injections

Prophylactic cleaning of teeth or implants where bleeding is anticipated

### Endocarditis Prophylaxis Not Recommended

Restorative dentistry† (operative and prosthodontic) with or without retraction cord‡

Local anesthetic injections (nonintraligamentary)

Intracanal endodontic treatment; post placement and buildup

Placement of rubber dams

Postoperative suture removal

Placement of removable prosthodontic or orthodontic appliances

Taking of oral impressions

Fluoride treatments

Taking of oral radiographs

Orthodontic appliance adjustment

Shedding of primary teeth

*Prophylaxis is recommended for patients with high- and moderate-risk cardiac conditions.

†This includes restoration of decayed teeth (filling cavities) and replacement of missing teeth.

‡Clinical judgment may indicate antibiotic use in selected circumstances that may create significant bleeding.

# PREVENTION OF BACTERIAL ENDOCARDITIS *(Continued)*

### Table 3. Recommended Standard Prophylactic Regimen for Dental, Oral, or Upper Respiratory Tract Procedures in Patients Who Are at Risk*

#### Endocarditis Prophylaxis Recommended

Respiratory Tract
- Tonsillectomy and/or adenoidectomy
- Surgical operations that involve respiratory mucosa
- Bronchoscopy with a rigid bronchoscope

Gastrointestinal Tract*
- Sclerotherapy for esophageal varices
- Esophageal stricture dilation
- Endoscopic retrograde cholangiography with biliary obstruction
- Biliary tract surgery
- Surgical operations that involve intestinal mucosa

Genitourinary Tract
- Prostatic surgery
- Cystoscopy
- Urethral dilation

#### Endocarditis Prophylaxis Not Recommended

Respiratory Tract
- Endotracheal intubation
- Bronchoscopy with a flexible bronchoscope, with or without biopsy†
- Tympanostomy tube insertion

Gastrointestinal Tract
- Transesophageal echocardiography†
- Endoscopy with or without gastrointestinal biopsy†

Genitourinary Tract
- Vaginal hysterectomy†
- Vaginal delivery†
- Cesarean section
- In uninfected tissues:
  - Urethral catheterization
  - Uterine dilatation and curettage
  - Therapeutic abortion
  - Sterilization procedures
  - Insertion or removal of intrauterine devices

Other
- Cardiac catheterization, including balloon angioplasty
- Implanted cardiac pacemakers, implanted defibrillators, and coronary stents
- Incision or biopsy or surgically scrubbed skin
- Circumcision

*Prophylaxis is recommended for high-risk patients, optional for medium-risk patients.
†Prophylaxis is optional for high-risk patients.

### Table 4. Prophylactic Regimens for Dental, Oral, Respiratory Tract, or Esophageal Procedures

| Situation | Agent | Regimen* | |
| --- | --- | --- | --- |
| | | Adults | Children |
| Standard general prophylaxis | Amoxicillin | 2 g P.O. 1 h before procedure | 50 mg/kg P.O. 1 h before procedure |
| Unable to take oral medications | Ampicillin | 2 g I.M./I.V. within 30 min before procedure | 50 mg/kg I.M./I.V. within 30 min before procedure |
| Allergic to penicillin | Clindamycin or | 600 mg P.O. 1 h before procedure | 20 mg/kg P.O. 1 h before procedure |
| | Cephalexin† or cefadroxil† or | 2 g P.O 1 h before procedure | 50 mg/kg P.O. 1 h before procedure |
| | Azithromycin or clarithromycin | 500 mg P.O. 1 h before procedure | 15 mg/kg P.O. 1 h before procedure |
| Allergic to penicillin and unable to take oral medications | Clindamycin or | 600 mg I.V. within 30 min before procedure | 20 mg/kg I.V. within 30 min before procedure |
| | Cefazolin† | 1 g I.M./I.V. within 30 min before procedure | 25 mg/kg I.M./I.V. within 30 min before procedure |

*Total children's dose should not exceed adult dose.

†Cephalosporins should not be used in individuals with immediate-type hypersensitivity reaction (urticaria, angioedema, or anaphylaxis) to penicillins

### Table 5. Prophylactic Regimens for Genitourinary/Gastrointestinal (Excluding Esophageal) Procedures*

| Situation | Agents* | Regimen† | |
| --- | --- | --- | --- |
| | | Adults | Children |
| High-risk‡ patients | Ampicillin plus gentamicin | Ampicillin 2 g I.M. or I.V. plus gentamicin 1.5 mg/kg (not to exceed 120 mg) within 30 min of starting the procedure; 6 h later, ampicillin 1 g I.M./I.V. or amoxicillin 1 g orally | Ampicillin 50 mg/kg I.M./I.V. (not to exceed 2 g) plus gentamicin 1.5 mg/kg within 30 min of starting the procedure; 6 h later, ampicillin 25 mg/kg I.M./I.V. or amoxicillin 25 mg/kg orally |
| High-risk‡ patients allergic to ampicillin/ amoxicillin | Vancomycin plus gentamicin | Vancomycin 1 g I.V. over 1-2 h plus gentamicin 1.5 mg/kg I.M./I.V. (not to exceed 120 mg); complete injection/infusion within 30 min of starting the procedure | Vancomycin 20 mg/kg I.V. over 1-2 h plus gentamicin 1.5 mg/kg I.M./I.V.; complete injection/infusion within 30 min of starting the procedure |
| Moderate-risk§ patients | Amoxicillin or ampicillin | Amoxicillin 2 g orally 1 h before procedure, or ampicillin 2 g I.M./I.V within 30 min of starting the procedure | Amoxicillin 50 mg/kg orally 1 h before procedure, or ampicillin 50 mg/kg I.M./I.V. within 30 min of starting the procedure |
| Moderate-risk§ patients allergic to ampicillin/amoxicillin | Vancomycin | Vancomycin 1 g I.V. over 1-2 h; complete infusion within 30 min of starting the procedure | Vancomycin 20 mg/kg I.V. over 1-2 h; complete infusion within 30 min of starting the procedure |

*Total children's dose should not exceed adult dose

†No second dose of vancomycin or gentamicin is recommended

‡High-risk: Patients are those who have prosthetic valves, a previous history of endocarditis (even in the absence of other heart disease, complex cyanotic congenital heart disease, or surgically constructed systemic pulmonary shunts or conduits).

§Moderate-risk: Individuals with certain other underlying cardiac defects. Congenital cardiac conditions include the following uncorrected conditions: Patent ductus arteriosus, ventricular septal defect, ostium primum atrial septal defect, coarctation of the aorta, and bicuspid aortic valve. Acquired valvar dysfunction and hypertrophic cardiomyopathy are also moderate risk conditions.

# PROPHYLAXIS FOR PATIENTS EXPOSED TO COMMON COMMUNICABLE DISEASES

| Disease | Exposure | Prophylaxis/Management |
|---|---|---|
| Invasive *Haemophilus influenzae* disease | Close contact with an infected child for more than 4 hours | Give rifampin 20 mg/kg orally once daily for 4 days (600 mg maximum daily dose) to entire family with at least one household contact less than 48 months old. Contraindication: Pregnant contacts. |
| Hepatitis A | Direct contact with an infected child, or sharing of food or utensils | Give 0.02 mL/kg immune globulin (IG) within 7 days of exposure. |
| Hepatitis B | Needlestick (used needle) Mucous membrane exposure with blood or body fluid Direct inoculation of blood or body fluid into open cut, lesion, or laceration | **Known source and employee status unknown: Test patient for HB₍s₎Ag and employee for anti-HB₍s₎.** If patient is HB₍s₎Ag negative and the patient does not have non-A, non-B hepatitis, do nothing. If patient is HB₍s₎Ag negative and has non-A, non-B hepatitis, offer ISG (optional). If patient is HB₍s₎Ag positive, give HBIG and hepatitis B vaccine within 48 hours of exposure. Employee antibody status may not be available for up to a week, so the above should be given as soon as patient's antigen status is known. Occasionally, the patient's antigen status will be unavailable for more than 24 hours. In these cases, HBIG should be given if the patient is high risk (ie, Asian immigrants, institutionalized patients, homosexuals, intravenous drug abusers, hemodialysis patients, patients with a history of hepatitis). If the employee is anti-HB₍s₎ negative, give the second and third doses of hepatitis B vaccine. **Known source and employee documented anti-HB₍s₎ positive:** If source has non-A, non-B hepatitis, offer ISG (optional). If employee is believed to be anti-HB₍s₎ positive due to vaccination, has received 3 doses of vaccine, and has not had an anti-HB₍s₎ test done, draw serum for anti-HB₍s₎ |
| Measles | 15 minutes or more in the same room with a child with measles from 2 days before the onset of symptoms to 4 days after the appearance of the rash | Children who have not been vaccinated and have not had natural infection should be isolated from the 7th through the 18th day after exposure and/or for 4 days after the rash appears. Those who have not been vaccinated should be vaccinated within 72 hours of exposure if no contraindication exists, or receive immune globulin (IG) 0.25 mL/kg I.M. for immunocompetent individuals and 0.5 mL/kg (maximum 15 mL) for immunosuppressed individuals. Children who are younger than 15 months of age should be revaccinated at 15 months of age but at least 3 months after receipt of vaccine or IG. Older individuals who have received IG should be vaccinated 3 months later. |
| Meningococcal disease | Household contact or direct contact with secretions | Household, day care center, and nursery school children should receive rifampin prophylaxis for 2 days. Dosages are given every 12 hours for a total of 4 doses. Dosage is 10 mg/kg/dose for children ages 1 month to 12 years (maximum 600 mg/dose), 5 mg/kg/dose for infants less than 1 month of age, and 600 mg/dose for adults. Contraindication: Pregnant contacts **Because prophylaxis is not always effective, exposed children should be monitored for symptoms. Employee exposure: Anyone who develops a febrile illness should receive prompt medical evaluation. If indicated, antimicrobial therapy should be administered.** |

| Disease | Exposure | Prophylaxis/Management |
|---------|----------|------------------------|
| Pertussis | Housed in the same room with an infected child or spent 15 minutes in the playroom with the infected child | **Prophylaxis:**<br>Contacts less than 7 years old who have had at least 4 doses of pertussis vaccine should receive a booster dose of DTP, unless a dose has been given within the past 3 years, and should receive erythromycin 40-50 mg/kg/day orally for 14 days.<br>Contacts less than 7 years old who are not immunized or who have received less than 4 doses of DTP should have DTP immunization initiated or continued according to the recommended schedule. Children who have received their third dose 6 months or more before exposure should be given their fourth dose at this time.<br>Erythromycin should also be given for 14 days.<br>Contacts 7 years of age and above should receive prophylactic erythromycin (maximum of 1 g/day) for 10-14 days.<br>All exposed patients should be watched closely for respiratory symptoms for 14 days after exposure has stopped because immunity conferred by the vaccine is not absolute and the efficacy of erythromycin in prophylaxis has not been established. |
| Tuberculosis | Housed in the same room with a child with contagious tuberculosis (tuberculosis is contagious if the child has a cough plus AFB seen on smear plus cavitation on CXR) | Place PPD immediately and 10 weeks after exposure. Start on INH. Consult Infectious Diseases if seroconversion occurs. |
| Varicella-zoster | 1 hour or more in the same room with a contagious child from 24 hours before vesicles appear to when all vesicles are crusted, which is usually 5 to 7 days after vesicles appear.<br>In household exposure, communicability is 48 hours before vesicles appear. | **Immunocompetent** children who have not been vaccinated or had natural infection, should have titers drawn only if they will still be hospitalized for more than 10 days after exposure. If titers are negative, they should be isolated from 10 to 21 days after exposure and/or until all lesions are crusted and dry. If VZIG was given the child should be isolated from 10 to 28 days after exposure.<br>**Immunocompromised** children who have not been vaccinated or had natural infection should first have titers drawn, and then receive VZIG (varicella-zoster immune globulin) **1 vial/10 kg I.M.** up to a maximum of 5 vials as soon as possible but at most 96 hours after exposure. Fractional doses are not recommended. If titers are positive, nothing further need be done. If titers are negative, the child should be isolated from 10 to 28 days after exposure and should be monitored very carefully for the appearance of vesicles so that treatment can be initiated. VZIG is available from the Blood Bank. |

# SUSPECTED ORGANISMS BY SITE OF INFECTION FOR EMPIRIC THERAPY

**Urinary Tract**

  Community acquired — *E. coli*, other gram-negative rods, *S. aureus*, *S. epidermidis*, *S. faecalis*

  Nosocomial — Resistant gram-negative rods, enterococci

**Respiratory Tract**

  Pneumonia

    Community acquired

      normal adult — *S. pneumoniae*, virus, *Mycoplasma* (atypical)

      normal child — *S. pneumoniae*, *H. influenzae*

      aspiration — Aerobic and anaerobic mouth flora

      alcoholic — *S. pneumoniae*, *Klebsiella*, anaerobes (below the belt)

      COPD — *S. pneumoniae*, *H. influenzae*

    Nosocomial

      aspiration — Mouth anaerobes, gram-negative aerobic rods, *S. aureus*

      neutropenic — Fungi, gram-negative aerobic rods, *S. aureus*

      HIV-infected — Fungi, *P. carinii*, *Legionella*, *Nocardia*, *S. pneumoniae*

  Epiglottis — *H. influenzae*

  Acute sinusitis — *S. pneumoniae*, *H. influenzae*, *M. catarrhalis* (*B. catarrhalis*)

  Chronic sinusitis — Anaerobes, *S. aureus*

  Bronchitis, otitis — *S. pneumoniae*, *H. influenzae*, *M. catarrhalis* (*B. catarrhalis*)

  Pharyngitis — Group A streptococci

**Skin and Soft Tissue**

  Cellulitis — Group A streptococci, *S. aureus*

  I.V. site — *S. aureus*, *S. epidermidis*

  Surgical wound — *S. aureus*, gram-negative rods

  Diabetic ulcer — *S. aureus*, gram-negative aerobic rods, anaerobes

  Furuncle — *S. aureus*

**Intra-abdominal** — Anaerobes (*B. fragilis*), *E. coli*, enterococci

**Cardiac**

  Endocarditis

    subacute — *S. viridans*

    acute

      I.V. drug user — *S. aureus*, gram-negative aerobic rods, *S. faecalis*, fungi

      prosthetic valve — *S. epidermidis*

**Gastric**

  Gastroenteritis — *Salmonella*, *Shigella*, *H. pylori*, *C. difficile*, ameba, *G. lamblia*, viral, *E. coli*

**Bone/Joint**

  Osteomyelitis/septic arthritis — *S. aureus*, gram-negative aerobic rods

**Central Nervous System**

  Meningitis

    <2 mo — *E. coli*, group B streptococci, *Listeria*

    2 mo to 12 y — *H. influenzae*, *S. pneumoniae*, *N. meningitidis*

    adult and nosocomial — *S. pneumoniae*, *N. meningitidis*, gram-negative aerobic rods

    postneurosurgery — *S. aureus*, gram-negative rods

# TUBERCULOSIS

### Tuberculin Skin Test Recommendations*

Children for whom immediate skin testing is indicated:

- Contacts of persons with confirmed or suspected infectious tuberculosis (contact investigation); this includes children identified as contacts of family members or associates in jail or prison in the last 5 years

- Children with radiographic or clinical findings suggesting tuberculosis

- Children immigrating from endemic countries (eg, Asia, Middle East, Africa, Latin America)

- Children with travel histories to endemic countries and/or significant contact with indigenous persons from such countries

Children who should be tested annually for tuberculosis†:

- Children infected with HIV or living in household with HIV-infected persons

- Incarcerated adolescents

Children who should be tested every 2-3 years†:

- Children exposed to the following individuals: HIV-infected, homeless, residents of nursing homes, institutionalized adolescents or adults, users of illicit drugs, incarcerated adolescents or adults, and migrant farm workers. Foster children with exposure to adults in the preceding high-risk groups are included.

Children who should be considered for tuberculin skin testing at ages 4-6 and 11-16 years:

- Children whose parents immigrated (with unknown tuberculin skin test status) from regions of the world with high prevalence of tuberculosis; continued potential exposure by travel to the endemic areas and/or household contact with persons from the endemic areas (with unknown tuberculin skin test status) should be an indication for repeat tuberculin skin testing

- Children without specific risk factors who reside in high-prevalence areas; in general, a high-risk neighborhood or community does not mean an entire city is at high risk; rates in any area of the city may vary by neighborhood, or even from block to block; physicians should be aware of these patterns in determining the likelihood of exposure; public health officials or local tuberculosis experts should help clinicians identify areas that have appreciable tuberculosis rates

**Children at increased risk of progression of infection to disease:** Those with other medical risk factors, including diabetes mellitus, chronic renal failure, malnutrition, and congenital or acquired immunodeficiencies deserve special consideration. Without recent exposure, these persons are not at increased risk of acquiring tuberculosis infection. Underlying immune deficiencies associated with these conditions theoretically would enhance the possibility for progression to severe disease. Initial histories of potential exposure to tuberculosis should be included on all of these patients. If these histories or local epidemiologic factors suggest a possibility of exposure, immediate and periodic tuberculin skin testing should be considered. An initial Mantoux tuberculin skin test should be performed before initiation of immunosuppressive therapy in any child with an underlying condition that necessitates immunosuppressive therapy.

---

*BCG immunization is not a contraindication to tuberculin skin testing.

†Initial tuberculin skin testing is at the time of diagnosis or circumstance, beginning as early as at age 3 months.

## TUBERCULOSIS *(Continued)*

### Tuberculosis Therapy

| Specific Circumstances/ Organism | Comments | Regimen |
|---|---|---|
| **Category I. Exposure** (Household members and other close contacts of potentially infectious cases) (Exposee tuberculin test negative)* | | |
| Neonate | Fx essential | INH (10 mg/kg/d) for 3 months, then repeat tuberculin test (TBnT). If mother's smear negative and infant's TBnT negative and chest x-ray (CXR) are normal, stop INH. In the United Kingdom, BCG is then given (*Lancet*, 1990, 2:1479), unless mother is HIV-positive. If infants repeat TBnT is positive and/or CXR abnormal (hilar adenopathy and/or infiltrate), administer INH + RIF (10-20 mg/kg/d) (or streptomycin) for a total of 6 months. If mother is being treated, separation from mother is not indicated. |
| Children <5 y | Rx indicated | As for neonate first 3 months. If repeat TBnT is negative, stop. If repeat TBnT is positive, continue INH for a total of 9 months. If INH is not given initially, repeat TBnT at 3 months; if positive, treat with INH for 9 months (see Category II below). |
| Older children and adults | No Rx | Repeat TBnT at 3 months, if positive, treat with INH for 6 months (see Category II below) |
| **Category II. Infection Without Disease** (Positive tuberculin test)* | | |
| Regardless of age (see INH Preventive Therapy) | Rx indicated | INH (5 mg/kg/d, maximum: 300 mg/d for adults, 10 mg/kg/d not to exceed 300 mg/d for children). Results with 6 months of treatment are nearly as effective as 12 months (65% vs 75% reduction in disease). *Am Thoracic Society* (6 months), *Am Acad Pediatrics*, 1991 (9 months). If CXR is abnormal, treat for 12 months. In HIV-positive patient, treatment for a minimum of 12 months, some suggest longer. Monitor transaminases monthly (*MMWR Morb Mortal Wkly Rep* 1989, 38:247). |
| Age <35 y | Rx indicated | Reanalysis of earlier studies favors INH prophylaxis for 6 months (if INH-related hepatitis case fatality rate is <1% and TB case fatality is ≥6.7%, which appears to be the case, monitor transaminases monthly (*Arch Int Med*, 1990, 150:2517). |
| INH-resistant organisms likely | Rx indicated | Data on efficacy of alternative regimens is currently lacking. Regimens include ETB + RIF daily for 6 months. PZA + RIF daily for 2 months, then INH + RIF daily until sensitivities from index case (if available) known, then if INH-CR, discontinue INH and continue RIF for 9 months, otherwise INH + RIF for 9 months (this latter is *Am Acad Pediatrics*, 1991 recommendation). |
| INH + RIF resistant organisms likely | Rx indicated | Efficacy of alternative regimens is unknown; PZA (25-30 mg/kg/d P.O.) + ETB (15-25 mg/kg/d P.O.) (at 25 mg/kg ETB, monitoring for retrobulbar neuritis required), for 6 months unless HIV-positive, then 12 months; PZA + ciprofloxacin (750 mg P.O. bid) or ofloxacin (400 mg P.O. bid) x 6-12 months (*MMWR Morb Mortal Wkly Rep*, 1992, 41(RR11):68). |

INH = isoniazid; RIF = rifampin; KM = kanamycin; ETB = ethambutol

SM = streptomycin; CXR = chest x-ray; Rx = treatment

See also guidelines for interpreting PPD in "Skin Testing for Delayed Hypersensitivity" in the Appendix.

*Tuberculin test (TBnT). The standard is the Mantoux test, 5 TU PPD in 0.1 mL diluent stabilized with Tween 80. Read at 48-72 hours measuring maximum diameter of induration. A reaction ≥5 mm is defined as positive in the following: positive HIV or risk factors, recent close contacts, CXR consistent with healed TBc. ≥10 mm is positive in foreign-born in countries of high prevalence, injection drug users, low income populations, nursing home residents, patients with medical conditions which increase risk (see above, preventive treatment). ≥15 mm is positive in all others (*Am Rev Resp Dis*, 1990, 142:725). Two-stage TBnT: Use in individuals to be tested regularly (ie, healthcare workers). TBn reactivity may decrease over time but be boosted by skin testing. If unrecognized, individual may be incorrectly diagnosed as recent converter. If first TBnT is reactive but <10 mm, repeat 5 TU in 1 week, if then ≥10 mm = positive, not recent conversion (*Am Rev Resp Dis*, 1979, 119:587).

# OVERDOSE AND TOXICOLOGY INFORMATION

### General Stabilization of the Patient

The recommended treatment plan for the poisoned patient is not unlike general treatment plans taught in advanced cardiac life support (ACLS) or advanced trauma life support (ATLS) courses. In this manner, the initial approach to the poisoned patient should be essentially similar in every case, irrespective of the toxin ingested, just as the initial approach to the trauma patient is the same, irrespective of the mechanism of injury. This approach, which can be termed as routine poison management, essentially includes the following aspects.

- Stabilization: ABCs (airway, breathing, circulation; administration of glucose, thiamine, oxygen, and naloxone)

- History, physical examination leading toward the identification of class of toxin (toxidrome recognition)

- Prevention of absorption (decontamination)

- Specific antidote, if available

- Removal of absorbed toxin (enhancing excretion)

- Support and monitoring for adverse effects

### Laboratory Evaluation of Overdose

**Unknown ingestion:** Electrolytes, anion gap, serum osmolality, arterial blood gases, serum drug concentration

**Known ingestion:** Labs tailored to agent

### History and Physical Examination

While the history and physical examination is the cornerstone of clinical patient management, it takes on special meaning with regard to the toxic patient. While taking a history may be a more direct method of the determination of the toxin, quite often it is not reliable. Information obtained may prove minimal in some cases and could be considered partial or inaccurate in suicide gestures and addicts. A quick physical examination often leads to important clues about the nature of the toxin. These clues can be specific symptom complexes associated with certain toxins and can be referred to as "toxidromes".

### Prevention of Absorption

Toxic substances can enter the body through the dermal, ocular, pulmonary, parenteral, and gastrointestinal routes. The basic principle of decontamination involves appropriate copious irrigation of the toxic substances relatable to the route of exposure. For example, with ocular exposure, this can be done with normal saline for 30-40 minutes through a Morgan therapeutic lens. With alkali exposures, the pH should be checked until the runoff of the solution is either neutral or slightly acidic. Skin decontamination involves removal of the toxin with nonabrasive soap. This should especially be considered for organophosphates, methylene chloride, digoxin, radiation, hydrocarbons, and herbicide exposure. Separate drainage areas should be obtained for the contaminated runoff.

Since >80% of incidents of accidental poisoning in children occur through the gastrointestinal tract, a thorough knowledge of gastric decontamination is essential. There are essentially four modes of gastric decontamination, of which three are physical removal (emesis, gastric lavage, and whole bowel irrigation). Activated charcoal associated with a cathartic is the fourth mode of preventing absorption.

Emesis with syrup of ipecac: Adults: 30 mL. **Note:** Ipecac use is becoming less frequently recommended since <30% of the stomach is usually emptied and its use may delay the use of activated charcoal.

### Enhancement of Elimination

Only recently has this aspect of poison management received more than cursory attention in practice and in the literature. The standard practice for enhancement of elimination consisted primarily of forced diuresis in order to excrete the toxin. However, the past 10 years experience has produced a radical change in the approach to this and therefore, a more focused methodology to eliminating absorbed toxins. Essentially, there are three methods by which absorbed toxins may be eliminated: recurrent adsorption with multiple dosings of activated charcoal, use of forced diuresis in combination with possible alkalinization of the urine, and use of dialysis or charcoal hemoperfusion.

# OVERDOSE AND TOXICOLOGY INFORMATION *(Continued)*

## Specific Treatment

| Drug or Drug Class | Signs/Symptoms | Treatment/Comments |
|---|---|---|
| Acetaminophen | Generally asymptomatic | Assess severity of ingestion; adult doses ≥140 mg/kg are thought to be toxic. Obtain serum concentration ≥4 hours postingestion and use acetaminophen nomogram to evaluate need for acetylcysteine. Gastric decontamination within 2-4 hours after ingestion. May administer activated charcoal for one dose, this may decrease absorption of acetylcysteine if given within 1 hour of acetylcysteine. For unknown ingested quantities and for significant ingestion give acetylcysteine orally (diluted 1:4 with juice or carbonated beverage); initial: 140 mg/kg then give 70 mg/kg every 4 hours for 17 doses. I.V. protocols are used in some institutions. |
| Alpha-adrenergic blocking agents | Hypotension, drowsiness | Give activated charcoal, additional treatment if symptomatic; use I.V. fluids, dopamine, or norepinephrine to treat hypotension. Epinephrine may worsen hypotension due to beta effects. |
| Aminoglycosides | Ototoxicity, nephrotoxicity, neuromuscular toxicity | Hemodialysis or peritoneal dialysis may be useful in patients with decreased renal function; calcium may reverse the neuromuscular toxicity. |
| Anticholinergics, antihistamines | Coma, hallucinations, delirium, tachycardia, dry skin, urinary retention, dilated pupils | For life-threatening arrhythmias or seizures. Adults: 2 mg/dose physostigmine, may repeat 1-2 mg in 20 minutes and give 1-4 mg slow I.V. over 5-10 minutes if signs and symptoms recur (relatively contraindicated if QRS >0.1 msec). |
| Barbiturates | Respiratory depression, circulatory collapse, bradycardia, hypotension, hypothermia, slurred speech, confusion, coma | Repeated oral doses of activated charcoal given every 3-6 hours will increase clearance. Adults: 30-60 g. Assure GI motility, adequate hydration, and renal function. Urinary alkalinization with I.V. sodium bicarbonate will increase renal elimination of longer-acting barbiturates (eg, phenobarbital). Charcoal hemoperfusion may be required in severe overdose. |

## Specific Treatment (continued)

| Drug or Drug Class | Signs/Symptoms | Treatment/Comments |
|---|---|---|
| Benzodiazepines | Respiratory depression, apnea (after rapid I.V.), hypoactive reflexes, hypotension, slurred speech, unsteady gait, coma | Dialysis is of limited value; support blood pressure and respiration until symptoms subside. Flumazenil: Initial dose: 0.2 mg given I.V. over 30 seconds. If further response is desired after 30 seconds, give 0.3 mg over another 30 seconds. Further doses of 0.5 mg can be given over 30 seconds at 1-minute intervals up to a total of 3 mg. Continuous infusions may be used in rare instances since duration of benzodiazepines is longer than flumazenil. |
| Beta-adrenergic blockers | Hypotension, bronchospasm, bradycardia, hypoglycemia, seizures | Activated charcoal; treat symptomatically; glucagon, atropine, isoproterenol, dobutamine, or cardiac pacing may be needed to treat bradycardia, conduction defects, or hypotension. Continuous infusion of glucagon has been used in long-acting beta-blocker overdosage. |
| Carbamazepine | Dizziness, drowsiness, ataxia, involuntary movements, opisthotonos, seizures, nausea, vomiting, agitation, nystagmus, coma, urinary retention, respiratory depression, tachycardia, arrhythmias | Use supportive therapy, general poisoning management as needed. Use repeated oral doses of activated charcoal given every 3-6 hours to decrease serum concentrations. Charcoal hemoperfusion may be needed. Treat hypotension with I.V. fluids, dopamine, or norepinephrine. Monitor EKG. Diazepam may control convulsions but may exacerbate respiratory depression. |
| Cardiac glycosides | Hyperkalemia may develop rapidly and result in life-threatening cardiac arrhythmias, progressive bradyarrhythmias, second or third degree heart block unresponsive to atropine, ventricular fibrillation, asystole | Obtain serum drug level, induce emesis or perform gastric lavage. Give activated charcoal to reduce further absorption. Atropine may reverse heart block. Digoxin immune Fab (digoxin specific antibody fragments) is used in serious cases. Each 40 mg of digoxin immune Fab binds with 0.6 mg of digoxin. |
| Cholinergic | Nausea, vomiting, diarrhea, miosis, CNS depression, excessive salivation, excessive sweating, muscle weakness | Suction oral secretions, decontaminate skin, atropinize patient. Atropine dose must be individualized. Adults: Initial atropine dose: 1 mg; titrate dose upward. Pralidoxime (2-PAM) may need to be added for moderate to severe intoxications. |
| Heparin | Severe hemorrhage | 1 mg of protamine sulfate will neutralize approximately 90 units of heparin sodium (bovine) or 115 units of heparin sodium (porcine) or 100 units of heparin calcium (porcine). |
| Hydantoin derivatives | Nausea, vomiting, nystagmus, slurred speech, ataxia, coma | Gastric lavage or emesis; repeated oral doses of activated charcoal may increase clearance of phenytoin. Use 0.5-1 g/kg (30-60 g/dose) activated charcoal every 3-6 hours until nontoxic serum concentration is obtained. Assure adequate GI motility, supportive therapy. |

## OVERDOSE AND TOXICOLOGY INFORMATION *(Continued)*

### Specific Treatment *(continued)*

| Drug or Drug Class | Signs/Symptoms | Treatment/Comments |
|---|---|---|
| Iron | Lethargy, nausea, vomiting, green or tarry stools, hypotension, weak rapid pulse, metabolic acidosis, shock, coma, hepatic necrosis, renal failure, local GI erosions | If immediately after ingestion and not already vomiting, give ipecac or lavage with saline solution. Give deferoxamine mesylate I.V. at 15 mg/kg/hour in cases of severe poisoning (serum iron >350 µg/mL) until the urine color is normal, the patient is asymptomatic, or a maximum daily dose of 8 g is reached. Urine output should be maintained >2 mL/kg/hour to avoid hypovolemic shock. |
| Isoniazid | Nausea, vomiting, blurred vision, CNS depression, intractable seizures, coma, metabolic acidosis | Control seizures with diazepam. Give pyridoxine I.V. equal dose to the suspected overdose of isoniazid or up to 5 g empirically. Give activated charcoal. |
| Nonsteroidal anti-inflammatory drugs | Dizziness, abdominal pain, sweating, apnea, nystagmus, cyanosis, hypotension, coma, seizures (rarely) | Induce emesis. Give activated charcoal via NG tube. Fluid therapy is commonly effective in managing the hypotension that may occur following an acute NSAIDs overdose, except when this is due to an acute blood loss. Seizures tend to be very short-lived and often do not require drug treatment; although, recurrent seizures should be treated with I.V. diazepam. Since many of the NSAIDs undergo enterohepatic cycling, multiple doses of charcoal may be needed to reduce the potential for delayed toxicities. Provide symptomatic and supportive care. |
| Opioids and morphine analogs | Respiratory depression, miosis, hypothermia, bradycardia, circulatory collapse, pulmonary edema, apnea | Establish airway and adequate ventilation. Give naloxone 0.4 mg and titrate to a maximum of 10 mg. Additional doses may be needed every 20-60 minutes. May need to institute continuous infusion, as duration of action of opiates can be longer than duration of action of naloxone. |
| Phenothiazines | Deep unarousable sleep, anticholinergic symptoms, extrapyramidal signs, diaphoresis, rigidity, tachycardia, cardiac dysrhythmias, hypotension | Activated charcoal; do **not** dialyze. Use I.V. benztropine mesylate 1-2 mg/dose slowly over 3-6 minutes for extrapyramidal signs. Use I.V. fluids and norepinephrine to treat hypotension. Avoid epinephrine which may cause hypotension due to phenothiazine-induced alpha-adrenergic blockade and unopposed epinephrine $B_2$ action. Use benzodiazepines for seizure management and to decrease rigidity. |

## Specific Treatment *(continued)*

| Drug or Drug Class | Signs/Symptoms | Treatment/Comments |
|---|---|---|
| Salicylates | Nausea, vomiting, respiratory alkalosis, hyperthermia, dehydration, hyperapnea, tinnitus, headache, dizziness, metabolic acidosis, coma, hypoglycemia, seizures | Induce emesis or gastric lavage immediately. Give several doses of activated charcoal, rehydrate, and use sodium bicarbonate to correct metabolic acidosis and enhance renal elimination by alkalinizing the urine. Control hyperthermia by cooling blankets or sponge baths. Correct coagulopathy with vitamin K I.V. and platelet transfusions as necessary. Hypoglycemia may be treated with I.V. dextrose. Seizures should be treated with I.V. benzodiazepines (diazepam 5-10 mg I.V.). Give supplemental potassium after renal function has been determined to be adequate. Monitor electrolytes; obtain stat serum salicylate level and follow. |
| Tricyclic antidepressants | Agitation, confusion, hallucinations, urinary retention, hypothermia, hypotension, tachycardia, arrhythmias, seizures | Give activated charcoal ± lavage. Use sodium bicarbonate for QRS >0.1 msec; alkalinization by hyperventilation has been used in patients on mechanical ventilation; I.V. fluids and norepinephrine may be used for hypotension; benzodiazepines may be used for seizure management. |
| Warfarin | Internal or external hemorrhage, hematuria | For moderate overdoses, give oral, S.C., or I.D., or slow I.V. (I.V. associated with anaphylactoid reactions) phytonadione; usual dose: 2.5-10 mg, adjust per prothrombin time. For severe hemorrhage, give fresh frozen plasma or whole blood. See Warfarin monograph. |
| Xanthine derivatives | Vomiting, abdominal pain, bloody diarrhea, tachycardia, extrasystoles, tachypnea, tonic/clonic seizures | Give activated charcoal orally. Repeated oral doses of activated charcoal increase clearance. Use 0.5-1 g/kg (30-60 g/dose) of activated charcoal every 1-4 hours (depending on the severity of ingestion) until nontoxic serum concentrations are obtained. Assure adequate GI motility, supportive therapy. Charcoal hemoperfusion or hemodialysis can also be effective in decreasing serum concentrations and should be used if the serum concentration approaches 90-100 mcg/mL in acute overdoses. |

# ANIMAL AND HUMAN BITES

## Wound Management

**Irrigation:** Critically important; irrigate all penetration wounds using 20 mL syringe, 19 gauge needle and >250 mL 1% povidone iodine solution. This method will reduce wound infection by a factor of 20. When there is high risk of rabies, use viricidal 1% benzalkonium chloride in addition to the 1% povidone iodine. Irrigate wound with normal saline after antiseptic irrigation.

**Debridement:** Remove all crushed or devitalized tissue remaining after irrigation; minimize removal on face and over thin skin areas or anywhere you would create a worse situation than the bite itself already has; do not extend puncture wounds surgically — rather, manage them with irrigation and antibiotics.

**Suturing:** Close most dog bites if <8 hours (<12 hours on face); do not routinely close puncture wounds, or deep or severe bites on the hands or feet, as these are at highest risk for infection. Cat and human bites should not be sutured unless cosmetically important. Wound edge freshening, where feasible, reduces infection; minimize sutures in the wound and use monofilament on the surface.

**Immobilization:** Critical in all hand wounds; important for infected extremities.

**Hospitalization/I.V. Antibiotics:** Admit for I.V. antibiotics all significant human bites to the hand, especially closed fist injuries, and bites involving penetration of the bone or joint (a high index of suspicion is needed). Consider I.V. antibiotics for significant established wound infections with cellulitis or lymphangitis, any infected bite on the hand, any infected cat bite, and any infection in an immunocompromised or asplenic patient. Outpatient treatment with I.V. antibiotics may be possible in selected cases by consulting with infectious disease.

## Laboratory Assessment

**Gram's Stain:** Not useful prior to onset of clinically apparent infection; examination of purulent material may show a predominant organism in established infection, aiding antibiotic selection; not warranted unless results will change your treatment.

**Culture:** Not useful or cost effective prior to onset of clinically apparent infection.

**X-ray:** Whenever you suspect bony involvement, especially in craniofacial dog bites in very small children or severe bite/crush in an extremity; cat bites with their long needle like teeth may cause osteomyelitis or a septic joint, especially in the hand or wrist.

## Immunizations

**Tetanus:** All bite wounds are contaminated. If not immunized in last 5 years, or if not current in a child, give DPT, DT, Td, or TT as indicated. For absent or incomplete primary immunization, give 250 units tetanus immune globulin (TIG) in addition.

**Rabies:** In the U.S. 30,000 persons are treated each year in an attempt to prevent 1-5 cases. Domestic animals should be quarantined for 10 days to prove need for prophylaxis. High risk animal bites (85% of cases = bat, skunk, raccoon) usually receive treatment consisting of:

- human rabies immune globulin (HRIG): 20 units/kg I.M. (unless previously immunized with HDCV)
- human diploid cell vaccine (HDCV): 1 mL I.M. on days 0, 3, 7, 14, and 28 (unless previously immunized with HDCV - then give only first 2 doses)

Consult with Infectious Disease before ordering rabies prophylaxis.

## Bite Wounds and Prophylactic Antibiotics

**Parenteral vs Oral:** If warranted, consider an initial I.V. dose to rapidly establish effective serum levels, especially if high risk, delayed treatment, or if patient reliability is poor.

### Dog Bite:

1. Rarely get infected (~5%)
2. Infecting organisms: Coagulase-negative staph, coagulase-positive staph, alpha strep, diphtheroids, beta strep, *Pseudomonas aeruginosa*, gamma strep, *Pasteurella multocida*
3. Prophylactic antibiotics are seldom indicated. Consider for high risk wounds such as distal extremity puncture wounds, severe crush injury, bites occurring in cosmetically sensitive areas (eg, face), or in immunocompromised or asplenic patients.

**Cat Bite:**
1. Often get infected (~25% to 50%)
2. Infecting organisms: *Pasteurella multocida* (first 24 hours), coagulase-positive staph, anaerobic cocci (after first 24 hours)
3. Prophylactic antibiotics are indicated in all cases.

**Human Bite:**
1. Intermediate infection rate (~15% to 20%)
2. Infecting organisms: Coagulase-positive staph, alpha, beta, gamma strep, *Haemophilus*, *Eikenella corrodens*, anaerobic streptococci, *Fusobacterium*, *Veillonella*, bacteroides.
3. Prophylactic antibiotics are indicated in almost all cases except superficial injuries.

See attached table for prophylactic antibiotic summary.

### Bite Wound Antibiotic Regimens

| | Dog Bite | Cat Bite | Human Bite |
|---|---|---|---|
| **Prophylactic Antibiotics** | | | |
| Prophylaxis | No routine prophylaxis, consider if involves face or hand, or immunosuppressed or asplenic patients | Routine prophylaxis | Routine prophylaxis |
| Prophylactic antibiotic | Amoxicillin | Amoxicillin | Amoxicillin |
| Penicillin allergy | Doxycycline if >10 y or co-trimoxazole | Doxycycline if >10 y or co-trimoxazole | Doxycycline if >10 y or erythromycin and cephalexin* |
| **Outpatient Oral Antibiotic Treatment** (mild to moderate infection) | | | |
| Established infection | Amoxicillin and clavulanic acid | Amoxicillin and clavulanic acid | Amoxicillin and clavulanic acid |
| Penicillin allergy (mild infection only) | Doxycycline if >10 y | Doxycycline if >10 y | Cephalexin* or clindamycin |
| **Outpatient Parenteral Antibiotic Treatment** (moderate infections – single drug regimens) | | | |
| | Ceftriaxone | Ceftriaxone | Cefotetan |
| **Inpatient Parenteral Antibiotic Treatment** | | | |
| Established infection | Ampicillin + cefazolin | Ampicillin + cefazolin | Ampicillin + clindamycin |
| Penicillin allergy | Cefazolin* | Ceftriaxone* | Cefotetan* or imipenem |
| **Duration of Prophylactic and Treatment Regimens** | | | |
| Prophylaxis: 5 days | | | |
| Treatment: 10-14 days | | | |

*Contraindicated if history of immediate hypersensitivity reaction (anaphylaxis) to penicillin.

# BREAST-FEEDING AND DRUGS

Adapted from American Academy of Pediatrics Committee on Drugs:
"Transfer of Drugs and Other Chemicals Into Human Milk,"
*Pediatrics*, 1994, 93:137-50.

The following questions and options should be considered when prescribing drug therapy to lactating women (1) Is the drug therapy really necessary? Consultation between the pediatrician and the mother's physician can be most useful. (2) Use the safest drug, for example, acetaminophen rather than aspirin for analgesia. (3) If there is a possibility that a drug may present a risk to the infant, consideration should be given to measurement of blood concentrations in the nursing infant. (4) Drug exposure to the nursing infant may be minimized by having the mother take the medication just after she has breast-fed the infant and/or just before the infant is due to have a lengthy sleep period.

In tables 1-6, the fact that a pharmacologic or chemical agent does not appear on the lists is not meant to imply that it is not transferred into human milk or that it does not have an effect on the infant; it only indicates that there were no reports found in the literature.

### Table 1. Drugs That Are Contraindicated During Breast-Feeding

| Drug | Reason for Concern, Reported Sign or Symptom in Infant, or Effect on Lactation |
| --- | --- |
| Bromocriptine | Suppresses lactation; may be hazardous to the mother |
| Cocaine | Cocaine intoxication |
| Cyclophosphamide | Possible immune suppression; unknown effect on growth or association with carcinogenesis; neutropenia |
| Cyclosporine | Possible immune suppression; unknown effect on growth or association with carcinogenesis |
| Doxorubicin* | Possible immune suppression; unknown effect on growth or association with carcinogenesis |
| Ergotamine | Vomiting, diarrhea. convulsions (doses used in migraine medications) |
| Lithium | One-third to one-half therapeutic blood concentration in infants |
| Methotrexate | Possible immune suppression; unknown effect on growth or association with carcinogenesis; neutropenia |
| Phencyclidine (PCP) | Potent hallucinogen |
| Phenindone | Anticoagulant; increased prothrombin and partial thromboplastin time in one infant; not used in the United States |

*Drug is concentrated in human milk

### Table 2. Drugs of Abuse: Contraindicated During Breast-Feeding*

| | |
| --- | --- |
| Amphetamine† | Marijuana |
| Cocaine | Nicotine (smoking) |
| Heroin | Phencyclidine |

*The Committee on Drugs strongly believes that nursing mothers should not ingest any compounds listed in Table 2. Not only are they hazardous to the nursing infant, but they are also detrimental to the physical and emotional health of the mother. This list is obviously not complete; no drug of abuse should be ingested by nursing mothers even though adverse reports are not in the literature.

†Drug is concentrated in human milk

### Table 3. Radioactive Compounds That Require Temporary Cessation of Breast-Feeding*

| Drug | Recommended Time for Cessation of Breast-Feeding |
|---|---|
| Copper 64 ($^{64}$Cu) | Radioactivity in milk present at 50 h |
| Gallium 67 ($^{67}$Ga) | Radioactivity in milk present for 2 wk |
| Indium 111 ($^{111}$In) | Very small amount present at 20 h |
| Iodine 123 ($^{123}$I) | Radioactivity in milk present up to 36 h |
| Iodine 125 ($^{125}$I) | Radioactivity in milk present for 12 d |
| Iodine 131 ($^{131}$I) | Radioactivity in milk present 2-14 d, depending on study |
| Radioactive sodium | Radioactivity in milk present 96 h |
| Technetium-99m ($^{99m}$Tc), $^{99m}$Rc macroaggregates, $^{99m}$Tc O4 | Radioactivity in milk present 15 h to 3 d |

*Consult nuclear medicine physician before performing diagnostic study so that radionuclide that has shortest excretion time in breast milk can be used. Before study, the mother should pump her breast and store enough milk in freezer for feeding the infant; after study, the mother should pump her breast to maintain milk production but discard all milk pumped for the required time that radioactivity is present in milk. Milk samples can be screened by radiology departments for radioactivity before resumption of nursing.

### Table 4. Drugs Whose Effect on Nursing Infants Is Unknown But May Be of Concern

Psychotropic drugs, the compounds listed under antianxiety, antidepressant, and antipsychotic categories, are of special concern when given to nursing mothers for long periods. Although there are no case reports of adverse effects in breast-feeding infants, these drugs do appear in human milk and thus conceivably alter short-term and long-term central nervous system function.

| Antianxiety | Antidepressant | Antipsychotic |
|---|---|---|
| Diazepam | Amitriptyline | Chlorpromazine |
| Lorazepam | Amoxapine | Chlorprothixene |
| Midazolam | Desipramine | Haloperidol |
| Perphenazine | Dothiepin | Mesoridazine |
| Prazepam* | Doxepin | |
| Quazepam | Fluoxetine | **Miscellaneous** |
| Temazepam | Fluvoxamine | Chloramphenicol |
| | Imipramine | Metoclopramide* |
| | Trazodone | Metronidazole |
| | | Tinidazole |

*Drug is concentrated in human milk

### Table 5. Drugs That Have Been Associated With Significant Effects on Some Nursing Infants and Should Be Given to Nursing Mothers With Caution*

| Drug | Reported Effect |
|---|---|
| Aspirin (salicylates) | Metabolic acidosis (one case) |
| Clemastine | Drowsiness, irritability, refusal to feed, high-pitched cry, neck stiffness (one case) |
| Mesalamine | Diarrhea (one case) |
| Phenobarbital | Sedation; infantile spasms after weaning from milk-containing phenobarbital, methemoglobinemia (one case) |
| Primidone | Sedation, feeding problems |
| Sulfasalazine (salicylazosulfapyridine) | Bloody diarrhea (one case) |

*Measure blood concentration in the infant when possible.

## BREAST-FEEDING AND DRUGS *(Continued)*

### Table 6. Maternal Medication Usually Compatible With Breast-Feeding

Acebutolol
Acetaminophen
Acetazolamide
Acitretin
Acyclovir*
Alcohol (ethanol)
Allopurinol
Amoxicillin
Antimony
Atenolol
Atropine
Azapropazone (apazone)
Aztreonam
B₁ (thiamine)
B₆ (pyridoxine)
B₁₂
Baclofen
Barbiturate
Bendroflumethiazide
Bishydroxycoumarin
  (Dicumarol®)
Bromide
Butorphanol
Caffeine
Captopril
Carbamazepine
Carbimazole
Cascara
Cefadroxil
Cefazolin
Cefotaxime
Cefoxitin
Cefprozil
Ceftazidime
Ceftriaxone
Chloral hydrate
Chloroform
Chloroquine
Chlorothiazide
Chlorthalidone
Cimetidine*
Cisapride
Cisplatin
Clindamycin
Clogestone
Clomipramine
Codeine
Colchicine
Contraceptive pill with
  estrogen and
  progesterone
Cycloserine
D (vitamin)
Danthron
Dapsone

Dexbrompheniramine
  maleate with
  d-isoephedrine
Digoxin
Diltiazem
Dipyrone
Disopyramide
Domperidone
Dyphylline*
Enalapril
Erythromycin*
Estradiol
Ethambutol
Ethanol
Ethosuximide
Fentanyl
Flecainide
Flufenamic acid
Fluorescein
Folic acid
Gold salts
Halothane
Hydralazine
Hydrochlorothiazide
Hydroxychloroquine*
Ibuprofen
Indomethacin
Iodides
Iodine
Iodine (povidone-iodine/
  vaginal douche)
Iopanoic acid
Isoniazid
K₁ (vitamin)
Kanamycin
Ketorolac
Labetalol
Levonorgestrel
Lidocaine
Loperamide
Magnesium sulfate
Medroxyprogesterone
Mefenamic acid
Methadone
Methimazole (active
  metabolite of carbi-
  mazole)
Methocarbamol
Methyldopa
Methprylon
Metoprolol*
Metrizamide
Mexiletine
Minoxidil

Morphine
Moxalactam
Nadolol*
Nalidixic acid
Naproxen
Nefopam
Nifedipine
Nitrofurantoin
Norethynodrel
Norsteroids
Noscapine
Oxprenolol
Phenylbutazone
Phenytoin
Piroxicam
Prednisone
Procainamide
Progesterone
Propoxyphene
Propranolol
Propylthiouracil
Pseudoephedrine*
Pyridostigmine
Pyrimethamine
Quinidine
Quinine
Riboflavin
Rifampin
Scopolamine
Secobarbital
Senna
Sotalol
Spironolactone
Streptomycin
Sulbactam
Sulfapyridine
Sulfisoxazole
Suprofen
Terbutaline
Tetracycline
Theophylline
Thiopental
Thiouracil
Ticarcillin
Timolol
Tolbutamide
Tolmetin
Trimethoprim and sulfa-
  methoxazole
Triprolidine
Valproic acid
Verapamil
Warfarin
Zolpidem

*Drug is concentrated in human milk.

## Antimicrobial Agents Taken by Mothers That Are Not Compatible With Breast-Feeding or Are Cause for Concern

| Maternal Antimicrobial Agent | Reported Sign or Symptom in Infant or Possible Cause for Concern | Committee on Drugs Evaluation |
|---|---|---|
| Chloramphenicol | Possible idiosyncratic bone marrow suppression | Unknown effect |
| Metronidazole | *In vitro* mutagen; may discontinue breast-feeding 12-24 hours to allow excretion of dose when single-dose therapy is given to mother | Unknown effect |
| Ciprofloxacin | Theoretically may affect cartilage development of weight-bearing joints; case report of pseudomembranous colitis in a 2-month old nursing infant | Not evaluated |
| Norfloxacin, ofloxacin, lomefloxacin, cinoxacin, enoxacin | Theoretically may affect cartilage development of weight-bearing joints | Not evaluated |
| Isoniazid | None; acetyl metabolite also secreted; may be hepatotoxic | Usually compatible with breast-feeding |
| Nalidixic acid | Hemolysis in infant with G-6-PD* deficiency | Usually compatible with breast-feeding |
| Nitrofurantoin | Hemolysis in infant with G-6-PD* deficiency | Usually compatible with breast-feeding |
| Sulfapyridine | Caution in infant with jaundice or G-6-PD* deficiency, and in ill, stressed, or premature infant | Usually compatible with breast-feeding |
| Sulfisoxazole | Caution in infant with jaundice or G-6-PD* deficiency, and in ill, stressed, or premature infant | Usually compatible with breast-feeding |

*Glucose-6-phosphate dehydrogenase.

Adapted from the *1997 Red Book – Report of the Committee on Infectious Diseases*, 24th ed.

## Antimicrobial Agents Listed by the American Academy of Pediatrics (AAP) Committee on Drugs as Usually Compatible With Breast-Feeding*

| | |
|---|---|
| Acyclovir | Dapsone†‡ |
| Amoxicillin | Erythromycin§ |
| Aztreonam | Kanamycin |
| Cefadaroxil | Moxalactam |
| Cefazolin | Pyrimethamine |
| Cefotaxime | Quinine |
| Cefoxitin | Rifampin |
| Ceprozil | Streptomycin |
| Ceftazidime | Sulbactam |
| Ceftriaxone | Tetracycline‡¶ |
| Chloroquine | Ticarcillin |
| Clindamycin | Trimethoprim-sulfamethoxazole |

*American Academy of Pediatrics Committee on Drugs, The Transfer of Drugs and Other Chemicals Into Human Milk, *Pediatrics*, 1994, 93:137-50.
†Sulfonamide detected in infant's urine.
‡While not listed as such by the Committee on Drugs, some experts recommend that the drug should be avoided in lactating women.
§Concentrated in human milk.
¶Negligible absorption by infant.
Adapted from the *1997 Red Book – Report of the Committee on Infectious Diseases*, 24th ed.

# CONSTIPATION, TREATMENT OPTIONS

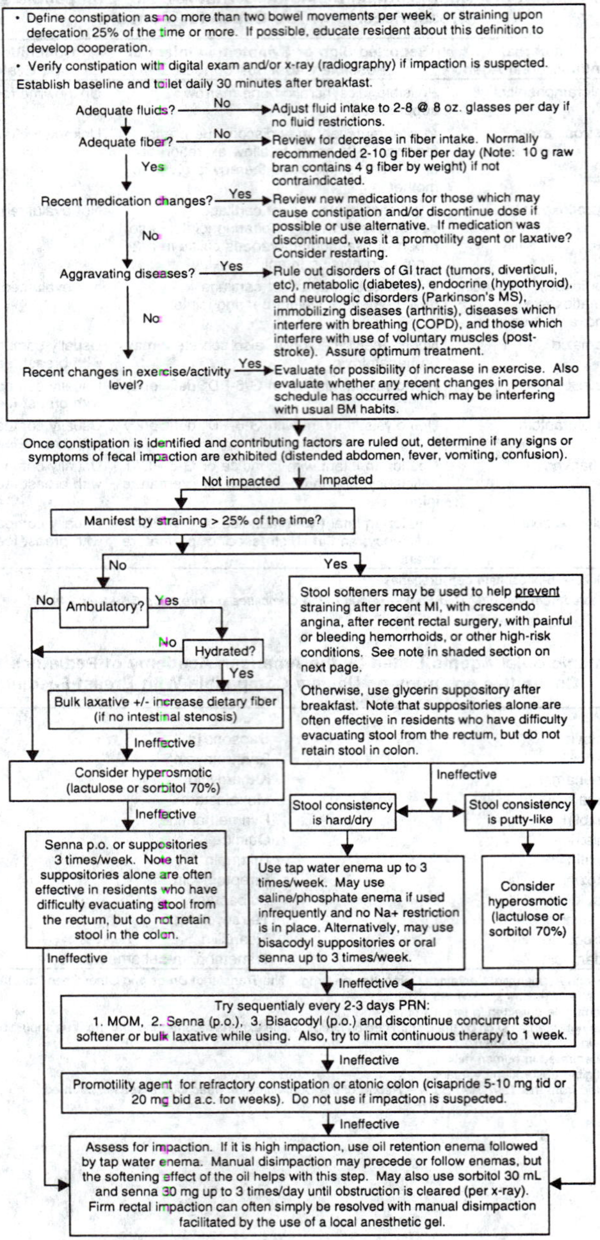

- Define constipation as no more than two bowel movements per week, or straining upon defecation 25% of the time or more. If possible, educate resident about this definition to develop cooperation.
- Verify constipation with digital exam and/or x-ray (radiography) if impaction is suspected.

Establish baseline and toilet daily 30 minutes after breakfast.

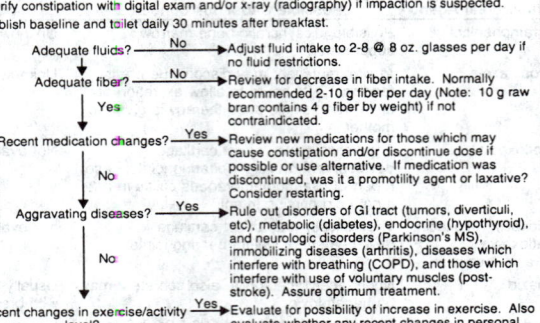

Adequate fluids? —No→ Adjust fluid intake to 2-8 @ 8 oz. glasses per day if no fluid restrictions.

Adequate fiber? —No→ Review for decrease in fiber intake. Normally recommended 2-10 g fiber per day (Note: 10 g raw bran contains 4 g fiber by weight) if not contraindicated.

Yes

Recent medication changes? —Yes→ Review new medications for those which may cause constipation and/or discontinue dose if possible or use alternative. If medication was discontinued, was it a promotility agent or laxative? Consider restarting.

No

Aggravating diseases? —Yes→ Rule out disorders of GI tract (tumors, diverticuli, etc), metabolic (diabetes), endocrine (hypothyroid), and neurologic disorders (Parkinson's MS), immobilizing diseases (arthritis), diseases which interfere with breathing (COPD), and those which interfere with use of voluntary muscles (post-stroke). Assure optimum treatment.

No

Recent changes in exercise/activity level? —Yes→ Evaluate for possibility of increase in exercise. Also evaluate whether any recent changes in personal schedule has occurred which may be interfering with usual BM habits.

Once constipation is identified and contributing factors are ruled out, determine if any signs or symptoms of fecal impaction are exhibited (distended abdomen, fever, vomiting, confusion).

Not impacted / Impacted

Manifest by straining > 25% of the time?

No / Yes

**No branch:**

No — Ambulatory? — Yes

No — Hydrated? — Yes

Bulk laxative +/- increase dietary fiber (if no intestinal stenosis)

Ineffective

**Yes branch:**

Stool softeners may be used to help <u>prevent</u> straining after recent MI, with crescendo angina, after recent rectal surgery, with painful or bleeding hemorrhoids, or other high-risk conditions. See note in shaded section on next page.

Otherwise, use glycerin suppository after breakfast. Note that suppositories alone are often effective in residents who have difficulty evacuating stool from the rectum, but do not retain stool in colon.

Ineffective

Consider hyperosmotic (lactulose or sorbitol 70%)

Ineffective

Senna p.o. or suppositories 3 times/week. Note that suppositories alone are often effective in residents who have difficulty evacuating stool from the rectum, but do not retain stool in the colon.

Ineffective

Stool consistency is hard/dry

Use tap water enema up to 3 times/week. May use saline/phosphate enema if used infrequently and no Na+ restriction is in place. Alternatively, may use bisacodyl suppositories or oral senna up to 3 times/week.

Stool consistency is putty-like

Consider hyperosmotic (lactulose or sorbitol 70%)

Ineffective

Try sequentially every 2-3 days PRN:
1. MOM, 2. Senna (p.o.), 3. Bisacodyl (p.o.) and discontinue concurrent stool softener or bulk laxative while using. Also, try to limit continuous therapy to 1 week.

Ineffective

Promotility agent for refractory constipation or atonic colon (cisapride 5-10 mg tid or 20 mg bid a.c. for weeks). Do not use if impaction is suspected.

Ineffective

Assess for impaction. If it is high impaction, use oil retention enema followed by tap water enema. Manual disimpaction may precede or follow enemas, but the softening effect of the oil helps with this step. May also use sorbitol 30 mL and senna 30 mg up to 3 times/day until obstruction is cleared (per x-ray). Firm rectal impaction can often simply be resolved with manual disimpaction facilitated by the use of a local anesthetic gel.

One should expect gradual rather than immediate results from a newly instituted laxative regimen. Additionally, nondrug interventions should be maintained during pharmacologic treatment of constipation as this is one of the cornerstones of long-term management.

**CONSTIPATING DRUGS**
Anticholinergics (antiparkinsons)
Antihistamines
Opiates
MAOIs
Tricyclic Antidepressants
Aluminum
Calcium (supplements & antacids)
Iron
Phenothiazines
Diuretics
Clonidine
Guanabenz
Guanfacine
Disopyramide
Irritant laxatives (with cathartic colon)
Anticonvulsants

**OPIOID-INDUCED CONSTIPATION**
Stimulant laxatives such as senna or bisacodyl in combination with a stool softener such as docusate sodium often serve as an effective first-line regimen. Senna p.o. up to 4 tablets 2-3 times/day may be needed. Next, bisacodyl tablets p.o. at bedtime and up to 2-3 times/day if needed. If desired, use docusate to augment the effect of one or both medications, especially if stool is hard. If impaction can be ruled out, use bisocodyl suppository followed by fleet enema (if needed). If impaction is suspected, see last step of pathway.

**STOOL SOFTENERS**
Stool softeners have no laxative action and are not helpful in alleviating chronic constipation and may cause fecal incontinence. Short-term use is appropriate to minimize straining caused by hard stools following rectal surgery or recent MI or when defecation causes hemorrhoidal pain, rectal bleeding, crescendo angina, or other high risk conditio.

**SALINE LAXATIVES**
Regular use of saline laxatives is not recommended because their risks outweigh the benefits of the laxative. Saline laxatives are only indicated for acute bowel evacuation for diagnostic procedures. Also, note that use of Milk of Magnesia in renally impaired residents can result in Mg++ toxicity (hypotension, muscle weakness, EKG changes, CNS changes).

**COMBINATION LAXATIVES**
Use of products containing two or more laxatives is not advised because of a lack of documented therapeutic benefit over use of a single ingredient. Additionally, risks may outweigh benefits.

**References**

Alessi CA and Henderson CT, "Constipation and Fecal Impaction in the Long-Term Care Patient," *Clin Geriatr Med,* 1988; 4:571-88.

Burke C, "Avoiding Problems of GI Dysmotility in Patients Treated for Chronic Pain," *ASCP* 1995 Symposia Highlights, 7-8.

Castle SC, "Constipation: Endemic in the Elderly," *Med Clin N Am* 1989; 73:1497.

Harari D, Gurwitz JH, and Minaker KL, "Constipation in the Elderly," *JAGS,* 1993; 41:1130-40.

Izard MW and Ellison FS, "Treatment of Drug Induced Constipation with a Purified Senna Derivative," *Conn Med,* 1962; 26:589.

Lange RL and DiPiro JT, *Pharmacotherapy,* 2nd ed, Norwalk, CT: Appleton & Lange, 1993.

Maguire LC, Yon JL, and Miller E, "Prevention of Narcotic-Induced Constipation," *N Eng J Med,* 1981; 305:1651.

Rousseau P, "Managing Constipation in the Elderly Population," *Fam Practice Recertification,* 1990; 12:76-95.

Szurszewski JH, Holt PR, and Schuster M, "Proceedings of a Workshop Entitled Neuromuscular Function and Dysfunction of the Gastrointestinal Tract in Aging," *Dig Dis Sci,* 1989; 34:1135.

Wrenn K, "Fecal Impaction," *N Engl J Med,* 1989; 321:658-61

# DISCOLORATION OF FECES
## DUE TO DRUGS

**Black**
Acetazolamide
Aluminum hydroxide
Aminophylline
Amphetamine
Amphotericin B
Bismuth salts
Chlorpropamide
Clindamycin
Corticosteroids
Cyclophosphamide
Cytarabine
Digitalis
Ethacrynic acid
Ferrous salts
Fluorouracil
Hydralazine
Hydrocortisone
Iodide-containing drugs
Melphalan

Methotrexate
Methylprednisolone
Phenylephrine
Potassium salts
Prednisolone
Procarbazine
Sulfonamides
Tetracycline
Theophylline
Thiotepa
Triamcinolone
Warfarin

**Blue**
Chloramphenicol
Methylene blue

**Green**
Indomethacin
Medroxyprogesterone

**Yellow/Yellow-Green**
Senna

**Orange-Red**
Phenazopyridine
Rifampin

**Pink/Red**
Anticoagulants
Aspirin
Barium
Heparin
Oxyphenbutazone
Phenylbutazone
Tetracycline syrup

**White/Speckling**
Antibiotics (oral)
Barium

# DISCOLORATION OF URINE
## DUE TO DRUGS

**Black/Brown/Dark**
Cascara
Chloroquine
Ferrous salts
Metronidazole
Nitrofurantoin
Quinine
Senna

**Blue**
Triamterene

**Blue-Green**
Amitriptyline
Methylene blue

**Orange/Yellow**
Heparin
Phenazopyridine
Rifampin
Sulfasalazine
Warfarin

**Red/Pink**
Daunorubicin
Doxorubicin
Heparin
Ibuprofen
Oxyphenbutazone
Phenylbutazone
Phenytoin
Rifampin
Senna

# DRUGS IN PREGNANCY

## MEDICATIONS KNOWN TO BE TERATOGENS

Alcohol
Androgens
Anticonvulsants
Antineoplastics
Diethylstilbestrol
Isotretinoin

Iodides
Live vaccines
Misoprostol
Tetracycline
Warfarin

## MEDICATIONS SUSPECTED TO BE TERATOGENS

Antithyroid drugs
Benzodiazepines
Estrogens
Fluoroquinolones

Lithium
Oral hypoglycemic drugs
Progestogens
Tricyclic antidepressants

## MEDICATIONS WITH NO KNOWN ADVERSE EFFECTS IN PREGNANCY*

Acetaminophen
Cephalosporins
Corticosteroids
Docusate sodium
Erythromycin

Multiple vitamins
Narcotic analgesics
Penicillins
Phenothiazines
Thyroid hormones

*These drugs appear to have minimal risk when used judiciously in usual doses under the supervision of a medical professional.

Adapted from DiPiro JT, Talbert RL, Hayes PE, et al, "Therapeutic Considerations During Pregnancy and Lactation," *Pharmacotherapy: A Pathophysiologic Approach*, 2nd ed, New York, NY: Elsevier, 1992.

# FACTORS AFFECTING PLASMA LEVELS OBTAINED FOR COMMON DRUGS

| Agent | Increased Levels | Decreased Levels |
|---|---|---|
| Aminoglycosides (amikacin, gentamicin, tobramycin) | Renal dysfunction, reduced volume of distribution (VD) | Pregnancy and early postpartum, ascites, burns |
| Carbamazepine | Enzyme inhibitors (eg, erythromycin, INH, propoxyphene) | Pregnancy, enzyme inducers (eg, phenytoin) |
| Digoxin | Renal dysfunction, severe CHF, hypothyroidism, drug intoxins | Malabsorption, hyperthyroidism |
| Lidocaine | CHF, liver disease, severe renal failure | |
| Lithium | NSAIDs, thiazide diuretics | Theophylline, pregnancy (2nd and 3rd trimester) |
| Nortriptyline | | Pregnancy, other states with increased VD |
| Phenytoin | Liver disease, disulfiram, INH | Renal failure (measure free levels), alcohol |
| Procainamide | Renal dysfunction, severe CHF, slow acetylator (NAPA/PA = 0.8 with normal renal function) | Fast acetylators (NAPA/PA = 1.2 with normal renal function) |
| Quinidine | Severe CHF, liver disease | Enzyme inducers (eg, phenytoin, Pb, rifampin) |
| Theophylline | CHF, liver disease, cor pulmonale, prolonged fever associated with viral illness, enzyme inhibitors (eg, cimetidine, cipro, verapamil, erythromycin) | Smoking, age <16, enzyme inducers (eg, rifampin, phenobarbital, carbamazepine, phenytoin) |
| Valproic acid | Liver cirrhosis, hypoalbuminemia | Induction of liver enzymes (Pb, phenytoin) |

# FEVER DUE TO DRUGS

| Most Common | Less Common | |
|---|---|---|
| Cephalosporins | Allopurinol | Hydralazine |
| Iodides | Antihistamines | Hydroxyurea |
| Isoniazid | Azathioprine | Ibuprofen |
| Methyldopa | Barbiturates | Mercaptopurine |
| Penicillins | Bleomycin | Nitrofurantoin |
| Phenytoin | Carbamazepine | Para-aminosalicylic acid |
| Procainamide | Cimetidine | Pentazocine |
| Quinidine | Cisplatin | Procarbazine |
| Streptomycin | Clofibrate | Propylthiouracil |
| Sulfas | Colistimethate | Sulindac |
| Vancomycin | Diazoxide | Streptozocin |
| | Folic acid | Triamterene |

Tabor PA, "Drug-Induced Fever," *Drug Intell Clin Pharm*, 1986, 20(6):413-20.

# FOOD-DRUG INTERACTIONS, KEY SUMMARY

| Drug | Food | Interaction |
|---|---|---|
| Acetaminophen | Watercress | Decreased levels of oxidative metabolites (mercapturate) of acetaminophen |
| Aspirin Azithromycin Captopril Didanosine Fosfomycin Isoniazid Mercaptopurine Methotrexate Methyldopa Penicillin G and V Phenobarbital Propantheline Rifampin Riluzole Tetracycline Valsartan | Any food | Decreased absorption |
| Carbamazepine Cefuroxime Hydralazine Lithium Metoprolol Propranolol | Any food | Increased absorption |
| Cyclosporine | Many foods | Decreased absorption |
| Acitretin Albendazole Atovaquone Beta-carotene Cyclosporine Etretinate Griseofulvin Halofantrine Isotretinoin Mefenamic acid Phenytoin Vitamin A Vitamin D Vitamin E Vitamin K | Dietary fat | Increased absorption |
| Biphosphonates (ie, etidronate, alendronate, tiludronate) | Foods with high mineral content (ie, milk) | Reduced absorption |
| Griseofulvin | High-fat meal | Faster absorption; increased serum levels by 50% |
| Misoprostol | High-fat meal | Reduced peak by delaying absorption |
| Pilocarpine (tablets) Zidovudine | High-fat meal | Reduced absorption |
| Cyclosporine Felodipine Nifedipine Nimodipine Nisoldipine Nitrendipine Verapamil | Grapefruit juice (naringen) | Increased absorption; increased oral bioavailability |
| Caffeine | Grapefruit juice (naringen) | Possibly prolongs caffeine's half-life |
| Coumarin | Grapefruit juice (naringen) | Delayed urinary excretion of 7-hydroxy-coumarin |
| Midazolam (oral) | Grapefruit juice (naringen) | Delayed absorption; increased bioavailability |
| Quinidine | Grapefruit juice (naringen) | Delayed absorption of quinidine; inhibits metabolism of quinidine |
| Terfenadine | Grapefruit juice (naringen) | Increases terfenadine bioavailability (can increase Q-T interval on EKG); increased absorption |
| Erythromycin stearate | Any food | Increased or decreased absorption |
| Furosemide | Any food | Decreased rate of absorption, potentially decreasing effect |
| Mercaptopurine | Any food | Decreased bioavailability by 30% |
| Isoniazid | Tuna, mackerel, salmon (dark meat fish) | Increased risk for scombroid fish poisoning |

| Drug | Food | Interaction |
|------|------|-------------|
| Levodopa | High-protein diet | Decreased absorption |
| Digoxin<br>Lovastatin | High fiber meal | Decreased absorption |
| Lithium | Sodium | Enhanced elimination requiring higher doses |
| Methyldopa | Iron | Reduced absorption |
| MAO inhibitors<br>Isocarboxazid<br>Phenelzine<br>Procarbazine<br>Tranylcypromine | High-protein foods that have undergone aging, fermentation, pickling, or smoking; aged cheeses, red wines, pods of broad beans and fava beans; bananas, raisins, avocados; caffeine-containing beverages, beer, ale, and chocolate | Elevated blood pressure |
| Phenobarbital<br>Phenytoin | High doses of vitamin $B_6$ (pyridoxine) and folic acid | Decreased absorption |
| Levodopa | Vitamin $B_6$ (pyridoxine) | Reduces blood level |
| Diprafenone<br>Felodipine<br>Hydralazine<br>Metoprolol<br>Nitrofurantoin<br>Propranolol | Any food | Increased bioavailability |
| Phenobarbital<br>Phenytoin<br>Theophylline<br>Warfarin | Charcoal-broiled foods | Increased metabolism requiring higher doses |
| Ketoconazole | Acidic beverages (pH <2.5, ie, Coca-Cola Classic®) | Increased absorption |
| Phenytoin | Most foods<br>Pudding | Absorption increased by 25%<br>Absorption decreased by 50% |
| Quinolones (eg, ciprofloxacin)<br>Minocycline<br>Tetracycline | Iron, calcium, aluminum, zinc, magnesium (eg, dairy products) | Decreased absorption |
| Quinidine | High salt (>400 mEq/day) | Increased first-pass hepatic elimination |
| Warfarin | Diets rich in vitamin K such as cauliflower, spinach, broccoli, turnip greens, liver, beans, rice, pork, fish, and some cheeses | Antagonism of effect |

Reprinted with permission from Saltiel E, "Food-Drug Interactions," *New Developments in Medicine & Drug Therapy*, Glenview, IL: Physicians & Scientists Publishing Co, Inc, 1994, 3(4):61.

D'Arcy PF, "Nutrient-Drug Interactions," *Adverse Drug React Toxicol Rev*, 1995, 14(4):233-54.

# HCFA GUIDELINES FOR UNNECESSARY DRUGS IN LONG-TERM CARE FACILITIES

## Procedures: §483.25(1)(1)

Consider drug therapy "unnecessary" only after determining that the facility's use of the drug is:

- in excessive dose (including duplicate drug therapy)
- for excessive duration
- without adequate monitoring
- without adequate indications of use
- in the presence of adverse consequences which indicate the dose should be reduced or discontinued, or
- any combination of the reasons above

Allow the facility the opportunity to provide a rationale for the use of drugs prescribed outside the preceding guidelines. The facility may not justify the use of a drug prescribed outside the proceeding guidelines solely on the basis of "the doctor ordered it." This justification would render the regulation meaningless. The rationale must be based on sound risk-benefit analysis of the resident's symptoms and potential adverse effects of the drug.

Examples of evidence that would support a justification of why a drug is being used outside these guidelines but in the best interests of the resident may include, but are not limited to:

- a physician's note indicating for example, that the dosage, duration, indication, and monitoring are clinically appropriate, **and the reasons why they are clinically appropriate**; this note should demonstrate that the physician has carefully considered the risk/benefit to the resident in using drugs outside the guidelines

- a medical or psychiatric consultation or evaluation (eg, geriatric depression scale) that confirms the physician's judgment that use of a drug outside the guidelines is in the best interest of the resident

- physician, nursing, or other health professional documentation indicating that the resident is being monitored for adverse consequences or complications of the drug therapy

- documentation confirming that previous attempts at dosage reduction have been unsuccessful

- documentation (including MDS documentation) showing resident's subjective or objective improvement, or maintenance of function while taking the medication

- documentation showing that a resident's decline or deterioration is evaluated by the interdisciplinary team to determine whether a particular drug, or a particular dose, or duration of therapy, may be the cause

- documentation showing why the resident's age, weight, or other factors would require a unique drug dose or drug duration, indication, monitoring, and

- other evidence the survey team may deem appropriate

If the survey team determines that there is a deficiency in the use of antipsychotics, cite the facility under either the "unnecessary drug" regulation or the "antipsychotic drug" regulation, but not both.

**Note:** The unnecessary drug criterion of "adequate indications for use" does not simply mean that the **physician's order** must include a reason for using the drug (although such order writing is encouraged). It means that the **resident** lacks a valid clinical reason for use of the drug as evidenced by the survey team's evaluation of some, but not necessarily all, of the following: resident assessment, plan of care, reports of significant change, progress notes, laboratory reports, professional consults, drug orders, observation and interview of the resident, and other information.

# HERBALS THAT MAY ALTER METABOLISM AND GI ABSORPTION OF DRUGS

| Herbal Medications That May Alter Metabolism | Herbals Medications That May Alter GI Absorption |
|---|---|
| Virginia snakeroot, Serpenteria (*Aristolochia serpenteria*) | California buckeye (*Aesculus californica*) |
| Indian root, Raiz del indio (*Aristolochia watson* | Ohio buckeye (*Aesculus glabra*) |
| Sagebrush (*Artemisia tridentata*) | Horse chestnut (*Aesculus hippocastanum*) |
| Common barberry (*Berberis vulgaris*) | Aloe |
| Button bush (*Cephalanthus*) | Uva, ursi, mananzanita, bearberry (*Arctostaphylos*) |
| Greater celandine (*Chelidonium*) | Cayenne, African bird peppers (*Capsicum*) |
| Balmony, turtlehead (*Chelone*) | Sodium copper chlorophyllin, chlorophyll |
| Fringetree (*Chionanthus*) | Mormon tea, American ephedra, canutillo (*Ephedra viridis*) |
| Wahoo, Burning bush (*Euonymus*) | Rhamnus frangula, buckthorn |
| Goldenseal (*Hydrastis*) | Maravilla (*Mirabilis multifulorum*) |
| Blue flag (*Iris versicolor*) | Wager ash, hop tree (*Ptelea*) |
| Veronicastrum, Culver's root (*Leptandra*) | California buckthorn (*Rhamnus californica*) |
| Oregon grape, Algerita (*Mahonia*) | Buckthorn (*Rhamnus frangula*) |
| American mandrake (*Podophyllum*) | Cascara sagrada (*Rhamnus purshiana*) |
| | Senna |
| | Yucca |

# NATURAL/HERBAL PRODUCTS AND DIETARY SUPPLEMENTS

Adapted from Wynn RL, Meiller TF, and Crossley HL, *Drug Information Handbook for Dentistry*, 4th ed, Hudson, OH: Lexi-Comp, Inc, 1998.

Medical problem: " I have a toothache."

2000 BC response: "Here, eat this root."

1000 AD: "That root is heathen; here, say this prayer."

1850 AD: "That prayer is superstitious; here, drink this potion."

1940 AD: "That potion is snake oil; here, swallow this pill."

1985 AD: "That pill is ineffective; here, take this new antibiotic."

2000 AD: "That antibiotic is artificial; here, eat this root."

Adapted from an anonymous Internet communication.

## INTRODUCTION

For centuries, Eastern and Western civilizations have attributed a large number of medical uses to plants and herbs. Over time, modern scientific methodologies have emerged from some of these remedies. Conversely, some of these agents have fallen into less popularity as more medical knowledge has evolved. In spite of this dichotomy, herbal and natural therapies for treatment of common medical ailments have become exceedingly popular. In America, people consistently seek out natural products that may be able to offset some perceived ailment or may assist in the prevention of an ailment. One area that has consistently drawn patients interested in herbal or natural remedies has been the area of weight loss. There are numerous systemic considerations when some of the natural products that have been attributed weight loss powers are utilized. Many of these products are sold under the blanket of dietary supplements and, therefore, avoid some of the more stringent Food and Drug Administration legislation. In 1994, that legislation was modified to include herbs, vitamins, minerals, and amino acids that may be taken as dietary supplements and that information must be available to patients taking them. The real concern, however, lies in the fact that health claims need not be approved by the FDA, but the advertisements must include a disclaimer saying that the product has not yet been fully evaluated. Claims of medicinal use/value are often drawn from popular use, not necessarily from scientific studies. The safety, however, when these agents are taken in combination with other prescription drugs is of concern and medical risk might result. Many of these natural products may have real medicinal value but caution on the part of the clinician is prudent. It is impossible within this chapter to cover all of the popular natural products. The chapter, therefore, has been limited to brief reviews of some of the most popular dietary supplements, herbs, and natural remedies currently being used by patients you might treat and what we know about the effects of some of these agents on the body's various systems. An extensive reading list is provided.

## TOP 20 MOST POPULAR NATURAL PRODUCTS

### ALFALFA

Alfalfa has been touted as a natural laxative, an antifungal, a liver detoxifier, a diuretic, and a food additive useful in treating kidney stones and urinary infections. Alfalfa is an important animal feed worldwide and its chemical constituents are well known. However, studies have concluded that alfalfa contains nothing of significant therapeutic value in the amounts generally recommended. The seed contains L-canabanine which has been implicated in pancytopenia in humans and may induce systemic lupus in monkeys. Allergic reactions have been provoked in some users.

## ALOE VERA

Products derived from this plant have been used for centuries. Aloe is popularly used as a cure-all and it has been advertised for use in treating acne, burns, and minor wounds. Although the FDA does not recognize the uses of aloe for the treatment of any specific condition, there is evidence to suggest that fresh aloe gel is an effective agent in wound healing. Data to support these claims are inconclusive, however, and the use of aloe by patients should not interfere with care.

## BILBERRY

Bilberry, also known as blueberry, is recommended by herbalists for use in connection with vascular and blood disorders and in treating varicose veins, thromboses, diarrhea, and angina. Preliminary studies have indicated that bilberry may have some benefit in aiding visual acuity, however, there is little clinical evidence to support the widespread usage. Potential interactions with over-the-counter prescription medications are unknown at this time.

## CAYENNE

Most cooks know of the chemical cayenne that is the active ingredient in chili pepper and lends itself to the strong taste of this herb. Cayenne has been known for many years to stimulate digestion and to promote sweating; sometimes assisting, therefore, in reducing fever. Cayenne contains an ingredient known as capsaicin which is the active ingredient in many over-the-counter and prescription forms of cream to treat arthritis. Capsaicin appears to alter the action of the compound associated with pain, the mechanism of which has not been completely studied.

## CHAMOMILE

This agent is often found in the form of dried leaves that can be used to create a tea. The tea is taken internally and has been recommended by naturalists as a cure for stomach pain, menstrual discomfort, and stress. Chamomile teas appear to have some unknown mechanism of immune activation, perhaps due to the presence of flavonoids in the compound.

## CRANBERRY

Cranberry has been used for centuries as an agent to assist in treatment of urinary tract infections. Cranberry juices contain a pH-altering chemical which may be of use in treating these infections. It is now thought that the cranberry actually prevents bacteria from adhering to the lining of the bladder and urinary tract. Again, this agent is rich in flavonoids, citric acids, and vitamin C.

## ECHINACEA

Echinacea is reported to have uses for treatment of colds, flu, bacterial and fungal infections, and even cancer. AIDS patients are sometimes advised by their peers to take echinacea. To date, pharmacological components and their actions on the human body are unclear. However, complex polysaccharides are found in the agent and seem to hold some promise as compounds for immunostimulation. In general, echinacea appears to be relatively safe but clinical information is lacking.

## EPHEDRA

Also known as ma-huang, ephedra has been used in China for more than 4000 years to treat symptoms of upper respiratory infections and asthma. Ephedra can be used as a nasal decongestant and has recently gained new popularity as a weight loss product. This agent, when used in combination with St John's Wort, apparently has effects on serotonin levels similar to the drug fenfluramine which was recently taken off the market. This combination of drugs has been known as natural fen-phen. Ephedra has also been recommended as an aphrodisiac.

## FEVERFEW

Feverfew has a long history of use in traditional and cult medicine as a treatment for fever, headache, and menstrual irregularities. More recently, it has been suggested for migraine headaches, arthritis, and insect bites. Be aware that

## NATURAL/HERBAL PRODUCTS AND DIETARY SUPPLEMENTS
*(Continued)*

patients may self-medicate with feverfew in an effort to treat migraine head-aches. One study of commercially available feverfew products has found that there is a lactone present that appears to have some activity. However, there are no long-term toxicology studies to indicate or refute this claim.

### GARLIC
Garlic and related products have been used for thousands of years. It is gener-ally considered by herbalists and naturalists as a cure-all. When garlic is crushed, it produces allicin which possesses some antibiotic, antiplatelet, anticholesterol properties. In addition, other sulfur-containing compounds are found in garlic and these produce some antithrombotic properties. For the most part, the consumption of moderate amounts of garlic is harmless. Large doses, however, are likely to stimulate heartburn and gastric or intestinal disorders.

### GINGER
Ginger has been taken for centuries due to its calming effects on an upset stomach. The stem of the rhizome from a tropical plant has been used to make the ginger root. Today it is widely used for morning sickness, seasickness, and motion sickness. Ginger may have some effect on cholesterol levels although further study is necessary. The presence of essential oils in ginger may be the active ingredients in this agent.

### GINKGO BILOBA
Ginkgo supplements are claimed by herbalists to help with the aging process and with mental acuity. The most popular of these agents is used as an extract to promote improved blood flow to a portion of the body. Clinical research has not proven that these claims are or are not true.

### GINSENG
Ginseng is commonly used as a substance to support general good health and has also been marketed in some countries as an aphrodisiac. As with the majority of herbal agents, there are few clinical studies. However, commercial products vary widely and the clinician may be aware that ginseng could produce some side effects.

### GREEN TEA
Green tea has been widely used in Asia to treat numerous ailments. This tea is derived from leaves and delicate leaf buds of an evergreen bush. It is thought that green tea has some antioxidant effect, as well as containing compounds and flavonoids as with many of the other herbs.

### KAVA
Kava is one of the most popular herbs on today's market. It is extracted from a root and is used to promote sleep and relaxation in anxious patients. This agent appears to be extremely safe, however, the full effect of the active ingredient know as kavalactones, is unknown. They appear to have an effect on the neural transmitter activity in the central nervous system.

### LICORICE
Licorice has been used for centuries to treat intestinal disorders and stomach distress. There appears to be some activity of licorice on patients who suffer from mild preulcerous conditions in the GI tract. Again, the flavonoids appear to be an active component.

### PSYLLIUM
Psyllium has been used by herbalists and natural product advocates to promote regular intestinal function, primarily as an agent to assist in constipation and in GI distress.

### ST JOHN'S WORT
St John's wort has become popular in the treatment of depression, anxiety, and even in AIDS. While some of the constituents seem to show a minimal amount of

antidepressant activity, other components may suggest that St John's wort is ineffective in treating these illnesses.

## SAW PALMETTO

Saw palmetto was an official drug used for a variety of ailments, mainly associated with urogenital disorders. It has actually been shown to have some efficacy in managing benign prostate hypertrophy. The drug, however, has not yet passed any of the rigid FDA requirements prior to being able to substantiate this claim.

## VALERIAN

Valerian has, for centuries, made claims of being a natural tranquilizer, a relaxant for pain and muscle spasms, as well as promoting restful sleep. Be aware that some patients may be drawn to use valerian in an effort to reduce TMD dysfunction or muscle pain.

Herbalists have often used these natural products singularly or in combination to achieve a therapeutic effect. Some of the natural agents have been combined for assisted weight loss or for reduction of more serious ailments such as high blood pressure or cardiovascular disease. One such combination recommends ephedra and St John's wort as a "natural fen-phen". These agents are not directly related to fenfluramine, but are thought to also act on serotonin levels in the brain. Be aware that there are some known interactions of these agents with drug therapies that may be used. However, our knowledge is extremely limited in this extent.

# EFFECTS ON VARIOUS SYSTEMS

## CENTRAL NERVOUS SYSTEM

### (Aconite, Ginseng, Xanthine derivatives)

Aconite and hawthorn have potentially sedating effects, and aconite also contains various alkaloids and traces of ephedrine. Some documented central nervous system (CNS) effects of aconite include sedation, vertigo, and incoordination. Hawthorn has been reported to exert a depressive effect on the CNS leading to sedation.

Ginseng, ma-huang, and xanthine derivatives can exert a stimulant effect on the central nervous system. Some of the CNS effects of ginseng include nervousness, insomnia, and euphoria. The action of ma-huang is due to the presence of ephedrine and pseudoephedrine. Ma-huang exerts a stimulant action on the CNS similar to decongestant/weight loss products (Dexatrim®, etc) thus causing nervousness, insomnia, and anxiety. Kola nut, green tea, guarana, and yerba mate contain varying amounts of caffeine, a xanthine derivative. Stimulant properties exerted by these herbs are expected to be comparable to those of caffeine, including insomnia, nervousness, and anxiety.

Products containing aconite and hawthorn should be used with caution in patients with known history of depression, vertigo, or syncope. Ginseng or xanthine derivatives should be avoided in patients with history of insomnia or anxiety. Use of natural products with these components may contribute to a worsening of a patient's pre-existing medical condition. Patients taking CNS-active medications should avoid or use extreme caution when using preparations containing any of the above components. These components may interact directly or indirectly with CNS-active medications causing an increase or decrease in overall effect.

**NATURAL/HERBAL PRODUCTS AND DIETARY SUPPLEMENTS**
*(Continued)*

# CARDIOVASCULAR SYSTEM

## CONGESTIVE HEART FAILURE

### (Diuretics, Xanthine derivatives, Licorice, Ginseng, Aconite)

*Alisma plantago*, bearberry (*Arctostaphylos uva-ursi*), buchu (*Barosma betulina*), couch grass, dandelion, horsetail rush, juniper, licorice, and xanthine derivatives exert varying degrees of diuretic action. Many patients with congestive heart failure (CHF) are already taking a diuretic medication. By taking products containing one or more of these components, patients already on diuretic medications may increase their risk for dehydration.

Ginseng and licorice can potentially worsen congestive heart failure and edema by causing fluid retention. Aconite has varying effects on the heart that itself could lead to heart failure. Patients with CHF should be advised to consult with their healthcare provider before using products containing any of these components.

## HYPERTENSION/HYPOTENSION

### (Diuretics, Ginkgo Biloba, Ginseng, Hawthorn, Ma-huang, Xanthine derivatives)

The stimulant properties of ginseng and ma-huang could worsen pre-existing hypertension. Elevated blood pressure has been reported as a side effect of ginseng. Although ma-huang contains ephedrine, a known vasoconstrictor, ma-huang's effect on blood pressure varies between individuals. Ma-huang can cause hypotension or hypertension. Due to its unpredictable effects, patients with pre-existing hypertension should use caution when using natural products containing ma-huang. Providers should caution patients with labile hypertension against the use of ginseng.

The diuretic effect of xanthine derivatives and other diuretic components could increase the effects of antihypertensive medications, increasing the risk for hypotension. Hawthorn and ginkgo biloba can cause vasodilation increasing the hypotensive effects of antihypertensive medication. Patients susceptible to hypotension or patients taking antihypertensive medication should use caution when taking products containing xanthine derivatives or diuretics. Patients with pre-existing hypertension or hypotension who wish to use products containing these components should be closely monitored by a healthcare professional for changes in blood pressure control.

## ARRHYTHMIAS

### (Ginseng)

It has been reported that ginseng may increase the risk of arrhythmias, although it is unclear whether this effect is due to the actual ingredient (ginseng) or other possible impurities. Patients at risk for arrhythmias should be cautioned against the use of products containing ginseng without first consulting with their healthcare provider.

# GASTROINTESTINAL SYSTEM

## PEPTIC ULCER DISEASE

### (Betaine Hydrochloride, White Willow)

Betaine hydrochloride is a source of hydrochloric acid. The acid released from betaine hydrochloride could aggravate an existing ulcer. White willow, like aspirin, contains salicylates.

Aspirin has been known to induce gastric damage by direct irritation on the gastric mucosa and by an indirect systemic effect. As a result, patients with a history of peptic ulcer disease or gastritis are informed to avoid use of aspirin and other salicylate derivatives. These precautions should also apply to white willow. Patients with a history of peptic ulcer disease or gastritis should not use products containing white willow or betaine hydrochloride as either could exacerbate ulcers.

## INFLAMMATORY BOWEL DISEASE

### (Cascara Sagrada, Senna, Dandelion)

Cascara sagrada and senna are stimulant laxatives. Their laxative effect is exerted by stimulation of peristalsis in the colon and by inhibition of water and electrolyte secretion. The laxative effect produced by these herbs could induce an exacerbation of inflammatory bowel disease. Patients with a history of inflammatory bowel disease should avoid using products containing cascara sagrada or senna, and use caution when taking products containing dandelion which may also have a laxative effect.

## OBSTRUCTION/ILEUS

### (Glucomannan, Kelp, Psyllium)

Glucomannan, kelp, and psyllium act as bulk laxatives. In the presence of water, bulk laxatives swell or form a viscous solution adding extra bulk in the gastrointestinal tract. The resulting mass is thought to stimulate peristalsis. In the presence of an ileus, these laxatives could cause an obstruction.

If sufficient water is not consumed when taking a bulk laxative, a semisolid mass can form resulting in an obstruction. Any patient who wishes to take a natural product containing kelp, psyllium, or glucomannan should drink sufficient water to decrease the risk of obstruction. This may be of concern in particular disease states such as CHF or other cases where excess fluid intake may influence the existing disease presentation. Patients with a suspected obstruction or ileus should avoid using products containing kelp, psyllium, or glucomannan without consent of their primary healthcare provider.

# HEMATOLOGIC SYSTEM

## ANTICOAGULATION THERAPY & COAGULATION DISORDERS

### (Horsetail Rush, Ginseng, Ginkgo Biloba, Guarana, White Willow)

Horsetail rush, ginseng, ginkgo biloba, guarana, and white willow can potentially affect platelet aggregation and bleeding time. Ginkgo biloba, ginseng, guarana, and white willow inhibit platelet aggregation resulting in an increase in bleeding time. Horsetail rush, on the other hand, may decrease bleeding time. Patients with coagulation disorders or patients on anticoagulation therapy may be sensitive to the effects on coagulation by these components and should, therefore, avoid use of products containing any of these components.

# ENDOCRINE SYSTEM

## DIABETES MELLITUS

### (Chromium, Glucomannan, Ginseng, Hawthorn, Ma-huang, Periploca, Spirulina)

Ma-huang and spirulina both may increase glucose levels. This could cause a decrease in glucose control, thereby, increasing a patient's risk for hyperglycemia. Patients with diabetes or glucose intolerance should avoid using ma-huang and spirulina containing products.

Chromium, ginseng, glucomannan, periploca (*gymneme sylvestre*), and hawthorn should be used with caution in patients being treated for diabetes. These ingredients may reduce glucose levels increasing the risk for hypoglycemia in patients who are already taking a hypoglycemic agent. Patients with diabetes who wish to use products containing these ingredients should be closely monitored for fluctuations in blood glucose levels.

## NATURAL/HERBAL PRODUCTS AND DIETARY SUPPLEMENTS
*(Continued)*

## OTHER

### PHENYLKETONURIA

### (Aspartame, Spirulina)

Patients with phenylketonuria should not use products containing aspartame or spirulina. Aspartame, a common artificial sweetener, is metabolized to phenylalanine, while spirulina contains phenylalanine.

### GOUT

### (Diuretics, White Willow)

Patients with a history of gout should avoid using natural products containing components with diuretic action or white willow. By increasing urine output, ingredients with diuretic action may concentrate uric acid in the blood increasing the risk of gout in these patients. White willow, like aspirin, may inhibit excretion of urate resulting in an increase in uric acid concentration. The increase in urate levels could cause precipitation of uric acid resulting in an exacerbation of gout.

## Natural/Herbal Products

| Herb | Use(s) | Administration | Adverse Effects | Clinical Considerations |
|---|---|---|---|---|
| ALOE | External: Burns/sunburn, wounds, skin irritation; antimicrobial, moisturizer Internal: Laxative, general healing | External: Aloe vera gel, applied liberally Internal: Aloe vera juice (not recommended, but if used, no more than 1 quart/day should be consumed) | External: Contact dermatitis Internal: Painful intestinal contractions | External: May delay healing of deep, vertical (surgical) wounds Internal: Loss of intestinal potassium with resulting decrease in serum potassium which may potentiate effects of cardiac glycosides and antiarrhythmics; decreased serum potassium is potentiated by concurrent use of thiazides, steroids, licorice, and other potassium-wasting drugs; avoid if pregnant |
| BILBERRY | Eye disorders (including day and night vision), cataracts, macular degeneration, diabetic retinopathy | 20-40 mg 3 times/day (calculated as anthocyanidin); bilberry tea | None reported | Inhibits platelet aggregation (monitor patients on antiplatelet drugs and warfarin); lowers blood glucose (monitor patients with diabetes mellitus |
| CAYENNE | External: Pain disorders, including shingle, stump pain, diabetic neuropathy, cluster headache, osteoarthritis, and rheumatoid arthritis Internal: Stomach protectant, thermogenesis | External: 0.025% to 0.075% capsaicin-containing preparation 4 times/day Internal: Liberally or as tolerated in diet | External: Initial transient, local burning Internal: Stomach upset, diarrhea, burning during bowel movements | Remove cayenne from hands with vinegar; eat bananas to decrease GI irritation from ingesting cayenne; protects stomach against NSAID damage by stimulating GI secretions of mucus if given 30 minutes before NSAID; reduces platelet aggregation and increases fibrinolytic activity; monitor patients on antiplatelet drugs and warfarin |
| CHAMOMILE | Antispasmodic: Upset stomach and indigestion Sedative: Sleep, nerve calming Anti-inflammatory: Skin problems and muscle stiffness | Tea or compress: Steep 2 tsp of fresh or dried flowers in 1 pint boiling water for 20 minutes; drink 3-4 cups/day | Hypersensitivity: Sneezing, dermatitis, and anaphylaxis; large amounts may cause GI upset | May be ingested regularly for accumulation and subsequent effect; potential for delaying concomitant drug absorption from the gut |
| DONG QUAI | Amenorrhea, dysmenorrhea, and menopause (especially hot flashes) | Powdered root or tea: 1-2 g 3 times/day Tincture (1:5): 1 teaspoonful 3 times/day Fluid extract: 1 mL (1/4 teaspoonful) 3 times/day | Sunburn from Angelica archangelica sp.; decreases blood pressure; possible CNS stimulation | Some species are phototoxic, resulting in rash or extreme sunburn (phototoxicity may be useful in patients with psoriasis); possible synergism with calcium channel blockers; inhibits platelet aggregation (monitor warfarin patients) |
| ECHINACEA | General infectious conditions from virus, bacteria, and Candida sp.; influenza, colds, upper respiratory tract infections, and urogenital infections; also snake bites | Fluid extract (1:1): 1-2 mL 3 times/day (1/4-1/2 teaspoonful) Solid extract (6.5:1): 300 mg 3 times/day | Tingling sensation on tongue; fever from freshly pressed juice; cross-sensitivity in patients allergic to sunflower seeds | Continual use not recommended; avoid in patients with autoimmune disease (eg, rheumatoid arthritis and lupus) or leukemia |

# NATURAL/HERBAL PRODUCTS AND DIETARY SUPPLEMENTS
*(Continued)*

## Natural/Herbal Products *(continued)*

| Herb | Use(s) | Administration | Adverse Effects | Clinical Considerations |
|---|---|---|---|---|
| FEVERFEW | Prophylactic for migraine headache; relieves fever and arthritis | 25-100 mg dry powdered leaf capsules (standardized to 0.25-0.5 mg parthenolide)/day or 2-3 leaves/day | Aphthous ulcers may result from chewing leaves | May take 4-6 months to see an effect; do not discontinue abruptly; reduces platelet aggregation and increased fibrinolytic activity (monitor patients on antiplatelet drugs and warfarin); avoid in pregnant women (uterine stimulant) and children <2 years |
| GARLIC | Broad spectrum antimicrobial; lowers blood pressure and serum cholesterol | 10 mg of allicin or a total allicin potential of 4000 mcg/day or 1 clove (4 g) of fresh garlic/day | Generally nontoxic but may cause GI irritation | Inhibits platelet aggregation and increases fibrinolytic activity (monitor patients on antiplatelet drugs and warfarin); increased serum insulin levels which may decreased blood glucose (monitor blood glucose) |
| GINGER | Motion sickness, morning sickness, postoperative nausea, arthritis, muscular pain, and migraine headache | Powdered ginger root: Nausea and vomiting; 250 mg 4 times/day Arthritis: 125-1000 mg 4 times/day | GI discomfort with high doses (>6 g) if taken on an empty stomach | Inhibits platelet aggregation (monitor patients on antiplatelet drugs and warfarin); increased calcium uptake by heart muscle may alter calcium channel blocker effect; fresh ginger root may yield better results: 1-2 g of powder = approximately 1/4-inch slice |
| GINKGO | Vascular insufficiency resulting in short-term memory loss, vertigo, headache, and tinnitus; depression, intermittent claudication, early Alzheimer's disease, senility, diabetic retinopathy | 40 mg 3-4 times/day; use standardized leaf extract containing 24% ginkgo heterosides | Rare with ginkgo biloba extract; most common are GI discomfort and headache | Response may be seen in 2-3 weeks, but take consistently for 12 weeks to improve prospects of positive clinical outcome |
| GINSENG (Panax; American, Chinese, Korean) | Antifatigue, antistress, regulates blood pressure (dose dependent), enhances immune function, menopausal symptoms, general adaptogen | Take 1-3 times/day; use product standardized to provide 10 mg of ginsenoside and Rg1:Rb2 ratio of 1:2 | Breast tenderness in women; nervousness and excitation that decreased with continued use or decreased dose; generally low toxicity from high-quality, standardized product | Use cyclically with 2 weeks on, followed by 2 weeks off; decreased platelet adhesiveness (monitor patients taking anticoagulants); variable effects on INR; high doses may inhibit immune function in early stages of infection; hypoglycemia effect (monitor patients with diabetes) |
| GINSENG (Siberian) | Adaptogen, antistress, lowers serum cholesterol, decreases blood pressure (increases blood pressure if low), decreases anginal symptoms, increases sense of well being, chronic fatigue syndrome, immune system booster | Take 1-3 times/day; 2-4 mL fluid extract (1:1) or 100-200 mg solid extract (20:1) containing 0.1% eleutheroside E | High doses (>4.5-6 mL 3 times/day) may induce insomnia, irritability, and anxiety; skin eruptions, diarrhea; headache; hypertension; pericardial pain in rheumatic heart patients | Estrogenic effect - do not use any form of ginseng during pregnancy; same clinical considerations as for panax ginseng |

# Natural/Herbal Products *(continued)*

| Herb | Use(s) | Administration | Adverse Effects | Clinical Considerations |
|---|---|---|---|---|
| GOLDEN SEAL | Bacterial and fungal infections of the mucous membranes, GI infections that cause diarrhea, liver cirrhosis, inflamed gallbladder, and eye infections | 250–500 mg 3 times/day; use product standardized to contain 8% to 12% berberine | Do not use during pregnancy; nausea, vomiting; CNS stimulant; may interfere with colon's ability to manufacture B vitamins | Use in conjunction with standard antimicrobial therapy; hypoglycemic effect (monitor patients with diabetes); prophylactic use for traveler's diarrhea (give 1 week before, during, and 1 week after travel); use for no longer than 2 months at a time |
| HAWTHORN | Atherosclerosis, high blood pressure, mild-to-moderate CHF, rheumatoid arthritis, and periodontal disease | Take 3 times/day: 1-2 mL hawthorn fluid extract (1:1) Standardized on procyanidine: 1-1.5 g freeze-dried hawthorn berries | None reported with low doses; high doses may induce hypotension and sedation | Increases body's utilization of vitamin C; inhibits angiotensin-converting enzyme (ACE) and may result in decreased dose requirement of ACE inhibitor drug; potentiates cardiac glycosides resulting in decrease in dose requirements; may take up to 2 weeks to see an effect; do not discontinue abruptly |
| LaPACHO (Pau d'arco) | Used to treat bacterial, fungal, viral, and parasitic infections, especially intestinal and vaginal candidiasis | Standardized to provide 1.5-2 g of lapachol/day as a tea or extract | None reported from whole bark | Purchase standardized product from reputable companies, as many products contain no active ingredients (lapachol or quinones) |
| LICORICE | Internal: Glycyrrhetinic acid (GA); Antiviral for cold symptoms and HSV-1, HSV-2, Addison's disease, inflammation External: GA, eczema, canker sore, HSV | Fluid extract (1:1): 2-4 mL Solid extract (4:1): 250-500 mg DGL for peptic ulcer disease: 2-4 380 mg chewable tables 20 minutes before meals | Lethargy to quadriplegia; aldosterone-like effects (increased sodium and water retention; decreased potassium and hypertension with >100 mg/day for more than 6 weeks) | Aldosterone-like effects may be prevented with high potassium/low sodium diet; avoid in patients with hypertension, renal or liver failure, cardiovascular disease, or current cardiac glycoside therapy; potentiates the action of prednisone and prednisolone and increases levels of endogenous corticosteroids; also potentiates topical steroids |
| MILK THISTLE | Liver disease, including cirrhosis and chronic hepatitis; gallstones, psoriasis, liver protectant from toxins (eg, death cup mushroom) | 140 mg silymarin 3 times/day, or 100-200 mg of phosphatidylcholine-bound silymarin twice daily | Possible loose stools as result of increased bile flow; mild allergic reaction | Prevent loose stools by ingesting psyllium and oat bran; phosphatidylcholine-bound silymarin is more effective |
| PEPPERMINT | Internal: Irritable bowel syndrome (IBS) External: Symptoms of common cold, arthritis, and other musculoskeletal problems | Tea: 1-2 tsp dried leaves in 1 cup water Enteric-coated capsules: 1-2 capsules (0.2 mL/capsule) 3 times/day for IBS Topical: 3-4 times/day | Internal: Skin rash, heart burn, muscle tremor External: Contact dermatitis | May potentiate esophageal reflex by relaxing esophageal sphincter; caution in patients with hiatal hernia External: Avoid concomitant use of topical menthols and heating pads (increases likelihood of contact dermatitis) |

1143

**NATURAL/HERBAL PRODUCTS AND DIETARY SUPPLEMENTS**
*(Continued)*

## Natural/Herbal Products *(continued)*

| Herb | Use(s) | Administration | Adverse Effects | Clinical Considerations |
|------|--------|----------------|-----------------|--------------------------|
| ST JOHN'S WORT | Mild to moderate depression, anxiety, antiviral | 300 mg 3 times/day of standardized 0.3% hypericin extract; take with meals | Rare in humans; possibility of photosensitivity with higher doses | Take with food to prevent GI upset; avoid concomitant use with SSRIs; avoid foods and drugs that interact with MAOIs, including cheese, wine, beer, levodopa, and 5-hydroxytryptophan |
| SAW PALMETTO | Benign prostatic hyperplasia (BPH) | 160 mg twice daily of standardized fat-soluble saw palmetto extract containing 85% to 95% fatty acids and sterols | Low, headache reported | Effect seen in patients in 4-6 weeks; no demonstrated effect on serum prostate-specific antigen levels; antiestrogen effect, avoid during pregnancy and in patients with breast cancer |
| VALERIAN | Sedative to treat insomnia; treatment of anxiety and stress | 150-300 mg of valerian extract (0.8% valeric acid) 30-45 minutes before bedtime | Rare morning drowsiness, headache, excitability, uneasiness, cardiac disturbances | Usually reduces morning sleepiness; may potentiate effects of other CNS depressants; decrease caffeine intake and daytime naps and increase exercise to improve results |

# TREATMENT OF SEXUALLY TRANSMITTED DISEASES

| Type or Stage | Drug of Choice | Dosage | Alternatives |
|---|---|---|---|
| *CHLAMYDIA TRACHOMATIS* | | | |
| **Urethritis, cervicitis, conjunctivitis, or proctitis (except lymphogranuloma venereum)** | | | |
| | Azithromycin or | 1 g oral once | Ofloxacin[2] 300 mg oral bid x 7 days; erythromycin 500 mg oral qid x 7 days |
| | Doxycycline[1,2] | 100 mg oral bid x 7 days | |
| **Infection in pregnancy** | | | |
| | Erythromycin[3] | 500 mg oral qid x 7 days[4] | Amoxicillin 500 mg oral tid x 10 days; azithromycin[5] 1 g oral once |
| **Neonatal** | | | |
| Ophthalmia | Erythromycin | 12.5 mg/kg oral or I.V. qid x 14 days | |
| Pneumonia | Erythromycin | 12.5 mg/kg oral or I.V. qid x 14 days | Sulfisoxazole[6] 100 mg/kg/d oral or I.V. in divided doses x 14 days |
| **Lymphogranuloma venereum** | | | |
| | Doxycycline[1,2] | 100 mg oral bid x 21 days | Erythromycin[3] 500 mg oral qid x 21 days |
| GONORRHEA[7] | | | |
| **Urethral, cervical, rectal, or pharyngeal** | | | |
| | Cefpodoxime 200 mg as a single dose; ceftriaxone | 125 mg I.M. once | Cefixime 400 mg oral once; ciprofloxacin[2] 500 mg oral once; ofloxacin[2] 400 mg oral once; spectinomycin 2 g I.M. once[8] |
| **Ophthalmia (adults)[9]** | | | |
| | Ceftriaxone | 1 g I.M. once, plus saline irrigation | |
| **Bacteremia, arthritis, and disseminated[10,11]** | | | |
| | Ceftriaxone | 1 g I.V. daily x 7-10 days, or for 2-3 days, followed by cefixime 400 mg oral bid or ciprofloxacin 500 mg oral bid to complete 7-10 days total therapy | Ceftizoxime or cefotaxime, 1 g I.V. q8h for 2-3 days or until improved, followed by cefixime 400 mg oral bid or ciprofloxacin 500 mg oral bid to complete 7-10 days total therapy |
| **Neonatal** | | | |
| Ophthalmia | Cefotaxime or | 25 mg/kg I.V. or I.M. q8-12h x 7 days, plus saline irrigation | Penicillin G[12] 100,000 units/kg/d I.V. in 4 doses x 7 days, plus saline irrigation |
| | Ceftriaxone | 125 mg I.M. once, plus saline irrigation | |
| Bacteremia, arthritis, and disseminated | Cefotaxime | 25-50 mg/kg I.V. q8-12h x 7-14 days | Penicillin G[12] 75,000-100,000 units/kg/d I.V. in 4 doses x 7-14 days |
| **Children (<45 kg)** | | | |
| Urogenital, rectal, and pharyngeal | Ceftriaxone | 125 mg I.M. once | Spectinomycin[13] 40 mg/kg I.M. once; amoxicillin[12] 50 mg/kg oral once, plus probenecid 25 mg/kg (max: 1 g) oral once |

# TREATMENT OF SEXUALLY TRANSMITTED DISEASES
(Continued)

| Type or Stage | Drug of Choice | Dosage | Alternatives |
|---|---|---|---|
| Bacteremia, arthritis, and disseminated | Ceftriaxone or | 50-100 mg/kg/d (max: 2 g) I.V. x 7-14 days | Penicillin G[12] 150,000-250,000 units/kg/d I.V. x 7-14 days |
| | Cefotaxime | 50-200 mg/kg/d I.V. in 2-4 doses x 7-14 days | |
| **SEXUALLY ACQUIRED EPIDIDYMITIS** | | | |
| | Ofloxacin | 300 mg bid x 10 days | Ceftriaxone 250 mg I.M. once, followed by doxycycline[1] 100 mg oral bid x 10 days |
| **PELVIC INFLAMMATORY DISEASE** | | | |
| **Hospitalized patients** | Cefoxitin or | 2 g I.V. q6h | Clindamycin 900 mg I.V. q8h plus gentamicin 2 mg/kg I.V. once, followed by gentamicin 1.5 mg/kg I.V. q8h until improved, followed by doxycycline 100 mg oral bid to complete 14 days[14] |
| | Cefotetan either one, plus | 2 g I.V. q12h | |
| | Doxycycline[2] followed by | 100 mg I.V. q12h, until improved | |
| | Doxycycline[2] | 100 mg oral bid to complete 14 days | |
| **Outpatients** | Cefoxitin, plus | 2 g I.M. once | Ofloxacin[2] 400 mg oral bid x 14 days, plus metronidazole 500 mg oral bid x 14 days or clindamycin 450 mg oral qid x 14 days |
| | Probenecid or | 1 g oral once | |
| | Ceftriaxone, either one followed by | 250 mg I.M. once | |
| | Doxycycline[2] | 100 mg oral bid x 14 days | |
| **VAGINAL INFECTION** | | | |
| **Trichomoniasis** | | | |
| | Metronidazole[15] | 2 g oral once | Metronidazole 375 mg or 500 mg oral bid x 7 days |
| **Bacterial vaginosis** | | | |
| | Metronidazole gel 0.75% | 5 g intravaginally bid x 5 days | Metronidazole 500 mg oral bid x 7 days |
| **Vulvovaginal candidiasis** | | | |
| | Topical butoconazole, clotrimazole, miconazole, terconazole, or tioconazole[17] | | Metronidazole 2 g oral once[16]; fluconazole 150 mg oral once |
| **SYPHILIS** | | | |
| **Early** (primary, secondary, or latent <1 y) | | | |
| | Penicillin G benzathine | 2.4 million units I.M. once[18] | Doxycycline[2] 100 mg oral bid x 14 days |
| **Late** (more than 1 year's duration, cardiovascular, gumma, late-latent) | | | |
| | Penicillin G benzathine | 2.4 million units I.M. weekly x 3 wk | Doxycycline[2] 100 mg oral bid x 4 wk |
| **Neurosyphilis[19]** | | | |
| | Penicillin G | 2-4 million units I.V. q4h x 10-14 days | Penicillin G procaine 2.4 million units I.M. daily, plus probenecid 500 mg qid oral, both x 10-14 days |

| Type or Stage | Drug of Choice | Dosage | Alternatives |
|---|---|---|---|
| **Congenital** | | | |
| | Penicillin G or | 50,000 units/kg I.M. or I.V. q8-12h for 10-14 days | |
| | Penicillin G procaine | 50,000 units/kg I.M. daily for 10-14 days | |
| **CHANCROID**[20] | | | |
| | Erythromycin[3] or | 500 mg oral qid x 7 days | Ciprofloxacin[2] 500 mg oral bid x 3 days |
| | Ceftriaxone or | 250 mg I.M. once | |
| | Azithromycin | 1 g oral once | |
| **HERPES SIMPLEX** | | | |
| **First episode genital** | | | |
| | Acyclovir | 400 mg oral tid x 7-10 days | Acyclovir 200 mg oral 5 times/d x 7-10 days |
| **First episode proctitis** | | | |
| | Acyclovir | 800 mg oral tid x 7-10 days | Acyclovir 400 mg oral 5 times/d x 7-10 days |
| **Recurrent** | | | |
| | Acyclovir[21] | 400 mg oral tid x 5 days | |
| **Severe** (hospitalized patients) | | | |
| | Acyclovir | 5 mg/kg I.V. q8h x 5-7 days | |
| **Prevention of recurrence**[22] | | | |
| | Acyclovir | 400 mg oral bid | Acyclovir 200 mg oral 2-5 times/d |

[1]Or tetracycline 500 mg oral qid or minocycline 100 mg oral bid.

[2]Contraindicated in pregnancy.

[3]Erythromycin estolate is contraindicated in pregnancy.

[4]In the presence of severe gastrointestinal intolerance, decrease to 250 mg qid and extend duration to 14 days.

[5]Safety in pregnancy not established.

[6]Only for infants older than 4 weeks.

[7]All patients should also receive a course of treatment effective for *Chlamydia*.

[8]Recommended only for use during pregnancy in patients allergic to beta-lactams. Not effective for pharyngeal infection.

[9]An oral fluoroquinolone, such as ciprofloxacin for 3-5 days, probably would also be effective, but experience is limited.

[10]If the infecting strain of *N. gonorrhoeae* has been tested and is known to be susceptible to penicillin or the tetracyclines, treatment may be changed to penicillin G 10 million units I.V. daily, amoxicillin 500 mg orally qid, doxycycline 100 mg orally bid, or tetracycline 500 mg orally qid.

[11]Endocarditis requires at least 3-4 weeks of parenteral therapy.

[12]If infecting strain of *N. gonorrhoeae* has been tested and is known to be susceptible.

[13]Not effective for pharyngeal infection.

[14]Or clindamycin 450 mg oral qid to complete 14 days.

[15]Metronidazole should be avoided during the first trimester of pregnancy; 2 g oral (single dose) may be given after the first trimester.

[16]Higher relapse rate, but useful for patients who may not comply with multiple-dose therapy.

[17]For preparations and dosage, see *The Medical Letter*, 36:81, 1994; avoid single-dose therapy.

[18]Some experts recommend repeating this regimen after 7 days, especially in patients with HIV infection.

[19]Patients allergic to penicillin should be desensitized.

[20]All regimens, especially single-dose ceftriaxone, are less effective in HIV-infected patients.

[21]Not highly effective for treatment of recurrences, but may help some patients if started early.

[22]Preventive treatment should be discontinued for 1-2 months once a year to reassess the frequency of recurrence.

# TYRAMINE CONTENT OF FOODS

| Food | Allowed | Minimize Intake | Not Allowed |
|---|---|---|---|
| Beverages | Milk, decaffeinated coffee, tea, soda | Chocolate beverage, caffeine-containing drinks, clear spirits | Acidophilus milk, beer, ale, wine, malted beverages |
| Breads/cereals | All except those containing cheese | None | Cheese bread and crackers |
| Dairy products | Cottage cheese, farmers or pot cheese, cream cheese, ricotta cheese, all milk, eggs, ice cream, pudding (except chocolate) | Yogurt (limit to 4 oz per day) | All other cheeses (aged cheese, American, Camembert, cheddar, Gouda, gruyere, mozzarella, parmesan, provolone, romano, Roquefort, stilton |
| Meat, fish, and poultry | All fresh or frozen | Aged meats, hot dogs, canned fish and meat | Chicken and beef liver, dried and pickled fish, summer or dry sausage, pepperoni, dried meats, meat extracts, bologna, liverwurst |
| Starches — potatoes/rice | All | None | Soybean (including paste) |
| Vegetables | All fresh, frozen, canned, or dried vegetable juices except those not allowed | Chili peppers, Chinese pea pods | Fava beans, sauerkraut, pickles, olives, Italian broad beans |
| Fruit | Fresh, frozen, or canned fruits and fruit juices | Avocado, banana, raspberries, figs | Banana peel extract |
| Soups | All soups not listed to limit or avoid | Commercially canned soups | Soups which contain broad beans, fava beans, cheese, beer, wine, any made with flavor cubes or meat extract, miso soup |
| Fats | All except fermented | Sour cream | Packaged gravy |
| Sweets | Sugar, hard candy, honey, molasses, syrups | Chocolate candies | None |
| Desserts | Cakes, cookies, gelatin, pastries, sherbets, sorbets | Chocolate desserts | Cheese-filled desserts |
| Miscellaneous | Salt, nuts, spices, herbs, flavorings, Worcestershire sauce | Soy sauce, peanuts | Brewer's yeast, yeast concentrates, all aged and fermented products, monosodium glutamate, vitamins with Brewer's yeast |

# PHARMACOLOGIC INDEX

## ANTIFUNGAL AGENT, TOPICAL *(Continued)*

## ANTIFUNGAL AGENT, VAGINAL

## ANTIFUNGAL/CORTICOSTEROID

## ANTIGOUT AGENT

## ANTIHISTAMINE

## ANTIHISTAMINE/ANTITUSSIVE

## ANTIHISTAMINE/DECONGESTANT/ANALGESIC

## ANTIHISTAMINE/DECONGESTANT/ANTICHOLINERGIC

## ANTIHISTAMINE/DECONGESTANT/ANTITUSSIVE

## ANTIHISTAMINE/DECONGESTANT COMBINATION

## ANTINEOPLASTIC AGENT, ANTIMETABOLITE *(Continued)*

## ANTINEOPLASTIC AGENT, MISCELLANEOUS

## ANTIPARASITIC AGENT, TOPICAL

## ANTI-PARKINSON'S AGENT (ANTICHOLINERGIC)

## ANTI-PARKINSON'S AGENT (COMT INHIBITOR)

## ANTI-PARKINSON'S AGENT (DOPAMINE AGONIST)

## ANTI-PARKINSON'S AGENT (MONOAMINE OXIDASE INHIBITOR)

## ANTIPLATELET AGENT

## ANTIPROTOZOAL

## ANTIPSORIATIC AGENT

## ANTIPSYCHOTIC AGENT, BENZISOXAZOLE

## ANTIPSYCHOTIC AGENT, BUTYROPHENONE

## ANTIPSYCHOTIC AGENT, DIBENZODIAZEPINE

## ANTIPSYCHOTIC AGENT, DIBENZOTHIAZEPINE

## ANTIPSYCHOTIC AGENT, DIBENZOXAZEPINE

## ANTIPSYCHOTIC AGENT, DIHYDOINDOLINE

## ANTIPSYCHOTIC AGENT, DIPHENYLBUTYLPERIDINE

## ANTIPSYCHOTIC AGENT, PHENOTHAZINE, PIPERAZINE

## ANTITUSSIVE *(Continued)*

## ANTITUSSIVE/DECONGESTANT

## ANTITUSSIVE/DECONGESTANT/EXPECTORANT

## ANTITUSSIVE/EXPECTORANT

## ANTIVIRAL AGENT

## ANTIVIRAL AGENT, OPHTHALMIC

## ANTIVIRAL AGENT, TOPICAL

## AROMATASE INHIBITOR

## BARBITURATE

## BENZODIAZEPINE

## BETA BLOCKER, BETA$_1$ SELECTIVE

## BETA BLOCKER, NONSELECTIVE

## BETA BLOCKER (WITH INTRINSIC SYMPATHOMIMETIC ACTIVITY)

## BETA$_1$/BETA$_2$ AGONIST

## BETA$_2$ AGONIST

## TOPICAL SKIN PRODUCT *(Continued)*

## TOPICAL SKIN PRODUCT, ACNE

## TOPICAL SKIN PRODUCT, ANTIBACTERIAL

## TOXOID

## TRACE ELEMENT

## TRACE ELEMENT, PARENTERAL

## UREA CYCLE DISORDER (UCD) TREATMENT AGENT

## URICOSURIC AGENT

## URINARY ACIDIFYING AGENT

## URINARY TRACT PRODUCT

## VACCINE

## VASODILATOR

## VASOPRESSIN ANALOG, SYNTHETIC

## VITAMIN

## VITAMIN D ANALOG

## VITAMIN, FAT SOLUBLE

## VITAMIN, WATER SOLUBLE

## XANTHINE OXIDASE INHIBITOR

# ALPHABETICAL INDEX

# ALPHABETICAL INDEX

# ALPHABETICAL INDEX

ALPHABETICAL INDEX

# ALPHABETICAL INDEX

# ALPHABETICAL INDEX

# *Other titles offered by Lexi-Comp . . .*

### *DRUG INFORMATION HANDBOOK* 7th Edition 1999-2000

by Charles Lacy, PharmD; Lora L. Armstrong, BSPharm; Morton P. Goldman, PharmD; and Leonard L. Lance, BSPharm

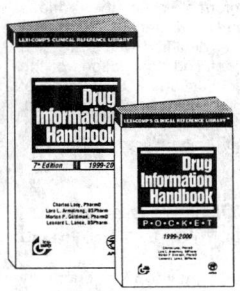

Specifically compiled and designed for the healthcare professional requiring quick access to concisely stated comprehensive data concerning clinical use of medications.

*The Drug Information Handbook* is an ideal portable drug information resource, containing 1200 drug monographs. Each monograph typically provides the reader with up to 29 key points of data concerning clinical use and dosing of the medication. Material provided in the Appendix section is recognized by many users to be, by itself, well worth the purchase of the handbook.

All medications found in the *Drug Information Handbook*, 7th Edition are included in the abridged Pocket edition.

### *PEDIATRIC DOSAGE HANDBOOK* 6th Edition 1999-2000

by Carol K. Taketomo, PharmD; Jane Hurlburt Hodding, PharmD; and Donna M. Kraus, PharmD

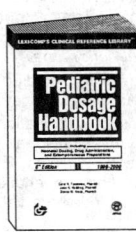

Special considerations must frequently be taken into account when dosing medications for the pediatric patient. This highly regarded quick reference handbook is a compilation of recommended pediatric doses based on current literature as well as the practical experience of the authors and their many colleagues who work every day in the pediatric clinical setting.

*The Pediatric Dosage Handbook* 6th Edition includes neonatal dosing, drug administration, and extemporaneous preparations for 640 medications used in pediatric medicine.

### *GERIATRIC DOSAGE HANDBOOK* 4th Edition 1998/99

by Todd P. Semla, PharmD; Judith L. Beizer, PharmD; and Martin D. Higbee, PharmD

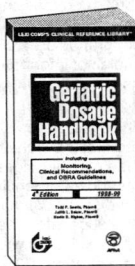

Many physiologic changes occur with aging, some of which affect the pharmacokinetics or pharmacodynamics of medications. Strong consideration should also be given to the effect of decreased renal or hepatic functions in the elderly as well as the probability of the geriatric patient being on multiple drug regimens.

Healthcare professionals working with nursing homes and assisted living facilities will find the 745 drug monographs contained in this handbook to be an invaluable source of helpful information.

## To order call toll free: 1-800-837-LEXI (5394)

### DRUG-INDUCED NUTRIENT DEPLETION HANDBOOK 1999-2000

by Ross Pelton, RPh, PhD, CCN; James B. LaValle, RPh, DHM, NMD, CCN; Ernest B. Hawkins, RPh, MS; Daniel L. Krinsky, RPh, MS

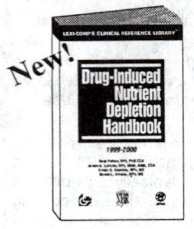

A complete and up-to-date listing of all drugs known to deplete the body of nutritional compounds.

Alphabetically organized and provide extensive cross-referencing to related information in the various sections of the book. Nearly 150 generic drugs that cause nutrient depletion are identified which are also cross-referenced to more detailed descriptions of the nutrients depleted and their actions. Symptoms of deficiencies, and sources of repletion are also included. This book also contains Studies and Abstracts section, a valuable Appendix, and Alphabetical & Pharmacological Indices.

### DRUG INFORMATION HANDBOOK FOR ONCOLOGY 1999-2000

by Dominic A. Solimando, Jr, MA; Linda R. Bressler, PharmD, BCOP; Polly E. Kintzel, PharmD, BCPS, BCOP; Mark C. Geraci, PharmD, BCOP

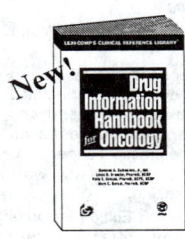

This comprehensive and easy-to-use oncology handbook was designed specifically to meet the needs of anyone who provides, prescribes, or administers therapy to cancer patients.

Presented in a concise and uniform format, this book contains the most comprehensive collection of oncology-related drug information available. Organized like a dictionary for ease of use, drugs can be found by looking up the *brand or generic name*!

This book contains 253 monographs, including over 1100 Antineoplastic Agents and Ancillary Medications.

Also containing up to 33 fields of information per monograph including: Use, U.S. Investigational, Bone Marrow/Blood Cell Transplantation, Vesicant, Emetic Potential. A Special Topics Section, Appendix, and Therapeutic Category & Key Word Index are valuable features to this book as well.

### DRUG INFORMATION HANDBOOK FOR PSYCHIATRY 1999-2000

by Matthew A. Fuller, PharmD; Martha Sajatovic, MD

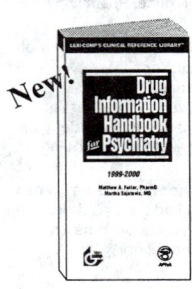

The source for comprehensive and clinically relevant drug information for the mental health professional. Alphabetically arranged by generic and brand name for ease-of-use. Containing monographs on 1,063 generic drugs and up to 34 key fields of information including; effect on mental status and effect on psychiatric treatment.

A special topics/issues section includes; psychiatric assessment, overview of selected major psychiatric disorders, clinical issues in the use of major classes of psychotropic medications, psychiatric emergencies, special populations, diagnostic and statistical manual of mental disorders (DSM-IV), and suggested reading. Also contains a valuable appendix section as well as a therapeutic category index and a alphabetical index.

## To order call toll free: 1-800-837-LEXI (5394)

## ANESTHESIOLOGY & CRITICAL CARE DRUG HANDBOOK 1999-2000

by Andrew J. Donnelly, PharmD; Francesca E. Cunningham, PharmD;
and Verna L. Baughman, MD

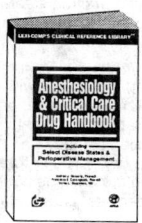

Contains over 512 generic medications with up to 25 fields of information presented in each monograph. It also contains the following Special Issues and Topics: Allergic Reaction, Anesthesia for Cardiac Patients in Noncardiac Surgery, Anesthesia for Obstetric Patients in Nonobstetric Surgery, Anesthesia for Patients With Liver Disease, Chronic Pain Management, Chronic Renal Failure, Conscious Sedation, Perioperative Management of Patients on Antiseizure Medication, Substance Abuse and Anesthesia.

The Appendix includes: Abbreviations & Measurements, Anesthesiology Information, Assessment of Liver & Renal Function, Comparative Drug Charts, Infectious Disease-Prophylaxis & Treatment, Laboratory Values, Therapy Recommendation, Toxicology, *and much more . . .*

## DRUG INFORMATION HANDBOOK FOR NURSING 2nd Edition 1999/2000

by Beatrice B. Turkoski, RN, PhD; Brenda R. Lance, RN, MSN; Mark F. Bonfiglio, PharmD

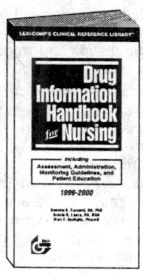

Advanced Practice Nurses, Registered Professional Nurses, and upper-division nursing students involved with drug therapy will find that this handbook provides quick access to drug data in a concise easy-to-use format.

Over 3950 U.S., Canadian, and Mexican medications are covered in the 998 generic drug monographs each containing up to 46 key points of information. The handbook contains basic pharmacology concepts and nursing issues such as patient factors that influence drug therapy (ie, pregnancy, age, weight, etc) and general nursing issues (ie, assessment, administration, monitoring, and patient education). The appendix contains over 200 pages of valuable information and the indices consist of Canadian/Mexican Brand Names, Controlled Substances, and Therapeutic Category.

## DRUG INFORMATION HANDBOOK FOR THE ALLIED HEALTH PROFESSIONAL 6th Edition 1999-2000

by Leonard L. Lance, BSPharm; Charles Lacy, PharmD; and Morton P. Goldman, PharmD

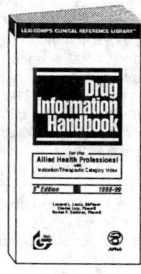

Working with clinical pharmacists, hospital pharmacy and therapeutics committees, and hospital drug information centers, the authors have assisted hundreds of hospitals in developing institution specific formulary reference documentation.

The most current basic drug and medication data from those clinical settings have been reviewed, coalesced, and cross-referenced to create this unique handbook. The handbook offers quick access to abbreviated monographs for 1384 generic drugs.

This is a great tool for physician assistants, medical records personnel, medical transcriptionists and secretaries, pharmacy technicians, and other allied health professionals.

# To order call toll free:  1-800-837-LEXI (5394)

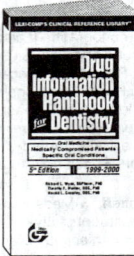
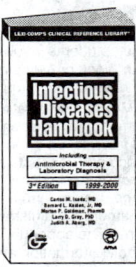
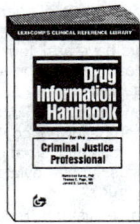

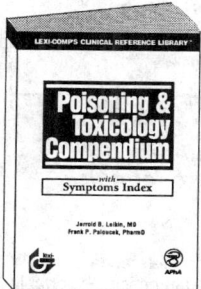
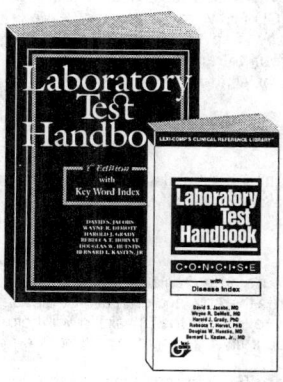
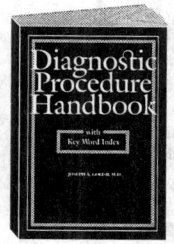

## "Lexi-Comp's Clinical Reference Library™ (CRL) has established the new standard for quick reference information"

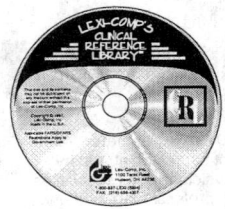

Lexi-Comp offers the Clinical Reference Library™ (CRL™), a series of clinical databases, as portable handbooks or integrated as part of a CD-ROM that also includes clinical decision support modules. CRL™ is delivered with a powerful search engine on a single CD-ROM and can be used with Microsoft® Windows™ release 3.1 or higher. In addition to our CD-ROM for Windows™, Lexi-Comp's databases can also be licensed for distribution on your Intranet, or used with your palmtop, Newton, or Windows™ CE device.

### Clinical Decision Support Modules

The Clinical Decision Support Modules are unique and significant to the power offered by Lexi-Comp's Clinical Reference Library™ on CD-ROM. These modules are also directly linked to CRL™'s databases.

 **Patient Analysis** - Users can specify a patient's drug profile and automatically analyze the data for drug interactions, duplicate therapy, and drug allergy alerts. Printing this medication summary report for review by the physician will help decrease adverse drug events, increase productivity, and improve patient care.

 **Stedman's Electronic Medical Dictionary™** - Instant access to the full functionality of a medical dictionary, including over 100,000 medical definitions, phrases, pronunciations, and related terms.

 **Calculations** - Instant access to the following calculations: Body Surface Area, Ideal Body Mass for Pediatrics and Adults, Estimated Creatinine Clearance (Cockroft & Gault), and Temperature Conversion.

 **Drug Identification** - This powerful module allows rapid identification of medications based on one or more of the following descriptors: use, pattern, shape, scoring, markings, form, coatings, color, generic name, and manufac-turer name. Color images are displayed for visual verification.

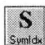 **Symptoms Analysis** - Enter symptoms presented by a patient to receive separate lists of medicinal, nonmedicinal, and biological agents associated with the selected symptoms.

## To order call toll free:  1-800-837-LEXI (5394)

Lexi-Comp, Inc.
1100 Terex Road
Hudson, Ohio 44236-4438

## BUSINESS REPLY MAIL

FIRST-CLASS MAIL    PERMIT NO 689    HUDSON, OH

POSTAGE WILL BE PAID BY ADDRESSEE

**LEXI-COMP, INC.**
*DIH for Physician Assistants* Reply Card
1100 Terex Road
Hudson, OH 44236-9915

# Thank you for purchasing Lexi-Comp's _Drug Information Handbook for Physician Assistants_

Return this postage-paid card so we can keep you up-to-date on all the latest products, promotions and upgrades.

☒ **Please put me on your "Mailing List".**

☒ **Please put me on your "Standing Order List" to automatically receive the new edition each year.**

Please print name of book _____

☒ **Please send me information on quantity discounts.**

Name (First) _____ (Last) _____

Title _____

Company _____

Address _____

City _____ State/Province _____

Zip/Postal Code _____ Country _____

Telephone: ( ___ ) _____ Fax: ( ___ ) _____

E-Mail Address _____

## OTHER AREAS OF INTEREST:

☐ Anesthesiology & Critical Care
☐ Diagnostic Procedures
☐ Drug Information
☐ Drug Information for Allied Health
☐ Drug Information for Cardiology*
☐ Drug Information for Dentistry
☐ Drug Information for Nursing
☐ Drug Information for Psychiatry
☐ Drug-Induced Nutrient Depletion Handbook

* 1999 targeted release

☐ Geriatric Dosage
☐ Natural Products Information*
☐ Drug Information for Oncology
☐ Natural Therapeutics*
☐ Infectious Diseases
☐ Laboratory Test
☐ Pediatric Dosage
☐ Poisoning & Toxicology
☐ Drug Information for Advanced Practice Nursing*

## ALSO INTERESTED IN THE FOLLOWING:

☐ Lexi-Comp's Formulary/Lab Custom Publishing Service
☐ Lexi-Comp's Clinical Reference Library™ on CD-ROM
( ___ Academic ___ Personal ___ Institutional)
☐ Lexi-Comp's CRL™ on a hand-held device